心脏电生理：
从细胞到临床

第四版

主　编 **DOUGLAS P. ZIPES, MD**
Distinguished Professor of Medicine, Pharmacology, and Toxicology
Director, Krannert Institute of Cardiology
Director, Division of Cardiology
Indiana University School of Medicine

JOSÉ JALIFE, MD
Professor and Chair
Department of Pharmacology
Professor of Medicine and Pediatrics
Director, Institute for Cardiovascular Research
SUNY Upstate Medical University
Syracuse, New York

主　译　郭继鸿　李学斌
副主译　浦介麟　张幼怡　张　萍　刘元生　杨延宗

北京大学医学出版社
Peking University Medical Press

Cardiac Electrophysiology: From Cell To Bedside, 4th edition.
Douglas P. Zipes, Jose Jalife
ISBN-13: 978-0-7216-0323-0
ISBN-10: 0-7216-0323-8
Copyright © 2004 by Elsevier Inc. All rights reserved.

Authorized Simplified Chinese translation from English language edition published by the Proprietor.
978-981-259-541-6
981-259-541-4

Elsevier（Singapore）Pte Ltd.
3 Killiney Road，#08-01 Winsland House I，Singapore 239519
Tel：(65) 6349-0200，Fax：(65) 6733-1817
First Published 2008
2008年初版

Simplified Chinese translation Copyright © 2008 by Elsevier（Singapore）Pte Ltd and Peking University Medical Press. All rights reserved.

Published in China by Peking University Medical Press under special agreement with Elsevier（Singapore）Pte Ltd. This edition is authorized for sale in China only, excluding Hong Kong SAR and Taiwan. Unauthorized export of this edition is a violation of the Copyright Act. Violation of this Law is subject to Civil and Criminal Penalties.

本书简体中文版由北京大学医学出版社与Elsevier（Singapore）Pte Ltd在中国大陆境内合作出版。本版仅限在中国境内（不包括香港特别行政区及台湾）出版及标价销售。未经许可之出口，是为违反著作权法，将受法制之制裁。

北京市版权局著作权合同登记号：图字：01-2006-1175

图书在版编目（CIP）数据

心脏电生理：从细胞到临床．第4版/（美）齐普斯（Zipes，D. P.），（美）贾莱夫（Jalife，J.）原著；郭继鸿、李学斌译．—北京：北京大学医学出版社，2007.5
书名原文：Cardiac Electrophysiology: From Cell To Bedside
ISBN 978-7-81071-994-0

Ⅰ. 心⋯ Ⅱ. ①齐⋯②贾⋯③郭⋯④李⋯ Ⅲ. 心脏—电生理学 Ⅳ. R331.3

中国版本图书馆CIP数据核字（2006）第121927号

心脏电生理：从细胞到临床

主　　译：郭继鸿　李学斌
出版发行：北京大学医学出版社（电话：010-82802230）
地　　址：(100083)北京市海淀区学院路38号　北京大学医学部院内
网　　址：http://www.pumpress.com.cn
E - mail：booksale@bjmu.edu.cn
印　　刷：北京佳信达艺术印刷有限公司
经　　销：新华书店
责任编辑：冯智勇　药蓉　曹霞　王智敏　　责任校对：杜悦　　责任印制：郭桂兰
开　　本：889mm×1194mm　1/16　　印张：71　　插页：15　　字数：2392千字
版　　次：2008年1月第1版　2008年1月第1次印刷
书　　号：ISBN 978-7-81071-994-0
定　　价：312.00元

版权所有，违者必究
（凡属质量问题请与本社发行部联系退换）

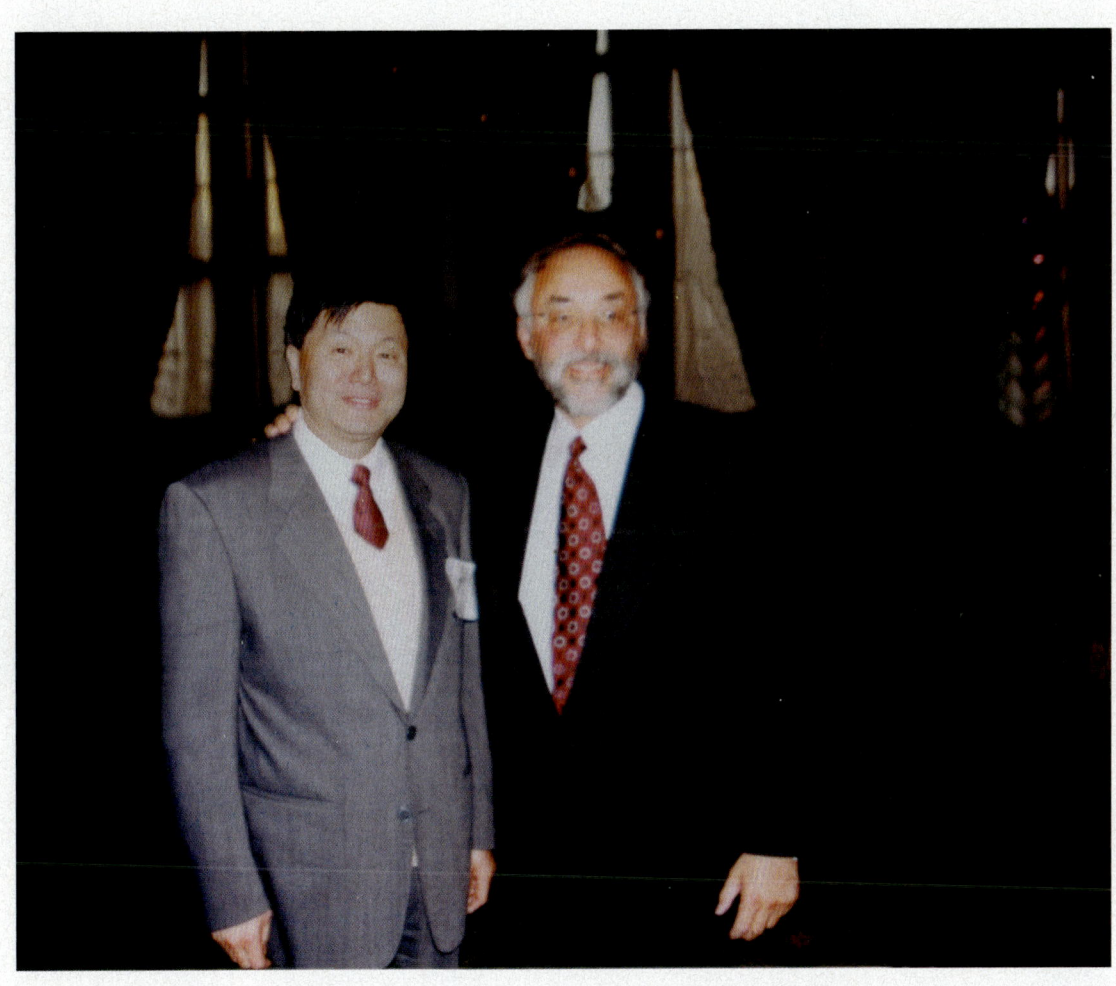

珍贵的留念：Zipes 与郭继鸿

译者前言

"前言"总位于书的最前面，但实际都是整书收笔时撰写的最后点缀。相当于一项浩大工程竣工时的备忘录，将工程立项的初衷，工程的精采夺目之处，有关工程的轶闻轶事都札记在案，留给读者和后人。

本书选题之时，略有踌躇和争议，当时Josephson的《临床心脏电生理学：技术与理论》的中译版刚面世不久，仅几个月2000册就畅销一空，此时再重组兵马将帅挥师翻译另一部心脏电生理学的巨著，唯恐触犯重复选题之大忌。但是翻开本书马上就意识到，这两本书的内容、风格、学术意义迥然不同。一个是繁华的"Downtown"中心矗立的摩天大厦，一个则是洒满耀眼珍珠、风景宜人的避暑海滩。前者是Josephson一人执笔捉刀，就一个主题，一泻千里，冲击成一本深不可测、举世无双的Bible（圣经）。而后者则是Zipes统辖百员战将就120个专题，铺天盖地，气势磅礴，打造出一部铁壁铜墙、令人仰视的心律失常的"百科全书"。这120个精选的专题，每个专题都可以或已经独立成书，而此时却由120位该专题的世界级大师各怀英雄绝技，一气呵成盖世佳篇，堆秀于本书。本书第一版于1990年问世，当时仅是一本纪念Zipes的老师Moe诞辰100周年学术会议的论文集，但经过主编的精心策划与谋略，使本书成为心律失常领域最重要的专著与工具书。难能可贵的是，第三版心律失常和心脏电生理的内容中基础与临床各自掺半，每章内容都是前沿与精粹并举，深邃与直白相伴，真正意义上体现了从细胞到临床、从理论到实践这一主题，是心律失常领域一本盖世绝伦的"百科全书"，让你通读本书时，顿生"夺之，必能得天下"之感。还需强调的是，限于篇幅，本版有些章节采取以分析和荟萃第三版以来该专题的进展为主线，而前版中已经阐述的基本概念、方法学等内容部分已被删减而未重述，读者需要了解这些内容时还需查阅第三版或其他相关文献。

再说本书主帅Zipes，他是目前美国，乃至全世界最负盛名、最具权威的心脏病学大师，心律失常和心脏电生理学的超级教授。如同当年的White一样，担任着美国心脏病学领域像JACC主席等多种最重要的学术领军位置和头衔。如果美国总统的亲自接见与会晤还不能证明他学术成就的显赫，那么Braundwald教授在《Braundwald心脏病学》第七版面世之时，将第一主编让位给Zipes，而自己退居该书第四主编的事实足以证明Zipes教授在世界心脏病学界的顶级位置。可以想象，本书能聚集这么多位的学术权威，共铸如此权威的专著，非Zipes莫属。Zipes教授与中国人民十分友好，几年前他访问了中国，除在北京等地做了精彩的学术报告外，还访问了西藏拉萨市医院。

本书决定翻译出版后，云集国内近百名精兵强将，奋勇上阵，势如破竹，众志成城。本书包括120个心律失常的专题，由于全书总篇幅的限制，各章原著者都竭力精练语言，高度浓缩内容，使部分的英文表述较难理解，造成直译或意译都颇棘手和艰难。翻译过程中，这些难点都经反复讨论和争辩，反复推敲和商榷。鉴于专业和翻译的水平，肯定本书正式出版时仍将存在理解不够、翻译不妥之处，敬请同道慷慨斧正。

本书翻译过程中，几位年轻有为的学者一直奋战在第一线。李学斌教授在繁忙的临床工作重压之下，仍不负众望，废寝忘食，出色完成了主译工作。浦介麟教授英中文水平双全，他认真伏案，逐句推敲，不愧是一位真正的学者。翻译此书时，张幼怡教授已任北京大学心血管病基础研究所所长之职，重任和繁忙都未能影响她对本书的一丝不苟，显示出一位年轻大师的风范。张萍教授受命于全书关键性的环节工作，摇鼓督战，兢兢业业。刘元生教授身为急诊科主任，业务与行政之事贯缠全身，但仍能静心笔耕，专注操笔，难能可贵。杨延宗教授是国内著名的心脏电生理学专家，又兼院长重职，他能捧印出山，执著参与使本书蓬荜生辉。本书的秘书王云龙博士为本书的出版做了大量的工作。还应当感谢北京大学医学出版社的王凤廷副社长，没有他的慧眼识珠，果断定夺，则根本无此书之谈。

我十分喜欢居里夫人的一句话："科学家的神圣任务就是要点燃科学道路上的路灯"。Zipes 先生点燃了心脏电生理和心律失常领域中这盏明亮的灯，而我们只是将这一火种传递到中国。

郭继鸿

二〇〇七年十月一日

译者名单

主　译：郭继鸿　李学斌
副主译：浦介麟　张幼怡　张　萍　刘元生
　　　　　杨延宗

译　者（按姓氏笔画排序）

丁燕生	北京大学第一医院
万　征	天津医科大学总医院
马克娟	北京阜外医院
马建新	解放军305医院
王　龙	北京大学人民医院
王　斌	北京航天中心医院
王云龙	北京安贞医院
王立群	北京大学人民医院
王建安	浙江医科大学第二附属医院
王洪涛	北京阜外医院
王祖禄	解放军沈阳军区总医院
叶志荣	福建泉州市第一医院
任晓庆	北京阜外医院
刘　彤	天津医科大学第二附属医院
刘　莹	大连医科大学附属第一医院
刘元生	北京大学人民医院
刘书旺	北京大学第三医院
刘少稳	复旦大学附属中山医院
孙志奇	黑龙江大庆油田总医院
孙宝贵	上海市第一人民医院
许　原	北京大学人民医院
许　静	天津胸科医院
余　飞	北京大学第三医院
吴　兵	福建泉州市第一医院
吴永全	上海同济大学同济医院
吴立荣	贵州医学院附属医院
张　伟	广西桂林市人民医院
张　灵	解放军263医院
张　涛	北京大学人民医院
张　萍	北京大学人民医院
张　惠	北京大学第三医院
张幼怡	北京大学第三医院
张海澄	北京大学人民医院
张敏丽	北京大学第三医院
李　宁	北京阜外医院
李　春	北京大学人民医院
李　鼎	北京大学人民医院
李广平	天津医科大学第二附属医院
李学斌	北京大学人民医院
李继文	北京大学人民医院
杨延宗	大连医科大学附属第一医院
杨俊娟	北京大学第一医院
杨新春	北京朝阳医院
肖　晗	北京大学第三医院
邹建刚	江苏省人民医院
陈　彧	北京大学人民医院
陈　琪	解放军301医院
陈明龙	江苏省人民医院
周益锋	北京中日友好医院
易　忠	北京航天中心医院
林　荣	福建泉州市第一医院
林治湖	大连医科大学附属第一医院
郑强荪	第四军医大学西京医院
侯爱军	河北邯郸市中心医院
姚　焰	北京阜外医院
姜　建	四川大学华西医院
洪　江	上海市第一人民医院
赵战勇	北京安贞医院
赵新然	北京阜外医院

钟幼民	北京大学人民医院	黄织春	内蒙古医学院附属医院
徐　宁	北京大学第三医院	龚开政	北京大学第三医院
浦　奎	解放军254医院	温尚煜	黑龙江大庆油田总医院
浦介麟	北京阜外医院	葛堪忆	北京大学第三医院
贾中伟	解放军254医院	楚英杰	河南省人民医院
郭成军	北京安贞医院	蒲晓群	中南大学湘雅医院
郭继鸿	北京大学人民医院	解基严	北京大学人民医院
高连君	大连医科大学附属第一医院	蔡思宇	浙江大学第二附属医院
黄卫斌	福建厦门市中山医院	滕思勇	北京阜外医院
黄文新	广西桂林医学院附属医院	黎　辉	黑龙江大庆油田总医院

序 言

对于基础研究的科学家、基础和临床心脏电生理学家以及心内科医生来说，全新改版的《心脏电生理学：从细胞到临床》第四版仍是学习和洞悉心脏电生理学及最新进展的可靠宝库。来自不同专业领域的精英撰写了本书各章精湛丰富的内容。本书就像副标题"从细胞到临床"暗示的两方面内容。本版坚守往版确定的作为本领域完备参考书的传统。前51章为心脏电生理学基础研究的内容，后69章是心律失常临床方面的内容。通过本书读者可以了解世界顶尖专家的最新研究进展。

基础研究新的章包括：如HCN的分子和结构基础，张力激活和内流放大通道。收缩-兴奋反馈新章介绍了心脏机械活动调节电学功能的方式。神经再生和心律失常章介绍了心肌梗死后交感神经再生所导致的神经重构进而引起心肌组织的电重构，并形成室速或室颤的触发因子。关于心房颤动的两章介绍了肺静脉中局灶电活动引发的房颤发作，以及左房后部及肺静脉区域的局灶折返引起的急性房颤的持续和向右房的扩布。有关室颤一章讨论了强的内流放大钾通道与室颤可能有关的转子稳定中的作用。有关心律失常的基因敲除和转基因动物模型的新章，回顾了建立鼠模型和研究电学功能的方法并分析了目前与心脏电生理学有关的遗传模型。另一方面，在药物遗传学与心律失常的章中讨论了基因组中多个DNA变异对药物反应的调节模式。临床相关新章包括Brugada综合征、儿茶酚胺和短联律间期室速以及植入式Holter的临床应用等。此外，介绍了新的标测技术并详细介绍了最新非传统的抗心律失常药物，以及房颤导管消融的最新研究成果和房颤发生中肺静脉的作用。

总之，读者将了解心脏电活动的分子和细胞基础，心律失常的机制，如何检测猝死的高危患者，如何评价患者病情，如何使用电学、手术或药物治疗。显然，本书的独特性在书的副标题中已经得到体现，读者在本书可获得心脏电生理学基础和临床方面的各种知识。这是《心脏电生理学：从细胞到临床》一书最重要的特点。

临床心脏电生理学仍在持续不断地快速发展，因此，不久的将来，读者将会发现本版书中许多概念是错误的。但我们相信本书对心脏电生理学感兴趣的人来说未来数年间仍是有用的参考书。

我们的妻子Joan Zipes，Paloma Jalife一如既往的坚定支持是本书得以成功完成的基础，在此深表感谢。本书各章作者的杰出工作使本书得以出版，并在此对他们卓有成效的工作深表感谢。感谢Laurie LeBouef和Janet Hutcheson所做的秘书工作。最后感谢在Elsevier公司工作的Anne Lenehan及其同事的耐心和帮助，并使本书能够送到全世界的心脏电生理学家手中。

Douglas P. Zipes
José Jalife

著者名单

MICHAEL J. ACKERMAN, MD, PHD
Assistant Professor of Medicine, Pediatrics, and Molecular Pharmacology, Mayo Medical School; Director, Long QT Syndrome Clinic and Sudden Death Genomics Laboratory, Mayo Clinic, Rochester, Minnesota
    Intracellular Signaling and Regulation of Cardiac Ion Channels

FELIPE AGUEL
Research Fellow, Department of Biomedical Engineering, Johns Hopkins University School of Medicine, Baltimore, Maryland
    Modeling Cardiac Defibrillation; Rotors and Spiral Waves in Two Dimensions

CESAR ALBERTE-LISTA, MD
Assistant Professor of Medicine, University of Wisconsin; Director of Electrophysiology Laboratory, W. S. Middleton Veterans Affairs Hospital; Staff Physician, Division of Cardiology, University of Wisconsin Hospital and Clinics, Madison, Wisconsin
    Differential Diagnosis of Wide QRS Complex Tachycardia

MATTHIAS ANTZ
II. Medizinische Abteilung, Allgemeines Krankenhaus St. Georg, Hamburg, Germany
    Catheter Ablation of Atrioventricular Reentry

CHARLES ANTZELEVITCH, PHD
Executive Director/Director of Research, Gordon K. Moe Scholar, Masonic Medical Research Laboratory, Utica, New York
    Drug-induced Channelopathies; The Brugada Syndrome

JUSTUS M. B. ANUMONWO, PHD
Assistant Professor, Department of Pharmacology, SUNY Upstate Medical University, Syracuse, New York
    Biophysical Properties of Inward Rectifier Potassium Channels

RISHI ARORA, MD
Assistant Professor of Medicine, Northwestern University School of Medicine, Northwestern Memorial Hospital, Northwestern Medical Faculty Foundation, Chicago, Illinois
    Differential Diagnosis of Wide QRS Complex Tachycardia

PETER H. BACKX, DVM, PHD
Professor of Physiology and Medicine, Faculty of Medicine, University of Toronto; Senior Scientist, Division of Molecular and Cellular Medicine, University Health Network, Toronto, Ontario, Canada
    Voltage Regulated Potassium Channels

JEFFREY R. BALSER, MD, PHD
Chairman, Department of Anesthesiology, Professor of Anesthesiology and Pharmacology, Vanderbilt University School of Medicine, Nashville, Tennessee
    Biophysics of Normal and Abnormal Cardiac Sodium Channel Function

KAREN BECKMAN, MD
Professor, Department of Medicine, Cardiovascular Section, The University of Oklahoma Health Sciences Center, Oklahoma City, Oklahoma
    Electrophysiologic Characteristics of Atrioventricular Nodal Reentrant Tachycardia: Implications for the Reentrant Circuits

DAVID G. BENDITT, MD, FACC, FRCP(C)
Professor of Medicine, Co-Director, Cardiac Arrhythmia Center, Cardiovascular Division, Department of Medicine, University of Minnesota, Minneapolis, Minnesota
    Head-up Tilt Table Testing

EDWARD J. BERBARI, PHD
Professor of Biomedical Engineering and Medicine, Indiana University, Purdue University, Indianapolis, Indianapolis, Indiana
    High-resolution Electrocardiography

OMER BERENFELD, PHD
Research Assistant Professor, Institute for Cardiovascular Research, Department of Pharmacology, SUNY Upstate Medical University, Syracuse, New York
    Theory of Reentry; Mechanisms of Maintenance of Atrial Fibrillation

DONALD M. BERS, PHD
Professor and Chair, Department of Physiology, Loyola University, Chicago, Stritch School of Medicine, Maywood, Illinois
   Cardiac Calcium Channels

ERIC C. BEYER, MD, PHD
Professor, Department of Pediatrics, Chief, Section of Pediatric Hematology/Oncology and Stem Cell Transplantation, University of Chicago, Chicago, Illinois
   Homomeric and Heteromeric Gap Junctions

MARTIN BIEL
Department Pharmazie, Zentrum für Pharmaforschung, Pharmakologie für Naturwissenschaftler, Ludwig-Maximilians-Universität, München, Germany
   HCN Channels: From Genes to Function

NEIL E. BOWLES, PHD
Assistant Professor, Pediatrics (Cardiology), Baylor University College of Medicine, Houston, Texas
   Human Molecular Genetics and the Heart

MARK R. BOYETT, BSC, PHD
Professor of Physiology, School of Biomedical Sciences, University of Leeds, Leeds, United Kingdom
   Cellular Mechanisms of Sinoatrial Activity

JOSEP BRUGADA, MD, PHD
Associate Professor of Medicine, University of Barcelona; Director of the Arrhythmia Unit, Cardiovascular Institute, Hospital Clinic, Barcelona, Spain
   The Brugada Syndrome

PEDRO BRUGADA, MD, PHD
Professor of Cardiology, OLV Hospital, Aalst, Belgium
   The Brugada Syndrome

RAMON BRUGADA, MD, FACC
Director, Molecular Genetics Program, Masonic Medical Research Laboratory, Utica, New York
   The Brugada Syndrome

NENAD BURSAC, PHD
Assistant Professor, Department of Biomedical Engineering, Duke University, Durham, North Carolina
   Rotors and Spiral Waves in Two Dimensions

ALFRED E. BUXTON, MD
Professor of Medicine, Brown University Medical School; Director of Arrhythmia Services and Clinical Electrophysiology Laboratory, Rhode Island and Miriam Hospitals, Providence, Rhode Island
   Results of Clinical Trials of Automatic External Defibrillators and Implantable Cardioverter-Defibrillators in Patients at Risk for Sudden Death

MICHAEL E. CAIN, MD
Tobias and Hortense Lewin Professor of Medicine, Director, Cardiovascular Division, Washington University School of Medicine; Director, Cardiovascular Division, Barnes-Jewish Hospital, St. Louis, Missouri
   Class III Antiarrhythmic Drugs: Amiodarone, Ibutilide, and Sotalol

HUGH CALKINS, MD
Professor of Medicine, Johns Hopkins University School of Medicine; Director of the Arrhythmia Service and Clinical Electrophysiology Laboratory, Johns Hopkins Hospital, Baltimore, Maryland
   Syncope

DAVID J. CALLANS, MD
Associate Professor, Division of Cardiovascular Medicine, University of Pennsylvania Health System, Philadelphia, Pennsylvania
   Sinus Rhythm Abnormalities; Ventricular Tachycardia in Patients with Coronary Artery Disease

RICCARDO CAPPATO, MD
Director, Center of Clinical Arrhythmia and Electrophysiology, Istituto Policlinico San Donato, Milan, Italy
   Catheter Ablation of Atrioventricular Reentry

SHEILA J. CARROLL, MD
Post-Doctoral Fellow, Pediatric Cardiology, College of Physicians and Surgeons of Columbia University, New York, New York
   KCNQ1/KCNE1 Macromolecular Signaling Complex: Channel Microdomains and Human Disease

AGUSTIN CASTELLANOS, MD, FACC, FAHA
Professor of Medicine, Division of Cardiology, University of Miami School of Medicine; Director, Clinical Electrophysiology, University of Miami/Jackson Memorial Medical Center, Miami, Florida
   Sudden Cardiac Death; Parasystole

LAN S. CHEN, MD
Associate Professor of Clinical Neurology, Keck School of Medicine, University of Southern California; Director, Clinical Neurophysiology Program, Childrens Hospital Los Angeles, Los Angeles, California
   Nerve Sprouting and Cardiac Arrhythmias

PENG-SHENG CHEN, MD
Pauline and Harold Price Chair in Cardiac Electrophysiology Research, Division of Cardiology, Department of Medicine, Cedars-Sinai Medical Center; Professor of Medicine, David Geffen School of Medicine, University of California, Los Angeles, Los Angeles, California
   Nerve Sprouting and Cardiac Arrhythmias

SHIH-ANN CHEN, MD
Professor of Medicine, National Yang Ming University, School of Medicine; Director of Cardiac Electrophysiology Laboratory, Taipei Veterans General Hospital, Taipei, Taiwan
   Catheter Ablation of Atrial Tachycardia

XIONGWEN CHEN
Temple University School of Medicine, Philadelphia, Pennsylvania
   Pharmacology of L-Type and T-Type Channels in the Heart

DAVID E. CLAPHAM, MD, PHD
Professor of Neurobiology, Aldo R. Castañeda Professor of Cardiovascular Research, Harvard Medical School; Investigator, Howard Hughes Medical Institute; Director of Cardiovascular Research, Children's Hospital Boston, Boston, Massachusetts
   Intracellular Signaling and Regulation of Cardiac Ion Channels

JACQUES CLÉMENTY, MD
Professor of Cardiology, University of Bordeaux II, Hôpital Cardiologique du Haut-Lévêque, Bordeaux-Pessac, France
   Catheter Ablation of Atrial Fibrillation: Triggers and Substrate

HARRY J. CRIJNS, MD, PHD
Professor of Cardiology, University of Maastricht; Professor and Chairman of the Department of Cardiology, University Hospital, Maastricht, The Netherlands
   Ventricular Tachycardia in Patients with Hypertrophy and Heart Failure

EMILE G. DAOUD, MD
MidOhio Cardiology and Vascular Consultants, MidWest Research Foundation, Riverside-Methodist Hospital, Columbus, Ohio
   Bundle Branch Reentry

MITHILESH K. DAS, MD, MRCP, FACC
Assistant Professor of Medicine, Krannert Institute of Cardiology; Assistant Professor of Clinical Medicine, Roudebush VA Medical Hospital, Methodist Hospital, University Medical Center, Wishard Hospital, Indianapolis, Indiana
   Differential Diagnosis of Wide QRS Complex Tachycardia

MARIO DELMAR, MD, PHD
Professor of Pharmacology, SUNY Upstate Medical University, Syracuse, New York
   Molecular Organization and Regulation of the Cardiac Gap Junction Channel Connexin43; Prospects for Pharmacologic Targeting of Gap Junction Channels

DARIO DIFRANCESCO, PHD
Department of Biomolecular Sciences and Biotechnology, Laboratory of Molecular Physiology and Neurobiology, University of Milano, Milano, Italy
   Pacemaker Channels and Normal Automaticity

JOHN P. DIMARCO, MD, PHD
Professor of Medicine, Cardiovascular Division, Director, Clinical Electrophysiology Laboratory, University of Virginia Health System School of Medicine, Charlottesville, Virginia
   Adenosine and Digoxin

HALINA DOBRZYNSKI, BSC, PHD
Research Fellow, University of Leeds, School of Biomedical Sciences, Leeds, United Kingdom
   Cellular Mechanisms of Sinoatrial Activity

HEATHER S. DUFFY, PHD
Research Associate, Department of Neuroscience, Albert Einstein College of Medicine, Bronx, New York
   Molecular Organization and Regulation of the Cardiac Gap Junction Channel Connexin43; Prospects for Pharmacologic Targeting of Gap Junction Channels

IGOR R. EFIMOV, PHD
Associate Professor of Biomedical Engineering, Physiology, and Biophysics, Case Western Reserve University, Cleveland, Ohio
   Mechanisms of AV Nodal Excitability and Propagation

JOACHIM R. EHRLICH, MD
Department of Medicine, Division of Cardiology, J.W. Goethe University, Frankfurt, Germany
   Atrial Fibrillation

NABIL EL-SHERIF, MD
Cardiology Division, Department of Medicine, SUNY Downstate Medical Center, Brooklyn, New York
   Torsade de Pointes

KENNETH A. ELLENBOGEN, MD
Kontos Professor of Medicine, MCV/VCU School of Medicine; Director, Clinical Electrophysiology Laboratory, Medical College of Virginia, Richmond, Virginia
   Atrial Tachycardia

ANDREW E. EPSTEIN, MD, FACC, FAHA
Professor of Medicine, Division of Cardiovascular Disease, University of Alabama at Birmingham, Birmingham, Alabama
   Ventricular Fibrillation

CENGIZ ERMIS, MD
EP Fellow, University of Minnesota, Minneapolis, Minnesota
   Head-up Tilt Table Testing

SABINE ERNST, MD
Director of Magnetic Navigation, II. Medizinische Abteilung, St. Georg General Hospital, Hamburg, Germany
   Catheter Ablation of Atrioventricular Reentry

N. A. MARK ESTES III, MD
Professor of Medicine, Tufts University School of Medicine; Director of Cardiac Arrythmia Service,

Tufts-New England Medical Center, Boston, Massachusetts
: New Antiarrhythmic Drugs

VLADIMIR G. FAST, PHD
Associate Professor, Department of Biomedical Engineering, University of Alabama at Birmingham, Birmingham, Alabama
: Cellular Mechanisms of Defibrillation

VADIM V. FEDOROV, PHD
Senior Research Scientist, Laboratory of Heart Electrophysiology, Institute of Experimental Cardiology, Moscow, Russia
: Cholinergic Atrial Fibrillation

GUY FONTAINE, MD, PHD
Research Director, Department of Rhythmology, Institut de Cardiologie, Hôpital de la Salpetriere, Paris, France
: Ventricular Tachycardia in Arrhythmogenic Right Ventricular Cardiomyopathies

SARA FORESTI, MD
Research Fellow, Electrophysiology, Department of Cardiology, Policlinico S. Matteo IRCCS, Oklahoma City, Oklahoma
: Electrophysiologic Characteristics of Atrioventricular Nodal Reentrant Tachycardia: Implications for the Reentrant Circuits

PAUL FORNES, MD, PHD
Associate Professor of Forensic Sciences, Medical School Cochin Port Royal, University of Paris (V); Associate Professor of Pathology, Department of Pathology, Hôpital Européen Georges Pompidou, Paris, France
: Ventricular Tachycardia in Arrhythmogenic Right Ventricular Cardiomyopathies

ROBERT FRANK, MD
Director, Department of Rhythmology, Institut de Cardiologie, Hôpital Pitié-Salpétrière, Paris, France
: Ventricular Tachycardia in Arrhythmogenic Right Ventricular Cardiomyopathies

MICHAEL R. FRANZ, MD, PHD, FACC
Professor of Medicine and Pharmacology, Department of Cardiology, Georgetown University Medical Center; Director of Electrophysiology, Department of Cardiology/Medicine, Veteran Affairs Medical Center, Washington, D.C.
: Monophasic Action Potential Recording

JOSEPH M. GALVIN, MB, BCH, MRCPI, FACC
Senior Lecturer in Medicine, Royal College of Surgeons in Ireland; Consultant Cardiologist, Co-Director, Cardiac Unit, James Connolly Memorial Hospital, Dublin, Ireland
: Ventricular Tachycardia in Patients with Dilated Cardiomyopathy

ALAN GARFINKEL, PHD
Professor of Medicine (Cardiology) and Physiological Science, University of California, Los Angeles, Los Angeles, California
: Nonlinear Dynamics of Excitation and Propagation in Cardiac Muscle

ANNE M. GILLIS, MD
Professor of Medicine, University of Calgary; Medical Director or Pacing and Electrophysiology, Calgary Health Region, Calgary, Alberta, Canada
: Class I Antiarrhythmic Drugs: Quinidine, Procainamide, Disopyramide, Lidocaine, Mexiletine, Flecainide, and Propafenone

MICHAEL R. GOLD, MD, PHD
Michael Assey Professor of Medicine; Chief of Cardiology; Medical Director, Heart and Vascular Center, Medical University of South Carolina, Charleston, South Carolina
: Newer Applications of Pacemakers

JEFFREY GOLDBERGER, MD
Associate Professor, Department of Cardiology, The Feinberg School of Medicine, Northwestern University, Chicago, Illinois
: Impact of Nontraditional Antiarrhythmic Drugs on Sudden Cardiac Death

RICHARD A. GRAY, PHD
Associate Professor, Department of Biomedical Engineering, University of Alabama at Birmingham, Birmingham, Alabama
: Global Mechanisms of Defibrillation

WOLFRAM GRIMM, MD
Professor of Internal Medicine and Cardiology; Director of the Electrophysiology Laboratory, Department of Cardiology, Philipps University, Marburg, Germany
: Accelerated Idioventricular Rhythm and Bidirectional Ventricular Tachycardia

WILLIAM J. GROH, BS, MD, MPH
Associate Professor of Medicine, Indiana School of Medicine, Indiana University; Associate Professor of Medicine, Methodist Hospital, Cardiology Department; Wishard Hospital, Cardiology Department; VA Medical Center, Cardiology Department, Indianapolis, Indiana
: Arrhythmias in Patients with Neurologic Disorders

DAVID E. HAINES, MD
Director, Heart Rhythm Center, William Beaumont Hospital, Royal Oak, Michigan
: The Biophysics and Pathophysiology of Lesion Formation during Radiofrequency Catheter Ablation

MICHEL HAÏSSAGUERRE, MD
Professor of Cardiology, University of Bordeaux II, Hôpital Cariologique du Haut-Lévêque, Bordeaux-Pesssac, France

Catheter Ablation of Atrial Fibrillation: Triggers and Substrate

CARLOS HARO, BS
Research Assistant, Department of Biomedical Engineering, Tulane University, New Orleans, Louisiana
Modeling Cardiac Defibrillation

DAVID L. HAYES, MD
Professor of Medicine, Mayo Medical School; Consultant, Division of Cardiovascular Diseases and Internal Medicine, Mayo Clinic, Rochester, Minnesota
Implantable Pacemakers

VOLODYA HAYRAPETYAN, PHD
Research Associate, Krannert Institute of Cardiology, Indiana University, Indianapolis, Indiana
Homomeric and Heteromeric Gap Junctions

JEAN-LOUIS HEBERT, MD, PHD
Assistant Professor, Faculty of Medicine, University of Paris XI; Chief, Cardiac Catheterization Laboratory, Department of Cardiovascular and Lung Physiology, University Hospital of Bicêtre, Le Kremlin-Bicêtre, Paris, France
Ventricular Tachycardia in Arrhythmogenic Right Ventricular Cardiomyopathies

CRAIG S. HENRIQUEZ, PHD
W. H. Gardner Jr. Associate Professor of Biomedical Engineering and Computer Science, Department of Biomedical Engineering, Duke University, Durham, North Carolina
Three-dimensional Propagation in Mathematical Models

STEFAN HERRMANN, PHD
Assistant, Institut für Pharmakologie und Toxikologie, Technical University München, München, Germany
HCN Channels: From Genes to Function

GERHARD HINDRICKS, MD
University Leipzig, Heart Center; Co-Director, Department of Electrophysiology, Leipzig, Germany
Catheter Ablation of Atrial Flutter

MÉLÈZE HOCINI, MD
Clinical and Research Associate, Hôpital Cardiologique du Haut-Lévêque, Bordeaux-Pessac, France
Catheter Ablation of Atrial Fibrillation: Triggers and Substrate

FRANZ HOFMANN
Professor and Chair in Pharmacology, Institut fur Pharmakologie und Toxikologie, Technical University München, München, Germany
HCN Channels: From Genes to Function

STEFAN H. HOHNLOSER, MD, FACC, FESC
Professor of Medicine, Department of Medicine, Division of Cardiology, J. W. Goethe University, Frankfurt, Germany
T-Wave Alternans

HARUO HONJO, MD
Associate Professor, Department of Humoral Regulation, Research Institute of Environmental Medicine, Nagoya University, Nagoya, Japan
Cellular Mechanisms of Sinoatrial Activity

STEVEN R. HOUSER, PHD, FAHA
Laura H. Carnell Professor of Physiology, Director, Cardiovascular Research Center, Temple University School of Medicine, Philadelphia, Pennsylvania
Pharmacology of L-Type and T-Type Channels in the Heart

LARRY V. HRYSHKO, BSC, PHD
Associate Professor of Physiology, Institute of Cardiovascular Sciences, St. Boniface Hospital Research Centre, University of Manitoba, Winnipeg, Manitoba, Canada
Membrane Pumps and Exchangers

EDWARD W. HSU, PHD
Assistant Professor, Department of Biomedical Engineering, Duke University, Durham, North Carolina
Three-dimensional Propagation in Mathematical Models

JIAN HUANG, MD, PHD
Assistant Professor of Medicine, Department of Medicine, University of Alabama at Birmingham, Birmingham, Alabama
Defibrillation Waveforms

JEAN-SÉBASTIEN HULOT, MD
Fellow, Service de Pharmacologie, Hôpital de la Salpetriere, Paris, France
Ventricular Tachycardia in Arrhythmogenic Right Ventricular Cardiomyopathies

GARY D. HUTCHINS, PHD
John W. Beeler Professor, Vice Chairman for Research, Department of Radiology, Indiana University School of Medicine, Indianapolis, Indiana
Neurocardiac Imaging

RAYMOND E. IDEKER, MD, PHD
Professor of Cardiology, Department of Medicine, University of Alabama at Birmingham, Birmingham, Alabama
Defibrillation Waveforms

ALBERTO INTERIAN, JR, MD
Professor of Medicine, Associate Chief, Division of Cardiology and Electrophysiology, University of Miami School of Medicine, Miami, Florida
Sudden Cardiac Death

SEI IWAI, MD
Assistant Professor of Medicine, Division of Cardiology, New York Presbyterian Hospital, Cornell University Medical Center, New York, New York
Ventricular Tachycardia in Patients with Structurally Normal Hearts

WARREN M. JACKMAN, MD
Professor of Medicine, George Lynn Cross Research Professor, Director, Clinical Electrophysiology, Co-Director, Cardiac Arrhythmia Research Institute, University of Oklahoma Health Sciences Center, Oklahoma City, Oklahoma
> Electrophysiologic Characteristics of Atrioventricular Nodal Reentrant Tachycardia: Implications for the Reentrant Circuits

PIERRE JAÏS, MD
Research Associate, University of Bordeaux II; Staff Physician, Hôpital Cardiologique du Haut-Lévêque, Bordeaux-Pessac, France
> Catheter Ablation of Atrial Fibrillation: Triggers and Substrate

JOSÉ JALIFE, MD
Professor and Chair, Department of Pharmacology; Professor of Medicine and Pediatrics, Director, Institute for Cardiovascular Research, SUNY Upstate Medical University, Syracuse, New York
> Dynamics and Molecular Mechanisms of Ventricular Fibrillation in Normal Hearts

CRAIG T. JANUARY, MD, PHD
Professor of Medicine and Physiology, University of Wisconsin Hospital and Clinics, Madison, Wisconsin
> Pharmacology of the Cardiac Sodium Channel

CHRISTOPHER R. JOHNSON, PHD
Director, School of Computing, Director, Scientific Computing and Imaging Institute, Distinguished Professor of Computer Science, University of Utah, Salt Lake City, Utah
> Three-dimensional Propagation in Mathematical Models

MARK E. JOSEPHSON, MD
Chief, Cardiovascular Division, Herman Dana Professor of Medicine, Harvard Medical School; Director, Harvard-Thorndike Electrophysiology Institute and Arrhythmia Service, Boston, Massachusetts
> Ventricular Tachycardia in Patients with Coronary Artery Disease

XAVIER JOUVEN, MD, PHD
Epidemiologist, University of Paris V; Cardiologist, Electrophysiologist, Hôpital Européen Georges Pompidou, Paris, France
> Ventricular Tachycardia in Arrhythmogenic Right Ventricular Cardiomyopathies

ALAN H. KADISH, BA, MD
Chester and Deborah C. Cooley Professor of Medicine, Feinberg School of Medicine, Northwestern University; Senior Associate Chief, Division of Cardiology, Department of Medicine, Northwestern Memorial Hospital, Chicago, Illinois
> Impact of Nontraditional Antiarrhythmic Drugs on Sudden Cardiac Death

JONATHAN M. KALMAN, MBBS, PHD, FACC
Professor of Medicine, Director of Cardiac Electrophysiology, Royal Melbourne Hospital, Melbourne, Australia
> Catheter Ablation of Atrioventricular Nodal Reentrant Tachycardia

TIMOTHY J. KAMP, MD, PHD
Associate Professor of Medicine and Physiology, University of Wisconsin Medical School, Madison, Wisconsin
> Pharmacology of the Cardiac Sodium Channel

ROBERT S. KASS, PHD
David Hosack Professor of Pharmacology and Chairman, Columbia University, College of Physicians and Surgeons, New York, New York
> KCNQ1/KCNE1 Macromolecular Signaling Complex: Channel Microdomains and Human Disease

HAROLD L. KENNEDY, MD, MPH, FACC, FESC
Professor, Department of Medicine, Division of Cardiology, University of South Florida, Tampa, Florida; Chief of Medicine, Chief of Cardiology and Cardiovascular Research, Bay Pines VA Medical Center, St. Petersburg, Florida
> Use of Long-term (Holter) Electrocardiographic Recordings

RICHARD E. KERBER, MD
Professor of Medicine, University of Iowa Hospitals and Clinics, University of Iowa College of Medicine; Staff Physician, University of Iowa Hospitals and Clinics, Iowa City, Iowa
> Transthoracic Cardioversion and Defibrillation

ANANT KHOSITSETH, MD
Fellow, Pediatric Cardiology, Mayo Graduate School of Medicine, Mayo Clinic, Rochester, Minnesota
> Intracellular Signaling and Regulation of Cardiac Ion Channels

MICHAEL J. KILBORN
Clinical Senior Lecturer, University of Sydney; Staff Cardiologist, Royal Prince Alfred Hospital, New South Wales, Australia
> Electrocardiographic Manifestations of Supernormal Conduction, Concealed Conduction, and Exit Block

ANDRÉ G. KLÉBER, MD
Professor of Physiology, Department of Physiology, University of Bern, Bern, Switzerland
> Intercellular Communication and Impulse Propagation

GEORGE J. KLEIN, MD
Head, Division of Cardiology, University of Western Ontario, London, Ontario, Canada
> The Use of Implantable Loop Recorders; Wolff-Parkinson-White Syndrome

BRADLEY P. KNIGHT, MD
Associate Professor of Medicine, Director of Cardiac Electrophysiology, Center for Advanced Medicine, University of Chicago, Chicago, Illinois
   Atrioventricular Reentry and Variants

ITSUO KODAMA, MD
Professor, Department of Circulation, Research Institute of Environmental Medicine, Nagoya University, Nagoya, Japan
   Cellular Mechanisms of Sinoatrial Activity

HANS KOTTKAMP, MD
Professor of Medicine, Department of Electrophysiology, University of Leipzig Heart Center, Leipzig, Germany
   Catheter Ablation of Atrial Flutter

ANDREW D. KRAHN, MD
Associate Professor, Division of Cardiology, University of Western Ontario; Cardiologist, London Health Sciences Centre, London, Ontario, Canada
   The Use of Implantable Loop Recorders

JAN P. KUCERA, MD
Senior Research Assistant, Department of Physiology, University of Bern, Bern, Switzerland
   Cardiac Tissue Architecture Determines Velocity and Safety of Propagation

KARL-HEINZ KUCK, MD
Chief Cardiologist, St. Georg General Hospital, II Med. Abteilung, Kardiologie, Electrophysiologie, Hamburg, Germany
   Catheter Ablation of Atrioventricular Reentry

JOHN D. KUGLER, MD
Chief, Joint Division of Pediatric Cardiology, University of Nebraska College of Medicine/Creighton University School of Medicine; D.B and Paula Varner Professor of Pediatrics, University of Nebraska College of Medicine; Director, Cardiology, Children's Hospital, Omaha, Nebraska
   Catheter Ablation in Pediatric Patients

CHI-TAI KUO, MD
Associate Professor in Medicine, Chang-Gung University, Taoyuan, Taiwan; Professor in Cardiology, Chief of the First Cardiovasular Division, Department of Medicine, Chang-Gung Memorial Hospital, Linkou, Taiwan
   Exercise-induced Cardiac Arrhythmias

JUNKO KUROKAWA, PHD
Associate Research Scientist, Department of Pharmacology, College of Physicians and Surgeons of Columbia University, New York, New York
   KCNQ1/KCNE1 Macromolecular Signaling Complex: Channel Microdomains and Human Disease

MAX J. LAB, MD
Professor Emeritus and Senior Research Investigator, Division of Medicine, National Heart and Lung Institute, London, United Kingdom
   Mechanoelectric Transduction/Feedback: Prevalence and Pathophysiology

WEN-TER LAI, MD
Professor of Internal Medicine, Kaohsiung Medical University; Chief, Cardiovascular Center, Chung Ho Memorial Hospital, Kaohsiung, Taiwan
   Exercise-induced Cardiac Arrhythmias

CLAIRE LARSON, BS
Research Assistant, Department of Biomedical Engineering, Tulane University, New Orleans, Louisiana
   Modeling Cardiac Defibrillation

KENNETH R. LAURITA, PHD
Assistant Professor of Medicine & Biomedical Engineering, The Heart & Vascular Research Center, MetroHealth Campus of Case Western Reserve University, Cleveland, Ohio
   Restitution, Repolarization, and Alternans as Arrhythmogenic Substrates

RALPH LAZZARA, MD
Natalie O. Warren Professor of Medicine, George Lynn Cross Research Professor, University of Oklahoma Health Sciences Center; Director, Cardiac Arrhythmia Research Institute, Oklahoma City, Oklahoma
   Electrophysiologic Characteristics of Atrioventricular Nodal Reentrant Tachycardia: Implications for the Reentrant Circuits

BRUCE B. LERMAN, MD
H. Altschul Master Professor of Medicine, Chief, Division of Cardiology, Director, Cardiac Electrophysiology Laboratory, Cornell University Medical Center, New York Presbyterian Hospital, New York, New York
   Ventricular Tachycardia in Patients with Structurally Normal Hearts

DEBORAH L. LERNER, MD
Instructor in Pediatrics, Division of Critical Care Medicine, Washington University School of Medicine, St. Louis, Missouri
   Gap Junction Distribution and Regulation in the Heart

SAMUEL LÉVY, MD
Professor of Cardiology, University of Marseille, School of Medicine; Chief of Division of Cardiology, Hôpital Nord, Marseille, France
   Implantable Atrial Defibrillators for Atrial Fibrillation

RONALD A. LI, PHD
Assistant Professor of Medicine, Institute of Molecular Cardiobiology, Johns Hopkins University School of Medicine, Baltimore, Maryland
   Sodium Channels

DAVID LIN, MD
Assistant Professor, University of Pennsylvania, Hospital of the University of Pennsylvania, Philadelphia, Pennsylvania
 Sinus Rhythm Abnormalities

DEBORAH LOCKWOOD, BM, BCH, MA
Assistant Professor of Medicine, Cardiovascular Division, Oklahoma University Health Sciences Center, Oklahoma City, Oklahoma
 Electrophysiologic Characteristics of Atrioventricular Nodal Reentrant Tachycardia: Implications for the Reentrant Circuits

BARRY LONDON, MD, PHD
Director, Cardiovascular Institute; Chief, Division of Cardiology, University of Pittsburgh, Cardiovascular Institute, Pittsburgh, Pennsylvania
 Mouse Models of Cardiac Arrhythmias

FEI LÜ, MD, PHD
Assistant Professor of Medicine, University of Minnesota; Director of Clinical Cardiac Electrophysiology Laboratory, Fairview University Medical Center, Minneapolis, Minnesota
 Head-up Tilt Table Testing

ANDREAS LUDWIG, MD
Associate Professor, Institut für Pharmakologie und Toxikologie, Technical University München, München, Germany
 HCN Channels: From Genes to Function

JONATHAN C. MAKIELSKI, MD
Senior Associate Chair for Research; Professor, Department of Medicine and Physiology, University of Wisconsin, Madison, Wisconsin
 Pharmacology of the Cardiac Sodium Channel

MAREK MALIK, MD, PHD
Department of Cardiological Sciences, St. George's Hospital Medical School, London, United Kingdom
 Heart Rate Variability and Baroreflex Sensitivity

EDUARDO MARBÁN, MD, PHD
Professor of Medicine, Physiology, and Biomedical Engineering, Chief of Cardiology, Johns Hopkins Hospital, Johns Hopkins University, Baltimore, Maryland
 Sodium Channels

FRANCIS E. MARCHLINSKI, MD
Professor of Medicine, University of Pennsylvania School of Medicine; Director, Cardiac Electrophysiology, University of Pennsylvania Health System, Philadelphia, Pennsylvania
 Accelerated Idioventricular Rhythm and Bidirectional Ventricular Tachycardia

VIAS MARKIDES, MB (HONS), BS (HONS), MRPC (UK)
Consultant Cardiologist, St. Mary's and Royal Brompton & Harefield NHS Trusts, Waller Cardiac Department, St. Mary's Hospital, London, United Kingdom
 Mapping

STEVEN M. MARKOWITZ, MD
Associate Professor of Clinical Medicine, Cornell University Medical Center, New York Presbyterian Hospital, New York, New York
 Ventricular Tachycardia in Patients with Structurally Normal Hearts

BARRY J. MARON, MD
Director, Hypertrophic Cardiomyopathy Center, Minneapolis Heart Institute Foundation, Minneapolis, Minnesota
 Ventricular Arrhythmias in Hypertrophic Cardiomyopathy

AGUSTÍN D. MARTÍNEZ
Research Associate, Department of Pediatrics, University of Chicago, Chicago, Illinois
 Homomeric and Heteromeric Gap Junctions

MARK A. MCGUIRE, MB, BS, PHD, FRACP
Clinical Associate Professor of Medicine, University of Sydney; Senior Staff Cardiologist, Director of Cardiac Arrhythmia Service, Royal Prince Alfred Hospital, New South Wales, Australia
 Electrocardiographic Manifestations of Supernormal Conduction, Concealed Conduction, and Exit Block

GERHARD MEISSNER, PHD
Professor, Departments of Biochemistry and Biophysics and Cell and Molecular Physiology, School of Medicine, University of North Carolina, Chapel Hill, North Carolina
 Sarcoplasmic Reticulum Ion Channels

WILLIAM M. MILES, MD
Voluntary Professor of Medicine, University of Miami School of Medicine, Miami, Florida; Consulting Electrophysiologist, Southwest Florida Heart Group, Fort Myers, Florida
 Assessment of the Patient with a Cardiac Arrhythmia

JOHN M. MILLER, MD
Professor of Medicine; Director, Clinical Cardiac Electrophysiology, Krannert Institute of Cardiology, Indianapolis, Indiana
 Differential Diagnosis of Wide QRS Complex Tachycardia

MICHAEL A. MILLER, PHD
Assistant Research Scientist, Division of Imaging Science, Department of Radiology, Indiana University School of Medicine, Indianapolis, Indiana
 Neurocardiac Imaging

SUNEET MITTAL, MD
Assistant Professor of Medicine, Division of Cardiology, New York Presbyterian Hospital, Cornell University Medical Center, New York, New York

Ventricular Tachycardia in Patients with Structurally Normal Hearts

FEDERICO MOLEIRO, MD
Full Professor (Cardiology), Experimental Cardiology Lab, Central University of Venezuela, Caracas, Venezuela
Parasystole

SVEN MOOSMANG, MD
Assistant Professor/Postdoc, Institut für Pharmakologie und Toxikologie, Technical University München, München, Germany
HCN Channels: From Genes to Function

FRED MORADY, MD
Professor of Medicine, McKay Professor of Cardiovascular Diseases, University of Michigan; Director, Clinical Electrophysiology Laboratory, University of Michigan Health System, Ann Arbor, Michigan
Atrioventricular Reentry and Variants

ALONSO P. MORENO, PHD
Associate Professor of Medicine, Krannert Institute of Cardiology, Indiana University School of Medicine, Indianapolis, Indiana
Homomeric and Heteromeric Gap Junctions

ARTHUR J. MOSS, MD
Professor of Medicine (Cardiology), Director, Heart Research Follow-up Program, University of Rochester School of Medicine and Dentistry, Rochester, New York
Long QT Syndrome—Therapeutic Considerations

ROBERT J. MYERBURG, MD
Professor of Medicine and Physiology, Director, Division of Cardiology, University of Miami School of Medicine D-39; Chief, Cardiology Service, Jackson Memorial Hospital, Miami, Florida
Sudden Cardiac Death; Parasystole

HIROSHI NAKAGAWA, MD, PHD
Associate Professor of Medicine Research, University of Oklahoma Health Sciences Center, Cardiac Arrhythmia Research Institute, Oklahoma City, Oklahoma
Electrophysiologic Characteristics of Atrioventricular Nodal Reentrant Tachycardia: Implications for the Reentrant Circuits

CARLO NAPOLITANO, MD, PHD
Adjunct Professor, School of Cardiology, University of Pavia; Research Coordinator, Molecular Cardiology Laboratories, IRCCS Fondazione S. Maugeri, Pavia, Italy
Genetics of Long QT, Brugada, and Other Channelopathies; Catecholaminergic Polymorphic Ventricular Tachycardia and Short-coupled Torsades de Pointes

STANLEY NATTEL, BSC, MDCM
Professor of Medicine, Paul David Chair in Cardiovascular Electrophysiology, University of Montreal; Director, Research Center, Montreal Heart Institute, Montreal, Quebec, Canada
Atrial Fibrillation

JEANNE M. NERBONNE, PHD
Professor, Department of Molecular Biology and Pharmacology, Washington University School of Medicine, St. Louis, Missouri
Heterogeneous Expression of Potassium Channels in the Mammalian Myocardium

VLADIMIR P. NIKOLSKI, PHD
Researcher, Department of Biomedical Engineering, Case Western Reserve University, Cleveland, Ohio
Mechanisms of AV Nodal Excitability and Propagation

JEFFREY E. OLGIN, MD
Associate Professor of Medicine, Chief, Cardiac Electrophysiology Service, University of California, San Francisco, San Francisco, California
Electrophysiology of the Pulmonary Veins: Mechanisms of Initiation of Atrial Fibrillation

HAKAN ORAL, MD
Assistant Professor, Internal Medicine, Director, Arrhythmia Research, University of Michigan, Ann Arbor, Michigan
Junctional Rhythms and Junctional Tachycardia

KENICHIRO OTOMO, MD, PHD
The University of Oklahoma Health Sciences Center, Oklahoma City, Oklahoma
Electrophysiologic Characteristics of Atrioventricular Nodal Reentrant Tachycardia: Implications for the Reentrant Circuits

GAVIN Y. OUDIT, MSC, MD
Clinician Investigator Program, Internal Medicine Resident, Faculty of Medicine, Division of Cardiology, University Health Network, Heart & Stroke/Richard Lewar Centre of Excellence, University of Toronto, Toronto, Ontario, Canada
Voltage-regulated Potassium Channels

FEIFAN OUYANG, MD
II. Medizinische Abteilung, St. Georg General Hospital, Hamburg, Germany
Catheter Ablation of Atrioventricular Reentry

PIERRE L. PAGÉ, MD
Professor of Surgery, Université de Montréal, Cardiac Surgeon, Hôpital du Sacré-Coeur de Montréal, Quebec, Canada
Surgery for Cardiac Arrhythmias

CARLO PAPPONE, MD, PHD
Professor of Cardiology, Director, Cardiac Electrophysiology and Pacing Unit, Department of Cardiology, University Vita-Salute, San Raffaele University Hospital, Milan, Italy
Pulmonary Vein Isolation for Atrial Fibrillation

EUGENE PATTERSON, PhD
Associate Professor, University of Oklahoma Health Sciences Center, Oklahoma City, Oklahoma
  Electrophysiologic Characteristics of Atrioventricular Nodal Reentrant Tachycardia: Implications for the Reentrant Circuits

ARKADY M. PERTSOV, PhD
Professor, Department of Pharmacology, SUNY Upstate Medical University, Syracuse, New York
  Scroll Waves in Three Dimensions

NICHOLAS S. PETERS, MD
Professor of Cardiology, Head of Cardiac Electrophysiology, Imperial College and St. Mary's Hospital, London, United Kingdom; Director of Electrophysiology Research, American Cardiovascular Research Institute, Atlanta, Georgia
  Mapping

ROBERT W. PETERS, BA, MD
Professor of Medicine, University of Maryland School of Medicine; Chief of Cardiology, VA Medical Center, Baltimore, Maryland
  Newer Applications of Pacemakers

SILVIA G. PRIORI, MD, PhD
Associate Professor of Cardiology, University of Pavia; Director of Molecular Cardiology, Salvatore Maugeri Foundation, Pavia, Italy
  Genetics of Long QT, Brugada, and Other Channelopathies; Catecholaminergic Polymorphic Ventricular Tachycardia and Short-coupled Torsades de Pointes; Long QT Syndrome—Genotype-Phenotype Considerations

CATHERINE PROST-SQUARCIONI, MD, PhD
Laboratoire d'Histologie et de Thérapie Génique, UFR Léonard de Vinci, Hôpital Avicenne, Bobigny, France
  Ventricular Tachycardia in Arrhythmogenic Right Ventricular Cardiomyopathies

ERIC N. PRYSTOWSKY, MD
Consulting Professor of Medicine, Duke University Medical Center, Durham, North Carolina; Director, Clinical Electrophysiology Laboratory, St. Vincent Hospital, Indianapolis, Indiana
  Wolff-Parkinson-White Syndrome

BONNIE B. PUNSKE, PhD
Research Assistant Professor of Medicine and Bioengineering, Nora Eccles Harrison Cardiovascular Research and Training Institute (CVRTI), University of Utah, Salt Lake City, Utah
  Body Surface Potential Mapping

ZHILIN QU, PhD
Assistant Professor of Medicine (Cardiology), David Geffen School of Medicine at University of California, Los Angeles, Los Angeles, California
  Nonlinear Dynamics of Excitation and Propagation in Cardiac Muscle

RAFAEL J. RAMIREZ, PhD
Department of Physiology, Heart & Stroke/Richard Lewar Centre of Excellence, University of Toronto, Toronto, Ontario, Canada
  Voltage-regulated Potassium Channels

ILARIA RIVOLTA, PhD
Department of Molecular Cardiology, Salvatore Maugeri Foundation, Pavia, Italy
  Genetics of Long QT, Brugada, and Other Channelopathies

RICHARD B. ROBINSON, PhD
Professor, Department of Pharmacology, Columbia University, New York, New York
  Molecular and Cellular Bases of β-Adrenergic and α-Adrenergic Modulation of Cardiac Rhythm

DAN M. RODEN, MD
Professor of Medicine and Pharmacology, Director, Division of Clinical Pharmacology, Vanderbilt University School of Medicine, Nashville, Tennessee
  Pharmacogenomics of Cardiac Arrhythmias and Impact on Drug Therapy

STEPHAN ROHR, MD
Department of Physiology, University of Bern, Bern, Switzerland
  Cardiac Tissue Architecture Determines Velocity and Safety of Propagation

SALVATORE ROSANIO, MD, PhD, FACC
Associate Professor of Medicine, University of Texas Medical Branch; Director of Electrophysiology Research, Division of Cardiology, Department of Internal Medicine, John Sealy Annex Hospital, Galveston, Texas
  Pulmonary Vein Isolation for Atrial Fibrillation

MICHAEL R. ROSEN, MD
Gustavus A. Pfeiffer Professor of Pharmacology, Professor of Pediatrics, Director, Center for Molecular Therapeutics, Columbia University, New York, New York
  Molecular and Cellular Bases of β-Adrenergic and α-Adrenergic Modulation of Cardiac Rhythm

DAVID S. ROSENBAUM, MD
Associate Professor of Medicine, Biomedical Engineering, Developmental Biology, Physiology and Biophysics, Director, Heart and Vascular Research Center, Case Western Reserve University, MetroHealth Campus, Cleveland, Ohio
  Restitution, Repolarization, and Alternans as Arrhythmogenic Substrates

LEONID V. ROSENSHTRAUKH, DSc, PhD
Professor of Physiology, Director, Department of Physiology, Director, Laboratory of Heart Electrophysiology, Institute of Experimental Cardiology, Moscow, Russia
  Cholinergic Atrial Fibrillation

BRADLEY J. ROTH, PHD
Associate Professor, Department of Physics, Oakland University, Rochester, Michigan
   Two-dimensional Propagation in Cardiac Muscle

YORAM RUDY, PHD
The M. Frank and Margaret C. Rudy Professor of Cardiac Bioelectricity, Director, Cardiac Bioelectricity Research and Training Center, Professor of Biomedical Engineering, Physiology and Biophysics, and Medicine, Case Western Reserve University, Cleveland, Ohio
   Ionic Mechanisms of Cardiac Electrical Activity: A Theoretical Approach

JEREMY N. RUSKIN, BS, PHD
Associate Professor of Medicine, Harvard Medical School; Director, Cardiac Arrhythmia Service, Massachusetts General Hospital, Boston, Massachusetts
   Ventricular Tachycardia in Patients with Dilated Cardiomyopathy

FREDERICK SACHS, PHD
U. B. Distinguished Professor of Biophysics, Center for Single Molecule Biophysics, Department of Physiology and Biophysics, SUNY, Buffalo, New York
   Heart Mechanoelectric Transduction

JEFFREY E. SAFFITZ, MD, PHD
Paul E. Lacy and Ellen Lacy Professor of Pathology, Department of Pathology, Washington University School of Medicine, St. Louis, Missouri
   Gap Junction Distribution and Regulation in the Heart

PRASHANTHAN SANDERS, MBBS (HONS), PHD, FRACP
Clinical Associate and Postdoctoral Research Fellow, Hôpital Cardiologique du Haut-Lévêque, Bordeaux-Pessac, France
   Catheter Ablation of Atrial Fibrillation: Triggers and Substrate

MICHAEL C. SANGUINETTI, PHD
Professor, Department of Physiology, University of Utah, Salt Lake City, Utah
   Gating of Cardiac Delayed Rectifier K+ Channels

NADIR SAOUDI, MD
Professor of Cardiology, Chef de Service, Centre Hospitalier Princesse Grace, Principauté de Monaco
   Parasystole

BENJAMIN J. SCHERLAG, PHD
Professor of Medicine, Helen Webster Professor of Cardiac Arrhythmias, George Lynn Cross Research Professor, University of Oklahoma Health Sciences Center, Cardiac Arrhythmia Research Institute, Oklahoma City, Oklahoma
   Electrophysiologic Characteristics of Atrioventricular Nodal Reentrant Tachycardia: Implications for the Reentrant Circuits

PETER J. SCHWARTZ, MD
Chairman, Cattedra Di Cardiologia, University of Pavia; Director, School for the Board in Cardiology; Chairman, Blood, Lung, and Heart Department, Chief, Coronary Care Unit, IRCCS Policlinico S. Matteo, Pavia, Italy
   Long QT Syndrome—Genotype-Phenotype Considerations; Prolonged Repolarization and Sudden Infant Death Syndrome

DAVID SCHWARTZMAN, MD
Associate Professor of Medicine, Atrial Arrhythmia Center, Univesity of Pittsburgh, Pittsburgh, Pennsylvania
   Atrioventricular Block and Atrioventricular Dissociation

OLIVER R. SEGAL, MRCP
Cardiology Research Fellow, St. Mary's Hospital and Imperial College of Medicine, London, United Kingdom
   Mapping

DIPEN C. SHAH, MD, DNB (CARD)
Assistant Professor, Service de Cardologie, Hôpital Cantonal Universitaire de Geneve, Geneva, Switzerland
   Catheter Ablation of Atrial Fibrillation: Triggers and Substrate

OLEG F. SHARIFOV, MD, PHD
Fellow, Department of Biomedical Engineering, University of Alabama at Birmingham, Birmingham, Alabama
   Cholinergic Atrial Fibrillation

KALYANAM SHIVKUMAR, MD, PHD
Director, UCLA Cardiac Arrhythmia Center and Electrophysiology Program, David Geffen School of Medicine at University of California, Los Angeles, Los Angeles, California
   Implantable Cardioverter-Defibrillator: Clinical Aspects

JEFFREY SIMMONS, MD
Assistant Professor of Clinical Medicine, Veterans Medical Center, Miami, Florida
   Sudden Cardiac Death

BRAMAH N. SINGH, MD, PHD, FRCP
University of California, Los Angeles, Cardiology Division, VA Medical Center West Los Angeles, Los Angeles, California
   β-Blockers and Calcium Channel Blockers as Antiarrhythmic Drugs

ALLAN C. SKANES, MD
Director, Electrophysiology Laboratory, London Health Sciences Center, London, Ontario, Canada
   The Use of Implantable Loop Recorders

TIMOTHY W. SMITH, DPHIL, MD
Assistant Professor of Medicine, Washington University School of Medicine; Staff Electrophysiologist,

Barnes-Jewish Hospital, St. Louis, Missouri
> Class III Antiarrhythmic Drugs: Amiodarone, Ibutilide, and Sotalol

KYOKO SOEJIMA, MD
Instructor in Medicine, Harvard Medical School; Cardiovascular Division, Brigham and Women's Hospital, Boston, Massachusetts
> Catheter Ablation of Ventricular Tachycardia

PAUL L. SORGEN, PhD
Assistant Professor, Department of Biochemistry and Molecular Biology, University of Nebraska Medical Center, Omaha, Nebraska
> Molecular Organization and Regulation of the Cardiac Gap Junction Channel Connexin43

DAVID C. SPRAY, PhD
Professor of Neuroscience and Medicine, Department of Neuroscience, Albert Einstein College of Medicine, Bronx, New York
> Molecular Organization and Regulation of the Cardiac Gap Junction Channel Connexin43; Prospects for Pharmacologic Targeting of Gap Junction Channels

MIDUTURU SRINIVAS, PhD
Instructor in Neuroscience, Department of Neuroscience, Albert Einstein College of Medicine, Bronx, New York
> Prospects for Pharmacologic Targeting of Gap Junction Channels

KENNETH M. STEIN, MD
Associate Professor of Medicine, Division of Cardiology, New York Presbyterian Hospital, Cornell University Medical Center, New York, New York
> Ventricular Tachycardia in Patients with Structurally Normal Hearts

SUSAN F. STEINBERG, MD
Associate Professor of Pharmacology, Columbia University, New York, New York
> Molecular and Cellular Bases of β-Adrenergic and α-Adrenergic Modulation of Cardiac Rhythm

WILLIAM G. STEVENSON, MD
Assistant Professor, Harvard Medical School; Director, Clinical Cardiac Electrophysiology Program, Brigham and Women's Hospital, Boston, Massachusetts
> Catheter Ablation of Ventricular Tachycardia

JULIANE STIEBER, MD
Assistant Professor, Institut für Pharmakologie und Toxikologie, Technical University München, München, Germany
> HCN Channels: From Genes to Function

MARCO STRAMBA-BADIALE, MD, PhD
Head, Pediatric Arrhythmias Center, IRCCS, Istituto Auxologico Italiano, Milan, Italy
> Prolonged Repolarization and Sudden Infant Death Syndrome

S. ADAM STRICKBERGER, MD
Director, Arrhythmia Research Program, Washington Hospital Center, Washington, D.C.
> Junctional Rhythms and Junctional Tachycardia

RUEY J. SUNG, MD
Professor of Medicine, National Cheng Kung University, School of Medicine, Tainan, Taiwan
> Exercise-induced Cardiac Arrhythmias

MICHAEL O. SWEENEY, MD
Cardiac Arrhythmia Service, Cardiovascular Division, Brigham and Women's Hospital, Boston, Massachusetts
> Sinus Node Dysfunction

CHARLES D. SWERDLOW, MD
Clinical Professor of Medicine, University of California, Los Angeles, Cedars Sinai Medical Center, Los Angeles, California
> Implantable Cardioverter-Defibrillator: Clinical Aspects

BRUNO TACCARDI, MD, PhD
Research Professor of Internal Medicine, University of Utah School of Medicine, Co-Director, Nora Eccles Harrison CVRTI, Salt Lake City, Utah
> Body Surface Potential Mapping

STEVEN M. TAFFET, PhD
Professor, Department of Pharmacology, SUNY Upstate Medical University, Syracuse, New York
> Molecular Organization and Regulation of the Cardiac Gap Junction Channel Connexin43

CHING-TAI TAI, MD
Professor of Medicine, National Yang-Ming University School of Medicine; Attending Physician, Taipei Veterans General Hospital, Taipei, Taiwan
> Catheter Ablation of Atrial Tachycardia

DANIEL THOMAS, MD
Professor, Chu Pitié Salpetriere Université Paris VI; Professor, Institut de Cardiologie, Hôpital de la Salpetriere, Paris, France
> Ventricular Tachycardia in Arrhythmogenic Right Ventricular Cardiomyopathies

GORDON F. TOMASELLI, MD
Professor, Department of Medicine, Johns Hopkins University, Baltimore, Maryland
> Sodium Channels

FERNANDO TONDATO, MD, PhD
Cardiac Electrophysiology Fellow, American Cardiovascular Research Institute, Norcross, Georgia
> Mapping

JEFFREY A. TOWBIN, MD
Professor, Departments of Pediatrics (Cardiology) and Molecular and Human Genetics, Baylor College of Medicine; Chief, Pediatric Cardiology, Foundation Chair in Pediatric Cardiac Research, Texas Children's Hospital, Houston, Texas
Human Molecular Genetics and the Heart; The Brugada Syndrome

JOSEPH V. TRANQUILLO
Graduate Student, Department of Biomedical Engineering, Duke University, Durham, North Carolina
Three-dimensional Propagation in Mathematical Models

NATALIA A. TRAYANOVA, PHD
Professor, Department of Biomedical Engineering, Tulane University, New Orleans, Louisiana
Modeling Cardiac Defibrillation

JOHN K. TRIEDMAN, MD
Associate Professor of Pediatrics, Harvard Medical School; Senior Associate in Cardiology, Children's Hospital, Boston, Massachusetts
Atrial Arrhythmias in Congenital Heart Disease

MARTIN TRISTANI-FIROUZI, MD
Associate Professor, Pediatric Cardiology, University of Utah School of Medicine, Salt Lake City, Utah
Gating of Cardiac Delayed Rectifier K+ Channels

CHIN-FENG TSAI, MD
Assistant Professor of Medicine, Division of Cardiology, Department of Medicine, Chung Shan Medical University Hospital, Taichung, Taiwan; Krannert Institute of Cardiology, Indianapolis, Indiana
Catheter Ablation of Atrial Tachycardia

LESLIE TUNG, PHD
Associate Professor, Department of Biomedical Engineering, Johns Hopkins University, School of Medicine, Baltimore, Maryland
Rotors and Spiral Waves in Two Dimensions

GIOIA TURITTO, MD
Associate Professor of Medicine, Director, Coronary Care Unit and Electrophysiology Laboratory, SUNY Downstate Medical Center, Brooklyn, New York
Torsade de Pointes

GEORGE F. VAN HARE, MD
Associate Professor; Director, Pediatric Arrythmia Center, Pediatric Cardiology, Stanford University, Palo Alto, California
Ventricular Tachycardia in Patients Following Surgery for Congenital Heart Disease

DAVID R. VAN WAGONER, BS, PHD
Associate Professor, Department of Molecular Medicine, Cleveland Clinic Lerner College of Medicine of Case Western Reserve University; Associate Staff, Department of Cardiovascular Medicine, Cleveland Clinic Foundation, Cleveland, Ohio
Electrical Remodeling and Chronic Atrial Fibrillation

MARC A. VOS, PHD
Department of Medical Physiology, UMC Utrecht, Utrecht, The Netherlands
Ventricular Tachycardia in Patients with Hypertrophy and Heart Failure

GREGORY P. WALCOTT, MD
Assistant Professor of Cardiology, Department of Medicine, University of Alabama at Birmingham, Birmingham, Alabama
Defibrillation Waveforms

ALBERT L. WALDO, MD
The Walter H. Pritchard Professor of Cardiology, Professor of Medicine, and Professor of Biomedical Engineering, Director, Clinical Cardiac Electrophysiology Program, Case Western Reserve University School of Medicine, University Hospitals of Cleveland, Cleveland, Ohio
Atrial Flutter: Mechanisms, Clinical Features, and Management

ZULU WANG, MD
The University of Oklahoma Health Sciences Center, Oklahoma City, Oklahoma
Electrophysiologic Characteristics of Atrioventricular Nodal Reentrant Tachycardia: Implications for the Reentrant Circuits

KENNETH M. WEINBERG, MD
Electrophysiology Fellow, The Feinberg School of Medicine, Northwestern University, Chicago, Illinois
Impact of Nontraditional Antiarrhythmic Drugs on Sudden Cardiac Death

DAVID WEINSTEIN, PHD
Technical Manager, Department of Computer Science, Scientific and Computing Institute, University of Utah, Salt Lake City, Utah
Three-dimensional Propagation in Mathematical Models

MARCEL WELLNER, MD
Senior Research Scientist, Institute for Cardiovascular Research, SUNY Upstate Medical University, Syracuse, New York
Theory of Reentry

BRUCE L. WILKOFF, MD
Director of Cardiac Pacing and Tachyarrhythmia Devices, Professor of Medicine, Cleveland Clinic Lerner College of Medicine, The Cleveland Clinic Foundation, Cleveland, Ohio
Implantable Cardioverter-Defibrillator: Technical Aspects

MARK A. WOOD, MD
Associate Professor, Internal Medicine/Cardiology, Medical College of Virginia, Richmond, Virginia
  Atrial Tachycardia

JIANYI WU, MD
Assistant Scientist, Krannert Institute of Cardiology, Indiana University, Indianapolis, Indiana
  Mechanisms of Initiation of Ventricular Tachyarrhythmias; Differential Diagnosis of Wide QRS Complex Tachycardia

JIASHIN WU, PHD
Assistant Professor Krannert Institute of Cardiology, Indianapolis, Indiana
  Mechanisms of Initiation of Ventricular Tachyarrhythmias

D. GEORGE WYSE, MD, PHD
Professor, Faculty of Medicine, University of Calgary; Cardiac Electrophysiologist, Calgary Health Region/The Libin Cardiovascular Institute of Alberta, Calgary, Alberta, Canada
  Results of Clinical Trials on Atrial Fibrillation

KATHRYN A. YAMADA, PHD
Research Associate Professor of Medicine, Washington University School of Medicine, St. Louis, Missouri
  Gap Junction Distribution and Regulation in the Heart

BIN YE, PHD
Department of Medicine, University of Wisconsin School of Medicine, Madison, Wisconsin
  Pharmacology of the Cardiac Sodium Channel

RAYMOND YEE, BMDSC, MD, FRCPC, FACC
Professor of Medicine, University of Western Ontario; Director of Arrhythmia Service, London Health Sciences Center-University Campus, London, Ontario, Canada
  The Use of Implantable Loop Recorders; Wolff-Parkinson-White Syndrome

ALEXEY V. ZAITSEV, PHD
Research Assistant Professor, Department of Pharmacology, SUNY Upstate Medical University, Syracuse, New York
  Mechanisms of Ischemic Ventricular Fibrillation: Who's the Killer?

WOJCIECH ZAREBA, MD, PHD
Associate Professor of Medicine (Cardiology), Associate Director, Heart Research Follow-up Program, University of Rochester School of Medicine and Dentistry, Rochester, New York
  Long QT Syndrome—Therapeutic Considerations

GUOQIANG ZHONG, MD
Post-doctoral Fellow, Krannert Institute of Cardiology, Indiana University, Indianapolis, Indiana
  Homomeric and Heteromeric Gap Junctions

DOUGLAS P. ZIPES, MD
Distinguished Professor, Krannert Institute of Cardiology, Indiana University School of Medicine, Indianapolis, Indiana
  Mechanisms of Initiation of Ventricular Tachyarrhythmias; Assessment of the Patient with a Cardiac Arrhythmia; Neurocardiac Imaging

目 录

第一部分 离子通道功能的结构与分子基础

第 1 章　钠通道 …………………………（1）
第 2 章　钙通道 …………………………（10）
第 3 章　电压调节性钾通道 ……………（19）
第 4 章　细胞内信号系统与心脏离子通道的
　　　　调节 ……………………………（33）
第 5 章　膜泵和离子交换 ………………（42）
第 6 章　肌浆网离子通道 ………………（51）
第 7 章　HCN 通道：从基因到功能 ……（60）
第 8 章　心脏缝隙连接蛋白 43 的分子组成
　　　　和调节 …………………………（67）

第二部分 心脏离子通道的生物物理学

第 9 章　正常和异常钠通道的生物物理学
　　　　……………………………………（77）
第 10 章　心脏门控延迟整流钾通道 ……（88）
第 11 章　机械电转换 ……………………（95）
第 12 章　起搏通道和正常的自律性 ……（102）
第 13 章　内向整流钾通道的生物物理学
　　　　　特性 ……………………………（110）
第 14 章　同源和异源缝隙连接通道 ……（118）

第三部分 心脏离子通道的分子间作用和药理学

第 15 章　心脏钠通道药理学 ……………（125）
第 16 章　心脏 L 型和 T 型钙电流的药理学
　　　　　……………………………………（131）
第 17 章　KCNQ1/KCNE1 大分子信号复合
　　　　　物：通道微结构与人体疾病 …（140）
第 18 章　药物诱发的通道病 ……………（147）
第 19 章　缝隙连接通道药理学靶点的前景
　　　　　……………………………………（154）

第四部分 离子通道与细胞电生理学

第 20 章　哺乳动物心肌钾通道的异源性
　　　　　表达 ……………………………（165）
第 21 章　心脏缝隙连接的分布和调节 …（177）
第 22 章　窦房结活动的细胞机制 ………（188）
第 23 章　房室结的兴奋性及其传导机制
　　　　　……………………………………（200）
第 24 章　细胞间的交流和电冲动的传导
　　　　　……………………………………（210）
第 25 章　心脏组织结构决定冲动传导的速
　　　　　度和安全性 ……………………（220）
第 26 章　致心律失常的基础：恢复、复极
　　　　　和交替 …………………………（229）
第 27 章　机械电转换/反馈：普遍性及
　　　　　病理生理学意义 ………………（238）

第五部分 心脏兴奋的模型

第 28 章　心脏电活动的离子机制：理论
　　　　　探索 ……………………………（251）
第 29 章　心肌中电激动的二维传导 ……（262）
第 30 章　数学模型中电激动的三维传导
　　　　　……………………………………（268）
第 31 章　心脏除颤模型 …………………（277）

第六部分 心脏电活动的中枢调节

第 32 章　β 和 α 肾上腺素受体调节心脏节
　　　　　律的分子和细胞基础 …………（285）
第 33 章　神经的新生与心律失常 ………（293）
第 34 章　胆碱能性心房颤动 ……………（300）

第七部分 非线性动力学、螺旋波和心脏节律

第 35 章 折返理论 …………………… (313)
第 36 章 心肌兴奋和传导的非线性动力学
　　　　 ……………………………… (323)
第 37 章 二维空间的旋转子和螺旋波 … (332)
第 38 章 三维空间的回旋波 …………… (340)

第八部分 心律失常发生的机制

第 39 章 肺静脉的电生理特性：房颤发生
　　　　 的机制 …………………… (351)
第 40 章 心房颤动的维持机制 ………… (359)
第 41 章 电重构与慢性心房颤动 ……… (371)
第 42 章 室性快速性心律失常的发生机制
　　　　 ……………………………… (376)
第 43 章 正常心脏心室颤动的动力学与
　　　　 分子机制 ………………… (386)
第 44 章 缺血性心室颤动的机制：谁是凶
　　　　 手？ ……………………… (395)
第 45 章 除颤的细胞机制 ……………… (403)
第 46 章 除颤的总体机制 ……………… (413)
第 47 章 除颤波形 ……………………… (422)

第九部分 分子遗传学和药物基因组学

第 48 章 心律失常的小鼠模型 ………… (429)
第 49 章 人类分子遗传学与心脏 ……… (440)
第 50 章 长 QT 综合征、Brugada 综合征
　　　　 和其他离子通道疾病的遗传学 … (459)
第 51 章 心律失常的药物基因组学及对
　　　　 药物治疗的影响 ………… (468)

第十部分 临床心律失常：机制、表现和处理

第 52 章 窦性心律失常 ………………… (475)
第 53 章 房室阻滞和房室分离 ………… (481)
第 54 章 心房扑动机制、临床表现和治疗
　　　　 ……………………………… (486)
第 55 章 房性心动过速 ………………… (494)
第 56 章 心房颤动 ……………………… (505)
第 57 章 交界区心律和交界区心动过速
　　　　 ……………………………… (517)
第 58 章 房室折返及变异形式 ………… (521)
第 59 章 房室结折返性心动过速的电生理
　　　　 学特征：折返环路的意义 …… (530)
第 60 章 先天性心脏病的房性心律失常
　　　　 ……………………………… (550)
第 61 章 冠心病相关性室性心动过速 …… (561)
第 62 章 扩张型心肌病的室性心律失常
　　　　 ……………………………… (567)
第 63 章 致心律失常性右室心肌病的室性
　　　　 心动过速 ………………… (580)
第 64 章 肥厚型心肌病的室性心律失常
　　　　 ……………………………… (593)
第 65 章 心脏肥大和心力衰竭的室性心动
　　　　 过速 ……………………… (600)
第 66 章 先天性心脏病术后的室性心动过
　　　　 速 ………………………… (611)
第 67 章 Brugada 综合征 ……………… (618)
第 68 章 儿茶酚胺敏感性多形性室速和短
　　　　 联律间期性尖端扭转型室速 … (626)
第 69 章 神经系统疾病与心律失常 …… (633)
第 70 章 长 QT 综合征：基因型与表现型
　　　　 的相关性 ………………… (644)
第 71 章 长 QT 综合征的治疗策略 …… (654)
第 72 章 非器质性心脏病室性心动过速
　　　　 ……………………………… (662)
第 73 章 束支折返性室速 ……………… (675)
第 74 章 尖端扭转型室速 ……………… (679)
第 75 章 加速性室性自主心律和双向性室
　　　　 性心动过速 ……………… (692)
第 76 章 心室颤动 ……………………… (697)
第 77 章 心室复极延长与婴儿猝死综合征
　　　　 ……………………………… (703)
第 78 章 心脏性猝死 …………………… (712)

第十一部分 心电图的识别

第 79 章 超常传导、隐匿传导和传出阻滞
　　　　 的心电图表现 …………… (723)
第 80 章 并行心律 ……………………… (728)
第 81 章 宽 QRS 波心动过速的鉴别诊断
　　　　 ……………………………… (736)

第十二部分 诊断与评价

- 第82章 心律失常的评估 …………… (747)
- 第83章 运动性心律失常 …………… (752)
- 第84章 动态心电图的应用 ………… (759)
- 第85章 植入式"Holter" ……………… (773)
- 第86章 高分辨心电图 ……………… (778)
- 第87章 体表电位标测 ……………… (788)
- 第88章 直立倾斜试验 ……………… (797)
- 第89章 心率变异性与压力反射敏感性 …………………………………… (809)
- 第90章 单相动作电位的记录 ……… (817)
- 第91章 T波电交替 ………………… (824)
- 第92章 心脏神经成像 ……………… (833)
- 第93章 心脏标测 …………………… (842)

第十三部分 临床综合征：认识、临床过程和处理

- 第94章 预激综合征 ………………… (853)
- 第95章 窦房结功能障碍 …………… (862)
- 第96章 晕厥 ………………………… (867)
- 第97章 心房颤动的临床试验 ……… (877)
- 第98章 有猝死风险患者的自动体外除颤器和植入式心脏复律除颤器临床试验结果 …………………… (883)

第十四部分 心律失常的药物和非药物治疗

- 第99章 Ⅰ类抗心律失常药物：奎尼丁、普鲁卡因胺、丙吡胺、利多卡因、美西律、氟卡胺和普罗帕酮 … (893)
- 第100章 抗心律失常药物：β受体阻滞剂和钙通道阻滞剂 …………… (900)
- 第101章 Ⅲ类抗心律失常药物：胺碘酮、依布利特和索他洛尔 ………… (913)
- 第102章 腺苷与地高辛 ……………… (922)
- 第103章 非传统抗心律失常药物对心脏性猝死的影响 ………………… (930)
- 第104章 新的抗心律失常药物 ……… (939)
- 第105章 经胸心脏复律与电除颤 …… (945)
- 第106章 植入式心脏复律除颤器：技术与现状 ……………………… (949)
- 第107章 植入式心脏复律除颤器的临床应用 …………………………… (958)
- 第108章 植入式心房除颤器治疗心房颤动 …………………………… (973)
- 第109章 植入式起搏器 ……………… (977)
- 第110章 起搏器的新应用 …………… (988)
- 第111章 射频导管消融术中损伤形成的生物物理学及病理生理学基础 …………………………… (995)
- 第112章 心房颤动触发灶和基质的导管射频消融术 …………………… (1004)
- 第113章 心房颤动的肺静脉隔离 …… (1015)
- 第114章 心房扑动的导管消融 ……… (1029)
- 第115章 房性心动过速的导管消融 … (1035)
- 第116章 房室结折返性心动过速的导管消融 ……………………… (1044)
- 第117章 房室折返性心动过速的导管消融 ………………………… (1052)
- 第118章 室性心动过速的导管消融 … (1060)
- 第119章 儿童患者的导管消融 ……… (1071)
- 第120章 心律失常的外科治疗 ……… (1078)

ID
第一部分
离子通道功能的结构与分子基础

第 1 章

钠 通 道

Ranald A. Li，Gordon F. Tomaselli，Eduardo Marbán

本章目录

- 钠通道的进化与遗传学 ………………… 1
- 功能单元 ……………………………………… 3
- 钠通道表达和功能的调节 ……………… 6
- 结论 …………………………………………… 7

本章主要回顾过去半个世纪来对钠通道结构和功能的研究进展，尤其是心脏钠通道。读者亦可参考各相关主题[4-9]，以便更好地理解。

一、钠通道的进化与遗传学

(一) 钠通道的进化与系统发育

电压门控钠通道是一种关键的蛋白质，它负责调节心肌、骨骼肌、神经细胞及其他可兴奋组织的动作电位的初始上升相。在心脏组织中，电压门控钠通道具有特别重要的作用：首先，钠通道的开放形成体表心电图上的 QRS 波群，它通过调节去极化电冲动在心肌中的扩散来决定兴奋的传导，保证心室的同步收缩；其次，在临床治疗中，钠通道是多种药物作用的靶点，如利多卡因和其他 I 类抗心律失常药物。最后，钠通道功能的再生和丧失均可引起多种遗传性疾病，如长 QT 综合征（LQTS）、Brugada 综合征和心脏传导性疾病。钠通道的发现在生理学的发展史上具有里程碑的意义。1952 年，Hodgkin 和 Huxley[1]以乌贼的轴突为实验对象，阐明了钠通道的基本特性，并通过仔细分析通道开放和关闭的门控动力学及离子如何穿越通道的滤过过程提出了现代通道学理论。此外，钠通道还是第一个被克隆的电压门控性离子通道[2]，从而开创了应用异源体系表达离子通道和在分子水平操纵离子通道的时代。由于钠通道被克隆的时间恰好与应用膜片钳记录单个细胞电生理学方法的改进相近，所以，膜片钳被用来记录单个通道的电生理特征，从而使离子通道的研究发生革命性的改变[3]。

在人类和其他脊椎动物，钠通道被发现存在于所有可兴奋组织中。这些信号分子被认为首先出现在水母的种系发育中，它们确保生物体通过分散的神经网络有效地传递电信号，但最近在更初级的原核生物中也有发现。在真核生物中，钠通道是高度保守的，并且在进化中它的中心选择压力得以保留，这样，钠通道就自然地解决了大型生物体内信号协调和交流的难题。而且，钠通道在轴突和肌肉中的分布特别密集，常常是该组织中数目最多的离子通道。以哺乳动物的心肌细胞为例，每个心肌细胞表达十万多个钠通道，而浦肯野纤维细胞表达的钠通道更丰富，达到一百多万个，然而，在该心肌细胞中仅有约 2 万个 L-型钙通道和更少的电压依赖钾通道表达。

钠通道的主要分子特征揭示了它的系统起源或组织来源。钠通道由多种亚基组成（见后面章），但只有成孔的 α-亚基是维持通道功能所必需的。图 1-1A 显示了真核生物钠通道 α-亚基结构图，它由约 2000 个氨基酸组成，包含四个同源的结构域（DⅠ~DⅣ），它们通过胞内连接体相连。每个结构域含有 6 个跨膜片段（S1~S6），其结构与电压门控钾通道的 α-亚基相似（见第 3 章）。四个同源的结构域顺时针排列组成一个中心孔。值得注意的是，钙通道有相似的整体结构,但结构域间有显著区别(见第 2 章)。因为单细胞生物可表达钾通道和钙通道,所以有可能是先有原始的相对简单的单个结构域钾通道,后来可通过基因复制进化为钙通道。钠通道可能以相似方式形成,或更可能来自原始钙通道的突变。与近来的发现相符合,一个命名为 NaChBac 的原核生物离子通道由含六个跨膜片段的单一结构域组成,它与电压门控钙离子通道有极其相似的序列,特别在成孔区,(见图 1-1C),它具有电压依赖性和钠离子选择性,对钙通道阻滞剂硝苯地平敏感[10]。

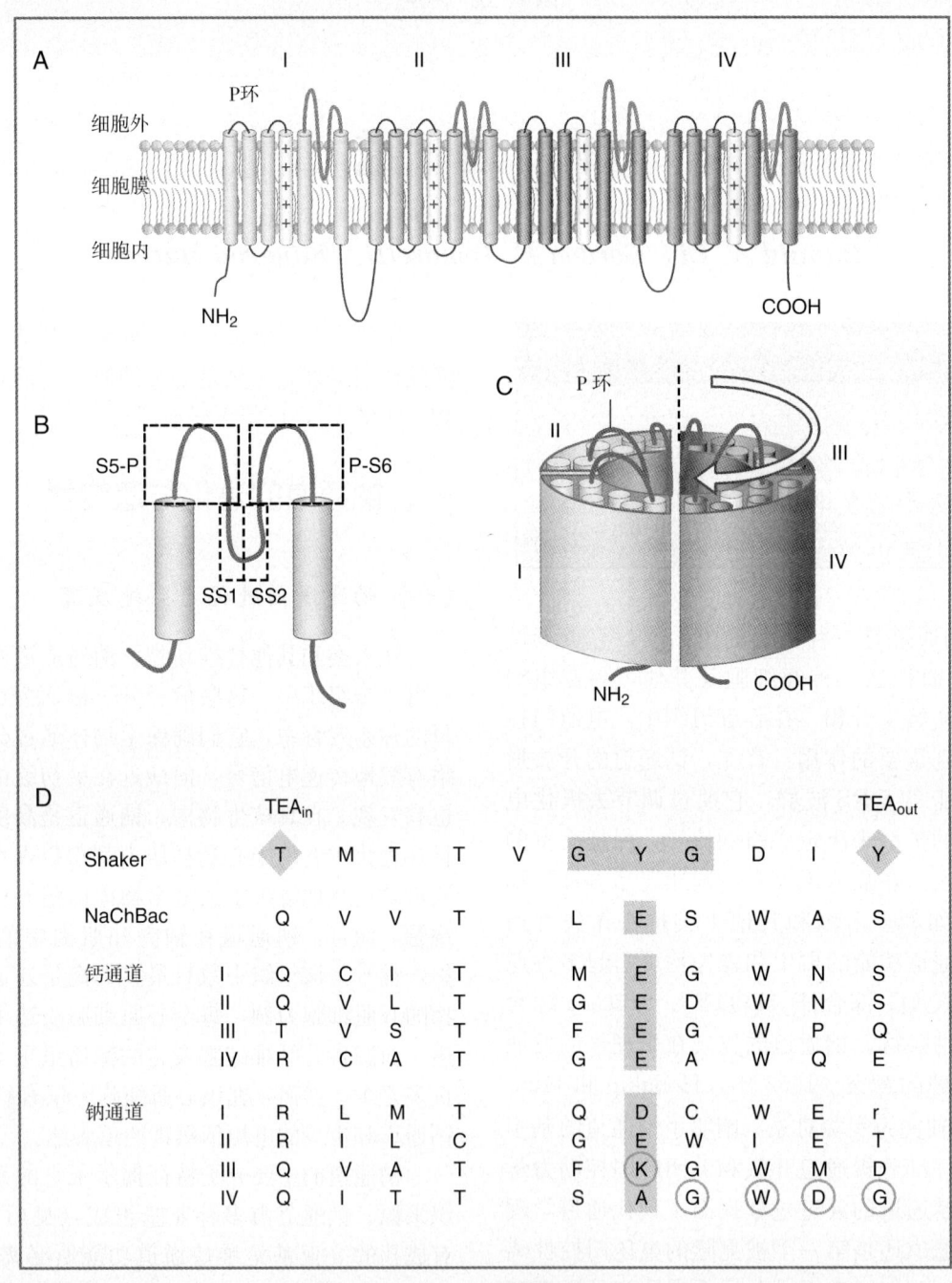

图 1-1 Na$^+$ 通道 α 亚基的示意图 A:推测的跨膜结构布局;带电荷的 S4 片段以白色表示,折返的 S5-S6 连接组成 S5-P,P-环(SS1 和 SS2)及 P-S6 用灰色表示。B:图示 S5 和 S6 跨膜片段,和折返的 S5-S6 连接体。S5-S6 连接组成 S5-P、P-环(SS1 和 SS2)及 P-S6。C:顺时针分布的 4 个结构域。D:K 通道(Shaker B)的孔区、心脏 L-型 Ca 通道的四个结构域、原核 Na 通道(NaChBac)、心脏 Na 通道的四个结构域的基本氨基酸组成。上部的残基显示的哺乳动物电压依赖 Na 通道是高度保守的。菱形区显示四乙基铵离子与 K 通道的外部和内部结合位点;盒形轮廓代表选择性滤过区,但是决定 Na 通道选择性的结构是盒子外边的残基(划圈的)

进化论的观点贯穿于各种主题中。离子通道被认为属于电压门控阳离子通道超家族：首先，它的结构有标准组件，由四个同源的亚基（如钾通道）或四个同源结构域组成（如哺乳动物的钠和钙通道）。其次，如图1-1A~C所示，这些蛋白质折叠缠绕形成中心性离子传导孔，与孔连接的区域（也称P-环区），其序列高度保守，以保证同一离子通道家族具有相似的离子选择性（如水母、电鳗、果蝇和人类的钠通道有相似的P-环区），而不同的离子通道家族具有不同的离子选择性（如钠和钾通道有不同的P-环区，见图1-1D）。离子通道孔区具有许多重要功能，如离子的选择性和传导性，并决定离子通道的药物反应性[4,7,9]，这一特性非常类似于酶的激活中心。第三，一般地，通道的开放呈电压依赖性这一门控过程，即"激活"，这一特征是高度保守的。因为在第四个跨膜片段（S4）上，每三个氨基酸包含一个带正电荷的碱性氨基酸（图1-2），去极化时它们从细胞膜内移向膜表面，引起一系列的构象变化，导致通道开放[5,8]。

（二）遗传学

哺乳动物基因组至少包含9种电压门控钠通道基因。不像钾通道和钙通道具有多种亚型，各种电压门控钠通道在跨膜和胞外区有50%以上的同源性，功能特征基本相似，它们的差异主要在于连接四个结构域胞内部分序列。各种钠通道的表达与发育有关，并具有组织特异性。例如心肌表达的钠通道α-亚基，它不但在成人心肌上大量表达，而且在胚胎期的骨骼肌也有表达。同样的，脑表达的钠通道α-亚基也被发现定位于心肌的横管部，可能在心肌的兴奋-收缩耦联环节中起一定的作用[12]。人类心肌钠通道hNa$_v$1.5（以前称hH1）定位于3号染色体的短臂（3p21-24）。心肌钠通道基因（SCN5A）的基因组结构已被破译，它包含28个外显子，基因组跨越80kb，第16号内含子包含一个二核苷酸重复序列多态性。

二、功能单元

（一）滤过性

依据以往的定义，透过/渗透是指所有离子通道孔的特性。渗透的基本特征和结构已在十年前被阐明。S5-S6以发夹样连接组成空腔的外部结构并有选择滤过作用，分为三个区域：S5-P、P-环（它的下降和上升区分别称为SS1和SS2）和P-S6（见图1-1B）[7]。尽管有各种证据表明钠通道孔区螺旋与KcsA晶体结构相似[13]，但钠通道和钾通道的孔区仍有许多结构和功能上的差异。例如，钾通道孔道能容纳多个钾离子，待滤过的钾离子须与孔道内的连接位点结合[14]，组成孔区的氨基酸羰基端形成孔道内的连接位点。很多研究显示，钠通道（也包括钙通道）的P-环氨基酸残基的侧链可能使孔道线性化[4]。钠通道的P-S6连接区可增加孔道外口部的有效钠离子浓度以提高单个钠通道的传导，而且P-S6连接区凹进细胞膜形成内陷仅次于P-环的凹陷[15]，但钾通道没有形成这种凹陷[14]。比对各个结构域的S5-S6间连接部分的氨基酸序列，发现它们之间是不同的（见图1-1D）。但钾通道的孔区由四个相同的P片段组成一个钾离子选择性孔隙，钠通道和钾通道的结构基础决定了它们具有不同的离子选择性滤过特性。进一步研究表明钠通道四个结构域的P-环对孔区的贡献存在不对称性，其中两个P-环对钠离子的选择起主导作用，位于第三结构域（Ⅲ）上的赖氨酸（hNa$_v$1.5第1418位）是区别钠和钙离子的关键，而与第四结构域（Ⅳ）P-环相邻多种残基（hNa$_v$1.5第1711至1714位）的突变可导致对单价离子的非选择性[16]。尽管钠和钾通道表现一些共有特征，但它们各自孔道的结构和功能却不相同，反映了钠离子（或钙离子）经过了复杂的进化。

现在还不清楚独特的P-环结构怎样与大多数溶液相互作用，并保证钠通道快速而特异地滤过钠离子[17]，钠通道对钠离子的滤过率是其他阳离子的100倍或更多，每个独立通道的滤过量>10^7个离子/秒。如上所述，孔道不对称性对决定哺乳动物电压门控钠通道渗透特性有重要作用，但原核的NaCHBac对钠离子的选择性超过钙离子，表明孔道不对称性也不是钠通道对钠离子的选择性所必需。NaCHBac孔道有四个谷氨酸，很明显这种氨基酸有利于该通道滤过钙离子[17]，但这种结构不能确保NaCHBac对钙离子的高度选择性。早期推测孔道的离子选择性部分具有严格的结构，至今仍未明确通道滤过的本质。对这一过程，目前认为钠通道可能像许多酶那样表现出高度的结构柔性，P片段内的成对半胱氨酸能形成二硫键。但是，如果它在分子内无实际的移动度，一些特殊结构也不能生成[18,19]。这种移动在数毫秒内发生，末端可跨动数十埃。有趣的是，由内部的二硫键连接成的通道比由2个还原性巯基形成的通道有较少的选择性[18]，暗示结构柔性对选择离子的迁移起重要作用（虽还未确定）。孔道运动也与缓慢失活和药物的结合有关[19,20]。

(二) 门控：激活与失活

Hodgkin 和 Huxley[1]的最初贡献之一是提出钠通道在开放过程中（激活状态）各种空间构象的转变，而在去极化期间（失活状态）通道关闭，钠通道生成另一空间构象。m 门构成激活的基础，b 门控制失活，推测 m 门和 b 门的开关呈电压依赖性且功能相对独立[1]。4 个携带阳性电荷的 S4 片段现被广泛认为是电压感受器。在激活过程中，每一个 S4 片段所包含的几个碱性氨基酸残基经含水缝隙穿越细胞膜，此缝隙向细胞膜内凹陷，其厚度小于双分子层，导致蛋白内孔的更狭窄（见图 1-2）[21]。每个 S4 片段在通道激活中的作用不同，一些带电荷残基比那些"同源"残基起更重要的作用。而且，在多个 S4 片段的电荷转换突变并不是对孔道产生简单的附加影响，因为各位点间还有一些协同性，S4 片段的电荷转换突变对门控的影响程度与突变位点有关[22]。应用定向荧光标记试验标记 S4/结构域Ⅳ，发现 S4/结构域Ⅳ在去极化期间出现电压依赖性移相位对于其他区仅滞后一个相位，同时激活速度减慢，暗示 S4/结构域Ⅳ的移动不是通道开放所必需[23]。而且，位于Ⅲ和Ⅳ结构域的电压敏感器负责钠通道的快速失活[24]（见下面）。门控电流和体外致突变研究揭示了激活和失活过程是耦联的，推测激活和失活耦联可能由 S4/Ⅳ区介导[25]。确实，电流衰减的时程大体上反映了电压依赖性激活过程[21]。

如果这些 S4 是电压敏感器，那么激活门在哪里呢？这个关键问题仍未弄清。孔道门被认为位于孔道内侧面，这样可保持孔道相连的氨基酸残基与外源试剂的相互作用，而不管通道呈开放、关闭或失活状态。有可能移动扭曲了 S4-S5 之间的连接部分，随后导致由 S6 组成的胞膜内孔如门样开放和关闭（类似与钾通道）。考虑这些可能，一些钠通道阻滞剂（例如携带电荷的利多卡因同源物 QX-314）仅当内孔开放时从细胞内环境进入通道，或当通道关闭时陷入胞浆侧的孔隙内。其他的研究也显示 S6 的突变可改变钠通道门控和局麻药的阻滞程度[9]。结合钾通道的发现，推测 S6 在电压变化时可能以"紧缩"的方式关闭胞内孔[26]，S6 就成为物理激活门的主要参与者。

通道的失活是一个非常复杂的过程，甚至比 Hodgkin 和 Huxley 曾经推想的过程更复杂[1]。不像先前讨论的激活模式相对单一，而通道的失活模式存

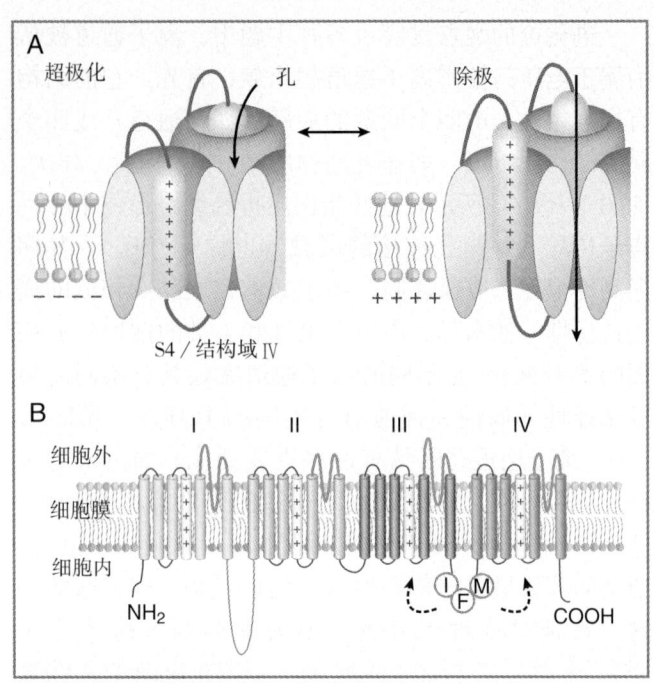

图 1-2 图解表述 Na^+ 通道 α-亚基插入 S4 电压感受器（A）和Ⅲ-Ⅳ区间连接（B），它促成快速失活，粗线表示推测的Ⅲ-Ⅳ区间受体

在多种形式。通过分析通道在超负相电位的恢复动力学可以得出一些时间参数，如通道从传统的快速失活中恢复需数十毫秒，而从慢速和超慢速失活中恢复需数十秒或更长。快速失活过程由位于Ⅲ和Ⅳ之间的细胞内连接部分调控，其中关键的残基被标记为 IFM，见图 1-2。应用 NMR 光谱技术确定了Ⅲ-Ⅳ连接区的三维结构[26]，它可能作为一个"塞子"嵌入由Ⅲ和Ⅳ区域的 S4-S5 在细胞质内形成的环[28,29]，正如Ⅳ S6 区末端的氨基酸残基一样[30]。这种推测恰好符合严密的实验结果，因为通道的快速失活能被胞浆内的蛋白酶阻断。大量的证据表明分布于通道各处的突变可影响通道的失活，与失活有关的关键部位是Ⅲ-Ⅳ连接区。目前对缓慢失活的结构基础还缺乏了解，大量遗传性疾病的研究表明：Brugada 综合征、家族性先天性肌强直及其他骨骼肌病被认为是抑制了缓慢失活[31,32]。另外，已报道多种孔道的突变可影响缓慢和超缓慢失活[33,34]。如钾通道 C 型失活一样，这些门控过程可能涉及外孔空间结构的动态重排，因为外孔空间结构影响孔道的结构柔性[19]，而孔道阻滞剂 μ-conotoxin 能抑制这些异常的门控过程[33]。

(三) 药物结合

局麻药（LA）作为抗心律失常和抗惊厥药被用来

治疗多种钠通道疾病（包括LQT3），它是通过影响钠离子通道的失活及失活后再生的动作电位。LAs通过优先结合开放的失活钠离子通道（即所谓的使用性依赖；LA的阻滞程度随通道去极化或反复的脉冲，或两种均发生时加强），从而抑制钠离子流和细胞的兴奋性[3]。LA受体集中定位在细胞内孔部，Ⅲ和Ⅳ区的S6为药物结合位点，药物可优先与该部位结合[9]。单通道记录显示内膜灌流QX-314可拮抗跨膜区（内部到结合点的）70%的电荷[35]，相应地，细胞外Cd^{+2}与半胱氨酸替代的P-环残基结合可中和约20%的电荷[15,16]。这些实验表明外部孔腔和细胞内孔部的LA受体结构非常近似，而且，多种P-环残基会影响LA阻滞效应[36,37]。

一些证据表明，LAs可充当通道失活门控的变构效应子[38]。当它们结合通道时，促进通道失活。无论这种药物的特殊作用模式是否正确，显然，门控同LA阻滞效应的相互作用是很明显的，以至于很难用一种"受体"对S6的作用来解释。根据先前的讨论，将位于S6和P区的受体位点突变后，门控动力学的变化未受药物的影响。此外，通道边远部的突变也能改变LA阻滞效应[39,40]。除去以上这些限制，S6和P区在药物对多种通道的影响中起关键作用，至少有一部分不依赖于门控的变化。

（四）神经毒素

钠通道是一些神经毒素的主要受体。神经毒素有高亲和力和专一性，能改变钠通道的特性，为研究这些蛋白质的结构与功能之间的关系提供了宝贵的工具。药理竞争研究和诱变作用已确定了一些神经毒素受体位点。其中，从河豚鱼中分离的含胍盐杂环河豚毒素，为我们理解钠通道特性作出了特别有意义的贡献。外表涂抹毫摩浓度TTX能闭塞神经和骨骼肌的孔道，阻断钠的传导，但阻断心肌上钠通道则需要更高的浓度（约10^{-5}摩）。结构域Ⅰ的P区存在一个特殊变异氨基酸残基（相当于$Na_v1.5$的第373位氨基酸残基，见图1-1D），常被用于描述亚基对TTX的敏感性；如该位点为芳香族氨基酸，则钠通道对TTX表现高亲和力，若该位点缺乏芳香族氨基酸，则钠通道对TTX表现为抵抗性[4]。有趣的是，该部位的氨基酸残基也调节LA在细胞外的通路，影响LA分子接近心肌通道内部的药物受体[41]。另外，组成孔道的氨基酸残基也结合TTX和相关的胍赤潮STX（赤潮海藻毒素），提示TTX/STX的受体分布位于通道的外表面[42]。

其他选择性结合钠通道的天然毒素，包括芋螺毒素（μ-CTX），一种从海螺毒液（Conus geograpbus）中分离的抑制肽。μ-CTX阻滞钠离子通道孔的部位与TTX/STX有部分重叠。然而，μ-CTX的高亲和力源于多种弱毒素与通道相互作用产生的累积效应，应用μ-CTX研究通道孔的价值比简单的TTX/STX更大（TTX/STX的分子量约300、μ-CTX的分子量约2600）[11,43-47]。尽管探索μ-CTX与钠通道的作用本质非常困难，但μ-CTX能提供更多钠通道的结构和药理学信息。μ-CTX末端有三个二硫键，结构稳定，这一特性使它特别适于对钠通道外口的探索。现在最好的钠通道α亚基三维图像是由20Å分辨率的电子显微镜重建的[48]，但毒素与通道相互作用后，可应用物理方法（如NMR光谱法和X线晶体成像术）建立高分辨率结构图。根据μ-CTX的典型三维结构和它们在特定点易变异的事实，以及观察到的通道-毒素间的相互作用，揭示了钠通道的4个内部区域是按顺时针形式分布的[11,45]。

同TTX/STX一样，μ-CTX可优先阻滞骨骼肌钠通道，它对骨骼肌钠通道的亲和力比心肌钠通道的高两个数量级。然而，对TTX/STX敏感的脑钠通道却对μ-CTX不敏感。结构域Ⅰ的P区存在一个特殊变异氨基酸残基常被用于描述亚基对TTX的敏感性，但该部位氨基酸的变异不会影响μ-CTX的亲和力[44]。结构域Ⅱ的S5-P连接区多个氨基酸残基的变异均可影响亚基对μ-CTX的敏感性；另外，同骨骼肌和神经源性钠通道相比，心肌源性钠通道还有其他区域可影响通道与μ-CTX的结合[47]。综上所述，通过研究毒素对孔道特异性阻滞效应，为我们了解孔道的结构、功能和药理特性提供了巨大帮助，为未来设计作用于离子通道药物提供了依据。

海葵（例如，anthopleurin海葵素A和B）、蝎子和一些蜘蛛毒素结合位于Ⅳ区的S4电压敏感元N-末端S3-S4连接部分，减慢钠电流衰减（失活）[49]。这些毒素好象通过结合通道外向激活时的ⅣS4区而发挥他们的生物作用，从而阻止通道的结构变化，而此变化是激活通道转化为失活态的必需[50]。尽管先前提到，神经毒素最具典型特征，但其他从各种生物中分离的钠通道毒素（例如，veratridine藜芦定，brevetoxin腰鞭毛虫毒素，batrachotoxin蛙毒，ciguatoxin鱼肉毒素，和grayanotoxine灰安毒素）通过其他机制改变钠离子通道的功能也有被描述。

三、钠通道表达和功能的调节

本章已着重描述了 α 亚基的基本结构和对功能有重要影响的特殊氨基酸残基,但还有许多其他因素参与形成钠通道的功能多样性,下面将讨论这些因素。

(一) 转录调节

实际上,通过在基因水平调节通道基因的转录就能控制细胞的兴奋性。钠通道表达是一个动态的过程,受发育水平和组织类型的调节。电活动形式能影响转录活性,例如,癫痫发作改变钠通道基因在脑部的表达水平。在去神经化的骨骼肌中,心肌钠通道亚型被诱导表达,而成熟骨骼肌钠通道亚型的表达被短暂地抑制。长期应用阻断钠通道的抗心律失常药物,心肌能增加钠通道 mRNA 的稳定表达水平,将在一定程度上抵消药物对通道的阻滞效应。

控制钠通道基因表达的机制刚刚有所了解。脑组织Ⅱ型钠通道($Na_v1.2$)的表达受 RE-1 沉默转录因子(REST)调控,限于神经元中表达。REST 含有 C2H2 锌指结构,与果蝇阻遏子 Kruppel 同源,能同 $Na_v1.2$ 通道调控区的特异的沉默元件(RE-1)结合。REST 在大多数组织中都有发现,但它在神经元上缺乏,故 $Na_v1.2$ 亚型能够表达。在朗飞(Ranvier)结上,神经元(neuronal)通道通过与钠离子通道 β 亚基之间的相互作用来募集锚蛋白[51]。但心肌钠离子通道亚型的调控表达机制仍不清楚。

(二) 辅助亚基

辅助 β 亚基是神经和骨骼肌钠通道功能的重要调节器,尽管它们对心肌钠通道的作用还不清楚。到目前为止,已证实有三种不同的 β 亚基($β_1$,$β_2$,$β_3$)和至少一种选择性剪接体($β_{1a}$)可与钠通道 α 亚基相连[52]。α 亚基与 β 亚基的比例在各通道亚型中有变化,免疫沉淀实验显示,脑组织钠通道为异源三聚体,$α:β_1:β_2=1:1:1$;骨骼肌亚型为异源二聚体,$α:β_1=1:1$。如图 1-3A 所示,$β_1$ 以非共价键与 α 连接,$β_2$ 则以二硫键与之相连。纯化的心肌通道未发现包含 α+β 的复合结构。

不像 α 亚基,钠通道 β 亚基与钾和钙通道无结构相关性。而且,三种 β 亚基序列不是同源的($β_1$ 和 $β_3$ 约有 45% 的序列相同;$β_2$ 分别与 $β_1$ 和 $β_3$ 有约 18% 和 13% 的序列相同),但它们被预测有相似的跨膜结构:

每个 β 亚基包含一个小的 C-末端、一条跨膜片段和一个包含几个糖基化位点的 N-末端(见图 1-3A)。另外,所有三个 β 亚基细胞外部分含有免疫球蛋白样折叠结构,与神经系统的细胞粘附分子(CAM)相似。确实,β 亚基已经表现出 CAM 样功能,与细胞外基质(如粘蛋白-C,tenascin-C 和粘蛋白-R)和细胞骨架信号分子相互作用调节细胞迁移、细胞的聚集、锚蛋白的补充和钠通道的生物合成、细胞分布和转运[53,54]。因此,钠通道 β 亚基具有多种功能。

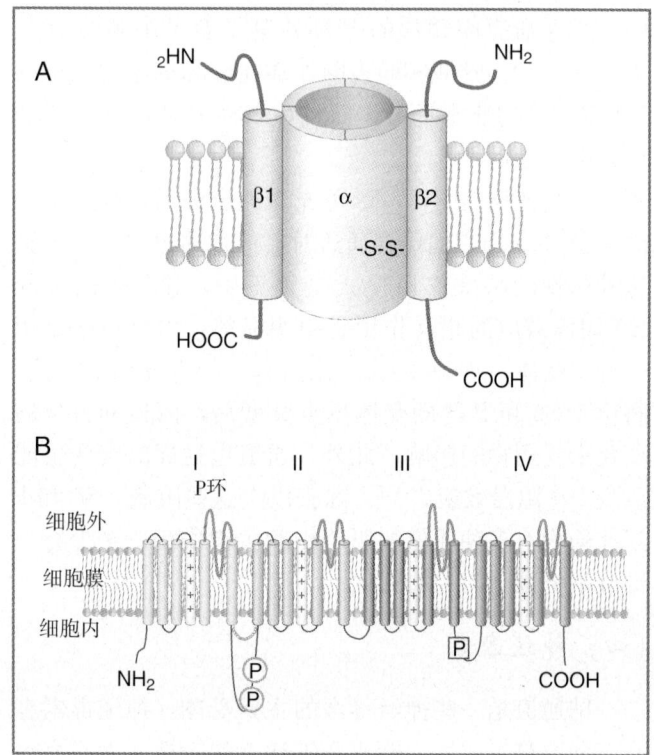

图 1-3 Na 通道亚基和磷酸化位点 A:Na 通道最大的亚基成分。注意不是所有 Na 通道含有任何一个或两个 β 亚基,但 α 亚基是功能必需的。B:图解说明 α 亚基重要的磷酸化位点。它们位于Ⅲ-Ⅳ连接部分和Ⅰ-Ⅱ连接部分的长变异段;连接部分的长度是亚型特异的。圆形的磷酸化位点是 PKA 依赖的(心脏亚型),方形的是 PKC 依赖的

尽管神经或骨骼肌 α 亚基在卵母细胞中表达时能形成有功能的通道,但表达的电流代表更慢的激活和失活以及电压依赖性差别,不同于天然细胞。这些亚型和 β 亚基共表达产生明确的功能,电流密度和细胞膜电容增加,激活和失活加速,稳态失活曲线负向漂移,类似于天然细胞的电流特征[52]。遗传突变研究已进一步确定 β 亚基的免疫球蛋白样结构域和 α 亚基的结构域Ⅳ P-S6 环,作为关键的区域负责功能的调节[55,56]。在药理学上,β 亚基的共表达也改变钠通道对 LA 的敏感性[57],推测这种变化可能与钠通道的门

控有关。

尽管β亚基对脑和骨骼肌钠通道有明显的调节作用（$β_1$突变与发热和癫痫的关系已有报道[58]），但心肌亚型β亚基的功能意义（及对心脏的生理学作用）仍存在争议，并有许多互相矛盾的结果被报道。关于β亚基在心脏上表达和优势尚无一致认识。一些研究表明$β_1$、$β_{1a}$、$β_2$和$β_3$存在于心脏[52]，但其他研究未检出这些辅助亚基[59]。然而，一些研究表明α和β亚基共表达时并未对心肌通道产生功能和药理学方面的影响，但另一些研究表明β亚基对心肌通道去极化和超极化方向的电压依赖性激活和/或失活有显著作用[57,60-63]。尽管有分歧，但心肌离子通道的基因突变引起遗传性LQT3和BS，其机制可能与α和β亚基在心脏中相互作用被破坏有关[63,64]。显然，进一步的实验需要阐明心肌钠通道β亚基的功能。

（三）翻译后修饰：磷酸化

钠通道受磷酸化调节是一个复杂的过程，涉及不同的激酶和磷酸酶。钠通道α亚基根据Ⅰ-Ⅱ连接部分的长度分为长（神经和心肌）和短（骨骼肌和鳗鱼）两个亚型。神经亚型有一个相当大的细胞内连接部分位于Ⅰ-Ⅱ区间，它包括5个一致的位点即蛋白激酶A（PKA）依赖的环磷酸腺苷（cAMP）（见图1-3B）。PKA调节神经和心肌钠通道的表达功能。脑组织通道Ⅰ-Ⅱ连接部分的磷酸化减少电流振幅，而不改变通道的门控动力学[65,66]。

心肌钠通道有8个PKA磷酸化点位于Ⅰ-Ⅱ连接体内，而神经钠通道则不同。心肌钠通道体外研究表明，cAMP依赖的磷酸化位点仅在两个丝氨酸上（$hNa_v1.5$的S525和S528）[67]。与神经通道相反，心肌钠通道经PKA磷酸化后电流增加，表明磷酸化能调节特殊亚型的功能[67,68]。推测内质网停滞信号的出现与PKA介导的电流增强有关[69]。定位在细胞膜的分子调节钠通道的机制已被提出，如G蛋白可直接调节钠电流，但G蛋白促进和抑制钠电流的研究结果均有报道。所以，钠通道磷酸化的重要性和G蛋白的直接效应尚未弄清，为了避免混乱，今后应从生理学角度谨慎解释涉及异源表达体系的研究结果。

与PKA相比，蛋白激酶C（PKC）可调节所有哺乳动物钠通道亚型的功能[70-72]。PKC的效应是极大地促进Ⅲ-Ⅳ失活连接体内一个高度保守的丝氨酸（S1503）磷酸化（见图1-3B）。PKC降低通道的最大传导率，并改变门控动力学。PKC能均匀地减慢肉眼可见的神经钠电流的衰减。PKC对骨骼肌和心肌通道的影响也有描述，包括加速电流衰减[70]和稳态失活曲线的负向漂移[72]。磷酸化对钠通道的功能调节作用已被涉及，经磷酸酶（如神经钙蛋白和磷酸酶2A）对α亚基的去磷酸化作用同样调节钠通道的功能[73]。目前，β亚基的磷酸化尚未被发现。

（四）翻译后修饰：糖基化

所有钠通道亚基均被糖基化修饰。β亚基、脑和肌肉α亚基被大量的糖基化，糖成分超过总量40%（eel electroplax鳗鱼电板α亚基）。相反，心肌α亚基的糖成分仅占总量5%。糖基化生物合成途径已经明确。简言之，新生的多肽穿过内质网膜进入腔内，N-连接区发生糖基化是通过选择N-X-S/T序列将糖类翻译转换为天门冬酰胺。进一步的糖基化加工发生在通道蛋白被转运到高尔基体和随后的胞浆膜时。唾液酸，N-连接糖（碳水化合物）的重要成分，在通道外侧产生局部负电荷区，预计它能影响电压依赖门控（状态）。例如，用唾液淀粉酶处理骨骼肌通道并除去唾液酸，通道的稳定失活态向正向漂移[74]。翻译后糖基化也是维持钠通道在神经元和雪旺细胞膜表达所必需。由于衣霉素能减少STX连接到神经母细胞位点的数目，故衣霉素能抑制钠通道糖基化。衣霉素也抑制棕榈酸盐、硫酸盐和连接$β_2$亚基的二硫键，阻止神经元钠通道的装配。翻译后糖基化影响通道蛋白翻转的阻力和细胞内外的相互作用。运用转基因技术表明唾液酸化作用在心力衰竭中有潜在致心律失常的风险[75]。

四、结　论

生理学家和心脏学家们有许多理由关注钠通道。通过研究神经轴突钠通道的特性建立了后来所有对兴奋性研究的基础。钠通道在电鳗体内的大量分布，保证了首个电压门控离子通道的克隆。同时，膜片钳技术的发展，让我们能较好的确定特定组织结构的分子生物学特性。这些结果极大地丰富了我们关于钠通道结构和功能间的关系。这项工作对我们理解心肌钠通道也产生积极影响。对Ⅲ-Ⅳ连接在失活过程中重要性的认识，促使Wang和他的同事[76]将长QT综合征的致病基因首先定位在3号染色体，并开展了对心肌钠通道的遗传检测。以后对SCN5A基因突变的分析揭示，另外的突变形成了多种长QT综合征和Brugada综合征。根据心律失常抑制实验，钠通道作为抗心律失常药首选作用靶点的前景有巨大影响，随着我们在理解结构和功能间关系、基因和这些关键信号蛋白的分子药理学的进步，根据它们明显的致心律失常作用，能促进我们以钠通道为目标发展更具效率和选择性的药物。

（浦介麟　王洪涛　滕思勇　译）

参 考 文 献

1. Hodgkin AL, Huxley AL: A quantitative description of membrane current and its application to conduction and excitation in nerve. J Physiol 117:500–544, 1952.
2. Noda M, Shimizu S, Tanabe T, et al: Primary structure of electrophorus electricus sodium channel deduced from cDNA sequence. Nature 312:121–127, 1984.
3. Hille B: Ionic channels of excitable membranes, 3rd ed. Sunderland, MA, Sinauer Associates, Inc., 2001.
4. Marban ET, Yamagishi T, Tomaselli GF: Structure and function of voltage-gated sodium channels. J Physiol 508(3):647–657, 1998.
5. Bezanilla F: The voltage sensor in voltage-dependent ion channels. Physiol Rev 80(2):555–592, 2000.
6. Goldin AL, Barchi RL, Caldwell JH, et al: Nomenclature of voltage-gated sodium channels. Neuron 28(2):365–368, 2000.
7. Fozzard HA, Hanck DA: Structure and function of voltage-dependent sodium channels: Comparison of brain II and cardiac isoforms. Physiologic Rev 76(3):887–926, 1996.
8. Yellen G: The moving parts of voltage-gated ion channels. Q Rev Biophys 31(3):239–295, 1998.
9. Catterall WA: Molecular mechanisms of gating and drug block of sodium channels. Novartis Found Symp 241:206–218, 2002.
10. Ren D, Navarro B, Xu H, et al: A prokaryotic voltage-gated sodium channel. Science 294(5550):2372–2375, 2001.
11. Li RA, Ennis IL, French RJ, et al: Clockwise domain arrangement of the sodium channel revealed by mu-conotoxin (GIIIA) docking orientation. J Biol Chem 276(14):11072–11077, 2001.
12. Maier SK, Westenbroek RE, Schenkman KA, et al: An unexpected role for brain-type sodium channels in coupling of cell surface depolarization to contraction in the heart. Proc Natl Acad Sci USA 99(6):4073–4078, 2002.
13. Yamagishi T, Li RA, Hsu K, et al: Molecular architecture of the voltage-dependent Na channel: functional evidence for alpha helices in the pore. J Gen Physiol 118(2):171–182, 2001.
14. Doyle DA, Morais Cabral J, Pfuetzner RA, et al: The structure of the potassium channel: molecular basis of K^+ conduction and selectivity. Science 280(5360):69–77, 1998.
15. Li RA, Velez P, Chiamvimonvat N, et al: Charged residues between the selectivity filter and S6 segments contribute to the permeation phenotype of the sodium channel. J Gen Physiol 115(1):81–92, 1999.
16. Chiamvimonvat N, Perez-Garcia MT, Ranjan R, et al: Depth asymmetries of the pore-lining segments of the Na^+ channel revealed by cysteine mutagenesis. Neuron 16(5):1037–1047, 1996.
17. Ellinor PT, Yang J, Sather WA, et al: Ca^{2+} channel selectivity at a single locus for high-affinity Ca^{2+} interactions. Neuron 15(5):1121–1132, 1995.
18. Tsushima R, Li R, Backx P: P-loop flexibility in Na^+ channel pores revealed by single- and double-cysteine replacements. J Gen Physiol 110(1):59–72, 1997.
19. Benitah JP, Chen Z, Balser JR, et al: Molecular dynamics of the sodium channel pore vary with gating: Interactions between P-segment motions and inactivation. J Neurosci 19(5):1577–1585, 1999.
20. Ong BH, Tomaselli GF, Balser JR: A structural rearrangement in the sodium channel pore linked to slow inactivation and use dependence. J Gen Physiol 116(5):653–662, 2000.
21. Yang N, George AL Jr, Horn R: Molecular basis of charge movement in voltage-gated sodium channels. Neuron 16(1):113–122, 1996.
22. Kontis KJ, Rounaghi A, Goldin AL: Sodium channel activation gating is affected by substitutions of voltage sensor positive charges in all four domains. J Gen Physiol 110:391–401, 1997.
23. Chanda B, Bezanilla F: Tracking voltage-dependent conformational changes in skeletal muscle sodium channel during activation. J Gen Physiol 120(5):629–645, 2002.
24. Cha A, Ruben PC, George AL Jr, et al: Voltage sensors in domains III and IV, but not I and II, are immobilized by Na^+ channel fast inactivation [see comments]. Neuron 22(1):73–87, 1999.
25. Chen LQ, Santarelli V, Horn R, Kallen RG: A unique role for the S4 segment of domain 4 in the inactivation of Na channels. J Gen Physiol 108:549–556, 1996.
26. Yellen G: The voltage-gated potassium channels and their relatives. Nature 419(6902):35–42, 2002.
27. Rohl CA, Boeckman FA, Baker C, et al: Solution structure of the sodium channel inactivation gate. Biochemistry 38(3):855–861, 1999.
28. McPhee JC, Ragsdale DS, Scheuer T, Catterall WA: A critical role for the S4-S5 intracellular loop in domain IV of the sodium channel alpha-subunit in fast inactivation. J Biol Chem 273(2):1121–1129, 1998.
29. Smith MR, Goldin AL: Interaction between the sodium channel inactivation linker and domain III S4-S5. Biophys J 73(4):1885–1895, 1997.
30. McPhee JC, Ragsdale DS, Scheuer T, Catterall WA: A mutation in segment IVS6 disrupts fast inactivation of sodium channels. Proc Nat Acad Sci USA 91(25):12346–12350, 1994.
31. Hayward L, Brown R Jr, Cannon S: Slow inactivation differs among mutant Na channels associated with myotonia and periodic paralysis. Biophys J 72(3):1204–1219, 1997.
32. Balser JR: The cardiac sodium channel: gating function and molecular pharmacology. J Mol Cell Cardiol 33(4):599–613, 2001.
33. Todt H, Dudley SC Jr, Kyle JW, et al: Ultra-slow inactivation in mu1 Na^+ channels is produced by a structural rearrangement of the outer vestibule. Biophys J 76(3):1335–1345, 1999.
34. Tomaselli GF, Chiamvimonvat N, Nuss HB, et al: A mutation in the pore of the sodium channel alters gating. Biophys J 68(5):1814–1827, 1995.
35. Gingrich KJ, Beardsley D, Yue DT: Ultra-deep blockade of Na^+ channels by a quaternary ammonium ion: Catalysis by a transition-intermediate state? J Physiol (Lond) 471:319–341, 1993.
36. Sunami A, Dudley SC, Jr, Fozzard HA: Sodium channel selectivity filter regulates antiarrhythmic drug binding. Proc Natl Acad Sci USA 94(25):14126–14131, 1997.
37. Kambouris NG, Hastings LA, Stepanovic S, et al: Mechanistic link between lidocaine block and inactivation probed by outer pore mutations in the rat micro1 skeletal muscle sodium channel. J Physiol 512(3):693–705, 1998.
38. Balser JR, Nuss HB, Orias DW, et al: Local anesthetics as effectors of allosteric gating. Lidocaine effects on inactivation-deficient rat skeletal muscle Na channels. J Clin Invest 98(12):2874–2886, 1996.
39. Kambouris NG, Nuss HB, Johns DC, et al: A revised view of cardiac sodium channel "blockade" in the long QT syndrome. J Clin Invest 105(8):1133–1140, 2000.
40. Li RA, Ennis IL, Tomaselli GF, Marban E: Structural basis of differences in isoform-specific gating and lidocaine block between cardiac and skeletal muscle sodium channels. Mol Pharmacol 61(1):136–141, 2002.
41. Sunami A, Glaaser IW, Fozzard HA: A critical residue for isoform difference in tetrodotoxin affinity is a molecular determinant of the external access path for local anesthetics in the cardiac sodium channel. Proc Natl Acad Sci USA 97(5):2326–2331, 2000.
42. Perez-Garcia MT, Chiamvimonvat N, Marban E, Tomaselli GF: Structure of the sodium channel pore revealed by serial cysteine mutagenesis. Proc Natl Acad Sci USA 93(1):300–304, 1996.
43. Li RA, Ennis IL, Velez P, et al: Novel structural determinants of mu-conotoxin (GIIIB) block in rat skeletal muscle (mu1) Na^+ channels. J Biol Chem 275(36):27551–27558, 2000.
44. Li RA, Tsushima RG, Kallen RG, Backx PH: Pore residues critical for mu-CTX binding to rat skeletal muscle Na^+ channels revealed by cysteine mutagenesis. Biophys J 73(4):1874–1884, 1997.
45. Dudley SC Jr, Chang N, Hall J, et al: mu-Conotoxin GIIIA interactions with the voltage-gated Na(+) channel predict a clockwise arrangement of the domains. J Gen Physiol 116(5):679–690, 2000.
46. Chang NS, French RJ, Lipkind GM, et al: Predominant interactions between mu-conotoxin Arg-13 and the skeletal muscle Na^+ channel localized by mutant cycle analysis. Biochemistry 37(13):4407–4419, 1998.
47. Li RA, Ennis IL, Xue T, et al: Molecular basis of isoform-specific micro-conotoxin block of cardiac, skeletal muscle, and brain Na^+ channels. J Biol Chem 278(10):8717–8724, 2003.

48. Sato C, Ueno Y, Asai K, et al: The voltage-sensitive sodium channel is a bell-shaped molecule with several cavities. Nature 409(6823):1047–1051, 2001.
49. Rogers JC, Qu Y, Tanada TN, et al: Molecular determinants of high affinity binding of alpha-scorpion toxin and sea anemone toxin in the S3-S4 extracellular loop in domain IV of the Na+ channel alpha subunit. J Biol Chem 271(27):15950–15962, 1996.
50. Cestele S, Qu Y, Rogers JC, et al: Voltage sensor-trapping: Enhanced activation of sodium channels by beta- scorpion toxin bound to the S3-S4 loop in domain II. Neuron 21(4):919–931, 1998.
51. Malhotra JD, Koopmann MC, Kazen-Gillespie KA, et al: Structural requirements for interaction of sodium channel beta 1 subunits with ankyrin. J Biol Chem 277(29):26681–26688, 2002.
52. Isom LL: Sodium channel beta subunits: Anything but auxiliary. Neuroscientist 7(1):42–54, 2001.
53. Srinivasan J, Schachner M, Catterall WA: Interaction of voltage-gated sodium channels with the extracellular matrix molecules tenascin-C and tenascin-R. Proc Natl Acad Sci USA 95(26):15753–15757, 1998.
54. Xiao ZC, Ragsdale DS, Malhotra JD, et al: Tenascin-R is a functional modulator of sodium channel beta subunits. J Biol Chem 274(37):26511–26517, 1999.
55. McCormick KA, Isom LL, Ragsdale D, et al: Molecular determinants of Na+ channel function in the extracellular domain of the beta1 subunit. J Biol Chem 273(7):3954–3962, 1998.
56. Qu Y, Rogers JC, Chen SF, et al: Functional roles of the extracellular segments of the sodium channel alpha subunit in voltage-dependent gating and modulation by beta1 subunits. J Biol Chem 274(46):32647–32654, 1999.
57. Makielski JC, Limberis JT, Chang SY, et al: Coexpression of b₁ with cardiac sodium channel a subunits in oocytes decreases lidocaine block. Mol Pharmacol 49:30–39, 1996.
58. Wallace RH, Wang DW, Singh R, et al: Febrile seizures and generalized epilepsy associated with a mutation in the Na+-channel beta1 subunit gene SCN1B. Nat Genet 19(4):366–370, 1998.
59. Grosson CL, Cannon SC, Corey DP, Gusella JF: Sequence of the voltage-gated sodium channel beta1-subunit in wild-type and in quivering mice. Brain Res Mol Brain Res 42(2):222–226, 1996.
60. Qu Y, Isom LL, Westenbroek RE, et al: Modulation of cardiac Na+ channel expression in Xenopus oocytes by beta 1 subunits. J Biol Chem 270(43):25696–25701, 1995.
61. Nuss HB, Chiamvimonvat N, Perez-Garcia MT, et al: Functional association of the beta 1 subunit with human cardiac (hH1) and rat skeletal muscle (mu 1) sodium channel a subunits expressed in Xenopus oocytes. J Gen Physiol 106:1171–1191, 1995.
62. Wright SN, Wang SY, Xiao YF, Wang GK: State-dependent cocaine block of sodium channel isoforms, chimeras, and channels coexpressed with the beta1 subunit. Biophys J 76(1):233–245, 1999.
63. An RH, Wang XL, Kerem B, et al: Novel LQT-3 mutation affects Na+ channel activity through interactions between alpha- and beta1-subunits. Circ Res 83(2):141–146, 1998.
64. Makita N, Shirai N, Wang DW, et al: Cardiac Na(+) channel dysfunction in Brugada syndrome is aggravated by beta(1)-subunit. Circulation 101(1):54–60, 2000.
65. Smith RD, Goldin AL: Phosphorylation at a single site in the rat brain sodium channel is necessary and sufficient for current reduction by protein kinase A. J Neurosci 17(16):6086–6093, 1997.
66. Cantrell AR, Tibbs VC, Yu FH, et al: Molecular mechanism of convergent regulation of brain Na(+) channels by protein kinase C and protein kinase A anchored to AKAP-15. Mol Cell Neurosci 21(1):63, 2002.
67. Murphy BJ, Rogers J, Perdichizzi AP, et al: cAmp-dependent phosphorylation of two sites in the alpha subunit of the cardiac sodium channel. J Biol Chem 271(46):28837–28843, 1996.
68. Frohnwieser B, Chen LQ, Schreibmayer W, Kallen RG: Modulation of the human cardiac sodium channel alpha-subunit by cAMP-dependent protein kinase and the responsible sequence domain. J Physiol 498(2):309–318.
69. Zhou J, Shin HG, Yi J, et al: Phosphorylation and putative ER retention signals are required for protein kinase A-mediated potentiation of cardiac sodium current. Circ Res 91(6):540–546, 2002.
70. Bendahhou S, Cummins TR, Potts JF, et al: Serine-1321-independent regulation of the mu 1 adult skeletal muscle Na+ channel by protein kinase C. Proc Nat Acad Sci USA 92(26):12003–12007, 1995.
71. Murray KT, Hu NN, Daw JR, et al: Functional effects of protein kinase C activation on the human cardiac Na+ channel. Circ Res 80(3):370–376, 1997.
72. Qu Y, Rogers JC, Tanada TN, et al: Phosphorylation of S1505 in the cardiac Na+ channel inactivation gate is required for modulation by protein kinase C. J Gen Physiol 108(5):375–379, 1996.
73. Chen TC, Law B, Kondratyuk T, Rossie S: Identification of soluble protein phosphatases that dephosphorylate voltage-sensitive sodium channels in rat brain. J Biol Chem 270(13):7750–7756, 1995.
74. Bennett E, Urcan MS, Tinkle SS, et al: Contribution of sialic acid to the voltage dependence of sodium channel gating. A possible electrostatic mechanism. J Gen Physiol 109(3):327–343, 1997.
75. Ufret-Vincenty CA, Baro DJ, Lederer WJ, et al: Role of sodium channel deglycosylation in the genesis of cardiac arrhythmias in heart failure. J Biol Chem 276(30):28197–28203, 2001.
76. Wang Q, Shen J, Splawski I, et al: SCN5A mutations associated with an inherited cardiac arrhythmia, long QT syndrome. Cell 80(5):805–911, 1995.

第 2 章

钙 通 道

Donald M. Bers

本章目录

- 钙通道的类型 …………………… 10
- 钙通道的分子特征 ………………… 11
- 钙通道选择性和通透性 …………… 11
- 钙通道门控 ………………………… 13
- 经钙通道流入的钙离子数量 ……… 16

钙通道是心脏电生理特征的基本成分，也是心脏兴奋-收缩耦联的关键启动因子。由跨膜钙离子内流激活的肌浆网（SR）钙释放通道将在第 6 章介绍。更多关于心脏钙通道与兴奋-收缩耦联的详细内容及文献，可参见 Bers 及其同事的文章[1,2]。

一、钙通道的类型

至少有 10 个钙通道基因，它们以几种不同的术语命名（表 2-1）。其中一些主要在神经元表达，在心肌表达的两个主要类型钙通道是 L 型和 T 型[1,3]。L-型钙通道（LTCCs）的特征是：巨大的单通道传导率（≈25pS 在 110 mMBa），长时间稳定开放（以 Ba 为负荷载体），对 1,4-dihydropyridines 二氢吡啶类钙拮抗剂（DHPs；见 16 章）敏感，激活需更强的去极化（如在较正的膜电位，Em）。T-型通道（TTCCs）的特征是：较小的传导率（≈8pS 在 110mM Ba），暂时的开放，对 DHPs 不敏感和激活需较负的 Em（表 2-2）。心脏上的 L 和 T 型钙通道有更进一步的区别，L 型钙电流（I_{Ca}）主要由 α_{1C} 引起（较少由 α_{1D} 引起），T 型 I_{Ca} 由 α_{1G} 和 α_{1H} 引起。现在，$Ca_v1.2$ 已被认为是更正式的术语，但 L 型和 T 型仍被广泛用于两组（$Ca_v1.x$ 和 $Ca_v3.x$）通道。

功能性 $I_{Ca,L}$ 出现在所有心肌细胞中，而心脏 $I_{Ca,T}$ 主要在心房细胞和心脏浦肯野细胞（图 2-1）[4,5]。静息 E_m 为 −20mV 时，$I_{Ca,L}$ 和 $I_{Ca,T}$ 的大小相似（见图 2-1B），但 E_m 为 0mV 时，$I_{Ca,L}$ 的峰值比 $I_{Ca,T}$ 大 3 倍。图 2-1C 表示总的 I_{Ca} 在四种不同类型细胞中的电流-电压关系。在负的 E_m（约 −40mV）出现明显的峰值反应 $I_{Ca,T}$。浦肯野细胞含大量 $I_{Ca,T}$，在起搏细胞和一些心房细胞中也有效多数量的 $I_{Ca,T}$[3,6]。成熟心室肌中 $I_{Ca,T}$ 的数目，在豚鼠为中量，但在牛蛙、小牛、猫、兔子、大鼠和雪貂上未检测到[3,8-10]。新生鼠心室肌细胞表达 $I_{Ca,T}$[11-13]，显著的 $I_{Ca,T}$ 可在猫[8]和鼠[14]心室肥大的进展中重新出现。心脏肌细胞上仅表现 T 和 L 型 I_{Ca}，但在心内神经元中可表达 N-、P/Q-或 R-型电流[15]。

在起搏和传导细胞中 $I_{Ca,T}$ 的相对突出和它激活的膜电位在起搏范围内，显示了 $I_{Ca,T}$ 在心房起搏中的作用[6,16]。因 $I_{Ca,T}$ 相对小且失活迅速，钙电流总量中 $I_{Ca,T}$ 的数量要小于 $I_{Ca,L}$ 的数量，在多数心室肌细胞中可忽略不计。它们可反映不同的功能作用，$I_{Ca,L}$ 更多地涉及触发 SR 的钙释放和 SR 钙的再储存，而不是起搏。

当 $I_{Ca,L}$ 的电荷载体是 Ca 时，失活迅速（见图 2-4 和钙依赖性晚失活），且 $I_{Ca,L}$ 动力学中会有 $I_{Ca,T}$ 混杂。但是当 Ba 是电荷载体时，$I_{Ca,L}$ 和 $I_{Ca,T}$ 能被更好地区别，因为 $I_{Ca,L}$ 失活特别慢（图 2-1 和 2-4）。若钙电流中主要是 $I_{Ca,T}$，也可依靠不同的 E_m 依赖性来区分。（图 2-1）。

表 2-1 钙通道类型

异构体	基因名称	通道名称	类型	组织
L-type				
α_{1S}	CACNA1S	$Ca_v1.1$	L	骨骼肌
α_{1C}	CACNA1C	$Ca_v1.2$	L	心，脑肺平滑肌腺体
α_{1D}	CACNA1D	$Ca_v1.3$	L	神经心
α_{1F}	CACNA1F	$Ca_v1.4$	L	?
α_{1A}	CACNA1A	$Ca_v2.1$	P/Q	神经
α_{1B}	CACNA1B	$Ca_v2.2$	N	神经
α_{1E}	CACNA1E	$Ca_v2.3$	R	神经心
T-type				
α_{1G}	CACNA1G	$Ca_v3.1$	T	神经心浦肯野纤维
α_{1H}	CACNA1H	$Ca_v3.2$	T	心，肾肝
α_{1I}	CACNA1I	$Ca_v3.3$	T	肝

表 2-2 L 型和 T 型钙通道的特性

	L-型	T-型
激活范围		
5 mM Ca^{2+}	−30mV 以上	−60mV 以上
110 mM Ba^{2+}	−10mV 以上	−50mV 以上
失活范围	−40mV 以上	−90～−60mV
Ca^{2+} 依赖	是	否
电压依赖	慢	快
尾电流失活	快	慢
电导		
110mM Ba^{2+}	25 pS	8pS
110mM Ca^{2+}	8 pS	8pS
150mM Na, EDTA	80 pS	50 pS
平均开放时间	典型<1ms	短，1～2ms
动力学	多次爆发/脉冲	单次脉冲一次爆发（失活）
药物敏感性		
二氢吡啶类	是	否
镉	高	低
镍	低	高
异丙肾上腺素	是	否
离体膜片	失去活性	保留活性

以 $I_{ca,T}$ 为主的心脏各型细胞中，横管系（T 管）较少。还未明确 T 管中是否存在 TTCCs，但心脏和骨骼肌中 LTCCs 是密集的。若无其他详细说明，下面讨论的钙通道和 I_{ca} 是指心肌细胞的 LTCCs 或 $I_{ca,L}$。

二、钙通道的分子特征

构成骨骼肌钙通道的五种蛋白亚基（α_1，α_2，β，γ，δ）的氨基酸序列都已明确。骨骼肌 α_1 亚基（α_{1S}）不同于心脏 α_1 亚基克隆（α_{1C}）[22]。α_1 亚基包括通道、药物受体和主要的调节位点，它的结构类似于 E_m-依赖的钠通道和钾通道（图 2-2）。α_{1C} 有四个同源结构域（Ⅰ到Ⅳ），每个区有 6 个跨膜片段（S_1-S_6，S_4 带电，是主要的电压感受器）和 S_5 与 S_6 之间的孔区，还有一个长长的羧基尾段。α_{1C} 的剪接变异体和 α_{1D} 也在心脏有表达[23,24]，但 α_{1D} 对 α_{1C}（或剪接变异体）的功能影响还不清楚。

α_2 亚基和 δ 亚基由同一 $\alpha_2\delta$ 基因产生[25]。$\alpha_2\delta$ 蛋白分开（但 α_2-δ 仍经二硫化物连接相互作用），且 δ 蛋白将复合物固定在细胞膜上（图 2-2）。也有不同的 $\alpha_2\delta$ 变异体（α_{2a} 主要在骨骼肌，α_{2b} 在脑组织，α_{2c} 和 α_{2d} 在心脏）。$\alpha_2\delta$ 和 α_{1C} 共表达能增加 DHP 受体结合位点、门控电流和 I_{ca}[26-28]。因此 $\alpha_2\delta$ 可有助于形成功能性肌纤维膜通道，但它也可改变钙通道门控[29]。γ 亚基是骨骼肌钙通道的重要部分[19,20]，但缺乏心脏有 γ 亚基的确切证据。

β 亚基也有多种基因（β_1-β_4），但心脏的主要亚型是 β_2，有其他的剪接变异体[2]。β_2 与 α_{1C} 共表达能使电流增加 10 倍，加速激活和失活动力学，改变稳态失活和极大增加高亲和力 DHP 连接位点的数目[30-32]。β 亚基可以是一个分子伴侣蛋白，帮助新生的 α_{1C} 分子适当折叠并到达肌纤维膜[33]。α_1 和 β 亚基间特异性作用结构域已被阐明（图 2-2）[34,35]。

如图 2-2 所示，α_{1C} 亚基上的其他位点也可能是与心脏兰尼定受体（ryanodine receptor, RyR）作用的位点、磷酸化位点（Ser-1928）、EF-手型和 IQ 模体（涉及钙依赖性失活），以及与主要的钙通道阻滞剂结合的位点（ⅢS$_5$、ⅢS$_6$ 和 ⅣS$_6$）。心脏的 α_{1C}、$\alpha_2\delta$ 和 β_2 亚基分别约是 200、175、60kD。

三种 TTCCs，α_{1G}、α_{1H} 和 α_{1I}，与 LTCCs 有相似结构（如Ⅰ-Ⅳ 结构域、S1-S6 跨膜片段和一个孔环）[36-38]。S4 和孔环区的序列是高度保守的，尽管在 P-环区有重要的不同（"EEEE"位点是重要的，因为透过 TTCCs 有氨基酸序列 SKD 对应 TFE 在Ⅲ 结构域）。全部序列都已明确的仍是少数。

三、钙通道选择性和通透性

钙通道孔最窄处直径约 6Å（因 tetramethylam-

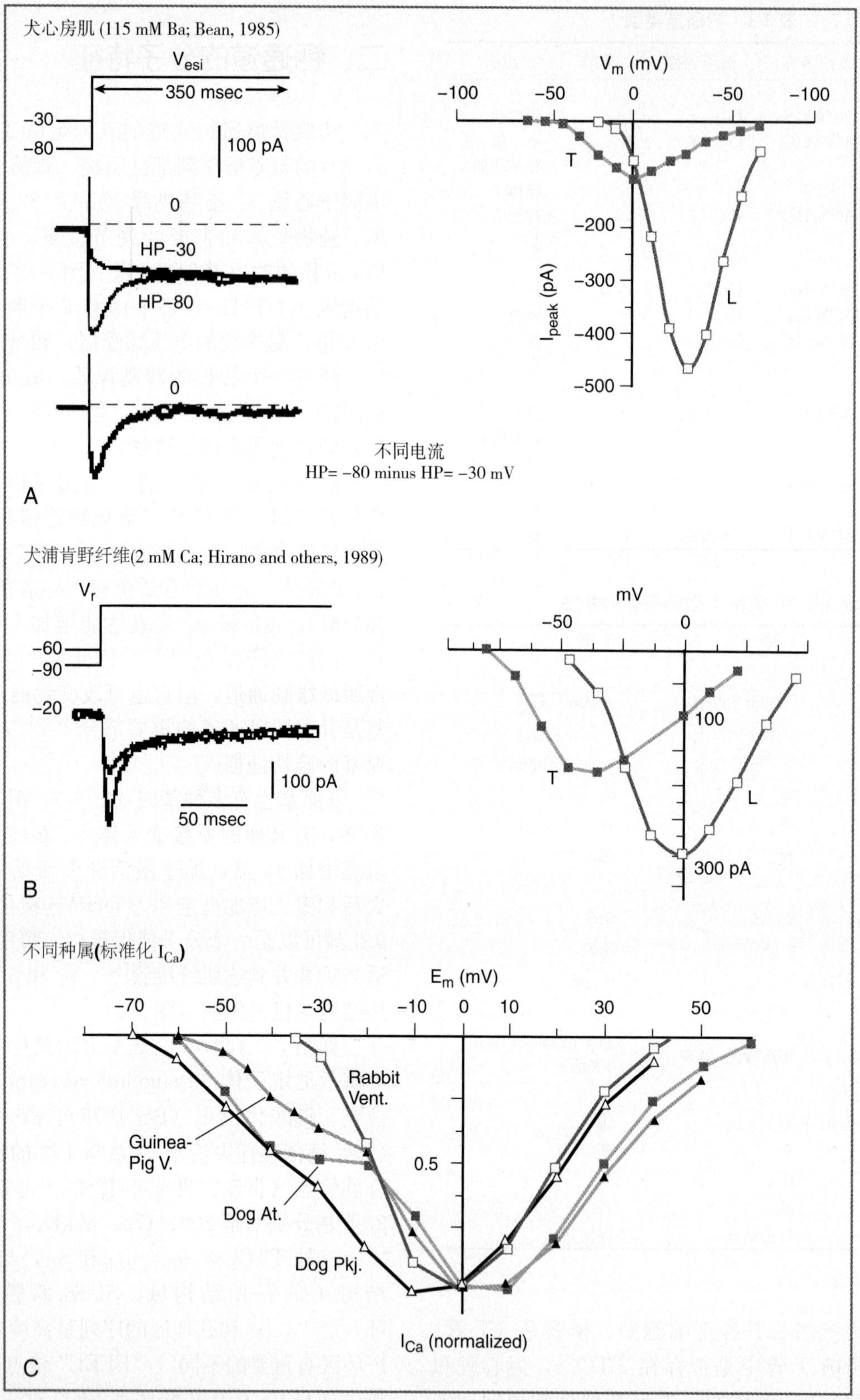

图 2-1　心脏 L-和 T-型 Ca 通道电流　A：由 E_m 阶跃到所示的钳制电位（holding potential，HP）引出的 Ba 电流（115 mM Ba）。不同的电流提示是 $I_{ca,T}$，HP＝30mV 时，激活的是 $I_{ca,L}$。B：与 A 相似的刺激程序，但在狗的浦肯野细胞以 2mM Ca 作为载流离子。A 和 B 间 E_m 转换是由于 2mM Ca 和 115 mM Ba 的表面电位不同。C：多种来源的标准化的 I_{Ca}，在－40mM 的峰值是由于 $I_{ca,T}$ 和组织及物种的不同（A，引自 Bean BP：Classes of calcium channels in vertebrate cells. Annu Rev Physiol 51：367-384，1989；B，引自 Hirano Y, Fozzard HA, January CT：Characteristics of L- and T-type Ca^{2+} currents in canine cardiac purkinje cells. AM J Physiol Heart Circ Physiol 256：H1478-H1492，1989；C，引自 Bears DM：Excitation-Contraction Coupling and Cardiac Contractile Force，2nd ed. Dordrecht，Netherland，Kluwer Academic Publishers，2001.）

能），这解释了已知的 I_{ca}。通过 LTCCs 的钡电流要大于钙电流，但钡电流更易被钴阻滞。这与钡与通道的结合相一致（比钙弱的亲和力），所以钴阻滞钡更有效率。这也能解释钡比钙的高流量，因为钡不会更多的"粘"在通道里，它会更快的通过。

四、钙通道门控

（一）表面电位和激活

心脏 I_{ca} 能被去极化迅速激活，到达峰电位约 2~7 毫秒（图 2-1），依赖温度和 E_m。钙通道激活需依靠 E_m，但像所有电压依赖通道一样，也对表面电位的变化敏感。表面电位产生于细胞膜表面固定的负电荷。图 2-3 显示变化的表面电位（ψ_o 和）怎样影响细胞膜内的电荷区（ψ_m），它是通道电压的感应器所感应的。在此图中，它的情况接近生理性钙和离子强度时，I_{ca} 激活阈值（$E_m = -40mV$）。对应于体表电荷密度的体表电位为 0.3~1.0 个电荷/nm^2。这与磷脂酸和糖的表面浓度等价，与实验的估计相一致。这种巨大的 ψ_o 优先反映负电荷的磷脂在心肌细胞内肌膜小叶的分布和细胞内较低的 2 价阳离子浓度。2 价阳离子能高效地筛选表面电荷，因其能被负 ψ_o 聚集并结合于负电荷位点，并中和它们。

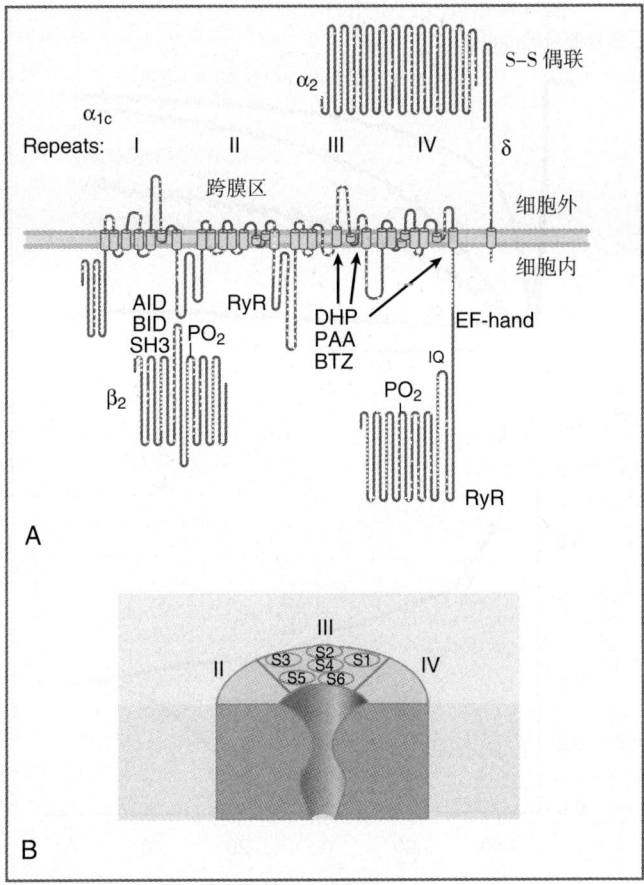

图 2-2 心脏 L-型 Ca 通道的亚基结构 A：α_1 亚基有四个结构域（Ⅰ-Ⅳ），每区有 6 个跨膜片段（S_1-S_6）和一个孔环。Ca 通道拮抗剂（1, 4-二氢吡啶，[DHP]）；苯基烷基胺类，[PAA]；benzothiazepines [BAZ]）结合ⅢS$_5$、ⅢS$_6$ 和ⅣS$_6$ 区。指出了 α_1 亚基间和植物碱（RyR）的可能作用位点，重要的磷酸化位点（PO$_4$），EF-手型区和能与钙调蛋白结合 IQ 模体。β_2 亚基是细胞质的，能被磷酸化（PO$_4$）和与 α_1 在 α-作用和 β-作用结构域（AID 和 BID）相互作用。B：A 剖面图表示 α_1 亚基是如何环绕中心孔（引自 E. Perez-Reyes；From Bers DM: Excitation-Contraction Coupling and Cardiac Contractile Force, 2nd ed. Dordrecht, Netherlands, Kluwer Academic Publishers, 2001.）

monium 四钾铵能穿过）[39]。虽然如此，钙通道对小的单价阳离子的选择性差异可大于 1000 倍（表 2-3），因此尺寸不是选择性的关键因素。钙通道选择性的关键因素，是孔道中的谷氨酸环（locus EEEE 位），四个 P-环各自组成一个 E[43-45]。完全缺乏二价阳离子，钙通道可传递非常大的钠或锂电流（表 2-3）。但是这种电流能被细胞外钙（$K_i \approx 1\mu M$）或镁（$K_i \approx 50~\mu M$）阻断。这能用二价阳离子与孔道的（EEEE 部）高度亲和力解释。以更高浓度[Ca]（如百万浓度）和驱动力，第二个钙能取代结合的钙而通过孔道（钠则不

表 2-3 L 型钙通道的选择性*

离子	P_{ion}/P_{cs}（某离子通透性/铯的通透性）	单通道电导†	未水化时的半径（Å）
Ca^{2+}	4200	9	0.99
Sr^{2+}	2800	9	1.13
Ba^{2+}	1700	25	1.35
Li^+	9.9	45	0.60
Na^+	3.6	85	0.95
K^+	1.4	—	1.33
Cs^+	1.0	—	1.69
Mg^{2+}	~0		0.65

* 选择性以通透性比值表示，数据来自 Hess 等的反转电位测量及 Tsien 的数据；

† 来自 Hess 等在 110mM 2 价阳离子和 150mM 1 价离子条件下的测量数据（后者 pH 为 9.0，以限制质子对通道的阻断）

在 $E_m = -40mV$ 时，图 2-3，跨双层膜电位或 $\psi_m = -60mV$。如果细胞外[Ca]增加，以至 ψ_o 几被消除，而在同样的 $E_m = -40mV$，ψ_m 进一步极化（-88mV）。因此，通道蛋白感受更负的电位，需要更大的去极化才能到达通道激活阈值。这就是为何图

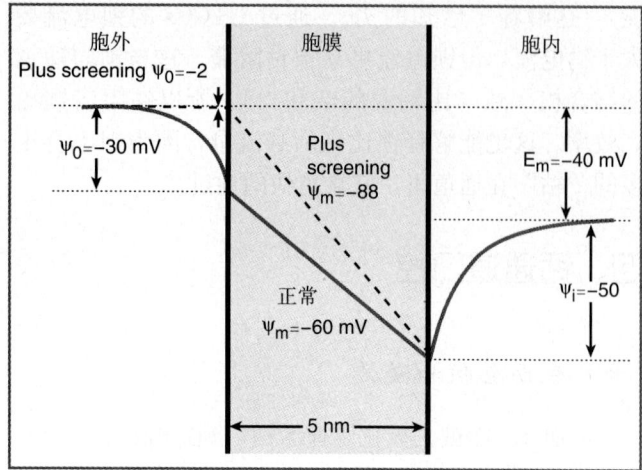

图 2-3 表面电位和通道门控 在高的细胞外二价离子浓度，外部表面电荷被屏蔽，因而在同样 E_m 情况下减小ψ_0和使跨双层膜电位（ψ_m）更负。而且，需要更大的去极化 E_m 才能达到同样的ψ_m（引自 Bers DM：Excitation-Contraction Coupling and Cardiac Contractile Force, 2nd ed. Dordrecht, Netherlands, Kluwer Academic Publishers, 2001.）

2-1A 中 115mM Ba，比 2-1B 中 2mM Ca 的电流-电压关系改变为更大的去极化 E_m。这种影响适用于所有 E_m-依赖性通道和 E_m 依赖性失活。它解释了低 [Ca] 时细胞兴奋性的增加。相反地，高 [Ca]。稳定 E_m-依赖性通道，降低兴奋性（图 2-5A 中曲线右移）。

（二）I_{Ca} 失活

钙通道的失活具有时间、E_m 和 [Ca]$_i$ 依赖性[46-48]。图 2-4A 示通过钙通道的非选择性单价电流（无二价阳离子时测到的 I_{NS}）的失活是非常缓慢的（$t_{1/2}$＞500ms），反映纯粹的 E_m 依赖性失活。在图 2-4A 中，I_{Ba} 的失活（$t_{1/2}$＝161ms）比 I_{NS} 更快，这可能反映 Ba 可以适当地模拟钙依赖性失活。当钙离子是电荷载体（charge carrier），电极内液中用 10mM（EGTA）络合瞬时钙离子（和 SR 钙释放），失活仍很快（$t_{1/2}$＝37ms）。这或许反映了钙依赖性失活决定于钙离子本身经通道的进入。EGTA 是一种缓慢的钙离子缓冲液，并不能阻止靠近钙通道口局部的 [Ca]$_i$ 的增加。正常的兴奋-收缩（E-F）耦联时，也有钙离子从 SR 释放，这进一步提高了钙通道附近局部的 [Ca]$_i$。图 2-4A 中最高的 I_{Ca} 轨迹是在正常的钙转运时产生的，I_{Ca} 失活更迅速（$t_{1/2}$＝17ms）。这强调了 SR 钙释放在生理状态下对 I_{Ca} 失活也起主要的作用。实际上，在动作电位（AP）钳制试验中，正常 SR 钙释放使通过 $I_{Ca,L}$ 的钙离子内流降低 50%[49]。

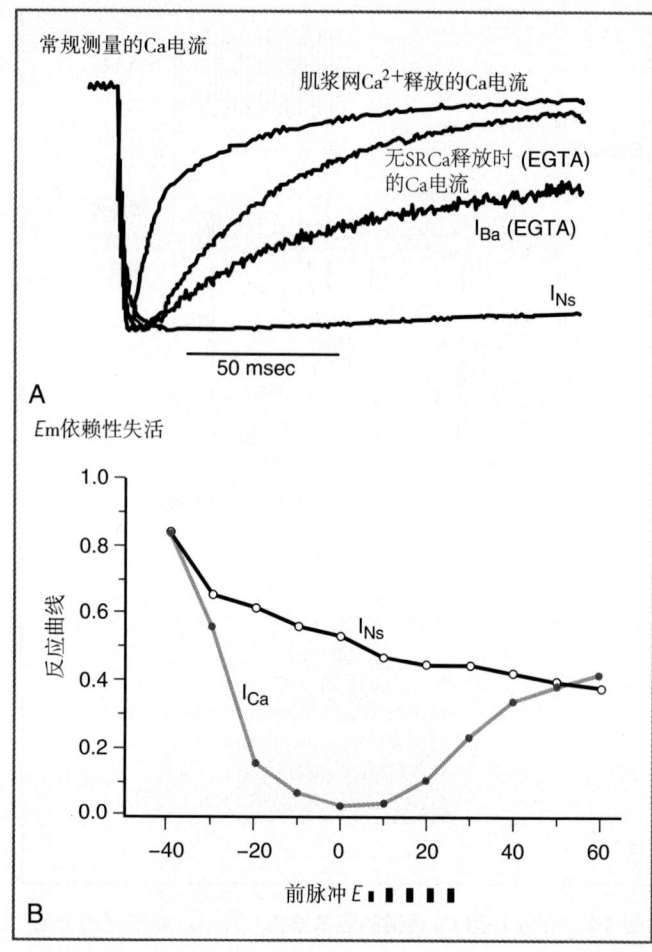

图 2-4 心脏 Ca 通道失活 A：0 mV（除了 I_{NS} 在 −30mV 时记录，以获得相似的激活状态和ψ_m）时常规测量的 Ca、Ba、Na 电流（I_{Ca}，I_{Ba}，I_{NS}）。I_{Ca} 是在穿孔膜片钳技术条件下（含有正常的 SR Ca 释放）和穿孔膜片钳技术（10mM 的 EGTA 以络合整体瞬时 Ca 离子）条件下记录。I_{Ba} 也是在穿孔膜片钳技术条件下（电极内液含 10mM EGTA）记录的。细胞外的 [Ca] 和 [Ba] 都是 2mM。I_{NS} 是在无二价阳离子条件下（内外液都有 10mM 乙烯二胺四乙酸 EDTA），[Na]$_o$ 为 20mM，[Na]$_i$ 为 10mM 时测量的。峰电流在标准化后便可以进行动力学比较。电流从顶部到底部下降的 $t_{1/2}$ 是 17、37、161 和大于 500ms。B：用豚鼠心室肌细胞，在 500ms 指令 E_m 脉冲后，记录的通过 Ca 通道（−10mV）的 I_{NS} 和 I_{Ca} 高度。I_{NS} 失活是 E_m 依赖的，其他 Ca 失活归因于 Ca-依赖性失活（A 引自 Bers DM：Excitation-Contraction Coupling and cardiac Contractile Force, 2nd ed. Dordrecht Netherlands, Kluwer Academis Publishers, 2001；B 引自 Hadley RW, Hume JR：An intrinsic potential-dependent inactivation mechanism associated with calcium channels in guinea-pig myocytes. J Physiol 389：205-222, 1987.）

图 2-4B 示 E_m 依赖性失活是 E_m 的一个功能[48]。即使在＋60mV，I_{NS} 的失活在 500ms 后也是不完全

的。在巨大的正向 E_m（几乎没有钙流入）下，I_{Ca} 失活和 I_{NS} 失活之间无区别（更纯粹的 E_m 依赖性）。其他 E_m 调节的 I_{Ca} 失活有同样 E_m 依赖的内向 I_{Ca} 振幅（最大约在 0mV，见图 2-1C）。快速钙依赖性失活是完全依赖于一个 AP 时间跨度的失活。

I_{Ca} 的钙离子依赖性失活提供一种反馈控制，来限制进一步的 Ca 进入。Ca_i 依赖性失活的一个显著特征是，即使当 [Ca]$_i$ 被 EGTA 或 BAPTA 很大程度地缓冲，收缩停止时，它仍迅速出现。这表明经 I_{Ca} 流入的钙离子一定通过局部活动引起了失活，或许在它与细胞内钙离子混合之前。Hofer 及其同事[50]在单个钙离子通道电流的基础上估计了 [Ca]$_i$ 为 4μM 的 K_i。

现已清楚，调钙蛋白是钙依赖性 I_{Ca} 失活的关键[51-54]。调钙蛋白表现出在钙通道激活或局部 [Ca]$_i$ 升高之前与静息的钙通道预结合（在 $α_{1C}$ 羧基末端 IQ 模体附近，见图 2-2）。当通道开放和局部 [Ca] 升高后，更多的钙离子与调钙蛋白结合（它有四个钙结合点），与钙通道的 IQ 模体产生强烈的相互作用，继而引起失活。

如果电压钳制脉冲（或 APs）非常长，在细胞质钙瞬时释放的过程中 I_{Ca} 会大量地失活，但当 [Ca]$_i$ 下降时可部分恢复[55]。这种长 APs 内 LTCCs 的再激活可促发致心律失常性早期后除极（EAD）[56]。

兔心室肌细胞 I_{Ca} 稳态激活和可用性（或失活）的曲线如图 2-5A 所示。钙通道激活变量（$d_∞$）在 −40mV 开始增加且在 0mV 达到最大。它的失活变量（$f_∞$）在 −45mV 开始下降且在 −15mV 接近 0。这两条曲线的少量重叠提示"窗口电流"。在大约 −28mV，传导率≈最大值（$d_∞×f_∞$）的 1%，因此在这一 E_m 时产生稳态 I_{Ca}，约为最大值的 1%。在 AP 复极化间期，随着 E_m 进入图 2-5A 的阴影区，可能（特别在长 AP 间期）一些 I_{Ca} 从失活恢复并引起净除极。这是 EAD 产生机制的基本假说。

钙通道失活后，从失活中恢复也是 [Ca]$_i$ 和 E_m 依赖的。图 2-5B 示恢复在 −50E_m 时比 −90E_m 时慢很多。这意味着，钙通道的恢复仅当 AP 复极化接近完成时变得非常快。在 −50mV 时，我们可见到失活通道的频率依赖性加速（如在 1Hz）。这就能用试验性程序依赖方式和生理性的频率依赖方式降低 I_{Ca}。

（三）钙依赖 I_{Ca} 易化或 I_{Ca} 阶梯

从 −40mV 的钳制电位，随着起搏频率增加有一

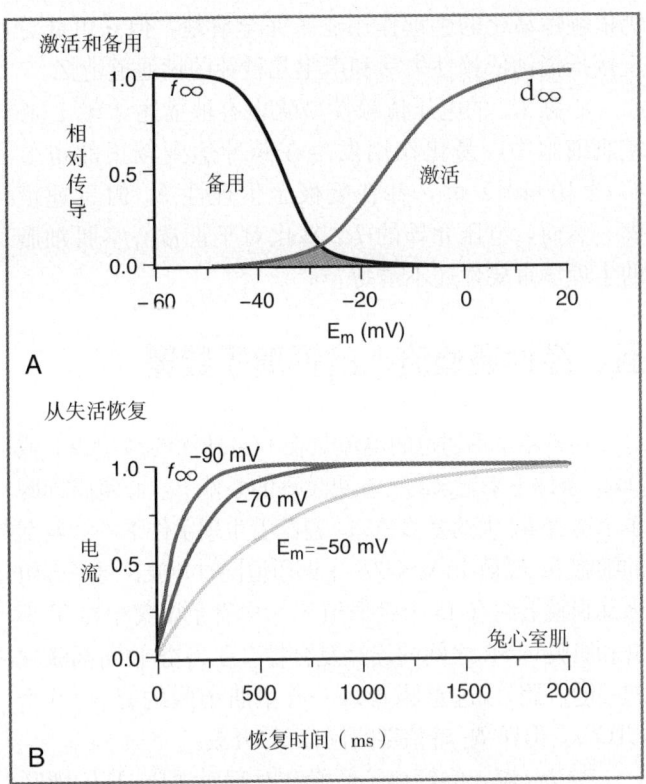

图 2-5 心脏 Ca 通道激活、备用和从失活恢复 A：I_{Ca} 利用率的测量是从 −90mV 去极化到指令 E_m 2秒，然后在 E_m=0mV 时检测剩余可用的 I_{Ca}（[Ca]$_o$=2mM）。此结果是稳态失活或可用性曲线。激活是通过测量根据欧姆定律（G=$I/\triangle V$）得到的驱动力（E_m-Erev）产生的峰电流。B：兔心室 I_{Ca} 从失活恢复是时间和 E_m 依赖的。用2秒到 +10mV 的脉冲诱发失活，然后 E_m 被保持在指定的电压水平不同的时间，直到用 0mV 脉冲来测量可用的 I_{Ca}。（A 引自 Yuan W, Ginsburg KS, Bers DM: Comparison of sarcolemmal calcium channel current in rabbit and rat ventricular myocytes. J Physiol 493：733-746，1996；B 引自 Bers DM: Excitation-Contraction Coupling and cardiac Contractile Force, 2nd ed. Dordrecht, Netherlands, Kluwer Academis Publishers, 2001.）

个进行性的 I_{Ca} 振幅下降[57,58]。这种负向 I_{Ca} 阶梯可能反映了钙通道在脉冲刺激之间失活的不完全恢复（在 −40mV）。相反在生理性的 E_m（−80mV），I_{Ca} 振幅有一个脉冲依赖的进行性增加和显著缓慢的失活[58,59]。这种正相的 I_{Ca} 阶梯是钙离子依赖性的（Ba 电流不会发生），发生时甚至没有 SR 的钙释放，它受钙调蛋白依赖性激酶Ⅱ依赖的磷酸化调节[60-63]。钙流入对随后的 I_{Ca} 的易化影响，完全不同于上面描述的 Ca_i 依赖性失活，但可同时存在。钙调蛋白依赖的激酶Ⅱ涉及调节 I_{Ca} 易化，也被定位在钙通道[54]。这种

钙依赖性易化的生理作用还未完全清楚，但它可部分直接抵消钙依赖性失活和产生几秒钟的钙通道记忆。

心脏 I_{Ca} 的电压依赖性易化也有被描述[65-67]。心室肌细胞中，易化作用发生在脉冲达到较正的电位（$>+100mV$）时，并在复极至生理性 E_m 时迅速消失。然而，电压介导的 I_{Ca} 易化对于正常心室肌细胞的生理学重要性还不清楚。

五、经钙通道流入的钙离子数量

通常单个钙通道的电流是在非生理性的高[Ca]或[Ba]条件下来记录的。在更生理的条件下，心室肌细胞单个通道 I_{Ca} 大约是 0.2pA，意味着生理条件下一个典型的细胞 I_{Ca} 峰值 1nA≈5000 个钙通道同时开放。每平方微米细胞膜上约有 15 个钙通道[68]，尽管主要集中在 T 小管和肌膜与 SR 之间的连接复合物（在兴奋-收缩耦联中起关键作用）。这意味着每一心室肌细胞约有 30 万个 LTCCs，但在 I_{Ca} 峰值期间仅有 3% 开放。

经 I_{Ca} 流入的钙离子数量和时程对 AP、E-C 耦联和钙依赖性肌丝激活有功能上的重要意义。在一个到 0mV 的电压钳方波脉冲期间，I_{Ca} 波形能被整合来推断：钙离子流入细胞浆约 $10\mu M$（这相当于三角形的峰值 $I_{Ca}=1nA$，120ms 长，在一个有 30pL 细胞浆的肌细胞）。然而，在 AP 期间钙离子的内流可能和方波脉冲引起的钙内流有显著的不同。图 2-6 比较方波脉冲和 AP 波形，用作电压钳中的指令电位[10,49,69,70]。在 AP 钳间期的 I_{Ca} 峰值比方波脉冲的要低和发生晚。这是因为在 AP 峰值（$+50mV$）钙通道激活迅速，但刚开始钙离子的驱动力尚低，因 E_m 接近 I_{Ca} 的反转电位（≈$+60mV$）。当 E_m 下降，I_{Ca} 驱动力的增加要比通道的失活快，在 AP 晚期产生一个巨大的电流。兔心室 I_{Ca} 在 AP 期间也比一个方波脉冲期间持续更久。图 2-6 中下部的小格表示钙离子流入的动态数。鼠心室肌细胞中，同样 200ms 方形脉冲期间钙流入数量高于兔的[10]。这决定于 I_{Ca} 激活和失活的不同。然而，鼠心室 AP 是非常短暂的，而某些种类兔心室肌 AP 钙流入波形远高于鼠的（$21\mu M$ 和 $14\mu M$）。

图 2-6 的 I_{Ca} 结果过高估计了生理性钙内流，因为 I_{Ca} 是在以 EGTA（它能减少钙依赖性失活 I_{Ca}）透析的细胞中测量到的。我们也在 25℃ 和 35℃ 及存在正常的 SR 钙释放的条件下，测量了兔心室肌细胞 AP 钳间期的 I_{Ca}，并阻断所有其他电流包括 $I_{Na/Ca}$ 及 $I_{Cl(Ca)}$ [49]。对于稳态（和收缩）AP 钳，I_{Ca} 峰值在

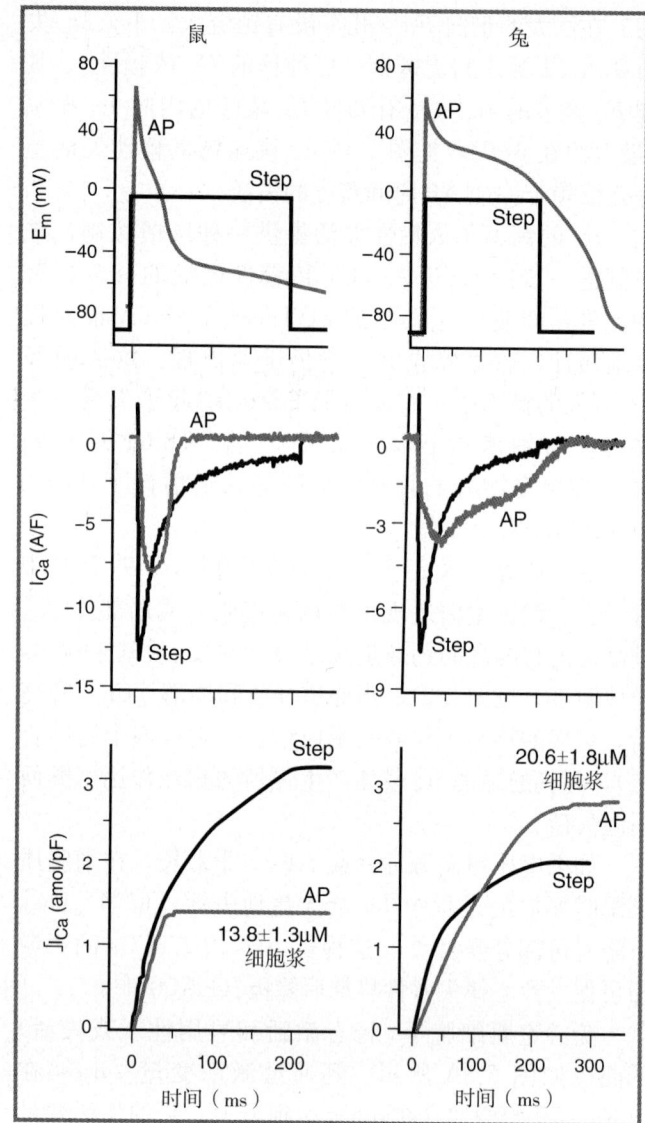

图 2-6 在方波脉冲和动作电位下的 I_{Ca}　鼠和兔心室肌（25℃）经电压钳记录的方波阶跃（step）或动作电位（AP）波形。其他的电流都被阻滞，如以铯替代 K 和以四乙铵替代 Na，细胞用 10mM EGTA 渗析以抑制瞬时 Ca。AP 钳间期 Ca 流出的连续部分以平均值表示（引自 Yuan W, Ginsburg KS, Bers DM: Comparison of sarcolemmal calcium channel current in rabbit and rat ventricular myocytes. J Physiol493：733-746.）

35℃ 比 25℃ 时要更早更高，但两种温度下总的钙内流却大致相同。我们测量在 APs 期间，当 SR 被再储满（先前的排空后）且收缩恢复到静止时，I_{Ca} 如何变化。当收缩和 SR 的钙释放变大时，I_{Ca} 在 AP 期间失活更迅速并完全失活（尤其在 AP 晚期降低 I_{Ca}）。在 25℃ 和 35℃，当 SR 由排空变为静止负载态，总的 I_{Ca} 由 $12\mu M$ 减到 $6\mu M$。这表明，I_{Ca} 的失活决定于 SR 的钙释放，两种温度下减少钙净内流约 50%。

由 SR 钙释放诱发的 I_{ca} 失活的动力学也提供了 SR 钙释放的时间信息[49,70]。我们推断，LTCC 感觉局部 SR 钙释放流量，在 25℃时 5ms 达到峰值（或 35℃时 2.5ms）。这比整个细胞内钙瞬时上升速率高很多，但并不奇怪，我们认为 SR 经 RyR 受体释放钙非常靠近 LTCC。这也表明，钙敏感性离子流是细胞内局部 [Ca]$_i$ 的优秀感应元。

总而言之，L-型 I_{ca} 是钙进入细胞的主要途径（与渗漏、Na/Ca 交换、I_{caT} 相比）。I_{ca} 在心脏电生理中起关键作用，影响 AP 构型和致心律失常作用（经 EADs）。I_{ca} 也是 E-C 耦联、整个细胞钙调节和传导的中心环节。AP 期间 I_{ca} 的动力学和幅度是控制经 SR 钙释放和促进 SR 钙再储存的关键因素。

（浦介麟 王洪涛 滕思勇 译）

参 考 文 献

1. Bers DM: Excitation-Contraction Coupling and Cardiac Contractile Force, 2nd ed. Dordrecht, Netherlands, Kluwer Academic Publishers, 2001.
2. Bers DM, Perez-Reyes E: Ca channels in cardiac myocytes: Structure and function in Ca influx and intracellular Ca release. Cardiovasc Res 42:339-360, 1999.
3. Bean BP: Classes of calcium channels in vertebrate cells. Annu Rev Physiol 51:367-384, 1989.
4. Bean BP: Two kinds of calcium channels in canine atrial cells. Differences in kinetics, selectivity, and pharmacology. J Gen Physiol 86:1-30, 1985.
5. Hirano Y, Fozzard HA, January CT: Characteristics of L- and T-type Ca^{2+} currents in canine cardiac Purkinje cells. Am J Physiol Heart Circ Physiol 256:H1478-H1492, 1989.
6. Hagiwara N, Irisawa H, Kameyama M: Contribution of two types of calcium currents to the pacemaker potentials of rabbit sino-atrial node cells. J Physiol 359:233-253, 1988.
7. Mitra R, Morad M: Two types of calcium channels in guinea-pig ventricular myocytes. Proc Natl Acad Sci U S A 83:5340-5344, 1986.
8. Nuss HB, Houser SR: T-type Ca^{2+} current is expressed in hypertrophied adult feline left ventricular myocytes. Circ Res 73:777-782, 1993.
9. Yuan W, Bers DM: Ca-dependent facilitation of cardiac Ca current is due to Ca-calmodulin-dependent protein kinase. Am J Physiol Heart Circ Physiol 267:H982-H993, 1994.
10. Yuan W, Ginsburg KS, Bers DM: Comparison of sarcolemmal calcium channel current in rabbit and rat ventricular myocytes. J Physiol 493:733-746, 1996.
11. Wetzel GT, Chen F, Klitzner TS: Ca^{2+} channel kinetics in acutely isolated fetal, neonatal, and adult rabbit cardiac myocytes. Circ Res 72:1065-1074, 1993.
12. Gaughan JP, Hefner CA, Houser SR: Electrophysiological properties of neonatal rat ventricular myocytes with α_1-adrenergic-induced hypertrophy. Am J Physiol Heart Circ Physiol 275:H577-H590, 1998.
13. Cribbs LL, Martin BL, Schroder EA, et al: Identification of the T-type calcium channel (Ca$_V$3.1d) in developing mouse heart. Circ Res 88:403-407, 2001.
14. Martínez ML, Heredia MP, Delgado C: Expression of T-type Ca^{2+} channels in ventricular cells from hypertrophied rat hearts. J Mol Cell Cardiol 31:1617-1625, 1999.
15. Jeong SW, Wurster RD: Calcium channel currents in acutely dissociated intracardiac neurons from adult rats. J Neurophysiol 77:1769-1778, 1997.
16. Lipsius SL, Hüser J, Blatter LA: Intracellular Ca release sparks atrial pacemaker activity. News Physiol Sci 16:101-106, 2001.
17. Tanabe T, Takeshima H, Mikami A, et al: Primary structure of the receptor for calcium channel blockers from skeletal muscle. Nature 328:313-318, 1987.
18. Ellis SB, Williams ME, Ways NR, et al: Sequence and expression of mRNAs encoding the α_1 and α_2 subunits of a DHP-sensitive calcium channel. Science 241:1661-1664, 1988.
19. Ruth P, Röhrkasten A, Biel M, et al: Primary structure of the β subunit of the DHP-sensitive calcium channel from skeletal muscle. Science 245:1115-1118, 1989.
20. Jay SD, Ellis SB, McCue AF, et al: Primary structure of the γ subunit of the DHP-sensitive calcium channel from skeletal muscle. Science 248:490-492, 1990.
21. Bosse E, Regulla S, Biel M, et al: The cDNA and deduced amino acid sequence of the γ subunit of the L-type calcium channel from rabbit skeletal muscle. FEBS Lett 267:153-156, 1990.
22. Mikami A, Imoto K, Tanabe T, et al: Primary structure and functional expression of the cardiac dihydropyridine-sensitive calcium channel. Nature 340:230-233, 1989.
23. Takimoto K, Li D, Nerbonne JM, Levitan ES: Distribution, splicing and glucocorticoid-induced expression of cardiac α_{1C} and α_{1D} voltage-gated Ca^{2+} channel mRNAs. J Mol Cell Cardiol 29:3035-3042, 1997.
24. Wyatt CN, Campbell V, Brodbeck J, et al: Voltage-dependent binding and calcium channel current inhibition by an anti-α_{1D} subunit antibody in rat dorsal root ganglion neurones and guinea-pig myocytes. J Physiol 502:307-319, 1997.
25. Jay SD, Sharp AH, Kahl SD, et al: Structural characterization of the dihydropyridine-sensitive calcium channel α_2-subunit and the associated δ peptides. J Biol Chem 266:3287-3293, 1991.
26. Wei XY, Pan S, Lang WH, et al: Molecular determinants of cardiac Ca^{2+} channel pharmacology—Subunit requirement for the high affinity and allosteric regulation of dihydropyridine binding. J Biol Chem 270:27106-27111, 1995.
27. Singer D, Biel M, Lotan I, et al: The roles of the subunits in the function of the calcium channel. Science 253:1553-1557, 1991.
28. Bangalore R, Mehrke G, Gingrich K, et al: Influence of L-type Ca channel α_2/δ-subunit on ionic and gating current in transiently transfected HEK 293 cells. Am J Physiol Heart Circ Physiol 270:H1521-H1528, 1996.
29. Felix R: Voltage-dependent Ca^{2+} channel $\alpha_2\delta$ auxiliary subunit: Structure, function and regulation. Receptors Channels 6:351-362, 1999.
30. Perez-Reyes E, Castellano A, Kim HS, et al: Cloning and expression of a cardiac/brain β subunit of the L-type calcium channel. J Biol Chem 267:1792-1797, 1992.
31. Neely A, Wei X, Olcese R, et al: Potentiation by the β subunit of the ratio of the ionic current to the charge movement in the cardiac calcium channel. Science 262:575-578, 1993.
32. Mitterdorfer J, Froschmayr M, Grabner M, et al: Calcium channels: The β-subunit increases the affinity of dihydropyridine and Ca^{2+} binding sites of the α_1-subunit. FEBS Lett 352:141-145, 1994.
33. Gao TY, Chien AJ, Hosey MM: Complexes of the α_{1C} and β subunits generate the necessary signal for membrane targeting of class C L-type calcium channels. J Biol Chem 274:2137-2144, 1999.
34. de Waard M, Pragnell M, Campbell KP: Ca^{2+} channel regulation by a conserved β subunit domain. Neuron 13:495-503, 1994.
35. Pragnell M, de Waard M, Mori Y, et al: Calcium channel β-subunit binds to a conserved motif in the I-II cytoplasmic linker of the α_1-subunit. Nature 368:67-70, 1994.
36. Perez-Reyes E, Cribbs LL, et al: Molecular characterization of a neuronal low-voltage-activated T-type calcium channel. Nature 391:896-900, 1998.
37. Cribbs LL, Lee JH, Yang J, et al: Cloning and characterization of α1H from human heart, a member of the T-type Ca^{2+} channel gene family. Circ Res 83:103-109, 1998.
38. Lee JH, Daud AN, Cribbs LL, et al: Cloning and expression of a novel member of the low voltage-activated T-type calcium channel family. J Neurosci 19:1912-1921, 1999.
39. McCleskey EW, Almers W: The Ca channel in skeletal muscle is a large pore. Proc Natl Acad Sci U S A 82:7149-7153, 1985.
40. Hess P, Lansman JB, Tsien RW: Calcium channel selectivity for divalent and monovalent cations. Voltage and concentration dependence of single channel current in ventricular heart cells. J Gen Physiol 88:293-319, 1986.
41. Tsien RW, Hess P, McCleskey EW, Rosenberg RL: Calcium channels: Mechanisms of selectivity, permeation and block. Ann Rev

Biophys Chem 16:265–290, 1987.
42. Prod'hom B, Pietrobon D, Hess P: Direct measurement of proton transfer rates to a group controlling the dihydropyridine-sensitive Ca^{2+} channel. Nature 329:243–246, 1987.
43. Ellinor PT, Yang J, Sather WA, et al: Ca^{2+} channel selectivity at a single locus for high-affinity Ca^{2+} interactions. Neuron 15:1121–1132, 1995.
44. Chen XH, Bezprozvanny I, Tsien RW: Molecular basis of proton block of L-type Ca^{2+} channels. J Gen Physiol 108:363–374, 1996.
45. Chen XH, Tsien RW: Aspartate substitutions establish the concerted action of P-region glutamates in repeats I and III in forming the protonation site of L-type Ca^{2+} channels. J Biol Chem 272:30002–30008, 1997.
46. Lee KS, Marbán E, Tsien RW: Inactivation of calcium channels in mammalian heart cells: Joint dependence on membrane potential and intracellular calcium. J Physiol 364:395–411, 1985.
47. Kass RS, Sanguinetti MC: Inactivation of calcium channel current in the calf cardiac Purkinje fiber. Evidence for voltage- and calcium-mediated mechanisms. J Gen Physiol 84:705–726, 1984.
48. Hadley RW, Hume JR: An intrinsic potential-dependent inactivation mechanism associated with calcium channels in guinea-pig myocytes. J Physiol 389:205–222, 1987.
49. Puglisi JL, Yuan W, Bassani JWM, Bers DM: Ca^{2+} influx through Ca^{2+} channels in rabbit ventricular myocytes during action potential clamp: Influence of temperature. Circ Res 85:e7–e16, 1999.
50. Höfer GF, Hohenthanner K, Baumgartner W, et al: Intracellular Ca^{2+} inactivates L-type Ca^{2+} channels with a Hill coefficient of approximately 1 and an inhibition constant of approximately 4 µM by reducing channel's open probability. Biophys J 73:1857–1865, 1997.
51. Zühlke RD, Reuter H: Ca^{2+}-sensitive inactivation of L-type Ca^{2+} channels depends on multiple cytoplasmic amino acid sequences of the α_{1C} subunit. Proc Natl Acad Sci U S A 95:3287–3294, 1998.
52. Peterson BZ, DeMaria CD, Yue DT: Calmodulin is the Ca^{2+} sensor for Ca^{2+}-dependent inactivation of L-type calcium channels. Neuron 22:549–558, 1999.
53. Qin N, Olcese R, Bransby M, et al: Ca^{2+}-induced inhibition of the cardiac Ca^{2+} channel depends on calmodulin. Proc Natl Acad Sci U S A 96:2435–2438, 1999.
54. Zühlke RD, Pitt GS, Deisseroth K, et al: Calmodulin supports both inactivation and facilitation of L-type calcium channels. Nature 399:159–162, 1999.
55. Sipido KR, Callewaert G, Carmeliet E: Inhibition and rapid recovery of Ca^{2+} current during Ca^{2+} release from sarcoplasmic reticulum in guinea pig ventricular myocytes. Circ Res 76:102–109, 1995.
56. January CT, Riddle JM: Early afterdepolarizations: Mechanism of induction and block. A role for L-type Ca^{2+} current. Circ Res 64:977–990, 1989.
57. Tseng GN: Calcium current restitution in mammalian ventricular myocytes is modulated by intracellular calcium. Circ Res 63:468–482, 1988.
58. Hryshko LV, Bers DM: Ca current facilitation during post-rest recovery depends on Ca entry. Am J Physiol Heart Circ Physiol 259:H951–H961, 1990.
59. Zygmunt AC, Maylie J: Stimulation-dependent facilitation of the high threshold calcium current in guinea-pig ventricular myocytes. J Physiol 428:653–671, 1990.
60. Yuan W, Bers DM: Ca-dependent facilitation of cardiac Ca current is due to Ca-calmodulin-dependent protein kinase. Am J Physiol Heart Circ Physiol 267:H982–H993, 1994.
61. Anderson ME, Braun AP, Schulman H, et al: Multifunctional Ca^{2+}/calmodulin-dependent protein kinase mediates Ca^{2+}-induced enhancement of the L-type Ca^{2+} current in rabbit ventricular myocytes. Circ Res 75:854–861, 1994.
62. Xiao RP, Cheng H, Lederer WJ, et al: Dual regulation of Ca^{2+}/calmodulin-dependent kinase II activity by membrane voltage and by calcium influx. Proc Natl Acad Sci U S A 91:9659–9663, 1994a.
63. Dzhura I, Wu Y, Colbran RJ, et al: Calmodulin kinase determines calcium-dependent facilitation of L-type calcium channels. Nat Cell Biol 2:173–177, 2000.
65. Pietrobon D, Hess P: Modal gating of L-type calcium channels. Biophys J 57:24a, 1990.
66. Sculptoreanu A, Rotman E, Takahashi M, et al: Voltage-dependent potentiation of the activity of cardiac L-type calcium channel α_1 subunits due to phosphorylation by cAMP-dependent protein kinase. Proc Natl Acad Sci U S A 90:10135–10139, 1993.
67. Kamp TJ, Hu H, Marbán E: Voltage-dependent facilitation of cardiac L-type Ca channels expressed in HEK-293 cells requires β-subunit. Am J Physiol Heart Circ Physiol 278:H126–H136, 2000.
68. Lew WYW, Hryshko LV, Bers DM: Dihydropyridine receptors are primarily functional L-type Ca channels in rabbit cardiac myocytes. Circ Res. 69:1139–1145, 1991.
69. Grantham CJ, Cannell MB: Ca^{2+} influx during the cardiac action potential in guinea pig ventricular myocytes. Circ Res 79:194–200, 1996.
70. Linz KW, Meyer R: Control of L-type calcium current during the action potential of guinea-pig ventricular myocytes. J Physiol. 513:425–442, 1998.

第 3 章

电压调节性钾通道

Gavin Y. Oudit, Rafael J. Ramirez, Peter H. Backx

本章目录	
■ 电压门控钾通道的生理特性	19
■ 电压门控钾通道的组成亚基	22
■ 瞬时外向电流（I_{to}）	26
■ 延迟整流电流	28
■ 电压调节内向整流钾电流（I_{k1}）	29
■ 背景钾电流	30
■ 电压调节性钾通道与心脏病	30
■ 致谢	30

在心脏组织，内向除极电流和外向复极电流综合作用形成动作电位。尽管在超极化期的钠（Na^+）/钙（Ca^{2+}）交换体和 Na^+/K^+ ATP 酶的驱动也产生少量的外向电流，但通过钾通道产生的外向钾电流仍是形成复极化电流的主要来源（见图 3-1）。心脏钾通道分为三大类：电压门控钾通道（Kv）（I_{to}, $I_{Kur}/I_{K,slow}$, I_{Kr}, I_{Ks}），内向整流性钾通道（I_{K1}, I_{KACh}, I_{KATP}）和背景钾电流通道（TASK-1, TWIK-1/2）（见图 3-1 和表 3-1）。电压调节性钾通道（Kv 和 I_{K1}）的表达水平、方式和生理特性会在心房和心室间、心脏不同部位（窦房结和浦氏纤维）、心室心肌的不同层面（心外膜心肌、中层心肌和心内膜心肌）以及正常和异常心肌细胞之间出现变化，这些可从相应心肌细胞的动作电位的变化得到验证。心脏电压调节性钾通道是一种大分子结构，有四个成孔的 α 亚基和细胞骨架中的辅助亚基以及胞浆中的信号复合物分子共同装配而成。由于辅助亚基和信号复合物会出现变化，所以该通道的结构是动态变化的（图 3-1 和 3-2）。在心脏组织，电压调节性钾通道的功能变化引起心肌细胞电学和收缩特性的改变，这些通道还是许多药物作用的分子靶点。而且，这些通道的突变引起许多心血管疾病，其中包括长 QT 综合征。

一、电压门控钾通道的生理特性

电压门控钾通道（Kv）是由 4 个 α 亚基形成的四聚体。每个 α 亚基由 6 个跨膜亚单元（S1-S6）组成，其 N 端和 C 端均位于胞膜内侧。S1-S4 亚单元负责通道感知电压的变化，S5-S6 亚单元间形成通道的孔区（见图 3-2 和 3-3）。细胞膜的电压水平决定 Kv 通道呈开放传导（激活）状态或非传导状态。非传导状态包括灭活（关闭）和失活状态。一般情况下，关闭的 Kv 通道激活或开放是对膜除极化的一种反应，随后通道会进入失活状态，呈时间依赖性。通道在复极化阶段重新进入关闭状态。由于通道空间构象变化引起通道呈电压和时间依赖性功能改变称为门控。不同的 Kv 通道具有不同的分子构成和电压门控方式。

（一）激活门控机制

Kv 通道激活（开放）的重要特征是通道的电压感受器与通道的激活（开放）相连。电压感受器被认为是保守的第 4 个跨膜亚单元（S4），因为在 S4 的氨基酸组成中，每隔 3 个氨基酸均为携带正电荷的精氨酸或赖氨酸残基（见图 3-3A），尽管在其他单元中也包含这种氨基酸。电流模式可预测随后的膜除极情况，电压感受器（S4 和 S3b 亚单元）的阳离子、亲水性的"浆"与螺旋-转折-螺旋结构相互作用驱动钾离子通过脂质膜到达膜外（～20Å）[1,1a]。有趣的是，

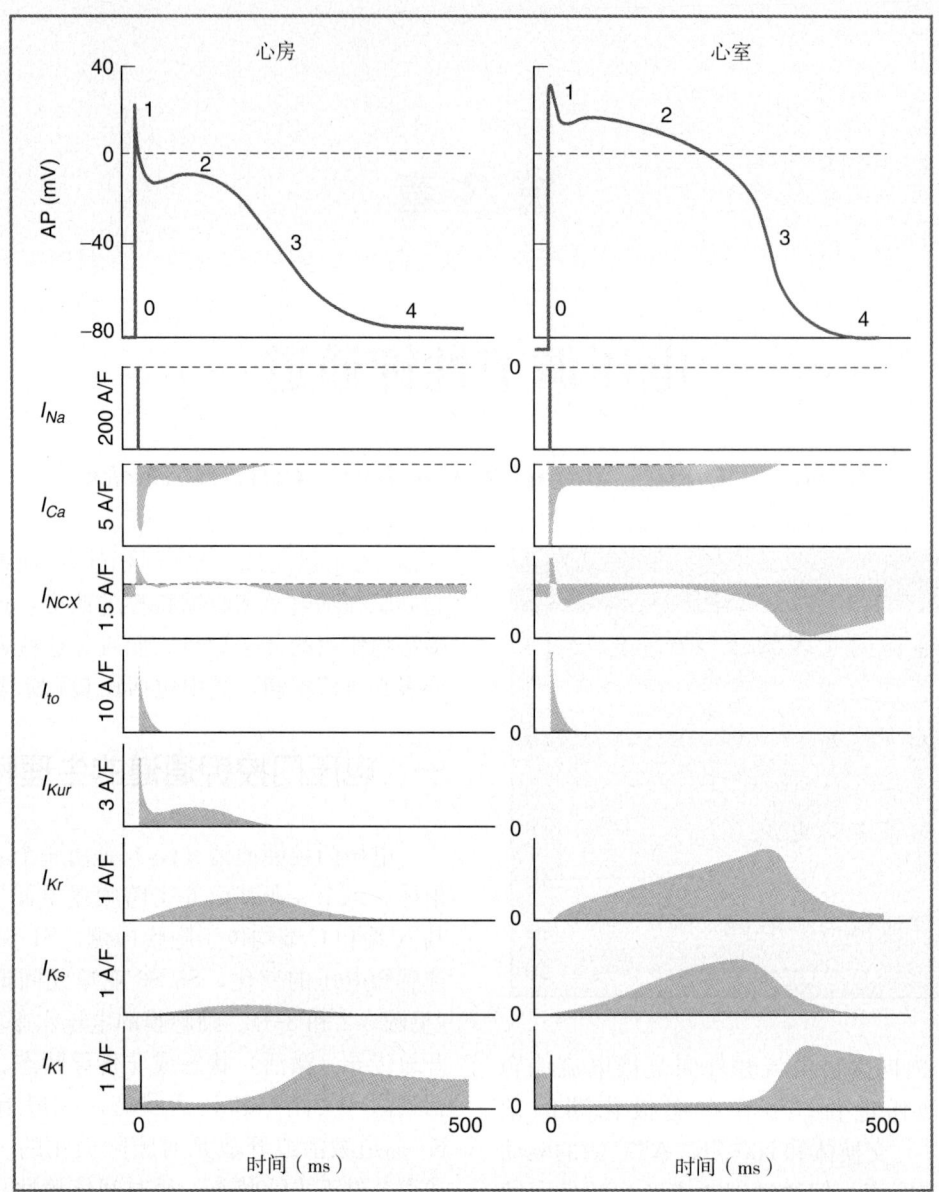

图 3-1 心脏动作电位（AP）波形 上组来自心房（左）和心室（右）肌细胞。标记除了 AP 的 5 个时程：0：AP 的超射代表了膜触极；1：早期复极；2：平台期；3：晚期复极；4：静息（舒张）期。AP 的变化直接与跨膜离子流总数呈比例（下组）。内向电流使膜除极，而外向电流使膜复极。与心房 AP 相比，心室 AP 间期明显长，平台期高以及膜静息电位更负。心房肌细胞超快速整流钾电流（I_{Kur}）使 AP 平台期低，心室肌细胞更大的内向整流钾电流（I_{K1}）使 3 相复极更快，静息膜电位更负

起搏通道（I_f/I_h）在超极化状态下激活是同通道胞膜面的收缩相连[2]。S4 亚单位的位移引起 S5 和 S6 跨膜 α 螺旋的移动，形成"激活门"，从而引起孔道开放[1,1a]。

位于孔内部的 S5 和 S6 螺旋形成弯曲的构象，形成门的铰链区，引导位于孔区内膜面的水合离子进入选择性的通透区（见图 3-3B）[1,3]，这种构象不仅促进钾离子通过跨膜区传导，也允许大的阳离子和失活粒子进入位于内膜面孔区内。S6 跨膜区嵌入膜内形成穿越束，负责一些 Kv 通道的闸门关闭。S6 穿越束螺旋驱动由高度保守的甘氨酸残基所组成的铰链区开放，该铰链区允许钾离子从开阔的孔区进入高选择性的通透区[1,3]。S6 穿越束也有高度保守的脯氨酸残基（PxP 或 PxG）组成，也是建立电压感受器与通道开放之间联系的关键成员之一。

表 3-1 心肌钾离子通道 α 亚单位

电流	描述	基因	AP 期	激活机制	克隆	分子组成
$I_{to,f}$	快失活一过性外向钾电流	KCND2 KCND3	Phase 1	电压 （去极化）	K_v4.2/4.3	单孔，6 个跨膜亚单位，四聚体
$I_{to,s}$	慢失活一过性外向钾电流	KCNA4 KCNA7 KCNC4	Phase 1	电压 （去极化）	K_v1.4/1.7/3.4	单孔，6 个跨膜亚单位，四聚体
I_{Kur}	超快延迟整流	KCNA5 KCNC1	Phase 2	电压 （去极化）	K_v1.5/3.1	单孔，6 个跨膜亚单位，四聚体
I_{Kr}	快速延迟整流	KCNH2	Phase 3	电压 （去极化）	HERG	单孔，6 个跨膜亚单位，四聚体
I_{Ks}	缓慢延迟整流	KCNQ1	Phase 3	电压 （去极化）	K_vLQT1	单孔，6 个跨膜亚单位，四聚体
I_{K1}	强内向整流	KCNJ2 KCNJ12	Phase 3 and 4	电压 （去极化）	Kir 2.1/2.2	单孔，2 个跨膜亚单位，四聚体
I_{KATP}	ADP 激活的 K^+ 通道*	KCNJ11	Phase 1 and 2	↑ADP/ATP 比率（ATP 损耗）	Kir 6.2	单孔，2 个跨膜亚单位，四聚体
I_{KACh}	M_2 受体门控钾通道†	KCNJ3 KCNJ5	Phase 4	乙酰胆碱	Kir 3.1/3.4	单孔，2 个跨膜亚单位，四聚体
I_{Kp}	背景电流钾通	KCNK1/6 KCNK3 KCNK4	All phases	代谢 参数 细胞膜张力	TWIK-1/2 TASK-1 TRAAK	双孔，4 个跨膜亚单位，二聚体
I_n	起搏电流通道‡	HCN2 HCN4	Phase 4	电压 （超极化）	HCN2/4	单孔，6 个跨膜亚单位，四聚体

* 弱内向整流
† 心房及结细胞上的 2 型 M 受体
‡ 心肌细胞与结细胞上存在非选择性的 HCN2 和 HCN4
SUR2A，由 kir6-2 亚单位形成的八聚体

（二）选择性滤过和渗透孔道

钾通道驱动钾离子以有限的扩散率选择性通过脂质双层膜，而其他阳离子基本不能滤过。钾通道的孔区是由 S5 和 S6 跨膜区以及 S5 和 S6 连接区（P 环）共同组成的，每个亚基呈对称性排列，中间部分形成孔区，正如 KcsA 钾通道的结构一样（见图 3-3A）。孔长度约 45Å，从内至外由 4 部分组成：胞浆段通道，在激活期间开放；水化的中心区，为孔最宽阔部位（约 10Å）；狭窄的选择性滤过区和宽而浅的细胞外孔腔（见图 3-3B）。狭窄的选择性滤过区大部分由氨基酸残基的羧基骨架构成（从内到外）：苏氨酸-X-甘氨酸-酪氨酸-甘氨酸（TXGYG 或"标签顺序"），伴随着氧原子从内向外面对离子的传导通路，X 代表任何一种氨基酸，GYG 序列是维持 K^+ 选择性的固有序列[4]（见图 3-3）。来源于 4 个 α 亚基的标签序列上的碳氧原子在空间上呈均衡排列，有利于通道对钾离子选择性滤过，尽管通道其他功能部位的空间变化也能改变通道的选择性，但这种调节仍然通过标签序列的空间改变来实施。

（三）失活门控学

失活是电压门控钾通道的基本特性，该过程是通道从开放状态变为关闭状态，空间构象转换为非传导性的稳定状态。一般来讲，失活通道不能重新开放，除非膜电位处于复极状态，允许通道恢复到关闭状态（见图 3-4F）。对于电压门控钾通道，失活过程与三种空间构象有关，分别是 N 型、C 型、U 型失活。

1. N 型失活模式（球链门控模式）

N 型失活模式最先见于描述 Shaker Kv 通道，发现其满足球链门控机制的许多原则，包括它的快速动力学方式。在 N 型失活模型中，N 端功能域（失活"球"拴在"链"上）连接到位于内孔区上的受体位点，因而阻塞了孔道[5]，如同先前描述的乌贼神经元的 Na^+ 电流[6]。失活功能域可存在于成孔的 α 亚基或某些 β 亚基上。如果 β 亚基的 T1 功能域（T1$_4$β$_4$）位于孔区的内侧（见图 3-3C），通道的失活似乎与 α 亚基的两侧功能域有关，因为 α 亚基的胞浆端功能域开放可让钾离子绕过位于孔区胞内侧的 β 亚基，从侧面

表 3-2 钾离子门控通道的附加亚单位

亚单位	基因	分子结构	CBD	电流	表面表达	激活和失活
KChAP	KChAP	细胞内 (85 kDa)	否	I_{to} ($K_v4.3$)* ↑	↑	↔ROA, ↓ROI, ↔RFI
KChiP2**‡	KCNIP2	细胞内 (220—270AA)	是	I_{to} ($K_v4.3$) ↑	↑	↓ROI§, ↑RFI, DVA
Frequenin		细胞内 (22 kDa)	是	I_{to} ($K_v4.2$)§ ↑	↑	↓ROI§, ↑RFI
Neuronal Ca^{2+} Sensor-1		细胞内 (25 kDa)	是	I_{to} ($K_v4.3$) ↑	↑	↓ROI, ↔RFI, DVA
β subunit1 ($K_v\beta1.2$)‡	KCNAB1	细胞内	否	I_{to} ($K_v1.4$) ↓	NR	↑ROI, ↓RFI
				I_{Kur} ‖	NR	NR
β subunit1 ($K_v\beta1.3$)‡	KCNAB1	细胞内 (419 AA)	否	I_{Kur} ↔	NR	↑ROI, HVA
β subunit3 ($K_v\beta3$)	KCNAB2	细胞内 (408 AA)	否	I_{to} ($K_v1.4$)	NR	↑ROI
				I_{to} ($K_v4.3$)	↑	↑ROI, ↓RFI
				I_{Kur} ↔	NR	↑ROI, HVA
MiRP1**	KCNE2	单跨膜区域	否	I_{Kr} ↓	DVA	
				I_{Ks}	NR	↓ROA
		(123 AA)		I_{to} ($K_v4.3$)	NR	↓ROI
MinK	KCNE1	单跨膜区域 (ECN-尾) (129-130 AA)	否 否	I_{Kr} ↑ I_{Ks} ↑	↔ ↔	HVA ↓ROA

* 效果被 $K_v\beta1.2$ 所抑制
** 主要表达于浦肯野纤维
＋拼接的变体
‡ 人类中存在的单核苷酸多态性
§ 依赖于 Ca^{2+}
‖ 被 KchAP 表达所拮抗
↑增加, ↔不变, ↓降低
AA, 氨基酸; CBD, 钙结合区域; DVA, 电压激活的除极改变; EC, 细胞外; HVA, 电压激活的超极化; NR, 未见报道; RFL, 失活后恢复; ROA, 激活速度; POI, 失活速度

进入孔区[7]。尽管有内孔阻塞的证据,但由于 N 端与通道相互作用的过程引起了通道空间构象的改变,导致另一种失活模式也常常起作用,这种失活模式是 C-型失活。

2. C 型失活模式（选择性区域的分子转换）

C 型失活为第 2 种失活模式,其机制与孔区外口的空间变化有关。N 型失活过程可加剧 C 型失活的进展,但截除 Kv1.x 通道 N 端（球）的变异通道仍保留 C 型失活。C 型失活对细胞外钾浓度和孔区外口至孔区的突变很敏感,细胞外钾浓度的升高或蓄积可引起 C 型失活。正常情况下,C 型失活过程慢于 N 型失活,可反复调整通道的电活性,而它对钾浓度的敏感性限制它对细胞外高钾的生理反应性。

3. U 型失活模式

除了 N 型和 C 型失活外,Kv1.x 通道还有另外一种失活模式,称为 U 型失活。随着刺激间期的延长,通道呈 U 型电压依赖性失活[8,9]。特别是在 0mV 水平长时间除极时,通道会进入 U 型失活,并快速恢复到关闭状态。而且,胞外的 TEA（四乙胺）和高钾浓度[8,9]可提高通道 U 型失活的比例。尽管目前尚不明确 U 型失活所产生的空间变化情况,但位于胞浆内 Kv 通道的 T1 功能域似乎参与了这一失活模式。越来越多的证据表明 U 型失活有重要的生理功能[8,9]。

二、电压门控钾通道的组成亚基

(一) 成孔 α 亚基

电压调节性钾通道是由 4 个成孔的 α 亚基组装成四聚体,并与辅助性调节亚基相互作用形成有功能的钾通道。随着对果蝇的 Kv 亚家族的识别（Shaker, Shab, Shaw, Shal）,也在哺乳类动物中发现了相应

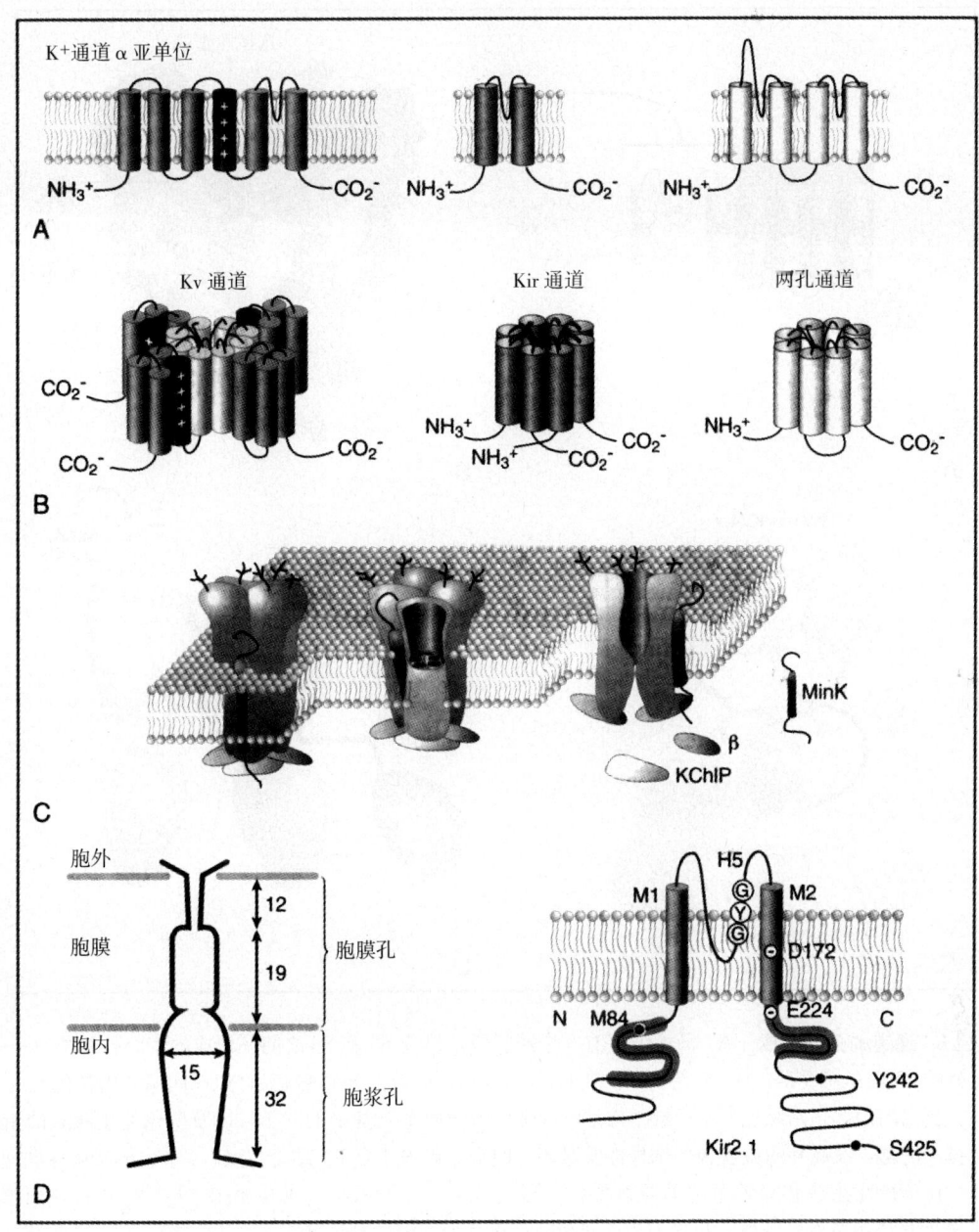

图 3-2 心脏 K^+ 通道的分子构成 A：Kv、Kir 和两孔 α 亚单位是分别有 6、2、4 个跨膜段的完整膜蛋白。B：α 亚单位作为四聚体或二聚体构成 K^+ 选择性孔。C：辅助亚基，如细胞内 Kvβ 亚基、Kv 通道相互作用蛋白（KChIP2）和 Mink，也有助于形成功能性心脏钾通道。D：显示关键氨基酸残基的 Kir2.1 拓扑学结构图（M1 和 M2 跨膜段和连接 H5 成孔环）；D172（天冬氨酸）和 E224（谷氨酸）残基对 Kir2.x 通道形成强的内向电流很重要（右）。根据 Nishida 模型的通道离子转导途径的几何图：选择性滤过器，12Å；内孔，19Å；胞浆孔，32Å（胞浆孔的最大直径是 15Å）（左）。（A-C，来自 Nerbonne 等, Circ Res 89：944-956, 2003; D, 来自 Lopatin 等, J Mol Cell Cardiol 33: 625-638, 2001）

的亚家族，分别为 Kv1.x（KCNA）、Kv2.x（KCNB）、Kv3.x（KCNC）和 Kv4.x（KCND），但研究显示 Kv5、Kv6、Kv8 和 Kv9 单独表达，不产生电流，推测这种通道可能调节其他 Kv 通道的功能。成孔的 α 亚基有 6 个跨膜功能域（S1-S6），N 端和 C 端均位于胞浆内。大多数研究认为，只有属于同一亚家族成员的 Kvα 亚基能相互作用，组装异源多聚体，形成有功能的通道。当然，异源多聚体的形成有赖于 N 端 120 个高度保守的氨基酸，命名为 T1 或 Nab 结构域。来源于 Kv1.x 和 Kv4.x 亚家族的 4 个 α 亚基装配成有功能的通道，分别产生瞬时外向钾电流的慢成分（$I_{to,s}$）和快成分（$I_{to,f}$）（见图 3-2 和 3-3A）（见表 3-1）[10,11]。

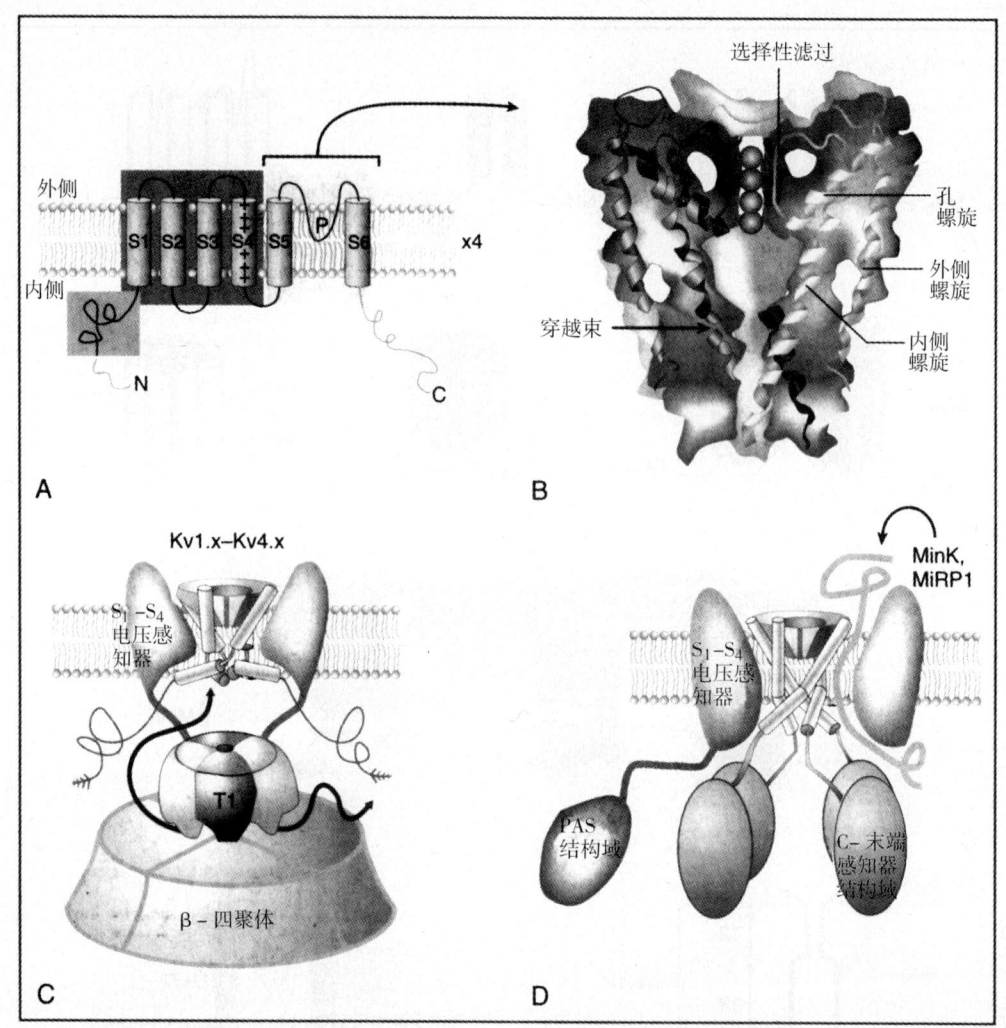

图 3-3 电压门控 K$^+$ 通道的分子构成 A：每个亚基有 6 个跨膜段，伴有 S5 和 S6 之间环形成的窄的孔区部分——选择性滤过器，以及带正电荷的 S4 电压感受器。B：细菌 KcsA 钾通道伴有与 S5 同源的外侧螺旋和与 S6 同源的内侧螺旋是电压门控钾通道成孔区的原型。蛋白的内部是暗绿色，第二层结构是由丝带代表的四个亚基中的三个，以及灰色的接触水的蛋白表面。从上方可见到窄的选择性滤器，及有孔螺旋支撑的选择性滤器环。四个球代表 4 个 K$^+$ 结合位点。4 个内部螺旋穿到通道底部收缩通道（"穿越束"）。在选择性滤器和穿越束之间是水灌注"腔"。C：Kv1.x-Kv4.x 亚家族在 N 末端具有"四聚体化结构域"（T1），它决定亚基四聚体组装的特异性，也作为蛋白间相互作用及细胞内信号传导的平台。C 端有一个 PDZ 结合区，它决定通道的物理定位及与大的信号复合物的联系。D：电压门控 KvLQT1 和 HERG 通道也是四聚体结构，但有不同的功能域，特征是缺乏 T1 结构域，在 C 端有感受器结构域。HERG 通道的 N 端有一个 PAS 功能域。（经 Yellen G 允许：Nature，419；35-42，2002，版权 2002，MacMillan 出版社）

Kv1.5α 亚基组装成 Kv1.5 通道，形成超速延迟整流钾电流（I_{Kur}），其拓扑结构同形成 I_{to} 电流的 Kv1.4 和 Kv4.x 亚基相似（见图 3-2 和 3-3A）（见表 3-1）[12,13]。表达 I_{to} 电流的 Kv 通道在肌纤维上分布不一致，具有组织特异性，在心房肌，Kv4.2 表达在肌纤维的周边和闰盘，而在心室肌主要表达在纵管系统。Kv 通道的 C 端含有膜定位信号，糖基化位点，也负责与 β 亚基相互作用，产生相应功能。

Kv 通道 α 亚基成员还包括 HERG（*KCNH2*）和 KvLQT1（*KCNQ1*）亚家族[15-17]。同 Kv1-4.x 亚家族一样，它们也为膜蛋白，含有 6 个跨膜亚单元，N 端和 C 端均位于胞膜内，S4 亚单元携带正电荷，具有电压感受器作用（见图 3-2 和 3-3A）。然而，与 Kv1-4.x 亚家族不同，HERG 和 KvLQT1 含有一些不同的功能域，它们缺乏 T1 功能域，在 C 端出现感受器功能域（见图 3-3D）。HERG Kvα 亚基组装成同源四聚体，与 β 亚基作用形成延迟整流钾电流快速部分（I_{Kr}），同样 KvLQT1Kvα 亚基组装成同源四聚体，与

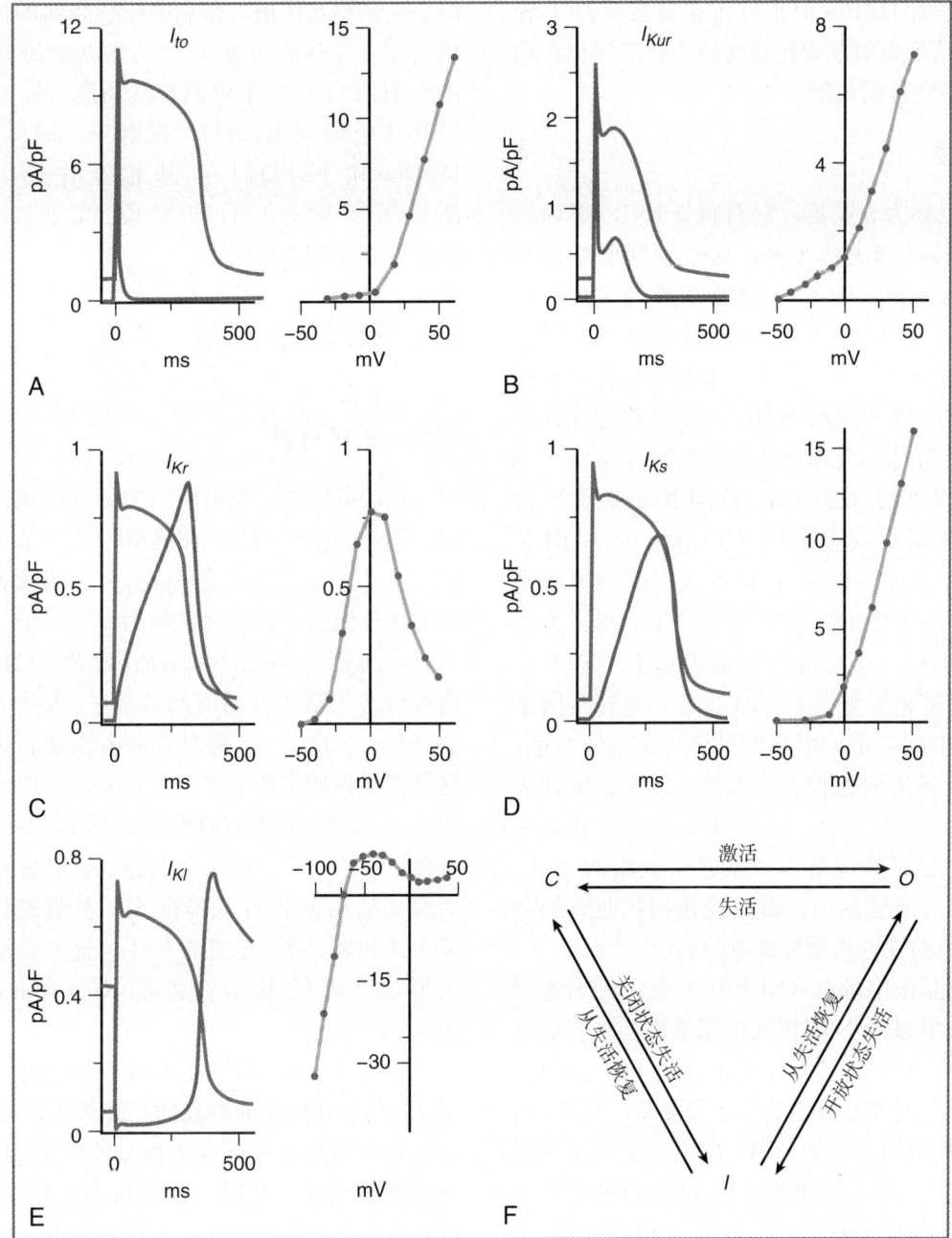

图 3-4 电压调控钾通道的电流-电压关系 A~E 组显示的是 AP 期间主要钾电流的时间曲线,以及稳态电流-电压关系(A-E,右图)。A:心室瞬时外向 K^+ 电流(I_{to})。B:心房超快速延迟整流钾电流(I_{kur})。C:心室快速延迟整流钾电流(I_{kr})。D:心室缓慢延迟整流钾电流(I_{ks})。E:心室内向整流钾电流(I_{K1})。F:离子通道的活性可用不同构成状态间蛋白的转变来描述。通道从非传导关闭态(C)到开放态(O)激活允许离子渗透。开放和关闭通道都能进入非传导失活态(I)。通道由开放到关闭态可看作通道的去活化

β亚基作用形成延迟整流钾电流缓慢部分(I_{Ks})[16,17]。另外,HERG 亚基有较大 N 端,其结构类似于 PAS 功能域,该结构参与转导[15,16]。相比较而言,Kv-LQT1 亚基的 N 端较短,缺乏 PAS 功能域[1,15],此外,HERG 的 C 端还包含一个环核苷酸连接功能域(CNBD)。在心脏组织,HERG 基因可检测 3 个 RNA 剪接体,即 2 个 N 端和 1 个 C 端剪接变异体,它们不形成有功能的通道,但可以调节 HERG 通道的门控动力学[16,18];KvLQT1 的 N 端截短异构体(或异构体 2)也在心脏表达,以负显性抑制方式调节 I_{Ks} 电流[17];但目前尚不清楚这些剪接变异体在体内如何调节延迟整流性钾电流[16,18]。编码 I_{to} 电流的钾通道主要

分布在闰盘区，而 HERG 似乎分布在肌浆膜和 T 管膜上[18]，这些结果表明在哺乳动物的心脏组织存在调节不同钾通道膜定位的机制。

(二) 辅助亚基

辅助亚基也称为 β 亚基，它们调节 Kv1.4-Kv4.x 亚家族的生理特性和表达水平，这些辅助亚基包括 KChAP、KChIPs 和其他 Ca^{2+} 敏感性蛋白（见表3-2）。$Kv\beta_1$、$Kv\beta_2$ 和 $Kv\beta_3$ 是三种高度同源的亚家族，在体内有多个剪接体[19,20]。每个 β 亚基均包含一个保守的核心区域和一个可变的 N 端，与电压门控性钾通道的活性位点相互作用发挥氧化还原酶的效应[7,20]。β 亚基可形成四聚体的对称结构，或同 Kvα 亚基 N 端的 T1 功能域作用形成多聚体（$T1_4\beta_4$）（见图3-3C）[7]。$Kv\beta_{1.2}$、$Kv\beta_{1.3}$ 和 $Kv\beta_3$ 均在人心脏组织中表达，而 $Kv\beta_3$ 在心室的表达水平明显高于心房，大约呈 2 倍关系，$Kv\beta_{1.2}$ 在心房和心室表达水平基本一致[19,21]。Kv 通道相关蛋白 C（KChAP）是转录因子连接蛋白家族中的一员，也能调节 Kv 通道的功能，增加特异的 Kv 通道的胞膜表达水平，而不影响其他通道的特性[10]（见表3-2）。KChAP 以类似于伴侣分子的作用模式发挥其调节 Kv 通道亚家族的功能。KChAP 是一种可溶性蛋白，瞬时连接到靶通道的 N 端，以转录非依赖性方式增加通道的表达[10,36]。

Kv 通道相互作用蛋白（KChIPs）是一种钙连接蛋白，同 Kv4α 亚基的 N 端相互作用重构心脏表达电流的某些特性，并改变它们的电流密度和失活动力学[10,22]。$KChIP_2$ 是在心脏表达的主要亚基，与 Kv 通道共定位在心脏组织，也能与 Kv 通道产生免疫共沉淀[22]（见表3-2）。在心肌组织，$KChIP_2$ 有两个剪接体，主要表达在 T 管和核上[23]。Kv4.2 和 $KChIP_2$ 共表达时可增加前者的表达电流密度，表明 $KChIP_2$ 可增加或稳定 Kv4.2 在细胞膜的表达水平，并调节其生理特性，增加心脏快速 $I_{to,f}$ 电流[22,24]。其他两种 KChIP 相关的 Ca^{2+} 连接蛋白是 frequenin 和神经元钙敏感蛋白-1，它们均在心脏表达，并增加 I_{to} 的电流密度，改变其失活动力学特性[10,25,26]（见表3-2）。

同样，HERG 和 KvLQT1 亚家族也受辅助亚基的调节，它们属于 KCNE 家族，包括 Mink、Mink 相关肽 1（MiRP1）、MiRP2 和 MiRP3，分别由 KCNE1、KCNE2、KCNE3 和 KCNE4 基因编码，Mink、MiRP1 和 MiRP2 均在心脏表达[15-17,27]（见表3-2）。这些蛋白均为跨膜蛋白，包含位于胞外的 N 端，它们同 α 亚基相互作用，影响电压感受器的位置或直接作用改变 α 亚基的功能[1,16,17]。最初的研究表明 MiRP1 能同 HERG 相互作用调节其功能，最近的研究表明 MiRP1 也能同 KvLQT1 作用[17]。同样，Mink 能同 HERG 和 KvLQT1 亚基相互作用并调节其功能[16,17,28]。因此，可以推测 KCNE 亚基可能同不同家族的 α 亚基相互作用。

三、瞬时外向电流（I_{to}）

(一) 生理特性

在心脏组织，I_{to} 电流由两部分组成：Ca^{2+} 激活的氯（Cl^-）电流（I_{to2}）和典型的 Ca^{2+} 非依赖性钾电流（I_{to1}）。$I_{to,f}$ 为快速 I_{to} 的简称，$I_{to,s}$ 为缓慢 I_{to} 的简称，均为快速激活，其时间常数为 2～10ms，但失活速率不一，前者 τ_i 为 25～80ms，后者 τ_i 为 80～200ms，前者稳态失活后复活时间常数 τ_{rec} 大约为 25～80ms，后者为 1～2s[10,29]。瞬时外向电流是心房和心室肌细胞早期复极的主要电流。人和犬心房肌细胞的 I_{to} 电流为 $I_{to,f}$，因为这种电流同 Kv4.3 通道的失活后复活的特性一致[10,11,30]；而人和犬心室肌细胞的 I_{to} 电流的失活后复活回归符合双幂模式，表明表达 $I_{to,f}$ 电流的 Kv4.3 和表达 $I_{to,s}$ 电流的 Kv1.4 通道参与心室 I_{to} 电流的形成，可能 Kv1.7 和或 Kv3.4 也起一定的作用[10-12,29,30]。

尽管 $I_{to,f}$ 和 $I_{to,s}$ 在心脏组织分布有一定的差异，但 $I_{to,s}$ 与动作电位时程长的心脏部位有关，如在间隔、左室心内膜和基底部的心肌细胞检测到 $I_{to,s}$，而 $I_{to,f}$ 电流则出现在心外膜、右室和心尖部心肌细胞[10,29]。同右室心外膜心肌相比，左室心外膜心肌细胞的 I_{to} 锋电流密度更小[32]。在心外膜心肌细胞，I_{to} 几乎以最大的电流用于复极，在正常心率范围内，这种复极电流密度与刺激频率基本无关，而且心外膜下心肌细胞的 I_{to} 电流的快速恢复特性类似人类心房肌细胞。由于 $I_{to,f}$ 电流占主导作用，I_{to} 复极电流密度与刺激频率基本无关，I_{to} 电流对动作电位图形的影响与心脏不同部位来源的心肌细胞有关，而且与心室肌细胞复极化是同步的，这样可以调节不同部位心肌细胞的收缩性[10]。由于 I_{to} 影响心肌细胞的复极化早期相，也明显影响 L 型 Ca^{2+} 电流的大小，进而调节兴奋-收缩耦联和心肌细胞的收缩性[33]。因此，I_{to} 电流通过影响其他离子流体现其功能的多样性，这些离子流包括 L 型

Ca^{2+} 电流和可能的 Na^+-Ca^{2+} 交换电流[10,33]。出生后心肌细胞发生的电重构与 I_{to} 电流的增加有关，同时，Kv4.x 表达水平的上调也缩短了动作电位时程[10]。因此，I_{to} 表达水平的改变（Kv4.2 mRNA 和蛋白表达）可能控制心脏电生理的周期性变化，并影响心律失常的形成[33a]。

（二）瞬时外向电流（I_{to}）的分子基础

在哺乳动物的心脏组织中，表达电流具有 I_{to} 特性的离子通道包括 Kv1.4、Kv1.7、Kv3.4、Kv4.2 和 Kv4.3（见表 3-1）[10,11,31]，而 Kv4.3 有 2 种剪接体，其差异在于编码产物是否在 C 端含有 19 个氨基酸[34]。基于失活模式不同，心脏 I_{to} 电流被分为缓慢成分 $I_{to,s}$ 和快速成分 $I_{to,f}$，前者由 Kv1.4 及可能由 Kv1.7 和/或 Kv4.3 形成，后者由 Kv4.2 和 Kv4.3 形成。在人类和犬心房和心室肌细胞，$I_{to,f}$ 由 Kv4.3 形成，而在其他物种，包括大鼠和小鼠，Kv4.2 是产生 $I_{to,f}$ 的主要通道。Kvβ 亚基能同 Kv1.4、Kv1.5 和 Kv4.3α 亚基特异性作用，调节后者的生理特性、稳定性和细胞膜表达[10,19,35]。Kvβ₂ 亚基能增加 Kv1.4 通道失活[19]，相反 Kvβ₁ 和 Kvβ₃ 亚基能增加 Kv4.3 通道的蛋白表达和电流密度，而不影响其门控动力学（见表 3-2）[10,35]。Kvβ₁ 和 Kvβ₃ 包含蛋白激酶 A（PKA）和蛋白激酶 C（PKC）的磷酸化位点，能调节它们与 Kvα 亚基的相互作用。MiRP1 是 I_{Kr} 的内生 β 亚基，但它能增加 Kv4.3 的表达电流，适度减慢 Kv4.3 的失活（见表 3-2）[35]。

KChIP 能增加 Kv 通道亚家族的表达，而不改变其门控和电压敏感性等特征，这种 Kv 通道为 Kv4.3，但它不增加 Kv1.5、Kir2.2、HERG 或 KvLQT1 的电流[36]。来源于心脏组织的 KChIP 和 Kv4.3 能产生免疫共沉淀，表明是心脏 I_{to} 电流的一个重要调节亚基[36]。Kvβ1.2 抑制由 KChIP 产生的效应，表明不同亚基在调节 I_{to} 电流时也存在相互作用（见表 3-2）[21]。Kv4.3 和 KChIP₂ 共同作用影响人和犬心脏组织不同部位的 $I_{to,f}$ 电流密度[37]，KChIP₂ 表达缺失引起 I_{to} 电流密度下降，并导致 I_{to} 跨壁梯度消失，动作电位延长，室性心律失常增加[24]。尽管传统上认为 I_{to} 是非 Ca^{2+} 依赖性电流，但 I_{to} 电流受 KChIP₂ 和其他连接蛋白（frequenin 和神经元 Ca^{2+} 敏感因子-1）的调节，表明自然的 I_{to} 也受细胞内 Ca^{2+} 的调节[10,23,26]。

基于失活特性的差异，心脏 I_{to} 电流被分为快速成分 $I_{to,f}$ 和缓慢成分 $I_{to,s}$。除了失活特征的差异外，他们在心脏不同部位的表达和活性水平也存在着广泛的差异[10,29,38]。N 型和 C 型失活是 Kv1.4、Kv1.7 和 Kv3.4 通道的失活模式，且这些失活模式与动力学特征相关[5]。大量的事实证明，C 型失活模式控制 Kv1.4 通道的失活后恢复活性，而 N 型失活模式则控制 Kv1.4 通道的进入失活状态的速率[5]。相比较而言，Kv4.x 亚家族成员则显示快速进入失活状态和快速从失活状态中恢复活性，这些特征可能与该通道具有独特的 C 型和 N 型失活模式有关[5,39]。

（三）调节

各种内分泌和/或旁分泌系统调节 I_{to} 的表达水平和电流密度，例如，用含血管紧张素Ⅱ（Ang-Ⅱ）的培养液培养犬心外膜心肌细胞，I_{to} 电流密度降低，犬心外膜心肌细胞特有的 $I_{to,f}$ 的变为心内膜心肌细胞特有 $I_{to,s}$，但没有改变 Kv1.4 或 Kv4.3 mRNA 表达水平[38]。相反，用含血管紧张素Ⅱ受体 1 型阻断剂氯沙坦的培养液培养犬心内膜心肌细胞，发现心内膜心肌细胞的 $I_{to,s}$ 成分减少，转化为心外膜心肌细胞特有的 $I_{to,f}$ 成分[38]。这些实验表明 I_{to} 可受多种病理生理因子调节，且这种调节并不是通过改变相关通道的表达水平来实现的。据此推测 I_{to} 的变化可能是 I_{to} 通道氧化还原状态的变化和巯基的修饰或 Ang-Ⅱ介导的 NADPH 氧化酶系统的激活（NADPH 系统与氧化条件的变化有关）[40]。α-肾上腺素激动剂能通过 PKC 依赖性和 PKC 非依赖性途径降低各物种来源的成年心房、心室和浦氏纤维细胞的 I_{to} 电流[10,41]。其中，兔心房肌细胞 I_{to} 电流对 α-肾上腺素激动剂的刺激反应是通过 PKC 依赖性途径降低 Kv1.4 通道介导的 I_{to} 电流实现的[42]，而心肌细胞 I_{to} 电流的变化则是通过 PKC 依赖性途径降低 Kv4.3 通道介导的 I_{to} 电流实现的[34]。

用含肾上腺素激动剂和 Ang-Ⅱ 的培养液长期培养心室肌细胞发现该心肌细胞 I_{to} 降低，与 Kv4.2 和 Kv4.3 表达水平降低有关，但 Kv1.4 表达水平升高[10,43]。然而，肾上腺素降低 Kv4.3 mRNA 的稳定性，Kv4.3 mRNA 的降解增加，从而降低了 Kv4.3 mRNA 的表达水平，与 Ang-Ⅱ 降低 Kv4.3 mRNA 表达水平的机制一致[43]。提高 α-肾上腺素激动剂和 Ang-Ⅱ受体激动剂的浓度可以下调 I_{to} 电流和钾通道的表达水平，该病理机制常见于心脏性疾病[10]。而且，增加和降低酪蛋白激酶的活性也分别降低和增加 Kv1.4 通道的失活速率[44]。类固醇激素如甲状腺素和醛固酮也影响 I_{to} 电流，甲状腺素水平低下则降低 I_{to}

电流密度，延长 AP，Kv4.2 表达水平降低，Kv1.4 表达水平增加；而甲状腺素水平升高则增加 I_{to} 电流密度，Kv4.2 和 Kv4.3 表达水平增加，Kv1.4 表达水平降低[41,45-47]。围生期甲状腺素的大量释放影响出生后 AP 时程和电重构，改变 Kv1.4、Kv4.2 和 Kv4.3 的转录和翻译水平[10,45]。同甲状腺素相比，醛固酮则通过受体特异性下调心室肌细胞 I_{to} 电流[48]。

四、延迟整流电流

（一）生理作用

同其他心脏钾电流相比，心脏延迟整流钾电流的产生相对较晚，包括三种成分，分别为 I_{kur}、I_{kr} 和 I_{ks}，每一种电流均呈电压和时间依赖性（见图 3-1 和 3-4B-D）。一般而言，延迟整流电流负责心肌细胞和浦氏纤维的 2 相和 3 相复极[16,17]。例如 I_{kr} 和 I_{ks} 的缓慢灭活有利于通道在 3 相复极的晚期仍具有传导性。不同部位的心室肌细胞，不同房室来源的心肌细胞以及不同物种的心肌细胞，动作电位的形态均不同，这种差异与 I_{kur}、I_{kr} 和 I_{ks} 通道的表达不同有关[12]。同心室肌细胞相比，典型心房肌细胞动作电位时程短，与快速激活、缓慢失活的 I_{kur} 通道的高水平表达有关（见图 3-1，3-4A）[9,12]。尽管心房 I_k 也包含 I_{kr} 和 I_{ks}，但 I_{kr} 在左房表达量多于右房细胞，以至于左房的动作电位时程更短[12]。在心室，I_{kr} 较多表达在心外膜和心尖部心肌细胞，且在这些部位的心肌细胞具有更短的动作电位[49]。由于 I_{ks} 电流密度降低，中层心肌细胞的动作电位时程相对较长[12]。同 I_{ks} 相比，I_{kr} 快速激活并具有明显的内向整流特性。这些特性源于 I_{kr} 的快速失活，在正向膜电位水平，I_{kr} 的失活速率甚至快于其激活速率[16]。因此，I_{kr} 在动作电位的平台期具有较低的传导性，但在 3 相复极期，其传导性明显增加（见图 3-1 和 3-4C）。相反，由于 I_{ks} 具有缓慢激活和缓慢灭活的特性，在动作电位平台期仍缓慢增加，但在 3 相复极期仍保留激活特性（见图 3-1 和 3-4D）[17]。在心率增快时，心房和心室肌细胞的动作电位缩短与 I_{ks} 和 I_{kr} 的缓慢灭活有关[16,50]。因此，当心脏的舒张期缩短时，这些仍处于激活状态的通道有利于快速复极化[16,50]。通过研究各种先天性和获得性长 QT 综合征的发病机制，可以明确延迟整流性通道的重要性。

（二）延迟整流电流（I_k）的分子基础

在人和犬的心房肌细胞均可检测到 I_{kur} 电流，分别由 Kv1.5 和 Kv3.1 通道产生。在其他物种，如鼠类的心房和心室肌细胞均可产生类似延迟整流电流，包括 Kv1.5 编码的 $I_{k,slow1}$ 和 Kv2.1 编码的 $I_{k,slow2}$。Kvβ1.2 和 Kv1.5 亚基在心脏组织免疫共沉淀表明 Kvβ1.2 能抑制 Kv1.5 的表达电流，而 KChIP 能在一定程度上削弱 Kvβ1.2 对 Kv1.5 的抑制效应。Kvβ1.3 和 Kvβ3 亚基通过 N 型失活模式可加速 Kv1.5 通道快速失活，而且 Kvβ1.3 和 Kvβ3 使人源性 Kv1.5 通道的电压激活曲线向下漂移（超极化），表明这些通道复合体能在较负性的膜电位水平被激活[19]。Kv1.5 和辅助性 Kvβ 亚基相互作用也能增加 I_{kur} 对细胞内氧化还原状态的敏感性[20]。Kv1.5 通道的失活模式代表了 Kv1.x 家族的典型失活特征。快速的 U 型失活模式也见于 Kv1.x 家族，其中包括 Kv1.5 通道，推测这种失活模式由位于 KvβN 端的 T1 功能域与 Kv1.5 的成孔区相互作用所致[9]。

在心肌细胞，HERG 同 Mink 相关肽 1（也称 MiRP1）共同装配形成通道复合物，这种复合物赋予 HERG 更多的门控动力学特征，降低通道的传导性被 Ⅲ 类抗心律失常药物 E4031 双相抑制，这些特性均见于自然心肌细胞中的 I_{kr}（见表 3-1 和 3-2）[16,51]。MiRP1 在心肌浦肯野纤维优先表达。HERG 或 MiRP1 基因突变可导致 I_{kr} 的功能缺陷，分别引起长 QT 综合征 2 型和 6 型[15-17,51]。同其他离子通道相比，HERG 易被药物阻滞，导致获得性 LQTS，可能与该通道具有独特的孔结构和功能有关[5,16]。HERG 通道的快速失活与孔区外口的空间变化有关，类似于 C 型失活，而与 N 型失活无关，因为截短 HERG 的 N 端基本不影响失活。然而，HERG 通道失活不完全符合 C 型失活模式，具有几种独特的特征，可能与孔区特异的氨基酸组成有关，如 HERG 在标签序列上缺乏苏氨酸，另外，HERG 通道 PAS 功能域可能在影响通道的灭活速率方面发挥效应[15]。

心脏 I_{ks} 电流由 KCNQ1 和 Mink 装配形成（见表 3-1 和 3-2）[17,27]，KCNQ1 与 Mink 的共表达水平受 pH 值的负向调节，Mink 可以改变 KCNQ1 通道对阻滞剂和温度的敏感性。KCNQ1 也能同 MiRP1 和 KCNE3 相互作用，且它们均在心房和心室中表达[27]，另外，HERG 也能同 Mink 共装配[16]。KCNQ1 和 Mink 基因突变影响 I_{ks} 电流水平，导致长 QT 综合征 1 型和 5 型[15,17]。Mink 定位在心室肌细胞 Z 线周围的 T 管，通过连接蛋白连接到肌纤维成分上，以伸展依赖性方式调节 I_{ks}，形成机械-电反馈系统[52]。KCNQ1 通门控特性包括激活相对缓慢,失活相对延迟且不完全,并呈电压非依赖性失活。然而,当 Mink 同 KCNQ1 相互作用时,激活会更慢,失活似乎消失,但通道的传导性增加[17](见表 3-2)。

(三) 调节

β-肾上腺素和 α-肾上腺素激动剂可分别通过蛋白激酶 A 和 C 途径增加 I_{kur} 电流,而酪氨酸蛋白激酶的 Src 家族的激活则降低 I_{kur} 电流,其机制是对 Kv1.5 通道 N 端的 Src 同源体 3(SH3)的功能域磷酸化[44]。类固醇激素如糖皮质激素、甲状腺素和雄激素均能改变 Kv1.5 的转录水平。甲状腺机能亢进能上调心房肌细胞的 Kv1.5 表达水平,从而缩短动作电位。尽管甲状腺机能减退能降低 Kv1.5 表达,而糖皮质激素增加 Kv1.5 表达,但目前仍不清楚心房肌细胞 Kv1.5 表达是否改变[47,54]。男性激素降低 Kv1.5 表达,降低 I_{kur} 电流密度,可解释心房的复极化具有性别差异性。Kv1.5 和 I_{kur} 周期性上调和心房动作电位时程在夜间周期性缩短可解释阵发性房颤为什么多发生于夜间[33a]。HERG 受蛋白激酶 A 和 cAMP 调节,前者可使 HERG 的 N 端和 C 端的氨基酸磷酸化,后者可与 C 端的 CNBD 功能域相互作用[16]。PKA 活化降低 HERG 电流,而 cAMP 连接到 HERG 通道上,增加 HERG 电流,其净效应是降低 HERG 电流[56]。PKA 和 cAMP 对 HERG 通道的不同效应也表现在通道的激活曲线的电压漂移。然而,当 HERG 同 MiRP1 或 Mink 共表达时,cAMP 对 HERG 的调节净效应是增加电流,如果,HERG 的 CNBD 区突变会使 HERG 的功能丧失,导致 LQT2[16,56,57]。

相反,α-肾上腺素激动降低 HERG 电流,但这种效应能被过量的 4,5-二磷酸磷脂酰肌醇(PIP2)所阻断,表明 α-肾上腺素通过 G 蛋白耦联受体刺激磷脂酶 C(PLC),导致内源性 PIP2 耗竭,HERG 电流降低。PIP2 对 HERG 通道的影响主要是改变通道的门控动力学而不影响单通道的传导性[58]。另外,内皮素-1 降低人心室肌细胞的 I_{kr}(延长动作单位),可能与局部 PIP2 耗竭有关,这些结果也间接支持 PIP2 与 HERG 通道相互作用[58,59]。β-肾上腺素激动也通过 PKA 途径对 KCNQ1 磷酸化而增加 I_{ks} 电流,这一过程中需要一些蛋白参与形成大分子复合物,包括蛋白激酶 A、蛋白磷酸酶 1 和靶蛋白 yotiao 等[60]。β-肾上腺素可增加 I_{kr} 和 I_{ks} 电流,缩短动作电位时程(APD),从而将肾上腺素系统与动作电位联系在一起。另外,PKC 也能调节 I_{ks} 电流[17]。甲状腺素能改变编码 I_{ks} 电流的亚基的表达水平,低甲状腺素血症增加 KCNQ1 和 Mink 的表达,而高甲状腺素血症则降低 KCNQ1 和 Mink 的表达[47]。

五、电压调节内向整流钾电流(I_{K1})

(一) 生理作用和内向整流机制

由于 I_{k1} 通道在正向膜电位水平时不传递外向钾电流,故 I_{k1} 通道具有内向整流特性(见图 3-4E),它在心脏动作电位的复极晚期(即 3 相)发挥主要作用,并维持静息膜电位(即 4 相)(见图 3-1)。I_{k1} 通道分布具有心腔差异性,它在心室肌细胞高度表达,而在心房肌细胞表达较少(见图 3-1),这与 Kir2.x 亚基的差异性表达相关[12,62],I_{k1} 电流所具有强大内向整流特性非常必要,因为它可以阻止外向钾电流,避免抵消细胞膜除极过程中通过电压门控性钠通道所产生的大量的内向钠离子流。I_{k1} 整流性与 Mg^{2+} 和多胺(腐胺、精胺和亚精胺)阻塞 Kir2.x 孔区有关。这些微粒从胞浆内进入通道的孔区后阻塞通道的内孔,但在 3 相复极化过程中,这种阻滞作用被解除,Kir2.x 恢复对 K^+ 外向通透性(见图 3-1 和 3-4E)[61]。因此,Kir2.x 通道的功能也呈电压依赖性,尽管它没有 Kv 通道所特有的 S1 至 S4 序列单元。

(二) 内向整流钾电流的分子机制

内向整流钾通道家族至少由 7 个成员组成,分别为 Kir1 至 Kir7 或 KCNJ1 至 KCNJ16[11,61]。该通道的成孔 α 亚基与 Kv 亚基不同,有两个跨膜亚单位组成,称为 M1 和 M2,M1 和 M2 之间为成孔区,两端为 N 端和 C 端结构(见图 3-2D)[61]。因此,内向整流钾通道的结构类似于 Kv 通道的 S5、S6 和 P-环。在 Kir 家族中,Kir2.x 亚家族通道具有最强的内向整流特性,其中 Kir2.1 至 Kir2.4 编码心脏 I_{k1} 电流[11,62,63]。在心脏组织,Kir2.1、Kir2.2 和 Kir2.3 似乎共同装配形成异源四聚体,影响心脏 I_{k1} 通道的传导性。同 Kv 通道相反,最接近跨膜区的 C 端和 M2 的序列似乎决定了 Kir 通道能形成同源多聚体和异源多聚体结构[66]。合适的蛋白折叠有利于 Kir2.x P-环末端的氨基酸(如 Kir 的 122cys 和 154cys)在亚基内部形成二硫键,保证了 Kir2.x 的功能[67]。Kir2.x 选择性滤过区在空间结构的稳定性也有赖于 P-环区内两个保守氨基酸的静电作用[68]。细胞内多胺和 Mg^{2+} 对 Kir 内向整流性的影响程度取决于 M2 功能域和最接近跨膜区的 C 端是否存在携带负电荷的氨基酸残基（见图 3-2D）[61]，除此之外，也受细胞内 Ca^{2+} 和细胞内骨架成分调节[69]。Kir 通道的孔道向胞浆内伸展，长度约 60Å，可允许胞浆内的多胺或 Mg^{2+} 进入孔道（见图 3-2D）[70]。除了 Kir2.x 外，心肌组织还存在 3 种内向整流较弱的钾通道，分别为 TWIK-1 背景钾通道（KCNK1）、I_{KACh} 通道（KCNJ3，5）（见第 4 章）和 I_{KATP} 通道（KCNJ11）（见 13 章）（见表 3-1）。

（三）调节

β-肾上腺素受体激动剂和应用药物水解 PKA 亚基均可降低人心室肌细胞的 I_{k1} 电流[71]。由于 PKA 水解使 Kir2.1 C 末端的丝氨酸磷酸化，因此应用这类药物可抑制 Kir2.1 所产生的电流[72]。α-肾上腺素受体激动剂可降低人心房肌细胞的 I_{k1} 电流[73]，可能通过 PKC 途径对 Kir2.1b 通道的丝氨酸和苏氨酸残基或 Kir2.3 通道的苏氨酸残基磷酸化而实现[65,74]。除了肾上腺素系统能影响 I_{k1} 电流外，AT1 受体激动剂、血管紧张素 II 也能下调心脏 I_{k1} 电流[75]。据报道 PIP2 与 I_{k1} 的活性有关，PIP2 缺失可致 I_{k1} 电流消失，而补充含 PIP2 的脂质体可恢复 I_{k1} 通道的活性[76]。心脏磷脂酶 C 和磷酸肌醇 3-激酶系统的活化可耗竭胞膜中的 PIP2，从而限制 Kir2.x 通道的功能[76,77]，但 Kir2.x 通道的 C 端和 N 端的碱性氨基酸似乎决定这两种系统对通道的抑制程度[76,77]（据推测 PIP2 带负电荷的磷脂基团面向膜的胞浆面可保持通道的活性）[76,77]。确实，Kir2.1 基因突变干扰 PIP2 和 Kir2.1 通道的相互作用，导致功能丧失，引起 Anderson 综合征（LQT7）[77,78]。而且，PIP2 同 Kir2.x 亚基的相互作用也有利于亚基的组装形成功能性通道[66,78]。

六、背景钾电流

除了 I_{k1} 电流外，其他背景钾电流也有利于动作电位的复极化，建立舒张期静息膜电位。该通道由两个 α 亚基组成一个串联重复序列，每个序列含 4 次跨膜功能域和一个成孔区，人心脏组织至少存在 3 个成员，分别为 TWIK-1/2（KCNK1/6）、TASK-1（KCNK3）和 TRAAK（KCNK4）（见表 3-1，图 3-2A 和 3-2B）[62,79,80]，这些通道产生半瞬时非失活的电流。TWIK-1 通道最明显的特征是具有较弱的内向整流性，在 -60mV 和 0mV 之间产生明显的外向电流[62,79]。它能被 PKC 系统激活，但细胞内酸中毒可抑制该通道的功能[79]。相反，TASK-1 和 TRAAK 电流基本无内向整流性，在动作电位的除极化期间，它们的活性更大。在生理范围内，TASK-1 电流对细胞外 pH 值的波动非常敏感，而 TRAAK 是机械敏感性通道，受花生四烯酸和多不饱和脂肪酸调节[79]。这些特性提示这些通道可能参与心肌细胞代谢和心肌细胞力学变化[62,79]。

七、电压调节性钾通道与心脏病

电压调节性钾通道在心肌的兴奋性方面具有广泛的作用，钾通道活性的变化可产生房性和室性心律失常，甚至可以削弱终末期心脏病心肌的收缩力[10,33,81,82]。尽管钾通道功能的改变可表现为两种机制，即功能再生或功能丧失，但大部分改变为钾电流的降低，其原因包括成孔 α 亚基和/或 β 亚基表达下降、调节途径改变或细胞代谢变化[10,24,40,81,83]。先天性长 QT 综合征的病理基础是 I_{kr}（LQT2 和 LQT6）、I_{ks}（LQT1 和 LQT5）[15,51] 和 I_{k1}（LQT7）电流降低[77,78]。Kv4.2/4.3[10,83]、HERG[16]、KCNQ1、KChIP2[24] 和 Mink[16] 的表达下调，与 I_{to}、I_{kr} 和 I_{ks} 的降低有关[16,84]。仅有的功能再生性钾离子通道病增加 I_{ks} 电流，缩短 AP，增加折返，引起家族性房颤。

电压调节性钾通道的下调可延长 AP，增加了心律失常发生的危险性，其机制包括早期后除极（EADS）和延迟后除极（DADS）[15,82]。而且，电流区域性改变增加心肌复极的弥散度，引起传导的单向阻滞，有利于折返性心律失常的发生[15,24]。在大多数物种如人和犬类，快速的早期复极是必须的，它有利于同步释放钙，补充足够的钙，使细胞内钙瞬时升高[33]。另一方面，1 相复极化速率减慢可降低 $I_{Ca,L}$ 电流，减少肌浆网对钙释放，从而削弱心脏病的钙循环[33]。因此，电压调节性钾通道对心脏功能的影响不能仅孤立地考察钾通道的功能，而应该结合其他离子通道或交换体在生理和病理条件下综合分析其功能。

八、致谢

由于版面空间有限，我们对未能引用该领域的更多优秀文献表示道歉。

我们的研究受加拿大健康研究所基金（P.H.B）

以及 Tiffin Trust 及心脏 & 中风/Richard Lewar centre（HSRLS）基金资助。G. Y. O 也接受了加拿大健康研究所以及加拿大心脏 & 中风基金会资助。R. J. R 受到了加拿大心脏 & 中风基金会资助。

（滕思勇　浦介麟　译）

参 考 文 献

1. Yellen G: The voltage-gated potassium channels and their relatives. Nature 419:35–42, 2002.
1a. Jiang Y, Ruta V, Chen J, et al: The principle of gating charge movement in a voltage-dependent K+ channel. Nature 423:42–48, 2003.
2. Mannikko R, Elinder F, Larsson HP: Voltage-sensing mechanism is conserved among ion channels gated by opposite voltages. Nature 419:837–841, 2002.
3. Jiang Y, Lee A, Chen J, et al: The open pore conformation of potassium channels. Nature 417:523–526, 2002.
4. Doyle DA, Morais Cabral J, Pfuetzner RA, et al: The structure of the potassium channel: Molecular basis of K+ conduction and selectivity. Science 280:69–77, 1998.
5. Rasmusson RL, Morales MJ, Wang S, et al: Inactivation of voltage-gated cardiac K+ channels. Circ Res 82:739–750, 1998.
6. Bezanilla F, Armstrong CM: Inactivation of the sodium channel. I. Sodium current experiments. J Gen Physiol 70:549–566, 1977.
7. Gulbis JM, Zhou M, Mann S, MacKinnon R: Structure of the cytoplasmic beta subunit-T1 assembly of voltage-dependent K+ channels. Science 289:123–127, 2000.
8. Klemic KG, Kirsch GE, Jones SW: U-type inactivation of Kv3.1 and Shaker potassium channels. Biophys J 81:814–826, 2001.
9. Kurata HT, Soon GS, Eldstrom JR, et al: Amino-terminal determinants of U-type inactivation of voltage-gated K+ channels. J Biol Chem 277:29045–29053, 2002.
10. Oudit GY, Kassiri Z, Sah R, et al: The molecular physiology of the cardiac transient outward potassium current (I$_{to}$) in normal and diseased myocardium. J Mol Cell Cardiol 33:851–872, 2001.
11. Nerbonne JM, Nichols CG, Schwarz TL, Escande D: Genetic manipulation of cardiac K(+) channel function in mice: What have we learned, and where do we go from here? Circ Res 89:944–956, 2001.
12. Schram G, Pourrier M, Melnyk P, Nattel S: Differential distribution of cardiac ion channel expression as a basis for regional specialization in electrical function. Circ Res 90:939–950, 2002.
13. Nitabach MN, Llamas DA, Araneda RC, et al: A mechanism for combinatorial regulation of electrical activity: Potassium channel subunits capable of functioning as Src homology 3-dependent adaptors. Proc Natl Acad Sci U S A 98:705–710, 2001.
14. Takeuchi S, Takagishi Y, Yasui K, et al: Voltage-gated K(+)Channel, Kv4.2, localizes predominantly to the transverse-axial tubular system of the rat myocyte. J Mol Cell Cardiol 32:1361–1369, 2000.
15. Keating MT, Sanguinetti MC: Molecular and cellular mechanisms of cardiac arrhythmias. Cell 104:569–580, 2001.
16. Tseng GN: I(Kr): The HERG channel. J Mol Cell Cardiol 33:835–849, 2001.
17. Kurokawa J, Abriel H, Kass RS: Molecular basis of the delayed rectifier current I(ks) in heart. J Mol Cell Cardiol 33:873–882, 2001.
18. Pond AL, Nerbonne JM: ERG proteins and functional cardiac I(Kr) channels in rat, mouse, and human heart. Trends Cardiovasc Med 11:286–294, 2001.
19. Deal KK, England SK, Tamkun MM: Molecular physiology of cardiac potassium channels. Physiol Rev 76:49–67, 1996.
20. Pongs O, Leicher T, Berger M, et al: Functional and molecular aspects of voltage-gated K+ channel beta subunits. Ann N Y Acad Sci 868:344–355, 1999.
21. Kuryshev YA, Wible BA, Gudz TI, et al: KChAP/Kvbeta1.2 interactions and their effects on cardiac Kv channel expression. Am J Physiol Cell Physiol 281:C290–299, 2001.
22. An WF, Bowlby MR, Betty M, et al: Modulation of A-type potassium channels by a family of calcium sensors. Nature 403:553–556, 2000.
23. Deschenes I, DiSilvestre D, Juang GJ, et al: Regulation of Kv4.3 current by KChIP2 splice variants: a component of native cardiac I(to)? Circulation 106:423–429.
24. Kuo HC, Cheng CF, Clark RB, et al: A defect in the Kv channel-interacting protein 2 (KChIP2) gene leads to a complete loss of I(to) and confers susceptibility to ventricular tachycardia. Cell 107:801–813, 2001.
25. Guo W, Malin SA, Johns DC, et al: Modulation of Kv4-encoded K(+) currents in the mammalian myocardium by neuronal calcium sensor-1. J Biol Chem 277:26436–26443, 2002.
26. Nakamura TY, Pountney DJ, Ozaita A, et al: A role for frequenin, a Ca2+-binding protein, as a regulator of Kv4 K+-currents. Proc Natl Acad Sci U S A 98:12808–12813, 2001.
27. Chen YH, Xu SJ, Bendahhou S, et al: KCNQ1 gain-of-function mutation in familial atrial fibrillation. Science 299:251–254, 2003.
28. Tinel N, Diochot S, Borsotto M, et al: KCNE2 confers background current characteristics to the cardiac KCNQ1 potassium channel. Embo J 19:6326–6330, 2000.
29. Nabauer M, Beuckelmann DJ, Uberfuhr P, Steinbeck G: Regional differences in current density and rate-dependent properties of the transient outward current in subepicardial and subendocardial myocytes of human left ventricle. Circulation 93:168–77, 1996.
30. Wang Z, Feng J, Shi H, et al: Potential molecular basis of different physiological properties of the transient outward K+ current in rabbit and human atrial myocytes. Circ Res 84:551–561, 1999.
31. Han W, Bao W, Wang Z, Nattel S: Comparison of ion-channel subunit expression in canine cardiac Purkinje fibers and ventricular muscle. Circ Res 91:790–797, 2002.
32. Di Diego JM, Sun ZQ, Antzelevitch C: I(to) and action potential notch are smaller in left vs. right canine ventricular epicardium. Am J Physiol 271:H548–561, 1996.
33. Sah R, Ramirez RJ, Oudit GY, et al: Regulation of cardiac excitation-contraction coupling by action potential repolarization: Role of the transient outward potassium current (I(to)). J Physiol 546:5–18, 2003.
33a. Yamashita T, Sekiguchi A, Iwasaki YK, et al: Circadian variation of cardiac K+ channel gene expression. Circulation 107:1917–1922, 2003.
34. Po SS, Wu RC, Juang GJ, et al: Mechanism of alpha-adrenergic regulation of expressed hKv4.3 currents. Am J Physiol Heart Circ Physiol 281:H2518–2527, 2001.
35. Deschenes I, Tomaselli GF: Modulation of Kv4.3 current by accessory subunits. FEBS Lett 528:183–188, 2002.
36. Kuryshev YA, Gudz TI, Brown AM, Wible BA: KChAP as a chaperone for specific K(+) channels. Am J Physiol Cell Physiol 278:C931–941, 2000.
37. Rosati B, Pan Z, Lypen S, et al: Regulation of KChIP2 potassium channel beta subunit gene expression underlies the gradient of transient outward current in canine and human ventricle. J Physiol 533:119–125, 2001.
38. Yu H, Gao J, Wang H, et al: Effects of the renin-angiotensin system on the current I(to) in epicardial and endocardial ventricular myocytes from the canine heart. Circ Res 86:1062–1068, 2000.
39. Bahring R, Boland LM, Varghese A, et al: Kinetic analysis of open- and closed-state inactivation transitions in human Kv4.2 A-type potassium channels. J Physiol 535:65–81, 2001.
40. Oudit GY, Trivieri MG, Backx PH: Sulfhydryl modulation of K+ currents: a possible cross-link between oxidative stress and altered cardiovascular function. J Mol Cell Cardiol 35(1):1–4, 2003.
41. Shimoni Y: Hormonal control of cardiac ion channels and transporters. Prog Biophys Mol Biol 72:67–108, 1999.
42. Murray KT, Fahrig SA, Deal KK, et al: Modulation of an inactivating human cardiac K+ channel by protein kinase C. Circ Res 75:999–1005, 1994.
43. Zhang TT, Takimoto K, Stewart AF, et al: Independent regulation of cardiac Kv4.3 potassium channel expression by angiotensin II and phenylephrine. Circ Res 88:476–482, 2001.
44. Nitabach MN, Llamas DA, Thompson IJ, et al: Phosphorylation-dependent and phosphorylation-independent modes of modulation of shaker family voltage-gated potassium channels by SRC family protein tyrosine kinases. J Neurosci 22:7913–7922, 2002.
45. Wickenden AD, Kaprielian R, Parker TG, et al: Effects of development and thyroid hormone on K+ currents and K+ channel gene expression in rat ventricle. J Physiol (Lond) 504:271–286, 1997.
46. Wickenden AD, Kaprielian R, You XM, Backx PH: The thyroid hormone analog DITPA restores I(to) in rats after myocardial infarction. Am J Physiol Heart Circ Physiol 278:H1105–1116, 2000.
47. Le Bouter S, Demolombe S, Chambellan A, et al: Microarray analysis

reveals complex remodeling of cardiac ion channel expression with altered thyroid status: Relation to cellular and integrated electrophysiology. Circ Res 92(2):234–242, 2003.
48. Benitah JP, Perrier E, Gomez AM, Vassort G: Effects of aldosterone on transient outward K+ current density in rat ventricular myocytes. J Physiol 537:151–160, 2001.
49. van Ginneken AC, Veldkamp MW: Implications of inhomogeneous distribution of IKS and IKr channels in ventricle with respect to effects of class III agents and beta-agonists. Cardiovasc Res 43:20–22, 1999.
50. Gintant GA: Two components of delayed rectifier current in canine atrium and ventricle: Does IKs play a role in the reverse rate dependence of class III agents? Circ Res 78:26–37, 1996.
51. Abbott GW, Sesti F, Splawski I, et al: MiRP1 forms IKr potassium channels with HERG and is associated with cardiac arrhythmia. Cell 97:175–187, 1999.
52. Furukawa T, Ono Y, Tsuchiya H, et al: Specific interaction of the potassium channel beta-subunit MinK with the sarcomeric protein T-cap suggests a T-tubule-myofibril linking system. J Mol Biol 313:775–784, 2001.
53. Yue L, Feng J, Wang Z, Nattel S: Adrenergic control of the ultra-rapid delayed rectifier current in canine atrial myocytes. J Physiol 516:385–398, 1999.
54. Takimoto K, Levitan ES: Glucocorticoid induction of Kv1.5 K+ channel gene expression in ventricle of rat heart. Circ Res 75:1006–1013, 1994.
55. Brouillette J, Trepanier-Boulay V, Fiset C: Effect of androgen deficiency on mouse ventricular repolarization. J Physiol 546:403–413, 2003.
56. Cui J, Melman Y, Palma E, et al: Cyclic AMP regulates the HERG K(+) channel by dual pathways. Curr Biol 10:671–674, 2000.
57. Satler CA, Walsh EP, Vesely MR, et al: Novel missense mutation in the cyclic nucleotide-binding domain of HERG causes long QT syndrome. Am J Med Genet 65:27–35, 1996.
58. Bian J, Cui J, McDonald TV: HERG K(+) channel activity is regulated by changes in phosphatidyl inositol 4,5-bisphosphate. Circ Res 89:1168–1176, 2001.
59. Magyar J, Iost N, Kortvely A, et al: Effects of endothelin-1 on calcium and potassium currents in undiseased human ventricular myocytes. Pflugers Arch 441:144–149, 2000.
60. Marx SO, Kurokawa J, Reiken S, et al: Requirement of a macromolecular signaling complex for beta adrenergic receptor modulation of the KCNQ1-KCNE1 potassium channel. Science 295:496–499, 2002.
61. Lopatin AN, Nichols CG: Inward rectifiers in the heart: An update on I(K1). J Mol Cell Cardiol 33:625–638, 2001.
62. Wang Z, Yue L, White M, et al: Differential distribution of inward rectifier potassium channel transcripts in human atrium versus ventricle. Circulation 98:2422–2428, 1998.
63. Zobel C, Cho HC, Nguyen T, et al: Molecular dissection of the inward rectifier potassium current (IK1) in rabbit cardiomyocytes: Evidence for heteromeric coassembly of Kir2.1 and Kir2.2. J Physiol 550:365–372, 2003.
64. Preisig-Muller R, Schlichthorl G, Goerge T, et al: Heteromerization of Kir2.x potassium channels contributes to the phenotype of Andersen's syndrome. Proc Natl Acad Sci U S A 99:7774–7779, 2002.
65. Karle CA, Zitron E, Zhang W, et al: Human cardiac inwardly-rectifying K+ channel Kir(2.1b) is inhibited by direct protein kinase C-dependent regulation in human isolated cardiomyocytes and in an expression system. Circulation 106:1493–1499, 2002.
66. Tinker A, Jan YN, Jan LY: Regions responsible for the assembly of inwardly rectifying potassium channels. Cell 87:857–868, 1996.
67. Cho HC, Tsushima RG, Nguyen TT, et al: Two critical cysteine residues implicated in disulfide bond formation and proper folding of Kir2.1. Biochemistry 39:4649–4657, 2000.
68. Yang J, Yu M, Jan YN, Jan LY: Stabilization of ion selectivity filter by pore loop ion pairs in an inwardly rectifying potassium channel. Proc Natl Acad Sci U S A 94:1568–1572, 1997.
69. Mazzanti M, Assandri R, Ferroni A, DiFrancesco D: Cytoskeletal control of rectification and expression of four substates in cardiac inward rectifier K+ channels. Faseb J 10:357–361, 1996.
70. Nishida M, MacKinnon R: Structural basis of inward rectification: Cytoplasmic pore of the G protein-gated inward rectifier GIRK1 at 1.8 A resolution. Cell 111:957–965, 2002.
71. Koumi S, Backer CL, Arentzen CE, Sato R: Beta-adrenergic modulation of the inwardly rectifying potassium channel in isolated human ventricular myocytes: Alteration in channel response to beta-adrenergic stimulation in failing human hearts. J Clin Invest 96:2870–2881, 1995.
72. Wischmeyer E, Karschin A: Receptor stimulation causes slow inhibition of IRK1 inwardly rectifying K+ channels by direct protein kinase A-mediated phosphorylation. Proc Natl Acad Sci U S A 93:5819–5823, 1996.
73. Sato R, Koumi S: Modulation of the inwardly rectifying K+ channel in isolated human atrial myocytes by alpha 1-adrenergic stimulation. J Membr Biol 148:185–191, 1995.
74. Zhu G, Qu Z, Cui N, Jiang C: Suppression of Kir2.3 activity by protein kinase C phosphorylation of the channel protein at threonine 53. J Biol Chem 274:11643–11646, 1999.
75. Rials SJ, Xu X, Wu Y, et al: Restoration of normal ventricular electrophysiology in renovascular hypertensive rabbits after treatment with losartan. J Cardiovasc Pharmacol 37:317–323, 2001.
76. Rohacs T, Chen J, Prestwich GD, Logothetis DE: Distinct specificities of inwardly rectifying K(+) channels for phosphoinositides. J Biol Chem 274:36065–36072, 1999.
77. Lopes CM, Zhang H, Rohacs T, et al: Alterations in conserved Kir channel-PIP2 interactions underlie channelopathies. Neuron 34:933–944, 2002.
78. Ai T, Fujiwara Y, Tsuji K, et al: Novel KCNJ2 mutation in familial periodic paralysis with ventricular dysrhythmia. Circulation 105:2592–2594, 2002.
79. Lesage F, Lazdunski M: Molecular and functional properties of two-pore-domain potassium channels. Am J Physiol Renal Physiol 279:F793–801, 2000.
80. Ozaita A, Vega-Saenz de Miera E: Cloning of two transcripts, HKT4.1a and HKT4.1b, from the human two-pore K+ channel gene KCNK4: Chromosomal localization, tissue distribution and functional expression. Brain Res Mol Brain Res 102:18–27, 2002.
81. Nabauer M, Kaab S: Potassium channel down-regulation in heart failure. Cardiovasc Res 37:324–334, 1998.
82. Pogwizd SM, Bers DM: Na/Ca exchange in heart failure: Contractile dysfunction and arrhythmogenesis. Ann N Y Acad Sci 976:454–465, 2002.
83. Kaab S, Dixon J, Duc J, et al: Molecular basis of transient outward potassium current downregulation in human heart failure: A decrease in Kv4.3 mRNA correlates with a reduction in current density. Circulation 98:1383–1393, 1998.
84. Tsuji Y, Opthof T, Kamiya K, et al: Pacing-induced heart failure causes a reduction of delayed rectifier potassium currents along with decreases in calcium and transient outward currents in rabbit ventricle. Cardiovasc Res 48:300–309, 2000.

第 4 章

细胞内信号系统与心脏离子通道的调节

Anant Kbositsetb, David E. Clapbam, Micbael J. Ackerman

本章目录

- 以 $I_{K.ACh}$ 为例来说明 G 蛋白对离子通道的细胞内调节 ……………… 33
- 交感神经系统激活调节离子通道的功能 ……………………………………… 36
- 总结 …………………………………………… 39

细胞膜分隔细胞与外界杂乱的世界,其由脂质双层组成,脂质层内镶嵌离子通道和复合的可溶性分子,包括蛋白质等。为了便于细胞与外界联系,细胞已建立了一套复杂的信号转导系统。对于兴奋性细胞,细胞膜上的离子通道负责电信号的转导,控制大脑思维、心脏跳动和肌肉收缩。心脏离子通道的功能紊乱可引起多种原发性心律失常综合征(心脏离子通道病),包括长 QT 综合征(LQTS)、Brugada 综合征、儿茶酚胺敏感性多形性室性心动过速(CPVT),甚至一些婴儿猝死综合征(SIDS)[1]。

电生理学家们已在过去五十年内阐明了心脏大多数离子通道的生理特性。仅在过去的二十年中,应用克隆和致突变等研究方法明确了离子通道的基本分子结构,找到了影响离子通道渗透性、电压感受性和通道失活的功能域(见图 4-1A)。与孔区相结合的毒物也称为分子塞(calipers),被用于估测通道的孔径(图 4-1B)[2]。最近,Doyle 及其同事提出了细菌钾通道高分辨率结构图,能够明察选择性滤孔的细节部分(图 4-1C 和 4-1D)[3],而且 Yellen 已详细描述了离子通道的内部工作方式。

本章将重点介绍关于离子通道调节方面的最新进展。神经递质和激素直接控制或通过信号转导机制改变离子通道的功能。因为这种调节方式多样化,本章将介绍 G 蛋白、环磷腺苷-蛋白激酶 A (PKA) -磷酸化以及由离子通道组成的大分子信号复合体。离子通道是一种高效率的结构,沿化学梯度选择性地快速转运离子,其速率达每通道每秒 1 千万个离子。因此,基于上述特点,我们毫不惊奇于它的可调节性。同其他蛋白质一样,离子通道作为大分子信号复合体的一部分被识别。

一、以 $I_{K.ACh}$ 为例来说明 G 蛋白对离子通道的细胞内调节

心脏 K^+ 通道的激活可使细胞膜电位超极化至 $-60mV$,在这种膜电位水平,几乎没有去极化通道开放,电信号被衰减。从迷走神经释放的乙酰胆碱激活位于窦房结和房室结起搏细胞(甚至贯穿整个心房组织)的毒蕈碱受体 2 型,随后,与受体相连的 G_α 激活 $I_{K.ACh}$,产生内向整流性钾电流,心率随之减慢,房室传导时间延缓[5]。因此,据于上述理论,临床上已开发了作用于受体、G 蛋白和通道的药物,用以终止房室折返性心动过速(图 4-2)。

受体(异源三聚体)、G 蛋白和离子通道共同定位在膜上,G 蛋白耦联受体(GPCRs)为 7 次跨膜结构的膜蛋白,配基如乙酰胆碱与受体特定位点连接,启动受体的构象变化,受体在细胞内的功能域可同 $G_{\alpha\beta\gamma}$ 复合物相互作用,在 G_α 亚基上催化 GTP 转化为 GDP。由于 $G\alpha$ 和 $G_{\beta\gamma}$ 之间的亲和力弱,$G_{\beta\gamma}$ 作为效应器进一步发挥作用。尽管 $G_{\beta\gamma}$ 是由两个分离的蛋白组

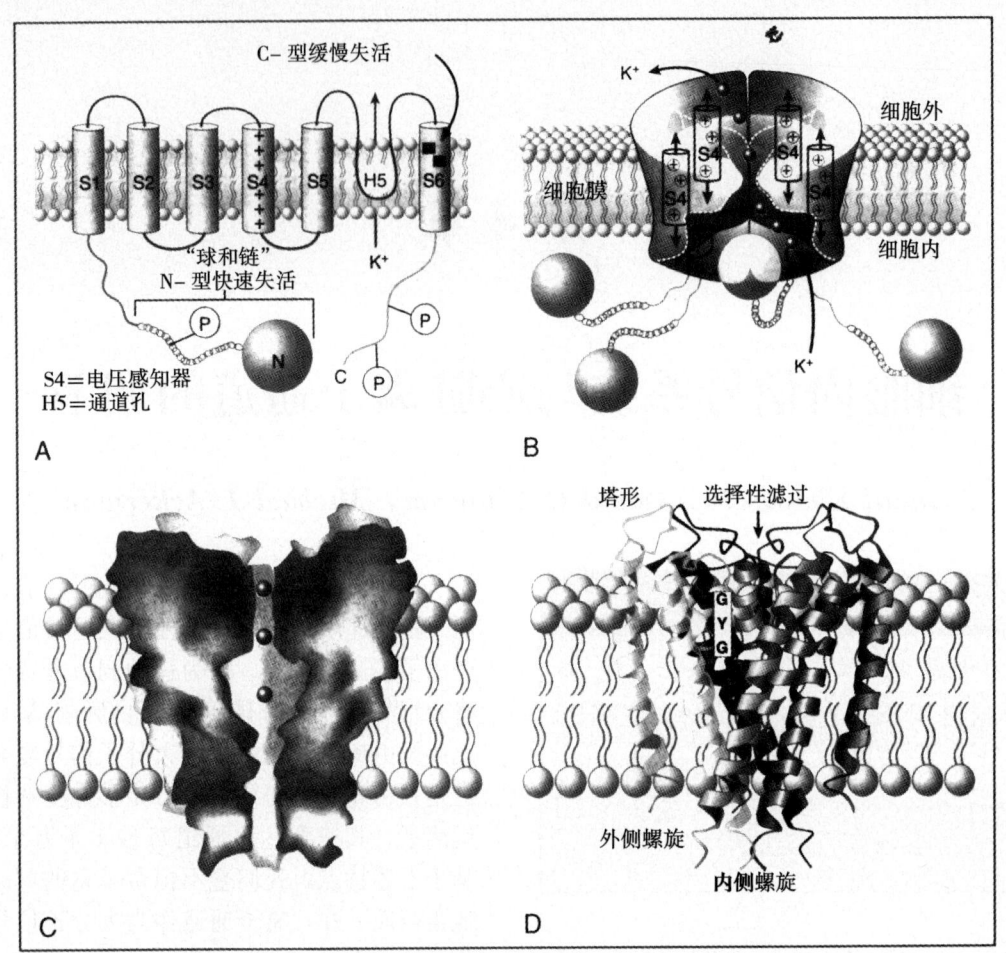

图 4-1 心脏离子通道基本的分子结构 A：离子通道的线性拓扑异构学。6 个跨膜亚单元（6TM）形成钠、钙和钾通道的孔结构。跨膜段标记为 S1-S6。N 端的"球和链"模拟的是参与 N 型失活的蛋白质区域。S4 电压感受器的正电圆圈代表着携带正电的赖氨酸和精氨酸残基。通道孔区（H5 或 P-环）的关键残基位于跨膜的 S5 和 S6 段之间。Na 和 Ca 通道基因编码有 4 个基本亚单位串联形成的单体蛋白，而电压激活钾通道（Kv）基因编码只有一个亚单位的蛋白。翻译后 4 个这样的亚单位装配成 B 图的钾通道。Kir 基因编码插有 H5 的两个跨膜段构成的单一亚单位。B：电压门控钾通道的四聚体结构。钾通道有 A 图显示的 4 个单独的亚单位组装而成。孔区结构是根据高亲和力蝎毒素数据以及核磁共振分子图像建立的[2]。宽的前庭（大约 2.8～3.4nm 宽，0.4～0.8nm 深）形成一个收缩的孔。C：S. lividans 的钾选择性通道（KcsA）的 X 光晶体学结构。显示的是 KcsA 的三维分子表面。孔区的轮廓是根据距孔中央最近的范德华蛋白接触构建的。三个 K⁺ 在选择性滤过器中排队通过。D：S. lividans 的钾选择性通道（KcsA）3.5Å 分辨率的 X 光晶体学结构。显示了 α 螺旋结构和排除钠和其他二价离子的选择性滤器，以及信号 GYG 序列（甘氨酸，酪氨酸，甘氨酸）。孔区最窄部分来自氨基酸的碳氧原子代替了钾离子周围的 H_2O 分子。中央腔的钾离子电荷被水形成的极化环境以及 4 个螺旋的偶极所稳定。跨膜 α 螺旋的细胞内端可能构成了通道激活门（A 和 B 引自 Ackerman MJ, Clapham DE: Ion channels: Basic science and clinic disease. N Engl J Med 336: 1575-1586, 1997; C 和 D 引自 Doyle DA, Morais Cabral J, Pfuetzner RA, et al: The structure of the K channel: Molecular basis of K conduction and selectivity. Science 280: 69-77, 1998.）

成，但这两个蛋白总是作为一个功能单位起作用。目前已知人基因组存在 21 个 $G_α$、5 个 $G_β$ 和 13 个 $G_γ$ 基因，它们的表达产物可形成 1300 多种异源三聚体，然而，细胞实际存在的数量是有限的，具体数量尚不明确[6]。

离子通道与激活的 G 蛋白间相互作用是离子通道最简单的调节模式。目前发现有数种神经递质与 $G_{αβγ}$ 相连，激活或抑制通道的功能，这些递质包括毒蕈碱、生长激素、μ-阿片、$α_2$-肾上腺素激动剂和腺苷。目前，我们最了解的是心脏 G 蛋白调控的内向整流性钾通道（GIRK）。人类基因组中包括 4 种 GIRK 基因（GIRK1-4 或 Kir3.1-3.4），编码的四种蛋白质相互

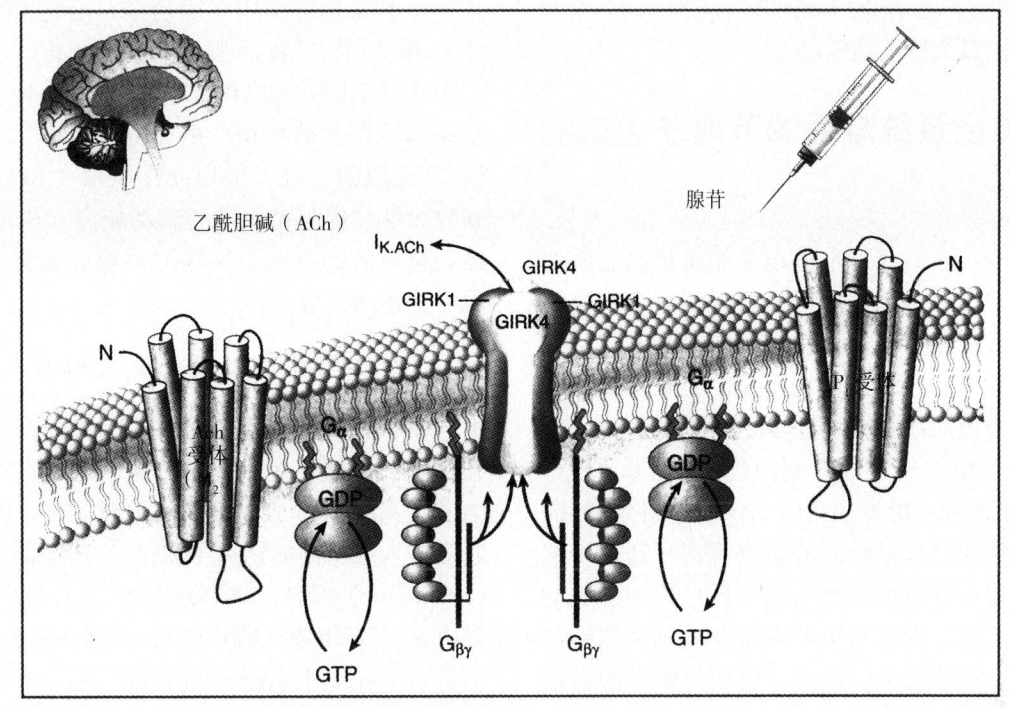

图 4-2　心脏内向整流钾通道，$I_{K.ACh}$ 的 $G_{\beta\gamma}$ 直接激活作用　乙酰胆碱（迷走神经释放）和肾上腺素（静脉内注射以终止房室折返性心动过速）都能激活 $I_{K.ACh}$。与它们相应的 G 蛋白耦联受体结合；M2 受体，显示了它的 7 个跨膜域，或 1 型嘌呤能受体激活百日咳毒素敏感 G 蛋白。$G_{\beta\gamma}$ 亚基直接与 $I_{K.ACh}$ 通道特异的 N 端和 C 端区域结合。$I_{K.ACh}$ 是由 2-G 蛋白-门控内向整流 K^+（GIRK）1 和 2-GRIK4 亚基构成的异源四聚体。RGS 蛋白加速 $G_{\alpha i}$-GTP 酶活性使 $I_{K.ACh}$ 通道具有快速动力学特征

作用形成异源四聚体复合物。在心脏组织中，只有 GIRK1 和 GIRK4 形成通道，而在神经系统中，这 4 种蛋白质均参与通道的形成。GIRK1 还称为 KDNJ3，由 501 个氨基酸组成，基因定位于 2q24.1。而 GIRK4 也称为 KDNJ5，由 419 个氨基酸组成，基因定位于 11q24。GIRK 亚基由两个跨膜功能域和一个成孔区组成（见图 4-1C 和 4-1D），每个亚基的成孔区均位于跨膜区 S1 和 S2 之间，由特定的氨基酸组成，称为 P 区。位于 P 区的氨基酸组成对钾离子有选择性的滤过作用，估计该通道对钾离子的滤过率是其他离子的 1000 倍。在生理条件下，钾离子只能通过这些离子通道排出细胞，使细胞膜超极化，膜电位位于更负的水平。

正如图 4-2 所描述的，乙酰胆碱与毒蕈碱 2 型受体结合或腺苷与毒蕈碱 1 型受体结合后激动 $G_{\alpha i\beta\gamma}$。$G_{\alpha i}$ 与 GTP 相连，而 $G_{\alpha i}$ 和 $G_{\beta\gamma}$ 在功能上是相互分离的，$G_{\beta\gamma}$ 与 GIRK 四聚体的胞内功能域相连（每个 $G_{\beta\gamma}$ 与 GIRK 通道的每个亚基相连）。应用体外重组技术，发现 6 个重组的 $G_{\beta\gamma}$ 亚基激活毒蕈碱门控的钾通道，产生 $I_{K.ACh}$ 电流，其半激活浓度波动于 3～30nM[7]。$G_{\beta\gamma}$ 直接连接在 GIRK1 和 GIRK2 亚基的 N 端和 C 端区域，激活 GIRK 通道，产生 $I_{K.ACh}$[8]。GIRK 通道至少有 3 个位点影响 $G_{\beta\gamma}$ 与 GIRK 的连接及随后 $G_{\beta\gamma}$ 对 GIRK 通道的激活；而 $G_{\beta 1}$ 亚基至少有 8 个氨基酸残基决定 $G_{\beta\gamma}$ 与 GIRK 的相互作用[9-1]。$G_{\beta\gamma}$ 由 7 个刀片型的螺旋桨样的蛋白质组成，每个 $G_{\beta\gamma}$ 的刀刃表面可能与 GIRK 亚基的 C 端的 α 螺旋相互作用。$G_{\beta\gamma}$ 位于胞浆内的延伸部位与 S2 跨膜区直接连接，推测 $G_{\beta\gamma}$ 作为控制杆调节通道的功能。

令人感兴趣的是，在神经和心房肌细胞中，受体介导的 GIRK 通道的灭活速率比体外表达系统中记录到的要快 20～40 倍，产生这种差异的原因可能与受体相关的其他蛋白质、G 蛋白和通道复合物分子的形成有关。各种 G 蛋白信号分子（RGS 蛋白），包括 RGS1、RGS3 或 RGS4 重建了 $I_{K.ACh}$ 通道的快速门控动力学特征[12]。因为，当受体激活时，RGS 蛋白加速 GDP 与 G_α 复合物解离。RGS3 和 RGS4 在心脏和脑组织中高度表达。到目前为止，尚未发现引起心律失常的 GIRK 通道的突变，但是，GIRK 通道是药物和迷走神经介导的分子靶点，利用此特点可终止室上性心动过速。

$G_{\beta\gamma}$ 既激活 GIRK 通道，也能调节其他离子通道，

这些机制最早在神经系统中阐明。$G_{\beta\gamma}$ 抑制 N 型和 P/Q 型钙通道，保留持续钠电流[13]。

二、交感神经系统激活调节离子通道的功能

尽管心脏有一套自我调节的电学系统控制心脏的电生理活动，但这一活动也同时受其他器官和系统的调节，如搏斗或逃跑时，交感神经兴奋刺激心脏，提高心率和心肌收缩力，增加心输出量。心脏对肾上腺素的变时和变力效应涉及下列过程，包括 G 蛋白耦联受体，G 蛋白三聚体的释放，刺激性 G_α 亚基（$G_{\alpha s}$）介导的 PKA 激活和心脏靶通道经 cAMP 介导磷酸化，这一瀑布式的反应过程最终对心脏许多离子通道磷酸化，如起搏通道在除极期间的大量开放可增加心脏的自律性，提高心率；而钙通道的大量开放则增加钙离子内流，增加心脏收缩力，同时，电压依赖性钾通道受调节后增加 3 相复极而缩短动作电位时程，增加心率。

（一）心脏超极化激活的环核苷酸门控通道的细胞内调节

超极化激活的起搏电流 I_f，也称 I_h 电流，是控制心脏起搏活性的成分之一。在窦房结组织，当膜电位低于 $-40\sim-50\text{mV}$ 时，I_f 通道开始激活，I_f 由超极化激活的环核苷酸门控通道基因（HCN）编码[14-8]。该家族由 4 个成员组成，分别是 HCN1 至 HCN4[15,16]，而 HCN2 和 HCN4 在心脏高度表达，并形成有功能的四聚体。HCN2 基因定位在 19p13.3，编码产物 HCN2 赋予心脏起搏通道快速激活动力学特征，而 HCN4 基因定位于 15q24-q25，编码产物 HCN4 赋予心脏起搏通道缓慢激活动力学特征[21,23]。HCN4 由 1203 个氨基酸组成，与 HCN2 的差异在于胞浆内的 N 端和 C 端，HCN2 的 C 端多余的 250 个氨基酸组成可解释它的缓慢激活动力学特征。

环核苷酸门控的非选择性通道是在克隆犬受体相关的环鸟苷单磷酸（环磷鸟苷）门控通道时发现的，而心脏 I_f 起搏通道具有环核苷酸门控的非选择性通道的部分特征[23]。HCN2 由 889 个氨基酸组成，含 6 个跨膜的功能域，其结构类似于电压门控钾通道（见图 4-1），但它含有一个环核苷酸连接功能域（CNBD），这一结构类似于 HERG 钾通道，另外，它还有一个 P 环，对钾和钠离子均有滤过作用[24]。

交感神经在心脏的分布较副交感神经的分布更广泛，肾上腺素可作用于窦房结、心房和心室组织。β 肾上腺素受体激活腺苷酸环化酶，产生 cAMP，cAMP 与 HCN2 和 HCN4 直接连接，使 HCN 通道在复极化后期开放更快、更充分[15,16,25,26]。cAMP 提高 HCN 通道的活性，增加动作电位 4 相自动除极，增加自律性，提高窦房结的激动能力。相反，副交感神经兴奋激活毒蕈碱受体则抑制腺苷酸环化酶的活性，阻滞上述激活效应。

（二）电压门控的 L 型钙通道的细胞内调节

在心脏组织，最主要的钙电流由电压门控的 L 型和 T 型钙通道产生，而由 L 型钙通道流入细胞内的钙离子是完成兴奋-收缩耦联的重要成分，因为，L 型钙通道进入细胞内的钙离子激活位于肌浆网上的兰尼定（ryanodine）受体（钙释放通道）。L 型钙通道孔区部分由 α_1 亚基组成（Cav1.2），该基因称为 CACNA1C，定位于 12q13.3，编码产物包括 2157 个氨基酸，由 4 个亚单位相互连接，每个亚单位含 6 个跨膜的功能域（6TM）[27,28]。P 环位于每个亚单位的 S5 和 S6 之间，这四个亚单位之间的 P 环形成通道的孔区。P 环含有带负电荷的谷氨酸残基，可连接钙离子并赋予通道对钙离子的选择性滤过[29]。

三个不同的辅助亚基（α_2/δ，β 和 γ 亚基图 4-3）同 α_1 亚基相连，控制通道的膜定位和/或调节通道的活性。α_1 亚基赋予通道的离子选择性和对电压调节的敏感性；β 亚基影响电流的大小和失活动力学特性；α_2/δ 亚基促进和加速通道的激活而 γ 亚基则将稳态失活曲线的膜电位水平转换至更负的膜电位水平[30]。

交感神经兴奋促进 cAMP/PKA 介导 Cav1.2 通道磷酸化。cAMP-PKA 使 $I_{Ca,L}$ 的 α_1 亚基磷酸化，随后，通道电压依赖性激活电压负向漂移，通道的活性提高。cAMP-PKA 通过激酶 A 锚定蛋白（AKAP15）定位于 T 管，形成通道复合物，配体蛋白通过 Cav1 特异的亮氨酸拉链结构域连接到心脏 Cav1.2 通道的 C 末端（见图 4-3）[31]。

（三）KCNQ1/KCNE1-I_{Ks} 通道的细胞内调节

心脏动作电位平台期的形成是由于内向电流和外向电流激烈竞争的结果，增加钾电流或降低钙电流缩短动作电位时程。交感神经系统的兴奋可增加 cAMP-PKA 的活性，而 cAMP-PKA 使形成动作电位平台期的钾通道磷酸化，同时，HCN 通道的活性也增加，这一过程可解释心脏对肾上腺素的正性变时效应。

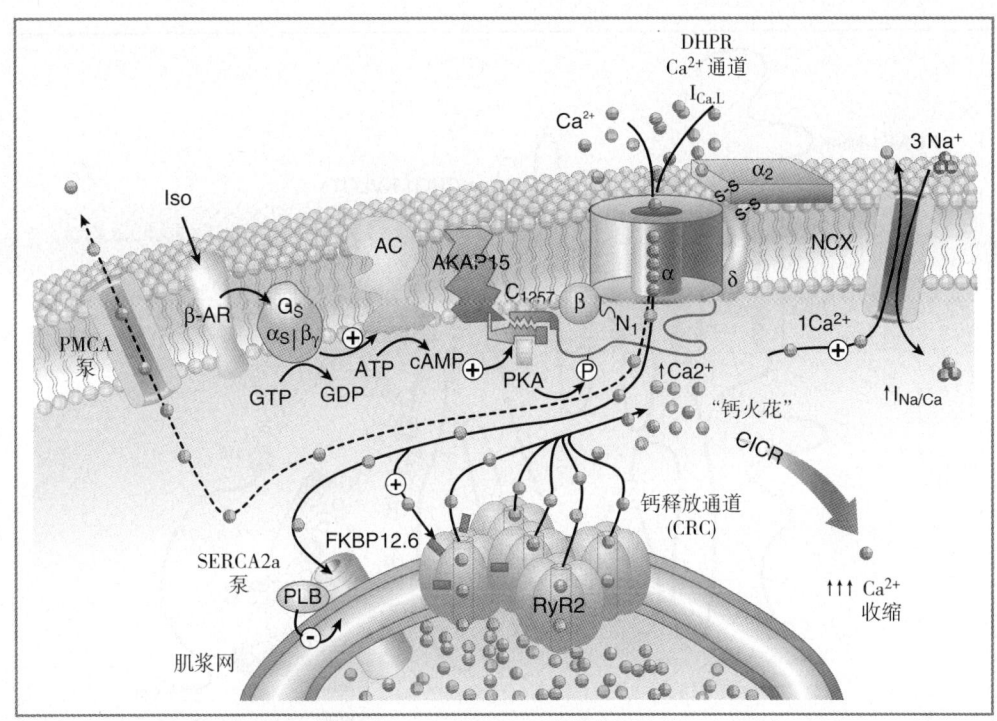

图 4-3 PKA 和 AKAP15 对 L 型钙通道的细胞内调节 交感神经系统的激活能触发增加 ICa.L 的级联反应事件：肾上腺素与 7 个跨膜域的 GPCR 连接，$G_{\alpha s}$ 与 $G_{\beta \gamma}$ 分离，引起环磷酸腺苷（cAMP）依赖性蛋白激酶 A 激活。连在 Cav1.2α 亚基细胞内 C 末端的 A-激酶锚定蛋白（AKAP15）使通道容易被蛋白激酶 A 磷酸化，增加钙内流。背景是钙诱导钙释放途径（CICR）的其他成分

心脏动作电位时程与 KCNQ1/KCNE1 通道复合物的功能密切相关。KCNQ1 基因定位在 11p15.5，编码产物由 676 个氨基酸组成，含 6 个跨膜的功能域，组成电压门控性钾通道（见图 4-1A）。约 25% 的遗传性 LQTS 由 KCNQ1 突变所致[32]。KCNQ1 与辅助亚基 KCNE1（Mink）、PKA、PKA 调节亚基（RII）、蛋白磷酸酶（PP1）和通道相互作用蛋白（Yotiao）[33]一起形成大分子复合物。Yotiao 是另一种 A 激酶锚定蛋白，连接 PKA 与 α 亚基（KCNQ1）。正如 AKAP15 与 Cav1.2 相互作用模式一样，Yotiao 与 KCNQ1 利用亮氨酸拉链结构域与 C 末端相互作用（图 4-4），而 PKA 连接到 Yotiao 上，并对位于 KCNQ1N 端第 27 位的丝氨酸磷酸化。有趣的是，KCNQ1 突变 G589D 破坏了 Yotiao 与 KCNQ1 相互作用的功能域，而不能形成巨分子复合物，导致了长 QT 综合征[33]。

（四）KCNH2（HERG）-I_{kr} 通道的细胞内调节

HERG 也称 KCNH2，定位在 7q35-36，编码产物由 1159 个氨基酸组成，约 20%~25% LQTS 由 HERG 突变所致，且许多突变均表现为膜转运缺陷[34-36]。HERG 通道具有独特的功能，影响动作电位 3 相复极和 2 相平台期的时程[37]。HERG 通道的 P 环氨基酸组成为 YFxxxxxxxxGFG，而大多数钾通道的 P 环的氨基酸组成包含 GYG 标签。推测这一结构使 HERG 通道具有较窄的内孔和较易变形的外孔，且这种结构特征能解释钠离子为什么能阻塞 HERG 通道[38]。另外，由于 HERG 通道孔区包含两个高度保守的脯氨酸残基，通道的内孔较其他钾通道大，这样使 S6 跨膜区扭曲，降低了内孔的孔径[39]。HERGS6 功能域包含两个芳香族氨基酸，分别是第 652 位的酪氨酸和第 656 位的苯丙氨酸，而其他钾通道则不具备这些氨基酸。这两种氨基酸残基均面对内孔，以 π 堆积力同更大的芳香类药物相互作用，干扰 HERG 通道的正常功能[40]。因此，HERG 通道独特的内孔结构使 HERG 通道能容纳和捕捉更大的药物，阻塞 HERG 通道，产生获得性 LQTS 和药源性猝死。

HERG 含有较长的 N 端和 C 端，N 端前 135 个氨基酸序列与 PAS 结构域类似，而 PAS 结构域被证明在原核细胞中作为光和化学感受器调节多种生物化学过程[42]。而 HERG 通道 N 端的 PAS 结构域可减慢 HERG 通道的灭活，推测正常的 N 端可连接到激活门[42,43]，因此，位于 PAS 结构域的突变可加速 HERG 灭活，使通道快速进入关闭状态，导致 LQT_2。

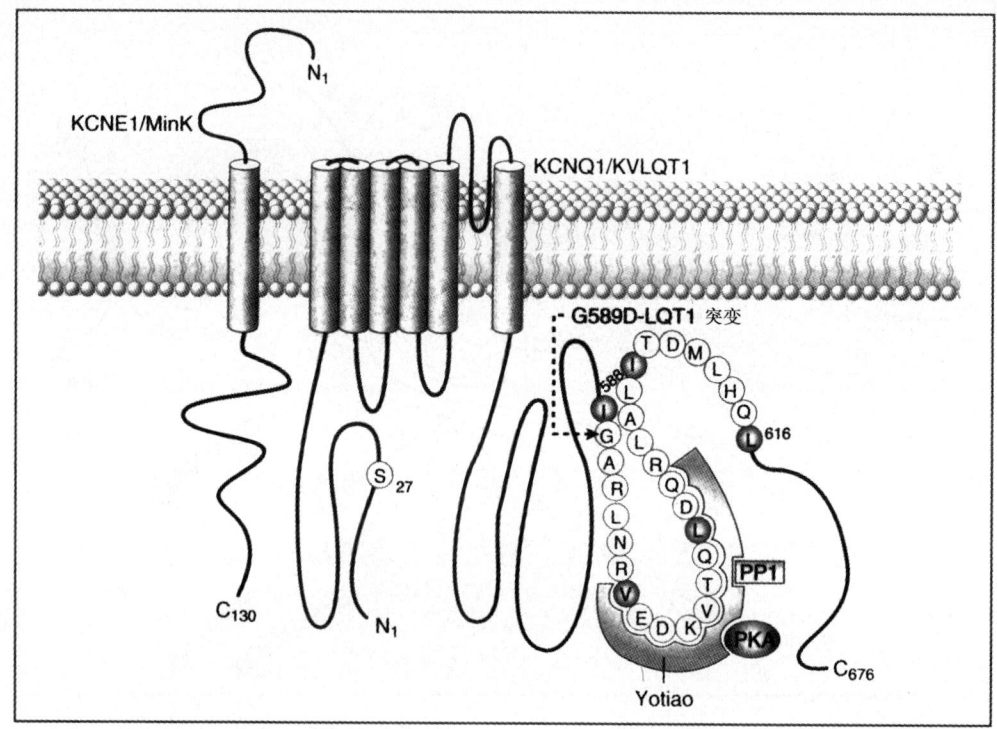

图 4-4 KCNQ1/KCNE1 通道（I_{ks}）的 cAMP-PKA 依赖性调节 显示了由 I_{ks} 通道复合物介导的 SNS 激活效应的分子因素。如图 4-3 所示，SNS 兴奋引起 PKA 激活，这里，PKA 结合另一种 A 激酶锚定蛋白，Yotiao。Yotiao 连在 KCNQ1 胞浆内 C 末端的亮氨酸拉链结构上。这一蛋白复合物使 N 端的丝氨酸残基（S27）磷酸化，导致 I_{ks} 增加。I_{ks} 通道的 β 亚基是有单一跨膜段的 KCNE1

交感神经兴奋时，cAMP 与 HERG 通道 C 末端 CNBD 相连，增加 I_{kr} 电流[44]。而 PKA 则使 HERG 通道的激活曲线向右侧偏移（或正向漂移），降低 I_{kr} 电流[45]。4,5-二磷酸磷脂酰肌醇同 HERGC 末端相互作用，改变 I_{kr} 电流密度和门控动力学[46]。最后，HERG 相互作用蛋白，简称为 GM130，在 HERG 的 C 端的末段与 HERG 通道相互作用参与通道在高尔基体内的转运和定位[47]。

（五）心脏钠离子通道的细胞内调节

心脏钠离子通道负责动作电位的快速除极，并激活钙、钾和氯离子通道。SCN5A 基因位于 3p21-24，编码产物包含 2016 个氨基酸残基，其结构类似于电压门控性钙通道，由 4 个亚单位组成，每个亚单位包含 6 个跨膜的功能域和 1 个成孔区（见图 4-5）。SCN5A 突变可引起 LQTS 和 Brugada 综合征，前者表现为功能再生，而后者表现为功能丧失。约 5% LQTS 和 20%Brugada 综合征源于 SCN5A 突变。

SCN1B 定位于 19q13.1，其编码产物同电压门控钾通道 α 亚基相互作用，改变后者的锋电流，加速钠通道的激活和失活，改变电压依赖性失活曲线[50]。除了 β1 亚基改变钠通道的激活外，细胞内钙离子浓度升高也调节钠通道的激活，在 SCN5A 的 C 端有钙离子感受器，能同钙调蛋白结合。CaM 分子量为 17kD，包含 4 个 "EF" 手，为钙连接功能域，能结合钙离子[53]。Ca^{2+}/CaM 调节钠通道的缓慢失活。有证据表明，机械刺激能激活 SCN5A 编码的钠通道[56]。通常，细胞内骨架成分介导通道与兴奋-收缩耦联装置之间的联系。如 SCN5A 可能通过 syntrophin 与肌动蛋白耦联（见图 4-5）[57-59]。Syntrophin（肌营养不良性相关蛋白，DAPS）是一个多基因家族，其编码产物含有同源的蛋白结构成分，最近，有研究发现 syntrophinγ_2 通过 PDZ 功能域与 SCN5A 的 C 末端 10 个氨基酸［该部位为 PDZ 连接结构域，E（S/T）XV］相互作用直接调节 SCN5A 的门控动力学[58]。目前已发现位于 SCN5A 的 IQ 功能域（1908～1927 位）和 C 末端的突变可引起心律失常，因此，有理由推测位于钙调蛋白或 syntrophin 的相应突变可引起遗传性心律失常。

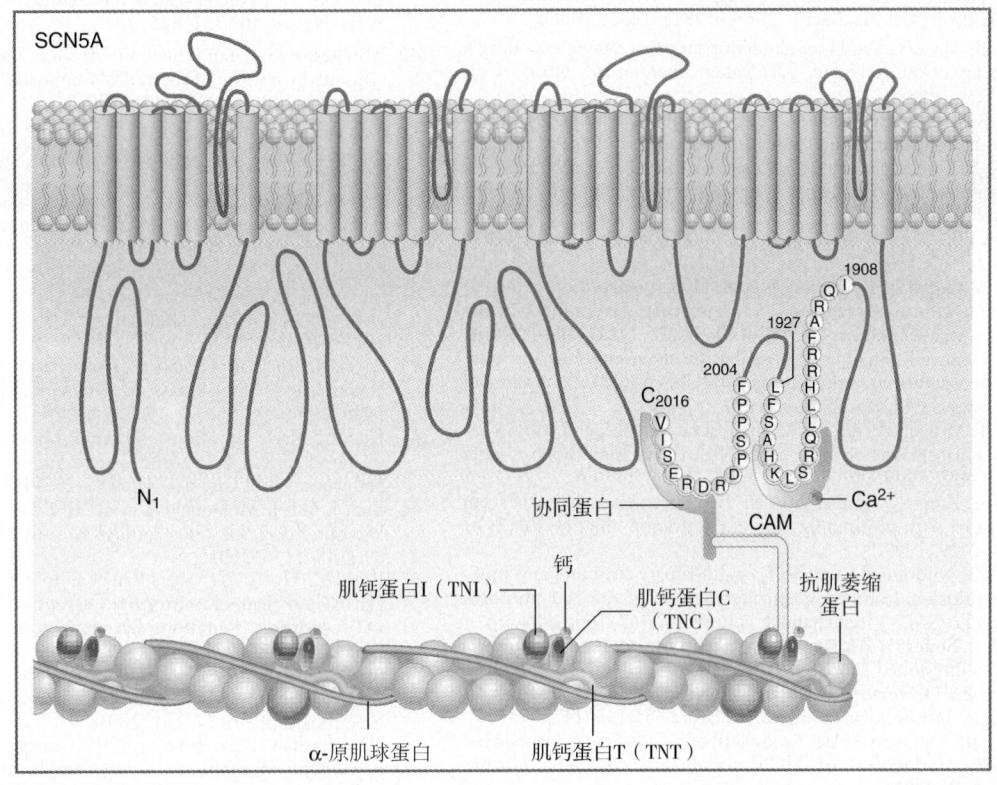

图 4-5 SCN5A 钠通道（I_{Na^+}）相互作用蛋白和细胞内调节　显示的是 SCN5A 钠通道的线性拓扑异构学。"IQ 结构域"（氨基酸 1908-1927）提供了钙调蛋白结合位点，末端 PDZ 结构域（ESIV）提供了 syntrophin 结合位点。从 syntrophin 及其与肌小节上肌动蛋白和细丝复合物的间接耦联所见，SCN5A 可能是机械敏感性通道

三、总结

离子通道能感受膜电位毫伏水平的变化，开放数毫秒，并精确地选择性滤过相应的离子，快速改变膜电位。总之，这种复杂的电活动控制 Ca^{2+} 流入心肌细胞，使心脏收缩，发挥泵血功能。位于窦房结和心肌细胞内的通道具有多种功能，协调工作，以严格保证心肌活动的同步性。另外，通道的功能还必须随生理状态的改变而改变。因此，我们综述了几种关键的细胞内调节机制，阐述心脏离子通道在各种状态下的门控动力学特征。

（浦介麟　滕思勇　译）

参 考 文 献

1. Ackerman MJ, Clapham DE: Ion channels: Basic science and clinical disease. N Engl J Med 336:1575–1586, 1997.
2. Aiyar J, Withka JM, Rizzi JP, et al: Topology of the pore-region of a K+ channel revealed by the NMR-derived structures of scorpion toxins. Neuron 15:1169–1181, 1995.
3. Doyle DA, Morais Cabral J, Pfuetzner RA, et al: The structure of the potassium channel: Molecular basis of K+ conduction and selectivity. Science 280:69–77, 1998.
4. Yellen G: The voltage-gated potassium channels and their relatives. Nature 419:35–42, 2002.
5. Wickman K, Nemec J, Gendler SJ, Clapham DE: Abnormal heart rate regulation in GIRK4 knockout mice. Neuron 20:103–114, 1998.
6. Clapham DE, Neer EJ: G protein beta gamma subunits. Annu Rev Pharmacol Toxicol 37:167–203, 1997.
7. Wickman KD, Iniguez-Lluhl JA, Davenport PA, et al: Recombinant G-protein beta gamma-subunits activate the muscarinic-gated atrial potassium channel. Nature 368:255–257, 1994.
8. Huang CL, Jan YN, Jan LY: Binding of the G protein betagamma subunit to multiple regions of G protein-gated inward-rectifying K+ channels. FEBS Lett 405:291–298, 1997.
9. He C, Zhang H, Mirshahi T, Logothetis DE: Identification of a potassium channel site that interacts with G protein betagamma subunits to mediate agonist-induced signaling. J Biol Chem 274: 12517–12524, 1999.
10. He C, Yan X, Zhang H, et al: Identification of critical residues controlling G protein-gated inwardly rectifying K(+) channel activity through interactions with the beta gamma subunits of G proteins. J Biol Chem 277:6088–6096, 2002.
11. Mirshahi T, Robillard L, Zhang H, et al: Gbeta residues that do not interact with Galpha underlie agonist-independent activity of K+ channels. J Biol Chem 277:7348–7355, 2002.
12. Doupnik CA, Davidson N, Lester HA, Kofuji P: RGS proteins reconstitute the rapid gating kinetics of gbetagamma-activated inwardly rectifying K+ channels. Proc Natl Acad Sci U S A 94: 10461–10466, 1997.
13. Ma JY, Catterall WA, Scheuer T: Persistent sodium currents through brain sodium channels induced by G protein betagamma subunits. Neuron 19:443–452, 1997.
14. Santoro B, Grant SG, Bartsch D, Kandel ER: Interactive cloning

with the SH3 domain of N-src identifies a new brain specific ion channel protein, with homology to eag and cyclic nucleotide-gated channels. Proc Natl Acad Sci U S A 94:14815–14820, 1997.
15. Santoro B, Liu DT, Yao H, et al: Identification of a gene encoding a hyperpolarization-activated pacemaker channel of brain. Cell 93:717–729, 1998.
16. Ludwig A, Zong X, Jeglitsch M, et al: A family of hyperpolarization-activated mammalian cation channels. Nature 393:587–591, 1998.
17. Gauss R, Seifert R, Kaupp UB: Molecular identification of a hyperpolarization-activated channel in sea urchin sperm. Nature 393:583–587, 1998.
18. Clapham DE: Not so funny anymore: Pacing channels are cloned. Neuron 21:5–7, 1998.
19. Moroni A, Gorza L, Beltrame M, et al: Hyperpolarization-activated cyclic nucleotide-gated channel 1 is a molecular determinant of the cardiac pacemaker current I(f). J Biol Chem 276:29233–29241, 2001.
20. Shi W, Wymore R, Yu H, et al: Distribution and prevalence of hyperpolarization-activated cation channel (HCN) mRNA expression in cardiac tissues. Circ Res 85:e1–6, 1999.
21. Vaccari T, Moroni A, Rocchi M, et al: The human gene coding for HCN2, a pacemaker channel of the heart. Biochim Biophys Acta 1446:419–425, 1999.
22. Ludwig A, Zong X, Stieber J, et al: Two pacemaker channels from human heart with profoundly different activation kinetics. EMBO J 18:2323–2329, 1999.
23. Kaupp UB, Niidome T, Tanabe T, et al: Primary structure and functional expression from complementary DNA of the rod photoreceptor cyclic GMP-gated channel. Nature 342:762–766, 1989.
24. Kaupp UB, Seifert R: Molecular diversity of pacemaker ion channels. Annu Rev Physiol 63:235–257, 2001.
25. DiFrancesco D, Tortora P: Direct activation of cardiac pacemaker channels by intracellular cyclic AMP. Nature 351:145–147, 1991.
26. Wainger BJ, DeGennaro M, Santoro B, et al: Molecular mechanism of cAMP modulation of HCN pacemaker channels. Nature 411:805–810, 2001.
27. Mikami A, Imoto K, Tanabe T, et al: Primary structure and functional expression of the cardiac dihydropyridine-sensitive calcium channel. Nature 340:230–233, 1989.
28. Wakamori M, Mikala G, Schwartz A, Yatani A: Single-channel analysis of a cloned human heart L-type Ca2+ channel alpha 1 subunit and the effects of a cardiac beta subunit. Biochem Biophys Res Commun 196:1170–1176, 1993.
29. Yang J, Ellinor PT, Sather WA, et al: Molecular determinants of Ca2+ selectivity and ion permeation in L-type Ca2+ channels. Nature 366:158–161, 1993.
30. Hersel J, Jung S, Mohacsi P, Hullin R: Expression of the L-type calcium channel in human heart failure. Basic Res Cardiol 97:I4–10, 2002.
31. Hulme JT, Ahn M, Hauschka SD, et al: A novel leucine zipper targets AKAP15 and cyclic AMP-dependent protein kinase to the C terminus of the skeletal muscle Ca2+ channel and modulates its function. J Biol Chem 277:4079–4087, 2002.
32. Splawski I, Shen J, Timothy KW, et al: Genomic structure of three long QT syndrome genes: KVLQT1, HERG, and KCNE1. Genomics 51:86–97, 1998.
33. Marx SO, Kurokawa J, Reiken S, et al: Requirement of a macromolecular signaling complex for beta adrenergic receptor modulation of the KCNQ1-KCNE1 potassium channel. Science 295:496–499, 2002.
34. Trudeau MC, Warmke JW, Ganetzky B, Robertson GA: HERG, a human inward rectifier in the voltage-gated potassium channel family. Science 269:92–95, 1995.
35. Warmke JW, Ganetzky B: A family of potassium channel genes related to eag in Drosophila and mammals. Proc Natl Acad Sci U S A 91:3438–3442, 1994.
36. January CT, Gong Q, Zhou Z: Long QT syndrome: Cellular basis and arrhythmia mechanism in LQT2. J Cardiovasc Electrophysiol 11:1413–1418, 2000.
37. Miller C: The inconstancy of the human heart. Nature 379:767–768, 1996.
38. Tseng GN: I(Kr): The HERG channel. J Mol Cell Cardiol 33:835–849, 2001.
39. del Camino D, Holmgren M, Liu Y, Yellen G: Blocker protection in the pore of a voltage-gated K+ channel and its structural implications. Nature 403:321–325, 2000.
40. Mitcheson JS, Chen J, Sanguinetti MC: Trapping of a methanesulfonanilide by closure of the HERG potassium channel activation gate. J Gen Physiol 115:229–240, 2000.
41. Mitcheson JS, Chen J, Lin M, et al: A structural basis for drug-induced long QT syndrome. Proc Natl Acad Sci U S A 97:12329–12333, 2000.
42. Morais Cabral JH, Lee A, Cohen SL, et al: Crystal structure and functional analysis of the HERG potassium channel N terminus: A eukaryotic PAS domain. Cell 95:649–655, 1998.
43. Chen J, Zou A, Splawski I, et al: Long QT syndrome-associated mutations in the Per-Arnt-Sim (PAS) domain of HERG potassium channels accelerate channel deactivation. J Biol Chem 274:10113–10118, 1999.
44. Kiehn J: Regulation of the cardiac repolarizing HERG potassium channel by protein kinase A. Trends Cardiovasc Med 10:205–209, 2000.
45. Kiehn J, Karle C, Thomas D, et al: HERG potassium channel activation is shifted by phorbol esters via protein kinase A-dependent pathways. J Biol Chem 273:25285–25291, 1998.
46. Bian J, Cui J, McDonald TV: HERG K(+) channel activity is regulated by changes in phosphatidyl inositol 4,5-bisphosphate. Circ Res 89:1168–1176, 2001.
47. Roti EC, Myers CD, Ayers RA, et al: Interaction with GM130 during HERG ion channel trafficking: Disruption by type 2 congenital long QT syndrome mutations—Human ether-a-go-go-related gene. J Biol Chem 277:47779–47785, 2002.
48. Antzelevitch C: Molecular biology and cellular mechanisms of Brugada and long QT syndromes in infants and young children. J Electrocardiol 34:177–181, 2001.
49. Viswanathan PC, Bezzina CR, George AL Jr, et al: Gating-dependent mechanisms for flecainide action in SCN5A-linked arrhythmia syndromes. Circulation 104:1200–1205, 2001.
50. Isom LL, De Jongh KS, Catterall WA: Auxiliary subunits of voltage-gated ion channels. Neuron 12:1183–1194, 1994.
51. Balser JR: The cardiac sodium channel: Gating function and molecular pharmacology. J Mol Cell Cardiol 33:599–613, 2001.
52. Tan HL, Kupershmidt S, Zhang R, et al: A calcium sensor in the sodium channel modulates cardiac excitability. Nature 415:442–447, 2002.
53. Tang W, Sencer S, Hamilton SL: Calmodulin modulation of proteins involved in excitation-contraction coupling. Front Biosci 7:d1583–1589, 2002.
54. Peterson BZ, Lee JS, Mulle JG, et al: Critical determinants of Ca(2+)-dependent inactivation within an EF-hand motif of L-type Ca(2+) channels. Biophys J 78:1906–1920, 2000.
55. Zuhlke RD, Pitt GS, Deisseroth K, et al: Calmodulin supports both inactivation and facilitation of L-type calcium channels. Nature 399:159–162, 1999.
56. Holm AN, Rich A, Miller SM, et al: Sodium current in human jejunal circular smooth muscle cells. Gastroenterology 122:178–187, 2002.
57. Gee SH, Madhavan R, Levinson SR, et al: Interaction of muscle and brain sodium channels with multiple members of the syntrophin family of dystrophin-associated proteins. J Neurosci 18:128–137, 1998.
58. Ou Y, Strege P, Miller SM, et al: Syntrophin gamma 2 regulates SCN5A gating by a PDZ domain-mediated interaction. J Biol Chem 278:1915–1923, 2003.
59. Schultz J, Hoffmuller U, Krause G, et al: Specific interactions between the syntrophin PDZ domain and voltage-gated sodium channels. Nat Struct Biol 5:19–24, 1998.
60. Ahn AH, Yoshida M, Anderson MS, et al: Cloning of human basic A1, a distinct 59-kDa dystrophin-associated protein encoded on chromosome 8q23-24. Proc Natl Acad Sci U S A 91:4446–4450, 1994.
61. Ahn AH, Kunkel LM: Syntrophin binds to an alternatively spliced exon of dystrophin. J Cell Biol 128:363–371, 1995.
62. Blake DJ, Weir A, Newey SE, Davies KE: Function and genetics of dystrophin and dystrophin-related proteins in muscle. Physiol Rev 82:291–329, 2002.

63. Suzuki A, Yoshida M, Ozawa E: Mammalian alpha 1- and beta 1-syntrophin bind to the alternative splice-prone region of the dystrophin COOH terminus. J Cell Biol 128:373–381, 1995.
64. Piluso G, Mirabella M, Ricci E, et al: Gamma1- and gamma2-syntrophins, two novel dystrophin-binding proteins localized in neuronal cells. J Biol Chem 275:15851–15860, 2000.
65. Ahn AH, Freener CA, Gussoni E, et al: The three human syntrophin genes are expressed in diverse tissues, have distinct chromosomal locations, and each bind to dystrophin and its relatives. J Biol Chem 271:2724–2730, 1996.

第 5 章

膜泵和离子交换

Larry V. Hrysbko

本章目录
■ Na^+-K^+-三磷酸腺苷酶 ········· 42
■ 肌膜 Ca^{2+}-三磷酸腺苷酶 ········ 44
■ 钠-氢交换 ··············· 45
■ 钠-钙交换 ··············· 46
■ 概要 ················· 48

心肌细胞的电活性反映了离子通道门控独特的周密协调,它激活和控制心脏的传导。而且,通道门控的细微差别允许心输出量和心率宽幅变化并提供固有的保护机制以防止发生电紊乱。因离子通道执行各自的任务,必须存在离子梯度以保证发出电信号。此外,为保证健康细胞的功能,细胞内的离子环境必须仔细保持以优化发生的多种反应过程。很大部分是由细胞膜上的泵和离子交换负责保持离子梯度和细胞内的离子环境。比较离子通道,关于膜泵和离子交换运作的信息非常少,这主要是由于目前还不能准确评价个体转运分子的活性和/或缺乏调节它们行为的药理学工具。因而对于膜泵和离子交换体来说,利用药物来研究结构与功能的关系,进而又进一步促进对药物的发展,并能得到很好的应用。不过,有清楚的例子和期望表明,通过修饰这些转运分子家族,可以作为一种治疗手段,展示出了一定的前景。

全面综述所有细胞膜泵和适当离子交换的心脏生理学及病理生理学将大大超过本章容量。因而,我们综述四种受到研究团体主要关注的膜泵和离子交换。这些大部分典型的离子泵和离子交换是临床感兴趣的题目。读者会经常涉及近期和广泛的综述文章,而不会阅读原著。膜离子泵如肌膜的钠(Na^+)-钾(K^+)-三磷酸腺苷(ATP)酶和钙离子(Ca^{2+})-ATP 酶将被讨论。膜离子交换,如肌膜的 Na^+-Ca^{2+} 交换和 Na^+-H^+ 交换会被描述。值得注意的是,这些选择性膜泵和离子交换离不开一定方式的运转,这对理解心脏生理学及病理生理学是重要的。

从历史的观点看,膜泵和离子交换药理试剂的范围是从那些已经利用几个世纪的试剂到在实验室表现出可观前景的新试剂。在它们中,有几种正在用于治疗多种心脏病的临床试验。再者,用于离子通道的药理工具却很少,这妨碍了我们了解特殊的转运机制和发现药物必需的偶然途径。然而从理论上来说,通过操作不同的离子泵和交换体可提供相似于或超过通过修饰离子通道进行治疗的可能性。

一、Na^+-K^+-三磷酸腺苷酶

(一) 生理学

镁离子(Mg^{2+})激活的 Na^+-K^+-ATP 酶组成心肌膜的 Na^+ 泵,一个酶负责保持这些细胞内的 Na^+ 和 K^+ 浓度梯度。这种功能对正常细胞运转是极为重要的,因为存在这些离子梯度是构成电激活、细胞容量和 pH 调节的基础,并为大量的再次激活转运过程提供能量。生理条件下转运过程是生电的,由于在泵出 3 个 Na^+ 的同时只有 2 个 K^+ 进入细胞,这就产生了一个外向电流。因此,Na^+ 泵的正常转运模式帮助保持心肌细胞的静息电位,它的短期抑制会导致一个几毫伏的轻微去极化[1]。尽管离子经 K^+ 通道(一小部

分经 Na^+ 通道）外流对心肌静息电位产生巨大影响，但更重要的是这些过程完全依靠 Na^+ 泵建立的离子梯度。抑制 Na^+ 泵能明显延长心肌的动作电位，引起超极化电流的直接减少[1]。而且，细胞内 Ca^{2+} 水平的改变引起的额外电生理影响是复杂的。Na^+ 泵在心肌细胞中特别重要，因为它的运作是调节细胞内 Na^+ 水平和之后心肌收缩的关键。细胞内 Na^+ 水平的细微变化会对心肌收缩产生显著的影响，因为它的水平直接影响心肌 Na^+-Ca^{2+} 交换的活性[2]。

（二）转运机制

Post-Albers 的 Na^+-K^+-ATP 酶离子转运模型已被普遍接受，并经独特的实验工具证实。这种转运模式的细节和构成实验的基础已有广泛论述[1,3,4]，这里仅做简要重述。细胞内 Na^+（Na_i^+）可结合该酶的 E_1 构象，因该构象具有离子结合的位点，并可同 Mg^{2+}-三磷酸腺苷结合。钠结合可引起 ATP 水解、酶的磷酸化以及结合 Na^+ 的封闭效应，使 Na^+ 不再靠近另一水域。该酶可从这种构象转变到 E_2 构象，该构象的离子结合位点朝向细胞外区，Na^+ 结合也就不再发生。酶的后一种构造被认为形成一个狭窄、高密度的进入通道，来自这一通道的 Na^+ 不结合/释放形成反应循环中的生电步骤[5,6]。磷酸化的酶（E_2P）此时结合细胞外的 K^+，并最终导致封闭这些离子、酶去磷酸化和结合位点重新朝向细胞内。细胞内 ATP 然后刺激释放 K^+，接着便可进入下一转运循环。相反的反应也能被实验性地诱出，生理条件下 Na^+ 泵仍被认为专门转运 Na^+ 流出和 K^+ 流入，然而，有趣的是，海产毒素、水蝎毒素能转换 Na^+ 泵成蛋白样通道，并且这种离子通道表现非常类似配体-门控离子通道的概念也得于迅速发展。

（三）生物化学和分子生物学

Na^+-K^+-ATP 酶是 P-型 ATP 酶超家族的成员，它是由一个 α 亚基和一个 β 亚基组成的。异源二聚体第三个 γ 亚基也被确认，尽管在心肌组织它的表达缺乏（人类）或极少（鼠和 xenopus），并且它不像 Na^+-K^+-ATP 酶复合物的基本成分[7]。有趣的是，有关的 FXYD 家族蛋白成员如 phospholemman（受磷蛋白），可促进 γ 亚基在心肌的作用[8,9]。三种亚基都表现不同的亚型。α 和 β 亚基已被确定有 4 种以上亚型[3]。尽管功能激活需两种亚基都出现，任何 α 和 β 亚基的结合均能产生功能性 Na^+ 泵。在心肌细胞，有许多完全不同种类亚型表达。在人心房和心室组织，$α_1$、$α_2$ 及 $α_3$ 亚型都有表达（与 $β_1$ 亚基结合），并存在心腔组织表达的特异性[10]。此外，在心肌组织中不同形式的亚型的区域性表达可特异到个体心肌细胞[11]。尽管几个研究已确定不同亚型化合物的不同功能，但仍未了解它的特殊性和定位。

各种 α 亚基约有 1000 氨基酸组成（分子量约为 110kD），引导离子转运并有 ATP 酶活性。它们是洋地黄类化合物的受体。水酶分析法和化学标记研究表明，拥有 10 个跨膜片段和面向细胞内的氨基端及羧基端。α 亚基通过蛋白生物化学和结构、功能研究已确定了多种重要功能区和残基。简单地说，ATP 结合和水解受跨膜片段 4 和 5 之间巨大细胞质区和高度保守天门冬氨酸序列调节，它被认为是特殊的磷酸化目标。阳离子结合发生在跨膜片段内，主要由受跨膜片段 5 和 6 内含羧基的残基介导。对 P-型 ATP 酶研究的巨大进展来自获得了肌浆网 Ca^{2+}-ATP 酶（SERCA）泵的高分辨晶体结构，后者也是一个与 P-型 ATP 酶相关的家族成员[12]。SERCA 执行功能的几个基本规则可直接延伸到 Na^+-K^+-ATP 酶，包括由离子闭塞和 ATP 水解引起的巨大构象变化[3,13]。

在心肌细胞，发现主要是 $β_1$ 亚基与各种 α-亚基联合。它是典型的 II 膜蛋白，有单一的跨膜片段，一个细胞内氨基端，它的主要部分位于细胞外。β 亚基的功能作用仍很不清楚。清楚的是它需 α 亚基激活并在运输和修正这些亚基的膜插入上起一定作用（确定这些功能的研究产生了许多线索）。例如，β 亚基变异或改变它的二硫化物桥（三个出现它的细胞外区域）均能改变 Na^+ 泵的功能性质。此外，由 α 亚基决定的酶构象变化可改变 β 亚单位蛋白酶清除位点，这就提示这些蛋白之间的构象变化是耦联的[3]。

（四）药理学

心肌 Na^+-K^+-ATP 酶被作为药理干预的靶标已有两个多世纪，很长时间未承认它的存在。特别是，这期间，洋地黄和各种心肌苷被用于治疗充血性心衰。目前，心肌苷继续用于治疗心功能不全，也广泛用于控制特殊室上性心律失常（如房颤）的心室率。尽管很长时期不断重新评估联合应用心肌苷的临床益处，同样对它治疗影响的科学基础也有持续的兴趣。

大约 40 年前，Na^+ 泵被确定作为心肌苷的目标蛋白。这些化合物通过调节 Na^+ 电化学梯度间接发挥其心肌变力效应。这又反过来调节肌膜 Na^+-Ca^{2+} 交换

体能移走细胞质中 Ca^{2+} 的能力。特别是，Na^+ 电化学梯度的降低可改变 Na^+-Ca^{2+} 交换的模式，导致 Ca^{2+} 的流出减少，Ca^{2+} 内流增加。在心脏舒张期，肌浆 Ca^{2+} 移动通过两种竞争转运机制实现，分别为进入肌浆网的再摄取和经 Na^+-Ca^{2+} 交换从细胞移出。因心肌苷减少 Na^+-Ca^{2+} 交换移动 Ca^{2+} 的净效率，所以经肌浆网的 Ca^{2+} 再摄取增加。在 Ca^{2+} 移动机制竞争平衡间的微小变化会被巨大放大，因舒张期 Ca^{2+} 水平也增加对心肌苷治疗的反应。心脏收缩期，巨大数量的 Ca^{2+} 从肌浆网中释放，加上舒张期提高的背景 Ca^{2+}。心肌收缩力对细胞内 Na^+ 相当敏感，当 Na^+ 水平有几毫摩尔的小变化收缩力，心肌收缩力就会显著增加[2]。而且，这些化合物的毒素经细胞内 Ca^{2+} 超载简单反映了预期心肌变力影响的实现。

已提出另一种心肌苷影响心肌收缩力的机制，包括直接调节肌浆网 Ca^{2+} 释放通道[14]和通过 Na^+ 通道诱导一种明显的 Ca^{2+} 传导[15]。但这些可能性仍存在高度争议，因有其他实验结果反对它们的重要性和存在。例如，已有显示心肌苷在缺乏 Na^+ 的细胞内无影响[2]，标志可能由于 Na^+ 依赖现象的原因。然而，这个结果也可能是种属特异性，因为在猫肌细胞缺乏 Na^+ 时也观察到心肌苷的变力效应[16]。在敲除 Na^+-Ca^{2+} 交换体的鼠的特殊心脏肌管，心肌苷未产生影响，表明 Na^+-Ca^{2+} 交换是这种变力作用所必需的[17]。

然而，尽管支持接受苷类作用概念的结果有很大争论，但它对其他物种的适用性也是未知的。总的说来，上述心肌苷的作用机制已被广泛接受，另外的可能机制仍需将来探索。

用心肌苷增加心肌收缩力已有相当的历史，但它还没有得到最佳的优化。最近的一个评估地高辛治疗心衰的临床试验发现，尽管它能明显减少住院率和心衰病情的进展，但未能改善死亡率[18]。另外，调查分析试验组数据[18]显示，对地高辛的治疗反应有性别差异，与用安慰剂治疗相比，女性用地高辛治疗增加 4.2% 的死亡率[19]。而且，地高辛的应用因其狭窄的治疗窗而受到限制，这也反映了其最佳血药浓度的个体差异。从科学的角度看，还需要对心肌苷有更深入的了解。例如，证据支持存在内生性苷样化合物的不断聚集[20]。低水平的内源性和外源性心肌苷可刺激而不是抑制 Na^+ 泵的概念已有人提出[21]。心脏损害易感性的明显性别差异正不断有人报道[19]。而且，通常考虑的离子通道如 Na^+ 泵、Na^+-Ca^{2+} 交换、Na^+ 水平在心衰期间都表现相当大的变化。考虑这些较少的例子，可以预期患者对强心苷的反应会有明显不同。因为心肌苷在心衰治疗中还具有重要作用，有必要加深我们对它的作用和最佳应用的理解。

二、肌膜 Ca^{2+}-三磷酸腺苷酶

（一）生理学

质膜 Ca^{2+} 泵在大部分真核细胞的 Ca^{2+} 移出时起十分重要的作用。肌膜 Ca^{2+}-ATP 酶是 P-型 ATP 酶超家族的一个成员，在心肌中这个酶移出细胞内 Ca^{2+} 与 Na^+-Ca^{2+} 交换系统平行。尽管 Ca^{2+} 流出是心肌细胞生存的必需，但令人奇怪的是，许多实验并不能证实肌膜 Ca^{2+}-ATP 酶的作用的试验失败了。这就是说，在大多数物种心肌组织舒张期的 Ca^{2+} 移动中，Ca^{2+}-ATP 酶看来并不是起决定性作用。

我们理解的许多 Ca^{2+}-ATP 酶在心肌舒张中的作用是由两种基本方法获得的。药理学在某些程度上受到限制是由于可用的工具药的局限性，其次现有药物的运用也未广泛展开。一般地，曙红和 Carboxyeosin 被用作抑制剂以证实这种作用[22,23]。这些药理学研究在已确定的肌膜 Ca^{2+}-ATP 酶的重要作用中是相当独特的，证实该酶负责 Ca^{2+} 移动的 24%～45%[24]。相比之下，研究肌膜 Ca^{2+}-ATP 酶对心脏舒张的作用是在抑制其他已知 Ca^{2+} 移动机制后推断的，它的作用几乎可忽略[25]。最后，在转基因鼠的肌膜 Ca^{2+} 泵双倍过度表达，对心脏的收缩和舒张没有明显影响。总而言之，研究结果有更大的差异性，需要进一步研究，但大多数证据并不支持这个转运系统有主要作用。值得一提的是，心肌同样过度表达 Na^+-Ca^{2+} 交换体对心脏生理功能并无明显不良影响，但它对心脏舒张的重要性已被大家所接受[26]。

肌膜 Ca^{2+}-ATP 酶两种生理作用之一最近已被提出。例如，在转基因，鼠过度表达这种泵的新生肌细胞，蛋白合成速率明显增加，暗示它在心肌细胞生长的作用[25]。最近有资料表明，Ca^{2+} 泵参与调节内皮素-1-介导的生长反应。Ca^{2+} 泵也参与组成电压依赖性 B-型 Ca^{2+} 通道，并已被证明可调节心肌细胞的程序死亡[27-29]。总的说，这种转运在心脏生理作用中的重要性仍相对模糊。有趣的是，敲除心脏 Na^+-Ca^{2+} 交换体这种与心肌细胞 Ca^{2+} 流出平行的机制，可导致胚胎性死亡，但此前心脏细胞可有节律的收缩[30]。尽管这些结果突出了 Na^+-Ca^{2+} 交换的重要性，仍不清楚，

在没有 Ca^{2+} 流出平行的机制存在时，这种节律收缩是怎样发生的。是否肌膜钙泵在特殊条件下能促进这种作用还不知道。

（二）生物化学和分子生物学

尽管肌膜和肌浆网 Ca^{2+}-ATP 酶都是 P-型 ATP 酶家族成员，它们的结构却完全不同。就是说，它们各自与其他 P-型 ATP 酶（如 Na^+-K^+-ATP 酶和 H^+-K^+-ATP 酶）有一定程度的相似。功能上，它们与转运循环时天冬氨酰磷酸盐媒介物的形成相关[31]。人类肌膜 Ca^{2+}-ATP 酶的四个非等位基因已被确定，并与广泛的可变剪接有关，它们组成巨大而独特的 Ca^{2+} 泵家族。这巨大多样性的生理基础还不知道，尽管在不同种剪切突变体间已观察到不同的功能和/或调节。据预测肌膜 Ca^{2+} 泵的拓扑结构模型有 10 个跨膜片段和细胞内有氨基和羧基端。有三个主要细胞内结构域组成蛋白质的大部分。第一个（位于跨膜片段 2 和 3 之间）作为"转导结构域"，主要参与转运有关的大范围的构象变化，并受磷脂酸的调节。第二个且最大的细胞内结构域位于跨膜片段 4 和 5 之间。它是 ATP 结合和酰基磷酸盐中间体形成的主要催化结构域。最后的细胞内区是该蛋白的羧基端，它是 Ca^{2+}/钙调蛋白调节的主要的调节点位[32-34]。

三、钠-氢交换

（一）生理学

调节细胞内 pH 对组织非常重要，特别是对那些耗能巨大的组织。以心肌为例，在反复的收缩行为期间代谢酸不断产生。为维持 pH 值，心脏肌膜上存在几种独立的调节机制，包括 Na^+-H^+ 交换体、Na^+-HCO_3^- 协同运输体、Cl^--OH^- 交换体和 Cl^--HCO_3^- 交换体。这些系统中，Na^+-H^+ 和 Na^+-HCO_3^- 交换负责减轻细胞内的酸中毒，后两种则增加细胞内的碱。在这部分将讨论 Na^+-H^+ 交换体，因它是现代药理学的一个有吸引力靶标。

Na^+-H^+ 交换体是离子转运计数器，它按化学比例交换一个细胞内质子和一个细胞外 Na^+。已确定 Na^+-H^+ 交换体的 7 个亚型（NHE1-7），心脏肌膜主要表达 NHE1。这个亚型对细胞内质子浓度增加而激活十分敏感，并且它的激活是由质子结合到一个 pH 感受器区域向诱导的构象变化来介导。而且，还有许多调节的机制可影响 NHE1 的 pH 敏感性，它们主要通过对调节该蛋白的巨大细胞内羧基端区域的磷酸化[35,36]。NHE1 构象变化能巨大改变多种生理反应，因这个亚型在哺乳动物细胞中广泛表达。

总之，生理条件下 NHE1 计数转运负责多数质子从心肌细胞流出。然而，临床感兴趣的是这种转运在病理生理下的运作，因为 NHE1 被证实在调节心脏局部缺血-再灌注损伤时起主要作用。特别对于缺血刺激，可有一个与无氧代谢转化有关的细胞内外的迅速酸化。细胞内酸化可独自引起与局部缺血有关的大面积收缩功能紊乱，因肌丝对 Ca^{2+} 敏感性和产生力量能力均受到显著削弱。尽管组织的缺血再灌注对挽救心肌很重要，这种反常的方法也会诱发额外的细胞损伤。随着再灌注，细胞外的 pH 迅速恢复，为 NHE1 恢复细胞内 pH 创造良好条件。随后，作为一种 Ca^{2+} 的转运机制，Na^+ 大量而迅速内流，可明显削弱心脏 Na^+-Ca^{2+} 交换的效率。这种短暂 Na^+ 电化学梯度减小，减少了 Na^+-Ca^{2+} 交换的前向（Ca^{2+} 流出）模式，Na^+-Ca^{2+} 交换的反相模式则加强。以上情况的加剧，能迅速导致细胞内 Ca^{2+} 超载，它与危险性心律失常和细胞死亡有关。因而，抑制 NHE1 是限制缺血心脏组织再灌注损害的非常有吸引力的方法。

（二）生物化学和分子生物学

心脏 Na^+-H^+ 交换是 NHE 家族的一个成员。目前有 7 种不同的亚型（NHE1-7）；后两个成员在细胞内发现[35,37]。NHE1 是心肌膜的主要亚型，并在其他型细胞也广泛表达。这个 110kD 的糖蛋白由大约 815 个氨基酸组成，包括 12 个跨膜片段区和位于细胞内的氨基、羧基端区[35,38]。这些跨膜区和它们相应的连接环组成蛋白的主要部分（近 500 氨基酸），参与调节激活相关的离子转运和质子传感。该蛋白的其他部分（≈315 个氨基酸）是个巨大的亲水羧基端区。NHE1 的功能、结构研究已证明一些次级区负责变构修饰 NHE1 的功能，通过多种信号级联。通过各种信号网络调节 NHE1 已有广泛的研究和综述，不再重复[35,36,39]。然而，几个最近的发现表现出对心脏病理生理的特殊作用。例如，NHE1 被认为对心脏肥大、纤维化和心室重构起重要作用[36,40]。而且，更多的证据表明，NHE1 涉及调节细胞增殖和肥大[35]。有趣的是，肌膜多磷酸肌醇（如 PIP_2）也可调节 NHE1 活性[38]，同观察到的心脏 Na^+-Ca^{2+} 交换有相似的反应，并在 ATP 损耗时更能影响它们的行为。

（三）药理学

有大量试验证据证明 NHE1 在再灌注引起的心肌损害中起作用。随着 NHE1 特异性抑制剂的出现，这些研究已用多种指数证明心脏保护，抵抗缺血损害。这些指数包括改善收缩力的恢复、减少梗死面积和过挛缩范围、减少离子失调和心律失常。基于上述证据，临床试验中评估 Na^+-H^+ 交换抑制剂目前正在迅速开展[36,41]。

有两种经典 NHE1 抑制剂，即氨咪氯胺（amiloride）（以及多种类似物如 ethypropylamiide 和 5-N-［menthylpropyl］amiloride）和 benzoylguanidines（及其多种类似物如 HOE694 和 HOE642）[39]。这些抑制剂对 NHE1 比其他 NHE 家族成员作用特异。这两种经典 NHE1 抑制物新的衍生物正不断被发现，利用它们进行研究的结果也进一步支持其有力的心肌保护作用。但两个最近评估 NHE1 抑制剂的临床试验显示有益的影响远低于预期。例如在 GUARDIAN 试验，观察 cariporide 对各种急性冠脉综合征的治疗效果，仅有一小部分病人被确定有益[41,42]。相似的，在 ESCAMI 试验 eniporide 作为急性心肌梗死再灌注的辅助治疗，并没观察到可改善临床结果或减少梗死面积。仅一小部分病人被确定心衰事件减少[41,43]。总之，将上述基础研究发现的治疗效果转化到临床试验中是困难的。然而，相当乐观的是有部分特殊病人被确定从这种方法获益。而且，从这些试验获得的信息或许对扩展和提高 NHE1 抑制剂的效用有价值。

四、钠-钙交换

（一）Na^+-Ca^{2+} 交换的生理作用

心脏 Na^+-Ca^{2+} 交换被认为是转运 Ca^{2+} 的主要机制，是心肌舒张的必需。在心脏连续搏动中这种交换可移出相同数量进入心肌细胞的 Ca^{2+}[44]。因 Ca^{2+} 内流水平调节控制心脏收缩，Na^+-Ca^{2+} 交换必须改变 Ca^{2+} 流出总量以与这些变化相一致。这种能力确保避免细胞内 Ca^{2+} 超载或 Ca^{2+} 耗竭。不同的物种和发育变化过程中，来自 L-型 Ca^{2+} 通道的活化 Ca^{2+} 与来自肌浆网的相比，有相当大的差异。而且，不管这些变异性有多大，在任何时期，Ca^{2+} 内流与 Ca^{2+} 流出必须相当，才能确保心脏的正常功能。

作为一种可逆的离子转运器，Na^+-Ca^{2+} 交换也可作为 Ca^{2+} 进入的机制。依靠存在的电化学梯度，这种交换能携带 Ca^{2+} 进入细胞，支持和增加心脏收缩。这种可逆 Na^+-Ca^{2+} 交换模式被认为协助兴奋-收缩耦联，并促进肌浆网中 Ca^{2+} 诱发的 Ca^{2+} 释放[45]。尽管这种机制的生理作用在过去几年被激烈争论，一致的意见正在出现。那就是，可逆的 Na^+-Ca^{2+} 交换对激活期的 Ca^{2+} 诱发的 Ca^{2+} 释放不是主要的。然而，它可直接影响肌浆网 Ca^{2+} 水平和控制细胞内 Ca^{2+} 水平，从而对心肌收缩力产生显著影响，特别在肌膜下位点附近，在那里 L-型 Ca^{2+} 通道和肌浆网释放通道紧密接近。离子交换器的这些作用直接影响心脏兴奋-收缩耦联的获益或效率[2,25,26]。

心脏舒张期，肌浆网和 Na^+-Ca^{2+} 交换系统竞争细胞质的 Ca^{2+}。已有试验证明这两个系统都有独立完成调节心脏舒张的能力[46]。肌浆网能以近于生理速度完成，而 Na^+-Ca^{2+} 交换独立作用时速度有所减少。这个发现有多个重要生理意义。最重要的是，两系统都有相当大的可逆能力实现心脏舒张期 Ca^{2+} 水平。其次，其他转运系统没有移动 Ca^{2+} 的多余能力，因为阻断肌浆网 Ca^{2+} 摄取和 Na^+-Ca^{2+} 交换，将严重削弱了心脏舒张。尽管线粒体和肌膜 Ca^{2+}-ATP 酶有助于降低细胞内 Ca^{2+} 水平，但在生理条件下可能并不是如此。特别是，肌浆网虽然能迅速独自舒张心肌，但因细胞内 Ca^{2+} 超载迅速发生，使这个过程不能连续进行。相反，Na^+-Ca^{2+} 交换能反复实现此过程，因它能从心肌细胞内前向移动 Ca^{2+}。这些关系和限制可能是构成心衰时 Na^+-Ca^{2+} 交换及肌浆网 Ca^{2+}-ATP 酶表达水平明显改变的基础。

（二）转运机制

Na^+-Ca^{2+} 交换是一种生电的离子计数转运，普遍认为以 $3Na^+：1Ca^{2+}$ 化学计量模式进行。因配对比例的结果，这种交换过程既影响膜电位也受膜电位影响。Na^+-Ca^{2+} 交换对心脏动作电位性质的贡献难以确定，因缺乏适当的抑制剂。在它运作的前向模式，Na^+-Ca^{2+} 交换产生内向电流将延长动作电位。除此之外，动作电位期间引导和激活 Na^+-Ca^{2+} 交换受多种因素的显著影响，包括肌膜下部 Ca^{2+} 和 Na^+ 动力的变化，电压的伴随变化，内在调节机制引起的动力变化。尽管它们对分析造成很大障碍，但对 Na^+-Ca^{2+} 交换运作动力学的理解正取得显著进步[2,25]。

最近研究已对 Na^+-Ca^{2+} 交换的化学计量提出疑问，证明可能是 4：1 或不定的化学计量[47,48]。如果另有研究支持这些发现，那我们理解的 Na^+-Ca^{2+} 交换的生理功能则值得考虑。特别是，这将深刻影响我们理解的 Ca^{2+} 流入和流出的配对数量，转运交换的比率，对动作电位性质的贡献，促进 Ca^{2+} 进入可逆性交换的可能性，以及调节更多有效的 Ca^{2+} 流入机制的必要性。多数现代发表的研究对原始的 3∶1 化学计量提供有力的支持[49]，暗示对这重要概念的重新认定目前还不需要。

目前已被广泛接受的 Na^+-Ca^{2+} 交换转运机制是一个连续的模式，单个离子-结合点位可反复暴露于细胞内膜和外膜表面。通过与 Na^+/Ca^{2+} 结合，该交换体和结合的离子便获得移位到对面膜表面位置的能力，随后结合的离子被释放，并且离子-结合点位可为下一次转运事件所利用。在这种模式的约束下，Na^+ 和 Ca^{2+} 都有能力竞争此单一结合点位。Na^+-Ca^{2+} 交换体的构造以及对转运离子亲和力的不同依赖于膜表面残余的离子结合点位。多个实验研究的结果均支持这个转运模式。而且，这些资料与同步转运并不一致，后者转运发生时 Na^+ 和 Ca^{2+} 必须被结合。例如，多组实验已证实离子流与交换体转运循环的部分反应有关[50,51]。同样，离子的亲和力受带相反电荷离子的浓度影响，这是连续转运模式的基本特征[50]。

多个团队试图测定 Na^+-Ca^{2+} 交换的周转率，并已报道了一个相当大范围的数值[26]。许多实验中，这些周转率是从研究检测交换的局部反应得出，因此这些数值未提供整个反应循环或生理条件下周转率的信息。目前，没有可靠的方法计数 Na^+-Ca^{2+} 交换。对 Na^+-Ca^{2+} 交换体生理周转率的正确评估对理解完成舒张期 Ca^{2+} 流出所需最小的 Na^+-Ca^{2+} 交换体密度有重要作用。而且，它们将提供了解 Na^+-Ca^{2+} 系统转运能力和本质的巨大前景，如通过激活调整机制调节它的功能。目前，我们对 Na^+-Ca^{2+} 交换流出如何与变化的 Ca^{2+} 内流配对仅有非常有限的了解。

（三）心脏 Na^+-Ca^{2+} 交换体 NCX1.1 的分子特性

Na^+-Ca^{2+} 交换体的原型，现在指的是 NCX1.1，在 1990 年被克隆。Na^+-Ca^{2+} 交换体超家族一般包括三个不同基因产物（NCX1，NCX2，NCX3）和大量剪切突变体[52]。交换体都有组织表达特异性，尽管心肌主要表达 NCX1.1。成熟 NCX1.1 蛋白由 938 个氨基酸组成，分子大小约 110kD。目前的拓扑结构模型显示 Na^+-Ca^{2+} 交换体有 9 个跨膜片段和一个位于跨膜片段 5-6 之间巨大的细胞质环，它组成此蛋白分子量的近一半[52-54]。多个重要功能结构域已被确定，这个交换体被自然分成离子转运跨膜区和细胞质调节区。在跨膜区内，两个折返环位于膜对面并对离子移动起重要作用。多个重要功能结构域已确定在巨大细胞质环内，包括高亲和力调节 Ca^{2+} 结合位点，该位点参与 Na_i^+-依赖失活（XIP 区），以及可变剪切区[52]。

（四）Na^+-Ca^{2+} 交换的调节

尽管 Na^+-Ca^{2+} 交换在心脏兴奋-收缩耦联中起关键作用，但这个转运系统的生理调节还知之甚少。一个需回答的主要问题是 Na^+-Ca^{2+} 交换系统是怎样调节使 Ca^{2+} 流出水平与 Ca^{2+} 流入变化相匹配。近期，两种形式的离子调节已被确定，这些自动调节机制受转运离子的自身调节。这些内在机制目前看来最能说明 Ca^{2+} 内流及 Ca^{2+} 流出的耦联，因为它们的运作能显著地改变功能性离子交换体的数量。Na_i^+-依赖或 I_1 调节的 Na^+-Ca^{2+} 交换描述了细胞质 Na_i^+ 促进交换体失活的能力，尽管这种反应仅在高浓度的细胞质 Na^+ 时发生。Ca^{2+}-依赖或 I_2 调节描述了细胞质 Ca^{2+} 对内向和外向交换电流的刺激影响，这种作用是在心肌内正常 Ca^{2+} 范围内观察到的[26,52]，在整个细胞记录以及孤立的膜钳片都非常明显，Ca^{2+} 依赖或 I_2 调节的作用使得 Na^+-Ca^{2+} 交换体能对 Ca^{2+} 流入水平的变化作出反应。

Na^+-Ca^{2+} 交换活性还受另外几个因素包括 pH、β肾上腺素刺激、ATP 水平和膜磷脂（特别是 PIP_2）的影响。在大多数时候这些调节反应是如何介导以及它们如何影响心脏的生理功能，仍不清楚。例如，已报道蛋白激酶 A 和 C 参与调节 Na^+-Ca^{2+} 交换体活性，还不确定这是否涉及交换体或其他未知靶标的磷酸化。PIP_2-介导的交换体调节涉及一种 Na^+-依赖或 I_1-依赖的交换体失活的减弱。然而，因为仍不知道 I_1 失活对正常心脏生理的作用，这种调节的适应性仍是模糊的。经 ATP 调节的 Na^+-Ca^{2+} 交换体看来涉及前述的 PIP_2-介导的机制。总之，我们对生理和病理生理中 Na^+-Ca^{2+} 交换的调节的了解非常少。

（五）Na^+-Ca^{2+} 交换在心脏病理生理中的作用

有充分的试验证据提示 Na^+-Ca^{2+} 交换体参与某些特殊类型的心脏损伤。其中，对 Na^+-Ca^{2+} 交换在缺血-再灌注损害中的作用了解得最清楚。缺血期，转变为无氧代谢且伴随代谢物排除的减少或缺失，这可导致心肌细胞酸化。在此期间，Na_i^+ 水平升高，其升高的程度据推测可能有模式和时间依赖性。在再灌注后，细胞外的pH迅速恢复，形成一个相当大的pH梯度。肌膜Na^+-H^+交换体在心肌缺血后恢复细胞内pH，进一步增加Na_i^+水平。随后跨膜Na_i^+电化学梯度的减少将减小经前向交换的Ca^{2+}流出的驱动力，并促进调节Ca^{2+}流入的反向交换力。依赖于上述损伤的严重性，Ca^{2+}流出能力的净减少能迅速产生Ca^{2+}超载和/或细胞死亡。根据这些情况，抑制Na^+-Ca^{2+}交换的反向模式是药理学干预进行再灌注治疗的相当有吸引力的靶标。

在多数心衰模型中，Na^+-Ca^{2+}交换水平被证明随着肌浆网Ca^{2+}-ATP酶水平相应的减少而增加。这种也常在人类心衰中观察到[55,56]。一个正在形成的概念是，可逆的Na^+-Ca^{2+}交换在维持心衰的心脏收缩中起重要作用，作为细胞内Ca^{2+}的下降的代偿。尽管Na^+-Ca^{2+}交换增加可促进收缩，但当前向Na^+-Ca^{2+}交换模式成为瞬时内向电流的主要部分时也有使心脏发生心律失常的危险[57]。根据这种情况，药理学的适当干涉策略是不容易的。在心肌苷治疗中，经间接抑制Na^+-Ca^{2+}交换来改善心肌收缩同它的促心律失常密不可分。

（六）Na^+-Ca^{2+}交换的药理学操作法

历史上，直接调控Na^+-Ca^{2+}交换体的功能是非常难懂的。以前利用的主要化合物同其他的离子转运系统比，完全缺乏对交换体的特异性。实验上，大多数抑制交换功能的方法是减少细胞内的Na^+和Ca^{2+}，或应用高浓度的Ni^{2+}或La^{3+}。然而，两个团队报道了一个新的isothiourea（异硫脲）化合物，现在叫KB-R7943[58,59]。深入研究了它的作用机制，并对其治疗潜能做了评估。但对它的作用位点、转运模式的选择、作用机制和亚型的选择还未有统一认识。相比之下，KB-R7943的心肌保护作用在多种心脏损伤模型中已被确定[26]。

最近，一个名为SEA0400非常有效的Na^+-Ca^{2+}交换抑制剂被提出。这个化合物能在心脏和神经细胞中以低的纳摩尔浓度抑制Na^+-Ca^{2+}交换活性[53,60]。这个化合物对多种不同的离子通道和转运体的作用已被检测，并且观察到对Na^+-Ca^{2+}交换体有相当的特异性。特别是它也影响Ca^{2+}状态和敲除NCX1.1鼠心脏肌管的兴奋性，提示它比单纯的交换抑制有更广谱的影响[61]。不过，近期一个比较SEA0400和KB-R7943对心脏保护影响的研究显示，SEA0400的效果很明确。特别是在一个冠状动脉结扎模型中，SEA0400被发现能减少梗死面积超过75%。无论在心肌缺血前或后应用。这种影响是浓度依赖的（EC_{50}=5.7nM），KB-R7943被观察到有相当低的功效，且功能恢复在高浓度时受损[62]。

控制Na^+-Ca^{2+}交换活性可能是减轻再灌注损害一个比较有希望的方法。尽管能完成的药理学工具数量目前有限，但初步结果显示与Na^+-H^+交换阻滞剂的影响相似。比较和对照缺血-再灌注损害的不同策略是有趣的。在两个事件中，目标都是阻断Na^+-Ca^{2+}反向交换防止细胞坏死后产生的Ca^{2+}超载。应用Na^+-H^+交换阻滞剂，可经阻止或减少Na_i^+积聚实现这一目标，尽管一个明显的结果是延长了酸中毒期。相反，抑制Na^+-Ca^{2+}反向交换模式，从酸中毒的恢复会正常进行，尽管Na_i^+会大幅升高直到被Na^+-K^+-ATP酶修正。如果Na^+-Ca^{2+}交换反向模式能被选择性抑制，急性（剧烈）的Ca^{2+}流入可被阻断，尽管Na^+-Ca^{2+}交换的前向模式会被短暂危害。其预期的结果可从合适增加收缩力到Ca^{2+}超载。显然，这样的构思过于简单化了再灌注损害的复杂多样的结果。不过，早期的结果已总体确定选择性调节Na^+-Ca^{2+}交换活性是一个有希望的心脏保护策略。虽然谨慎乐观，但用于这种方法的药理学工具仍模糊，且我们理解的主要差距也需要相应的工具。而且，从Na^+-H^+交换阻滞剂临床试验获得的经验证明，从试验到临床应用是有一定距离的。

五、概要

面对日益的人口老龄化，除了预防外，更多的心脏疾病需要用药物手段经济地治疗。在这方面，控制离子转运看来是有前景的，特别是能减少心肌梗死的危害。为实现这一目标需要更深入地了解各种离子泵和交换体及相应的功能化学调节剂的增加。近期在调节Na^+-H^+和Na^+-Ca^{2+}交换方面研究的进步及有希望的试验结果给我们以信心，需要进一步研究。

（王洪涛　滕思勇　浦介麟　译）

参 考 文 献

1. Glitsch HG: Electrophysiology of the sodium-potassium-ATPase in cardiac cells. Physiol Rev 81:1791–1826, 2001.
2. Bers DM: Excitation-contraction coupling and cardiac contractile force. London, UK, Kluwer Academic Publications, 2001.
3. Kaplan JH: Biochemistry of Na,K-ATPase. Annu Rev Biochem 71:511–535, 2002.
4. Scheiner-Bobis G: The sodium pump. Its molecular properties and mechanics of ion transport. Eur J Biochem 269:2424–2433, 2002.
5. Holmgren M, Wagg J, Bezanilla F, et al: Three distinct and sequential steps in the release of sodium ions by the Na^+/K^+-ATPase. Nature 403:898–901, 2000.
6. Hilgemann DW: Channel-like function of the Na,K pump probed at microsecond resolution in giant membrane patches. Science 263:1429–1432, 1994.
7. Therien AG, Blostein R: Mechanisms of sodium pump regulation. Am J Physiol Cell Physiol 279:C541–C566, 2000.
8. Crambert G, Fuzesi M, Garty H, et al: Phospholemman (FXYD1) associates with Na,K-ATPase and regulates its transport properties. Proc Natl Acad Sci U S A 99:11476–11481, 2002.
9. Therien AG, Pu HX, Karlish SJ, Blostein R: Molecular and functional studies of the gamma subunit of the sodium pump. J Bioenerg Biomembr 33:407–414, 2001.
10. Wang J, Schwinger RH, Frank K, et al: Regional expression of sodium pump subunits isoforms and Na^+-Ca^{++} exchanger in the human heart. J Clin Invest 98:1650–1658, 1996.
11. McDonough AA, Zhang Y, Shin V, Frank JS: Subcellular distribution of sodium pump isoform subunits in mammalian cardiac myocytes. Am J Physiol Cell Physiol 270:C1221–C1227, 1996.
12. Toyoshima C, Nakasako M, Nomura H, Ogawa H: Crystal structure of the calcium pump of sarcoplasmic reticulum at 2.6 Å resolution. Nature 405:647–655, 2000.
13. Kaplan JH, Hu YK, Gatto C: Conformational coupling: The moving parts of an ion pump. J Bioenerg Biomembr 33:379–385, 2001.
14. Jorgensen PL: Aspects of gene structure and functional regulation of the isozymes of Na,K-ATPase. Cell Mol Biol (Noisy-le-grand) 47:231–238, 2001.
15. Santana LF, Gomez AM, Lederer WJ: Ca^{2+} flux through promiscuous cardiac Na^+ channels: Slip-mode conductance. Science 279:1027–1033, 1998.
16. Nishio M, Ruch SW, Wasserstrom JA: Positive inotropic effects of ouabain in isolated cat ventricular myocytes in sodium-free conditions. Am J Physiol Heart Circ Physiol 283:H2045–H2053, 2002.
17. Reuter H, Henderson SA, Han T, et al: The Na^+-Ca^{2+} exchanger is essential for the action of cardiac glycosides. Circ Res 90:305–308, 2002.
18. The effect of digoxin on mortality and morbidity in patients with heart failure. The Digitalis Investigation Group. N Engl J Med 336:525–533, 1997.
19. Rathore SS, Wang Y, Krumholz HM: Sex-based differences in the effect of digoxin for the treatment of heart failure. N Engl J Med 347:1403–1411, 2002.
20. Schoner W: Endogenous cardiac glycosides, a new class of steroid hormones. Eur J Biochem 269:2440–2448, 2002.
21. Gao J, Wymore RS, Wang Y, et al: Isoform-specific stimulation of cardiac Na/K pumps by nanomolar concentrations of glycosides. J Gen Physiol 119:297–312, 2002.
22. Gatto C, Hale CC, Xu W, Milanick MA: Eosin, a potent inhibitor of the plasma membrane Ca pump, does not inhibit the cardiac Na-Ca exchanger. Biochemistry 34:965–972, 1995.
23. Choi HS, Eisner DA: The role of sarcolemmal Ca^{2+}-ATPase in the regulation of resting calcium concentration in rat ventricular myocytes. J Physiol 515:109–118, 1999.
24. Choi HS, Eisner DA: The effects of inhibition of the sarcolemmal Ca-ATPase on systolic calcium fluxes and intracellular calcium concentration in rat ventricular myocytes. Pflugers Arch 437:966–971, 1999.
25. Bers DM: Cardiac excitation-contraction coupling. Nature 415:198–205, 2002.
26. Hryshko LV: The cardiac Na^+-Ca^{2+} exchanger. In Page E, Fozzard HA, Solaro RJ (eds): Handbook of Physiology. Section 2: The Cardiovascular System. Vol. 1: The Heart, Chap 10. Oxford, UK, Oxford University Press, 2002, pp 388–419.
27. Henaff M, Antoine S, Mercadier JJ, et al: The voltage-independent B-type Ca^{2+} channel modulates apoptosis of cardiac myocytes. FASEB J 16:99–101, 2002.
28. Antoine S, Pinet C, Coulombe A: Are B-type Ca^{2+} channels of cardiac myocytes akin to the passive ion channel in the plasma membrane Ca^{2+} pump? J Membr Biol 179:37–50, 2001.
29. Pinet C, Antoine S, Filoteo AG, et al: Reincorporated plasma membrane Ca^{2+}-ATPase can mediate B-type Ca^{2+} channels observed in native membrane of human red blood cells. J Membr Biol 187:185–201, 2002.
30. Philipson KD: Na^+-Ca^{2+} exchange: Three new tools. Circ Res 90:118–119, 2002.
31. Carafoli E, Brini M: Calcium pumps: Structural basis for and mechanism of calcium transmembrane transport. Curr Opin Chem Biol 4:152–161, 2000.
32. Strehler EE, Zacharias DA: Role of alternative splicing in generating isoform diversity among plasma membrane calcium pumps. Physiol Rev 81:21–50, 2001.
33. Monteith GR, Roufogalis BD: The plasma membrane calcium pump—a physiological perspective on its regulation. Cell Calcium 18:459–470, 1995.
34. Penniston JT, Enyedi A: Modulation of the plasma membrane Ca^{2+} pump. J Membr Biol 165:101–109, 1998.
35. Putney LK, Denker SP, Barber DL: The changing face of the Na^+/H^+ exchanger, NHE1: Structure, regulation, and cellular actions. Ann Rev Pharmacol Toxicol 42:527–552, 2002.
36. Karmazyn M, Gan XT, Humphreys RA, et al: The myocardial Na^+-H^+ exchange. Structure, regulation, and its role in heart disease. Circ Res 85:777–786, 1999.
37. Numata M, Orlowski J: Molecular cloning and characterization of a novel $(Na^+,K^+)/H^+$ exchanger localized to the trans-Golgi network. J Biol Chem 276:17387–17394, 2001.
38. Aharonovitz O, Zaun HC, Balla T, et al: Intracellular pH regulation by Na^+/H^+ exchange requires phosphatidylinositol 4,5-bisphosphate. J Cell Biol 150:213–224, 2000.
39. Orlowski J: Na^+/H^+ exchangers. Molecular diversity and relevance to heart. Ann N Y Acad Sci 874:346–353, 1999.
40. Engelhardt S, Hein L, Keller U, Lohse MJ: Inhibition of Na^+/H^+-exchange prevents hypertrophy, fibrosis and heart failure in β_1-adrenergic receptor transgenic mice. Naunyn-Schmiedebergs Arch Pharmacol 365:343, 2002.
41. Avkiran M, Marber MS: Na^+/H^+ exchange inhibitors for cardioprotective therapy: Progress, problems and prospects. J Am Coll Cardiol 39:747–753, 2002.
42. Theroux P, Chaitman BR, Danchin N, et al: Inhibition of the sodium-hydrogen exchanger with cariporide to prevent myocardial infarction in high-risk ischemic situations. Main results of the GUARDIAN trial. Guard during ischemia against necrosis (GUARDIAN) Investigators. Circulation 102:3032–3038, 2000.
43. Zeymer U, Suryapranata H, Monassier JP, et al: The Na^+/H^+ exchange inhibitor eniporide as an adjunct to early reperfusion therapy for acute myocardial infarction. Results of the evaluation of the safety and cardioprotective effects of eniporide in acute myocardial infarction (ESCAMI) trial. J Am Coll Cardiol 38:1644–1650, 2001.
44. Bridge JH, Smolley JR, Spitzer KW: The relationship between charge movements associated with I_{Ca} and I_{Na-Ca} in cardiac myocytes. Science 248:376–378, 1990.
45. Leblanc N, Hume JR: Sodium current-induced release of calcium from cardiac sarcoplasmic reticulum. Science 248:372–376, 1990.
46. Bers DM, Bassani JW, Bassani RA: Competition and redistribution among calcium transport systems in rabbit cardiac myocytes. Cardiovasc Res 27:1772–1777, 1993.
47. Fujioka Y, Komeda M, Matsuoka S: Stoichiometry of Na^+-Ca^{2+} exchange in inside-out patches excised from guinea-pig ventricular myocytes. J Physiol 523(Pt 2):339–351, 2000.
48. Dong H, Dunn J, Lytton J: Stoichiometry of the cardiac Na^+/Ca^{2+} exchanger NCX1.1 measured in transfected HEK cells. Biophys J 82:1943–1952, 2002.
49. Hinata M, Yamamura H, Li L, et al: Stoichiometry of Na^+-Ca^{2+} exchange is 3:1 in guinea-pig ventricular myocytes. J Physiol 545:453–461, 2002.
50. Hilgemann DW, Nicoll DA, Philipson KD: Charge movement during Na^+ translocation by native and cloned cardiac Na^+/Ca^{2+} exchanger. Nature 352:715–718, 1991.
51. Niggli E, Lederer WJ: Molecular operations of the sodium-calcium

exchanger revealed by conformation currents. Nature 349:621–624, 1991.
52. Philipson KD, Nicoll DA: Sodium-calcium exchange: A molecular perspective. Annu Rev Physiol 62:111–133, 2000.
53. Tanaka H, Nishimaru K, Aikawa T, et al: Effect of SEA0400, a novel inhibitor of sodium-calcium exchanger, on myocardial ionic currents. Br J Pharmacol 135:1096–1100, 2002.
54. Iwamoto T, Uehara A, Imanaga I, Shigekawa M: The Na^+/Ca^{2+} exchanger NCX1 has oppositely oriented reentrant loop domains that contain conserved aspartic acids whose mutation alters its apparent Ca^{2+} affinity. J Biol Chem 275:38571–38580, 2000.
55. Hasenfuss G, Schillinger W, Lehnart SE, et al: Relationship between Na^+-Ca^{2+}-exchanger protein levels and diastolic function of failing human myocardium. Circulation 99:641–648, 1999.
56. Dipla K, Mattiello JA, Margulies KB, et al: The sarcoplasmic reticulum and the Na^+/Ca^{2+} exchanger both contribute to the Ca^{2+} transient of failing human ventricular myocytes. Circ Res 84:435–444, 1999.
57. Pogwizd SM, Schlotthauer K, Li L, et al: Arrhythmogenesis and contractile dysfunction in heart failure: Roles of sodium-calcium exchange, inward rectifier potassium current, and residual β-adrenergic responsiveness. Circ Res 88:1159–1167, 2001.
58. Iwamoto T, Watano T, Shigekawa M: A novel isothiourea derivative selectively inhibits the reverse mode of Na^+/Ca^{2+} exchange in cells expressing NCX1. J Biol Chem 271:22391–22397, 1996.
59. Watano T, Kimura J, Morita T, Nakanishi H: A novel antagonist, No. 7943, of the Na^+/Ca^{2+} exchange current in guinea-pig cardiac ventricular cells. Br J Pharmacol 119:555–563, 1996.
60. Matsuda T, Arakawa N, Takuma K, et al: SEA0400, a novel and selective inhibitor of the Na^+-Ca^{2+} exchanger, attenuates reperfusion injury in the in vitro and in vivo cerebral ischemic models. J Pharmacol Exp Ther 298:249–256, 2001.
61. Reuter H, Henderson SA, Han T, et al: Knock-out mice for pharmacological screening: Testing the specificity of Na^+-Ca^{2+} exchange inhibitors. Circ Res 91:90–92, 2002.
62. Magee WP, Deshmukh G, DeNinno MP, et al: Differing cardioprotective efficacy of the Na^+-Ca^{2+} exchanger inhibitors, SEA0400 and KB-R7943. Am J Physiol Heart Circ Physiol 284:H903–H910, 2003.

第 6 章

肌浆网离子通道

Gerbard Meissner

本章目录

- 肌浆网的离子渗透性 ·················· 51
- 心脏兴奋-收缩耦联的机制 ············ 51
- 心脏 Ca^{2+} 释放通道的结构和表达 ······ 52
- Ca^{2+} 释放通道的单价及二价离子传导性
  ····································· 52
- 内源的效应物对 Ca^{2+} 释放通道的调节
  ····································· 53
- 植物碱和咖啡因对 Ca^{2+} 释放通道的调节
  ····································· 56
- K^+，Na^+ 通道 ······················· 57
- H^+ 渗透性 ··························· 57
- Cl^- 通道 ···························· 57
- 总结 ································· 58
- 致谢 ································· 58

肌浆网（Sarcoplasmic reticulum，SR）是细胞内的膜样结构，它通过向肌浆迅速地释放钙离子和移出钙离子而调节心肌的收缩和舒张。钙离子释放通道（ryanodihe-reckptor）RyR2[1,2]和钙泵是两个主要的转运蛋白，负责钙离子的释放和摄取（图 6-1）。心脏 RyR2s 拥有巨大的蛋白结构（junctional processes，"接头过程"、"足"），它跨越狭窄的缝隙，使 SR 与细胞膜表面及其内陷（T-管）紧密接触。钙离子释放通道也被称为植物碱（斯里兰卡肉桂碱）受体，因它与植物碱有高度的亲和力并能特异地结合植物碱，以区别于另一种细胞内钙释放通道——三磷酸肌醇受体（IP_3R）。心脏 SR 膜上也包括 K^+、Na^+、Cl^- 和 H^+（OH^-）离子通道[4]。在 Ca^{2+} 的快速释放和摄取期间，单价离子穿过各自通道被认为可缓解 Ca^{2+} 的移动对 SR 膜电位的影响。

一、肌浆网的离子渗透性

借鉴研究骨骼肌 SR 的操作方法，对离体的心脏 SR 囊泡部分进行了研究，基本确定了心脏 SR 膜的离子渗透性。骨骼肌和心肌的均一化作用引起 SR 分裂成各种未知的囊泡群体，它们部分决定于糖密度梯度，离心沉淀为"轻"和"重"囊泡成分[5,6]。从哺乳动物肌肉，已基本推导出轻的囊泡在 SR 的非结合区、纵向区，重的囊泡在 SR 的结合区、终末池区（图 6-1）。两种类型囊泡都包含 Ca^{2+} 泵，并能容易的透过单价离子，说明单价离子通道广泛分布于骨骼肌和心脏 SR 膜。心脏 Ca^{2+} 释放通道集中分布在密度大的区间、受接头驱动的 SR 囊泡。

二、心脏兴奋-收缩耦联的机制

在心肌，一个动作电位触发 Ca^{2+} 迅速从 SR 中释放，这一过程涉及兴奋-收缩耦联机制。电压以及位于细胞膜和 T-管表面的二氢吡啶敏感性（L-型）Ca^{2+} 通道（二氢吡啶受体）介导了动作电位期间的 Ca^{2+} 内流[7]。细胞内 Ca^{2+} 浓度的增加能触发 SR Ca^{2+} 释放通道大量释放 Ca^{2+}，这个过程被称作"钙诱导的 Ca^{2+} 释放"。细胞内 Ca^{2+} 总量的瞬间增高被称作 Ca^{2+} 火花（Ca^{2+} sparks）。单个 L-型 Ca^{2+} 通道的开放显然足够引起由 4~6 个 RyR2 激活介导的一个 Ca^{2+} 火花，经

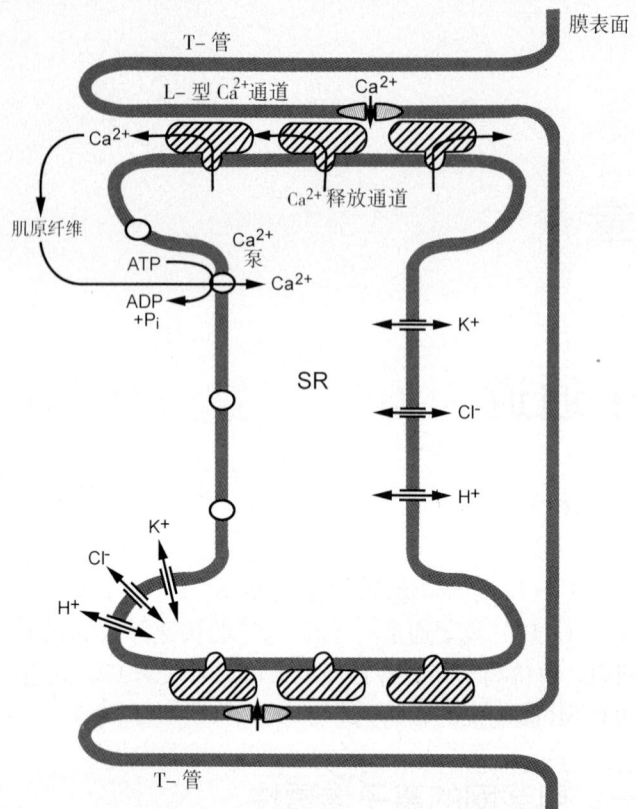

图 6-1 图解示肌细胞片段 图示膜表面、内陷部、横（T-）管和细胞内膜系统，肌浆网（SR）。Ca^{2+} 释放被表示受 SR Ca^{2+} 释放通道调节，同样的以"连接区"或"足"跨越 T-管与 SR 膜之间的间隙。Ca^{2+} 分离受 SR Ca^{2+} 泵或（Ca^{2+} + Mg^{2+}）腺苷三磷酸酶（ATP 酶）调节，单价离子通道被认为遍布于 SR，未显示出 SR 连接部分与表面膜和纵向 SR 连接区配对

完全地整合可形成开放和关闭的同时发生，称作耦联门控[9]。在哺乳动物心室，RyR2 基本位于细胞膜和 T-管表面附近，它为钙诱发的 Ca^{2+} 释放提供形态学基础。在哺乳动物心房，如鸟类心脏，许多 SR 上的 Ca^{2+} 释放通道远离 L-型 Ca^{2+} 通道，说明心室和心房的 SR Ca^{2+} 释放机制是不同的。

三、心脏 Ca^{2+} 释放通道的结构和表达

哺乳动物组织中有三种不同基因编码的 Ca^{2+} 释放通道，心脏的植物碱受体（或兰尼丁受体）是其中之一。RyR1 被发现在骨骼肌中高度分布。RyR2 主要分布在心脏、脑部，但其他组织有少量分布。RyR3 在包括骨骼肌、心肌细胞等各种组织中低水平表达，且不是横纹肌功能的必需[11]。然而，缺乏 RyR2 的变异鼠在胚胎期 10 天死亡，并有心脏管的形态学异常，说明 RyR2 对心脏的正常发育和功能具有重要意义[12]。

心脏 RyR2 的分子生物学特性以及由 Ca^{2+} 和其他分子参与的调节机制已在犬和兔的心脏上进行了广泛的研究。纯化的 RyR2 为一 30S 的蛋白复合物，由四个巨大（$M_r \approx 560000$）亚基紧密连接四个小亚基（FK506 连接蛋白，$M_r 126000$）组成[1]。一般地，膜结合的 RyR2 能被两性离子去污剂 Chaps 和高离子浓度溶液（1.0M NaCl）溶解；30S 通道复合物经蔗糖梯度离心进一步纯化[13]。经低温电子显微镜和三维构象已揭示一个巨大的、松散填充（$29 \times 29 \times 12$）nm 细胞质足部区和一个小的跨膜结构[14]（图 6-2）。

心肌细胞 cDNA 编码一约 5000 氨基酸的蛋白。从亲水图推断氨基酸序列，这个 $M_r \approx 560000$ 的多肽有两个主要结构域：(1) 一个羧基端成孔区，哺乳动物和非哺乳动物间有高度的序列相似性并穿越细胞膜 4~8 次，因此，四聚体的 RyR2 有 16~32 个跨膜片段。(2) 一个巨大的可变的膜外区，被认为与细胞质的足部结构相对应[2,15]。基本序列分析表明巨大的细胞质足部结构存在多个磷酸化位点和多个 Ca^{2+}、ATP 和钙调蛋白的结合位点。尚未发表的研究显示 Ca^{2+} 敏感位点、磷酸化位点和钙调蛋白结合区共同分享游离 Ca^{2+} 和钙调蛋白结合的 Ca^{2+}（N. Yamaguchi, L. Xuand G. Meissner，未发表的资料）。

四、Ca^{2+} 释放通道的单价及二价离子传导性

RyRs 是阳离子选择性的，它有极大的离子传导性，在 50mM Ca^{2+} 溶液中对二价阳离子的传导性为 100~150 pS，在 250mM K^+ 溶液中对单价阳离子传导性为 ≈ 750pS。它对 Ca^{2+} 的巨大传导率最初表现在以单通道记录融合脂质双分子层的骨骼肌和心肌细胞 SR 小囊泡。将纯化的 RyR2 复合物重建成平面脂质双分子层结构可在两方面简化通道的研究：首先，SR 的 K^+、Na^+ 和 Cl^- 通道在囊泡融合期能形成双分子层，但在纯化的 RyR2 标本中这些通道则不能形成双分子层。其次，因囊泡上常存在不止一条通道，用纯化的 RyR2 标本容易获得单一的释放通道。有几种方法建立单通道的活性，即直接应用两性离子去污剂 Chaps、纯化的 30S 通道复合物置于平面的脂质双分子层上或纯化的通道与脂质双分子层融合为蛋白脂质体。[18]两种方法均能产生相同的单通道传导性，但根

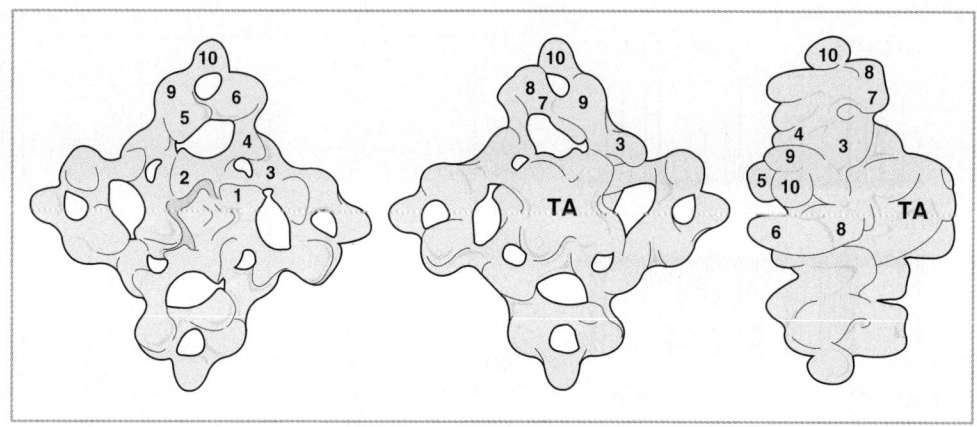

图6-2 电子显微镜对冰-水标本三维重建的心肌 Ca^{2+} 通道 用三个视野显示，一个视野显示T-管（左），一个视野显示SR内腔（中），一个视野显示跨膜区（右）。TA，跨膜集合（引自 Shama MR, Penczek P, Grassucci R, et al: Cryoelectron microscopy and image analysis of the cardiac ryanodine receptor. J Biol Chem 273: 18429-18434, 1998）

据我们的实验结果，在嵌入脂质双分子层之前不应用去污剂重构蛋白脂质体可再生更多的通道活性。

两种模型被用于描述心肌RyR2的离子传导性：基于Eying rate（注视速率）原理建立一个四屏障模型[19]和一个运用Poisson and Nernst-Planck方程建立的扩散模型[20]。这个四屏障模型设想中央存在一个高亲和力的结合位点，它能帮助二价阳离子而不是单价离子通过。这种模型预示在生理条件下，RyR2主要转运 Ca^{2+} 或被 Mg^{2+} 占据[19]。因此，RyR2不能有效地传导 K^+ 和 Na^+，避免在SR释放 Ca^{2+} 期间生成膜电位。如先前所述，SR释放 Ca^{2+} 期间的电荷补偿很可能由SR的单价离子通道的转运实现，RyR2对单价离子的高传导性适合用Poisson and Nernst-Planck方程的扩散模型解释[20]。这个扩散模型预计在通道过滤孔道（直径7Å，长10Å）有高度恒定的负电荷，在溶液浓度低于25mM时将富集高浓度的碱金属离子（浓度可达≈4M）。

五、内源的效应物对 Ca^{2+} 释放通道的调节

RyR2是一个配基门控性通道，能与多种分子发生相互作用。Ca^{2+} 门控通道的激活受多种分子调节，包括腺嘌呤核苷酸和 Mg^{2+}，蛋白-蛋白相互作用包括SR连接蛋白（triadin, junctin）、肌集钙蛋白（calsequestrin，一个SR内腔的高容量、低亲和力 Ca^{2+} 结合蛋白）、钙调蛋白（calmodulin，一个小的细胞浆钙结合蛋白）及蛋白激酶和磷酸脂酶[21,22]。而且，RyR2有大量的自由巯基基团，这说明活性氮和活性氧均可以调节活体内通道的活性（详细讨论见后）。

（一）Ca^{2+}、Mg^{2+}、H^+ 和腺嘌呤核苷酸的调节

采用三种互补技术研究了RyR2的调节：通过单通道合成到平面脂质双分子层来测量微电流，从SR的小囊泡测量微 Ca^{2+} 流量，和测量植物碱结合的 $[^3H]$。

图6-3示应用顺式 Ca^{2+}（SR内的）处理从犬心脏纯化的 Ca^{2+} 释放通道时记录的电流波动图。当胞质内游离 Ca^{2+} 浓度为 $1\mu M$ 时，可在双分子层的胞质腔内观察到稀少的和不能完全分辨的通道开放；当胞质内游离 Ca^{2+} 浓度增加到 $10\mu M$ 时可显著增加通道的开放概率；但 Ca^{2+} 浓度大于 $100\mu M$ 时通道活性反而下降。Ca^{2+} 依赖性通道激活呈双峰说明通道内存在高亲和力（激活）和低亲和力（失活）的 Ca^{2+} 结合位点，它们接近细胞液侧并推测位于RyR2巨大的细胞液内足部区域。除细胞浆的 Ca^{2+} 之外，SR腔内 Ca^{2+} 流过开放的RyR2，并通过细胞浆内的 Ca^{2+} 接近通道的激活和失活位点来调节通道的活性[23]（也见 Sitsapesan and Williams[24]）。

图6-4 描述犬心脏SR囊泡的 Ca^{2+} 依赖性 Ca^{2+}

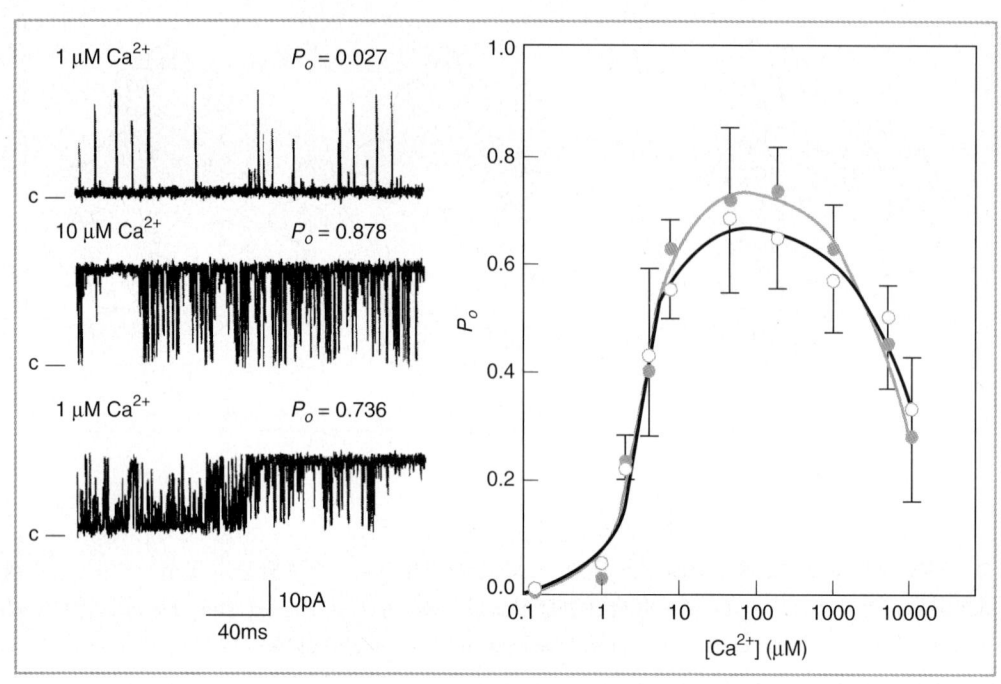

图 6-3 纯化的犬心脏 30S Ca^{2+} 释放通道的单通道记录图 显示顺式 Ca^{2+}（细胞质 SR）影响通道开放的概率（P_o）。单通道电流表现向上的偏差（c，关闭的通道），溶液为 0.25M KCl 和指定的游离顺式（细胞质）Ca^{2+} 浓度，钳制电压为 +35mV（实心图）和 -35mV（空心图）（引自 Xu L，Mann G，Meissner G：Regulation of cardiac Ca^{2+} release channel [ryanodine receptor] by Ca^{2+}, H^+, Mg^{2+}, and adenine nucleotides under normal and simulated ischemic conditions. Circ Res 79：1100-1109，1996.）

释放，它被 1mM[45] Ca^{2+} 填充[45]。Ca^{2+} 流出率由缺少或存在 Mg^{2+} 和 ATP（用非水解性 ATP 类似物 AMP-PCP）决定，它们是心脏上更好的离子刺激条件。在缺乏其他通道刺激物时，Ca^{2+} 依赖性 Ca^{2+} 释放没有变化。Mg^{2+} 增加至 3mM，将与 Ca^{2+} 竞争通道高亲和力的 Ca^{2+} 激活位点，减少[45] Ca^{2+} 的释放率。用 5mM 腺嘌呤核苷酸和 8mM Mg^{2+}（3mM 游离的 Mg^{2+}）作释放媒介时，激活心脏 RyR2 需要更大的 Ca^{2+} 浓度，且无 Ca^{2+} 失活被观察到，这种情况见于 1mM 游离的 Ca^{2+} 浓度时。

[3H] 标记 ryanodine 提供了第三个研究 RyRs 的调节方法。Ryanodine 是一种高度特效的植物碱，它依据肌肉的类型和活性，能引起肌肉挛缩或肌力下降[25]。尽管多个植物碱的结合位点及植物碱与 RyRs 间相互作用的复杂性已被描述，但 RyRs 在低浓度植物碱中的结合动力学相对简单。在这些条件下，[3H] 标记 ryanodine 是一种评价 RyR 活性敏感而方便的方法。一般而言，RyRs 的激活的基本条件包括微摩尔浓度的 Ca^{2+} 或毫摩尔浓度的 ATP，它们可增加 [3H] ryanodine 与通道的亲和力。图 6-5 示在三种不同 pH 值下的 Ca^{2+} 依赖性 [3H] ryanodine 与心脏 SR 囊泡的结合情况。在 pH 值 7.3 时，缺乏和存在 5mM MgAMPPCP，[3H] ryanodine 与心脏 SR 囊泡的结合呈 Ca^{2+} 依赖性，观察结果类似于单通道（见图 6-3）和 SR 囊泡/[45] Ca^{2+} 流出（见图 6-4）。在缺乏 Mg^{2+} 和 AMPPCP 下，当溶液的 pH 值由 7.3 变到 6.5 和 6.2 时，[3H] ryanodine 与通道的亲和力明显降低。在存在 Mg^{2+} 和 AMPPCP 下，当 Ca^{2+} 浓度波动在 1 至 10μM 间时，[3H] ryanodine 与通道的亲和力也对 pH 高度敏感。然而，Ca^{2+} 浓度波动在 0.1 至 1mM 时，过多的酸较少影响对 [3H] ryanodine 与通道的亲和力，因为当 Mg^{2+} 和 AMPPCP 存在时，过多的酸的主要减少 Ca^{2+} 与通道的高亲和力位点的结合。

从图 6-3 到图 6-5 可得出两个结论。首先，Mg^{2+} 和腺嘌呤核苷酸在调节心脏 Ca^{2+} 释放通道方面具有重要作用。其次，因缺血时间延长的心肌缺乏 ATP，心

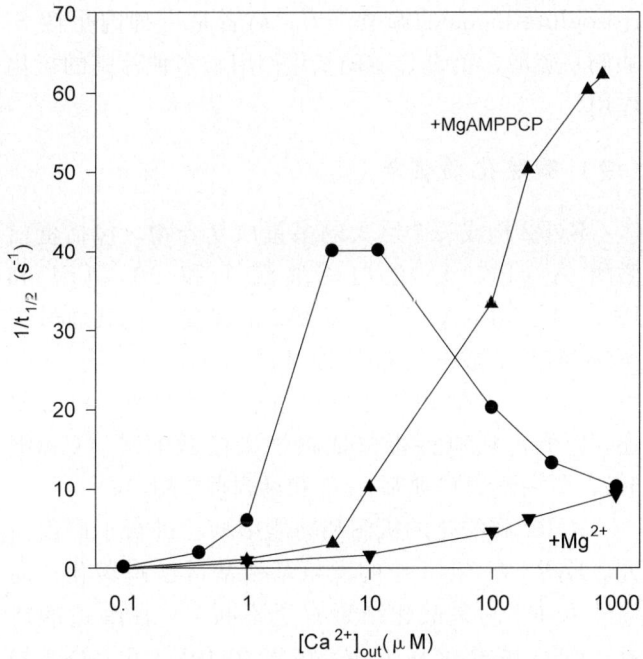

图 6-4 在存在和缺乏 Mg^{2+} 和 AMP-PCP 时，Ca^{2+} 激活的肌浆网 (SR)$^{[45]}Ca^{2+}$ 释放 心脏 SR 囊泡以 1mM $^{[45]}Ca^{2+}$ 填充和不同浓度游离的 Ca^{2+}（实心圆），和 3mM Mg^{2+}（向下的实心三角），或 8mM Mg^{2+} 加 5mM AMP PCP（其中 3mM 游离 Mg^{2+}）（向上的实心三角）[45]。Ca^{2+} 从 Ca^{2+} 释放囊泡流出的一半的时间（$t_{1/2}$）决定于 Ca^{2+} 浓度，并受 Mg^{2+}、腺嘌呤核苷酸和钙调蛋白调节（引自 Meissner G, Henderson JS: Rapid calcium release from cardiac sarcoplasmic reticulum vesiche is dependent on Ca^{2+} and is modulated by Mg^{2+}, adenine nucleotide, and calmodulin. J Biol Chem 262: 3065-3073, 1987.）

脏 SR Ca^{2+} 释放会显著改变；另外缺血性心脏的 pH 变小，通道对 Ca^{2+} 敏感性会降低。

（二）钙调蛋白的调节

钙调蛋白是一种胞浆的蛋白，分子量 16.7kD，它与 RyR2 直接作用或与其他调节 SR Ca^{2+} 释放的蛋白相互作用来影响 SR Ca^{2+} 释放。它主要调节肌纤维膜电压依赖 L-型 Ca^{2+} 通道/二氢吡啶受体、钙调蛋白依赖性蛋白激酶和钙调蛋白刺激的蛋白磷酸酶，即钙调蛋白依赖的磷酸酶（calcineurin）[26]。

在缺少 ATP 时，钙调蛋白抑制 RyR2，表明钙调蛋白直接调节 RyR2，而不是通过磷酸化[27]。不依赖 Ca^{2+} 的浓度，纯化的 RyR2 每个亚基以纳摩级亲和力结合一个钙调蛋白。遗传突变已表明，完整的 RyR2 像 RyR1[28]，有一个高亲和力的钙调蛋白结合区域（氨基酸序列 3581-3610），无钙以及 Ca^{2+} 结合形式的

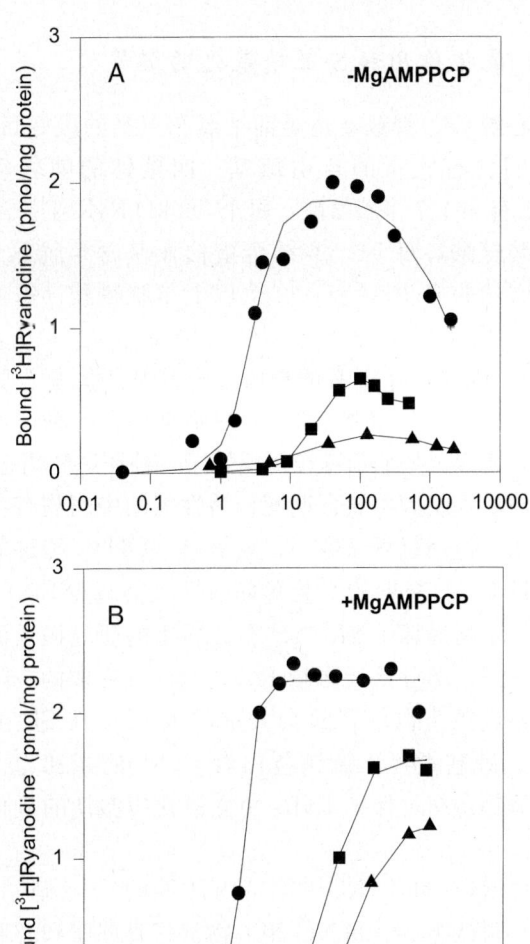

图 6-5 [^{3}H] ryanodine 与心脏肌浆网囊泡的结合依赖于 Ca^{2+} 和 pH 值 图 A：缺乏 5mM MgAMPPCP，以 0.1M KCl 溶液包含不同浓度的游离 Ca^{2+}，在 pH 7.3（实心图）、pH 6.5（实心方形）和 pH 6.2（实心三角）时 [^{3}H] ryanodine 与心脏肌浆网囊泡的结合图。图 B：存在 5mM MgAMPPCP，以 0.1M KCl 溶液包含不同浓度的游离 Ca^{2+}，在 pH 7.3（实心图）、pH 6.5（实心方形）和 pH6.2（实心三角）时 [^{3}H] ryanodine 与心脏肌浆网囊泡的结合图（引自 Xu L, Mann G, Meissner G: Regulation of cardiac Ca^{2+} release channel [ryanodine receptor] by Ca^{2+}, H^+, Mg^{2+}, and adenine nucleotides under normal and simulated ischemic conditions. Circ Res 79: 1100-1109, 1996.）

钙调蛋白均可共享这一结构域（N. Yamaguchi, L. Xu, andG. Meissner, 未发表的研究）。在微摩和毫摩 Ca^{2+} 浓度下，删除这个区域的 RyR2 可除去钙调蛋白的抑制。

（三）氧化作用和 S-亚硝基化的调节

心脏 Ca^{2+} 释放通道是活性氧和氮类的极好目标，因它们含有大量的自由巯基。四聚体的哺乳动物 RyR2 有 364 个半胱氨酸，每个 560kD RyR 亚基含 89 个半胱氨酸，每 FK506 结合蛋白亚基含半胱氨酸 2 个。天然的 RyR2，有 132 个以上半胱氨酸（每亚基 33 个）是自由的（J. Sun and G. Meissner，未发表的研究）。因此，在正常的心脏，在巯基还原复合物的作用下（主要是谷胱甘肽），细胞维持在一种还原性环境，所以大量的巯基很可能处于一种还原的状态。

缺血组织的再氧合期间，活性氧的中间物有广泛的形式，包括超氧（O_2^-）、氢氧基（OH^o）和过氧化氢（H_2O_2）。早期的实验解释活性氧类减少 SR Ca^{2+} 摄取，意指损坏了 SR Ca^{2+} 泵。后来的研究揭示活性氧的作用，部分是经影响 RyR2 的活性完成的，随着内源性调钙蛋白的释放会大量增加 Ca^{2+} 从 SR 的释放[27]。巯基氧可下调钙蛋白对 RyR2 的亲和力。反之，调钙蛋白可保护 RyRs 免受氧化应激期的氧化修饰。

RyR1[29] 和 RyR2[30] 都是内源性的硫-亚硝基物，因此，可认为 NO 和 NO 相关物都是骨骼肌和心肌细胞 E-C 耦联的生理调节剂。心肌细胞表达所有三种 NO 合酶（NOS）亚型：内皮 NOS（nNOS）、神经 NOS（nNOS）和可诱导的 NOS（iNOS）。它们都沿内皮排列，且全都能释放 NO。在正常心肌细胞，主要的亚型是 eNOS，靶目标是心肌细胞肌膜腔和内皮质膜腔的小窝蛋白。免疫电镜显示 nNOS 是离体心肌 SR 囊泡的标志，而在骨骼肌囊泡上未检测到[31]。这表明 SR 的 nNOS 是心肌细胞的特性。iNOS 在正常心脏缺乏或较少，但在病理状态下它的浓度可迅速增加[32]。

NO 是细胞功能的重要调节剂和实现许多心肌 E-C 耦联生理调节的关键[33-35]。在体外研究中，激活和抑制都有报告，说明 NO 对 RyRs 的分子调节有多种方式[33]。而且，构成骨骼肌和心肌植物碱受体 S-亚硝基化的机制不同。在 RyR1，有个单半胱氨酸（C3635），它位于钙调蛋白结合区，可受 NO 调节[1]。生理浓度 NO S-亚硝基化在肌肉（$Po_2 \sim 10mmHg$），依靠肌钙蛋白激活，但在周围氧分压 $Po_2 \sim 150mmHg$ 时则否。明显不同的是，NO 在低浓度或周围氧分压对 RyR2 几乎无影响（J. Sun and G. Meissner，未发表的研究）。反之，RyR1 和 RyR2 的激活都受 S-nitrosoglutathione 的调节[30,36]，后者是一种内生性 S-亚硝基硫醇，负责 S-亚硝基化作用和多种巯基的氧化作用。

（四）磷酸化的调节

RyR2 构成一个巨大的多蛋白复合物，包括蛋白激酶 A（PKA）、蛋白磷酸酶 1 和 2A（PP1 和 PP2A），和 PKA、PP1、PPA2 的锚蛋白，其通过亮氨酸/异亮氨酸的拉链结构基序与 RyR2 结合[37,38]。另外的蛋白激酶和磷酸酶对通道激活的调节已被描述。它们包括肌钙蛋白依赖性蛋白激酶 Ⅱ（CaMK Ⅱ），蛋白激酶 C 亚基 α、β 和钙调磷酸酶[1]。

RyR2 磷酸化的机制和功能影响已进行了广泛研究。RyR2 在 2943 位的丝氨基残基可被磷酸化；而体外 RyR2 的磷酸化结果有所不同[1]。在晚近的研究，PKA 磷酸化从 RyR2 解离 FKBP12.6，并增加低传导态的出现[38]。在心衰时，RyR2 大分子复合物 PP1、PPA2 水平降低而不是 PKA 活性增加可导致 RyR_2 超磷酸化和形成"泄漏"通道。这些资料受到 Jiang 和他的同事的研究结果挑战，他们观察到心衰时 Ca^{2+} 暂时下降和 SRCa^{2+} 摄取的减少，但 RyS 正常。

六、植物碱和咖啡因对 Ca^{2+} 释放通道的调节

在影响 SR Ca^{2+} 释放的大量药物和化学修饰反应中，植物碱和咖啡因因它们广泛用于评价 SR 调控细胞质 Ca^{2+} 的功能而著名[40,41]。单通道测量提供了腺苷和咖啡因最直接的作用，即显示植物碱调节 RyR2 的传导和门控行为，但咖啡因仅激活 RyR2，不调节传导。在图 6-6A，展示了植物碱调节前后的单 K^+ 传导、Ca^{2+} 激活、心脏 Ca^{2+} 释放通道。当通道进入长的持续稳定传导期，加 $2\mu M$ 植物碱 2 分钟后，它的门控动力学和传导被迅速改变。后来加入 $100\mu M$ 植物碱导致通道迅速关闭。通道低传导和完全关闭状态的典型性质是，对其他的配基如 Ca^{2+}、ATP 或 Mg^{2+} 对通道门控状态的影响不敏感（见图 6-3 到 6-5）。

与植物碱相反，咖啡因增加两个次高值 Ca^{2+} 激活心脏 RyR2 的开放时间，不改变单通道的传导率（见 6-6B）。咖啡因通过使 RyR2 对 Ca^{2+} 的激活更敏感来激活它（见 Liu 和他的同事[42] 及引文），且不降低它们对 Mg^{2+} 和 ATP 调节的敏感性。像植物碱一样，咖啡因被广泛用于评价 SR 和内质网对调控细胞的 Ca^{2+}

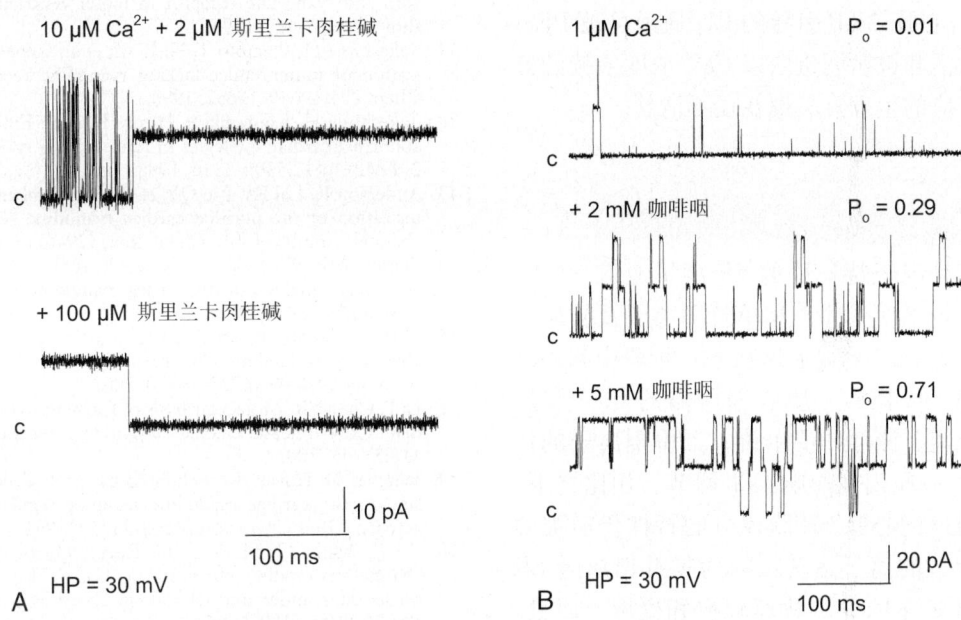

图 6-6 植物碱（斯里兰卡肉桂碱）和咖啡因对纯化和再生的犬心脏 Ca^{2+} 释放通道的影响　通道电流表现向上的偏差（c，闭合的通道），是在均衡的 0.25 M KCl、pH 7.35 包含必需的游离细胞质 Ca^{2+} 浓度介导的条件下记录的。A：上部的描迹表示出未受调节的通道一半的次级传导状态和通道开放概率（P_o）～1，是在加入 $2\mu M$ 胞质的植物碱。下部的描迹表示加入 $100\mu M$ 胞质的植物碱 1 分钟后从次级状态到完全闭合状态的过渡。B：两个纯化的心脏 Ca^{2+} 释放通道在缺乏（上面的描迹）和存在 2mM（中间的描迹）和 5mM 胞质咖啡因时记录的情况（From Xu L, Tripathy A, Pasek DA, et al：Potential for pHarmacology of ryanodine receptor/calcium release channel Ann NY Acad Sci 853：130-148，1998）

浓度的作用。应用咖啡因可提供多种便利，它能迅速和可逆地引起 Ca^{2+} 释放。咖啡因的两个限制是：激活需相当高的浓度，特异性不如植物碱。

七、K^+，Na^+ 通道

SR 上存在 K^+ 和 Na^+ 传导通道，首先在分离的兔骨骼肌 SR 囊泡证实，这是经核素流和膜电位及通过囊泡整合通道成平面双分子层实现的[4]。相似的单价阳离子传导通道随后在心脏的 SR 囊泡[4]和平面双分子层[43]上发现。同位素流、光散射和采用犬轻、重心脏 SR 囊泡进行膜电位的测量都表明，通道以超过 $50/\mu m^2$ 的密度遍及分布于 SR 细胞膜。

在平面脂质双分子层上，心脏 SR K^+ 通道表现慢-门控动力学及 101 和 157pS 两种传导率（在 500mM K^+）[44]。通道能被无机离子阻滞，包括 Cs^+，一个慢透过离子；和 Ca^{2+}，一个非透过离子。当毫摩尔浓度的 Ca^{2+} 出现在细胞质侧或 SR 腔侧或平面质双分子层两侧，Ca^{2+} 可阻滞通道。腔内毫摩尔浓度 Ca^{2+} 阻滞心脏 SR K^+ 通道是有趣的，因为 SR Ca^{2+} 释放期间的 Ca^{2+} 浓度减少可增加 K^+ 在心脏 SR 膜的穿透性。

八、H^+ 渗透性

在兔骨骼肌和犬心脏 SR 存在有效的 H^+ 渗透系统，是从存在非渗透性离子 $Tris^+$ 和 $Pipes^-$ 时通过由低到高 pH 值转运 SR 囊泡证实的[4]。兔骨骼肌 SR 囊泡的停流（stop-flow）测量法产生一个 pH 平衡半时（half-time）约 6ms，经过计算它相当于一个 H^+（OH^-）以 11cm/s 渗透[45]。通过观察 SR Ca^{2+} 泵可催化 1 个 Ca^{2+}：nH^+（n=1～1.5）的交换反应，可得到 H^+ 渗透通路生理功能的一些线索[46]。H^+-渗透通路可促进 Ca^{2+} 摄取期从 SR 流出的 H^+ 的返回过程。

九、Cl^- 通道

阴离子渗透 SR 膜的最初证据是由一些观察得到的，如氟化物、草酸盐、正磷酸盐或焦磷酸盐通过急速地转运 SR 囊泡内的 Ca^{2+} 来加强 ATP 激发的 Ca^{2+} 摄取。核素流和光散射实验证实了在骨骼肌和心脏囊泡上存在阴离子渗透通路[4]。利用平面脂质双分子层的单通道记录法已显示骨骼肌和心肌 SR 包含阴离子

通道，有传导磷酸盐阴离子[47]和腺嘌呤核苷酸包括ATP[48]的能力。心脏ATP引导的Cl^-通道可被PKA依赖的磷酸化激活和被钙调蛋白以Ca^{2+}浓度依赖的方式抑制。这些反应的生理意义现在还不清楚。

十、总结

心肌表达多种组织特异性的SR离子通道。包括Ca^{2+}释放通道（植物碱受体）和单价阳离子及阴离子选择性通道。心脏Ca^{2+}释放通道在E-C耦联中起关键作用，是通过从SR释放心肌收缩所需的Ca^{2+}实现的。通道已被分离、测序，受单价、二价阳离子的传导性以及Ca^{2+}、一些内在影响因素调节。相比之下，组成单价离子通道的心肌SR膜成分的特性仍需被确定。这些通道调节的离子运动被认为是补偿通过SR膜的电荷，从而支持Ca^{2+}的快速释放和摄取。而且，近期的证据表明，调节单价离子通道活性方法的细节还不十分清楚。

十一、致谢

作者感谢Daniel Pasek提供图6-1。对NIH基金ARI8687和HL27430的支持表示衷心的感谢。

（马克娟　浦介麟　译）

参 考 文 献

1. Meissner G: Regulation of mammalian ryanodine receptors. Front Biosci 7:2072–2080, 2002.
2. Franzini-Armstrong C, Protasi F: Ryanodine receptors of striated muscles: A complex channel capable of multiple interactions. Physiol Rev 77:699–729, 1997.
3. East JM: Sarco(endo)plasmic reticulum calcium pumps: recent advances in our understanding of structure/function and biology. Mol Membr Biol 17:189–200, 2000.
4. Meissner G: Monovalent ion and calcium ion fluxes in sarcoplasmic reticulum. Mol Cell Biochem 55:65–82, 1983.
5. Meissner G: Isolation and characterization of two types of sarcoplasmic reticulum vesicles. Biochim Biophys Acta 389:51–68, 1975.
6. Jones LR, Cala SE: Biochemical evidence for functional heterogeneity of cardiac sarcoplasmic reticulum vesicles. J Biol Chem 256:11809–11818, 1981.
7. Wier WG, Balke CW: Ca2+ release mechanisms, Ca2+ sparks, and local control of excitation-contraction coupling in normal heart muscle. Circ Res 85:770–776, 1999.
8. Wang SQ, Song LS, Lakatta EG, et al: Ca2+ signalling between single L-type Ca2+ channels and ryanodine receptors in heart cells. Nature 410:592–596, 2001.
9. Marx SO, Gaburjakova J, Gaburjakova M, et al: Coupled gating between cardiac calcium release channels (ryanodine receptors). Circ Res 88:1151–1158, 2001.
10. Carl SL, Felix K, Caswell AH, et al: Immunolocalization of sarcolemmal dihydropyridine receptor and sarcoplasmic reticular triadin and ryanodine receptor in rabbit ventricle and atrium. J Cell Biol 129:672–682, 1995.
11. Takeshima H, Ikemoto T, Nishi M, et al: Generation and characterization of mutant mice lacking ryanodine receptor type 3. J Biol Chem 271:19649–19652, 1996.
12. Takeshima H, Komazaki S, Hirose K, et al: Embryonic lethality and abnormal cardiac myocytes in mice lacking ryanodine receptor type 2. EMBO J 17:3309–3316, 1998.
13. Anderson K, Lai FA, Liu QY, et al: Structural and functional characterization of the purified cardiac ryanodine receptor-Ca2+ release channel complex. J Biol Chem 264:1329–1335, 1989.
14. Sharma MR, Penczek P, Grassucci R, et al: Cryoelectron microscopy and image analysis of the cardiac ryanodine receptor. J Biol Chem 273:18429–18434, 1998.
15. Du GG, Sandhu B, Khanna VK, et al: Topology of the Ca2+ release channel of skeletal muscle sarcoplasmic reticulum (RyR1). Proc Natl Acad Sci USA 99:16725–16730, 2002.
16. Li P, Chen SR: Molecular basis of Ca2+ activation of the mouse cardiac Ca2+ release channel (ryanodine receptor). J Gen Physiol 118:33–44, 2001.
17. Witcher D, Kovacs RJ, Schulman H, et al: Unique phosphorylation site on the cardiac ryanodine receptor regulates calcium channel activity. J Biol Chem 266:11144–11152, 1991.
18. Xu L, Mann G, Meissner G: Regulation of cardiac Ca2+ release channel (ryanodine receptor) by Ca2+, H+, Mg2+, and adenine nucleotides under normal and simulated ischemic conditions. Circ Res 79:1100–1109, 1996.
19. Tinker A, Lindsay AR, Williams AJ: Cation conduction in the calcium release channel of the cardiac sarcoplasmic reticulum under physiological and pathophysiological conditions. Cardiovasc Res 27:1820–1825, 1993.
20. Chen DP, Xu L, Tripathy A, et al: Selectivity and permeation in calcium release channel of cardiac muscle: Alkali metal ions. Biophys J 76:1346–1366, 1999.
21. MacKrill JJ: Protein-protein interactions in intracellular Ca2+-release channel function. Biochem J 337:345–361, 1999.
22. Marks AR: Ryanodine receptors, FKBP12, and heart failure. Front Biosci 7:970–977, 2002.
23. Xu L, Meissner G: Regulation of cardiac muscle Ca2+ release channel by sarcoplasmic reticulum lumenal Ca2+. Biophys J 75:2302–2312, 1998.
24. Sitsapesan R, Williams AJ: Regulation of current flow through ryanodine receptors by luminal Ca2+. J Membr Biol 159:179–185, 1997.
25. Sutko JL, Airey JA, Welch W, et al: The pharmacology of ryanodine and related compounds. Pharmacol Rev 49:53–98, 1997.
26. Anderson ME: Calmodulin and the Philosopher's stone. Changing Ca2+ into arrhythmias. J Cardiovasc Electrophysiol 13:195–197, 2002.
27. Balshaw DM, Yamaguchi N, Meissner G: Modulation of intracellular calcium-release channels by calmodulin. J Membr Biol 185:1–8, 2002.
28. Yamaguchi N, Xin C, Meissner G: Identification of apocalmodulin and Ca2+-calmodulin regulatory domain in skeletal muscle Ca2+ release channel, ryanodine receptor. J Biol Chem 276:22579–22585, 2001.
29. Eu JP, Sun J, Xu L: The skeletal muscle calcium release channel: Coupled O2 sensor and NO signaling functions. Cell 102:499–509, 2000.
30. Xu L, Eu JP, Meissner G, et al: Activation of the cardiac calcium release channel (ryanodine receptor) by poly-S-nitrosylation. Science 279:234–237, 1998.
31. Xu KY, Huso DL, Dawson TM, et al: Nitric oxide synthase in cardiac sarcoplasmic reticulum. Proc Natl Acad Sci USA 96:657–662, 1999.
32. Arstall MA, Sawyer DB, Fukazawa R, et al: Cytokine-mediated apoptosis in cardiac myocytes. The role of inducible nitric oxide synthase induction and peroxynitrite generation. Circ Res 85:829–840, 1999.
33. Eu JP, Xu L, Stamler JS, et al: Regulation of ryanodine receptors by reactive nitrogen species. Biochem Pharmacol 57:1079–1084, 1999.
34. Ziolo MT, Katoh H, Bers DM: Positive and negative effects of nitric oxide on Ca2+ sparks: Influence of beta-adrenergic stimulation. Am J Physiol 281:H2295–H2303, 2001.
35. Petroff MG, Kim SH, Pepe S, et al: Endogenous nitric oxide mechanisms mediate the stretch dependence of Ca2+ release in cardiomy-

36. Sun J, Xu L, Eu JP, et al: Nitric oxide, NOC-12 and S-nitrosoglutathione modulate the skeletal muscle calcium release channel/ryanodine receptor by different mechanisms: An allosteric function for O_2 in S-nitrosylation of the channel. J Biol Chem 278:8184–8189, 2003.
37. Marx S, Reiken S, Hisamatsu Y, et al: Phosphorylation-dependent regulation of ryanodine receptors: A novel role for leucine/isoleucine zippers. J Cell Biol 153:699–708, 2001.
38. Marx S, Reiken S, Hisamatsu Y, et al: PKA phosphorylation dissociates FKBP12.6 from the calcium release channel (ryanodine receptor): Defective regulation in failing hearts. Cell 101:365–376, 2000.
39. Jiang MT, Lokuta AJ, Farrell EF, et al: Abnormal Ca2+ release, but normal ryanodine receptors, in canine and human hearts. Circ Res 91:1015–1022, 2002.
40. Zucchi R, Ronca-Testoni S: The sarcoplasmic reticulum Ca2+ channel/ryanodine receptor: Modulation by endogenous effectors, drugs and disease states. Pharmacol Rev 49:1–51, 1997.
41. Xu L, Tripathy A, Pasek DA, et al: Potential for pharmacology of ryanodine receptor/calcium release channel. Ann NY Acad Sci 853:130–148, 1998.
42. Liu W, Pasek DA, Meissner G: Modulation of Ca2+-gated cardiac muscle Ca2+-release channel (ryanodine receptor) by mono- and divalent ions. Am J Physiol 274:C120–C128, 1998.
43. Tomlins B, Williams AJ, Mongomery RAP: The characterization of a monovalent cation- selective channel of mammalian cardiac muscle sarcoplasmic reticulum. J Membr Biol 80:191–199, 1984.
44. Liu QY, Strauss HC: Blockade of cardiac sarcoplasmic reticulum K+ channel by Ca2+: Two-binding-site model of blockade. Biophys J 60:198–203, 1991.
45. Nunogaki K, Kasai M: Determination of the rate of rapid pH equilibration across isolated sarcoplasmic reticulum membranes. Biochem Biophys Res Comm 140:934–940, 1986.
46. Levy D, Seigneure M, Bluzat A, et al: Evidence for proton countertransport by the sarcoplasmic reticulum Ca2+-ATPase during calcium transport in reconstituted proteoliposomes with low ionic permeability. J Biol Chem 265:19524–19534, 1990.
47. Laver DR, Lenz GK, Dulhunty AF: Phosphate ion channels in sarcoplasmic reticulum of rabbit skeletal muscle. J Physiol 535:715–728, 2001.
48. Kawano S, Kuruma A, Hirayama Y, et al: Anion permeability and conduction of adenine nucleotides through a chloride channel in cardiac sarcoplasmic reticulum. J Biol Chem 274:2085–2092, 1999.

第 7 章

HCN 通道：从基因到功能

Andreas Ludwig, Juliane Stieber, Moosmang, Stefan Herrmann, Martin Biel, Franz Hofmann

本章目录

- HCN 通道的分子基础 ·············· 60
- HCN 通道的结构-功能关系 ········· 61
- HCN 离子通道复合物的形成 ········ 62
- HCN 通道在心脏的表达 ············ 63
- 心脏 HCN 通道和天然 I_f ·········· 63
- 鼠 HCN2 的敲除 ··················· 63
- 总结 ······························ 65

心脏的起搏细胞表现为独有的动作电位形式，与心房和心室肌细胞不同，它们有一个缓慢的除极过程，从而产生自主激活，这一过程至少由 3 种阳离子通道相互作用产生，即 HCN 通道（超极化激活的环核苷酸门控通道）、T-和 L-型钙离子（Ca^{2+}）通道。研究心脏起搏电流的分子基础对基础研究人员和临床医生同样有意义，因为通过调节这些离子通道来控制心率和节律是重要的干预措施。这一章节主要介绍 HCN 通道，它产生 I_f 电流（也称为 I_h 或 I_q）。I_f 在心脏和脑负责产生起搏活动，因此被命名为"起搏电流"。另外，此电流还具有其他功能，包括在脑内对震荡活性（Oscillatory activity）、兴奋性及可塑性的控制。在过去的几年里，随着 I_f 电流分子基础被确定，对 HCN 通道分子构成及功能的了解也显著增加。

一、HCN 通道的分子基础

人们对 I_f 通道的电生理特性已经有了很好的了解（见参考文献 1 和 2）。这一通道不同于大多数电压依赖性离子通通的一个显著特点是，它的激活依赖于膜的超极化而不是膜的除极。它对钾离子（K^+）和钠离子（Na^+）通透，对 K^+ 的选择性是 Na^+ 的 4 倍。在窦房结细胞最大舒张电位（大约 -60～-75mV），I_f 通道产生内向电流使膜除极达到 T 型和 L 型钙离子通道激活电位（图 7-1）。环腺嘌呤单核苷酸（cAMP）调节 I_f 通道电压激活特性，cAMP 与通道的直接结合改变激活曲线，使其趋于激活电压，通道开放更完全，此外，还加速了通道的激活。cAMP 对通道的这种作用（图 7-1）可以解释 β 肾上腺素受体激动剂增加心率的反应（提高了细胞内 cAMP 水平）[3]。同样，胆碱受体激动剂通过降低 cAMP 水平可以阻止通道的开放，降低心率[4]。

最近，一些研究小组成功地克隆出编码 I_f 通道的 cDNAs[5-10]，通道被命名为超极化激活的环核苷酸门控阳离子通道（HCN）。在哺乳动物，确定了 4 种不同的基因，HCN1～HCN4，克隆 cDNA 的种属由小写字母代表（如：hHCN 指人 HCN2 通道），在海胆和 heliotbis virescens 中发现了亲缘相近的基因 spHCN[11] 和 HvCNG[12]。4 种哺乳动物基因在心脏和脑组织表达[5,6,8]，但是，不同 HCN 构型在不同类型心脏和神经细胞中表达有很大的不同。

HCN 通道家族属于电压门控阳离子通道超家族，与环核苷酸门控通道（CNG）和 eag 钾离子通道家族亦有一定的关系。HCN 通道由 6 个跨膜部分组成（S1～S6），包括带正电荷的 S4 部分，作为电压敏感器（图 7-2）[14,15]，在第 5 和 6 跨膜段之间是离子转运的孔区，蛋白的羧基端具有环核苷酸结合域（CNBD），因此，HCN 通道既有电压门控结构特性又有环核苷酸门控特性，这与通道被膜电位和 cAMP 双调节相一致。

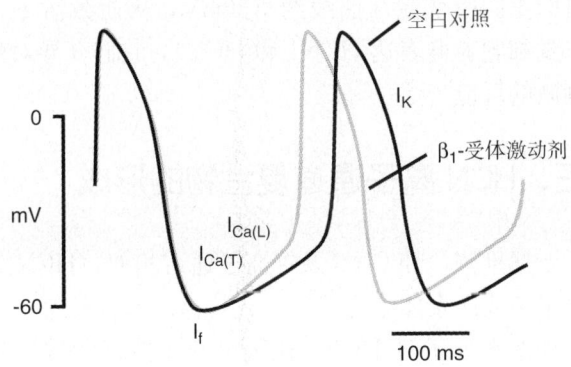

图 7-1 窦房结动作电位 在空白对照（黑色）和存在 β_1-肾上腺受体激动剂（灰色）下的窦房结细胞动作电位。显示了触发窦房结起搏活动的 4 种电流：I_f，超极化激活阳离子电流；$I_{Ca(T)}$，T 型 Ca^{2+} 电流；$I_{Ca(L)}$，L 型 Ca^{2+} 电流；I_k，延迟整流 K^+ 电流

HCN1 到 HCN4 之间密切相关，氨基酸序列达 60% 相似，6 个跨膜段和 CNBD 高度保守，相似序列达 80%～90%，相反，通道的氨基和羧基端各不相同。

二、HCN 通道的结构-功能关系

在异源表达系统，每种 HCN 构型产生一种超极化激活电流（HCN1[8]，HCN2[5,6]，HCN3[16]，HCN4[6,9,10]），它们具有天然 I_f 的典型特征，即被超极化膜电位激活，被铯（Cs^+）阻断。然而，由 4 种构型产生的电流的激活动力学、激活电压和 cAMP 调节程度是不同的。

（一）激活动力学

根据 HCN 通道的激活速度，可以清楚地区别 4 种构型，HCN1 最快被激活（激活时间常数 τ 在 −70 到 −140mV 电位范围内是 30ms 和 300ms 之间），HCN2 和 HCN3 位于中间（τ 在 200ms 到 500ms），HCN4 最慢（τ 在 300ms 到几秒）。通道开放速度主要依赖于膜电位，超极化电位越大，开放越快。影响 HCN 通道门控动力学的另一个重要因素是温度。

（二）激活的电压依赖性

报道的每种通道的半激活电位（$V_{1/2}$）存在很大差异，例如，HCN4 的 $V_{1/2}$ 值从 −75 到 −110mV[6,9,10]，已清楚显示这种差异至少部分是由于使用不同的脉冲程序[10,17]，短的电压脉冲不能激活通道达到稳定状态，预测的 $V_{1/2}$ 值偏向于负值，此外，实验用溶液的离子构成能影响电流的特征。因此，在比较天然通道和克隆通道的生理特性时应考虑上述参数。在相同条件下 4 种 HCN 通道的 $V_{1/2}$ 值并无显著差别[16]。

HCN 通道的超极化门控活动在两种模型中被描述[18,19]。一种模型认为，HCN 通道在静息膜电位处于失活态，超极化使通道从失活态转变为开放态（失活恢复），在这一模型中，S4 段不依赖超极化移动。另一模型认为，S4 段感受膜电位变化，超极化时向内移动，除极时向外移动，这意味着 HCN 通道 S4 段的活动方向与除极激活通道一样，然而，在 HCN 通道，S4 的内向移动将开放激活门，而在除极激活通道这一移动是关闭门。支持第二种模型的直接实验证据来自于对 spHCN 的 S4 段半胱氨酸残基电压依赖易感性的研究[15]，它显示 S4 段超极化时向内移动，除极时向外移动。由于 HCN 通道和超极化激活通道的开放对电压的反应相反，那么两者的电压感受器和激活门之间的耦联机制一定不同。

HCN 通道连接第 4 和第 5 跨膜段的细胞内连接子上，丙苷酸移码突变表明这一区域对于 S4 段的移动与激活门的开放及关闭之间的耦联非常重要[20]，激活门本身可能位于通道孔区细胞内侧[21,22]。

（三）离子选择性

HCN 通道孔区携带 GYG 氨基酸模体，形成了 K^+ 通道上的选择通透装置，但与这些通道相反，

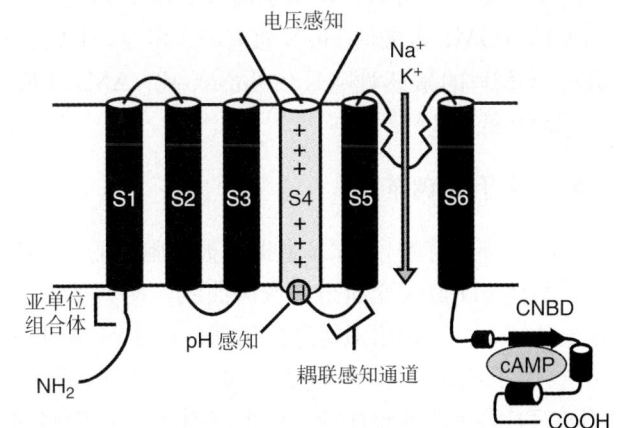

图 7-2 超极化激活环核苷酸门控离子通道（HCN）的主要结构 柱形图示 6 个跨膜段 S1～S6。正电荷充电的 S4 段是通道的电压感受器。⑪、CNBD（环核苷酸结合域）分别代表通道 pH 值感受器和位于 S4 段与 S4-S5 连接子间组氨酸残基。细胞浆 S4-S5 连接子对于 S4 移动与激活门开放和关闭间的耦联非常重要

HCN 通道对 K⁺ 有低选择性（$P_{Na}/P_K = 0.15 \sim 0.25$）[5,8,11]，这意味着 HCN 通道在生理状态下携带除极的 Na⁺ 电流。对于 HCN 通道孔区存在 GYG 模体，为什么对 K⁺ 却是低选择性还不清楚。除了 GYG 模体，其他区域可能联合决定着离子选择特性。

（四）环核苷酸的调节

4 种 HCN 构型通过羧基端的 CNBD 来介导 cAMP 的调节作用，这一结构域与 cAMP 和环鸟嘌呤单核苷酸（cGMP）依赖性蛋白激酶[23]、cAMP-鸟嘌呤核苷酸交换因子 Epac[24] 及 CNG 离子通道的 CN-BDs 有 40%左右的同源性[13]。cAMP 改变激活电压为正向电压从而触发 HCN 通道的激活，cAMP 还可提高通道的激活速度。然而，4 种 HCN 通道对 cAMP 的反应程度各不相同，cAMP 对 HCN2 和 HCN4 的调节能力强（$V_{1/2}$ 被改变约$+10 \sim +15mV$）；相反，HCN1 的激活曲线被环核苷酸改变得很少[25-27]。

有实验显示去除 CNBD 区域，通道的激活电压转为正向，这与 cAMP 对野生型通道的作用相似，说明在无 cAMP 结合状态下，CNBD 通过将电位控制在超极化电位以下来阻止通道的激活，cAMP 与 CNBD 的结合减少了这种阻滞作用，HCN1 和 HCN2 通道被阻滞程度的不同可以解释两者对 cAMP 反应性的差别，HCN1 被 CNBD 轻度阻滞（去除 CNBD，向正向电压转变很小），而 HCN2 被阻滞的程度较大（去除 CN-BD，向正向电压转变很大）。因此，HCN2 对 cAMP 的反应程度大，而 HCN1 只轻度被 cAMP 影响。除了 cAMP，cGMP 也激活 HCN 通道[5]，但是，HCN2 通道对 cGMP 的敏感性（$K_a = 6\mu M$）比 cAMP（$K_a = 0.5\mu M$）低约 10 倍。

（五）质子的调节

除了环核苷酸，HCN 通道还被细胞内的 pH 值调节。酸性 pH 值改变通道的激活曲线，使其偏向超极化电位以下，从而阻滞通道的激活。位于 S4 段和 S4-S5 连接子间的一个保守的组氨酸残基（HCN2 的 His321）是 pH 敏感性的主要决定因素[30]。细胞内质子对通道活性的作用可以调节丘脑延迟或脑干神经元，对控制心脏 HCN 通道也同样重要。缺血时，细胞 pH 可以降至 6.0 甚至更低，心脏传导系统 HCN 通道活性被质子阻滞会破坏节律的产生，引起（缓慢）性心律失常。

与细胞内质子的作用相比，强酸性的细胞外溶液可向正向改变激活曲线约$+30mV$，从而激活 I_b。一味觉细胞亚群表达 HCN1 和 HCN4，它们介导对酸性刺激的反应[31]。

三、HCN 离子通道复合物的形成

据推测，和 CNG 及钾离子通道相似，HCN 亚单位组装成四聚体结构[32,33]。支持这一假设的第一个实验证据来自于对 HCN1 孔区突变显性抑制效应的研究[34]，突变的离子通道以剂量依赖形式抑制了联合表达的野生型 HCN1。这一结果符合 HCN 通道为四聚体结构的假设。通道氨基末端保守区域间的相互作用被认为对亚单位的联合表达非常重要[35,36]。

由于在单细胞型中构建了几种 HCN 异构体（如：在窦房结细胞构建了 HCN2+4[16]，在海马 CA1 神经元细胞构建了 HCN1、HCN2 和 HCN4，在丘脑延迟神经元细胞构建了 HCN2+4[17,37]），因此人们产生了 HCN 亚单位是否能形成异源异构体的疑问。在蟾蜍卵母细胞上构建 HCN1+HCN2 样结构和联合表达单一的 HCN1 和 HCN2 亚单位都产生了一种电流，它的特点介于 HCN1 和 HCN2 同源聚合体电流之间，这一结果与具有天然生理特性的异源聚合通道相一致。而且，HCN1 孔区突变通过显性抑制作用抑制了联合表达的 HCN2，表明 HCN 亚单位确实能够形成异源聚合复合物[34]。

同源聚合体仅在 HCN1 和 HCN2 间被构建，考虑到 HCN 异构体间高度的同源性，其他 HCN 亚单位的联合构建也是可行的，但还没有相关研究。

HCN 通道异源聚合体上亚单位间的定量关系还不清楚，可能是 2:2，因为 HCN 通道属于 P 环超家族通道成员，一般认为 P 环结构通道具有围绕中心孔区的四折叠聚合结构[39]。然而，三种不同实验方法一致显示在这一家族中，与 HCN 通道相邻的 CNG 通道以 3:1 的关系形成异源聚合体[40-42]。

一个公认的问题是，HCN 异源聚合体不仅能在异源表达系统形成，是否也能在体内形成。一个表达几种 HCN 基因的天然细胞有可能只产生同源聚合通道，那么不同的 HCN 构型复合物可能在不同的细胞被表达（如：体细胞、神经元和神经轴突）。值得注意的是，几种细胞类型已被确定只表达单一的 HCN 构型（例如：小脑球细胞、视网膜光感受器细胞只显示唯一的 HCN1 信号）[16,37]，这支持天然 HCN 通道可能也存在同源聚合体的假设。

HCN 通道的辅助亚单位可能是 minK-相关多肽 MiRP1（KCNE2）。MiRP1 与 HCN1 或 HCN2 联合表达增加了 HCN 电流密度，加速了通道的激活[43]。但是，在天然通道复合物上也未显示有 MiRP1 与 HCN 的联合。

四、HCN 通道在心脏的表达

已发现 HCN1、HCN2 和 HCN4 在成人心脏表达，在心脏的不同部位亚单位的表达形式不同，并具有某种种属特异性。迄今在所有研究的种属中，HCN4 在窦房结细胞表达程度最高，它占全部 HCN 信号的 80% 以上[16,44]。在鼠的窦房结细胞，其他的 HCN mRNA 是 HCN2 mRNA；原位杂交实验仅发现很少量的 HCN1[16]。在兔的窦房结细胞，HCN1 的表达显著高于鼠的[25,44]。

在犬的心脏浦氏纤维，也发现了 HCN4 转录产物和其蛋白[45]。在这些细胞，HCN4 mRNA 的表达显著高于 HCN2，并未发现 HCN1 的表达。相比之下，与兔的窦房结细胞一样，兔的浦氏纤维表达 HCN4 和 HCN1[44]。

在心房和心室肌细胞也发现了 HCN 通道的转录产物。在非起搏细胞，主要存在 HCN2，在鼠、犬和人的工作心肌细胞还存在少量的 HCN[6,16,45]。

五、心脏 HCN 通道和天然 I_f

如前所述，文献中 I_f 与重构的 HCN 电流特性间的比较因采用不同的电流实验参数而受阻，从所报道的窦房结 I_f 的 $V_{1/2}$ 值（-65～-92mV）和激活时间常数的范围较大可看出这一点，这种差别部分与实验的设置不同有关。图 7-3 为相同条件下 HEK293 细胞 HCN 通道和窦房结 I_f 通道的对比。显然，窦房结 I_f 主要为 HCN4 电流，天然电流略快的激活动力学特性符合窦房结 I_f 由 HCN4（主要，缓慢激活）和 HCN2（少量，快速激活）联合活性产生的假设。在一些种属，如兔，有必要进行基因敲除实验（见后）来共同确定心脏 I_f 的分子基础。

尽管存在实验的差别，但很明显心室肌细胞比窦房结细胞 I_f 的电流密度低，有更负的 $V_{1/2}$ 值（-95～-135mV）[33]。据报道缺血性心脏病病人的心室肌细胞与对照组相比，有两倍高的 I_f 电流密度，激活曲线向正向电位改变[46,47]，从而增加了缺血心脏 I_f 通过产生病理除极电流引起心律失常发生的可能性。

心室细胞和窦房结 I_f 的 $V_{1/2}$ 值的不同不足以被这些区域 HCN2 和 HCN4 表达差异所揭示，因为这两种通道的电压依赖性非常相似[16]。其他的细胞因素（除了 cAMP 或质子）和辅助亚单位可能影响 HCN 异构体的电压依赖性，对新生儿和成人心室肌细胞过度表达 HCN2 的研究显示了这一点[48]，已知新生儿心肌细胞 I_f 的激活电压不像成人细胞那样负，然而成人和新生儿细胞过度表达 HCN2 通道，激活电压却有相同的差别（+20mV），这一差别并不来自于内源性 cAMP 水平的不同，因此，心肌细胞的发育状态对 HCN2 异构体的电压依赖性有很强的决定性。

六、鼠 HCN2 的敲除

据我们所知，我们实验室首先发表了关于 HCN 通道基因去除鼠系的生成和分析的文章[49]。我们用以 Cre/loxP 为基础的方法，敲除了 HCN2 通道。HCN2 缺乏鼠比野生型同产鼠小，活动和捕捉能力减弱，此外，还发生窦性心律失常。HCN2 的缺乏并不引起其他 HCN 通道表达的升高，表明不同 HCN 构型在功能上并不是多余的。接下来主要讨论这些鼠的心脏表型。

HCN2 缺乏鼠心电图显示为 RR 间期有很大不同的窦性心律失常，在静息时明显，运动时消失。P 波、QRS 波和 PQ 间期没有变化。有趣的是，野生鼠和基因敲除鼠在静息和自发活动时心率没有差别，β 受体激动剂和阿托品对心率升高的程度在 HCN2$^{-/-}$ 鼠和野生型鼠一样。I_f 的主要作用是调节心率对交感神经刺激的反应[1]。实验结果表明对于 β 受体激动剂的变时作用 HCN2 并不是必需的。

两种不同的实验显示心律失常确实是由于窦房结缺陷引起。首先，从 HCN2 缺乏鼠分离的心房存在心律失常搏动，说明心脏存在自主缺陷；第二，心肌细胞特异性去除 HCN2 的鼠与整体缺乏 HCN2 的鼠有相同的窦性心律失常，说明窦性心律失常是由窦房结功能障碍引起，并不依赖于所提到的 HCN2$^{-/-}$ 神经缺陷。

从 HCN2 敲除鼠分离的窦房结细胞与野生型的相比，它们的 I_f 大约减少了 30%（图 7-4B），此外，激活的电流显著减慢。这些结果提供了以下证据：（1）HCN2 产生部分 I_f，（2）窦房结 I_f 的主要成分是由比 HCN2 门控更慢的通道产生，可能是 HCN4。

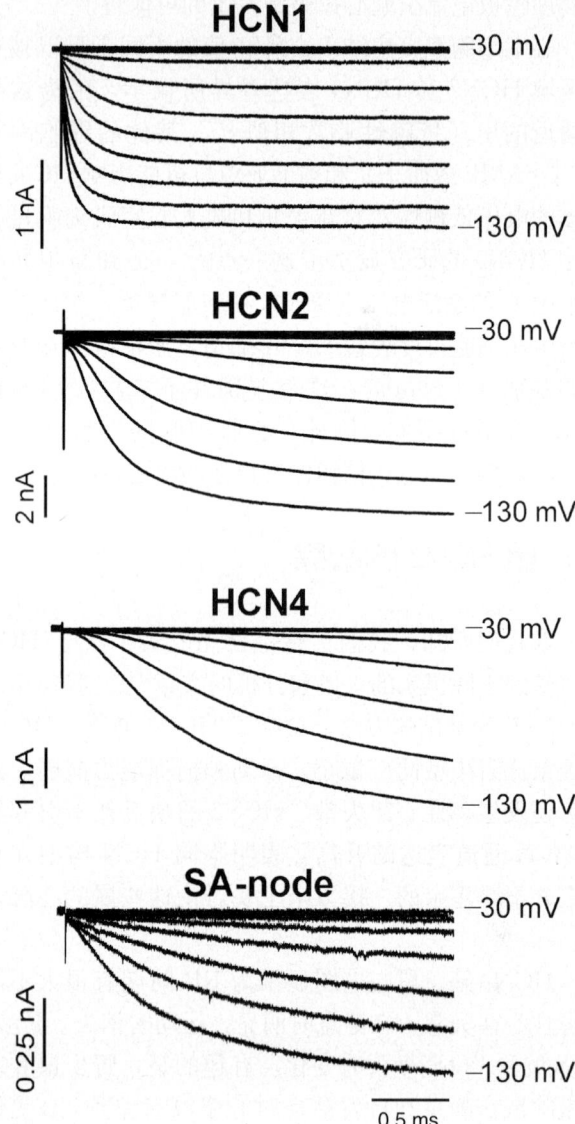

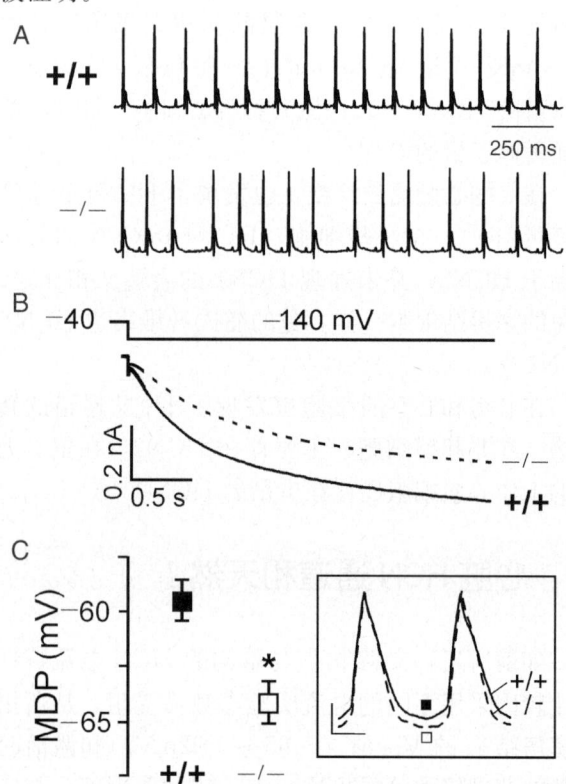

12mV，说明这些细胞在静息时，HCN2 被激活增强，静息电位处于过除极水平，HCN2 在窦房结细胞也有同样的功能，HCN2 敲除细胞的最大舒张电位比野生型的负 5mV（图 7-4C）。因此，HCN2 在窦房结可能主要是控制静息膜电位。以下机制主要解释 HCN2 缺陷鼠的心律失常：HCN2 的缺失使膜超极化，可能破坏动作电位有规律的产生，过度的超极化（如：K^+ 通道活性升高）不能被很快的限制，从而导致下一个动作电位产生延迟。

HCN2 缺陷鼠的表型意味着在人类，HCN2 功能缺陷将引起运动失常性癫痫和窦房结功能障碍，但还未被证明。

图 7-3　HCN 通道和窦房结通道间的对比　记录的表达在 HEK293 细胞上鼠 HCN1、人 HCN2、人 HCN4 通道电流及鼠窦房结细胞 I_f 电流。电流在室温、相同条件下全细胞电压记录。钳制电位 −40mV，电压从 −30 到 −130mV 范围。使用溶液如下：细胞外液：120NaCl，20KCl，$MgCl_2$，$2CaCl_2$，10 4-(2-hydroxyethyl)-1-piperazineethanesulfonic acid (HEPES)，10glucose，$2BaCl_2$，$2MnCl_2$，$0.3CdCl_2$，pH 7.4；电极内液：10 NaCL，30 KCl，90 L-aspartic acid monopotassium (K-Asp)，1 $MgSO_4$，10 HEPES，5 [ethylenebis (oxyethylenenitrilo)] tetraacetic acid (EDTA)，3 Mg-ATP，pH 7.4。窦房结细胞是从野生型成鼠分离的梭形细胞

HCN2 敲除鼠的丘脑皮质神经元 I_f 几乎完全消失。这些神经元的静息膜电位比野生型细胞大约负

图 7-4　HCN 缺陷鼠的心脏表型　A：野生型和 HCN2-缺陷型鼠静息心电图（Ⅱ导联）。B：窦房结细胞 I_f 电流，野生型（实线）和 $HCN2^{-/-}$（虚线）鼠分离的窦房结细胞的平均电流曲线，从钳制电位 −40～−140mV 的全细胞膜片钳记录。C：由窦房结细胞自发动作电位决定的最大舒张电位（MDP），星号代表 $P<0.05$。插图是野生型和 HCN2 缺陷型细胞的动作电位。刻度方块：200msec，20mV（引自 Ludwig A，Zong X，Stieber J，et al：Absence epilepsy and sinus dysrhythmia in mice lacking the pacemaker channel HCN2. EMBO J 22：216-224，2003. C European Molecular Biology Organization.）

HCN4 的生理作用

近来的文献中描述了特发性窦性心动过缓和变时无能病人 HCN4 的杂合突变。突变导致 HCN4 通道缺乏 CNBD 结构域,对 cAMP 不敏感,改变了失活动力学机制。联合表达实验显示突变通道对野生型通道有显性抑制效应。不幸的是,并没有获得有关突变引起疾病的遗传连锁数据,然而,实验结果支持 HCN4 是窦房结起搏的主要成分这一假设。对鼠 HCN4 通道的定点敲除技术无疑简化了对此通道生理功能的研究。

七、总结

编码超极化激活阳离子通道的 4 个基因已经确定,HCN 的构型和组织特异性的差异能部分解释各种兴奋细胞 I_f 的不同生理特性。其他一些因素,如同源聚合体和辅助亚单位可能造成了 I_f 的多样性。基因敲除实验已经开始用于确定整体动物 HCN 通道的生理功能。联合遗传、生化和生理学方法的深入研究将阐明不同 HCN 构型与 I_f 生理功能间的关系。

(浦介麟　马克娟　译)

参 考 文 献

1. DiFrancesco D: Pacemaker mechanisms in cardiac tissue. Annu Rev Physiol 55:455–472, 1993.
2. Pape HC: Queer current and pacemaker: The hyperpolarization-activated cation current in neurons. Annu Rev Physiol 58:299–327, 1996.
3. DiFrancesco D, Tortora P: Direct activation of cardiac pacemaker channels by intracellular cyclic AMP. Nature 351:145–147, 1991.
4. DiFrancesco D, Ducouret P, Robinson RB: Muscarinic modulation of cardiac rate at low acetylcholine concentrations. Science 243:669–671, 1989.
5. Ludwig A, Zong X, Jeglitsch M, et al: A family of hyperpolarization-activated mammalian cation channels. Nature 393:587–591, 1998.
6. Ludwig A, Zong X, Stieber J, et al: Two pacemaker channels from human heart with profoundly different activation kinetics. EMBO J 18:2323–2329, 1999.
7. Santoro B, Grant SG, Bartsch D, Kandel ER: Interactive cloning with the SH3 domain of N-src identifies a new brain specific ion channel protein, with homology to eag and cyclic nucleotide-gated channels. Proc Natl Acad Sci U S A 94:14815–14820, 1997.
8. Santoro B, Liu DT, Yao H, et al: Identification of a gene encoding a hyperpolarization-activated pacemaker channel of brain. Cell 93:717–729, 1998.
9. Ishii TM, Takano M, Xie LH, et al: Molecular characterization of the hyperpolarization-activated cation channel in rabbit heart sinoatrial node. J Biol Chem 274:12835–12839, 1999.
10. Seifert R, Scholten A, Gauss R, et al: Molecular characterization of a slowly gating human hyperpolarization-activated channel predominantly expressed in thalamus, heart, and testis. Proc Natl Acad Sci U S A 96:9391–9396, 1999.
11. Gauss R, Seifert R, Kaupp UB: Molecular identification of a hyperpolarization-activated channel in sea urchin sperm. Nature 393:583–587, 1998.
12. Krieger J, Strobel J, Vogl A, et al: Identification of a cyclic nucleotide- and voltage-activated ion channel from insect antennae. Insect Biochem Mol Biol 29:255–267, 1999.
13. Biel M, Zong X, Ludwig A, et al: Structure and function of cyclic nucleotide-gated channels. Rev Physiol Biochem Pharmacol 135:151–171, 1999.
14. Vaca L, Stieber J, Zong X, et al: Mutations in the S4 domain of a pacemaker channel alter its voltage dependence. FEBS Lett 479:35–40, 2000.
15. Mannikko R, Elinder F, Larsson HP: Voltage-sensing mechanism is conserved among ion channels gated by opposite voltages. Nature 419:837–841, 2002.
16. Moosmang S, Stieber J, Zong X, et al: Cellular expression and functional characterization of four hyperpolarization-activated pacemaker channels in cardiac and neuronal tissues. Eur J Biochem 268:1646–1652, 2001.
17. Santoro B, Chen S, Luthi A, et al: Molecular and functional heterogeneity of hyperpolarization-activated pacemaker channels in the mouse CNS. J Neurosci 20:5264–5275, 2000.
18. Santoro B, Tibbs GR: The HCN gene family: Molecular basis of the hyperpolarization-activated pacemaker channels. Ann N Y Acad Sci 868:741–764, 1999.
19. Biel M, Schneider A, Wahl C: Cardiac HCN channels: structure, function, and modulation. Trends Cardiovasc Med 12:206–212, 2002.
20. Chen J, Mitcheson JS, Tristani-Firouzi M, et al: The S4–S5 linker couples voltage sensing and activation of pacemaker channels. Proc Natl Acad Sci U S A 98:11277–11282, 2001.
21. Shin KS, Rothberg BS, Yellen G: Blocker state dependence and trapping in hyperpolarization-activated cation channels: Evidence for an intracellular activation gate. J Gen Physiol 117:91–101, 2001.
22. Rothberg BS, Shin KS, Phale PS, Yellen G: Voltage-controlled gating at the intracellular entrance to a hyperpolarization-activated cation channel. J Gen Physiol 119:83–91, 2002.
23. Pfeifer A, Ruth P, Dostmann W, et al: Structure and function of cGMP-dependent protein kinases. Rev Physiol Biochem Pharmacol 135:105–149, 1999.
24. de Rooij J, Zwartkruis FJ, Verheijen MH, et al: Epac is a Rap1 guanine-nucleotide-exchange factor directly activated by cyclic AMP. Nature 396:474–477, 1998.
25. Moroni A, Gorza L, Beltrame M, et al: Hyperpolarization-activated cyclic nucleotide-gated channel 1 is a molecular determinant of the cardiac pacemaker current I_f. J Biol Chem 276:29233–29241, 2001.
26. Ulens C, Tytgat J: Functional heteromerization of HCN1 and HCN2 pacemaker channels. J Biol Chem 276:6069–6072, 2001.
27. Wainger BJ, DeGennaro M, Santoro B, et al: Molecular mechanism of cAMP modulation of HCN pacemaker channels. Nature 411:805–810, 2001.
28. Wang J, Chen S, Siegelbaum SA: Regulation of hyperpolarization-activated HCN channel gating and cAMP modulation due to interactions of COOH terminus and core transmembrane regions. J Gen Physiol 118:237–250, 2001.
29. Munsch T, Pape HC: Modulation of the hyperpolarization-activated cation current of rat thalamic relay neurones by intracellular pH. J Physiol 519(Pt 2):493–504, 1999.
30. Zong X, Stieber J, Ludwig A, et al: A single histidine residue determines the pH sensitivity of the pacemaker channel HCN2. J Biol Chem 276:6313–6319, 2001.
31. Stevens DR, Seifert R, Bufe B, et al: Hyperpolarization-activated channels HCN1 and HCN4 mediate responses to sour stimuli. Nature 413:631–635, 2001.
32. Biel M, Ludwig A, Zong X, Hofmann F: Hyperpolarization-activated cation channels: A multi-gene family. Rev Physiol Biochem Pharmacol 136:165–181, 1999.
33. Ludwig A, Zong X, Hofmann F, Biel M: Structure and function of cardiac pacemaker channels. Cell Physiol Biochem 9:179–186, 1999.
34. Xue T, Marban E, Li RA: Dominant-negative suppression of HCN1- and HCN2-encoded pacemaker currents by an engineered HCN1 construct: Insights into structure-function relationships and multimerization. Circ Res 90:1267–1273, 2002.
35. Proenza C, Tran N, Angoli D, et al: Different roles for the cyclic nucleotide binding domain and amino terminus in assembly and expression of hyperpolarization-activated, cyclic nucleotide-gated channels. J Biol Chem 277:29634–29642, 2002.
36. Tran N, Proenza C, Macri V, et al: A conserved domain in the NH2 terminus important for assembly and functional expression of pacemaker channels. J Biol Chem 277:43588–43592, 2002.
37. Moosmang S, Biel M, Hofmann F, Ludwig A: Differential distribu-

tion of four hyperpolarization-activated cation channels in mouse brain. Biol Chem 380:975–980, 1999.
38. Chen S, Wang J, Siegelbaum SA: Properties of hyperpolarization-activated pacemaker current defined by coassembly of HCN1 and HCN2 subunits and basal modulation by cyclic nucleotide. J Gen Physiol 117:491–504, 2001.
39. Doyle DA, Morais Cabral J, Pfuetzner RA, et al: The structure of the potassium channel: molecular basis of K$^+$ conduction and selectivity. Science 280:69–77, 1998.
40. Weitz D, Ficek N, Kremmer E, et al: Subunit stoichiometry of the CNG channel of rod photoreceptors. Neuron 36:881–889, 2002.
41. Zheng J, Trudeau MC, Zagotta WN: Rod cyclic nucleotide-gated channels have a stoichiometry of three CNGA1 subunits and one CNGB1 subunit. Neuron 36:891–896, 2002.
42. Zhong H, Molday LL, Molday RS, Yau KW: The heteromeric cyclic nucleotide-gated channel adopts a 3A:1B stoichiometry. Nature 420:193–198, 2002.
43. Yu H, Wu J, Potapova I, et al: MinK-related peptide 1: A beta subunit for the HCN ion channel subunit family enhances expression and speeds activation. Circ Res 88:E84–E87, 2001.
44. Shi W, Wymore R, Yu H, et al: Distribution and prevalence of hyperpolarization-activated cation channel (HCN) mRNA expression in cardiac tissues. Circ Res 85:e1-6, 1999.
45. Han W, Bao W, Wang Z, Nattel S: Comparison of ion-channel subunit expression in canine cardiac Purkinje fibers and ventricular muscle. Circ Res 91:790–797, 2002.
46. Cerbai E, Sartiani L, DePaoli P, et al: The properties of the pacemaker current I_f in human ventricular myocytes are modulated by cardiac disease. J Mol Cell Cardiol 33:441–448, 2001.
47. Hoppe UC, Jansen E, Sudkamp M, Beuckelmann DJ: Hyperpolarization-activated inward current in ventricular myocytes from normal and failing human hearts. Circulation 97:55–65, 1998.
48. Qu J, Barbuti A, Protas L, et al: HCN2 overexpression in newborn and adult ventricular myocytes: Distinct effects on gating and excitability. Circ Res 89:E8–E14, 2001.
49. Ludwig A, Budde T, Stieber J, et al: Absence epilepsy and sinus dysrhythmia in mice lacking the pacemaker channel HCN2. EMBO J 22:216–224, 2003.
50. Schulze-Bahr E, Neu A, Friederich P, et al: A mutation in the cardiac pacemaker channel gene causes sinus node dysfunction. Circulation 104:II-192, 2001.

第 8 章

心脏缝隙连接蛋白 43 的分子组成和调节

Mario Delmar, *Heatber S. Duffy*, *Paul L. Sorgen*, *Steven M. Taffet*, *David C. Spray*

本章目录

- 缝隙连接的结构 67
- 连接子和连接蛋白 68
- 连接蛋白亚单位的膜拓扑学 69
- 连接蛋白 43 的分子结构 69
- pH 值对 Cx43 调节的结构基础：超出了初级结构 73
- 总结和未来的方向 74

缝隙连接为相邻细胞间进行直接的细胞-细胞通讯提供了路径，这些通道具有许多生物功能，例如电传导、胚胎发育、细胞生长。在人类，它们的组成蛋白发生突变与无症状性耳聋、Charcot-Maric-Tooth 综合征、眼齿指发育不良[1]及遗传性白内障[2,3]有关。在心脏，缝隙连接对动作电位的传播[4,5]及正常的心脏胚胎发育[6]是非常重要的。本章，我们总结心脏缝隙连接的结构及我们目前所知的通道功能，预想在某一天对结构功能分析获得的信息将转化为分子的合理设计，以提高或是干预通道的功能，为调节心脏电紧张和代谢的同步提供新的工具。

一、缝隙连接的结构

直到 19 世纪中期，多数组织学家认为心肌是一个合胞体，在细胞间有原生质桥允许电活动在心脏快速传递。当电子显微镜首次用于研究心脏组织时，清楚地发现细胞是个个体单位，两端边界是闰盘，Weidmann 等[7]的研究与之相比，发现心脏的电传播远远超出单个细胞长度，最初对这一矛盾的回答来自于对心脏电子显微图的仔细分析[8,9]。Sjostrand 和同事[9]在 1958 年的文章中提出闰盘内存在特殊的表面，描述为"三条黑线和两条插入的低密度线"，将其命名为纵向连接面，与先前确定的螯虾的大神经元相似[10]。正是这一结构提供了细胞间直接通讯途径，可以解释组织的同步化行为。对心肌细胞的测量表明闰盘上细胞膜间的平均距离是 240Å[11]，而在其他位点间的距离则降到大约 150Å，这表明膜的外叶相邻很近，事实上达到了融合，形成了紧密相连区域。Dewey 与 Barr[12]将这一融合描述为"连接"，指出融合的两侧都存在电子稠密物质。1967 年，Revel 和 Karnovsky[13]用薄片电子显微镜和氢氧化镧染色在鼠的心脏闰盘上显示了紧密相对的膜间区域（图 8-1A 和 B）[13]。他们发现这些区域并不是融合，相反是一个可测量的"缝隙"，约 18Å，将相对的质膜外叶分开（图 8-1C）。图像进一步显示相对的膜间有一个结构桥接在一起，氢氧化镧不能通过这一结构。En Face 显示这一连接是一些颗粒或亚单位呈六边形的聚集束（图 8-1D），在每一个颗粒的中心是直径 10Å 以下的电子通透孔，他们推测每个亚单位组成"空的棱柱"，形态上与细胞间电子流的转移有关[7]。后来，Revel 将连接区的"缝隙"称为缝隙连接[14,15]。McNutt 和 Weinstein 用冷冻电子显微镜进一步研究了这些颗粒的详细结构，确认了在心脏缝隙连接内每个亚单位以六边形方式排列（图 8-1E）。对膜"侧边"的其他研究表明，个体颗粒在相对的膜上以洞的形式被匹配起来，从一个双边对另一个双边分布[16]。

Caspar[17] 和 Makowski[18] 应用低角度 X 线衍射技术在肝组织对缝隙连接进行了深入研究。他们发现每个形态单位符合一对六聚体,每个六聚体又与每个膜有关。Makowski[19]首次显示孔并不是完美的圆柱形,而是存在窄的细胞外空间。Unwin 和 Zampighi[20] 分离肝的缝隙连接,用电子显微镜分析了它们的三维结构,通过倾斜连接膜以投射电子光柱形成不同的图像,用 Fourier 分析形成轮廓图。这些和其他一些研究[19,21]总结出每个六边形的排列代表一个单一的半通道,六边形中心相当于通道的孔。

后来,用原子力显微镜对缝隙连接通道进行了详细的测量[22,23],发现膜通道从脂质膜的细胞外表面伸出 1.4nm,原子力显微探针深入孔内达 0.7nm,细胞外侧孔的大小估计约为 3.8nm。Perkins[24] 和 Unger[25,26] 及他们的同事用电子晶体光谱研究获得了每个半通道或完整缝隙连接的详细结构(详细介绍见后)。缝隙连接孔的最新测量达到 7.5Å[26]。

总之,从 Weidmann 最初研究发现心脏的电紧张传播还不足 50 年的时间,细胞间通信的高级结构和分子图就已经出现。由于它和心脏电生理有关,本章将简短描述缝隙连接蛋白的特征,着重介绍心脏最丰富的连接蛋白 Cx43 的结构。文献中有相关缝隙连接生物学方面的精彩综述[3]。

二、连接子和连接蛋白

随着分子克隆技术的发展,确定了编码连接蛋白的基因,同时也将蛋白的结构、功能和它们的分子特征联系起来。一般认为,缝隙连接是一种蛋白亚单位即连接蛋白的寡聚体。6 个连接蛋白分子聚集形成连接子结构(或"半通道"),Makowski 和他的同事[18] 及 Unwin 和 Zampighi[20] 报道这一结构是单一的六体形。两个相对的细胞各提供一个连接子,在细胞外间隙部分形成一个缝隙连接通道。

人类基因组共有 20 个不同的连接蛋白亚型[27],最普遍的分类是根据连接蛋白 DNA 顺序预测的蛋白分子量进行的(如:连接蛋白 43 [Cx43] 预测的分子量是 43kD)。每种连接蛋白亚型在特定的组织表达,大多数组织表达一种以上的连接蛋白。连接蛋白的多样性在功能上还不能被完全解释,但是每种连接蛋白可能都有它表达的组织所必要的特性。事实上,鼠的遗传调节表明某一种连接蛋白的表达缺乏时,将引起这一亚型特有的表型,而且,用另一种亚型蛋白代替并不能完全挽救这种表型[28,29]。例如,敲除 Cx43 基因引起心脏的形态异常,用 Cx32 基因代替 Cx43 基因不能阻止心脏缺陷的发生[28]。镜下,通过基因插入 Cx46 代替 Cx50 纠正了细胞分化缺陷,阻止了级联反应,但并没有恢复正常的生长[29]。连接蛋白特异性是否是由于某种缝隙连接允许通过的分子,或是细胞内某种连接蛋白与之反应的分子,还是一些其他因子,还不确定。然而,有可能的是连接蛋白功能的分化与特异的分子结构及特殊亚型的调节功能有关。

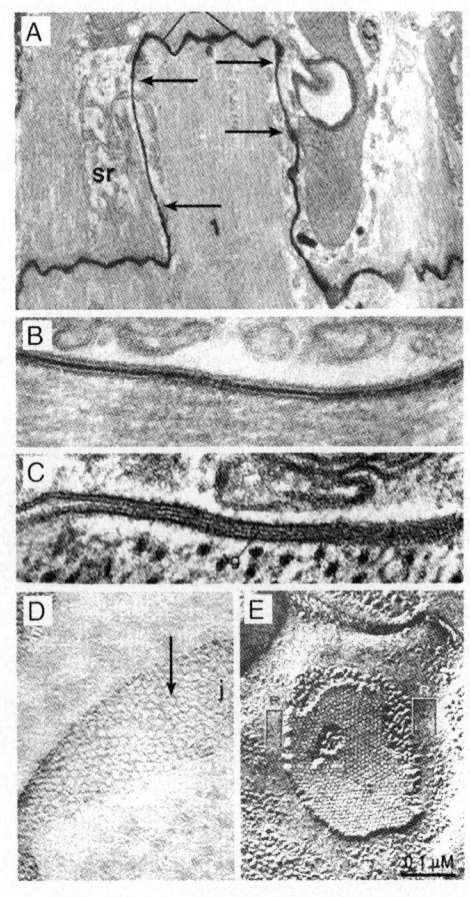

图 8-1 A:镧染色心脏纵面观显示闰盘的分布,包括相邻的膜附着区(平行箭头间)。B:"缝隙"连接交叉部分的高倍镜图像(200 000×)显示呈三条密度线的相邻的膜附着面。C:鼠心脏镧染色阻断显示在连接区(g)正常细胞空间降低到大约 20Å。D:鼠心脏连接 En face 薄片图像显示六边形亚单位,后来发现是缝隙连接的半通道。E:心脏缝隙连接的冷冻图像证明连接内颗粒的存在,以六边形排列,形成心肌细胞间连接(A~D,引自 Revel JP, Karnovsky MJ: Hexagonal array of subunits in intercellular junctions of the mouse heart and liver. J Cell Biol 33:C7-C12, 1967. E, 引自 McNutt NS, Weinstein RS: The ultrastructure of the nexus. A correlated thin-section and freeze-cleave study. J Cell Biol 47:666-668, 1970.)

三、连接蛋白亚单位的膜拓扑学

亲水性分布图和其他方法研究表明，一旦连接蛋白被组装，将在细胞膜穿过 4 次，形成 4 个跨膜结构域（TM1-TM4），2 个细胞外环（EL1-EL2）及 3 个细胞内区域：氨基末端、细胞浆环和羧基末端（NT、CL、CT，见图 8-2）。以拓扑异构学分析[30-32]，主要序列的特性和其他数据为基础，许多研究将某一连接蛋白的主要结构和它的功能与调节联系起来，这些实验对理解缝隙连接的生物学特性提供了重要的资料。然而，由于构成功能结构域的残基不一定必须邻近主要序列，因此主要结构和功能间的关联研究受限。而且，大量的功能结构域在空间上保留着相似的结构，尽管氨基酸相似性的水平有限。理解分子功能内在机制的每一步都需要确定结构域的二级和四级结构。最近，为确定连接蛋白结构域的高级结构进行了大量努力，在此，我们将讨论 Cx43 的功能相关性方面，总结近来深入探讨它的结构和功能所做的工作。

四、连接蛋白 43 的分子结构

Cx43 是心脏最丰富的缝隙蛋白，它的存在和正确的调节对于心肌梗死发生致死性心律失常[33]以及正常心脏的胚胎发育都非常重要[6,34]，Cx43 对心脏动作电位传导的重要性已被广泛认识。如果 Cx43 通道关闭或不存在，那么正常心脏的传导就会被破坏，引起致死性心律失常[4,5,35]。Cx43 通道由大量的激酶调节[36]，其他一些蛋白如 ZO-1[37]、微管蛋白、src[39]、小窝蛋白（carveolin）[40]、β-连锁蛋白[41]或 p120-连锁蛋白[42]与 Cx43 以非共价形式相互关联，这些蛋白相互作用的功能还不清楚，可能是调节细胞内通信，在 Cx43 表达组织，例如心脏，对于细胞内外信号耦联可能起重要作用。以下对 Cx43 不同结构域的当前认识做一概述。

（一）连接蛋白 43 通道孔区

研究微结构方法学的发展使我们对缝隙连接通道作为单一的功能/结构体有了初步认识：如上所述，早期研究表明缝隙连接作为半通道，是 6 个部分的聚合体，中央是一个孔区[20,21]。一些研究人员对早先的发现进一步加以确定并延伸[22,23,43]。主要的进步来自于 Unger 和他的同事的研究[26]。他们采用电子晶体

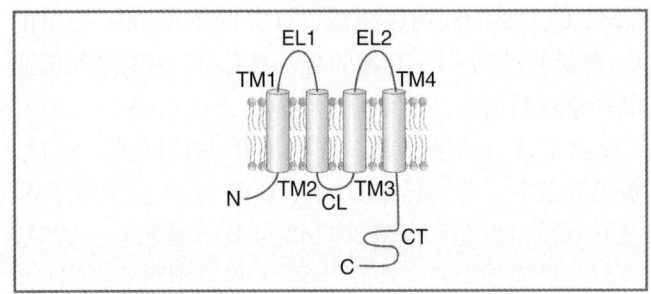

图 8-2　连接蛋白亚单位的拓扑学　圆柱体代表磷脂双分子层。N：氨基末端；C：羧基末端；CL：细胞质环路；TM1 至 TM4：转膜结构域 1~4；EL1-2：细胞外环路 1 和 2

图来描述由缺乏羧基末端的 Cx43 亚单位构成的缝隙连接通道的三维结构。组装的缝隙连接通道在膜平面 7.5Å 和垂直方向 21Å 的位置可以被观察到，研究清楚地展现了 α 螺旋状的 24 个跨膜域的电子密度。如图 8-3 所示，这 24 个跨膜 α 螺旋由 4 个跨膜域重复 6 次组成（标记 A 到 D），这与连接子由 6 个连接蛋白寡聚而成、每个有 4 个跨膜结构域的说法是一致的。Unger 和同事的研究图像进一步揭示孔区细胞外缝隙边缘很窄，40~15Å。这种狭窄是由于与通道平行的跨膜域（图 8-3 右侧组 C 标记）倾斜所致（最初由 Makowski[18]用低角度 X 线衍射分析发现，Unwin 和 Zampighi[20]的数据也提到）。Unwin 的研究图像显示的孔区结构与开放的通道相一致还是与关闭的通道相一致还不清楚。Unger 及同事的资料还表明 Cα 螺旋延伸超过双层结构进入细胞浆，如果 C 结构域与第三个跨膜结构域相符（见后），则可能表明细胞浆环的部分仍是 α 螺旋，这与我们用核磁共振观察到的结构域相一致。Unger 及同事的重要研究为我们从结构观点理解缝隙连接提供了基本框架，然而值得注意的是，研究者需要缩短 Cx43 羧基末端来获得孔区足够的形象，因此，除了细胞浆环的一小部分，这一结构中并没有包括细胞内结构的特点。

（二）通道孔区主要序列与高级结构的关系

研究电子低温晶体学显示的孔区结构与通过拓扑结构确定的连接蛋白结构域之间的关系很困难。主要序列中的跨膜域（TM1-TM4，见图 8-2）是结构中的哪一段结构域（A-D，见图 8-3）？研究人员试图通过半胱氨酸扫描突变[44,45]和分子模型[46]来回答这一问题，结果是完全不一致。Zhou 和他的同事[44]得出结论：（1）第一个跨膜域构成孔内结构；（2）一个以上的跨膜域沿孔排列。最近，Skerrett 和同事总结出

TM3 是主要的孔内结构域,且等同于 Unger 提出的 Cα 螺旋超结构[26]。有趣的是,对 Cx43 主要序列低温晶体学资料的分子模型分析得到了不同结果[46],图 8-4 显示了这一研究结果。颜色的排列是绿色、红色、黄色和蓝色,分别标记 D、C、B′和 A′。当序列 TM1 与 C 螺旋(红色)一致,TM2 与 B′(黄色)一致时,模型为低能量形式,螺旋 D 和 A′将分别对应 TM4 和 TM3。然而,重要的是这些模型结果仍需斟酌,因为它有不合理的特点,如一些通道周围的充电残基与膜脂质相接触,如图 8-5 所示。总之,迄今功能和分子模型分析并没有得出主要序列和高级结构间联系的统一结论,一些差异可能是由于研究的连接蛋白通道不同(Zhou 和同事[44]研究 Cx32-Cx43 的突变,Skerrett 和同事[45]研究 Cx32 缝隙连接,Nunn 和其他人[46]研究缩短的 Cx43 缝隙连接),一些差异可能是由于方法的局限性,还可能是由于研究的通道采取的开关模式不同(见 Skerrett 和同事的讨论[45])。随着人们回答这一问题所作出的努力,不久可能会有更明了的缝隙连接通道图形出现。

(三) 细胞外结构域

细胞外环对两个半通道间相互作用的稳定很重要,当形成通道时,相互作用通过二硫键加以稳定[47]。并不意外的是,在连接蛋白家族的不同成员间,这些结构域有高度的序列同源性。主要序列分析也得出细胞外环存在反平行 β-片状结构,内部通过二硫键稳定,与两个连接子尾部相分离,这有待通过直接结构分析证实。

(四) 细胞内结构域

如前所述,Unger 和他的同事[26]对超结构的研究是在缺乏羧基端结构域的模型上进行的,然而,这一区域是通道调节的基础。虽然点特异性突变研究为 Cx43 参与通道调节的不同区域提供了重要信息,但是完整结构图还需要探讨这些结构域的高级构型。Tivvitts 和其他研究者用 X 线衍射分析发现,连接蛋白细胞浆部分"似乎很有弹性"和"局部可能有次序性的二级结构,但因没有更长范围的序列,通过衍射数据很难总结这一结构的特点"。下面我们将介绍最近通过 NMR 获得的数据,它为解决细胞内结构提供了最初的方法。

1. 核磁共振

解决高级结构的另一方法是应用 NMR。这一技术通过收集定位在强的外部磁场内的核分子来测量振动电磁场的分子相互作用,从而可以得出多肽和小蛋白样分子的特点。分子的 NMR 波谱不仅由存在的原子类型决定还由他们的空间相互关系决定,通过一系列实验和推导分析,可以构建分子的三维结构。在 Macomber 的书中对 NMR 的原理和应用作了很好的解释[49]。以下介绍应用 NMR 得出的各种连接蛋白节段的结构。

2. 氨基末端

有关连接蛋白氨基端结构的唯一信息来自于 Purnick 和他的同事的研究[50]。这些作者运用 NMR 研究连接蛋白 26 前 15 个氨基酸对应多肽的结构,总结出两个部分有高级结构(可能是 α 螺旋),被一个弯曲的"铰链"分开,通过结构和功能分析,作者猜测氨基端形成通道的前庭,参与电压门控。由于连接蛋白高度的异源性,这些数据不能直接推导到 Cx43。未来的研究将决定由一个连接蛋白确定的结构在其他连接蛋白是否是保守的,即使在基本序列不同的情况下。

3. 细胞浆环

我们最近承担了 Cx43 的 CL 的 NMR 分析[53]。

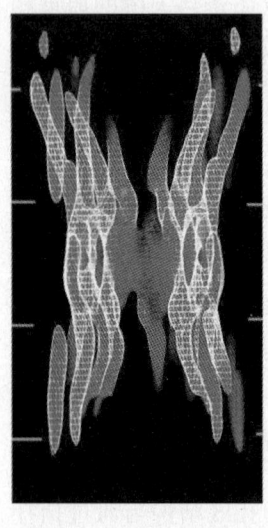
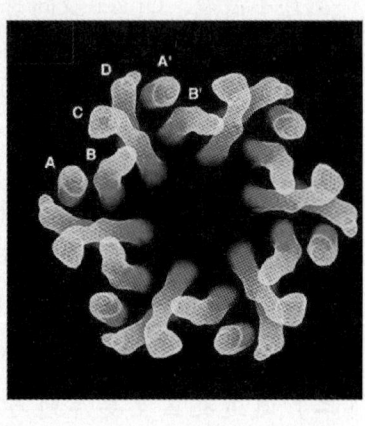

图 8-3 通过电子晶体学得到的 Cx43 超微结构　平面距离是 7.5Å,垂直距离是 21Å。左图显示的是整个通道的侧面观,红线代表脂质双分子层,红星代表那些孔径被估计最小的点。右图代表横切面的形状,通道由六个面组成,每个面又由四个相同密度区组成,每个密度区代表一个转膜区(引自 Unger VM, Kumer NM, Gilula NB, Yeager, MR: Three dimensional structure of a recombinant gap junction membrane channel. Science 283: 1176-1180, 1999)(见彩图 1)

低pH值对Cx43L2进行了详细的结构分析。一系列NMR实验和弯角动力学结构计算形成了图8-7所示结构,上方是Cx43L2氨基酸序列,红色为α螺旋部分的序列,H126和H142咪唑环位置在结构中标出。有趣的是,有更强螺旋特点的两部分含有组氨酸,参与Cx43L2和Cx43羧基端的相互作用(见后)。

4. 羧基端结构

自从Cx43主要序列被首次报道,就认为羧基端结构可能参与通道的调节,给出了假设的磷酸化位点数量。而且,结构域的缩短阻止了细胞内酸化下通道的关闭[52]。最近又显示Cx43与细胞内大量的蛋白相连,包括ZO-1、src、caveolin、β-连锁蛋白、p120-连锁蛋白和微管蛋白。Cx43的蛋白结合域,至少对微管蛋白和ZO-1来说存在于羧基端部位。因此,清楚地理解Cx43调节的结构-功能相关性需要得到羧基端高级结构的特点。

对心脏缝隙连接结构的研究表明在垂直于膜平面轴上,通道的大小约为250Å,当CT结构被缩短时,

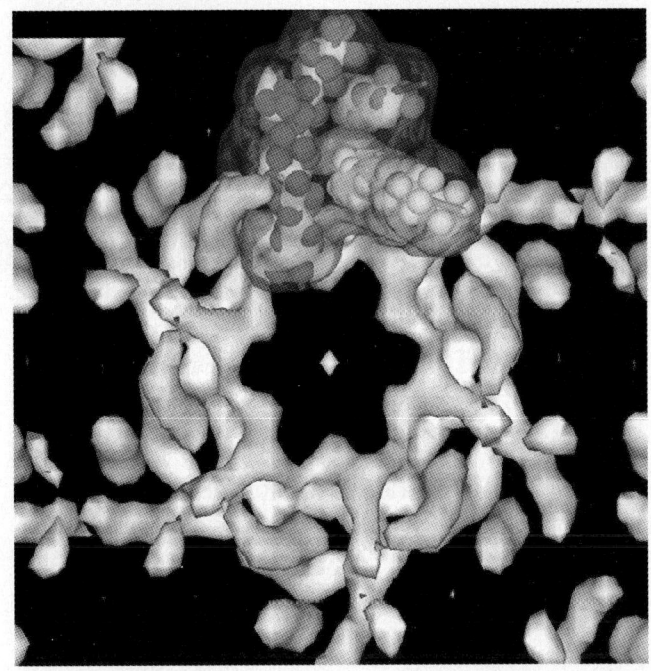

图8-4 **Cx43通道的分子模型** 以电子晶体光谱获得的Cx43通道超微结构为基础(图8-3),将主要序列的氨基酸排列成超微结构确定的跨膜域。模型构建了低能量构型,根据这一模型,Unger26确定的主要序列与α螺旋间的关系是:TM4,螺旋C2(绿色);TM1,螺旋C(红色);TM2,螺旋B′(黄色);TM3,螺旋A′(蓝色)。然而,这一模型仍存在局限性,一些特殊点似乎不合理(见图8-5)(引自Nunn RS, Macke TJ, Olson AJ, Yeager M: Transmembrane alpha-helices in the gap junction membrane channel: Systematic search of packing models based on the pair potential function. Microsc Res Tech 52: 344-351, 2001.)(见彩图2)

拓扑学预测表明完整的CL结构包括从氨基酸95到105[32]。和结构分析一样,功能分析也很容易,我们把结构域分成两部分,一部分从氨基酸95到114,另一部分(定位Cx43L2)从119到144,因为功能分析表明Cx43L2区域在通道调节中起作用,我们重点解决Cx43L2的结构。一个重要的发现是溶剂的酸化对Cx43L2多肽的结构组成有明显影响,如图8-6中¹H核极化效应光谱(NOESY)所示。NOESY确定特殊的通过空间的极性转移,因此提供蛋白结构序列的类型和范围,如不存在通过空间的极性转移表明缺乏组成结构,与NOESY光谱相对应,但不脱离对角线关系。pH值从8.0(图8-6A)降到5.8(图8-6B)引起内部残基交叉峰有很大升高(也就是轮廓可从对角线确定),图8-6B数字1到26代表Cx43从119到144氨基酸信号,这些数据表明空间的相互作用与酸化后的二级结构(α螺旋)组成相一致,因此我们在

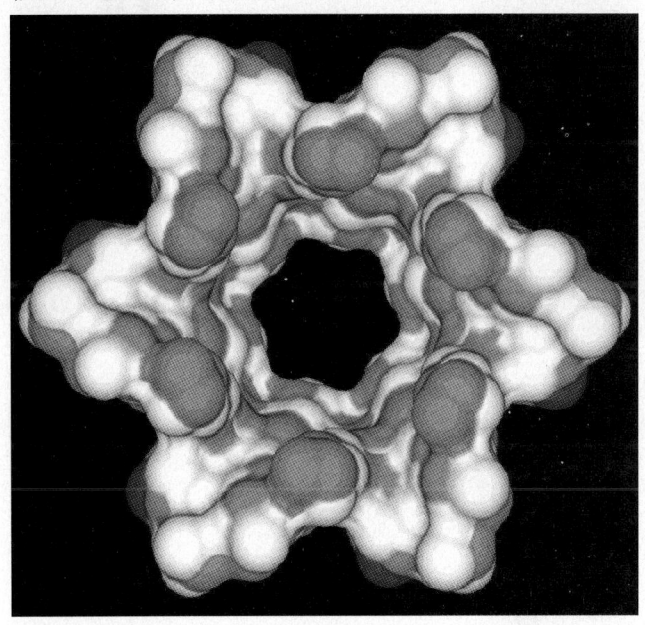

图8-5 **连接子模型的上面观** 球代表氨基酸,直径10Å。排列颜色如下:红色,Asp Glu;蓝色,Arg Lys;绿色,Tyr Phe Trp;黄色,Met Cys;白色,Gly Ala Val Leu Ile Pro。这一模型代表了低能量构型。然而,特征仍不合理,例如,充电残基与脂质相连(引自Nunn RS, Macke TJ, Olson AJ, Yeager M: Transmembrane alpha-helices in the gap junction membrane channel: Systematic search of packing models based on the pair potential function. Microsc Res Tech 52: 344-351, 2001.)(见彩图3)

同样的测量大小为 150Å[26,53]。然而，由于这一结构的有限分辨率，不能得到进一步的分子结构信息。

我们运用 NMR 研究羧基端结构[51,54]，最近在蛋白数据库公布了共振队列。在细菌内产生重建的 Cx43CT，通过谷胱甘肽柱纯化，再过滤浓缩。结构分析表明高级结构的两个区域，可能是 α 螺旋，夹在随机缠绕的两侧中间。令人注意的发现是溶剂 pH 从 8.0 到 5.8 的改变并没有引起结构发生预测的重要调整。而且，我们实验室未公布的数据表明 CT 结构为二聚体，从而得出一个值得关注的可能是六聚体的连接子实际可能是"二聚体的三聚体"[55,56]。我们早期的结果表明二聚体的一个区域可能包括脯氨酸富集区，作为 src 上 SH3 结构的结合域，还包含三个丝氨酸中的两个，被分裂素激活蛋白（MAP）激酶磷酸化，结合 src 和/或 MAP 磷酸化是否调节二聚体产生功能作用还不清楚。最后，我们在 ZO-1 第二个 PDZ 结构存在下获得了 Cx43CT 的共振峰。先前数据显示了氨基酸 371 到 382 的结构重排，因此有可能 ZO-1 的结合与丝氨酸富集区结构有关，它含有大量的潜在的磷酸化位点，这一发现提供了一种可能，即 Cx43CT-ZO-1 的关联与通道的正确调节有关。

总之，最近的进展使我们对心脏缝隙连接主要成分的 Cx43 分子结构有了初步了解，获得了与通道功能相关的结构信息。缝隙连接调节的各个方面远远超出本章节的范围，因此我们将重点讨论细胞内 pH 值对 Cx43 的调节。

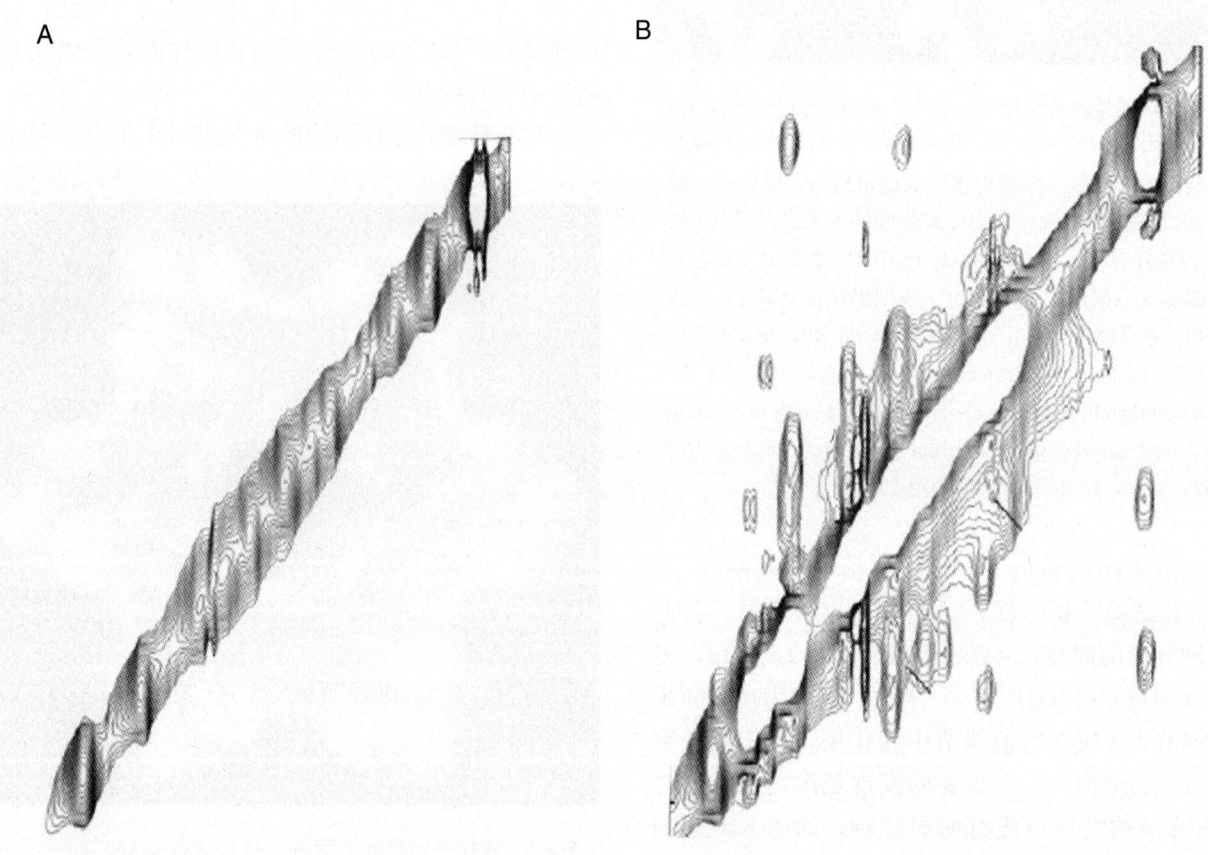

图 8-6 与 Cx43 119 到 144 序列对应的合成多肽的 ^{1}H 核极化效应光谱 在 pH8.0（A）和 pH5.8（B）的光谱，高 pH 值存在有限的结构顺序，信号不能从对角线充分分离，酸化导致高级结构形成，B 上小的数值相当于多肽的氨基酸排列，数字排列是位置 1 相当于 Cx43 氨基酸 119（引自 DuffyHS, Sorgen PL, Girvin ME, et al：pH-dependent intramolecular binding and structure involving Cx43 cytoplasmic domains. J Biol Chem 277：36706-36714，2002.）

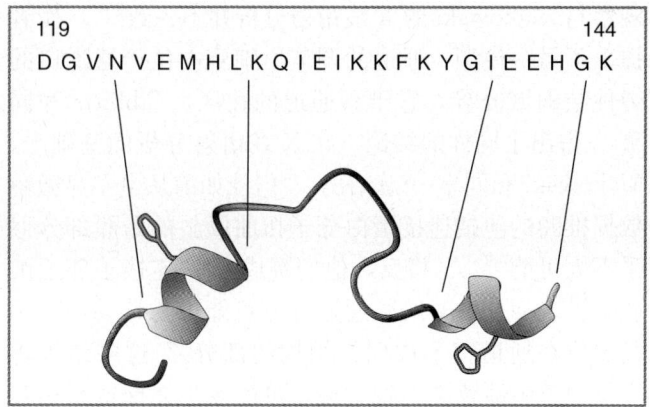

图8-7 连接蛋白43中氨基酸119-144的结构通过低pH值条件下核磁共振技术得以明确 氨基酸序列如顶线所示，使用单字母编码，两个α螺旋区域间被一段不定型结构分隔。这部分区域被假定为作为该通道化学门控期间羧基末端的受体（引自Duffy HS, Sorgen PL, Girvin ME, er al：pH-dependent intramolecular binding and structure involving Cx43 cytoplasmic domains. J Biol Chem 277：36706-36714，2002)

五、pH值对Cx43调节的结构基础：超出了初级结构

（一）Cx43的pH值门控：心脏电生理意义

实验证据强烈支持这一观点：缝隙连接对于动作电位的传导非常重要。而且，在遗传改变鼠上获得的证据表明，心室Cx43成分的有效增加显著提高了心室颤动的危险性[4]，因此低阻抗途径的破坏被认为是心律失常的潜在原因。文献积累的证据表明，心肌缺血和梗死导致细胞内pH值下降[57]。因此，酸化诱导的Cx43通道的关闭可能是发生缺血相关心律失常的重要机制[57,58]。我们实验室已经在酸化诱导Cx43关闭的结构基础方面进行了长期的研究。

以下我们将用pH门控一词指酸化诱导缝隙连接关闭过程。此词在缝隙连接领域广泛应用，但并非指低pH值诱导的缝隙连接关闭代表了通道的关闭，如Hodgkin-Huxley模式中所描述的情况。尽管存在这种可能，但还没有相关显示。

（二）Cx43的pH门控：一个"球-链样"模型

羧基端作为pH门控的调节域的首次确定来自于我们实验室进行的研究，显示Cx43氨基酸257的缩短（M257突变）阻止了酸化诱导的失耦联[52]，接下来的研究表明，如果CT端作为分离部分被联合表达，失耦联能恢复[59]。基于这些和其他数据，我们推断Cx43的pH门控与门控的"球-链样"模型是一致的，这一模型，最初用于钠离子通道的电压门控研究，后来显示Shaker[61]和其他钾离子通道的N型失活，说明通道的阻断是系在"链"上的细胞内粒子与孔上受体相互作用的结果。因此我们推断Cx43的pH门控发挥着粒子-受体相互作用功能，其中CT结构作为门控粒子。在正常pH下，门控粒子将远离孔区，通道开放；酸化时，粒子与孔上蛋白分离区域（受体）相结合，通道关闭。值得注意的是粒子-受体模型与胰岛素和胰岛素样生长因子[62]及src[63]对Cx43的调节结果相一致。我们实验室的进一步研究表明，一些其他连接蛋白（不是全部）有同样的pH门控模型。事实上，Cx40的CT结构能调节缩短的Cx43通道，Cx43的CT结构也能挽救缩短的Cx40通道对pH敏感性[64]。当酸化时，对于通道的关闭，这些异源结构的相互作用可能比同源结构的相互作用更有效[64]。球-链样机制似乎代表了Cx43和Cx40残基的存在状态[65,66]。

以上列出的结果强烈支持这样的假设，即羧基端结构域与孔上"受体"结合对Cx43通道进行调节，然而，仍存在的问题是，这种相互作用是直接还是通过介质发生的。而且，无论结合是直接的还是间接的，门控粒子受体的定位和结构仍不清楚。像阐述这些问题的第一个方法一样，我们最近运用了镜共振光谱学新方法体外确定Cx43是否发生分子内直接相互作用。考虑到它和本章的相关性，我们将对这一研究Cx43上蛋白-蛋白相互作用的方法学作一简短介绍。

（三）镜面共振光谱学

镜面共振光谱学利用光波通过两种不同衍射指数的介质时方向的改变进行研究，当波从高衍射指数物质向低衍射指数物质传导时，有一个特殊的角度能使波被完全反射（完全内部反射；图8-8A）。然而，电磁场穿透低衍射物质，这一"渐逝区"（evanescence field）随距离呈指数消失，如果高衍射物质（n_2）两侧都被低衍射物质（n_1）包围（"镀上"），光将被成功的完全内部反射限制在高衍射物质内（图8-8B）。这种"波导"只在一个离散角度θ时发生，这对系统的物理参数极其敏感。这种生物感受器的原理是结合在或邻近镀层物质表面的蛋白改变了θ值，根据此原理，配体（这里指Cx43CT）被固定在小容器的表面，加入一个潜在的结合体。如果两种分子确实结合，会

显示 θ 值发生改变（以秒弧为单位）。这种方法可对蛋白-蛋白相互作用进行实时测量，并对结合动力学进行直接测量。从浓度依赖性曲线，可计算出解离常数[51]。

（四）CT 结构域与细胞浆环片段结合的体外演示：结构满足功能？

我们应用共振镜技术检测 Cx43CT 是否以 pH 依赖形式与 Cx43 的其他细胞内区域相结合（见 Duffy 和同事[51]对结果的详细描述）。重组的 Cx43CT 以共价方式在感受器表面与羧甲基葡聚糖基质相结合，暴露于不同的合成肽，它们与 Cx43 细胞内区域相对应。在所有的检测多肽中，只有与细胞浆环的第二半（Cx43L2）相对应的多肽才有结合现象。图 8-9A 是用 100μM 的 Cx43L2 肽进行实验显示的代表曲线，平面图描绘的是共振信号振幅（以秒弧为单位）的时间函数。灰色曲线的溶液 pH 值是 6.5。为了检测对 pH 值的依赖相关性，Cx43L2-Cx43CT 结合实验在 pH 7.4（图 8-9A 黑色曲线）被重复。清晰地发现，溶液的 pH 值升到 7.4 时引起反应幅度显著下降，这些数据表明低 pH 值增加 Cx43L2 多肽对 Cx43CT 的亲和力。当反应在 pH 7.4 进行时，其他的检验多肽和重组的 Ca^{2+} 结合钙调蛋白也不能与 Cx43CT 相结合（资料未显示）。

图 8-9B 显示了 $CX43L_2$ 的浓度与结合幅度之间的相关性。图中的数据是对在 pH 6.5 到 pH 为 7.4 记录到的最适削减轨迹（subtracted traces）。Cx43CT-Cx43L2 相互作用的 kD 值是 24M，其是由削减轨迹的浓度依赖曲线所估测到的。在 pH 7.4 时的结合曲线幅度太小而不能达到最适，因此，在这些条件下，kD 值并不能被计算出来。综上所述，这些结果说明，羧基端结构域与 Cx43 胞浆环的第二半部分的结合是有选择性的，且依赖于 pH 值及浓度。

（五）Cx43 孔区结构及 pH 门控

以上资料表明 pH 门控是羧基端结构作为门控粒子与作为受体的细胞浆第二半环相互作用的结果（图 8-10）。关于这种相互作用是否通过引起孔区结构转化或通过在未发生改变的孔区加"塞子"来破坏细胞-细胞间通讯仍有很多问题。1980 年 Unwin 和 Zampighi 提出了 Cx43 模型，后来用于研究钙对缝隙连接的调节，表明通道的开放和关闭是通过蛋白亚单位沿着它们的直线轴进行协调的倾斜滑动的结果。然而，这一

观察与 Makowski 的 X 线衍射分析并不一致[18]。作者提出了另一模型，通道的调节由细胞内位于通道口的弹性结构域介导，它干预通道的孔区，Tibbitts 和同事[43]得出了同样的结论。在 X 线衍射分析的基础上，Makowski 和同事[18]总结出："门控如前从电子显微镜数据推断的包括连接蛋白分子扭曲倾斜的跨膜部分似乎不太可能[43]。"相反，他们赞成[20]"连接子邻近细胞浆膜表面和面对跨膜通道部分可能更易移动，特别是定位在通道口形成门控结构的部分。"这些结果将支持通道阻滞化学门控学说，可能发生在球链型相互作用中。Unger 和同事[26]的高级结构只提供了一种构型，是否还存在另外一种结构与通道的不同传导状态相对应还不清楚。

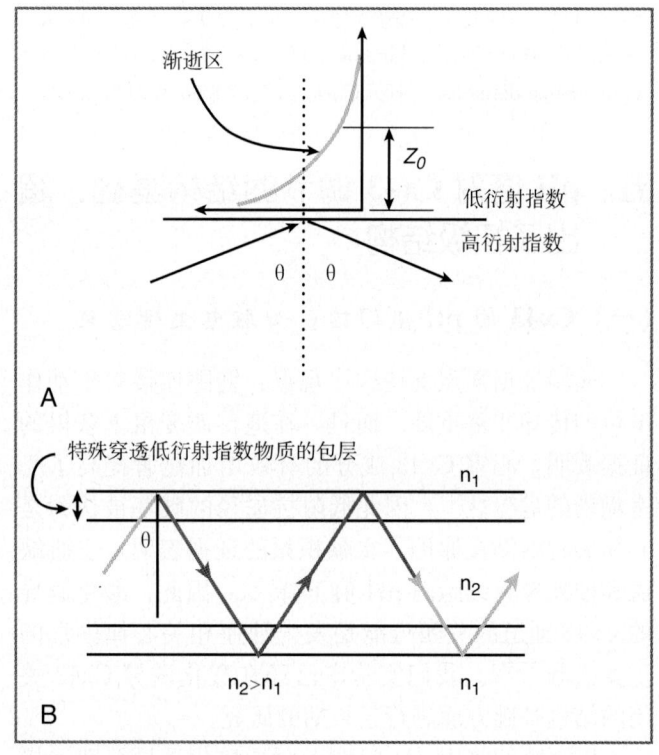

图 8-8 镜面共振光谱学原理 光以一特殊关键的角度，从高指数到低指数物质边缘时被反射，反射波在表面产生了穿透距离 Z_0 的渐逝电磁场。（A），光能在不同衍射指数物质间被限制（指导）；（B），指导的发生角度是表面分子构成的功能，如果新的分子进入渐逝区，共振角度将改变。这一方法被用于确定固定于表面的配体和加入容器的物质间的连接（引自 the lasys Web site at www. affinity-sensor.com）

六、总结和未来的方向

这一章，我们总结了关于缝隙连接结构和功能研

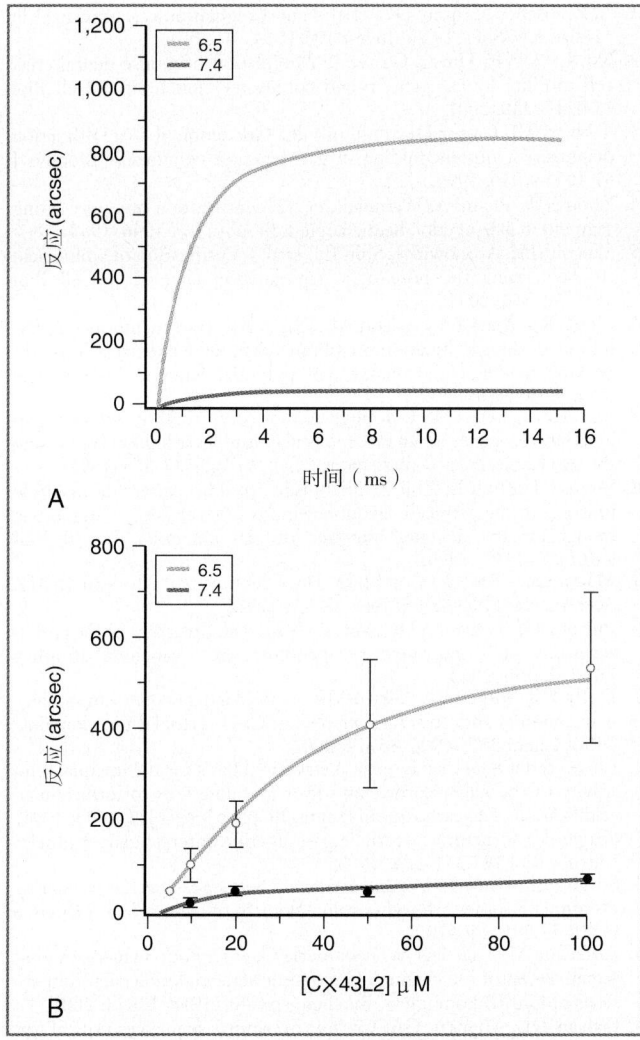

图 8-9 镜面共振光谱学显示 Cx43 羧基端结构与相当于细胞浆环第二半部分（氨基酸 119 到 144）的多肽相结合 A：Cx43CT 固定于容器时获得的曲线。黑线是溶液 pH 值 7.4 时记录的曲线，灰色是 pH 值 6.5 时的曲线。数据显示结合的振幅和动力学有 pH 值依赖性。B：在 pH 6.5（灰色）和 pH 7.4（黑色）时 Cx43CT 与 Cx43L2 的结合存在浓度依赖性。在所有的浓度测试中，酸化使结合幅度显著升高。我们推断这种细胞内的结合可能通过引起细胞内酸化介导心脏缝隙连接通道的关闭（引自 Duffy HS，Sorgen PL，Girvin ME，et al：pH-dependent intramoleular binding and structure involving Cx43 cytoplasmic domains. J Biol Chem 277：36706-36714，2002.）

究的重要发现。距证实心脏电传播已经 50 余年[7]，缝隙连接的第一个显微镜观察也已 40 余年[8,9]，今天，超结构研究已经达到分子水平，我们对功能的理解扩展到整体器官，学到了很多，同时还有更多问题没有回答。随着科学和技术的发展，有可能进行结构更高的研究和对不同方法得到的信息进行整合。而

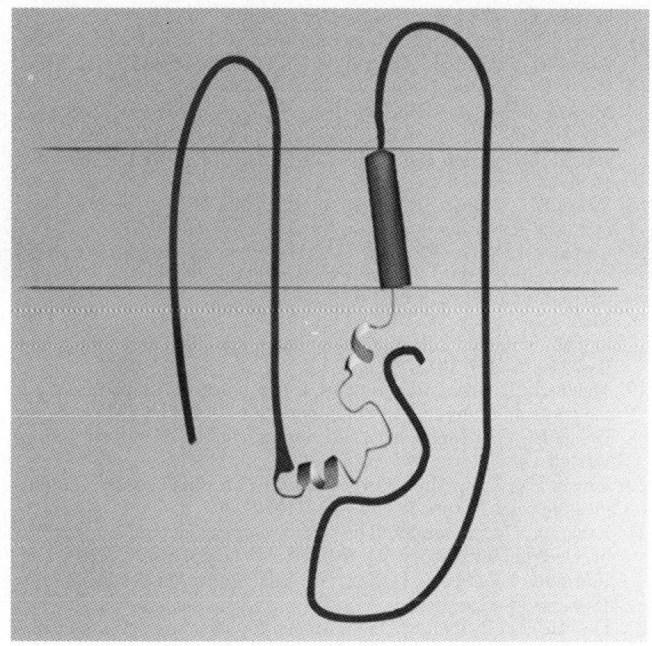

图 8-10 Cx43 分子的拓扑学分布显示了主要序列内 Cx43L2 的位置，我们推测 pH 门控导致作为门控颗粒的羧基端与作为受体的 Cx43L2 区间发生相互作用

且，缝隙连接领域有可能达到以合理的结构为基础进行药物设计阶段。这对于我们理解健康和疾病时通道门控的特有功能结果方面迈出了有意义的一步。

（浦介麟　马克娟　译）

参 考 文 献

1. Paznekas WA, Boyadjiev SA, Shapiro RE, et al: Connexin 43 (GJA1) mutations cause the pleiotropic phenotype of oculodentodigital dysplasia. Am J Hum Genet 72:408–418, 2002.
2. White TW, Paul DL: Genetic diseases and gene knockouts reveal diverse connexin functions. Annu Rev Physiol 61:283–310, 1999
3. Harris AL: Emerging issues of connexin channels: biophysics fills the gap. Q Rev Biophys 34:325–472, 2001.
4. Gutstein DE, Morley GE, Tamaddon H, et al: Conduction slowing and sudden arrhythmic death in mice with cardiac-restricted inactivation of connexin43. Circ Res 88:333–339, 2001.
5. Vaidya D, Tamaddon HS, Lo CW, et al: Null mutation of connexin43 causes slow propagation of ventricular activation in the late stages of mouse embryonic development. Circ Res 88:1196–1202, 2001.
6. Reaume AG, De Sousa PA, Kulkarni S, et al: Cardiac malformation in neonatal mice lacking connexin43. Science 267:1831–1834, 1995.
7. Weidmann S: The electrical constants of Purkinje fibers. J Physiol 118:348–360, 1952.
8. Sjöstrand FS, Andersson E: Electron microscopy of the intercalated discs of cardiac muscle tissue. Experientia 10:369–370, 1954.
9. Sjöstrand FS, Andersson-Cedergren E, Dewey MM: The ultrastructure of the intercalated discs of frog, mouse and guinea pig cardiac muscle. J Ultrastruct Res 1:271–287, 1958.
10. Robertson JD: Ultrastructure of two invertebrate synapses. Proc Soc Exp Biol Med 82:219–223, 1953.
11. Davson H: A Textbook of General Physiology. Boston, Little, Brown, 1964, pp 843–866.
12. Dewey MW, Barr L: Intercellular connections between smooth muscle cell: The nexus. Science 137:670–672, 1962.

muscle cell: The nexus. Science 137:670–672, 1962.
13. Revel JP, Karnovsky MJ: Hexagonal array of subunits in intercellular junctions of the mouse heart and liver. J Cell Biol 33: C7–C12, 1967.
14. Revel JP: In Proceedings of the 26th Meeting of the Electron Microscopy Society of America, Baton Rouge, LA, Claitor's, 1968, p 40.
15. McNutt NS, Weinstein RS: The ultrastructure of the nexus. A correlated thin-section and freeze-cleave study. J Cell Biol 47:666–688, 1970.
16. Steere RL, Sommer JR: Stereo ultrastructure of nexus faces exposed by freeze-fracturing. J Microsc (Paris) 15:205–218, 1972.
17. Caspar DLD, Goodenough DA, Makowski L, Phillips WC: Gap junction structures: I. Correlated electron microscopy and X ray diffraction. J Cell Biol 74:605–628, 1977.
18. Makowski L, Caspar DLD, Phillips WC, Goodenough DA: Gap junction structures: II. Analysis of the X-ray diffraction data. J Cell Biol 74:629–645, 1977.
19. Makowski L: Structural domains in gap junctions: Implications for the control of intercellular communication. In Bennett MVL, Spray DC (eds): Gap Junctions. Cold Spring Harbor, NY, Cold Spring Harbor Laboratory, 1985, pp 5–12.
20. Unwin PN, Zampighi G: Structure of the junction between communicating cells. Nature 283:545–549, 1980.
21. Zampighi GA, Simon SA: The structure of gap junctions as revealed by electron microscopy. In Bennett MVL, Spray DC (eds): Gap Junctions. Cold Spring Harbor, NY, Cold Spring Harbor Laboratory, 1985, pp 13–22.
22. Hoh JH, Lal R, John SA, et al: Atomic force microscopy and dissection of gap junctions. Science 253:1405–1408, 1991.
23. Hoh JH, Sosinsky GE, Revel JP, Hansma PK: Structure of the extracellular surface of the gap junction by atomic force microscopy. Biophys J 65:149–163, 1993.
24. Perkins G, Goodenough D, Sosinsky G: Three-dimensional structure of the gap junction connexon. Biophys J 72:533–544, 1997.
25. Unger VM, Kumar NM, Gilula NB, Yeager M: Projection structure of a gap junction membrane channel at 7 Å resolution. Nat Struct Biol 4:39–43, 1997.
26. Unger VM, Kumar NM, Gilula NB, Yeager MR: Three-dimensional structure of a recombinant gap junction membrane channel. Science 283:1176–1180, 1999.
27. Willecke K, Eiberger J, Degen J, et al: Structural and functional diversity of connexin genes in the mouse and human genome. J Biol Chem 383:725–737, 2002.
28. Plum A, Hallas G, Magin T, et al: Unique and shared functions of different connexins in mice. Curr Biol 10:1083–1091, 2000.
29. White TW: Unique and redundant connexin contributions to lens development. Science 295:319–320, 2002.
30. Yancey SB, John SA, Lal R, et al: The 43-kD polypeptide of heart gap junctions: Immunolocalization, topology, and functional domains. J Cell Biol 108:2241–2254, 1989.
31. Laird DW, Revel JP: Biochemical and immunochemical analysis of the arrangement of connexin43 in rat heart gap junction membranes J Cell Sci 97:109–117, 1990.
32. Yeager M, Gilula NB: Membrane topology and quaternary structure of cardiac gap junction ion channels. J Mol Biol 223:929–948, 1992.
33. Kanno S, Saffitz JE: The role of myocardial gap junctions in electrical conduction and arrhythmogenesis. Cardiovasc Pathol 10: 169–177, 2001.
34. Lo CW, Wessels A: Cx43 gap junctions in cardiac development. Trends Cardiovasc Med 8:264–269, 1998.
35. Lerner DL, Yamada KA, Schuessler RB, Saffitz JE: Accelerated onset and increased incidence of ventricular arrhythmias induced by ischemia in Cx43-deficient mice. Circulation 101:547–552, 2000.
36. Lampe PD, Lau AF: Regulation of gap junctions by phosphorylation of connexins. Arch Biochem Biophys 384:205–215, 2000.
37. Toyofuku T, Yabuki M, Otsu K, et al: Direct association of the gap junction protein connexin-43 with ZO-1 in cardiac myocytes. J Biol Chem. 273:12725–12731, 1998.
38. Giepmans BN, Hengeveld T, Postma FR, Moolenaar WH: Interaction of c-Src with gap junction protein connexin-43. Role in the regulation of cell-cell communication. J Biol Chem 276:8544–8549, 2001.
39. Giepmans BN, Verlaan I, Hengeveld T, et al: Gap junction protein connexin-43 interacts directly with microtubules. Curr Biol 11:1364–1368, 2001.
40. Schubert AL, Schubert W, Spray DC, Lisanti MP: Connexin family members target to lipid raft domains and interact with caveolin-1. Biochemistry 41:5754–5764,

41. Ai Z, Fischer A, Spray DC, et al: Wnt-1 regulation of connexin43 in cardiac myocytes. J Clin Invest 105:161–171, 2001.
42. Xu X, Li WE, Huang GY, et al: Modulation of mouse neural crest cell motility by N-cadherin and connexin43 junctions. J Cell Biol 154:217–230, 2001.
43. Tibbitts TT, Caspar DL, Phillips WC, Goodenough DA: Diffraction diagnosis of protein folding in gap junction connexons. Biophys J 57:1025–1036, 1990.
44. Zhou XW, Pfahnl A, Werner R, et al: Identification of a pore lining segment in gap junction hemichannels. Biophys J 72:1946–1953, 1997.
45. Skerrett IM, Aronowitz J, Shin JH, et al: Identification of amino acid residues lining the pore of a gap junction channel. J Cell Biol 159:349–360, 2002.
46. Nunn RS, Macke TJ, Olson AJ, Yeager M: Transmembrane alpha-helices in the gap junction membrane channel: Systematic search of packing models based on the pair potential function Microsc Res Tech 52:344–351, 2001.
47. Rahman S, Evans WH: Topography of connexin32 in rat liver gap junctions. Evidence for an intramolecular disulphide linkage connecting the two extracellular peptide loops J Cell Sci 100:567–578, 1991.
48. Foote CI, Zhou L, Zhu X, Nicholson BJ: The pattern of disulfide linkages in the extracellular loop regions of connexin 32 suggests a model for the docking interface of gap junctions. J Cell Biol 140:1187–1197, 1998.
49. Macomber RS: A Complete Introduction to Modern NMR Spectroscopy. New York, John Wiley, 1998.
50. Purnick PE, Benjamin DC, Verselis VK, et al: Structure of the amino terminus of a gap junction protein. Arch Biochem Biophys 381:181–190, 2000.
51. Duffy HS, Sorgen PL, Girvin ME, et al: pH-dependent intramolecular binding and structure involving Cx43 cytoplasmic domains. J Biol Chem 277:36706–36714, 2002.
52. Liu S, Taffet S, Stoner L, et al: A structural basis for the unequal sensitivity of the major cardiac and liver gap junctions to intracellular acidification: The carboxyl tail length. Biophys J. 64:1422–1433, 1993.
53. Yeager M: Structure of cardiac gap junction intercellular channels. J Struct Biol 121:231–245, 1998.
54. Sorgen PL, Duffy HS, Cahill SM, et al: Sequence-specific resonance assignment of the carboxyl terminal domain of connexin43. J Biomol NMR 23:245–246, 2002.
55. Safferling M, Tichelaar W, Kummerle G, et al: First images of a glutamate receptor ion channel: Oligomeric state and molecular dimensions of GluRB homomers. Biochemistry 40:13948–13953, 2001.
56. Galvan DL, Mignery GA: Carboxyl-terminal sequences critical for inositol 1,4,5-trisphosphate receptor subunit assembly. J Biol Chem 277:48248–48260, 2002.
57. Cascio WE: Myocardial ischemia: What factors determine arrhythmogenesis? J Cardiovasc Electrophysiol 12:726–729, 2001.
58. Peters NS, Coromilas J, Severs NJ, Wit AL: Disturbed connexin43 gap junction distribution correlates with the location of reentrant circuits in the epicardial border zone of healing canine infarcts that cause ventricular tachycardia. Circulation 95:988–996, 1997.
59. Morley GE, Taffet SM, Delmar M: Intramolecular interactions mediate pH regulation of Cx43 channels. Biophys J 70:1294–1302, 1996.
60. Armstrong CM, Bezanilla F: Inactivation of the sodium current. II. Gating current experiments. J Gen Physiol 70:567–590, 1977.
61. Zagotta WN, Hoshi T, Aldrich RW: Restoration of inactivation in mutants of Shaker potassium channels by a peptide derived from ShB. Science 250:568–571, 1990.
62. Homma N, Alvarado JL, Coombs W, et al: A particle-receptor model for the insulin-induced closure of connexin43 channels. Circ Res 83:27–32, 1998.
63. Zhou L, Kasperek EM, Nicholson BJ: Dissection of the molecular basis of pp60 (v-src) induced gating of connexin 43 gap junction channels. J Cell Biol 144:1033–1045, 1999.
64. Stergiopoulos K, Alvarado JL, Mastroianni M, et al: Hetero-domain interactions as a mechanism for the regulation of connexin channels. Circ Res 84:1144–1155, 1999.
65. Moreno AP, Chanson M, Anumonwo J, et al: Role of the carboxyl terminal of connexin43 in transjunctional fast voltage gating. Circ Res 90:450–457, 2002.
66. Anumonwo JMB, Taffet SM, Gu H, et al: The carboxyl terminal domain regulates the unitary conductance and voltage dependence of connexin40 gap junction channels. Circ Res 88:666–673, 2001.
67. Unwin PN, Ennis PD: Two configurations of a channel-forming membrane protein. Nature 307:609-613, 1984.

第二部分
心脏离子通道的生物物理学

第 9 章

正常和异常钠通道的生物物理学

Jeffrey R. Balser

本章目录

- 快速门控过程：结构与功能的同步化 ········· 78
- 慢失活：孔隙的协调重排 ········· 79
- 长 QT 综合征的突变机制：门控作用使钠离子流增强 ········· 80
- Brugada 综合征：门控突变使钠离子流减少 ········· 81
- 心脏传导性疾病：一种生物物理的代偿作用？ ········· 82
- 钠通道内的钙信号：结构与功能的新的主题 ········· 82
- 遗传性心律失常对抗心律失常药物机制的提示 ········· 82
- 慢失活和 P 段：一种使用依赖性机制 ········· 83
- 未来：动态的钠通道结构 ········· 84

电压门控性钠通道（I_{Na}）为一类跨细胞膜蛋白质，为心脏动作电位快速超射期的离子流，是主要的心肌传导的离子流。因此，钠通道与遗传和获得性心脏兴奋性紊乱性疾病有关，是发病过程中起关键性作用的分子。正在进行的研究显示钠通道结构的数据，揭示其生物物理功能可以更加精细调整心脏的兴奋性，及进一步治疗心律失常构建框架蓝图。

关于钾通道区域孔隙的精细晶体结构的可视性资料越来越明确[1]，钠通道的小片段的结构的资料也逐步明确[2,3]。当科学家们发现这些立体结构后，动力学分析可以提供精细的功能模型，以演示这些较大的孔隙结构蛋白由于膜电位的改变如何在不到 1ms 时间内快速改变其结构组成（这一过程称为门控）。

由于遗传学研究表明电兴奋紊乱与心脏钠通道突变密切相关，对病变通道进行功能研究揭示了一些独特的门控缺陷的病理学机制。值得注意的是抗心律失常药物无论是水溶性（salutary）还是毒性作用均与钠通道门控的动态结构密切相关，因此设计要求既针对 Na 通道结构又要针对药物动力学来开发药物。

本章阐述了已有正常和异常心脏钠通道功能的理论观点，对钠通道的结构进行了详细的描述，对第一章的内容进一步延伸，并且对与通道功能动力学相关的结构-功能之间的关系进行详细的阐述，以便对后面（第 49 章和 50 章）的遗传性钠通道突变的致心律失常机制的通道功能动力学和第 15 章、第 51 章的钠通道阻滞剂的分子药理学机制进行铺垫。同时本章的阐述和引用（citations）是有选择性的，读者可以参考更多详细的与治疗有关的专题，包括第二信使和酶对钠通道的调节，阳离子渗透的详细过程及辅助亚基的调节[4-7]。

一、快速门控过程：结构与功能的同步化

通过对通道蛋白的克隆与表达，我们理解了钠通道结构如何与门控功能相关联。TTX"敏感"的人心脏钠通道（hH1）由 SCN5A 基因编码，包含一个大的α亚基，α亚基包括四个同构亚基或称同构域（从 I-IV；如图 9-1A），通过细胞浆连接片段依次连接在一起。在过去的 20 余年，定向突变基因学与膜片钳电生理技术相结合，及最近应用氨基酸荧光染色定位方法确定了在电压依赖性门控功能的特定氨基酸部位及动态变化[5,9]。

图 9-1B 显示了除极时细胞膜钠通道的主要门控状态。在除极化时，通道处于"激活"的状态，包括有关的 4 个带电的 S4 片段（如图 9-1A 示）的外向运动，导致通道孔隙开放[10]。几乎在同时，除极导致钠通道快速去激活（如图 9-1B），通道的明显的关闭状态还依赖于 S4 感受器外向运动，但主要依赖于Ⅲ和Ⅳ结构域的变化（分别为 D3S4 和 D4S4；这里的阐述将在全篇文章中引用）[9,11]。除了 S4 片段的外向运动外，快速去激活状态的重要结构改变为Ⅲ-Ⅳ的连接点的变化（linker）（如图 9-1A），它可以阻断孔隙内部的一个"lid"。因为它结合的部位位于或接近内部的前方[13]。一个三联体疏水基团位于（IFM）Ⅲ-Ⅳ连接体的中央区附近（如图 9-1A），可能包含一个"latch"，使 lid 在一个关闭的位置位于孔隙内部上方。

快速去激活态通常情况下在激活态稍后即开始。这有两种结果，首先，它包括在通道关闭前一个短暂的钠离子内流时间（如图 9-1C），其次，尽管在去激

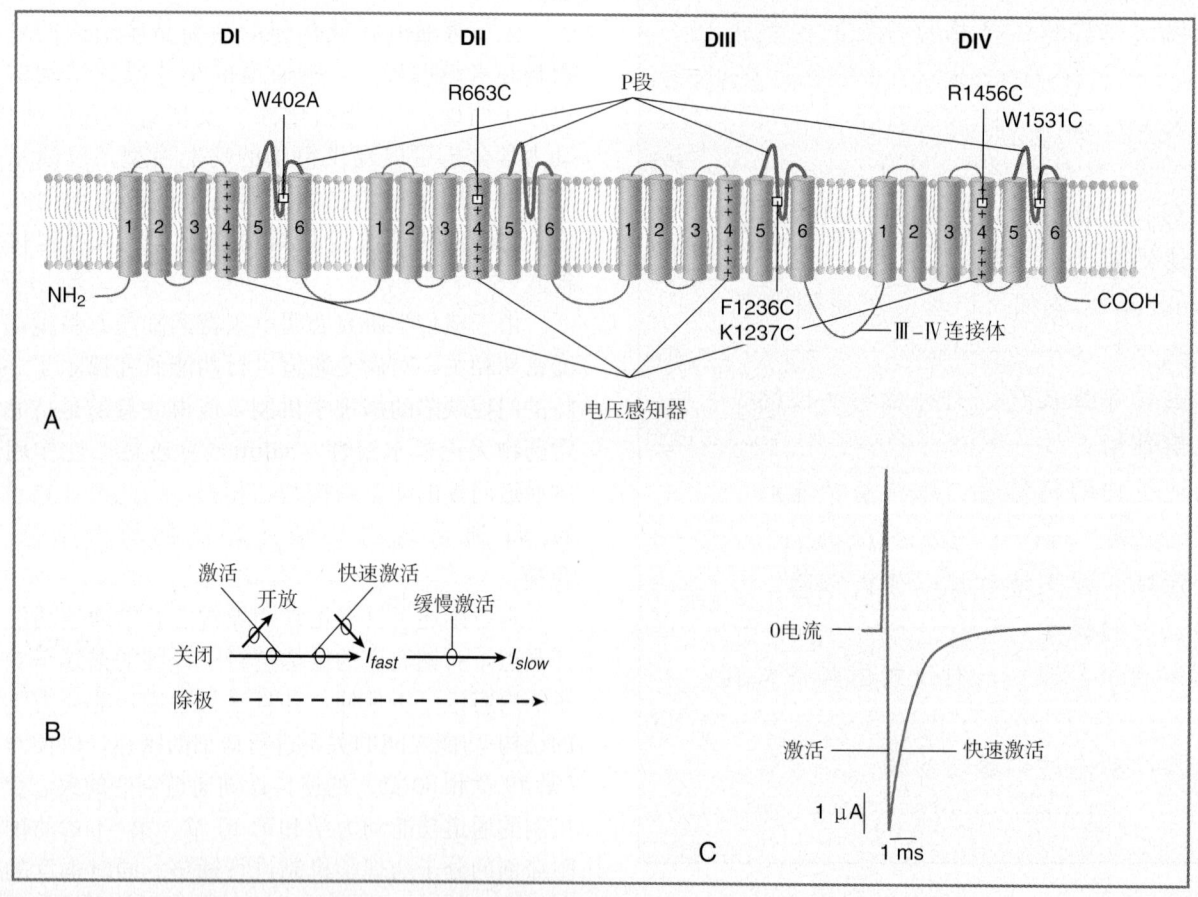

图 9-1 钠通道 A：电压门控钠通道的布局。每个单独的结构域的 S4 包含阳离子的赖氨酸及精氨酸残基，监测跨膜区域的变化。S5 和 S6 连接体的外面突出部分为 P 段，共同组成孔隙的外侧部分。第Ⅲ-Ⅳ连接体在快速失活中发挥主要作用，文章中讨论的不同的氨基酸残基根据最初的大鼠骨骼肌的克隆进行编号[8]。B：简单地图解钠通道门控结构根据膜除极化发生改变。激活和快速失活几乎同时发生，因此通道有时没有经过开放即达到快速失活状态（Ifast）（关闭状态的失活状态），持续的除极引起通道处于稳定的慢失活状态（Islow）。C：从培养的（HEK-293）全细胞电流记录表达了重组的人心脏的钠通道的电流。通过即刻的除极引发电流，类似于心脏动作电位的刺激，值得注意的是电流快速增加（与结合门控同步）然后在通道处于快速失活时衰减

活之前大多数钠通道处于开放状态,但确实有一小部分去激活态离子通道从未开放过(如图 9-1B),这部分通道被称为"关闭状态的去激活状态",是一种基本的门控状态,被认为是心脏钠离子通道有别于其他类型钠离子通道的关键所在。神经和肌肉组织的钠通道很少处于关闭状态的去激活态,这样可以使相应的组织在大多数除极时的静息膜电位下保持可兴奋性。另外,关闭状态的去激活态受与原发性心律失常综合征的遗传突变的调节有关,并且通道在突变时会改变对抗心律失常药物的反应(后面将进行讨论)[14,15]。

二、慢失活:孔隙的协调重排

尽管快速失活 Na^+ 通道能够在两次刺激之中的超极化间期中快速恢复(10ms 以内),在延长的除极时程中,Na^+ 通道逐渐进入慢失活状态(总称为 I_S,见图 9-1B),这种更稳定、不能传导的状态持续时间可显著不同,从几百毫秒至几秒不等。在与心脏动作电位时程相关的时间里,心肌 Na^+ 通道形成一种中间动态化合物。尽管快失活似乎主要包括细胞浆结构、定位突变和 chimric 分析,都提示 P 段在慢失活中发挥关键作用[22-25],直线位于每个结构域内的 S5 和 S6 段之间的连接体顺序折向细胞膜内并在孔隙外排列成线(如图 9-1A)。

在钾离子通道,缓慢 C 型失活包括 P 段的动态性重新排列,这样明显地改变了通道的通透性。在缓慢失活相,对位于钠通道的外部的孔隙进行研究发现了动态变化的形式[28,29],提示在钾通道的缓慢 C 型失活与钠通道缓慢失活之间具有类似之处。包括在 Ⅲ-Ⅳ 区域内的 P 段的半胱氨酸的替代(如图 9-1A,K1237C-W1513C,及图 9-2)形成了一个内部结合的二硫化物,当暴露于氧化物催化剂时则阻断了孔隙[28]。二硫化物的结合依赖于通道的除极化,在中等长度的时程(200ms,图 9-2A)的去极化反应最快,提示相比较在快失活态(IF)或缓慢失活态(IS)在中间 IM 失活态时 P 段的半胱氨酸可以距离更近(如图 9-2B)[23]。已有观点认为钠通道的孔隙在门控和渗透性方面具有高度灵活性,甚至可以认为钠通道具有类似于酶的特性。

正如 S4 片段具有使膜蛋白转变为快速失活态的门控结构一样,D4S4 传感器似乎在慢失活中具有类似的功能。同样的,钾通道的结构-功能模式与钠通道的结构-功能变化相类似。最近应用膜片钳和电压钳荧光测定方法发现在慢失活(C 型失活)相钾通道孔隙外部直接与 S4 电压敏感器相互作用[32]。在钠通道,半胱氨酸与位于 D4S4 的第三个外部的精氨酸相结合使慢失活门控作用增强(R1456C;如图 9-1A)[33]。

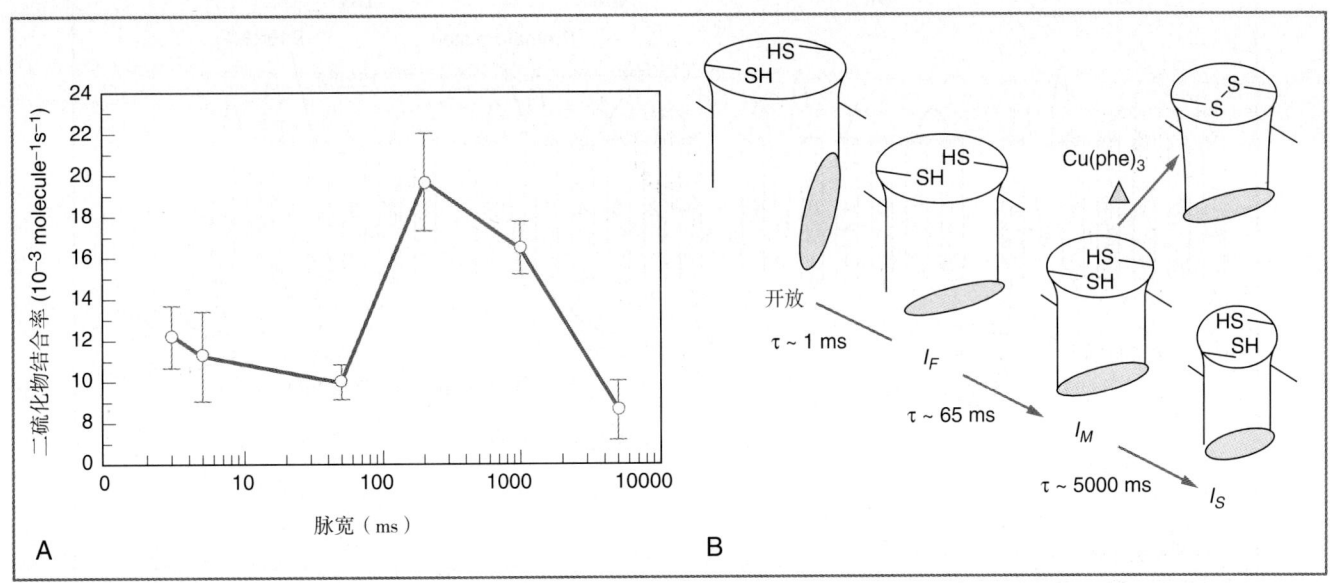

图 9-2 在孔隙外部的二硫键由 100μM 的 Cu(phe)催化 A:钠通道在蟾蜍卵母细胞表达的 K1237C-W1531C 通道在脉冲频率为 0.05Hz 时可产生钠离子流,钠电流减少的频率反映了结构域之间二硫化物结合率(纵坐标)。脉冲时程(横坐标)从 3ms 至 5ms 变化改变了二硫键结合率:二硫键在中间脉宽时最强。B:图表演示了当除极周长扩大时序贯的 3 种失活状态(快速\中间\缓慢:I_F, I_M, I_S)。进入 3 种失活状态的时间常数通过试验方案[23]和文献[30]中获得。图表显示处于中间 IM 状态时,1237 和 1531 半胱氨酸空间上最适合形成二硫键(引自 Benicah JP, Chen Z. BalserJ, et al:钠通道孔隙门控改变的分子动力学:P 段运动与失活的相互作用。J Neurosci 19:1577-1585. 1999.)

但这一作用会由于第一结构域内的 P 段上由丙氨酸替代而拮抗其作用（W402A；如图 9-1A）[33]，已知这一替代作用可抑制 IM 组成的慢失活部分[34]，所以快失活相和慢失活相均通过激发电压敏感的 S4 段的结构变化导致几种门控结构的组合变化，通过控制孔隙对钠离子的通透性来调控一系列时程。

三、长 QT 综合征的突变机制：门控作用使钠离子流增强

心脏钠通道突变与常染色体显性表现形式的长 QT 综合征（LQT3）（如图 9-3）有关，导致的心电图 QT 间期延长与特异的多形性室性心动过速（尖端扭转室速）。这些突变持续地干扰快失活过程[36-38]，除极化过程中通道重复开放，使动作电位平台期引起一种小的持续的 Na^+ 流（图 9-1A），这种额外的内向离子流原发的一种获得性钠通道功能，使细胞复极延迟并使患者易于发生多形性室速。令人惊奇的是这种持续的钠离子流与快速除极时的峰值钠离子流相比非常微弱（约为 0.5%～2%）[18,37,38]，不管怎样，在这种持续的电流，动作电位延长和致心律失常兴奋性之间的联系已通过大量的实验模型得到证实，表明钠通道功能与心脏的兴奋性呈高度非线性关系。

与Ⅲ-Ⅳ连接部位在快速失活期的作用相一致，第一次报道的 LQT3 突变为这个区域缺失 3 种碱基（1505 至 1507△KPQ；如图 9-3）[36]，其他 3 个突变位于通道的细胞浆面附近（N1325S，R1644H，及 T1645M）[36,37,40]，并且可能影响快速失活时的Ⅲ-Ⅳ连接体的运动或结合力，有多个部位与快速失活的门控机制有关，Na 通道的其他部位的突变对门控过程也很重要，也会导致 LQT3。位于带电的 S4 段的 2 种 SCN5A 突变（T1304M 及 R1623Q；如图 9-3）[40,41]使快失活不稳定[42,43]。值得注意的是，通过荧光定位研究这些位于感受器部位（D3S4 和 D4S4）的突变很可能与快速失活有关[9]，在高度保守的邻近 COOH 的终末端羧基部位也潜藏着许多 LQT3 突变（如图 9-3），与上面描述的快失活门控中这些部位的作用相一致。COOH 末端的结构机制如何影响快速失活尚不清楚，通过对许多 COOH 基末端电荷中和的同时并未表现为更严重或叠加的作用，提示这种酸基作为一种大的带电基团可能未参与快速失活。然而，邻近的 COOH 基末端可能与孔隙内的位点相互作用，这些位点不带电荷或者对与孔隙关闭有关的其他门控区域发生变构效应。

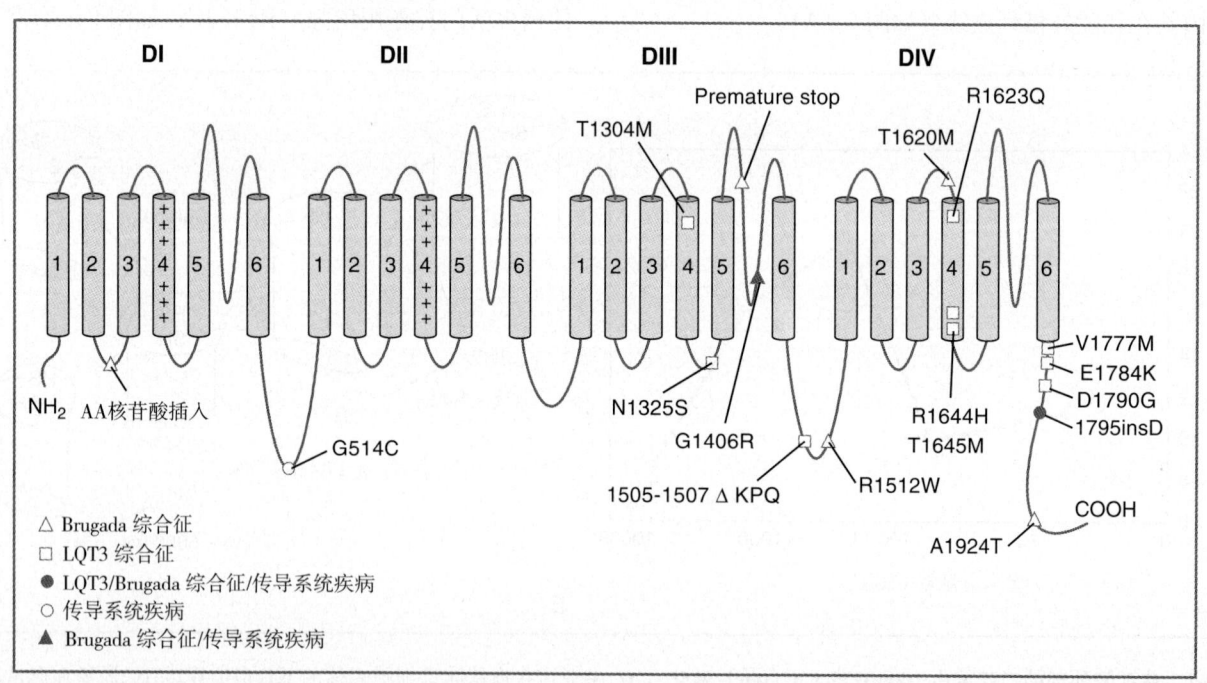

图 9-3　心脏钠通道的遗传性突变　钠通道结构在图中演示，与图 9-1 和文中描述的与 LQT 综合征（LQT3）和 Brugada 综合征有关突变形式相同（据人心脏钠通道进行编号为 hH1）。演示的突变只代表与这些遗传性综合征有关的 SCN5A 突变的一小部分。突变倾向于簇集和围绕着 S4 片段、第Ⅲ-Ⅳ连接体、COOH 末端、Ⅲ-Ⅳ连接体及 P 环，与这些部位在通道门控中的重要作用有关

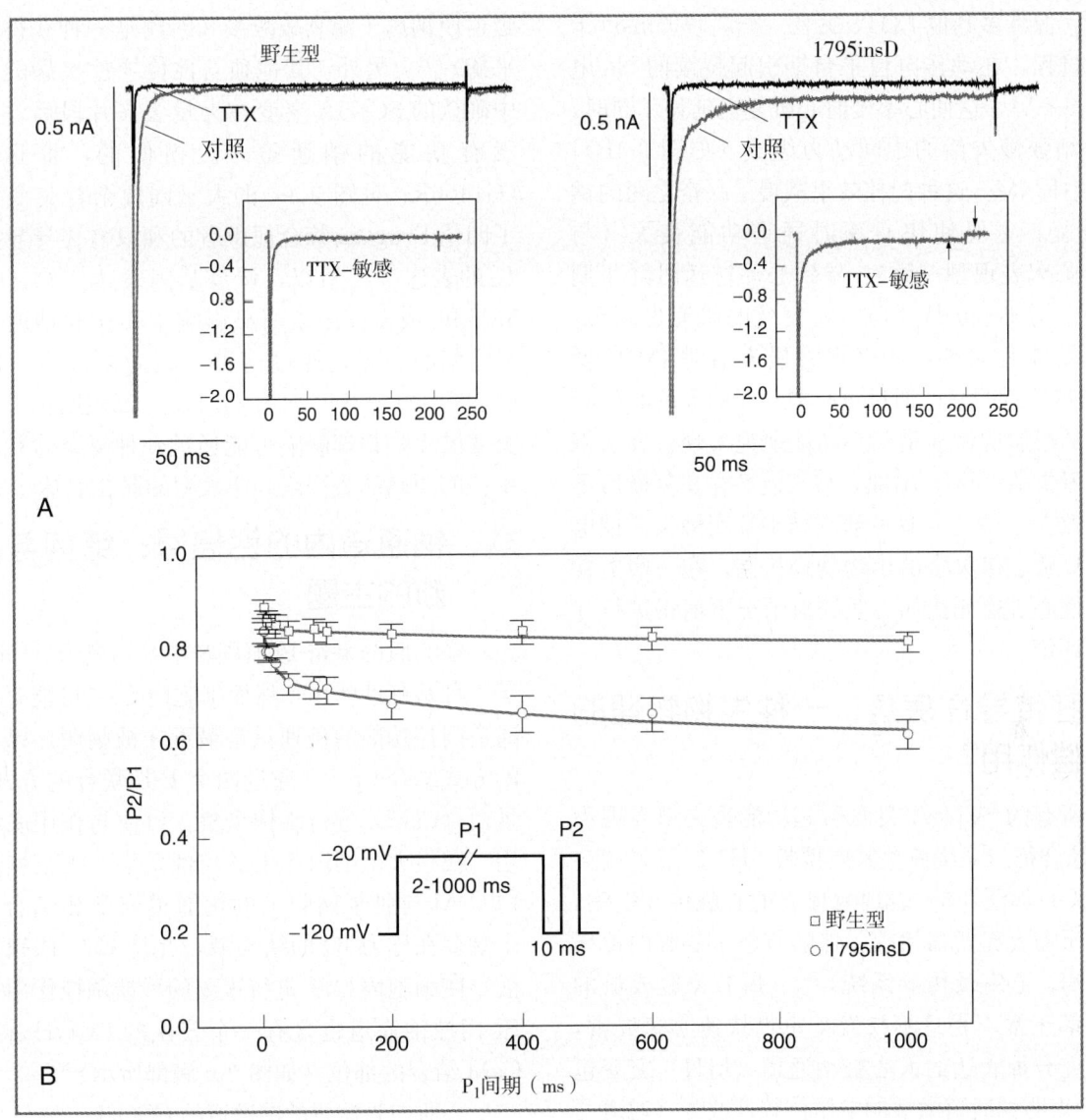

图 9-4 COOH 末端的突变改变了 2 种门控过程及引发了 LQT3 和 Bruguda 综合征[17] A：1795insD 突变引起持续的内向电流部分，与其他 LQT3 突变相似（比如 ΔKPQ）。每幅图演示了 TTX 敏感电流（30μM），通过滤过获得，并且演示了突变后明显增大的 TTX 敏感电流（箭头所示）。B：一种增强的失活的缓慢动力学组成部分在 1795insD 突变中也能看到。在应用电压钳制刺激参数下可观察到慢失活过程，同时通道在不同的时间间期（P1）除极然后从 10ms 的快失活恢复，而不是从慢失活恢复。由 P2 脉冲诱发的残余的钠电流反映了在 P1 脉冲引发的中间慢失活程度（IM）。突变增加了慢失活成分的幅值（修改自 Veldkamp MW, Viswanathan PC, BezzINa C, et al：Two distinct congenital arrythmias evoked by a ysfunctional Na^+ channel. Circ Res 86：E91-E97，2000.）

四、Brugada 综合征：门控突变使钠离子流减少

Brugada 综合征为一种典型的特发性室性心律失常性疾病，最近确认为 SCN5A 突变，与 LQT3 患者不同，这种疾病患者表现为典型的心电图表现，包括右束支阻滞和 V1～V3 的 ST 段抬高、发作特发性室速和室颤，在第 50 章和 67 章将详细讨论 Brugada 综合征的细胞和离子通道的生物生理机制。与 LQT3 突变相反，Brugada 综合征突变表现为 Na 通道功能的丧失。

进一步研究发现了功能获得和丧失之间的联系，这些不同的心律失常综合征有许多相似之处，可由于心率依赖性同时并存 LQT3 和 Brugada 综合征，在心率慢时 QT 间期延长，在运动时 ST 段明显抬高[17,45]。

LQT3 是由于功能获得引发，而 Brugada 综合征是由于功能丧失引起，与此相一致，COOH 末端突变（1795insD）对 Na 通道的失活动力学组成具有相反的

作用效应。像许多其他LQT3突变一样，1795insD干扰快失活过程，在动作电位平台期引起持续的Na电流（如图9-4A），这使心率慢时心脏复极延长。同时，1795insD增强慢失活的中间动力组成（如图9-4B）；在图9-2中称IM，这种门控效果减慢了兴奋之间的钠通道的恢复，主要使快心率时通道功能丧失（与1795insD临床表现型一致），导致心动过速时舒张期相对缩短。对Brugada T1620M突变的研究也发现，除了通道功能丧失外，还表现为慢失活时IM的增强[46]。值得注意的是，通过对心梗5天的犬的心外膜梗死边缘的心肌的钠通道门控功能研究发现，失活恢复延迟及慢失活（IM）增加，与该模型存在复极后不应答相一致[47]。总之，这些研究结果证明慢失活钠电流增强是导致心律失常的生物物理机制，在一些更常见的继发性心脏猝死比如心肌缺血情况下值得进行仔细的研究评价。

五、心脏传导性疾病：一种生物物理的代偿作用？

不是所有的SCN5A突变引起功能丧失都表现为Brugada综合征。一个荷兰家族携带hH1 I-II连接突变（G514C；如图9-3）表现为独立的心脏传导疾病，有两个孩子需要起搏器治疗，伴随有整个心脏的传导缓慢（心房、心室及传导系统）[48]。所有家庭成员的心脏结构都正常，并且不易发生室性快速心律失常，膜片钳研究异种表达的人心脏钠通道（hH1）突变包括G514C表明钠通道激活的电压依赖性改变（通道开放需要更高的除极电压），反映了其他Brugada综合征突变有关的功能丧失缺陷[49]。但是，在电压依赖性失活（一种获得性功能缺陷）时，一种平行除极改变"平衡的"原发激活缺陷，引起钠电流的减少程度降低。在一种心脏动作电位传导的计算模型（图9-5）这种轻度的功能丧失不足以引起明显的与Brugada综合征的动作电位除极缺陷[49]，但是可以预示心脏传导延迟约15%可以引起缓慢型心律失常表现型[48]。应该注意在Brugada/LQT3中相似的1795insD携带者也可表现为传导性障碍，与钠通道功能丧失和传导性疾病之间的因果关系相一致。

尽管携带G514C的功能丧失通过对抗门控缺陷得以补偿，在这种或其他遗传性传导疾病综合征中也可能存在其他平衡机制。在两种其他家族性传导障碍疾病（G278S及D1595N），这种通道突变表现为钠通道慢失活增加（一种功能丧失），还有由于快速失活的延迟使钠离子流衰减减慢（因此是一种获得性功能的平衡）[50]。另外，其他独立性传导性疾病的两个家族中确认的SCN5A突变在大量丢失片段后，生成完全没有功能的钠通道[51]。相似的，III区域P段（G1406R；见图9-3）的大量同源杂合突变完全消除了四位Brugada综合征患者的和只有传导异常患者的I_{Na}的表达[52]。所以，调节基因表达产物、等位基因外显和/或发育因素明显影响了心律和钠通道功能外显之间的关系，通过何种方式尚未确定。这些例子（1795insD，G1406R和G514C）都表明钠通道的单一突变的生物物理缺陷可能通过一种复杂途径激发一种单一的明确的表型或心律表型的联合表达。

六、钠通道内的钙信号：结构与功能的新的主题

在心肌的兴奋-收缩耦联中，钙离子（Ca^{2+}）发挥了一种基础性作用，然而细胞内Ca^{2+}可能直接调节钠通道门控功能的机理只是最近才被阐明。以共同作用的方式结合Ca^{2+}（通过四个E-F联合的方式），钙调蛋白（CaM）进行结构重整，以便与作用底物相互作用，在很大范围内产生适应性反应。钙依赖性钙调蛋白CaM与肌浆网膜上的钙通道末端相结合，COOH末端存在称为IQ的结构域，允许Ca^{2+}依赖性通道失活，使细胞内Ca^{2+}进行重要的反馈调控作用[53,54]。电压-门控钠通道也含有一个公认的COOH末端IQ的CaM结合的部位（如图9-6底部所示）[55]。

心肌与骨骼肌的钠通道的COOH末端与CaM的特异性结合发生相互作用对钠通道的门控功能具有重要影响[56,57]。在心肌的钠通道，这种结合作用明显增强了慢失活过程（如图9-6，左）并且因此在有突变时在导致Brugada综合征和传导性疾病时产生协同作用（前面已描述）。针对于IQ结构域的突变可干扰CaM的结合[56,57]并以抑制Ca^{2+}/CaM依赖调节的方式与人类钠通道结合，这种结合影响了通道的门控和动力学调控。这种细胞Ca^{2+}与钠通道功能之间的关系还未完全阐明，并且可能在一些常见的获得性钙失调性心脏疾病（心衰和缺血）中对细胞兴奋性具有重要影响。

七、遗传性心律失常对抗心律失常药物机制的提示

遗传性SCN5A突变对钠通道功能提供了很多有意义的信息，这些通道突变也提供了许多有用的针对抗心律失常的分子药理学研究机制。在第15章中对

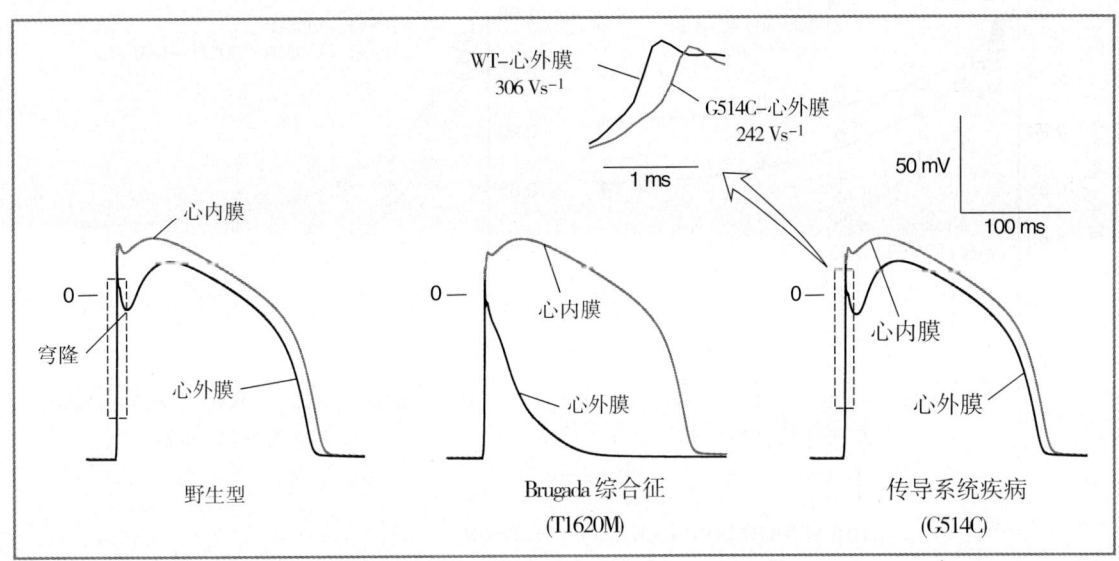

图 9-5 模拟 Brugada 综合征与传导性疾病的动作电位的模型（所示为心外膜和心内膜的动作电位） 左图：野生型动作电位，较大短暂的钾电流（Ito）形成了心外膜"穹隆"；中图：T1620M，激活门控被折衷，而快失活增强，引起了钠电流的明显减低，这导致心外膜早除极但心内膜并非如此，导致产生跨膜电压梯度及 Brugada 综合征[49]。右图：G514C，图中激活门控被折衷（类似于 T1620M），而快失活减弱，后者可能使钠电流增加及使激活缺陷得以补偿，钠电流减低的绝对值比 T1620M 减少的程度小，因此心外膜动作电位的平台期仍得以保持，尽管动作电位超射（虚线框内）延迟。虚线框：动作电位超射期（框内包括野生型和 G514C 动作电位）通过放大的时间区域显示突变减慢的动作电位超射速率（dV/dtmax），由此减慢了心肌传导（引自 tan HL，Bink-Boelkens MTE，BezzINa CR，et al：A sodium channel mutation causes isolated cardiac conduction disease. Nature 409：1043-1047，2001.）

钠通道的药理学研究做了详细的阐述。但是，这部分将提供一些实例说明异常钠通道门控功能改变如何表现为遗传性心律失常，进而从根本上影响了药物治疗效果。

钠通道阻滞剂在治疗 LQT3 患者时有效[58,59]，具有治疗作用的钠通道阻滞剂，比如利多卡因的结合位点主要位于 S6 片段的细胞浆部分的氨基酸部位（如图 9-7C，左）。同时在 LQT3 突变时持续的病理性电流可以被利多卡因或其类似物抑制（如图 9-4A）[37,61]。通过对 LQT3 的药物作用研究确定利多卡因可以对 LQT3 突变孔隙的开放结构优先结合，或者甚至有可能对开放通道的快失活具有"修复"作用[42,62]。但是，对 R1623Q 的 LQT3 突变的研究出乎意料地揭示了利多卡因对持续电流的作用机制[14]。对无药物情况下研究发现 R1623Q 通道的关闭态的失活确实增加（如图 9-1B）[14]。相反，在突变所致开放态下的失活异常更加明显[42]，应用大量的 Markov 模型，证明利多卡因的结合可能增强了异构效应使关闭状态的通道失活[14]。

尽管 Na 通道阻滞剂可能对 LQT3 突变引起的持续电流有益处，近期研究表明氟卡胺——一种有效的 Na 通道阻滞剂，在许多携带 LQT3 突变的患者中引发 Brugada 波样的 ST 段抬高，与此有关的药理学敏感性可能同时有治疗效果（通过抑制持续性电流）和致心律失常危险（由于抑制了峰值钠电流）的作用。在离体水平的研究结果支持这一结论，研究表明至少两种 LQT3 突变综合征的突变（1795insD 和 ΔKPQ）表现为明确的关闭状态的失活[15,64]，并且两种形式的突变均表现为：在钳制的关闭状态的失活电位时，氟卡胺的阻断作用增强[15]，所以，关闭状态的失活门控是一种钠通道门控机制，当进行调整时，可能进一步影响药物治疗的临床作用。

八、慢失活和 P 段：一种使用依赖性机制

很久以前即观察到，钠电流在重复引发的动作电位过程中逐渐减小（使用依赖性），并且在钠通道阻滞剂应用时，这种效果应更加明显。近期研究表明，应用半胱氨酸标记的快失活门控结构（比如Ⅲ-Ⅳ连接体）已经证明，与以前的假设相反，使用依赖性不是由于钠通道陷于快失活状态[15]。同时，在许多调节慢失活（突变和阳离子替代）的因素作用下对钠通道使

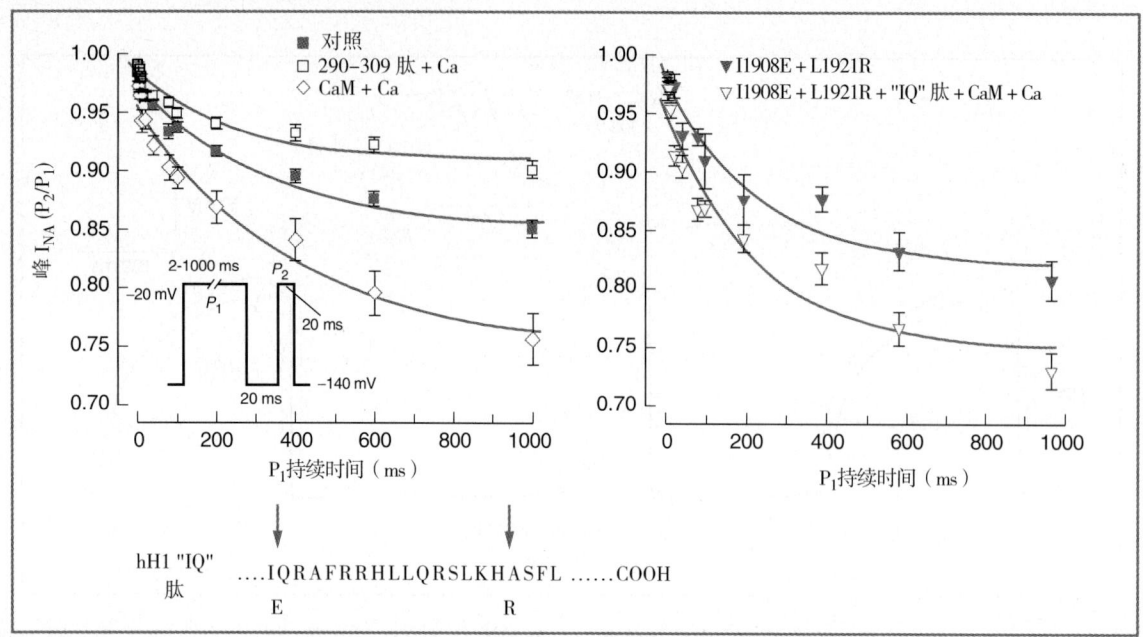

图9-6 钙离子和钙调蛋白（CaM）激酶调节心脏钠通道慢失活 左图：在培养的（HEK-293）细胞中表达的野生型心脏钠通道的慢失活测定方法与图9-4B中应用的一致（参见插图中电压钳制参数），在细胞内含有钙离子为一种钙调蛋白激酶肽抑制剂（290～309肽），也暴露于细胞内，抑制慢失活；相反，CaM在钙离子存在时使慢失活增强，与Brugada综合征见到的相似。右图：hH1钠通道突变在公认的COOH末端"IQ"区域有两个关键残基（下面）进行修饰（I1908E+L1921R）。这种双重突变会使通道抵抗CaM引起慢失活（未显示）；但是CaM的慢失活门控效应通过细胞内液野生型"IQ"肽段得以恢复（空白的倒三角形）

用依赖性研究表明在去极化刺激之间通道的缓慢恢复可能包括钠通道阻滞剂与慢失活结构状态的相互作用。许多更直接的试验，近期研究应用合成的半胱氨酸（F1236C，参见图9-1A），作为一种P段慢失活活动的标记证明这种基因的共价调节通过甲磺硫代硫酸获得状态状态依赖性乙胺盐（MTSEA），一系列简短的5S的去极化刺激比更长（100ms）的脉宽（如图9-7A）足以使通道开放及引起快失活（但不引起慢失活），产生更多快速MTSEA调节（图9-7B），提示慢失活抑制了去极化引起的半胱氨酸端链接近MTSEA。重要的是，利多卡因进一步抑制由于这些持续的（100ms）除极而不是短暂的（5s）除极引起的去极化依赖的巯基修饰（图9-7A和B）。在P段附加部位基因（k1237）与利多卡因NH2末端的静电吸引作用提示S6基因形成了位于P段近端的利多卡因受体[68]。因此，有人假设结构的重新调整，钠通道P段移入使利多卡因和孔隙的相互作用更加稳定。BS在一些特殊家族中慢失活增强时（比如T1620M和1795insD）[17,46]造成门控缺陷使Brugada表现型恶化[15]。

九、未来：动态的钠通道结构

通过观察图9-3提示，非随机收集BS传导性疾病及LQT3位点，比如T1620M（BS）位于第Ⅳ结构域S3和S4之间连接体的外侧，只有3个基因的COOH末端朝向S4精氨酸（R1623Q；LQT3）。已观察到R1623Q对快失活[42,43]的门控效应及T1620M对快失活和慢失活的作用[11,36,69]，类似的收集LQT3和BS突变在Ⅲ-Ⅳ连接部位显示（如图9-3）。尽管失活恢复减慢[70,71]，并且位于ΔKPQ LQT3缺失的5个残基，许多LQT3和Brugada突变在COOH末端的酪氨酸（Y1795）突变为半胱氨酸或组氨酸分别引发了LQT3或BS，并且在离体水平引起对门控失活的功能获得性或功能丢失性作用，这与活体表现型相一致[72]。

令人惊奇的是这些邻近的突变产生相反的作用并且多功能部位强调了将来研究重点是确定三维蛋白结构。目前对通道结构的特点的研究仅限于可溶性胞浆部分的结构域。对Ⅲ-Ⅳ连接体的分离进行这种核的磁共振性溶液结构的研究揭示一种稳定折叠的核心包含一个α螺旋带有NH2-末端序列的帽状结构，形成了

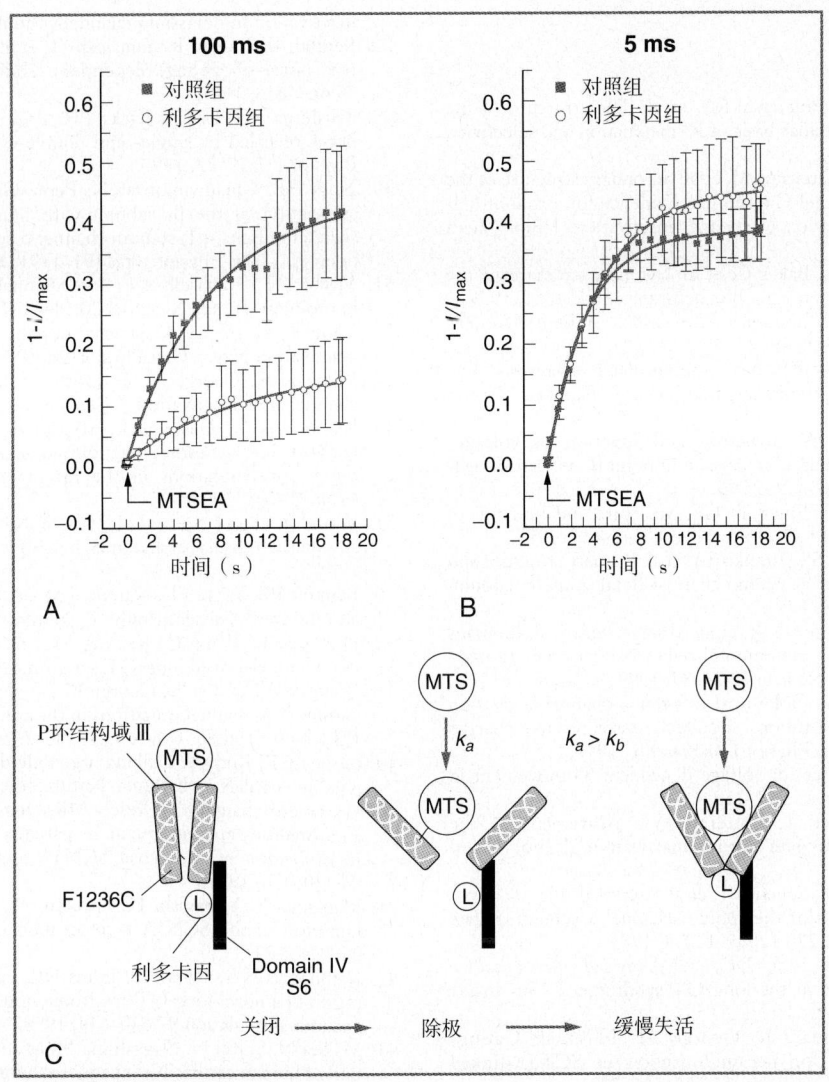

图9-7 F1236C通道的MTSEA变型由慢失活调节及使用依赖性利多卡因阻断 A：HEK-293细胞表达F1236C通道进行短时（5ms）或中等长度（100ms）除极刺激时，峰值钠电流（与前MTSEA有关）对应于累积的除极时间作图，在无利多卡因时，MTSEA变型在短时程时更快，提示在慢失活时使1236半胱氨酸更不易接近（对比图形的升支及实心符号，图A和B）。另外，利多卡因（100μM）明显地降低了除极-依赖性MTSEA变化速率，但脉宽为100ms，而不是5ms（空白的符号）。C：在慢失活和利多卡因（L）阻断时P段选择性滤过概念模型及MTS接近度。模型提示当通道开放时设计的接近选择性滤过处的P环上半胱氨酸处于暴露状态，但在慢失活时暴露程度减低，提示选择性滤过部分在慢失活时重整。利多卡因在与细胞浆面选择性滤过区的假定的S6结构域上的受体结合时可能同时在慢失活时进行重整的P段更加稳定并由此增加使用依赖性（修改自Ong BH, Tomaselli GF, Basler JR: A structural rearrangement in the sodium channel pore linked to slow INactivation and use dependence. J Gen Physiol 116：653-661，2000.）

一个模型，模型里稳定折叠的核心包括一个闩样结构（3个疏水残基；IFM如图9-1A），以一个灵活的铰链为枢纽，进而在快失活门控阶段阻断孔隙结构。可溶性COOH末端结构域还被提纯并具有环形二相色性。揭示高度有序的α螺旋近端区域对失活门控发挥重要作用[2]。尽管钠通道的完全的晶体状结构研究在较低水平，近期从低温电子显微镜获得的低分辨率（19Å）三维立体密度图揭示了沿细胞浆及细胞膜外表面的胞膜内凹陷及孔穴的令人惊奇的复杂工作网络[73]。这种复杂的前向遮挡结构在暴露于疏水与亲水性微环境时包含杂乱的折叠环和螺旋，与单个结构域快速转换。这种结构将用来解释一个看来细微的氨基酸替代，尽管很接近，在重要的片段也可引起蛋白功能与心脏兴奋性的相反的改变。

（赵新然　浦介麟　译）

参 考 文 献

1. Doyle DA, Cabral JM, Pfuetzner RA, et al: The structure of the potassium channel: Molecular basis of K⁺ conduction and selectivity. Science 280:69–77, 1998.
2. Cormier JW, Rivolta I, Tateyama M, et al: Secondary structure of the human cardiac Na⁺ channel C terminus: Evidence for a role of helical structures in modulation of channel inactivation. J Biol Chem 277:9233–9241, 2002.
3. Rohl CA, Boeckman FA, Baker C, et al: Solution structure of the sodium channel inactivation gate. Biochemistry 38:855–861, 1999.
4. Balser JR: Structure and function of the cardiac sodium channels. Cardiovasc Res 42:327–338, 1999.
5. Catterall WA: From ionic currents to molecular mechanisms: The structure and function of voltage-gated sodium channels. Neuron 26:13–25, 2000.
6. Fozzard HA, Hanck DA: Structure and function of voltage-dependent sodium channels: Comparison of brain II and cardiac isoforms. Physiol Rev 76:887–926, 1996.
7. Marban E, Yamagishi T, Tomaselli GF: Structure and function of voltage-gated sodium channels. J Physiol 508:647–657, 1998.
8. Trimmer JS, Cooperman SS, Tomiko SA, et al: Primary structure and functional expression of a mammalian skeletal muscle sodium channel. Neuron 3:33–49, 1989.
9. Cha A, Ruben PC, George AL Jr, et al: Voltage sensors in domains III and IV, but not in I and II, are immobilized by Na⁺ channel fast inactivation [see comments]. Neuron 22:73–87, 1999.
10. Kontis KJ, Rounaghi A, Goldin AL: Sodium channel activation gating is affected by substitutions of voltage sensor positive charges in all four domains. J Gen Physiol 110:391–401, 1997.
11. Yang N, Horn R: Evidence for voltage-dependent S4 movement in sodium channels. Neuron 15:213–218, 1995.
12. Kellenberger S, Scheuer T, Catterall WA: Movement of the Na⁺ channel inactivation gate during inactivation. J Biol Chem 271:30971–30979, 1996.
13. McPhee JC, Ragsdale DS, Scheuer T, et al: A critical role for transmembrane segment IVS6 of the sodium channel a subunit in fast inactivation. J Biol Chem 270:12025–12034, 1995.
14. Kambouris NG, Nuss HB, Johns DC, et al: A revised view of cardiac sodium channel blockade in the long-QT syndrome. J Clin Invest 105:1133–1140, 2000.
15. Viswanathan PC, Bezzina CR, George AL Jr, et al: Gating-dependent mechanisms for flecainide action in SCN5A-linked arrhythmia syndromes. Circulation 15:542–544, 2001.
16. Sheets MF, Kyle JW, Hanck DA: The role of the putative inactivation lid in sodium channel gating current immobilization. J Gen Physiol 115:609–620, 2000.
17. Veldkamp MW, Viswanathan PC, Bezzina C, et al: Two distinct congenital arrhythmias evoked by a multidysfunctional Na⁺ channel. Circ Res 86:E91–E97, 2000.
18. Wei J, Wang DW, Alings M, et al: Congenital long-QT syndrome caused by a novel mutation in a conserved acidic domain of the cardiac Na⁺ channel. Circulation 99:3165–3171, 1999.
19. Cannon SC: Slow inactivation of sodium channels: More than just a laboratory curiosity. Biophys J 71:5–7, 1996.
20. Cummins TR, Sigworth FJ: Impaired slow inactivation in mutant sodium channels. Biophys J 71:227–236, 1996.
21. Shander GS, Fan Z, Makielski JC: Slowly recovering cardiac sodium current in rat ventricular myocytes: Effects of conditioning duration and recovery potential. J Cardiovasc Electrophysiol 6:786–795, 1995.
22. Balser JR, Nuss HB, Chiamvimonvat N, et al: External pore residue mediates slow inactivation in m1 rat skeletal muscle sodium channels. J Physiol 494:431–442, 1996.
23. Benitah JP, Chen Z, Balser J, et al: Molecular dynamics of the sodium channel pore vary with gating: Interactions between P-segment motions and inactivation. J Neurosci 19:1577–1585, 1999.
24. Todt H, Dudley SC Jr, Kyle JW, et al: Ultra-slow inactivation in mu1 Na⁺ channels is produced by a structural rearrangement of the outer vestibule. Biophys J 76:1335–1345, 1999.
25. Vilin YY, Makita N, George AL Jr, et al: Structural determinants of slow inactivation in human cardiac and skeletal muscle sodium channels. Biophys J 77:1384–1393, 1999.
26. Liu Y, Jurman ME, Yellen G: Dynamic rearrangement of the outer mouth of a K channel during gating. Neuron 16:859–867, 1996.
27. Kiss L, LoTurco J, Korn SJ: Contribution of the selectivity filter to inactivation in potassium channels. Biophys J 76:253–263, 1999.
28. Benitah JP, Ranjan R, Yamagishi T, et al: Molecular motions within the pore of voltage-dependent sodium channels. Biophys J 73:603–613, 1997.
29. Tsushima RG, Li RA, Backx PH: P-loop flexibility in Na⁺ channel pores revealed by single- and double-cysteine replacements. J Gen Physiol 110:59–72, 1997.
30. Nuss HB, Chiamvimonvat N, Perez-Garcia MT, et al: Functional association of the β_1 subunit with human cardiac (hH1) and rat skeletal muscle (m1) sodium channel α subunits expressed in Xenopus oocytes. J Gen Physiol 106:1171–1191, 1995.
31. Marban E, Tomaselli GF: Ion channels as enzymes: Analogy or homology? Trends Neurosci 20:144–147, 1997.
32. Loots E, Isacoff EY: Molecular coupling of S4 to a K⁺ channel's slow inactivation gate. J Gen Physiol 116:623–635, 2000.
33. Mitrovic N, George AL Jr, Horn R: Role of domain 4 in sodium channel slow inactivation. J Gen Physiol 115:707–718, 2000.
34. Kambouris N, Hastings L, Stepanovic S, et al: Mechanistic link between local anesthetic action and inactivation gating probed by outer pore mutations in the rat m1 sodium channel. J Physiol 512:693–705, 1998.
35. Wang Q, Shen J, Splawski I, et al: SCN5A mutations associated with an inherited cardiac arrhythmia, long QT syndrome. Cell 80:805–811, 1995.
36. Bennett PB, Yazawa K, Naomasa M, et al: Molecular mechanism for an inherited cardiac arrhythmia. Nature 376:683–685, 1995.
37. Dumaine R, Wang Q, Keating MT, et al: Multiple mechanisms of Na⁺ channel-linked long-QT syndrome. Circ Res 78:916–924, 1996.
38. Wang DW, Yazawa K, George AL, et al: Characterization of human cardiac Na⁺ channel mutations in the congenital long QT syndrome. Proc Natl Acad Sci U S A 93:13200–13205, 1996.
39. Clancy CE, Rudy Y: Linking a genetic defect to its cellular phenotype in a cardiac arrhythmia. Nature 400:566–569, 1999.
40. Wattanasirichaigoon D, Vesely MR, Duggal P, et al: Sodium channel abnormalities are infrequent in patients with long QT syndrome: Identification of two novel SCN5A mutations. Am J Med Genet 86:470–476, 1999.
41. Matsuoka R, Yamagishi H, Furutani M, et al: A de novo missense mutation of the SCN5A gene in long QT syndrome. Circulation 96:I-56, 1997.
42. Kambouris NG, Nuss HB, Johns DC, et al: Phenotypic characterization of a novel long QT syndrome mutation in the cardiac sodium channel. Circulation 97:640–644, 1998.
43. Makita N, Shirai N, Nagashima M, et al: A de novo missense mutation of human cardiac Na⁺ channel exhibiting novel molecular mechanisms of long QT syndrome. FEBS Lett 423:5–9, 1998.
44. Brugada P, Brugada J: Right bundle branch block, persistent ST segment elevation and sudden cardiac death: A distinct clinical and electrocardiographic syndrome. A multicenter report. J Am Coll Cardiol 20:1391–1396, 1992.
45. Bezzina C, Veldkamp MW, van Den Berg MP, et al: A single Na⁺ channel mutation causing both long-QT and Brugada syndromes. Circ Res 85:1206–1213, 1999.
46. Wang DW, Makita N, Kitabatake A, et al: Enhanced sodium channel intermediate inactivation in Brugada syndrome. Circ Res 87:e37–e43, 2000.
47. Pu J, Balser JR, Boyden PA: Lidocaine action on Na⁺ currents in ventricular myocytes from the epicardial border zone of the infarcted heart. Circ Res 83:431–40, 1998.
48. Tan HL, Bink-Boelkens MTE, Bezzina CR, et al: A sodium channel mutation causes isolated cardiac conduction disease. Nature 409:1043–1047, 2001.
49. Dumaine R, Towgin JA, Burgada P, et al: Ionic mechanisms responsible for the electrocardiographic phenotype of the Brugada syndrome are temperature dependent. Circ Res 85:803–809, 1999.
50. Wang DW, Viswanathan PC, Balser JR, et al: Clinical, genetic, and biophysical characterization of SCN5A mutations associated with atrioventricular conduction block. Circulation 105:341–346, 2002.
51. Schott JJ, Alshinawi C, Kyndt F, et al: Cardiac conduction defects associate with mutations in SCN5A. Nat Genet 23:20–21, 1999.
52. Kyndt F, Probst V, Potet F, et al: Novel SCN5A mutation leading either to isolated cardiac conduction defect or Brugada syndrome in a large French family. Circulation 104:3081–3086, 2001.
53. Lee A, Wong ST, Gallagher D, et al: Ca²⁺/calmodulin binds to and modulates P/Q-type calcium channels [see comments]. Nature 399:155–159, 1999.

54. Zuhlke RD, Reuter H: Ca^{2+}-sensitive inactivation of L-type Ca^{2+} channels depends on multiple cytoplasmic amino acid sequences of the α1C subunit. Proc Natl Acad Sci U S A 95:3287-3294, 1998.
55. Mori M, Konno T, Ozawa T, et al: Novel interaction of the voltage-dependent sodium channel (VDSC) with calmodulin: Does VDSC acquire calmodulin-mediated Ca^{2+}-sensitivity? Biochemistry 39:1316-1323, 2000.
56. Deschenes I, Neyroud N, DiSilvestre D, et al: Isoform-specific modulation of voltage-gated Na^+ channels by calmodulin. Circ Res 90:E49-E57, 2002.
57. Tan HL KS, Zhang R, Stepanovic S, et al: A calcium sensor in the sodium channel modulates cardiac excitability. Nature 416:59-61, 2002.
58. Benhorin J, Taub R, Goldmit M, et al: Effects of flecainide in patients with new SCN5A mutation: Mutation-specific therapy for long-QT syndrome? Circulation 101:1698-706, 2000.
59. Shimizu W, Antzelevitch C: Sodium channel block with mexiletine is effective in reducing dispersion of repolarization and preventing torsade de pointes in LQT2 and LQT3 models of the long-QT syndrome. Circulation 96:2038-2047, 1997.
60. Ragsdale DS, McPhee JC, Scheuer T, et al: Molecular determinants of state-dependent block of Na^+ channels by local anesthetics. Science 265:1724-1728, 1994.
61. An RH, Bangalore R, Rosero SZ, et al: Lidocaine block of LQT-3 mutant human Na channels. Circ Res 79:103-108, 1996.
62. Wang DW, Yazawa K, Makita N, et al: Pharmacological targeting of long QT mutant sodium channels. J Clin Invest 99:1714-1720, 1997.
63. Priori SG, Napolitano C, Schwartz PJ, et al: The elusive link between LQT3 and Brugada syndrome: The role of flecainide challenge. Circulation 102:945-947, 2000.
64. Chen T, Sheets MF: Enhancement of closed-state inactivation in long QT syndrome sodium channel mutations delta KPQ. Am J Physiol Heart Circ Physiol 283:H966-H975, 2002.
65. Vedantham V, Cannon SC: The position of the fast-inactivation gate during lidocaine block of voltage-gated Na^+ channels. J Gen Physiol 113:7-16, 1999.
66. Chen Z, Ong B-H, Kambouris NG, et al: Lidocaine induces a slow inactivated state in rat skeletal muscle sodium channels. J Physiol 524:37-49, 2000.
67. Ong BH, Tomaselli GF, Balser JR: A structural rearrangement in the sodium channel pore linked to slow inactivation and use dependence. J Gen Physiol 116:653-661, 2000.
68. Sunami A, Dudley SC Jr, Fozzard HA: Sodium channel selectivity filter regulates antiarrhythmic drug binding. Proc Natl Acad Sci U S A 94:14126-14131, 1997.
69. Chahine M, George AL, Zhou M, et al: Sodium channel mutations in paramyotonia congenita uncouple inactivation from activation. Neuron 12:281-294, 1994.
70. Deschenes I, Baroudi G, Berthet M, et al: Electrophysiological characterization of SCN5A mutations causing long QT (E1784K) and Brugada (R1512W and R1432G) syndromes. Cardiovasc Res 46:55-65, 2000.
71. Rook MB, Alshinawi CB, Groenewegen WA, et al: Human SCN5A gene mutations alter cardiac sodium channel kinetics and are associated with the Brugada syndrome. Cardiovasc Res 44:507-517, 1999.
72. Rivolta I, Abriel H, Tateyama M, et al: Inherited Brugada and long QT-3 syndrome mutations of a single residue of the cardiac sodium channel confer distinct channel and clinical phenotypes. J Biol Chem 276:30623-30630, 2001.
73. Sato C, Ueno Y, Asai K, et al: The voltage-sensitive sodium channel is a bell-shaped molecule with several cavities. Nature 409:1047-1051, 2001.

第 10 章

心脏门控延迟整流钾通道

Micbael C. Sanguinetti，Martin Tristani-Firouzi

本章目录

- 单通道的分子基础 88
- 门控 91

多种电压门控通道影响着肌细胞动作电位的构型和时程，但是从平台期至复极主要是受到延迟整流 K^+ 通道激活的影响。在心脏，延迟整流 K^+ 电流（I_K）至少由三种不同的电流组成——I_{kur}、I_{kr} 和 I_{ks}，这三种电流因为激活速度不同，并且因其特异的阻断剂敏感性不同而相互区别[1-4]。激活速度的顺序是：I_{kur}（超速）>I_{Kr}（快速）>I_{Ks}（缓慢）。

就像其名字所示，超速激活的延迟整流 K^+ 电流 I_{kur} 是 I_K 中激活速度最快的[5]。这一电流也被称作是稳态电流（I_{SS}）、维持电流（I_{SUS}）、持续稳定电流（I_{Kp}）。I_{kur} 的特征是快速激活（10ms，0mV），缓慢的部分失活，对 4-aminopyridine 敏感。这一特异性在不同的物种有所变化，提示了宏观电流其通道分子基础的多样性。在人类，I_{kur} 是心房复极主要的延迟整流电流[5]，但是在心室却不存在[8]。在人类以外的哺乳动物，I_{kur} 在心室动作电位复极过程中发挥重要作用[9,10]。

I_{kr} 命名起源于豚鼠心脏 I_K 的成分，可以被 E-4031 和 D-sotalol 阻断。I_{kr} 的整流性来自于一个在动作电位平台期起始时出现并随着复极完成逐渐增大的外向电流（图 10-1）。I_{kr} 电流的缓慢失活也有助于窦房结细胞缓慢的舒张期去极化。

I_{KS} 在膜电位去极化超过 -30mV 时被激活，最大半激活电压为 +20mV，对特异的阻断剂 chromanol 293B[12] 和 benzodiazepine L-735，821 敏感[13]。I_{ks} 的激活速度比其他已知的 K^+ 电流更慢，需要极长时间的膜电位除极以达到稳定的水平，这在体内不能获得。因为 I_{ks} 的激活率慢，所以它对复极净电流的贡献是在心肌动作电位平台期的最后。在图 10-2 中给出了 I_{kur}、I_{kr} 及 I_{ks} 全细胞和单通道电流典型的例子。

三种不同的延迟整流 K^+ 电流对心肌复极的作用，在不同的物种、心脏的不同部位以及不同心率时有所不同。例如，I_{kr} 密度在心尖部最大，而 I_{ks} 在兔的心室底部占优势[14]。Luo 和 Rudy 在豚鼠心室上建立的离子流模型，提供了一个关于三种 I_K 成分在一个心肌细胞上相对密度的代表性的例子（见图 10-1）。

Nerbonne 综述了关于心脏延迟整流 K^+ 电流生理和药理学的特性[16]，我们也在早先进行了描述[17]。这些特性的摘要在表 10-1 中列出。这里我们描述了心脏延迟整流 K^+ 通道的分子基础和应用克隆的通道来确定其电压门控机制和结构基础的最新研究。

一、单通道的分子基础

（一）超速激活的延迟整流通道

多个 Kv 家族成员的生物物理特性的交迭，加上 Kvβ 调节亚单位造成的异质性，使得明确 I_{kur} 的分子基础变得复杂。尽管有这些困难，但有证据支持 Kv1.5 在心房产生 I_{kur}。Kv1.5 克隆最初来自大鼠和人类的心室，编码一个与野生的 I_{kur} 有相似的生物物理和药理学特征的通道。试验应用针对 Kv1.5 的反义寡核苷酸找到 Kv1.5 构成 I_{kur} 的证据。通过反义寡核苷酸技术功能性的敲除 Kv1.5，可以选择性的抑制培

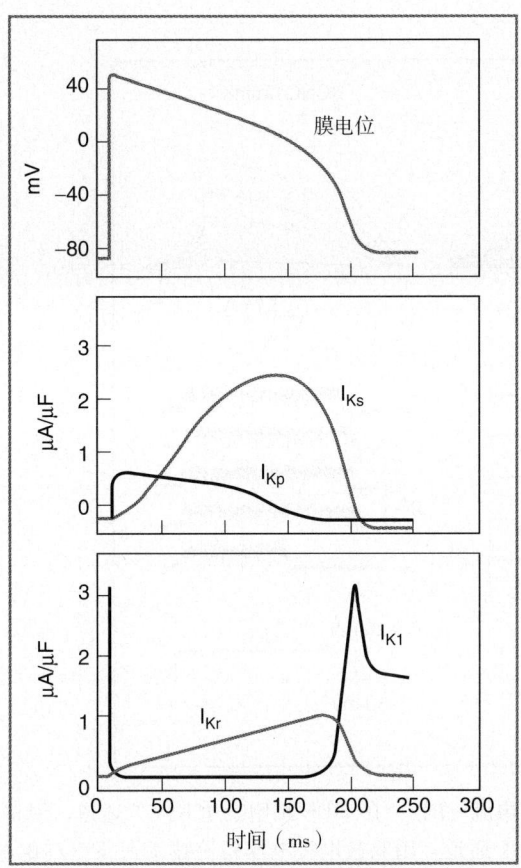

图10-1 模拟引起心肌动作电位复极的钾电流 豚鼠心室肌模型,在大部分物种I_{kur}代替I_{Kp}(引自 Zeng J, Laurita KR, Rosenbaum DS, et al. Two components of the delayed rectifier K$^+$ current in ventricular myocytes of the guinea pig type. Theoretical formulation and their role in repolarization Circ Res 77:140-152,195.)

养的人、大鼠、小鼠心房肌细胞50%~70%的I_{kur}电流[18-20]。用这种技术不能完全的去除I_{kur},提示在I_{kur}起源上的异源性。实际上,在小鼠的心房肌细胞上,针对Kv2.1的反义核苷酸也能抑制一种快速激活的维持的I_k成分。基因靶向方法进一步支持Kv1.5和I_{kur}的分子联系。功能性的敲除Kv1.5,导致了小鼠心室肌快速激活的对4-AP敏感的I_k成分的消除[21]。Kv1.5α亚单位能与和Kvβ亚单位共组装,就可以对其进一步调节,并可以部分解释I_{kur}在不同物种间特性的异质性。Kv1.5和Kvβ1.3共表达引起激活过程向超极化方向增加13mV,去激活过程减慢3倍,并显著加速通道的失活[22]。Kvβ1.3也能降低与多种通道阻滞剂连接的亲和力[23]。Kvβ亚单位对Kv1.5的调节作用有细胞特异性和种属特异性可以解释报道的I_{kur}特性的差异,或者是Kv1.5和其他Kv1α亚单位的异源多聚体组装造成了I_{kur}特性的多样性。

(二) 快速激活的延迟整流通道

基于 eag K$^+$ 通道的序列多态性,HERG被首先从人的海马克隆出来[24]。HERG在卵母细胞的异源表达可引起与心脏I_{kr}电流特征相似的电流,包括I-V关系的整流性、单通道电导和门控的电压依赖性[25,26]。因而推测HERG编码了介导心脏I_{kr}电流的同源四聚体通道的α亚单位。在异源表达系统,HERG亚单位可以和由KCNE1编码的minK[27]或与minK相关的起调节作用的β亚单位(minK相关蛋白1,MiRP1,由KCNE2编码[28])共同装配,minK可以增加电流密度,但是对HERG通道的生物物理特性没有显著的影响。但是minK优先与KCNQ1结合,而HERG优先和MiRP1结合[28],所以在心肌细胞中一般地不可能形成minK-HERG复合物。异源表达研究显示,与单独的HERG相比,HERG/MiRP1通道单通道电导降低,去激活的速度减慢,被特异性药物的阻断作用更快,而这些改变更接近于心肌上I_{kr}通道的特点。然而Weerapura和其同事的一系列研究却不支持MiRP1为HERG调节亚单位。他们报告在同样的记录条件下,HERG的生理和药理特性和豚鼠的I_{kr}相似,存在的差异并没有因为与MiRP1共表达而有显著的改变。还发现MiRP1可以和其他的离子通道亚单相位互作用,包括瞬时外向K$^+$通道Kv4.2[30],超极化激活的阳离子通道HCN2[31]。MiRP1和这些通道有比和HERG连接更大的亲和力。MiRP1在窦房结有高水平的表达,在心房也有显著的表达,但在心室的表达水平非常低[31]。因而,minK或MiRP1作为HERG调节单位的生理作用还不确定。

(三) 缓慢激活的延迟整流通道

当minK作为一个公认的离子通道亚单位从大鼠肾脏被克隆出来后,它在卵母细胞上表达时可以引发一种缓慢的K$^+$电流,和I_{ks}的特征相似。但是人类的minK只有129个氨基酸,只有一个单独的跨膜结构域,因此不大可能单独构成一个功能性的通道。而且将minK转染到哺乳动物细胞时不能引发电流。Keating等[33]在对一个LQT相关基因的定位寻找研究中发现了假定的minK蛋白伴侣。这个蛋白首先被命名为KvLQT1,后来被重命名为KCNQ1,有676个氨基酸,6个跨膜结构域,和一个成孔的环,是典型的电压门控K$^+$通道α亚单位。将KCNQ1和minK共同在哺乳细胞表达可以引发I_{ks}电流,在卵母细胞可以比单

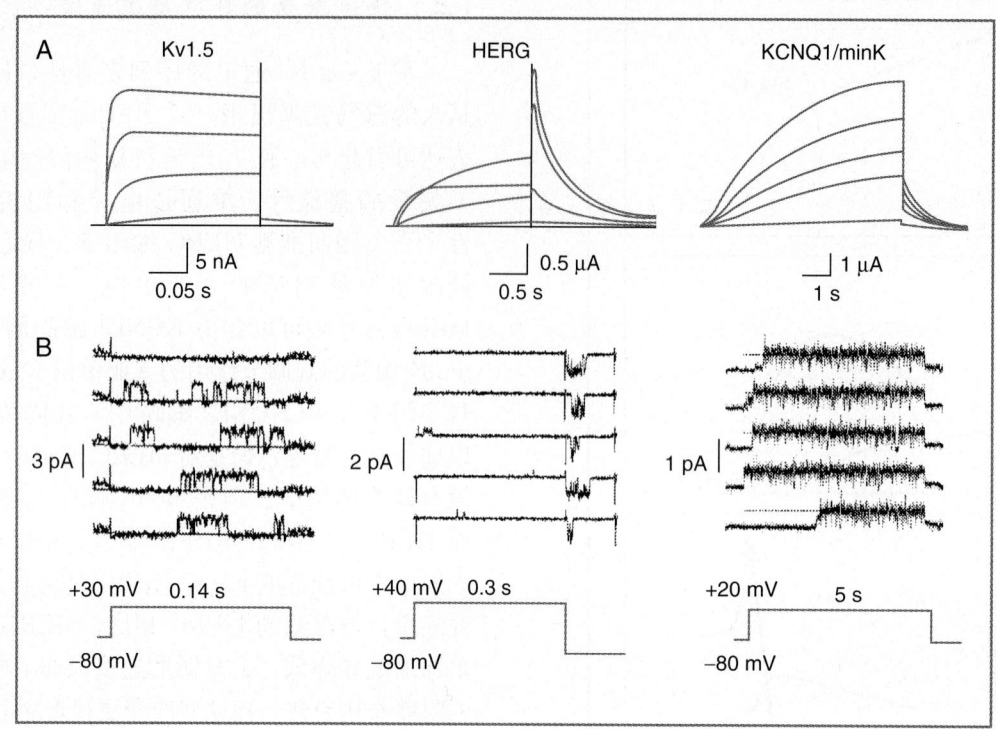

图 10-2 心脏延迟整流 K⁺ 通道的典型例子：全细胞电流（A）和单通道电流（B） 在 HEK 细胞表达 Kv1.5 通道，用膜片钳技术记录全细胞电流[66]。在蟾蜍卵母细胞表达 HERG 和 KCNQ1/minK 通道，用双微电极电压钳制技术记录全细胞电流。Kv1.5 和 HERG 单通道电流的记录用细胞贴附模式，KCNQ1/rat minK 单通道电流的记录用内面向外模式。在图的底部给出相应的电压程序

独的表达 minK 增加 I_{ks} 电流的幅度[34-36]。在没有 minK 的时候，KCNQ1 亚单位可以共同组装成同源多聚体通道，但是与 minK 共同组装可以提高单通道的电导，减慢激活的速度和去失活。KCNQ1/minK 异源多聚体通道也比 KCNQ1 对一些阻滞剂更敏感，如 chromanol 293B[37]。异源多聚体也可以改变通道对一些激动剂的敏感性。例如，benzodiazepine R-L3 可以增加 KCNQ1 通道的电流幅度并减慢门控作用，但对 KCNQ1/minK 通道无此作用[38]。

表 10-1 人类心脏延迟整流钾电流的生理和药理特性

特性	电流		
	I_{kur}	I_{kr}	I_{ks}
分子基础	Kv1.5	HERG+MiRP1	KCNQ1+minK
名称	KCNA5	KCNH2+KCNE2	KvLQT1+KCNE1
阻滞剂	4-氨基吡啶	Dofetilide，E4031，MK-499	Chromanol 293B，L-735821
激活 $V_{1/2}$	−4mV	−30 mV	+20 mV
0 mV 激活速度	10ms	200ms	800ms
失活 $V_{1/2}$	−25 mV	−80mV	N/A
0 mV 失活速度	250，3000ms	10ms	N/A
单通道电导	17pS	2pS	4.5pS

在组装成一个有功能的通道时，minK 亚单位的数量以及它与 KCNQ1 亚单相位互作用的位点还不十分清楚。有一个基于野生型和突变体亚单位的相互作用研究，得出结论在每个通道中有两个 minK 亚单位[32]。然而 KCNQ1-minK 结合蛋白的特性研究提示，异源多聚体通道的化学计量可能不是一个固定的数字[39]。KCNQ1-minK 相互作用的结构基础也不知道。Mink 基因的 Cys-Scanning 诱变及巯基反应性 Cd^{2+} 引起的 KCNQ1/minK 通道阻断的改变提示 minK 位于 KCNQ1/minK 通道复合物的选择决定性孔区的邻近区域，或与 S6 结构域的残基相互作用，因而不可能构成孔道的一部分[41]。突变形成研究提示了 minK Thr-58 在改变 KCNQ1 通道门控中的重要作用[42]。

二、门控

（一）电压感受器和门控作用

类似于其他电压门控 K^+（Kv）通道，Kv 1.5、HERG 和 KCNQ1 都有一个对膜电位敏感的感受器，一个可以在电压感受器运动时开放的激活门，一个选择性孔道可以允许 K^+ 透过，而不是 Na^+、Ca^{2+} 等其他阳离子。所有的 Kv 通道都有 6 个 α 螺旋跨膜结构域。许多研究，大部分是应用 Drosopbila Shaker 通道，显示第四个结构域（S4）是压力感受器，它的每三个氨基酸残基中含一个碱性残基。膜去极化导致 S4 外向转换或旋转，这可能引起了细胞内激活门开放。最近有人通过电压钳制荧光计研究了 HERG 门控中 S4 的作用。用荧光探针在 S4 结构域末端连续的几个氨基酸残基的氨基端进行标记,荧光的改变就可以反映电流的时间和电压依赖特征。通过荧光,这些残基显示了快、慢电压依赖性改变。快荧光成分的动力学，和通道失活后恢复重新开放的动力学相关联。慢荧光成分和 HERG 通道激活和去激活动力学以及激活的电压依赖性高度相关。

最近通过晶体学研究细菌 K^+ 通道，通道结晶存在开放构型（MthK 通道）或关闭构型（KcsA 通道），是了解激活门控的结构基础[44-46]。在关闭构型，沿着通道孔线形排列的 4 个内部螺旋（相当于 Kv 通道的 S6 结构域），向着细胞膜倾斜，相互交叉贴近细胞质的界面，形成一个狭窄的孔道（激活门），阻止离子的通过。通道开放涉及内部螺旋向外直接地开放，因而增大了孔道的直径。允许螺旋开放的关键枢纽点可能是一个位于内部螺旋结构上的甘氨酸位点[45,46]。这一甘氨酸（Gly）残基在大多数的 Kv 通道中都是保守的，Kv1.5 和 HERG 通道的激活可能也有类似的构型改变。但是 KCNQ1 在对应其他 Kv 通道的 Gly 位点上是一个 Ala 残基，这一残基更有利于维持 α 螺旋的结构。大多数 Kv 通道的 S6 结构域在靠近激活门的位置还包含一个 Pro-Val-Pro 模体。假定是 Pro-Val-Pro 模体破坏 S6 结构域的 α 螺旋结构，可能在许多 Kv 通道中是激活门一个关键的成分[47,48]，但是这一模体在 HERG 中并不存在。在 KCNQ1 中，这一序列是 Pro-Ala-Gly，但它在门控中有和 Pro-Val-Pro 模体在 Shaker K^+ 通道中类似的作用。尽管通过对 Shaker 通道门控的研究，以及两种细菌 K^+ 通道结构的研究使得对于通道结构和功能的理解已经取得了惊人的进展，但是从这些研究中获得的一些关于门控的规则并不能直接应用到心脏延迟整流电流上来。

缓慢的通道激活速率（通道开放），经常伴随着缓慢的通道去激活（通道关闭）。但是，去除 HERG 氨基末端的 354 个氨基酸，可以加速通道的去激活，但是不会引起相应的激活的改变。HERG 氨基末端的晶体结构显示一个碱性的螺旋-环-螺旋结构，是一种典型的 Per-Arnt-Sim 结构域，这在许多信号传导蛋白中是蛋白与蛋白相互作用的关键结构域[49]。在 HERG 中 Per-Arnt-Sim 结构域对通道去激活的影响还不清楚，但是它可能是与一系列的蛋白或 HERG 的其他区域相互作用来减慢通道的关闭。

（二）电压感受器-激活门耦联

电压感受器的运动必须要和通道开放耦联，但是这一过程的结构基础还没有完全弄清楚。它可能通过 Kv 通道复合体大量结构域的协调的运动，或者通过不连续区域的相互作用来完成。例如，除极可以引起全面的电压感受器的重新排布，以此影响到 S5、S6 结构域来开放通道[47]。或者，电压感受器的运动可能通过特异性氨基酸与激活门相耦联。例如，因为 S4-S5 链的存在，或许是这一区域调节了电压感受器和激活门之间的耦联。S4-S5 链的突变，改变许多 Kv 通道的激活和门控电荷运动[50-52]。靠近 HERG 的 S4 结构域的点突变 D540K 使得通道关闭状态不稳定，允许电压依赖性的通道在膜超极化时再开放[53]。D540K 突变导致的关闭状态不稳定提示在 S4-S5 链和激活门之间存在相互联系。S6 结构域 C 末端区域突变形成显示，带阳性电荷的残基（Arg-665）在超极化引起的

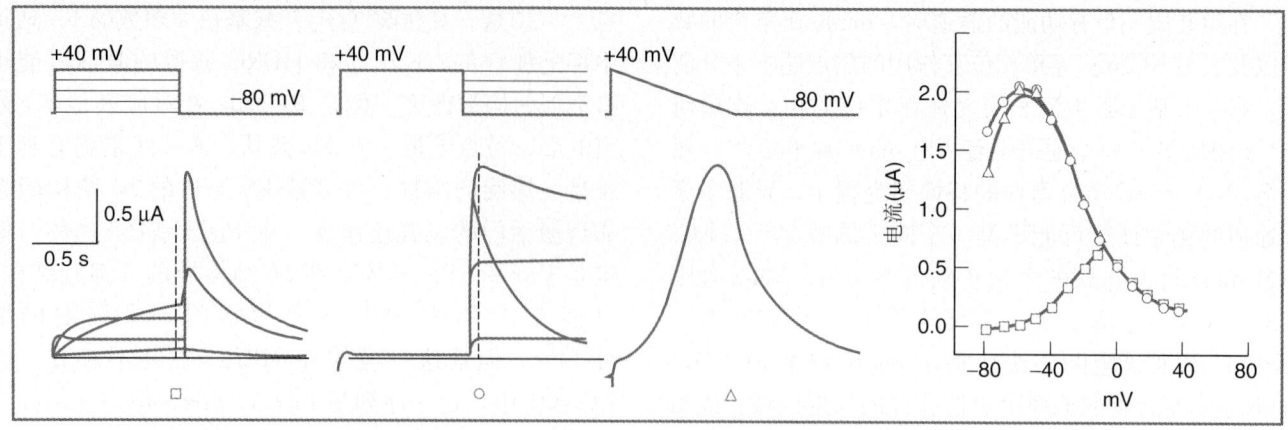

图10-3 HERG通道在电压钳制下的I-V依赖关系 通道表达在蟾蜍卵母细胞，用双电极电压钳技术记录全细胞电流。在虚线标出的时间点取电流值作I-V曲线

通道激活中是必须的。提示S4-S5链和S6之间的静电排斥可以介导D540K HERG通道的再开放。因此，至少在HERG通道，在电压感受器和激活门之间的耦联可能部分的是由S4-S5链传导。

（三）快速失活引起I_{kr}的整流

不像大多数的Kv通道，HERG显示出内向整流性，是在心脏动作电位的平台期限制外向K^+电流电导的重要特性。不像典型的内向整流K^+通道，整流性来自细胞内多聚氨基酸的阻断，HERG内向整流性的机制是通道快速失活（tau<20ms）。因为HERG通道失活的速率要比通道激活的速率快，经常用一种特殊的三倍脉冲电压钳制程序来评估通道电压依赖性失活。先给一个正电位的脉冲（例如+40mV）使通道快速激活和失活，然后给一个短的可变电位的预脉冲（例如10ms），使通道部分的从失活恢复，而没有明显的去激活。最后给予一个正电位的测量脉冲，来测量在预脉冲电位时开放的通道的比例[54,55]。用这种方法测量的HERG通道半失活电压在-80～-90mV之间，大约比通道的半激活电压负70mV。另一种来测量I_{Kr}电压依赖性失活的方法，是测量最大激活I-V关系。当膜电位非常负的时候，电导的斜率是恒定的，但是当膜电位上升到-90mV时，电导斜率逐渐变小。在传导斜率最大时每一个测量电位的电流和K^+驱动力（测量电位减去反转电位）可以用来计算整流的因子，在兔的结细胞半最大电压接近-60mV，而在蟾蜍卵母细胞表达的HERG通道的半电压为-50mV。

相对于I_{Kr}的失活速度，它的激活速度较慢，因而I_{Kr}-V关系随着脉冲的时程变化，形状也是不典型的

延迟整流K^+电流。在大多数已经发表的研究中，I_{Kr}-V关系是由与通道激活到稳定水平所需时间相关的短脉冲（例如：0.5～2s）引起的电流决定的。例如，用1s长的脉冲来测量时，I_{Kr}-V关系曲线的峰值大约是0mV，但是如果脉冲的时间足够长到使通道开放到稳定状态，峰值大约为-60mV。I_{Kr}-V关系对刺激程序的依赖见图10-3，这是在Xenopus卵母细胞表达的HERG通道。为了确定最大激活的I_{Kr}-V关系，先将细胞膜去极化到+40mV 1秒钟，足够长的时间使通道完全激活。测量复极化到不同水平（-120～+30mV，阶越10mV）产生的尾电流的峰值。得到的I-V关系是在每一个电位水平，与失活通道相比开放通道的相对数量。测量I_{Kr}-V关系的第三种方法是，给一个+40mV的脉冲紧跟一个缓慢的斜坡刺激使跨膜电位恢复到保持电压水平，在这一例子中是-80mV。用这一方案粗略地勾画出动作电位的形状，接近完全激活的I-V关系曲线，明显的不同于用1s去极化方案获得的I_{Kr}-V关系曲线。

HERG通道失活的结构基础还不明确，但是通过突变研究已经明确，影响失活的残基位于靠近孔道外部开口的位置，类似于其他C型失活机制的通道。N型失活是由于通道蛋白氨基末端占据了通道孔的部位，而C型失活是由于选择性滤过形成了狭窄的孔道结构。靠近孔道的两个残基同时突变（G628C, S631C）[54]或者单点突变（S620T）[56]，使通道无失活，并且使I-V关系曲线（图10-3）由钟形变成线形。另一个孔的突变S631A引起电压依赖性失活+100mV的变化，而对电压依赖性激活没有显著的影响[57]。Shaker通道的半胱氨酸重组试验提示，孔道外部开口部位的重新组装介导了通道的C型失

活[47,58]。先前描述的孔道突变的作用支持 HERG 通道失活是由狭窄的选择性滤过机制这一理论。HERG 通道门控对 $[Na^+]_o$、$[Ca^{2+}]_o$ 异常敏感。外部 Na^+ 阻断外向电流，机制是 Na^+ 和外部的 K^+ 竞争结合靠近外部孔道的结合位点，这也可以解释升高 $[K^+]_o$ 尽管降低了 K^+ 的驱动力却可以增加外向 K^+ 流的矛盾现象[25]。$[Ca^{2+}]_o$ 小的改变可以使通道电压依赖性激活向膜电位更高的方向移动，这种影响归因于静息或激活的通道靠近 S4 电压敏感区的两个外部残基 Glu518 和 Glu519 对 Ca^{2+} 亲和力不同[60]。

（四）Mink 改变 KCNQ1 的门控

Mink 导致了 KCNQ1 通道三种生物学特性的改变：1）Mink 提高了单通道的电导，2）减慢电流激活的速率，3）抑制通道失活。单独在蟾蜍卵母细胞异源性表达的 KCNQ1 通道开放和关闭都非常迅速，这妨碍了对通道开放程度和时间的测量。Yang[61] 以及 Sesti[62] 等报告，KCNQ1/minK 单通道的电导（γ）比 KCNQ1 同源多聚体通道的电导大 4～6 倍。例如，在正常细胞外 $[K^+]$ 溶液中单独的 KCNQ1 通道的 γ 为 0.7pS，而 KCNE1 和人的 minK 在蟾蜍卵母细胞共表达的通道的 γ 为 4.5pS（见图 10-2）[61]。MinK 可能减慢电压感受器反应的速度，或 S4 激活门控耦联的速度，也或者使两者同时减慢从而减慢 KCNQ1 通道的激活。MinK 抑制 KCNQ1 通道失活的机制尚未明确。从观察膜除极引起的 KCNQ1 通道激活的过程来看，通道的失活不明显，但可以从尾电流的分析获得。膜复极引起 KCNQ1 通道的电导在通道去激活之前暂时增加，在尾电流上形成"钩形"部分，对此进行测量可以间接的分析 KCNQ1 通道失活的性质。KCNQ1 通道最大失活的半电压为 $-18mV$，在最大值处电流下降约 35%[63]。不像其他 Kv 通道的失活，KCNQ1 通道的失活发生在一段延迟之后。在 $+40mV$ 这段延迟大约为 75ms。如果通道先暂时恢复到开放状态，则即刻发生失活的过程没有延迟，并且速度要快 10 倍。这就说明 KCNQ1 通道至少有两种开放状态，转变到失活状态是与第二种开放状态相联系的，是非电压依赖性的[64]。KCNQ1 通道失活的分子机制还不清楚，但是与典型的 C 型失活相比，KCNQ1 通道的失活不依赖细胞外的 $[K^+]$[64]。KCNQ1/minK 通道的尾电流缺乏钩形的形态，并不显示出失活。但是 Push 及其同事认为这可能是因为 Iks 通道失活比 KCNQ1 通道更慢。

与 KCNQ1 通道相比，KCNQ2 通道不表现出失活。研究两者的差异可以确定 KCNQ1 所特有的可以促进失活门控的残基。通过 KCNQ1-KCNQ2 混合通道将失活相关的节段定位在 S5 跨膜结构域和孔链区[65]。进一步的突变形成试验揭示了 KCNQ1 的类似 KCNQ2 残基的 Gly-272 或 Val-307 的改变，可以阻止通道失活。而且通过将 KCNQ2 相应残基进行突变可以造成通道的失活。KCNQ1 特定的突变可以增强通道内在的失活过程。例如，L273F 种可以引起 LQT 综合征的突变，可以增加 KCNQ1 失活的速度和程度，降低心脏的 Iks[65]。需要进一步的研究来明确是否 KCNQ1 通道的失活涉及选择性滤过机制，就像假定的其他 C 型失活的 Kv1.5 或 HERG 通道。

（李　宁　浦介麟　译）

参 考 文 献

1. Sanguinetti MC, Jurkiewicz NK: Two components of cardiac delayed rectifier K+ current: Differential sensitivity to block by class III antiarrhythmic agents. J Gen Physiol 96:195–215, 1990.
2. Clay JR, Ogbaghebriel A, Paquette T, et al: A quantitative description of the E-4031-sensitive repolarization current in rabbit ventricular myocytes. Biophys J 69:1830–1837, 1995.
3. Liu D-W, Antzelevitch C: Characteristics of the delayed rectifier current (I_{Kr} and I_{Ks}) in canine ventricular epicardial, midmyocardial, and endocardial myocytes: A weaker I_{Ks} contributes to the longer action potential of the M cell. Circ Res 76:351–365, 1995.
4. Gintant GA: Two components of delayed rectifier current in canine atrium and ventricle (Does I_{Ks} play a role in the reverse rate dependence of class III agents?). Circ Res 78:26–37, 1996.
5. Wang Z, Fermini B, Nattel S: Sustained depolarization-induced outward current in human atrial myocytes: Evidence for a novel delayed rectifier K+ current similar to Kv1.5 cloned channel currents. Circ Res 73:1061–1076, 1993.
6. Boyle WA, Nerbonne JM: A novel type of depolarization-activated K+ current in isolated adult rat atrial myocytes. Am J Physiol 260:H1236–H1247, 1991.
7. Yue DT, Marban E: A novel cardiac potassium channel that is active and conductive at depolarized potentials. Pflugers Arch 413:127–133, 1988.
8. Li G-R, Feng J, Yue L, et al: Evidence for two components of delayed rectifier K+ current in human ventricular myocytes. Circ Res 78:689–696, 1996.
9. Yue L, Feng J, Li G, Nattel S: Characterization of an ultrarapid delayed rectifier potassium channel involved in canine atrial repolarization. J Physiol (Lond) 496(Pt 3):647–662, 1996.
10. Backx PH, Marban E: Background potassium current active during the plateau of the action potential in guinea pig ventricular myocytes. Circ Res 72:890–900, 1993.
11. Shibasaki T: Conductance and kinetics of delayed rectifier potassium channels in nodal cells of the rabbit heart. J Physiol 387:227–250, 1987.
12. Busch AE, Suessbrich H, Waldegger S, et al: Inhibition of I_{Ks} in guinea pig cardiac myocytes and guinea pig I_{sK} channels by the chromanol 293B. Eur J Physiol 432:1094–1096, 1996.
13. Salata JJ, Jurkiewicz NK, Sanguinetti MC, et al: The novel class III antiarrhythmic agent, L-735,821 is a potent and selective blocker of I_{Ks} in guinea pig ventricular myocytes. Circulation 94:I529, 1996.
14. Cheng J, Kamiya K, Liu W, et al: Heterogeneous distribution of the two components of delayed rectifier K+ current: A potential mechanism of the proarrhythmic effects of methanesulfonanilide class III agents. Cardiovasc Res 43:135–147, 1999.
15. Luo C-h, Rudy Y: A dynamic model of the cardiac ventricular action

potential (I. simulations of ionic currents and concentration changes). Circ Res 74:1071–1096, 1994.
16. Nerbonne JM: Molecular basis of functional voltage-gated K+ channel diversity in the mammalian myocardium. J Physiol (Lond) 525(Pt 2):285–298, 2000.
17. Sanguinetti MC, Tristani-Firouzi M: Delayed and inward rectifier potassium channels. In Zipes DP, Jalife J (eds): Cardiac Electrophysiology from Cell to Bedside, 3rd ed. Philadelphia, WB Saunders, 2000, pp 79–86.
18. Bou-Abboud E, Nerbonne JM: Molecular correlates of the calcium-independent, depolarization-activated K+ currents in rat atrial myocytes. J Physiol 517:407–420, 1999.
19. Bou-Abboud E, Li H, Nerbonne JM: Molecular diversity of the repolarizing voltage-gated K+ currents in mouse atrial cells. J Physiol 529(Pt 2):345–358, 2000.
20. Feng J, Wible B, Li G, et al: Antisense oligodeoxynucleotides directed against Kv1.5 mRNA specifically inhibit ultrarapid delayed rectifier K+ current in cultured adult human atrial myocytes. Circ Res 80:572–579, 1997.
21. London B, Guo W, Pan X, et al: Targeted replacement of KV1.5 in the mouse leads to loss of the 4-aminopyridine-sensitive component of I(K,slow) and resistance to drug-induced qt prolongation. Circ Res 88:940–946, 2001.
22. England SK, Uebele VN, Kodali J, et al: A novel K$^+$ channel b-subunit (hKvb1.3) is produced via alternative mRNA splicing. J Biol Chem 270:28531–28534, 1995.
23. Gonzalez T, Navarro-Polanco R, Arias C, et al: Assembly with the Kvbeta1.3 subunit modulates drug block of hKv1.5 channels. Mol Pharmacol 62:1456–1463, 2002.
24. Warmke J, Drysdale R, Ganetzky B: A distinct potassium channel polypeptide encoded by the *Drosophila eag* locus. Science 252:1560–1564, 1991.
25. Sanguinetti MC, Jiang C, Curran ME, Keating MT: A mechanistic link between an inherited and an acquired cardiac arrhythmia: *HERG* encodes the I_{Kr} potassium channel. Cell 81:299–307, 1995.
26. Trudeau M, Warmke JW, Ganetzky B, Robertson GA: HERG, a human inward rectifier in the voltage-gated potassium channel family. Science 269:92–95, 1995.
27. McDonald TV, Yu Z, Ming Z, et al: A minK-HERG complex regulates the cardiac potassium current I_{Kr}. Nature 388:289–292, 1997.
28. Abbott GW, Sesti F, Splawski I, et al: MiRP1 forms IKr potassium channels with HERG and is associated with cardiac arrhythmia. Cell 97:175–187, 1999.
29. Weerapura M, Nattel S, Chartier D, et al: A comparison of currents carried by HERG, with and without coexpression of MiRP1, and the native rapid delayed rectifier current. Is MiRP1 the missing link? J Physiol 540:15–27, 2002.
30. Zhang M, Jiang M, Tseng GN: minK-related peptide 1 associates with Kv4.2 and modulates its gating function: Potential role as beta subunit of cardiac transient outward channel? Circ Res 88:1012–1019, 2001.
31. Yu H, Wu J, Potapova I, et al: MinK-Related peptide 1: A beta subunit for the HCN ion channel subunit family enhances expression and speeds activation. Circ Res 88:E84–E87, 2001.
32. Wang K-W, Goldstein SAN: Subunit composition of minK potassium channels. Neuron 14:1303–1309, 1995.
33. Wang Q, Curran ME, Splawski I, et al: Positional cloning of a novel potassium channel gene: KVLQT1 mutations cause cardiac arrhythmias. Nat Genet 12:17–23, 1996.
34. Barhanin J, Lesage F, Guillemare E, et al: KvLQT1 and IsK (minK) proteins associate to form the I_{Ks} cardiac potassium channel. Nature 384:78–80, 1996.
35. Sanguinetti MC, Curran ME, Zou A, et al: Coassembly of KvLQT1 and minK (IsK) proteins to form cardiac I_{Ks} potassium channel. Nature 384:80–83, 1996.
36. Yang WP, Levesque PC, Little WA, et al: KvLQT1, a voltage-gated potassium channel responsible for human cardiac arrhythmias. Proc Natl Acad Sci USA 94:4017–4021, 1997.
37. Lerche C, Seebohm G, Wagner CI, et al: Molecular impact of MinK on the enantiospecific block of I(Ks) by chromanols. Br J Pharmacol 131:1503–1506, 2000.
38. Salata JJ, Jurkiewicz NK, Wang J, et al: A novel benzodiazepine that activates cardiac slow delayed rectifier K+ channels. Mol Pharmacol 53:220–230, 1998.
39. Wang W, Xia J, Kass RS: MinK-KvLQT1 fusion proteins, evidence for multiple stoichiometries of the assembled IsK channel. J Biol Chem 273:34069–34074, 1998.
40. Tai KK, Goldstein SAN: The conduction pore of a cardiac potassium channel. Nature 391:605–608, 1998.
41. Tapper AR, George AL Jr: Location and orientation of minK within the IKs potassium channel complex. J Biol Chem 276:38249–38254, 2001.
42. Melman YF, Krumerman A, McDonald TV: A single transmembrane site in the KCNE-encoded proteins controls the specificity of KvLQT1 channel gating. J Biol Chem 277:25187–25194, 2002.
43. Smith PL, Yellen G: Fast and slow voltage sensor movements in HERG potassium channels. J Gen Physiol 119:275–293, 2002.
44. Doyle DA, Morais Cabral J, Pfuetzner RA, et al: The structure of the potassium channel: Molecular basis of K+ conduction and selectivity. Science 280:69–77, 1998.
45. Jiang Y, Lee A, Cadene M, et al: The open pore conformation of potassium channels. Nature 417:523–526, 2002.
46. Jiang Y, Lee A, Chen J, et al: Crystal structure and mechanism of a calcium-gated potassium channel. Nature 417:515–522, 2002.
47. Yellen G: The moving parts of voltage-gated ion channels. Q Rev Biophys 31:239–295, 1998.
48. del Camino D, Holmgren M, Liu Y, Yellen G: Blocker protection in the pore of a voltage-gated K+ channel and its structural implications. Nature 403:321–325, 2000.
49. Morais Cabral JH, Lee A, Cohen SL, et al: Crystal structure and functional analysis of the HERG potassium channel N terminus: A eukaryotic PAS domain. Cell 95:649–655, 1998.
50. Schoppa NE, McCormack K, Tanouye MA, Sigworth FJ: The size of gating charge in wild-type and mutant *Shaker* potassium channels. Science 255:1712–1715, 1992.
51. Slesinger PA, Jan YN, Jan LY: The S4-S5 loop contributes to the ion-selective pore of potassium channels. Neuron 11:739–749, 1993.
52. Shieh C-C, Klemic KG, Kirsch GE: Role of transmembrane segment S5 on gating of voltage-dependent K+ channels. J Gen Physiol 109:767–778, 1997.
53. Sanguinetti MC, Xu QP: Mutations of the S4-S5 linker alter activation properties of HERG potassium channels expressed in Xenopus oocytes. J Physiol 514:667–675, 1999.
54. Smith PL, Baukrowitz T, Yellen G: The inward rectification mechanism of the HERG cardiac potassium channel. Nature 379:833–836, 1996.
55. Spector PS, Curran ME, Zou A, et al: Fast inactivation causes rectification of the I_{Kr} channel. J Gen Physiol 107:611–619, 1996.
56. Ficker E, Jarolimek W, Kiehn J, et al: Molecular determinants of dofetilide block of HERG K+ channels. Circ Res 82:386–395, 1998.
57. Zou A, Xu QP, Sanguinetti MC: A mutation in the pore region of HERG K+ channels reduces rectification by shifting the voltage dependence of inactivation. J Physiol 509:129–138, 1998.
58. Liu Y, Jurman ME, Yellen G: Dynamic rearrangement of the outer mouth of a K+ channel during gating. Neuron 16:859–867, 1996.
59. Numaguchi H, Johnson JP Jr, Petersen CI, Balser JR: A sensitive mechanism for cation modulation of potassium current. Nat Neurosci 3:429–430, 2000.
60. Johnson JP Jr, Balser JR, Bennett PB: A novel extracellular calcium sensing mechanism in voltage-gated potassium ion channels. J Neurosci 21:4143–4153, 2001.
61. Yang Y, Sigworth FJ: Single-channel properties of IKs potassium channels. J Gen Physiol 112:665–678, 1998.
62. Sesti F, Goldstein SA: Single-channel characteristics of wild-type IKs channels and channels formed with two minK mutants that cause long QT syndrome. J Gen Physiol 112:651–663, 1998.
63. Tristani-Firouzi M, Sanguinetti MC: Voltage-dependent inactivation of the K+ channel KvLQT1 is eliminated by association with minK subunits. J Physiol 510:37–45, 1998.
64. Pusch M, Magrassi R, Wollnik B, Conti F: Activation and inactivation of homomeric KvLQT1 potassium channels. Biophys J 75:785–792, 1998.
65. Seebohm G, Scherer CR, Busch AE, Lerche C: Identification of specific pore residues mediating KCNQ1 inactivation. A novel mechanism for long QT syndrome. J Biol Chem 276:13600–13605, 2001.
66. Zhang S, Kehl SJ, Fedida D: Modulation of Kv1.5 potassium channel gating by extracellular zinc. Biophys J 81:125–136, 2001.
67. Fedida D, Wible B, Wang Z, et al: Identity of a novel delayed rectifier current from human heart with a cloned K+ channel current. Circ Res 73:210–216, 1993.
68. Kiehn J, Lacerda AE, Brown AM: Pathways of HERG inactivation. Am J Physiol 277:H199–H210, 1999.

第 11 章

机械电转换

Frederick Sacbs

在进化过程中需要根据代谢引起的渗透压变化控制细胞体积，因而生物压力敏感性进化比较早[1,2]。在细菌[3,4]、Archea[4,5]和真核细胞中都有压力敏感的离子通道。当自由生长的有机体需要对障碍或捕食者作出反应时，对特定的机械换能的需要就会增加。例如，草履虫就有两种机械敏感系统。一种钙离子通透系统集中在后端，可以使其加速（逃离捕食者），还有一种钾离子通透系统集中在它的前端，可以使其后退避开障碍物。因此在多细胞生物中保持这种遗传特质并不奇怪，并且还适应于感受触觉、听觉、自动的肌肉反馈，和种种的对空腔器官的感受器，例如对血压敏感的感受器。

超过了神经系统，机械敏感性在所有的细胞都得到了保持，并发挥不同的功能，从骨沉积到通过肾素和尿钠肽激素系统来控制血容量。在心脏系统，容易看到这种机械电的耦联，例如心率对神经张力敏感[6]，以及心腔扩张引起的心律失常[7-9]。

当机械压力改变换能器的能量时就会发生机械换能。在机械压力领域，如果一个分子有大小不同的状态，则在每一个状态有不同的能量。例如，肌动蛋白和微管蛋白等多聚肽的组装是机械敏感的，对它们进行牵张会引起它们解离。在心脏，肌钙蛋白和钙离子的结合是压力敏感的[10]。从心脏经典的张力-速度关系，从原子能显微镜和激光 trap 研究以及基本的物理学推测，可以得知分子发动机对机械压力敏感的特性。

本章重点讲述压力敏感的离子通道，但是同样的思路可以应用于其他的酶。基本的物理学原理是，力（F）作用于物体上并作用了一段距离（x）即 $U=\int Fdx$，如果力是个常数即 Fx。当改变是急剧的，可以看作是作用在面积上而不是长度上的，这种能量用术语表达就是膜的张力（T），这种在平面上的改变 $\Delta U=T\Delta A$。认为离子通道是位于膜上半径为 r 的圆柱体（图 11-1）。如果关闭的通道有向外的半径 r_c，开放的通道半径为 r_o，膜张力为 T，那么通道的变化将产生能量 $\Delta U=T\pi \cdot (r_o^2-r_c^2)$。按照 Boltzmann 方程，通道开放的概率（假设通道只有两种状态，开放或关闭）由以下公式 $Po=Pc \cdot \exp(\Delta U/kT)$ 得出，这里 Pc 是通道关闭的概率，k_BT 是 Boltzmann 时间常数和绝对温度。k_BT 是需要知道的一个有用的数学常数，因为它代表分子在温度 T 时的平均能量。通过设定的这些等级参数就可以判断是否一个给定的能量是有意义的，用两个常用的单位，$k_BT=25$meV（毫电子伏特）或 4.1pN-nm。设定膜张力的等级参数，使脂质膜溶解的张力大约是 10dyne/cm $=10^{-2}$N/m $=$ 10mN/m^2。

在我们这种简单的柱状通道例子中，如果 $r_c=2.5$nm，$r_o=3$nm，那么一个小的张力 1mN/m 可以使开放的通道比关闭的通道处于较低的能量状态。这可以通过公式得出 $\Delta U=10^{-3}\times 3.14\times (9\times 10^{-18}-6.25\times 10^{-18})=0.86\times 10^{-20}$Nm（J）$=8.6$pN-nm，或 2.1 k_BT。从 Boltzmann 方程可知 $Po/Pc=\exp(2.1k_BT/k_BT)=8.1$。因此张力使得通道开放的概率是关闭状态的 10 倍。这是张力激活的离子通道（stretch-activited channel，SAC）的基本特性。

SAC 的原型结构是来自细菌的 MscL。图 11-1 显示了通道开放和关闭状态模型，现在的模型是基于 x 线、自旋标记物和分子模型的数据[12-15]。通道是个五聚体，每一单体有两个螺旋状的跨膜段。在静息时，这些螺旋与胞膜成一定的角度倾斜排列。当通道开放

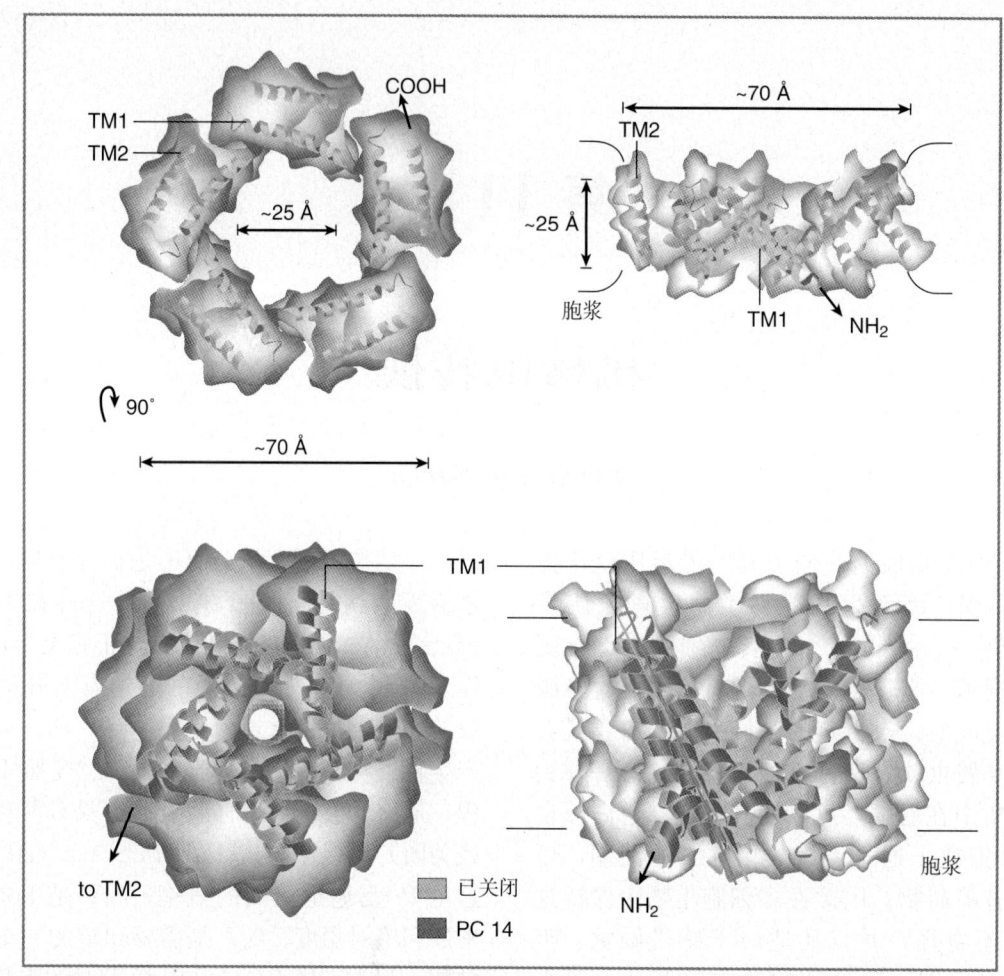

图 11-1 开放和关闭状态的 MscL 上图显示了对牵张敏感引起的直径的较大变化。侧面的图显示当通道开放时其厚度变薄,这就在脂质双层膜和通道的厚度之间产生疏水性的不协调。这就引起膜变厚来适应通道的开放状态,然后再变薄来适应通道关闭状态

时,这些螺旋扭曲使通道开放就像照相机的光圈。注意这种通道关闭和开放之间直径的较大改变。尽管通道有一个较大的非选择性电导(3nS 在生理盐溶液),对于门控能量来说,孔直径的改变不是一个重要的成分。起主要作用的是外部的直径改变。MscL 有多个传导状态,但是仅有的显著地张力依赖性速率是向前的速率即从关闭状态到最小的亚能级[16]。其他的亚能级可能代表孔内 C 末端残基的内部的重组。

像个安全的阀门适合成为一个通道,MscL 强烈地倾向于关闭状态,仅在张力接近膜溶解时才开放。可以重组 MscL 进入人工的双层膜的技术允许克隆这一通道,并且可以校准绝对的敏感度,因为张力是被限制于双层膜的[16]。尽管 MscL 已经明确的被作为真核细胞通道的原型,但看起来并没有序列或生理上的同源性。即使是在 *Escherichia coli* 通道之间也没有同源性。最近,Rees 的实验室解决了第二个 MSC 的结构,叫做 MscS (mechanosensitive channel small)[17]。这个通道是个七聚体,每个单体有三个跨膜螺旋。

在原位研究压力敏感性通道使得研究复杂化。在真核细胞机械压力可以通过双层膜、细胞外基质和细胞骨架散布(图 11-2),因此激活一个通道精确的压力不能清楚的确定。虽然如此,我们还是得到了一些 MscS 的数据。

最有特征的真核细胞 SACs 是双孔(2P)结构域钾通道(图 11-3)[18]。这些通道可以被膜片中张力激活,或者两性的分子如溶血脂质和花生四烯酸激活。可以被两性分子激活最早是在 MscL 观察到的[19],并且出现于使局部双层膜弯曲的压力处。这些两性分子优先溶解入膜中的一层,并向相邻的部分扩张,像两性金属的温度调节装置,使双层膜弯曲。引起的张力

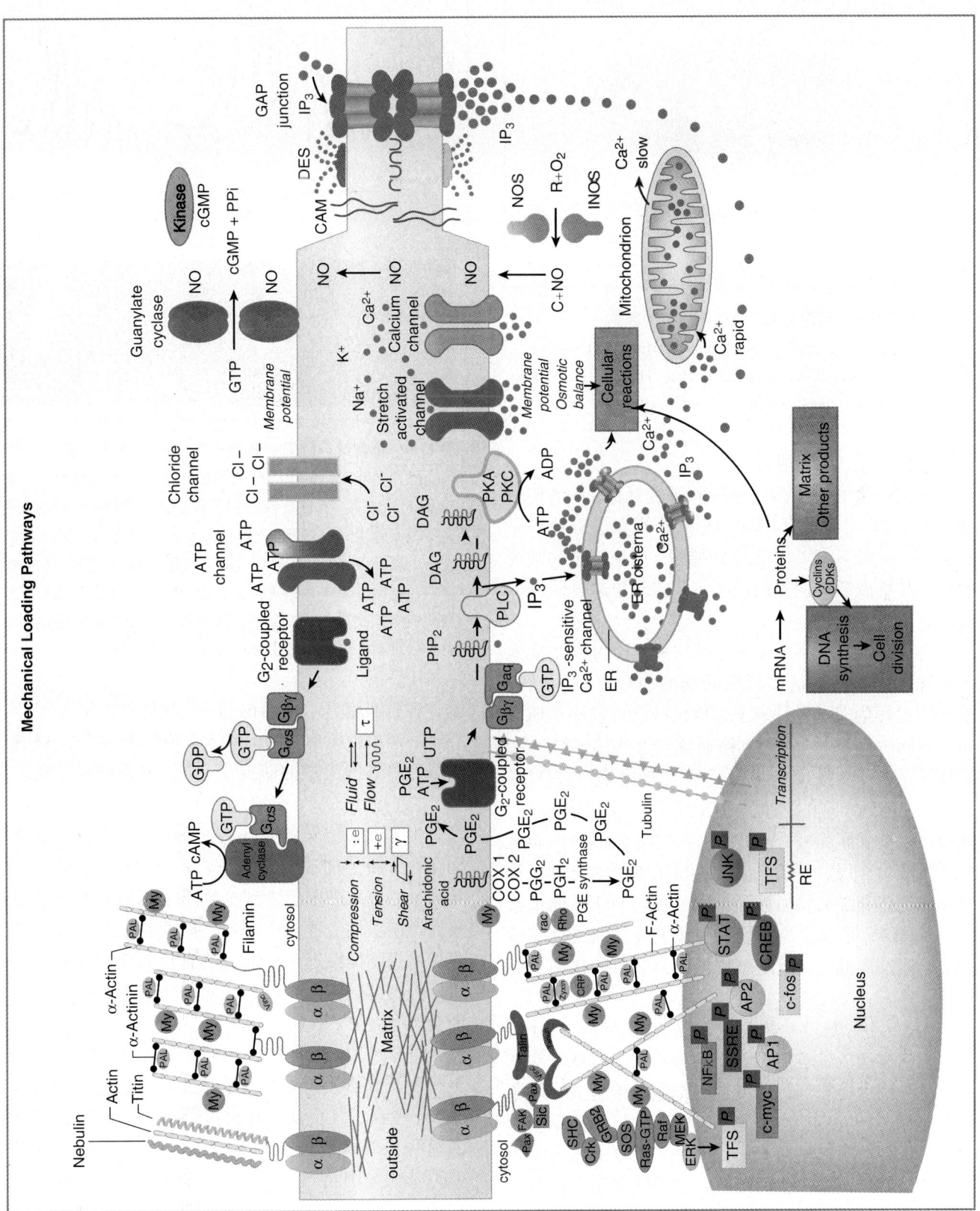

图 11-2 细胞质中一些对压力反应的化合物的示意图。缝隙连接也是张力敏感的(引自 Bans Aj, LeeG, Graff R, el: Mechanical forces and signaling in cknnective tissue cells: celluar mechanisms of detection transduction, and response to mechanical deformation. Current Oponions in Orthopaedics, 12: 389-396, 2001. Property of Flexcll Corp.)

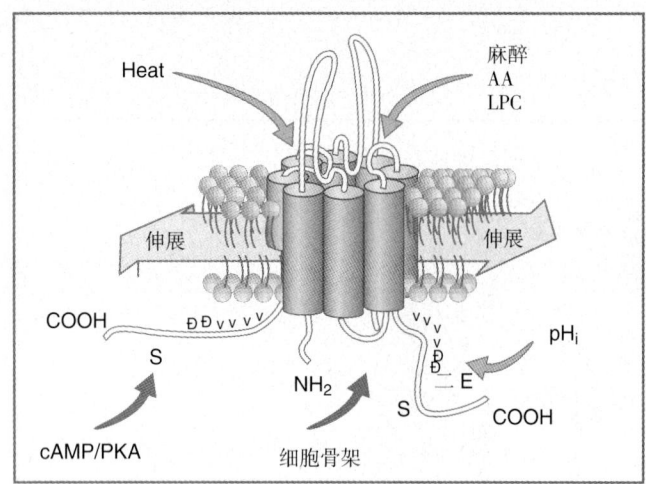

图 11-3 TREK-1 可能的结构及影响门控的因素 （Courtesy of Eric Honore，PHD，Institut de Pharmacologie Moleculaire et Cellulaire，CNRS，Institut Paul Hamel，660 route des Lucioles，Sophia Antipolis，06560，valbonne，France）

围绕层膜的中点激活通道。

研究得最好的 MSCs 是钾离子选择性 2P 结构域通道[18]。2P 通道的 TREK-1 形式出现在心脏特别是心房[20]。TREK 可以被花生四烯酸、临床剂量的常规麻醉剂和机械牵张强烈的激活，假定都是通过同样的激活方式[18]。

这种假定是来自一个论点即这些通道可以在缺血区被静止的激活，这些区域的细胞崩解释放两性分子[21,22]。因为非选择性离子通道也可以被这些物质激活，在同一细胞上开放两种通道产生复杂的影响。TREK-1 也可以被细胞内的环腺苷单磷酸（cAMP）抑制[20]，提示与自主神经系统的耦联。抑制这些 K^+ 通道可以使细胞除极，提高 Ca^{2+} 电流，协同肾上腺素的正性变力作用。一般来讲，机械敏感的通道可以被电压、配体和膜的张力激活。实际上，TREK 通道被 Aplysia 的 S 通道同源克隆，后者被分类到复合胺或 cAMP 门控的通道，但是被机械压力调节的作用更有效[23]。

SACs 不总是单一的对压力改变有反应，它还表现出失活和适应，有点像 Na^+ 通道[24-26]。这种时间依赖性的起因可能在通道本身或与细胞骨架有关。为了说明正性机械反应动力学的复杂性，图 11-4 显示了一个膜片区域，重复给予吸引的脉冲。重复的压力使得膜片变柔软（产生更大的改变在给予同样压力微分的区域）。但是让这一膜片静息 20 秒它将恢复初始时的硬度水平。

表达在心脏的 SACs 随年龄和物种变化。成年大

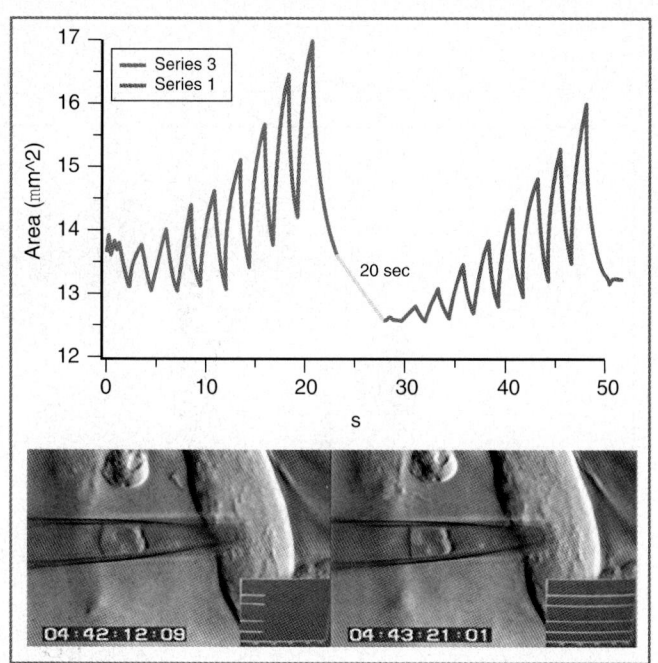

图 11-4 重复给予吮吸刺激使皮质膜的僵硬度降低（上图）
当膜片变软时，给予同样的刺激脉冲影响的区域增大。在 20 秒的静息期，僵硬度恢复到正常。这种僵硬度可逆的变化提示细胞骨架完整性的变化，因为这种变化不是脂质的特性。下图细胞贴附式膜片图像，有负压（左），无负压（右）。左面分界面是脂质膜。右边分界面是皮质与细胞质分离的地方。膜片上的细胞器、膜和玻璃电极之间的锐角显示由于膜粘附在电极上而引起的在膜上的静息张力

鼠心房肌细胞显示主要的是 K^+ 选择性 SACs[20,27,28]，只有一例报告阳离子的 SACs 在成年组织[28]。对成年大鼠心房细胞大量的研究中，Niu 和 Sachs 发现，只有 K^+ 选择性 SACs 可能是 TREK-1 家族。看起来并没有报告说在成年的工作心肌细胞有 SACs，尽管它们存在于新生的或胎儿组织。Zeng 及其同事[25]从成年大鼠心室肌细胞记录到全细胞电流但是不能记录到单通道的活性。他们认为是这些通道位于 T 管，因此膜片电极不能接近。这里可能有目的性的放大这一位置因为内部的膜比质膜在收缩时将有更大的变形，可能会折叠起来。

牵张可以以不同的方式增大背景和瞬时的 Ca^{2+} 水平[30,31]。最直接的方式就是通过 Ca^{2+} 通透性的阳离子 SACs 增加 Ca^{2+}。这种现象可以在平滑肌细胞通过单通道的 Ca^{2+} 电流或荧光看到[32]，或者通过心肌细胞 Ca^{2+} 荧光（图 11-5）。这种在心肌细胞的由机械力引起的 Ca^{2+} 流动，可以被非选择性的 SACs 阳离子抑制剂阻断[2,33]，例如 Gd^{3+} 和链霉素[34]。

细胞钙离子可以被机械地调节，通过其他方式而

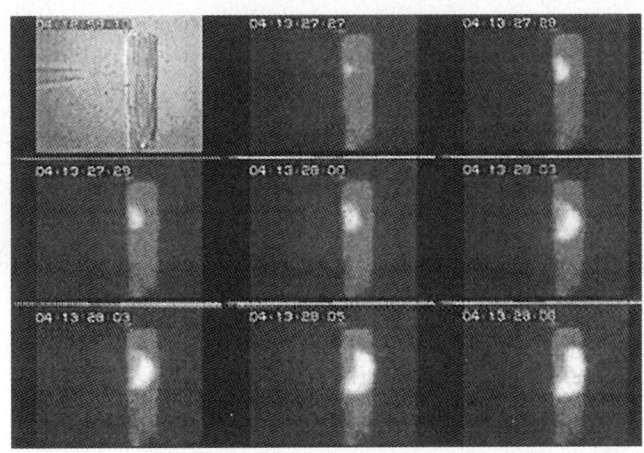

图 11-5 用抛光过的电极轻压成年大鼠心室肌细胞,引起 Ca^{2+} 波 细胞用 Fluo-3AM 染色。去除细胞外的 Ca^{2+} 或添加 Gd^{3+} 可以阻断这种 Ca^{2+} 波

不通过 SACs。细胞膨胀可以给膜压力激活 MSCs。细胞肿胀通常会引起细胞 Cl^- 传导的增大,但是继于阳离子 SACs 激活之后。可能是通过局部的 Ca^{2+} 流动激活 Cl^- 通道[35-38]。因为 Cl^- 通透性比阳离子的通透性大得多,阳离子通道电流会被掩盖。

SACs 激活在导致血流动力学不稳的心律失常中显得比较重要。充血性心力衰竭时由于细胞慢性的张力增高,慢性激活一种肿胀激活的阳离子电流[39]。这种电流可以被高张地收缩降低,或者被阳离子 SACs 阻断剂例如 Gd^{3+} 和 GsMtx-4 阻断[40]。

尽管 Ca^{2+} 通过 SACs 流动是最直接的改变细胞内 Ca^{2+} 的方式,牵张也通过其他途径影响 Ca^{2+} 水平。Na^+ 经过阳离子 SACs 内流,通过 Na^+-Ca^{2+} 交换增加肌浆网下 Ca^{2+}。电压依赖性的通道本身,包括 Ca^{2+} 通道也对牵张敏感[41]。电压依赖性的 K^+ 通道和 Na^+ 对机械压力敏感[42],提示我们可以同样来假设 L 型 Ca^{2+} 通道。压力可以直接激活 maxi Ca/K 通道,或通过 Ca^{2+} 通透性 SACs 的耦联。另一个机械力改变 Ca^{2+} 的机制不通过膜。牵张收缩蛋白会引起结合 Ca^{2+} 的释放[44],暴露钙结合位点会有相反的作用[45]。所有这些成分的相互作用导致了复杂的动力学,因而对这些现象很好的解释需要大量的计算机模型[46-48]。

对心脏牵张的一个典型的影响是心律失常的启动[6,49],血流动力学障碍是最常见的心律失常的表现。在一个很好的试验例子中,图 11-6 显示在心室周期性的球囊扩张可以引起同步的起搏活动。与牵张能引起内向电流一致,猛地击打胸壁会引起室颤或心震荡(commotio cordis)。可以解释每年发生的一些年轻运动员的死亡事件[52]。在患者身上观察到的另一相反的作用是 Valsava 动作可以终止纤维颤动[6]。甚至还有报道说一例患者在救护车碰撞时发生了心脏复率。

心脏对变形的反应可以非常快速(<10ms)[9],而且不需要发生代谢变化。牵张可以提高心率的能力可能是调节心脏充盈反馈环的一部分。心腔越充盈,收缩的可能性越大。这种牵张对心率的影响是心肌细胞内在的特性,不需要神经支配,尽管有全身整体水平的压力感受器反射。

因为分配在纤维方向的各向异性和细胞的不均一性[48],使得压力在心脏的分配是复杂的。但是理解机械电换能将机械力的不均一性转变为电的不均一性是非常重要的。例如,考虑梗死区域的收缩问题(图 11-7)。收缩时的高压力趋向于在薄弱区域引起膨出[47]。除极时,薄弱区边缘的可兴奋细胞在最大收

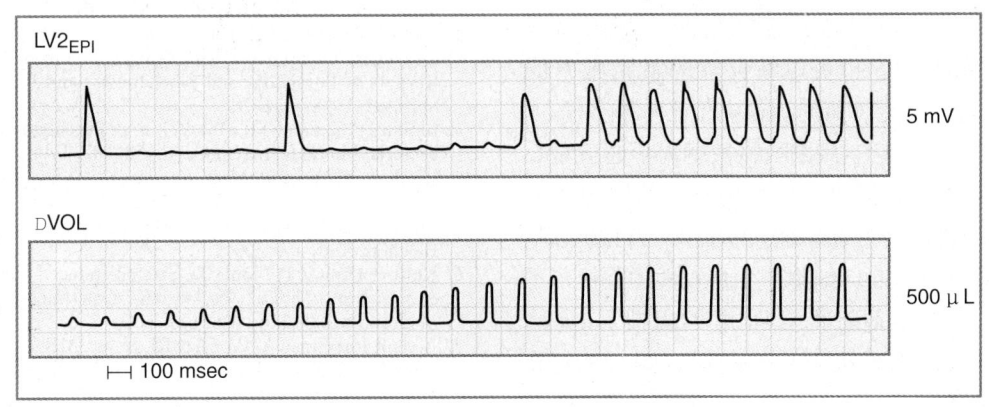

图 11-6 兔心室由于牵张引起的期外收缩 期外收缩发生的概率随心室内球囊体积增大而增加(上图记录动作电位,下图是球囊体积的变化)。快速的扩张比缓慢扩张更有效,提示离子通道本身或细胞骨架的动力学改变(引自 Franz MR, Cima R, Wang D, et al: Electrophysiologic Effects of Myocardial Stretch and Mechanical Determinants of Stretch-Activated Arrhythmias. Circulation, 1992; 86: 968-978)

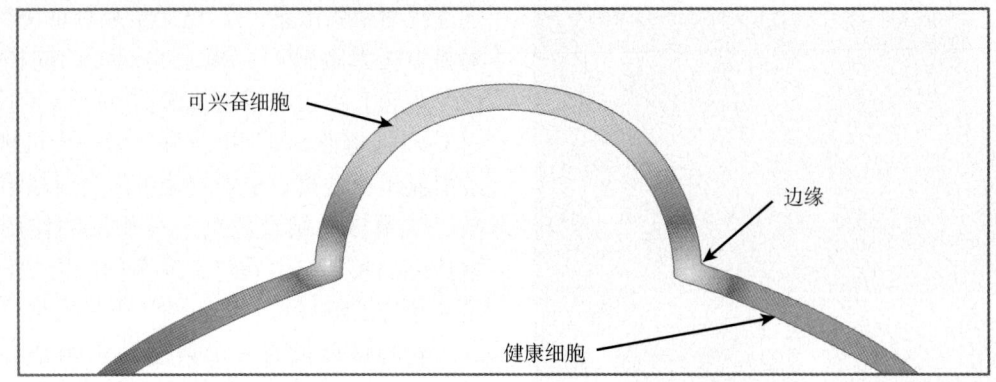

图 11-7　在收缩期室壁梗死区的变化　损伤区高的压力和薄弱的收缩力在边界区域产生牵张，可以在复极时产生兴奋电流

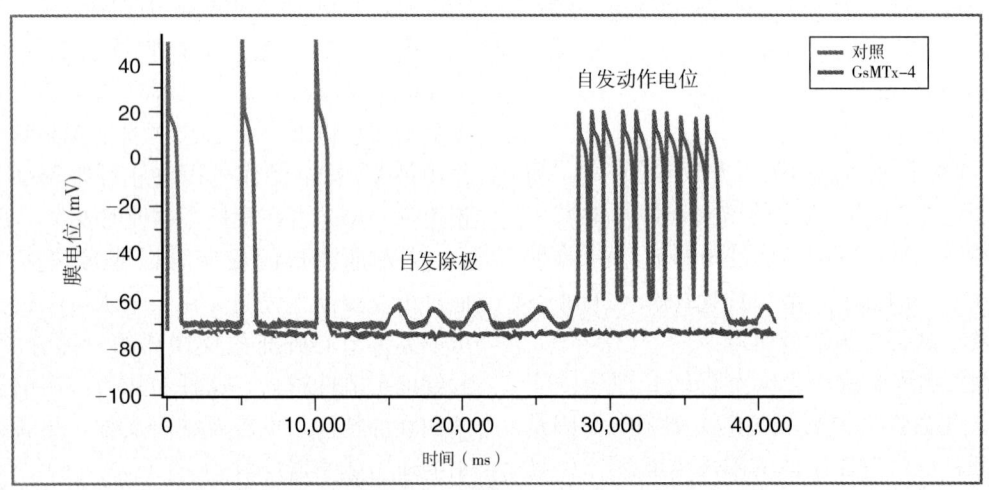

图 11-8　在兔的充血性心力衰竭模型，心室细胞自发性后除极可以被 1μM 的 GsMtx-4 阻断　（引自 Clemo HF, Baumgarten CM: The role of a volume-sensitive cation current in the genesis of spontaneous depolarizations and triggered activity in the heart: A potential cause of lethal arrhythmia. J Physiol 544, 2002）

缩压时产生兴奋电流，这被称为所谓的"易损区"。

如果存在机械敏感性离子通道，它将参与压力诱发的心律失常。有一个例子，从狼蛛毒液分离出的一种缩氨酸 GsMtx-4，可以特异性的阻断一些阳离子 SACs[38,53]。在兔模型它也可以特异性的阻断压力促进的房颤[54]，同时对无负荷的动作电位不影响[38]。

缺乏特异性的药理学，判断机械敏感离子通道对心脏生理和病理的作用是困难的。利用特异的试剂例如 GsMtx-4，我们就能够开始观察确切的作用。当心肌细胞被快速的刺激起搏减慢时，细胞产生自发性的除极，不能被 K^+ 或 Ca^{2+} 通道试剂阻断[55,56]，但可以被 GsMtx-4 阻断（图 11-8）。如果我们从字面上理解 GsMtx-4 的特异性，可能是快速的起搏使 SR 超载，引起 Ca^{2+} 释放[58]，局部收缩伴 SACs 激活。显然关于 SACs 对心脏的作用还有待研究，同时也有越来越多有效的工具可以利用。

（浦介麟　李　宁　滕思勇　译）

参　考　文　献

1. Hamill OP, Martinac B: Molecular basis of mechanotransduction in living cells. Physiol Rev 81:685–740, 2001.
2. Sachs F, Morris CE: Mechanosensitive ion channels in non specialized cells. In Blaustein MP, Greger R, Grunicke H, et al (eds): Reviews of Physiology and Biochemistry and Pharmacology. Berlin, Springer, 1998, pp 1–78.
3. Blount P, Sukharev SI, Moe PC, et al: Mechanosensitive channels of bacteria. Methods Enzymol 294:458–482, 1999.
4. Kloda A, Martinac B: Molecular identification of a mechanosensitive channel in archaea. Biophys J 80:229–240, 2001.
5. Martinac B: Mechanosensitive channels in prokaryotes. Cell Physiol Biochem 11:61–76, 2001.
6. Kohl P, Hunter P, Noble D: Stretch-induced changes in heart rate and rhythm: Clinical observations, experiments and mathematical models. Prog Biophys Mol Biol 71:91–138, 1999.
7. Bode F, Katchman A, Woosley RL, Franz MR: Gadolinium decreases stretch-induced vulnerability to atrial fibrillation. Circulation 101:2200–2205, 2000.
8. Franz MR: Mechano-electrical feedback in ventricular myocardium. Cardiovasc Res 32:15–24, 1996.

9. Zabel M, Koller BS, Sachs F, Franz MR: Stretch-induced changes in the isolated heart: Importance of the timing of stretch and implications for stretch-activated ion channels. Cardiovasc Res 32:120–130, 1996.
10. Tavi P, Han C, Weckstrom M: Mechanisms of stretch-induced changes in [Ca^{2+}]i in rat atrial myocytes: Role of increased troponin C affinity and stretch-activated ion channels. Circ Res 83:1165–1177, 1998.
11. Perozo E, Kloda A, Cortes DM, Martinac B: Physical principles underlying the transduction of bilayer deformation forces during mechanosensitive channel gating. Nat Struct Biol 9:696–703, 2002.
12. Chang G, Spencer RH, Lee AT, et al: Structure of the MscL homolog from Mycobacterium tuberculosis: A gated mechanosensitive ion channel. Science 282:2220–2226, 1998.
13. Perozo E, Kloda A, Cortes DM, Martinac B: Physical principles underlying the transduction of bilayer deformation forces during mechanosensitive channel gating. Nat Struct Biol 9:696–703, 2002.
14. Perozo E, Cortes DM, Sompornpisut P, et al: Open channel structure of MscL and the gating mechanism of mechanosensitive channels. Nature 418:942–948, 2002.
15. Betanzos M, Chiang CS, Guy HR, Sukharev S: A large iris-like expansion of a mechanosensitive channel protein induced by membrane tension. Nat Struct Biol 9:704–710, 2002.
16. Sukharev S, Sigurdson W, Kung C, Sachs F: Energetic and spatial parameters for gating of the bacterial large conductance mechanosensitive channel, MscL. J Gen Physiol 113:525–539, 1999.
17. Bass RB, Strop P, Barclay M, Rees DC: Crystal structure of Escherichia coli MscS, a voltage-modulated and mechanosensitive channel. Science 298:1582–1587, 2002.
18. Patel AJ, Lazdunski M, Honore E: Lipid and mechano-gated 2P domain K(+) channels. Curr Opin Cell Biol 13:422–428, 2001.
19. Perozo E, Kloda A, Cortes DM, Martinac B: Physical principles underlying the transduction of bilayer deformation forces during mechanosensitive channel gating. Nat Struct Biol 9:696–703, 2002.
20. Terrenoire C, Lauritzen I, Lesage F, et al: A TREK-1-like potassium channel in atrial cells inhibited by beta-adrenergic stimulation and activated by volatile anesthetics. Circ Res 89:336–342, 2001.
21. Ruwhof C, van Wamel JT, Noordzij LA, et al: Mechanical stress stimulates phospholipase C activity and intracellular calcium ion levels in neonatal rat cardiomyocytes. Cell Calcium 29:73–83, 2001.
22. Caldwell RA, Baumgarten CM: Plasmalogen-derived lysolipid induces a depolarizing cation current in rabbit ventricular myocytes. Circ Res 83:533–540, 1998.
23. Vandorpe DH, Small DL, Dabrowski AR, Morris CE: FMRFamide and membrane stretch as activators of the Aplysia S-channel. Biophysical J 66:46–58, 1994.
24. Bett GCL, Sachs F: Activation and inactivation of mechanosensitive currents in the chick heart. J Membr Biol 173:237–254, 2000.
25. Zeng T, Bett GCL, Sachs F: Stretch-activated whole-cell currents in adult rat cardiac myocytes. Am J Physiol Heart Circ Physiol 278:H548–H557, 2000.
26. Hamill OP, McBride Jr DW: Rapid adaptation of single mechanosensitive channels in Xenopus oocytes. Proc Natl Acad Sci U S A 89:7462–7466, 1992.
27. Pleumsamran A, Kim D: Membrane stretch augments the cardiac muscarinic K+ channel activity. J Membr Biol 148:287–297, 1995.
28. Zhang YH, Youm JB, Sung HK, et al: Stretch-activated and background non-selective cation channels in rat atrial myocytes. J Physiol (Lond) 523(pt 3):607–619, 2000.
29. Niu W, Sachs F: Dynamic properties of stretch-activated K+ channels in adult rat atrial myocytes. Prog Biophys Mol Biol 82(1-3):121–135, 2003.
30. Tatsukawa Y, Kiyosue T, Arita M: Mechanical stretch increases intracellular calcium concentration in cultured ventricular cells from neonatal rats. Heart Vessels 12:128–135, 1997.
31. Salmon AH, Mays JL, Dalton GR, et al: Effect of streptomycin on wall-stress-induced arrhythmias in the working rat heart. Cardiovasc Res 34:493–503, 1997.
32. Zou H, Lifshitz LM, Tuft RA, et al: Visualization of Ca2+ entry through single stretch-activated cation channels. Proc Natl Acad Sci U S A 99:6404–6409, 2002.
33. Hamill OP, McBride DW: The pharmacology of mechanogated membrane ion channels. Pharmacol Rev 48:231–252, 1996.
34. Gannier F, White E, Lacampagne A, et al: Streptomycin reverses a large stretch induced increase in [Ca]i in isolated guinea pig ventricular myocytes. Circ Res 28:1193–1198, 1994.
35. Hu H, Sachs F: Mechanically activated currents in chick heart cells. J Membr Biol 154:205–216, 1996.
36. Clemo HF, Stambler BS, Baumgarten CM: Persistent activation of a swelling-activated cation current in ventricular myocytes from dogs with tachycardia-induced congestive heart failure. Circ Res 83:147–157, 1998.
37. Suchyna TM, Johnson JH, Clemo HF, et al: Identification of a peptide toxin from Grammostola spatulata spider venom that blocks stretch activated channels. J Gen Physiol 115:583–598, 2000.
38. Suleymanian MA, Clemo HF, Cohen NM, Baumgarten CM: Stretch-activated channel blockers modulate cell volume in cardiac ventricular myocytes. J Mol Cell Cardiol 27:721–728, 1995.
39. Clemo HF, Stambler BS, Baumgarten CM: Persistent activation of a swelling-activation cation current in ventricular myocytes from dogs with tachycardia-induced congestive heart failure. Am J Physiol 251:C197–C208, 1999.
40. Clemo HF, Baumgarten CM: Swelling-activated Gd3+-sensitive cation current and cell volume regulation in rabbit ventricular myocytes. J Gen Physiol 110:297–312, 1997.
41. Calabrese B, Tabarean IV, Juranka P, Morris CE: Mechanosensitivity of N-type calcium channel currents. Biophys J 83:2560–2574, 2002.
42. Gu CX, Juranka PF, Morris CE: Stretch-activation and stretch-inactivation of Shaker-IR, a voltage-gated K+ channel. Biophys J 80:2678–2693, 2001.
43. Kawakubo T, Naruse K, Matsubara T, et al: Characterization of a newly found stretch-activated KCa,ATP channel in cultured chick ventricular myocytes. Am J Physiol 276:H1827–H1838, 1999.
44. Nickerson DP, Smith NP, Hunter PJ: Cardiac electromechanics. Philos Trans R Soc Lond Math Phys Eng Sci 359:1159–1172, 2001.
45. Niggel J, Suchyna TM, Sigurdson W, Sachs F: Mechanically induced calcium movements in astrocytes and C-6 glioma cells. J Membr Biol 174:121–134, 2000.
46. Sachs F: Modeling mechanical-electrical transduction in the heart. In Mow VC, Guliak F, Tran ST, Hochmuth RM (eds): Cell Mechanics and Cellular Engineering. New York, Springer Verlag, 1994, pp 308–328.
47. Rice JJ, Winslow RL, Dekanski J, McVeigh E: Model studies of the role of mechano-sensitive currents in the generation of cardiac arrhythmias. J Theor Biol 190:295–312, 1998.
48. Vetter FJ, McCulloch AD: Mechanoelectric feedback in a model of the passively inflated left ventricle. Ann Biomed Eng 29:414–426, 2001.
49. Kohl P, Sachs F: Mechanoelectric feedback in cardiac cells. Proc R Soc Lond Math Phys Eng Sci 359:1173–1185, 2002.
50. Franz MR, Cima R, Wang D, et al: Electrophysiological effects of myocardial stretch and mechanical determinants of stretch-activated arrhythmias [published erratum appears in Circulation 86:1663, 1992]. Circulation 86:968–978, 1992.
51. Bett GCL, Sachs F: Whole-cell mechanosensitive currents in rat ventricular myocytes activated by direct stimulation. J Membr Biol 173:255–263, 2000.
52. Maron BJ, Gohman TE, Kyle SB, et al: Clinical profile and spectrum of commotio cordis. JAMA 287:1142–1146, 2002.
53. Oswald RE, Suchyna TM, McFeeters R, et al: Solution structure of peptide toxins that block mechanosensitive ion channels. J Biol Chem 277:34443–34450, 2002.
54. Bode F, Sachs F, Franz MR: Tarantula peptide inhibits atrial fibrillation during stretch. Nature 409:35–36, 2001.
55. Nuss HB, Kaab S, Kass DA, et al: Cellular basis of ventricular arrhythmias and abnormal automaticity in heart failure. Am J Physiol Heart Circ Physiol 277:H80–H91, 1999.
56. Jones DL, Petrie JP, Li HG: Spontaneous, electrically, and cesium chloride induced arrhythmia and afterdepolarizations in the rapidly paced dog heart. Pacing Clin Electrophysiol 24:474–485, 2001.
57. Clemo HF, Baumgarten CM: The role of a volume-sensitive cation current in the genesis of spontaneous depolarizations and triggered activity in the failing heart: A potential cause of lethal arrhythmia. J Physiol 544, 2002.
58. Schlotthauer K, Bers DM: Sarcoplasmic reticulum Ca2+ release causes myocyte depolarization: Underlying mechanism and threshold for triggered action potentials. Circ Res 87:774–780, 2000.

第 12 章

起搏通道和正常的自律性

Dario DiFrancesco

本章目录

- 心脏窦房结起搏细胞电流的特性 …… 102
- 自主神经系统对心率的调节涉及起搏电流 …… 103
- HCN 亚型对窦房结起搏通道的作用… 104
- 心脏的变时性调节：有多少种机制？ …… 104
- F 通道阻滞剂的心率减低作用 ……… 106
- 总结 …… 108
- 致谢 …… 108

一、心脏窦房结起搏细胞电流的特性

窦房结区的起搏细胞通过其特有的能产生自发性动作电位的能力来起搏心脏。即使将窦房结区的心肌与心脏的其他部位完全分离，其自发性起搏的能力依然持续。这是基于起搏细胞动作电位有一特殊的时相（4 相），舒张期（或起搏）除极。在一个动作电位的终末期，起搏除极缓慢的将膜电位升至可以发动一次新的动作电位的阈电位，因此引起可反复的激动。

舒张期除极的机制是什么？在 70 年代晚期的一个重要发现回答了这个问题，Brown，DiFrancesco 和 Nobil 在兔的窦房结发现了一种新的电流[1]。因为这种电流（被称为 funny，I_f）呈内向且在舒张期超极化时（大约 $-60 \sim -45$ mV）缓慢激活，所以被认为与舒张期起搏细胞动作电位除极的产生有关（图 12-1A，B）。而且当刺激 β 受体时 I_f 电流增大（图 12-1D），这可以解释儿茶酚胺诱导的结细胞自主性活动加速。

在浦肯野纤维也早就观察到一种起搏电流，但是那是一种外向 K^+ 电流，可以在舒张期电压范围内去激活（I_{k2} 电流[2]）。浦肯野纤维的 I_{k2} 电流和窦房结的 I_f 电流在很多方面类似，两种电流不同的离子特征一直让人迷惑，直到 1981 年对 I_{k2} 电流成分重新阐述[3,4]。这两种电流实际上是同样的，而因为交叉存在"K^+ 损耗"，10 多年来一直错误地认为 I_{k2} 是一种单纯的 K^+ 电流。这显示出在不同的心脏细胞起搏成分的相似性，也开始了对窦房结细胞和浦肯野纤维 I_f 特性的研究[5]。

在窦房结细胞，I_f 电流在大约 $-40/-50$ mV 超极化时激活，在 -100 mV 时完全激活（图 12-1E）。最大激活 I-V 曲线几乎呈线形，由于混合了对 K^+ 和 Na^+ 的通透性反转电位大约是 $-10/-20$ mV[6]。因为 I_f 电流的激活范围与舒张期除极交叉，提示此电流在动作电位的终末期激活会参与形成 4 相除极的内向电流。在浦肯野纤维，I_f 电流的特性也基本明确，其激活曲线的位置比结细胞的左移。在后面我们将讨论，在心脏的不同部位，可能是 I_f 通道的分子组成特性不同造成其功能的差异。

I_f 电流作为起搏除极主要机制的重要性还存在争议，主要是因为其电流激活窗口电压的可变性，在一些情况下激活的电压太负似乎不能参与细胞的动作电位。但是关于 I_f 激活曲线可变性原因的讨论可以在以前的文章中见到[5,8]。在对心脏以及发育中的心脏细胞 I_f 特性的研究中发现独立的证据证明在起搏活动中有超极化激活的电流。I_f 电流的表达与自发性的活动有关，这不仅在哺乳动物的心脏细胞（窦房结或房室结的细胞表达 I_f 电流可以自发性搏动，而不表达 I_f

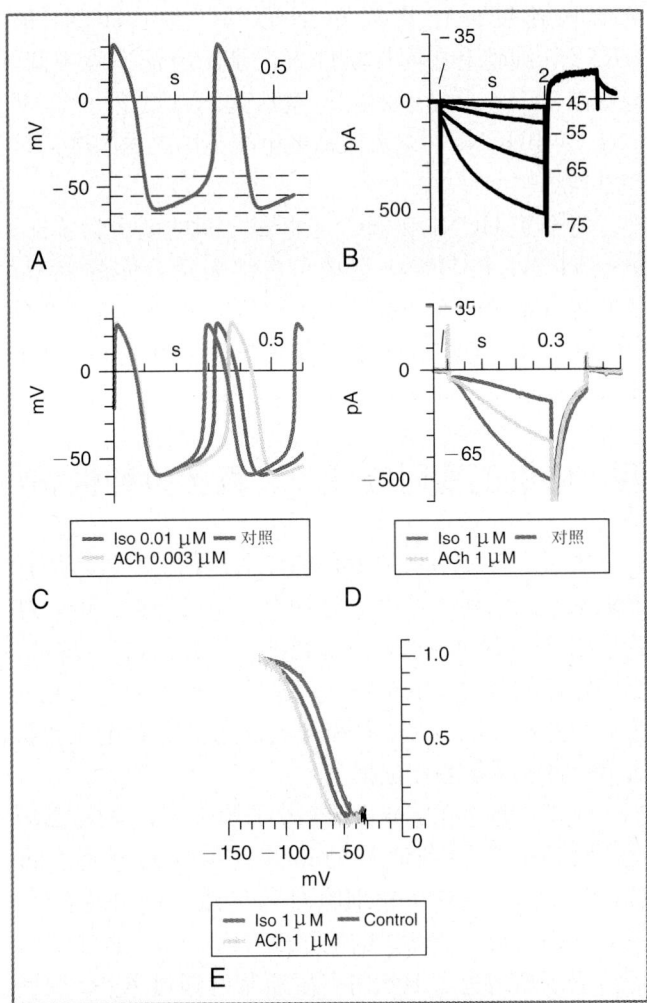

图12-1 A：从单个的兔窦房结心肌细胞记录到的自发性动作电位 B：从保持电压－35mV到指示电压超极化激活的 I_f 电流，相对应的电压也在图A中显示。从超极化后到－15mV，引起内向Ca^{2+}和外向K^+电流的激活。C~E:低剂量自主神经介质对起搏节率的调节。C：通过调节舒张期除极的速度，单个窦房结细胞的自发性活性可以被Iso（0.01μM）加速，被ACh（0.003μM）减慢，而不改变动作电位的形状和时程。D：在单个的窦房结细胞，从保持电压－35mV到－65mV，I_f 电流可以被Iso（1μM）增大，被ACh（1μM）减小。E：β肾上腺素能刺激可以使激活曲线右移，增加舒张期除极的I_f 电流的数量，加速除极，而毒蕈碱刺激的作用与之相反

电流的成年心室肌细胞则不能自发性搏动），在发育中的鸡胚心室细胞，zebra鱼的心脏也可见到。而 I_f 电流表达缺乏与心动过缓突变的缓慢心率相关[10]。培养的大鼠心室肌细胞中也存在 I_f 电流与自发性活动的关系，实际上来自新生鼠的培养细胞可以记录到 I_f 电流激活的电位接近生理电位，比来自成年大鼠的培养细胞激活的电压要高，后者接近静息电位[11,12]。在小鼠心室肌细胞的发育过程中也有类似的直接的联系[13]。而且在培养的胚胎大鼠心室肌细胞过度表达HCN2（一种野生型心脏起搏通道分子，详见下文）可以引起潜在的自发性节率的增加，和显著的舒张期除极坡度的增大[12]。在表达超极化激活电流（I_h）的神经元细胞中也可以观察到起搏活动[14]。最后，关于 I_f 电流和起搏关系的证据在于观察到部分的阻断 I_f 电流引起心率减慢。这一点在后面还将讨论。

二、自主神经系统对心率的调节涉及起搏电流

自主神经的活动可以清楚的显示 I_f 电流和起搏的关系。心脏的窦房结有丰富的交感和副交感神经末梢，两者分别有正性和负性变时效应。β肾上腺素性和胆碱性的变时效应可以在分离的可自发性搏动的窦房结细胞上进行复制。当给予低剂量的β受体激动剂或乙酰胆碱，由于分别加速或减速舒张期除极的速率而改变自发性的频率，但对于动作电位的形状或时程几乎没有改变，这也提示特异性的影响了 I_f 电流。

HCN通道有几种不同特性的亚型存在，它们相互依赖并影响通道的活性，是其在不同组织表达细胞功能差异的基础[5,14]。实际上，HCN亚型在心脏和神经组织有不同的表达模式[34,35]，与其在相应组织的特定的功能相对应。

不同亚型有不同特性的分子基础是什么？它们在核心区域有高度的同源性（图12-2），可能差异集中在C末端、N末端或者两者同时有序列的本质改变。与这一假说一致的是，位于C末端的CNBD可以通过对通道的抑制作用来影响动力学，这种作用可以被cAMP结合部分的去除[32,36]。

HCN通道动力学的电压依赖性可以用一个变构体的模型来描述[31]，假设通道是个四聚体，每一个亚型有一个电压感受器（位于S4结构域），当任意一个可变的电压感受器呈现开放的构型，通道开放（图12-2D）。用变构体的模型，可以从对电压感受器动力学和开/关转变联合的贡献来解释单独的HCN亚型的动力学特性。在超极化时通道开放，可以看作是以下共同的贡献：（1）电压感受器迅速的从关闭到开放状态，紧接着（2）变构体大约10倍的减慢通道关闭→开放转变。变构体模型基本的假设是当四个电压感受器中的任意一个转变为开放状态，通道开放的可能性增大。

Altomare及其同事[31]的变构体模型，用一个整

体的模式解释了所有的三种心脏亚型 HCN1、HCN2、HCN4 的主要动力学特性及其差异。例如，按照这一模型 HCN2 激活曲线越负的部分是由感受器的电压依赖性引起的，因而对所有亚型其开/关转换的电压依赖性是相似的。也就是说，HCN1 相对于 HCN2、HCN4 激活快是由于电压感受器和开/关转换的速度快。

变构体的开/关转换不仅易于解释 HCN 电压依赖性的改变，也可以解释 cAMP 介导的通道调节：由 cAMP 结合引起的电压改变，是因为 cAMP 对通道开放状态比关闭状态亲和力大[37]。

三、HCN 亚型对窦房结起搏通道的作用

了解不同亚型的特性对于确定哪种亚型对给定组织中的原始通道起作用有重要的意义。与电生理特性一起，Northern blot 分析、RNase 保护分析、亚型特异性抗体免疫标记可以用来研究 HCN 亚型的分布情况。在心脏组织有 HCN 的强烈表达。最初用 Northern blot 法发现在心脏和脑有 HCN2 的表达，HCN1 主要在脑中表达[23,24]。因为逆转录 PCR（RT-PCR）提示在心房、心室、窦房结都有 HCN2 表达[23]，这些数据表明 HCN2 是心脏中的基本的亚型。但是进一步的研究用 RNase 保护分析显示在窦房结有 HCN4 高度的表达，而仅有痕量的 HCN2[38]。有趣的是 HCN1 也在窦房结和浦肯野纤维中存在[38]，在窦房结细胞可以用免疫标记的方法检测到蛋白水平的 HCN1[39]。

在图 12-3，用特异性的抗-HCN1 抗体免疫定位，显示在从兔窦房结区用酶解分离的单独的起搏细胞。这一区域的细胞，有典型的细胞学特征，包括发育差的收缩系统，稀少紊乱的条纹和大空泡，可以通过与神经细丝抗体反应鉴定，这在周围的心房细胞是不表达的[39]。

在图 12-3 中抗 HCN1 抗体标记不连续的区域，提示通道在膜上局部的分隔，与野生的 f 通道组装在膜上的"热点"部位而不是均一的在起搏细胞膜上表达这一概念一致[22]。

试验证据显示许多亚型在窦房结和其他心脏组织参与形成野生的 f 通道。因为野生通道的特性不总是与单个表达在野生组织的亚型一致，有可能不同的亚型能组装成异源多聚体 f 通道。在图 12-4A，从保持电压 -35mV 到 -95mV，记录兔的窦房结细胞 I_f 的活化速度介于在表达 rbHCN1 或 rbHCN4 的 HEK293 细胞上在同样条件下记录的电流速度中间。像在图 12-4B 中显示的，I_f 激活时间常数介于 rbHCN1 或 rbHCN4 在电流激活的电压范围之内的激活时间常数。

有介于 HCN1 和 HCN4 电流之间的动力学特征，加上 HCN1 和 HCN4 是在窦房结表达最多的亚型，这些证据都表明在天然的心脏起搏区域的 f 通道是由 HCN1 和 HCN4 亚单位组装成的异源多聚体，但是化学计量的亚单位的比例还要进一步研究。

四、心脏的变时性调节：有多少种机制？

关于 I_f 电流在心脏起搏的产生和调节中的作用长期以来已经明确[1,5,40,41]。像在上文中已经列出的，这些作用基于 I_f 电流的基本的特性：具有内在的可维持缓慢除极的能力，对于肾上腺素能和胆碱能变时性刺激的敏感性，以及在心脏和神经细胞表达 I_f 电流和具有节律性相关的独立证据。

最近，基于在节律性活动中肌膜下 Ca^{2+} 的正常转运，对于心率活动调节的其他机制的研究也有进展[42,44]。这一机制依赖细胞内 Ca^{2+} 激活的内向 Na^+-Ca^{2+} 交换电流。在动作电位除极之前，Ca^{2+} 通过 T 型 Ca^{2+} 离子通道进入细胞内引发肌浆网通过 RyRs 受体释放 Ca^{2+}，后者激活 Na^+-Ca^{2+} 交换电流[45]。有人认为这同样也是 β 肾上腺素能刺激引起正性变时效应的机制[46]，证据是 β 肾上腺素能刺激引起心率和 Ca^{2+} 震荡的平行增大，而去除 Ca^{2+} 转运（通过用 ryanodien 或耗竭 Ca^{2+} 储存）可以使心率减慢并削弱 β 受体介导的对心率的调节[46,47]。

然而有很多观察的结果反对这一观点——通过 RyRs 释放 Ca^{2+} 在起搏节律的调节中起主要作用。例如，中度的 β 受体刺激通过使舒张期早期和晚期除极的斜率增大来加速节律，这是 I_f 电流增加（图 12-1）而不是 Ca^{2+} 释放介导的作用，因为后者主要集中在舒张期除极的最后阶段[42,44]。要反对 RyR 介导的机制，包括腺苷酸环化酶-cAMP-I_f 通路，需要解释由于低 ACh 浓度引起的心率减慢，这也涉及与 β 受体刺激时对应的对舒张早期除极的改变（图 12-1）[20]。而且使用特异性 I_f 阻断剂如 zatebradine，ZD-7299，或者 ivabradine 可以使起搏心率减慢[48-52]，这也提示 I_f 电流在起搏过程中起到基本的作用。

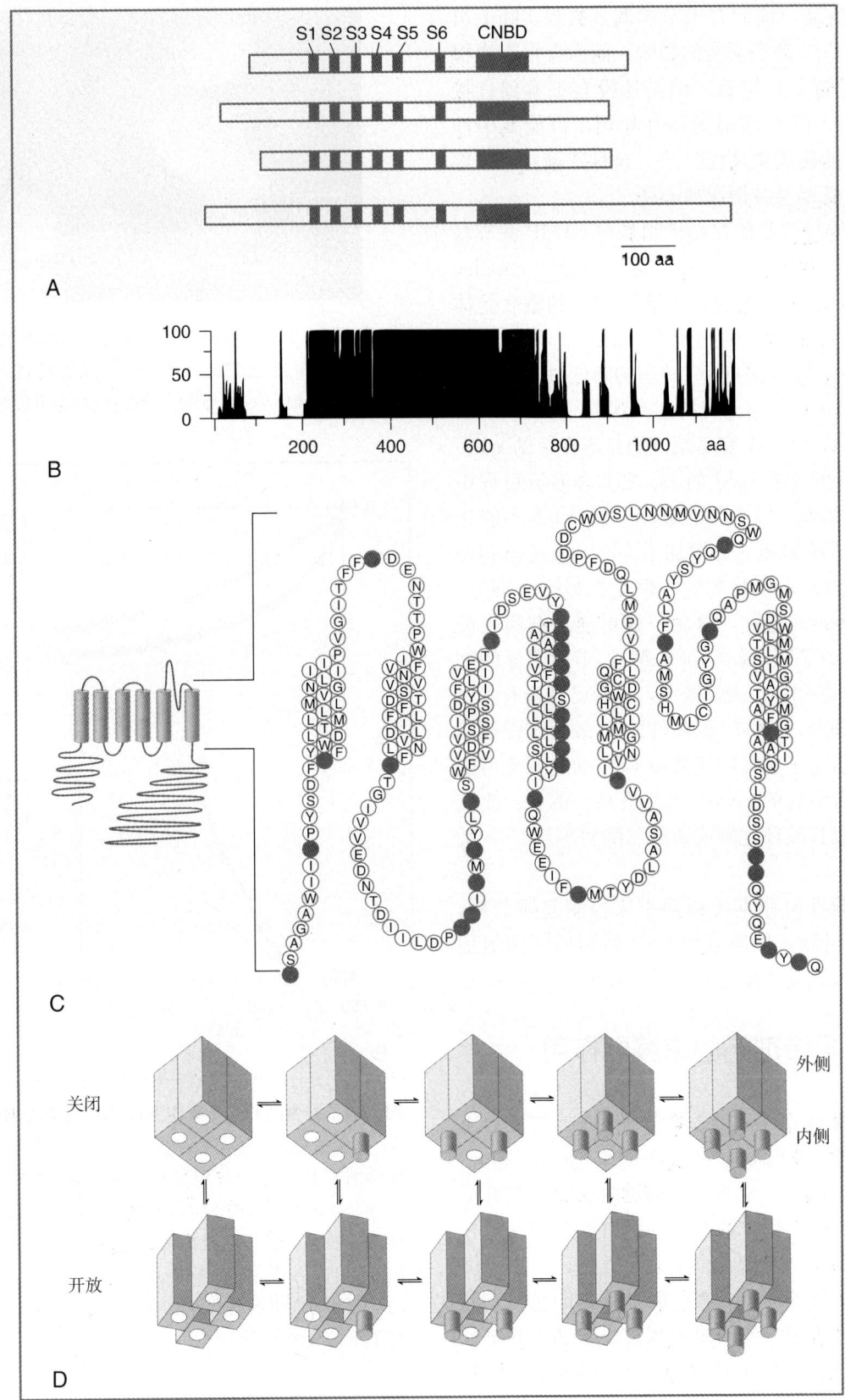

图 12-2 HCN 通道 A：HCN 通道拓扑示意图（从上到下分别是 HCN1～HCN4 亚型），显示了 S1～S6 跨膜结构域和环核苷酸结合区（CNBD）。B：各亚型核心区域序列有高度同源性（从 S1～CNBD）而 C 末端和 N 末端有更较多的变异。C：兔的 HCN4 跨膜结构域线形氨基酸序列。在放大的部分，实心圆圈代表的是带阳性电荷的残基。D：HCN4 通道门控模型变构体。通道是一个四聚体，每一个亚基都有一个电压感受器（圆柱体），当任意一个感受器在超极化时进入开放状态，通道开放的可能性增大。所有四个亚基协调改变构型（从关闭到开放或者相反）

应该注意的是，基于 I_f 的节律调节机制实际上可能收到细胞内 Ca^{2+} 动态平衡的影响，因为有报告说提高 Ca^{2+} 浓度会增大 I_f 电流。但是还没有观察到直接快速的关于 Ca^{2+} 和 I_f 通道的相互作用，可能其中涉及了 Ca^{2+} 依赖的磷酸化过程[54,55]。这种依赖性可以部分的解释 Ca^{2+} 耗竭会减慢起搏心率[56]。

I_f 依赖性的起搏节律控制机制是在 cAMP 调节基础上的，cAMP 直接激活通道。通过给予 ryanodien 抑制 β 受体介导的心率加速，可能影响了刺激 β 受体后 cAMP 激活 I_f 通道的某一步骤，因此反映出 I_f 机制的削弱，而不是直接的 Ca^{2+} 转运的降低对心率的调节[57]。在图 12-5 中的结论支持这一观点。

在图 12-5A，将一个窦房结细胞暴露在 3 的 ryanodine 中，分别在给予 $1\mu M$ 的 Iso 之前和灌流过程中记录自发性的活动。与前面的数据一致，Iso 不能正常的使自发性活动加速（只增加了 2%），β 受体刺激和自发性活动的关系也是如此。但是在另一个细胞，在暴露于 ryanodine 之后，灌流一种可透过细胞膜的 cAMP 类似物（CPT-Camp，$300\mu M$），节律明显的加快约 20%（图 12-5B）。这就提示，尽管已经没有 β 受体介导的节律调节，cAMP 依赖性的 I_f 激活过程依然起作用。这就否定了正常的胞浆中 Ca^{2+} 动态变化可能影响 β 受体刺激引起的 cAMP 水平升高，例如：改变 cAMP 通路上腺苷酸环化酶或磷酸二酯酶等对 Ca^{2+} 敏感的因素。

尽管通过改变舒张期除极斜率来控制起搏节律，是基于 I_f 调节机制，但肌浆网 Ca^{2+} 转运的作用更适合于在舒张期末促进产生更安全的动作电位。

五、F 通道阻滞剂的心率减低作用

I_f 和心率调节之间的功能联系使得 f 通道成为重要的药理学靶点。降低心率的试剂（如：zetabradine，ZD7288，invabradine）能引起心动过缓反应而没有反面的影响收缩力的作用。这些药物都有潜在的治疗作用。例如：心绞痛时减慢心率是有益处的，因为可以降低工作心肌对氧的需求，因而降低缺血的风险，同时没有负性肌力作用。许多使用减慢心率试剂的研究已经发现了它们作用的分子基础。这些研究已经清楚的显示这些试剂是通过选择性的抑制 I_f 来起作用[48-51]。部分阻断引起 I_f 减低导致起搏活性减慢，是通过降低舒张期除极的斜率，与 ACh 作用的方式类似（图 12-1）。

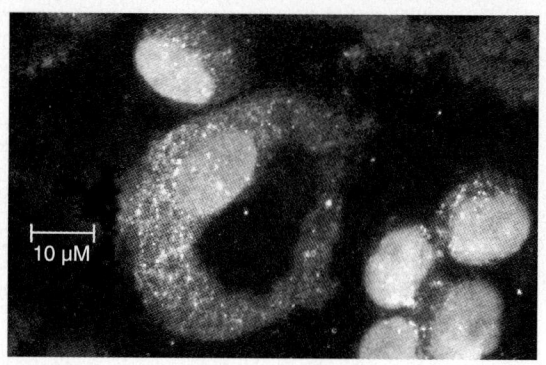

图 12-3 抗 HCN1 抗体标记兔的窦房结细胞 亮点染色对应的是红色荧光抗 HCN1。多克隆抗体针对一个 KLH-共轭 19aa 缩氨酸，选择性的在 mHCN1 的 C 末端

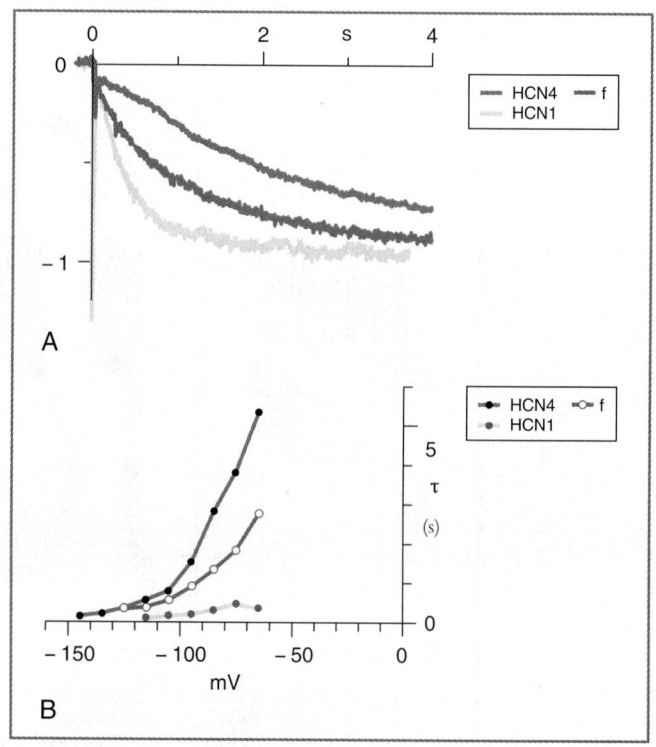

图 12-4 野生的 f 通道和 HCN1，HCN4 亚型激活动力学比较
A：从保持电压-35mV，超极化到-95mV，在单独的兔窦房结细胞和在两个分别异源性表达 rbHCN1、rbHCN4 的 HEK293 细胞记录到正常的电流。记录对所有的细胞都是同样的。细胞外液和电极内液的离子浓度按照 Viscomi 的方法[32]。B：A 中同样细胞在从-145～-65mV 超极化范围内，激活时间常数的电压依赖性。在初始化延迟后，图线进行了单指数修正[31]

UL-FS 49 对 I_f 通道的阻断显示出使用依赖性，阻断作用相对较慢（几十秒），发生在通道开放时，作用在通道的细胞内部分[50]。这种使用依赖性的特性

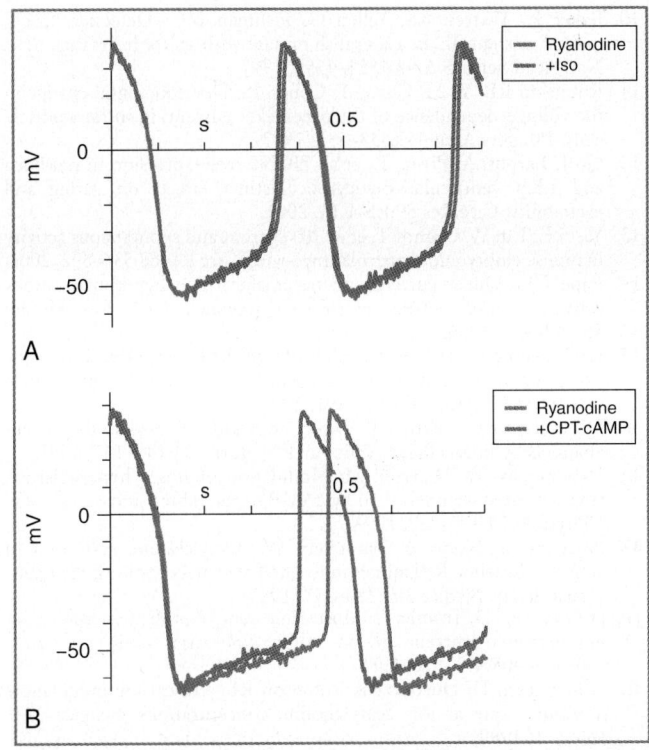

图12-5 Ryanodine 抑制 Iso (1μM) 引起的自律性加速，但不改变 cAMP 引起的加速 (CPT-cAMP 300μM)。A：在 Iso 灌流前和灌流中，从长时间（134秒）暴露于 Ryanodine 的窦房结细胞记录的活动。B：在 CPT-cAMP 灌流前和灌流中，从长时间（321秒）暴露于 Ryanodine 的另一个窦房结细胞记录到的活动。Iso 引起的速率改变是 2%（从 2.70 到 2.74Hz），CPT-cAMP 引起的加速为 20%（从 2.09 到 2.50Hz）

在治疗方面很有作用，因为它对开放频率高的通道的阻断作用更明显，意味着药物对快速性节律更有效。对 I_f 最大激活 I-V 关系阻断的电压依赖性提示，药物分子进入通道孔达到电的膜厚度的 39%[50]。

Ivabradine（一种最近发展的降低心率的分子）对天然通道的阻断作用也有了细节的研究[52]。在窦房结细胞药物在细胞内的作用是一种特异性的 f 通道阻滞剂（IC_{50} = 1.5～2.8μM）[51,52]。发现了以下特征：(1) ivabradine 是一种开放通道的阻断剂，即阻断和阻断的去除发生在通道开放状态，因而需要膜超极化；(2) 超极化促成阻断的去除；(3) 当电压超过了电流的翻转电位时阻断作用才有明显的电压依赖性，这说明从内向电流转变成外向电流对阻断作用有强烈的影响；(4) 需要内向电流来减轻阻断作用。因为当用 Cs^+ 阻断内向电流后，超极化并不能去除阻断作用；(5) 在 Na^+ 取代试验，阻断的程度和流过通道的电流的大小有关而不是与电压大小有关（图12-6）。

这些数据显示 ivabradine 引起电流依赖性而不是电压依赖性的 f 通道阻滞作用，导致内向整流性，很像细胞内的多价阳离子对内向整流 K^+ 通道的作用。这些特征揭示 f 通道的透过是一种多离子、单列通过的过程[52]。来源于 ivabradine 对 I_f 通道阻滞特异性的使用依赖性，使它对心率降低能力在自发性心率快时

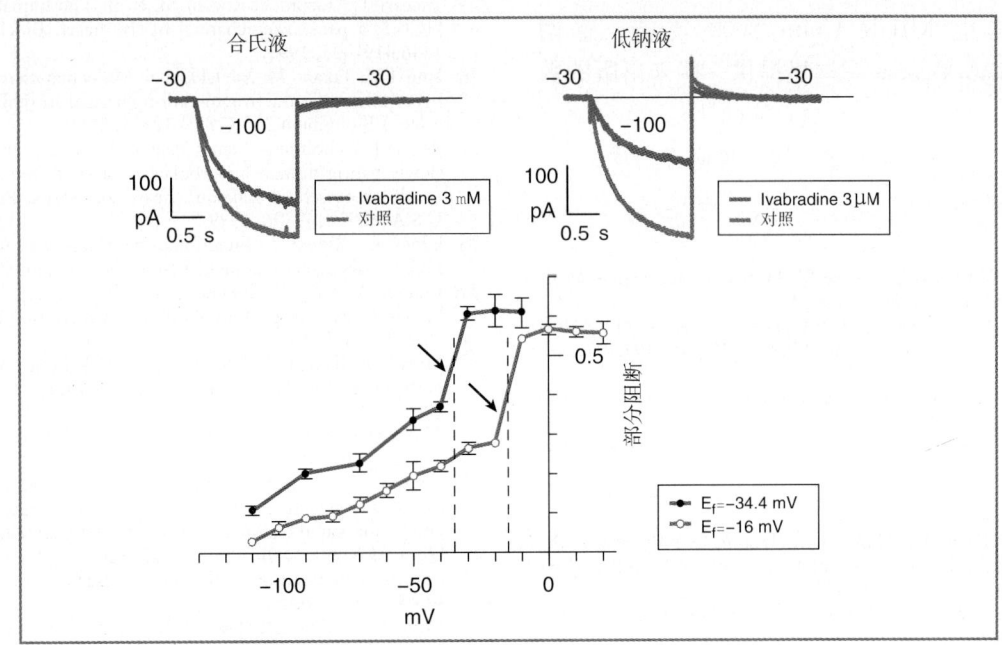

图12-6 Ivabradine 阻断 I_f 对电流驱动力的依赖性。A：从两个细胞记录的电流曲线显示了 3μM Ivabradine 对不同程度的稳态阻断作用，细胞外钠浓度分别为 140mM（左图），和 35mM（右图）。刺激程序为每6秒给予激活/去激活（-100/-30mV）刺激。在正常钠外液部分阻断作用大约为 24%，在钠浓度降低的外液阻断作用为 54%。B：比较在正常台式液（空心圆圈）和 35mM Na^+ 外液（实心圆圈）中平均的电压依赖性的部分阻断作用。垂直的虚线对应的是 I_f 在两种条件下的反转电位，在正常台式液 E_f = -16.0mV，35mM Na^+ 外液 E_f = -34.4mV。箭头指示的是阻断曲线上相应 E_f 值的交点（修改自 Baruscotti M, Difrancesco D: Current-dependent block of rabbit sino-atrial node If channels by ivabradine J Gen Physiol 120: 1-13, 2002.）

更强，这可能对临床治疗有用。

六、总结

从最初发现的 20 多年来，funny 电流已经在心脏和脑中被详细的描述，在细胞功能多样性基础上已经确定了它的作用。尽管还没有完全详尽的对涉及起搏功能所有的过程的理解，有许多证据提示，在心脏窦房结细胞，I_f 的机制是最适于产生自发性激活并调节自主神经传导对节律的控制。f 通道是天然的控制心率药物的作用靶点，尤其是选择性降低心率的药物（例如特异性的 I_f 抑制剂 ivabradine），对于减慢心率有益的疾病具有潜在的治疗作用。

克隆 HCN 通道，确定在心脏组织表达的不同 HCN 亚型和在窦房结特异性的表达，为了解 f 通道特性的分子基础提供了新的途径。希望在不久的将来，对于与 f 通道动力学和通透特性相关的分子位点，联系 cAMP 连接、电压超极化和通道门控的过程等问题，结构功能研究将提供更好的理解。此外，发展新的药物能与确定的结合位点相互作用，具有更好的组织特异性将成为可能。

七、致　谢

这项工作由 MIUR Cofin 2000 支持，感谢 C. Altomare 和 A. Bucchi 在这里提供一些未出版的数据。

（浦介麟　李　宁　滕思勇　译）

参 考 文 献

1. Brown HF, DiFrancesco D, Noble SJ: How does adrenaline accelerate the heart? Nature 280:235–236, 1979.
2. Noble D, Tsien RW: The kinetics and rectifier properties of the slow potassium current in calf Purkinje fibres. J Physiol 195:185–214, 1968.
3. DiFrancesco D: A new interpretation of the pace-maker current in calf Purkinje fibres. J Physiol 314:359–376, 1981.
4. DiFrancesco D: A study of the ionic nature of the pace-maker current in calf Purkinje fibres. J Physiol 314:377–393, 1981.
5. DiFrancesco D: Pacemaker mechanisms in cardiac tissue. Annu Rev Physiol 55:455–472, 1993.
6. DiFrancesco D, Ferroni A, Mazzanti M, Tromba C: Properties of the hyperpolarizing-activated current (if) in cells isolated from the rabbit sino-atrial node. J Physiol 377:61–88, 1986.
7. Irisawa H, Brown HF, Giles W: Cardiac pacemaking in the sinoatrial node. Physiol Rev 73:197–227, 1993.
8. DiFrancesco D: The contribution of the 'pacemaker' current (if) to generation of spontaneous activity in rabbit sino-atrial node myocytes. J Physiol 434:23–40, 1991.
9. Satoh H, Sperelakis N: Developmental changes and modulation through G-proteins of the hyperpolarization-activated inward current in embryonic chick heart. Ann NY Acad Sci 707:413–416, 1993.
10. Baker K, Warren KS, Yellen G, Fishman MC: Defective "pacemaker" current (Ih) in a zebrafish mutant with a slow heart rate. Proc Natl Acad Sci U S A 94:4554–4559, 1997.
11. Robinson RB, Yu H, Chang F, Cohen IS: Developmental change in the voltage-dependence of the pacemaker current, if, in rat ventricle cells. Pflugers Arch 433:533–535, 1997.
12. Qu J, Barbuti A, Protas L, et al: HCN2 overexpression in newborn and adult ventricular myocytes: Distinct effects on gating and excitability. Circ Res 89:E8–E14, 2001.
13. Yasui K, Liu W, Opthof T, et al: I(f) current and spontaneous activity in mouse embryonic ventricular myocytes. Circ Res 88:536–542, 2001.
14. Pape HC: Queer current and pacemaker: The hyperpolarization-activated cation current in neurons [review]. Annu Rev Physiol 58:299–327, 1996.
15. DiFrancesco D, Tromba C: Inhibition of the hyperpolarization-activated current (if) induced by acetylcholine in rabbit sino-atrial node myocytes. J Physiol 405:477–491, 1988.
16. DiFrancesco D, Tortora P: Direct activation of cardiac pacemaker channels by intracellular cyclic AMP. Nature 351:145–147, 1991.
17. DiFrancesco D, Mangoni M: Modulation of single hyperpolarization-activated channels (i(f)) by cAMP in the rabbit sino-atrial node. J Physiol 474:473–482, 1994.
18. Sakmann B, Noma A, Trautwein W: Acetylcholine activation of single muscarinic K channels in isolated pacemaker cells of the mammalian heart. Nature 303:250–253, 1983.
19. DiFrancesco D, Tromba C: Muscarinic control of the hyperpolarization-activated current (if) in rabbit sino-atrial node myocytes. J Physiol 405:493–510, 1988.
20. DiFrancesco D, Ducouret P, Robinson RB: Muscarinic modulation of cardiac rate at low acetylcholine concentrations. Science 243:669–671, 1989.
21. DiFrancesco D, Tromba C: Acetylcholine inhibits activation of the cardiac hyperpolarizing-activated current, if. Pflugers Arch 410:139–142, 1987.
22. DiFrancesco D: Characterization of single pacemaker channels in cardiac sino-atrial node cells. Nature 324:470–473, 1986.
23. Santoro B, Liu DT, Yao H, et al: Identification of a gene encoding a hyperpolarization-activated pacemaker channel of brain. Cell 93:717–729, 1998.
24. Ludwig A, Zong X, Jeglitsch M, et al: A family of hyperpolarization-activated mammalian cation channels. Nature 393:587–591, 1998.
25. Vaccari T, Moroni A, Rocchi M, et al: The human gene coding for HCN2, a pacemaker channel of the heart. Biochim Biophys Acta 1446:419–425, 1999.
26. Ishii TM, Takano M, Xie LH, et al: Molecular characterization of the hyperpolarization-activated cation channel in rabbit heart sinoatrial node. J Biol Chem 274:12835–12839, 1999.
27. Seifert R, Scholten A, Gauss R, et al: Molecular characterization of a slowly gating human hyperpolarization-activated channel predominantly expressed in thalamus, heart, and testis. Proc Natl Acad Sci U S A 96:9391–9396, 1999.
28. Ulens C, Tytgat J: Functional heteromerization of HCN1 and HCN2 pacemaker channels. J Biol Chem 276:6069–6072, 2001.
29. Ludwig A, Zong X, Stieber J, et al: Two pacemaker channels from human heart with profoundly different activation kinetics. EMBO J 18:2323–2329, 1999.
30. Moroni A, Barbuti A, Altomare C, et al: Kinetic and ionic properties of the human HCN2 pacemaker channel. Pflugers Arch 439:618–626, 2000.
31. Altomare C, Bucchi A, Camatini E, et al: Integrated allosteric model of voltage gating of HCN channels. J Gen Physiol 117:519–532, 2001.
32. Viscomi C, Altomare C, Bucchi A, et al: C terminus-mediated control of voltage and cAMP gating of hyperpolarization-activated cyclic nucleotide-gated channels. J Biol Chem 276:29930–29934, 2001.
33. Qu J, Altomare C, Bucchi A, et al: Functional comparison of HCN isoforms expressed in ventricular and HEK 293 cells. Pflugers Arch 444:597–601, 2002.
34. Santoro B, Tibbs GR: The HCN gene family: Molecular basis of the hyperpolarization-activated pacemaker channels [review]. Ann NY Acad Sci 868:741–764, 1999.
35. Kaupp UB, Seifert R: Molecular diversity of pacemaker ion channels. Annu Rev Physiol 63:235–257, 2001.
36. Wainger BJ, DeGennaro M, Santoro B, et al: Molecular mechanism of cAMP modulation of HCN pacemaker channels. Nature 411:805–810, 2001.

37. DiFrancesco D: Dual allosteric modulation of pacemaker (f) channels by cAMP and voltage in rabbit SA node. J Physiol 515:367–376, 1999.
38. Shi W, Wymore R, Yu H, et al: Distribution and prevalence of hyperpolarization-activated cation channel (HCN) mRNA expression in cardiac tissues. Circ Res 85:e1–e6, 1999.
39. Moroni A, Gorza L, Beltrame M, et al: Hyperpolarization-activated cyclic nucleotide-gated channel 1 is a molecular determinant of the cardiac pacemaker current I(f). J Biol Chem 276:29233–29241, 2001.
40. Noble D: The surprising heart: A review of recent progress in cardiac electrophysiology. J Physiol 353:1–50, 1984.
41. Accili EA, Proenza C, Baruscotti M, DiFrancesco D: From funny current to HCN channels: 20 years of excitation. News Physiol Sci 17:32–37, 2002.
42. Huser J, Blatter LA, Lipsius SL: Intracellular Ca2+ release contributes to automaticity in cat atrial pacemaker cells. J Physiol 524(pt 2):415–422, 2000.
43. Ju YK, Allen DG: The mechanisms of sarcoplasmic reticulum Ca2+ release in toad pacemaker cells. J Physiol 525:695–705, 2000.
44. Bogdanov KY, Vinogradova TM, Lakatta EG: Sinoatrial nodal cell ryanodine receptor and Na(+)-Ca(2+) exchanger: Molecular partners in pacemaker regulation. Circ Res 88:1254–1258, 2001.
45. Lipsius SL, Huser J, Blatter LA: Intracellular Ca2+ release sparks atrial pacemaker activity. News Physiol Sci 16:101–106, 2001.
46. Vinogradova TM, Bogdanov KY, Lakatta EG: beta-Adrenergic stimulation modulates ryanodine receptor Ca(2+) release during diastolic depolarization to accelerate pacemaker activity in rabbit sinoatrial nodal cells. Circ Res 90:73–79, 2002.
47. Rigg L, Heath BM, Cui Y, Terrar DA: Localisation and functional significance of ryanodine receptors during beta-adrenoceptor stimulation in the guinea-pig sino-atrial node. Cardiovasc Res 48:254–264, 2000.
48. Goethals M, Raes A, van Bogaert PP: Use-dependent block of i_f in isolated rabbit sinoatrial node cells by zatebradine. J Physiol 467:59P, 1993.
49. BoSmith RE, Briggs I, Sturgess NC: Inhibitory actions of ZENECA ZD7288 on whole-cell hyperpolarization activated inward current (If) in guinea-pig dissociated sinoatrial node cells. Br J Pharmacol 110:343–349, 1993.
50. DiFrancesco D: Some properties of the UL-FS 49 block of the hyperpolarization-activated current (i(f)) in sino-atrial node myocytes. Pflugers Arch 427:64–70, 1994.
51. Bois P, Bescond J, Renaudon B, Lenfant J: Mode of action of bradycardic agent, S 16257, on ionic currents of rabbit sinoatrial node cells. Br J Pharmacol 118:1051–1057, 1996.
52. Bucchi A, Baruscotti M, DiFrancesco D: Current-dependent block of rabbit sino-atrial node I(f) channels by ivabradine. J Gen Physiol 120:1–13, 2002.
53. Zaza A, Maccaferri G, Mangoni M, DiFrancesco D: Intracellular calcium does not directly modulate cardiac pacemaker (I_f) channels. Pflugers Arch 419:662–664, 1991.
54. Chang F, Cohen IS, DiFrancesco D, et al: Effects of protein kinase inhibitors on canine Purkinje fibre pacemaker depolarization and the pacemaker current I_f. J Physiol 440:367–384, 1991.
55. Accili EA, Redaelli G, DiFrancesco D: Differential control of the hyperpolarization-activated current I_f by cAMP gating and phosphatase inhibition in rabbit sino-atrial node myocytes. J Physiol 500:643–651, 1997.
56. Li J, Qu J, Nathan RD: Ionic basis of ryanodine's negative chronotropic effect on pacemaker cells isolated from the sinoatrial node. Am J Physiol 273:H2481–H2489, 1997.
57. DiFrancesco D, Robinson RB: beta-Modulation of pacemaker rate: Novel mechanism or novel mechanics of an old one? Circ Res 90:E69, 2002.

第 13 章

内向整流钾通道的生物物理学特性

Justus M. B. Anumonwo

本章目录

- Kir 通道结构和分子特性 111
- Kir 通道的整流机制 114
- 总结 115

心脏内向整流钾（Kir）通道的作用为稳定静息膜电位，决定兴奋阈值，调节动作电位的复极相[1-3]。内向整流呈现这样一种现象：其电导性在超极化时增强，而在膜电位超过钾平衡电位（Ek）时减弱。导致整流的原因是，除极引起细胞内阳离子向通道的胞浆口运动，从而阻塞了离子的渗透通路（见 Nichols et al[4] 和 Lopatin and Nichols[1]）。内向整流二极管样的特性构成了 Kir 通道的关键性生物物理学特征，即在细胞静息状态下保持良好的电导性以稳定细胞膜电位，并且在动作电位的平台期防止细胞丢失过多的钾离子。

过去三十年的研究，已发现心脏有三种重要 Kir 通道：乙酰胆碱激活 K^+ 电流（$I_{K,ACh}$），ATP 敏感 K^+ 电流（$I_{K,ATP}$），及经典内向整流钾电流（I_{K1}）。本章先简要讨论心肌细胞上 Kir 通道的一般特性，然后描述不同种属相关通道的分子生物物理学特性。本章的其他一些内容则摘自最近出版的多篇优秀综述[1,5,6]。

1. 乙酰胆碱激活 K^+ 电流（$I_{K,ACh}$）

顾名思义，$I_{K,ACh}$ 由迷走神经释放的乙酰胆碱激活。乙酰胆碱通过心肌细胞上的毒蕈碱受体（M2）发挥效应。尽管它为乙酰胆碱门控 K^+ 通道，但其他物质如 α_2-肾上腺受体拮抗剂、生长激素抑制因子和腺苷等刺激也起反应。$I_{K,ACh}$ 通道主要在窦房结和心房细胞上表达，当其被激活后，$I_{K,ACh}$ 允许 K^+ 外流，导致细胞膜超极化而减慢心率。$I_{K,ACh}$ 的电导性与 I_{K1} 相似，大约 30~40 pS[7,8]。

2. ATP 敏感 K^+ 电流（$I_{K,ATP}$）

$I_{K,ATP}$ 通道的主要作用是使细胞兴奋性与细胞代谢状态相匹配。通道可被存在于胞浆内的腺苷酸快速而可逆性终止，其抑制效能依次为 AMP 最弱，ADP 中等，ATP 最强。在心脏，核苷酸效应 IC_{50} 分别为 AMP 10 mM，ADP 250 μM，ATP 20 μM。在平衡液（150 mM K^+），心肌细胞的单元电导率是 70~90 pS[9]，平均开放时间大约 1 毫秒[10]。在心脏应激状态下，如低氧和缺血时，$I_{K,ATP}$ 通道激活，导致钾外流及动作电位间期（APD）缩短。而 APD 缩短则可降低心肌收缩力，这对功能减退的心肌是有利的。

3. 经典内向整流 K^+ 电流（I_{K1}）

在心房肌、心室肌和蒲肯野纤维细胞，静息钾离子电导率主要取决于非电压依赖内向整流 K^+ 电流，即 I_{K1}。经深入研究，认为 I_{K1} 在结细胞（窦房结和房室结）上不存在，或很少表达。最近一篇文献已论述了其一般特性[1]。I_{K1} 整流作用取决于细胞内一些离子，特别是 Mg^{2+} 和多胺对通道孔的阻滞。I_{K1} 通道也可被 Cs^+ 和 Ba^{2+} 所阻滞，所阻滞部位是通道孔的细胞外口。一些研究均表明 I_{K1} 单元电导率为细胞外钾离子浓度的平方根。

不同的研究小组所报告的通道整体电导值变化很大。Sakmann 和 Trube[11] 广泛研究了豚鼠心室肌细胞 I_{K1} 特性，报告其电导率值为 27 pS。Kurachi[12] 报告

I_{K1} 通道的整体电导率 40 pS，平均开放时间长达 100 ms。而在另一个豚鼠心室肌细胞 I_{K1} 通道的研究中，Shioya 及同事[13] 报告整体电导率值为 33～34 pS。对这些数值的不同其原因尚不清楚，可能的原因是所研究的组织细胞不同及种属不同所引起的，这个问题将在以后的章节中进一步讨论。

一、Kir 通道的结构和分子特性

Kir 离子通道家族包含一大组 K^+ 通道，它们在结构和功能上不同于电压门控性（kv）钾通道[14-16]。在对果蝇基因克隆后应用电压门控性（kv）钾通道亚单位同形扫描，并未发现任何 Kir 通道。1993 年取得了突破性进展，三家不同的实验室应用表达克隆，首次获得并描述了 Kir 通道的特征[17-19]。目前，Kir 通道家族至少有七个成员（图 13-1；表 13-1）。一般来说，Kir 通道拥有 40% 的氨基酸成分，而其亚族成员则高达 60% 以上。

Kir 通道为四聚体，每个亚基有二个跨膜区域。Kir 通道的小孔段（H5 或 P 区）通常有 K^+ 通道标记序列，Gly-Tyr/Phe-Gly 序列[5]。证据表明，一些 Kir 通道包含同价同效基因复合物（相同 Kir 亚单位）或异侧复合物（相关 Kir 亚单位）。Kir4 和 Kir5 在脑部组成内向整流电流，而 Kir1，Kir2，Kir3 和 Kir6 则在心脏表达。比较而言，对 Kir2，Kir3，Kir6 通道了解的信息较多，这些通道均在心脏表达，特别是 Kir2 亚家族，是本章节后面部分讨论的重点。

在讨论具有二个跨膜区域的 Kir 通道亚单位时，值得注意的是 Lesage 和其同事[20] 首先克隆了另一组内向整流 K^+ 通道，从而形成了两类 Kir 通道系列。此通道称为 TWIK-1，被认为其二聚体形成较弱内向整流特性的通道。这些通道在心房、心室组织均表达，以心室表达为著。TWIK 通道对 Ba^{2+} 的敏感性弱，其整流特性有 Mg^{2+} 依赖性。与经典 Kir 通道相比，对 TWIK 知之甚少。然而，越来越多的证据表明这些通道主要构成了心脏的背景电流（限于篇幅，本章不再进一步讨论 TWIK 通道）。

（一）与 $I_{K,ACh}$ 有关的 Kir3 亚家族

Kir3 亚型被认为是调节 $I_{K,ACh}$（见 Nerbonne 和同事[6] 综述）。此通道经膜界通路直接和 M2 受体结合，并且其结合机制涉及百日咳毒素敏感的 GTP 结合蛋白 G。当 G 蛋白的 βγ 亚单位结合到 Kir3.x 通道上时

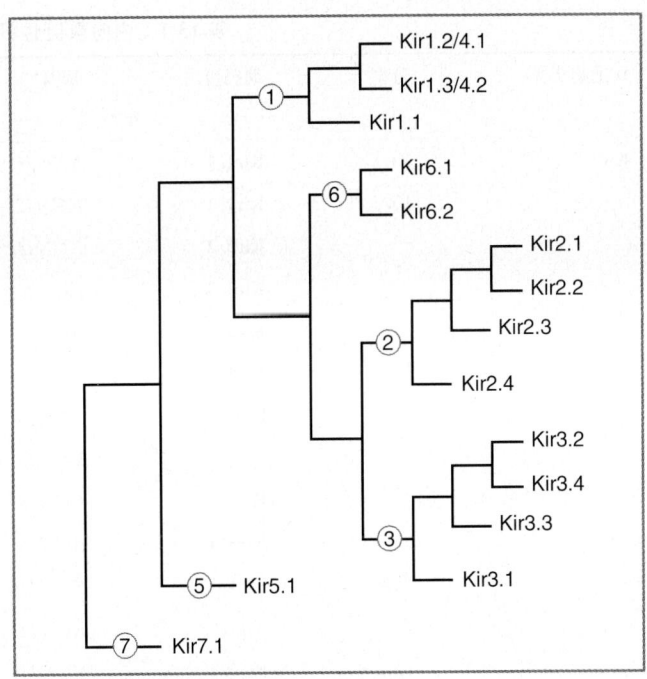

图 13-1 人类内向整流钾通道亲缘关系树枝图 （引自 Reimann F，Ashcroft FM：inwardly rectifying potassium channels. Curr Opin Cell Biol 11：503-508，1999.）

即可激活 $I_{K,ACh}$ 通道[21]。

Kir3.x 通道在 $I_{K,ACh}$ 中的作用已在从 Kir3.4 靶点基因敲除小鼠中得以支持。动物实验表明敲除 Kir3.4 靶点基因则缺乏任何可测量到的 $I_{K,ACh}$[22]。那么 Kir3 通道亚型在 $I_{K,ACh}$ 通道复合体中是怎样组合的？证据表明在心脏由 Kir3.1 和 Kir3.4 蛋白所组成的 $I_{K,ACh}$ 通道为同价同效基因通道复合体，其化学计量组成为 1：1（Kir3.1 和 Kir3.4 通道也被称为 GIRK1，GIRK4）。GIRK 代表 G 蛋白耦联的内向整流 K^+ 通道。但本章仍使用术语 Kir3.x。还有证据表明，在 Kir3 的两个亚型中，Kir3.4 对通道处理和细胞表面定位至关重要，而且与 G 蛋白 βγ 亚单位的连接点也位于 Kir3.4 上。

（二）$I_{K,ATP}$ 通道：Kir6 亚家族复合体和磺脲类受体

证据表明，$I_{K,ATP}$ 的分子相关成分是 Kir6 亚家族和编码磺脲类受体的 ATP 连接盒状蛋白[23]。异多亚基复合物由 Kir6.2 和 SUR2A 组成，但不清楚此通道复合物的哪个亚单位具备 ATP 敏感性。Kir6.2 蛋白在复合物中的作用业已建立：在 Kir6.2$^{-/-}$ 小鼠则缺乏 $I_{K,ATP}$ 通道活性[24,25]。Kir6.1 也在心脏表达，实验表明如在心室肌细胞存在反义 SUR1 则 $I_{K,ATP}$ 功能降低。

表 13-1　内向整流性钾通道 α 亚单位蛋白多样性

K通道类型	分型	编码蛋白	基因	染色体		心肌通道电流
				人	鼠	
Kir	Kir1	**Kir1.1**	KCNJ1	11q25		?
	Kir2	**Kir2.1**	KCNJ2	17q23	11	I_{k1}
		Kir2.2	KCNJ12	17p11.2	11	I_{k1}
		Kir2.3	KCNJ4	22U		?
		Kir2.4	KCNJ14	19q13.4		?
	Kir3	**Kir3.1**	KCNJ3		2	$I_{K,ACh}$
		Kir3.2	KCNJ6	21q22		
			KCNJ7		16	
		Kir3.3	KCNJ9	1q21	1	
		Kir3.4	KCNJ5	11q25	9	$I_{K,ACh}$
	Kir4	Kir4.1	KCNJ10	1q21	1	
		Kir4.2	KCNJ15	21q22	16	
	Kir5	Kir5.1	KCNJ16	17q25		
	Kir6	**Kir6.1**	KCNJ8	12p11.1	6	
		Kir6.2	KCNJ11	11p15		$I_{K,ATP}$

引自 Nerbonne JM, Nichols CG, Schwarz TL, Escande D: Genetic manipulation of cardiac K⁺ channel function in mice: What have we learned, and where do we go from here? Circ Res 89: 944-956, 2001

(三) Kir2 亚家族

Kir2 亚家族成员 (Kir2.1-Kir2.4, 即 Kir2.x) 接近 60% 序列同源, 其一个重要区别是尾部的长度不一, Kir2 通道亚单位的结构示意图见图 13-2。Kir2 亚型表达有其组织和种属特异性区别[26-29]。Kir2 亚家族成员中有高度的序列同源性, 在心肌细胞表达有重要生物物理特性和调控特性, 概述于表 13-2 中。

1. Kir2.1 通道

Kubo 和同事[17]使用克隆表达技术, 在小鼠巨噬细胞族分离了编码 428 个氨基酸蛋白的 cDNA。此蛋白编码内向整流钾通道, 为 IRK1 (Kir2.1) 的翻版, 它每个亚单位有 2 个跨膜区段, 40% 的序列与 ATP 调节 K 通道相似[18]。此通道选择性通过 K 离子, 传导 K⁺ 平衡电位下的内向 K⁺ 电流, 还允许少许外向电流, 其在卵母细胞膜片钳的单元电导率为 23pS。Kir2 通道整流机制大部分已在表达 Kir2.1 通道的异种体进行过研究, 并在后面章节进一步阐述。Kubo 和同事[17]也报告了电压和时间依赖性通道, 它可被细胞外 Na⁺、Cs⁺ 和 Ba²⁺ 所阻断, 其特性提示为开放的阻滞通道。细胞外 Cs⁺ 阻滞骤然下降, 表明在通道孔内有多个阳离子结合位点。

在另一项研究中, Ishihara[30]在小鼠成纤维母细胞确定了 Kir2.1 通道时间依赖性外向电流的特性。特别研究了 Mg²⁺、四甲烯二胺和内源性精胺存在条件下的外向电流特性。从去极化电位到复极化可导致外向电流的时间依赖性改变: 外向电流开始短暂增加,

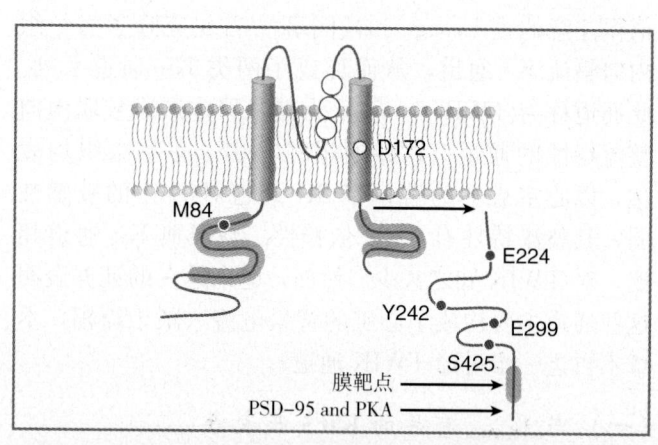

图 13-2　Kir2 通道亚单位膜局部解剖示意图　在通道功能和调节中的重要部位被标识。D172, E224、E299 为通道整流重要位点; G-Y-G: 钾通道标记序列; PKA: 蛋白激酶 A; Y242: 酪氨酸激酶磷酸化位点

表 13-2 单独的 kir2.X 通道亚型的生物物理学及调节特性

性质	Kir2.1	Kir2.2	Kir2.3
单一传导（pS）	25	35	10
钡阻断，IC_{50}（μm）	3.2	0.5	10.3
花生四烯酸作用，EC_{50}	不敏感	不敏感	447
质子阻滞（pK_a）	4.95	—	6.6

然后下降。开始的增加是由于二价离子（Mg^{2+}，四甲烯二胺）阻滞的暂时解除，而再降低则是由于精胺的阻滞。因此，平台期 Mg^{2+} 的作用对心脏复极电位至关重要。

最近，Liu 与合作研究人员[27]研究了豚鼠 Kir2.1 通道的整体电导率和药理阻滞作用，它在 HEK293 细胞和卵母细胞异源表达。他们报告在 K^+ 平衡液中（140mM）的总电导率是 30.6pS。所需半量最大阻滞（IC_{50}）的钡浓度在 −100mV 时为 3.24μM。

总之，这些资料显示在心脏表达的 Kir2 亚家族中，Kir2.1 通道有中度的电导特性，对 Ba^{2+} 有敏感性。值得注意的是，一些研究经常观察到 Kir2.1 通道不同的整体电导率值。然而，这些值不同于宿主心肌细胞上 I_{k1} 的总电导率值。一个可能性是 Kir2.1 通道蛋白与表达系统的其他蛋白互相作用，而导致总电导率值的改变[27,31]。

2. Kir2.2 通道

与 Kir2.1 通道比较，所知 Kir2.2 亚基的信息较少。已在小鼠[32]和大鼠[33]脑细胞进行了 Kir2.2 通道的分子克隆和功能表达。在后者研究中，此通道的氨基酸序列，命名为 RB-IRK2，与小鼠 Kir2.1 通道有 70% 序列相同。鼠类 Kir2.2 通道为 427 个氨基酸蛋白，在卵母细胞表达时，等摩尔 K^+ 浓度（140mM）下其电导率为 34.2pS[32]。在他们的实验条件下，Kir2.1 通道的整体电导率值较小，为 22.2pS。也有报告，与 Kir2.1 通道相比，Kir2.2 通道在超极化状态下大量失活。Koyama 和同事[33]也报告 Kir2.2 通道对 Cs^+ 和 Ba^{2+} 敏感，呈现时间和电压依赖性方式的通道阻滞。最近阐述了从豚鼠心脏克隆的 Kir2.2 通道的生物物理特性[27]。总电导率均值 40pS，通道对细胞外 Ba^{2+} 高度敏感。细胞外 Ba^{2+} 阻滞（0.51μM）的 IC_{50} 在 Kir2 亚家族中最低。研究还提示尽管豚鼠心肌细胞表达 Kir2.1、Kir2.2 和 Kir2.3 通道，但 Kir2.2 通道是内向整流电流的主要通道（见后面讨论）。

3. Kir2.3 通道

Makhina 和同事[34]研究了人类海马克隆的内向整流通道 HRK1（Kir2.3）的特性。研究报告其 60% 的序列与以前克隆的 Kir2.1 序列相似，编码 445 个氨基酸的蛋白。在卵母细胞异种表达后，从细胞膜片钳直接或噪音分析测量的总电导率平均为 10pS。研究报告 Kir2.3 通道可被细胞外 Ba^{2+}（$K_0=183μM$）和 Cs^+（$K_{-130mV}=30μM$）所阻滞。通道也可在细胞内阻滞，但细胞外无 TEA（$K_0=62μM$）。Morishige 与合作者[35]从小鼠脑 cDNA 程序库，确定了 Kir2.3 通道克隆的 MB-IRK3 的特点，它也是编码 445 个氨基酸的蛋白。研究还描述了细胞外 140mM K^+ 浓度下总电导率 10pS，并有明确的浓度与电压依赖性的由细胞外 Ba^{2+} 和 Cs^+ 导致的通道阻滞。同年，Perier 和同事[36]描述了从人类海马分离的，并在卵母细胞表达的强整流 Kir 通道的特性。与 Kir2.1 通道相比，此通道有 67% 的序列同源性。他们也报告 Kir2.3 电流可被细胞外 Ba^{2+} 和 Cs^+ 所阻滞。Cs^+ 阻滞分析表明在跨膜电域内 Cs^+ 结合位点的理论 δ 是 1.4。Perier 和同事[36]还报告 Kir2.3 通道的总电导率是 13pS，在负电位下，通道门电路动力学缓慢，开放时间长。通道电导率与通道整流依赖于细胞外 K 离子。

因此，尽管序列具有同源性，但每个 Kir2 亚基的特性却显著不同。可以肯定这些亚基的不同必定在局部环境下对 I_{k1} 有重要意义[29,37]，此作用正在本实验室被检测。

（四）与经典内向整流有关的 Kir2 亚家族

据认为 Kir2 亚家族成员主要与 I_{k1} 有关。Kir2.x 亚家族成员具有时间和电压依赖整流特性，这几乎与心脏自身的 I_{k1} 的特性相同[1]。在上述的四个 Kir2 亚家族成员中，仅 Kir2.1、Kir2.2 和 Kir2.3 在心肌细胞表达[27]。多克隆抗体免疫细胞化学分析表明，Kir2.4 仅在心脏神经细胞上表达[27]。在 I_{k1} 中 Kir2.1 和 Kir2.2 的作用通过基因敲除方法得到进一步证实[38]。从 $Kir2.1^{-/-}$ 小鼠心室肌细胞不能记录到可探测的 I_{k1}。然而，在 $Kir2.2^{-/-}$ 小鼠可观察到 I_{k1} 50% 的降低，提示有可能 Kir2.2 也参与 I_{k1}。Kir2.3 在 I_{k1} 的作用尚不清楚[6]。

Kir2.x 亚基在通道中的相互作用情况尚未充分了解。Kir2 通道家族在体内是以同源四聚体[39]还是异源四聚体[40,41]形式存在尚有争论。最近，另一项研究已提供证据表明 Kir2 通道为异基数[42]。研究者在 HEK293 细胞或非洲蟾蜍属卵母细胞，用成对 Kir2 通道（Kir2.x 和 Kir2.y）共表达为单一通道或连环体，并研究了 Ba^{2+} 阻滞的药理作用。有趣的是，他们发现卵母细胞 Kir2.1 和 Kir2.2 共表达后，其通道 Ba^{2+} 阻滞的 IC_{50} 与其独立表达的单通道的期望值明显不同。另外，应用双酵母杂交系统研究显示，不同 Kir2 通道亚基的 N-端和 C-端的确相互作用。

正如以前所提到的，报告的 I_{k1} 总电导率值变化很大，由 27 到 40pS 不等[11-13]。I_{k1} 总电导率值的不同是否由于这些组织/细胞中 Kir2.x 通道的表达不同？最近一篇试图回答这个问题的文献对 I_{k1} 的生物物理和分子特性做了研究[27]，应用细胞膜片钳技术在分离的心室肌细胞检测了三种单通道的电导率：34、23.8 和 10.7pS。Kir2 通道的总电导率，异源表达比在宿主细胞表达要高出 25%，在 Kir2.1、Kir2.2 和 Kir2.3 分别为 30.6、42.0 和 14.2pS。应用多细胞 RT-PCR 方法，研究人员检测了 Kir2.1、Kir2.2 和 Kir2.3 通道的一些信息。RNA 分析结果和本组的研究结果（见 Dhamoon 和同事[26,37]）表明，Kir2.1 比其他亚基的显色更为显著。然而，根据宿主心肌细胞 Ba^{2+} 阻滞的药理作用与在卵母细胞异源表达的作用相比，提示对宿主细胞 I_{k1} 的主要贡献者为 Kir2.2 亚基。RT-PCR 资料与通道活性之间的显著不同，可能是由于宿主环境下 Kir2 通道所形成的通道复合体不均质所引起。

二、Kir 通道的整流机制

内向整流概念由于电压依赖性胞浆颗粒阻塞通道孔而首先提出，此后的研究证实 Kir 通道的整流是由于细胞内阳离子，包括 Na^+、Mg^{2+} 和多胺所致的电压依赖性通道阻塞（Lopatin 和 Nichols 综述[1]）。此种通道阻塞的敏感性在不同的 Kir 亚家族表现不同[43]，尽管每种 Kir 通道都表现内向整流特性，但 Kir 通道被分为"强整流通道"（Kir2 和 Kir3）或"弱整流通道"（Kir1 和 Kir6）[1,4,5]。弱内向整流被细胞膜超极化所瞬间"激活"或打开，而强整流则是以时间依赖性方式所激活。在细胞膜超极化期间强内向整流的激活动力反映了时间依赖性而非通道阻滞特性。

1. Kir 通道的阳离子阻滞与内向整流

基于内向整流原始机制的提示，一些实验室开始研究 Kir 通道不同阳离子对离子渗透和整流的作用。Ciani 和 Ribalet[44] 在大鼠胰岛素瘤细胞膜上（RINm5F）研究了 ATP 敏感通道对离子的通透性。Horie 和同事[45] 应用开放的膜片钳构型，研究了豚鼠心室肌细胞 Na^+ 和 Mg^{2+} 对 ATP 敏感 K^+ 通道电压依赖性阻滞作用。从这些研究结果证实 Na^+ 和 Mg^{2+} 参与 ATP 敏感通道的内向整流。

在不同的心脏细胞上也研究了经典内向整流电流的多方面机制特点和细胞内阳离子的作用[46-48]。这些结果为细胞内 Mg^{2+} 对内向整流的作用提供了额外佐证。Matsuda 和同事[46] 应用膜片钳技术，控制细胞内部，记录整个细胞和单通道的外向电流。他们报告静息 K 电导率以欧姆为电位，通道的内向整流为生理浓度的细胞内 Mg^{2+} 所致的电压依赖性阻滞所引起。Vandenberg[47] 的研究也显示豚鼠心室肌细胞的内向整流依赖于细胞内 Mg^{2+}。应用细胞接触式膜片钳，内向整流单通道显示很强的整流作用：在接近 E_k 时电流明显下降，在正电位时测不到电流。因此可得出结论，整流是开放通道被内部 Mg^{2+} 快速阻滞所引起的。在另一个重要的研究中，Oliva 及其合作者[48] 在分离的犬蒲肯野细胞研究了内向整流机制。实验结果提示整流并非仅仅由于电压依赖性 Mg^{2+} 阻滞，或由于电压依赖性内向门控通道所导致。整流假定模型也被提出：随着电压依赖性门控出现，Mg^{2+} 阻塞通道同时发生。

伴随 Kir 通道克隆成功，在卵母细胞或哺乳动物细胞的表达通道上，细胞内 Mg^{2+} 在内向整流中的作用进一步被检验和证实。例如，Lu 和 MacKinnon[49] 在卵母细胞异种表达的 Kir1.1 通道上，检验了 Mg^{2+} 对内向整流的作用（图 13-3）。在细胞膜两侧等摩尔 K^+ 浓度（100mM）下用膜片钳记录电流。Mg^{2+} 引起浓度依赖性经过通道的外向电流阻滞。图 13-3 显示 Mg^{2+} 浓度增加引起外向电流降低，但通道的内向电流没有变化。

2. Kir 通道的多胺阻滞形成"内在"整流

这样内向整流中细胞内 Mg^{2+} 的通道阻滞作用被合理的建立起来。然而，在某些 Kir 通道，甚至在缺乏细胞内 Mg^{2+} 情况下也观察到一致的内向整流现象。而且 Oliva 及其合作者[48] 的工作提示存在额外的"内在"整流机制，它为电压不依赖性（而非细胞内 Mg^{2+} 依赖）。这个迷惑最终被 Lopatin 和合作者[50] 所解开，他们报告强内向整流器的"内在"整流是由于称作多胺（精胺、亚精胺、腐胺和尸胺）的细胞内有机阳离子所引起。他们认为所谓的内在整流是由于多胺引发的电压依赖性通道阻滞所致。与带有两个正电荷的腐胺或 Mg^{2+} 比较，带有四个和三个正电荷的精胺和亚精胺，对通道的阻滞作用更为迅速。

关于多胺（或 Mg^{2+}）诱导内向整流的结构基础，Lu 和 MacKinnon[49] 研究显示，在 Kir 通道第二跨膜节段一个位置的突变可改变 Mg^{2+} 敏感性。突变也可将弱整流通道（Kir1.1）转变为强整流通道（图13-4）。在 Kir2 亚家族成员，证据显示细胞内多胺和 Mg^{2+} 所致的强内向整流，取决于位于第二跨膜区域和羧基末端尾部的三个负电荷残基：D172[51]、E224[52]和 E299[53]（见图13-2）。有趣的是，所有 Kir2 通道亚基均有此三个残基。

3. Kir2 通道亚基的整流区别

与其序列同源相一致，所有 Kir2 通道都有三个重要的参与整流的残基。异源表达研究已证实 Kir2.x 通道总电导率，在正电位到 E_K 过程中强烈内向矫正[17,32,34]。然而本实验室研究出乎意料地显示，全细胞电流整流特性在三个亚基中是不同的[26,37]。使用从 -100 到 $+10 mV$ 的电压，在三个亚基中比较了钡敏感性外向电流轮廓。为比较 Kir2.x 通道外向电流的整流作用，使用了一个方便的术语，整流因子（R），定义为最大外向电流除以最大内向电流。对 Kir2.1 和 Kir2.3 通道，R 没有显著不同（0.61 ± 0.03 [n=6] vs 0.50 ± 0.08 [n=6]）。而 Kir2.2 的整流因子 R（0.37 ± 0.06 [n=6]）与 Kir2.1 和 Kir2.3 通道则显著不同（P=0.05）。还有，在 Kir2.x 亚基 0mV 时的电流明显不同。在电压为 0mV 时，Kir2.1 和 Kir2.2 通道没有外向电流，而 Kir2.3 通道则为最大外向电流的 39%。

这些早期发现的意义重大。例如，在不同的组织给予不同的 Kir2 表达类型。I_{k1} 的特性，特别是 I_{k1} 的整流主要取决于 Kir2 通道亚基的表达。在这种情况下，I_{k1} 依赖的细胞兴奋性和调节特性将取决于特殊 Kir2 通道亚基的表达。

三、总结

Kir 通道的生物物理和调节特性对于心脏电活动至关重要。大量实验证据清晰表明，一些 Kir 亚家族成员其主要分子机制奠定了在宿主心肌细胞内向整流电流的基础。例如，Kir2 亚家族成员主要参与经典内向整流电流。然而，一些重要问题仍没有答案。特别是关于 I_{k1}，是否有重要的辅助/调节蛋白以维持通道的结构完整性？此外，Kir2 亚基的生物物理和调节特性的不同是怎样影响组成 I_{k1} 的同质和异质通道复合物的？毫无疑问，这些问题将是近期研究的焦点。

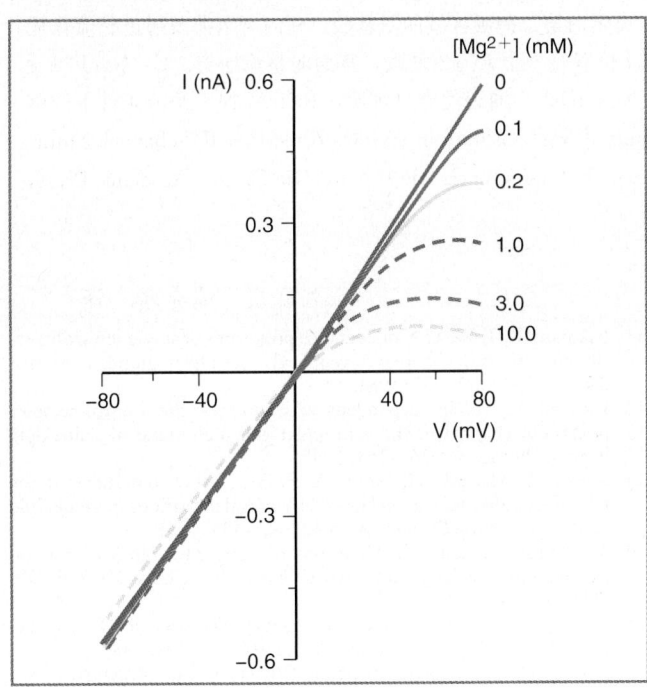

图 13-3 **细胞内 Mg^{2+} 对内向整流电流的影响** 细胞内镁离子引起浓度依赖性 Kir1.1 通道外向电流（而非内向电流）的抑制作用。细胞膜两侧等摩尔浓度（100mM KCl）下记录电流（引自 Lu Z, MacKinnon R: Electrostatic tuning of Mg^{2+} affinity in an inward-rectIfier K^+ channel. Nature 371: 243-246, 1994; and Ashcroft F: inwardly rectIfying K^+ channels. In Ion Channels and Disease. San Diego, Academic Press, 2000, pp 135-159.）

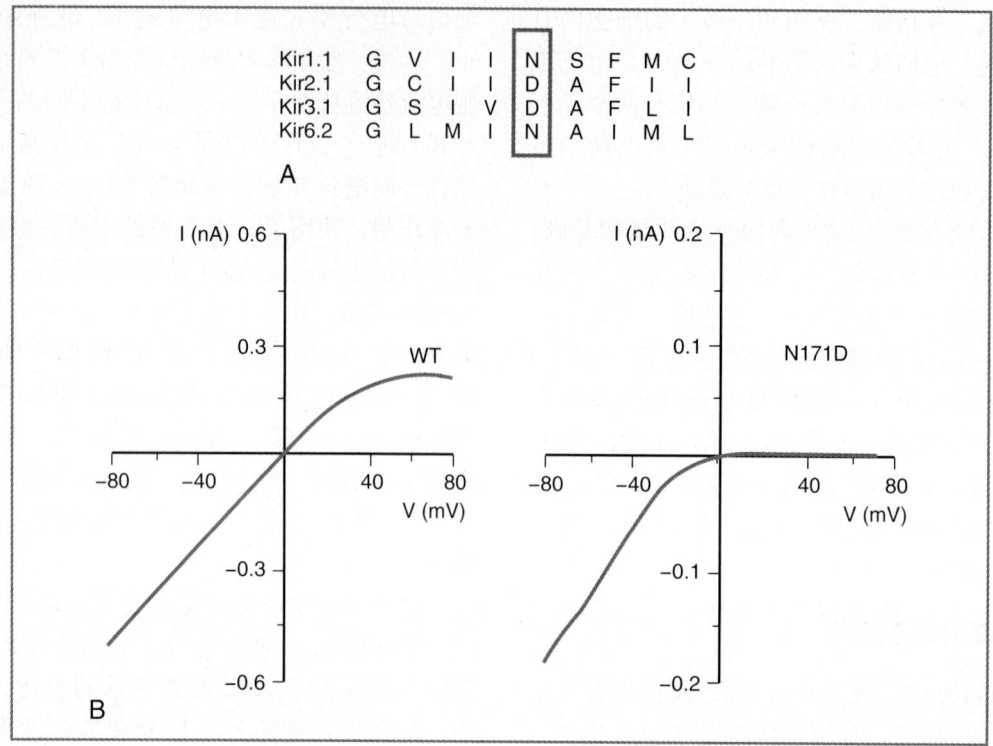

图 13-4 171 残基对 Kir 通道内向整流的作用 A：表上所列 Kir 通道蛋白第二跨膜区域的氨基酸。框内所示涉及通道整流作用的天门冬酰胺（N）/天冬氨酸（D）。B：在野生型 Kir1.1 蛋白，171 位置有一个天门冬酰胺，其为弱整流通道。C：N171 突变为天冬氨酸（D），弱整流通道变化为强整流通道。在表达野生型或突变 Kir1.1 通道的卵母细胞，100mM 钾平衡液条件下细胞膜片钳所记录的电流（引自 Lu Z，MacKinnon R：Electrostatic tuning of Mg^{2+} affinity in an inward-rectIfier K^+ channel. Nature 371：243-246，1994；and Ashcroft F：Inwardly rectIfying K^+ channels. In Ion Channels and Disease. San Diego，Academic Press，2000，pp 135-159.）

（任晓庆　浦介麟　译）

参 考 文 献

1. Lopatin AN, Nichols CG: Inward rectifiers in the heart: An update on I_{K1}. J Mol Cell Cardiol 33:625–638, 2001.
2. Shimoni Y, Clark RB, Giles WR: Role of an inwardly rectifying potassium current in rabbit ventricular action potential. J Physiol 448:709–727, 1992.
3. Hume JR, Uehara A: Ionic basis of the different action potential configurations of single guinea-pig atrial and ventricular myocytes. J Physiol 368:525–544, 1985.
4. Nichols CG, Makhina EN, Pearson WL, et al: Inward rectification and implications for cardiac excitability. Circ Res 78:1–7, 1996.
5. Reimann F, Ashcroft FM: Inwardly rectifying potassium channels. Curr Opin Cell Biol 11:503–508, 1999.
6. Nerbonne JM, Nichols CG, Schwarz TL, Escande D: Genetic manipulation of cardiac K+ channel function in mice: What have we learned, and where do we go from here? Circ Res 89:944–956, 2001.
7. Sakmann B, Noma A, Trautwein W: Acetylcholine activation of single muscarinic K+ channels in isolated pacemaker cells of the mammalian heart. Nature 303(5914):250–253, 1983.
8. Kurachi Y, Nakajima T, Sugimoto T: Acetylcholine activation of K+ channels in cell-free membrane of atrial cells. Am J Physiol 251(3 pt 2):H681–H684, 1986.
9. Ashcroft SJ, Ashcroft FM: Properties and functions of ATP-sensitive K-channels. Cell Signal 2:197–214, 1990.
10. Terzic A, Jahangir A, Kurachi Y: Cardiac ATP-sensitive K+ channels: Regulation by intracellular nucleotides and K+ channel-opening drugs. Am J Physiol 269(3 pt 1):C525–C545, 1995.
11. Sakmann B, Trube G: Conductance properties of single inwardly rectifying potassium channels in ventricular cells from guinea-pig heart. J Physiol 347:641–657, 1984.
12. Kurachi Y: Voltage-dependent activation of the inward-rectifier potassium channel in the ventricular cell membrane of guinea-pig heart. J Physiol 366:365–385, 1985.
13. Shioya T, Matsuda H, Noma A: Fast and slow blockades of the inward-rectifier K+ channel by external divalent cations in guinea-pig cardiac myocytes. Pflugers Arch 422:427–435, 1993.
14. MacKinnon R, Yellen G: Mutations affecting TEA blockade and ion permeation in voltage- activated K+ channels. Science 250:276–279, 1990.
15. Yool AJ, Schwarz TL: Alteration of ionic selectivity of a K+ channel by mutation of the H5 region. Nature 349:700–704, 1991.
16. Doyle DA, Morais CJ, Pfuetzner RA, et al: The structure of the potassium channel: Molecular basis of K+ conduction and selectivity. Science 280:69–77, 1998.
17. Kubo Y, Baldwin TJ, Jan YN, Jan LY: Primary structure and functional expression of a mouse inward rectifier potassium channel. Nature 362:127–133, 1993.
18. Ho K, Nichols CG, Lederer WJ, et al: Cloning and expression of an inwardly rectifying ATP-regulated potassium channel. Nature 362:31–38, 1993.
19. Dascal N, Schreibmayer W, Lim NF, et al: Atrial G protein-activated K+ channel: Expression cloning and molecular properties. Proc Natl Acad Sci U S A 90:10235–10239, 1993.
20. Lesage F, Guillemare E, Fink M, et al: TWIK-1, a ubiquitous human weakly inward rectifying K+ channel with a novel structure. EMBO J 15:1004–1011, 1996.
21. Logothetis DE, Kurachi Y, Galper J, et al: The beta gamma subunits

of GTP-binding proteins activate the muscarinic K⁺ channel in heart. Nature 325:321–326, 1987.
22. Wickman K, Nemec J, Gendler SJ, Clapham DE: Abnormal heart rate regulation in GIRK4 knockout mice. Neuron 20:103–114, 1998.
23. Inagaki N, Gonoi T, Clement JP, et al: Reconstitution of I_{KATP}: An inward rectifier subunit plus the sulfonylurea receptor. Science 270:1166–1170, 1995.
24. Miki T, Nagashima K, Tashiro F, et al: Defective insulin secretion and enhanced insulin action in KATP channel-deficient mice. Proc Natl Acad Sci U S A 95:10402–10406, 1998.
25. Suzuki M, Li RA, Miki T, et al: Functional roles of cardiac and vascular ATP-sensitive potassium channels clarified by Kir6.2-knockout mice. Circ Res 88:570–577, 2001.
26. Dhamoon AS, Bagwe S, Guha P, et al: Differential expression and whole-cell current rectification profiles of guinea pig Kir2.x channels. Biophys J 82(1):587a, 2002.
27. Liu GX, Derst C, Schlichthorl G, et al: Comparison of cloned Kir2 channels with native inward rectifier K⁺ channels from guinea-pig cardiomyocytes. J Physiol 532(pt 1):115–126, 2001.
28. Wang Z, Yue L, White M, et al: Differential distribution of inward rectifier potassium channel transcripts in human atrium versus ventricle. Circulation 98:2422–2428, 1998.
29. Melnyk P, Zhang L, Shrier A, Nattel S: Differential distribution of Kir2.1 and Kir2.3 subunits in canine atrium and ventricle. Am J Physiol Heart Circ Physiol 283:H1123–H1133, 2002.
30. Ishihara K: Time-dependent outward currents through the inward rectifier potassium channel IRK1. The role of weak blocking molecules. J Gen Physiol 109:229–243, 1997.
31. Nehring RB, Wischmeyer E, Doring F, et al: Neuronal inwardly rectifying K(+) channels differentially couple to PDZ proteins of the PSD-95/SAP90 family. J Neurosci 20:156–162, 2000.
32. Takahashi N, Morishige K, Jahangir A, et al: Molecular cloning and functional expression of cDNA encoding a second class of inward rectifier potassium channels in the mouse brain. J Biol Chem 269:23274–23279, 1994.
33. Koyama H, Morishige K, Takahashi N, et al: Molecular cloning, functional expression and localization of a novel inward rectifier potassium channel in the rat brain. FEBS Lett 341(2-3):303–307, 1994.
34. Makhina EN, Kelly AJ, Lopatin AN, et al: Cloning and expression of a novel human brain inward rectifier potassium channel. J Biol Chem 269:20468–20474, 1994.
35. Morishige K, Takahashi N, Jahangir A, et al: Molecular cloning and functional expression of a novel brain-specific inward rectifier potassium channel. FEBS Lett 346(2-3):251–256, 1994.
36. Perier F, Radeke CM, Vandenberg CA: Primary structure and characterization of a small-conductance inwardly rectifying potassium channel from human hippocampus. Proc Natl Acad Sci U S A 91:6240–6244, 1994.
37. Dhamoon AS, Sarmast F, Bagwe S, et al: Differential expression of individual Kir2.x isoforms determines differences in action potential shape and $[K]_o$ dependence if I_{K1} in atrial and ventricular myocytes. PACE 36:956, 2003.
38. Zaritsky JJ, Redell JB, Tempel BL, Schwarz TL: The consequences of disrupting cardiac inwardly rectifying K K⁺ current (I_{K1}) as revealed by the targeted deletion of the murine Kir2.1 and Kir2.2 genes. J Physiol 533(pt 3):697–710, 2001.
39. Tinker A, Jan YN, Jan LY: Regions responsible for the assembly of inwardly rectifying potassium channels. Cell 87:857–868, 1996.
40. Cohen NA, Sha Q, Makhina EN, et al: Inhibition of an inward rectifier potassium channel (Kir2.3) by G-protein betagamma subunits. J Biol Chem 271:32301–32305, 1996.
41. Fink M, Duprat F, Heurteaux C, et al: Dominant negative chimeras provide evidence for homo and heteromultimeric assembly of inward rectifier K⁺ channel proteins via their N-terminal end. FEBS Lett 378:64–68, 1996.
42. Preisig-Muller R, Schlichthorl G, Goerge T, et al: Heteromerization of Kir2.x potassium channels contributes to the phenotype of Andersen's syndrome. Proc Natl Acad Sci U S A 99:7774–7779, 2002.
43. Fakler B, Brandle U, Bond C, et al: A structural determinant of differential sensitivity of cloned inward rectifier K⁺ channels to intracellular spermine. FEBS Lett 356(2-3):199–203, 1994.
44. Ciani S, Ribalet B: Ion permeation and rectification in ATP-sensitive channels from insulin-secreting cells (RINm5F): Effects of K⁺, Na⁺ and Mg²⁺. J Membr Biol 103:171–180, 1988.
45. Horie M, Irisawa H, Noma A: Voltage-dependent magnesium block of adenosine-triphosphate-sensitive potassium channel in guinea-pig ventricular cells. J Physiol 387:251–272, 1987.
46. Matsuda H, Saigusa A, Irisawa H: Ohmic conductance through the inwardly rectifying K channel and blocking by internal Mg²⁺. Nature 325:156–159, 1987.
47. Vandenberg CA: Inward rectification of a potassium channel in cardiac ventricular cells depends on internal magnesium ions. Proc Natl Acad Sci U S A 84:2560–2564, 1987.
48. Oliva C, Cohen IS, Pennefather P: The mechanism of rectification of I_{K1} in canine Purkinje myocytes. J Gen Physiol 96:299–318, 1990.
49. Lu Z, MacKinnon R: Electrostatic tuning of Mg²⁺ affinity in an inward-rectifier K⁺ channel. Nature 371:243–246, 1994.
50. Lopatin AN, Makhina EN, Nichols CG: Potassium channel block by cytoplasmic polyamines as the mechanism of intrinsic rectification. Nature 372:366–369, 1994.
51. Stanfield PR, Davies NW, Shelton PA, et al: A single aspartate residue is involved in both intrinsic gating and blockage by Mg²⁺ of the inward rectifier, IRK1. J Physiol 478(pt 1):1–6, 1994.
52. Yang J, Jan YN, Jan LY: Control of rectification and permeation by residues in two distinct domains in an inward rectifier K⁺ channel. Neuron 14:1047–1054, 1995.
53. Kubo Y, Murata Y: Control of rectification and permeation by two distinct sites after the second transmembrane region in Kir2.1 K⁺ channel. J Physiol 531(pt 3):645–660, 2001.

第 14 章

同源和异源缝隙连接通道

Alonso P. Moreno, *Volodya Hayrapetyan*, *Guoqiang Zhong*,
Agustin D. Martinez, *Eric C. Beyer*

本章目录
- 心血管连接蛋白的多样性 ……… 118
- 细胞间联系的调节 ……… 119
- 异源寡聚缝隙连接通道 ……… 119
- 体内异源多聚离子通道的研究 ……… 119
- 连接蛋白共表达形成异源多聚离子通道的体外研究 ……… 120
- 总结 ……… 123

自从首先发现了心肌细胞间直接的联系，我们才直观的认识到心肌细胞间需要有高水平的细胞间联系来保持动作电位在整个心脏中恰当的传播。这种心肌细胞间直接的联系是建立在细胞间通道的基础之上，包括在质膜上特异性的缝隙连接结构。缝隙连接通道是由两个六聚体的半通道（连接子）构成。这些半通道是由一个或多个同源亚单位的连接蛋白家族成员组成。心脏的连接蛋白包括：连接蛋白 43（Cx43），连接蛋白 40（Cx40），连接蛋白 45（Cx45）。在血管上发现了另一个连接蛋白 37（Cx37）。在心血管细胞上可能还存在其他的连接蛋白，但是没有发表的确实数据。

连接蛋白数量或表达类型的改变能改变细胞间耦联的水平。但是直到最近，由连接蛋白表达改变引起的心脏缝隙连接传导的改变才在心血管领域受到了一点注意。测量显示心肌细胞间的传导非常高（代表了成百上千的缝隙连接通道），但是也提示电流的运动不能被限制在通道中通过，而且电流传导的速度和各向异性不可能充分的改变[1]。

但是来自对动物模型和人体组织研究的证据证明，在一些病理情况下连接蛋白的表达可以到非常低的水平。与其他一些去耦联的因素一起，可能引起室性心动过速或其他的心律失常。有多个报告显示，连接蛋白表达的改变作为重塑过程的一部分，与心脏的各种病理有关。由于 Cx43 在心肌细胞中的优势，因而它是研究最广泛的连接蛋白。从人体组织研究显示，Cx43 表达下降与严重的心肌病有关系[2,3]。Kitamura 及同事[4] 研究了一系列 31 个扩张性心肌病的患者，发现室性心动过速的发展与 Cx43 的表达以及缝隙连接斑的异源分配之间有关联。连接蛋白数量和分配的改变可能和慢性心律失常的发生有关：发现在房颤模型中有 Cx40 的分布[5]。

对转基因和基因敲除的小鼠的研究证实，需要表达合适水平的连接蛋白来维持心脏细胞间足够的联系。通过同源重组破坏 Cx40 和 Cx43 基因，分别使其在希氏束和心室中不表达，可以引起严重的传导异常[6-9]。定向去除 Cx43 的小鼠与野生型小鼠相比，显示有显著的传导减慢，在缺血时自发性室性心动过速的发生率增加[10]。

一、心血管连接蛋白的多样性

通过免疫组织化学研究，心脏连接蛋白的分布和表达显示出独特的模式。大量的不同，包括空间的分布，缝隙连接的大小，构成了心肌不同区域不同的传导特性，和传导系的各个部分。Cx43 基本是存在于心房和心室的工作心肌细胞（也在末梢的传导系统）[11]。在一些血管内皮尤其是有湍流的位置，也有 Cx43[12]。Cx40 存在于心房和传导系统[6,17,11]。Cx40 在心室发育的早期表达然后降低[13]。Cx40 是在体内表达最为广泛的心内膜连接蛋白[13]，但在将细胞培养时 Cx40 表达很快消失。Cx40 在一些血管平滑肌细胞表达[14]。在高血压和房颤的动物模型，Cx40 的表达增加[15,16]。在心脏的各个部分 Cx45 表达数量都相当低[11]，Cx45 的分布可能对定义传导系统的发育是重要的[17]，Cx45 也在血管平滑肌表达，可能对正常血管的生成是非常重要的[18]。在胚胎心脏发育的过程中，Cx45 的表达下降，在许多血管 Cx37 是内膜缝隙连接的重要成分[19]，但是它在心脏不表达。

在成熟的哺乳动物心脏特定的传导区域，也可能发现连接蛋白的异源和区域不平衡共表达，一些报告指出，连接蛋白在窦房结和界嵴之间的表达有清楚的分界。在窦房结的中心区域，主要是表达 Cx40 和 Cx43，在移行区共表达 Cx43 和 Cx45。这一区域紧靠界嵴，主要是表达 Cx43。连接蛋白的不同表达可能有助于限制心肌细胞间的联系，从而抑制心房肌细胞超极化侵入窦房结区，同时也保持细胞间足够的联系使得起搏兴奋的传播。

在许多心血管组织有多种连接蛋白的共表达，尽管表达一种连接蛋白就足以形成缝隙连接在细胞间联系，大多数细胞表达两种或以上的连接蛋白。当 Cx37，Cx40，Cx43，Cx45 在同一种细胞表达，通过双标记的荧光激光共聚焦显微镜或免疫电子显微镜显示，它们共同定位于同一分布区域[19,21]。连接蛋白共表达和形成异源的混合半通道，很可能是调节心血管细胞间联系的主要机制。

不同连接蛋白序列，形成的通道可能有不同的门控特性，或者对不同的分子和离子有通透性。连接蛋白特异的通道特性，可以通过转染细胞或卵母细胞表达连接蛋白来阐明。每一种连接蛋白构成的通道有不同的电导，Cx45 是 26pS 而人类 Cx37 大到 300pS[22]。缝隙连接通道对一定大小范围的第二信使和代谢物质有选择性。比较显微注射的荧光染料在细胞间传递显示，特定连接蛋白组成的通道对分子的通透性不同[22,23]。溶质的大小和电荷显示出对缝隙连接通道速率的影响，连接蛋白表达的不同引起对大分子选择通透性的不同，可以变化 10 倍或更多[24]。

二、细胞间联系的调节

改变连接蛋白的表达并不是唯一的调节细胞间联系的方法。其他的方法，如激活各种细胞中的信号通路也可以有效的改变缝隙连接的传导。大多数的连接蛋白都是磷酸化蛋白，调节蛋白激酶的活性可以改变缝隙连接的电导（通过改变通道开放的几率或通道募集）[25]。例如，激活蛋白激酶 C（通过佛波醇酯），继而使 Cx43 磷酸化，降低单元电导的分布[26]。缝隙连接也对细胞内低 pH 敏感（就像在急性缺血时引起的 pH 下降），引起通道关闭[27]。生物化学和形态学的研究也显示了，在缺血发生的 1 小时里，Cx43 去磷酸化，含有 Cx43 的缝隙连接丢失或重组[28,29]。质膜酸化时缝隙连接传导下降。Stergiopoulos 及其同事[29a]已经展示了不同连接蛋白对 pH 依赖性的不同。不同连接蛋白产生的缝隙连接的电导显示出对跨连接电压不同的依赖性。V_j（通常是电压依赖性的失活）可以用不同的 Boltzmann 方程的参数来描述。

三、异源寡聚缝隙连接通道

因为有大量的证据指出有多种连接蛋白在同一个细胞和连接共表达，所以就有可能在体内形成异源通道。缝隙连接的联系可能不仅被由一种连接蛋白构成的通道的通透性或门控来控制，也可能受到通道中多个不同亚单相位互作用的调节。

传统的缝隙连接模型显示，确定的通道由一种连接蛋白同源聚合形成（图 14-1A）。但是多种连接蛋白在同一细胞共表达将导致两种异源表达的缝隙连接：通道由两种不同的同源半通道形成（图 14-1B），或在每一个半通道中有两种连接蛋白（图 14-1 C）。由表达两种连接蛋白的细胞对来形成异源通道，将导致大量的通道多样性（因为可能有 196 种不同的缝隙连接通道组成形式）[30]。

四、体内异源多聚离子通道的研究

（一）生化分析

虽然免疫电子显微镜研究发现在同一细胞上有多种连接蛋白表达，但它们并不能在一个通道内混合出现。迄今，还没有生化研究总结心脏组织异源聚合离

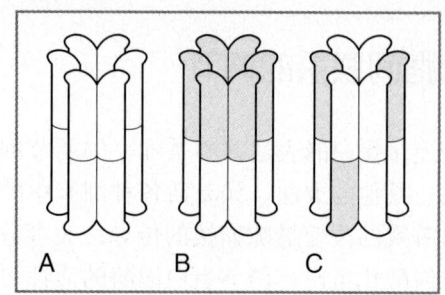

图 14-1 表达两种不同连接蛋白的细胞上连接蛋白的组合
A：只表达一种相同的连接蛋白的细胞配对形成同型通道，它由两个同源聚合半通道构成。B：表达不同连接蛋白的细胞配对形成一个异型通道，它由两个同源聚合半通道构成。C：两种连接蛋白共表达的细胞配对形成一个通道，它由异源聚合半通道构成

子通道的构成（大量不可溶的收缩蛋白的存在使缝隙连接的分离非常复杂，所以这方面的实验很困难）。然而，生化资料已用于根据亲和质谱的免疫共沉淀或共分离研究，以证明在晶状体和心脏等几种组织内同一半通道上存在联合表达的连接蛋白[31-33]。有可能这些结果被外推到心血管组织。

（二）在体电生理分析

尽管心肌细胞缝隙连接离子通道的记录和分析复杂难懂，但不断有大量文章对体内心血管细胞上存在功能性的异源多聚离子通道提供可靠的证据。在犬的心室肌细胞和内皮细胞上，多项整体传导性的记录表明 Cx43 和 Cx45 的联合表达诱导异源多聚离子通道的形成。

五、连接蛋白共表达形成异源多聚离子通道的体外研究

阐述心脏连接蛋白相互作用的另一种方法是用共表达连接蛋白的细胞系或构建连接蛋白能被导入和控制的细胞系，包括注射连接蛋白 RNA 的蟾蜍卵母细胞以及内源性表达一种或多种心脏连接蛋白和转染多种连接蛋白基因的培养细胞株[35-37]。对分别表达 Cx37、Cx40、Cx43 和 Cx45 的离子通道及其门控特性已进行了更广泛的研究，获得了有关各种连接子的门控和通透性特征。每种连接子的特点是不同的，它们在蟾蜍卵母细胞或哺乳动物细胞表达系统大量存在。Cx40 和 Cx43 共表达的一个例外是：蟾蜍卵母细胞表达研究发现 Cx40 和 Cx43 对构成异源通道是不相容的，但在稳定转染的肿瘤细胞上却存在功能性的 Cx40-Cx43 异源通道[36]。

（一）连接蛋白共表达的生化分析

许多试验方法用于研究连接蛋白的共表达。已构建了 Cx43 与其他心血管连接蛋白（Cx37、Cx40 或 Cx45）的任一种共表达的稳定转染细胞[30,38-40]。双标记免疫荧光显示在所有情况下，连接蛋白转运到附加膜上（如缝隙连接一样），并有确切相同的分布位置，表明共表达的细胞上缝隙连接包括两者连接蛋白。

共表达的心脏连接蛋白发生寡聚反应需要半通道（连接子）预先溶解，可从 100 000g 溶解在 1% 中性去污剂的细胞裂解液的上清中获得。溶解的连接子在 5%～25% 蔗糖梯度中的沉降速度能确定共表达的 Cx40 和 Cx43 的寡聚化[39]，还可通过 SDS 聚丙烯酰胺凝胶电泳和免疫印迹的化学交联确定[39]。他及同事[38]用共免疫沉淀方法发现了 Cx40 和 Cx43 的共寡聚化。亲和力纯化策略也已被用于研究异源聚合体的形成；Cx40 或 Cx45 被导入携有 Cx43 及羧基端 $(His)_6$ 顺序的 Hela-Cx43 $(His)_6$ 细胞[39,40]，$(His)_6$ 标签用于分离连接子。Triton X-100 上清液加入 Ni^{2+}-NTA 亲和层析柱对 $(His)_6$ 有很高的亲和力，因此能结合带此种标签的连接蛋白及相关蛋白，启动材料和柱成分通过免疫印迹分析。共表达的连接蛋白与 Cx43 $(His)_6$ 被洗脱，对照实验可确定共表达连接蛋白的相关特异性。

（二）共表达连接蛋白的电生理分析

异源配对

表达单一连接蛋白的稳定转染细胞进行配对用于研究 Cx43-Cx37、Cx43-Cx340 和 Cx43-Cx45 异源结合的特征[30,36,41]。所有的结合能形成功能性的异源通道，显示了非对称的 V_j-依赖性的门控特性。一些 V_j-依赖性的门控能被已知的连接蛋白半通道的特征解释；另外一些异源结合显示了新的特征，表明连接子的对接影响了它们的特性。例如，在除极冲动中，Cx43 连接子（Cx43-Cx45 细胞配对上）的失活与同源 Cx43 通道相比动力学明显减慢[41]。Cx32 的类似研究表明跨连接电压的门控作用可能只是由连接子上的一个连接蛋白引起[42]。异源配对上观察到的单通道事件在只表达一种连接蛋白的细胞上（同源聚合的/同型的通道）并没有观察到。

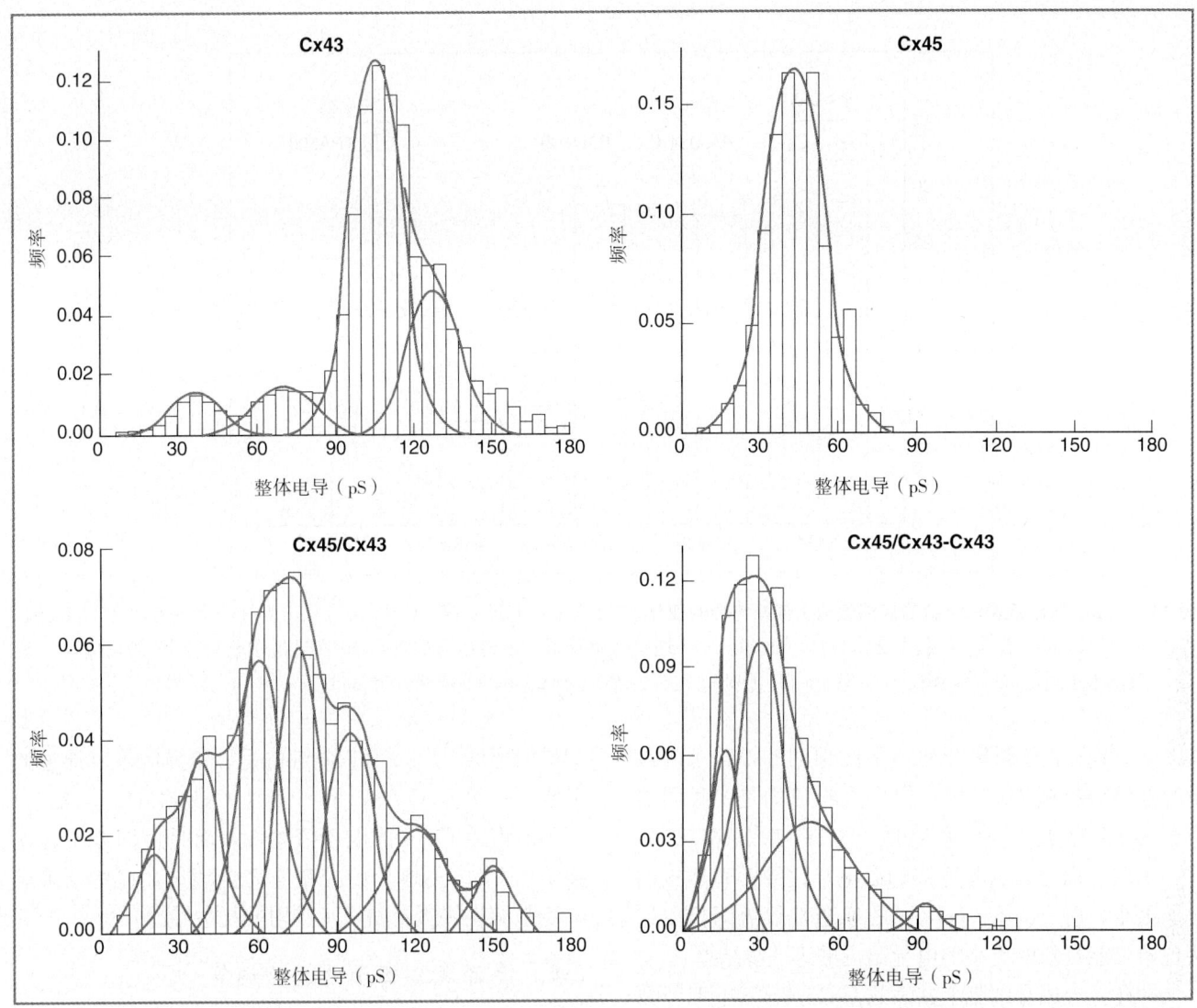

图 14-2 由连接蛋白 43（Cx43）和连接蛋白 45（Cx45）形成的同源聚合和异源聚合通道的整体电导分布　直方图代表了跨缝隙电压脉冲从 ±30～±60mV 时观察到的跃迁频率分布。Cx43 同源聚合通道（左上）有最大的电导 123pS，跃迁为 35、70、100pS。Cx45 同型通道的分布表明在 40pS 有一个峰。当表达 Cx45 和 Cx43 的细胞配对时，这些双异源聚合通道的分布有多个峰，主要在 60pS。单异源性通道（一个细胞表达 Cx45 和 Cx43，另一个细胞只表达 Cx43）的细胞配对时，电导分布显著降低，少于 40pS

（三）共表达（异源聚合）连接蛋白的结合

对于共表达连接蛋白的一些结合（Cx43-Cx37、Cx43-Cx45）来说，整体通道事件被测定[30,40]。许多现象与包含同源聚合半通道的细胞上所观察到的不同。许多传导事件与在随机组合的 192 个不同的异源聚合体上所预测的结果相一致。然而，当 Cx43 和 Cx40 共表达时，许多连接蛋白的异源结合是没功能的。没有观察到超出纯的同源型和异源型通道之间范围的更大或更小的通道。

连接的电导

我们最近观察到由 Cx43-Cx43/45 构成的单异源聚合通道的整体电导降低，在此，配对的细胞一个只表达 Cx43，另一个表达 Cx43 和 Cx45（Mono-43）。当 Cx43 和 Cx45 都表达时，配对的整体电导非常高或与同源型的通道同样高。但我们当前的结果表明单异源聚合 Cx43 通道的总的电导不符合预测的各电导之和，即假设整个通道的电导是由每种亚单位呈一定比例形成的。最糟糕的方案是，一个细胞表达 Cx43（同源聚合连接子），另一个细胞只表达 Cx45（很低的

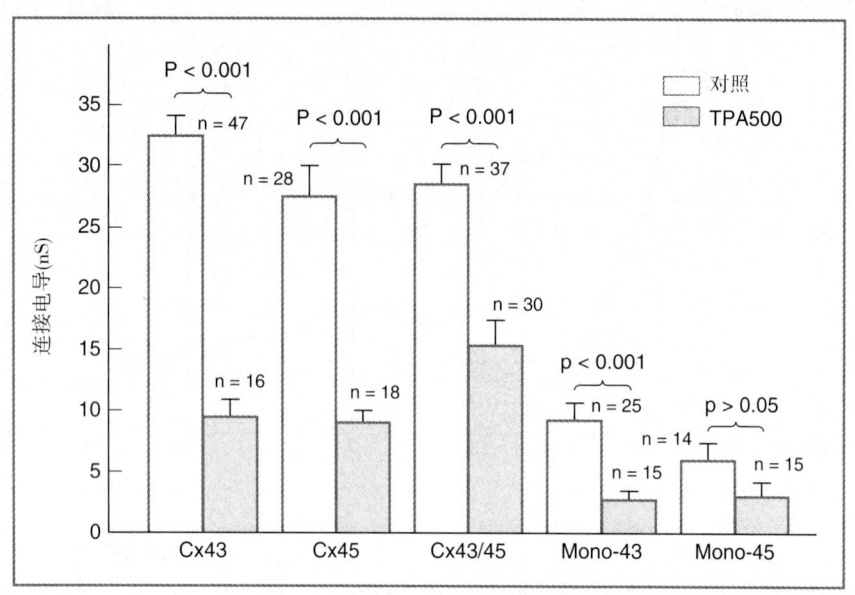

图 14-3 由不同连接蛋白结合形成的通道上连接电导的变化 Cx45 来自鸡的克隆，Cx43 来自鼠。所有的连接蛋白在 HeLa 细胞表达。Cx43 同型通道在细胞上通讯最好，而 Mono-45 通道通讯降低。值得注意的是 Cx45 通过失耦联对 TPA 的反应与 van Veen 及同事报道的 mCx45 相反[47]。Mono-43，Cx43-Cx45/Cx43；Mono-45，Cx45-Cx45/Cx43

Cx43），如在单异源聚合通道上所预测的，记录的最小的电导应接近 60pS[41]，但令人吃惊的是，我们的记录显示存在多种通道电导，一些低至 25pS（图 14-2），而且，这些连接的总电导比异源型连接的电导更小，对 Lucifer yellow 的通透性显著降低。这些现象可能是新的更小的电导出现的进一步结果。

同样，当成骨细胞上共表达 Cx43 和 Cx45 时，数据显示 Lucifer yellow 的通透性降低，再一次表明新形成的通道或是有更大的选择性或是孔径更小。异源聚合连接子可能有更小的孔，它们的选择性主要由 Cx45 的存在决定，我们的资料表明这些通道甚至比双异源聚合通道的选择性更大。

Cx43 和 Cx45 在心肌组织联合表达似乎是非随机分布的，如在窦房结，连接蛋白的表达有一定的区域性。这样，在正常组织可能存在边缘带（或与病变心肌表达下调的连接子相隔）为功能性的单异源聚合通道的存在提供适当的条件，有利于正常的或病理性的传导。

呈异源聚合构型的配对连接子诱导形成离子通道，其电压依赖性门控特性难以预测。我们最近发现 Cx43 和 Cx45 异源聚合通道的相互作用破坏了 Cx43 连接子的快速门控，这一现象的可能解释是当 Cx45 与 Cx43 相接后，负责快速门控的羧基端尾被破坏，如先前所示，当 Cx43 尾被去除时，快速门控将发生相似的降低[44]。令我们吃惊的是，单异源聚合通道的形成（一侧是 Cx43，另一侧是 Cx43/Cx45 共表达）并不能恢复 Cx43 的电压依赖性，而是使同源聚合连接子上 Cx43 的电压门控效应完全消失，这些结果进一步强调连接蛋白间相互作用的复杂性。

（四）异源聚合离子通道的调节

对心脏同型缝隙连接通讯的调节已进行了很多研究，或是在表达连接蛋白的肿瘤细胞上，或是在直接分离的心肌细胞上。一致显示蛋白激酶 C 被激活后（丝氨酸 368 起重要作用）[46]，Cx43 通道的总电导下降。蛋白激酶 C 对 Cx45 的门控似乎依赖于连接蛋白的物种。当鼠的同种型在 HeLa 细胞上表达时[47]，连接的电导增加，但对于鸡的 Cx45（cCx45），g_j 是降低的（图 14-3）。在这些实验中，结果显示对于 Cx43 和 chCx45，12-o-十四烷酰佛波醋酸酯-13（TPA）能降低连接的电导。根据我们的资料，对于异源聚合的连接，连接蛋白对磷酸化的门控作用变得不敏感（图 14-3）。

细胞内 pH 值的改变发生的门控作用是另一种类型的门控，受连接蛋白相互作用的强力影响。最近在卵母细胞上进行的研究清楚地表明当一个细胞既表达 Cx40 又表达 Cx43 时（pHa 7.0），这两种不同的连接蛋白对 pH 值（pHa～6.7）门控的敏感性不同，它们对细胞内的酸化作用变得不敏感，这些结果实质上表明连接蛋白的共表达能做为防止缺血失耦联的调节防御机制。

六、总结

心脏有多种不同的连接蛋白表达，有助于形成缝隙连接通道，这些通道对于心肌细胞间的电流和信号分子的通过非常重要。各种连接蛋白形成的通道具有不同的传导和调节特性，而且，它们之间能混合形成异源寡聚离子通道。在不同的心脏病理情况下，连接蛋白的表达发生改变，这将引起通过各种各样的心血管缝隙连接通道的细胞间通讯发生重大改变。

（浦介麟　李　宁　马克娟　译）

参 考 文 献

1. Jongsma HJ, Wilders R: Gap junctions in cardiovascular disease. Circ Res 86:1193–1197, 2000.
2. Dupont E, Matsushita T, Kaba RA, et al: Altered connexin expression in human congestive heart failure. J Mol Cell Cardiol 33:359–371, 2001.
3. Kaprielian RR, Gunning M, Dupont E, et al: Downregulation of immunodetectable connexin43 and decreased gap junction size in the pathogenesis of chronic hibernation in the human left ventricle. Circulation 97:651–660, 1998.
4. Kitamura H, Ohnishi Y, Yoshida A, et al: Heterogenous loss of connexin43 protein in nonishcemic dilated cardiomyopathy with ventricular tachycardia. J Cardiovasc Electrophys 13:865–870, 2002.
5. van der Velden HM, van Kempen MJ, Wijffels MC, et al: Altered pattern of connexin40 distribution in persistent atrial fibrillation in the goat. J Cardiovasc Electrophysiol 9:596–607, 1998.
6. Simon AM, Goodenough DA, Paul DL: Mice lacking connexin40 have cardiac conduction abnormalities characteristic of atrioventricular block and bundle branch block. Curr Biol 8:295–298, 1998.
7. van Rijen HV, van Veen TA, van Kempen MJ, et al: Impaired conduction in the bundle branches of mouse hearts lacking the gap junction protein connexin40. Circulation 103:1591–1598, 2001.
8. Kirchhoff S, Nelles E, Hagendorff A, et al: Reduced cardiac conduction velocity and predisposition to arrhythmias in connexin40-deficient mice. Curr Biol 8:299–302, 1998.
9. Gutstein DE, Morley GE, Tamaddon H, et al: Conduction slowing and sudden arrhythmic death in mice with cardiac-restricted inactivation of connexin43. Circ Res 88:333–339, 2001.
10. Lerner DL, Yamada KA, Schuessler RB, Saffitz JE: Accelerated onset and increased incidence of ventricular arrhythmias induced by ischemia in Cx43-deficient mice. Circulation 101:547–552, 2000.
11. Davis LM, Rodefeld ME, Green K, et al: Gap junction protein phenotypes of the human heart and conduction system. J Cardiovasc Electrophysiol 6:813–822, 1995.
12. Gabriels JE, Paul DL: Connexin43 is highly localized to sites of disturbed flow in rat aortic endothelium but connexin37 and connexin40 are more uniformly distributed. Circ Res 83:636–643, 1998.
13. Van Kempen KM, Vermeulen JL, Moorman AF, et al: Developmental changes of connexin40 and connexin43 mRNA distribution patterns in the rat heart. Cardiovasc Res 32:886–900, 1996.
14. Little TL, Beyer EC, Duling BR: Connexin43 and connexin40 gap junction proteins are present in arteriolar smooth muscle and endothelium in vivo. Am J Physiol 268:H729–H739, 1995.
15. Dupont E, Ko Y, Rothery S, et al: The gap-junctional protein connexin40 is elevated in patients susceptible to postoperative atrial fibrillation. Circulation 103:842–849, 2001.
16. Polontchouk L, Haefliger JA, Ebelt B, et al: Effects of chronic atrial fibrillation on gap junction distribution in human and rat atria. J Am Coll Cardiol 38:883–891, 2001.
17. Coppen SR, Severs NJ, Gourdie RG: Connexin45 (alpha6) expression delineates an extended conduction system in the embryonic and mature rodent heart. Dev Genet 24:82–90, 1999.
18. Kruger O, Plum A, Kim J, et al: Defective vascular development in connexin 45-deficient mice. Development 127:4179–4193, 2000.
19. Yeh HI, Rothery S, Dupont E, et al: Individual gap junction plaques contain multiple connexins in arterial endothelium. Circ Res 83:1248–1263, 1998.
20. Coppen SR, Kodama I, Boyett MR, et al: Connexin45, a major connexin of the rabbit sinoatrial node, is co-expressed with connexin43 in a restricted zone at the nodal-crista terminalis border. J Histochem Cytochem 47:907–918, 1999.
21. Kwong KF, Schuessler RB, Green KG, et al: Differential expression of gap junction proteins in the canine sinus node. Circ Res 82:604–612, 1998.
22. Veenstra RD, Wang HZ, Beblo DA, et al: Selectivity of connexin-specific gap junctions does not correlate with channel conductance. Circ Res 77:1156–1165, 1995.
23. Elfgang C, Eckert R, Lichtenberg-Frate H, et al: Specific permeability and selective formation of gap junction channels in connexin-transfected HeLa cells. J Cell Biol 129:805–817, 1995.
24. Valiunas V, Beyer EC, Brink PR: Cardiac gap junction channels show quantitative differences in selectivity. Circ Res 91:104–111, 2002.
25. Brink PR: Are gap junction channels a therapeutic target and if so what properties are best exploited? Curr Drug Targets 3:417–425, 2002.
26. Kwak BR, Hermans MM, De Jonge HR, et al: Differential regulation of distinct types of gap junction channels by similar phosphorylating conditions. Mol Biol Cell 6:1707–1719, 1995.
27. Morley GE, Taffet SM, Delmar M: Intramolecular interactions mediate pH regulation of connexin43 channels. Biophys J 70:1294–1302, 1995.
28. Beardslee MA, Lerner DL, Tadros PN, et al: Dephosphorylation and intracellular redistribution of ventricular connexin43 during electrical uncoupling induced by ischemia. Circ Res 87:656–662, 2002.
29. Huang XD, Sandusky GE, Zipes DP: Heterogeneous loss of connexin43 protein in ischemic dog hearts. J Cardiovasc Electrophysiol 10:79–91, 1999.
29a. Stergiopoulis K, Alvarado JL, Mastroianni M, et al: Hetero-domain interactions as a mechanism for the regulation of connexin channels. Circ Res 84:1144–1155, 1999.
30. Brink PR, Cronin K, Banach K, et al: Evidence for heteromeric gap junction channels formed from rat connexin43 and human connexin37. Am J Physiol 273:C1386–C1396, 1997.
31. Jiang JX, Goodenough DA: Heteromeric connexons in lens gap junction channels. Proc Natl Acad Sci U S A 93:1287–1291, 1996.
32. Bevans CG, Kordel M, Rhee SK, Harris AL: Isoform composition of connexin channels determines selectivity among second messengers and uncharged molecules. J Biol Chem 273:2808–2816, 1998.
33. Berthoud VM, Montegna EA, Atal N, et al: Heteromeric connexons formed by the lens connexins, connexin43 and connexin56. Eur J Cell Biol 80:11–19, 2001.
34. Elenes S, Rubart M, Moreno AP: Junctional communication between isolated pairs of canine atrial cells is mediated by homogeneous and heterogeneous gap junction channels. J Cardiovasc Electrophys 10:990–1004, 1999.
35. Moreno AP, Laing JG, Beyer EC, Spray DC: Properties of gap junction channels formed of connexin 45 endogenously expressed in human hepatoma (SKHep1) cells. Am J Physiol 268:C356–C365, 1995.
36. Valiunas V, Weingart R, Brink PR: Formation of heterotypic gap junction channels by connexins 40 and 43. Circ Res 86:E42–E49, 2000.
37. Barrio LC, Capel J, Jarillo JA, et al: Species-specific voltage-gating properties of connexin-45 junctions expressed in Xenopus oocytes. Biophys J 73:757–769, 1997.
38. He DS, Jiang JX, Taffet SM, Burt JM: Formation of heteromeric gap junction channels by connexins 40 and 43 in vascular smooth muscle cells. Proc Natl Acad Sci U S A 96:6495–6500, 1999.
39. Valiunas V, Gemel J, Brink PR, Beyer EC: Gap junction channels formed by coexpressed connexin40 and connexin43. Am J Physiol Heart Circ Physiol 281:H1675–H1689, 2001.

40. Martinez AD, Hayrapetyan V, Moreno AP, Beyer EC: Connexin43 and connexin45 form heteromeric gap junction channels in which individual components determine permeability and regulation. Circ Res 90:1100–1107, 2002.
41. Elenes S, Martinez AD, Beyer EC, Moreno AP: Heterotypic docking of Cx43 and Cx45 connexons blocks fast voltage gating of Cx43. Biophys J 81:1406–1418, 2001.
42. Oh S, Abrams CK, Verselis VK, Bargiello TA: Stoichiometry of transjunctional voltage-gating polarity reversal by a negative charge substitution in the amino terminus of a Cx32 chimera. J Gen Physiol 116:13–31, 2000.
43. Koval M, Geist ST, Westphale EM, et al: Transfected connexin45 alters gap junction permeability in cells expressing endogenous connexin43. J Cell Biol 130:987–995, 1995.
44. Moreno AP, Chanson M, Anumonwo J, et al: Role of the carboxyl terminal of connexin43 in transjunctional fast voltage gating. Circ Res 90:450–457, 2002.
45. Kwak BR, Saez JC, Wilders R, et al: Effects of cGMP-dependent phosphorylation on rat and human connexin43 gap junction channels. Pflugers Arch 430:770–778, 1995.
46. Lampe PD, TenBroek EM, Burt JM, et al: Phosphorylation of connexin43 on serine368 by protein kinase C regulates gap junctional communication. J Cell Biol 149:1503–1512, 2000.
47. van Veen TA, van Rijen HV, Jongsma HJ: Electrical conductance of mouse connexin45 gap junction channels is modulated by phosphorylation. Cardiovasc Res 46:496–510, 2000.
48. Gu H, Ek-Vitorin JF, Taffet SM, Delmar M: Coexpression of connexins 40 and 43 enhances the pH sensitivity of gap junctions: A model for synergistic interactions among connexins. Circ Res 86:E98–E103, 2000.

第三部分
心脏离子通道的分子间作用和药理学

第 15 章

心脏钠通道药理学

Jonathan C. Makielski, Bin Ye, Timothy J. Kamp, Craig T. January

本章目录

- 抑制 I_{Na} 的作用 ……………………… 125
- 抗心律失常药物的分类 ………………… 126
- 使用依赖性阻滞的分子机制 …………… 127
- 药物相互作用点的分子生物学 ………… 128
- 心脏钠离子通道本质上对抗心律失常药更加敏感吗 …………………… 128
- 延迟钠电流的阻滞 ……………………… 129
- 药物对通道转运的影响——新的抗心律失常药物作用 ………………… 129
- 钠离子通道阻滞药物的特异性 ………… 129

心脏钠离子通道是由 SCN5A 基因[1]编码的产物（Na$_V$1.5），作为 α 亚单位，联合 β 亚单位共同构成，主要存在于心脏，部分在脑和胃肠道系统，它只是编码其他组织中结构相似的电压依赖性钠通道基因家族中的一种，除此还有骨骼肌（Na$_V$1.4）和脑（Na$_V$1.1）组织的钠离子通道[2]。α 亚单位自身具备了通道的主要特征，例如 Na$^+$ 选择性、电压依赖性激活和失活，并具有多数药物和毒素的所有结合位点，然而，各种钠通道的药理学和毒理学特性并不一样。例如，心脏钠通道经典的功能是对河豚毒素的阻断作用相对不敏感。而由不同基因编码的 β 亚单位影响着通道的动力学和药理学特性。

通过钠通道的离子流（I_{Na}）决定着心房肌、浦肯野纤维和心室肌的兴奋性和传导性。钠的内流还调节着细胞内的钠和通过钠-钙交换泵调节细胞内钙，以及心肌的收缩力。钠通道的电压和时间依赖性调节能使通道在除极到阈电位（约 -70mV）以上在 1ms 内快速激活和开放，触发兴奋和传导。接着，该通道呈电压依赖性失活，电流通常在几毫秒内降低至峰值的 1% 以下，但仍有少量的电流伴随着持续的钙电流形成动作电位的平台期。复极后，钠通道一般从失活态快速恢复（10ms 内），准备再次开放。因此，钠通道阻滞剂通过抑制 I_{Na} 峰值来降低兴奋性和传导性，也可阻滞延迟钠电流以缩短动作电位时程，而增强延迟钠电流的药物和毒素可延长动作电位和不应期。

一、抑制 I_{Na} 的作用

尽管许多毒素和一些药物有增强 I_{Na} 作用，但抗心律失常药是降低 I_{Na} 的。这种抑制或阻滞作用分为两种类型：电张力性阻滞（tonic block）和使用依赖性阻滞（use-dependent block）。电张力性阻滞是延长的静息期或少量除极后在单次除极期间发生的阻断，使用依赖性阻滞是由更高频率的除极产生的。例如利多卡因阻断 I_{Na} 峰电流，电压钳记录到两种类型的阻滞（图 15-1）。在对照 I_{Na} 曲线记录后，应用利多卡因，并进行一系列除极电压钳记录。第一次除极引起的电流降低是电张力性阻断，经常被叫做第一次脉冲阻断，随着追加除极，发生了另一种阻断，如第 50 个除极记录的曲线所示，这种阻断叫做使用依赖性阻断，也叫额外阻断、频率依赖性阻断、电压依赖性阻断、状态依赖性阻断，以及还有一些命名强调这种阻断的其他特性或根据推测的分子机制[3]。使用依赖性阻断对抗心律失常作用非常重要，因为在快速型心律失常时心率越快，作用效果越显著，因此，使用依赖性阻断发生和恢复的方式对理解药物临

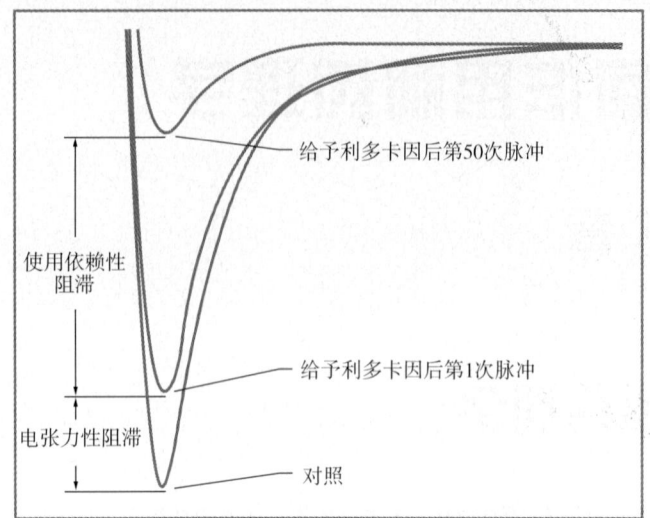

图 15-1 利多卡因阻滞的钠电流图 显示一系列脉冲中用药后第 1 次和第 50 次除极记录的 I_{Na} 和对照 I_{Na}。钳制电位 140mV；除极阶跃是 20mV

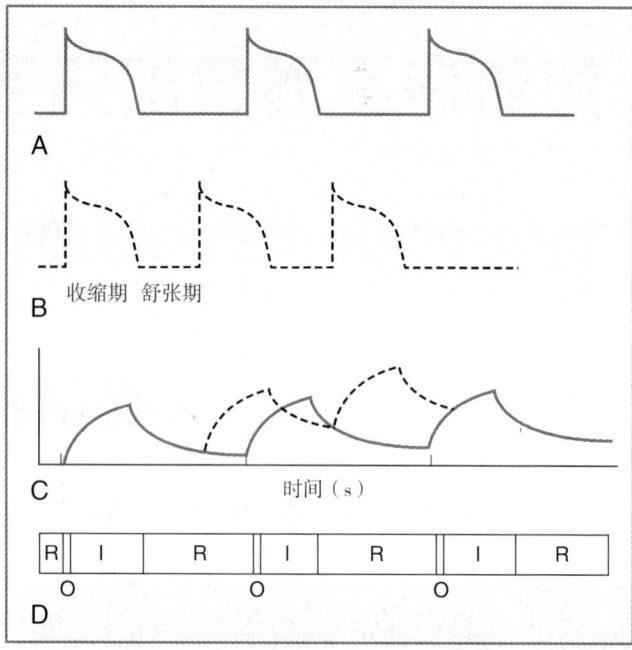

图 15-2 I_{Na} 的使用依赖性阻滞 A 和 B：两种频率下心室的动作电位。C：频率对使用依赖性阻滞的影响。除极时产生阻滞，复极时缓解。频率越快，阻滞积累越大。D：与 A 对应的通道状态模型

床特征很关键，这种阻断的基本的分子机制也很重要，但非常复杂。

使用依赖性阻滞之所以发生是因为阻断在除极时（电收缩）产生，复极后（电舒张）消失。图 15-2 显示在慢频率（图 15-2A）和快频率（图 15-2B）时三种心脏动作电位。除极时（图 15-2C）阻断呈指数形式发生，复极呈指数形式恢复。如果在下一次除极时阻断没有完全恢复，那么新的阻断将在比前一循环更高的水平上发生，从而阻断发生积累（图 15-2C 实线）。图 15-2B 显示在快频率时，由于药物阻断恢复的时间很短，第二次和第三次动作电位发生的阻断作用从更高的水平开始（图 15-2B）。另外，发生阻断的数量依赖于除极的频率，但也略微依赖于药物阻断特性的恢复，即快速恢复的药物比缓慢恢复的药物在下一次除极产生的阻断要少。而且，还要认识到恢复速率依赖于膜电压这样的参数，且通常有一些临床事件，如膜除极、缺血和酸中毒会减慢恢复，对于抗心律失常药非常重要，因此，抗心律失常药在疾病状态下可能存在更大的通道阻滞作用。阶段性离子通道阻滞学说没有对根本的分子机制做任何假设，本书的先前版本对这一过程作了大量描述，这在 Starmer 和 Grant[5] 的受体防卫假说中更为详细。关于使用依赖性阻滞的分子机制仍有争论，因为解释实验数据必须依赖模型，经常是同一数据使用不同的模型因而有不同的解释。有关 Na 通道[1] 药物阻断的许多讨论要从一种特殊模型来着手，如下面讨论的调节-受体模型，但须强调的是理解抗心律失常药物阻断作用的关键特征可以不参考这些模型。

二、抗心律失常药物的分类

Vaughan Williams 推荐了一种抗心律失常药物的分类方法，经过多年的调整和考验仍延用并被广泛采用。Ⅰ类药物（表 15-1）最初描述为是降低心脏动作电位超射速度、减慢传导速度的药物，发现其作用机制是 Na 电流阻滞作用。Harrison[6] 根据它们对心电图的影响、传导减慢以及动作电位时程进一步分为ⅠA 类、ⅠB 类、ⅠC 类。Campbell[7] 用动作电位超射速度实验显示使用依赖性阻断发生的动力学决定了分类，并能解释对 QRS 间期的影响。CAST（Cardiac Arrhythmia Suppression Trial）试验[8] 强调了这种分类的临床重要性，研究发现ⅠC 类药物发生阻断的动力学最慢，能增加心梗后伴少许心室异位起搏点患者的死亡率。在 Vaughan Williams 的分类中，把延长动作电位时程和 QT 间期的药物归属于Ⅲ类，这些药物一般阻断钾离子通道，在ⅠA 类药物中如奎尼丁也有钾通道阻滞作用，这是动作电位和 QT 间期延长最可能的机制。为什么伴中度使用依赖性的药物倾向于Ⅲ类药物的效应还不清楚。

表 15-1　HARRISON/CAMPBELL 调整的 VAUGHN WILLIAMS 分类

分类	药物	ECG 影响	Harrison	Campbell	依赖的状态
IA	奎尼丁 普鲁卡因胺 丙吡胺	延长 QT 间期	减慢传导 延长 APD	中度使用依赖性动力学	开放态
IB	利多卡因 美西律 托卡尼 胺碘酮	几乎无影响	在生理情况下对 传导和 APD 无影响	快速使用依赖性动力学	失活态
IC	氟卡胺 普罗帕酮	延长 QRS 间期	显著减慢传导	缓慢使用依赖性动力学	开放态

ECG, 心电图；ADP, 动作电位

三、使用依赖性阻滞的分子机制

使用依赖性的基本模型是由 Hille[9] 为研究神经组织以及 Hondeghem 和 Katzung[10] 为研究心脏组织作为受体调节模型而独立推导的（图 15-3）。这一模型假设药物对通道的亲和力是根据通道的动力学状态而不同。在心脏循环期间，Na 通道经历至少 3 种不同状态（见图 15-2D），在静息电位时，通道处于关闭或静息态和预开放态（R），除极时，通道变为开放态（O），转运离子，产生离子流。随着除极，通道逐渐变为失活态（I），不转运离子，但一直维持到膜复极，此时通道恢复为预开放态。如果某种药物对开放和/或失活态通道的亲和力大于静息态，那么该药物将在收缩期结合至通道，舒张期与通道分离。在受体调节模型上，确定药物易与开放态还是失活态（或两者）通道相互作用很有意义。其中，一些药物显示出随着一步步除极，与之俱增的结合时间被延长，这表明药物易与失活态结合，因为除极时维持着这一状态。另外一些药物不依赖于除极时程，被认为与通道开放态相互作用，因为瞬时开放态的持续时间不依赖于除极间期，当然，其他的解释是可能的。Na 通道动力学并不像三种状态模型这么简单。通道的确在进入开放过程中经历几种"预开放"瞬时态，药物能优先与这些状态结合，或药物与通道很快发生相互作用，在很短的除极过程中达到平衡，除极延长，作用消失。Na 通道门控体系也包括大量慢的和中等程度的失活态。快或慢失活态的分类可能对临床工作有用，因为一般情况下，开放态通道阻滞药物倾向于充正电荷，恢复动力学比失活态阻断剂慢（见图 15-1）。与静息态的相互作用将产生电紧张性阻断，在此我们不讨论这种情况，因为电紧张性阻断不是抗心律失常药物治疗剂量下的特征，但却是局部麻醉药的普遍特征。

受体防卫模型[11]是另一种解释使用依赖性阻断更为简单的模型。它推测受体亲和力是固定的，但随着通道状态的改变，受体的俘获和防卫功能产生了有差别的结合，从而在亲和力上存在明显不同。如同对这些假设模型所作的研究一样，则描述这种阻断和表现其特征的数学回归关系式的发展是很有价值的工作。此外，没有必要与受体调节假说相互排斥，更好的是可以相互补偿。然而，受体防卫模型自身也许不能解释所有的实验数据，如改变药物结合通道的门控[12]，这主要应用受体调节模型。

另一种普遍而没有被阐述的药物阻断模型假说是药物结合的通道被"填塞"，不能转运。也可能是药物结合有利于关闭状态。事实上，Khodorov 和同事[13]最初就指出 Na 通道的药物阻断是失活态的"稳定态"，后来有研究者在这一概念上不断变化来解释药物的作用[14]。另一种可能是药物降低了单通道的电导，但在很少发生这种情况的例子中，进一步的研究表明这是一种"闪烁式阻断"，通道快速开放和关闭，滤波时只是降低了电导。

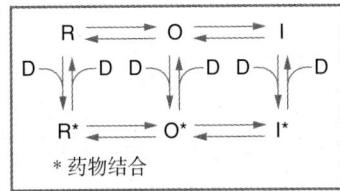

图 15-3　受体调节模型　这一模型假设药物对通道的亲和力因通道的动力学状态不同而不同。药物结合和不结合之间其通道的动力学状态能一由系列速度常数构成的模型表示

四、药物相互作用点的分子生物学

早先的研究间接地表明 Na 通道上存在药物相互作用位点,不仅药物可以与之作用,而且渗透的离子也可以进入,因为膜不通透的药物只能从内侧作用,而外部的 Na 能与药物相互竞争从外侧作用[15]。Na$_V$1.5 和其他 Na 通道序列的测定和克隆能通过改变假设的作用位点,表达携带突变的通道,来验证这一观点。心脏的 Na 通道有 4 个同源结构域(Ⅰ~Ⅳ),每个结构域有 6 个跨膜区(S1~S6),和 1 个 S5 和 S6 间的 "P" 区,如图 15-4 所示。特异性点突变最先指出了Ⅳ区 S6 在药物结合中的作用[16],后来的证据也表明了其他结构域 S6 的作用[17,18],Ⅲ和Ⅳ区间的连接子显示参与了通道的失活,并影响药物的相互作用[19],进一步研究发现Ⅲ和Ⅳ区间的连接子可能直接参与了位点的相互作用[20]而不是通过改变失活而起作用。Ⅰ[21]和Ⅲ[22]孔区结构也参与了抗心律失常药物的结合。Ⅲ区的 S4 和 S5 间的连接部参与了通道的失活[23],近来的证据表明心脏 Na 通道所有结构域的 S4 和 S5 间连接部对利多卡因的药物作用非常重要[24]。图 15-4 标出了药物作用位点的结构,画圈的是最强的作用点。值得注意的是这些位点同时也是参与失活的结构。失活的电压依赖性影响药物的阻断,失活的负向漂移将增加已显现的阻断,而正向的漂移则降低阻断,因此,改变失活的突变可能会被错误地解释为结合位点的直接效应,区分两者非常困难,但是当失活未被漂移或失活向阻断效应相反的方向漂移时,那么该突变可被认为在药物作用位点上。

β$_1$ 亚单位也影响利多卡因对通道的阻断作用[25]。β$_2$ 和 β$_3$ 亚单位的作用还不清楚。

五、心脏钠离子通道本质上对抗心律失常药更加敏感吗

虽然普遍使用的Ⅰ类抗心律失常药有神经毒性,但它们有相对的心脏选择性,药物和毒素对心脏 Na 通道与对其他电压依赖性 Na 通道家族成员在亲和力上的根本差异是否能解释这种临床选择性呢?事实上,心脏 Na 通道在药理学上被描述为"河豚毒素抵抗型" Na 通道,因为 Na$_V$1.5 对河豚毒的亲和力强度低于 Na 通道家族其他成员。对于临床上有效的抗心律失常药,如利多卡因,一旦失活动力学的差别被解释[26],那么对 Na 通道家族不同成员亲和力的差异就有了依据,有表明Ⅳ区 S6 上特异的氨基酸决定着这种差异[27]。然而,激活动力学效应也可以起作用[28]。在心脏,离子通道的重要区别是对外部非渗透药物的阻断作用有易感性,开始认为是在一个次要的药物结合位点上[29],后来表明在Ⅰ区 P 段和Ⅳ区 S6 段,心脏的氨基酸残基与脑的不同,从而使药物能渗透到通道内部位点[21]。

这些差异具有生物物理学意义,但实际上,药物在患者体内产生的效应是由组织和细胞的差异决定的,如心脏较长的动作电位效应、不同的静息电位和心率,而不是通道亲和力的根本差别。例如,上面提到的,由于维持着(失活)状态连接,利多卡因的作用效应随除极的延长而增加,因为心室的动作电位比心房组织长,因此利多卡因对心室的作用比对心房的强,而神经和肌肉组织的动作电位更短,因此药效更小。近来报道了心脏 Na 通道结构的不均一性,包括广泛的遗传多态性和普遍存在的剪接变异体[30],但在药理学上可能存在的差异还没有相关叙述。

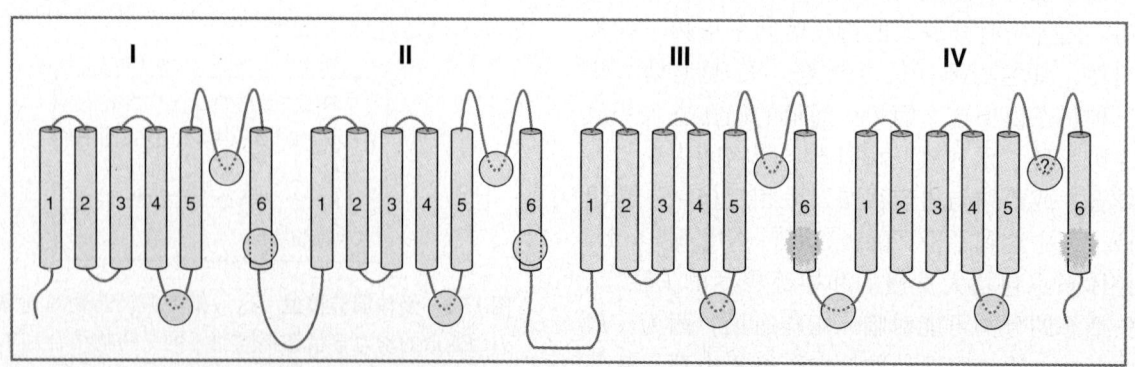

图 15-4 Na 通道蛋白结构和抗心律失常药相互作用靶点的分子模型 Ⅲ和Ⅳ识别区域 S6 位点的深色阴影区表示最强药物相互作用靶点;浅色阴影区也是药物与 Na 通道相互作用的靶点

六、延迟钠电流的阻滞

在长的除极期间存在着一个小的（<1%峰值）I_{Na}，许多年前发现这种延迟 I_{Na} 能被河豚毒素阻断，缩短动作电位时程[31]。延迟 I_{Na} 可能是动作电位延长以及遗传性（50 章）和获得性长 QT 综合征（LQT3）[32]的原因。LQT3 患者（ΔKPQ突变），用氟卡尼治疗，作用于延迟 I_{Na}，确实引起 QT 间期缩短[33]。对于 ΔKPQ 突变，使用氟卡尼治疗产生的对延迟 I_{Na} 的使用依赖性阻滞强于对 I_{Na} 峰电流的作用，这种阻断作用与野生型通道上的作用相比恢复得慢[34]。这些发现使我们认清氟卡尼阻断延迟 I_{Na} 的机制，在细胞和分子水平提出了开放通道阻滞的原理，这是治疗 LQT3 有效的药理学特性。然而，临床上对此方法应加以慎重，因为延迟 I_{Na} 降低的 Brugada 综合征与一些 LQT3 病例重叠发生，Brugada 综合征患者其延迟 I_{Na} 的进一步降低有潜在的危害。

七、药物对通道转运的影响——新的抗心律失常药物作用

哺乳动物细胞内离子通道蛋白翻译后的转运存在药物和温度依赖性调节（改善或"挽救"），对囊性纤维化病变的氯离子通道[35]和 HERG 钾离子通道已有相关研究报道[36]。对 Na 通道研究发现，美西律能升高鼠心肌上 Na 通道的信使 RNA[37]，美西律还能挽救 M1766L 突变引起的 Na 通道转运缺陷[38]，这是一个普遍效应，对于 Brugada 综合征的 G1743R 突变，药物也能挽救蛋白质的表达[39]。尽管研究还不成熟，但药物诱导的离子通道蛋白的转录后调节和挽救翻译后的生成及转运有潜力成为人类心脏疾病抗心律失常治疗的新方法。

八、钠离子通道阻滞药物的特异性

临床上大多数相关的 Na 通道药物缺乏对 Na 通道完全的选择性。Na 通道阻滞药物或 I 类药物（见表 15-1）经常被认为对 Na 通道的阻滞是它们体内治疗量的主要作用方式，但是许多药物也阻断其他通道和受体。已提出了 I A 类药物对钾离子通道有阻断作用，许多 Na 通道阻滞剂也能抑制钙离子通道（主要是 L 型），如普罗帕酮这样的药物还可作为 β-肾上腺素能受体阻断剂。胺碘酮经常被认为主要是 III 类抗心律失常药，却能显著影响 Na 通道，也阻断钙通道、钾通道和 β-肾上腺素能受体，细胞水平上还影响甲状腺活动。因此在评估 Na 通道阻滞剂的临床作用时必须也要考虑对其他通道和受体的影响。

（浦介麟　赵新然　滕思勇　译）

参 考 文 献

1. Goldin AL: Evolution of voltage-gated Na+ channels. J Exp Biol 205:575–584, 2002.
2. Maier SK, Westenbroek RE, Schenkman KA, et al: An unexpected role for brain-type sodium channels in coupling of cell surface depolarization to contraction in the heart. Proc Natl Acad Sci U S A 99:4073–4078, 2002.
3. Courtney KR: Mechanism of frequency-dependent inhibition of sodium currents in frog myelinated nerve by the lidocaine derivative GEA. J Pharmacol Exp Ther 195:225–236, 1975.
4. Campbell TJ, Wyse KR, Hemsworth PD: Effects of hyperkalemia, acidosis, and hypoxia on the depression of maximum rate of depolarization by class I antiarrhythmic drugs in guinea pig myocardium: differential actions of class Ib and Ic agents. J Cardiovasc Pharmacol 18:51–59, 1991.
5. Starmer CF, Grant AO: Phasic ion channel blockade. A kinetic model and parameter estimation procedure. Mol Pharmacol 28:348–356, 1985.
6. Harrison DC: Symposium on the perspectives on treatment of ventricular arrhythmias: Introduction. Am J Cardiol 52:1C–2C, 1983.
7. Campbell TJ: Subclassification of class I antiarrhythmic drugs: Enhanced relevance after CAST. Cardiovasc Drugs Ther 6:519–528, 1992.
8. The Cardiac Arrhythmia Suppression Trial (CAST) Investigators: Preliminary report: Effect of encainide and flecainide on mortality in a randomized trial of arrhythmia suppression after myocardial infarction. N Engl J Med 321:406–412, 1989.
9. Hille B: Local anesthetics: Hydrophilic and hydrophobic pathways for the drug-receptor reaction. J Gen Physiol 69:497–515, 1977.
10. Hondeghem LM, Katzung BG: Time- and voltage-dependent interactions of antiarrhythmic drugs with cardiac sodium channels. Biochim Biophys Acta 472:373–398, 1977.
11. Starmer CF, Grant AO, Strauss HC: Mechanisms of use-dependent block of sodium channels in excitable membranes by local anesthetics. Biophys J 46:15–27, 1984.
12. Hanck DA, Makielski JC, Sheets MF: Lidocaine alters activation gating of cardiac Na channels. Pflugers Arch 439:814–821, 2000.
13. Khodorov BI, Shishkova E, Peganov E, Revenko S: Inhibition of sodium currents in frog Ranvier node treated with local anesthetics. Role of slow sodium inactivation. Biochim Biophys Acta 433:409–435, 1976.
14. Balser JR, Nuss HB, Orias DW, et al: Local anesthetics as effectors of allosteric gating. Lidocaine effects on inactivation-deficient rat skeletal muscle Na channels. J Clin Invest 98:2874–2886, 1996.
15. Strichartz GR: The inhibition of sodium currents in myelinated nerve by quaternary derivatives of lidocaine. J Gen Physiol 62:37–57, 1973.
16. Ragsdale DS, Mcphee JC, Scheuer T, Catterall WA: Molecular determinants of state-dependent block of Na+ channels by local anesthetics. Science 265:1724–1728, 1994.
17. Yarov-Yarovoy V, Brown J, Sharp EM, et al: Molecular determinants of voltage-dependent gating and binding of pore-blocking drugs in transmembrane segment IIIS6 of the Na+ channel α subunit. J Biol Chem 276:20–27, 2001.
18. Yarov-Yarovoy V, Mcphee JC, Idsvoog D, et al: Role of amino acid residues in transmembrane segments IS6 and IIS6 of the Na+ channel α subunit in voltage-dependent gating and drug block. J Biol Chem 277:35393–35401, 2002.
19. Bennett PB, Valenzuela C, Chen LQ, Kallen RG: On the molecular nature of the lidocaine receptor of cardiac Na+ channels. Modification of block by alterations in the alpha-subunit III-IV interdomain. Circ Res 77:592, 1995.

20. Fan Z, George ALJ, Kyle JW, Makielski JC: Two human paramyotonia congenita mutations have opposite effects on lidocaine block of Na$^+$ channels expressed in a mammalian cell line. J Physiol 496:275-286, 1996.
21. Sunami A, Glaaser IW, Fozzard HA: A critical residue for isoform difference in tetrodotoxin affinity is a molecular determinant of the external access path for local anesthetics in the cardiac sodium channel. Proc Natl Acad Sci U S A 97:2326-2331, 2000.
22. Sunami A, Dudley SC Jr, Fozzard HA: Sodium channel selectivity filter regulates antiarrhythmic drug binding. Proc Natl Acad Sci U S A 94:14126-14131, 1997.
23. Smith MR, Goldin AL: Interaction between the sodium channel inactivation linker and domain III S4-S5. Biophys J 73:1885-1895, 1997.
24. Ye B: Structure-Function of the Cardiac Sodium Channel (SCN5A/Na$_V$1.5)—The Common Background Sequence and the Effects of Naturally Occurring (Pathogenic and Non-Pathogenic). and Designed Mutations [thesis]. Madison, University of Wisconsin, 2002.
25. Makielski JC, Limberis JT, Chang SY, et al: Coexpression of β1 with cardiac sodium channel α subunits in oocytes decreases lidocaine block. Mol Pharmacol 49:30-39, 1996.
26. Makielski JC, Limberis J, Fan Z, et al: Intrinsic lidocaine affinity for Na channels expressed in *Xenopus* oocytes depends on α (hH1 vs. rSkM1) and β1 subunits. Cardiovasc Res 42:503-509, 1999.
27. Weiser T, Qu Y, Catterall WA, Scheuer T: Differential interaction of R-mexiletine with the local anesthetic receptor site on brain and heart sodium channel alpha-subunits. Mol Pharmacol 56:1238-1244, 1999.
28. Nuss HB, Kambouris NG, Marban E, et al: Isoform-specific lidocaine block of sodium channels explained by differences in gating. Biophys J 78:200-210, 2000.
29. Alpert LA, Fozzard HA, Hanck DA, Makielski JC: Is there a second external lidocaine binding site on mammalian cardiac cells? Am J Physiol 257:H79-H84, 1989.
30. Ye B, Valdivia CR, Ackerman MJ, Makielski JC: A common human SCN5A polymorphism modifies expression of an arrhythmia causing mutation. Physiol Genomics 12:187-193, 2003.
31. Dudel J, Peper K, Rudel R, Trautwein W: Effect of tetrodotoxin on membrane currents in mammalian cardiac fibres. Nature 213:296-297, 1967.
32. Undrovinas AI, Maltsev VA, Sabbah HN: Repolarization abnormalities in cardiomyocytes of dogs with chronic heart failure: role of sustained inward current. Cell Mol Life Sci 55:494-505, 1999.
33. Windle JR, Geletka RC, Moss AJ, et al: Normalization of ventricular repolarization with flecainide in long QT syndrome patients with SCN5A:DeltaKPQ mutation. Ann Noninvasive Electrocardiol 6:153-158, 2001.
34. Nagatomo T, January CT, Makielski JC: Preferential block of late sodium current in the LQT3 DKPQ mutant by the class IC. Antiarrhythmic flecainide. Mol Pharmacol 200057:101-107, 2000.
35. Denning GM, Anderson MP, Amara JF, et al: Processing of mutant cystic fibrosis transmembrane conductance regulator is temperature-sensitive. Nature 358:761-764, 1992.
36. Zhou Z, Gong Q, January CT: Correction of defective protein trafficking of a mutant HERG potassium channel in human long QT syndrome. Pharmacological and temperature effects. J Biol Chem 274:31123-31126, 1999.
37. Duff HJ, Offord J, West J, Catterall WA: Class I and IV antiarrhythmic drugs and cytosolic calcium regulate mRNA encoding the sodium channel alpha subunit in rat cardiac muscle. Mol Pharmacol 42:570-574, 1992.
38. Valdivia CR, Ackerman MJ, Tester DA, et al: A novel SCN5A arrhythmia mutation, M1766L, with expression defect rescued by mexiletine. Cardiovasc Res 54:624-629, 2002.
39. Valdivia CR, Tester DA, Makielski JC, Ackerman MJ: Clinical, molecular, and functional characterization of a SCN5A Brugada syndrome mutation with expression defect rescued by mexiletine. Circulation 106:II-283, 2002.

第 16 章

心脏 L 型和 T 型钙电流的药理学

Xiongwen Chen, *Steven R. Houser*

本章目录

- L 型钙通道的结构与功能 131
- L 型钙通道的药物调节 132
- L 型钙通道的蛋白激酶和磷酸化调节 ... 136
- 心脏 T 型钙通道的药理学 138

心脏动作电位（AP）期间钙内流是一个重要的过程，因为钙内流使肌浆网（SR）内钙离子（Ca^{2+}）释放并因此使细胞浆 Ca^{2+} 增加以激发收缩。目前在心脏发现有两种电压依赖性钙通道，其中 L-型（长时间开放）钙通道（LTCC），是心脏细胞主要的钙通道，也是本章讨论的主要内容；关于 T-型（短暂开放）钙通道（TTCC）的功能特点知之甚少。

LTCC 存在于每个心肌细胞，并且这种钙通道的 Ca^{2+} 内流具有许多重要功能。在窦房结细胞，LTCC 的离子流（I_{Ca-L}）促进起搏的激活并且是 AP 超射期的主要电流。I_{Ca-L} 也是房室结（AV）细胞 AP 的超射期的电流，并且是该部位传导速度的决定因素。在心房、心室及希-浦纤维心肌细胞，钠电流是 AP 快速超射期的电流，在这些细胞，I_{Ca-L} 的缓慢激活主要与 AP 平台期的形成相关。

I_{Ca-L} 作为一种信使分子具有重要作用，它在兴奋-收缩耦联中发挥重要功能，LTCC 的 Ca^{2+} 内流对引发和调节 Ca^{2+} 从 SR 释放非常重要，并且是 Ca^{2+} 装载在 SR 的主要来源[45]。I_{Ca-L} 电流幅值是决定心搏周期长短的重要决定因素。如果 LTCC 的主要作用为激发心脏跳动、调节房室结 AP 的传导、AP 平台期的时程及心脏收缩性，那么对这些通道的功能进行调节将显著地影响心功能。

对心肌细胞的 TTCC 的功能作用知之甚少（见第 2 章）。已明确这种通道比 LTCC 少很多，而且并不是所有的成年心脏的心肌细胞都表达 TTCCs。这种通道的一个有趣的特点是受发育的调节。在婴儿或新生儿的心脏，多数心肌细胞具有功能性 TTCC，但是在成年心脏，通过 TTCC 的电流（I_{Ca-T}）通常不存在于心室肌细胞，但是可以在窦房结、房室结、浦肯野纤维和心房中发现。在这些细胞，I_{Ca-T} 常被认为与起搏电流和传导有关。此外，I_{Ca-T} 在肥厚心室肌中存在[4]，提示 TTCC 在肥厚心肌生成过程中重新表达，并且 I_{Ca-T} 可能具有重要的信号功能，这些想法相对地极少有人进行研究，在此不再进一步讨论。

一、L 型钙通道的结构与功能

（一）结构

第 2 章中对这些题目已进行了详细的描述，这里只讨论适当的内容以理解药物影响及改变 LTCC 结构的信号途径，后面将做讨论。心脏 LTCC 由 4 个亚基组成：α1、β、α2 及 δ。α1 亚基是组成孔隙的亚基，分子量约为 230kD；在 1989 年首先进行了克隆[5]，它的分子结构已清楚地阐明，通道的不同部分的功能作用也已进行了详细的研究[6,7]。LTCC 是一种具有 4 个（I～IV）相同结构域的较大膜蛋白，每个结构域有 6 个（从 1～6）跨膜片段。这种分子在膜内进行组合形成 Ca^{2+} 选择性孔隙，每个结构域的 S5 和 S6 段排列着通道孔隙。每个结构域的 S4 片段包括带电荷的氨基酸，该氨基酸被认为参与了通道的电压敏感性功能，分子的 NH_3 基和-COOH 尾端都在细胞内侧面并且对调节通道功能具有重要作用。

$α_1$ 亚基可以独立地调节 I_{Ca-L} 而不需要其他亚基的参与，但是有证据表明 LTCC 辅助亚基可调节 α 亚基的活动。β 亚基是一种小分子（51～71kD）蛋白质，没有跨膜结构域，这种胞浆内蛋白质影响了 LTCC 的活动，并且也似乎作为一种分子伴侣指引 α 亚基位于细胞膜表面的合适的部位。$α_2$ 和 δ 亚基来源于同一基因产物，经过不同的转录后剪接形成。这两种蛋白质通过二硫键彼此连接。δ 亚基具有跨膜片段锚定细胞外的 $α_2$ 亚基于细胞膜。$α_2$ 亚基与 $α_1$ 亚基相互作用影响其生物物理学特性（I_{Ca-L} 的激活时间）。

（二）功能

LTCC 的 Ca^{2+} 电流包括电压和 Ca^{2+} 依赖的通道结构的转换引起孔隙结构的 $α_1$ 亚基短暂地允许 Ca^{2+} 渗透入心肌细胞内。正常的静息电位为 -80mV，多数的 LTCC 处于关闭的可激活状态（随除极而开放），除极促使结构状态改变，使 $α_1$ 亚基孔隙开放，Ca^{2+} 顺电化学梯度移入细胞，其与许多其他电压敏感性离子通道相似，除极也可导致 LTCC 通道失活，所以通道的开放时间很短暂。LTCC 的失活比许多其他电压调节的离子通道失活要复杂，因为其同时具有电压和 Ca^{2+} 依赖性成分。LTCC 失活的 Ca^{2+} 依赖成分使大的 Ca^{2+} 电流的失活速率比 Ca^{2+} 电流小者的失活速率更快，这可能抑制 Ca^{2+} 超载。每个 AP 时，Ca^{2+} 在 LTCC 通道从关闭态变转为开放态时内流并且最终失活。药物和信号瀑布通过改变 LTCC 状态的转换影响 I_{Ca-L}。整个细胞的 I_{Ca-L} 的大小在任何条件下决定于将要开放的几率（P_o）与时间（t）、可开放的通道数量（N）及单通道的电流幅值（i）：$I_{Ca-L} = N(t) \times i \times P_o(t)$。

二、L 型钙通道的药物调节

（一）L 型钙通道的激动剂和拮抗剂

近来有 3 种重要而结构不同的化学药物被临床应用以改变 LTCC 的活动（二氢吡啶 [DHPs]、苯丙磺酸类 [PAAs] 及硫氮䓬类 [BTZs]）（如图 16-1）。普通的 DHP 衍生物包括阿莫地平、azidoping、Bay K8644、cGP28392、FRC-8653、H-16051、iodipine、硝苯地平、尼莫地平、nisodipine、尼群地平、PN200-110、S-202-791 及 YC-170。绝大多数二氢吡啶类药物是 LTCC 拮抗剂，是阻滞 L 型 Ca^{2+} 电流的。而（-）Bayk8644、CGP28392、FRC8653、H-160-51、（+）-S-202-791 和 YC-170 可以增强 LTCC，并且因此被称为 LTCC 激动剂。所有 PAAs 和 BTZs 为 LTCC 拮抗剂。PAAs 包括维拉帕米、D600、D888 及 D890。BTZs 有少数几个衍生物，最常用的为地尔硫䓬（DLT），这些 LTCC 激动剂和/或拮抗剂在 LTCCs 有特定的结合位点，通过应用膜-非渗透性、药物带的电荷、影像亲和标记和分子生物学技术产生缺失突变或嵌合的通道来确定这些特定结合位点，这些研究使 LTCC 通道的结构和功能研究有了很大进展[10]。

（二）药物结合部位

三类 LTCC 激动剂和拮抗剂的作用机制可以解释为经典的配体-受体模型。这一理论假设是，带电的或非带电的药物得以接近特异性结合位点，这些位点位于水溶性区域（细胞内或外面或孔隙内部）或溶解于膜的脂质区域，结合于 LTCC 的 $α_1$ 亚基的药物现在已经得以确定，由于这种与 $α_1$ 亚基的结合使得 AP 期间有 Ca^{2+} 进入心肌细胞内。

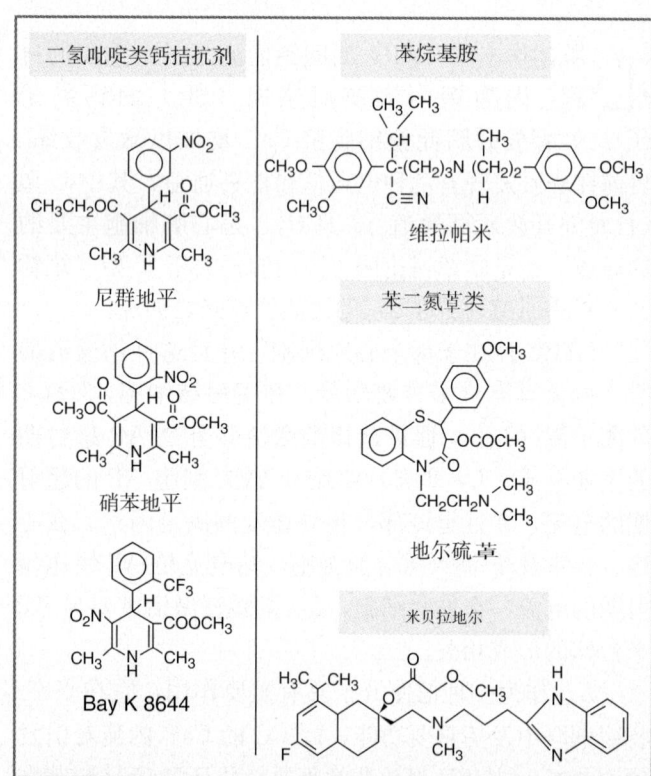

图 16-1 上图分别代表 L 型和 T 型 Ca^{2+} 通道的激动剂和拮抗剂的化学结构。其中，米贝拉地尔是 T 型 Ca^{2+} 通道拮抗剂，而其他药物是 L 型 Ca^{2+} 通道拮抗剂。Bay K8644 是 L 型 Ca^{2+} 通道的激动剂

LTCC 的带电或非带电的拮抗剂首先用于药物结合部位研究。这些研究表明,细胞外应用 DHPs 或 PAAs 的带电荷形式是无效的[11],而当应用非带电的药物片段时效果增加[12]。另外,细胞内应用带电荷的 DHPs 也是无效的,提示非带电的 DHPs 是较理想并且结合部位需要膜的脂质环境。不过细胞内应用带电荷的 PAAs 可有效地阻断 I_{Ca-L},提示 PAAS 以带电形式进入细胞浆结合到位点,而且其带电形式才能有效结合。地尔硫䓬能从细胞外和细胞内分别阻滞 I_{Ca-L},但是其带电荷的形式(四价形式)对 LTCC 的亲和力明显降低,这提示地尔硫䓬的非带电形式更有利于结合。

联合应用影像亲和标记技术和抗体扫描技术能确定三类拮抗剂中每种化合物的更为特异的结合区域[10](图 16-2)。DHP、PAA 及 BTZ 中每类药物都分别有自己的结合位点,并且一种药物的结合影响了其他药物的作用。影像亲和标记表明,DHP、PAAs 和 BTZ 的结合部位均位于 $α_1$ 亚基,ⅢS6 和 ⅣS6 为 BTZ 和 DHP 的结合区域。此外,应用合成的骨骼肌和心肌 LTCC 的嵌合通道试验发现,ⅢS5[13]也需要 DHP 与心脏 LTCC 结合,这些试验均表明这些药物通过与 LTCC 结合发挥作用,其结合部位在通道孔隙部位内部或附近(S5 和 S6 段)。并应用突变分析更进一步确定了与药物结合的必需氨基酸残基[10],其特定的氨基酸残基 Thr-1039 和 Gln-1043 位于 ⅢS5、Tyr-1152、Ile-1156,Met-1161 位于 ⅢS6,Asn-1472 位于 ⅣS6,这些位点似乎对 DHP 结合至关重要。近期还发现 $α_1$ 亚基的 ⅢS5-S6 连接体部位内的 Ser-1115 在 DHP 结合中具有重要作用[15]。PAA 结合的氨基酸残基包括位于 ⅣS6 的 Tyr-1463、Ala-1467、Ile-1470 和 Met-1464 及位于 ⅢS6 的 Tyr-1152、Ile-1153、Phe-1164 和 Val-1165。而对于 BTZ 结合,ⅣS6 部位的 Tyr-1463、Ala-1467 及 Ile-1470 非常重要。此外,近期研究表明 ⅣS5 与地尔硫䓬阻断 I_{Ca-L} 有关,这些研究都提示所有的三类 LTCC 激动剂和拮抗剂的结合都与 S6 片段有关,而 S6 段很可能参与了通道孔隙的形成;而且一般与 ⅣS6 有关,可以解释与不同的激动剂和拮抗剂结合的相互作用。

DHP 和 PAA 结合受细胞外 $[Ca^{2+}]$ 和其他阳离子影响:高的 Ca^{2+} 浓度抑制药物结合,提示药物结合的变构体模型包括一个或多个 Ca^{2+} 结合位点。这方面进一步研究能形成一种更新的生物化学模型,即假设 LTCC 选择性滤过区域有两个 Ca^{2+} 结合位点,一个对 Ca^{2+} 有高度亲和力,另一个具有相对低的亲和力。这种模型假设只有当高亲和力的位点被占据时,LTCC 处于一种非传导状态(失活状态),并且有利于 DHP 激动剂的结合。在 $[Ca^{2+}]_o$ 高时,低亲和力部位也被占据,则 LTCC 才具有渗透性。这种模型假设时,LTCC 激动剂影响了第二个钙离子结合以产生高传导状态,而且拮抗剂能稳定 Ca^{2+} 与高亲和力部位的结合[10]。

(三)L 型 Ca^{2+} 通道激动剂与拮抗剂的作用机制

应用单通道记录技术研究已充分证实,LTCC 的激动剂和拮抗剂都不会改变单通道 LTCC 的电流(I_{Ca-L})。这些研究指出,Ca^{2+} 激动剂和拮抗剂不改变各自的带电荷的通道的传导性,而是改变通道的开放与关闭能力。

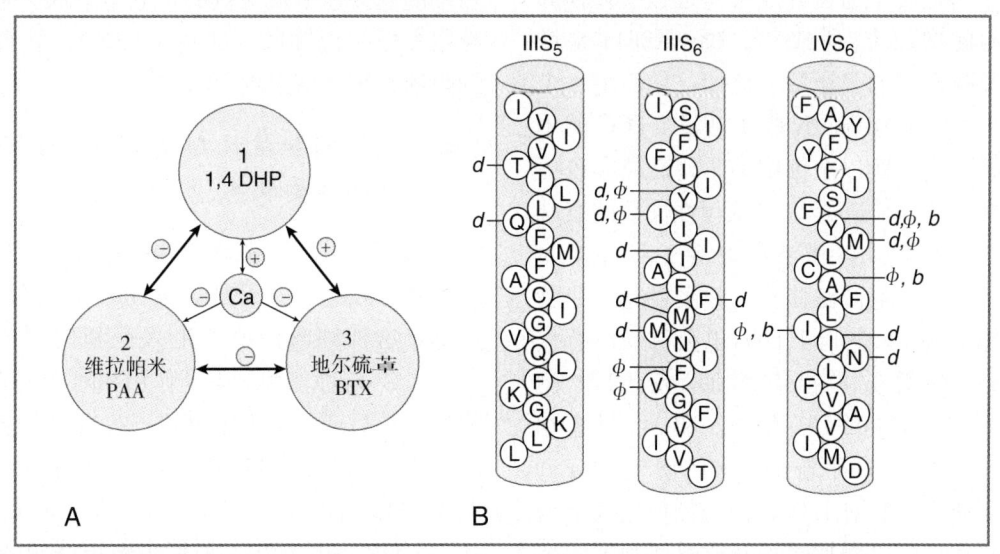

图 16-2 L 型 Ca^{2+} 通道的拮抗剂结合位点 A,DHP、PAA 和 BTZ 拮抗剂结合至 L 型 Ca^{2+} 通道位点间的相互作用。例如,DHP 结合至 L 型 Ca^{2+} 通道位点时能增强 BTZ 和 Ca^{2+} 间的结合。B,ⅢS₅、ⅢS₆ 和 ⅣS₆ 区域的拮抗剂结合位点,这些位点对 DHP(d)、PAA(ø)和 BTZ(b)是十分重要的

LTCC 拮抗剂部分地或全部地阻断整个细胞的 Ca^{2+} 电流（I_{Ca-L}），而没有减弱通过单通道 LTCCs（i_{Ca-L}）的电流幅度。应用 LTCC 拮抗剂部分阻断 i_{Ca-L}，但对通道的激活时间很少或没有影响，且 DHPs 通过在除极延长时减少通道开放来增加 I_{Ca-L} 的失活[17]。PAAs 和地尔硫䓬不改变 I_{Ca-L} 的衰减速率[18]。但是一些研究报告显示，当 Ba 离子（Ba^{2+}）作为电荷携带者或在高浓度拮抗剂存在时，能使通道失活增加[19]。

所有的三类拮抗剂使通道的失活状态更加稳定，这种作用减少了单通道水平的开放的能力[18]和可能性（P_o），并且减少了与通道激活有关的电荷运动（门控电荷）。在单通道水平，DHP 拮抗剂对通道开放和关闭几乎无作用[20]，但 PAAs（比如 D-600）[18]能显著缩短开放时间并使关闭态的时间延长。关于 BTZs 对单通道 LTCCs 的作用知之甚少，但是已经提出地尔硫䓬能减小 P_o 而对 I_{Ca-L} 幅值影响很小[21]。除此，所有的 Ca^{2+} 通道拮抗剂的一个重要特点是，其结合力（及有关作用）明显地受膜电位的影响，超极化时减少拮抗剂的结合。在超极化时，去除 D-600、地尔硫䓬和尼非地平的阻断作用的时间分别为 14.8s、2.2s 和 0.5s[22]。

在调节 LTCC 的活动时，DHP 药物的一个有趣的特点是：相似的分子结构可能是激动剂也可能是拮抗剂。其中研究最透彻的 LTCC 拮抗剂是 Bay K8644，具有（－）和（＋）立体异构体。Bay K8644（－）形式具有激动作用，可以增加 I_{Ca-L} 最大电流 2～4 倍[23]，这种作用是由于通道开放时间延长（被称为 2 型门控）并由此增加 P_o 所致[24]。Bay K8644 也增加 I_{Ca-L} 的激活及减慢它的去激活（比如，它产生一个即刻的尾电流）[24]。因为 Bay K8644 延长 LTCC 的单通道水平的开放时间，所以全细胞的 I_{Ca-L} 衰减应该更慢，但是，增加 I_{Ca-L} 加速了 Ca^{2+} 依赖性失活的衰减速率。Bay K8644 也使 I_{Ca-L} 激活和失活（d_∞ 和 f_∞）电压依赖性向更超极化电位偏移[23]。重要的是，尽管 Bay K8644 增加了 I_{Ca-L}，其对 LTCC 电荷活动没有作用，提示 LTCC 的总数量没有增加[25]。DHP 类 LTCC 激动剂（＋）-S-202-791 对 I_{Ca-L} 和 i_{Ca-L} 具有相似的作用[23]。最近对一种新的 DHP 激动剂 Bay Y5959 已进行了研究，它对 LTCC 的门控作用效果与 Bay K8644 不同，它可以增加平均开放时间和平均关闭时间，结果减少了 Ca^{2+} 电流的激活速率，增加了峰电流并减慢了复极时的 LTCC 去激活[26]。

在单通道水平对 LTCC 激动剂和拮抗剂的研究提出了"门控模式"理论（图 16-3），这一理论尚存争议[10]。根据这一理论，LTCC 激活或"门控"有三种不同的形式或"模式"，LTCC 的 0 模式为开始的失活态（不可利用），然后有一段无通道活动的较长时期。模式 1 是指 LTCC 门控的正常状态，其特点为在快速程序刺激时很短的开放时期（在除极之后）。模式 2 的门控状态的特点为长时间的开放[24]。对包含一个单个 LTCC 的膜进行重复的电压阶梯试验表明，不同模式的转换速率要比一个门控模式时的不同状态的转变（C_1、C_2、O 和 I 态）要慢得多。在正常条件下，模式 1 门控态最常见，伴随偶尔的模式 0 时期。在自然状态下模式 2 门控状态相对少得多，但可以由 DHP 类 LTCC 激动剂如 Bay K8644 和蛋白激酶 A（PKA）-依赖的磷酸化诱发。

（四）药物对 L 型 Ca^{2+} 通道的双重作用

药物调节 LTCC 的活动时会作为激动剂或拮抗剂，首次通过（－）Bay K8644[27]进行了描述。当（1）药物浓度很高；（2）应用于钳制膜电位为正电位时；及（3）试验脉冲的频率很高[28]时，这种分子对 I_{Ca-L} 有拮抗作用。进一步研究表明，立体异构体（－）-Bay K8644 和（＋）-S-202-791 为更具选择性的拮抗剂，并且只有细胞被钳制在正的膜电位时才产生拮抗作用[29]，这些结果提示[28]，药物结合的通道在除极后重新恢复到可利用状态的速率变慢。

LTCC 拮抗剂也能作为激动剂，尤其在低浓度时，在慢的起搏速率及更负的钳制电位时，通常这种作用是很短暂并温和的（30%～40%），并且似乎在观察到阻断作用之前出现[18]。

（五）激动剂和拮抗剂使 L 型 Ca^{2+} 通道产生结合的特定状态

所有的 LTCC 激动剂和拮抗剂都倾向于与特定的通道状态相结合（开放、关闭或失活状态）。对于激动剂，这种倾向性使产生兴奋和使用依赖性 I_{Ca-L} 阻断[23]。兴奋性依赖的阻断作用相对较弱，并且在长的静息电位后或从负的膜电位产生非常缓慢速率的除极时发生。兴奋性阻断效果依赖于膜电位。比如，在相对正的钳制电位（比如－50mV）时可以完全阻断 I_{Ca-L} 的 DHPs 的浓度却只能阻断正常静息电位－80mV 时 I_{Ca-L} 的 10%～20%。而在静息膜电位是－80mV 时，尼群地平与 LTCCs 结合的 K_D 为 730μmol/L，然

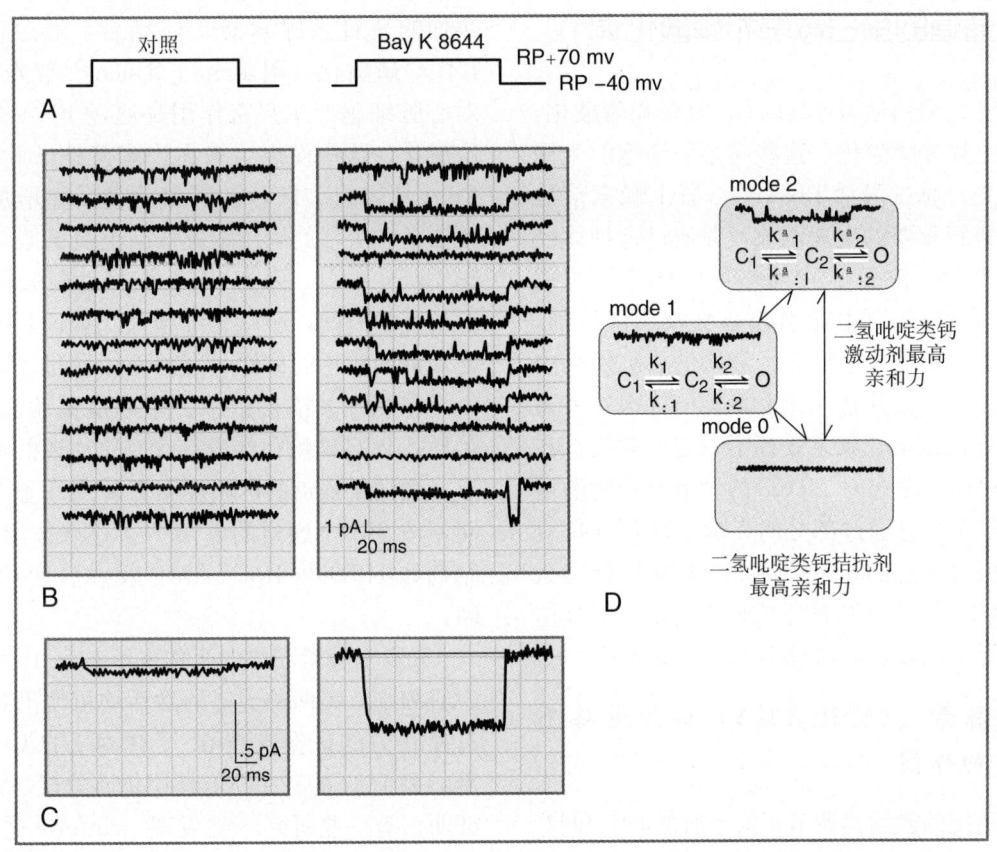

图 16-3 Bay K8644 是 L 型 Ca^{2+} 通道的激动剂，其对通道门控的影响　A，电压膜片钳记录的单通道电流图，静息膜电位为 $-60mV$；B，左图是未给 Bay K8644 时的单通道电流，右图是给予 $5\mu m$ Bay K8644 后的单通道电流。注意由 Bay K8644 诱发的非常长的开放时间；C，所有扫描的平均电流；D，L 型 Ca^{2+} 通道门控的模态理论。模式间转变的速率比不同状态间转换的速率慢得多。C_1 和 C_2 是两个关闭状态，O 是开放状态（引自：Bers DM：Excitationcontraction Coupling and Cardiac Contraetile Force, Znd ed. Dordrecht The Netherlands，Kluwer Academic，2001）

而在钳制膜电位为 $-10mV$ 时 K_D 为 $0.36nmol/L$[31]。这些研究结果与其他研究结果强有力地支持以下观点：即 DHPs 与失活态的 LTCC 具有最高的亲和力，并在除极化膜电位时增强。

反复除极能使抑制作用累积称为使用依赖性阻断。为增加脉冲时程、频率及正的钳制电位或条件电位时增强了 DHP、PAA 和 BZT 阻断剂的阻断效果，表明所有种类药物更倾向于与开放和/或失活状态的 LTCC 相结合，PAAs（如维拉帕米）似乎对开放态的 LTCC 最易结合（如需要电压脉冲诱发开放状态及随后阻断），因为其表现为比 DHPs 更强的使用依赖性[32]。

（六）L 型 Ca^{2+} 通道激动剂和拮抗剂的临床应用

LTCC 激动剂为正性肌力药物，目前还未在临床应用，但已证明对治疗心衰有价值。Bay K8644 没有正性肌力作用，但增加患者的死亡率。Bay K8644 的副作用包括增加周围血管阻力及收缩压增高、APs 延长，这可导致心律失常，并使神经 LTCC 兴奋性增加引起惊厥。由于 LTCC 的广泛分布和其功能特点，这些作用都是可以推理出来的。尽管有一些相对新的 DHP 激动剂如 Bay Y5959[6]，它似乎由于缺乏组织特异性，没有被广泛应用于临床。

相反，LTCC 拮抗剂长期用来治疗高血压、劳力性心绞痛及房性心律失常[33]。不过，在所有这些临床应用中，其益处看来是由于 LTCC 拮抗剂对开放态或失活态的 LTCC 有高度亲和力。抗高血压和抗心绞痛是利用了这样的事实，即平滑肌的静息电位比工作心脏更加趋向除极化，因此 LTCC 阻断和产生相应的血管舒张作用，并且没有显著的负性肌力作用。这种 Ca^{2+} 通道阻滞剂的使用依赖性特点（如维拉帕米）尤其在治疗房性心律失常时有效，这些问题在第 98 章进行了详细的讨论。

三、L 型钙通道的蛋白激酶和磷酸化调节

蛋白激酶使 L 型钙通道（LTCC）复合物磷酸化，蛋白磷酸化酶使其去磷酸化，这些与心肌细胞的生理和病理变化有关。通过激活 PKA 的 β 肾上腺素信号途径对 LTCC 进行重要的生理调节，并通过这种途径进行 LTCC 磷酸化，使 Ca^{2+} 内流增加、SRCa^{2+} 负荷增加、SR 内 Ca^{2+} 释放及由此引起心脏收缩性增加，这一信号瀑布的异常在充血性心力衰竭的心脏疾病中进行了详细的描述，尤其是 β 肾上腺素拮抗剂看来是通过影响 LTCC 的磷酸化状态发挥了一定的益处。在这里综述了通过信号瀑布对 LTCC 的调节、药物激活或阻断这些途径至少是通过部分的影响 LTCC 发挥对心脏的作用。值得注意的是，钙调蛋白依赖性蛋白激酶-Ⅱ（Ca MKⅡ）是 LTCC 的重要调节物质，但是这已在第 2 章进行了综述，在这里不再进一步阐述。

（一）β 肾上腺素（cAMP/PKA）信号通路对 LTCCs 的作用

交感神经系统的激活是调节正常心脏的心率和收缩力的一个重要机制。交感神经释放儿茶酚胺与细胞表面的 β 肾上腺素能受体结合，通过激活 PKA 使 LTCC 磷酸化（图 16-4）。Tsien[34] 首先提出，cAMP 对心脏细胞产生兴奋作用是通过 PKA 介导的 LTCC 磷酸化。这些设想后来在许多其他试验中得以证实。PKA 依赖的 LTCC 的磷酸化使 I_{Ca-L} 增加数倍，并且使激活和失活的电压依赖性向更负的膜电位偏移（如图 16-5，NF）。因为 PKA 依赖性磷酸化延长了单通道的开放时间，所以全细胞 I_{Ca-L} 应该衰减得更慢，但是如前面所述的那样，这种作用通过增加 I_{Ca-L} 而促进 Ca^{2+} 依赖性失活被抵消。单通道试验表明，PKA 依赖性 LTCC 磷酸化在没有改变单通道的传导性的情况下，增加了通道的可用性和 P_o，并引起 2 型门控状态而不改变单个通道的电导[23]。这些作用可被 PKA 抑制剂如 H-89 和 RpP-cAMP 及多肽素和 PKA-I 所阻断。

β 肾上腺素受体的两种主要亚型 β1 和 β2，存在于心肌细胞。该两种受体的激活均可使 LTCCs 磷酸化。有强有力的证据支持 β1 受体对 LTCCs 具有信使作用。关于 β2 的有关功能作用仍有争议，并且尚未充分证明。有一些研究[35] 已发现，zinterol 是一种 β2 肾上

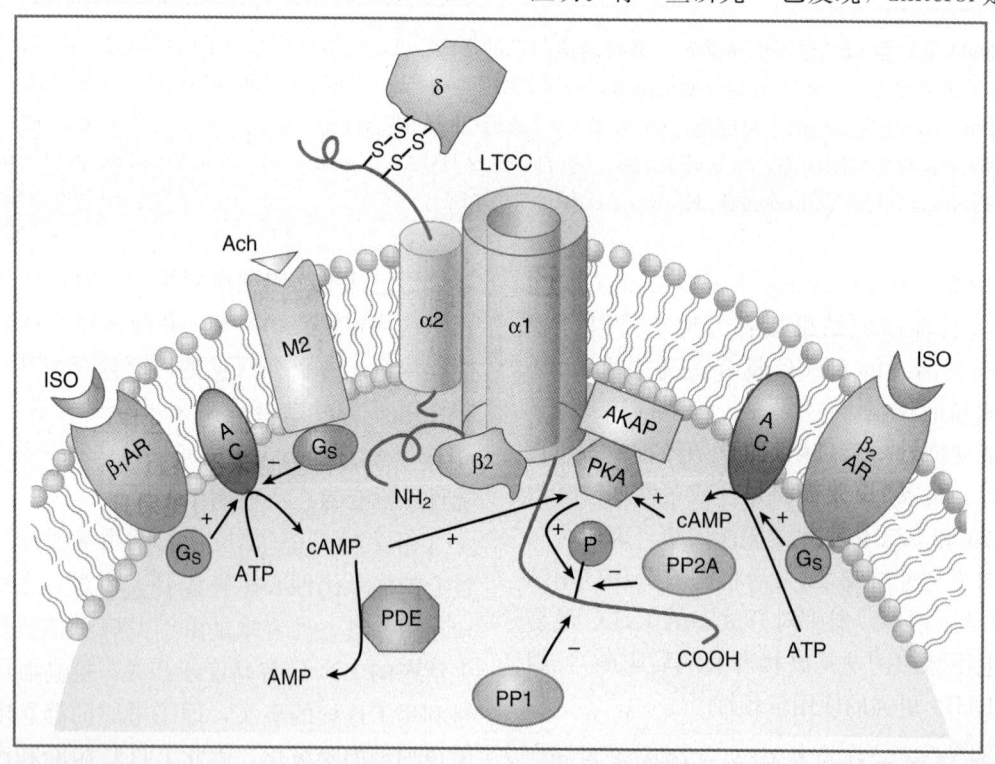

图 16-4　β 肾上腺素系统通过 CAMP/PKA 通路对 L 型 Ca^{2+} 通道调控的范例概略图　当激动剂（如异丙肾上腺素）结合到 β 肾上腺素能受体（β1 和 β2 肾上腺素能受体）时，相关的调节性 G 蛋白被激活，而抑制性 GBr 亚单位从 Gαs 解离。激活状态的 Gαs 再广泛激活腺苷酸环化酶（细胞膜上）。激活的腺苷酸环化酶催化产生 cAMP，然后局部的 cAMP 浓度显著增加，并激活蛋白激酶 ACPKA。PKA 通过激酶锚定蛋白（AKAPs）与 L 型 Ca^{2+} 通道紧密结合。此后，PKA 对 L 型 Ca^{2+} 通道进行磷酸化。该幅图显示 PKA 依赖性 α_1 亚单位 C 末端（COOH）磷酸化。β2 受体部位也存在 PKA 位点，但这些位点在图中为简单化而未标注。磷酸化的 L 型 Ca^{2+} 通道又被蛋白磷酸酶 2A 和蛋白磷酸酶Ⅰ（PPI）去磷酸化。cAMP 通过磷酸二酯酶（PDE）清除。此外，M_2 胆碱能受体的激活可以通过 G_i 蛋白抑制腺苷酸环化酶活化

腺素受体激动剂，能使 I_{Ca-L} 增加。但是 Nagykaldi 等最近提出，ziterol 对 I_{Ca-L} 的作用可被 β1 拮抗剂 CGP20712A 阻断而不被 β2 拮抗剂阻断。他们认为，zinterol 通过 β1 肾上腺受体发挥作用，因为它的特异性较低，其他的神经载体及激素如组胺、胰高血糖素、甲状旁腺素及血清素也可以通过 cAMP/PKA 信号通路调节 I_{Ca-L}，这些调节作用与通过 β 肾上腺素受体的信号通路相比要弱得多。

$α_{1c}$ 亚基的 Ser-1928 及 $β_{2a}$ 亚基的 Ser-478 和/或 Ser-479，被认为是 LTCC 通道的 PKA 磷酸化位点[37]，能使 I_{Ca-L} 增加[37]，但是通过直接的方法尚未证实这种假设。另外，$α_{1c}$ 的 C-末端定位的 Ser-1928 的作用尚有争议，因为这个部位的蛋白质可以被蛋白酶裂解或被剪接片段接合替代；有趣的是，研究发现 LTCC 裂解的细胞浆的 C 末端仍保留链接于被膜包埋的 α 亚基部分的功能[38]，有关 $α_1$ 亚基和 $β_{2a}$ 磷酸化调节 LTCCs 的机理作用远未确定。Naguro 等发现[39] 被称为大鼠脑型 $IIα_{1c}$（相当于心脏 $α_{1c}$ 的 Ser-1928）上的 Ser-1901 可以通过 PKA 磷酸化使 P_0 增加，并且其他 PKA 位点的磷酸化能使电压依赖性激活左移，这些结果对于心脏 Ca^{2+} 通道非常重要，因为这样可能开发出一些钙通道特异性药物，从而特异性地调节 LTCC 磷酸化。其他重要的结果包括 LTCC 的 PKA 磷酸化需要激酶 A-锚定蛋白（AKAPs）使 PKA 即刻锚定于 LTCCs 上。有一项研究表明，PKA-依赖性 $α_{1c}$ 磷酸化需要 AKAP，然而 $β_{2a}$ 亚基通过 PKA 发生磷酸化却不需要 AKAP。关于在病态心肌的磷酸化缺乏的这些分子物质的作用需要进行深入的研究。调节 LTCC 磷酸化状态并决定其激活状态和 I_{Ca-L} 大小的信号通路以 β 肾上腺素受体的信号通路为例在图 16-4 进行了详细的说明。

除以上提到的内容外，磷酸二酯酶使 cAMP 裂解为 AMP 及蛋白磷酸酶（PP1 和 PP2）使 LTCCs 去磷酸化，也影响了 LTCC 的磷酸化状态。对人的心肌衰竭细胞的研究表明，LTCC 的磷酸化状态增加，这是由于正常的去磷酸化的 LTCC 的磷酸酶活性较低；其他一些对正常心肌的研究表明，磷酸酶活性为心脏 LTCC 特性的重要决定因素[40]。

（二）心肌细胞内蛋白激酶 C（PKC）对 LTCC 的调节作用

与 PKA 的作用不同，PKC 对 I_{Ca-L} 的作用存在争

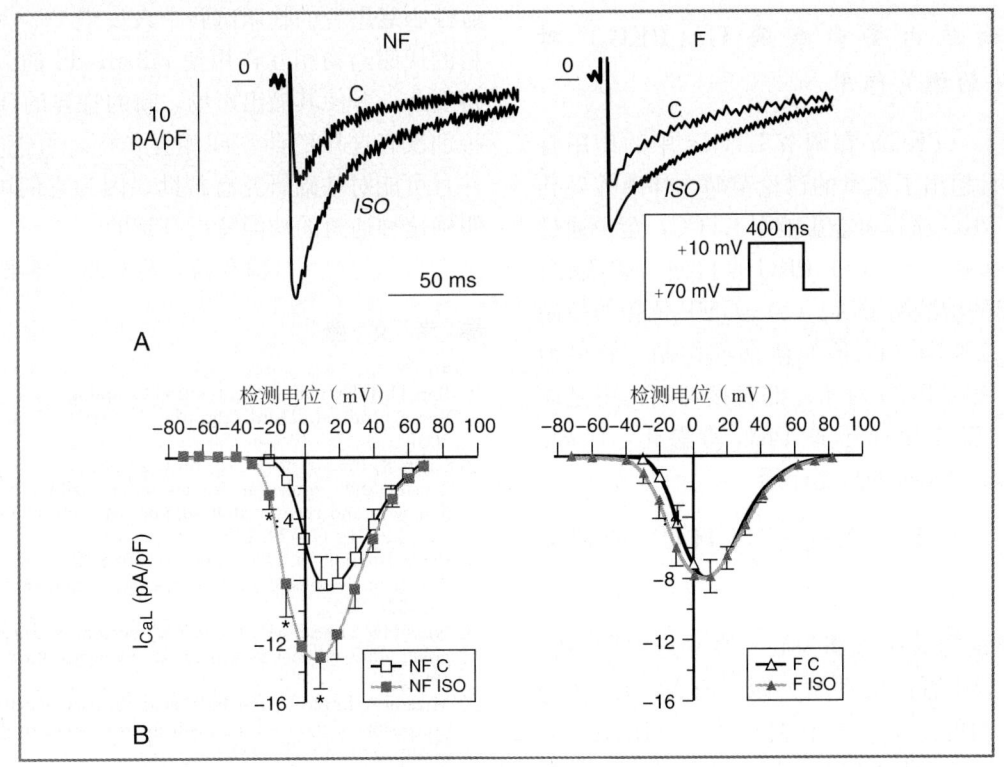

图 16-5　1μM 异丙肾上腺素对非衰竭（NF，n=12，N=6）和衰竭（F，n=9，N=4）的人心室肌细胞膜上 L 型 Ca^{2+} 通道的影响　A，加入 1μM 异丙肾上腺素前后的电流图。异丙肾上腺素能明显增加非衰竭的心室肌细胞的 L 型 Ca^{2+} 电流（190±15%），但对衰竭的心室肌细胞影响极小（124±12%）。B，异丙肾上腺素对非衰竭和衰竭心室肌细胞 L 型 Ca^{2+} 通道电压相关性的影响。异内肾上腺素能显著增加非衰竭的心室肌细胞的最大 L 型 Ca^{2+} 电流，但对衰竭的心室肌细胞影响极小（NF：1.57，F：1.08）（引自 Chen X. piacentino V 3rd, Furukawa S, et al: L-type Ca^{2+} channel density and regulation are altered in failing human ventricular myocytes and recover after support with mechanical assist devices，Cire Res 91：517-524，2002）

议,一些研究发现了 PKC 的激动作用,而其他一些研究则发现其抑制作用或双相作用[37]。在离体试验中,LTCC 的 α₁ 和 β₂ 亚基为 PKC 调节磷酸化的较好的作用底物,具有 2~3 个摩尔当量 α₁ 亚基的磷酸化及 1~2 个摩尔 β₂ 亚基的磷酸化[37]。PKC 的作用位点可能位于 N-末端(Thr-27 和 Thr-31),这些位点由于 PKC 的磷酸化表现为使 I_{Ca-L} 抑制[41]。其他的研究表明非 N-末端的 PKC 位点在去磷酸化状态下抑制 LTCC[43]磷酸酶活性,并且这些位点的磷酸化解除了这种抑制及使 LTCC 的 P_o 增加。

PKC 被认为可能调节许多激素和神经递质的电生理和收缩作用,包括 α-肾上腺素能激动剂、细胞内 ATP、血管紧张素Ⅱ、糖皮质激素、精氨酸-加压素、内皮素。在应用穿透性膜片钳情况下(无细胞分离),血管紧张素Ⅱ可能通过 PKC 磷酸化增强 I_{Ca-L}[43],但对断裂的膜片进行钳制时几乎没有作用。在正常的兔心室肌细胞,内皮素-1 对 I_{Ca-L} 具有双重作用,先抑制 I_{Ca-L} 然后使其增加。而且,内皮素-1 明显削弱 β 肾上腺素对 I_{Ca-L} 的刺激作用[44]。PKC 作为 LTCC 的调节因素是一个尚未解决的重要的研究课题,现在已清楚的是 PKC 对 LTCCs 的许多作用都明显地弱于 PKA。

(三) 心肌细胞内蛋白激酶 G (PKG) 对 LTCCs 的调节作用

蛋白激酶 G(PKG)在调节 LTCCs 中的作用有更多的争议并且超出了本章的讨论范畴。环磷酸鸟苷酸(cGMP)/PKG 途径可能影响了 LTCC,至少通过 3 种途径产生影响[37]:(1)PKG 直接使其磷酸化;(2)PKG 引起的磷酸酶激活;(3)cGMP 依赖的控制 cGMP 的磷酸二酯酶(PGEs)激活或抑制。简单地说,许多研究表明 PKG 对 I_{Ca-L} 的直接抑制作用是通过 cGMP 的刺激作用而不是 PKG 磷酸化,比如,cGMP 依赖的对 PDEⅢ的抑制作用。

(四) 病态心脏的 L 型钙通道 (LTCC) 的调节异常

对肾上腺素的反应减弱为心力衰竭进展期的特点,并且与心衰患者的活动耐力减低有关。I_{Ca-L} 对 β 肾上腺素激动剂的反应在心衰时减小[2](图 16-5),并且导致衰竭心脏的收缩储备下降,这些反应减弱的机制还不是非常确定,可能包括受体数目减少、腺苷环化酶活性降低(使 cAMP 生成减少)、增加 G_i 对 β 肾上腺受体的结合、增加 β 肾上腺受体激酶对肾上腺素反应的表达的去敏感、增加 PDE 活性、AKAP 增加或定位异常、增加信号通路的活性(如 cGMP/PKG 通路)拮抗 cAMP/PKA 通路[45]、磷酸酶活性减低导致 LTCC 磷酸化状态异常[46],这些过程都值得进一步研究。有趣的是近来有效的心力衰竭调节因素如 β 肾上腺受体阻断剂可能通过改变 PKA 目标蛋白如 LTCC 的磷酸化状态发挥了一些有益作用[2]。

四、心脏 T 型钙通道的药理学

目前尚没有高度特异的 T 型钙通道拮抗剂,mibefradil(也称作 Ro40-5967)是目前最特异的拮抗剂,但是它对 LTCC 有潜在的作用。在结构上,miberfradil 是四氢萘酚的一种衍生物,并且与三种经典的 LTCC 拮抗剂无关,它抑制 T 型钙电流并使稳态失活向更负电压偏移[47]。近期研究表明,mibefradil 能引起外周血管扩张及心率减慢,但不降低心衰患者的心肌收缩力。另外,mibefradil 抑制肾上腺髓质和皮质释放神经内分泌激素醛固酮及抑制交感神经释放去甲肾上腺素[48]。临床试验表明,mibefradil 是一种有效的抗心绞痛、抗高血压及抗缺血物质。但是,对充血性心衰患者的临床试验令人失望[49]。其中,没有预料的代谢药物相互作用使 mibefradil 的公认的益处变得复杂,并使其撤出市场。新的特异的 T 型钙通道拮抗剂没有这样的药物间相互作用,可能有临床用处,并且可能对基础研究有帮助,因为它们可能对进一步明确这种通道的功能特点有帮助。

(浦介麟 马克娟 滕思勇 译)

参 考 文 献

1. Bers DM: Excitation-Contraction Coupling and Cardiac Contractile Force, 2nd ed. Dordrecht, the Netherlands, Kluwer Academic, 2001.
2. Chen X, Piacentino V 3rd, Furukawa S, et al: L-type Ca²⁺ channel density and regulation are altered in failing human ventricular myocytes and recover after support with mechanical assist devices. Circ Res 91:517–524, 2002.
3. Qu Y, Boutjdir M: Gene expression of SERCA2a and L- and T-type Ca channels during human heart development. Pediatr Res 50:569–574, 2001.
4. Nuss HB, Houser SR: T-type Ca²⁺ current is expressed in hypertrophied adult feline left ventricular myocytes. Circ Res 73:777–782, 1993.
5. Mikami A, Imoto K, Tanabe T, et al: Primary structure and functional expression of the cardiac dihydropyridine-sensitive calcium channel. Nature 340:230–233, 1989.
6. Striessnig J: Pharmacology, structure and function of cardiac L-type Ca²⁺ channels. Cell Physiol Biochem 9:242–269, 1999.
7. Perez-Reyes E, Schneider T: Molecular biology of calcium channels. Kidney Int 48:1111–1124, 1995.
8. Anderson ME: Ca²⁺-dependent regulation of cardiac L-type Ca²⁺ channels: Is a unifying mechanism at hand? J Mol Cell Cardiol

33:639–650, 2001.
9. Catterall WA, Striessnig J: Receptor sites for Ca^{2+} channel antagonists. Trends Pharmacol Sci 13:256–262, 1992.
10. Mitterdorfer J, Grabner M, Kraus RL, et al: Molecular basis of drug interaction with L-type Ca^{2+} channels. J Bioenerg Biomembr 30:319–334, 1998.
11. Adachi-Akahane S, Amano Y, et al: Quaternary diltiazem can act from both sides of the membrane in ventricular myocytes. Jpn J Pharmacol 61:263–266, 1993.
12. Kass RS, Arena RJ. Influence of pH on Calcium channel block by amlodipine, a charged dihydropyridine compound. Implications for location of the dihydropyridine receptor. J Gen Physiol 93:1109–1127, 1989.
13. Grabner M, Wang Z, Hering S, et al: Transfer of 1,4-dihydropyridine sensitivity from L-type to class A (BI) calcium channels. Neuron 16:207–218, 1996.
14. Doring F, Degtiar VE, Grabner M, et al: Transfer of L-type calcium channel IVS6 segment increases phenylalkylamine sensitivity of α_{1A}. J Biol Chem 271:11745–11749, 1996.
15. Yamaguchi S, Okamura Y, Nagao T, et al: Serine residue in the IIIS5-S6 linker of the L-type Ca^{2+} channel α_{1C} subunit is the critical determinant of the action of dihydropyridine Ca^{2+} channel agonists. J Biol Chem 275:41504–41511, 2000.
16. Bodi I, Koch SE, Yamaguchi H, et al: The role of region IVS5 of the human cardiac calcium channel in establishing inactivated channel conformation: Use-dependent block by benzothiazepines. J Biol Chem 277:20651–20659, 2002.
17. Gurney AM, Nerbonne JM, Lester HA: Photoinduced removal of nifedipine reveals mechanisms of calcium antagonist action on single heart cells. J Gen Physiol 86:353–379, 1985.
18. McDonald T, Pelzer D, Trautwein W: Dual action (stimulation, inhibition) of D600 on contractility and calcium channels in guinea-pig and cat heart cells. J Physiol 414:569–586, 1989.
19. Lee KS, Tsien RW: Mechanism of calcium channel blockade by verapamil, D600, diltiazem and nitrendipine in single dialysed heart cells. Nature 302:790–794, 1983.
20. Brown AM, Kunze DL, Yatani A: Dual effects of dihydropyridines on whole cell and unitary calcium currents in single ventricular cells of guinea-pig. J Physiol 379:495–514, 1986.
21. Zahradnikova A, Zahradnik I: Interaction of diltiazem with single L-type calcium channels in guinea-pig ventricular myocytes. Gen Physiol Biophys 11:535–543, 1992.
22. Uehara A, Hume JR: Interactions of organic calcium channel antagonists with calcium channels in single frog atrial cells. J Gen Physiol 85:621–647, 1985.
23. McDonald TF, Pelzer S, Trautwein W, Pelzer DJ: Regulation and modulation of calcium channels in cardiac, skeletal, and smooth muscle cells. Physiol Rev 74:365–507, 1994.
24. Hess P, Lansman JB, Tsien RW: Different modes of Ca channel gating behaviour favoured by dihydropyridine Ca agonists and antagonists. Nature 311:538–544, 1984.
25. Josephson IR, Sperelakis N: Fast activation of cardiac Ca^{++} channel gating charge by the dihydropyridine agonist, BAY K 8644. Biophys J 58:1307–1311, 1990.
26. Bechem M, Goldmann S, Gross R, et al: A new type of Ca-channel modulation by a novel class of 1,4-dihydropyridines. Life Sci 60:107–118, 1997.
27. Bechem M, Schramm M: Calcium-agonists. J Mol Cell Cardiol 19(Suppl 2):63–75, 1987.
28. Hadley RW, Hume JR: Calcium channel antagonist properties of Bay K 8644 in single guinea pig ventricular cells. Circ Res 62:97–104, 1988.
29. Kamp TJ, Sanguinetti MC, Miller RJ: Voltage- and use-dependent modulation of cardiac calcium channels by the dihydropyridine (+)-202–791. Circ Res 64:338–351, 1989.
30. Sanguinetti MC, Kass RS: Voltage-dependent block of calcium channel current in the calf cardiac Purkinje fiber by dihydropyridine calcium channel antagonists. Circ Res 55:336–348, 1984.
31. Bean BP: Nitrendipine block of cardiac calcium channels: High-affinity binding to the inactivated state. Proc Natl Acad Sci U S A 81:6388–6392, 1984.
32. McDonald TF, Pelzer D, Trautwein W: Cat ventricular muscle treated with D600: Characteristics of calcium channel block and unblock. J Physiol 352:217–241, 1984.
33. Clusin WT, Anderson ME: Calcium channel blockers: Current controversies and basic mechanisms of action. Adv Pharmacol 46:253–296, 1999.
34. Tsien RW: Adrenaline-like effects of intracellular iontophoresis of cyclic AMP in cardiac Purkinje fibres. Nat New Biol 245:120–122, 1973.
35. Chen-Izu Y, Xiao RP, Izu LT, et al: G_i-dependent localization of β_2-adrenergic receptor signaling to L-type Ca^{2+} channels. Biophys J 79:2547–2556, 2000.
36. Nagykaldi Z, Kem D, Lazzara R, Szabo B: Canine ventricular myocyte β_2-adrenoceptors are not functionally coupled to L-type calcium current. J Physiol 520:271–280, 1999.
37. Keef KD, Hume JR, Zhong J: Regulation of cardiac and smooth muscle Ca^{2+} channels (Ca$_V$1.2a,b) by protein kinases. Am J Physiol Cell Physiol 281:C1743–1756, 2001.
38. Gao T, Yatani A, Dell'Acqua ML, et al: cAMP-dependent regulation of cardiac L-type Ca^{2+} channels requires membrane targeting of PKA and phosphorylation of channel subunits. Neuron 19:185–196, 1997.
39. Naguro I, Nagao T, Adachi-Akahane S: Ser^{1901} of α_{1C} subunit is required for the PKA-mediated enhancement of L-type Ca^{2+} channel currents but not for the negative shift of activation. FEBS Lett 489:87–91, 2001.
40. duBell WH, Lederer WJ, Rogers TB: Dynamic modulation of excitation-contraction coupling by protein phosphatases in rat ventricular myocytes. J Physiol (Lond) 493:793–800, 1996.
41. McHugh D, Sharp EM, Scheuer T, Catterall WA: Inhibition of cardiac L-type calcium channels by protein kinase C phosphorylation of two sites in the N-terminal domain. Proc Natl Acad Sci U S A 97:12334–12338, 2000.
42. Shistik E, Keren-Raifman T, Idelson GH, et al: The N terminus of the cardiac L-type Ca^{2+} channel α_{1C} subunit. The initial segment is ubiquitous and crucial for protein kinase C modulation, but is not directly phosphorylated. J Biol Chem 274:31145–31149, 1999.
43. Kurata S, Ishikawa K, Iijima T: Enhancement by arginine vasopressin of the L-type Ca^{2+} current in guinea pig ventricular myocytes. Pharmacol 59(1):21–33, 1999.
44. Watanabe T, Endoh M: Characterization of the endothelin-1–induced regulation of L-type Ca^{2+} current in rabbit ventricular myocytes. Naunyn Schmiedebergs Arch Pharmacol 360(6):654–664, 1999.
45. Port JD, Bristow MR: Altered beta-adrenergic receptor gene regulation and signaling in chronic heart failure. J Mol Cell Cardiol 33:887–905, 2001.
46. Schroder F, Handrock R, Beuckelmann DJ, et al: Increased availability and open probability of single L-type calcium channels from failing compared with nonfailing human ventricle. Circulation 98:969–976, 1998.
47. Pinto JM, Sosunov EA, Gainullin RZ, et al: Effects of mibefradil, a T-type calcium current antagonist, on electrophysiology of Purkinje fibers that survived in the infarcted canine heart. J Cardiovasc Electrophysiol 10:1224–1235, 1999.
48. Clozel JP, Ertel EA, Ertel SI: Voltage-gated T-type Ca^{2+} channels and heart failure. Proc Assoc Am Physicians 111:429–437, 1999.
49. Levine TB, Bernink PJ, Caspi A, et al: Effect of mibefradil, a T-type calcium channel blocker, on morbidity and mortality in moderate to severe congestive heart failure: The MACH-1 study. Mortality Assessment in Congestive Heart Failure Trial. Circulation 101:758–764, 2000.

第 17 章

KCNQ1/KCNE1 大分子信号复合物：通道微结构与人体疾病

Sheila J. Carroll, Junko Kurokawa, Robert S. Kass

本章目录

- β-AR 信号转导：通道蛋白局部调节的协调性 ……………………………… 140
- KCNE1 和 KCNQ1 的组装是 KCNQ1 磷酸化诱导的功能性改变 ……………… 142
- 遗传性 KCNE1 突变能破坏 SNS 对 I_{ks} 的功能性调节 ……………………………… 142
- SNS 介导的调节作用引起 I_{Ks} 通道解耦联：心律失常的新机制 ……………… 143

自主神经系统通过交感和副交感神经的活动对心率和心脏收缩的控制是心血管系统的基本特征。运动或情绪激动刺激交感神经系统（SNS），导致心率快速明显的增快，而且为了保证舒张期足够的充盈时间，伴随发生心室动作电位（APD）时程及对应的心电图（EKG）QT 间期的缩短。在 SNS 作用下，心脏电活动发生缺陷调节能够引起心律失常[1]。

SNS 对心脏电活动的控制是由 β-肾上腺素受体（β-ARs）介导的，它们通过环腺苷酸（cAMP）依赖性蛋白激酶 A（PKA）的磷酸化作用来调节相应离子通道的功能。PKA 的作用靶点包括调节细胞钙离子浓度的离子通道，它调整表面电信号的振幅和时间，从细胞内钙贮存库和肌浆网释放钙离子。PKA 依赖性磷酸化作用调节着 L 型钙离子通道的活动，使钙内流增加，从而使 AP 延长，并为接下来肌浆网吸收钙提高来源。同时 PKA 也激活细胞内肌浆网上主要的钙释放通道，2 型 RyR 受体（RyR2）[2]，该受体负责释放钙离子触发肌肉收缩。

交感神经刺激也能引起 cAMP 依赖性缓慢激活钾离子（K）通道电流 I_{Ks} 的增加。这种调节能增加复极电流，以应对 PKA 对 L 型钙离子通道的刺激作用[3]。SNS 刺激改变内向和外向电流间的平衡来调节心室的 APD 和 QT 间期。AP 间期直接控制细胞内的钙，细胞内外电流的平衡是交感神经活动调节钙稳态的重要机制。

离子通道蛋白的遗传性突变与心律失常有关，交感神经系统的作用能加剧这些心律失常。例如，编码 I_{Ks} 通道亚单位的基因，*KCNQ1* 和 *KCNE1*[4,5]，与遗传性长 QT 综合征（LQTS）有关，它是一种少见疾病，因为心室复极功能障碍，所以 EKG 上表现为 QT 间期延长，能引起多形性室性心动过速、晕厥、抽搐和猝死[6]。其中，编码 I_{Ks} 通道 α 亚单位的 *KCNQ1* 突变引起 LQT-1，编码 β 亚单位的 *KCNE1* 突变引起 LQT-5[7]。对于受累的患者，引起心律失常的触发点是基因特异性的，那些存在 *KCNQ1* 或 *KCNE1* 突变的患者，在 SNS 活动增强的情况下易发生致死性心律失常的危险性非常大[8]。在 SNS 与 *KCNQ1*/*KCNE1* 调节间的分子联系尚未清楚前，LQTS 发生心律失常的触发点机制有重要意义。

一、β-AR 信号转导：通道蛋白局部调节的协调性

β-AR 对主要离子通道蛋白的复杂调节作用借助于 cAMP 依赖性 PKA 和蛋白磷酸化酶[9,10]，与靶蛋

白、A-激酶锚蛋白（AKAPs）[11]相互作用来完成的。AKAPs 是一组结构多样性蛋白，具有和 PKA、蛋白磷酸化酶（PP1）、蛋白激酶 C（PKC）相结合的功能[12,13,14]。锚蛋白与蛋白的结合决定着它们的定位和底物的特异性，这使调节酶在细胞内作用底物部位有较高的浓度[15]。局部信号复合物的形成是信号的准确转导所必需的，当局部复合物破坏时会使反映部分失衡，但不是全部，旁路传导不受影响，其中一个机制是破坏了靶蛋白-中介蛋白-蛋白的相互作用，使局部复合物间解耦联。

（一）亮氨酸/异亮氨酸拉链协调蛋白-蛋白间的相互作用

Mark 和他的同事[2,17]首先阐述了心脏钙释放通道/RyR2 是由大分子信号复合物调节的，其中激酶和磷酸化酶对通道的作用是通过亮氨酸/异亮氨酸拉链（LIZ）介导的蛋白-蛋白相互作用完成的，表明这一结构是协调离子通道信号复合物的一个常见模体[17]。接下来的研究显示，至少两种由 PKA 调节的离子通道是这样的：L 型钙离子通道和 KCNQ1/KCNE1 钾离子通道[19]。

LIZ 呈 α-螺旋结构，早先被认为是介导转录因子与 DNA 结合的高度保守模体[20]，缠绕的螺旋是由反复重复的 (abcdefg)$_n$ 构成，疏水性残基出现在"a"和"d"部位，形成螺旋的疏水表面；而"b, c, e, f, g"是亲水残基，形成螺旋可溶水的暴露部分[21]。亮氨酸拉链（LZs）由于是柔软的侧链，所以其通常出现在"d"的位置，尽管亮氨酸可能被异亮氨酸、缬氨酸代替（如 mixed lineage 激酶-3）[22]。相邻螺旋体侧链间"e""g"部位的静电相互作用有助于两部分特异性结合[23]，如果不存在离子配对，带电荷的残基可能失去稳定性[24]。此外，"e""g"部位的残基在相邻结构阻隔的空间内发生有限的替代[25]。

（二）点特异性突变引起的复合物间解耦联

突变的产生被成功地用于研究蛋白间相互作用螺旋的结构特异性，例如 GCN4 DNA 结合域[26]、膜磷蛋白（phospholamban）[25]、肌球蛋白结合亚单位/cGKID[27]、RyR1 和 RyR2[17]、KCNQ1/KCNE1 通道[19]。当一个或多个"d"位置的亮氨酸或异亮氨酸被丙氨酸代替时会降低 LZ 介导蛋白-蛋白相互作用的能力，但并不破坏天然的 α 螺旋结构[26,28]。

KCNQ1/KCNE1 通道

目前已知 KCNQ1/KCNE1 通道形成大分子信号复合物，通过 KCNQ1 羧基端（C-）的 LZ 结构与靶蛋白 yotiao[29] 的结合来协调作用（图 17-1）[19]。PKA 和 PP1 与 yotiao 连接，直接集合成通道大分子复合物，主要由 KCNQ1 末端氨基酸残基 Ser[27] 的磷酸化反应调节[19]。在中国仓鼠卵巢细胞（CHO）上重构建 PKA 和 PP1 介导调节的 KCNQ1/KCNE1 电流需要 KCNQ1/KCNE1 和 yotiao 联合表达，并可被突变的 KCNQ1LZ 消除，因突变阻止了 yotiao 和通道的结合，消除了 Ser 的磷酸化[27]。

PKA 对 KCNQ1/KCNE1 通道复合物磷酸化作用的功能结果是，这些通道的活性显著升高、电压依赖性通道活性的超极化转变和舒张期通道由激活（开放）到静息（关闭）的缓慢变化。这些结果共同作用保证了在电压除极阶段，KCNQ1/KCNE1 通道在 SNS 刺激下比不刺激有更高的活性。结果，在 SNS 作用下，重要的复极过程被激活，钾离子电流抵消了 SNS 增高的钙电流，这些钙电流本身会引起 APD 延长[3]。

（三）疾病时 KCNQ1/KCNE 信号复合物解耦联

如同人工构建的突变体，如在 KCNQ1 LZ 的第二和第三"d"部位，内氨酸代替亮氨酸，将去除它与 yotiao 的相互作用，但不破坏 α 螺旋结构，遗传性突变也一样，破坏了 LZs，使信号分子与其底物解耦联。如前所述，LZ 上"e"和"g"部位残基由于相邻结构的空间限制，发生替换的范围有限[26]。因此，在 bKCNQ1 的 LZ 结构的"e"部位发生的 G589D 突变破坏了 yotiao 与 bKCNQ1 的靶向结合。在芬兰家系中发现，G589D 突变与 LQT-1 有关，另外，由于 KCNQ1-G589D 突变破坏了 KCNQ1 的 C 端 LZ 结构，从而使 β-肾上腺素能介导的通道调节作用失效。G589D 突变通过阻断 PKA 和 PP1 与通道 C 端的大分子复合物的靶向性形成，使通道调节功能障碍，此时受累患者表现为在精神和体力应激时 QT 间期调节功能障碍[31]，运动时易发生心律失常和心脏骤停的危险[30]。因此，KCNQ1 通道单一残基的遗传突变将破坏 KCNQ1/KCNE1 信号复合物，增加患者心律失常的风险。

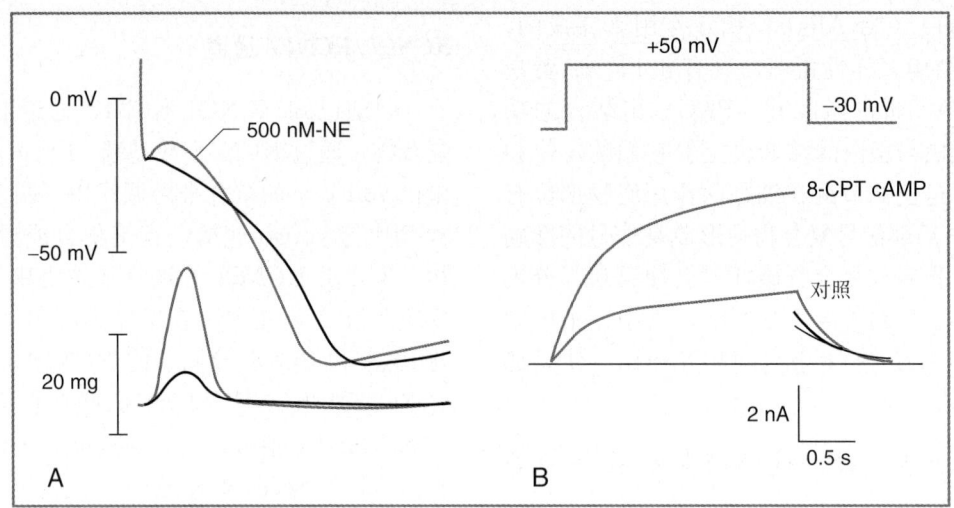

图 17-1 A：在分离的小牛浦肯野纤维，去甲肾上腺素（NE）提高了平台期高度，加强了收缩力，缩短了动作电位时程（APD）。（来自 Kass RS，Wiegers SE：The ionic basis of concentration-related effects of noradrenaline on the action potential of calf cardiac purkinje fibres. J Physiol 322：541-558，1982.）B：在分离的豚鼠心肌细胞，膜通透的环腺嘌呤核苷酸类似物 8（CPT）-cAMP 提高了缓慢外向钾电流。电流图是电压从钳制电位－30～＋50 mV 的记录电流，对照和 8-（CPT）-cAMP 为同一细胞。（来自 Walsh KB，Kass RS：Regulation of a heart potassium channel by protein kinase A and C. Science 242：67-69，1988）

二、KCNE1 和 KCNQ1 的组装是 KCNQ1 磷酸化诱导的功能性改变

β-AR 刺激引起的心室 APD 的缩短部分是由于缓慢外向钾离子电流（I_{Ks}）cAMP 依赖性增加引起的。任一 I_{Ks} 亚单位 KCNQ1 或 KCNE1 的突变都与遗传性 LQTS 有关（LQT-1 或 LQT-5）。Kurokawa 和他的同事研究发现，cAMP 介导的 *KCNQ1/KCNE1* 通道的功能性调节，即 cAMP 依赖性 *KCNQ1* 氨基端 PKA 磷酸化的结果，需要 KCNQ1 的表达伴随它的辅助亚单位 KCNE1 的表达。他们研究了 cAMP 和磷酸激酶阻滞剂冈田酸（okadaic 酸）（OA）对 CHO 细胞表达电流的影响，以探讨 *KCNE1* 在 *KCNQ1/KCNE1* 通道 cAMP 依赖性调节中的作用（图 17-2）。在表达 bKCNQ1、bKCNE1 和 yotiao 的 CHO 细胞的膜片钳实验中，cAMP 和 OA 能增加 *KCNQ1/KCNE1* 通道的活性，通过测量存在和不存在 cAMP 和 OA 时尾电流的幅度做定量分析发现通道活性几乎增加了两倍[19]。除了对电流振幅的影响外，cAMP/OA 还能引起通道激活的依赖电压向负向转变。然而，在表达 bKCNQ1 和 yotiao 而无 bKCNE1 的细胞上，细胞内 cAMP 和 OA 对 KCNQ1 通道的活性无显著影响。在这些实验中，KCNE1 对 KCNQ1 的磷酸化并不是必要的。

Kurokawa 和他的同事[32]在 *KCNQ1* 的 27 位残基上用天门冬氨酸代替丝氨酸，当与 *KCNE1* 联合表达时，发现 S37D 突变重建了 *KCNQ1* 磷酸化的大多数功能。相似的方法用于确定 Kir6.2 通道的 PKA 依赖性调节作用[32a]。尽管缺乏外源性 cAMP，但 S27D 突变还是增加了电流振幅约 2 倍，引起通道激活电压负向转变，然而，当无 *KCNE1* 联合表达时，S27D 既没有显著增加 *KCNQ1* 通道的活性，也没有改变激活电压。因此，*KCNQ1* 的磷酸化不依赖于 *KCNE1* 的联合表达，但是磷酸化的通道转化为有基本生理活性的通道时需要 *KCNE1* 的存在；当不存在 *KCNE1* 时，*KCNQ1* 的磷酸化对通道的活性无显著的影响。值得注意的是，在无 *KCNE1* 联合表达时，*KCNQ1* 的磷酸化不引起通道活性的超极化，这表明 PKA 依赖性 *KCNQ1* 的磷酸化是通过 27 位残基的电荷来调节通道活性，且残基的改变到通道的激活这一转变需要 *KCNQ1* 和 *KCNE1* 的联合表达。从蛋白的磷酸化转变为通道必要的生理功能是 *KCNE1* 辅助亚单位一个新的作用，在 LQT-5 中，这一作用被破坏，同时也是心血管疾病时脑到心脏的信号解耦联的一个机制。

三、遗传性 *KCNE1* 突变能破坏 SNS 对 I_{ks} 的功能性调节

与 LQT-5 有关的 *KCNE1* 突变即 D76N，能引起

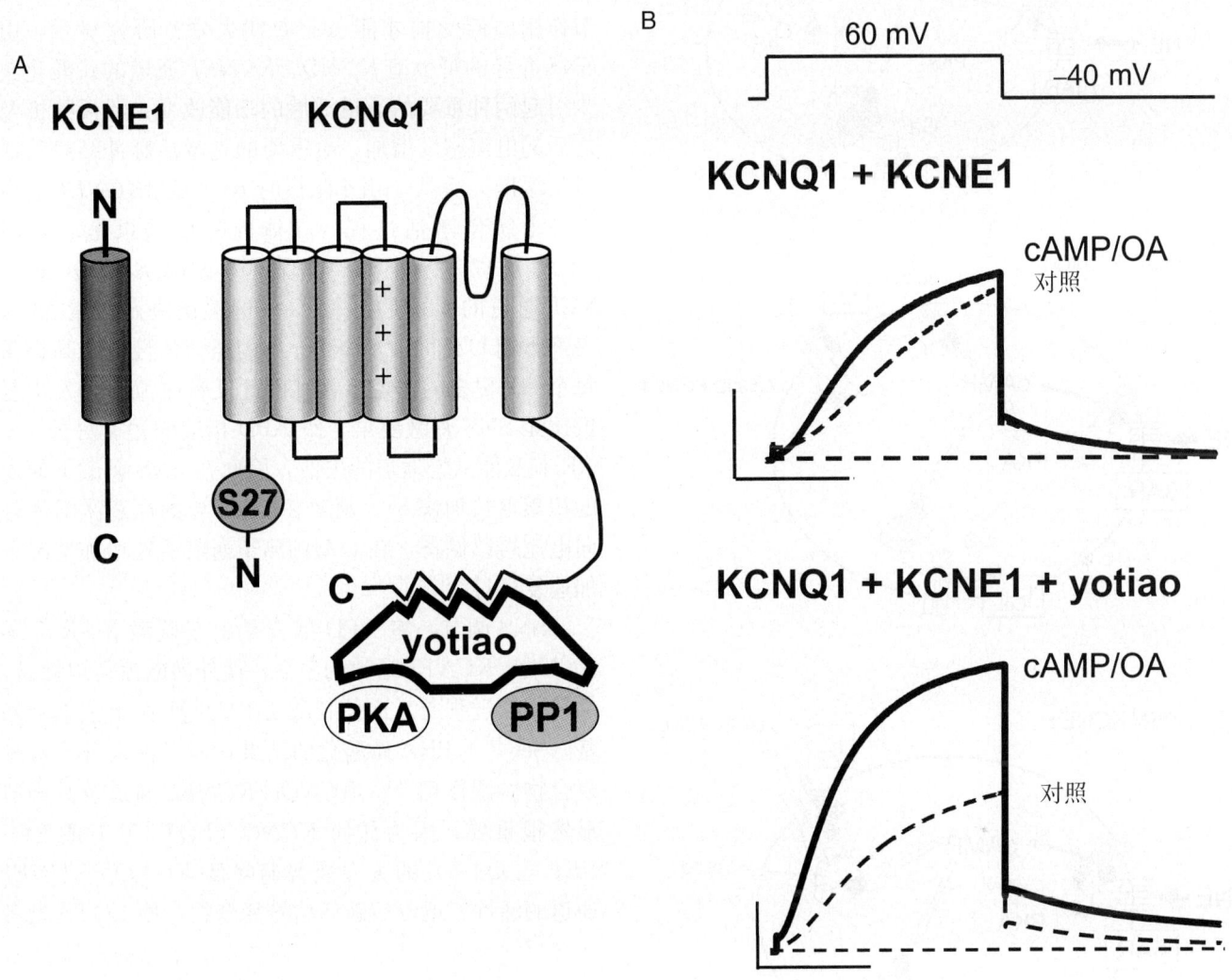

图17-2 A：KCNE1/KCNQ1/yotiao 大分子信号复合物。B：转染 KCNE1/KCNQ1（上组）和 KCNE1/KCNQ1/yotiao（下组）细胞记录的不存在（对照）和存在细胞内 cAMP/OA 时的膜电流。yotiao 细胞转染对表达电流的调节非常重要

cAMP 介导的 KCNQ1/KCNE1 通道调节的功能性破坏，尽管 KCNQ1 对 PKA 磷酸化作用仍存在反应。Kurokawa 和他的同事[32]发现，cAMP 介导的对 KCNQ1/KCNE1 通道的功能性调节，是 KCNQ1 N 端 PKA 磷酸化的结果，它需要 KCNQ1 和辅助亚单位 KCNE1 的联合表达（图17-3）。甚至像 D76N 这样的点突变也能严重破坏 KCNQ1 磷酸化的功能结果。这一突变减少了基础电流密度，即使在不存在 SNS 刺激时，表达它的细胞复极电流降低，出现细胞动作电位和 QT 间期延长。突变消除了 cAMP 对通道的功能性调节，结果是预想的复极延迟，在 SNS 刺激时更明显，表明突变导致 K$^+$ 通道活性储备不足，不能对抗 SNS 激活的 L 型钙离子通道。因此，随着交感活性的增高，ADP 控制不足。KCNE1 疾病相关突变改变了磷酸化通道复合物对 SNS 驱动的分子信号的生理性反应，但与 KCNQ1 C 端的 LZ 结构的突变一样[19]，通道复合物并没有与这些信号分子解耦联。

四、SNS 介导的调节作用引起 I_{Ks} 通道解耦联：心律失常的新机制

心脏至少有 3 种关键的离子通道（RyR2、L 型通道和 KCNQ1/KCNE1 通道）是 PKA 依赖性的调节作用，其调节作用需要组装 LZ 介导的大分子复合物，

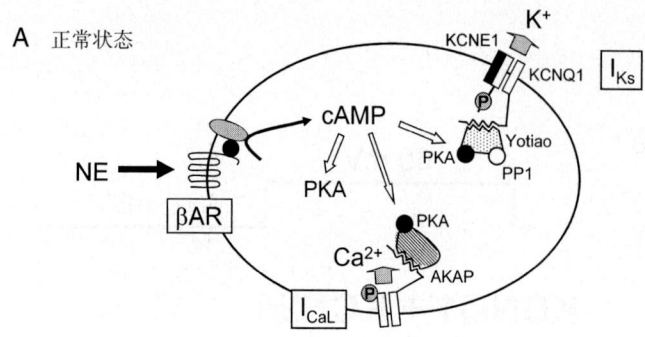
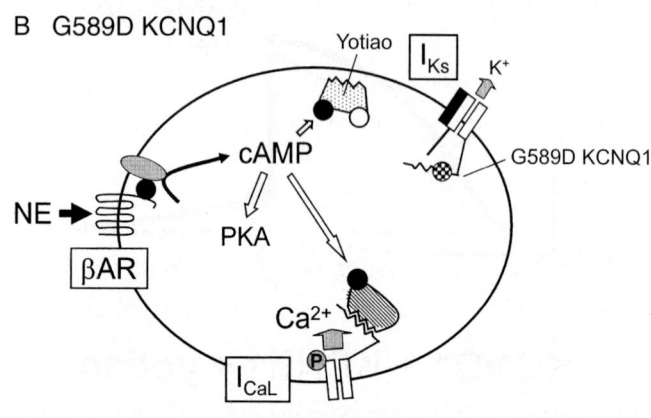
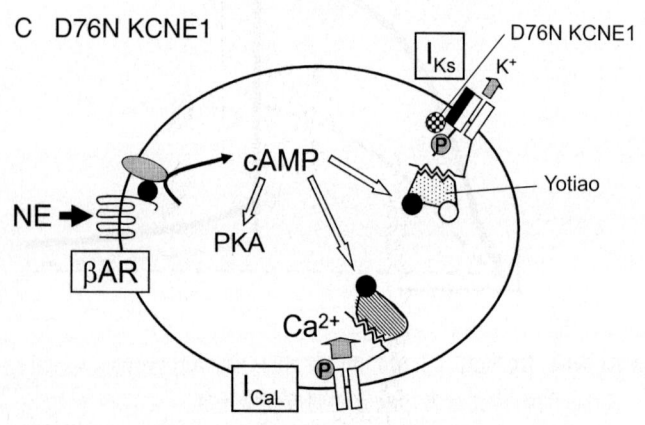

图 17-3 图解显示心肌细胞 L 型钙离子通道的信号微结构域和 KCNE1/KCNQ1/yotiao 复合物（E1/Q1） A：在野生型细胞，刺激 β-AR 能提高细胞内 cAMP，导致钙离子通道和钾离子通道的蛋白激酶 A（PKA）依赖性磷酸化。B：LQT-1 G589D 突变引起 yotiao 解耦联，阻止了 I_{ks} 通道的 β-AR 介导的磷酸化，但不影响 I_{CaL} 通道。C：LQT-5 D76N 突变并不能阻止 I_{ks} 通道的 PKA 磷酸化，但是消除了对 β-AR 刺激的功能性反应。LTCCs 不被这种突变影响

因此这组复合物的破坏能引起对 SNS 刺激反应的失衡（图 17-4）。LQT-1 突变 G589D，是与疾病有关的微结构域信号复合物破坏的第一个例子，KCNE1 的 D76N 突变是第二个新的局部离子通道调节受损机制。

然而，后面的例子是功能解耦联而不是生化结构的解耦联。

LZ 介导的对 I_{Ks}（KCNQ1/KCNE1 通道）的调节作用如何受损才能引起心律失常？研究显示，由 SNS 介导的野生型 KCNQ1/KCNE1 通道的磷酸化至少引起两种重要的通道活性的功能改变：激活除极及之后的电流密度增加，更重要的是激活脉冲结束后通道的缓慢失活[33]。由于除极时 KCNQ1/KCNE1 通道有一个缓慢激活过程（在体内除极结果是心室肌 AP），所以每一个 AP 过程中开放的 KCNQ1/KCNE1 通道的累积是心室 APD 的关键决定因素之一，最终影响 QT 间期。SNS 介导的通道活性的升高提供每个 AP 更多的通道活性，因此反转电流平衡发生复极比无 SNS 刺激要早，使 APD 相应缩短。另外，β-AR 刺激能减慢通道的失活，因此在 SNS 刺激下通道的积累增长加快[34]。刺激 β-AR 介导的通道激活使外向电流得以储备，在 L 型钙离子通道活性增加情况下加速复极过程[3]。

SNS 调节心室 APD 部分是由于刺激 β-AR 介导 KCNQ1/KCNE1 通道的激活，使外向电流得以储备，加速复极过程[3]。这种刺激是 KCNQ1 亚单位单个残基（Ser[27]）PKA 磷酸化的结果，与 C 端大分子信号复合物协调作用[19]。KCNQ1/KCNE1 通道及其调节显然很重要，因为任何 KCNQ（LQT-1）1 或 KCNE1（LQT-5）的突变能普遍降低 KCNQ1/KCNE1 通道的活性，或专门破坏信号复合物，使 LQTS 患者在交感活动增加时发生心律失常和猝死的危险性最大。

G589D 突变位于 KCNQ1 的 C 端 LZ 结构内，使 KCNQ1/KCNE1 通道与 SNS 介导的调节作用解耦联，但不影响 RyR2 或 L 型钙离子通道，这两种通道都具有被 SNS 活动调节的能力。因此，RyR2 通道和 L 型钙离子通道的活性都升高，但是没有正常的 SNS 刺激的复极钾离子通道电流的升高。KCNE1 的 D76N 突变严重破坏了 KCNQ1 磷酸化的生理性相关功能，它消除了 cAMP 对 KCNQ1/KCNE1 通道的功能性调节，降低了基础电流密度。预计这种突变即使在无 SNS 刺激时，将降低患者的复极电流，延长细胞 APs，引起 QT 间期延长。受累患者在交感活性增高时钾通道活性储备不足，不能抵消 SNS 对 L 型钙离子通道的刺激，因而不足以控制 APD。D76N 突变，并不是使通道与 SNS 介导的磷酸化作用解耦联，而是有效地破坏了通道对 SNS 活动的功能性反应，实质

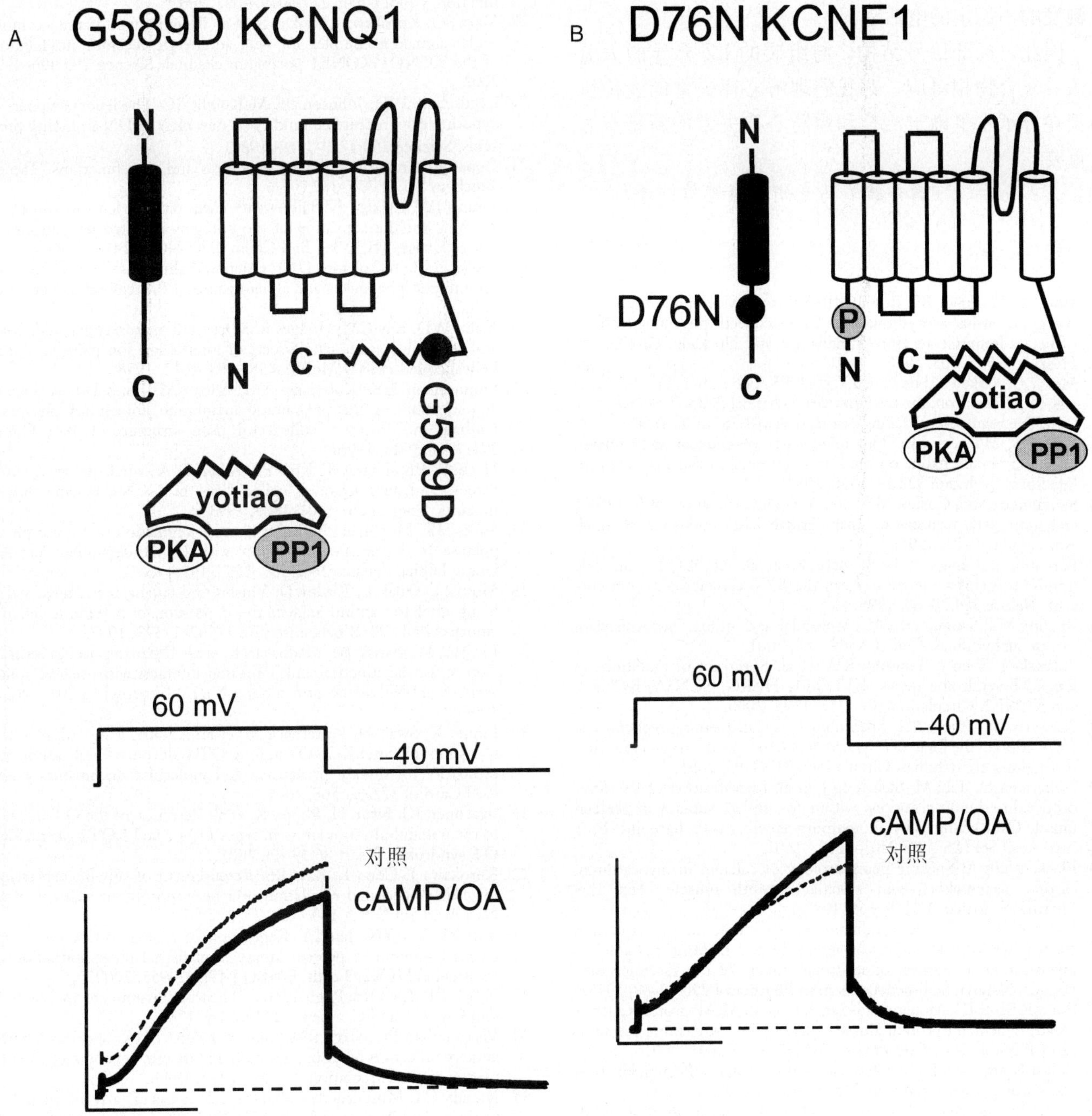

图 17-4 I_{ks}（*KCNQ1*/*KCNE1*）通道与 cAMP 依赖性调节作用解耦联的直接试验证据　A：G589D　LQT-3 突变与 KCNE1/KCNQ1/yotiao 信号复合物解耦联（上组）。下组：细胞转染 KCNE1/G589D（KCNQ1）/yotiao 的 CHO 细胞的电流对 cAMP/OA 无反应。B：联合表达 D76N KCNE1 和 KCNQ1/yotiao（上组）消除了电流对 cAMP/OA 的功能性反应（引自 Kurokawa J, Chen L, Kass RS: Requirement of subunit expression for cAMP-mediated regulation of a heart potassium channel. Proc Natl Acad Sci USA 100：2122-2127, 2003.）

上，最终的结果与 *KCNQ1* 的 G589D 突变相似：在 SNS 作用时离子电流失衡。

钙调机制的失衡使细胞易发生两种类型钙介导的心律失常：早后除极（EADs）[35,36] 和迟后除极（DADs）[37-39]，它们都能触发受累细胞发生心律失常。

KCNQ1/*KCNE1* 大分子信号复合物的点突变是引起疾病的两种新机制；LZ 突变引起的 I_{ks} 通道对 SNS 刺激反应的生理性破坏和 *KCNE1* 突变引起的功能性破坏。因此，*KCNQ1* LZ 结构或 *KCNQ1* 的辅助亚单位 *KCNE1* 上单个残基的遗传性突变能破坏脑和心脏

之间的信号传递，从而发生由钙介导的致心律失常事件触发的不稳定的电活动。

因此，局部信号结构，与组装的 LZ 介导的大分子信号复合物相对应，对我们理解心律失常的遗传机制及在分子水平确定治疗和预防心律失常的新靶点非常重要。

（浦介麟　马克娟　滕思勇　译）

参 考 文 献

1. Wit AL, Hoffman BF, Rosen MR: Electrophysiology and pharmacology of cardiac arrhythmias. IX. Cardiac electrophysiologic effects of beta adrenergic receptro stimulation and blockade. Part C. Am Heart J 90:795–803, 1975.
2. Marx SO, Reiken S, Hisamatsu Y, et al: PKA phosphorylation dissociates FKBP12.6 from the calcium release channel (ryanodine receptor): Defective regulation in failing hearts. Cell 101:365–376, 2000.
3. Kass RS, Wiegers SE: The ionic basis of concentration-related effects of noradrenaline on the action potential of calf cardiac purkinje fibres. J Physiol 322:541–558, 1982.
4. Sanguinetti MC, Curran ME, Zou A, et al: Coassembly of KvLQT1 and minK(IsK) proteins to form cardiac I(Ks) potassium channel. Nature 384:80–83, 1996.
5. Barhanin J, Lesage F, Guillemare E, et al: K(V)LQT1 and IsK (minK) proteins associate to form the I(Ks) cardiac potassium current. Nature 384:78–80, 1996.
6. Keating MT, Sanguinetti MC: Molecular and cellular mechanisms of cardiac arrhythmias. Cell 104:569–580, 2001.
7. Splawski I, Shen J, Timothy KW, et al: Spectrum of mutations in long-QT syndrome genes: KVLQT1, HERG, SCN5A, KCNE1, and KCNE2. Circulation 102:1178–1185, 2000.
8. Schwartz PJ, Priori SG, Spazzolini C, et al: Genotype-phenotype correlation in the long-QT syndrome: Gene-specific triggers for life-threatening arrhythmias. Circulation 103:89–95, 2001.
9. Nakayama H, Taki M, Striessnig J, et al: Identification of 1,4-dihydropyridine binding regions within the alpha1 subunit of skeletal muscle Ca2+ channels by photoaffinity labeling with diazepine. Proc Natl Acad Sci U S A 88:9203–9207, 1991.
10. Fleckenstein A: Specific pharmacology of calcium in myocardium, cardiac pacemakers, and vascular smooth muscle. Ann Rev Pharmacol Toxicol 17:149–166, 1977.
11. Bayer R, Hennekes R, Kaufmann R, Mannhold R: Iontorpic and electrophysiological actions of verapamil and D600 in mammalian myocardium: I. Pattern of inotropic effects of the racemic compounds. Naunyn Schmiedebergs Arch Pharmacol 290:49–68, 1975.
12. Potet F, Scott JD, Mohammad-Panah R, et al: AKAP proteins anchor cAMP-dependent protein kinase to KvLQT1/IsK channel complex. Am J Physiol Heart Circ Physiol 280:H2038–H2045, 2001.
13. Edwards AS, Scott JD: A-kinase anchoring proteins: Protein kinase A and beyond. Curr Opin Cell Biol 12:217–221, 2000.
14. Scott JD, Dell'Acqua ML, Fraser ID, et al: Coordination of cAMP signaling events through PKA anchoring. Adv Pharmacol 47:175–207, 2000.
15. Gray PC, Scott JD, Catterall WA: Regulation of ion channels by cAMP-dependent protein kinase and A-kinase anchoring proteins. Curr Opin Neurobiol 8:330–334, 1998.
17. Marx SO, Reiken S, Hisamatsu Y, et al: Phosphorylation-dependent regulation of ryanodine receptors: A novel role for leucine/isoleucine zippers. J Cell Biol 153:699–708, 2001.
18. Hulme JT, Ahn M, Hauschka SD, et al: A novel leucine zipper targets AKAP15 and cyclic AMP-dependent protein kinase to the C terminus of the skeletal muscle Ca2+ channel and modulates its function. J Biol Chem 277:4079–4087, 2002.
19. Marx SO, Kurokawa J, Reiken S, et al: Requirement of a macromolecular signaling complex for beta adrenergic receptor modulation of the KCNQ1-KCNE1 potassium channel. Science 295:496–499, 2002.
20. Landschulz WH, Johnson PF, McKnight SL: The leucine zipper: A hypothetical structure common to a new class of DNA binding proteins. Science 240:1759–1764, 1988.
21. Lupas A: Coiled coils: New structures and new functions. Trends Biochem Sci 21:375–382, 1996.
22. Leung IW, Lassam N: Dimerization via tandem leucine zippers is essential for the activation of the mitogen-activated protein kinase kinase kinase, MLK-3. J Biol Chem 273:32408–32415, 1998.
23. Walshaw J, Woolfson DN: Open-and-shut cases in coiled-coil assembly: Alpha-sheets and alpha-cylinders. Protein Sci 10:668–673, 2001.
24. Kohn WD, Kay CM, Hodges RS: Orientation, positional, additivity, and oligomerization-state effects of interhelical ion pairs in alpha-helical coiled-coils. J Mol Biol 283:993–1012, 1998.
25. Simmerman HK, Kobayashi YM, Autry JM, Jones LR: A leucine zipper stabilizes the pentameric membrane domain of phospholamban and forms a coiled-coil pore structure. J Biol Chem 271:5941–5946, 1996.
26. Harbury PB, Zhang T, Kim PS, Alber T: A switch between two-, three-, and four-stranded coiled coils in GCN4 leucine zipper mutants. Science 262:1401–1407, 1993.
27. Surks HK, Mochizuki N, Kasai Y, et al: Regulation of myosin phosphatase by a specific interaction with cGMP-dependent protein kinase Ialpha. Science 286:1583–1587, 1999.
28. Moitra J, Szilak L, Krylov D, Vinson C: Leucine is the most stabilizing aliphatic amino acid in the d position of a dimeric leucine zipper coiled coil. Biochemistry 36:12567–12573, 1997.
29. Lin JW, Wyszynski M, Madhavan R, et al: Yotiao, a novel protein of neuromuscular junction and brain that interacts with specific splice variants of NMDA receptor subunit NR1. J Neurosci 18:2017–2027, 1998.
30. Piippo K, Swan H, Pasternack M, et al: A founder mutation of the potassium channel KCNQ1 in long QT syndrome: Implications for estimation of disease prevalence and molecular diagnostics. J Am Coll Cardiol 37:562–568, 2001.
31. Paavonen KJ, Swan H, Piippo K, et al: Response of the QT interval to mental and physical stress in types LQT1 and LQT2 of the long QT syndrome. Heart 86:39–44, 2001.
32. Kurokawa J, Chen L, Kass RS: Requirement of subunit expression for cAMP-mediated regulation of a heart potassium channel. Proc Natl Acad Sci U S A 100:2122–2127, 2003.
32a. Lin YF, Jan YN, Jan LY: Regulation of ATP-sensitive potassium channel funciton b protein kinase A–mediated phosphorylation in transfected HEK293 cells. EMBO J 19:942–955, 2000.
33. Walsh KB, Kass RS: Regulation of a heart potassium channel by protein kinase A and C. Science 242:67–69, 1988.
34. Viswanathan PC, Shaw RM, Rudy Y: Effects of IKr and IKs heterogeneity on action potential duration and its rate dependence: A simulation study. Circulation 99:2466–2474, 1999.
35. January CT, Moscucci A: Cellular mechanisms of early afterdepolarizations. Ann N Y Acad Sci 644:23–32, 1992.
36. January CT, Riddle JM: Early afterdepolarizations: Mechanism of induction and block. A role for L-type Ca2+ current. Circ Res 64:977–990, 1989.
37. January CT, Fozzard HA: Delayed afterdepolarizations in heart muscle: Mechanisms and relevance. Pharmacol Rev 40:219–227, 1988.
38. Wit AL, Rosen MR: Pathophysiologic mechanisms of cardiac arrhythmias. Am Heart J 106:798–811, 1983.
39. Kass RS, Lederer JW, Tsien RW, Weingart R: Role of calcium ions in transient inward currents and aftercontractions induced by strophanthidin in cardiac Purkinje fibres. J Physiol 281:187–208, 1978.

第 18 章

药物诱发的通道病

Charles Antzelevitch

本章目录

- 药物诱发的与 LQTS 有关的通道疾病 …………………… 147
- 药物影响多种离子通道 ………… 149
- 遗传学对于药物诱发的 LQTS 的影响 ……………………………………… 152
- 致谢 …………………………… 152

药物诱发的对离子通道活性的调节，可以影响传导、促进复极化的离散、引起触发激动，因此能引起被动性或主动性心律失常的产生。钠通道和钙通道阻滞剂能抑制内向电流常减慢传导、降低兴奋性，并引起窦房阻滞和房室阻滞继发的缓慢性心律失常。同样，抑制内向电流也可以引起主动性心律失常：以单向阻滞和缓慢传导的形式形成基质产生折返，或者通过引起动作电位平台期丢失而显著缩短心外膜下动作电位所致。在后一种情况下，钠通道和钙通道阻滞可以引起透壁的或心外膜下复极离散，导致 2 相折返引起的期前收缩、ST 段抬高、多形性室性心动过速及所有 Brugada 综合征的电生理特征[1]。当抑制外向复极电流时，通常引起动作电位时程（APD）增加和早后除极（EAD），引起触发活动。因为 APD 延长通常是不一致的，所以抑制外向电流的药物通常能增加跨壁复极离散度（TDR），因而导致基质发生尖端扭转型室速（TdP），这是 LQTS 的特征表现[2]。本章重点讲获得性 LQTS，即最常见的药物诱发的通道病。

一、药物诱发的与 LQTS 有关的通道疾病

QT 间期是通过体表测量心室复极所需的时间。QT 间期延长发生在大部分心室肌细胞动作电位延长时，原因可能是一个或更多的复极电流减小、或内向电流增大、或两者同时改变。药物对 APD 的影响是由其改变内向和外向电流作用的平衡决定的。ADP 延长可以是药物对一个或多个离子通道、离子泵或交换体影响的结果。抑制快速激活延迟整流钾通道（I_{Kr}）是药物引起 QT 间期延长的最常见的原因[3]。在后面还要讨论，有许多药物阻断多个离子通道，因而引起更复杂的动作电位形态改变。

I_{Kr} 阻断和 QT 间期延长在近几年里吸引了极大的兴趣，因为它们可能和一些危及生命的心律失常有关，例如尖端扭转型室速[4]。有Ⅲ类作用的抗心律失常药物，通过阻断钾通道延长心脏的复极，首先列入这类与致心律失常综合征相关的药物。研究表明，用奎尼丁治疗的病人其 TdP 的发生率估计为 2.0%～8.8%[5-7]。DL-索他洛尔引起的心律失常发生率是 1.8%～4.8%。有一些新的Ⅲ类药物也有相近的发生率，如得菲利特[11]、依布利特[12]。

数量不断增加的非心血管药物，大多数是通过抑制 I_{Kr} 引起 TdP 或使其恶化[4]。这些药物包括 50 多种商品化的或用于研究的非心血管药物以及 20 多种心血管系统非抗心律失常作用的药物。最近几年里一些新药频繁出现这个问题，从而使许多制剂撤出市场（例如：prenylamine, terodiline, sertindole, grepafloxacin, terfenadine, astemizole, cisapride）。

药物诱发的 TdP 在很大程度上是复极离散增加的

结果，是继发于心室肌细胞内的电不均一性的放大[13-22]。在过去的十年里，有证据表明我们对心室肌细胞多样性的正确评价有显著的进展。大量的研究已经阐明了心室肌细胞电生理特性的区域性差异，以及不同的细胞类型对药理学试剂和病理状态的反应的不同（见 Antzelevitch 和 Dumaine[15] Antzelevitch 及同事[19]的综述）。在这些已经揭示的不均一性中，包括犬、猫、兔、大鼠、小鼠和人类心脏心内膜和心外膜心肌细胞电学和药理学的差异，以及位于心室深层结构的 M 细胞的电生理特征和药理学反应的差异。

M 细胞的特征是心率减慢时和（或）受延长 QT 间期的药物作用时其动作电位的延长比心外膜和心内膜细胞更多[23]。这些特征的离子基础包括存在一个较小的缓慢激活的延迟整流电流 I_{Ks}、一个较大的延迟钠电流（late I_{Na}）和一个较大的生电性的钠-钙交换电流（I_{Na-Ca}）。有报道在犬、豚鼠、兔、猪和人的心室里都有 M 特征的细胞[2]。

这三种类型心室肌细胞存在复极时程的差异，产生电压梯度，形成心电图上的 T 波。当发生 LQT 时，M 细胞的 APD 延长被认为是为心律失常的形成提供了基质。应用动脉灌注楔标本的研究，已经复制出获得性 LQTS 的试验模型（图 18-1）。这种楔模型能够产生并维持多种心律失常，包括 TdP。

单独阻断 I_{Ks} 可以使心室壁全层复极均一延长，但不引起心律失常（见图 18-1A）。当加用异丙肾上腺素时能导致心外膜和心内膜的 APD 缩短，而对 M 细胞的 APD 没有改变或改变很小，从而引起 TDR 的显著增大，形成自发性或刺激诱导的 TdP[24]。这些细胞的改变通常引起 LQT1 特征性的宽 T 波和长 QT 间期。在这种模型下，TdP 的形成对 β 肾上腺素的刺激非常敏感，这和先天性 LQTS 尤其是 LQT1 对自主神经刺激的高敏感性相一致[25]。

D-索他洛尔阻断 I_{Kr} 也会引起 M 细胞动作电位较大程度的延长，以及三种细胞动作电位 3 相的减慢，这将引起 T 波振幅降低、QT 间期延长、TDR 增大，形成自发性或刺激诱导的 TdP（见图 18-1B）。低钾血症进一步加重了 T 波振幅的降低，形成了低凹形的或双峰的外形，类似于在 LQT2 型综合征患者中常见的心电图表现[26,27]。

ATX-Ⅱ 使延迟钠电流增大，显著延长 QT 间期，T 波形成延迟，有的病例 T 波增宽，并通过延长 M 细胞的 APD 引起 TDR 的明显增加（见图 18-1C）。ATX-Ⅱ 延长心外膜和心内膜的 APD 相对强的作用导致了 T 波发生的延迟，这与 LQT3 型患者常观察到的

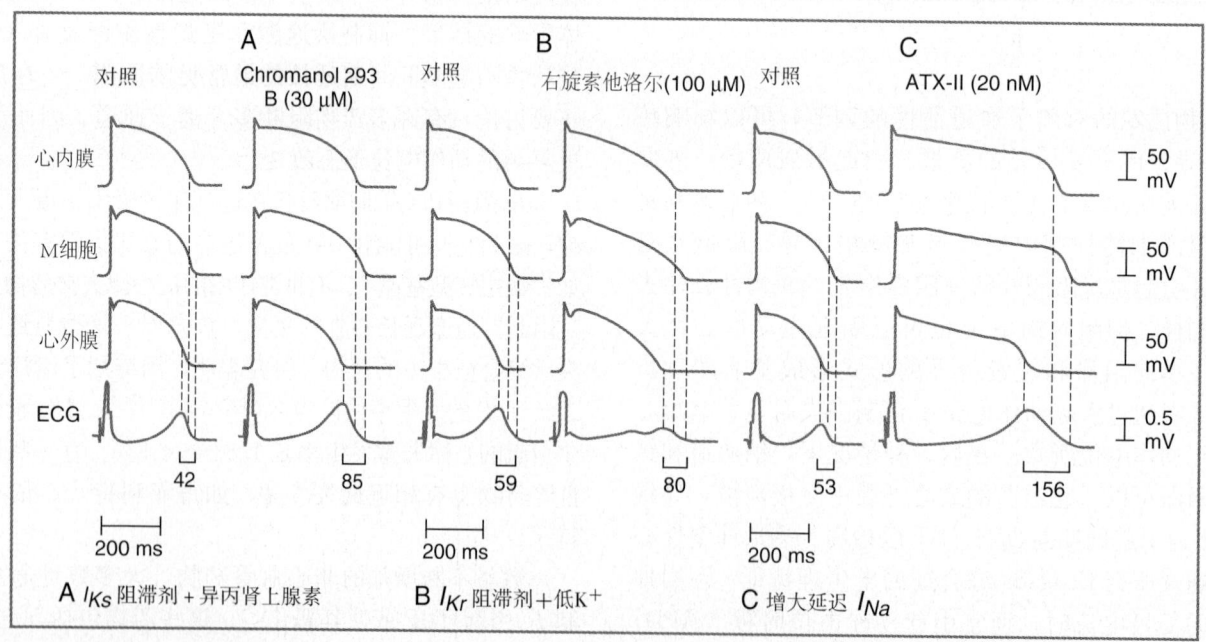

图 18-1 用犬的动脉灌注左室楔模型，记录跨膜动作电位和跨壁心电图，分别为对照和使用 I_{Ks} 阻断剂（A）、I_{Kr} 阻断剂（B）、增大延迟 I_{Na}（C）后的改变。图中同时记录了心内膜（Endo）、M 细胞和心外膜（Epi）的动作电位和跨壁 ECG。BCL=2000ms。在所有的例子中，ECG 的 T 波顶点和心外膜动作电位的复极一致，而 T 波的终末与 M 细胞动作电位的复极相一致。心内膜细胞的复极介于 M 细胞和心外膜细胞复极时间之间。整个心室壁复极的跨壁离散定义为 M 细胞和心外膜细胞复极时间的差异，在图中心电图下面的一行表示（引自 Shimizu W，Antzelevitch C：Cellular basis for the electrocardiographic features of the LQT1 form of the long QT syndrom：Effects of β-adrenergic agonists, antagonists and sodium channel blockers on transmural dispersion of repolarization and Torsades de Pointes. Circulation 9 8；2314-2322，1998；and Shimizu W，Antzelevitch C：Sodium channel block with mexiletine is effective in reducing dispersion of repolarization and preventing Torsade de pointes in LQT2 and LQT3 models of the long QT syndrom . Circulation 96；2038-2047，1997.）

T 波出现晚和等电位 ST 段的延长相一致。

在先天性或获得性 LQTS 中最常遇到的快速性心律失常是 TdP，是一种典型的多形性室性心律失常。TdP 最常见于使用了 I_{Kr} 阻断剂的患者，尤其是存在低钾血症、心率缓慢或长间歇等类似于使用 I_{Kr} 阻断剂的情况下，在分离的浦肯野纤维和 M 细胞能引起 EAD 和触发激活。一次 EAD 诱发的期前收缩被认为可以引起期前收缩引发的 TdP，但是心律失常的维持通常认为是由环路折返引起（见参考文献 2）。此外，在 wedge 模型，可以自发的或用电刺激诱导产生 TdP。图 12-8 显示了一个药物诱发 TdP 的例子，楔型灌流的是生理温度的台式液。如果灌注的是冷的液体，所有局灶的期外收缩活动就被抑制，不能观察到自发性的 TdP，但是心律失常很容易被单个发生在心外膜的期前收缩诱发，该部位心肌不应期最短。动作电位记录显示以 TDR 的形式持续存在一个折返基质。综合以上观察到的现象有力地证明了折返机制是 TdP 的基础。

尽管存在或不存在 QT 间期延长，多形性室性心律失常可以是局灶和折返机制二者导致的结果，已有的证据表明以下的假说，这两种机制可能是大多数 LQT 相关的 TdP 的基础（图 18-3）。这一假说假定在基础条件下，存在 TDR 形式的电不均一性。有一些药物通过抑制 I_{Kr}/I_{Ks} 或增强延迟 I_{Ca}/延迟 I_{Na} 来降低复极电流，放大这种内在的不均一性。凡能导致 I_{kr} 降低或延迟 I_{Na} 增强的情况，可以优先延长 M 细胞的动作电位，继而 QT 间期延长伴随着 TDR 的显著增大，这就形成了产生折返的易损窗。复极电流的降低也为在 M 细胞和浦肯野细胞发生 EAD 诱发的触发活动提供了前提。当触发活动落在易损期时，将引起期前收缩触发 TdP。在 I_{Kr} 阻断的情况下，β 受体激动剂进一步放大这种瞬时的跨壁电不均一性，但是在用 I_{Na} 促进剂的情况下则相反[28,29]。与此相比，降低 I_{Ks} 能引起整个心室壁 APD 均一的延长，导致 QT 间期延长但是并不增大 TDR。在这种情况下也不会产生自发的和程序电刺激引起的 TdP，除非使用 β 受体激动剂。除此，在缩短心外膜和心内膜 APD 的情况下，异丙肾上腺素可以显著增大 TDR，为 EAD 诱导的触发活动形成易损窗，进而发生 TdP。

二、药物影响多种离子通道

药物可以影响两种或更多的离子通道，例如奎尼丁、戊巴比妥、胺碘酮、ranolazine、azimilide 可以产

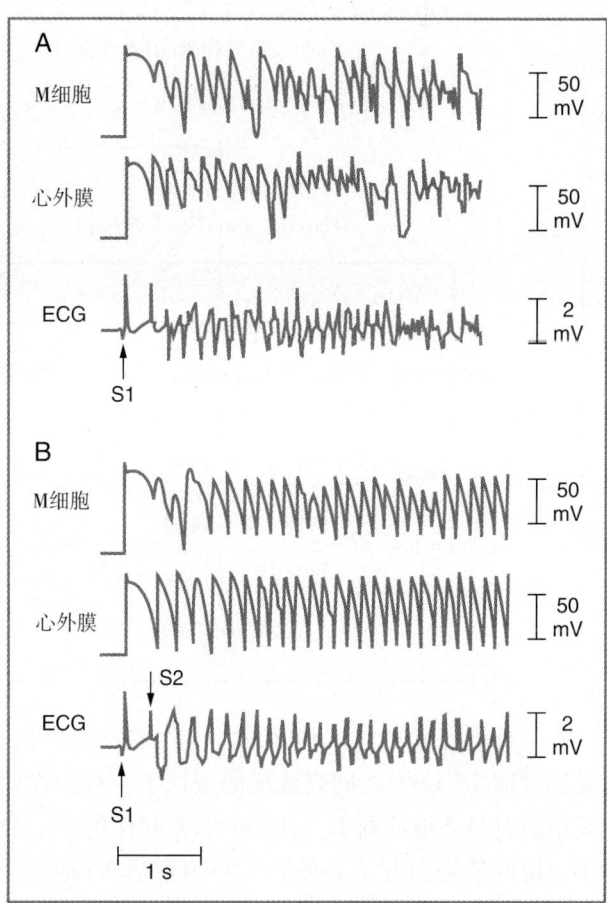

图 18-2　在犬动脉灌注的左室楔模型，自发性或电刺激诱发的具有 TdP 特征的多形性室性心动过速。A：自发性 TdP 发生在用 chromanol（30μmol/L）+异丙肾上腺素（100nmol/L）预处理的模型。一次自发性的期前收缩配对间期为 285ms，可能起源于心内膜下的浦肯野系统，引起了阵发性 TdP。B：灌注温度较凉（36℃）时失去期前收缩活动，可能是因为缺乏早后除极引起的触发活动。除此，发生在心外膜（不应期最短的部位）的单独期前收缩可以引起 TdP，证明折返旁路以复极跨壁离散的形式存在。S1-S1=2000ms（引自 Antzelevitch C，Shimizu W：Cellular mechanisms underlying the long QT syndrome. Curr Opin Cardiol 17：43-51，2002）

生更复杂的反应。低治疗浓度奎尼丁 3μmol/L～5μmol/L 可以使 M 细胞的 APD 显著延长但并不影响心外膜和心内膜的 APD，同时在这个浓度也可以显著地抑制 I_{Kr}。而较高浓度的奎尼丁可以进一步延长心内膜和心外膜的动作电位时程，同时可以阻断 I_{Ks}，但因为抑制了延迟 I_{Na} 可以缩短 M 细胞的 APD[30]。因此低浓度奎尼丁可以延长 QT 间期、增大 TDR，然而在较高浓度时 QT 间期延长并不伴有 TDR 增大。这可能解释为什么奎尼丁在低治疗浓度时会引起 TdP 但在高浓度或中毒剂量却不会引起 TdP[19,31]。

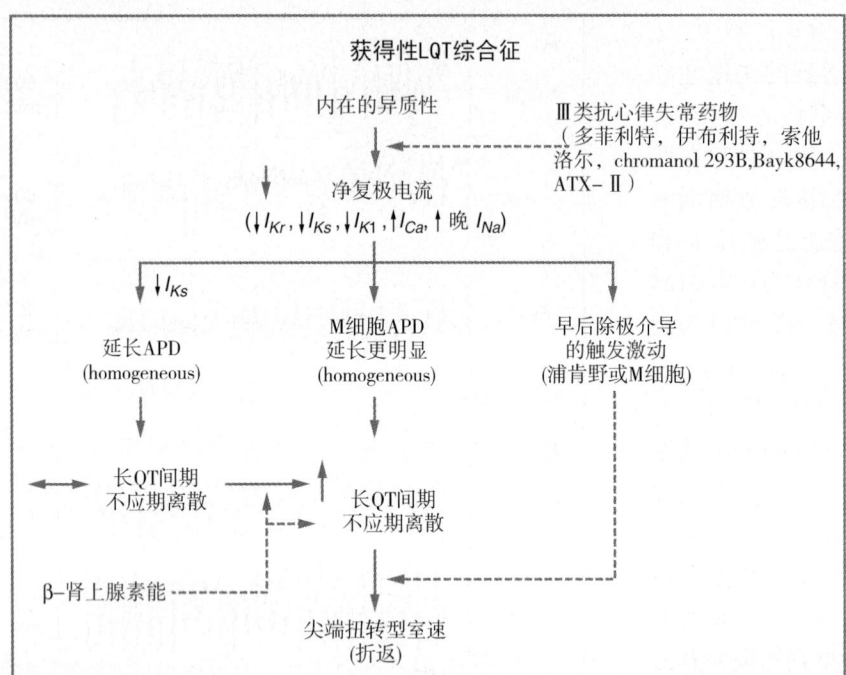

图 18-3 获得性 LQTS 产生 TdP 的细胞机制　APD：动作电位时程；EAD：早后除极

有一种延长 QT 间期却降低 TDR 的药物如戊巴比妥钠（图 18-4）[32]。同高浓度的奎尼丁一样，戊巴比妥钠通过显著地抑制 I_{Kr}、I_{Ks} 和 I_{Na} 来起作用[33]。这种多通道的阻滞引起了心外膜和心内膜 APD 延长大于 M 细胞，使得 TDR 明显变小。此外，药物对延迟 I_{Na}（和 I_{Ca}）的影响也抑制 D-索他洛尔对 M 细胞诱发的 EAD 活动。尽管戊巴比妥钠有延长 QT 间期的作用，但是不会引起 TdP[32]。由于它可以降低跨膜离散度并抑制 EAD 引起的触发活动，这种麻醉剂可以有效地抑制 D-索他洛尔引起的 TdP[18]。

胺碘酮是另一种能延长 QT 间期的药物，但仅在少数情况下会引起 TdP。胺碘酮是一种重要的抗心律失常药物，用于控制房性或室性心律失常。它除了有 β 受体阻断的特性外，还可以阻断心脏的钠通道、钾通道和钙通道。胺碘酮相对于其他Ⅲ类抗心律失常药物来讲，它的有效抗心律失常作用和低的致心律失常发生率，归因于它复杂的药理作用。胺碘酮长期使用时（口服每日 30～40mg/kg，使用 30～45 天），可明显延长狗心外膜和心内膜的 ADP，而对 M 区的 ADP 延长较少甚至轻度的缩短，因此降低 TDR[34]。此外，胺碘酮长期使用还可以抑制 I_{Kr} 阻断剂 D-索他洛尔引起的复极离散和 EAD 的作用。因此长期胺碘酮治疗可以改变心室肌细胞的电生理特性，使跨壁复极离散度降低，尤其是在离散增大的情况下。对于慢性房室阻滞的犬来说，胺碘酮是唯一不会引起 TdP 的Ⅲ类抗心律失常药物[35]。

Ranolazine 是一种试验性的抗心绞痛药物，已有研究表明其具有类似于胺碘酮的作用，可以改变离子和细胞活动[36]。同胺碘酮一样，Ranolazine 可以阻断延迟 I_{Na}（IC$_{50}$：5.9μmol/L）、I_{Kr}、I_{Ca}（IC$_{50}$：296μmol/L）。尽管它能有效地阻断 I_{Kr}，但它只是轻度延长 QT 间期，因为它同时有效地阻断了内向电流，尤其是延迟钠电流。虽然 Ranolazine 有延长 QT 间期的作用，但可以降低 TDR，抑制 D-索他洛尔诱发的 EAD 活动。而且在试验动物模型上，Ranolazine 并不能引起自发性的 TdP 以及程序刺激诱发的心律失常。但这些结果阐明，即使是有效的阻断 I_{Kr}，也不能就此一点证明该药物有致心律失常的作用。

最近的研究进一步证明了这一结论。在小鼠的心房瘤细胞（AT-1）和转染了人类 HERG 基因的 Ltk 细胞中，就一系列临床上具有诱发 TdP 风险的抗心律失常药物评价了 I_{Kr} 阻断的重要性[37]。结果提示并非所有引起 TdP 的药物都是有效的 I_{Kr} 阻断剂。I_{Kr} 阻断也不是发生 TdP 所必需的，这些药物的其他特性也参与了诱发 TdP。

虽延长 QT 间期而不引起 TdP 的抗心律失常药物有一个共同点就是可以抑制 I_{Ks}、I_{Kr}、I_{Na}（和/或 I_{Ca}），因此可以延长不应期而不增大 TDR，实际上在一些情况下还会降低跨膜离散度。

另一种可以延长 QT 间期而不增大 TDR 的药理学试剂是 I_{Ks} 阻断剂 chromanol 293B，可以使心室壁 APD 均一性延长[24]。尽管它可以延长 QT 间期，但

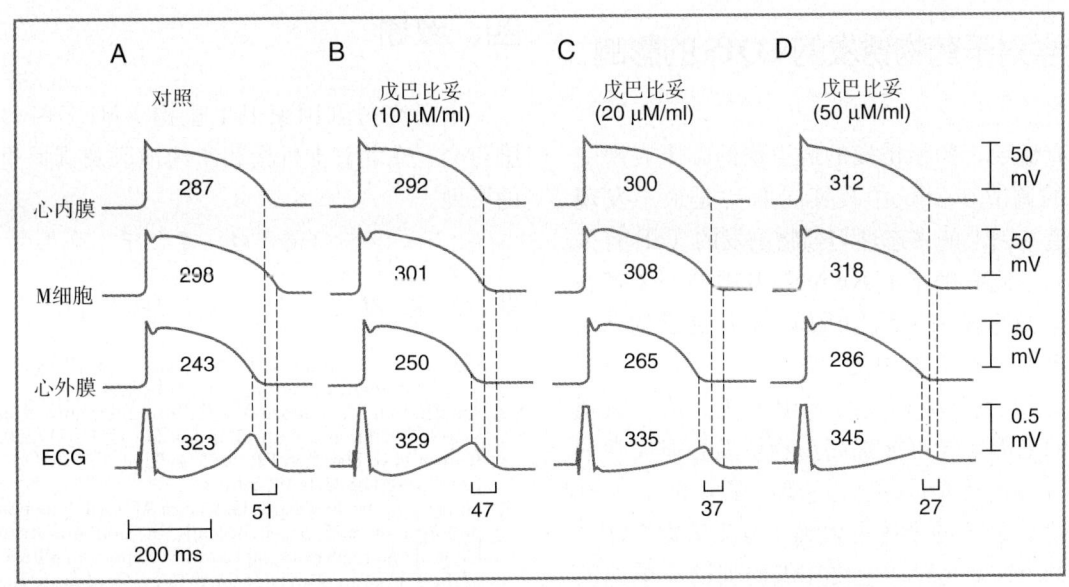

图 18-4 戊巴比妥钠对动作电位和心电图的剂量依赖性（10，20，50μg/ml）作用，在犬动脉灌注左室楔形模型上 图中显示：同时在心内膜（Endo）、M 细胞和心外膜（Epi）记录的动作电位和跨壁 ECG。BCL=2000ms。戊巴比妥延长 QT 间期，增大心外膜和心内膜细胞的 APD 比对 M 细胞明显，因此降低跨膜复极离散，以剂量依赖的方式使 T 波变平坦。每个动作电相位关的数字指的是 APD_{90} 的值。标记在心电图上的数字指的是 QT 间期。在心电图下一行的数字表示复极跨壁离散（引自 Shimizu W，McMahon B，Antzelevitch C：Sodium pentobarbital reduces transmural dispersion of repolarization and prevents Torsades de pointes in models of acquired and congenital long QT syndromes＞ J Cardiovasc Electrophysiol 10：156-164，1999.）

在试验模型中从未引起 TdP，不管是自发性的还是程序电刺激引起的。如增加一种 β 肾上腺素能药物就可以显著缩短心外膜和心内膜的 ADP，但不改变 M 细胞的 ADP，因而能引起显著的复极离散，这将会产生自发性或刺激诱发的 TdP。这些发现支持这个假说，即 LQT 首要的问题不是长的 QT 间期，而是复极的离散，后者经常伴随 QT 间期的延长。

如果 QT 间期延长和 I_{Kr} 阻断不是可靠的证据来推断药物有诱发 TdP 的倾向，那还有更好的替代指标吗？从前面的讨论中知道，TDR 可能是更为可靠的指标，但是怎样才能从体表心电图中量化这一参数呢？对动脉灌注心室楔形标本（wedge prepatation）的研究提示，从 T 波锋到终末的间期（T_{peak}-T_{end}）可以提供合理的 TDR 指标。

当 T 波向上时，心外膜复极反应最早，M 细胞动作电位是最晚的。心外膜动作电位完全复极化和 T 波的顶峰一致，M 细胞复极和 T 波的终末一致。因此可以说 M 细胞的动作电位时程决定了 QT 间期，而心外膜动作电位的时程决定了 QT 峰间期。从这些研究得到另一个有趣的发现是，T 波锋至终末的间期可以提供 TDR 的指标[19,26]。图 18-1 显示了在基础状态和 LQTS 时两者的关系[19,27,29]。

从胸前导联测量 T 波锋至终末的间期最有意义，因为它可以更准确地反映 TDR。在更复杂的负向、双向或三向的 T 波时，从 T 波的第一个成分的最低点到 T 波终末的间期可作为 TDR 心电图的近似值[38]。

有研究证实了把 T 波锋至终末间期作为跨膜离散度的指标和心律失常风险因子的有效性。这些研究报告显示，在各种已知的倾向于引起 TdP 的条件下，T 波锋至终末间期延长[2,39-47]。但需要进一步的研究来评价如电不均一性等这些非侵入性的参数，及其在估计心律失常风险的预后价值。

最近的研究包括心房灌注在内的研究提示，在 T 波锋值和终末之间的区域可能在较宽的条件下提供 TDR 的指标（Tsuboi 和 Antzelevitch 尚未发表的结果）。特别是 Van Opstal 及其同事最近报告显示，在慢性房室阻滞的犬，JT 区和心室间的复极离散相关，这是另一个发生 TdP 风险指标。

TDR 不应该与复极 QT 离散度搞混，这是提出的另一个尚有某些矛盾的危险因子。

三、遗传学对于药物诱发的 LQTS 的影响

最近研究显示，药物诱发的通道病的临床表现受到遗传因素的调节。Abbott 及其同事[49]是最早发现一个离子通道基因上的多态性与药物诱发的 TdP 有关的研究者之一。他们确定了 KCNE2 基因的一个多态性位点 T8A，这个基因编码 MiRP，是 I_{kr} 通道的 β 亚单位。这一多态性在人群中的比例是 1.6%，其与奎尼丁和新诺明/甲氧苄啶相关的 TdP 有关。这一发现提示，普通的基因变异可能提高药物诱发心律失常的风险。最近 Yang 及其同事[50]发现，在大约 10%～15% 的获得性 LQTS 的个体可以确定有先天性 LQTS 基因编码区的 DNA 变异，主要在编码辅助亚单位的基因上，进一步支持假说——即亚临床的突变和多态性可能易于产生药物诱发的 TdP。Splawski 及同事进一步发展了这一概念。在那些有升高的获得性 TdP 的风险的非洲人和美国黑人中，通过一个由药物诱发的心律失常的个体组成的人群，他们确定了一个在钠通道基因 SCA5N 上涉及丝氨酸和酪氨酸亚单位杂合的多态性（S1102Y）。这一多态性位点在有阵发性心律失常的 23 名患者中的比例是 57%，在对照组中为 13%。这一发现提示：应该确定这一多态性位点的携带者，并避免使用可增加致心律失常发生风险的药物治疗。因为用较低的花费就可以很快得到精确的结果，因此这项检查有可能得到广泛的应用。

基因变异也可以通过影响药物代谢来调节药物诱发的通道病。对于相对特异的 I_{Kr} 阻断剂，药物的血浆水平和 TdP 的发生率有明确的关系。负责药物代谢的酶其编码基因突变可以改变药物代谢动力学，引起血浆浓度较大的波动，因此产生显著的促心律失常作用[52,53]。例如，已经报道了在细胞色素酶 P4502D6（涉及一些 QT 延长药物代谢的酶）上有多个多态性位点，可以使其功能降低或失活；约有 5%～10% 的美国黑人和白人缺乏有功能的 P4502D6。研究显示，有大量的蛋白质（包括药物转运分子和其他药物代谢酶）参与药物的吸收、分布和清除。每一个基因的变异都有可能调节药物的浓度和作用。目前已经确定了细胞色素酶 P450 作用的多个底物和抑制剂。可以在网上（http://medicine.iupui.edu/flockhart/）找到一个综合的数据库。

四、致谢

本研究得到国家卫生机构（HL47678）、美国心脏协会、东北分支机构和纽约地区及佛罗里达州会员的资助。

（浦介麟 李 宁 滕思勇 译）

参 考 文 献

1. Antzelevitch C, Brugada P, Brugada J, et al: Brugada syndrome: A decade of progress. Circ Res 91:1114–1118, 2002.
2. Antzelevitch C, Shimizu W: Cellular mechanisms underlying the long QT syndrome. Curr Opin Cardiol 17:43–51, 2002.
3. Bednar MM, Harrigan EP, Anziano RJ, et al: The QT interval. Prog Cardiovasc Dis 43:1–45, 2001.
4. Haverkamp W, Breithardt G, Camm AJ, et al: The potential for QT prolongation and pro-arrhythmia by non-anti-arrhythmic drugs: Clinical and regulatory implications. Report on a Policy Conference of the European Society of Cardiology. Cardiovasc Res 47:219–233, 2000.
5. Selzer A, Wray HW: Quinidine syncope. Paroxysmal ventricular fibrillation occurring during treatment of chronic atrial arrhythmias. Circulation 30:17–26, 1964.
6. Roden DM, Woosley RL, Primm RK: Incidence and clinical features of the quinidine-associated long-QT syndrome: Implications for patient care. Am Heart J 111:1088–1093, 1986.
7. Kay GN, Plumb VJ, Arciniegas JG, et al: Torsade de Pointes: The long-short initiating sequence and other clinical features: Observations in 32 patients. J Am Coll Cardiol 2:806–817, 1983.
8. Haverkamp W, Martinez-Rubio A, Hief C, et al: Efficacy and safety of d,l-sotalol in patients with ventricular tachycardia and in survivors of cardiac arrest. J Am Coll Cardiol 30:487–495, 1997.
9. Lehmann MH, Hardy S, Archibald D, et al: Sex difference in risk of torsade de pointes with d,l-sotalol. Circulation 94:2535–2541, 1996.
10. Hohnloser SH: Proarrhythmia with class III antiarrhythmic drugs: Types, risks, and management. Am J Cardiol 80:82G–89G, 1997.
11. Kober L, Bloch Thomsen PE, Moller M, et al: Effect of dofetilide in patients with recent myocardial infarction and left-ventricular dysfunction: A randomised trial. Lancet 356:2052–2058, 2000.
12. Stambler BS, Wood MA, Ellenbogen KA, et al: Efficacy and safety of repeated intravenous doses of ibutilide for rapid conversion of atrial flutter or fibrillation. Ibutilide Repeat Dose Study Investigators. Circulation 94:1613–1621, 1996.
13. Antzelevitch C: Heterogeneity of cellular repolarization in LQTS. The role of M cells. Eur Heart J Suppl 3:K-2–K-16, 2001.
14. Antzelevitch C, Nesterenko VV, Muzikant AL, et al: Influence of transmural repolarization gradients on the electrophysiology and pharmacology of ventricular myocardium. Cellular basis for the Brugada and long-QT syndromes. Philos Trans R Soc Lond (Biol) 359:1201–1216, 2001.
15. Antzelevitch C, Dumaine R: Electrical heterogeneity in the heart: Physiological, pharmacological and clinical implications. In Page E, Fozzard HA, Solaro RJ (eds): Handbook of Physiology. The Heart. New York, Oxford University Press, 2001, pp 654–692.
16. Antzelevitch C, Shimizu W, Yan GX: Electrical heterogeneity and the development of arrhythmias. In Olsson SB, Yuan S, Amlie JP (eds): Dispersion of Ventricular Repolarization: State of the Art. New York, Futura Publishing Company, 2000, pp 3–21.
17. Antzelevitch C: Regional differences in electrophysiology of ventricular cells: Clinical implications for sudden cardiac death. In Aliot E, Clementy J, Prystowsky EN (eds): Fighting Sudden Cardiac Death: A Worldwide Challenge. Armonk, NY, Futura, 2000, pp 109–130.
18. Weissenburger J, Nesterenko VV, Antzelevitch C: Transmural heterogeneity of ventricular repolarization under baseline and long QT conditions in the canine heart in vivo. Torsades de Pointes develops with halothane but not pentobarbital anesthesia. J Cardiovasc Electrophysiol 11:290–304, 2000.
19. Antzelevitch C, Shimizu W, Yan GX, et al: The M cell. Its contribu-

tion to the ECG and to normal and abnormal electrical function of the heart. J Cardiovasc Electrophysiol 10:1124–1152, 1999.
20. Kozhevnikov DO, Yamamoto K, Robotis D, et al: Electrophysiological mechanism of enhanced susceptibility of hypertrophied heart to acquired torsade de pointes arrhythmias: Tridimensional mapping of activation and recovery patterns. Circulation 105:1128–1134, 2002.
21. Vos MA, van Opstal JM, Leunissen JD, Verduyn SC: Electrophysiologic parameters and predisposing factors in the generation of drug-induced Torsade de Pointes arrhythmias. Pharmacol Ther 92:109–122, 2001.
22. Akar FG, Yan GX, Antzelevitch C, Rosenbaum DS: Unique topographical distribution of M cells underlies reentrant mechanism of torsade de pointes in the long-QT syndrome. Circulation 105:1247–1253, 2002.
23. Sicouri S, Antzelevitch C: A subpopulation of cells with unique electrophysiological properties in the deep subepicardium of the canine ventricle: The M cell. Circ Res 68:1729–1741, 1991.
24. Shimizu W, Antzelevitch C: Cellular basis for the electrocardiographic features of the LQT1 form of the long QT syndrome: Effects of β-adrenergic agonists, antagonists and sodium channel blockers on transmural dispersion of repolarization and Torsade de Pointes. Circulation 98:2314–2322, 1998.
25. Schwartz PJ, Priori SG, Spazzolini C, et al: Genotype-phenotype correlation in the long-QT syndrome: Gene-specific triggers for life-threatening arrhythmias. Circulation 103:89–95, 2001.
26. Yan GX, Antzelevitch C: Cellular basis for the normal T wave and the electrocardiographic manifestations of the long QT syndrome. Circulation 98:1928–1936, 1998.
27. Shimizu W, Antzelevitch C: Sodium channel block with mexiletine is effective in reducing dispersion of repolarization and preventing Torsade de Pointes in LQT2 and LQT3 models of the long-QT syndrome. Circulation 96:2038–2047, 1997.
28. Li GR, Feng J, Yue L, Carrier M: Transmural heterogeneity of action potentials and Ito1 in myocytes isolated from the human right ventricle. Am J Physiol 275:H369–H377, 1998.
29. Shimizu W, Antzelevitch C: Differential effects of beta-adrenergic agonists and antagonists in LQT1, LQT2 and LQT3 models of the long QT syndrome. J Am Coll Cardiol 35:778–786, 2000.
30. Balser JR, Bennett PB, Hondeghem LM, Roden DM: Suppression of time-dependent outward current in guinea-pig ventricular myocytes. Actions of quinidine and amiodarone. Circ Res 69:519–529, 1991.
31. Anyukhovsky EP, Sosunov EA, Feinmark SJ, Rosen MR: Effects of quinidine on repolarization in canine epicardium, midmyocardium, and endocardium. II. In vivo study. Circulation 96:4019–4026, 1997.
32. Shimizu W, McMahon B, Antzelevitch C: Sodium pentobarbital reduces transmural dispersion of repolarization and prevents torsade de pointes in models of acquired and congenital long QT syndromes. J Cardiovasc Electrophysiol 10:156–164, 1999.
33. Sun ZQ, Eddlestone GT, Antzelevitch C: Ionic mechanisms underlying the effects of sodium pentobarbital to diminish transmural dispersion of repolarization [abstract]. Pacing Clin Electrophysiol 20:II-1116, 1997.
34. Sicouri S, Moro S, Litovsky SH, et al: Chronic amiodarone reduces transmural dispersion of repolarization in the canine heart. J Cardiovasc Electrophysiol 8:1269–1279, 1997.
35. van Opstal JM, Schoenmakers M, Verduyn SC, et al: Chronic Amiodarone evokes no Torsade de Pointes arrhythmias despite QT lengthening in an animal model of acquired long-QT syndrome. Circulation 104:2722–2727, 2001.
36. Zygmunt AC, Thomas GP, Belardinelli L, et al: Ranolazine produces ion channel effects similar to those observed with chronic amiodarone in canine cardiac ventricular myocytes [abstract]. Pacing Clin Electrophysiol 25:II-626, 2002.
37. Yang T, Snyders D, Roden DM: Drug block of I(kr): Model systems and relevance to human arrhythmias. J Cardiovasc Pharmacol 38:737–744, 2001.
38. Emori T, Antzelevitch C. Cellular basis for complex T waves and arrhythmic activity following combined I(Kr) and I(Ks) block. J Cardiovasc Electrophysiol 12:1369–1378, 2001.
39. Lubinski A, Lewicka-Nowak E, Kempa M, et al: New insight into repolarization abnormalities in patients with congenital long QT syndrome: The increased transmural dispersion of repolarization. Pacing Clin Electrophysiol 21:172–175, 1998.
40. Sarubbi B, Pacileo G, Ducceschi V, et al: Arrhythmogenic substrate in young patients with repaired tetralogy of Fallot: Role of an abnormal ventricular repolarization. Int J Cardiol 72:73–82, 1999.
41. Sarubbi B, Ducceschi V, Briglia N, et al: Compared effects of sotalol, flecainide and propafenone on ventricular repolarization in patients free of underlying structural heart disease. Int J Cardiol 66:157–164, 1998.
42. Tun A, Khan IA, Wattanasauwan N, et al: Increased regional and transmyocardial dispersion of ventricular repolarization in end-stage renal disease. Can J Cardiol 15:53–56, 1999.
43. Tanabe Y, Inagaki M, Kurita T, et al: Sympathetic stimulation produces a greater increase in both transmural and spatial dispersion of repolarization in LQT1 than LQT2 forms of congenital long QT syndrome. J Am Coll Cardiol 37:911–919, 2001.
44. Rudehill A, Sundqvist K, Sylven C: QT and QT-peak interval measurements. A methodological study in patients with subarachnoid haemorrhage compared to a reference group. Clin Physiol 6:23–37, 1986.
45. Pietila E, Fodstad H, Niskasaari E, et al: Association between HERG K897T polymorphism and QT interval in middle-aged Finnish women. J Am Coll Cardiol 40:511–514, 2002.
46. Viitasalo M, Oikarinen L, Swan H, et al: Ambulatory electrocardiographic evidence of transmural dispersion of repolarization in patients with long-QT syndrome type 1 and 2. Circulation 106:2473–2478, 2002.
47. Yoshiga Y, Shimizu A, Yamagata T, et al: Beta-blocker decreases the increase in QT dispersion and transmural dispersion of repolarization induced by bepridil. Circ J 66:1024–1028, 2002.
48. van Opstal JM, Verduyn SC, Winckels SK, et al: The JT-area indicates dispersion of repolarization in dogs with atrioventricular block. J Interv Card Electrophysiol 6:113–120, 2002.
49. Abbott GW, Sesti F, Splawski I, et al: MiRP1 forms IKr potassium channels with HERG and is associated with cardiac arrhythmia. Cell 97:175–187, 1999.
50. Yang P, Kanki H, Drolet B, et al: Allelic variants in long-QT disease genes in patients with drug-associated torsades de pointes. Circulation 105:1943–1948, 2002.
51. Splawski I, Timothy KW, Tateyama M, et al: Variant of SCN5A sodium channel implicated in risk of cardiac arrhythmia. Science 297:1333–1336, 2002.
52. Ford GA, Wood SM, Daly AK: CYP2D6 and CYP2C19 genotypes of patients with terodiline cardiotoxicity identified through the yellow card system. Br J Clin Pharmacol 50:77–80, 2000.
53. Roden DM: Pharmacogenetics and drug-induced arrhythmias. Cardiovasc Res 50:224–231, 2001.

第 19 章

缝隙连接通道药理学靶点的前景

Miduturn Srinivas, Heather Duffy, Mario Delmar, David C. Spray

本章目录

- 心血管缝隙连接介导的重要功能 …… 154
- 心脏缝隙连接也可能传递不恰当的信号 … 154
- 影响连接强度的内源性和外源性因素 …… 155
- 通过跨连接电压和低 pH 关闭通道比较 …… 155
- 通过药物关闭缝隙连接 …… 156
- 半通道及其作为药理学靶点的前景 …… 159
- 缝隙连接直接和间接的靶点，多肽和抗体的门控结构域 …… 159
- 抗体和多肽对细胞间交换的调节 …… 161
- 总结 …… 162

缝隙连接斑是细胞间电流流动产生心脏同步性收缩的形态学基础[1]。在正常情况下，心脏各部分的心肌细胞是高度联系的，形成一个功能性的统一体，在整个组织以协同的方式传播电信号（代谢信号也是一样）。这种通过缝隙连接交换离子和小分子的直接的细胞间交换称作"耦联"（coupling），反映了从一个细胞到另一个细胞的信号交换。由于通道关闭引起的信号传递的改变被称为"解耦联"（uncoupling）。因为正常心脏功能的重要性，通过使细胞解耦联或增加不恰当的细胞间耦联破坏这种系统，将导致潜在的致命事件。因此发展药理学工具，直接的增加、降低或维持在心肌细胞正常的耦联强度可以提高心脏的功能，抑制不恰当的信号传播，或者在不利的情况下维持心脏功能。

一、心血管缝隙连接介导的重要功能

缝隙连接通道负责介导基本的离子、代谢物和信号分子在细胞间传递。在进化过程中，缝隙连接信号在分割空间传递并跨过边界传导被认为是在分化过程中基本的顺序进程，甚至终末分化的成体细胞也需要通过缝隙连接来协调它们与相邻细胞之间的活动。在心脏，电流通过缝隙连接流动，从而同步起搏活动，协调收缩波的扩散，产生心脏输出。在血管，缝隙连接同步内皮反应，调节血管张力，甚至可能为内皮-平滑肌细胞间的交换提供直接通路。实验研究显示，通过连接蛋白敲除的小鼠表型证实，缝隙连接有着重要的结构性功能。例如 Cx43 敲除的小鼠出生时死于因神经嵴移入缺陷引起的右室肥大[3]，心律也有严重的紊乱[4]。

二、心脏缝隙连接也可能传递不恰当的信号

缝隙连接除了介导细胞间基本分子传递的重要性之外，这些细胞间通道也能传递不恰当的信号。在病理条件下，例如缺血性损伤时，凋亡信号可以从细胞到细胞的传播，增大细胞死亡的面积。这种从直接受损的细胞向其临近细胞传播的损伤叫做"旁观细胞致死"（bystander cell killing），并已经用于治疗的用途：由抗肿瘤试剂更昔洛韦在疱疹胸腺激酶转换细胞产生的凋亡信号可以经缝隙连接介导传播，可以增强抗肿瘤的治疗作用[6]。同样，在正常情况下受限的区域耦联强度增强可以在错误的方向传播电信号，包括在心脏形成旁路。在这种情况下关闭缝隙连接就可能

有益处。

最近大量的研究给出了降低缝隙连接在特效制药学上应用的例子：使用缝隙连接阻断剂可以限制在脑和心脏细胞死亡的程度[7]。尽管缺血时缝隙连接关闭被假设为适于器官存活的保护性机制，但有证据证实在这些情况下通道关闭可能是不完全的，即只是时程延长或降低通道开放时间，还会允许毒性物质通过而杀死邻近的细胞。此外，通过外源性药物治疗使快速地解耦联可能会更有效的限制这种旁观细胞致死效应，可能会增强局部损伤后的功能恢复。

当组织损伤不太严重的情况下，内源性的解耦联机制可能导致更严重的生理改变。例如，心脏暂时的缺血可能引起致心律失常的解耦联，这对心脏和神经系统的功能是有害的。但是在解耦联药剂存在的情况下和降低 Cx43 表达的小鼠，这种缺血损伤引起的保护性作用会降低[8,9]。而且，Cx43 杂合的小鼠脑梗死的大小比野生型和基因敲除的小鼠面积要大[10]。治疗的目标可能是 pH 或缝隙连接通道的亲脂性，在中度缺血的情况下，通过这些内源性分子来降低解耦联。

三、影响连接强度的内源性和外源性因素

鼠和人类的基因组序列已经给出了一个详尽的关于 20 种连接蛋白基因的列表[11]。在这些异构体中，只有 3 种在心肌细胞大量表达。其中，Cx40 存在于结组织、心房和浦肯野纤维；Cx45 存在于心脏的特异性传导系统；Cx43 连接工作心肌细胞[12]。

不是所有 20 种连接蛋白都有通道的特性和对门控刺激敏感，而且这些连接蛋白已经被详细的研究显示出大量的功能差异。缝隙连接可以由各种连接蛋白构成，可以被一定的因素关闭，包括 pH 和跨连接电压[13]。并且，磷酸化可能会增强或降低耦联，这依赖于激活哪一种激酶来决定。目前已经知道一定数量的药理学试剂可以阻断缝隙连接。这些药理学的解耦联剂包括一些长链的醇、挥发性的麻醉剂、甘草亭酸及其衍生物、oleamide、aminosulfonates、tetraalkylammonium 离子和抗疟药物奎宁。另外，最近的研究提示，一些氯离子通道阻滞剂也可以关闭缝隙连接通道[14,15]。

四、通过跨连接电压和低 pH 关闭通道比较

已经研究了关闭缝隙连接通道的两种门控机制：即通过改变跨连接电压和通过酸化细胞的胞浆。对表达缝隙连接通道的细胞应用大的跨连接电压阶越，能引起连接电流强烈的下降至非零的稳态水平（图 19-1A）。评价不同连接蛋白电压门控提示，对大多数的连接蛋白这种稳态传导在 0mV 平衡，并符合 Boltzmann 关系（图 19-1B）。但是，即使在最高的 V_j 维持水平，连接电流依然保持。这种残余的电流参与形成通道的亚传导状态（图 19-1C）。关于 V_j 对心脏连接蛋白连接电导影响的 Boltzmann 图形见图 19-1B。这三种心脏的连接蛋白有着惊人的不同：V_0，半失活电压，在 Cx43 是 +45mV，在 Cx45 大约是 +15mV。另外，对仅有很少缝隙连接的细胞进行单通道研究发现，V_j 脉冲使得缝隙连接通道从高电导变为低电导状态[16]。这种通过制药学靶向电压门控的效用是可疑的。尽管在这种亚状态下降低的通透性，实际可能对限制细胞间大的或高电荷的代谢物的分配是有用的，但是残余的亚传导状态不能被任何一种目前已知的解耦联剂所降低。是否这种电压感受器或电压门控与另一种门控机制相一致？

通过细胞内酸化门控，与改变跨连接电压相比会引起一些连接蛋白所构成缝隙连接完全的关闭，可能是一种可利用的药理学干预机制。细胞内酸化可以使检查的所有连接蛋白形成的缝隙连接的电导降低（图 19-2）。尽管对参与这一过程需要的有关分子还有争论，但大部分的数据支持质子对连接蛋白氨基酸残基有直接的滴定作用。尽管看起来所有的连接蛋白都构成 pH 敏感的通道，但是由不同连接蛋白构成缝隙连接通道的敏感性差异很大[17]。对心脏连接蛋白，酸化引起通道关闭的 pKa 值范围从 6.6～7.0（图 19-2B），提示这些连接蛋白可以在病理条件下被关闭。最早的关于 pH 敏感性的定量研究提示，关于细胞内 pH（pH_i）-缝隙连接电导（G_j）关系的 Hill 系数最高到 4，提示 4 或更多的合作位点牵涉到门控当中[18]。不同连接蛋白 pKa 的不同和 pH 敏感性斜率的不同，可能是由于连接蛋白胞膜结构域上滴定残基的数量不同或局部环境不同。

在该篇文章[1]的其他章节详述了后来用直接点突变进行的研究，提示 pH 门控可以归于一种"球-链"作用模式来关闭通道[19]。最近，分光镜研究用重新连接 Cx43 羟基末端（Cx43CT）和不同合成多肽的方法，提供了一种可能的机制来理解与 pH 门控相关的结构改变[20]。镜像回声研究证明，对应 Cx43 第二半胞质环的合成多肽可以和 Cx43CT 再结合，而且这种

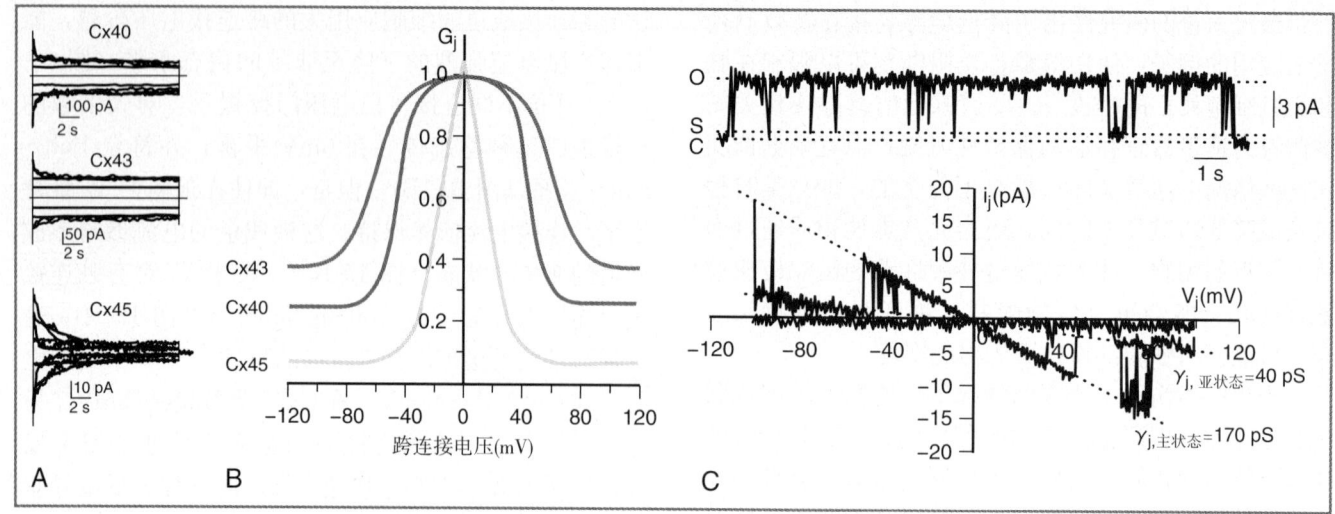

图 19-1 由 Cx40、Cx43、Cx45 构成的缝隙连接的跨连接电压敏感性 A：分别由指示的连接蛋白构成的缝隙连接，在电压 100mV、增益 20mV 记录的连接通道电流。注意 Cx45 对电压最敏感，Cx43 和 Cx40 都有一部分电流对电压不敏感，即使是维持在很高的电压。B：由不同的心脏连接蛋白构成的缝隙连接标准化的连接电导（G_j）与跨连接电压关系曲线。注意半失活电压在 Cx45、Cx40、Cx43 分别是 15mV、40mV、60mV。C：从一对表达 Cx40 的细胞作单通道记录，维持跨连接电压在 40mV（上图），跨连接电压范围从 −100mV～+100mV，速度为 10mV/s。注意在两个记录中都有一个主状态和亚状态电导，在高电压时，主要是亚状态电导为主

结合的亲和力在 pH 为 6.5 时要比 pH 为 7.0 时更高。除此，应用核磁共振方法的结构研究已经证实参与相互作用的 Cx43CT 和环区的结构特征。对于细胞浆环多肽和完整的环结构域，pH 值从 7.4～5.8 的改变将引起这两个亚结构域 α 螺旋的感应，每一个 α 螺旋含有一个组氨酸残基，其 pK 值大约为 6.8。

为了确定 Cx43CT 上与环多肽结合的位点，我们检测了是否合成的对应 Cx43CT 上特异结构域的多肽能阻断这种反应。最初的研究显示，Cx43CT 大部分羟基末端区域对应的多肽有浓度依赖的抑制作用。而且，也发现一种针对这种多肽的多克隆抗体可以强烈地阻断 Cx43CT 和细胞浆环多肽的相互作用。

这些结果为发现药理学治疗靶点提供了重要的方向。例如，设计一种药物直接地结合到 Cx43 胞浆环多肽区域，能抑制环与羟基末端结构域的连接作用，因而关闭通道。或者，胞浆环多肽区域或羟基末端结构域内邻近位点分子相互作用可以干扰 pH 引起的球-链结合作用，从而降低通道的 pH 敏感性。假设可利用这种高亲和力的分子将其靶向应用于心脏，则可以将副作用减低到最小。

五、通过药物关闭缝隙连接

很久以来就知道长链烷醇（辛醇和庚醇）可以降低神经的兴奋性和突触传递，早在 20 年前，就有报告说其在高浓度时可以降低分离的龙虾轴突电紧张的突触传递[21]。Johnston 和他的同事报告，在他们最初关于辛醇对灌注的小龙虾连接膜的作用研究中，这种试剂仅在细胞外使用有效。最近对于卵母细胞 Cx46 和 Cx50 半通道电流解耦联剂的报道中，Eskandari 及其同事认为这对 Cx50 同样有效，但辛醇对 Cx46 半通道没有影响。尽管在非洲蟾蜍的卵母细胞表达的连接蛋白通常对辛醇和庚醇的敏感性不如在哺乳动物细胞敏感，没有证据表明在哺乳动物细胞对不同连接蛋白构成的缝隙连接通道有强烈的选择性阻断。因为它们的解耦联作用迅速、稳定、可逆、无毒性，所以长链烷醇辛烷和庚烷在评价急性缝隙连接阻断作用中一直非常有用，例如对培养细胞间 Ca^{2+} 的传播。尽管其他的一些麻醉剂作用机制的假说涉及对膜的流动性的改变，但这种作用的机制一直不明。

（一）普通麻醉剂

普通麻醉剂解耦联作用的假说是通过与长链醇同样的或相关的机制，包括氟烷和异氟烷，在吸入性麻醉的剂量（1～3mmol/L）可以迅速并可逆地去耦联心肌细胞。在单通道记录的基础上，作用的机制涉及通过直接关闭到完全关闭状态降低开放的概率[22]，

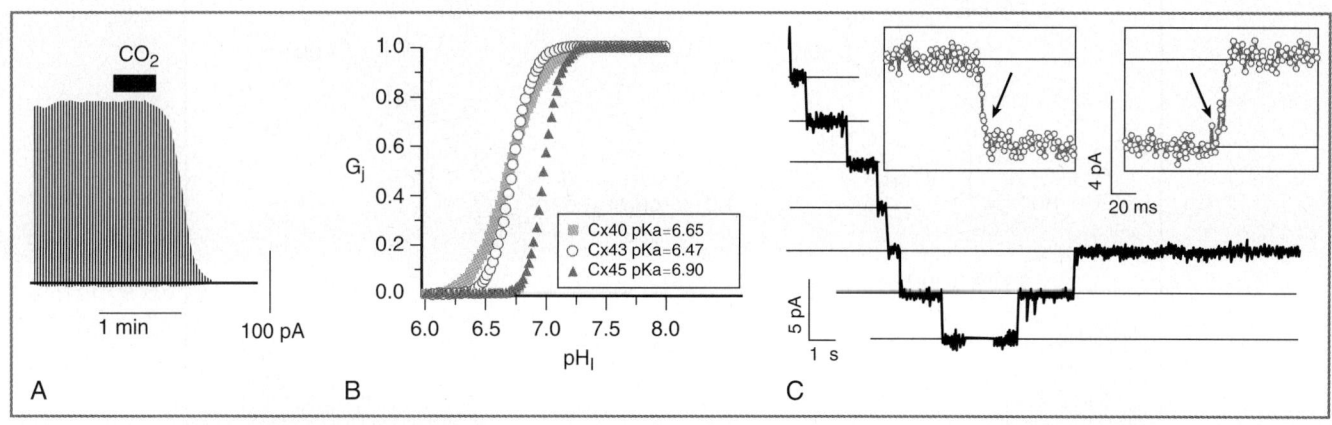

图 19-2 细胞内酸化可以关闭缝隙连接通道 A：在瞬时转染了大鼠 Cx43 的神经母细胞瘤细胞上记录的缝隙连接电流，对应的电压脉冲是 20mV。当应用饱和 CO_2 的液体时使连接的电导迅速下降到 0。B：在注射了心脏连接蛋白 mRNA 的一对蟾蜍卵母细胞中，测得的连接电导（G_j）对细胞内 pH（pH_i）的依赖性，当 pH 被由 CO_2 平衡的液体改变时，pH_i 由荧光指示剂来衡量。曲线代表满足 Hill 方程的拟合数据。C：在一对转染了 Cx43 的哺乳动物细胞上进行单通道记录，对应 CO_2 压力下的通道关闭情况。注意暴露于 CO_2 时阶梯样下降的电流，到电导为 0，以及阶梯样的恢复。插入的框显示的是短时间内采样记录的最后转变到 0 时的电流和最早再开放的通道；注意电流转变的减慢（箭头所示）

而且在随后的研究中也未能解决该问题。尽管这种高脂溶性提示其机制可能涉及疏水性脂蛋白表层的作用，但在连接蛋白分子中作用的位点还不清楚。

（二）甘草酸代谢

欧亚甘草糖包含抑制 11β 羟类固醇脱氢酶抑制剂，可以降解成可的松和氢化可的松。如过度吸收欧亚甘草会引起肾脏盐皮质激素受体异常高活性，导致机体由欧亚甘草诱发的高血压。欧亚甘草基本的活性成分是甘草苦酸，甘草苦酸代谢会激活盐皮质激素受体。Davidson 及同事[23]应用代谢协同化验发现，α 和 β 甘草苦酸（α,β GA）和生胃酮（结构见图 19-3）在低浓度 2μmol/L 可抑制人的成纤维细胞的耦联，并且即使在抑制剂存在的情况下共同培养三周，这种解耦联作用也是可逆的。两年后又进行了后续的试验，通过结构激活分析又确定了其他重要的激活衍生物[24]，但是 α、β GA 和生胃酮成为最广泛应用的这类解耦联化合物。GAs 和生胃酮对缝隙连接的作用看起来与它们抑制类固醇脱氢酶的作用无关，因为更重要的脱氢酶抑制剂 GA 通常是作为一种对耦联非特异作用的无活性对照。最初的报道发现醛固酮和糖皮质激素并不影响缝隙连接介导的耦联[23]。

通过 α、β GA 和生胃酮阻断缝隙连接通道比其他的解耦联剂需要更长的暴露时间（图 19-3）。尽管缺乏细节的研究，但目前缝隙连接通道各亚型对解耦联剂的敏感性没有差异[25]。虽然一些作者有资料解释连接蛋白磷酸化和亚单位聚集的变化，但除了这些制剂的有效性和无毒性，其作用机制还有许多没有被研究。

（三）抗疟药物

因为在治疗疟疾方面的效果，奎宁是世界上最广泛应用的药物之一。早在 17 世纪，耶稣会传教士们在秘鲁最早报道了奎宁的抗疟特性，在那里的安第斯土著人早就发现了这种有苦味的树汁具有治疗作用。这种树被林奈叫作金鸡纳（cincbona），来纪念第一个用奎宁治疗疟疾的欧洲人。奎宁广泛的传播应用 300 年证明了它没有毒副作用，尽管过量应用时会引起低血糖、急性听力丧失（特别是对高频的听力）和视觉紊乱（视觉迟钝和弱视）。

先前的研究提示奎宁能激活鱼视网膜的水平细胞的半通道，并加强表达一定连接蛋白的卵母细胞（如 Cx35 而不是 Cx43）缝隙连接半通道电流[26]。我们研究了关于奎宁对转染了各种连接蛋白的神经母细胞瘤细胞的作用，提示奎宁对一定缝隙连接通道构成的缝隙连接有重要的作用，例如由 Cx36 和 Cx50 构成的缝隙连接，EC_{50} 值分别为 32μmol/L 和 73μmol/L（图 19-4B），中度阻断 Cx45 缝隙连接。EC_{50} 值与阻断钾离子通道和容量激活的氯离子通道的有效浓度相同，接近在慢性抗疟治疗中的血浆浓度。重要的是，由其他连接蛋白构成的缝隙连接对奎宁不敏感，300μmol/L 的奎宁对由 Cx32、Cx43、Cx26 或 Cx40

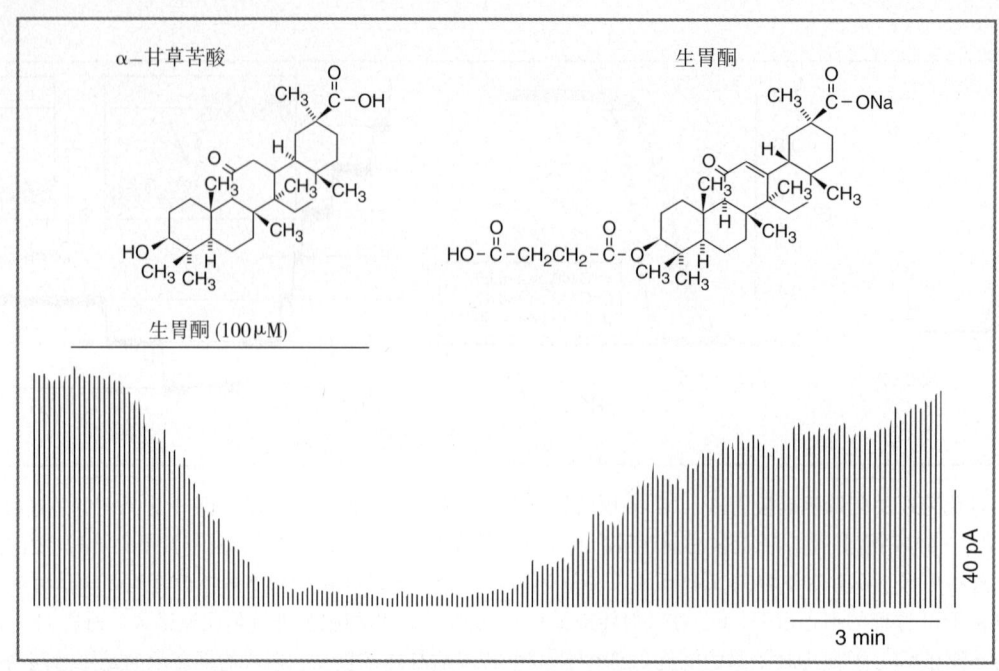

图 19-3 α甘草苦酸和生胃酮可逆性的降低缝隙连接电流　上图：α甘草苦酸和生胃酮的结构。下图：暴露于 100μmol/L 的生胃酮时使连接通道电流降低到接近 0 的水平，但可以缓慢而完全的恢复

构成的缝隙连接通道产生很小或没有阻断作用（图19-4C）。对 Cx50 转染的单通道研究揭示了奎宁的阻断作用是剂量依赖性降低通道开放的概率，并很慢地将通道从完全开放状态转变到完全关闭状态。这一机制不同于 K^+ 开放通道被局部麻醉剂的阻断。后者由于快速的从开放变到关闭状态，其通道整体的电导降低。有研究显示，用一种不能透过膜的奎宁的衍生物进行研究，胞内和胞外的 pH 值变化提示奎宁的阻断作用是从细胞浆接近的（可能在通道内部），起效的方式肯定是充电的[27]。

随后一系列没有发表的研究评价了其他奎宁衍生物的作用，研究显示，mefloquine（结构见图19-4A）是另一种广泛应用的抗疟药物，用来治疗多种药物抵抗的恶性疟原虫和间日疟原虫感染，其能更有效地降低缝隙连接传导的作用，由一些连接蛋白构成通道的 EC_{50} 值低于 1μM。另外，mefloquine 可以在一定浓度（10～30μmol/L）阻断心脏连接蛋白构成的通道。尽管没有必要去联系缝隙连接的作用，但有趣的是，mefloquine 治疗可加重神经精神学紊乱以及加重癫痫患者发作。

（四）芬那酸（Fenamates）

芬那酸是非甾体类消炎药，当使用至纳摩尔浓度时可以抑制环氧化酶（结构见图19-5C）。在高浓度 10～100μmol/L 时这种化合物是有效的各种膜离子通道阻滞剂[28]。Harks 及其助手最近用单电极电压钳方式来测量瞬时的电容并以此估计耦联强度，评价了芬那酸对培养的单层肾脏细胞系（NRK cells）的功效。FFA（flufenamic acid）、NFA（niflumic acid）、MFA（meclofenamic acid）的解耦联作用是迅速而强大的，但不是完全可逆的。如按阻断电和染料耦联有效性的顺序从强到弱依次为 MFA、NFA、FFA，EC_{50} 范围在 25～100μmol/L。Flufenamate 作用独立于试验中的其他解耦联机制，包括膜电位、蛋白激酶 C、环氧化酶激活、细胞内的 pH 和 Ca^{2+} 水平。通过研究母代和 Cx43 转染的 SKHep1 细胞，作者进一步证实芬那酸对 Cx45 和 Cx43 通道都有阻断作用。

我们在瞬时转染的 N2A 细胞，评价了芬那酸对连接蛋白构成的缝隙连接通道的作用（图19-5A，B），发现在双电压钳控制下，降低缝隙传导的 EC_{50} 值与在单层 NRK 细胞上的结构惊人的相似[14]。芬那酸对各种连接蛋白亚型没有选择性。在我们的研究中，芬那酸的作用位点与奎宁相同。因为芬那酸是一种弱酸（pKa≈6），我们认为调节细胞内外的 pH 将会影响其阻断作用。如提高不带电的位点浓度降低细胞外的 pH，会显著增加芬那酸的效力，提示这些药物通过其不带电形式接近它们的结合位点。但是与奎宁相比，调节细胞内部的 pH 值对这些药物的效力没有显著的影响，提示作用位点不在通道孔内。相对奎宁及

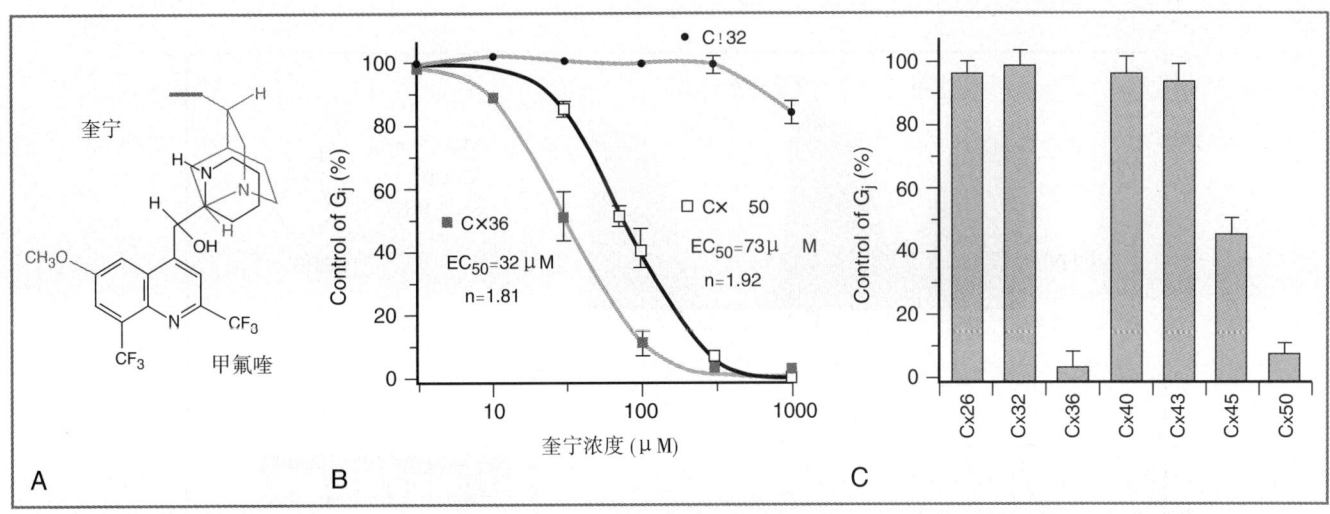

图19-4 奎宁及其衍生物可以选择性地阻断由一定连接蛋白构成的缝隙连接 A：奎宁及其更有效的类似物 mefloquine 的结构。B：奎宁对转染了三种连接蛋白的细胞间连接电导作用的量效关系。注意Cx32非常不敏感，而300μmol/L奎宁对Cx36和Cx50几乎完全阻断，EC_{50}值分别为32μmol/L和73μmol/L。C：300μmol/L奎宁对七种连接蛋白构成的缝隙连接的影响。有两种心脏连接蛋白对奎宁不敏感（Cx43和Cx40），而Cx45的电导被降低了50%。

其衍生物来说，芬那酸的通道阻滞作用似乎涉及急性的门控而不是开放通道的关闭（图 19-5D）。不像奎宁，芬那酸阻断作用的位点还不清楚，因为不带电的活性形式是亲脂性的，在疏水的或亲水的连接蛋白结构域都可以作用。

六、半通道及其作为药理学靶点的前景

最近有许多研究结果已经被解释为证据提供的，即连接蛋白半通道在一些病理情况下开放引发了思索——这些通道在病理条件下开放可能引起心脏和脑的离子失平衡[29-31]，并引起星形胶质细胞释放三磷酸腺苷（ATP）[32]。在历史上，最早的缝隙连接半通道可能有功能的报告，是来自大电导的阴离子通道的电生理记录[33,34]，如此大的电导只能是通过缝隙连接半通道形状的通道来流动的。现在普遍接受的观点是，这种大电导的阴离子通道最大可能是由电压依赖性阴离子通道形式的质膜组成[35]。在线粒体外膜发现了大量的这种异构体，而且，这种电压依赖性阴离子通道最近被认为在细胞凋亡性死亡中发挥关键的作用。除了被错误的认为是一种功能性的半通道外，电压依赖性阴离子通道在缝隙连接生理中也有另一个重要的作用，即因为它几乎同步的电压敏感性，构成了早期对缝隙连接电压敏感性生物物理分析的基础[36]。

有相当充足的证据表明，功能性缝隙连接半通道存在于鳐和硬骨鱼的水平细胞[26,37]。当一定的连接蛋白在卵母细胞外源性表达及细胞外 Ca^{2+} 活性降低时，就可以形成功能性半通道[38-40]。最近，有报道说，当细胞外钙离子降低或在细胞外液中加入奎宁时，哺乳动物细胞中Cx43和Cx45半通道可以开放[41,42]。另外，代谢抑制剂可以诱发心肌细胞的通道开放，引起细胞内钠和钙浓度的增加[29,30]，并增加星形胶质细胞对染料的摄取[31]。尽管这些通道被作为Cx43半通道的对应物来说明，半通道存在的基本的证据在于对Lucifer yellow和其他染料分子的非连接通透性，以及可以被非选择性阻断剂例如FFA和lanthanum所抑制。从这些研究历史提示，对这一问题有足够的谨慎。Beyer和Steinberg报告说，选择一种巨噬细胞系抵抗高浓度的ATP就会产生Cx43缺乏的细胞，并得出结论：Cx43半通道导致了暴露于毫摩尔的ATP中时连接的高通透性。而负责ATP诱导Lucifer yellow分子大小的染料分子透过的受体在5年后被克隆，同时也发现了P2X受体[44]。因此，尽管半通道可能是一个发展缝隙连接阻断剂诱人的靶点，但它在哺乳动物细胞的特性和功能还有待于进一步的了解。

七、缝隙连接直接和间接的靶点，多肽和抗体的门控结构域

在过去的几年里，越来越多的证据表明，缝隙连接蛋白可以和其他胞浆的或胞膜上的蛋白相互作用。尽管连接蛋白作为缝隙连接孔形成元素的理论无可置

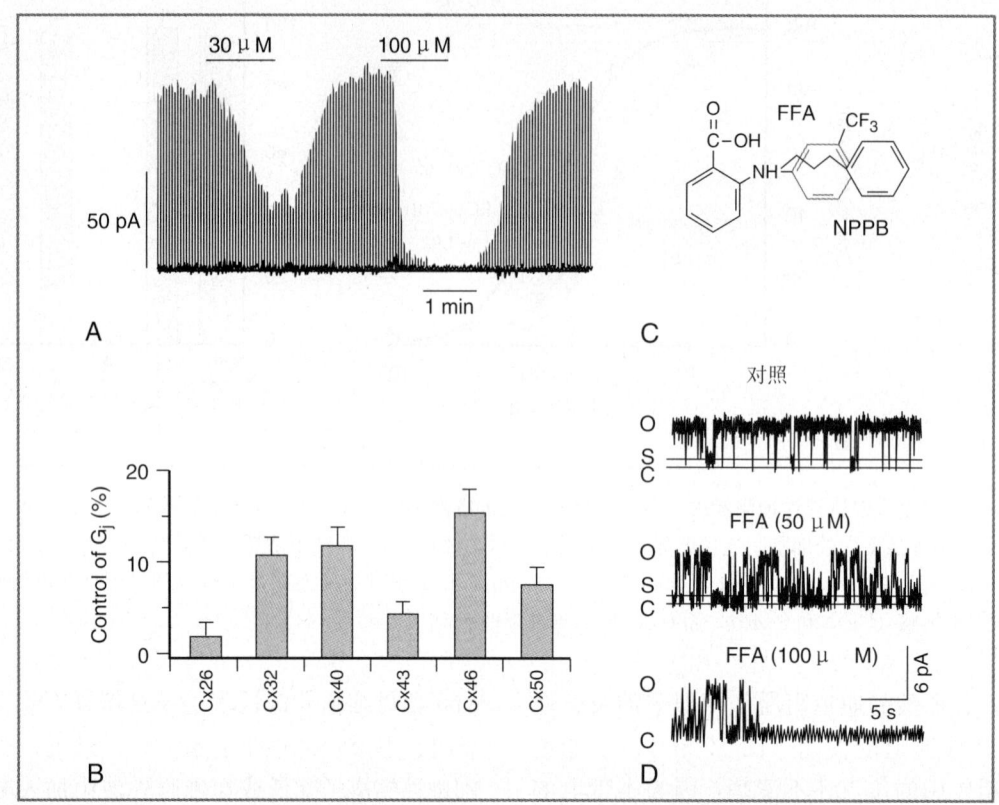

图 19-5 某些阴离子通道阻滞剂（芬那酸）对缝隙连接的阻断，但没有明显的连接蛋白特异性 A：FFA 可以迅速而可逆的降低 Cx26 连接通道的电导。B：在试验的转染细胞中，30μM 的 FFA 可以降低所有 6 种连接蛋白连接的电导，包括 Cx43 和 Cx40。C：两种有效的芬那酸 FFA 和 NPPB 的结构，强调了分子中相同的部分。D：单通道记录显示，在通道完全开放状态 (O)，使用 FFA 作用时间有剂量依赖性降低，在亚传导状态（S）和（C）所需要时间没有明显的增加（引自：Srinivas M，Hopperstad MG，Spray DC：Quinine blocks specific gap junction channel subtypes. Proc Natl Acad Sci USA 98：10942-10947，2001.）

疑，但目前显示该孔可以被其他附加的分子修饰，它们在信号转导和连接缝隙连接于细胞骨架方面起重要作用[45]，我们把这种复合物称为"连接（nexus）"（图 19-6）。这种连接复合物的成分被认为在不同的连接蛋白是不同的，而且在不同的细胞间联系和不同的生理或病理条件下也不同。Duffy 及同事[45]和 Delmar 等[1]总结了至目前和心脏连接蛋白相联系的蛋白。对于 Cx43 有 zonula occluding 1（ZO-1）、v-和 c-src、小窝蛋白-1、微管蛋白、β-连接素、p120 连接素。Cx45 可以和 ZO-1 相互作用。但还没有发现 Cx40 的蛋白伴侣。每个连接伴侣都涉及细胞的其他功能，例如形成紧密连接（ZO-1 和连接素）、信号传导通路（v-和 c-src 及连接素）、细胞骨架和脂质膜的功能（微管蛋白和小窝蛋白）。结果提示，缝隙连接可能被这些功能调节并在这些过程中起作用。

缝隙连接是信号从一个细胞传到下一个细胞的最理想的位点。连接复合物存在信号分子和细胞骨架又能提供可能的局部机制，使信号可以从连接蛋白传导到胞膜，并通过信号通路影响细胞的活动，也可能对损伤后的调节起作用。这可能是一种最全面的在细胞与其邻近细胞间传递信号的方法。显然，长期关闭细胞间的缝隙连接将产生节律异常，而在一些压力条件下，短暂的关闭缝隙连接对于防止异常信号向未经受压力的细胞传播是重要的。这些连接是如何关闭的还不清楚，除了通道的门控外，蛋白连接伴侣的存在为暂时关闭缝隙连接提供另一种机制。

尽管这些联系的作用在缝隙连接通道交换和功能上的作用还没有完全明确，但通过定点突变的方法可以确定它们在连接蛋白分子上的结合位点。当过度表达或在细胞内给予连接位点的类似物希望可以竞争性抑制连接蛋白与修饰蛋白的连接，进而破坏缝隙连接通道的传递功能。因为细胞浆结构域序列是连接蛋白特异性的，有希望这些抑制剂也可以是连接蛋白选择性的。

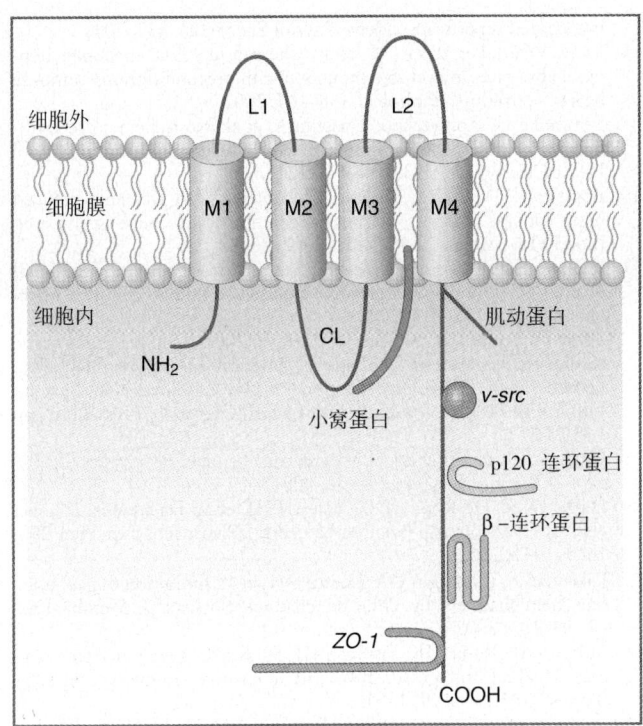

图 19-6 Cx43 连接复合物的成分 Cx43 的膜拓扑图显示有四个跨膜的结构域（M1、M2、M3、M4）、两个细胞外环（L1，L2）、三个胞浆内结构域、NH2 末端、一个细胞浆内环（CL）和一个羧基末端（COOH）。并显示了连接伴侣和大概的结合位置。小窝蛋白是在非特异性的位点与脂质双层膜相互作用，在图中显示了其他伴侣结合在羧基末端的各个位置

第一个被描述的 Cx43 的连接伴侣是 ZO-1，它是一种脚手架形蛋白质，最早是在紧密连接中发现的一种蛋白质[48]。ZO-1 是一个大的蛋白质分子，有多个位点，可以有亲同性和亲异性的相互作用[48]。相互作用位点有三个分离的 PDZ 结合结构域，其中一个 SH3 结构域、一个失活的鸟苷酸位点（GUK 结构域）和一个富含脯氨酸的尾巴[49]。ZO-1 和 Cx43 的结合通过第二个 PDZ 结合结构域和 Cx43 的羧基末端的相互作用，大概是为修饰蛋白提供了一个结合框。当截短形式的 ZO-1 导入心肌细胞以后，将对 Cx43 发挥负显性作用，维持 Cx43 在胞浆里而不是在胞膜上。这可以作为一种生理的机制从细胞膜上移开连接蛋白，引起暂时的解耦联。对于 Cx43PDZ 连接结构域的靶向药物，ZO-1 连接的氨基酸（至少是 379～382 个氨基酸），可以破坏与 ZO-1 的相互作用，也有可能改变通道的功能。

酪氨酸激酶 Src 和 Cx43 的相互作用，只有当细胞内源性的 c-src 激活或持续的 v-src 激活时才发生，

这也提示另一种引起 Cx43 抑制的可能方向。Src 与 Cx43 相互作用的结构域是 SH3 结构域，可以直接连接到 Cx43 羧基末端的 253～256、274～284 位点。这是一种小的结构域，大约 7kD，如果引入到靶细胞，预计可以引起缝隙连接通道的关闭。如果将这一结构域做得易改变，就可以在靶细胞引起缝隙连接通道暂时的关闭。

其他与心脏的三种缝隙连接有关的连接伴侣的功能还不清楚，尽管在每个研究中都支持连接伴侣有调节缝隙连接通道功能的作用。总的来说，制造连接伴侣类似的多肽和连接结构域类似物，来引起蛋白伴侣间结合的抑制，或用抗体直接破坏蛋白连接伴侣的连接，都可以为改变连接蛋白通道的功能提供选择。当新的研究明确了连接伴侣的作用及其作用机制，则直接针对特异性缝隙连接蛋白的药物将会增加。当找到新的作用靶点时，将有可能进一步对通道进行调控。

八、抗体和多肽对细胞间交换的调节

由于连接蛋白的氨基酸序列的不同，所以针对大多数连接蛋白可以产生特异性的单一抗体，其中一些抗体可以抑制功能性的耦联。除了针对细胞外环抗原决定簇产生的抗体外[50]，这些抗体显示出可以有效的结合到细胞浆的结构域。这些特定区域代表了应用于细胞内部抑制作用的主要问题。另外，针对细胞外结构域的特异性抗体，可以与缝隙连接通道外表面结合，并通过干扰连接子的入位或者破坏细胞外环状序列高亲和力的相互作用，发挥阻断作用。这种方法的缺点包括高抗体浓度及长暴露时间。但对这些试剂缺乏非特异性毒性的研究。

Dahl 及其同事介绍了另一个可选择的策略[51]，使用对应细胞外环序列的多肽来阻断细胞间的耦联。这种研究的合理性在于，细胞外环提供识别模体，这些多肽可以和与对应位点结合的连接蛋白相竞争。有许多研究应用小的肽段来阻断由不同连接蛋白介导的缝隙连接联系（详见 Berthoud 及同事的研究[52]）。这些研究指出，大多数有效的多肽涉及连接蛋白细胞外环 I 上保守的 QPG 和 SHVR 模体，以及细胞外环 II 上的 SRPTEK 模体（图 19-6）。这些多肽作用的机制涉及到阻止解离后相邻细胞间半通道复位。多肽抑制缝隙连接耦联的可能性归因于直接破坏缝隙连接的组装，或者与细胞内区域作用影响了通道的门控。但使用连接蛋白类似的多肽也存在许多缺点。尽管在许多

例子中，多肽可以选择性的完全关闭通道，但在大多数研究中这种通道的关闭仅仅是部分关闭。而且在大多数研究中，要取得阻断效果，就需要高浓度多肽和较长的孵育时间。同时，多肽的稳定性也限制了它的长期应用研究。

除了这种多肽可以与细胞外的环状结构域相结合来阻断缝隙连接通道外，有人提出其他的多肽也可以增强缝隙连接耦联。例如，抗心律失常六肽，最早是在筛查可以使培养的鸡心肌细胞产生同步跳动的化合物时确定的，并在研究中发现它可以增强哺乳动物心脏的耦联、抑制缺血/灌注过程中的解耦联。这些研究重要的原因是，不但发现了可以增强缝隙连接介导的细胞间传导的因素，而且还提供为确定这种有活性化合物的分析方法。在开放药物领域持续存在的一个主要局限性是缺乏高产量的筛查，因此新的突破还有待于新的筛查方法的研发。

九、总结

尽管在缝隙连接领域中分子水平的研究已有了很大进展，但近期对于调节或抑制门控敏感性、促进细胞间重要的信号转导或阻断不恰当信号转导的药理学试剂的研究方面，包括确定药物和分类方面的研究没有什么进展。不过，已经确定了一些高效的连接蛋白亚型选择性阻断剂，包括奎宁的衍生物、芬那酸。最近发现的连接蛋白分子内和分子间的相互作用也将提供重要的靶点。研究靶向多肽和另外的有活性化合物的衍生物将提供新的有疗效的药物，如生胃酮的低毒性和相对的高效性，可能使其成为目前对缝隙连接抑制的急性或慢性研究中最普遍使用的药物。

（浦介麟 李 宁 译）

参 考 文 献

1. Delmar M, Duffy HS, Sorgen P, et al: Molecular organization and regulation of the cardiac gap junction channel connexin43. In Zipes DP, Jalife J (eds): Cardiac Electrophysiology: From Cell to Bedside, 4th ed. Philadelphia, WB Saunders, 2004.
2. Plum A, Hallas G, Magin T, et al: Unique and shared functions of different connexins in mice. Curr Biol 10:1083–1091, 2000.
3. Lo CW, Wessels A: Cx43 gap junctions in cardiac development. Trends Cardiovasc Med 8:264–269, 1998.
4. Morley GE, Vaidya D, Jalife J: Characterization of conduction in the ventricles of normal and heterozygous Cx43 knockout mice using optical mapping. J Cardiovasc Electrophysiol 11(3):375–377, 2000.
5. Pitts JD: The discovery of metabolic co-operation. Bioessays 20(12):1047–1051, 1998.
6. Andrade-Rozental AF, Rozental R, Hopperstad MG, et al: Gap junctions: The "kiss of death" and the "kiss of life." Brain Res Rev 32:308–315, 2000.
7. Garcia-Dorado, D, Ruiz-Meana M: Propagation of cell death during myocardial reperfusion. News Physiol Sci 15:326–330, 2000.
8. Li G, Whittaker P, Yao M, et al: The gap junction uncoupler heptanol abrogates infarct size reduction with preconditioning in mouse hearts. Cardiovasc Pathol 11:158–165, 2002.
9. Schwanke U, Konietzka I, Duschin A, et al: No ischemic preconditioning in heterozygous connexin43-deficient mice. Am J Physiol Heart Circ Physiol 283:H1740–H1742.
10. Frantseva MV, Kokarovtseva L, Velazquez JLP: Ischemia-induced brain damage depends on specific gap junctional coupling. J Cereb Blood Flow Metab 22:453–462, 2002, 2002.
11. Willecke K, Eiberger J, Degen J, et al: Structural and functional diversity of connexin genes in the mouse and human genome. J Biol Chem 383(5):725–737, 2002.
12. Spray DC, Suadicani S, Srinivás M, et al: (2001). Gap junctions in the cardiovascular system. In Page E, Fozzard HA, Solaro RJ (eds): Handbook of Physiology. Section 2: The Cardiovascular System. Vol. 1: The Heart. New York, UK, Oxford University Press, 2002, pp 169–212.
13. Harris AL: Emerging issues of connexin channels: Biophysics fills the gap. Q Rev Biophys 34:325–472, 2001.
14. Harks EGA, De Roos ADG, Peters PHJ, et al: Fenamates: A novel class of reversible gap junction blockers. J Pharmacol Exp Ther 298:1033–1041, 2001.
15. Eskandari S, Zampighi GA, Leung DW, et al: Inhibition of gap junction hemichannels by chloride channel blockers. J Membr Biol 185:93–102, 2002.
16. Moreno AP, Rook MB, Fishman GI, Spray DC: Gap junction channels: Distinct voltage-sensitive and insensitive conductance states. Biophys J 67:113–119, 1994.
17. Stergiopoulos K, Alvarado JL, Mastroianni M, et al: Hetero-domain interactions a s a mechanism for the regulation of connexin channels. Circ Res 84(10):1144–1155, 1999.
18. Spray DC, Scemes E: Effects of pH (and Ca) on gap junction channels. In Kaila K, Ransom BR (eds): New York, Academic Press, 1998, pp 477–489.
19. Morley GE, Ek-Vitorin JF, Taffet SM, Delmar M: Structure of connexin43 and its regulation by pH_i. J Cardiovasc Electrophysiol 8(8):939–951, 1997.
20. Duffy HS, Sorgen PL, Girvin ME, et al: pH-dependent intramolecular binding and structure involving Cx43 cytoplasmic domains. J Biol Chem 276:8544–8549, 2002.
21. Johnston MF, Simon SA, Ramon F: Interaction of anaesthetics with electrical synapses. Nature 286:498–500, 1980.
22. Burt JM, Spray DC: Volatile anesthetics reversibly reduce gap junctional conductance between cardiac myocytes. Circ Res 65:829–837, 1989.
23. Davidson JS, Baumgarten IM, Harley EH: Reversible inhibition of intercellular junctional communication by glycyrrhetinic acid. Biochem Biophys Res Commun 134(1):29–36, 1986.
24. Davidson JS, Baumgarten IM: Glycyrrhetinic acid derivatives: A novel class of inhibitors of gap-junctional intercellular communication. Structure-activity relationships. J Pharmacol Exp Ther 246(3):1104–1107, 1988.
25. Spray DC, Rozental R, Srinivas M: Prospects for rational development of pharmacological gap junction channel blockers. Curr Drug Targets 3(6):455–464, 2002.
26. Malchow RP, Qian H, Ripps H: Evidence for hemi-gap junctional channels in isolated horizontal cells of the skate retina. J Neurosci Res 35:237–245, 1993.
27. Srinivas M, Hopperstad MG, Spray DC: Qunine blocks specific gap junction channel subtypes. Proc Natl Acad Sci U S A 98:10942–10947, 2001.
28. Schultz BD, Singh AK, Devor DC, Bridges RJ: Pharmacology of CFTR chloride channel activity. Physiol Rev 79:S109–S144, 1999.
29. John SA, Kondo R, Wang SY, et al: Connexin-43 hemichannels opened by metabolic inhibition. J Biol Chem 274:236–240, 1999.
30. Kondo RP, Wang SY, John SA, et al: Metabolic inhibition activates a non-selective current through connexin hemichannels in isolated ventricular myocytes. J Mol Cell Cardiol 32:1859–1872, 2000.
31. Contreras JE, Sanchez HA, Eugenin EA, et al: Metabolic inhibition induces opening of unopposed connexin 43 gap junction hemichannels and reduces gap junctional communication in cortical astrocytes in culture. Proc Natl Acad Sci U S A 99(1):495–500, 2002.
32. Cotrina ML, Kang J, Lin JH, et al: Astrocytic gap junctions remain open during ischemic condition. J Neurosci 18:2520–2537, 1998.

33. Schwarze W, Kolb HA: Voltage-dependent kinetics of an anionic channel of large unit conductance in macrophages and myotube membranes. Pflugers Arch 402:281–291, 1984.
34. Blatz AL, Magleby KL: Single voltage-dependent chloride-selective channels of large conductance in cultured rat muscle Biophys J 43:237–241, 1983.
35. Buettner R, Papoutsoglou G, Scemes E, et al: Evidence for secretory pathway localization of a voltage-dependent anion channel isoform. Proc Natl Acad Sci U S A 97:3201–3206, 2000.
36. Spray DC, Harris AL, Bennett MV: Voltage dependence of junctional conductance in early amphibian embryos. Science 204:432–434, 1979.
37. DeVries SH, Schwartz EA: Hemi-gap-junction channels in solitary horizontal cells of the catfish retina. J Physiol 445:201–230, 1992.
38. Paul DL, Ebihara L, Takemoto LJ, et al: Connexin46, a novel lens gap junction protein, induces voltage-gated currents in nonjunctional plasma membrane of *Xenopus* oocytes. J Cell Biol 115:1077–1089, 1991.
39. Pfahnl A, Dahl G: Localization of a voltage gate in connexin46 gap junction hemichannels. Biophys J 75:2323–2331, 1998.
40. Trexler EB, Bennett MV, Bargiello TA, Verselis VK: Voltage gating and permeation in a gap junction hemichannel. Proc Natl Acad Sci U S A 93(12):5836–5841, 1996.
41. Li H, Liu TF, Lazrak A, et al: Properties and regulation of gap junctional hemichannels in the plasma membranes of cultured cells. J Cell Biol 134(4):1019–1030, 1996.
42. Stout CE, Costantin JL, Naus CC, Charles AC: Intercellular calcium signaling in astrocytes via ATP release through connexin hemichannels. J Biol Chem 277(12):10482–10488, 2002.
43. Beyer EC, Steinberg TH: Evidence that the gap junction protein connexin-43 is the ATP-induced pore of mouse macrophages. J Biol Chem 266(13):7971–7974, 1991.
44. Surprenant A, Rassendren F, Kawashima E, et al: The cytolytic P2Z receptor for extracellular ATP identified as a P2X receptor (P2X7). Science 272(5262):735–738.
45. Duffy HS, Delmar M, Spray, DC Formation of the gap junction nexus: binding partners for connexins. J Physiol (Paris) 96(3–4): 243–249, 2002.
46. Spray DC, Duffy HS, Scemes E: Gap junctions in glia: Types, roles and plasticity. Adv Exp Med Biol 468:339–359, 1999.
47. Gutstein DE, Morley GE, Vaidya D, et al: Heterogeneous expression of gap junction channels in the heart leads to conduction defects and ventricular dysfunction. Circulation 104(10):1194–1199, 2001.
48. Stevenson BR, Siliciano JD, Mooseker MS, Goodenough DA: Identification of ZO-1: A high molecular weight polypeptide associated with the tight junction (zonula occludens) in a variety of epithelia. J Cell Biol 103(3):755–766, 1986.
49. Fanning AS, and Anderson JM: Protein-protein interactions: PDZ domain networks. Curr Biol. 6(11):1385–1388, 1996.
50. Hofer A, Dermietzel R: Visualization and functional blocking of gap junction hemichannels (connexons) with antibodies against external loop domains in astrocytes. Glia 24(1):141–154, 1998.
51. Dahl G, Werner R, Levine E, Rabadan-Diehl C: Mutational analysis of gap junction formation. Biophys J 62(1):172–180, 1992.
52. Berthoud VM, Beyer EC, Seul KH: Peptide inhibitors of intercellular communication. Am J Physiol Lung Cell Mol Physiol 279(4): L619–L622, 2000.
53. Dhein S: Peptides acting at gap junctions. Peptides 23(9):1701–1709, 2002.

第四部分
离子通道与细胞电生理学

第 20 章

哺乳动物心肌钾通道的异源性表达

Jeanne M. Nerbonne

本章目录

- 心肌电压门控外向 K^+ 电流的多样性 ··· 166
- 参与复极的其他种类心肌 K^+ 电流 ··· 168
- 电压门控 K^+ 通道中参与形成孔区的 α 亚单位的分子多样性 ··· 170
- 由 β 亚单位产生的电压门控 K^+ 通道的分子多样性 ··· 171
- 电压门控 K^+ 通道的亚单位和心脏瞬时外向 K^+ 通道之间的关系 ··· 171
- 电压门控 K^+ 通道的亚单位和心脏延迟整流 K^+ 通道之间的关系 ··· 173
- 其他心脏 K^+ 电流的分子构成 ··· 174
- 双孔结构 K^+ 通道 ··· 174
- 总结 ··· 175

在哺乳动物心肌中,动作电位的波形、时程,以及频率依赖性都具有显著的分布区域差异。这些差异影响了兴奋-收缩耦联以及心肌兴奋性的传播,并且这些差异还影响了心室复极的正常扩散。电生理研究表明,在哺乳动物的心肌中有多种类型的电压门控 K^+ 通道表达,并且这些通道的差异表达,参与了动作电位波形和不应期区域差异的形成。在一些病变心肌中,可发生电压门控 K^+ 电流的重构,从而影响兴奋的传播与节律,导致复极不均匀,成为了折返性心律失常的电生理基础。在确定了大量的电压门控 K^+ (voltage-gated K^+,Kv) 通道的孔区形成亚单位 (α 亚单位) 和附属亚单位 (β 亚单位) 后,逐步阐明了各种心肌电压门控 K^+ 通道的分子组成,也促进了对调控这些通道的特性和细胞表面功能性表达的分子机制研究。

哺乳动物心脏的动作电位波形,在不同部位有着很大的差异 (见图 20-1)。例如,在心房和心室肌,由电压门控 Na^+ 通道的内向电流组成的动作电位上升支速率很快 (见图 20-1),而在缺少电压门控 Na^+ 通道的结性组织 (如窦房结及房室结),主要由电压门控 Ca^{2+} 通道的内向 Ca^{2+} 电流组成的动作电位的上升支就明显相对缓慢 (见图 20-1)。除此之外,动作电位的高度、时程以及复极的时程也存在明显的区域差异 (见图 20-1)。上述这些差异主要反映出外向 K^+ 电流的功能性表达或特性在分布上的区域性差异,其次才是内向电流 (Na^+,Ca^{2+}),它们对心肌兴奋性的正常传播及心室复极的扩散均可产生重要影响。

对细胞的电生理研究已详细描述了主要的内向 (Na^+,Ca^{2+}) 和外向 (K^+) 电流的特性 (见图 20-1),这些电流参与了心肌细胞动作电位的形成。与 Na^+ 和 Ca^{2+} 电流相比,心肌 K^+ 电流具有多种类型的特点,并且在不同种 K^+ 电流中,电压门控 K^+ 电流数目最多,最具多样性 (见表 20-1)。目前已从心脏不同区域的细胞中,通过生理学或药理学的方法区分出了多种不同类型的电压门控 K^+ 通道 (见表 20-1),这些通道的差异表达对动作电位波形和不应期的区域性差异的形成具有十分重要的作用 (见图 20-1)[1,2]。另外,电压门控 K^+ 通道的密度、分布以及特性在许多心肌病变时都可发生明显改变,它们可影响兴奋的传导,降低节律性,从而促进致命性心律失常的发生[1]。因此,对调控这些通道的特性和

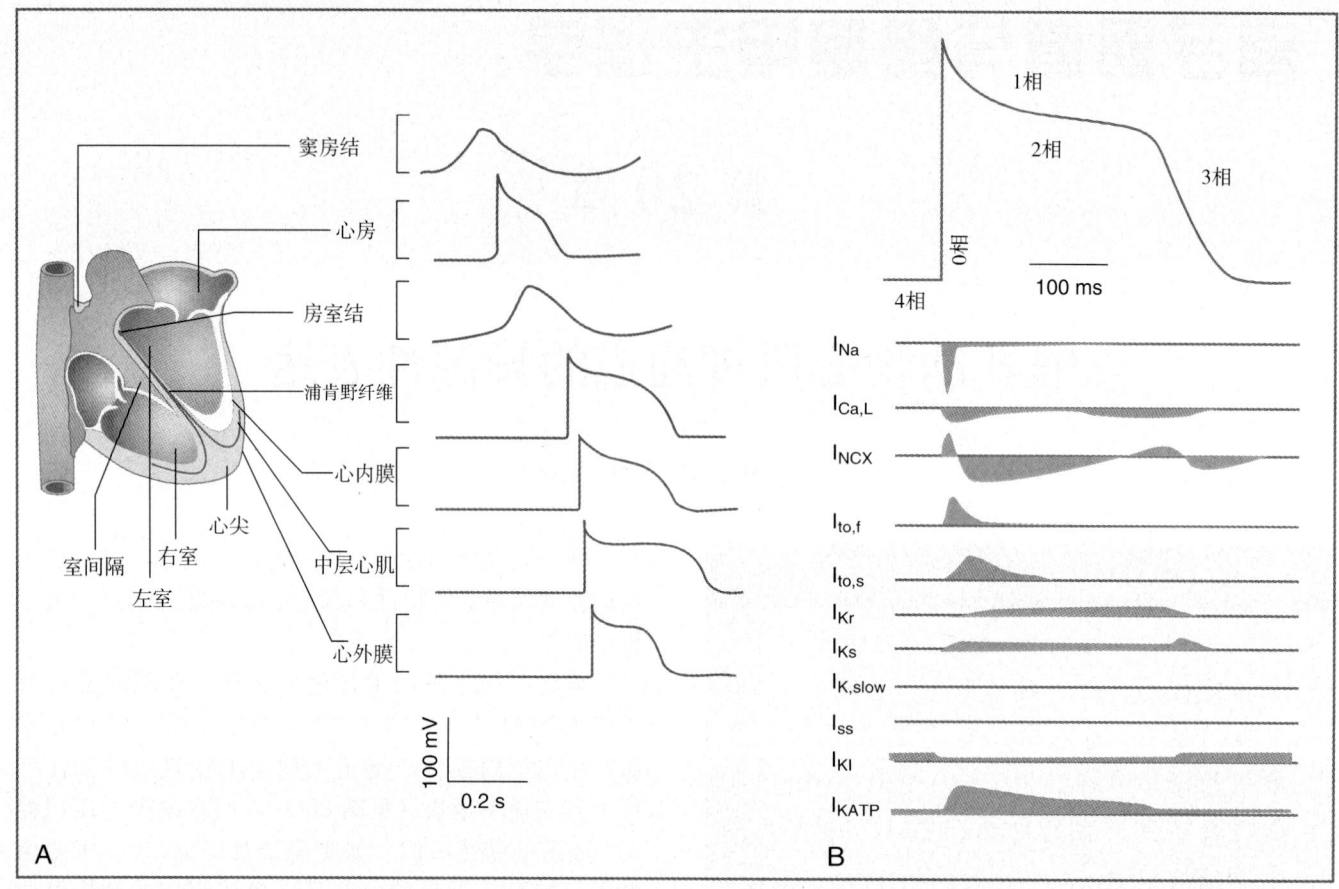

图 20-1 A：心脏不同区域动作电位波形的变化。值得注意的是，图中动作电位通过及时更替来反映兴奋传导的时间顺序。B：人类心室肌动作电位图和形成动作电位的离子电流。每种 K^+ 电流对形成动作电位波形的作用在不同种属，心肌的不同区域，以及不同类型的心肌细胞中都是不同的。ATP：三磷酸腺苷

功能表达的分子机制研究已成为广大学者关注的焦点。目前已明确了大量电压门控 K^+ 通道的参与形成孔区的 α 亚单位和附属 β 亚单位（见表 20-2）[3,4]，而且近年来，在确定这些亚单位和心肌细胞上表达的功能性电压门控 K^+ 通道之间的关系方面也取得了巨大进展[5,6]。这些研究揭示了电生理上不同类型的电压门控 K^+ 通道的分子内部联系确实是完全不同的[6]。重要的是，功能性电压门控 K^+ 通道的分子组成的确定，使得将来的研究能够集中在以下几个方面：阐明在正常心肌中，控制这些通道功能性表达的区域差异的分子机制；在心肌病变时，这些通道表达和/或特性被破坏的分子机制。本章综述了心肌电压门控 K^+ 通道的电生理特性和分子多样性，并重点阐述差异分布的 K^+ 通道，同时探讨调控 K^+ 通道区域表达的分子机制。

一、心肌电压门控外向 K^+ 电流的多样性

电压门控 K^+ 电流可影响动作电位的幅度和时程。在大多数的细胞中，目前已证实存在两大类电压门控 K^+ 电流：瞬时外向 K^+ 电流（I_{to}）和延迟外向整流 K^+ 电流（I_k）（见表 20-1）。瞬时电流 I_{to} 激活较快，主要参与早期复极（1 相）；而延迟整流 K^+ 电流（I_k）主要参与晚期复极（3 相）（见图 20-1）。这些是大的分类，然而实际上，在心脏细胞上有很多种类型的瞬时 K^+ 电流（I_{to}）和延迟整流 K^+ 电流（I_k）表达（见表 20-1）[5,6]。例如，电生理和药理学研究均已经明确证实存在两种瞬时外向 K^+ 电流，即 $I_{to,fast}$（$I_{to,f}$）和 $I_{to,slow}$（$I_{to,s}$），这些电流在分布上也存在差异[6]。快速激活和失活的瞬时外向 K^+ 电流（$I_{to,f}$）的特性是能够从稳态失活状态快速恢复，而 $I_{to,s}$ 则只能从失活状态

表 20-1　参与形成动作电位的阳离子电流

离子流	激活	失活	恢复	药理学	表达区域	心室的异源性表达
内向						
I_{Na}	快速	快速	快速	TTX	心房，心室，蒲肯野纤维	无
$I_{Ca(L)}$	快速	Ca^{2+}依赖的	快速	DHP	心房，心室，结区，浦肯野纤维	无
$I_{Ca(T)}$	快速	快速	快速	Cd^{2+}	心房，结区	无
I_f	快速	缓慢	快速	Cs^+	结区	无
外向						
$I_{to,f}$	快速	快速	快速	mM 4-AP HaTX HpTX	心房，心室，浦肯野纤维	有
$I_{to,s}$	快速	缓慢	缓慢	mM 4-AP	心室	有
I_{Kr}	中速	快速	缓慢	E-4031 Dofetillde	心室	有
I_{Ks}	非常慢	无	—	NE-10064 NE-10133	心室	有
I_{Kur}	快速	无	无	μM 4-AP	心房	无
I_{Kp}	快速	无	—	Ba^{2+}	心室	?
I_K	缓慢	缓慢	缓慢	mM TEA	心室	?
$I_{K,slow1}$	快速	缓慢	缓慢	mM 4-AP	心房，心室	无
$I_{K,slow2}$	快速	非常慢	缓慢	mM TEA	心房，心室	无
I_{ss}	缓慢	无	—	mM TEA	心房，心室	无
I_{KI}	—	—	—	Ba^{2+}	心房，心室	无
$I_{K,ATP}$	—	—	—	SUR	心房，心室	无

注：ATP，三磷酸腺苷；DHP, dihydropyridines，双氢吡啶；HaTX, hanatoxin；HpTX, heteropodatoxin；SUR, sulfonylureas，磺脲类；TEA, tetraethylammonium，四乙胺；TTX, tetrodotoxin，河豚毒素；4-AP, 4-aminopyridine，4-氨基吡啶

中缓慢地恢复[5,6]。另外，$I_{to,f}$可通过使用 Heteropoda 毒素 2 或 Heteropoda 毒素 3 将其与其他种电压门控外向 K^+ 电流（包括 $I_{to,s}$）区分开来。

在哺乳动物的心室，$I_{to,f}$ 和 $I_{to,s}$ 的分布都具有区域差异[6]。例如，在犬的左心室，心外膜和心肌中层细胞的 $I_{to,f}$ 密度大约是心内膜细胞的 5～6 倍（见图 20-2）[2]。在成年小鼠心室中，$I_{to,f}$ 密度也有很明显的区域差异，特别明显的是，$I_{to,f}$ 密度在右心室细胞比在左心室大，而在左心室细胞中，$I_{to,f}$ 密度在心尖部细胞又比在基底部的大[6-8]。在小鼠的心室间隔部，外向 K^+ 电流表达差异更明显：所有的室间隔细胞都表达 $I_{to,s}$，而几乎所有的（≈80%）室间隔细胞也都表达 $I_{to,f}$[6]。但是，室间隔细胞 $I_{to,f}$ 密度明显低于右心室或左心室细胞（P<0.001）[9]。在雪貂的左心室细胞中也有 $I_{to,f}$ 和 $I_{to,s}$ 的差异表达，并且仅在左室心内膜细胞有 $I_{to,s}$ 表达[9]。尽管存在分布上的表达差异，但 $I_{to,f}$ 和 $I_{to,s}$ 的特性在不同类型和不同种属的细胞中却非常相似，提示，这些通道（$I_{to,f}$ 和 $I_{to,s}$）最基本的分子结构很可能一样[6]。

电生理和药理学研究已经区分出多种类型的心脏延迟整流 K^+ 电流 I_k（见表 20-1），也证明了这些电流同样存在分布上的表达差异。例如在心房肌细胞，最主要的复极 K^+ 电流是快速激活而非失活的 K^+ 电流 I_{kur}（$I_{Kultrarapid}$），这种电流在心室肌细胞和结组织细胞均没有发现[6]。相比而言，在大多数心室肌细胞，有两种主要的延迟整流电流——I_{Kr}（$I_{K,rapid}$）和 I_{Ks}（$I_{K,slow}$），这两种电流在时间和电压依赖特性方面与 I_{kur} 截然不同[6]。I_{Kr} 和 I_{Ks} 在生物物理学特性方面也是不一样的：I_{Kr} 激活和失活都很快，表现出明显的内向整流，并且能被Ⅲ类抗心律失常药［包括多非利特（dofetilide）和索他洛尔（satalol）］特异性阻断[10]。相对而言，I_{Ks} 不具有内向整流，并且这种电流激活得很慢。最重要的是，近来研究证实这些离子通道内部的分子构成也都是不同的。

与瞬时外向 K^+ 电流相似，哺乳动物心室肌细胞 I_{Kr} 和 I_{Ks} 的表达也存在着显著的区域差异[1,2,6]。例如，如图 20-2 所示，犬的左室心外膜和心内膜细胞的 I_{Ks} 密度比中层心肌细胞的大[2]。在豚鼠左心室中也存在着 I_{Kr} 和 I_{Ks} 区域性差异表达[12]。例如，豚鼠左室游离

表 20-2　电压门控 K⁺ 通道（Kv）参与孔区形成的 α 亚单位种类

家族/亚家族		蛋白	基因	心脏离子流
Kv				
	Kv1	Kv1.1	KCNA1	
		Kv1.2	KCNA2	$I_{K,slow}$（大鼠）（IK, OTX）
		Kv1.3	KCNA3	
		Kv1.4	KCNA4	$I_{to,s}$
		Kv1.5	KCNA5	I_{Kur}（人/大鼠）
		Kv1.6	KCNA6	$I_{K,slow1}$（小鼠）
		Kv1.7	KCNA7	
	Kv2	**Kv2.1**	KCNB1	$I_{K,slow2}$（小鼠）
		Kv2.2	KCNB2	?
	Kv3	**Kv3.1**	KCNC1	I_{Kur}（犬）
		Kv3.2	KCNC2	
		Kv3.3	KCNC3	
		Kv3.4	KCNC4	
	Kv4	Kv4.1	KCND1	?
		Kv4.2	KCND2	$I_{to,f}$
		Kv4.3	KCND3	$I_{to,f}$
	Kv5	**Kv5.1**	KCNF1	?
	Kv6	Kv6.1	KCNG1	
		Kv6.2	KCNG2	
	Kv8	Kv8.1	KCN?	
	Kv9	Kv9.1	KCNS1	
		Kv9.2	KCNS2	
		Kv9.3	KCNS3	
EAG				
	eag	eag	KCNH1	
		ERG1	KCNH2	I_{Ks}
		ERG2	KCNH3	
		ERG3	KCNH4	
		elk		
KvLQT		**KvLQT1**	KCNQ1	I_{Ks}
		KCNQ2	KCNQ2	
		KCNQ3	KCNQ3	
		KCNQ4	KCNQ4	
		KCNQ5	KCNQ5	

注：黑体字代表其在心脏中表达

表 20-3　电压门控 K⁺ 通道附属亚单位

家族	亚单位	基因	心脏离子流
Kvβ	**Kvβ1**	KCNAB1	$I_{to,f}$?, $I_{K,slow1}$?
	Kvβ2	KCNAB2	?
	Kvβ3	KCNAB3	
KCNE	minK	KCNE1	I_{Ks}
	MiRP1	KCNE2	I_{Kr}?, $I_{to,f}$?, I_f?
	MiRP2	KCNE3	
	MiRP3	KCNE4	
KChAP	**KChAP**		$I_{to,f}$?, I_K?, $I_{K,slow1}$?, $I_{K,slow2}$?
KChIP	KChIP1	KCNIP1	
	KChIP2	KCNIP2	$I_{to,f}$
	KChIP3	KCNIP3	
NCS	**NCS-1**	FREQ	$I_{to,f}$或其他?
DPPX	DPPX	DPPX	$I_{to,f}$或其他?

注：黑体字代表其在心脏中表达。KChAP, K⁺ channel accessory protein, K⁺ 通道附属蛋白；KChIP, Kv channel interacting proteins, Kv 通道交互作用蛋白；NCS, neuronal Ca²⁺-sensing, 神经元 Ca²⁺ 感受器；DPPX, dipeptidyl aminopeptidase-like protein, 二肽基氨基肽酶样蛋白

壁的心外膜下心肌细胞的 I_{Kr} 密度就比中层心肌细胞和心内膜下心肌细胞的 I_{Kr} 密度大[12]。相对而言，在豚鼠左心室基底部和心内膜细胞的 I_{Kr} 和 I_{Ks} 密度就明显小于中层心肌细胞和心外膜细胞[12]。电压门控 K⁺ 电流密度分布的差异，导致了在心肌不同部位（如心房和心室，右心室和左心室，心尖和心室基底部）和心室壁的不同结构层次（心外膜、中层心肌和心内膜）记录到的动作电位在波形上的差异[1,2,5-8,11,12]。

在大鼠和小鼠心室细胞中，存在另一种特性与 I_{Ks} 和 I_{Kr} 完全不同的延迟整流 K⁺ 电流（见表 20-1）。这种新的延迟整流 K⁺ 电流也被归为 I_K，表示为 $I_{K,slow}$ 或 I_{ss}（见表 20-1）[6]。$I_{K,slow}$ 首先在小鼠心室肌细胞被发现，它是一种快速激活而缓慢失活的 K⁺ 电流，这种特性与该细胞上表达的 $I_{to,f}$、$I_{to,s}$ 和 I_{ss} 都不同[6]。另外，有报道，4-氨基吡啶（4-aminopyridine，4-AP）在微摩尔浓度水平就可选择性阻断 $I_{K,slow}$，但不能影响 $I_{to,f}$ 和 $I_{to,s}$[6,13]。然而，后续的研究发现，小鼠心室 $I_{K,slow}$ 存在两种不同的组分：$I_{K,slow1}$ 可以被微摩尔浓度的 4-AP 阻断，而 $I_{K,slow2}$ 可以被四乙铵（tetraethylammonium，TEA）选择性阻断[14-16]。另外研究表明，$I_{K,slow1}$ 和 $I_{K,slow2}$ 反映了其分子组成的差异[6,14-16]。与 $I_{to,f}$ 和 $I_{to,s}$ 的表达差异相比，$I_{K,slow1}$、$I_{K,slow2}$ 和 I_{ss} 在小鼠心房和心室肌细胞上的表达比较一致[6,14-17]。

二、参与复极的其他种类心肌 K⁺ 电流

除了电压门控 K⁺ 电流以外，内向整流 K⁺ 电流，尤其是心脏内向整流 K⁺ 电流 I_{k1} 和三磷酸腺苷（ATP）依赖的 K⁺ 电流（ATP dependent K⁺ current，I_{KATP}）也参与形成心肌动作电位[18,19]。虽然与电压门控 K⁺ 电流相比，这些电流在哺乳动物心脏上的表达看起来比较一致，但这些电流的密度在心脏的

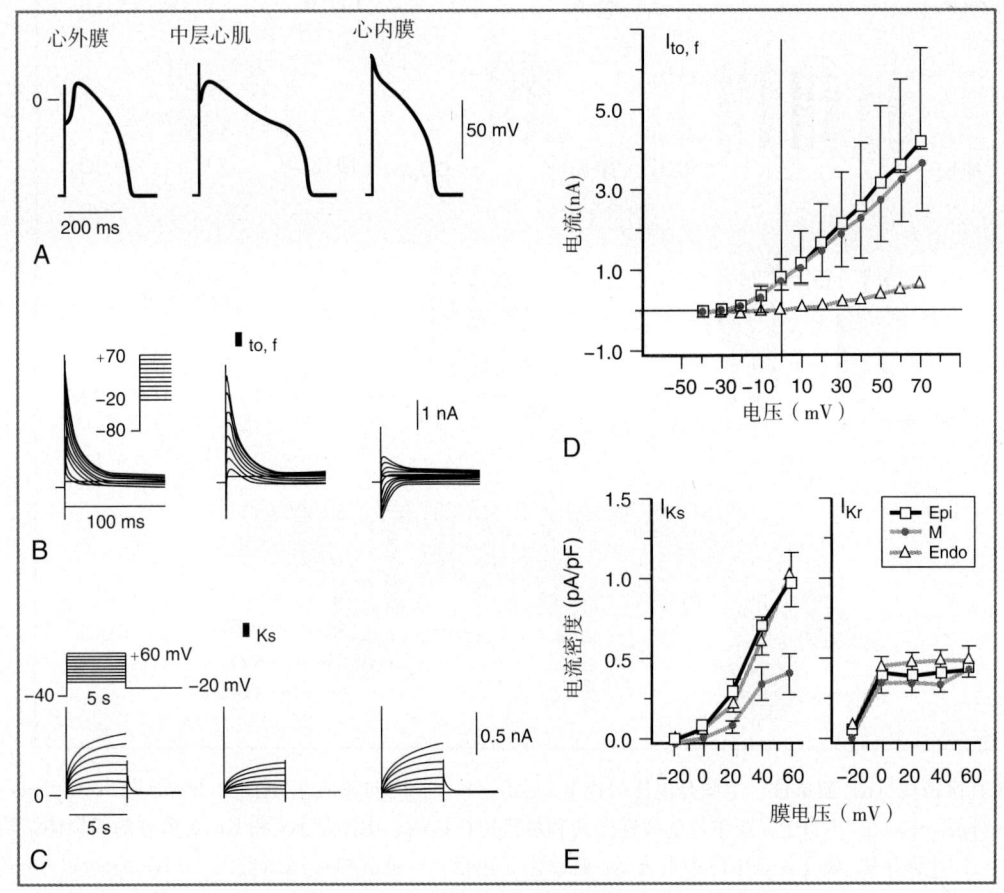

图20-2 犬心室肌细胞中动作电位波形和电压门控外向K^+电流分布的跨壁差异 A：分别在犬左心室、心外膜、中层心肌和心内膜心肌细胞记录到的代表性动作电位。B图和C图：分别是在犬心外膜、中层心肌和心内膜左室肌细胞记录到的瞬时外向电流（$I_{to,f}$）(B) 和缓慢延迟整流K^+离子流（I_{Ks}）波形。D：心外膜、中层心肌和心内膜细胞的瞬时外向电流（$I_{to,f}$）的平均峰离子流和电压的关系，结果以均数±标准差表示。E：I_{Ks}的密度（计算外向离子流尾端对E-4031不敏感成分），而非I_{Kr}，在中层心肌细胞中明显少于心外膜或心内膜左室肌细胞（ * $P<0.05$），结果以均数±标准差来表示（引自 Antzelevich C, Dumaine R：Electrical heterogeneity in the heart：Physiological, pharmacological and clinical implication. In：Page E, Fozzard HA, Solaro RJ [eds]：*Handbook of Physiology*, Section 2：The Cardiovascular System, Vol 1. New York, Oxford, 2002, pp 654-692.）

不同区域（如心房、心室和传导组织）还是有比较明显差异的。在心房和心室肌细胞中，I_{k1}在维持静息膜电位和平台期电位中都起着重要作用，并且它还参与了3相复极（见图20-1）。I_{k1}能维持心房和心室静息膜电位，是由于在负性膜电位的情况下这些通道的传导性较高[18]。尽管I_{k1}通道的电压依赖特性使得它在膜电位高于约-40mV时传导性很低，但I_{k1}通道确实参与了心室细胞动作电位平台期以及3相复极时的外向K^+电流（见图20-1），这是由于在除极时膜电位对K^+的驱动力很高[18]。

心肌ATP依赖的K^+通道是一种较弱的内向整流通道，它能被细胞内的ATP所抑制，而被二磷酸核苷激活[19]。在心室肌细胞中，缺血和缺氧时I_{KATP}的激活可通过动作电位时程的缩短来反映，提示它可能是细胞代谢和膜电位之间的一种内在联系[19]。I_{KATP}通道的开放可能参与了缺血预适应的心肌保护[20]。然而，不像心室电压依赖性K^+通道，I_{KATP}通道在左、右心室以及心室壁的各层细胞分布比较一致。而且，其表达的密度比其他膜K^+通道的密度大得多，这就提示可能只要有少量通道激活，动作电位时程就可出现显著地缩短。

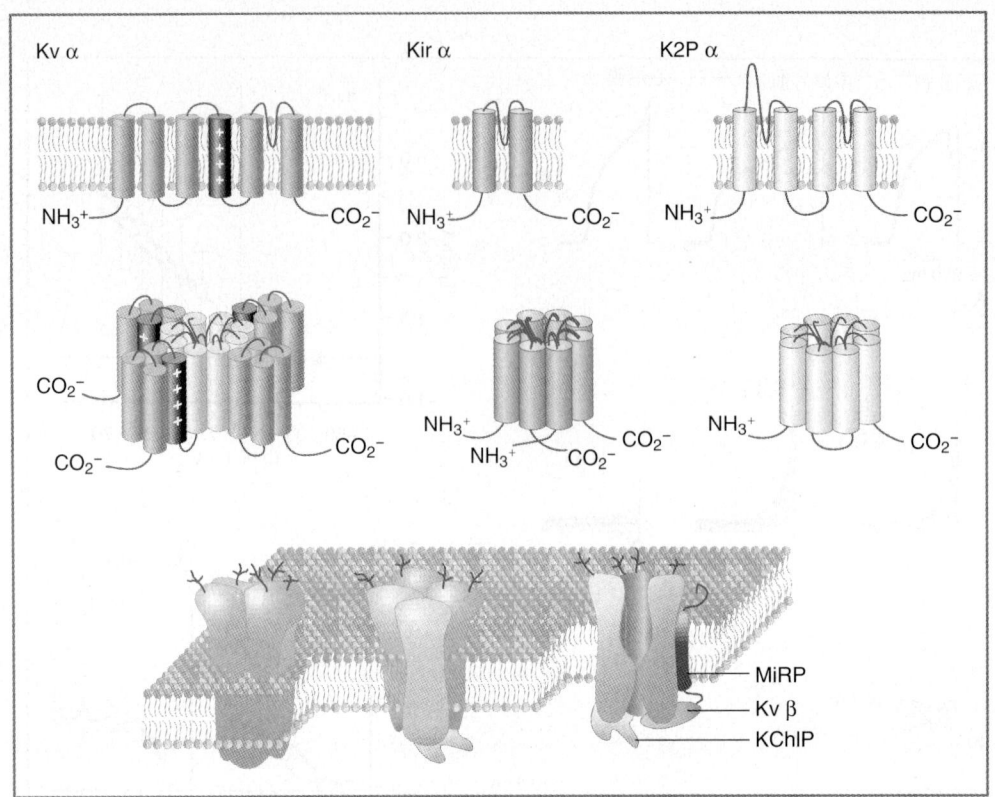

图 20-3　K^+ 通道孔区形成（α）亚单位　上图是电压门控 K^+ 通道（Kv）、内向整流 K^+ 通道（Inwardly rectifying, Kir）和双孔区 K^+ 通道（Two pore domain, K2P）α 亚单位的线性序列和跨膜拓扑结构。中图是 Kv 和 Kir 亚单位的四聚体结构和 K2P 亚单位的二聚体结构。下图是由 Kv 成孔 α 亚单位和附属 Kv 亚单位 [包括 Kv 通道相互作用蛋白 2（Kv channel interacting protein 2, KChIP2）、Kvβ 和 MiRP1] 组成功能性的电压门控 K^+ 通道示意图

三、电压门控 K^+ 通道中参与形成孔区的 α 亚单位的分子多样性

电压门控 K^+（Kv）通道中参与形成孔区的 α 亚单位是一种六次跨膜结构域蛋白（见图 20-3），其中第五和第六跨膜区参与形成 K^+ 通道孔[3]。由于 α 亚单位中带正电荷的第四跨膜区（见图 20-3）与电压门控 Na^+ 通道和 Ca^{2+} 通道的相应区域具有同源性，故可将这段跨膜区域归为电压门控通道的"S4"超家族[3,6]。然而，与电压门控 Na^+ 通道和 Ca^{2+} 通道不同的是，功能性电压门控 K^+ 通道有四个 α 亚单位（见图 20-3）。而且与心肌功能性电压门控 K^+ 通道的多样性相似的是，也存在多种 Kv α 亚单位（见表 20-1 和 20-2）。一些同源的 Kv α 亚单位的亚家族目前已经被鉴定出来，如 Kv1.x，Kv2.x，Kv3.x，Kv4.x，它们中大多数在哺乳动物心脏中都有表达（见表 20-2）。另外，功能性 K^+ 通道多样性的形成还可通过转录时不同剪切来完成，也可通过来自两种或多种属于同一 Kv 亚家族的 Kv α 亚单位蛋白形成异源及多源的多聚体来形成。

与 Kv1.x～Kv4.x α 亚单位的这些亚家族不同的是，Kv5.x～Kv9.x 亚家族成员的异源性表达本身并不能表现出功能性的电压门控 K^+ 通道[6]。将这些 α 亚单位（Kv5.1，Kv6.1，Kv8.1，Kv9.1）中的任何一种与 Shab（Kv2.x）亚家族成员联合注入细胞都会减弱 Shab（Kv2.x）引起的电流[6]。虽然这些研究提示，Kv5.x～Kv9.x 亚家族成员是 Kv2.x 亚家族的调节性 Kv α 亚单位，但这些"静止的"亚单位在功能性电压门控 K^+ 通道产生中的作用尚不清楚[6]。

哺乳动物 Kv α 亚单位的其他亚家族基因（见表 20-2）是随着一种蛋白 *human ether-a-go-go-related protein* HERG1（*KCNH2*）以及 KvLQT1（*KCNQ1*）的克隆而被发现的，其中 HERG1（KCNH2）一个位点突变可导致家族性长 QT 综合征（familial long QT syndrome, LQT2）；而 KvLQT1（KCNQ1）的一个位点突变可导致遗传性长 QT 综合征（inherited long QT syndrome, LQT1）[11]。ERG1

的异源性表达可表现出内向整流的电压门控 K^+ 电流，其特性与心脏 I_{Kr} 相似（见表 20-1）[11]。尽管有很多种 ERG（*KCNH*）亚家族成员（见表 20-2），但仅见到 ERG1 在心肌表达[6]。然而，在小鼠和人的心脏中已经明确 ERG1 的转录过程存在多种剪切形式，而且推测这种剪切形式可能在心脏 I_{Kr} 通道的形成中起作用[6,11]。与 ERG1 相比，KvLQT1 单独异源性表达表现出快速激活而不失活的 K^+ 电流，然而与 minK（见表 20-3）共同表达时，会产生缓慢激活的 K^+ 电流，这一电流形成了心脏延迟整流 I_{Ks} 的慢速部分[6,11]。*KCNQ* 亚家族的其他成员尽管不在哺乳动物心肌表达，但它们已经被克隆出来，并且证明它们具有导致良性家族性新生儿惊厥的突变位点[6]。*KCNQ2*/*KCNQ3* 共表达产生缓慢激活且不失活的选择性 K^+ 电流，这种通道的特性与神经元 M 通道类似[21]。

四、由 β 亚单位产生的电压门控 K^+ 通道的分子多样性

除了 Kv α 亚单位存在多样性外（见表 20-2），很多 Kv 通道的附属亚单位（Kv β）基因也已经被分离鉴定出来（见表 20-3）。这些 Kv β 亚单位基因中最先被明确的是 minK，它编码一个只具有单一的跨膜区的小分子蛋白（130 个氨基酸）[22]。有证据表明 minK 和 KvLQT1 共同形成功能性的心肌 I_{Ks} 通道[6,11,22]。minK 其他的同族成员，如 MiRP1（*KCNE2*）、MiRP2（*KCNE3*）和 MiRP3（*KCNE4*）也被陆续分离鉴定出来（见表 20-3），并且有证据提示 MiRP1 的功能是作为心脏 I_{Kr} 通道的 ERG1 的附属亚单位[23]。有趣的是，有报道发现 MiRP2 在哺乳动物骨骼肌中与 Kv3.4 组合在一起，并且在异源性表达系统中与 Kv4.x α 亚单位组合在一起[24,25]。这些观察提示了一种有趣的可能性，即 *KCNE* 附属亚单位能够与多种 Kv α 亚单位组合在一起，从而参与形成了多种类型的心肌电压门控 K^+ 通道。然而，还没有直接的实验证据支持这一假说，并且 *KCNE* 附属亚单位在功能性心脏电压门控 K^+ 通道或其他通道的形成中起着怎样的作用还需要进一步的明确[24-26]。

随着从大脑中分离鉴定出一种低分子量（≈45kD）的胞浆 β 亚单位，另一种类型的 Kv 附属亚单位也被发现了[4]。已经发现了有 4 种同源 Kv β 亚单位：Kvβ1、Kvβ2、Kvβ3 和 Kvβ4（表 20-3），它们在转录过程中也有多种剪切形式，其中 Kvβ1 和 Kvβ2 在心脏中表达[6]。Kv β 亚单位可与 Kv1 α 亚单位的胞内部分发生相互作用，而且研究还发现，Kv β 亚单位可影响 Kv α 亚单位编码的 K^+ 电流的特性以及 K^+ 通道在细胞表面的表达[4,6]。由于 Kv α 和 β 亚单位在内质网中是组合在一起的，功能性通道表达的增加提示 Kv β 亚单位可影响通道的组装、加工或稳定性，或者充当了伴侣蛋白[4,6]。然而，重要的是，我们还不知道在心肌中 Kv β1 和 Kv β2 亚单位与哪种 Kv α 亚单位联系在一起，并且这些 Kv β 亚单位在功能性 K^+ 通道的形成中起着怎样的作用还需要进一步明确[6]。在酵母双杂交系统中，利用 Kv2.1 的 N 末端作诱饵得到一种新的电压门控 K^+ 通道相关蛋白（K^+ channel accessory protein，KChAP）（见表 20-3）[27]。KChAP 与 Kv2.1（或 Kv2.2）共同表达可显著增加功能性 Kv2.x 的密度，而不会对电流的生物物理学特性产生太大的影响。这提示 KChAP 的功能可能是作为伴侣蛋白，而并非是一种亚单位[27]。总之，这些发现提示，KChAP 在决定多种心肌电压门控 K^+ 通道在细胞表面的功能性表达中可能起着重要作用[6]。然而目前还没有直接的实验证据支持这一假说。

近来分离得到的与 Kv 通道相互作用蛋白（Kv channel interacting proteins，KChIPs），也是在酵母双杂交系统中利用 Kv2.1 的 N 末端作诱饵得到的（见表 20-3）[28]。心脏中只有 KChIP2 表达，但 KChIP2 却存在多种剪切变异体[28-31]。有趣的是，KChIPs 属于神经元 Ca^{2+} 敏感性（NCS）蛋白的恢复蛋白（recoverin）家族[32]，并且包含 4 个 EF 手形区域[28]。然而，有别于其他的 NCS-1 蛋白，KChIP2（还有 KChIP3））N 末端缺少十四烷酰化位点[28]。当 KChIPs 与 Kv4 α 亚单位共表达时，它会增加 K^+ 电流的密度，减慢失活，增加失活状态下的恢复速度，并且改变激活的电压依赖性[28]。与之不同的是，当 KChIP 与 Kv1.4 或 Kv2.1 共表达时，并不影响它们编码的 K^+ 电流的特性或密度。这与认为 KChIPs 是特异性地调节 Kv4α 亚单位编码的 K^+ 通道的观点一致[28]。另外，尽管 KChIP 与 Kv4 α 亚单位的结合不是 Ca^{2+} 依赖的，但 EF 手形区域 2、3 和 4 的突变会使 KChIP1 对 Kv4 编码的 K^+ 电流的调节作用消失[28]。

五、电压门控 K^+ 通道的亚单位和心脏瞬时外向 K^+ 通道之间的关系

许多证据可提示，Kv4 亚家族的 Kvα 亚单位编码

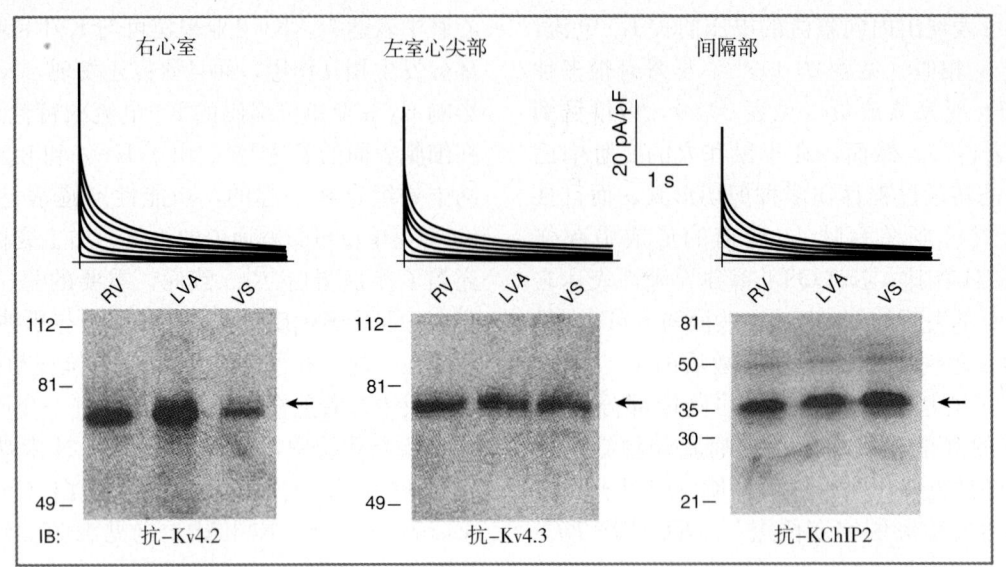

图 20-4 小鼠心室 $I_{to,f}$ 异源性表达的分子基础　上图：通过全细胞膜片钳技术记录到的离体小鼠心室肌细胞电流，结果表明右心室细胞峰值外向 K^+ 电流密度和 $I_{to,f}$ 密度都大于在左心室心尖部心肌细胞的相应离子流密度，而且峰值外向 K^+ 电流密度和 $I_{to,f}$ 密度在心室间隔部细胞明显较少。下图：成年小鼠心室肌细胞 Kv4.2、Kv4.3 和 KChIP2 表达的免疫印迹分析。从成年 C57BL6 小鼠的右心室、左心室心尖和间隔部分别取得总量相等的膜蛋白（50μg 每条带），上样于 8% 的 SDS-PAGE（十二烷基磺酸钠-聚丙烯酰胺凝胶电泳），然后转到 PVDF 膜，用抗 Kv4.2、抗 Kv4.3 和抗 KChIP2 的抗体进行免疫标记。在约 70kD 处有显示的条带（箭头所指）是 Kv4.2（左），约 75kD 处的条带是 Kv4.3（中），而约 35kD 处的条带是 KChIP2（右）。Kv4.3 和 KChIP2 在成年小鼠心室中是均一高表达，而 Kv4.2 蛋白表达与功能性的 $I_{to,f}$ 区域性异源表达（上图）相一致（引自 Guo W, Li H, London B, Nerbonne JM：Functional consequences of elimination of $I_{(to,f)}$ and $I_{(to,s)}$：Early afterdepolarizations, atrioventricular block, and ventricular arrhythmias in mice lacking Kv1.4 and expressing a dominant-negative Kv4 alpha subunit. Cir Res 2000；87：73-79. ；and Guo W, Li H, Aimond F, et al：Role of heteromultimers in the generation of myocardial transient outward K^+ currents. Cir Res 2002；90：586-593.）

心脏 $I_{to,f}$ 通道[6]。在大鼠和小鼠的心室肌细胞中，以其反义寡核苷酸（antisense oligodeoxynucleotides, AsODNs）拮抗 Kv4.2 或 Kv4.3 的作用，发现 $I_{to,f}$ 的密度下降了约 50%[5,6]。另外，在表达 Kv4.2 突变体 Kv4.2W362F（Kv4.2DN）的转基因小鼠中（Kv4.2 功能缺失），分离得到的心室和心房肌细胞没有 $I_{to,f}$[6]。生化和电生理研究进一步提示在成年小鼠的心室细胞中 Kv4.2 和 Kv4.3 是联系在一起的，并且在小鼠心室功能性的 $I_{to,f}$ 通道是异源性的[33]。考虑到 $I_{to,f}$ 特性的相似性（见表 20-1），似乎有理由认为 Kv4α 亚单位亦是其他种动物 $I_{to,f}$ 的基础。然而，在犬和人心脏中，由于未见有 Kv4.2 表达的报道，因此候选亚单位为 Kv4.3[34]。尽管 Kv4.3 存在剪切变异体，但 Kv4.3 蛋白的表达水平和它们在心脏功能性 $I_{to,f}$ 通道形成中起着怎样的作用都还需进一步研究。

在成年小鼠心室细胞中发现 KChIP2 能与 Kv4.2 及 Kv4.3 α 亚单位免疫共沉淀下来，这与 KChIP2 亚单位在 Kv4 编码的小鼠心室 $I_{to,f}$ 通道形成中起作用的观点相一致[33]。在犬和人类心脏中，在心室壁各层都有 KChIP2 的 mRNA 表达[29,30]，提示这可能是导致人类和犬的心室中心外膜和心内膜 $I_{to,f}$ 密度存在差异的基础（见图 20-2）[2,6]。尽管有报道发现在犬的心肌中，KChIP2 的蛋白表达并非平行于其 mRNA 的表达[30]。然而后续的研究显示，在犬的心室细胞中 KChIP2 的 mRNA 表达和蛋白质表达，以及 $I_{to,f}$ 密度的表达模式确实很相似[35]，这一发现也与下述观点一致，即在犬和人类的心室中，KChIP2 在决定功能性 $I_{to,f}$ 密度中起重要作用。然而，在大鼠和小鼠中并不存在 KChIP2 mRNA 或蛋白的表达（见图 20-4）[29,30]。另外，Kv4.2 的 mRNA 和蛋白的表达存在显著的区域性差异（见图 20-4），因此看来在啮齿类动物中，Kv4.2（而非 KChIP2）的差异表达是形成 $I_{to,f}$ 密度区域性变化的基础[33,36]。然而，近来的研究亦发现在雪貂的心室中，KChIP2 的一种剪切变异体，KChIP2b，在决定 $I_{to,f}$ 密度区域性差异中起作用[31]。尽管在成年小鼠的心室中发现，KChIP 相关蛋白 NCS-1 亦是均匀表达，但这种作为假定的 Kv 通道附属亚单位的蛋白表达模式还未在犬或人类的心脏中观察到，并且

NCS-1 在控制心肌功能性 $I_{to,f}$ 密度中起何作用尚未确定。同样，其他 Kv 附属亚单位，包括 MiRP1[25]、Kvβ1[38] 以及近来发现的 Kv4 特异性附属亚单位 DP-PX[39]，在心肌 $I_{to,f}$ 通道的形成和/或在决定 $I_{to,f}$ 密度区域性差异方面起着怎样的功能性作用还需要深入研究。（见表 20-3）。

在心室肌细胞中慢速瞬时外向 K^+ 电流，$I_{to,s}$，其动力学和药理学特性与 $I_{to,f}$ 完全不同（见表 20-1），这提示心室 $I_{to,s}$ 与 $I_{to,f}$ 各自的分子构成也是截然不同的。直接的实验证据支持了这一假说，即对特异性缺失 Kv1.4 基因小鼠（Kv1.4$^{-/-}$）的分离心肌细胞进行电生理实验，发现在间隔细胞测不到 $I_{to,s}$[40]。然而，在 Kv1.4$^{-/-}$ 小鼠的心室（和心房）肌细胞中，$I_{to,f}$、$I_{K,slow1}$、$I_{K,slow2}$ 以及 I_{ss} 的特性及密度与在野生型细胞中测量到的没有区别[40]。有趣的是，在 Kv4.2 基因缺失小鼠（$I_{to,f}$ 亦缺失）的心室中出现明显电重构，而 $I_{to,s}$ 和 Kv1.4 蛋白的上调可以解释这一现象[7]。考虑到慢速瞬时外向 K^+ 电流在其他种属的相似性以及时间和电压依赖的特性，尽管目前没有明确的实验证据，似乎有理由认为在雪貂、兔、犬和人的心室肌细胞中 Kv1.4 亦编码 $I_{to,s}$。

六、电压门控 K^+ 通道的亚单位和心脏延迟整流 K^+ 通道之间的关系

如前所述，ERG1 是 LQT2 的一个突变位点，并且 ERG1 的异源性表达表现出与心脏 I_{Kr} 类似的电压门控内向整流选择性 K^+ 通道[11]。尽管在小鼠和人的心脏中已经明确存在着独特 N 和 C 末端的 ERG1 的不同剪切体，但生化实验显示，在心室（大鼠、小鼠、人）中只表现一种 ERG1 全长蛋白质的功能，这提示 ERG1 的剪切体在功能性 I_{Kr} 通道的形成中并不起作用[41]。有研究发现心脏功能性 I_{Kr} 通道是个多聚体，由 ERG1 和 minK 组成，并且近来的研究发现在马的心室中，ERG1 和 minK 可以免疫共沉淀下来[42]。然而，只有在其他种属中也能发现类似的 ERG1 和 minK 之间的相互关系才能确定上述观点。

尽管 *KCNQ1*（LQT1 的突变位点）的异源性表达可导致快速激活而不失活的电压门控 K^+ 电流，但它与 minK 共表达会产生与心脏 I_{Ks} 类似的慢速激活的 K^+ 电流[11]。这些观察以及生化研究资料提示，异源性表达的 KvLQT1 与 minK 共同形成了心脏功能性的

表 20-4 内向整流 K^+ 通道（Kir）和双孔 K^+ 通道（K2P）的 α 亚单位

家族/亚家族	蛋白	基因	心脏离子流
Kir			
Kir1	**Kir1.1**	KCNJ1	?
Kir2	**Kir2.1**	KCNJ2	I_{k1}
	Kir2.2	KCNJ12	I_{k1}
	Kir2.3	KCNJ4	?
	Kir2.4	KCNJ14	?
Kir3	**Kir3.1**	KCNJ3	I_{KACh}
	Kir3.2	KCNJ6	
		KCNJ7	
	Kir3.3	KCNJ9	
	Kir3.4	KCNJ5	I_{KACh}
Kir4	Kir4.1	KCNJ10	
	Kir4.2	KCNJ15	
Kir5	Kir5.1	KCNJ16	
Kir6	**Kir6.1**	KCNJ8	
	Kir6.2	KCNJ11	I_{KACh}
K2P			
TWIK	**TWIK-1**	KCNK1	?
	TWIK-2	KCNK6	?
	TWIK-3	KCNK7	
	TWIK-4	KCNK8	
TREK	TREK-1	KCNK2	?
	TREK-2	KCNK10	
TASK	**TASK-1**	KCNK3	I_{Kp}?
	TASK-2	KCNK5	
	TASK-3	KCNK9	
	TASK-4	KCNK14	
	TASK-5	KCNK15	
TRAAK	**TRAAK-1**	KCNK4	
THIK	THIK-1	KCNK13	
	THIK-2	KCNK12	?
TALK	TALK-1	KCNK16	
	TALK-2	KCNK17	?

注：黑体字表示其在心脏中表达

I_{Ks}通道[11]。近来对马心室的研究提供了直接的生化证据，证明 KvLQT1 和 minK 可发生相互作用[41]。然而，还没有研究表明在人和犬的心肌中 KvLQT1 和 minK 是直接结合在一起的，而且功能性 I_{Ks} 通道的化学计量学特性也不明确。另外，控制功能性 I_{Ks} 通道细胞表面表达的分子机制，以及在人和犬的心室肌中存在的功能性 I_{Ks} 密度区域性差异的分子机制也都还不清楚。

与瞬时外向 K^+ 电流相似，应用分子遗传学的方法，结合生化和电生理手段，近年来在小鼠中进行的哺乳动物心肌功能性延迟整流 K^+ 通道多样性的分子基础的研究，使我们对此领域有了更深一步的认识。例如，Kv1 α 亚单位在小鼠心室 $I_{K,slow}$ 的形成中所起的作用随着研究的深入而被揭示。人们发现在 Kv1 α 亚单位表达缺失的转基因小鼠中（Kv1.1$^{-/-}$），其心室肌细胞的 $I_{K,slow}$ 特异性地减弱[13]。然而，随后研究发现在 Kv2.1 表达缺失的小鼠中，其心室肌细胞 $I_{K,slow}$ 也是下降的[14]。对此进一步的分析显示，野生型小鼠心室 $I_{K,slow}$ 存在两种截然不同的组分：一种称为 $I_{K,slow1}$，它对微摩尔浓度的 4-AP 敏感，是由 Kv1 α 亚单位编码，而另外一种，即 $I_{K,slow2}$，它由 Kv2 α 亚单位编码并且对 TEA 敏感[14]。随后的研究发现在 Kv1.5 缺失的小鼠中，其心室肌细胞中无 $I_{K,slow1}$，提示 Kv1.5 编码 $I_{K,slow1}$[15]。这些发现结合前面使用 Kv1.4$^{-/-}$ 动物（该种动物心室细胞无 $I_{to,s}$）的研究提示，Kv1 α 亚单位与 Kv4 α 亚单位不同，其成员 Kv1.4 和 Kv1.5 在成年小鼠心室并不相关。相反，在小鼠心室肌细胞中，功能性 Kv1 α 亚单位编码的 K^+ 通道是由 Kv1.4 α 亚单位（$I_{to,s}$）或 Kv1.5 α 亚单位（$I_{K,slow1}$）单一成分组成。然而，Kv 附属亚单位在功能性 $I_{to,s}$、$I_{K,slow1}$、$I_{K,slow2}$ 通道的产生中起何种作用以及控制这些通道表达的具体分子机制仍需要进一步研究。

七、其他心脏 K^+ 电流的分子构成

在心脏和其他细胞中，内向整流 K^+ 通道是由含多个亚家族的整流 K^+ 通道（Kir）的孔区形成 α 亚单位的基因来编码（见表 20-4），每个基因编码一个具有两次跨膜结构域的蛋白质，这些蛋白质再组装成四聚体形成 K^+ 选择性孔道（见图 20-3）。基于产生于异源性表达系统电流的特性，人们发现 Kir2 α 亚单位编码很强的心脏内向整流 I_{K1} 通道，并且 Kir2 亚家族的一些成员也在心肌上有表达[18]。关于 Kir2 α 亚单位在心脏 I_{K1} 通道形成中作用的研究是在缺失 Kir2.1（Kir2.1$^{-/-}$）或 Kir2.2（Kir2.2$^{-/-}$）小鼠心肌细胞上完成的[43]。尽管 Kir2.1$^{-/-}$ 小鼠表现有腭裂，并且出生后很快死亡，使我们无法对其成年动物进行电生理方面的研究，但小鼠新生期 Kir2.1$^{-/-}$ 心室肌细胞的电压膜片钳记录显示其 I_{K1} 是缺失的[43]。相对而言，来自成年 Kir2.2$^{-/-}$ 心室肌细胞的记录显示出其 I_{K1} 在数量上明显减少[43]。总之，这些结果提示，Kir2.1 和 Kir2.2 都参与了小鼠心室 I_{K1} 通道的形成，并且心脏的功能性 I_{K1} 通道是异源性的。很明显，进一步的研究应当集中在直接验证这一假说，并且阐述控制功能性 I_{K1} 通道区域性差异表达的分子机制。

在哺乳动物心脏中，I_{KATP} 通道在心肌缺血及预处理中发挥重要作用[19,20]。在异源性表达系统中，带有 ATP 结合盒式蛋白的 Kir6.x 亚单位可编码磺酰脲类受体（sulfonylurea receptors，SURx），它可同 Kir6.2 共表达而重组成 I_{KATP} 通道[44]。尽管药理学和 mRNA 表达研究提示，心肌细胞 I_{KATP} 通道是由 Kir6.2 和 SUR2A 编码的，但 Kir6.2 可能起主要作用，这是因为人们发现在 Kir6.2$^{-/-}$ 动物的心室肌细胞中测不到 I_{KATP}[45]。另外，心脏 I_{KATP} 通道活性在 SUR2$^{-/-}$ 心肌细胞中下降，而在 SUR1$^{-/-}$ 心肌细胞中不受影响，这提示 SUR2 发挥着重要作用[46,47]。有趣的是，在 SUR2$^{-/-}$ 心肌细胞中其余的 I_{KATP} 通道特性与那些产生于共表达 Kir6.2 和 SUR1 心肌细胞的 I_{KATP} 通道特性类似[46]，这提示 SUR1 可能可以和 Kir6.2 共组装在一起，从而产生功能性的心脏 I_{KATP} 通道。

尽管在 Kir6.2$^{-/-}$ 和野生型的心室肌细胞中，其动作电位波形观察不到区别，但在缺血或代谢阻断的状态下，野生型细胞中出现动作电位缩短，而 Kir6.2$^{-/-}$ 细胞却没有这种现象[45]，这一现象与以下假说一致，即心脏 I_{KATP} 通道在病理状态下，尤其是与代谢应激有关的病理状态下发挥着重要作用。有趣的是，在表达突变 I_{KATP} 通道（对 ATP 敏感性显著降低，下降 40 倍）的转基因动物中，动作电位时程大部分未受影响，这提示在体情况下存在其他的抑制机制调节心脏 I_{KATP} 通道活性[48]。因此，与强大的心肌内向整流 I_{K1} K^+ 电流类似，需要对心肌 I_{KATP} 通道的调控、功能发挥和区域性表达差异的分子机制进一步深入研究。

八、双孔结构 K^+ 通道

除了电压门控 K^+ 通道和内向整流 K^+ 通道（分别

见表20-2和20-4）形成孔区的α亚单位是四聚体外（见图20-3），一种有着四个跨膜段及双孔结构域的新型K⁺亚单位随着TWIK-1（two-pore, weakly inwardly rectifying K⁺ channel subunit-1）的克隆而被发现。两个孔区都参与了K⁺选择性孔道的形成，而且TWIK-1亚单位是一个二聚体[50]。大量双孔区K⁺通道（two-pore domain K⁺，KTP）α亚单位基因被发现，而且其中一些在哺乳动物心肌中表达（见表20-4）。KTP亚单位的异源性表达产生的电流，其生物物理特性以及对一些调节因子（包括pH和脂肪酸）的敏感性与其他K⁺电流截然不同[49]。

通过对KTPα亚单位的多样性（见表20-4）、亚单位表达分布的广泛性[49]，以及多种生理相关的刺激可调节KTP亚单位编码的通道特性的研究，揭示了KTP通道可能具有多种重要的功能。然而在其他种属细胞中，这些心肌的亚单位/通道的生理作用仍不明确[49]。有趣的是，在心脏中也发现存在TWIK相关K⁺通道亚单位-1（TWIK-related K⁺ channel subunit-1，TREK-1）和双孔、酸敏感K⁺通道亚单位-1（two-pore, acid-sensitive K⁺ channel-1，TASK-1）的表达，这些亚单位的异源性表达产生了瞬时、不失活的K⁺电流，这种电流表现出很弱的或没有电压依赖性[49]。尽管这些特性提示KTP亚单位可能参与了"背景"或"渗漏"K⁺通道的形成[50]，但是没有直接的实验证据支持这一假说。众多研究者都在致力于验证这一假说，明确心脏背景（K⁺）传导性的分子机制，并探索控制这些通道在哺乳动物心肌表达和发挥功能的分子机制。

九、总　　结

电生理研究已经区分出多种类型的电压门控内向和外向电流，它们参与了哺乳动物心肌细胞中动作电位的复极（见表20-1）。外向电流（K⁺）比内向电流（Na^+，Ca^{2+}）更多而且更多样。大多数心肌细胞表达了所有的电压门控和内向整流K⁺通道（见表20-1）。另外，其中一些K⁺通道在不同心肌细胞以及心室壁的不同层次的表达都有明显差异。分子克隆技术已经发现了多种电压门控（Kv）以及非电压门控（Kir和KTP）K⁺通道的孔区形成α亚单位（见表20-2和表20-4）和附属电压门控（Kv）β亚单位（见表20-3），这些亚单位参与形成了多种具有明显电生理差异的心脏K⁺电流（见表20-1），而且在对这些α亚单位参与形成大多数表达于哺乳动物心肌细胞的K⁺通道的研究方面，近年来已取得了巨大的进展（见表20-2和表20-4）。另外，在关于心肌K⁺电流异源性表达的分子机制方面进行的生化研究也为此提供了一些新的认识。例如，已证明$I_{to,f}$电流密度的区域性差异与成年小鼠心室中Kv4.2蛋白表达差异有关[33]，然而，KChIP2附属通道蛋白的差异表达看来也是犬和人心室中$I_{to,f}$密度在各层心肌存在差异的原因[29,35]。

与研究Kv和Kirα亚单位编码电压门控和内向整流心肌K⁺电流方面取得的进展相比，目前关于大多数Kv通道附属亚单位或KTP亚单位的功能所知其少（见表20-3和表20-4）。看来下一步研究的重点应该主要集中在阐明不同Kvβ亚单位和KTPα亚单位在心肌K⁺通道的产生中所发挥的作用，以及探讨调控心肌K⁺通道（由Kvα、Kvβ、Kirα和KTPα亚单位编码的心肌K⁺通道）的特性及细胞表面表达的分子机制。重要的是，大量研究已描述了功能性K⁺通道的表达在不同心肌病变时的改变，这些改变可反映通道特性的变化，以及通道分子组成的改变，或/和通道的基本亚单位组装过程的变化。有很多可能的分子机制（转录、翻译和翻译后水平的）参与到调节心肌K⁺通道在正常以及损伤或病变心肌中的功能表达和特性。似乎可以肯定的是未来的工作将主要集中于更细致地探讨这些机制。

（张幼怡　肖晗　龚开政　译）

参 考 文 献

1. Nerbonne JM, Guo W: Heterogeneous expression of voltage-gated potassium channels in the heart: Roles in normal excitation and arrhythmias. J Cardiovasc Electrophysiol 13:406-409, 2002.
2. Antzelevitch C, Dumaine R: Electrical heterogeneity in the heart: Physiological, pharmacological and clinical implications. In: Page E, Fozzard HA, Solaro RJ (eds): Handbook of Physiology, Section 2: The Cardiovascular System, Vol 1. New York, Oxford, 2002, pp 654-692.
3. Coetzee WA, Amarillo Y, Chiu J, et al: Molecular diversity of K⁺ channels. Ann NY Acad Sci 868:233-285, 1999.
4. Pongs O, Leicher T, Berger M, et al: Functional and molecular aspects of voltage-gated K⁺ channel β subunits. Ann NY Acad Sci 868:344-355, 1999.
5. Oudit GY, Kassiri Z, Sah R, et al: The molecular physiology of the cardiac transient outward potassium current (I_{to}) in normal and diseased myocardium. J Mol Cell Cardiol 33:851-872, 2001.
6. Nerbonne JM: Molecular analysis of voltage-gated K⁺ channel diversity and functioning in the mammalian heart. In Page E, Fozzard HA, Solaro RJ (eds): Handbook of Physiology, Section 2: The Cardiovascular System, Vol 1. New York, Oxford, 2002, pp 568-594.
7. Guo W, Li H, London B, Nerbonne JM: Functional consequences of elimination of $I_{to,f}$ and $I_{to,s}$: Early afterdepolarizations, atrioventricular block, and ventricular arrhythmias in mice lacking Kv1.4 and expressing a dominant-negative Kv4 alpha subunit. Circ Res 87:73-79, 2000.
8. Brunet S, Aimond F, Li H, et al: Expression of repolarizing voltage-gated K⁺ currents in adult mouse ventricles: Impact of anatomy and gender. J Physiol 2003 (submitted).

9. Brahmajothi MV, Campbell DL, Rasmussen RL, et al: Distinct transient outward potassium current (Ito) phenotypes and distribution of fast-inactivating potassium channel alpha subunits in ferret left ventricular myocytes. J Gen Physiol 113:581–600, 1999.
10. Jurkiewicz NK, Sanguinetti MC: Rate-dependent prolongation of cardiac action potentials by a methanesulfonanilide class III antiarrhythmic agent. Specific block of rapidly activating delayed rectifier K^+ current by dofetilide. Circ Res 72:75–83, 1993.
11. Keating MT, Sanguinetti MC: Molecular and cellular mechanisms of cardiac arrhythmias. Cell 104:569–580, 2001.
12. Bryant SM, Wan X, Shipsey SJ, Hart G: Regional differences in the delayed rectifier current (I_{Kr} and I_{Ks}) contribute to the differences in action potential duration in basal left ventricular myocytes in guinea-pig. Cardiovasc Res 40:322–331, 1998.
13. London B, Jeron A, Zhou J, et al: Long QT and ventricular arrhythmias in transgenic mice expressing the N terminus and first transmembrane segment of a voltage-gated potassium channel. Proc Natl Acad Sci U S A 95:2926–2931, 1998.
14. Xu H, Barry DM, Li H, et al: Attenuation of the slow component of delayed rectification, action potential prolongation, and triggered activity in mice expressing a dominant-negative Kv2 alpha subunit. Circ Res 85:623–633, 1999.
15. London B, Guo W, Pan XH, et al: Targeted replacement of Kv1.5 in the mouse leads to loss of the 4-aminopyridine-sensitive component of $I_{(K,slow)}$ and resistance to drug-induced QT prolongation. Circ Res 88:940–946, 2001.
16. Zhou J, Kodirov S, Murata M, et al: Regional upregulation of Kv2.1-encoded current, $I_{K,slow2}$, in Kv1DN mice is abolished by crossbreeding with Kv2DN mice. Am J Physiol Heart Circ Physiol 284:H491–H500, 2003.
17. Bou-Abboud E, Li H, Nerbonne JM: Molecular diversity of the repolarizing voltage-gated K^+ currents in mouse atrial cells. J Physiol 529:345–358, 2000.
18. Nichols CG, Lopatin AN: Inward rectifier potassium channels. Ann Rev Physiol 59:171–191, 1997.
19. Findlay I: The ATP sensitive potassium channel of cardiac muscle and action potential shortening during metabolic stress. Cardiovasc Res 28:760–761, 1994.
20. Grover GJ, Garlid KD: ATP-sensitive potassium channels: A review of their cardioprotective pharmacology. J Mol Cell Cardiol 32:677–695, 2000.
21. Wang HS, Pan Z, Shi W, et al: KCNQ2 and KCNQ3 potassium channel subunits: Molecular correlates of the M-channel. Science 282:1890–1893, 1998.
22. Abbott GW, Goldstein SA: A superfamily of small potassium channel subunits: Form and function of the MinK-related peptides (MiRPs). Q Rev Biophys 31:357–398, 1998.
23. Abbott GW, Sesti F, Splawski I, et al: MiRP1 forms I_{Kr} potassium channels with HERG and is associated with cardiac arrhythmia. Cell 97:175–187, 1999.
24. Abbott GW, Butler MH, Bendahhou S, et al: MiRP2 forms potassium channels in skeletal muscle with Kv3.4 and is associated with periodic paralysis. Cell 104:217–231, 2001.
25. Zhang M, Jiang M, Tseng GN: minK-related peptide 1 associates with Kv4.2 and modulates its gating function: Potential role as beta subunit of cardiac transient outward channel? Circ Res 88:1012–1019, 2001.
26. Yu H, Wu J, Potapova I, et al: MinK-related peptide 1: A beta subunit for the HCN ion channel subunit family enhances expression and speeds activation. Circ Res 88:E84–E87, 2001.
27. Wible BA, Yang Q, Kuryshev YA, et al: Cloning and expression of a novel K^+ channel regulatory protein, KChAP. J Biol Chem 273:11745–11751, 1998.
28. An WF, Bowlby MR, Betty M, et al: Modulation of A-type potassium channels by a family of calcium sensors. Nature 403:553–556, 2000.
29. Rosati B, Pan Z, Lypen S, et al: Regulation of KChIP2 potassium channel beta subunit gene expression underlies the gradient of transient outward current in canine and human ventricle. J Physiol 533:119–125, 2001.
30. Deschenes I, DiSilvestre D, Juang GJ, et al: Regulation of Kv4.3 current by KChIP2 splice variants: A component of native cardiac $I_{(to)}$? Circulation 106:423–429, 2002.
31. Patel S, Campbell DL, Morales MJ, Strauss HC: Heterogenous expression of KChIP2 isoforms in the ferret heart. J Physiol 539:649–656, 2002.
32. Burgoyne RD, Weiss JL: The neuronal calcium sensor family of Ca^{2+}-binding proteins. Biochem J 353:1–12, 2001.
33. Guo W, Li H, Aimond F, et al: Role of heteromultimers in the generation of myocardial transient outward K^+ currents. Circ Res 90:586–593, 2002.
34. Dixon JE, Shi W, Wang HS, et al: Role of the Kv4.3 K^+ channel in ventricular muscle. A molecular correlate for the transient outward current. Circ Res 79:659–668, 1996.
35. Rosati B, Grau F, Rodriguez S, et al: Concordant expression of KChIP2 mRNA, protein and transient outward current throughout the canine ventricle. J Physiol 548:815–822, 2003.
36. Dixon JE, McKinnon D: Quantitative analysis of potassium channel mRNA expression in atrial and ventricular muscle of rats. Circ Res 75:252–260, 1994.
37. Guo W, Malin SA, Johns DC, et al: Modulation of Kv4-encoded K^+ currents in the mammalian myocardium by neuronal calcium sensor-1. J Biol Chem 277:26436–26443, 2002.
38. Perez-Garcia MT, Lopez-Lopez JR, Gonzalez C: Kv β1.2 subunit coexpression in HEK-293 cells confers O_2 sensitivity to Kv4.2 but not to Shaker channels. J Gen Physiol 113:897–908, 1999.
39. Nadal MS, Ozaita A, Amarillo, et al: The CO26-related dipeptidyl aminopeptidase-like protien DPPX is a critical component of neuronal A-type K^+ channels. Neuron 37:449–461, 2003.
40. Guo W, Xu H, London B, Nerbonne JM: Molecular basis of transient outward K^+ current diversity in mouse ventricular myocytes. J Physiol 521:587–599, 1999.
41. Pond AL, Scheve BK, Benedict AT, et al: Expression of distinct ERG proteins in rat, mouse, and human heart. Relation to functional I(Kr) channels. J Biol Chem 275:5997–6006, 2000.
42. Finley MR, Li Y, Hua F, et al: Freeman LC. Expression and coassociation of ERG1, KCNQ1, and KCNE1 potassium channel proteins in horse heart. Am J Physiol Heart Circ Physiol 283:H126–H138, 2002.
43. Zaritsky JJ, Redell JB, Tempel BL, Schwarz TL: The consequences of disrupting cardiac inwardly rectifying K^+ current (I_{K1}) as revealed by the targeted deletion of the murine Kir2.1 and Kir2.2 genes. J Physiol 533:697–710, 2001.
44. Babenko AP, Aguilar-Bryan L, Bryan J: A view of sur/KIR6.X, KATP channels. Ann Rev Physiol 60:667–687, 1998.
45. Suzuki M, Li RA, Miki T, et al: Functional roles of cardiac and vascular ATP-sensitive potassium channels clarified by Kir6.2-knockout mice. Circ Res 88:570–577, 2001.
46. Pu J, Wada T, Valdivia C, et al: Evidence of KATP channels in native cardiac cells without SUR. Biophys J 80:625–626, 2001.
47. Seghers V, Nakazaki M, DeMayo F, et al: SUR1 knockout mice. A model for K(ATP) channel-independent regulation of insulin secretion. J Biol Chem 275:9270–9277, 2000.
48. Koster JC, Knopp A, Flagg TP, et al: Tolerance for ATP-insensitive K(ATP) channels in transgenic mice. Circ Res 89:1022–1029, 2001.
49. Lesage F, Lazdunski M: Potassium channels with two P domains. In Jan LY (ed): Current Topics in Membranes, Vol 46. San Diego, Academic Press, 1999, pp 199–222.
50. Goldstein SA, Bockenhauer D, O'Kelly I, Zilberberg N: Potassium leak channels and the KCNK family of two-P-domain subunits. Nat Rev Neurosci 2:175–184, 2001.

第 21 章

心脏缝隙连接的分布和调节

Jeffrey E. Saffitz, *Deborah L. Lerner*, *and Kathryn A. Yamada*

本章目录

- 缝隙连接在心脏中的分布及其与各向异性传导的关系 …………………… 177
- 缝隙连接蛋白在传导中的作用 …………………… 182
- 细胞间信息交流的调节 …………………… 183

心脏中电冲动的传导以及代谢和信号的交换，都需要细胞间进行离子和小分子物质的传递。该过程发生在缝隙连接，是一种特殊的肌质膜区域，包含一组紧密组装在一起的跨膜通道，这些通道锚定在细胞之间的空隙里，直接联系相邻细胞的胞浆组分。缝隙连接是一种动态的细胞器，与细胞外基质、细胞内骨架蛋白和信号蛋白都有联系，这些联系很可能又同时参与调节缝隙连接通道的分布、功能和开关。自从 15 年前第一个缝隙连接通道基因被克隆并测序以来，对电冲动传导的决定物质——缝隙连接的分子和结构特征均有了进一步的认识。本章主要集中介绍目前关于缝隙连接通道是怎样调节的，以及特异性缝隙连接的分布是怎样导致心脏不同组织中特异性的传导特性方面的知识。关于缝隙连接在心脏电生理中的作用的其他知识，可以参考本书的其他章节；关于连接蛋白的分子结构和功能请参见第 8 章；关于混合缝隙连接通道请参见第 14 章；关于心脏缝隙连接的药理学内容请参见第 19 章；而关于小鼠心律失常模型请参见第 48 章。

一、缝隙连接在心脏中的分布及其与各向异性传导的关系

（一）缝隙连接及其亚细胞环境

在缝隙连接处，细胞间电耦联部位与负责心肌细胞机械耦联的闰盘区之间存在着紧密的空间联系。缝隙连接通常位于或靠近工作的心房或心室肌细胞的末端，在那里形成最大的闰盘与邻近细胞相连[1]。尽管细胞外基质和细胞内骨架蛋白可能在调节缝隙连接通道结构和功能中起作用，但是关于它们在大分子复合体中的特异性相互作用所知甚少。在这些相互作用中，最具有特征性的是心脏缝隙连接通道蛋白即连接蛋白 43 (connexin43, Cx43) 和紧密连接蛋白-1 (zonula occludens protein-1, ZO-1)[2,3]，后者可能在发生心肌重构时心肌细胞间的相互联系中起作用[4]。然而，关于缝隙连接在胞内和肌质膜上的定位，仍需要深入了解。

（二）缝隙连接在细胞水平上的分布

用电镜观察平行于心肌细胞长轴的超薄切片，发现根据在心室肌闰盘中的定位可以把缝隙连接分为两组。第一组是由小的盘状连接组成，其定位于闰盘的粘附（褶皱的）区段，这一区段主要组成了粘合膜连接（又称中间连接）（见图 21-1A 空心箭头）；第二组是皱褶间区段，位于闰盘粘附部分的分支片段间（见图 21-1A 实心箭头）。在纵向面上，缝隙连接皱褶间的区段都是定向平行于细胞长轴，并且并列垂直于闰盘的粘附部分。如图 21-1A 所示，缝隙连接皱褶间的

区段长度可跨越多个肌小节的长度（Z带长度之间），这是因为每个典型的粘附区段盖住了1~3个肌小节，因此缝隙连接皱褶间的区段长度相当于多段肌小节的总长度[1]。

在垂直于细胞长轴的横断面做左心室心肌切片，可见大多数缝隙连接是一组看起来很小、各方向长度一致的盘状结构[1]。然而，对于一些缝隙连接，尤其是那些位于闰盘皱褶间区域的连接，从横断面比从纵向切面观察到的长度更长。例如，在组织长轴面上，平均缝隙连接剖面长度约为 $0.8\mu m$，只有大约3%的缝隙连接剖面长度大于 $3.0\mu m$（见直方图，图21-1B）。与此不同的是，在横切面上观察，缝隙连接剖面长度的分布是不对称的，结果使得平均剖面长度较大（$\sim 1.2\mu m$）。产生这一差别的主要原因来自于从横切面上所见到的那些较长的缝隙连接（见图21-1C）。这些长缝隙连接尽管不是很多，却在整个缝隙连接膜中占了很大比例（~40%）[1]。它们可能在细胞间的离子转运中起着重要作用。有趣的是，这些大的缝隙连接在邻近心梗愈合处的间质纤维化区会发生断裂。

心室肌细胞闰盘的三维模型最先是在1989年提出的，这一模型可显示出大皱褶间区段缝隙连接（见图21-1C矩形斑点状碎片）呈丝带样形状，位于闰盘皱褶间的细胞膜表面，它们的长轴垂直于细胞长轴。这一模型后来在心室肌细胞的免疫荧光共聚焦图像中得到证实（实验中采用了抗缝隙连接蛋白抗体染色）。当在切片上能观察到单个心肌细胞末端时，就可以看到丝带样的缝隙连接形成一个环，包绕在细胞周围。细胞末端内部包含大量斑点状的免疫荧光信号，它们大多数可能都是小盘状连接，位于闰盘的粘附部分。

在大末端闰盘上的缝隙连接，其空间分布非常适合心脏的功能需要。目前认为，位于细胞末端的大缝隙连接环更有利于促进细胞间离子转运，而且还可提供合适的电流负荷环境（current-to-load），从而也有利于增强传导的安全性（主要维持传导所需要的最小电流量和实际传导的电流量）。然而，由于脂质双分子层有很多高密度的蛋白质，含有缝隙连接的膜区域就比较坚硬，而且在剪切力作用下很容易破裂，这对于心肌细胞收缩来说可能很重要。大缝隙连接与闰盘里细胞间的粘附点离得很近，它们丝带样的形状垂直于细胞长轴，这些都是进化的结果，从而有利于保护缝隙连接免受剪切力的影响。因此，心室肌细胞缝隙连接在细胞上的排列方式，就决定了下述功能。

（三）缝隙连接在组织水平的分布

心脏是由多种具有完全不同结构和传导特性的组织组成。例如，冲动传导的速度和方向在心房和心室组织有很大差异，在心脏传导系统的结性组织和束支也都有较大的差异[1]。由于存在细胞大小和形状等组织特异性的差别，以及兴奋去极化和复极离子流表达形式的不同便产生了差异性的传导。然而，在缝隙连接处细胞间电联系的特殊模式也发挥着重要作用。就像以下例子显示的那样，形态学研究显示出不同心脏组织都是通过广泛分布的缝隙连接相连，这与它们的电传导特性相一致。

1. 缝隙连接在心室肌中的分布

尽管缝隙连接都聚集到心室肌细胞的末端，那里有最大的闰盘，而实际上缝隙连接在整个心室肌细胞表面都存在。用抗缝隙连接蛋白抗体染色分离的心肌细胞，总是可以看到这样的分布现象（见图21-2A）。缝隙连接的这种分布反映了心室肌细胞复杂的三维结构，心室肌每个细胞和它周围许多细胞都是以不同程度的头对尾、边对边方式相连（见图21-2B）。在犬的左心室游离壁上用三维形态的方法测量与单个心肌细胞相连的细胞数目，结果发现每个心室肌细胞平均有11个细胞与之相连（见图21-2C）。近一半的毗邻细胞与中心细胞的相连方式主要是边对边（见图21-2C Ⅰ型和Ⅱ型连接），而另一半则以头对尾的方式（Ⅲ型和Ⅳ型连接）[1,5]。通过比较实际和"有效的"长/宽比，可以发现心室肌细胞重叠程度十分明显。测量分离的犬心室肌细胞，实际的长/宽比值将近6:1，但组织心室肌细胞"有效的"长/宽比，即平行于细胞长轴的细胞数目和垂直于细胞长轴的细胞数目之比，只有3.4:1。这种高度重叠的细胞间联系方式与心室传导的中度各向异性（纵向传导和垂直传导速率之比为~3:1）相一致。激动波形沿着一层均匀的心室肌传导，无论是沿着长轴方向还是垂直于长轴方向，都会有很多机会经过细胞间连接，但是由于细胞是长形的，波形沿着垂直于长轴方向传导必定会经过更多的细胞间连接，从而遇到更多阻力，因而与沿着长轴方向传导的波形相比，传导速率会更慢。这些观察表明，心室中传导速率的各向异性主要是由心室肌的形状决定的，而不是取决于细胞间连接的各向异性分布。近来，Spach及其同事们[6]提出了支持这一结

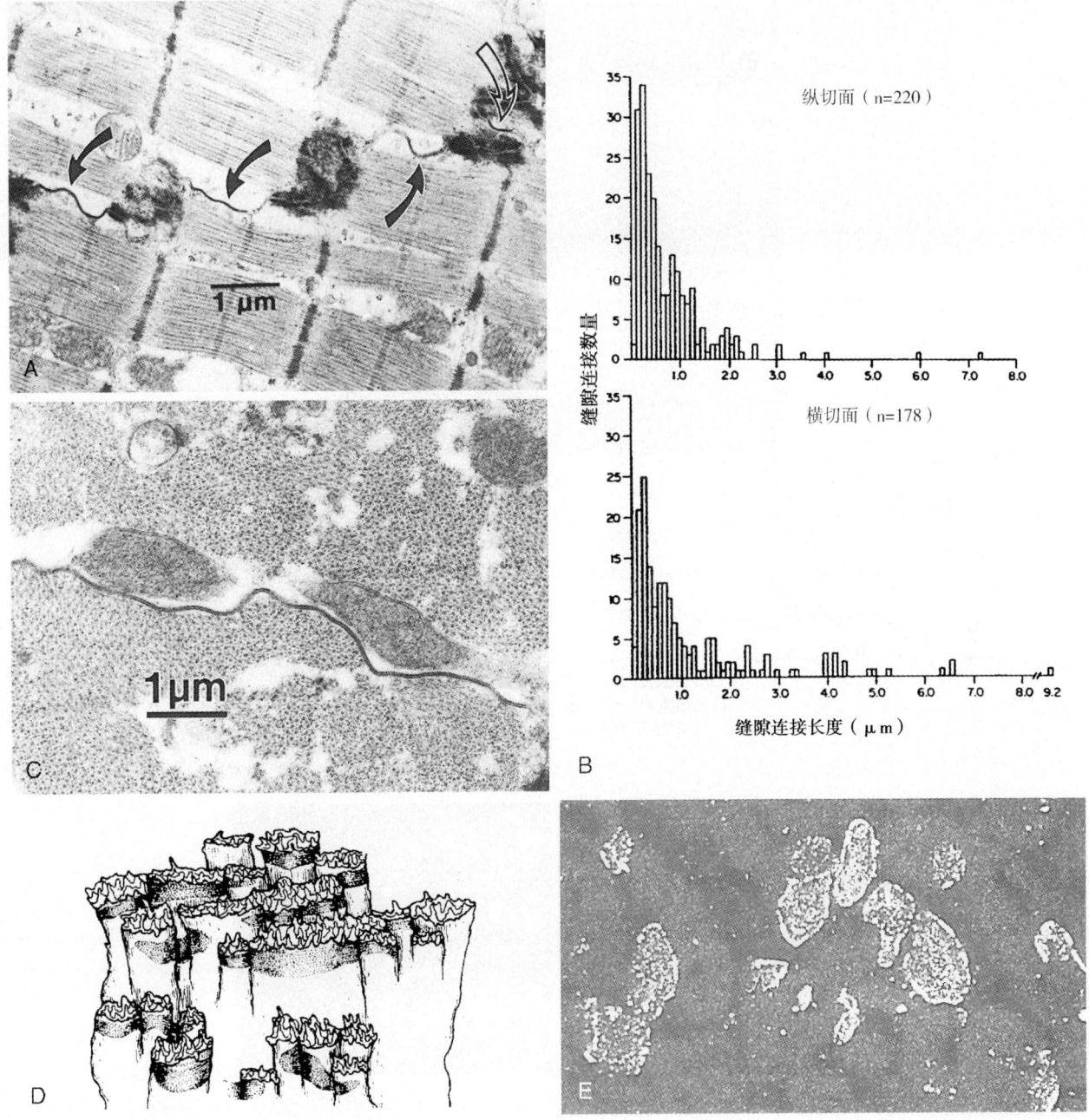

图 21-1 A：犬的连接两个心室肌细胞闰盘的透射电镜图。该组织切片切面平行于细胞长轴。闰盘包含了多个粘附结构，在电镜下可以看到电子密集的结构覆盖在肌小节的末端和肌小节的分支。在粘附连接和细胞长轴平面之间是皱褶间缝隙连接（实心箭头所示）。小的缝隙连接（空心箭头所示）位于粘附结构内。B：缝隙连接长度的直方图（分别从犬左心室肌的纵切面和横切面的超薄切片测得）。C：犬左心室肌横切面的投射电镜图，显示了长缝隙连接的侧面轮廓（长度约为 8μm）。D：示意图显示典型心肌细胞末端，大皱褶内缝隙连接（图中细胞膜表面点片状物质）和闰盘的粘附结构（图中手指样突出物）之间的关系。最大的缝隙连接是方形或丝带样形状。它们位于粘附结构分支之间的膜区域。大缝隙连接的长轴方向垂直于心肌细胞的长轴方向。因此 A 图中显示的皱褶间缝隙连接（实心箭头所示）是其短轴切面。E：心肌细胞末端大闰盘的合成共聚焦显微图像。图中用抗缝隙连接蛋白抗体显示的缝隙连接是白色的结构。在每个闰盘的周围是大缝隙连接环，在电镜横切面图像中所见的相应结构就是最大皱褶间连接。闰盘内部包含有很多小的缝隙连接，包括皱褶连接和小皱褶间连接。大体积的外周连接比小体积的内部连接数目少得多，但是由于它体积大，使得外周连接组成了整个缝隙连接膜区域最主要的成分（A，C，D 图引自 Hoyt RH，Cohen ML，Saffitz JE：Distribution and three-dimensional structure of intercellular junctions in canine myocardium. *Cir Res* 1989；64：565-574. B 图引自 Luke RA，Saffitz JE：Remodeling of ventricular conduction pathways in healed canine border zones. *J Clin Invest* 1991；87：1594-1602. E 图引自 Peters NS，Severs NJ，Rothery SM，et al：Spatiotemporal relation between gap junctions and fascia adherens junctions during postnatal development of human ventricular myocardium. *Circulation* 1994；90：713-725.）

180　第四部分　离子通道与细胞电生理学

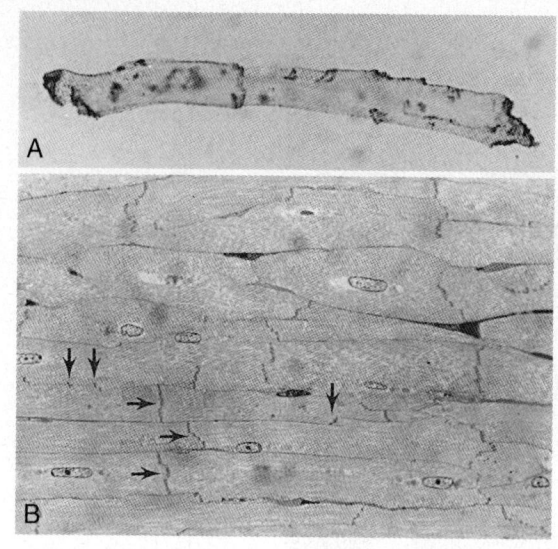

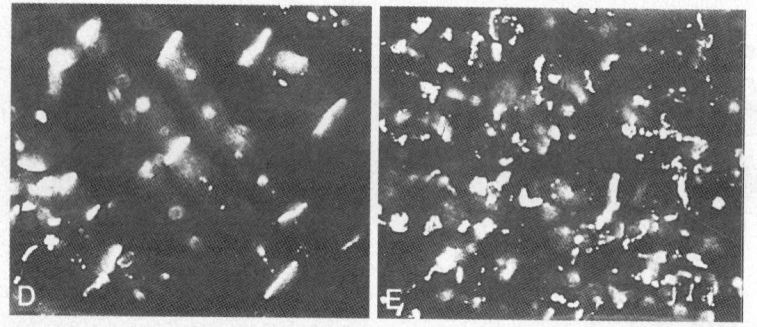

图 21-2　A：离体犬左心室肌细胞经抗缝隙连接蛋白抗体染色可见到缝隙连接在细胞表面的分布。最大的缝隙连接都集中在细胞末端，但是有大量小的缝隙连接分布于细胞的整个长轴上。B：1μm 厚的犬左心室切片显示出心室肌细胞的复杂排列。每个细胞通过闰盘和缝隙连接以头对尾（平行箭头）和边对边（垂直箭头）的方式连接。C：犬左心室、界嵴区和窦房结处的细胞连接的数目和空间定位图。括弧里的数字表示每种连接方式的百分比。结果都以均数±标准差表达，星号表示每种连接方式的数目，在心室或界嵴区与在窦房结的数目相比有显著差异（$P < 0.01$）。D 和 E：犬界嵴区（D）和左心室（E）缝隙连接分布的免疫组化图。界嵴区缝隙连接蛋白染色显示其分布方式与束支中连接心房肌细胞的闰盘的简单而平直的方式一致。相反，心室中缝隙连接的分布就复杂得多，多为边对边和头对尾的连接方式（A 图引自 Luke RA，Beyer EC，Hoyt RH，Saffitz JE：Quantitative analysis of intercellular connections by immunohistochemistry of the cardiac gap junction protein connexin 43. *Cir Res* 1989；65：1450-1457. B 图引自 Luke RA，Saffitz JE：Remodeling of ventricular conduction pathways in healed canine border zones. *J Clin Invest* 1991；87：1594-1602. C 图引自 Saffitz JE，Green KG，Schuessler RB：Structural determinants of slow conduction in the canine sinus node. *J Cardiovasc Electrophysiology* 1997；8：738-744. D 和 E 图摘自 Saffitz JE，Kanter HL，Green KG，et al：Tissue-specific determinants of anisotropic conduction velocity in canine atrial and ventricular myocardium. *Circ Res* 1994；74：1065-1070.）

论的证据，即在决定心室肌垂直传导方面，细胞形态比缝隙连接的各向异性分布更重要。

2. 界嵴区缝隙连接的分布

界嵴是心房肌分离出来的一个束支，它将产生于窦房结的冲动传到房室交界区。界嵴处的传导很快（~1 m/s），并且具有高度各向异性[1,5]。界嵴区长轴与垂直轴传导方向的速率之比（10∶1）与心室处（3∶1）的相比是很高的。心室肌细胞周围平均有11个细胞与之相连，而界嵴区的心肌细胞则不同，周围平均只有6个细胞相连（见图21-2C），细胞间连接方式多数是头对尾形式（60% Ⅳ型连接，19% Ⅲ型连接，见图21-2C）。界嵴区的细胞缺乏像心室肌细胞那样复杂的表面形态，心室肌细胞表面沿着长轴方向有很多缝隙连接，而界嵴区细胞表面长轴方向的缝隙连接相对较少[1,5]。界嵴区细胞的闰盘相对较直，而且都是位于细胞末端。用免疫染色的方法可以观察到，缝隙连接在心室肌和界嵴区的空间定位明显不同（如图21-2D和2E）。界嵴区特异性的缝隙连接排列方式可能造成了这一组织的一大特点，即在不同方向的传导速率有很大不同。

3. 窦房结缝隙连接的分布

窦房结缓慢而不均一的传导在很大程度上是由窦房结心肌细胞的电生理特性所决定的，但是形态学的研究表明，结构特征也起了很重要的作用[1,5,7]。重建缝隙连接可显示出犬窦房结另一副完全不同的"面貌"。典型的窦房结细胞周围，平均只有5个细胞与之相连（如图21-2C）[7]。在心房和心室肌细胞，缝隙连接通常集中于细胞末端，那里有最大的闰盘，但是在窦房结，缝隙连接几乎都在小的单个闰盘处，这些闰盘位于窦房结心肌细胞表面的任一方向。小闰盘和缝隙连接在细胞表面的这种排列使得小窦房结细胞可以复杂的分支方式定向，包括边对边和头对尾等各种定位。因此，74%的窦房结细胞间的连接是Ⅱ型和Ⅲ型的[1,7]。相反，63%的心室缝隙连接或者是以单纯的边对边（Ⅰ型）或者是单纯的头对尾方式（Ⅳ型），60%的界嵴区缝隙连接是单纯的头对尾方式（见图21-2C）。

通过比较超微结构的形态学参数，可发现在左心室、界嵴区和窦房结的缝隙连接分布有着明显的不同。每100μm的闰盘侧面长度中，缝隙连接的总数在心室和界嵴心肌细胞中分别是窦房结细胞的2.8倍和2.1倍[7]。

心室肌中平均每个缝隙连接的侧面长度是窦房结的4.8倍[7]。尽管界嵴区的平均缝隙连接侧面长度比心室肌要小很多，但仍比窦房结的缝隙连接大很多。由于在心室和界嵴区，每单位闰盘长度的缝隙连接总数和平均缝隙连接长度都比在窦房结大，所以在心室和界嵴心肌细胞中，每100μm的闰盘中缝隙连接累积的侧面长度就分别是在窦房结细胞的12.7倍和3.2倍[7]。因此，作为计算心肌细胞面积的一个函数，缝隙连接总长度在心室和界嵴区分别是在窦房结的27倍和5倍[7]。不仅窦房结细胞通过闰盘与周围相连的细胞数目比心室和界嵴区细胞要少，而且窦房结中心的细胞间连接数也较少，缝隙连接也格外小。

4. 其他心脏组织的缝隙连接

除了犬的窦房结外，还没有报道心脏传导系统的其他部位细胞间连接的空间定位。然而，有人在一些传导特性各异的心脏组织中比较了缝隙连接蛋白免疫反应信号的数目和分布[1,5]。例如，Cx43表达在犬的心房和心室组织比在房室结高得多[1,5]。犬房室结的Cx43信号呈斑点状，而且在结细胞之间散在分布。对犬窦房结Cx43的染色也观察到类似的现象[8]。经采用每平方毫米细胞核数目进行标准化后，估计心室肌Cx43免疫信号的相对密度大约是房室结的33倍[1]，这个比例与用超微结构测量方法得到的犬心室肌中每单位心肌细胞缝隙连接侧面长度是窦房结中的27倍的结果类似[7]。这些观察提供了又一证据支持这一假说，即窦房结和房室结组织缓慢而不均一的传导，至少部分是由于结细胞间缝隙连接非常小且散在分布所致。

在传导最快的心肌组织，即浦肯野纤维束中，人们发现其缝隙连接的分布很独特[1,5]。用免疫组化的方法分析犬心脏"假腱索"中的浦肯野纤维束内Cx43的分布，结果发现在整个浦肯野细胞的边界，缝隙连接染色形成了连续的染色带[1,5]。在牛心脏的浦肯野纤维束中也有类似的发现[1]。根据电缆理论，传导速率与传导电缆或纤维的有效半径的平方根成正比。因此浦肯野纤维周围分布的缝隙连接通道在功能上增加了传导束的半径，从而增加了传导速率，且不受激活膜特性的任何变化的影响。浦肯野纤维在束间典型的排列是，它和心室肌间有一层胶原组织，这样可以防止游离离子流入周围的心室组织，这种排列可能也加速了传导，如本章后文所讨论的，浦肯野纤维中那些特殊的缝隙连接蛋白的表达，在其快速传导中起决定性作用。

（四）心脏缝隙连接分布在不同发育期的变化

胚胎心脏和新生心脏的心室肌细胞是通过一些小的、弥散分布的缝隙连接相连，这点与成年心室肌细胞完全不同。在光镜下，用抗 N-cadherin 的抗体可显示人新生心脏上粘合膜连接（又称中间连接）的分布，结果发现粘合膜连接的分布和缝隙连接的分布很难区分。出生后随着心脏的逐渐成熟，缝隙连接和闰盘的粘合膜连接成分也都出现渐进的再分布，逐渐形成成年心脏的分布方式，即位于或接近细胞末端的大连接都与大闰盘联系在一起[1]。在人类的心脏，这种转变要到 6 岁才完成[1]。在鼠的心脏中，心室肌细胞缝隙连接的分布也有类似的变化[9]。

关于心室肌细胞周围与之相连的细胞数目以及头对尾连接和边对边连接的相对比例在新生心室肌和成年心室肌中是否有不同，目前尚不清楚。尽管在细胞水平上，缝隙连接的分布在新生心室肌和成年心室肌之间有明显不同，但它们各自细胞间的连接方式可能是类似的。例如，在传统的新生大鼠心肌细胞原代培养中，新生心肌细胞上有大量小的缝隙连接均匀分布在整个细胞表面，但是在那些紧密排列的单层细胞中，发现每个细胞周围相连的细胞数目与在成年犬左心室的切片中测量到的结果类似[10]。近来，Spach 及其同事们[6]强调，在决定各向异性的传导特性方面，细胞大小比缝隙连接的分布更具有决定性作用。在发育的不同阶段出现缝隙连接分布的不同，其电生理意义还不是很清楚。有趣的是，在心脏的病理状态下，缝隙连接的分布出现不同形式的重构，而重构后的分布形式类似于新生心脏（见后文）。

二、缝隙连接蛋白在传导中的作用

与大多数已分化细胞类似，每个心肌细胞表达多种连接蛋白[1,5,11]，连接蛋白家族的成员（connexin，Cx）形成了缝隙连接通道。功能迥异的心脏组织不仅仅是通过不同空间排列方式的缝隙连接相连，而且还表达三种心脏连接蛋白的不同组合：Cx43、Cx45、Cx40[1,5,11]。尽管心脏连接蛋白表达的表型在不同种属间会有差异，但是人们在小鼠、大鼠、犬、牛和人的心脏中观察到这种蛋白表达的形式还是相当一致的。一般而言，哺乳动物心室肌表达 Cx43 和 Cx45[1,5,11-13]，而心房肌和心脏传导系统表达 Cx43、Cx45 和 Cx40[1,5,8,12-14]。单个连接蛋白形成的通道具有特异的单一电导率、电压敏感性和通透性[1,11,15]。在心脏连接蛋白中，Cx40 通道具有最大的单一电导率（主要为 121pS 或 158pS），而 Cx45 通道电导率最小（29pS）[1,11,15,16]。在心房肌和浦肯野纤维中选择性的表达 Cx40，可能有助于这些组织的快速传导。Cx43 通道表现出多个电导率（50pS 和 90pS 是最常观察到的）[1,11,15]，而且 Cx43 通道对跨膜电相位对不敏感，对阴离子和阳离子以及不同大小电荷和分子量的荧光染料具有高度通透性[13]。相反，Cx40 和 Cx45 通道具有相对的阳离子选择性[15,16]。Cx45 的门控作用是电压依赖性的，采用经典的用于连接耦联染色的荧光黄（lucifer yellow）进行染色观察，结果发现通过 Cx40 通道远不像通过 Cx43 通道那样自由，而且不能通过 Cx45 通道。

现在已经可利用基因工程小鼠来进行连接蛋白表达的不同表型在心脏生理中的生物学意义研究。1995 年，Reaume 及其同事们[17-19]报道了 Cx43 缺失小鼠。Cx43 缺失突变纯合子的小鼠能发育成形，但是出生后很快死亡，主要是由于圆锥动脉干（conotruncus）的发育不良而导致右室流出道梗阻。然而，杂合子小鼠（Cx43$^{+/-}$）有正常的寿命，而且其心脏结构或收缩功能与野生型小鼠（Cx43$^{+/+}$）相比都没有明显异常[20]。Cx43$^{+/-}$小鼠的心脏包含近 50% 野生型水平的 Cx43[13,21,22]。尽管与早期报道的关于 Cx43$^{+/-}$小鼠 Cx43 低表达影响传导的结果不一致[21-23]，近来一项应用高时间分辨率的光电二极管光学标测系统（photodiode optical mapping system）研究的结果表明，在 Cx43$^{+/-}$小鼠心脏表面传导速度有 25%～30% 的减慢（见图 21-3）[24]。最近在对 Cx43 条件缺失的小鼠研究中，结果清楚地表明 Cx43 在心室传导和致心律失常方面起着主要作用[25]。在年轻的成年小鼠中，特异性地去除心脏的 Cx43 等位基因，结果导致小鼠严重的室性心动过速、室颤以及心源性猝死[25]。在 Cx43$^{+/-}$小鼠中 Cx45 的表达数量是正常的，但是仍然不能防止 Cx43 减半表达所致的传导减慢[21,22]。这些结果表明 Cx43 是主要的心室肌电耦联蛋白。

最初对 Cx43$^{+/-}$小鼠的研究中发现，心房表面

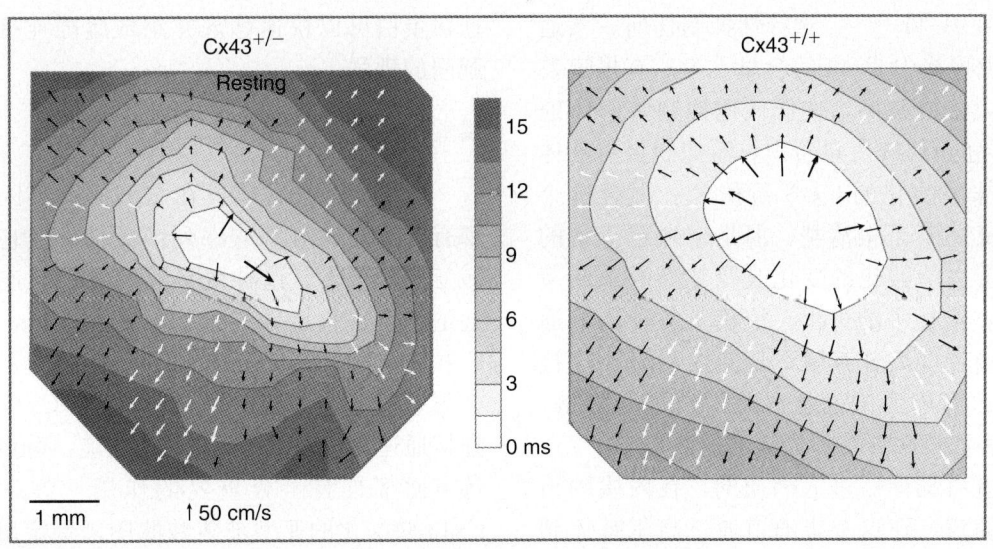

图21-3 成年离体灌注 Cx43$^{+/-}$ 小鼠（左）和 Cx43$^{+/+}$ 小鼠（右）的心室表面等时相图，描述从刺激点（每幅图近中心部位的白色区域）向外传播的顺序和形式 Cx43$^{+/-}$ 小鼠心脏传导速度较慢，因而等时线较为密集。传导速度的计算是所有局部速度向量（包括垂直于或平行于纤维方向，白色箭头所示）的平均值（引自 Eloff BC, Lerner DL, Yamada KA, et al：High resolution optical mapping reveals conduction slowing in connexin43 deficient mice. *Cardiovasc Res* 2001；51：681-690.）

的传导速率没有异常，心表面心电图的 P 波时程也没有改变[21]。Cx43$^{+/-}$ 小鼠的心房肌包含50%的野生型 Cx43，但是 Cx45 或 Cx40 含量都没有改变[22]。Cx43$^{+/-}$ 小鼠心房传导表型的缺失首次证明了 Cx40 是心房肌主要的电耦联蛋白。后来在 Cx40 缺失的小鼠中也证实了这一结论[26-28]。Cx40 缺失小鼠有正常的心室传导速率，但是它们表现出心房传导障碍和房性心律失常。这些观察提示，Cx43 和 Cx40 是决定心房和心室肌细胞间耦联的具有心腔特异性的分子机制，并且连接蛋白表达的不同表型使得不同心脏组织具有其特异的功能。在病理状态下，心脏连接蛋白表型可发生改变，但其病理生理意义目前正在研究中。改变连接蛋白亚型的表达，尤其是改变其空间表达的异源性，可能导致不连续传导和心律失常。

三、细胞间信息交流的调节

缝隙连接的形成是一个复杂的多步骤过程，而且受多种信号通路交互作用的调节。不像传统的离子通道那样表现出灵敏的离子选择性和严格的门控特性，缝隙连接通道对离子和小分子是非选择性地通透，并且在生理情况下，门控机制表现出相对小的电压敏感性[15]。心脏缝隙连接耦联的调节大部分是通过改变细胞表面缝隙连接通道的数目来进行。这种数目的改变通常发生得很快，在数分钟之内。而且有多种机制参与，使得心脏在各种需要改变细胞间联系的生理和病理状态下能够作出适应性的反应。

（一）心脏缝隙连接处细胞间耦联的调节

在正常情况下，心肌细胞之间耦联得非常好。心室肌的缝隙连接是生物学中最大的缝隙连接[29]。缝隙连接被认为是提供了很宽的安全界限，以保证离子转运能够在合适的时间和地点有效地激活心肌。目前正在致力于阐明心肌细胞是如何通过快速改变缝隙连接的功能性通道的数目来调节耦联，这种对通道数目的调节机制主要是翻译后的调节，包括了由连接蛋白磷酸化介导的通道蛋白的运输、组装和降解。

（二）连接蛋白组装和降解的细胞间通路

连接蛋白的运输以非常快的速率进出缝隙连接，半衰期仅 1～3 h[30]。因此，通过缝隙连接的连接蛋白的流动，必定是通过细胞表面正常表达功能性通道以及防止连接蛋白异常蓄积或丢失来调节[31]。例如，即使对连接蛋白的降解很微小地调节也会导致细胞间联系的快速变化。

决定心脏中连接蛋白循环的因素是什么尚不清楚。在培养细胞（包括心肌细胞）中进行的连接蛋白降解的研究以及在离体成年大鼠心脏中的研究都表明，Cx43的降解是通过溶酶体和蛋白酶体两条通路来进行（见图21-4）[30-32]。选择性抑制任何一条通路都会增加缝隙连接中Cx43的含量[30-32]。有报道发现在离体灌流大鼠心脏中，选择性地抑制溶酶体通路会导致磷酸化的Cx43大量蓄积，而抑制蛋白酶体通路则会导致非磷酸化的Cx43蓄积[30]。尽管这个结果的功能意义还不是很清楚，但是越来越清楚的是，通过连接蛋白磷酸化的变化改变其降解来调节连接蛋白在缝隙连接中的进出。依赖于各种调节通路的活性，连接蛋白离开浆膜下囊泡内的缝隙连接联合，或者转运到溶酶体或蛋白酶体内进行降解，或者回到细胞表面再次参与形成缝隙连接[33-36]。

各种连接蛋白翻译后进入内质网，在内质网组成六聚体的半通道，在这个半通道通过高尔基体到达膜表面之前，被称为连接子（connexons）[34,35]。连接子在囊泡中转运到胞膜的非结合区域[34,35]，然后迁移到缝隙连接斑块的周围，在那里与邻近细胞的半通道锚定在一起形成功能性的通道，然后组成缝隙连接斑块[34,36]。用绿色荧光蛋白在活体哺乳动物细胞中标记Cx43，时间推移成像法显示了荧光囊泡到达以及离开细胞表面的动态图像[33]。综合不同时间段看到的荧光标记Cx43的图像，清楚地表明有新的蛋白加入了缝隙连接周围[36]。连接蛋白持续从缝隙连接斑块周围流入中心，在那里又被组装入胞吞小泡内[36]。尽管细胞中大部分连接蛋白定位在缝隙连接，但仍有相当数量的连接蛋白位于高尔基体、非结合区胞膜以及细胞内囊泡中。这些非结合区的连接蛋白可以快速移入并组成缝隙连接，以加强细胞间的耦联[33]。

磷酸化对连接蛋白的调节

连接蛋白家族成员在它们的跨膜区和胞外区域都有着很高的氨基酸序列同源性，但它们的胞内区域变异却很大。这种变异导致了不同连接蛋白组成通道各自具有特异的生物物理特性[1]，尤其是胞内C末端包含了大部分的调节元件[37,38]。这一区域多个氨基酸残基的磷酸化对Cx43和Cx45组装成缝隙连接通道，以及对Cx43通道功能、分解和靶向降解等方面都具有十分重要的作用[38,39]。至少有5种Cx43磷酸化的亚型被磷酸肽图谱鉴定出来，但是在心肌细胞中磷酸化残基的具体数目和模式还不很清楚，很可能是依赖于生理或病理生理状态[38]。Cx43的磷酸化主要发生在丝氨酸残基，但是在那些表达活化的酪氨酸激酶的细胞中也有特异性的酪氨酸残基被磷酸化[38]。新合成的Cx43在它到达细胞膜前会被磷酸化，在加入到缝隙连接斑块时又一次地被磷酸化。Cx45的磷酸化亚型似乎比Cx43的少，但是关于Cx45磷酸化的功能含义却所知甚少。将特异性的丝氨酸残基进行直接的位点突变会导致Cx45通道循环动力学显著加快[39]。

Cx43能够被丝裂原激活蛋白激酶、蛋白激酶C和蛋白激酶A磷酸化其特异性的丝氨酸残基，而被

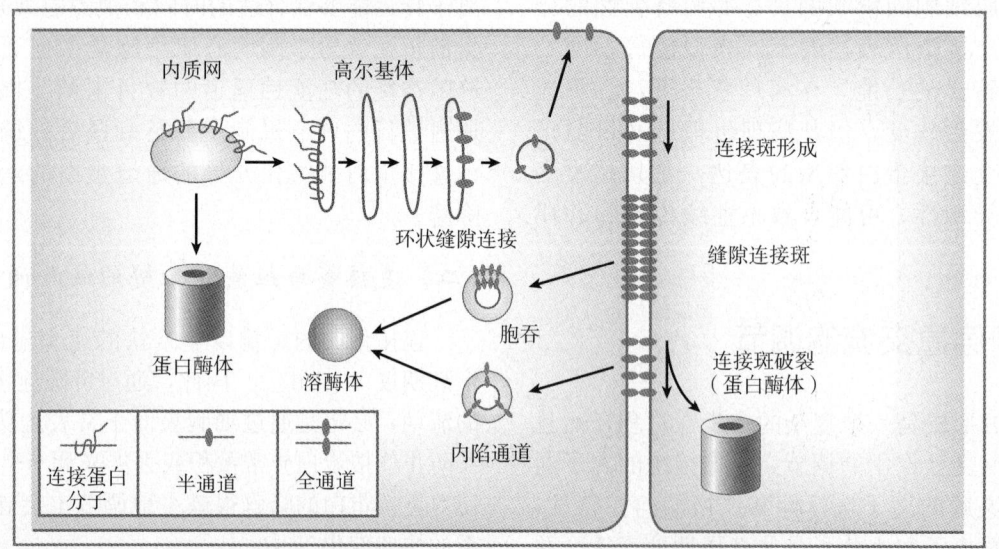

图21-4　连接蛋白细胞内降解通路模式图　（引自Saffitz JE，Laing JG，Yamada KA：Connexin expression and turnover. Implications for cardiac excitability. *Cir Res* 2000；86：723-728.）

v-src 和 c-src 磷酸化其酪氨酸残基[38]，但是获得这些信息的研究都是在转染细胞中或是在那些不能反映在体心肌细胞内环境的情况下进行的。正常心肌细胞中大多数的 Cx43 是在多个位点被磷酸化，结果在聚丙烯酰胺凝胶电泳时就出现，分子量在 43~46kD 之间的亚型占据了明显优势。大多数磷酸化 Cx43 位于缝隙连接中，但是令人惊讶的是，关于那些内源性的、推测可发生组成性激活的、负责维持高基础水平的磷酸化连接蛋白的激酶所知甚少。同样对那些在病理状态下催化连接蛋白磷酸化改变的特异性激酶和磷酸酶所知也不多。

（三）生理和病理状态下缝隙连接耦联的调节

在急性严重的细胞损伤时，心肌细胞会和周围细胞脱耦联。尽管这一反应被认为是限制损伤化学因子传播的一种适应性行为，但是它也会产生瞬时传导异常从而促发心律失常。在损伤不是很严重的情况下，心肌细胞典型的反应是肥大，此时会有基因表达的改变以及细胞和组织结构的重构，从而适应变化的需要。在生理性肥大或病理性肥大代偿期，细胞间联系一般是增强的，大多数是通过增加细胞表面连接蛋白的数目来实现的。然而，当肥大反应不足以适应代谢需要，最终出现了显性心力衰竭，这时连接蛋白的表达可发生明显下调，推测这种下调反映出细胞间联系的减少。心肌结构重构是与缝隙连接分布的重构密切相关。可能最具有代表性的例子是，已经证明，在心肌梗死边缘区连接蛋白表达的改变和缝隙连接的再分布与促进折返性心律失常发生的传导障碍有关[41]。

1. 急性缺血引起的细胞间耦联的改变

正常心脏中维持高水平的耦联是带有很大风险的，因为当心脏受到损伤时，损伤化学因子会从严重损伤区域传播到损伤较轻的区域，从而增加了心脏的损伤。因此，心肌细胞能够通过脱耦联快速地与周围损伤细胞分离是有很大好处的。典型的电学脱耦联发生在以下情况：严重的酸中毒，细胞内 Ca^{2+} 和两性分子（如溶血磷脂）的蓄积，这些情况都能直接导致缝隙连接通道的关闭[1]。然而，急性缺血时的脱耦联包含了连接蛋白功能和分布的复杂变化，人们推测这些变化是通过多种应激活化（stress-activated）通路介导的。随着脱耦联的开始，Cx43 发生了显著的去磷酸化，并且从缝隙连接处再分布到胞内位点（图 21-5)[42]。这些改变在再灌注的时候会发生逆转，而且与电耦联的恢复和收缩活性的恢复有关。

直到缺血性损伤的较晚期才会结束脱耦联。在实验模型中，缝隙连接脱耦联主要发生于缺血开始后的 15 min，直到缺血后 30 或 40 min 才结束，而此时细胞损伤已经进入不可逆阶段了[42]。因此，在相当长的间隔时间内，缺血细胞仍是存活的且具有电活性，但是传导较慢而且变得明显地不连续，这些改变都具有高度的致心律失常性。例如，急性冠状动脉结扎后，$Cx43^{+/-}$ 鼠的离体心脏比野生型鼠的心脏表现出更高的室性心动过速的发生率，而且心律失常的发生也明显较早[43]。结果提示，缺血开始时细胞间的耦联水平是致心律失常的潜在决定因素。而且，考虑到 $Cx43^{+/-}$ 小鼠在缺血时心律失常的发生较早和发生率较高，我们认为 $Cx43^{+/-}$ 小鼠在缺血时的脱耦联会较早达到一个临界水平。

2. 急性肥大反应时缝隙连接耦联的加强

对于中度的负荷增加心肌细胞的反应是代偿性的肥大，这种生长的特点是收缩蛋白合成增加，组装新的肌小节，以及伴随着传导速率增加的收缩功能改善[44]。似乎也伴随着连接蛋白表达的增加，而后者的

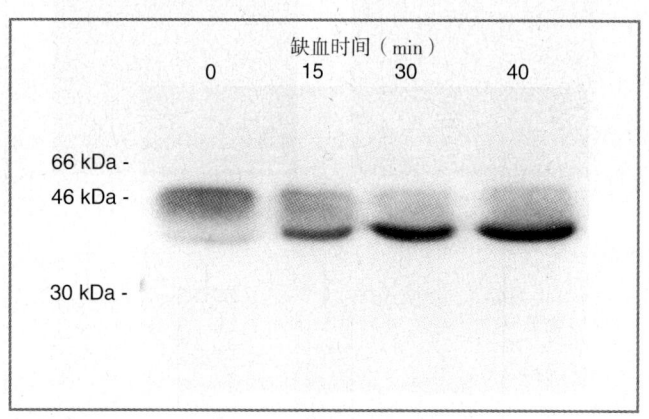

图 21-5 大鼠离体灌流心脏分别缺血（无灌流）0、15、30 或 40 min 时心室肌的连接蛋白 43（Cx43）的蛋白质免疫印记图 在缺血发生前，大多数 Cx43 显示两条带，分子量分别为 44 kD 和 46 kD。缺血时，较高分子量的条带信号减弱，而 41 kD 处的条带信号增强，说明存在进行性的 Cx43 去磷酸化。这一过程发生的时间与电脱耦联发生的时间一致（引自 Beardslee MA, Lerner DL, Tadros PN, et al: Dephosphorylation and intracellular redistribution of ventricular connexin43 during electrical uncoupling induced by ischemia. Cir Res 2000; 87: 656-662.)

增加会导致缝隙连接数目的增加，从而加强细胞间耦联。这些现象主要是在离体研究中得于描述和定义的。将新生大鼠心肌细胞与可透膜的环磷酸腺苷孵育24 h，结果发现 Cx43 表达和缝隙连接的数目增加，而且伴随着传导速率增快[45]。将培养的心室肌细胞与血管紧张素Ⅱ孵育6~24 h，同样也导致了 Cx43 表达和缝隙连接数目增加达2倍，而这一增加是与 Cx43 蛋白合成速率增加有关[46]。最近的研究表明，在培养的新生心室肌细胞中，线性的搏动牵张仅1 h 就可导致 Cx43 表达增加2倍，与此同时传导速率也会增加30%[47,48]。而培养心肌细胞中，与牵张引起的 Cx43 表达上调直接相关的信号通路是转化生长因子β、血管内皮生长因子和血管紧张素Ⅱ（见图21-6）[48]。

3. 慢性心脏疾病时缝隙连接耦联减少

室内传导阻滞是慢性心力衰竭最普遍的特征[44]，可能与（至少部分是）连接蛋白表达改变有关。在不同病因（包括缺血、高血压、血管异常和原发性心肌病）导致的末期心脏疾病的患者心脏中，缝隙连接上的 Cx43 表达均可发生下调[1]。这通常见于那些有活性但结构已发生改变的细胞，这些细胞表现出典型的冬眠心肌的退化特征[41,49]。末期心脏疾病时连接蛋白表达的下调也与位于细胞末端较大的缝隙连接选择性地丢失有关[49]。

目前对导致慢性心脏病时连接蛋白表达变化和缝隙连接重构的相关机制所知甚少。近来研究结果表明，丝裂原激活蛋白激酶家族成员之一的 JNK（c-Jun N-terminal kinase，JNK）可能参与了其相关的细胞内信号通路。JNK 可在缺血再灌注和血流动力学超负荷所致的心肌损伤时被激活。选择性地激活 JNK 通路，会导致新生心室肌细胞 Cx43 表达快速而明显地下调[50]。明确介导连接蛋白重构的特异性信号分子，有助于我们设计出新的治疗方案以防止慢性心脏病时心律失常的发生。

（张幼怡　肖晗　龚开政　译）

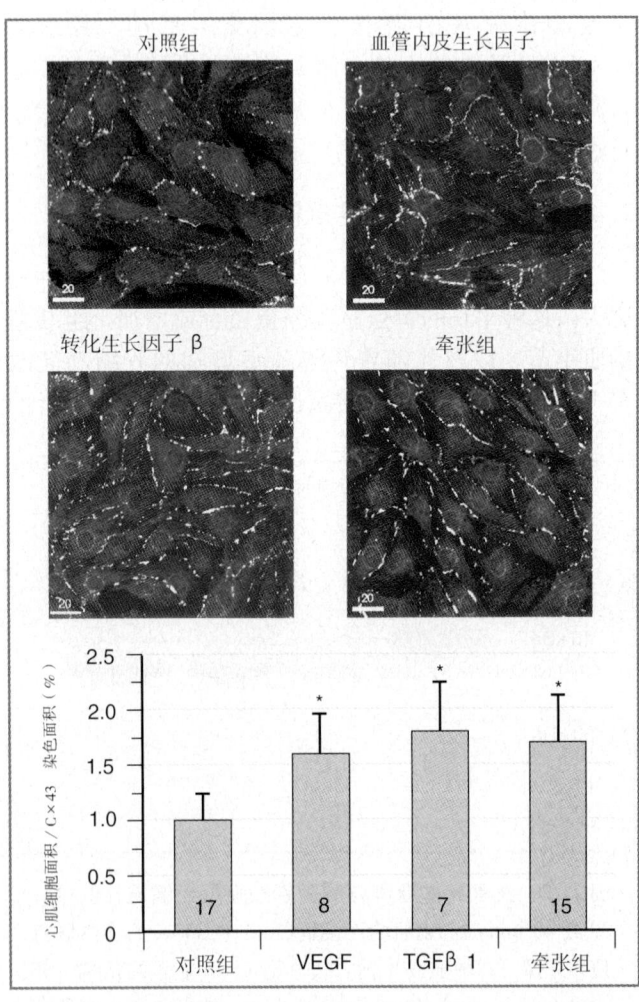

图 21-6　共聚焦图像和定量数据柱图　显示给予心肌细胞外源性血管内皮生长因子（vascular endothelial growth factor，VEGF）和转化生长因子β（transforming growth factor β，TGF-β），或搏动牵张1小时之后连接蛋白43（Cx43）表达增加（引自 Pimentel RC，Yamada KA，Kleber AG，Saffitz JE：Autocrine regulation of myocyte Cx43 expression by VEGF. Cir Res 2002；90：671-677.）

参 考 文 献

1. Saffitz JE, Yeager MJ: Intracardiac cell communication and gap junctions. In Spooner PM, Rosen MR (eds): Foundation of Cardiac Arrhythmias. Basic Concepts and Clinical Approaches. New York, Marcel Dekker, 2000, pp 171–204.
2. Toyofuku T, Yabuki M, Otsu K, et al: Direct association of the gap junction protein connexin-43 with ZO-1 in cardiac myocytes. J Biol Chem 273:12725–12731, 1998.
3. Toyofuku T, Akamatsu Y, Zhang H, et al: c-Src regulates the interaction between connexin-43 and ZO-1 in cardiac myocytes. J Biol Chem 276:1780–1788, 2001.
4. Barker RJ, Price RL, Gourdie RG: Increased association of ZO-1 with connexin43 during remodeling of cardiac gap junctions. Circ Res 90:317–324, 2002.
5. Saffitz JE, Yamada KA, Schuessler RB: Distribution and function of gap junction proteins in atrial-AV nodal conduction. In Mazgalev TN, Tchou PJ (eds): Atrial-AV Nodal Electrophysiology: A View from the Millenium. Armonk, Futura Publishing, 2000, pp 107–120.
6. Spach MS, Heidlage JF, Dolber PC, Barr RC: Electrophysiological effects of remodeling cardiac gap junctions and cell size: Experimental and model studies of normal cardiac growth. Circ Res 86:302–311, 2000.
7. Saffitz JE, Green KG, Schuessler RB: Structural determinants of slow conduction in the canine sinus node. J Cardiovasc Electrophysiol 8:738–744, 1997.
8. Kwong KF, Schuessler RB, Green KG, et al: Differential expression of gap junction proteins in the canine sinus node. Circ Res 82:604–612, 1998.
9. Angst BD, Khan LU, Severs NJ, et al: Dissociated spatial patterning of gap junctions and cell adhesion junctions during postnatal differ-

entiation of ventricular myocardium. Circ Res 80:88–94, 1997.
10. Fast VG, Darrow BJ, Saffitz JE, Kléber AG: Anisotropic activation spread in heart cell monolayers assessed by high-resolution optical mapping: role of tissue discontinuities. Circ Res 75:115–127, 1996.
11. Van Veen AA, van Rijen HV, Opthof T: Cardiac gap junction channels: Modulation of expression and channel properties. Cardiovasc Res 51:217–229, 2001.
12. Verheule S, van Kempen MJ, te Welscher PH, et al: Characterization of gap junction channels in adult rabbit atrial and ventricular myocardium. Circ Res 80:673–681, 1997.
13. Johnson CM, Kanter EM, Green KG, et al: Redistribution of connexin45 in gap junctions of connexin43-deficient hearts. Cardiovasc Res 53:921–935, 2002.
14. Coppen SR, Dupont E, Rothery S, Severs NJ: Connexin45 expression is preferentially associated with the ventricular conduction system in mouse and rat heart. Circ Res 82:232–243, 1998.
15. Veenstra RD: Size and selectivity of gap junction channels formed from different connexins. J Bioenerg Biomembr 28:317–337, 1996.
16. Beblo DA, Wang H-Z, Beyer EC, et al: Unique conductance, gating, and selective permeability properties of gap junction channels formed by connexin40. Circ Res 77:813–822, 1995.
17. Reaume AG, de Sousa PA, Kulkarni S, et al: Cardiac malformation in neonatal mice lacking connexin43. Science 267:1831–1834, 1995.
18. Huang GY, Wessels A, Smith BR, et al: Alteration in connexin 43 gap junction gene dosage impairs conotruncal heart development. Dev Biol 198:32–44, 1998.
19. Ya J, Erdtsieck-Ernste EBHW, de Boer PAJ, et al: Heart defects in connexin43-deficient mice. Circ Res 82:360–366, 1998.
20. Betsuyaku T, Kovacs A, Saffitz JE, Yamada KA: Cardiac structure and function in young and senescent mice heterozygous for a connexin43 null mutation. J Mol Cell Cardiol 34:175–184, 2002.
21. Guerrero PA, Schuessler RB, Davis LM, et al: Slow ventricular conduction in mice heterozygous for a Cx43 null mutation. J Clin Invest 99:1991–1998, 1997.
22. Thomas SA, Schuessler RB, Berul CI, et al: Disparate effects of deficient expression of connexin43 on atrial and ventricular conduction: Evidence for chamber-specific molecular determinants of conduction. Circulation 97:686–691, 1998.
23. Morley GE, Vaidya D, Samie FH, et al: Characterization of conduction in the ventricles of normal and heterozygous Cx43 knockout mice using optical mapping. J Cardiovasc Electrophysiol 10:1361–1375, 1999.
24. Eloff BC, Lerner DL, Yamada KA, et al: High resolution optical mapping reveals conduction slowing in connexin43 deficient mice. Cardiovasc Res 51:681–690, 2001.
25. Gutstein DE, Morley GE, Tamaddon H, et al: Conduction slowing and sudden arrhythmic death in mice with cardiac-restricted inactivation of connexin43. Circ Res 88:333–339, 2001.
26. Simon AM, Goodenough DA, Paul DL: Mice lacking connexin40 have cardiac conduction abnormalities characteristic of atrioventricular block and bundle branch block. Curr Biol 8:295–298, 1998.
27. Kirchhoff S, Nelles E, Hagendorff A, et al: Reduced cardiac conduction velocity and predisposition to arrhythmias in connexin40-deficient mice. Curr Biol 8:299–302, 1998.
28. Hagendorff A, Schumacher B, Kirchhoff S, et al: Conduction disturbances and increased atrial vulnerability in connexin40-deficient mice analyzed by transesophageal stimulation. Circulation 99:1508–1515, 1999.
29. Saffitz JE, Green KG, Kraft WJ, et al: Effects of diminished expression of connexin43 on gap junction number and size in ventricular myocardium. Am J Physiol Heart Circ Physiol 278:H1662–H1670, 2000.
30. Beardslee MA, Laing JG, Beyer EC, Saffitz JE: Rapid turnover of connexin43 in the adult rat heart. Circ Res 83:629–635, 1998.
31. Saffitz JE, Laing JG, Yamada KA: Connexin expression and turnover. Implications for cardiac excitability. Circ Res 86:723–728, 2000.
32. Laing JG, Tadros PN, Westphale EM, Beyer EC: Degradation of connexin43 gap junctions involves both the proteasome and the lysosome. Exp Cell Res 236:482–492, 1997.
33. Jordan K, Solan JL, Dominguez M, et al: Trafficking, assembly, and function of a connexin43-green fluorescent protein chimera in live mammalian cells. Mol Biol Cell 10:2033–2050, 1999.
34. Lauf U, Giepmans BNG, Lopez P, et al: Dynamic trafficking and delivery of connexins to the plasma membrane and accretion of gap junctions in living cells. Proc Natl Acad Sci U S A 99:10446–10451, 2002.
35. Martin PEM, Blundell G, Ahmad S, et al: Multiple pathways in the trafficking and assembly of connexin 26, 32 and 43 into gap junction intercellular communication channels. J Cell Sci 114:3845–3855, 2001.
36. Gaietta G, Deerinck TJ, Adams SR, et al: Multicolor and electron microspic imaging of connexin trafficking. Science 296:503–507, 2002.
37. Goodenough DA, Goliger JA, Paul DL: Connexins, connexons, and intercellular communication. Annu Rev Biochem 65:475–502, 1996.
38. Lampe PD, Lau AF: Regulation of gap junctions by phosphorylation of connexins. Arch Biochem Biophys 384:205–215, 2000.
39. Hertlein B, Butterweck A, Haubrich S, et al: Phosphorylated carboxy terminal serine residues stabilize the mouse gap junction protein connexin45 against degradation. J Membr Biol 162:247–257, 1998.
40. TenBroek E, Lampe PD, Solan JL, et al: Ser364 of connexin43 and the upregulation of gap junction assembly by cAMP. J Cell Biol 155:1307–1318, 2001.
41. Peters NS, Coromilas J, Severs NJ, Wit AL: Distributed connexin43 gap junction distribution correlates with the location of reentrant circuits in the epicardial border zone of healing canine infarcts that cause ventricular tachycardia. Circulation 95:988–996, 1997.
42. Beardslee MA, Lerner DL, Tadros PN, et al: Dephosphorylation and intracellular redistribution of ventricular connexin43 during electrical uncoupling induced by ischemia. Circ Res 87:656–662, 2000.
43. Lerner DL, Yamada KA, Schuessler RB, Saffitz JE: Accelerated onset and increased incidence of ventricular arrhythmias induced by ischemia in Cx43-deficient mice. Circulation 101:547–552, 2000.
44. Cooklin M, Wallis WRJ, Sheridan DJ, Fry CH: Changes in cell-to-cell electrical coupling associated with left ventricular hypertrophy. Circ Res 80:765–771, 1997.
45. Darrow BJ, Fast VG, Kléber AG, et al: Functional and structural assessment of intercellular communication: increased conduction veocity and enhanced connexin expression in dibutyryl cAMP-treated cultured cardiac myocytes. Circ Res 79:174–183, 1996.
46. Dodge SM, Beardslee MA, Darrow BJ, et al: Effects of angiotensin II on expression of the gap junction channel protein connexin43 in neonatal rat ventricular myocytes. J Am Coll Cardiol 32:800–807, 1998.
47. Zhuang J, Yamada KA, Saffitz JE, Kléber AG: Pulsatile stretch remodels cell-to-cell communication in cultured myocytes. Circ Res 87:316–322, 2000.
48. Pimentel RC, Yamada KA, Kléber AG, Saffitz JE: Autocrine regulation of myocyte Cx43 expression by VEGF. Circ Res 90:671–677, 2002.
49. Kaprielian RR, Gunning M, Dupont E, et al: Downregulation of immunodetectable connexin43 and decreased gap junction size in the pathogenesis of chronic hibernation in the human left ventricle. Circulation 97:651–660, 1998.
50. Petrich BG, Gong X, Lerner DL, et al: c-Jun N-terminal kinase activation mediates downregulation of connexin43 in cardiomyocytes. Circ Res 91:640–647, 2002.

第 22 章

窦房结活动的细胞机制

Itsuo Kodama,*Haruo Honjo*,*Halina Dobrzynski*,*Mark R. Boyett*

本章目录

- 参与起搏活动的离子通道 …………… 188
- 窦房结动作电位模型的建立 ………… 192
- 结构和功能的组合 …………………… 194
- 老年性窦房结功能障碍 ……………… 197
- 总结 …………………………………… 197

心脏有节律的跳动是源于一个小的特殊组织——窦房结的动作电位。随着近年来窦房结细胞电生理、分子生物学和显微形态学方面知识的丰富，窦房结在各种生理和病理状态下的起搏机制开始被全面地了解。本章主要讨论：(1) 参与窦房结细胞自发活动的离子活动及其分子基础和 (2) 窦房结中不同类型细胞经过复杂而精密的组织形成一个完整的、有力而且可靠的心脏起搏点。

一、参与起搏活动的离子通道

动作电位起源于窦房结的一小部分，主导起搏位点（leading pacemaker site）。它通常位于窦房结的中心。动作电位通常是从中心的主导起搏位点传播到窦房结的外围，然后进入界嵴的心房肌（因为房间隔可阻断传导）（图 22-1A）。窦房结的外围（窦房结靠近界嵴的区域）有时被称为"节周组织"或"过渡组织"。尽管窦房结外围组织的主要功能是传导来自窦房结中心、由主导起搏位点产生的动作电位，但是这些外围组织也存在自律性。在有些情况下，如自主神经激动时，主导起搏位点常常从窦房结中心移到外周[1]。因此，窦房结外围组织的起搏活性与处于中心位置的组织一样，也同样具有重要的生理功能。

运用膜片钳技术在主要起搏细胞（可能来自窦房结中心）上的实验研究，获得了大量关于参与窦房结起搏离子流的知识。在 1993 年的一篇综述中，Irisawa 及其同事[2]描述了窦房结起搏点去极化在不同时间多个电压依赖的离子流在背景电流存在情况下的相互作用。据他们所述，在前一动作电位衰退（失活）时，延迟整流 K^+ 电流（I_K）以时间和电压依赖的方式激活，并且在背景内向离子流存在的情况下，在最大舒张电位（maximum diastolic potential，MDP）之后产生最初的起搏点去极化。除了背景内向离子流，超极化激活离子流（I_f）的部分激活帮助起搏点去极化。在舒张期的后半部分，T 型 Ca^{2+} 电流（$I_{Ca,T}$）加速了起搏点的去极化。接近阈值时，自发动作电位由 L 型 Ca^{2+} 电流（$I_{Ca,L}$）触发。

在上述综述发表后的 10 年间，人们进行了更多的研究，发现这一情况比原来想象的更加复杂。目前在心脏中已经发现了两种延迟整流 K^+ 电流：快速激活电流，I_{Kr}；慢速激活电流，I_{Ks}[3]。尽管存在实质上的种属差异，I_{Kr} 和 I_{Ks} 都参与了窦房结起搏点的去极化[4-7]。也有证据表明 4-氨基吡啶（4-AP）敏感的 K^+ 电流也参与了窦房结动作电位[8,9]。在 1995 年，Guo 及其同事[10]在兔窦房结起搏细胞发现了一种新的内向离子流，命名为 I_{st}（持续内向离子流）。这种离子流亦在其他种属的窦房结中先后被发现[11]。近来有人提出，在基础状态和 β 肾上腺素受体激动情况下，肌浆网 Ca^{2+} 的释放在窦房结起搏活动中起着重要作用[12-14]。另外，应用转基因动物的研究，发现 $I_{Ca,L}$ 在窦房结起搏活动中可能也具有作用[15,16]。图 22-2 描绘

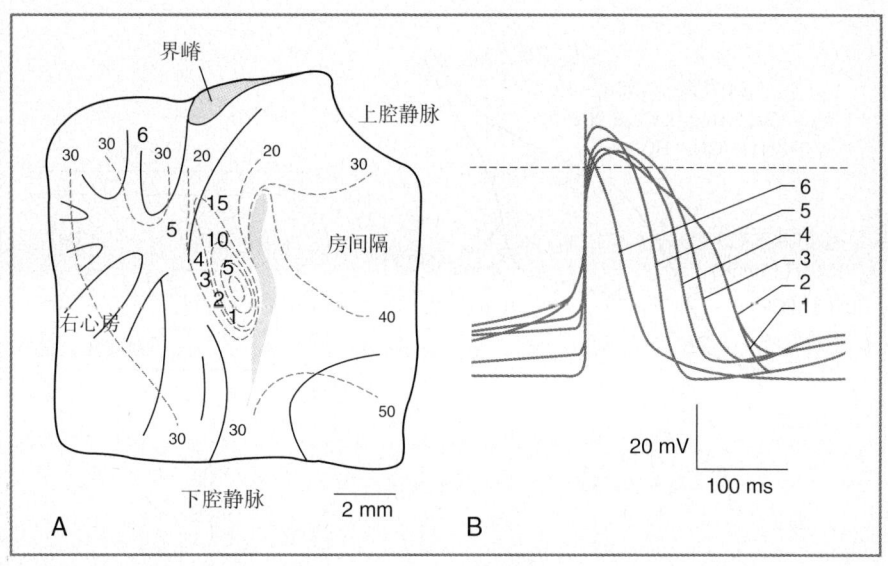

图 22-1 兔窦房结及其周围的激动顺序和自发动作电位 A：心内膜表面的激动顺序。激动时间的等时线是按每 5~10 s 绘制。面向房间隔的兴奋被阻断（阻断区由虚线区表示）。B：自发活动期间 1~6 位点的动作电位叠加记录（周长大约是 490 ms）（引自 Boyett MR et al：Downward gradient in action potential duration along conduction path in and around the sinoatrial node. *Am J Physiol* 1999；276：H686-H698.）

了参与窦房结起搏活动的所有离子通道和运载体[17]。目前大多数通道和运载体的分子基础已经明确（图 22-2）。

（一）延迟整流 K$^+$ 电流

在心脏中有两种不同的电生理和药理学特性的延迟整流 K$^+$ 电流（I_{Kr}，I_{Ks}）[3]。I_{Kr} 在较负的膜电位时被激活，它激活的时程相对较快。I_{Kr} 激活电压的特性显示其为内向整流电流。相比之下，I_{Ks} 在更正的膜电位时被激活，其激活的时程相对较慢，而且没有内向整流特性。I_{Kr} 可被Ⅲ类抗心律失常药（如多非利特 dofetilide，D-索他洛尔 D-sotalol，E-4031）特异性地阻断，然而 I_{Ks} 可被色原烷醇 293B（chromanol 293B）抑制。从兔、豚鼠、猪和小鼠分离到的窦房结细胞上都可发现这两种类型的 I_K，但它们在不同种属间的相对分布变异很大[4-7]。在兔窦房结起搏中 I_{Kr} 比 I_{Ks} 起着更重要的作用，因为起搏活动很容易被 I_{Kr} 的阻断剂抑制或取消，然而色原烷醇 293B 却不能影响起搏活动[4,6]。相反地，I_{Ks} 却是豚鼠和猪的窦房结细胞主要离子流成分[5,7]。在人的窦房结细胞，目前还没有资料显示 I_{Kr} 和 I_{Ks} 哪一个占主导地位。

目前已明确了心脏中 I_{Kr} 和 I_{Ks} 的分子基础。I_{Kr} 和 I_{Ks} 通道的孔区形成 α 亚单位分别是 ERG 和 KvLQT1。KvLQT1 与 β 亚单位 minK 相连形成 I_{Ks} 通道。ERG 可能和 minK 相关蛋白 MiRP1 相连形成 I_{Kr} 通道，但这一点还需要证实。有资料显示窦房结区域有 ERG 和 minK 的 mRNA 表达，但还需进一步确证[18,19]。

Lei 及其同事们[6]在兔窦房结细胞，通过测量细胞电容（cell capacitance，Cm）发现，I_{Kr} 和 I_{Ks} 的密度都和细胞的大小有关。细胞电容越大，离子流的密度就越大。这提示在兔窦房结，I_{Kr} 和 I_{Ks} 的密度存在区域差异；其密度在由小细胞组成的窦房结中心可能较低，而在由较大的细胞组成的窦房结外围较高。

（二）超极化激活离子流

超极化激活离子流（I_f）是一种时间依赖的内向离子流，它产生于窦房结起搏点超极化时[20]。这种离子流尽管在舒张期电位时最主要是 Na$^+$，但它本身可能同时包含有 K$^+$[20]。I_f 是由超极化产生的电压梯度所激活，但阈值电位在不同研究中有所不同（-40~-60mV）[20]。I_f 激活曲线的电压依赖性受细胞内环磷酸腺苷（cyclic adenosine monophosphate，cAMP）影响，β 肾上腺素受体激活使得 cAMP 增加，导致电压依赖性的正向移动，而胆碱受体激活使 cAMP 降低，导致电压依赖性的负向移动。

I_f 在窦房结起搏点去极化时产生的生理意义还是个有争议的问题。DiFrancesco[20]认为 I_f 在窦房结起搏过程尤其是被自主神经影响的情况下起着关键作

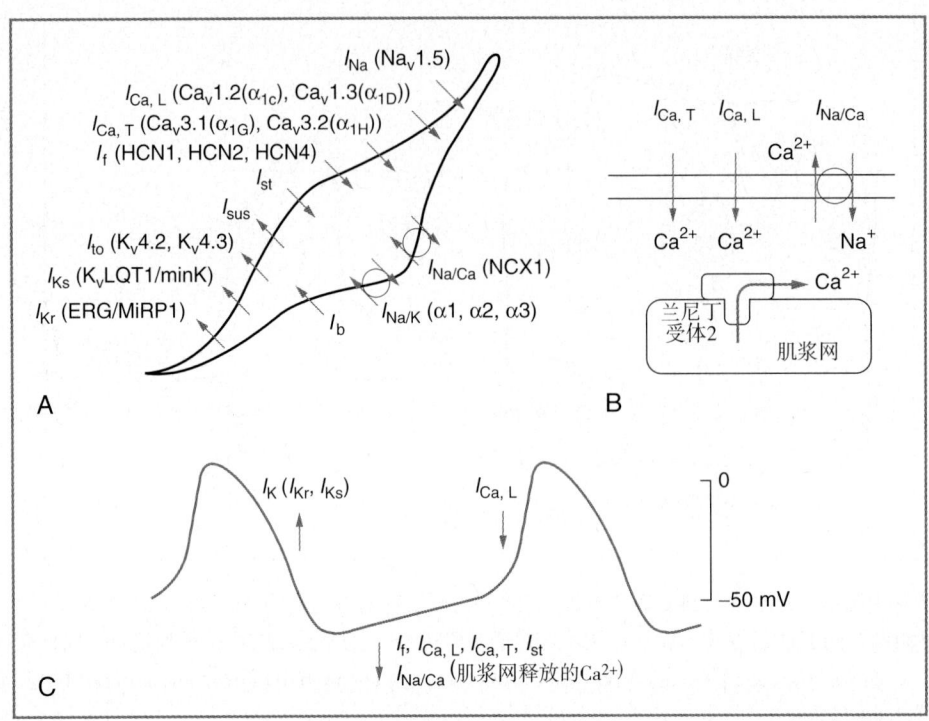

图 22-2　参与窦房结细胞起搏去极化和动作电位的离体通道和运载体　A：离子流、运载体和它们的分子基础。括弧内是通道和运载体的分子基础（克隆）。B：肌浆网 Ca^{2+} 的释放在起搏去极化中的作用。兰尼定受体（ryanodine receptor，RyR）为肌浆网 Ca^{2+} 释放通道。C：参与起搏去极化的离子流。向下的箭头表示内向（去极化）离子流；向上的箭头表示外向（复极化）离子流。起搏去极化包括外向离子流 I_K（I_{Kr}，I_{Ks}）的失活和其他内向离子流的激活（引自 Kodama I, Honjo H, Boyett MR et al: Are we lost in the labyrinth of the sinoatrial node pacemaker mechanism? *J Cardiovasc Electrophysiol* 2002；13：1303-1305.）

用，然而其他人认为 I_f 的作用可能是比较次要的[2,11]。I_f 的三种阻断剂（Cs^+，扎替雷定 zatebradine 和 ZD-7288）都能使兔窦房结的自发心率有中等程度的下降（12%～16%）[1]。然而在副交感神经/胆碱受体激动所致的负性变时效应和在交感神经/肾上腺素受体激动所致正性变时效应的情况下，I_f 阻断剂对窦房结影响的报道结果并不一致，有的抑制，有的没有影响[1,20]。

在使用小球块的兔窦房结组织实验中，发现用 Cs^+ 阻断 I_f 后，对窦房结外围组织起搏活动的抑制作用强于中心组织[1]。在离体单个兔窦房结细胞中发现，细胞电容越大，I_f 密度越大。这些观察提示 I_f 在窦房结外围组织中对起搏活动所起的作用可能比在窦房结中心组织中更重要，有人认为这可能是一种保护机制（见后讨论部分）。

随着超极化激活环化核苷酸门控（hyperpolarization-activated cyclic nucleotide gated，HCN）通道家族被克隆出来，我们才可能逐步明确 I_f 的分子特性。HCN 通道属于电压门控钾离子通道超家族，具有六次跨膜区，而且很可能组成四聚体。HCN 通道家族所有已知成员（HCN1～HCN4）在大脑中都有表达，而在心脏中只有 HCN1、HCN2 和 HCN4 表达[22]。原位杂交显示，窦房结中 HCN4 mRNA 比 HCN1 和 HCN2 的 mRNA 表达都高[22-24]。将克隆自兔窦房结的 HCN1 和 HCN4（rbHCN1，rbHCN4）转入哺乳动物细胞表达，发现其形成的 I_f 电生理特性与细胞本身的 I_f 类似，但不完全相同[23,24]。细胞本身的 I_f 激活动力学和 cAMP 引起的半激活电压的变化介于 rbHCN1 和 rbHCN4 之间。这就提出了以下两种可能：两种亚型可形成异源多聚体的天然 I_f 通道或是形成一个由多个同源多聚体的复合通道[23]。

（三）Ca^{2+} 离子流

窦房结起搏细胞所产生的动作电位的上升支几乎都是源于 $I_{Ca,L}$。近来认为它对起搏点去极化的贡献可能很小，因为 $I_{Ca,L}$ 的激活阈值电位通常高于－40mV，而起搏点的去极化通常发生在更负的电位。两个转基因动物的研究使这一观点变得更加矛盾[15,16]。L 型

Ca^{2+}通道（L-type Ca^{2+} channels，LTCCs）是一个具有多个亚单位的复合体，其中形成孔区的α_1亚单位具有不同异构体。在心血管系统中，形成LTCCs最多的异构体是α_{1C}（Cav1.2）。在心房肌细胞有α_{1D}（Cav1.3）形成的LTCCs，尽管表达量不高。Cav1.3缺陷小鼠（$\alpha_{1D}^{-/-}$）由于耳蜗内毛细胞上LTCCs的完全缺失，表现为耳聋[15]，此外，这种小鼠还表现出心动过缓和心律失常，提示α_{1D}-LTCCs在小鼠心脏中对形成正常的窦房结起搏活动十分重要[15]。近来通过与野生型小鼠的窦房结细胞相比，发现Cav1.3缺陷小鼠窦房结细胞的动作电位，具有较慢的自发激动速率和较慢的起搏去极化特性[16]。Cav1.3缺陷小鼠窦房结细胞的$I_{Ca,L}$激活曲线表现出向去极化方向的移动（$\sim$5mV）[16]。在哺乳动物细胞上异源性表达克隆的LTCCs，发现与α_{1C}-LTCCs相比，α_{1D}-LTCCs具有更负的电流激活范围，因而使α_{1D}-LTCCs能够在窦房结起搏细胞的正常起搏去极化过程中介导Ca^{2+}内流[16,25]。根据这些研究结果，Verheijck及其同事们[25]发现，在兔窦房结细胞中$I_{Ca,L}$可以在-60mV的电位被激活。

$I_{Ca,T}$在~-50mV激活，而在$-40\sim-90$mV间失活。因此，$I_{Ca,T}$能够参与窦房结细胞起搏去极化的后半部分[27]。表达$I_{Ca,T}$通道孔区形成亚单位的大量基因目前已经被克隆出来，而且在心脏中发现有两种异构体，即α_{1G}（Cav3.1）和α_{1H}（Cav3.2）[28]。Cav3.1 mRNA在小鼠窦房结中表达较为丰富，约是周围心房肌的30倍[28]。Cav3.2 mRNA在窦房结中表达也很丰富，但是其表达水平要低于Cav3.1 mRNA[28]。异源性表达的Cav3.1和Cav3.2通道的失活状态恢复过程有着不同的动力学特性；Cav3.1通道恢复时间常数（$\sim$120 ms）较Cav3.2通道（$\sim$400 ms）快[29]。兔窦房结细胞天然$I_{Ca,T}$恢复时间常数为$\sim$140 ms[27]，提示在窦房结中以Cav3.1为主。但是就Ni^{2+}的敏感性而言，天然$I_{Ca,T}$与Cav3.2类似，而与Cav3.1不同[30]。因此在窦房结中到底哪种$I_{Ca,T}$异构体占主导地位还需进一步明确。

（四）Na^+离子流

在窦房结细胞中是否存在Na^+电流（I_{Na}）以及Na^+电流是否参与起搏活动是长期以来有争议的问题。基于使用河豚毒素（tetrodotoxin，TTX）和硝苯地平（nifedipine）对兔窦房结组织的实验结果，Kodama及其同事们发现[31]，在窦房结外围组织是I_{Na}负责动作电位的上升支，而在窦房结中心则是$I_{Ca,L}$。在兔的窦房结单个细胞中，Honjo及其合作者们[21]发现I_{Na}具有明显的细胞大小依赖性；在细胞电容$\leqslant$30 pF的小细胞（推测来自窦房结中心组织）中，I_{Na}很小或可以忽略，但是在细胞电容$\geqslant$30 pF的大细胞（推测来自窦房结外围组织）中，存在有明显的I_{Na}（50$\sim$100 pA/pF）。

Baruscotti及其同事们[32]证实，在新生兔窦房结细胞中存在TTX敏感的I_{Na}，并在起搏去极化中起着重要作用。参照Honjo及其同事们的研究，推测I_{Na}可从窦房结中心组织细胞中消失。他们也发现，在出生后的头40天里I_{Na}也可以消失，从而推测认为在新生兔窦房结细胞中，I_{Na}可能是由神经元型通道产生[31]，但是其具体的分子基础尚需确定。

（五）持续的内向离子流

Noma及其合作者在兔、豚鼠和大鼠的自发激活窦房结细胞中发现了持续的内向离子流（I_{st}）[10,11]。I_{st}在典型的窦房结细胞起搏去极化电位范围（$-60\sim-40$ mV）激活，比$I_{Ca,L}$的激活阈值电位还要更负。I_{st}不像$I_{Ca,L}$，在去极化过程中没有明显的不应期。由于除去细胞外Na^+会使该种离子流抑制，而在无Ca^{2+}的溶液环境中则不影响它，说明这种离子流的载体是Na^+[11]。I_{st}与$I_{Ca,L}$具有共同的药理学特性：对TTX不敏感，能被有机的和无机的Ca^{2+}拮抗剂所阻断（维拉帕米、D600、尼卡地平、Ni^{2+}和Co^{2+}），能被Ca^{2+}激动剂Bay-K8644增强，而β肾上腺素受体激动能将I_{st}增加2倍[11]。有报道在豚鼠窦房结细胞可记录到全细胞的I_{st}[33]。I_{st}单通道的离子流幅度比传统的Na^+和L型Ca^{2+}离子流幅度要小，平均单位电导为13.3 pS，反转电位为+13 mV。I_{st}仅在自发跳动的细胞中观察得到，而在分离自同一窦房结的静息细胞中则观察不到，这一现象提示I_{st}在起搏活动中起着重要作用[11]。

关于I_{st}，虽然有对$I_{Ca,L}$组分有类似I_{st}离子流的报道，但只有一个研究组曾对I_{st}进行过明确地描述[11]。Verheijck及其同事们发现[26]，在兔的窦房结细胞中没有硝苯地平敏感的I_{st}样Na^+离子流。I_{st}的存在和它的生理重要性仍需进一步明确。在窦房结动作电位的数字模型中，I_{st}的参与导致了起搏频率的中度升高，这种升高程度依赖于I_{st}相对于其他参与的内向离子流的幅度。例如，在Zhang及其合作者[34]的外周细胞模型中，引入了I_{Na}和相对大的$I_{Ca,L}$、$I_{Ca,L}$和$I_{b,Na}$，

I_{st} 的贡献便可以忽略不计,而在中心细胞模型中,引入了相对较小的 $I_{Ca,L}$、$I_{Ca,L}$ 和 $I_{b,Na}$,当 I_{st} 增加两倍后,自发心率可增加 14%。

(六) 肌浆网 Ca^{2+} 释放的作用

肌浆网 Ca^{2+} 释放早已被认为与窦房结的起搏活动有关;人们推测由肌浆网 Ca^{2+} 释放导致的细胞内 Ca^{2+} 瞬变激活了内向 Na^+/Ca^{2+} 交换离子流 ($I_{Na/Ca}$),从而促进起搏点的去极化 (见图 22-2B)。Hüser 及其同事们[12]发现在猫心房起搏细胞的自发跳动过程中,在动作电位上升支之前有肌纤维膜下胞浆内 Ca^{2+} 的增加。在兔窦房结细胞的实验中,Bogdanov 及其同事们[13]研究表明,起搏点去极化过程中兰尼定(ryanodine)受体 Ca^{2+} 释放产生了肌纤维膜下胞浆内 Ca^{2+} 的增加,从而导致内向 $I_{Na/Ca}$。兰尼定消除了动作电位上升支之前的 Ca^{2+} 瞬变,并以剂量依赖方式抑制自发激动速率(IC_{50},2.6 μM)。兰尼定在高浓度的时候 (30~100 μM) 可将自发跳动消除。基于这些结果,Bogdanov 及其同事们推断,肌浆网 Ca^{2+} 释放可通过激活 $I_{Na/Ca}$ 在窦房结起搏活动中起重要作用 (图 22-2B)。来自同一工作组的研究表明,异丙肾上腺素 (0.1 μM) 可增加动作电位前的 Ca^{2+} 流幅度,加速起搏去极化,继而加速自发激动速率[14]。当兰尼定受体被兰尼定阻断其效应后,β 肾上腺素受体激动就不能增加 Ca^{2+} 幅度,也不能增加起搏活动的去极化速率和自发激动速率,仅能增加 $I_{Ca,L}$ 的幅度[14]。Vinogradova 及其同事们[14]推断,兰尼定受体的 Ca^{2+} 释放在 β 肾上腺素受体激动增加窦房结激动速率的过程中起着交换机的作用。

令人惊讶的是,近来的报告与之前的观察结果不一致。有资料显示,肌浆网 Ca^{2+} 释放在窦房结起搏活动中并没有起到如前人所说的那么重要的作用。在另一项研究中,分离兔和豚鼠的窦房结细胞,运用各种方法抑制 Ca^{2+} 瞬变后,都不能消除起搏活动,而仅仅只是降低了自发速率 21%~37%[35]。过去我们认为 β 肾上腺素受体激动对参与窦房结正性变时效应的多种离子流具有作用,如 $I_{Ca,L}$、I_{Kr}、I_{Ks} 和 I_f。在完整的兔窦房结组织中,我们观察到 30 μM 的兰尼定作用 60 min 仅使自发激动速率降低了 19%,而异丙肾上腺素 (0.03 μM) 的正性变时效应并不能被兰尼定阻断[34]。在主要起搏细胞的窦房结动作电位的数字模型中,结合了胞内 Ca^{2+} 处理,Kurata 及其同事们[36]发现,除去肌浆网 Ca^{2+} 释放仅仅能使自发心动周期增加 3.4%。导致上述肌浆网 Ca^{2+} 释放所起作用在结论上的不一致,可能与观察的窦房结细胞类型不同有关 (见后文讨论)。总之,肌浆网 Ca^{2+} 释放在调节窦房结起搏活动中的生理意义尚不明确。

(七) 4-氨基吡啶敏感的 K^+ 电流

Honjo 及其同事们[8]和 Lei 及其合作者[9]在兔的窦房结细胞中发现有 4-AP 敏感的 K^+ 电流,并全面描述了这种离子流的特征。该种离子流包括瞬时离子流和持续离子流两种组分:I_{trans} 和 I_{sus}。在其他心脏组织中,I_{trans} 的电生理和药理学特性与那些瞬时外向 K^+ 电流类似。而持续离子流组分可能是 I_{to} 的不失活组分或是 4-AP 敏感的超快速延迟整流 K^+ 电流,$I_{K,ur}$。I_{trans} 和 I_{sus} 的密度都与细胞电容有关,并且在较大细胞中离子流密度较大 (从窦房结外围组织细胞推测所得)。窦房结外围组织的 I_{trans} 和 I_{sus} 密度比窦房结中心组织的高,可能参与了从中心到外围组织动作电位时程下降梯度的形成 (见后文)[1]。我们在窦房结组织中的观察支持了这一假说,4-AP (5 mM) 引起的动作电位时程延长在外围组织要比在中心组织延长更多[1]。

(八) 其他离子流

除了上面所述的离子流之外,研究发现窦房结还有其他一些离子流存在,包括有 Na^+/K^+ 泵离子流 ($I_{Na/K}$),ACh 激活的 K^+ 电流 ($I_{K,ACh}$),ATP 敏感的 K^+ 电流,ATP 敏感的阳离子流,以及牵张激活的阴离子流[1,2]。由于窦房结细胞电容约为 30~60 pF,而它们在舒张期的膜电位去极化速率约为 0.03~0.1 V/s,故一个 1~6 pA 的净内向离子流足以使起搏点发生去极化。因此,无论是内向或外向离子流 (包括时间依赖和非时间依赖的) 的微小改变都很容易影响到窦房结起搏活动。

二、窦房结动作电位模型的建立

窦房结细胞的动作电位是上面所述多种离子流动态相互作用的结果。为了能定量、整体地解释这一复杂的相互作用,人们建立了各种能详尽反映其生物物理特性的兔窦房结细胞数字化模型。大多数模型都是代表"典型的"(或主要的) 窦房结动作电位。然而,Zhang 及其合作者[37]的实验发现,在兔窦房结中心和外周的细胞之间,动作电位的参数、离子流密度以及

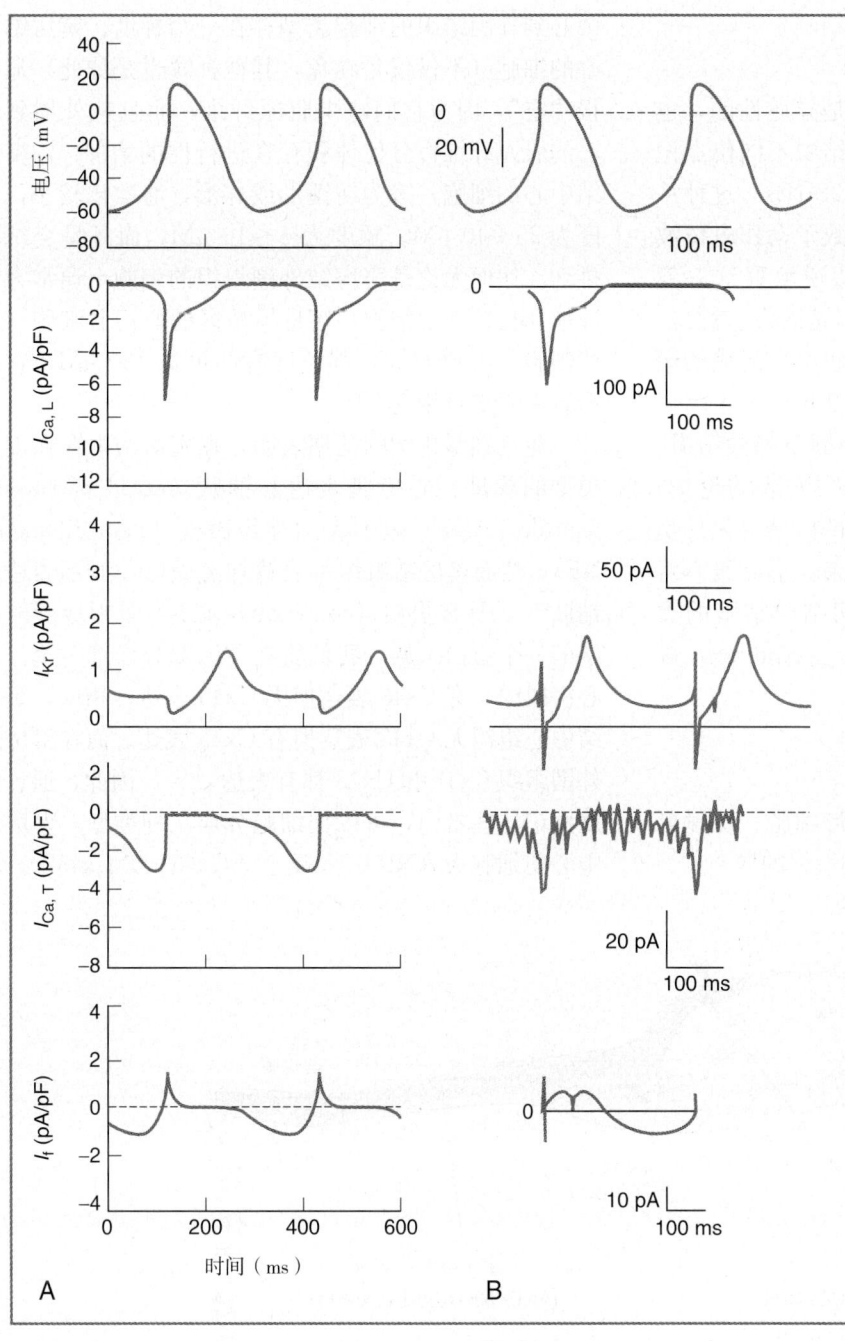

图 22-3 Kurata 和他的同事们建立的窦房结主要起搏细胞模型中自发动作电位及其时间依赖性离子流[35] A：动作电位的模型示踪信号，从上到下依次是 $I_{Ca,L}$、I_{Kr}、$I_{Ca,L}$。B：用膜片钳方法记录到的中心窦房结细胞的自发动作电位和离子流证实了该模型的有效性（引自 Kurata Y, Hisatome I, Imanishi S, et al: Dynamical description of sinoatrial node pacemaking improved mathematical model for primary pacemaker cell. *Am J Physiol* 2002；283：H2074-H2101.）

药理学反应都具有区域性差异。他们根据这一特性，分别建立了窦房结中心细胞和外周细胞的动作电位模型；并假定中心细胞比外周细胞小，而且离子流密度也依赖于细胞的大小。在兔窦房结组织的实验中可观察到，阻断 I_{Na}、$I_{Ca,L}$、4-AP 敏感的离子流，I_{Kr} 和 I_f 所产生的效应在中心和外围组织是不同的，这一现象在 Zhang 等人建立的模型中可再现。但这些模型最主要的局限性在于，它们都被假定胞内离子流是稳定不变的，而我们知道胞内 Ca^{2+} 的动态变化和胞内 Na^+、K^+ 浓度的变化对起搏活动都有着很重要的影响。因此，近来 Kurata 及其合作者[36]又建立了一种能反映兔窦房结单个"主要"起搏细胞的改良数字模型，该模型在建模过程中不仅纳入了目前对离子流（包括 I_{st} 和 $I_{K,ACh}$）的最新实验数据，还考虑到了肌浆网功能（Ca^{2+} 的摄取和释放）以及肌浆网下一小块特定区域的胞内离子稳态。这种模型可再现自发动作电位，还可观察到动作电位发生期类似膜片钳记录到的那些离子流（$I_{Ca,L}$、$I_{Ca,L}$、I_{Kr} 和 I_f），以及这些离子流的阻断剂对窦房结起搏活动的影响（见图 22-3）。

三、结构和功能的组合

已经明确在很多种属的窦房结都是异质性的，也就是有多种细胞成分组成的。在窦房结中不同位点记录到的动作电位波形差别非常大（图 22-1B）。这种从窦房结中心到周围组织的位置变化导致了动作电位波形在整个窦房结内的变异。有两种假说解释这一变化：梯度模型和镶嵌模型[1,38,39]。根据镶嵌模型假说，窦房结是由两种类型细胞（窦房结和心房）组成的镶嵌型结构，并且其电生理活性的区域变化是由于窦房结细胞/心房细胞比率从中心到外周不断下降的结果。这方面可参阅 Verheijck 及其同事们[39]发表的论文。而根据梯度模型假说[38]，电生理特性的区域变化是窦房结细胞特性从中心到外周变化的结果。下面我们将对这一观点的许多细节，比如兔窦房结中细胞的类型、电耦联、电学活性以及 Ca^{2+} 运作（handling）等进行阐述。

（一）细胞类型

窦房结的细胞有很多种形态（蛛形细胞、纺锤形细胞和长纺锤形细胞），反映了窦房结组织的异质性[1]。有充分的证据可证明，在兔的窦房结中，从中心到外围组织的细胞类型存在一个梯度。窦房结中心的细胞（不仅仅是在兔，其他种属也是如此）显得很"空"，因为它们缺少肌原纤维，而且从外周到中心的肌原纤维百分比体积存在进行性的增加[1]。窦房结中心的细胞，多为纺锤形或蛛形，通常比较小，长度为 25～40 μM，宽度为 4～10 μM，而且呈交织状排列。然而无论是窦房结外围组织的细胞（通常为纺锤形和长纺锤形细胞）还是界嵴区的心房肌细胞（杆状细胞）都比较大，其长度有的可达 150 μM，它们沿着界嵴平行排列[1,40]。

免疫细胞化学的证据表明，在窦房结中存在细胞类型的梯度：心房肌表达心钠肽（atrial natriuretic peptide，ANP）但不表达神经微丝（neurofilament，NF），然而窦房结组织可表达神经微丝，而不表达心钠肽[42]。连接蛋白（connexins，Cxs）是形成缝隙连接的一个蛋白家族，我们将在下一部分详细讨论。在心房肌中，有 Cx43 表达但无 Cx45 表达；相反，窦房结中心组织无 Cx43 表达但有 Cx45 表达。而在窦房结外围组织 Cx43 和 Cx45 都有表达[40,41]。因此，通过免疫标记这些蛋白，可以把细胞分成三种类型：窦房结中心的细胞为 ANP－/NF＋/Cx43－/Cx45＋，窦

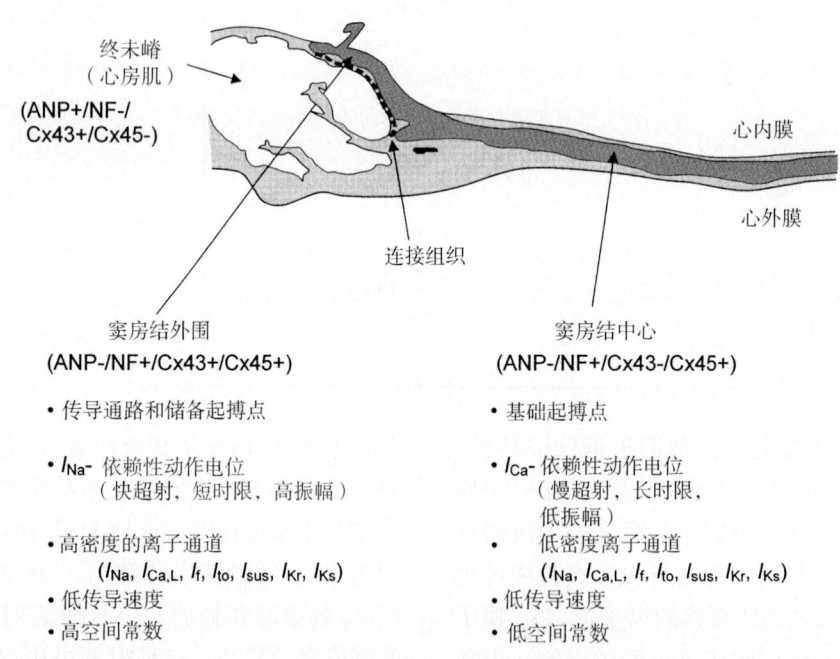

图 22-4 兔窦房结切片图（在通过界嵴区和腔静脉间区域之间切开） 窦房结内和周围的细胞类型鉴定是基于对 Cx43、Cx45、心钠肽（ANP）以及神经微丝（NF）抗体的免疫反应。窦房结外围和中心的电生理特性总结如下。（引自 Boyett MR, Dobrzynski H, Lancaster MK, et al: Sophisticated architecture is required for the sinoatrial node to perform its normal pacemaker function. J Cardiovasc Elecrophysical 2003; 14: 104-106.）

房结外围组织细胞为 ANP－／NF＋／Cx43＋／Cx45＋, 心房肌的细胞为 ANP＋／NF－／Cx43＋／Cx45－。Dobrzynski 及其同事也对此进行了研究见图 22-4（资料尚未发表），这是从界嵴到窦房结的切面示意图，描述了这三种类型细胞的分布情况。腔静脉间区域的窦房结组织可一直上升到界嵴与心内膜面的交界处，然而窦房结中心组织位于腔静脉之间的区域，外围组织位于界嵴处。

（二）电耦联

通过测量各种数据（例如成对细胞之间的空间常数和耦联电导性），得知窦房结中心的细胞间电耦联很弱，然而心房肌的细胞间电耦联却很好；估计窦房结外围组织的细胞间电耦联可能也很好[1]。这可解释为什么在窦房结中心动作电位的传导速率很低，而在外围组织和心房肌传导速率却较高[1]。这种电耦联的组织差异可能是 Cx 表达差异的结果：Cx43 是心脏中一种重要的缝隙连接蛋白，存在于工作的心房肌和心室肌的闰盘上。很多研究（少数例外）表明，在不同种属（兔，小鼠，大鼠，豚鼠，狗，牛和人）的窦房结中心无 Cx43 表达[42,43]。相反，在窦房结中心，Cx40、Cx45、可能还有 Cx46 都有表达[42,43]。运用免疫细胞化学的方法，在窦房结细胞上标记的 Cx40 和 Cx45 呈小的散点状分布，相反在工作心肌细胞上标记的 Cx43 表达很丰富且是有组织的分布[40,41]。这与电镜结果一致，在电镜下发现窦房结的缝隙连接很小且是散在分布[44]。在兔的单个窦房结细胞中，Honjo 及其合作者[40]发现在小细胞（假定是来自中心组织）中可高表达 Cx45, 但却无 Cx43 表达，而在大细胞（假定是来自外围组织）中也有较多 Cx45 表达（图 22-5A）。

从理论上讲，对于窦房结而言，很难既参与起搏活动又驱动心房肌，因为它有来自心房肌的抑制性超极化影响[45]。窦房结中心微弱的电耦联使得窦房结可免受这种抑制影响，从而使得窦房结中心能够起搏[45]。有人认为在窦房结外围组织中，存在电耦联良好的心房细胞和电耦联很弱的窦房结细胞之间的交错排列，从而使得窦房结能够驱动周围的心房肌[46]，但是这种观点尚有争议。运用免疫细胞化学的方法在不同种属（包括人类）中都发现存在这种交错排列[43]。

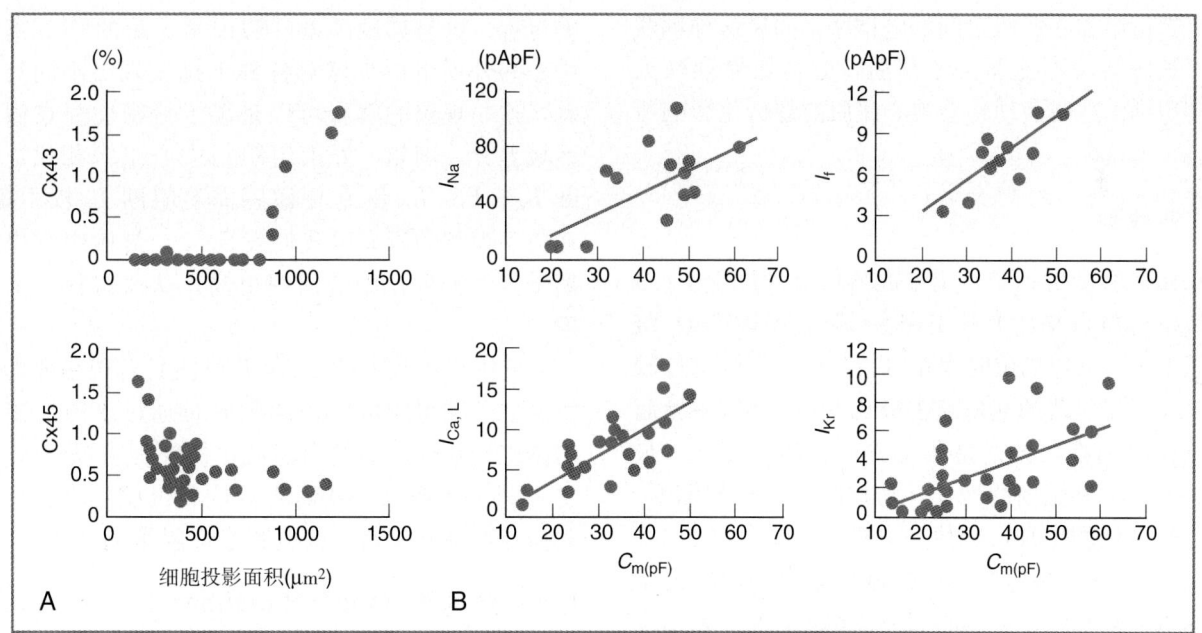

图 22-5 兔窦房结中离子流密度和连接蛋白的表达对细胞大小的依赖性 A：连接蛋白表达和细胞大小间的联系。纵轴为抗 Cx43 和抗 Cx45 的免疫阳性区域占总面积的百分比，横轴为细胞投影面积。Cx43 仅在较大的细胞（＞800 μm^2）中表达，而 Cx45 主要在小细胞中表达。数据来自于 Honjo 及其同事们的研究[40]。B：离子流密度和细胞大小的相关性。纵轴为 I_{Na}、I_f、$I_{Ca,L}$ 和 I_{Kr} 的密度，横轴为电容（Cm）。直线表示线性回归。数据来自于 Honjo 及其同事们的研究（I_{Na}，I_f）[21]，以及 Lei 等的研究（$I_{Ca,L}$，I_{Kr}）[6]。

间是，在兔的窦房结中，Coppen及其同事们[41]发现Cx43阳性的心房肌细胞和Cx43阴性的窦房结细胞之间的大多数边界都能清晰显示，两种组织间并不存在明显地广泛交错。相反，在窦房结外围组织，Cx43和Cx45都有表达。在兔单个窦房结细胞中所得到的数据也与上述结果一致——在大细胞（假定为外周组织细胞）中，Cx43和Cx45都有表达，并且它们常常共定位在同一缝隙连接斑块[40]。这些观察结果提出一种可能，即在窦房结中存在异型缝隙连接通道（heterotypic gap junction channels）（一种由连接蛋白Cx43组成，另一种由伴侣连接蛋白Cx45组成）或者是异源通道（heteromeric channels）（由Cx43和Cx45混合组成）。有报道发现在其他动物种属中有一种包含有Cx43和Cx45的类似过渡结构的物质[43]，位于中心（主导起搏位点）和心房肌之间，可能是一个具有中间耦联电导（intermediate coupling conductance）的区域。这种区域最先是由Joyner和van Capelle[45]提出来的，在他们的模型分析中，这一区域使得窦房结能够驱动周围的心房肌。

图22-4描述了在不同种属中，窦房结和邻近界嵴心房肌之间的连接组织屏障。这种连接组织屏障可能限制了窦房结和心房肌之间的电耦联，如果这种耦联太小，窦房结就不能驱动心房肌，但是如果耦联太大，窦房结的起搏活动将会被心房肌的超极化影响所抑制。

（三）电活动

在完整的窦房结中，主导起搏位点（位于中心）的动作电位特点是：上升支速率（$V_{max}<10V/s$）缓慢，幅度小，动作电位时程相对长，最大舒张电位较负，以及伴有显著的起搏点去极化[1,47]。当从主导起搏位点移向别处，无论是哪个方向，都有V_{max}（最高$>100V/s$）和幅度的增加，动作电位时程的缩短，最大舒张电位的增加，起搏点去极化减少（见图22-1B）[1,47]。分离自窦房结不同区域的组织小球保留了相似的电活动梯度；从中心到外围组织，V_{max}和幅度增加，动作电位时程缩短，最大舒张电位增加[1]。唯一不一致的地方是起搏点活性；从中心到外围组织，小球上的起搏点去极化和自发激动速率是增加的。来自邻近心房肌的电紧张的影响（electrotonic influence）可以用来解释这一矛盾。在完整组织中，外围窦房结细胞的起搏点去极化会被来自非起搏心房细胞（具有更负的舒张电位）的超极化离子流所减弱。靠近窦房结中心的细胞受这种电紧张的干扰较小，这是因为这些细胞离心房肌较远，并且细胞间的电耦联较弱[1]。

对组织小球的研究揭示窦房结及其周围电活动存在区域差异，而这种差异可能是窦房结内在电活动区域变化的结果（梯度模型）[1,38]，或是心房细胞和相邻均一窦房结细胞以不同方式混合的结果（镶嵌模型）[39]。如前文所论述的，在兔的窦房结中，从中心到外周，细胞的大小是逐渐增加的。我们通过测量细胞电容研究了兔窦房结电活性和细胞大小之间的关系[1,6,8,9,21]。结果表明动作电位参数和细胞大小之间高度相关；在较大细胞（假定来自窦房结外周组织）中，动作电位的V_{max}、幅度和最大舒张电位以及自发激动速率都比小细胞（假定来自窦房结中心组织）的大。大小窦房结细胞间动作电位的变化与外周和中心窦房结组织小球间的变化是一致的[1]。如前文所提到的，在离子流密度和细胞大小间也存在显著相关；较大细胞中，I_{Na}、$I_{Ca,L}$、I_{to}、I_{sus}、I_{Kr}、I_{Ks}和I_f的密度均比在小细胞中大（见图22-4和22-5B）[1,6,8,9,21]。这些观察结果提示从中心到外周的窦房结细胞在电学特性上有一个逐渐过渡的过程，这与梯度模型的假说是一致的[38]。窦房结中心和外周组织小球对各种干扰表现出不同的电活动，这一现象的解释可以是离子流密度存在假定的区域差异。例如，外围组织与中心组织相比，对阻断I_{Na}、I_{to}、I_{sus}和I_f更敏感而对阻断I_{Kr}较不敏感。在数字模型的研究中我们发现[37]，外围组织中这些离子流的密度比中心组织更高，从而解释了上述现象。

外围组织较大的I_{Na}和I_f可能具有很重要的功能意义。外围组织的窦房结细胞是通过缝隙连接与心房细胞耦联的。继发的超极化使外围组织细胞的I_{Na}和I_f进一步激活，从而将对抗和可能克服心房肌对起搏点激动和兴奋性的电紧张抑制作用。

（四）钙运作（Ca^{2+} Handling）

很多证据表明钙运作在窦房结的中心和外围组织间是不同的。如前文所述，$I_{Ca,L}$密度在窦房结的中心细胞可能较少。Musa及其合作者[48]在兔和豚鼠窦房结上，运用免疫标记的方法发现，从外周到中心，Cav1.2的表达呈下降趋势。同样，从中心到外周Na^+/Ca^{2+}交换器（Na^+/Ca^{2+} exchanger, NCX1），

肌浆网 Ca^{2+} 释放通道（SR Ca^{2+} release channel, RYR2）和肌浆网钙泵（SR Ca^{2+} pump, SERCA2）的表达也都是下降的。在窦房结中心细胞，免疫标记的兰尼定受体仅在细胞膜下出现。相反，在外周细胞兰尼定受体既定位于细胞膜下（对应连接型肌浆网），也定位于胞浆中［对应终末池（corbular）肌浆网或非连接型肌浆网］。中心细胞和外周细胞的肌浆网钙泵均散在分布于胞浆中。这些观察结果与电镜结果一致，电镜下观察到窦房结细胞（尤其是中心细胞）中的肌浆网也是散在分布的[1]。与这些发现相一致的是，Lancaster 和他的同事们观察到（资料尚未发表），在窦房结小细胞中（假定为中心细胞），胞内钙瞬变（Ca^{2+} transient）小且慢，而且基本不依赖于肌浆网 Ca^{2+} 释放；在窦房结大细胞中（假定为外周细胞），胞内钙瞬变大且快，而且强烈依赖于肌浆网 Ca^{2+} 释放。由于这些差别，可以认为胞内 Ca^{2+} 对起搏活性的调节在外周组织中更加重要。

四、老年性窦房结功能障碍

窦房结的异质性在窦房结老化过程中可能起着十分重要的作用。随着人年龄的增加，其固有心率下降，窦房传导时间增加。在老年人中，病态窦房结综合征是有症状心律失常最常见的原因：它可包括窦性心动过缓、窦性停搏、窦房传导阻滞或交替性心动过缓（alternating bradycardia）和房性心动过速。类似的这种年龄相关的改变在其他种属中也有发现[49]。在新生兔中，I_{Na} 离子流（TTX敏感的）在整个窦房结中都有表达，但是在成年兔中，I_{Na} 离子流在窦房结中心是缺失的，它仅在窦房结外周组织表达[21,32]。在兔和猫的窦房结中，Aling 和 Bouman[49] 发现，窦房结的整个面积并没有随着年龄而改变，但是整个面积中的上升支速率低的区域增加了，例如，窦房结外周组织的上升速率下降到类似于在中心组织的水平。这提示外周组织 Na^+ 通道存在年龄依赖的下调。Zhang 及其同事在一个包含有离子流密度区域差异的窦房结多细胞模型中观察到，除去窦房结外周组织的 I_{Na}，可减慢起搏活动并增加窦房传导时间，从而可能导致窦房结阻滞现象。这些变化与年龄相关的改变类似。有趣的是 Nav1.5 敲除的小鼠和 Na^+ 通道 β 亚单位敲除的小鼠都有病态窦房结综合征的表现[50]。Na^+ 通道看来可能不是窦房结随着年龄增加而丧失的唯一离子通道：Jone 等研究初步表明，豚鼠窦房结中心 Cx43 和 Cav1.2 缺失的面积随着年龄的增加而增加。这种 Cx43 和 Cav1.2 的缺失可能有助于解释随着年龄增加出现的固有心率下降和窦房传导减慢。Cav1.3 敲除小鼠亦表现出病态窦房结综合征[15]。

五、总　结

本章介绍了窦房结是怎样完成其起搏活动并驱动周围心房肌这两大功能的。现在不断有新的资料来揭示这一复杂机制，而其中最重要的进展是认识到了正是多种不同离子流的完美组合使得窦房结在各种生理和病理情况下能够发挥良好的起搏功能。目前发现窦房结的起搏活动中存在大量的离子活动，例如多种内向离子流参与了起搏去极化，这些离子机制在窦房结的起搏活动中发挥重要作用。窦房结是一个复杂且不均一的组织，这对它在很多方面发挥正常功能起着决定性作用。首先，窦房结可通过以下方式保护它不受到周围心房肌超极化的影响，例如，通过结缔组织限制了两种组织间的接触面积，窦房结内电耦联的弱化，两种组织在边界区交错排列，以及窦房结外围组织上存在的高密度 I_{Na} 和 I_f。其次，窦房结可以驱动周围心房肌，这是借助于 I_{Na}、窦房结外周存在的良好电耦联以及两种组织交界区的交错排列来实现这一功能。第三，在不同情况下，窦房结可以通过移动起搏点来继续发挥其起搏功能，这部分是基于离子通道和 Ca^{2+} 运作蛋白表达存在区域性差异来完成的。最后，窦房结为了保护它不受周围心房肌动作电位的影响，很可能通过以下两种机制：一是离子通道以一种特别的方式表达，从而导致窦房结中心的动作电位时程最长；另一机制为窦房结面向房间隔存在一个阻滞区。

（张幼怡　肖晗　龚开政　译）

参 考 文 献

1. Boyett MR, Honjo H, Kodama I: The sinoatrial node, a heterogeneous pacemaker structure. Cardiovasc Res 47:658–687, 2000.
2. Irisawa H, Brown HF, Giles W: Cardiac pacemaking in the sinoatrial node. Physiol Rev 73:197–227, 1993.
3. Sanguinetti MC, Tristani-Firouzi M: Delayed and inward rectifier potassium channels. In Zipes DP, Jalife J (eds): Cardiac Electrophysiology From Cell to Bedside, 3rd ed. Philadelphia, WB Saunders, 2000, pp 79–86.
4. Ono K, Ito H: Role of rapidly activating delayed rectifier K$^+$ current in sinoatrial pacemaker activity. Am J Physiol 269:H453–H462, 1995.
5. Ono K, Shibata S, Iijima T: Properties of the delayed rectifier potassium current in porcine sino-atrial node cells. J Physiol (Lond) 524:51–62, 2000.
6. Lei M, Honjo H, Kodama I, et al: Heterogeneous expression of the delayed-rectifier K$^+$ currents $i_{K,r}$ and $i_{K,s}$ in rabbit sinoatrial node cells. J Physiol (Lond) 535:703–714, 2001.
7. Matsuura H, Ehara T, Ding WG, et al: Rapidly and slowly activating components of delayed rectifier K$^+$ current in guinea-pig sino-atrial node pacemaker cells. J Physiol (Lond) 540:815–830, 2002.
8. Honjo H, Lei M, Boyett MR, et al: Heterogeneity of 4-aminopyridine-sensitive current in rabbit sinoatrial node cells. Am J Physiol 276:H1295–H1304, 1999.
9. Lei M, Honjo H, Kodama I, et al: Characterisation of the transient outward K$^+$ current in rabbit sinoatrial node cells. Cardiovasc Res 46:433–441, 2000.
10. Guo J, Ono K, Noma A: A sustained inward current activated at the diastolic potential range in rabbit sino-atrial node cells. J Physiol (Lond) 483:1–13, 1995.
11. Mitsuiye T, Shinagawa Y, Noma A: Sustained inward current during pacemaker depolarization in mammalian sinoatrial node cells. Circ Res 87:88–91, 2000.
12. Hüser J, Blatter LA, Lipsius SL: Intracellular Ca^{2+} release contributes to automaticity in cat atrial pacemaker cells. J Physiol (Lond) 524:415–422, 2000.
13. Bogdanov KY, Vinogradova TM, Lakatta EG: Sinoatrial nodal cell ryanodine receptor and Na$^+$-Ca^{2+} exchanger: Molecular partners in pacemaker regulation. Circ Res 88:1254–1258, 2001.
14. Vinogradova TM, Bogdanov KY, Lakatta EG: β-Adrenergic stimulation modulates ryanodine receptor Ca^{2+} release during diastolic depolarization to accelerate pacemaker activity in rabbit sinoatrial nodal cells. Circ Res 90:73–79, 2002.
15. Platzer J, Engel J, Schrott-Fischer A, et al: Congenital deafness and sinoatrial node dysfunction in mice lacking class D L-type Ca^{2+} channels. Cell 102:89–97, 2000.
16. Zhang Z, Xu Y, Song H, et al: Functional roles of Ca$_v$1.3 (?$_{1D}$) calcium channel in sinoatrial nodes: Insight gained using gene-targeted null mutant mice. Circ Res 90:981–987, 2002.
17. Kodama I, Honjo H, Boyett MR: Are we lost in the labyrinth of the sinoatrial node pacemaker mechanism? J Cardiovasc Electrophysiol 13:1303–1305, 2002.
18. Wymore RS, Gintant GA, Wymore RT, et al: Tissue and species distribution of mRNA for the I$_{Kr}$-like K$^+$ channel, erg. Circ Res 80:261–268, 1997.
19. Kupershmidt S, Yang T, Anderson ME, et al: Replacement by homologous recombination of the minK gene with lacZ reveals restriction of minK expression to the mouse cardiac conduction system. Circ Res 84:146–152, 1999.
20. DiFrancesco D: Pacemaker mechanisms in cardiac tissue. Annu Rev Physiol 55:455–472, 1993.
21. Honjo H, Boyett MR, Kodama I, et al: Correlation between electrical activity and the size of rabbit sino-atrial node cells. J Physiol (Lond) 496:795–808, 1996.
22. Shi W, Wymore R, Yu H, et al: Distribution and prevalence of hyperpolarization-activated cation channel (HCN) mRNA expression in cardiac tissues. Circ Res 85:e1–e6, 1999.
23. Moroni A, Gorza L, Beltrame M, et al: Hyperpolarization-activated cyclic nucleotide-gated channel 1 is a molecular determinant of the cardiac pacemaker current I_f. J Biol Chem 276:29233–29241, 2001.
24. Ishii TM, Takano M, Xie LH, et al: Molecular characterization of the hyperpolarization-activated cation channel in rabbit heart sinoatrial node. J Biol Chem 274:12835–12839, 1999.
25. Koschak A, Reimer D, Huber I, et al: α1D (Cav1.3) subunits can form L-type Ca^{2+} channels activating at negative voltages. J Biol Chem 276:22100–22106, 2001.
26. Verheijck EE, van Ginneken ACG, Wilders R, et al: Contribution of L-type Ca^{2+} current to electrical activity in sinoatrial nodal myocytes of rabbits. Am J Physiol 276:H1064–H1077, 1999.
27. Hagiwara N, Irisawa H, Kameyama M: Contribution of two types of calcium currents to the pacemaker potentials of rabbit sino-atrial node cells. J Physiol (Lond) 395:233–253, 1988.
28. Bohn G, Moosmang S, Conrad H, et al: Expression of T- and L-type calcium channel mRNA in murine sinoatrial node. FEBS Lett 481:73–76, 2000.
29. Klöckner U, Lee JH, Cribbs LL, et al: Comparison of the Ca^{2+} currents induced by expression of three cloned alpha1 subunits, α1G, α1H and α1I, of low-voltage-activated T-type Ca^{2+} channels. Eur J Neurosci 11:4171–4178, 1999.
30. Lee JH, Gomora JC, Cribbs LL, et al: Nickel block of three cloned T-type calcium channels: Low concentrations selectively block α1H. Biophys J 77:3034–3042, 1999.
31. Kodama I, Nikmaram MR, Boyett MR, et al: Regional differences in the role of the Ca^{2+} and Na$^+$ currents in pacemaker activity in the sinoatrial node. Am J Physiol 272:H2793–H2806, 1997.
32. Baruscotti M, DiFrancesco D, Robinson RB: Na$^+$ current contribution to the diastolic depolarization in newborn rabbit SA node cells. Am J Physiol 279:H2303–H2309, 2000.
33. Mitsuiye T, Guo J, Noma A: Nicardipine-sensitive Na$^+$-mediated single channel currents in guinea-pig sinoatrial node pacemaker cells. J Physiol (Lond) 521:69–79, 1999.
34. Zhang H, Holden AV, Boyett MR: Sustained inward current and pacemaker activity of mammalian sinoatrial node. J Cardiovasc Electrophysiol 13:809–812, 2002.
35. Honjo H, Inada S, Lancaster MK, et al: Sarcoplasmic reticulum Ca^{2+} release is not a dominating factor in sinoatrial node pacemaker activity. Circ Res 92:e41–e44, 2002.
36. Kurata Y, Hisatome I, Imanishi S, et al: Dynamical description of sinoatrial node pacemaking: Improved mathematical model for primary pacemaker cell. Am J Physiol 283:H2074–H2101, 2002.
37. Zhang H, Holden AV, Kodama I, et al: Mathematical models of action potentials in the periphery and center of the rabbit sinoatrial node. Am J Physiol 279:H397–H421, 2000.
38. Zhang H, Holden AV, Boyett MR: Gradient model versus mosaic model of the sinoatrial node. Circulation 103:584–588, 2000.
39. Verheijck EE, Wessels A, van Ginneken ACG, et al: Distribution of atrial and nodal cells within the rabbit sinoatrial node: Models of sinoatrial transition. Circulation 97:1623–1631, 1998.
40. Honjo H, Boyett MR, Coppen SR, et al: Heterogeneous expression of connexins in rabbit sinoatrial node cells: Correlation between connexin isotype and cell size. Cardiovasc Res 53:89–96, 2002.
41. Coppen SR, Kodama I, Boyett MR, et al: Connexin45, a major connexin of the rabbit sinoatrial node, is co-expressed with connexin43 in a restricted zone at the nodal-crista terminalis border. J Histochem Cytochem 47:907–918, 1999.
42. Boyett MR, Dobrzynski H, Lancaster MK, et al: Sophisticated architecture is required for the sinoatrial node to perform its normal pacemaker function. J Cardiovasc Electrophysiol 14:104–106, 2003.
43. Boyett MR, Honjo H, Zhang H et al: The sinoatrial node: Gap junction distribution and impulse propagation. In De Mello WC, Janse MJ (eds): Heart Cell Coupling and Impulse Propagation in Health and Disease. Boston, Kluwer Academic Publishers, 2002, pp 207–234.
44. Saffitz JE, Green KG, Schuessler RB: Structural determinants of slow conduction in the canine sinus node. J Cardiovasc Electrophysiol 8:738–744, 1997.
45. Joyner RW, van Capelle FJL: Propagation through electrically coupled cells: How a small SA node drives a large atrium. Biophys J 50:1157–1164, 1986.

46. ten Velde I, de Jonge B, Verheijck EE, et al: Spatial distribution of connexin43, the major cardiac gap junction protein, visualizes the cellular network for impulse propagation from sinoatrial node to atrium. Circ Res 76:802–811, 1995.
47. Boyett MR, Honjo H, Yamamoto M, et al: Downward gradient in action potential duration along conduction path in and around the sinoatrial node. Am J Physiol 276:H686–H698, 1999.
48. Musa H, Lei M, Honjo H, et al: Heterogeneous expression of Ca^{2+} handling proteins in rabbit sinoatrial node. J Histochem Cytochem 50:311–324, 2002.
49. Alings AM, Bouman LN: Electrophysiology of the ageing rabbit and cat sinoatrial node: A comparative study. Eur Heart J 14:1278–1288, 1993.
50. Papadatos GA, Wallerstein PMR, Head CEG, et al: Slowed conduction and ventricular tachycardia after targeted disruption of the cardiac sodium channel gene *SCN5A*. Proc Natl Acad Sci U S 99:6210–6215, 2002.

第 23 章

房室结的兴奋性及其传导机制

Igor R. Efimov and Vladimir P. Nikolski

本章目录

- 序言 ………………………………… 200
- 房室交界区结构/功能关系的悖论 … 200
- 房室交界区形态和电生理的异质性… 201
- 房室交界区电生理异质性的分子基础… 201
- 成像技术整合解剖学及电生理学的方法 ………………………………… 202
- 房室结折返的荧光成像 …………… 203
- 房室交界区自律性的荧光成像 …… 206
- 房室结的光学相干断层成像 ……… 206
- 房室交界区双路径电生理学的连接蛋白假说 ………………………………… 207
- 结论 ………………………………… 208

一、序 言

Douglas Zips 在他最近一本书的序言中这样描述房室结（atrioventricular node，AV node）的重要性，"房室结是心脏的'灵魂'，对其解剖和电生理学特性的很好理解是打开了解心脏解剖和电活动的钥匙"。这本书向我们提供了对心房-房室结电生理学最新最全面的"新千年的见解"[1]。他总结认为，尽管近一个世纪以来有多如繁星的聪明头脑在心脏电生理方面进行了大量的科学探索，但房室结仍然是"一个谜中之谜"[1]。虽然这本向我们展示了一个世纪以来房室结研究成果的巨著才仅仅出版两年，我们还是希望读者能从本章了解到更新的研究进展：运用最新的成像模式的结果，使房室传导理论变得更加清楚，同时也为我们提供了大量新的见解，值得进一步的研究。这些成像模式包括：（1）运用电压敏感的染料对电活性的快速荧光成像（fast fluorescent imaging）；（2）结构光学相干断层成像（structural optical coherence tomography imaging）；（3）蛋白表达的高分辨率免疫组化成像。

二、房室交界区结构/功能关系的悖论

自从 Tawara[2] 发现房室结以来，就始终让新一代的研究者为之着迷，同时它也是解剖学家和电生理学家们激烈争论的焦点。这些争论主要集中在几个主要的论题，这些论题反映了房室结电生理特性的双重性，即它既是一个冲动"传导器"（conductor）又是一个"振荡器"（oscillator）。这些论题包括：（1）何时房室结开始传导冲动[3]，何时它作为一个振荡器接受来自心房输入的电张力（electrotonic）调节[4]，或机械调节[5]？（2）房室结折返、双路径以及隐性房室传导的解剖和功能的基础是什么[6-8]？

房室交界区高度复杂性给整个20世纪的解剖学界带来了巨大的挑战。科学家们对房室交界区组成的几个主要成分各执己见。Janse 及其同事们[9] 认为"对房室交界区的组织目前缺乏一个共同的命名法则"。争论主要集中在：房室传导轴的解剖起源是由后向前[6]还是由下向上[10]，致密房室结（compact AV node）本身具体的解剖定位和形态定义[10]；是否存在专门的传导束[6,10-13]、纤维或是路径到达房室结；是否存在解剖意义上的 Koch 三角[10,13]；以及是否存在峡部[13]。我们通常已将峡部作为房室结折返消融的

靶点[14]，而且就电生理的观点而言，它确实存在。由于对房室传导部解剖的最基本问题缺乏统一认识，电生理学家在对房室传导进行临床评估以及治疗房室结折返性心动过速时，就不得不在这两种完全不同的"解剖"和"电标测"方法中作出选择[14]。解剖学方法是以慢路径的解剖标志为靶点，如位于冠状窦口和三尖瓣之间的峡部。"电标测"方法是以慢路径上的特异性慢频电位标记为靶点[15,16]。

外科手术和电生理治疗方法可反映房室交界区的一些结构和功能。然而到目前为止，在临床实践中还不能同时采用上述两种方法进行操作，这就导致二者所得到的结论在某种程度上有些不一致。Meijler 和 Janse[4]为此而感叹并精辟地总结道："我们面临的是一个矛盾的状况，即最典型的结性动作电位却没有找到最典型的结细胞与之相关联"。因此，尽管对房室结进行了一个世纪的解剖学、电生理学和临床研究，引用 Zipes 的话，房室结仍然是"一个谜中之谜"。

三、房室交界区形态和电生理的异质性

20 世纪史无前例的技术革新，使得我们对房室传导的电生理特性的了解有了巨大的进步。与临床研究相似，在基础心脏生理实验室也同时存在两种研究方法：解剖学[2]和电生理学[14,17]。曾有人尝试结合两种研究方法，但得到的结果却非常有限[18]。无论是哪种方法，目前都已提供了大量证据证明了房室交界区具有复杂的形态和电生理异质性。

最先描述房室结的是 Tawara[2]，但其解剖定义尚有争论。基于形态学的研究结果，Anderson 和 Ho 坚持认为房室结的范围只是纤维环外的一种结性组织[10]。相反，其他研究人员认为房室结存在一个前封闭后开放的区域[19]，甚至有人认为，如 Billette[20]指出"房室结包含所有参与形成心房-希氏束间期以及与那些具有频率依赖和双径特性相关的所有结构"。我们同意 Billette 的定义，认同他将房室结定义为异质性结构，即由致密房室结以及房室结周围延伸区域组成，还包含 Koch 三角区的组织。

根据 Bharati[13]组织学的观点，房室结分三层：(1) 表层或心内膜下层，(2) 中间层，(3) 最深层。这三层结构与房室结部观察到的三种不同电生理反应相关联。基于微电极记录到的动作电位形态，将房室结分为以下三种截然不同的区域[21,22]：(1) 房结区 (atrionodal, AN)，(2) 真正的结区或紧密结区 (true nodal or compact nodal, N)；(3) 结-希区 (nodo-His, NH)。N 区反应以动作电位超射上升速率相对较慢和幅度小为特征。AN 和 NH 动作电位分别表现为 N 区和心房肌之间 (AN) 以及 N 区和希氏束之间 (NH) 的过渡形态。我们通常相信，在形态上"典型的"结细胞和电生理典型的结细胞 (N cells) 之间存在关联。然而，仍然没有令人信服的证据证明这种相关性。Billette[23]更进一步地向我们展示了房室结最全面的微电极记录，从而根据动作电位的形态、兴奋性和不应期将房室结分为 6 种不同的细胞类型。更重要的是，Billette 的资料向我们提供了令人信服的证据，表明几乎遍及整个 Koch 三角都存在各种不同电生理特性的细胞类型，这就再次强调了整个房室交界区，已远远超出了单纯的 N 区，在其结构-功能的完整性上具有不可分割性。近来形态学[6]和电生理学[12,24]证据表明了结后延伸部的存在，这一部位在一些情况下可以达到冠状窦以及甚至可以与界嵴直接相连，这些证据还可以解释在离紧密房室结较远的位置上仍存在结细胞和过渡细胞。然而，对房室结单纯的形态学分析并不能解释房室结复杂的电生理活动。近来在分子生物学和细胞生物学研究方面取得的进展，为我们提供了一些深刻的了解，将用于解释正常和病理状态下的房室传导。

四、房室交界区电生理异质性的分子基础

房室结是数字化心脏病学的"灰姑娘"，它是心脏一种主要的细胞类型或主要结构，但是到目前为止，房室结的特征还不能在一个精确数字模型的框架中被确定。相比之下，窦房结在这方面显得更为幸运，目前对窦房结已建立了大量数字化模型[25]。一些尝试以数字化的方式解释房室传导的研究都是基于对已有的窦房结模型进行经验性的修改。有分子生物学数据提示，房室结的电生理异质性是由离子通道和缝隙连接表达的异质性造成的[19]。

（一）钠通道

Petrecca 及其同事们[26]提供了有力的证据表明，在致密房室结区和分离的卵圆形细胞（此种细胞表现出 N 型电生理反应）中钠离子通道表达水平较低，而

且缺乏显著的 I_{Na} 离子流。I_{Na} 的缺乏解释了为什么结细胞动作电位的上升支上升缓慢且对河豚毒素有抵抗的特性。另外，他们还提出证据表明，缺乏 I_{Na} 的细胞也缺乏瞬时外向离子流（I_{to}），但具有显著的奇特离子流（I_F），这与记录到的 N 细胞具有起搏能力是一致的[28]。另一方面，AN 和 NH 型的过渡细胞有更丰富的 I_{Na} 表达[19,26]，这解释了这些细胞具有快速的超射速率和传导速度。

（二）钙通道

钙通道在房室结的传导中起着重要作用[27,29]，在缺乏钠通道的情况下它可能负责冲动传导。L 型和 T 型钙通道、$I_{Ca,L}$ 和 $I_{Ca,L}$ 都可在房室结见到[31]。这些通道的药理学特性已经被详细地描述。然而，到目前为止还没有钙离子通道表达的立体成像。这样的数据是非常重要的，众所周知，房室结的特性是钙离子依赖的，所以钙通道表达的异质性很可能有助于阐明房室结结构/功能之间的联系。

（三）钾通道

钾通道在房室结上的表达也显得很不均一。瞬时外向离子流 I_{to} 与 I_{Na} 类似，主要表达于房室结的过渡层，而在 N 区表达却很少[30]。Noma 及其同事们[29]进行了一个经典的研究，表明延迟整流离子流 I_K 是房室结主要的去极化离子流。近来的研究表明，快速组分 I_{Kr} 即使不是延迟整流钾离子流唯一的，也是占主导地位的成分[32,33]。与窦房结不同的是，很少有证据表明在房室结里存在慢速组分，I_{Ks}[33]。内向整流钾通道的作用目前仍不清楚。有资料提示 I_{K1} 通道在维持心房和心室细胞静息电位中起着重要作用。然而，I_{K1} 通道在房室结中几乎是缺失的[19]。另一方面，大量对房室结进行迷走干预的实验资料提示，$I_{K,Ach}$ 可能具有一定的作用。而 Noma 及其同事[29]以及其他研究者证实了起搏"奇特"离子流 I_F 的存在及其重要作用。

（四）缝隙连接通道

缝隙连接通道在房室传导中具有重要的作用。在哺乳动物心脏可检测到的缝隙连接蛋白主要有三种异构体（isoforms）：连接蛋白 43（connexin43, Cx43）、Cx40 和 Cx45，它们存在的特定区域已被标记出来。目前已有资料提示，这三种异构体都在 Koch 三角中有表达，而且在房室传导中发挥着重要作用。在致密房室结（N 区）中，Cx43[26,36,37] 表达水平很低。Cx43 负责几乎所有心肌细胞与细胞之间的联系，尤其是心房和心室肌。另一方面，房室结的过渡层，包括 AN 和 NH 区，有较高水平的 Cx43 表达。我们的资料提示，Cx43 表达的空间异质性可能与房室结的双路径电生理特性、细胞-细胞联系通路的形成有关，从而形成了慢快两种传导通路[38]。也有报道发现另外两种连接蛋白亚型在致密房室结（Cx45）和 NH 区（Cx40 和 Cx45）传导中起作用[37]。

五、成像技术整合解剖学及电生理学的方法

迄今为止，研究房室结结构/功能关系的最大障碍是不能同时评价离子通道异质性的表达、形态结构和三维空间的电生理反应。组织学和免疫组化的结果很难和只用有限数量电极得到的电生理结果相比对。近来，随着电压敏感染料荧光成像技术（Fluorescent imaging with voltage-sensitive dyes）的应用，为房室传导研究[39]搭建了一座解剖与电生理之间的桥梁[24,40-42]。

在过去十年里，使用电压敏感染料荧光成像技术给心脏电生理的研究带来了一场革命[43]。这一技术可以获得各种空间尺度（从亚细胞的亚结构到整个心脏）的跨膜电压的高分辨率成像[43]。在最初运用荧光成像对房室传导进行研究时，我们发现在正常窦性心律时，房室结远端区域收集到的光学信号包含两种不同的成分，我们推测这可能与解剖学家所描述的房室结的两种不同层组织的激活相对应[2,6,10,13]。我们后来的研究为这一假说提供了一些证据[40]。同时使用微电极和光学记录的方法，我们发现荧光成像记录到的两种光学信号成分确实与微电极在不同层（表层和中间层）记录到的跨膜电压动作电相位一致[13]。这两层有着截然不同的形态和电生理特性。表层由过渡 AN 细胞组成，这些细胞表达钠通道和 Cx43，而中间的紧密房室结层不表达钠通道，而且细胞间的耦联依赖于低电导的 Cx45。结果，这两层有着完全不同的动作电位形态，恰好分别与 AN 和 N 区相对应。这两层在传导速率上也有很大区别，分别是 30~70 cm/s 和 2~10 cm/s。

目前正在致力发展能根据荧光信号对电活动进行精确的三维解剖图像重建技术。在不久的将来可能可以提供快速发展的散漫光断层成像（diffusive optical tomography，DOT）[44]和光学相干断层成像（optical coherence tomography，OCT）[45]等方法（讨论见后）。同时，我们的房室结实验也对荧光技术对组织的探测深度有了新的评价。此前其他一些研究组的结果提示，光学信号能提供组织表面以下100～500μm的信息。我们对拥有不同层的房室结的研究表明，这种荧光技术探测深度可达到1～2 mm[39-42]。这种多相光学信号形态可以很容易用具有高度异质层的房室结近端电活动的"纵向分离"（longitudinal dissociation）现象来解释，该现象是由Mines首先报道的[46]。

图23-1描绘的是具有纵向分离-双向信号形态特征性标志的一个例子，这些光学信号是在兔房室结逆向传导时记录到的[24]。实验中给希氏束一个单独提前H1H2起搏刺激，希氏束距离观察视野（6×6 mm）右边界仅几微米。图23-1A向我们描述了整个准备过程和观察视野。在房室传导束上选择了四个记录位点。来自这些位点的信号见图23-1B。位点1是房室结的后/下位，位点2～4是在致密房室结区域。图23-1B描绘了按照基本刺激顺序的以300ms为间隔的基本起搏H1A1，以及配对间期为100ms的早搏刺激H2A2。希氏束和界嵴的电描记图也在图中表示。来自四个位点的光学印记是相互重叠的。除了位点1，所有的印记都包含了在基本起搏和早搏时记录到的双成分动作电位，这表明了纵向分离的存在。两种成分之间的延迟在早搏传导时较基本起搏传导时有所增加，这提示房室结不同层具有不同的频率依赖性。图23-1C表示的是这些数据的可能解释。该图是房室结传导轴上的垂直剖面图，它与图23-1A描述的4个选择记录位点的位置相连。每个光电二极管记录两层（房室结和过渡区域）或一层（过渡区域）组织的平均电活性。结果，2号和4号位点的记录包括了紧密房室结（白色结构）激活的第一成分以及过渡细胞表面AN层（灰色结构）激活的第二成分。黑色结构代表的是分隔心房和远端房室结及希氏束的连接组织。所有对兔的房室传导的前传和逆传的研究都记录了这样一个多相信号形态图。

我们利用灌流电压敏感染料的缓慢扩散估计了两种成分起源的深度[24]。在这个研究中，使用1μM的di-4-ANEPPS，这个浓度是之前使用浓度的1/10～1/20[39]。在最初的5～10 min，仅有组织表层被染色，因为染料是缓慢扩散进入更深层组织。结果，在染色开始时，仅有第二（较晚）成分的光学反应被观察到。在逆向传导过程中，这一成分代表房室结的AN表层的激活。更深层房室组织（第一或较早成分）的激活仅在染色20 min后才可分辩。在40 min时停止给予染料，然后开始冲洗。第一成分的幅度仍然继续增加，这是因为从表层到深层的染料还在继续扩散。同时，第二和第一峰的差别开始下降，反映了染料从表层被清洗掉[24]。结果，灌流染料的扩散方向与形成双成分光学信号两层的解剖定相位一致。

六、房室结折返的荧光成像

首先对房室结折返进行清楚而巧妙描述的是Mines[46]，他描述了折返发生前的纵向分离以及由此导致了折返的发生。半个多世纪以后，Coumel及其同事们[47]以及Janse及其同事们[48]分别在人和兔中记录并证实了折返是由早搏刺激引起的。Janse等用10个微电极观察到了兔房室结折返期间的电位。31年后的今天，尽管有过很多努力，但仍然没有人能够重复Janse[48]这项极其困难的研究，也没人能重复其结果，进行房室结折返时的跨膜电位的描绘。微电极记录到

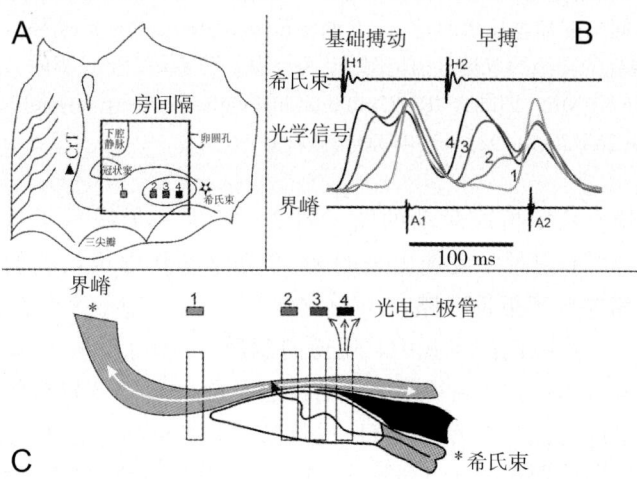

图23-1 逆向传导时的光学信号图像 A：标本上4个记录位点的定位图。B：分别于基础搏动（H1H1=300 ms）和早搏（起始于希氏束，H1H2=100 ms）时记录到的光学信号与电学图。图上的数字分别对应相应的记录位点（如A图和C图所示）。C：沿着房室传导轴和结后延伸部的Koch三角横切面（详见正文）（引自Nikolski V, Efimov I: Fluorescent imaging of a dual-pathway atrioventricular-nodal conduction system. *Circ Res* 2001；88：E23-30.）

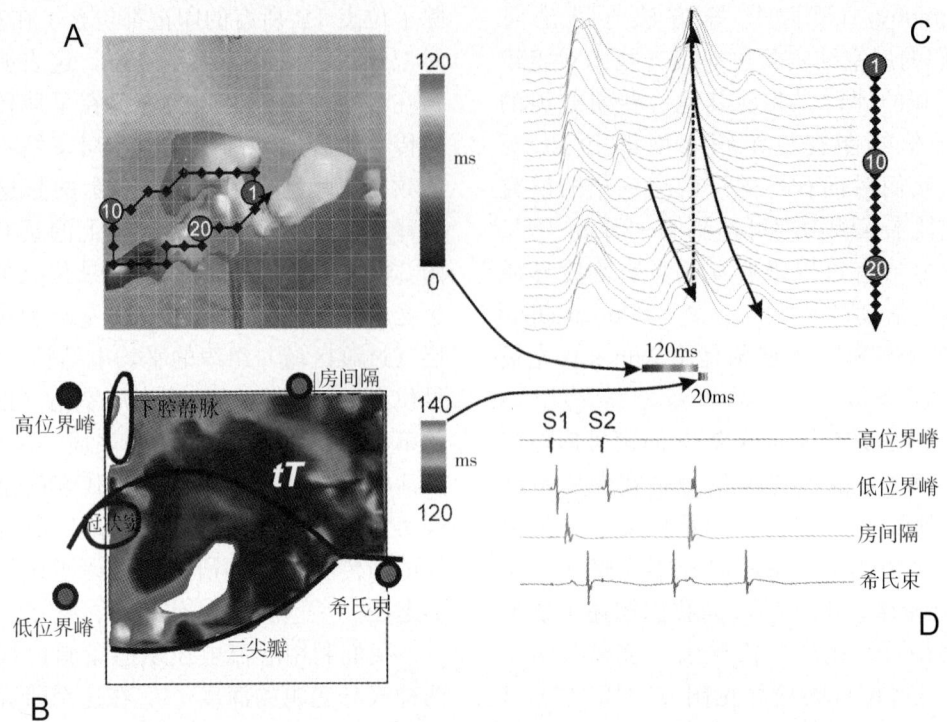

图 23-2　来自界嵴的早搏刺激引起的典型（慢-快）房室结折返　A：单个早搏冲动引起的折返时的传导彩图。它只显示了折返的前 120 ms，描绘了结后延伸部，致密房室结，以及快路径的激活。该图是与标本图像重叠在一起的（见图 B 相应标志）。蓝色菱形指示的位点，其相应光学记录见图 C。B：折返传导的延续部分：过渡区房结层 20 ms 的激活。该区的显微图像亦在图中显示出来。我们可以发现 A、B 两图的激活时间有明显差别。C：折返通路上的动作电位光学记录：实线箭头指示的是慢路径和快路径的传导。虚线箭头指示的是表面过渡层的快传导。下方的时间尺度标志显示的是 A、B 两幅传导图中相应的时间间隔。D：于最后一次基本刺激（S1），早搏刺激（S2）和折返搏动时记录到的传统的双极电描记图。记录了从高位界嵴、低位界嵴、房间隔到希氏束（引自 Nikolski VI, Jones SA, Lancaster MK, Boyett MR, Efimov IR: Cx43 and dual-pathway electrophysiology of the atrioventricular node and atrioventricular nodal reentry. *Cir Res* 2003；92：469-475.）（见彩图 4）

目前为止仍然是细胞电生理的金标准，但也为对心脏进行具有空间分辨率的电学标测带来了巨大挑战。

现在，我们能够通过对房室结动作电位的荧光标测技术来显示出详细的房室结折返图。图 23-2 是一幅描绘所谓的"典型"房室结折返（慢/快折返）的图，该图反映了这样一个事实，即折返激动前传是通过慢路径，而逆传则是通过快路径。与多位点微电极记录不同，此项工作只抓住几个位点，光学技术能给我们提供整个房室结折返时的数以百计的记录[23,48]。图 23-2A 是一幅冲动经慢、快路径传导的彩色图，传导时间为 120 ms。下面一幅图是反映表层 AN 的快速激活（图 23-2B），在该层传导同样的距离仅需 20 ms，因此会将激动从快路径传回到慢路径，使激动重新经慢路径传导，从而可形成环路。据我们所知，这幅图是第一幅完整的反映典型（慢/

快）房室折返激动的图。图 23-2C 进一步展示了从 256 个记录中挑选出来的 24 个光学动作电位，它们都选自于折返环路。

在我们的实验中，用逆向刺激（retrograde stimulation）方法获得了类似的折返记录。图 23-3 描绘的是由希氏束起搏（H1H1 的周长为 300 ms）产生稳定逆向传导的模式（见图 23-A1），以及折返或回波搏动（echobeat）和早搏刺激（H1H2=160ms）产生的稳定逆向传导的模式。本图是用三维堆积条图（Stackplot）A1-B1-C1-D1（左）和同时记录的电描记图 A2-B2-C2-D2（右）来显示折返。

在基础搏动时（图 23-3 A1 和 23-3 A2），冲动从希氏束进入房室结，接着分成两个小波。一个向右，向 Todaro 腱（快通路出口）的方向传导；另一个向左，沿着房室结后延伸。经快路径传导，到达 AN 层突破点较早，从而快速激活心房的慢路径，因此消

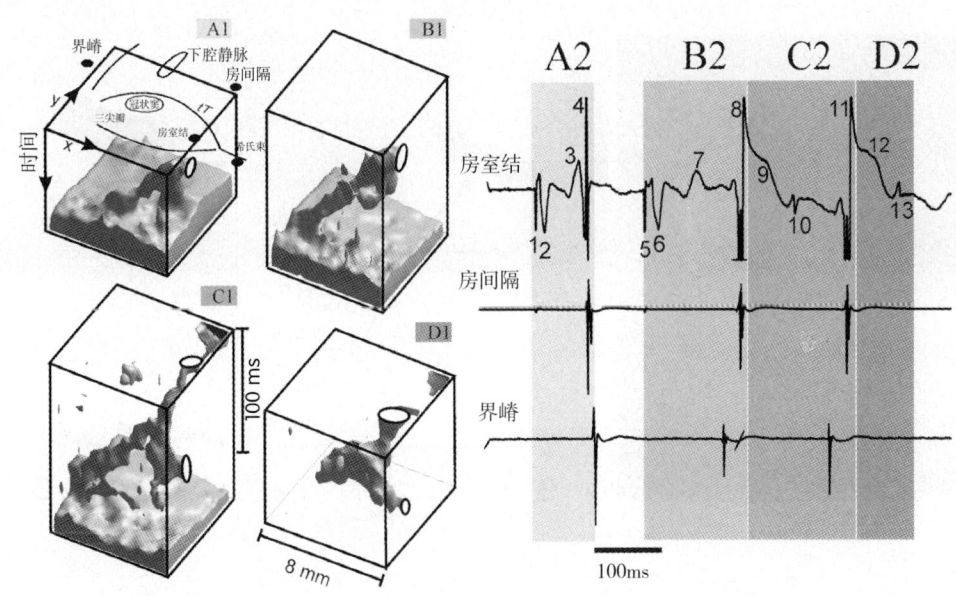

图 23-3 非典型（快-慢）的房室结折返：堆积条图（Stack-plot）和电描记图 左：经过房室结双径传导的空间-时间图。数据来自于包括 Koch 三角的标本（如图 23-5A 所示）。该图记录了 4 个后续的搏动，其相应的电描记图见右侧图。左侧图表中不同的高度反映的是分析时间的不同时程。将连续记到的荧光信号的时间倒数（dF/dt）二维图整合在一起，建立了三维图像[24]。然后，不同表面用密度阈值来表示，为了保证沿通路传导的连续性，该密度阈值是经过时间校正的。白色椭圆形表示的是三维图的入口和出口。A1，基础搏动时的快路径（右分支）逆向传导。B1，早搏（代偿间歇为 160ms）时的慢路径（左分支）逆向传导。C1，快-慢房室结折返搏动，包括经由快路径前传和经由慢路径的逆传。D1，折返自我终止时的快路径前传和减弱的慢路径逆传。右：记录基本逆向传导和房室结折返的双极电描记图。记录位点如图 23-2A1 所示。电信号记录的时间间隔 A2-B2-C2-D2 与堆积条图的时间间隔 A1-B1-C1-D1 相对应。最上一条信号是 Koch 三角顶端的双极电描记图。记录了以下几种反应：A2，基础搏动。房室结的电描记图的几个标记分别为（1）希氏束激活/刺激伪象，（2）房室结激活，（3）快路径开始的标志，它紧随并被（4）房结过渡层的反应所掩盖。我们注意到在下方的房间隔和界嵴的电描记图先后有两个激动信号（房间隔在前，界嵴在后），这可能是由于快路径的突破所造成的。B2，早搏。此时房室结电描记图记录的几个标记为（5）希氏束刺激伪象，（6）房室结激活，（7）快要消失的快路径，（8）心房过渡层的反应。我们可以注意到在界嵴和房间隔电描记图中，激动信号的顺序发生了逆转（即界嵴在前，房间隔在后），这个可能是因为突破位点从快路径转到慢路径。C2，房室结折返搏动。房室结电描记图记录的几个标记为（9）快路径和房室结，（10）希氏束激活，（11）房结过渡层。界嵴-房间隔激动信号顺序未变（同早搏）。D2，慢路径内房室结折返的终止。房室结电描记图记录的标记为（12）快路径和房室结，（13）希氏束。我们可以看到此时没有界嵴和房间隔的激动信号（引自 Nikolski V, Effmov I: Fluorescent imaging of a dual-pathway atrioventricular-nodal conduction system. *Cir Res* 2001；88：E23-E30.）

除了慢路径的逆向冲动。

在早搏配对间期为 160ms 时（见图 23-3B1、B2），快路径仍处于不应期，结果传导只通过慢路径，然后快速激活心房。双极电描记图记录到的快路径电位幅度在早搏时较基本搏动时小，这一现象支持了递减传导的概念，递减传导产生减弱的不充分的驱动力，如在传导衰竭（conduction failure）中见到的一样，从而激活 AN 层细胞。

在冲动沿着慢路径缓慢传导时，之前阻滞的快通路又能充分恢复。因此，在从慢路径出口出来并激活了整个心房表面 AN 层，兴奋再次通过快路径进入房室结（见图 23-3 C1 上平面的白椭圆形）。然后兴奋分成两个小波。一个小波向右传导，通过致密房室结然后离开视野场向希氏束方向传导（见图 23-3 C1 的另一白椭圆）。希氏束激活的光学信号与图 23-3 中电描记图 C2 的第 10 个搏动同时发生。与此同时，另一小波向左传导，经慢路径逆向扩散，再次到达慢路径在冠状窦下峡部的突破点。接下来，心房快速激动，激

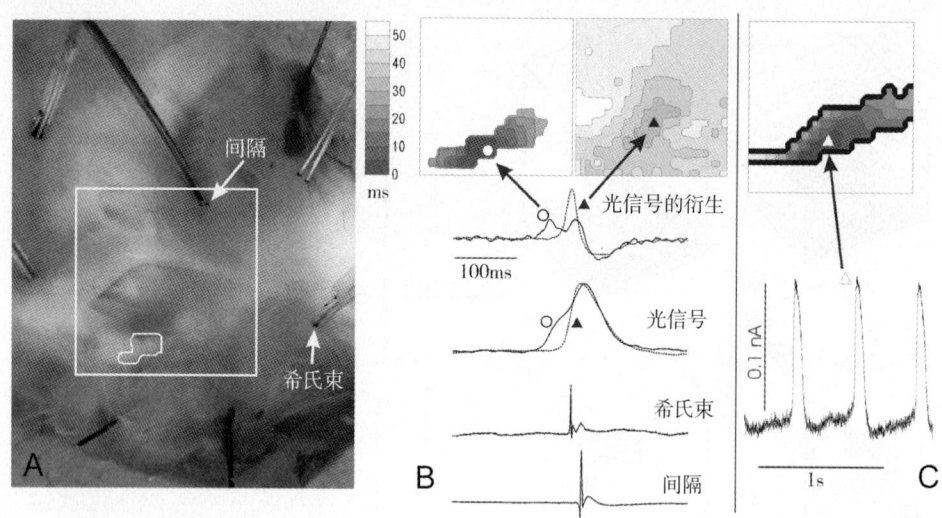

图 23-4 房室结的自律性 A：标本图像。白色四方形内的是光学成像系统的视野范围。白色曲线圈内的部位是交界性心律时的最早激动部位。B：房室结较深细胞层的激动标测图，以及从较深层突破之后，结后延伸部（左图）和表面房室层（右图）的激动图像。本图描绘的是起搏部位（白圆圈）和表层突破点（黑三角）的光学信号及其最初衍生信号，另外还有希氏束和房间隔的双极电记录。相对应的记录位点见图 A 箭头所指处。C：具有逆向传导阻滞的标本在房室交界区自发性节律时的激动图像。只有较深层的细胞层被激动。记录曲线描绘的是起搏位点（白色三角）处未过滤的光学信号

动再次前传到快路径（图 23-3 D1 顶部的白椭圆）并且分成两个小波。再一次，一个波穿过了房室结并激动了朝向希氏束方向的视野（图 23-3 D1 的另一个椭圆），后者与图 23-3D2 中的第 13 个搏动同时发生。另一波折返回慢路径然后很快消失。因此，折返是自限性的。不像人的心脏，兔的心脏很少出现持续的房室结折返引起的心动过速。通常而言，当折返被诱发，无论是逆传还是前传早搏刺激的，我们都只能观察到单个折返搏动。

七、房室交界区自律性的荧光成像

自从首次发现房室结具有自律性以来，很多研究者就在寻找主要起搏位点。他们发现冲动形成的位点是在致密房室结[28]或在 NH 区[49]。荧光成像给我们一个独特的机会来定位心跳起源的位点。我们的数据表明这样的位点不仅在致密房室结或 NH 区能发现，在房室结后延伸区也有发现。

图 23-4 描绘的是：将窦房结手术去除后，房室结具有自发起搏活性时，房室结区的光学图。在图 23-4 A 和 23-4 B 显示的标本中，房室结驱动心房和希氏束。如图 23-4 A 所示，冲动起源于冠状窦下的峡部。然后缓慢地沿着结后延伸区向两个方向传导，直到冲动到达 Koch 三角中间的突破点，接下来心房快速激动（如图 24 B 右图）。利用光学标记示踪及其衍生技术在图 23-4 B 中向我们列出了在起源位点（圆形和实心的标记）和突破位点（三角和斜线的标记）记录到的光学动作电位。我们可以看到最早兴奋的解剖位置是在房室结后束的延伸区。在一些标本中，我们将房室结和心房完全分离，持续观察了房室结的电活动 3~4 h。图 23-4 C 描绘的就是这种电活动。尽管心房和房室结间的联系已经完全切断，房室结后延伸区仍可继续保持强有力的起搏活动，这种起搏通过房室结延伸区、致密房室结安全地传导，最后到达希氏束。然而，我们并没有观察到向心房的传导。下面的光学标记，清楚地展示了舒张期去极化和结样动作电位。我们仅能在这种房室结和心房分离的标本中观察到清楚的房室结电位，否则因为来自表面房室结的光学动作电位将会掩盖大部分的结性动作电位。

八、房室结的光学相干断层成像

尽管用电压敏感的染料进行荧光成像取得了令人瞩目的成功，但是这项技术在认识心脏组织的三维结

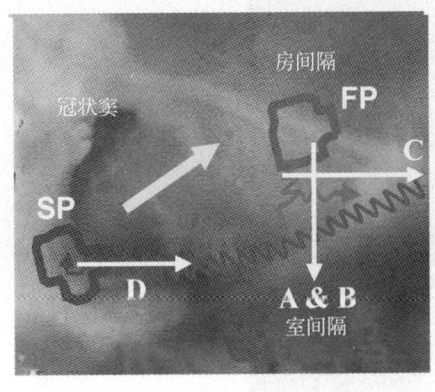
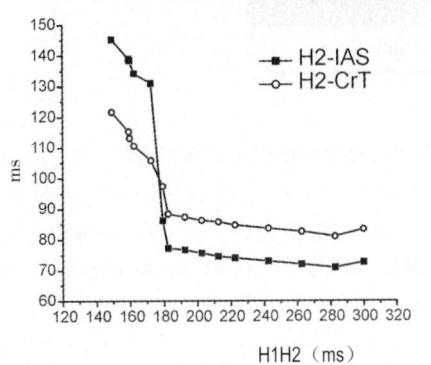
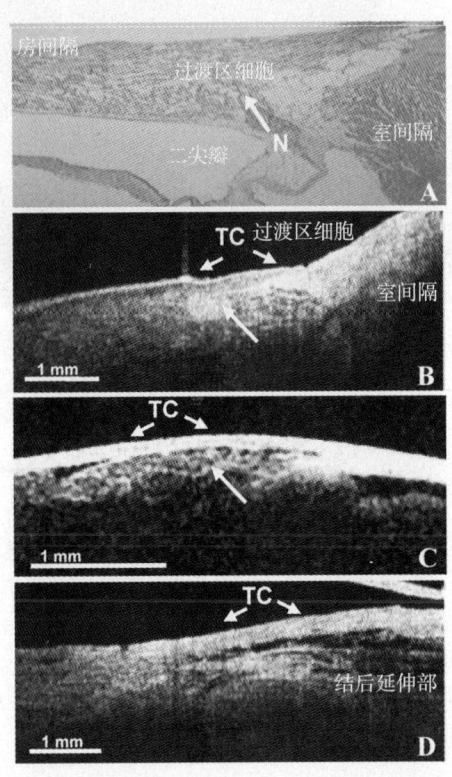

图 23-5 光学相干断层（Optical Coherence Tomography，OCT）成像显示了在早搏刺激下（具有不同代偿间歇，表现在传导曲线上是呈"跳跃性"的改变），突破点发生转移的双路径传导　左上图：标本图像以及对应于慢（SP）快（FP）径传导的不同代偿间歇时的突破位点图像。双路径是由荧光成像来确定的[24]。左下图：由希氏束产生逆向刺激时的传导曲线，表现了早搏刺激 H2 和房间隔（IAS）及界嵴区（CrT）的激动（双极电极记录）之间存在延迟。我们注意到传导曲线中存在明显的跳跃，尤其是黑色曲线，它反映的是希氏-隔传导延迟。这种传导曲线中的跳跃，反映了从快路径到慢路径突破位点的转移[24]。右图：沿着左图所示标本的纵切面图，包括从上到下组织的组织学（彩色）和 OCT（灰色）图像（引自 Gupta M, Rolins AM, Izatt JA, Efimov IR: Imaging of the atrioventricular node using optical coherence tomography. *J Cardiovasc Electrophysiol* 2002；13：95.）（见彩图 5）

构方面仍然有局限性。我们的数据能够清晰地显示来自组织更深层的光学信号，但是我们还不能对这些产生特殊光学动作电位各层进行精确的解剖定位，也还不能在三维空间重建电活动。近来我们介绍了一种新的光学成像模型，OCT，它可能为我们提供所需要的三维图像。图 23-5 展示的是首次尝试用 OCT 对房室结区进行形态的三维重建。如右图所示，OCT 图像能够让我们清楚地看到房室交界区深达 1 mm 或更多的不同解剖结构。OCT 的优势在于，这项技术可以使得临床电生理实验室能够使用经导管 OCT 成像技术。例如可开发一种携带 OCT 图像仪的导管进行射频消融。这种导管将可以让我们精确定位慢路径的解剖位置（见图 23-5D），并且安全地消融靶点。到目前为止，OCT 技术只能用于那些未使用过任何染料和对比剂的组织进行结构的三维成像。因此，到目前为止，使用这项技术描绘跨膜电压或其他电生理参数还暂时不可行。然而，可吸收染料目前正在研究中，我们希望具有功能三维成像的 OCT 能够在五年内用于房室结和慢路径的血管内标测。

九、房室交界区双路径电生理学的连接蛋白假说

免疫组织化学研究结果提供了大量信息，使我们对房室传导和结合部的节律形成了一种认识，即各种蛋白的表达（包括离子通道、受体、缝隙连接、信号分子等）都具有高度异质性。特别是我们最近证实了功能性折返通路存在分叉的分子基础[24,38]。

我们用免疫标记的方法标记 Cx43，发现 Cx43 阳性的束支分布是从冠状窦到房室结，周围是 Cx43 阴

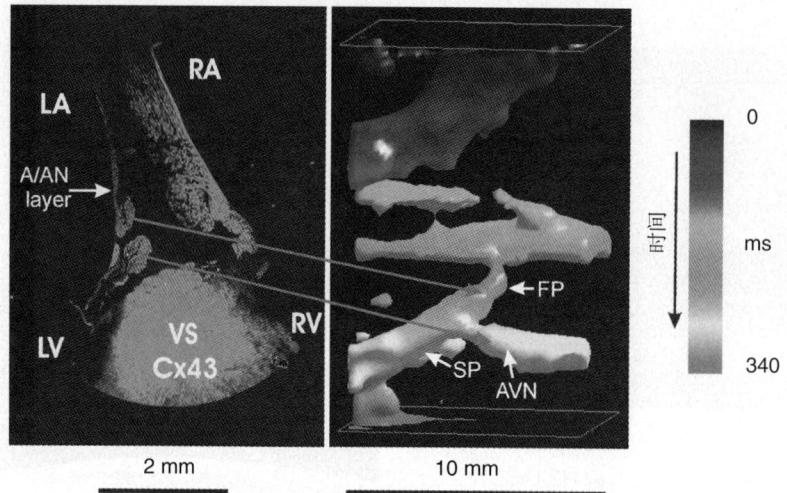

图 23-6 与 Cx43 免疫标记相对应的、在 Koch 三角于早搏刺激和折返时的光学电位衍生的堆积条图　右图是房室结区在早搏刺激和折返时传导的三维空间时相图（光学电位信号首次衍生的堆积条图也显示出来）。左图的组织切片图显示 Cx43 标记阳性的束支对应于光学标测的激动路径。详见正文 AV：房室；RA and LA：右房和左房；RV and LV：右室和左室；SP and FP：慢快通路束支；VS：室间隔（引自 Nikolski VP, Jones SA, Lancaster MK, et al：Cx43 and the dual-pathway electrophysiology of the atrioventricular node and atrioventricular nodal reentry. *Cir Res* 2003；92：469-475.）

性组织。这一结果与荧光数据结合起来，提示这些 Cx43 阳性的束支是双路径和折返的基础。在一些标本中，观察到 Koch 三角中部慢路径也存在分叉（见图 23-2 和 23-3）。免疫标记的方法发现这种功能定义的分叉传导通路与分叉的 Cx43 阳性的束支相关。图 23-6 是用堆积条图展示了这种分叉传导通路，呈现了早搏和折返搏动时房室结区的折返通路。对 Cx43 进行免疫标记（见图 23-6，左图），Cx43 阳性的束支在空间上与光学信号显示的激动通路相关，图中相对应的是快路径（上）束支和慢路径（下）束支。

这些房室结资料与以前在窦房结观察到的 Cx43 阳性的束支一致[51,53]，较早的研究提示这些束支可加强来自小窦房结区传导的安全性，有助于大心房对抗不合宜的电源-电流接收器（source-sink）的关系（关于电源-电流接收器方面的内容请参阅第 25 章，译者注）。对连接蛋白异构体的进一步研究旨在明确它们在房室交界区传导和起搏活动中的作用。

十、结　论

荧光成像使我们能真实地看到房室结折返的整个通路和结性节律时起搏点的位置，在这方面取得了令人瞩目的成功，同时通过前传和逆传双路径传导的激动也证明了这一新成像技术的巨大应用价值。仅仅在几年时间里对房室结研究所取得的进展[39-42]被进一步开发出大量新的方法，包括 OCT 和 DOT。我们相信这些电压敏感成像方法新的衍生技术将使我们能够真实地看到房室交界区电活动以及心脏其他组织的实时三维成像。这种新的方法使得我们能够重建房室结内各种传导模式的完整三维波形。

与此同时，免疫组化的快速发展使得我们不断发现很多令人瞩目的机制，如心房心室在正常和病理状态下传导的各种分子机制。要想更深入了解房室结复杂的异质性三维结构，可能还需要产生一个理论基础来发展房室结数学模型。在不久的将来，这样一个模型将会用于探索房室结结构及功能的关系。我们相信这是谜中最主要的一部分，而这个谜正是由参加国际研究项目"真实心脏"的心脏电生理学家提出的。

（张幼怡　徐宁　龚开政　译）

参　考　文　献

1. Mazgalev TN, Tchou PJ (eds): Atrial-AV Nodal Electrophysiology: A View from the Millenium. Armonk, NY, Futura, 2000.
2. Tawara S: Das Reizleitungssystem des Saugetierherzens: Eine Anatomische-Histologische Studie Uber Das Atrioventrikularbundel Und Die Purkinjeschen Faden. Jena, Verlag von Gustav Fischer, 1906.
3. Lewis T, Master AM: Observations upon conduction in the mammalian heart: AV conduction. Heart 12:209–269, 1925.

4. Meijler FL, Janse MJ: Morphology and electrophysiology of the mammalian atrioventricular node. Physiol Rev 68:608–647, 1988.
5. Scherf D, Cohen J: The Atrioventricular Node and Selected Cardiac Arrhythmias. New York, Grune and Stratton, 1964.
6. Noue S, Becker AE: Posterior extensions of the human compact atrioventricular node: A neglected anatomic feature of potential clinical significance. Circulation 97:188–193, 1998.
7. Moe GK, Preston JB, Burlington H: Physiologic evidence for a dual A-V transmission system. Circ Res 4:357–375, 1956.
8. Langendorf R: Concealed A-V conduction: The effect of blocked impulses on the formation and conduction of subsequent impulse. Am Heart J 35:542–552, 1948.
9. Janse MJ, Loh P, de Bakker JM: Is the Atrium Involved in AV Nodal Reentry. In Mazgalev TN, Tchou PJ (eds): Atrial-AV Nodal Electrophysiology: A View from the Millenium. Armonk, NY, Futura, 2000.
10. Anderson RH, Ho SY: The Atrial Connection of the Specialized Axis Responsible for AV Conduction. In Mazgalev TN, Tchou PJ (eds): Atrial-AV Nodal Electrophysiology: A View from the Millenium. Armonk, NY, Futura, 2000.
11. Racker DK: Atrioventricular node and input pathways: A correlated gross anatomical and histological study of the canine atrioventricular junctional region. Anat Rec 224:336–354, 1989.
12. Medkour D, Becker AE, Khalife K, Billette J: Anatomic and functional characteristics of a slow posterior AV nodal pathway: Role in dual-pathway physiology and reentry. Circulation 98:164–174, 1998.
13. Bharati, S: Anatomic-Morphologic Relations Between AV Nodal Structure and Function in the Normal and Diseased Heart. In Mazgalev TN, Tchou PJ (eds): Atrial-AV Nodal Electrophysiology: A View from the Millenium. Armonk, NY, Futura, 2000.
14. Shah D, Haissaguerre M, Gaita F: Slow pathway ablation for atrioventricular nodal reentry. J Cardiovasc Electrophysiol 13:1054–1055, 2002.
15. Haissaguerre M, Gaita F, Fischer B, et al: Elimination of atrioventricular nodal reentrant tachycardia using discrete slow potentials to guide application of radiofrequency energy. Circulation 85:2162–2175, 1992.
16. Jackman WM, Beckman KJ, McClelland JH, et al: Treatment of supraventricular tachycardia due to atrioventricular nodal reentry, by radiofrequency catheter ablation of slow-pathway conduction. N Engl J Med 327:313–318, 1992.
17. Watanabe Y, Dreifus LS: Inhomogeneous conduction in the A-V node: A model for re-entry. Am Heart J 70:505–514, 1965.
18. Anderson RH, Janse MJ, van Capelle FJ, et al: A combined morphological and electrophysiological study of the atrioventricular node of the rabbit heart. Circ Res 35:909–922, 1974.
19. Petrecca K, Shrier A: Spatial Distribution of Ion Channels, Receptors, and Innervation in the AV node. In Mazgalev TN, Tchou PJ (eds): Atrial-AV Nodal Electrophysiology: A View from the Millennium. Armonk, NY, Futura, 2000.
20. Billette J: What is the atrioventricular node? Some clues in sorting out its structure-function relationship. J Cardiovasc Electrophysiol 13:515–518, 2002.
21. Hoffman BF, Paes de Carvalho A, de Mello WC: Transmembrane potentials of single fibers of the atrio-ventricular node. Nature 181:66–67, 1958.
22. Paes de Carvalho A, de Almeida DF: Spread of activity through the atrioventricular node. Circ Res 8:801–809, 1960.
23. Billette J: Atrioventricular nodal activation during periodic premature stimulation of the atrium. Am J Physiol 252:H163–H177, 1987.
24. Nikolski V, Efimov I: Fluorescent imaging of a dual-pathway atrioventricular-nodal conduction system. Circ Res 88:E23–E30, 2001.
25. Demir SS, Clark JW, Giles WR: Parasympathetic modulation of sinoatrial node pacemaker activity in rabbit heart: A unifying model. Am J Physiol 276:H2221–H2244, 1999.
26. Petrecca K, Amellal F, Laird DW, et al: Sodium channel distribution within the rabbit atrioventricular node as analysed by confocal microscopy. J Physiol 501:263–274, 1997.
27. Zipes DP, Mendez C: Action of manganese ions and tetrodotoxin on atrioventricular nodal transmembrane potentials in isolated rabbit hearts. Circ Res 32:447–454, 1973.
28. Paes de Carvalho A, de Mello WC, Hoffman BF (eds): The Specialized Tissues of the Heart. Amsterdam, Elsevier, 1961.
29. Noma A, Irisawa H, Kokobun S, et al: Slow current systems in the a-v node of the rabbit heart. Nature 285:228–229, 1980.
30. Munk AA, Adjemian RA, Zhao J, et al: Electrophysiological properties of morphologically distinct cells isolated from the rabbit atrioventricular node. J Physiol 493:801–818, 1996.
31. Liu Y, Zeng W, Delmar M, Jalife J: Ionic mechanisms of electronic inhibition and concealed conduction in rabbit atrioventricular nodal myocytes. Circulation 88:1634–1646, 1993.
32. Howarth FC, Levi AJ, Hancox JC: Characteristics of the delayed rectifier K current compared in myocytes isolated from the atrioventricular node and ventricle of the rabbit heart. Pflugers Arch 431:713–722, 1996.
33. Habuchi Y, Han X, Giles WR: Comparison of the hyperpolarization-activated and delayed rectifier currents in rabbit atrioventricular node and sinoatrial node. Heart and Vessels 9(Suppl): 203–206, 1995.
34. Mazgalev T, Dreifus LS, Michelson EL, Pelleg A: Vagally induced hyperpolarization in atrioventricular node. Am J Physiol 251: H631–H643, 1986.
35. Clemo HF, Belardinelli L: Effect of adenosine on atrioventricular conduction. I: Site and characterization of adenosine action in the guinea pig atrioventricular node. Circ Res 59:427–436, 1986.
36. Coppen SR, Severs NJ: Diversity of connexin expression patterns in the atrioventricular node: Vestigial consequence or functional specialization? J Cardiovasc Electrophysiol 13:625–626, 2002.
37. Gourdie RG, Severs NJ, Green CR, et al: The spatial distribution and relative abundance of gap-junctional connexin40 and connexin43 correlate to functional properties of components of the cardiac atrioventricular conduction system. J Cell Sci 105:985–991, 1993.
38. Nikolski VP, Jones SA, Lancaster MK, et al: Cx43 and the dual-pathway electrophysiology of the atrioventricular node and atrioventricular nodal reentry. Circ Res 92:469–475, 2003.
39. Efimov IR, Fahy GJ, Cheng YN, et al: High resolution fluorescent imaging of rabbit heart does not reveal a distinct atrioventricular nodal anterior input channel (fast pathway) during sinus rhythm. J Cardiovasc Electrophysiol 8:295–306, 1997.
40. Efimov IR, Mazgalev TN: High-resolution three-dimensional fluorescent imaging reveals multilayer conduction pattern in the atrioventricular node. Circulation 98:54–57, 1998.
41. Choi BR, Salama G: Optical mapping of atrioventricular node reveals a conduction barrier between atrial and nodal cells. Am J Physiol 274:H829–H845, 1998.
42. Wu J, Wu J, Olgin J, et al: Mechanisms underlying the reentrant circuit of atrioventricular nodal reentrant tachycardia in isolated canine atrioventricular nodal preparation using optical mapping. Circ Res 88:1189–1195, 2001.
43. Rosenbaum DS, Jalife J (eds): Optical Mapping of Cardiac Excitation and Arrhythmias. Armonk, NY, Futura, 2002.
44. Arridge SR: Optical tomography in medical imaging. Inverse Probl 15:R41–R93, 1999.
45. Huang D, Swanson EA, Lin CP, et al: Optical coherence tomography. Science 254:1178–1181, 1991.
46. Mines GR: On dynamic equilibrium in the heart. J Physiol 46:349–383, 1913.
47. Coumel P, Carbol C, Fabiato A, et al: Tachycardie permanente par rythme reciproque. Arch Mal Coeur Vaiss 60:1830–1864, 1967.
48. Janse MJ, Capelle FV, Freud GE, Durrer D: Circus movement within the AV node as a basis for supraventricular tachycardia as shown by multiple microelectrode recording in the isolated rabbit heart. Circ Res 28:403–414, 1971.
49. Watanabe Y, Dreifus LS: Sites of impulse formation within the atrioventricular junction of the rabbit. Circ Res 22:717–727, 1968.
50. Gupta M, Rollins AM, Izatt JA, Efimov IR: Imaging of the atrioventricular node using optical coherence tomography. J Cardiovasc Electrophysiol 13:95, 2002.
51. Kwong KF, Schuessler RB, Green KG, et al: Differential expression of gap junction proteins in the canine sinus node. Circ Res 82:604–612, 1998.
52. Joyner RW, van Capelle FJ: Propagation through electrically coupled cells: How a small SA node drives a large atrium. Biophys J 50:1157–1164, 1986.
53. Coppen SR, Kodama I, Boyett MR, et al: Connexin45, a major connexin of the rabbit sinoatrial node, is co-expressed with connexin43 in a restricted zone at the nodal-crista terminalis border. J Histochem Cytochem 47:907–918, 1999.

第 24 章

细胞间的交流和电冲动的传导

André G. Kléber

本章目录

- 细胞间耦联在均匀传播中的作用 …… 210
- 细胞间耦联在缓慢传导中的作用 …… 213
- 细胞间耦联与不均匀传播 ………… 216
- 总结 …………………………… 217

窦房结发放冲动以后，电冲动在心房肌和心室肌快速传播，引起心肌协调的兴奋并产生收缩效应。对电冲动传播过程的认识有助于了解正常的心脏功能以及心律失常的发生机制。通常认为心律失常的机制是冲动的产生和传导异常。电冲动传播的紊乱，特别是传导缓慢和传导阻滞被认为是折返激动的基础，成为大多数快速型心律失常的触发和维持机制。

电冲动传播的主要决定因素包括：能产生动作电位的心肌细胞的电生理特性，细胞网络中提供细胞间功能性电连接的缝隙连接，以及能够对激动波波锋形状和方向产生重要影响的、二维和三维各向异性的肌小梁和心脏组织层[1,2]。

本章主要集中探讨连接蛋白在正常和缓慢传播中的作用。它涉及的知识包括心脏缝隙连接的结构特性、分子特性、生物物理和药理学特性以及连接蛋白在心脏不同区域分布的差异性。这些知识都将在本书相关章节进行详细的阐述（具体可参阅本书第 8 章、第 14 章、第 19 章和第 21 章）。虽然有必要用一个章节来专门讨论缝隙连接在电冲动传播中的作用，但更为重要的是应该认识到上述决定电冲动传播的因素之间可发生相互作用。因此，由缝隙连接介导的细胞间耦联的变化，对电冲动传播的影响还依赖于其他决定因素的状态[1,2]。

一、细胞间耦联在均匀传播中的作用

（一）单细胞链（single cell chain）

单细胞链是一种简单的模型，可以用于理解心脏电冲动传播的原理，了解缝隙连接在冲动传播中所起的作用。目前，已经在计算机模型[1,3,4]或者构建的心脏细胞株上开展了单细胞链的研究[5]。图 24-1 显示了培养的乳鼠心脏细胞电冲动传播过程中细胞兴奋性的测量结果。实验采用高分辨率的跨膜电位光学标测技术测量电冲动穿过两个毗邻细胞所需时间，并与一个单细胞沿其主轴方向的激动时间进行比较。图 24-1 A-B 显示了在一个细胞胞浆中两个位点及毗邻细胞的第三个位点上动作电位上升支的测量结果[5]。图 24-1 C 给出了细胞内和细胞间传导时间的直方图，电冲动通过某一单个细胞边界并继续前行 30 μm 距离平均时间是 118 μs。相比之下，电冲动在胞浆中传播 30 μm 只需 38 μs。从这些数据可以计算出传导通过头尾相连细胞的连接处的平均时间为 80 μs。这些结果提示，电冲动通过细胞间连接的传导时间与沿细胞主轴激动一个细胞所需时间在同一个数量级。这些实验证实了以前使用 Luo-Rudy I 模型（LRdI）在合成的细胞链上进行的计算机模拟，计算的豚鼠心室动作电位[1]。在考虑到冲动在胞浆内可传导 100μm 的距离并能通过一个仅 80Å（1Å＝0.1 nm）宽的缝隙连接进行细胞间传导之后，这些理论及实验研究证实，即使在正常情况下，电冲动传播在细胞水平上也是一个不连续的过程。

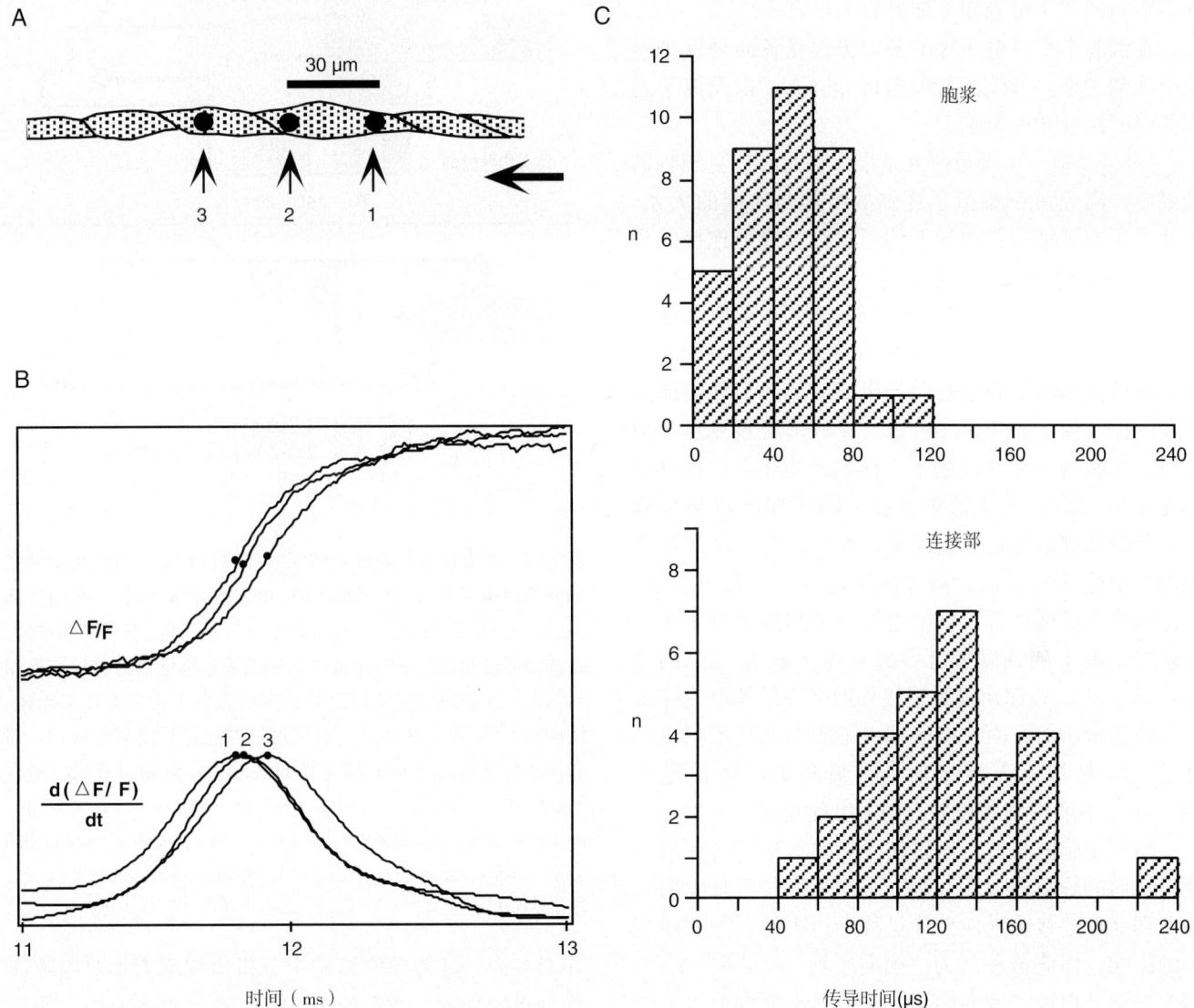

图 24-1 在单个细胞链的电传播　A：由乳鼠心肌构成的一种合成的细胞链微观图。在细胞链上以 1、2、3 标志表示光敏二极管位置，单个环形二极管直径大小为 6.5 μm，它们之间的间距为 30 μm。B：在位置 1~3 的动作电位上升支的光学记录，这是采用电压敏感染色标记的荧光变化（ΔF/F）改变来测量（上面的曲线），下面的曲线是首次衍生的荧光变化（ΔF/F dt），数字 1~3 显示局部激动时间的最大值，单位为 ms。C：胞浆中（点 1 与 2 之间，顶图）以及连接部传导时间的直方图（点 2 与 3 之间，底图）。这两种平均传导时间的差异大约是 80μs，可反映跨越头尾细胞连接的平均传播时间（引自 Fast VG, Kleber AG: Microscopic conduction in culture strands of neonatal rat heart cells measured with voltage-sensitive dyes. *Circ Res* 1993；73：914-925.）

（二）各向异性的细胞网络

心脏组织的大部分是由长形心肌细胞组成，心肌细胞与结缔组织基质和微血管共同形成了具有各向异性的细胞网络。在大多数正常心脏组织中，缝隙连接位于细胞的末端，而侧面连接较少。侧面连接的密度在心室肌相对较高，而在心室传导系统及心房界嵴较低。在乳鼠心室肌及邻近梗死区的重构组织，缝隙连接沿细胞的周边以一定的间距规律地进行分布（可参阅第 21 章参考文献 1）。这种特殊的心脏构造造成了电的各向异性，即电冲动传播速度 θ 以及其他电生理参数依赖于冲动传播的方向。了解这些正常的心脏电生理功能很重要，它们已被应用于解释折返的触发及维持机制[1,2]。

在宏观水平，即传播速度测量跨过几个心肌细胞长度，平均各向异性速率比值（定义为纵向速率与横向速率的比值，$V_L:V_T$）的范围从心房界嵴的 8.9 和心室肌的 2.7 可到培养细胞的 2.0[2]。

在细胞水平，电生理的各向异性受各向异性细胞的形状和大小，缝隙连接的数量和分布，以及离子通道各向异性分布的影响。

图 24-2 是一个理论研究结果。在犬心室肌细胞的网络中，高分辨率模拟了详细的结构与功能的关系，以此说明心脏细胞各向异性的形状以及缝隙连接的离散分布对冲动传播及跨膜动作电位上升支速率变化（dV/dt_{max}）的影响。网络中的每个细胞都是由多达 36 个兴奋元件组成。这种由于细胞边界以及细胞表面缝隙连接分布的不连续性，产生了细胞间多种传播速度及动作电位上升支的 dV/dt_{max}。许多资料显示，通过整个细胞的传播速度是不一样的。实际上，流过缝隙连接后（即超出了缝隙连接）的局部电流是弥散的，此时局部的传播速度降低。相反，当冲动接近细胞间缝隙连接的时候，局部传播速度 θ 会有所增加。这是因为在这些位置有轴向电流与细胞边界发生了部分碰撞，关于部分碰撞可参阅参考文献 1、2。同样的，dV_m/dt_{max} 在超出缝隙连接外的那些局部电流弥散的部位是最小的，而在能表现出细胞内电紧张电流的部位（即在缝隙连接之前）是最高的，这就导致 dV_m/dt_{max} 沿着冲动传播的方向上出现波动[1,6,7]。

与单细胞链相比，细胞在天然的细胞网络中也可通过侧面的缝隙连接相互耦联。侧面耦联可减少由细胞两端缝隙连接在纵向传导过程中产生的不连续所带来的影响，因此被称之为"侧面平均"（见图 24-1）。侧面平均是由通过侧面的缝隙连接的小部分电流产生的，它可以减少因为细胞头尾连接造成的电传导的不连续。因此，在合成的细胞网络中，细胞的侧向排列以及形成的侧面连接可以减少单细胞链通过细胞头尾连接的平均传导时间，可缩短到总传导时间的 50%，而在 5 个细胞宽度的细胞链里，这种传导时间的缩短可达总传导时间的 20%。如图 24-2 所示，这种冲动纵向传播及 dV_m/dt_{max} 的变化不仅可反映出细胞头尾连接产生的结构不连续性，还可反映出由于侧面缝隙连接产生的"侧面平均"作用。

如前面提到的，缝隙连接大多分布在细胞两端，在大部分心脏组织中沿着细胞侧面边界分布较稀少。然而，在乳鼠心脏组织里，缝隙连接围绕细胞周边有规律的呈点状间隔分布[8]。在心肌梗死周边的重构心肌，也观察到了类似的分布模式[9]。最近，Spach 及其同事[10]进行了一项理论研究，旨在从缝隙连接的分

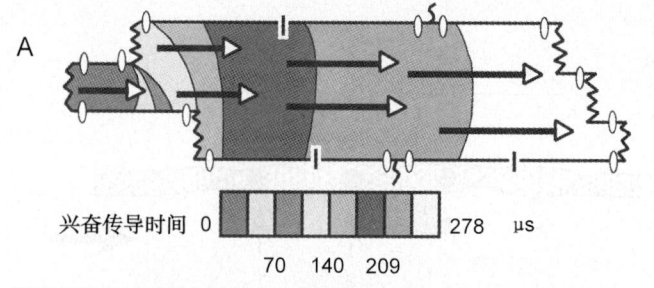

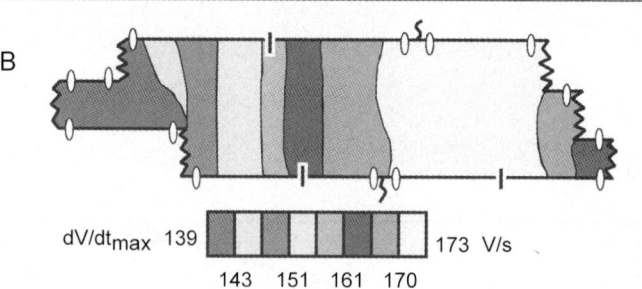

图 24-2 在各向异性网络中的纵向传播过程中，对细胞间兴奋顺序的模拟（A）以及细胞内 dV/dt_{max} 的分布（B） 纵向传播从图左到图右。注意，等时线的间距与 dV/dt_{max} 是紧密对应的。在冲动通过左边的缝隙连接进入细胞后，细胞内的传导变得相对缓慢，在朝向细胞尾部缝隙连接的方向上传导会逐步加速。同样地，dV/dt_{max} 在冲动通过头尾缝隙连接后变得相对低，而在冲动传导通过细胞末端连接部之前会立即相对升高（引自 Spach MS, Heidlage JF: The stochastic nature of cardic propagation at a microscopic level-electrical description of myocardial architecture and its application to conduction. *Circ Res* 1995; 76: 366-380.）

布对各向异性传导的影响中分析出细胞大小对缝隙连接分布的影响，结果见图 24-3。在这项研究中，作者根据实验数据，首次模拟了成年犬心室肌细胞和乳鼠心室肌细胞的细胞网络中的冲动传播（分别如图 24-3 中的 a 柱和 d 柱所示）。然后，他们制造了两个合成的细胞网络，一个是成年犬心室肌的大细胞，具有乳鼠心脏组织样的缝隙连接分布（见图 24-3 b 柱）；另一个是乳鼠心室肌的小细胞，具有成年狗心室肌样的缝隙连接分布（见图 24-3c 柱）。尽管在纵向传播上四种模式显示出了类似的电活动，但是在横向传播中四种模式却是十分不同的。重要的是，细胞的大小是沿传播轴在细胞间出现的激动延迟以及 dV_m/dt_{max} 的重要决定因素。然而，尽管缝隙连接的分布方式不同，但是对传导速度的影响却不大。这种细胞大小对传导速度的影响在随后的实验研究中被进一步证实。研究发现，各向同性乳鼠心肌细胞培养系，即由非线性排列的非伸长型细胞构成，其平均传导速度低于各向异性

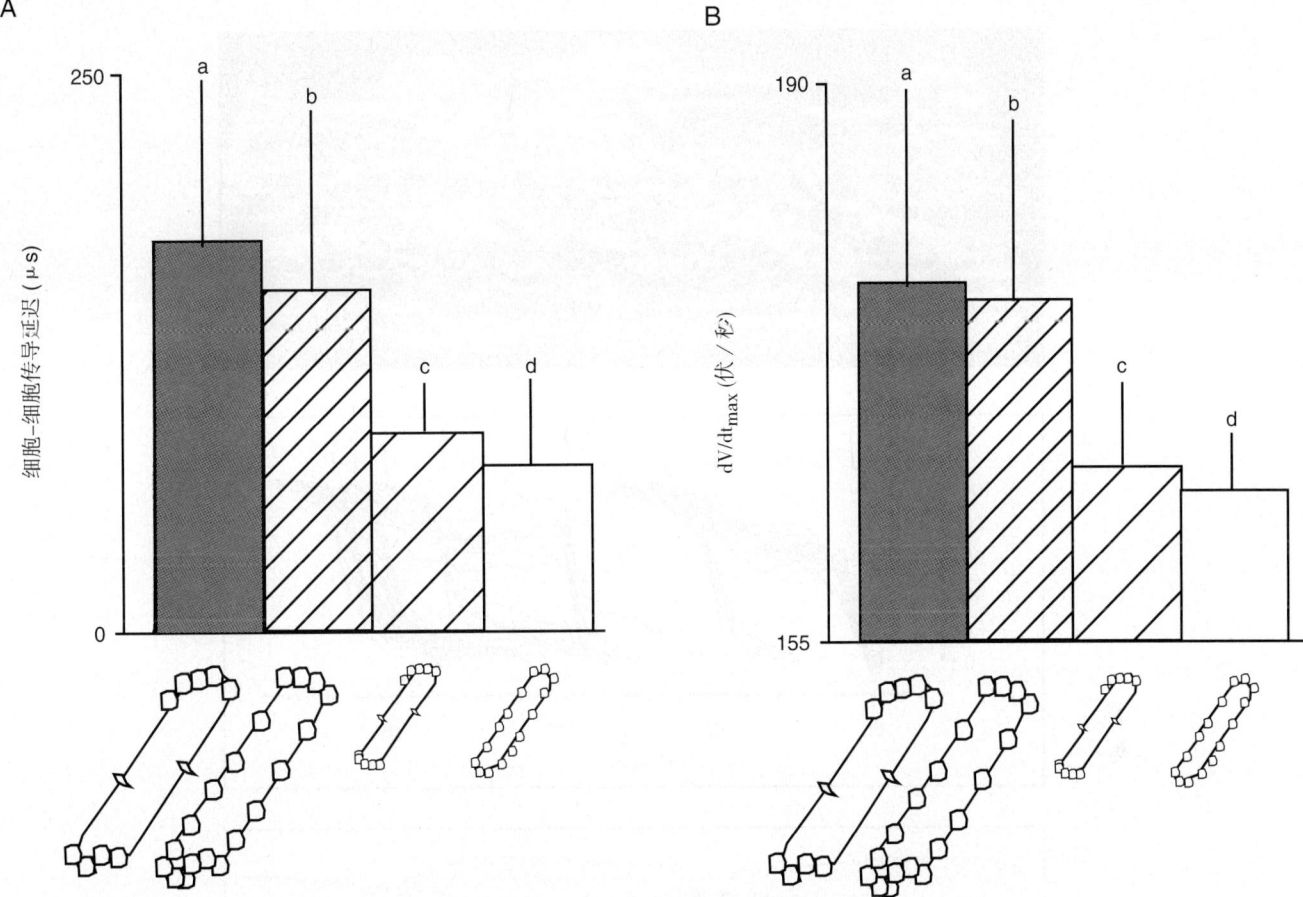

图 24-3 在横向传播中,细胞大小以及缝隙连接分布模式对细胞-细胞间传播延迟(A)以及动作电位上升支速度(B)的影响

a 柱是来自正常成年犬心肌细胞模型的模拟值,其缝隙连接主要位于细胞纵向末端。d 柱为在细胞周边具有规律分布的缝隙连接的正常乳鼠心肌细胞的模拟值。b 柱对应的是具有成年犬心肌细胞大小而伴有乳鼠心肌细胞缝隙连接分布模式的一个虚拟细胞的模拟值。c 柱对应的是具有乳鼠心肌细胞大小而伴有成年犬心肌细胞缝隙连接分布模式的一个虚拟细胞的模拟值。注意,细胞大小与缝隙连接分布模式比较而言,对所有参数具有更大的影响作用(引自 Spach MS, Heidlage JF, Dolber PC, Barr RC: Electrophysiological effects of remodeling cardiac gap junctions and cell size: Experimental and model studies of normal cardiac growth. *Circ Res* 2000; 86: 302-311.)

细胞培养系的纵向传导速度,后者是由各向异性排列的伸长型细胞组成[8]。

二、细胞间耦联在缓慢传导中的作用

(一) 传播的安全系数 (safety factor, SF)

电冲动传导的经典原理是通过局部的环行电流引起心肌细胞的顺序兴奋,而这种局部环行电流主要是由已兴奋细胞和静息细胞之间产生的电压梯度引起的,并可通过细胞间的阻抗进行估算。这一原理被用来定义传导的安全系数(SF),它是一个重要的参数,可为我们提供关于传播速度对离子通道、细胞间耦联以及细胞几何形态的依赖程度等重要信息。SF 可通过以下公式进行计算[3]:

$$SF = \frac{\int_A I_c dt \cdot + \cdot \int_A I_{out} dt}{\int_A I_{in} \cdot dt} \quad A \mid Q_m > 0 \quad [1]$$

原则上,当细胞参与电冲动传播过程($Q_m > 0$)时,这个方程与电流在 A 期流动的时间积分率(也就是电负荷)相对应。这个公式的分母对应于细胞的电流负荷,是细胞接受上游组织的电流并通过激活 I_{Na} 来使自己去极化达到兴奋的阈值所产生的电流。这个公式的分子是细胞通过激活离子通道产生的电流负荷。这个负荷分为两个部分:细胞为了自身除极产生的电流($Q_c = \int I_c dt$)以及为下游细胞去极化产生的电流($Q_{out} = \int I_{out} dt$)。如果一个细胞兴奋产生的电流负荷(即分子)超过了产生激动所必需的电流负荷

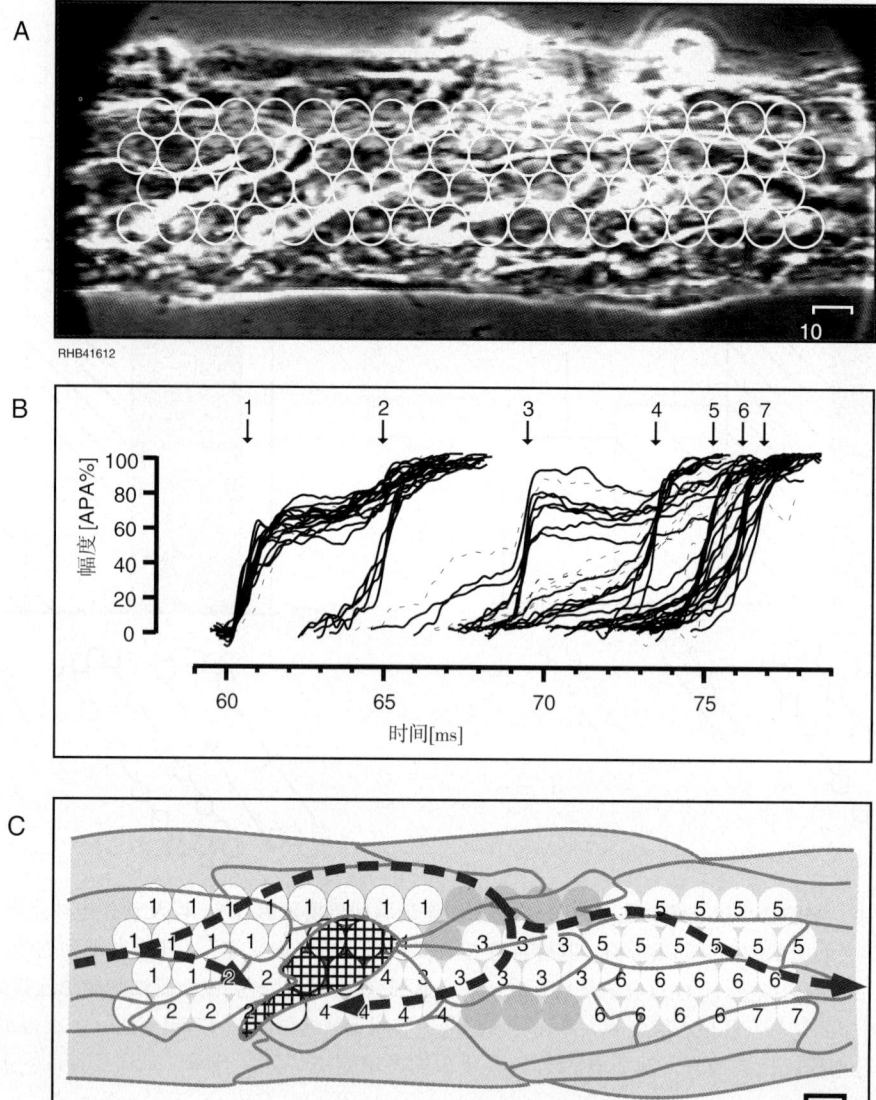

图 24-4 在一个合成的乳鼠心肌细胞链上,当出现显著的细胞间脱耦联情况下的动作电位传播(棕榈烯酸 10μM) A:合成的乳鼠心肌细胞链的一段显微照片。白色的圆圈显示的是每个光敏二极管的位置。链宽约为 60 μm。B:在 A 中每一个二极管记录的动作电位显示了各组间成簇的上升支。每一组的激动几乎是同时发生的,组间的传播延迟大约在 5 ms 左右。C:几乎同时发生的各组动作电位与细胞形态叠加后的示意图。注意,一到三个细胞几乎同时激动,矩形阴影标记的是细胞发生了完全传导阻滞。B 与 C 的比较可显示出在细胞边界处的传导延迟 (引自 Rohr S, Kucera JP, Kleber AG: Slow conduction in cardiac tissue. I: Effects of a reduction of excitability versus a reduction of electrical coupling on microconduction. *Circ Res* 1998;83:781-794.)

(即分母),传播就会成功发生。这个传播安全系数的概念对于定义和解释细胞间耦联在传播中的作用是十分有用的。对于正常的传导速度,SF 大约是 1.5,也就是说,它代表一个细胞通过去极化离子通道产生的总的电流负荷超过了从上游传导到这个细胞的电流负荷的 50%[3]。

(二) 急性细胞间脱耦联所致的传导减慢

在缺血、缺氧、细胞内酸中毒以及解耦联药物作用(例如酒精和脂肪酸)等情况下,可发生急性的细胞间脱耦联[2]。图 24-4 显示了解耦联药物棕榈油酸(palmitoleic acid)(10 μM)对合成的乳鼠心脏细胞束的作用。细胞(平均宽度为 80 μm)在用普通灌流液进行表面灌流的情况下，电冲动以 47 cm/s 的速度进行传播，这一速度在完整心脏的心室肌细胞的传导速度范围之内。应用解耦联药物之后，发生了完全的传播阻滞，并且在洗去药物之后传播速度仍非常缓慢（1 cm/s）（图 24-4 B-C）。如图 24-4 B 所示，在非常慢的传导速度时自发动作电位因几毫秒的延迟可被分成许多不同的串。图 24-4 C 显示在合成的细胞束，沿着细胞排列，在不同的测量位置都出现同时发生的动作电位，上面标识的数字代表动作电位簇的个数。这种激动的模式是十分典型的不连续传导。单个细胞或者是成串的两三个细胞几乎同时激动，在细胞边界，也就是在缝隙连接存在的部位明显延迟。这类传导的实验研究与先前在单细胞链上进行的模拟传导的理论研究相一致[1,3]。如前面提到的，安全系数对于解释由细胞间脱耦联所致的慢速传导的机制是十分有用的：电连接的减少，局部环行电流以及上述公式中分母的减少。同时，细胞的电脱耦联可以阻止局部电流向下游传导。作为第三个因素，流进下游的局部电流的减少可以造成下游膜的电容负荷减小，产生多个单细胞的同时兴奋，就可通过图 24-4 B 显示的那些成串的动作电位来证实。这种成串的集合，伴随动作电位上升支的速度增加，增大了公式 24-1 中的分子。总之，细胞间脱耦联过程中的传播安全系数就增加了[1,3]，只有在细胞间脱耦联达到一个极限水平时，轴电流减少才会成为一个制约因素。在这种情况下，安全系数可迅速变小，出现传导阻滞。然而，非常慢的传导只有在细胞间脱耦联达到非常显著的水平才会发生。缝隙连接电导的减少要大于 100 倍才能产生如图 24-4 所示的结果。在细胞间脱耦联过程中，安全系数的变化以及传播速度的减低与抑制去极化膜电流中观察到的变化有着显著的不同。因此，抑制钠离子内向电流可引起安全系数快速减低和传导阻滞，传导速度比缝隙连接脱耦联时慢一个数量级[3]。需要强调的是，非常慢速的传播以及安全系数的增加不只发生在显著的细胞间脱耦联过程中，在明显的结构重构中也会发生（参阅第 25 章）。

细胞间脱耦联导致的传导缓慢与传导过程中离子通道受累有关。在正常传导以及心房肌和心室肌的正常电生理情况下，传播都是由内向钠离子电流 I_{Na} 来驱动的。如果通过细胞边界时有明显的传导延迟存在，当前一串膜电位已经去极化达到平台（plateau）水平时，此串膜位点就可发生去极化（见图 24-4 B）。因此，L 型钙离子通道电流 $I_{ca(L)}$ 形成主要的电流负荷促使下游的膜位点串发生去极化。从钠离子依赖的传导转换到钙离子依赖的传导在类似模拟实验中也被证实（见第 25 章）[11]，而且也被 Shaw 和 Rudy[3] 的连接脱耦联的理论所证实。在细胞间脱耦联达到一个显著的水平时，L 型钙离子电流对传播的贡献要超过 I_{Na} 的好几倍。

20 世纪 50 年代早期，首次证实了闰盘作为低电阻的细胞间连接[1]，Sperelakis 和 McConnell[12] 进一步发展了关于电冲动的"电场机制"传递的假说，也就是无连接蛋白介导电耦联的细胞间传递，作为一种代偿或替代机制来解释电传播。近来一项理论研究提出，这种机制是由于细胞间的狭窄裂隙产生的电场来介导的，并且与闰盘附近的细胞间裂隙内 Na^+ 通道有关[13]。然而，目前还缺乏这一机制的实验证据，也就是需要证实在闰盘处存在成簇的 Na^+ 通道以及大量的细胞间裂隙。所有用解耦联药物来使连接蛋白完全脱耦联的实验中，可观察到缝隙连接蛋白非依赖的传播阻滞。

（三）小鼠心肌细胞间低耦联水平时的电冲动传播

解耦联药物的应用产生了从正常耦联状态到完全脱耦联状态的快速转换，在某种程度上限制了对细胞间耦联状态与传播之间关系的实验分析。近年来，应用针对连接蛋白的基因工程小鼠进行电传播及心律失常的研究结果也陆续发表[14]。在心室肌细胞中，连接蛋白 43（connexin43，Cx43）是一种最主要的缝隙连接蛋白。杂合子的 Cx43 缺失会造成缝隙连接处 Cx43 表达减少大约 50% 左右，但传播速度 θ 的变化报道各异。有的研究观察在体鼠心脏的传播速度 θ 有 20%~30% 的减少，甚至也有报道 θ 没有减少[14-17]。在完全敲除 Cx43 基因（Cx43$^{-/-}$）的成年小鼠进行电生理传播的研究目前还没有，因为 Cx43 完全敲除小鼠（Cx43$^{-/-}$）在出生后很快死于心脏畸形[18]。心脏特异性敲除 Cx43 的小鼠在杂合子动物没有表现出有 θ 的明显减少[16]。在 Cx43$^{-/-}$ 的 CKO 动物可观察到缝隙连接处 Cx43 表达显著减少（大约 95%），同时伴随有 θ 平均减少幅度达 50%。还需要指出的是，Cx43 的嵌合体老鼠（即 Cx43 突变缺失）会随着心室的 Cx43 突变缺失程度的增加，致死性心律失常的发生也随之增加。同样，心房及心室传导系统由于 Cx40 的缺失可导致传播速度上的改变[19]。上述实验研究结果与连接蛋白在闰盘的表达是一致的。然而，关于遗传性缝隙连接蛋白的缺失对传导的影响还有一些争议。另外，这种连接蛋白缺失的致心律失常发生机制目前还不是很清楚，还需要进一步的实验研究。

三、细胞间耦联与不均匀传播

在那些所谓的阻抗不匹配发生的位点，心脏正常的电生理传播多是不均匀的，也就是说一块相对较小组织要激活一块更大的组织，反之亦然。这种不匹配的产生可能是因为心脏组织结构的不连续，或者是因为电波在连续电传播介质中遇到了功能性障碍物后发生了偏移（形成了螺旋波以及螺旋波折返[1]）。因此，不均匀性传播在结构连续或者是结构不连续的组织中都是一种普遍存在的现象。在过去的几年里研究表明，不均匀性传播对理解房室结功能以及心律失常发生都是十分重要的。由于在这本书的第 25 章里，对不连续结构引起的不均匀性传播已有过阐述，本部分主要集中讨论细胞间耦联状态在不均匀传导中的作用。这种作用在一些简单的结构不连续模型中已进行了详细的探讨，如从中心点峡部到急剧组织扩张（expansion）[1]。在急剧组织扩张的情况下，细胞间耦联变化的效应在图 24-5 中有所显示。图 24-5 A 显示的是兴奋元件从一个小细胞链到达一个大块组织的排列情况，它们在 x 和 y 方向是通过电阻进行相连的，这些电阻可用来计算通过一块急剧扩张组织的传播情况。扩张部的顺向传播（图 24-5B），也就是从小细胞链到大块组织，其产生取决于下游电流的不匹配。这种不匹配是由于下游小模拟链（small simulated strand）细胞产生的电流与下游在扩张部大细胞块激动所需要的电流不相匹配（参阅第 25 章）[1,2]。扩张部的弥散局域电流产生的弯曲等时线超出了扩张部[11,20]。在那些很小直径的小细胞链，其曲率半径因为太小以至于不能顺向传播[20]。图 24-5 C 显示了无论是模型中所有的激动元件（图 24-5C，虚线）还是大块的组织（图 24-5C，实线）脱耦联均会导致 h_c 下降，并在一条细胞链宽度的传播中恢复传导，这对于正常水平的细胞间耦联，通常会显示出单向的传播阻滞。这一发现也在乳鼠心肌细胞的合成组织实验中被证实[21]。在图 24-5 D 显示了这一潜在机制。大块组织在 y 方向的兴奋元件之间阻抗的增加降低了临界直径 h_c，然而，对于在 x 方向阻抗的增加却不会产生这种作用。这表明所有的细胞间脱耦联综合效应将导致

扩张部局部下游电流的侧面弥散的减少。这些结果的发现以及与在一个细胞链的均匀传导比较可以得出几个结论，如图 24-6 所示。在均匀性传导中，细胞间耦联水平需要非常大的变化才能产生缓慢传导（细胞间阻抗增加 100 倍以上[3]）。换句话说，传导速度对于细胞间耦联的改变不是十分敏感。在非连续性传导中，正常情况下，很小的细胞间耦联的变化对于传导阻滞的形成都有很重要的作用。还有，在非连续组织中细胞间脱耦联可以"稳定"传导，因为它可将单向阻滞逆转为双向传播。

因为单向阻滞以及传播速度的减慢都可以促进产生折返性心律失常，细胞间脱耦联作为一个独立的致心律失常因素，其作用是不可能被预测的。实际上，要进行这样的预测，整合所有那些致心律失常的相互依赖因素的知识是非常有必要的，这些因素包括：离子通道状态，细胞间耦联状态，组织结构特点。因为这种相互依赖是复杂的，也是非线性关系的，计算机模型对全面理解这些所有的复杂相互作用提供了一个很好的工具。

对于图 24-5 描述的结构不连续性，在超出组织形态发生急剧变化的部位之外，弯曲的兴奋波的半径减少到临界值以下的位点可立即发生传导阻滞。重要的是，弯曲的心脏激动波的出现无论是在不连续结构传播中，还是在功能性折返的螺旋波中（也就是在电连续介质中发生的折返兴奋）都是一种普遍现象[1,22,23]。螺旋波的曲率朝向它核心方向出现降低，并且螺旋波在曲率的临界半径之下出现中断，在那里弥散的局部兴奋电流就不能再引起下游兴奋。这个被称为"奇异相"（phase singularity）的点就界定了一个螺旋波核心的轨迹[23,24]。图 24-5 显示了类似于细胞间脱耦联影响非连续传播的情况，支持传播的最小曲率半径依赖于细胞间耦联的程度[25]。对于螺旋波的描述可以分为螺旋波的起始，螺旋波的移动及稳定，以及螺旋波的解散三个部分。Pertsov 及其同事[23]的研究揭示了在局部阻抗物旁（对应局部的解耦联组织）螺旋波的漂移及锚定。他们观察到，螺旋波在心室外膜的微血管处锚定。在细胞培养中观察到由于细胞间脱耦联，螺旋波的解散增加[26]，并且在模拟二维到三维激动的理论研究中也可观察到这种现象[27]。在涉及螺旋波的实验性心律失常，尤其是心房纤颤及心室颤动中，关于细胞间脱耦联的作用还需要进一步研究。

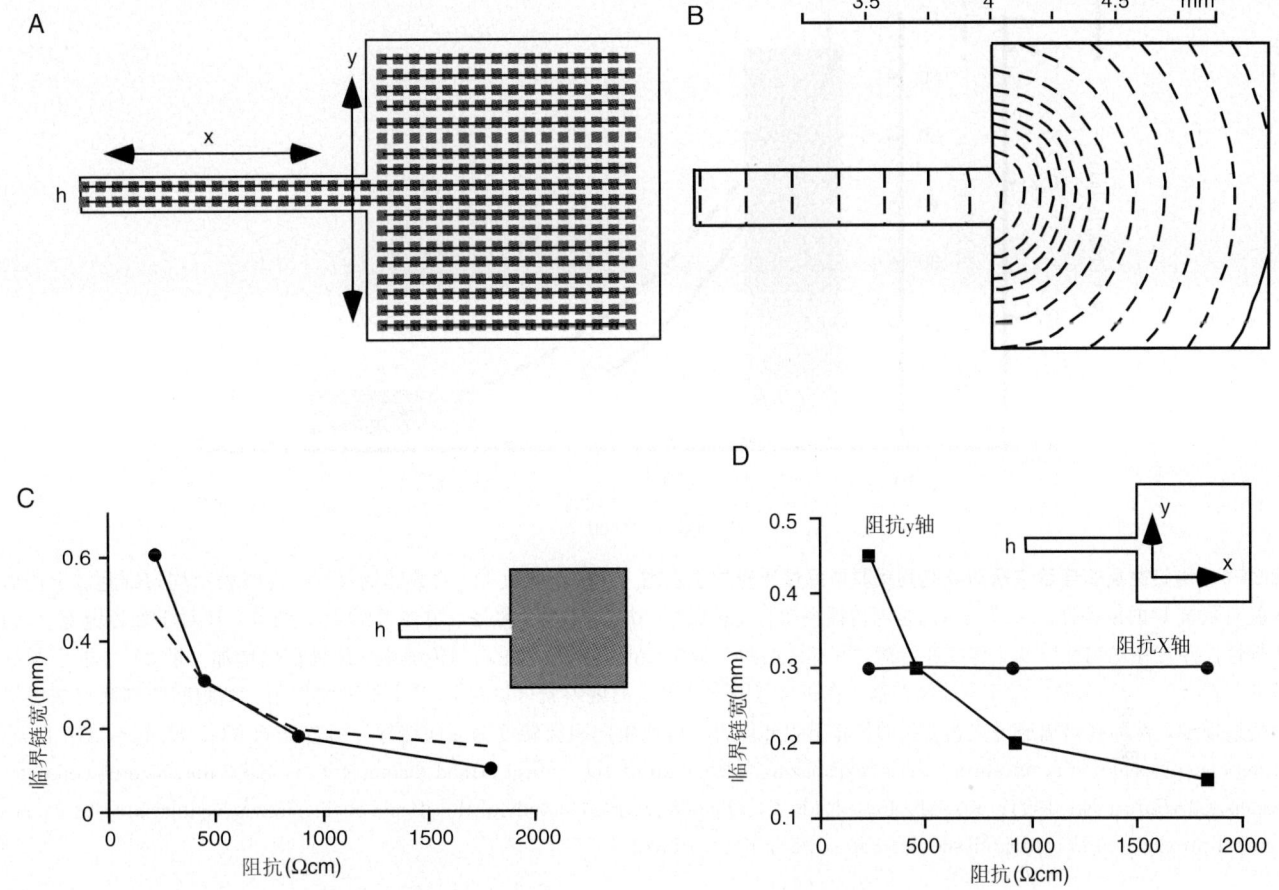

图 24-5 计算传播通过不连续组织时细胞间脱耦联的效应 A：由可兴奋元件组成的计算机模型（动作电位以 Beeler Reuter 或者 Luo-Rudy I 模型计算）。模拟从一个小的心肌细胞链到一个大块组织的兴奋传播。可兴奋元件在 x 和 y 方向上通过电阻相连，模拟了缝隙连接。h 表示链的宽度。B：模拟顺向传播模式（从一个小的心肌细胞链到一个大块组织）。注意，等时线被标记成曲线，超出了扩张部，等时线间距为 0.3 ms。通过等时线可以想象在这种突然的转变中出现了传播速度减慢。减少链的宽度 h 可导致传播等时线曲率的下降，最终在临界链宽 h_c 的位置发生了单向传导阻滞（数据未显示）。C：临界链宽对细胞间耦联的依赖性。链上和大块组织耦联阻抗的增加可使 h_c 下降（虚线），其中最主要是因为大块组织的阻抗增加（实线）。D：细胞间阻抗在 x 和 y 方向上单独变化的作用。注意，C 图显示的效应主要是由 y 方向上的细胞间阻抗的增加所引起的，而在 x 方向上的增加几乎没有作用。这表示局部电流侧向弥散的变化，是解释在不连续组织中细胞间脱耦联对传播效应的主要机制（引自 Fast VG, Kleber AG：Block of impulse propagation at an abrupt tissue expansion：evaluation of the critical strand diameter in 2- and 3- dimensional computer models. *Cardiovasc Res* 1995；30：449-459.）

四、总　结

由缝隙连接形成的细胞间耦联以多种方式影响电冲动的传播。在均一组织里，缝隙连接电导性的减少可以减慢传播的速度。传播的安全系数会由于细胞间耦联的减少而增加，并导致传播速度非常缓慢，可达 1cm/s。而当细胞间阻抗增大 100 倍而发生传播阻滞时，这种安全系数的增加才会停止。中等程度的脱耦联对于在均一组织中电冲动传播影响很小，例如重构的心脏组织（参阅第 21 章）。严重细胞间脱耦联时，L 型钙通道的电流负荷对于驱动传播是十分必要的。在非连续结构中，细胞间脱耦联可以逆转单向传导阻滞到双向传导，并稳定传播，在正常的耦联阻抗水平发生小的变动时也可以观察到这种效应。

因为细胞间耦联的稳定和不稳定效应可能同时存在，电冲动传播也依赖于所有因素的相互作用，所以对于细胞间脱耦联、离子通道的状态以及大体组织结构的了解对于解释在疾病状态下缝隙连接蛋白表达变化对心律失常的作用是非常有必要的。

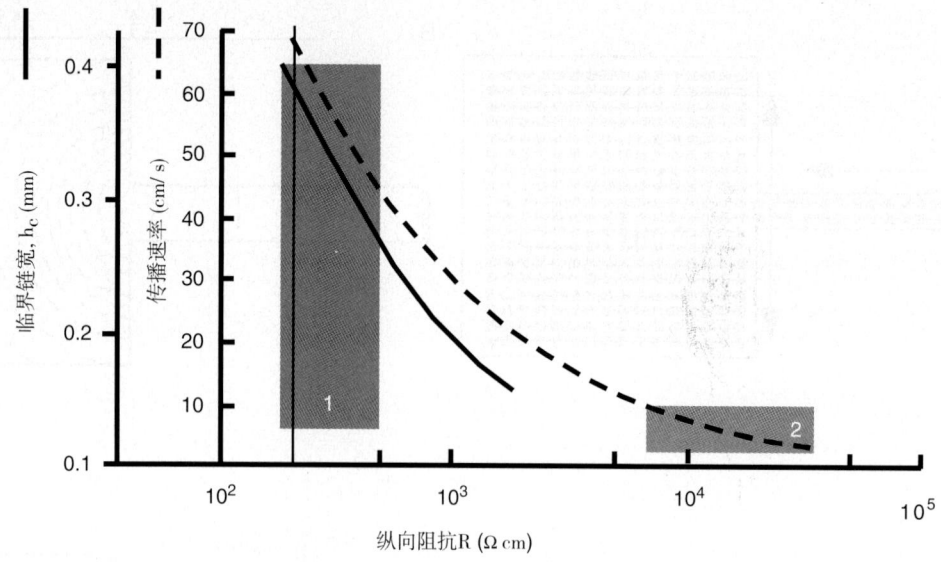

图 24-6 均匀性及非连续传播对细胞间耦联依赖性比较的示意图 （纵向阻抗 R，对数比例尺） 虚线表示均匀细胞链上传播速度对阻抗 R 的依赖性。实线表示的是当传播突然跨越扩张组织时（非连续传播，可参考图 24-5 细节）R 对于临界链宽 h_c 的依赖性。注意在均匀性以及非连续性传播之间存在的两个最主要的差别是，在均匀传播中，R 呈百倍增加（框 2）才能引起缓慢的传播（θ＜10 cm/s）；对于不连续传播，在正常范围下的很小的偏差就可以对 h_c 产生很大的作用。细胞间脱耦联可减慢均匀传播速度，然而在传播通过突然变化的扩张组织部位时，可使单向阻滞转变为双向传导（引自 Fast VG，Kleber AG：Block of impulse propagation at an abrupt tissue expansion：evaluation of the critical strand diameter in 2- and 3-dimensional computer models. *Cardiovasc Res* 1995；30：449-459；Rudy Y，Quan W：a model study of the effects of the discrete cellular atructure on electrical propagation in cardiac tissue. *Circ Res* 1987；61：815-823.）

（张幼怡 龚开政 徐 宁 译）

参 考 文 献

1. Kléber AG, Rudy Y: Basic mechanisms of cardiac impulse propagation and reentrant arrhythmias. Phys Rev. In press.
2. Kléber AG, Janse MJ, Fast VG: Normal and abnormal conduction in the heart. In Page E, Fozzard HA, Solaro RJ, eds: The Handbook of Physiology. New York, Oxford University Press, 2002.
3. Shaw RM, Rudy Y: Ionic mechanisms of propagation in cardiac tissue. Roles of the sodium and L-type calcium currents during reduced excitability and decreased gap junction coupling. Circ Res 81:727-741, 1997.
4. Rudy Y: The cardiac ventricular action potential. In Page E, Fozzard HA, Solaro RJ, eds: Handbook of Physiology. New York, Oxford University Press, 2002.
5. Fast VG, Kléber AG: Microscopic conduction in cultured strands of neonatal rat heart cells measured with voltage-sensitive dyes. Circ Res 73:914-925, 1993.
6. Spach MS, Barr RC: Effects of cardiac microstructure on propagating electrical waveforms. Circ Res 86:e23-e28, 2000.
7. Spach MS, Heidlage JF: The stochastic nature of cardiac propagation at a microscopic level—electrical description of myocardial architecture and its application to conduction. Circ Res 76:366-380, 1995.
8. Fast VG, Kléber AG: Anisotropic conduction in monolayers of neonatal rat heart cells cultured on collagen substrate. Circ Res 75:591-595, 1994.
9. Peters NS: New insights into myocardial arrhythmogenesis: Distribution of gap-junctional coupling in normal, ischaemic and hypertrophied human hearts. Clin Sci (Colch) 90:447-452, 1996.
10. Spach MS, Heidlage JF, Dolber PC, Barr RC: Electrophysiological effects of remodeling cardiac gap junctions and cell size: Experimental and model studies of normal cardiac growth. Circ Res 86:302-311, 2000.
11. Rohr S, Kucera J: The calcium inward current can play a critical role for the success of impulse propagation across abrupt expansions of cardiac tissue in presence of the sodium inward current. Biophys J 72:754-766, 1997.
12. Sperelakis N, McConnell K: Electric field interactions between closely abutting excitable cells. IEEE Eng Med Biol Mag 21:77-89, 2002.
13. Kucera JP, Rohr S, Rudy Y: Localization of sodium channels in intercalated disks modulates cardiac conduction. Circ Res 91:1176-1182, 2002.
14. Reaume AG, de Sousa PA, Kulkarni S, et al: Cardiac malformation in neonatal mice lacking connexin43. Science 267:1831-1834, 1995.
15. Eloff BC, Lerner DL, Yamada KA, et al: High resolution optical mapping reveals conduction slowing in connexin43 deficient mice. Cardiovasc Res 51:681-690, 2001.
16. Gutstein DE, Morley GE, Tamaddon H, et al: Conduction slowing and sudden arrhythmic death in mice with cardiac-restricted inactivation of connexin43. Circ Res 88:333-339, 2001.
17. Guerrero PA, Schuessler RB, Davis LM, et al: Slow ventricular conduction in mice heterozygous for a connexin43 null mutation. J Clin Invest 99:1991-1998, 1997.
18. Ya J, Erdtsieck-Ernste EB, de Boer PA, et al: Heart defects in connexin43-deficient mice. Circ Res 82:360-366, 1998.
19. Verheule S, van Batenburg CA, Coenjaerts FE, et al: Cardiac conduction abnormalities in mice lacking the gap junction protein connexin40. J Cardiovasc Electrophysiol 10:1380-1389, 1999.
20. Fast VG, Kléber AG: Cardiac tissue geometry as a determinant of unidirectional conduction block: Assessment of microscopic excitation spread by optical mapping in patterned cell cultures and in a computer model. Cardiovasc Res 29:697-707, 1995.
21. Rohr S, Kucera JP, Fast VG, Kleber AG: Paradoxical improvement of impulse conduction in cardiac tissue by partial cellular uncoupling. Science 275:841-844, 1997.
22. Van Capelle FJL, Durrer D: Computer simulation of arrhythmias in

a network of coupled excitable elements. Circ Res 47:453–466, 1980.
23. Pertsov AM, Davidenko JM, Salomonsz R, et al: Spiral waves of excitation underlie reentrant activity in isolated cardiac muscle. Circ Res 72:631–650, 1993.
24. Fast VG, Kléber AG: Role of wavefront curvature in propagation of cardiac impulse. Cardiovasc Res 33:258–271, 1997.
25. Zykov VS, Morozova OL: Speed of spread of excitation in two-dimensional excitable medium. Biofizika 24:739–744, 1979.
26. Bub G, Shrier A, Glass L: Spiral wave generation in heterogeneous excitable media. Phys Rev Lett 88:058101, 2002.
27. Fenton F, Hastings H, Evans S: Multiple mechanisms of spiral wave break up in a model of cardiac electrical activity. Chaos 12:852–892, 2002.

第 25 章

心脏组织结构决定冲动传导的速度和安全性

Stephan Rohr & Jan P. Kucera

本章目录
■ 概述 …………………………………… 220
■ 心脏组织结构与冲动传播 …………… 221
■ 单分支结构的冲动传导 ……………… 222
■ "推拉"概念 …………………………… 222
■ 沿多分支结构的冲动传播 …………… 223
■ 意义和深思 …………………………… 227
■ 致谢 …………………………………… 228

无论在生理或病理的情况下，从大体结构，如房室结可减慢传导速度并保持传导安全，到微观的亚细胞结构的膜蛋白，如在本书其他章节已详细描述的缝隙连接或离子通道，心脏的电冲动传导受其组织结构的影响。许多研究表明，在电相互联系的可兴奋细胞构建的三维网络中，心肌细胞的微观组织结构是心肌电冲动传播速度和安全的主要决定因素。在这一章节里，将主要介绍在多细胞组织中传导的安全性以及传导速度等方面的新观点，特别重点介绍沿着多分支结构传播的内容。

一、概 述

心肌组织冲动传导的安全性以及传导速度取决于心肌组织间三维网络结构电传导的主动和被动特性（active and passive properties）。在这个网络中，任意时间点的传导特性都依赖于兴奋区域的去极化电流（相当于电源，current source）与激动邻近静息组织所需电流（相当于电流接收器，current sink）之间的平衡。显然，电源容量比电流接受器越大，则传导的安全系数就越大[1]。关于安全系数的概念可参考第 24 章。一个早已众所周知的，可用来显示组织结构对这种关系影响的例子就是，在浦肯野纤维和心室组织之间连接部的传导。在这个连接部，相对小的电源（浦肯野纤维）与相对较大的电流接受器（庞大的心室组织）在容量上的不平衡可导致顺向传导的延迟或者是阻滞（浦肯野纤维→心室），而逆向传导却往往不会被影响。因此，这种电源到接受器的大小不匹配足可以诱导单向传导阻滞，因此有助于折返激动的产生。

那么电源和电流接受器各自大小的主要决定因素是什么呢？它们又是如何影响传导的安全性呢？

（一）主动的膜特性

通常说来，电源的大小取决于去极化电流（钠内向电流 [I_{Na}] 和钙内向电流 [$I_{Ca,L}$]）以及处于动作电位的上升支和平台的复极化电流之间的平衡。关于内向电流，很久以前就已清楚，钠内流 I_{Na} 在快速传导中起着十分关键的作用，而且与传播的速度和安全性呈正相关关系[2]。而且，在近期的计算机模拟试验中发现，钠通道的亚细胞结构分布模式也有可能影响冲动的传播[3]。这些计算机仿真模拟还显示出如同以往免疫组化研究的结果[4,5]，发现钠通道主要分布于闰盘，它们在缝隙连接脱耦联的时候有可能提高传导的速度以及安全性，且只有闰盘的裂隙具有很高的基础阻抗时才可能观察到这种作用。当这种阻抗可以被忽略时，这种效应将会十分微弱。这与另一个计算机仿真模拟研究所显示的结果一致，即钠通道的重分布对于动作电位上升支最大速率以及横向传播的局部传导延迟没有很大影响[6]。已经在实验[7]和计算机仿真模拟[1,2]中证明，另外一种主要的内向电流 $I_{Ca,L}$，对电源的大小也有一定贡献。尽管其激活动力学慢于钠离子流，但在慢速传导的安全性以及局部传导延迟中可以产生一定的作用，也就是这种电流对于下游的去极化是有帮助的。除了上述内向电流，电源的大小还受动作电位上升支和平台期的复极电流的影响。这些电流的增加，例如激活三磷酸腺苷依赖钾离子流（$I_{K,ATP}$），被认为可以减小电源的大小，同时增加电流接受器的大小，这是因为电流接受器要达到激活阈值所需的电流是增加的。因此，在缺氧的计算机仿真模拟中已经证实，$I_{K,ATP}$ 的激活可以在 I_{Na} 高度抑制的情况下导致传导阻滞[8]。

（二）被动的膜特性

心肌组织的消极性可影响传导的速度和安全性，它包括各个心肌细胞的输入阻抗，心肌细胞间的电耦联的程度，以及由心肌细胞构成的特殊三维细胞网络结构。关于电耦联，已经证明，进行性缝隙连接脱耦联可伴有传导速度的减低，就像在计算机模拟中显示的一样，可增加传导的安全系数[2]。缝隙连接耦联的减少与细胞膜活性减低的效应进行定量比较显示，前者（1cm/s）比单独减低细胞膜活性可更多地减慢冲动的传导（10~15cm/s）[2,9]。最后，心肌细胞构成的独特三维立体网络结构是传导速度以及安全性的重要调节者，因为这个可兴奋细胞的特殊网络结构可决定电流接受器的大小，这可通过在任何时空点上的传播波形看出，这一点在后面还将被详细探讨。

二、心脏组织结构与冲动传播

为了探讨心脏组织结构在冲动传播中的重要功能，解析在正常及病理状态下所看到的心脏组织结构的复杂性，就像图25-1显示的那样，将其还原成一个简单的几何图形来理解是非常有帮助的。本节将会对三个基本的结构基序在其单独或联合时的情况进行阐述。

（一）均匀的各向异性组织

在通常的情况下，心肌组织是由杆状心肌细胞组成，心肌细胞平行排列并且组成致密的纤维束。在杆状心肌细胞纵向上具有很强电耦联性，但是在横向上相对较弱。这种心肌细胞纤维的平行排列早期被认为是组成心肌各向异性传导的基础，即在心肌沿细胞方向的传导比横跨细胞间的传导速度要快得多。但是，Spach及其合作者们[6]发现，上升支的最大速度在横向传导时要大于纵向传导，这一特征可能与缝隙连接在肌纤维横向和纵向的分布不同有关。最近，同一个研究小组研究显示，上升支速度在不同方向的差异也受单个心肌细胞大小的影响，因此在心肌组织中，冲动传导的特征与更细微的细胞结构单位密切相关[6]。

（二）组织扩张

第二个基础结构涉及急剧的组织扩张（如被前文提及的浦肯野纤维），这在过去几十年中一直吸引着众多研究者的注意。在愈合的梗死组织中也同样存在这种特征性结构。在梗死组织的边缘，存活心肌组织与瘢痕组织以一种高度复杂的方式混合形成复杂的组织结构。有研究显示在这种组织中，冲动传导与否依赖于组织扩张的形状[10,11]、$I_{Ca,L}$[7] 以及电耦联的程度[12]。

（三）分支性的组织结构

在生理条件下，形成分支是心脏组织很普遍的现象，只是程度有所不同，可从心室快速传导系统形成束支，也可以在单个心肌细胞水平形成分支。后者可看成为单分支（见图25-1），因此心肌的组织结构是多分支结构的一个典型例子。在最近的组织学研究中表明，"心室肌细胞并不是均一连接的组织，而是有独特三维立体结构的层状肌细胞结构"[13]。形成这种结构的肌层平均来说有四个细胞的厚度。这些片层结构通过一到两个细胞厚的桥结构连接在一起（图25-6B）。在二维结构中，这种结构可以被描述为格子样的结构，如图25-1。因此在生理情况下，出现分支的频率比较高（约等于 $6/mm^2$）[13]，随着年龄增加以及心肌肥大纤维化增多，这种频率可能会有所降低。这将会增加心肌组织的各向异性传导及慢速不连续传导（即"Z"字形传导）的比例[14]，从而有助于形成折返激动。

尽管关于均一或不均一的各向异性组织冲动传导的研究报道很多，但是在复杂分支组织内对传导特性的系统性研究并不多。近来，随着研究技术的发展才得以实现。这些技术包括（1）心肌细胞培养技术；（2）对组织标本冲动传导进行高分辨率的光学标测。下面将综合已有的实验结果以及计算机模拟试验的结果，对正常或兴奋性降低情况下多分支复杂组织结构

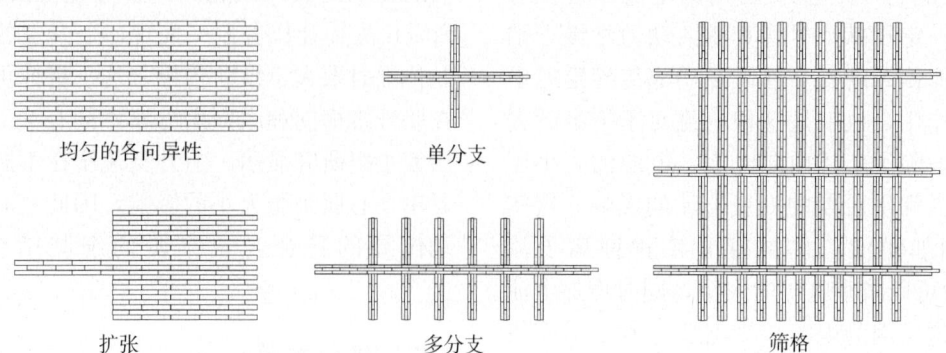

图 25-1 心脏细胞组织结构的典型示意图 发生在年轻而健康工作的心肌细胞中的阻滞，均匀的各向异性组织是其基础结构。心室与浦肯野纤维的连接部可作为组织急剧扩张的一个例子。在浦肯野纤维网络中可以看到单分支，然而，尤其是作为筛格（lattice）组成形式的多分支结构可看成心室肌里邻近心肌层之间的一个分支模型

的冲动传导特征进行阐述。

三、单分支结构的冲动传导

单分支结构的冲动传导特征可见图 25-2[15]。图 25-2 A 中相差图显示了所观察组织的中心部分。视野中心可见一个 10 mm 长的心肌细胞主干（水平方向）上分出两个 460 μm 长的分支结构。像这种结构的新生大鼠心室肌的细胞培养体系是通过光刻技术（photolithographic technique）获得的[16]。从视野左边的几毫米外处有一个刺激电极，它以固定的频率对标本发放刺激，使得冲动到达分支节点前已经处于稳定状态。采用高时空分辨率的光学成像技术，结合电压敏感染料可显示冲动传导通过分支点的特征[17]。如图 25-2 B 所示，分支的两边，即作为局部电流的接收器，沿主干冲动传导的延迟在对照时为 1.5 ms，而在细胞外钾离子升高的情况下为 4.7 ms（$[K^+]_o$ = 14.8 mM，这时传导主要由 $I_{Ca,L}$ 来介导）[8,9]。而且，尤其在细胞外钾离子升高的情况下，沿分支传导的速度比沿主干的速度要快。分支和主干的传导速度的差异取决于分支的长度，而且如果长度大于空间常数（单层培养的心肌细胞的 λ 大约为 400 μm）时，这种差异就会消失。如同预测的一样，标本内总的传导速度在分支长度超过 λ 之前会随分支长度增加而减低。

当分支的长度在 λ 范围内，分支要比发出分支的节点处的下游部分激动要早，提示分支很可能对主干提供去极化电流，有助于冲动的跨节点传导。这个假说被联合应用钠离子通道阻滞剂河豚毒素以及钙通道阻滞剂硝苯地平导致分支无兴奋性的实验所证实。如图 25-3 C 所示，这一干预可导致跨节点冲动传导的失败，由此可以证明分支产生的内向电流对于沿主干传导的顺利进行是十分重要的。

四、"推拉"概念

关于分支内向电流促进传导顺利通过分支节点的研究，提示分支有两方面的作用：起初，它表现为电流接受器靠近激动波而将去极化电流从主干"拉开"，从而诱发一个局部传导延迟。然后，基于它们的快速激动特点，又转变为主干的电源，由此"推动"激动向下游传导。通过用细胞培养实验中得到的资料进行参数的校正，用计算机模拟实验对这种"推拉"效应在跨单分支节点传导的作用进行评价[18]。一个模拟的通过单个分支节点的传导特征如图 25-3 A 所示，左图是短支，右图是长支，后者其长度大于 λ。这些模拟不仅产生实验数据，也可以对"推拉"的效应进行量化研究（图 25-3 Ad）。模拟刺激激活短支以后，初始的"拉过来"的电流（I_{pull}）被一个轻度低于最大程度的"推开"电流（I_{push}）紧随其后。相比之下，在激活长分支的过程中，只有 I_{pull} 的程度稍强一些，因为分支和主干的激动产生的速度是相同的，因此排除了这两种结构间的主要电压梯度。实质上，结果表明分支不仅可作为电流接受器，而且在去极化时可转变为电源，因此从原则上讲，可促进下游的去极化。为什么说是从原则上讲呢？如图 25-3 B 结果所示，在一个单个分支节点的局部激动延迟在 I_{push} 存在（实线）和缺失（虚线）情况下都依赖于分支的长度，I_{push} 对单分支节点下游的激活的作用几乎是可以忽略不计的。这可被以下事实来解释，I_{push} 的最大值发生在 I_{Na} 很大空间范围（已过了分支节点）激活的时候，造成

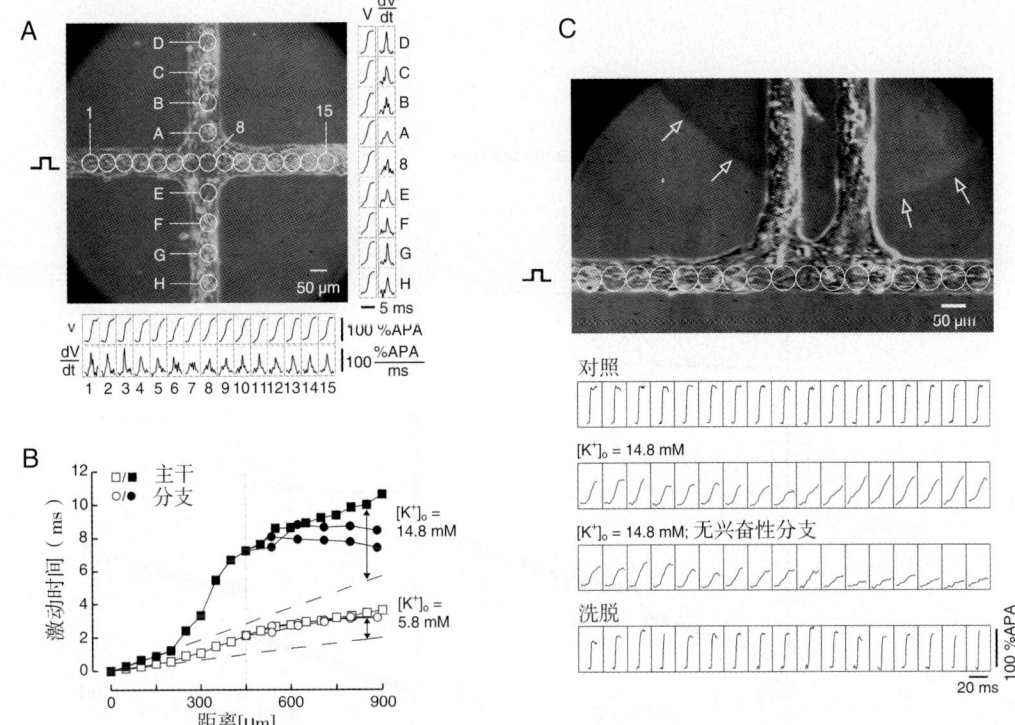

图 25-2 冲动传导通过单个分支结点的传导特征 A：培养的乳鼠心室肌细胞单细胞层组织标本的相差图，可以看到一个单分支结点（主干长度为 10 mm，分支长度为 460 μm）。主干在左边被给予 2 Hz 的刺激，动作电位的一些参数经采用电压敏感染料在白色圆环指示的位置进行光学标测。分支和主干的动作电位的上升支和 dV/dt 分别在图的右下方显示。B：在正常状况下（$[K^+]_o$=5.8mM）以及激动减低（$[K^+]_o$=14.8mM）下的激动状况。在分支结点前的主干（方形）方向的激动延迟以及分支（圆形）的快速激活与 $[K^+]_o$ 升高有关。C：在无兴奋分支的结点处冲动传导失败。如相差图中所示，两个分支结点在同一个方向上接受实验液体表面灌注（给药边界如箭头所示）。在第三排的信号提示，分支结构在河豚毒素以及尼非地平联合灌注的情况下 $[K^+]_o$ 的上升可以导致分支结点的传导失败（引自 Kucera JP，Kleber AG，Rohr S：Slow conduction in cardiac tissue Ⅱ：Effects of branching tissue geometry. *Circ Res* 1998；83：795-805.）

I_{push} 的作用可以忽略不计。然而，分支的激活，即使其并不促进传导通过分支节点，但是对于分支节点总的传导延迟却有着十分重要的作用。如果分支被失活而不能兴奋（图 25-3 B），在全长分支传导延迟都将增加。而且，在 $[K^+]_o$ 的上升期，当分支长度大于 700 μm 时传导就出现失败，这与实验观察到的现象相一致（图 25-2 C）。因此，旁边分支的激活，即使它"推的"效应在通过分支节点的时候没有增加传导，但是对于减少由分支产生分支节点处的电负荷却是十分重要的。即使当更多电流接受器沿主干增加的时候，I_{push} 也没能使传导通过单个的分支节点产生明显的变化。

五、沿多分支结构的冲动传播

冲动沿多分支结构传播的特征如图 25-4 所示。标本包括一个 10mm 长的主干（水平方向），每 300 μm 伸出一个 360μm 长的侧向分支。以 2 Hz 的频率刺激标本，在这一结构的末端至少 1mm 的区域内的冲动传导被光学方法记录下来。在正常的 $[K^+]_o$，传导速度大约是 29cm/s，当 $[K^+]_o$ 升高时，速度大约下降到 9cm/s。这些数值比在同一条件下的线性细胞链获得的数据要小（在正常 $[K^+]_o$ 大约 45cm/s，$[K^+]_o$ 的升高时大约 16cm/s）。如图 25-4 B 所示，沿这样多分支结构冲动传导的特征是在每一个分支节点前冲动传导发生延迟。在这些延迟之后跟随着侧分支的快速激动，从而沿主干产生激动使冲动通过分支节点。对于短的侧面分支，这一现象可以被通过来自既定分支节点的电紧张里有"盲端"的存在来解释，其可以产生一个去极化阈下电流的局部限制（"反射"）。当有一个大的电负荷诱导产生下游组织去极化时，可诱导一个分支节点的快速激活。令人惊讶的是，类似的激

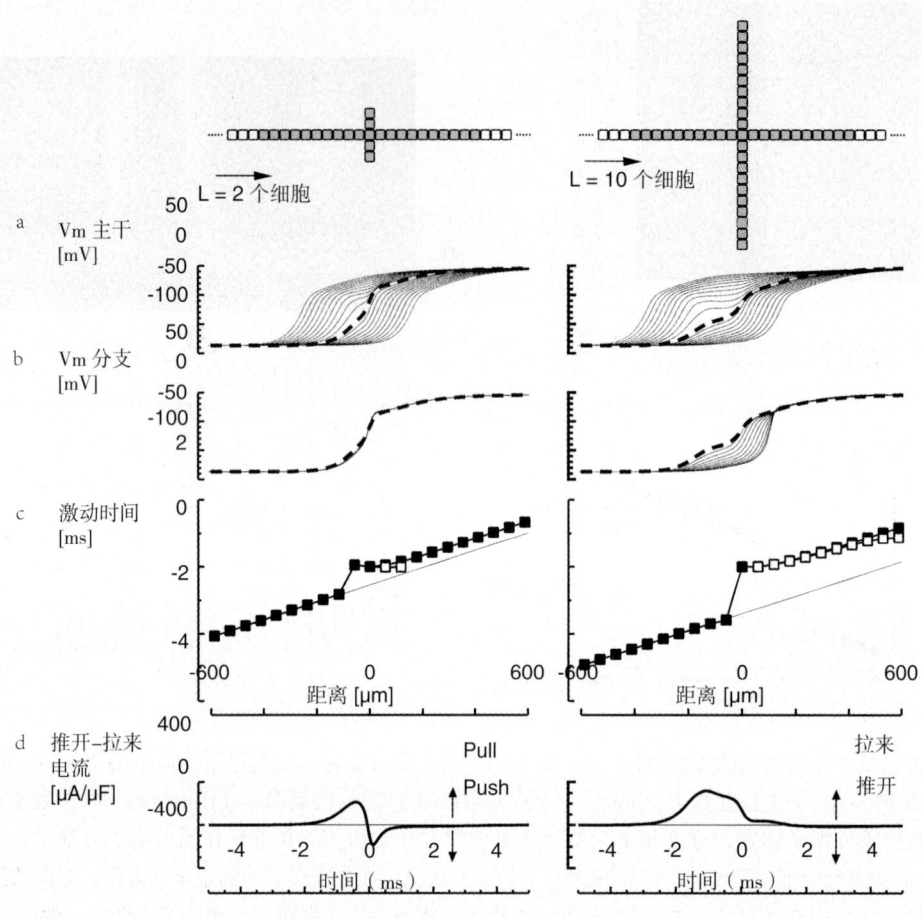

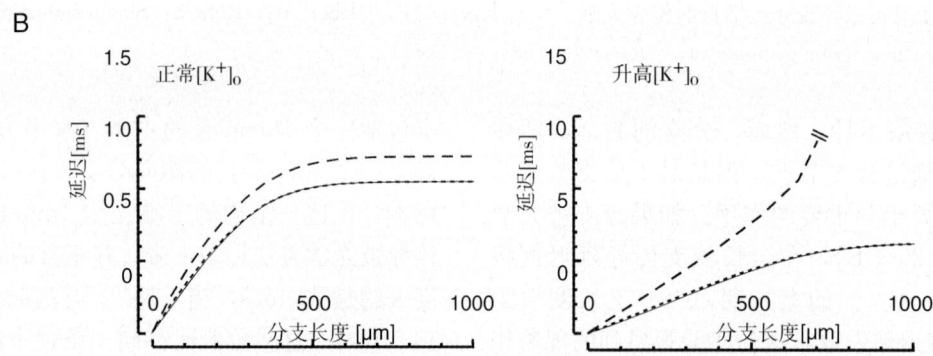

图 25-3 冲动传导通过单个分支节点的计算机模拟实验 A：冲动传导通过单个短分支结构以及长分支结构的特征。a，动作电位沿主干的上升支显示在电紧张负荷存在情况下的典型双向扭转。b，在模拟刺激情况下，短分支的激活是同时发生的，而长分支的激活显示，跨膜电压空间变化模式与沿主干通过分支结点时的情况类似。c，如同所预期的一样，激活的延迟与主干的长度有关。对比图 25-2 的数据，可以看出，在刺激下突然发生延迟是因激动时间是衍生于 dV/dt_{max} 的时间点，用实验获得数据中 50% 的复极时间来替代。d，从分支结点流向侧支的电流（"拉来"电流，I_{pull}），以及从分支向结点返回的电流特征（"推开"电流，I_{push}）。对于长分支结构而言，I_{pull} 更大，I_{push} 显示出相反的特征。B：左图显示在单分支节点 I_{push} 对传导延迟的效应。传导延迟对分支（实线）长度的依赖，很少被移动 I_{push} 改变（虚线）。相比之下，分支不兴奋可诱导传导延迟的明显增加，在 $[K^+]_o$ 升高的情况下（右图），分支长度大于 700 μm 时可发生传导阻滞（引自 Kucera JP, Rudy Y：Mechanistic insights into very slow conduction in branching cardiac tissue：A model study. *Circ Res* 2001；89：799-806.）

活序列在一些非常长的分支（大于或等于λ）也被观察了。这一现象很有可能被分支以及既定节点的下游组织之间的电张力负荷差异所解释：如果分支间的间隔≤λ时，对于施加于既定节点的电张力负荷在下游方向就要大于两个分支，因此后者会有一个更快被激活的倾向。为了验证这一假设，将短的（150μm）和长的（300μm）分支间隔所造成分支提前激活节段的长度进行了比较。如同所预期的一样，短间隔在下游方向，于较大电张力负荷诱导下，侧支初始节段的提前激动的距离大约是130μm，相比之下，长间隔所对应的是95μm。

如图25-4 C所示的分支间隔300μm和图25-4 D的分支间隔150μm的不同结构，增加分支结构的长度和减少分支之间的间隔都可以引起传导速度的降低，在分支长度为1 mm并且分支间隔150μm的情况下，正常对照的传导速度大约是17 μm/s，这一速度在线性细胞链兴奋性降低期的速度范围之内，即在$[K^+]_o$=14.8 mM情况下，$I_{Ca,L}$依赖的慢速传导。在给予复杂分支结构的表面灌流导致高$[K^+]_o$时兴奋性减低，同时可观察到传导速度的急剧减低。这一干预导致了非常慢的传导速度（≈1cm/s），相当于在线性细胞链观察到的缝隙连接脱耦联时的传导速度[9]。然而与后者比较，在多分支组织的兴奋性降低期间缓慢传导更能对抗传导阻滞，因此可产生一个较高的安全系数。

对分支组织与具有相似传导速度的线性细胞系二者传导的安全系数比较，结果可见图25-5 A。在这幅图中，采用对既定的分支结构的传导安全系数与一个传导速度近似的线性细胞链的安全系数进行标准化后，得到了一个传导的相对安全系数，线性细胞系的减慢传导或通过在正常$[K^+]_o$时减少I_{Na}或者在高$[K^+]_o$时通过完全去除I_{Na}再加上逐步减少$I_{Ca,L}$来模拟实现。在这些图中可以看出，增长分支结构诱导的传导速度的减低，除了特别短的分支结构，安全系数总是比同样传导速度的线性细胞链的传导系数要大。在那个最长的以及伴235μm的分支间隔的分支与表现相同程度减慢传导的线性细胞链比较，传导的安全

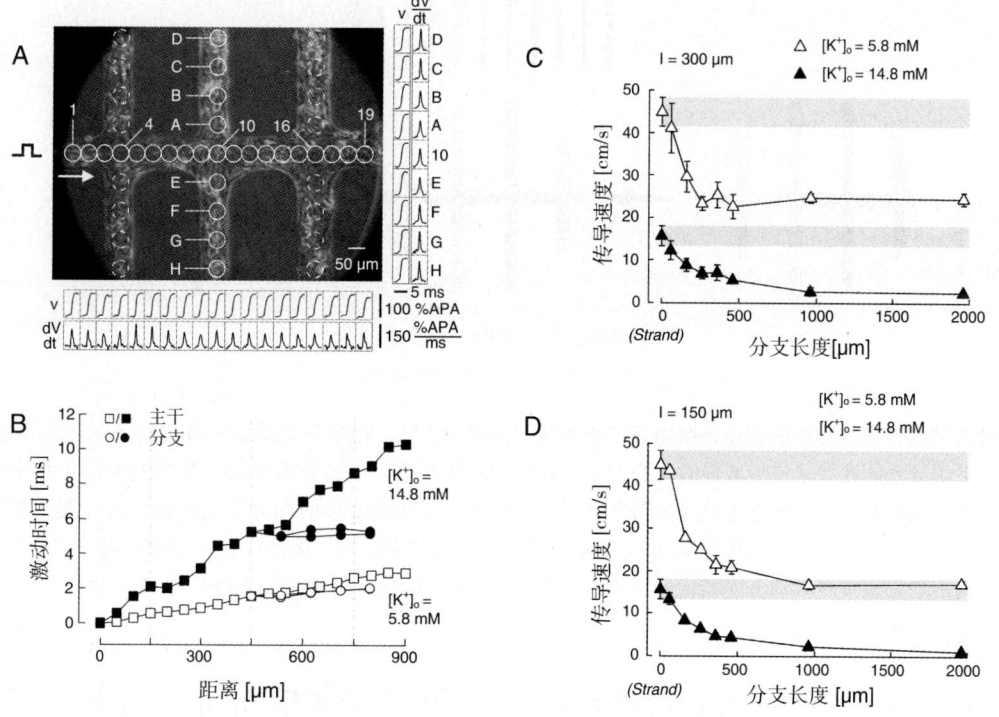

图25-4 沿多分支结构的冲动传导特征 A：主干（水平方向）在每300μm的地方分出一个360μm分支的细胞生长模式的相差示意图。主干在左边给予2 Hz的刺激，冲动传导的特征用光学方法在白色圆环指示的位置进行测量。在分支和主干动作电位的上升支和dV/dt分别在图的右边和图的下面显示。B：在通常状况下（$[K^+]_o$=5.8 mM）和兴奋性减低（$[K^+]_o$=14.8 mM）情况下的激动传播。在主干（方形）分支点前方有激动延迟，在分支（圆形）有快速激活，在通过既定节点后对下游产生了激活作用。C：传导速度在通常情况$[K^+]_o$（空心图例）以及$[K^+]_o$升高（实心图例）的情况下与分支间隔300μm的分支长度有关。D：如图C所示，分支间隔变为150μm的情况（引自Kucera JP, Kleber AG, Rohr S: Slow conduction in cardiac tissue Ⅱ: Effects of branching tissue geometry. *Circ Res* 1998；83：795-805.）

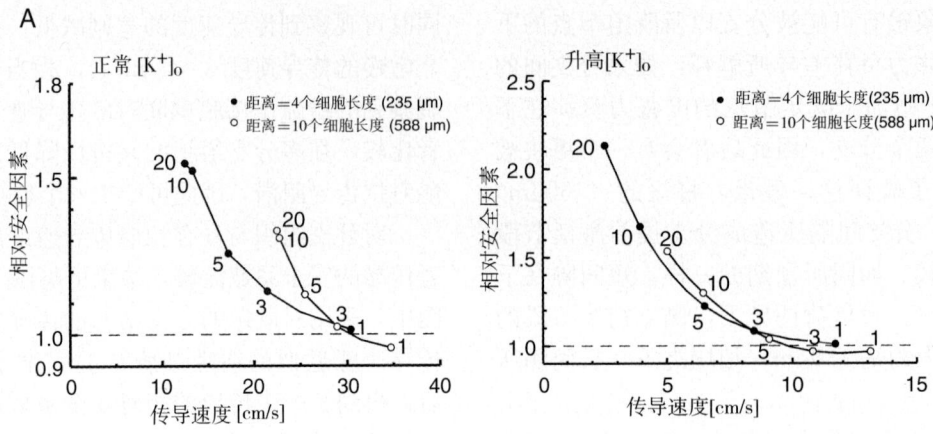

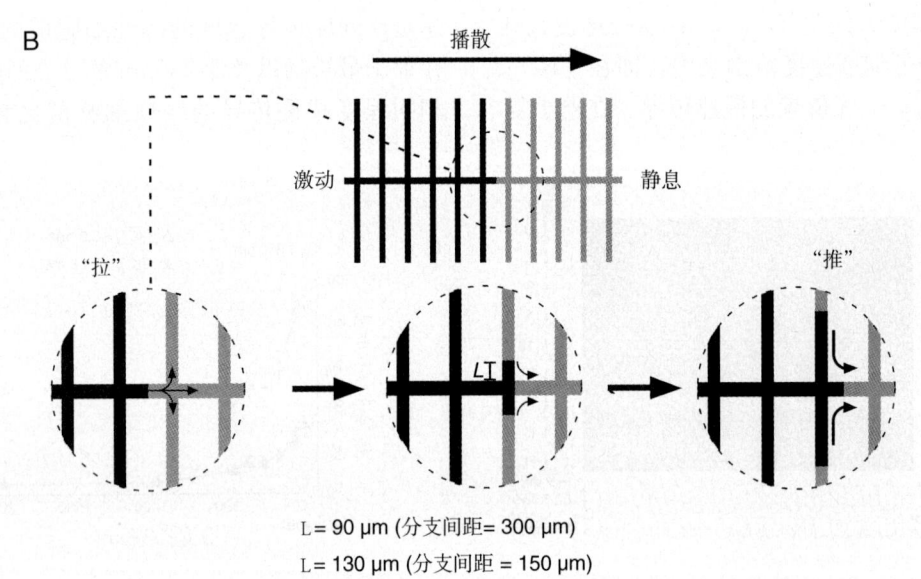

图 25-5　在多分支结构传导过程中的安全系数以及"推和拉"的概念　A：在多分支结构中分支间隔宽（空心图例）和窄（实心图例）的情况下诱导功能性冲动传导减慢时的相对安全系数。曲线旁边标记的数值显示了多个细胞长度的分支长度（1个细胞大约 60μm）。在普通兴奋（右）状态下以及兴奋性减低（左）状况下冲动传导的相对安全系数。B："推和拉"效应示意图。从激动波到达两个分支的中点开始，去极化波（I_{pull}）先沿着主干进入分支结构，由此引起传导的减慢（"拉"的效应）。电张力负荷在空间上的不均分布首先激动分支结构的距离 L。这些预先激动的区域为下游的去极化提供动力（I_{push}），因此使得激动向下游传导（"推"的效应）

系数增大了一倍。这种传导相对安全系数的增加是由于 I_{push} 的作用，因为抑制这种电流，传导不仅减慢，而且在高 $[K^+]_o$ 时，在那些分支间距离小于 400μm 的结构也不能发生传导。

为什么 I_{push} 调整传导的效率在单分支结构（几乎没有效果）以及多分支结构（增大传导的速度以及安全系数）是不同的呢？如前面论及单分支结构所指出的那样，单分支结构的 I_{push} 产生太晚以至于对下游组织激活没有显著的作用。而在多分支结构中情况有所不同，因为通过分支节点时传导减慢，使得 I_{push} 可以及时发展并且可以促进下游组织激活。图 25-5 B 显示的是冲动利用"推和拉"的效应沿多分支复杂结构传导的基本特征示意图。当激动波运动到两个分支的中点位置时，从这个点开始，去极化的电流同时流向下游以及侧向分支，因此引起了局部传导的减慢（I_{pull}）。因为侧向分支（较小）以及下游组织间（较

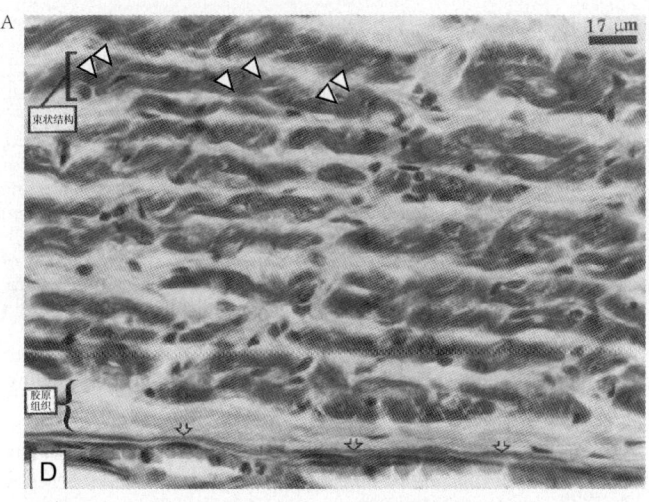
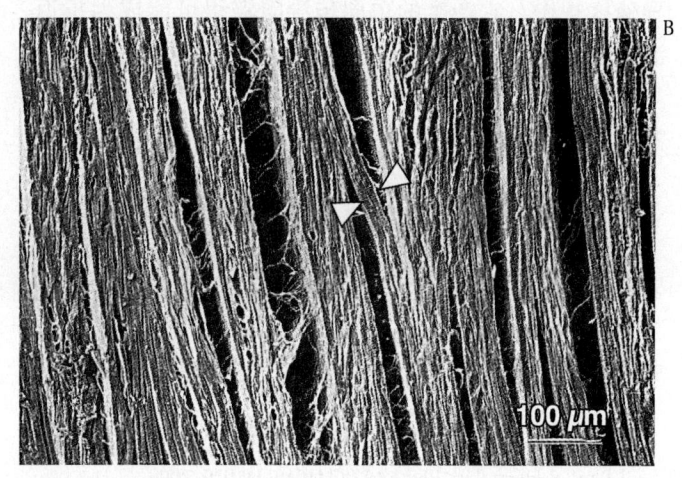

图 25-6 心脏组织结构中多分支结构可能影响传导的一个例子 A：犬的心脏房室束的近端组织学图片显示缠绕在一起的心肌纤维结构（成对的箭头指示），构成可被胶原组织（CT）分隔的一级束状结构，箭头所示结构为血管边缘（引自 Racker DK, Kadish AH：Proximal atrioventriculr bundle, atrioventricular node, and distal atrioventricular bundle are distinct anatomic structures with unique histologicasl characteristics and innervations. *Circulation* 2000；101：1049-1059.）B：犬心室组织正切面观可以看到心肌细胞层状排列，靠分支（箭头指示）将两个邻近的片层连接在一起（引自 LeGrice IJ, Smaill BH, Chai LZ, et al：Laminar structure of the heart：ventricular myocyte arrangement and connective tissue architecture in the dog. *AM J Physiol Heart Circ Physiol* 1995；38：H571-582.）

大）呈递出的电张力负荷的不平衡，侧向分支先于下游组织产生激动的这段距离为 L，它与下游负荷的大小有关。从这些已预先激动的组织产生的去极化电流可接着返回主干并推动激动通过分支节点。

六、意义和深思

基于冲动沿多分支结构传导的基本特征（例如传导速度很慢但同时十分安全），提出了一个问题，即在整体心脏这种传导发生在什么地方呢？

在生理情况下，这种缓慢而安全的传导是房室结的一个标志。分支组织可能参与房室结传导的证据有三条：（1）在房室结的电生理研究中发现，房室结的激动通常由心房或心室的激动来诱导。这种现象可用在分支结构模型中分支会产生所谓的"死亡终点"通路来解释。（2）最近对于房室结的组织学研究发现[19]，它是由 8 条纤维互相缠绕而组成的麻花状结构（图 25-6 A）。一些初级肌纤维肌束在二级肌束又被隔开，最后被胶原包绕成鞘。基于这一独特的组织学特点，可以推测这些心肌纤维在盘绕形成一个线状的心肌细胞主干的过程中必然会发出分支，这些分支可再次互相拧绕。或者是，在二级肌束中就包含了这种多分支结构，那些拧绕的一级肌束作为分支，二级肌束则是主干。在这种情况下，拧绕是形成多分支结构的基本机制，使得那些分支可以排列得很致密，进而沿主干的非分支区的传导速度降低。显然，这个假说需要更多的组织学研究证据，从而揭示这些拧绕的心肌纤维束的三维细胞结构。（3）沿分支结构传导的计算机模拟显示，它们是有效的频率过滤器，因此而形成了房室结的典型特征，以保护心室，减少房性心动过速对心室的影响[20]。

关于分支组织存在的第二个例子涉及心室壁的细胞结构。在对犬心室的大体和微观结构的分析中，LeGrice 及其同事报道[13]，肌纤维被排列成大约四个心肌细胞厚度的心肌层，它们互相重叠构成心室壁。如图 25-6 B 所示，这些片层被细胞间桥联结在一起。这一结构可用一个模型来模拟，这个模型由多个分支的链组成，链上的分支互相联结形成了肌层，从而形成了一个筛格（lattice），在这样一个筛格里，分支间的间距（即邻近肌层之间的距离）是十分短的，然而分支的长度却很长。这种组织结构的排列，侧边电联结的稀少以及心肌细胞的形状对生理及病理状态下各向异性传导的影响程度还需要进一步的研究。

最后要指出的是，在梗死区域边缘，当存活心肌被瘢痕组织"浸润"的时候可能会形成多分支组织结构。在这一区域，分支结构联合急剧扩张的组织很可能仅仅只占一个很小的微区域，但由于分支结构的传导速度很慢，它产生的单向传导阻滞很可能成为折返激动的解剖学基础。

七、致　谢

这一研究由瑞士国家科学基金提供支持。

（张幼怡　龚开政　徐　宁　译）

参　考　文　献

1. Wang Y, Rudy Y: Action potential propagation in inhomogeneous cardiac tissue: Safety factor considerations and ionic mechanism. Am J Physiol Heart Circ Physiol 278:H1019–H1029, 2000.
2. Shaw RM, Rudy Y: Ionic mechanisms of propagation in cardiac tissue: Roles of the sodium and L-type calcium currents during reduced excitability and decreased gap junction coupling. Circ Res 81:727–741, 1997.
3. Kucera JP, Rohr S, Rudy Y: Localization of sodium channels in intercalated disks modulates cardiac conduction. Circ Res 91:1176–1182, 2002.
4. Cohen SA: Immunocytochemical localization of rH1 sodium channel in adult rat heart atria and ventricle: Presence in terminal intercalated disks. Circulation 94:3704–3709, 1995.
5. Rohr S, Flückiger R, Cohen SA: Immunocytochemical localization of sodium and calcium channels in cultured neonatal rat ventricular cardiomyocytes [abstract]. Biophys J 76: A366, 1999.
6. Spach MS, Heidlage JF, Dolber PC, Barr RC: Electrophysiological effects of remodeling cardiac gap junctions and cell size: Experimental and model studies of normal cardiac growth. Circ Res 86:302–311, 2000.
7. Rohr S, Kucera JP: Involvement of the calcium inward current in cardiac impulse propagation: Induction of unidirectional conduction block by nifedipine and reversal by Bay K 8644. Biophys J 72:754–766, 1997.
8. Shaw RM, Rudy Y: Electrophysiologic effects of acute myocardial ischemia: A mechanistic investigation of action potential conduction and conduction failure. Circ Res 80:124–138, 1997.
9. Rohr S, Kucera JP, Kléber AG: Slow conduction in cardiac tissue. I: Effects of a reduction of excitability versus a reduction of electrical coupling on microconduction. Circ Res 83: 781–794, 1998.
10. Rohr S, Salzberg BM: Characterization of impulse propagation at the microscopic level across geometrically defined expansions of excitable tissue: Multiple site optical recording of transmembrane voltage (MSORTV) in patterned growth heart cell cultures. J Gen Physiol 104:287–309 1994.
11. Fast VG, Kléber AG: Cardiac tissue geometry as a determinant of unidirectional conduction block: Assessment of microscopic excitation spread by optical mapping in patterned cell cultures and in a computer model. Cardiovasc Res 29:697–707, 1995.
12. Rohr S, Kucera JP, Fast VG, Kléber AG: Paradoxical improvement of impulse conduction in cardiac tissue by partial cellular uncoupling. Science 275:841–844, 1997.
13. LeGrice IJ, Smaill BH, Chai LZ, et al: Laminar structure of the heart: ventricular myocyte arrangement and connective tissue architecture in the dog. Am J Physiol Heart Circ Physiol 38:H571–H582, 1995.
14. De Bakker JMT, Van Capelle FJL, Janse MJ, et al: Slow conduction in the infarcted human heart—zigzag course of activation. Circulation 88:915–926, 1993.
15. Kucera JP, Kléber AG, Rohr S: Slow conduction in cardiac tissue. II: Effects of branching tissue geometry. Circ Res 83:795–805, 1998.
16. Rohr S, Flückiger-Labrada R, Kucera JP: Photolithographically defined deposition of attachment factors as a versatile method for patterning the growth of different cell types in culture. Pfluegers Arch 446:125–132, 2003.
17. Rohr S, Kucera JP: Optical recording system based on a fiber optic image conduit: Assessment of microscopic activation patterns in cardiac tissue. Biophys J 75:1062–1075, 1998.
18. Kucera JP, Rudy Y: Mechanistic insights into very slow conduction in branching cardiac tissue: A model study. Circ Res 89:799–806, 2001.
19. Racker DK, Kadish AH: Proximal atrioventricular bundle, atrioventricular node, and distal atrioventricular bundle are distinct anatomic structures with unique histological characteristics and innervation. Circulation 101:1049–1059, 2000.
20. Meijler FL, Jalife J: AV node function during atrial fibrillation. In Mazgalev TN, Tchou PJ (eds.): Atrial-AV Nodal Electrophysiology: A View from the Millennium. Armonk, NY, Futura, 2000, pp. 251–268.

第 26 章

致心律失常的基础：恢复、复极和交替

Kenneth R. Laurita & David S. Rosenbaum

本章目录
- 心肌细胞间复极电流的不均一性 …… 229
- 复极交替 ……………………………………… 231
- 细胞间耦联使复极同步化 ……………… 234
- 总结 ……………………………………………… 236

在折返激动的经典描述中，Schmitt 和 Erlanger[1] 认为，不同电生理特性的传导通路是构成折返激动的基础。在这种情况下，当冲动沿某一条浦肯野纤维通路发生传导失败，形成单向阻滞时（图 26-1 A），却能成功地通过邻近的另一通路传导下去（图 26-1 B），并沿着心肌继续前传，当事先传导受阻的浦肯野纤维通路离开了不应期恢复传导时，前传的冲动可重新返回这条通路，从而形成一个完整的折返环。在有不同传导通路的其他心脏组织中也会发生类似的情况，如房室结、旁路以及束支。在这些组织发生的折返环一般都有解剖学基础。而大多数心律失常的发生却没有解剖学基础，而是由发生心律失常心肌组织的电生理特性所决定。尽管折返激动的原理都很类似，但功能性折返却较为复杂，因为它不由解剖学特性所决定，而是取决于兴奋、纤维定向以及心肌复极等功能性变化因素。

对于解剖性折返和功能性折返来说，单向阻滞都是必需的。然而对于功能性折返环，复极不均匀（或离散，dispersion）是产生单向阻滞的一个首要条件。通常来讲，复极不均匀与传导阻滞有着直接的关系。如果一个早搏刺激落在复极不均匀的区域，那么在复极延迟的地方，冲动就不能够继续传导。一条传导阻滞路径的产生依赖于延迟复极的空间分布及延迟程度，围绕这条阻滞区域，冲动只能进入细胞的完全复极（可兴奋）区域进行传播。许多重要的研究已经证实，复极不均匀与心律失常的易损性之间存在着紧密的联系[2-5]。基于 Moe 等[2] 的最初假说，复极不均匀对于纤维性颤动是必需的。在 Moe 等的关于纤维性颤动的计算机模拟模型中，基于心肌不应期的异质性所产生的多子波（multiple wave fronts），其形成与消失都是随机分布的。功能性折返激动还有另外一种与复极不均匀无关的机制。例如，由心肌纤维结构的异质性形成的"各向异性折返（anisotropic reentry）"，这些组织的传导安全系数及其速度在方向上的差异决定了折返环的形成，而不是取决于复极不均匀[6,7]，或者是一个螺旋波的转动及弯曲导致了"电源"（current source）与"电流接受器"（current sink）的明显不匹配，从而导致即便是已经充分复极的组织冲动也不能传播[8]，关于"电源"与"电流接收器"的概念可参阅本书第 25 章。然而，尽管 Moe 等的研究已经过去了 50 多年，但是复极的不均匀性是如何导致功能性折返的产生以及引起心源性猝死，目前还是没有完全研究清楚。从我们以及其他研究小组的研究结果看，复极可出现显著的不均匀性，并且其发生不是随机的，看起来这种复极不均匀性在早期复极与延迟复极的不同区域存在一个梯度。这一章主要讨论几个独特的可增加复极离散、促进心律失常发生的机制。

一、心肌细胞间复极电流的不均一性

许多研究一直集中在平行排列的心室肌层之间的离子通道的多样性上，它可导致心室出现不同功能的区域[9-11]。例如，参与早期复极的瞬时外向离子流

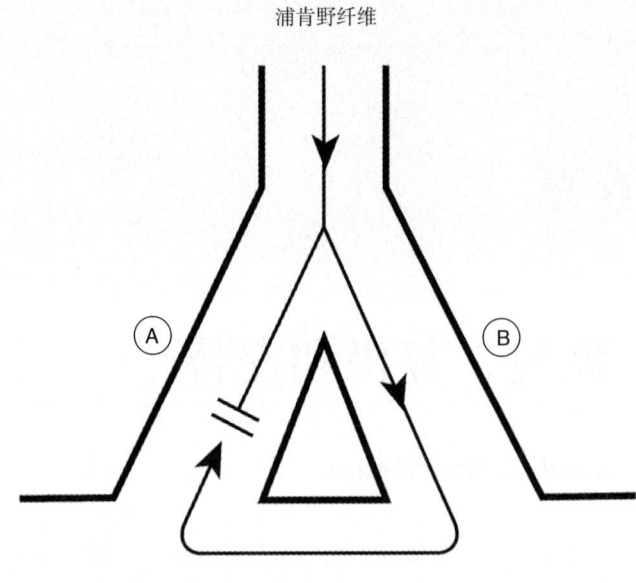

图 26-1 折返激动环在浦肯野纤维形成的示意图 当一个冲动沿浦肯野纤维传导并在通路 A 处被阻滞，冲动可以继续沿通路 B 向下传导，进入心肌。最后，冲动会折返回原先发生阻滞的 A 通路，从而完成一个折返激动环

(I_{to})几乎都是在心外膜表达，而不是心内膜[9,10]。相比之下，存在于心肌中层的 M 细胞低表达延迟整流(I_{Ks})的缓慢成分[12]。在单独的心室肌细胞层也有可能发生离子通道表达的不均匀。通过光学标测技术，我们研究显示，豚鼠心外膜的复极不均匀主要是由复极电流的异质性引起[13]。但是，正常存在于整个心室的离子通道表达的异质性，并不会产生明显的复极不均匀而诱发心律失常。

在某些病理情况下，有可能显著增加膜内的复极电流不均匀性，因此导致复极的离散。例如，先天长 QT 综合征（long QT syndrome，LQTS）是一种少见的临床疾病，但其临床症状有时非常危险棘手，目前发现它存在与心肌复极有关的特殊离子通道的基因突变[14-16]。LQTS 病人可发生由尖端扭转性室性心动过速引起的晕厥以及心源性猝死[17]，已证实，复极的离散是这类患者的一个危险因素[18]。在过去的 10 年里，证明它存在几个离子通道蛋白的突变，使得我们对 LQTS 有了更深的了解。例如，与最常见的 LQT1 有关的染色体缺陷是 KVLQT1，它可与 MinK 共同组装成产生 I_{Ks} 的离子通道[19]。而

与 LQT3 有关的离子通道基因突变，已经被认为与 SCN5A 有关，其编码一个 I_{Na} 的 α 亚单位[15]。与 LQT2 有关的基因突变被认为与 HERG 有关，它负责产生 I_{kr}[14]。内向电流与外向电流之间精细的平衡决定着复极的发生，电流微妙的变化就可对心肌复极时间产生严重的影响[20]。在这种情况下，这些离子通道的异常表达，再联合 M 细胞自身微弱的 I_{Ks}，就可显著增强复极的离散度，从而成为功能性折返激动产生的基础。

在模拟 LQTS 有关的基因突变实验中，主要是中层心肌细胞（即 M 细胞）复极的延长，导致形成长 QT 间期以及与 LQTS 有关的复极跨膜梯度[21-23]。图 26-2 显示了一个测量自动脉灌流犬左室楔形标本的跨膜心室复极梯度的例子，一边显示的是正常对照，另一个作为 LQT2 的实验模型[23]。在正常情况下，复极的梯度是非常小的，相比之下，在 LQT2 的情况下，因为 M 细胞延长的动作电位时程（action potential duration，APD），使中层心肌的一个区域发生延迟复极。结果与对照比较，尽管细胞间耦联是正常的，而复极梯度却平均增加了 300%。在不同的实验中尽管形成的最大 APD 延长有所变化，但都是发生在中层心肌，在中间心肌层与心外膜心肌层之间形成了最大的复极跨膜梯度。我们[23]以及其他的研究小组[21,22]已经证实，发生在这种高复极梯度时的早搏能直接导致单向传导阻滞和尖端扭转性室速。而且，LQT2 型的复极梯度在形成功能性线性传导阻滞中具有重要的作用，这种阻滞区在尖端扭转性室速发作中可出现大小和形状的变化，这再次肯定了复极梯度在功能性传导折返中的作用。有趣的是，在延迟复极中很难观察到环状"岛"（也就是 M 细胞）。这些复极的环状模式可能提供给折返激动一个更有利的基础，因为它们可允许部分早搏无限制地通过心外膜层传播到心内膜层，从而形成一个完整的折返激动环。

各向异性的复极电流所产生的较大复极梯度并不只限于心室肌。临床研究表明，由迷走神经兴奋引起的心房纤维颤动（简称房颤）的发生主要依赖于不应期的缩短以及不均匀（离散），这主要有利于形成大的折返环[24]。在心房组织内，副交感神经释放的乙酰胆碱（acetylcholine，ACh）作用于 M 型 ACh 受体，通过一种 G 蛋白耦联机制，打开一个内向延迟钾通道（$I_{K,ACh}$），从而诱发 APD 的缩短。因为心房肌内迷走神经分布的区域不同[25]，APD 缩短的程度也不一致，导致了组织内不应性离散度的增加。迷走神经刺激大

早搏来确定,而另外一条恢复曲线可由一个短间期搏动来确定[36]。这就意味着这种恢复的异质性可随心跳的不同产生(即时间上的异质性),并且基于先前搏动的情况,也可产生空间上的异质性。图 26-4 A 显示了跨过心脏表面两个位点产生的成对恢复曲线,实线表示的恢复是在奇数搏动后产生(短 APD),而虚线表示的恢复是在偶数搏动后产生(长 APD)。心室尖方向恢复曲线几乎看不到(图 26-4,B 位点)。与之对比的是,在心室基底部(图 26-4B),恢复曲线的差别很大。图 26-4 A 显示了一个穿过整个标测区 Δ-恢复(也就是恢复异质性的瞬间变化)的空间异质性。因此,在交替的过程中,电恢复时间(是随心跳的不同有所不同)和空间上的异质性[37]。

电恢复在时间和空间上的异质性可以解释心脏上复杂、可预测和可再现的不协调复极方式。由于用实验的方法去区分电恢复的时空异质性的不同作用是十分困难的,计算机模拟研究已用来阐述在不协调交替机制中,这两种异质性它们各自的作用及其相互作用。计算机利用实验中得到的电恢复曲线来模拟计算 APD 和舒张间期(diastolic interval,DI)[37]。舒张间期是由起搏周长减去前一个 APD 所得,并且作为一个输入到合适电恢复曲线里的参数而测定下一个跳动的 APD。例如,在长的 APD(也就是偶数搏动)之后,下一个 DI 被计算出来,并且使用奇数搏动的恢复曲线来测定出下一个 APD(即奇数跳动的)。接着奇数跳动的 APD 又被用来测定出下一个 DI,再用偶数搏动的恢复曲线去测定下一个 APD(即偶数跳动的)。计算机模拟的结果在图 26-4 B 显示,两个细胞电恢复在时间异质性上明显不同,靠上的那个有很大的 Δ-恢复,而靠下的那个只有小的 Δ-恢复。这种模拟的结果揭示了不协调交替的机制。从电恢复图(图 26-4 左)和时间序列图(图 26-4 右)可观察到,在电恢复异质性大的细胞,APD 随心跳发生交替。此时,于 215ms 引入一个提前刺激(见图 26-4 B,底行)只会引起交替的程度暂时降低,但是不足以逆转交替的时相(也就是长-短-长 APD 序列)。因为电恢复曲线分离较大(也就是电恢复有很大的时间异质性),这个细胞不可能发生时相上的逆转。对于电恢复异质性小的细胞,APD 也随心跳发生交替,但与前述异质性大的细胞相比较,这种交替程度较小。但是,在 215ms 的提前刺激可逆转交替的时相,这是由于它使偶数搏动更短于奇数搏动(即长-短-更短 APD 序列)。因为在这个细胞上,恢复曲线只要有很小的不同,就可发生时相上的逆转。因此,一个细胞若发生时相的逆转,它可直接导致不协调交替的发生。重要的是,缺乏电恢复时空异质性的模拟实验并不能够显示出不协调交替。这种时相逆转的机制也许可以解释不协调交替是如何形成,乃至产生功能性折返的基础。

APD 恢复对认识交替这个过程提供了一些重要见解。然而,复极交替更详细的内在机制还需要进一步阐明。很有可能,不协调交替的机制与引起首次交替时细胞复极有关。对分离的心肌细胞的研究表明,细胞内钙循环在 APD 交替中起到十分重要的作用。例如,心肌细胞实验显示,在电压膜片钳或者动作电位钳下,没有电压交替时也可发生钙的瞬时交替[38]。这些资料显示,复极交替对于钙瞬时交替的发生不是必需的,而且,重要的是钙循环可能参与复极的交替。为了证明钙循环是整体心脏 APD 交替发生的基础这个假说,我们利用光学标测技术在整体心脏上同时对细胞内钙以及跨膜电位进行了测定[39]。发现在起搏诱导交替的豚鼠模型中,即使存在空间上不协调交替,复极交替与钙瞬时交替也是平行发生的(图 26-5 A)[40]。另外,复极交替与钙瞬时交替的心率阈值几乎是相同的。尽管细胞内钙以及跨膜电位之间的相互关系还不是很清楚,就好比"鸡"和"蛋"的关系一样,但这些资料提示了钙瞬时交替与复极交替之间存在重要的联系。然而,那些最早发生交替的位点却给我们提供了重要线索。在靠近左室基底部经常发生交替(见图 26-5 B 阴影线区)。有趣的是,这个位置与对豚鼠进行基础起搏时出现心外膜 APD 最长(右室基底)的位置或者最短(左室心尖部)的位置不同。我们先前已经证实了在正常的豚鼠心脏,恢复动力学最快的位置是基线 APD 最长的地方[13]。然而,我们的数据也显示,在 APD 最长的地方并不是交替发生的地方(见图 26-5 B,柱图)。这与恢复是一种复极交替的机制的观点相矛盾。相反,我们采用新的光学标测技术来测量钙瞬变振幅在空间上的异质性,发现在钙释放和再摄取的地方,交替发生是减少的[41]。这些数据进一步证明了复极交替是由细胞内钙介导的。但是,需要指出的是,这并没有排除 APD 恢复的作用。钙释放与 APD 都不是互相排斥的,而且因为跨膜电位与细胞内钙之间的相互作用,事实上,APD 恢复应该已反映出控制钙循环的机制。恢复的时空异质性很可能用来解释不协调的发生,它的形成取决于钙释放的异质性(图 26-3)。值得注意的是,确实存在细胞内钙释放的空间异质性[42],并且在心力衰

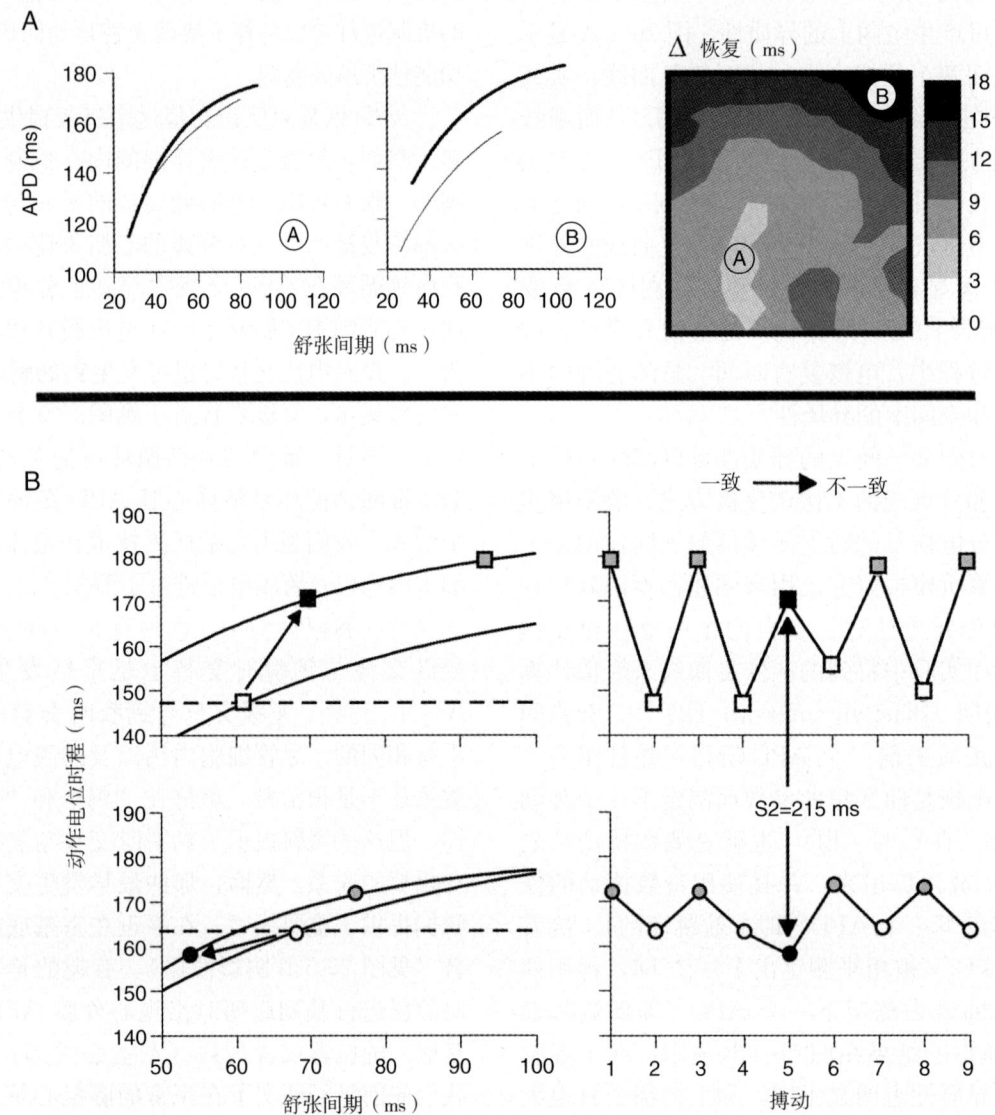

图 26-4 恢复的时间和空间异质性 A：在跨过心尖（位置 A）到心室基底部（位置 B）两个代表性位置在交替期奇数搏动和偶数搏动的恢复曲线。通过轮廓图可以显示出，Δ-恢复的变化（奇数和偶数恢复曲线的差异）遍及整个标测阵列。B：使用来自实验的恢复曲线（左）在一个恢复时间异质性高（上）以及低（下）位点上计算机的模拟结果。稳态交替由白色及灰色的图形表示。注意，当一个提前刺激应用于一个短的提前配对间期，在一个小的 Δ-恢复位点就可以造成时相逆转，但不是在 Δ-恢复大的地方，后者可导致不协调交替

竭时，钙循环的异常[43]、T 波交替以及心律失常的易损性[44]都是增加的。

三、细胞间耦联使复极同步化

细胞间耦联在生理性电传导中的作用是毋庸置疑的。但是，细胞内耦联在相邻细胞同步化复极以及复极离散中的重要性可能并不是很明显。从理论上来讲，局部膜电流以及邻近细胞间的电张力电流共同负责跨膜电位。事实上，计算机模拟实验已经证实，细胞间耦联的进行性减少可以减少电张力电流，并且还可显示出膜复极电流的内在跨膜异质性[45,46]。还需要指出的是，对犬左室楔形标本的实验表明，在耦联比较好的心肌，APD 在跨越不同细胞类型（心外膜层，

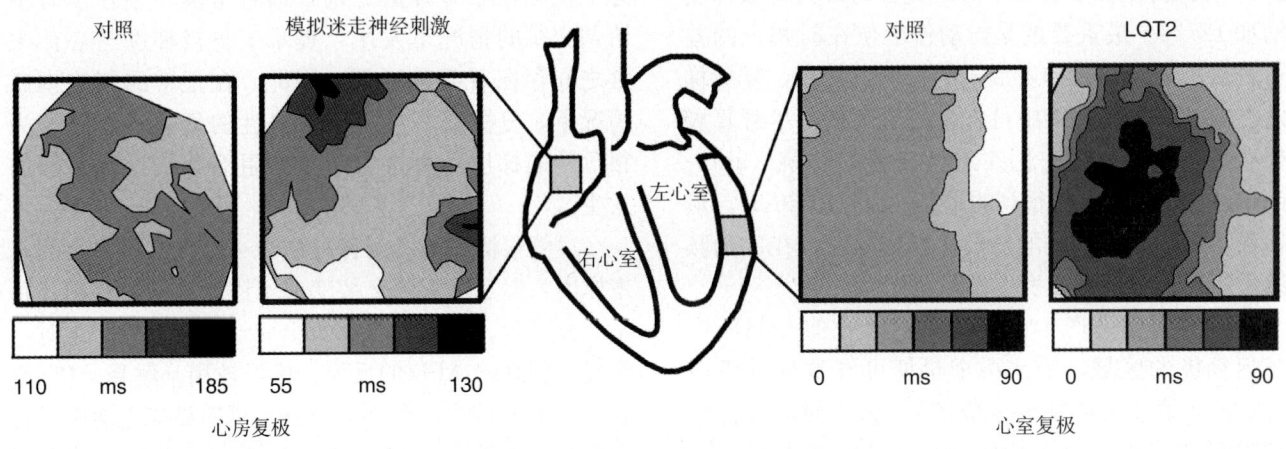

图 26-2 在对照以及有内在复极电流的不均一性增强情况下，心房（左）和心室（右）的复极示意图　在正常情况下，心房和心室的复极梯度相对小。但是，在模拟迷走神经刺激的情况下（IPS）以及长 QT 综合征 2 型（LQT2）时，心房和心室的复极梯度都明显增加

大增加了早搏诱发的房颤[26]，提示复极不均匀诱导的单向传导阻滞是房颤的一个重要机制。然而，一直以来，以高空间分辨率在细胞水平证实迷走神经介导房颤的机制是很难的，主要是没有一个良好的迷走神经刺激模型可用于在体实验。

我们已经证明，在离体灌流的犬右心房，迷走神经兴奋导致的心房复极梯度足以导致单向传导阻滞以及作为房性心律失常的发生机制[26]。采用高分辨率标测技术研究表明，心内副交感迷走神经对心房梳状肌区的复极模式可产生影响（图 26-2 右）。正常情况下（对照）的平均复极时间明显长于迷走兴奋时的平均复极时间。在迷走神经激动的情况下，最大复极梯度比起对照可明显增加（平均 160%）。这些数据证明，在右心房游离壁，迷走激动可显著增加复极的离散度。而且，这个梯度差异足以可以导致单向传导阻滞以及大的折返激动。这个结果与先前在犬心进行双侧颈神经根刺激诱发房性心动过速的实验结果相一致[27]。有趣的是，迷走神经刺激的心房复极的最大梯度（13±3 ms/mm）[26]与 LQT2 时心室的最大复极梯度（12±2 ms/mm）相当[23]。然而与 LQTS 模型不同的是，迷走激动可通过缩短心房不应期而显著缩短心房平均复极时间。这也许可以解释为什么在 LQTS 模型中，折返激动与纤颤相比更容易形成，也更容易自发终止。

二、复极交替

从上述讨论可以知道心脏内离子通道病理性表达可产生复极的离散（不均匀），这在功能性折返发生的机制中起到关键性的作用。这种复极的离散在一些生理性干扰，如早搏、自主神经张力失衡或者缺血时可发生。发生的机制之一就是复极交替，即每隔一次心跳，复极的时程就发生一次周期性的变化（可表现在动作电位或心电图的 T 波）。这有很重要的临床意义[28]，因为从心电图上可看到 T 波交替就意味着患者处于室性心律失常发生的易损期，在许多病理情况下容易出现室性心律失常[29-31]。使用光学标测技术，我们已经证明复极交替是一种通过复极梯度促进功能性折返产生的独特机制。

以常规的周长（Cycle length）进行刺激的时候，复极交替可引起级联的心电事件发生，导致折返性室颤（ventricular fibrillation，VF）[32,33]。首先，在一个阈值心率之上，所有细胞随心跳（beat-to-beat）出现的膜复极交替都是发生在同一个时相（也就是一致性交替），其典型表现为心电图上毫伏水平的 T 波交替。协调性交替现象只与复极离散度的交替有关，而且这种复极离散度的交替并不伴有复极梯度方向的改变。另外，对于这种随心跳进行的电冲动的传播也不会发生本质上的改变。当起搏频率进一步增加到邻近心肌细胞也开始向相反的时相发生交替时，便产生了一个很危险的心率。由于这些细胞具有时相上的紊乱，因此被认为是不协调交替[34]。如图 26-3 所示，不协调交替在脉冲传导和复极模式及顺序上产生一些重要变化。首先，复极等时线（repolarization isochrone line）非常拥挤可形成陡峭的复极梯度（见图 26-

3 底)。对比协调性交替，不协调交替的最大复极梯度可增加 127%。最重要的是，动作电位在时相上的差异可直接影响到这些梯度形成的程度。其次，复极梯度的方向在一次次心跳中可发生完全翻转。尽管复极的模式是复杂的，但它们在这种交替的心跳（alternate beat）发生上有着很高的重复性（见图 26-3）。最后，当与先前心跳产生的复极梯度逆向时，在冲动频率减慢后，传导就开始发生交替变化。

在不协调交替产生的情况下，由先前心跳所产生延迟复极的区域，引入一个早搏可导致传导阻滞（见图 26-3 第 3 个心跳的复极图）。脉冲便沿线性功能性阻滞区的两边向下传导，并且从标测图显示以外的区域折返回来，形成了折返性室颤的第一个自发性心跳。重要的是，在这些实验里，不协调交替总是发生在心室纤颤之前，而且室颤不会在没有不协调交替的情况下发生，提示了复极梯度与心律失常之间存在着某种联系。因此，在正常的细胞耦联情况下，复极交替可从相对良性的复极梯度转变为很危险的梯度，直接参与单向阻滞和折返性室颤的发生。

尽管很清楚复极交替可作为一个致心律失常的基本原因，但是从协调交替变成不协调交替的机制还是不十分清楚。电恢复（electrical restitution），是对一个提前刺激的 APD 的反应，已经被用来解释 APD 交替的发生机制[35]。然而，电恢复可明显受先前有无过早搏动（也就是心脏记忆）的影响，而且它在有无 APD 交替是不同的。例如，在有交替的时候，恢复曲线（restitution curve）可通过一个伴随长间期搏动的

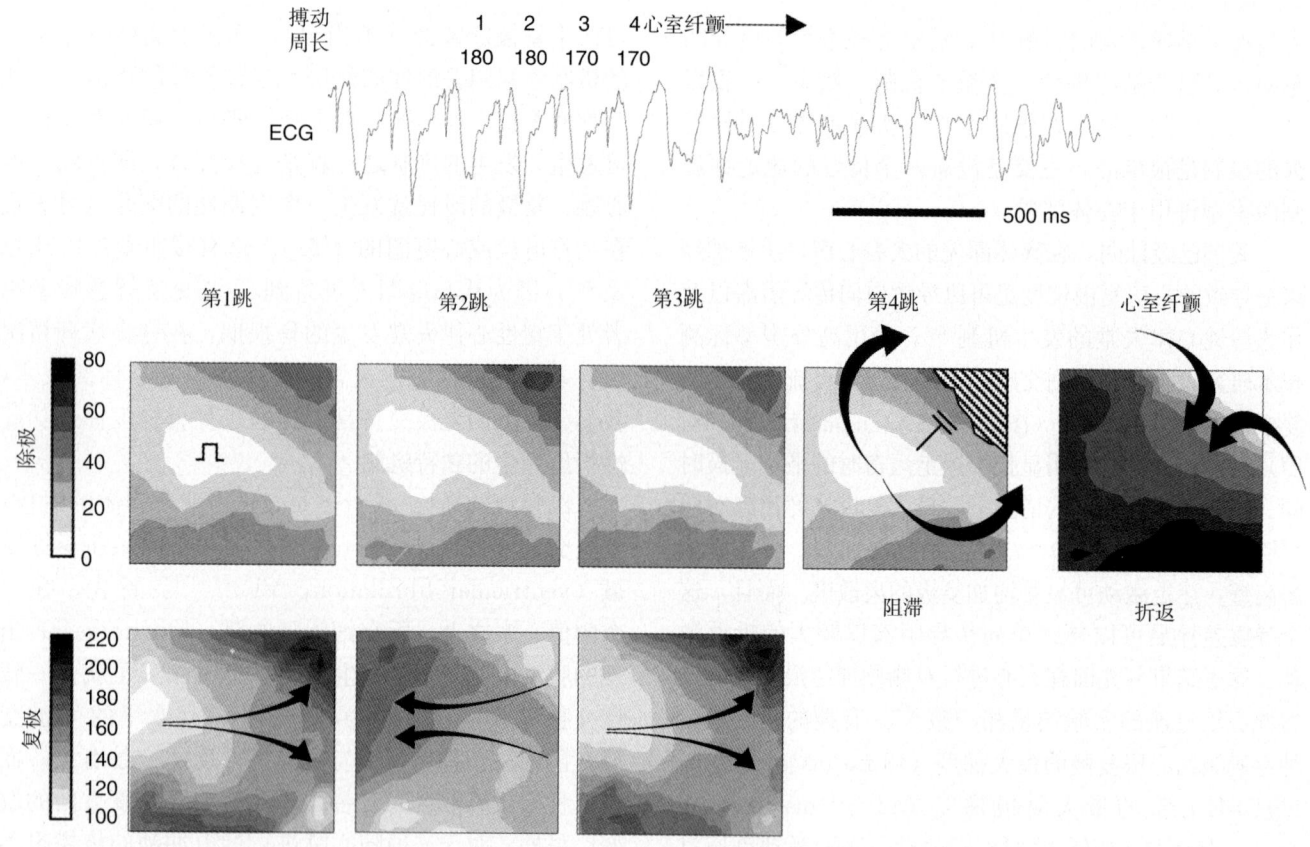

图 26-3 举例说明折返性心室纤维颤动（VF）的发生与复极交替相关　豚鼠心外膜的去极化和复极模式示意图（时间以 ms 表示）。当起搏频率加快的时候，不协调交替增强了，复极梯度的方向随着心跳（beat-to-beat）产生了完全翻转，更重要的是，这种陡峭的梯度在协调交替的时候并不会出现（资料未显示）。这些梯度为折返的产生创造了适宜的基础，因为刺激周长的轻度缩短（第四跳）使得对着复极梯度方向的局部传导失败，这种复极梯度是由先前心跳产生的（第三个搏动复极图的右上角）。不协调交替对于单向阻滞的发生是必需的，随之便可发生折返性心室颤动。在图上方显示的心电图（ECG）可作为参考（引自 Laurita KR, Pastore JM, Rownbaum DS：Maping arrhythmia substrates related to repolarization：I. Dispersion of repolarization. In Rosenbaum D, Jalife J [ed]：Optical Mapping of Cardiac Excitation and Arrhythias Armonk NY，Futura Publishing Co，2001：p205-225.）

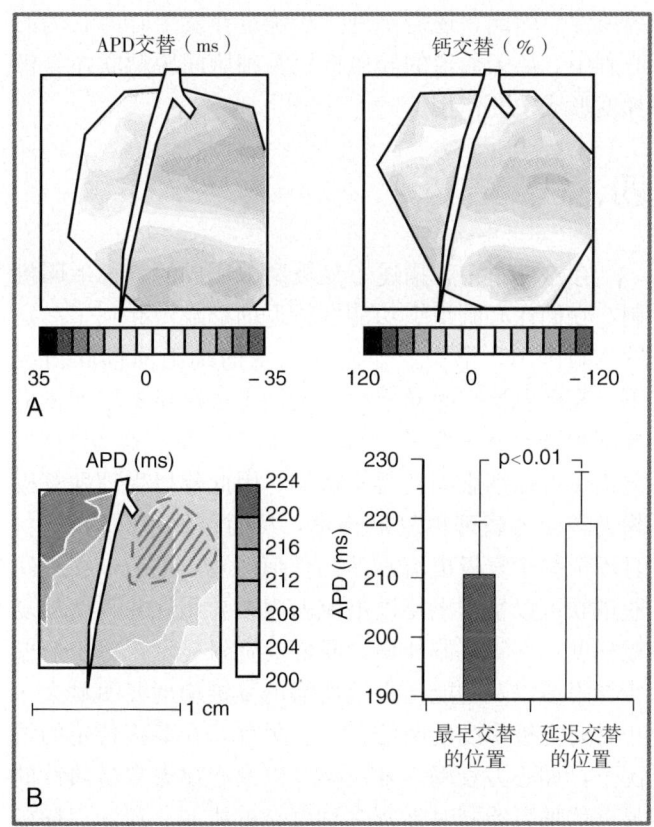

图 26-5 A：在 375 bpm 的起搏频率下，豚鼠心脏左前降支对应的心外膜面的动作电位时程（APD）（左）及钙瞬变交替（右）的标测图。红色指示两个连续搏动的 APD 及钙瞬变强度的增加，而蓝色表示降低。APD 交替和 CaF 交替在空间上都显示出不协调，邻近区域发生相反的时相交替。APD 梯度的方向是从右室基底部指向左室心尖，与左室前降支成直角（B左）。APD 以及钙瞬时交替可经常性的发生在左室基底部，且不依赖于起搏位置。重要的是，在 APD 最长或者最短的地方都不会发生交替。在所有的实验中都被观察相似的结果（B）。在 150 bpm 基础起搏频率下，最早发生交替位置（左室基底部）的 APD 显著短于最迟发生交替位置的 APD（右室基底部）（原书无彩图，译者注）

中层，心内膜层）的差异比游离的同一细胞类型的 APD 的差异要小[23,47]。我们综合计算机模拟以及实验研究结果，提出邻近细胞间的电张力电流可以减弱 APD 缩短，因此减少复极的离散[48]。同样，细胞间耦联可以显著影响复极梯度。

在生理与病理情况下，当考虑到跨过透壁肌层之间的电耦联的不均匀时，细胞间耦联与复极梯度之间的关系就变得更加复杂。例如，Yan 和同事们[47]使用细胞外电极，测量了动脉灌流的犬心楔形组织标本的跨膜组织阻抗。结果他们发现，心外膜层与心外膜下层之间的组织阻抗比与中层和心内膜层都大。跨膜 APD 也是不均匀的，在表层下的肌层组织中，APD 明显增加。跨膜组织间的阻抗与 APD 之间的紧密联系提示，细胞间耦联以及预先存在的离子通道的内在异质性，在跨膜复极梯度的形成中起到十分重要的作用。这些资料提供了有价值的细胞间耦联和复极梯度之间关系的认识。但是，因为在心脏整体中测量细胞间耦联的作用十分困难，这就使得很难得出太多的结论。

我们研究小组已经发明了在整体心肌应用光学标测技术测量细胞间耦联的方法[49]。使用电压敏感染料，能够以很高的分辨率测量到亚阈值刺激的跨膜电位的空间分布。亚阈值反应在空间上的衰变可为一个指数，由此计算出的心脏空间常数可以作为细胞间耦联的一个敏感指标。我们已经用这种方法测量了犬心楔形组织标本跨膜细胞间耦联。图 26-6 A 显示了八个不同标本的跨膜空间常数（λ_{TM}）。在心外膜下层的 λ_{TM} 显著短于深层的 λ_{TM}。而用共聚焦免疫荧光方法定量检测的缝隙连接蛋白 43（Cx43）的表达，也显示出了类似的模式（图 26-6B）。心外膜下层缝隙连接蛋白 43 的表达明显少于其他层。在心外膜下层深部测量跨膜传导速度以及动作电位上升支所用时间（数据未列出）的结果与心外膜下层深部细胞间耦联的急剧降低相一致。在同一种实验模型中，λ_{TM} 以及缝隙连接蛋白 43 表达的跨膜异质性与 APD 的跨膜模式的比较可以见图 26-6 C。最长的 APD 发生在中层心肌，其次是心外膜下层的深部，而且有趣的是，在细胞间耦联减低（图 26-6A-B）的心外膜下层与心外膜下层深部之间存在 APD 最大的跨膜梯度（图 26-6 D）。细胞大小以及细胞外基质的组织学分析并不能解释 λ_{TM} 的异质性。因此，这些资料提示在有正常耦联的心肌组织，缝隙连接蛋白 43 的异质性表达能够解释参与维持跨膜复极梯度的电生理功能的异质性。

在正常情况下，细胞间耦联的跨膜异质性并不认为能够显著增加复极的梯度，因为心脏在正常情况下并不倾向发生心律失常。而且，需要指出的是，即使存在明显的细胞间脱耦联，如果没有复极电流空间上异质性的存在，复极梯度是可以忽略不计的。但是，在某些细胞间脱耦联的情况下，这种良性的内在复极异质性可转变为致心律失常的复极梯度。例如，在减少细胞间耦联的情况下，不协调交替更容易出现[50]。同样，在心力衰竭和缺血的情况下，细胞间脱耦联的发生可以使心律失常增加[51,52]。使用光学标测技术，我们已经揭示衰竭心肌可出现跨膜复极梯度的显著增加，而且足以引起折返性室性心律失常[53]。但是，也有可能在心力衰竭时出现加重的心脏复极电流的空间异质性。因此，还需要进一步确定在发生心力衰竭的心脏中，离子通道的异质性以及细胞间脱耦联在复极梯度形成中的作用。

四、总结

在这一章中，描述了复极离散形成的三种不同机制，它们在心脏组织功能性折返的形成中起到了一定的基础作用。第一，即使在正常的细胞间耦联情况下，复极电流空间异质性的增加也可以显著增加复极梯度和致心律失常的易损性。第二，在T波交替时，复极交替在细胞间变得不协调，因此使得生理性复极梯度转变为病理性复极梯度，从而导致室颤的发生，且不依赖于复极电流表达的任何改变。最后，细胞间脱耦联可以暴露出复极电流的内在异质性并且增加复极梯度。不管机制如何，我们的资料显示，对于形成传导阻滞以及功能性折返所需的复极梯度要明显大于正常时复极梯度的两倍[13,54]。另外，在某些特定的情况下，如心力衰竭，复极梯度以及心律失常易损性的显著增加可能同时涉及多种复杂的机制。在这三种机制中，光学标测技术起到了十分重要的作用，因为：（1）它能以高准确度以及高分辨率对复极化梯度进行定量；（2）有助于理解复极梯度增加的细胞机制；（3）证明这些梯度与单向传导阻滞和折返激动之间有直接因果关系。

（张幼怡　龚开政　徐　宁 译）

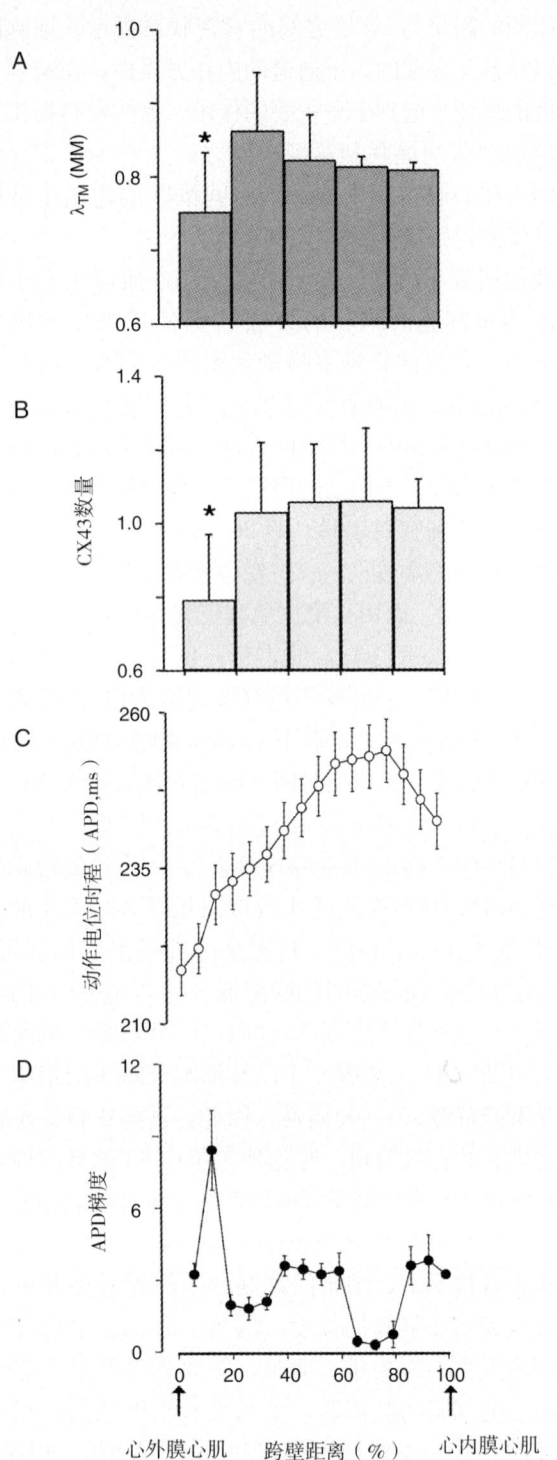

图26-6　A：与深层心肌比较，心外膜下跨膜空间常数出现显著的减低。（*$P<0.05$）B：同样地，与深层心肌比较心外膜下的缝隙连接蛋白43（Cx43）的表达也显著减低。C：动作电位时程（APD）的分布以及在起搏周长为2000 ms时，穿过犬左室壁的APD的情况分布。APD从表层到内层的变化是一个完整的过程。D：APD的衍化图显示，在跨心外膜表层13%～20%的距离可产生最大的APD梯度。（引自Poelzing S, Akar FG, Baron E, Rosenbaum DS: Heterogeneous connexin43 expression produces electrophysiologic heterogeneities across the ventricular wall. *Am J Physiol* 2004; 286: H2001-H2009.）

参 考 文 献

1. Schmitt FO, Erlanger J: Directional differences in the conduction of the impulse through heart muscle and their possible relation to extrasystolic and fibrillatory contractions. Am J Physiol 87:326–347, 1928.
2. Moe GK, Rheinboldt WC, Abldskov JA: A computer model of atrial fibrillation. Am Heart J 67:200–220, 1964.
3. Han J, Moe G: Nonuniform recovery of excitability in venticular muscle. Circ Res 14:44–60, 1964.
4. Allessie A, Bonke FI, Schopman FJG: Circus movement in rabbit atrial muscle as a mechanism of tachycardia: The role of nonuniform recovery of excitability in the occurrence of unidirectional block as studied with multiple microelectrodes. Circ Res 39:169–177, 1976.
5. Laurita KR, Girouard SD, Akar FG, Rosenbaum DS: Modulated dispersion explains changes in arrhythmia vulnerability during premature stimulation of the heart. Circulation 98:2774–2780, 1998.
6. Wit A, Allessie M, Bonke F, et al: Electrophysiologic mapping to determine the mechanism of experimental ventricular tachycardia intiated by premature impulses. Am J Cardiol 49:166–185, 1982.
7. Spach MS, Dolber PC: The relation between discontinuous propagation in anisotropic cardiac muscle and the "vulnerable period" of reentry. In Zipes DP, Jalife J (eds): Cardiac Electrophysiology and Arrhythmias. Orlando: Grune & Stratton, 1985, pp 241–251.
8. Davidenko J, Cabo C, Jalife J: Wave-front curvature leads to slow conduction and block in two-dimensional cardiac muscle. In Spooner P, Joyner R, Jalife J (eds): Discontinuous Conduction in the Heart.

Armonk, NY: Futura Publishing, 1997, pp 295–320.
9. Litovsky SH, Antzelevitch C: Transient outward current prominent in canine ventricular epicardium but not endocardium. Circ Res 62:116–126, 1988.
10. Fedida D, Giles WR: Regional variations in action potentials and transient outward current in myocytes isolated from rabbit left ventricle. J Physiol (Lond) 442:191–209, 1991.
11. Sicouri S, Antzelevitch C: A subpopulation of cells with unique electrophysiological properties in the deep subepicardium of the canine ventricle: The M cell. Circ Res 68:1729–1741, 1991.
12. Liu D-W, Antzelevitch C: Characteristics of the delayed rectifier current (I_{Kr} and I_{Ks}) in canine ventricular epicardial, midmyocardial, and endocardial myocytes: A weaker I_{Ks} contributes to the longer action potential of the M cell. Circ Res 76:351–365, 1995.
13. Laurita KR, Girouard SD, Rosenbaum DS: Modulation of ventricular repolarization by a premature stimulus: Role of epicardial dispersion of repolarization kinetics demonstrated by optical mapping of the intact guinea pig heart. Circ Res 79:493–503, 1996.
14. Curran ME, Splawski I, Timothy KW, et al: A molecular basis for cardiac arrhythmia: *HERG* mutations cause long QT syndrome. Cell 80:795–803, 1995.
15. Wang Q, Shen J, Splawski I, et al: *SCN5A* mutations associated with an inherited cardiac arrhythmia, long QT syndrome. Cell 80:805–811, 1995.
16. Wang Q, Curran ME, Splawski I, et al: Positional cloning of a novel potassium channel gene: *KVLQT1* mutations cause cardiac arrhythmias. Nat Genet 12:17–23, 1996.
17. Dessertenne F: La tachycardie ventriculaire a duex foyers opposes variables. Arch Mal Coeur 59:263–272, 1966.
18. Priori SG, Napolitano C, Diehl L, Schwartz PJ: Dispersion of the QT interval: A marker of therapeutic efficacy in the idiopathic long QT syndrome. Circulation 89:1681–1689, 1994.
19. Sanguinetti MC, Curran ME, Zou A, et al: Coassembly of K_vLQT1 and minK (IsK) proteins to form cardiac I_{Ks} potassium channel. Nature 384:80–83, 1996.
20. Sanguinetti MC: Dysfunction of delayed rectifier potassium channels in an inherited cardiac arrhythmia. Ann NY Acad Sci 868:406–413, 1999.
21. Shimizu W, Antzelevitch C: Cellular basis for the ECG features of the LQT1 form of the long-QT syndrome: Effects of beta-adrenergic agonists and antagonists and sodium channel blockers on transmural dispersion of repolarization and torsade de pointes. Circulation 98:2314–2322, 1998.
22. El-Sherif N, Caref EB, Yin H, Restivo M: The electrophysiological mechanism of ventricular arrhythmias in the long QT syndrome: Tridimensional mapping of activation and recovery patterns. Circ Res 79:474–492, 1996.
23. Akar FG, Yan GX, Antzelevitch C, Rosenbaum DS: Unique topographical distribution of m cells underlies reentrant mechanism of torsade de pointes in the long-QT syndrome. Circulation 105:1247–1253, 2002.
24. Liu L, Nattel S: Differing sympathetic and vagal effects on atrial fibrillation in dog: Role of refractoriness heterogeneity. Am J Physiol 273:H805–H816, 1997.
25. Chiou CW, Eble JN, Zipes DP: Efferent vagal innervation of the canine atria and sinus and atrioventricular nodes: The third fat pad. Circulation 95:2573–2584, 1997.
26. Hirose M, Carlson MD, Laurita KR: Cellular mechanisms of vagally mediated atrial tachyarrhythmia in isolated arterially perfused canine right atria. J Cardiovasc Electrophysiol 13:918–926, 2002.
27. Wang J, Liu L, Feng J, Nattel S: Regional and functional factors determining induction and maintenance of atrial fibrillation in dogs. Am J Physiol 271:H148–H158, 1996.
28. Rosenbaum DS, Jackson LE, Smith JM, et al: Electrical alternans and vulnerability to ventricular arrhythmias. N Engl J Med 330:235–241, 1994.
29. Salerno JA, Previtali M, Panciroli C, et al: Ventricular arrhythmias during acute myocardial ischemia in man. The role and significance of R-ST-T alternans and the prevention of ischemic sudden death by medical treatment. Eur Heart J 7:63–75, 1986.
30. Platt SB, Vijgen JM, Albrecht P, et al: Occult T wave alternans in long QT syndrome. J Cardiovasc Electrophysiol 7:144–148, 1996.
31. Walker ML, Rosenbaum DS: Repolarization alternans: Implications for the mechanism and prevention of sudden cardiac death. Cardiovasc Res 57:599–614, 2003.
32. Pastore JM, Girouard SD, Laurita KR, et al: Mechanism linking T-wave alternans to the genesis of cardiac fibrillation. Circulation 99:1385–1394, 1999.
33. Laurita K, Pastore J, Rosenbaum D: Mapping arrhythmia substrates related to repolarization: 1. Dispersion of repolarization. In Rosenbaum D, Jalife J (eds): Optical Mapping of Cardiac Excitation and Arrhythmias. New York, NY: Futura Publishing, 2001, pp 205–225.
34. Hirata Y, Toyama J, Yamada K: Effects of hypoxia or low pH on the alteration of canine ventricular action potentials following an abrupt increase in driving rate. Cardiovasc Res 14:108–115, 1980.
35. Koller M, Riccio M, Gilmour R: Dynamic restitution of action potential duration during electrical alternans and ventricular fibrillation. Am J Physiol 275:H1635–H1642, 1998.
36. Rubenstein DS, Lipsius SL: Premature beats elicit a phase reversal of mechanoelectrical alternans in cat ventricular myocytes: A possible mechanism for reentrant arrhythmias. Circulation 91:201–214, 1995.
37. Pastore JM, Rosenbaum DS: Spatial and temporal heterogeneities of cellular restitution are responsible for arrhythmogenic discordant alternans [abstract]. Circulation 100:I-51, 1999.
38. Hüser J, Wang YG, Sheehan KA, et al: Functional coupling between glycolysis and excitation-contraction coupling underlies alternans in cat heart cells. J Physiol (Lond) 524:795–806, 2000.
39. Laurita KR, Singal A: Mapping action potentials and calcium transients simultaneously from the intact heart. Am J Physiol 280:H2053–H2060, 2001.
40. Pruvot EJ, Katra RP, Rosenbaum DS, Laurita KR: Role of calcium cycling versus restitution in the mechanism of repolarization alternans. Circ Res 94:1083–1090, 2004.
41. Katra RP, Pruvot E, Laurita KR: Intracellular calcium handling heterogeneities in intact guinea pig hearts. Am J Physiol 286:H648-H656, 2004.
42. Laurita KR, Katra RP, Wible B, et al: Transmura heterogeneity of calcium handling in canine. Circ Res 92:668–675, 2003.
43. O'Rourke B, Kass DA, Tomaselli GF, et al: Mechanisms of altered excitation-contraction coupling in canine tachycardia-induced heart failure. I. Experimental studies. Circ Res 84:562–570, 1999.
44. Klingenheben T, Zabel M, D'Agostino RB, et al: Predictive value of T-wave alternans for arrhythmic events in patients with congestive heart failure. Lancet 356:651–652, 2000.
45. Viswanathan PC, Shaw RM, Rudy Y: Effects of I_{Kr} and I_{Ks} heterogeneity on action potential duration and tts rate dependence: A simulation study. Circulation 99:2466–2474, 1999.
46. Lesh MD, Pring M, Spear JF: Cellular uncoupling can unmask dispersion of action potential duration in ventricular myocardium: A computer modeling study. Circ Res 65:1426–1440, 1989.
47. Yan GX, Shimizu W, Antzelevitch C: Characteristics and distribution of M cells in arterially perfused canine left ventricular wedge preparations. Circulation 98:1921–1927, 1998.
48. Laurita KR, Girouard SD, Rudy Y, Rosenbaum DS: Role of passive electrical properties during action potential restitution in the intact heart. Am J Physiol 273:H1205–H1214, 1997.
49. Akar F, Roth B, Rosenbaum D: Optical measurement of cell-to-cell coupling in intact heart using subthreshold electrical stimulation. Am J Physiol 281:H533–H542, 2001.
50. Pastore JM, Rosenbaum DS: Role of structural barriers in the mechanism of alternans-induced reentry. Circ Res 87:1157–1163, 2000.
51. Peters NS: New insights into myocardial arrhythmogenesis: Distribution of gap-junctional coupling in normal, ischaemic and hypertrophied human hearts. Glaxo/MRS Young Investigator Prize. Clin Sci 90:447–452, 1996.
52. Peters NS, Green CR, Poole-Wilson PA, Severs NJ: Reduced content of connexin43 gap junctions in ventricular myocardium from hypertrophied and ischemic human hearts. Circulation 88:864–875, 1993.
53. Akar FG, Rosenbaum DS: Transmural electrophysiological heterogeneities underlying arrhythmogenesis in heart failure. Circ Res 93:638–645, 2003.
54. Laurita KR, Rosenbaum DS: Interdependence of modulated dispersion and tissue structure in the mechanism of unidirectional block. Circ Res 87:922–928, 2000.

第 27 章

机械电转换/反馈：普遍性及病理生理学意义

Max J. Lab

本章目录

- 机械电换能器在多种细胞广泛存在 …… 238
- 机械电转换在多种属、多组织及电生理学上广泛存在 …………………… 240
- 机械电转换的病理生理学改变-临床表现，是心律失常的基本机制 ………… 242
- 治疗方法 …………………………… 246
- 理论上的深思 ……………………… 246

机械电转换（mechanoelectric transduction）是一个广泛存在的生物物理学现象，它是指将机械刺激转换成电信号的过程。而"反馈"是生物物理学控制调节的一个重要机制，具有重要的病理生理意义。目前发现了越来越多的机械电转换现象，一个新的概念正在逐渐形成：即机械电转换现象在心脏生理及病理生理学中的实际作用可能比预想的更大。这并不奇怪，心脏最基本的生理功能是机械性的，大部分病理改变都会引起机械方面的紊乱。电是驱动维持生命的机械泵的动力。因此，机械电转换/反馈从细胞到临床都已构成一种重要的保护方式。本章首先重点讲述转换的概念，然后从理论上及病理生理学方面阐述它的普遍意义。由于篇幅的限制，我们不再罗列以前发表的资料，而是集中对其进行概略式的阐述。一些学者已经对此现象做了大量的综述，其中一些很具有代表性[1-14]。本章所引用的参考文献大多都是比较新的，但在为了强调某个概念时也引用了早期文献。

一、机械电换能器在多种细胞广泛存在

（一）短期（急性）机械敏感通道（被动，舒张）

已经证明，在许多组织包括心脏，都存在特异性机械门控或牵张激活通道（stretch activated channels, SACs, 见图 27-1A）[15]，也可参阅本书第 11 章。膜的牵张增加了通道的开放几率，以此来接纳带电离子，从而对膜电位产生影响。在整体心脏上，通过记录单相动作电位（monophasic action potentials, MAP）获得对细胞电生理特性的定性认识，通道的电生理特性在整体心脏上是相同的。需要注意的是，有一类反向电位（reversal potential）[6]，如果给予过早牵张会产生复极化倾向，而迟一点的牵张可导致去极化。反向电位本身不会发生什么改变。SAC 阻断剂被广泛用于研究机械传导现象，但是对使用这些阻断剂的实验结果解释要慎重。链霉素作为阻断剂，其在整体心房上的作用就存在异质性[16]。

还有其他几种通道看来也是机械敏感型的[14]，包括 ATP 依赖的钾通道（K_{ATP} 见图 27-1A 9 点钟位置）、L-型钙通道（L-type Ca channel, LTCC）、钠通道以及串联孔钾通道（tandem pore potassium, 2-PK, 见图 27-1A 8 点钟位置）如 TREK-1 和 IKAA，以及离子交换器（ion exchanger）（见图 27-1 A 3 点钟位置）。后面会有证据表明，机械压力/张力通过与之级联的磷酸激酶 A 及钙通道可对 β 肾上腺素受体产生影响（见图 27-1 A 11 点钟位置）。毒蕈碱型乙酰胆碱受

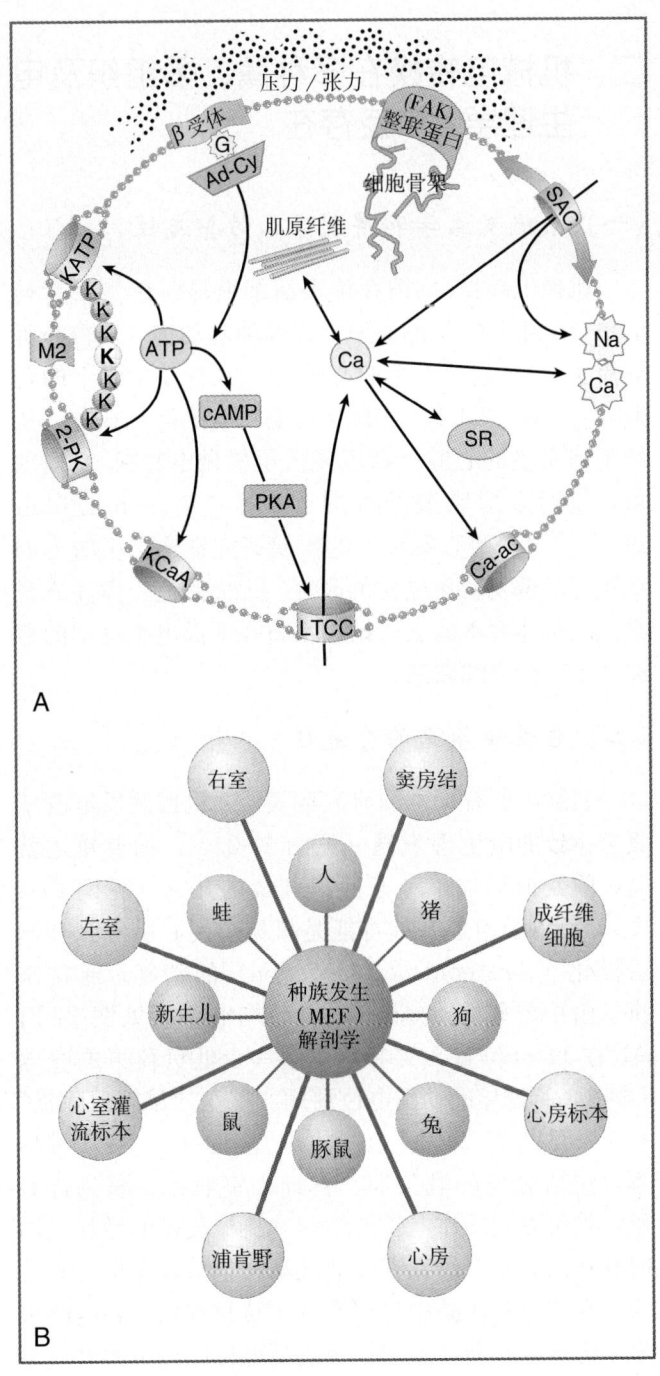

图 27-1 机械电转换在细胞学、系统发生学和解剖学上普遍存在 A：启动机械电转换/反馈的细胞换能器图示。机械压力/张力（顶部）通过细胞外基质（如图散点所示）传导到细胞膜上，这些机械力的变化会通过整合素及粘着斑激酶（focal adhesion kinases, FAK）调节换能器然后传到细胞内部及细胞骨架上（1 点钟的位置）。在膜上分布着多种可以影响电的机械敏感型通道或受体。比如牵张激活通道（SACs，2 点钟位置）开放接纳 Na^+ 和 Ca^{2+}，前者通过影响 Na^+/Ca^{2+} 交换（3 点钟位置）进而影响动作电位，后者通过增加肌浆网负荷来增加胞内 Ca^{2+} 浓度。其他可以快速影响电的机械敏感型通道，包括三磷酸腺苷（adenosine triphosphate, ATP）依赖的 K^+ 通道（K_{ATP}，10 点钟位置），L-型钙通道（L-type Ca channel, LTCC，6 点钟位置）和串联孔钾通道（tandem pore potassium，2-PK，8 点钟位置）。机械改变可以影响一些受体及它们的 G 蛋白。β 肾上腺素受体可以被环磷酸腺苷（cyclic adenosine monophosphate, cAMP）、腺苷酸环化酶（adenyl cyclase, AC）和 ATP 激活（机械敏感型的毒蕈碱型 G 蛋白门控乙酰胆碱受体，M_2，在 9 点钟位置，与细胞内 K^+ 靠近）。机械性的诱导 ATP 改变也可以对其他通道产生影响，包括牵张激活的 KCa-ATP 通道（KCaA，在 7 点钟位置）、2-PK、TREK-1（与 2-PK 一起位于 8 点钟位置）。肌纤维的机械改变（中心位置）对胞内 Ca^{2+} 的影响是至关重要的。除了影响 Na^+/Ca^{2+} 交换之外，它还可以影响前面提到的一些通道以及其他 Ca^{2+} 活化的通道（Ca-ac 位于 5 点钟方向）。B：系统发生学和解剖学上的普遍性。在系统发生学上（内部组），从两栖动物、哺乳动物到人类都存在机械电转换/反馈。从解剖学上来看（外部组），几乎所有动物亚门的心脏都存在机械电转换/反馈。

体（M_2）也是机械敏感型的，它在图 27-1 A 9 点钟位置，属于内向整流 K^+ 通道超家族，存在于心房和窦房结上，GIRK1~4（也称 Kir3.1~3.4）可以被 G 蛋白和机械牵张调节。

机械刺激诱导 ATP 改变的证据正在逐渐增多[14]，包括 Ca^{2+} 活化的 K^+ 通道（KCa），类似于牵张激活的 KCa-ATP 通道。大 K^+ 通道（111±3.0 pS），如 TREK-1，在成年大鼠的心室肌细胞上被发现不仅是机械敏感的，也可以被细胞内低 pH 或细胞内 ATP 激活。

（二）短期（急性）-主动（收缩期）肌原纤维/钙的相互作用充当换能器

主动的肌原纤维收缩也有一种转换机制（见图 27-1A，肌原纤维）。等张（缩短）肌虽然产生的力量逐渐减小，但与被牵张/等长肌相比动作电位时程（action potential duration, APD）和钙瞬变时程（duration calcium transient）较长。这看起来有些违反直觉，缩短肌肉伴随力的下降，但这可减少肌钙蛋白-C对钙的结合，在产生力低时增加细胞内钙。钙的升高可能影响几种跨膜电流从而延长APD，例如通过钠/钙交换（见图27-1A 双向箭头）和钙活化电流（见图27-1A 5点位置）。这些钙离子相关的内容可参阅已发表的综述[17]。

（三）长期-细胞信号级联反应是机械换能器的作用机制

机械刺激也可以启动环磷酸腺苷（cyclic adenosine monophosphate，cAMP）等多种二级信号转导级联反应（见图27-1 A 中心偏左的位置）[14]。先前已对一些机械-化学敏感通道，如通道运载而非特异性牵张激活的离子电流进行了详细的论述[18]。其他受体也可提供换能器，这些受体首先通过肌醇三磷酸（inositol triphosphate，IP3）和肌浆网钙释放调节胞内钙，其次通过磷脂C（phospholipase C，PLC）促进膜转位（membrane translocation）调节Na^+/H^+交换，进而通过Na^+/Ca^{2+}交换调节细胞内钙浓度。细胞钙浓度的改变产生了电的变化。

（四）细胞骨架的作用，包括张力整合体（Tensegrity）

机械传导可以由胞内细胞骨架调节，细胞骨架通过粘着斑复合体插入细胞膜（见图27-1A 1点位置）[6,14]。部分细胞骨架与离子通道的功能有关。许多刺激与机械电化学通道共用信号通路，从而产生复合反应。细胞骨架形成的机械工程，成为了细胞内和细胞间生物化学信息交流的基础。任何与细胞骨架相关的膜通道都可能引起胞内外信息的交流，而且压力-张力也可以通过细胞骨架传到通道上。但是，细胞骨架在机械传导中的确切作用尚不清楚。它可以通过脂质膜屏蔽张力传递而激活或者关闭（splint）通道。在生理情况下，机械交联系统（mechanical interconnecting system）有预应力（prestress）存在，形成张力整合体参与维持机械的平衡和稳定。细胞间力的传导主要集中在细胞膜粘着斑复合体上，这部分细胞膜附着于细胞外基质，且含有整合素和与胞内肌动蛋白（细胞骨架的主要成分）结合的蛋白质。这样就构成了一个很清晰的从细胞外基质到细胞内胞浆结构的力学传导通路。

二、机械电转换在多种属、多组织及电生理学上广泛存在

（一）系统发生学和解剖学上的普遍性

机械电转换/反馈在许多活细胞都存在[15]，青蛙的单个细胞到完整的心室，以及哺乳动物（原位心脏灌流实验），包括人类的心脏[14]。系统发生学上的普遍性可见图27-1 B。实际上心脏所有的解剖成分，从细胞到完整的心腔，都表现出了机械电转换/反馈现象，包括心房肌成纤维细胞、窦房结[19]和心房组织[3,16,20]。一些心室标本的实验研究证实，机械力的变化可以诱发动作电位的改变。表面灌流、灌注或者是原位整体标本的实验结果都将在下面电生理学的普遍性中进行详细叙述。

（二）电生理学上的普遍性

实际上所有标本的研究都表明，机械诱发电改变具有一致的电生理表现（见图27-2）[6]。简要重述就是，膜变形增加了离子通道开放的几率（见图27-2左），而离子通道开放可能是机械诱发心脏舒张和阈去极化（threshold depolarization）的基础。通常来讲，由一个较大负荷诱导的动作电位（见图27-2；AP在11点位置，实心）比起一个低负荷下的收缩（虚线）所诱导的动作电位要短。这与"早期后除极"相关（见图27-2；AP在1点位置，实心）。在多种标本，包括分离的乳头肌、青蛙心室肌条、灌流蛙心脏，均可看到动作电位的缩短和机械负荷的增加是同时存在的。几个研究室在哺乳动物包括人完整心脏灌流及在体心脏实验中也观察到了这种现象。心电图可显示机械电反馈，用来记录表面电位。它是通过一组导线将细胞动作电位通过心脏的多相传导所产生的电矢量之和进行显示。随着负荷的降低，心电图QT间期延长（见图27-2 心电图，2点位置）。在评价复极电生理的不均匀性上，T波比QT间期更直接。复极是从心外膜到心内膜，从基底部到心尖部，与去极化的路线正好相反。因而产生了同向的向量，表现为心电图上不规则的直立T波。心肌内的收缩也是不均匀的，所以机械电反馈可能起调节作用。机械负荷可以改变T波（见图27-2 心电图，2点位置）。这可能是调节区域性力学不均匀性的容积变化（见图27-3B）[21]。当然也有一些关于T波随着容积改

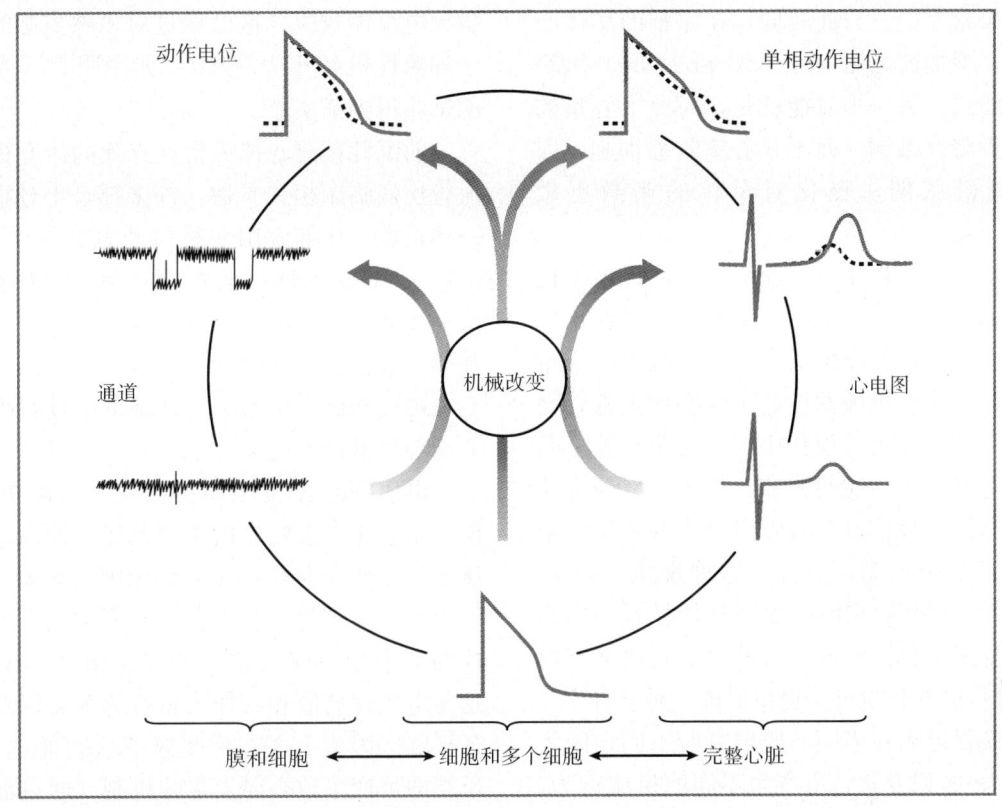

图 27-2 概括电生理学上的普遍性（电生理记录如图所示） 实验研究显示机械导致的电位改变（环底部表示未施压/牵张，环顶部表示施压/牵张后）所表现出的电生理特性基本是一致的。膜和细胞（左）-机械敏感通道，摒弃单个无意义的信号（水平记录，8 点位置），膜变形（如微吸管吸入、渗透性肿胀、细胞膨胀）可增加通道开放的几率（记录呈音阶式改变，10 点位置）。细胞和多个细胞（中央）-静息（舒张期）膜电位。正常的动作电位如图 6 点所示。微电极和抽吸电极分别产生动作电位（APs）和单相动作电位（MAPs），如图 11 点和 1 点所示。连续的或瞬时的牵拉使心肌去极化（实线的记录）。AP, 大负荷缩短了细胞的动作电位（11 点位置实线所示）。在整体心脏（右），心室的单相动作电位（1 点位置）表示出相当的变化，包括后除极。图中还显示了心电图（ECG），正常的心电图（4 点位置），负荷改变后 QT 间期和 T 波的变化（2 点位置，实线心电图，参见文内）

变而改变的单纯物理学解释。心电图的 U 波也可能会被机械改变调节，可能与早期后除极相关。

总之，观察到的这些现象是非常一致的，当然也有个别例外。尽管高机械负荷通常都缩短复极时相，有一些研究却显示高机械负荷可以延长复极时相。可能的解释就是发生在动作电位末尾的早期后除极实际上延长了动作电位。如果在 QT 间期出现一个粗钝的 U 波，则会使 QT 间期产生明显的延长。这样，不一致性可能仅仅只是表面现象。

（三）解释的缺陷

机械干扰导致电假象

机械电反馈的概念曾经受到质疑，尤其在整体心脏上。方法学上可测量机械变量（力量、长度和压力）和电生理变量（通道开放的几率、细胞内的动作电位、单相动作电位和心电图）。实验标本的任何机械变量改变都会改变电发生器和记录电极之间的关系。这是机械诱导电假象的根源，可能涉及到所有的标本。但是，由机械变化导致的电变化通常都很类似，且在不同的实验条件下，结果都比较一致。一个有影响力的研究表明，机械变化导致电生理改变通常与潜在的期前收缩以及心律失常的发生有关，后者更常见。虽然大多数实验都消除了假象的影响，但是对于一些特殊实验的解释仍然要慎重。在整体心室，由牵张诱发心律失常的报道比离体灌流实验中机械诱发心律失常的报道更常见。如果这是真的，除上述的机制以外，是否还有其他因子对整体心室起调节作用呢？内源性的儿茶酚胺可能是其中一种，它是一种天然的增加舒张期去极化阈值的物质。在整体心脏上，心得安可以抑制牵张诱发的心律失常，多巴酚丁胺则可以促进心律失常[6,14]。与此相同，在完整的离体心脏灌流实验中，增加流出压（outflow pressure）可释放更多的儿茶酚胺。另一种可能就是，对整个心室的牵拉可激活浦肯野纤维网，而不是心室收缩细胞，因为浦肯野纤维舒张期去极化对牵拉的刺激更敏感。

系统发生学、解剖学和电生理学的共性提示了机械电转换的生理作用[6,7]。首先，窦房结控制着正常心脏的心率，在去除神经支配的右心房，压力改变也可以调节心率，这就是机械调控的窦性心律失常，而通常窦性心律失常都只用外周和中枢反射来解释。其次，存在机械电对机械功能的调节。整体心脏的等长收缩就描述了这样一种情况，心腔内压力的逐步缓慢上升，可导致后负荷的急剧升高。这种现象（anrep效应）一直用心室局部血流的改变同时伴随着心内膜缺血的缓慢恢复来解释。然而，机械改变导致细胞内钙和/或动作电位的变化也可能提供另外一种解释[17]。

机械电转换很可能在不同心肌层有所不同，因为完整心脏的压力/容积变化，可产生不同的机械行为。在系统压力变化时，随着复极向量变化，心电图T波也发生改变，这在心室不同部位会产生不同的电生理效应。

三、机械电转换的病理生理学改变-临床表现，是心律失常的基本机制

在反馈环中一个适时的机械干扰会引起临床上与此相关的早搏，这不仅仅只在原位左心室，而且也可在右心室和心房[3,22]。机械电反馈越来越被认为是导致心源性猝死的重要机制之一。心源性猝死通常源于心律失常[11,12,23]。虽然这一部分讨论的心律失常主要与心室有关，但心房纤颤是人类（和马）最常见的心律失常，并且也可能致残和致死[24]。在心室发生的这些机制和相关因素也能运用于心房。心房扩大可能是导致房颤的必需因素[3]。

在临床上，心脏急性牵张所诱发的现象在前面已经阐述了，但是慢性牵张通常是许多心脏疾病的基础。在这些情况下，心肌细胞中那些对力的传导起重要作用的细胞骨架会发生显著改变[25]。细胞骨架（肌动蛋白和肌小管成分[26]）和离子通道的密切关系已经被阐述，它可导致心力衰竭和扩张性心肌病早期动作电位的延长。

在临床上需要强调的是，病理条件似乎可以放大机械电反馈效应。这已通过对多种类型的实验标本给予外源性机械压力/张力，如牵张[27-35]或渗透性压力的试验得到证实[36]。

前瞻性预测心律失常性猝死的研究提出了一些心血管疾病临床相关参数，许多都是十分抽象的，包括一些指数，比如应用非线性动力学的"混沌"（chaos）、心率变异性；电生理现象，比如晚电位（late potential）、QT离散、电交替；机械指标，如射血分数等。它们甚至还包括一些社会心理因素，这可能与自主神经功能失调有关。此前的综述曾提到上述这些方面与机械因素有关[12]。

电生理的异质性和去极化（后除极和舒张期除极）是心律失常发生的主要基础。而且这些在某种程度上与心律失常性猝死的临床因素有关。为了支持这一论点必须满足一些条件。不同的病因可产生各种各样的电生理心律失常机制（见图27-3A和表27-1），这与电生理离散和心律失常性猝死，以及提到的各种各样临床因素有关。但是这些病因通过机械电转换/反馈即可产生致心律失常的机制（通过促进机械电相互作用的离散），也可引起相关的临床表现。下一部分将讨论这些相关因素，并提示心脏的异常负荷也具有很重要作用。

（一）由机械电转换/反馈诱发心律失常的病理-电生理机制

目前已经认识到有几种电生理机制可以促进、诱发、维持心律失常（见图27-3A和表27-1）[6,9]。单个细胞的机制，如后除极以及触发；多细胞机制，如复极的离散，它是产生波长改变和折返的基础。这些机制很多都涉及钙的异常变化[37]。只要机械电反馈在多种临床相关因素与机械学上提供任何联系，那么就可以用这些机制来解释心律失常的发生。表27-1列举了已知的与机械学有关的致心律失常机制。

后除极在心律失常的发生上是很重要的，机械诱导的后除极看来可以达到阈值并诱发期前收缩（见图27-3A）。动作电位上的"小峰"表示早期后除极，但更合适的术语应该是"机械激活的去极化"或者"牵张导致的去极化"，因为它们产生的机制可能不同。空间上的电生理异质性是发生心律失常病理学的重要因素，这种异质性可以促使心肌不同区出现异常的电流动（见图27-3A "i"），从而产生异常的去极化，尤其是在病变心脏更易发生。在许多心脏病理情况下，

27 机械电转换/反馈：普遍性及病理生理学意义 243

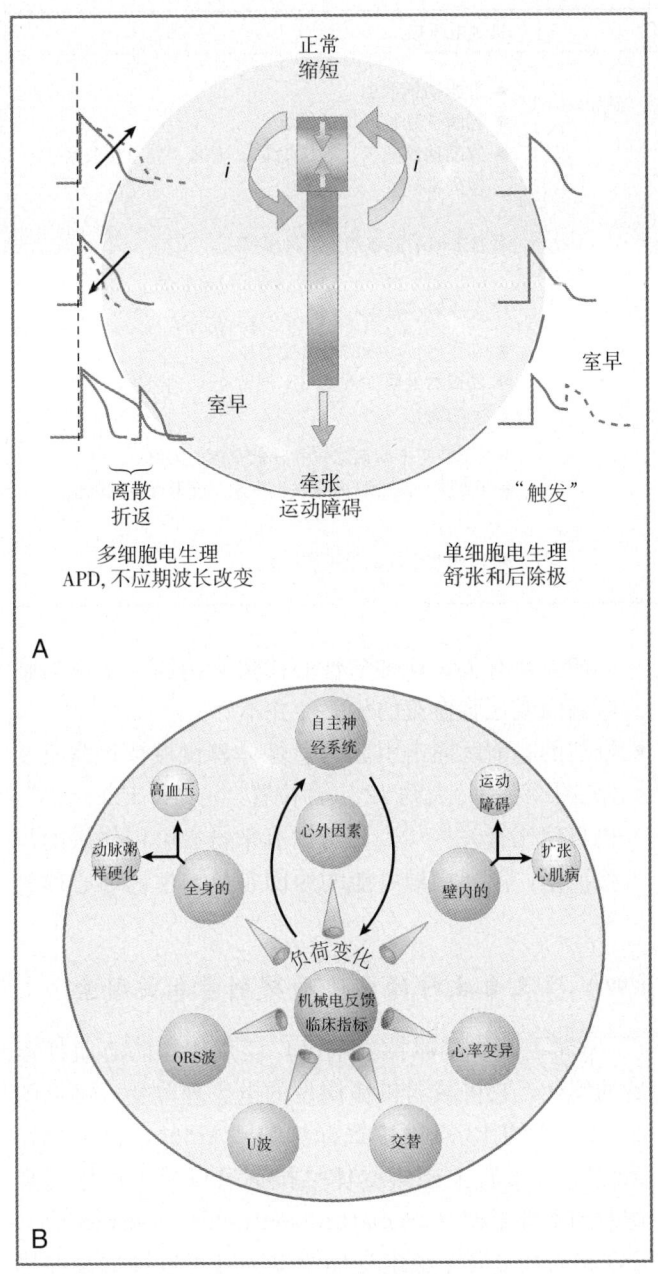

图 27-3 机械电转换/反馈和病理学共性 A：心律失常的电生理机制涉及机械电的异质性。图中央表示心肌的两个节段。正常的节段（顶端）在连续给予负荷时出现正常收缩，并产生正常的动作电位（2 点位置）。如果是弱的（如缺血）节段（底部）收缩，它的缩短将产生延长（虚线）的动作电位（叠加于 10 点位置）。在弱的牵张节段，动作电位（和不应期）缩短（虚线，9 点位置）。牵张的节段也可以产生后除极（3 点位置）和室性早搏。复极化时间是离散的，在节段之间产生电流（箭头和 [i]），这些离散也叠加在图中动作电位上（8 点位置）。不应期的离散将产生波长的改变和折返（左侧底部），并伴随着室性早搏的发生。B：机械电反馈（MEF 中央）与已知的猝死临床指标。这些负荷的改变可以是：（i）全身性的（systemic）（10 点位置），比如高血压和动脉狭窄；（ii）壁内的（2 点位置），例如扩张性心肌病或者二尖瓣病变时心房扩张；（iii）心脏外的因素（12 点位置），例如撞击心脏。自主神经系统（12 点位置上）也可以与负荷异常改变相互作用。与机械电反馈有关的心电图学的相关因素有（见文章）：心电图指标如显示在 8 点位置的 QRS 波和 7 点位置的 U 波，以及对心电图进行测量的一些指标，如显示在 5 点位置的交替和 4 点位置的心率的变异性

一些部位的压力和张力往往比其他部位大，好像一部分牵拉另一部分（见图 27-3 A 中央）。在心室，这些机械力上的不均匀会通过机械电反馈引起复极离散（见图 27-3A 左侧部分）。机械力学的变化可以引起心肌不应期和兴奋性的改变。当然，不是所有的研究都能得到很有说服力的证据，但这可能与导联的位置有关：机械电反馈也存在异质性。在心律失常时，传导速度的改变会导致折返。尽管机械可以导致相似的变化，但结果并不是非常确定的[9]，这还需要加以分辨。

（二）临床相关因素和机械电转换/反馈类似表现

在此讨论与心律失常有关的临床相关因素与机械电因素之间存在的可能联系，这些联系可以贯穿上述其中一些或所有的电生理机制。许多相关因素看来是很明显的，如力学测量有力地支持心律失常与机械电反馈的相关性。另一些相关因素不是很明显，但虽然如此，那些真实的、自发的、尚未阐明的相关因素可能更为重要。

表 27-1 心脏病理改变与机械电反馈诱发心律失常的机制的对比

致心律失常机制	心脏病变	机械电反馈
细胞内钙改变	● 舒张期钙增加（钙负荷） ● 钙转移延长和/或收缩期钙减少（例如）	● 舒张期钙增加 ● 钙瞬变延长（等张收缩） ● 收缩期钙减少（等长收缩）；伸展＋钙（负荷增加心律失常）
后除极	产生室性早搏的特征	看起来似乎能够产生室性早搏
不应期	改变（如，缩短）	改变（如，缩短）
电生理异质性（和异常的电流）	产生复极离散（电生理重构）	● 动作电位时程的离散度增加 ● 复极的异质性改变（T 波改变——电生理离散的一个功能）
兴奋性的改变 （波长改变，促发折返）	大量的资料表明存在改变	● （急性）不应期缩短和降低室颤的阈值 ● （慢性）使心脏更易发生室颤（降低纤颤的阈值）
传导性改变（波长改变，促发折返）	大量的资料表明存在改变	● 产生改变（结果不统一）

（三）机械相关因素

- 发生扩张伴低射血分数的心脏（如心力衰竭时，见图 27-3B，在大约 2 点钟）和猝死相关，尽管有争议认为并不是所有心脏性猝死都是由心律失常引起的，猝死的患者中可能有一半是心律失常引起。室早并不能用来预测猝死，但心力衰竭时的左室射血分数仍是猝死的一个有力预测指标。心力衰竭时大部分抗心律失常药很可能并不能控制心律失常，部分药物甚至会促进猝死的发生。这使人们对评价疗效指标的有效性提出了质疑。相似的是，二尖瓣病变可出现心房的扩张，和心衰一样都易产生房性心动过速[3]。

- 室壁运动异常（dyskinesia）在缺血区非常显著，这种运动障碍可见图 27-3B，在大约 2 点钟位置发生了"壁内的，intramural"的"运动障碍，Dys"。此外，心律失常性猝死和室壁运动异常有关[38]。在另外一项研究中偶然观察到，植入式起搏器发出超速抑制控制室速的过程中可通过减轻异常的室壁运动而减少机械电反馈[39]。长期的停搏可导致机械电反馈的增强，促发心律失常。所有的机械因素均参与室壁力学的改变，但更重要的是，在心肌重塑和修复过程中，导致区域性机械功能异质性，这很可能也促发心律失常。

- 在实验中或某些临床疾病时，全身性的负荷改变（见图 27-3B，大约 11 点钟位置"全身性，systemic"）如高血压（Hypt）和主动脉缩窄（AS），也和心律失常有关，这种室性心律失常的高发生率与临床病因或冠脉血流的相关性并不好。

- 剧烈的心前区撞击引起的急性体外机械性负荷改变（见图 27-3B，大约 12 点钟位置"心外，Excardis"）也与猝死有关[40,41]。尽管没有来自心脏创伤后的尸检证据，但死亡最可能的原因是机械性诱导心律失常。

（四）涉及自主神经系统的解剖学相关因素

β 肾上腺素受体拮抗剂已广泛用于预防心肌梗死后的猝死，它可减弱机械诱发的电生理改变，可见图 27-3B，大约 12 点钟位置标注的"Auton，自主神经系统"[14]。β 肾上腺素受体拮抗剂可以减少机械因素诱发的室性早搏（premature ventricular contractions, PVCs），而 β 肾上腺素受体激动剂却可以增加室性早搏。溴苄铵（bretylium tosylate）不仅可以临床治疗心律失常，还可抑制牵张诱发的心律失常。它可以使恢复曲线变平（关于"恢复曲线"可参阅第 26 章相关部分），达到抗心律失常的目的[42]。

除此之外，心脏交感神经的减少（enervation）也是不均匀的。这一点似乎很重要，因为已证实心交感神经分布减少是特发性扩张型心肌病患者发生心源性死亡的一个重要预测指标。这种交感神经的不均匀减少将会加剧机械电耦联的异质性。

（五）电生理学的相关因素

- 心室除极波（QRS 波群）的改变（见图 27-3B，在大约8点钟位置）可反映传导异常,当右室显著扩大并伴有QRS波延长时有较高的心律失常发生率[6,12,43]。在法洛（Fallot's）四联症被修补后,长期的右室容量负荷增加,舒张功能异常,以及QRS波延长,这些都是互相关联的,其中QRS波延长是预测致命性心室心律失常的一个敏感指标。

- 心电图中异常的U波（见图27-3B,在大约7点钟位置）可能与心律失常有关,特别当患者有长QT综合征（long QT syndrome,LQTS）和尖端扭转性室性心动过速（或伴低钾血症[4]）时。U波可能与心动周期晚期不均匀复极有关,但也有证据提示机械性改变也可引起U波。

- 心率变异性的降低（见图27-3B,在大约4点钟位置）与心室扩张和心肌衰竭相关,甚至在左心室扩张的早期,尚未出现心衰的阶段,夹闭（splint）窦房结可以降低心率变异性,这可能是抑制了随呼吸引起的动态改变,达到减少变异性的高频成分。在心衰晚期可出现伴有舒张末期高压力负荷的心室扩张,这种舒张末期的高压力负荷可影响到右心房,这将牵拉窦房结并减少心率变异性的高频成分。

- 在实验性心肌缺血和临床心肌缺血时,心室纤颤发生前可出现电生理交替（见图27-3B,"交替,altns"在大约5点钟位置）,而且,这方面的证据也越来越多[44]。心力衰竭和缺血（也会表现出负荷改变）可以调节或者产生电机械性改变。重要的是,这些电交替和机械性改变都是异质性的[45]。其中,在机械性改变中,机械电反馈也将出现异质性并促发心律失常。

（六）与电解质紊乱（低钾血症）有关的因素

电解质缺失被认为是一种危险因素,对患者进行利尿治疗可导致低钾血症,而低钾血症可以导致心律失常[9,14]。低钾血症与实验性机械转导有关,因为在离体心脏灌流中,低钾可以促进机械因素诱导心律失常。

急性缺血时,缺血局部钾离子增加,这可以导致运动障碍,表现为心脏收缩时受损区域膨出和伸展。先驱性的实验研究表明,在实验性冠脉结扎后,可通过外源性和机械性阻止或限制心肌的异常伸展,结果使得缺血局部的高钾明显降轻（参见Nazir SA, Dick D, Lab MJ. 在1997年意大利Trento举行的国际机械电反馈会议论文：Myocaardial stetch contributes to extracellular K+ accumulation in acute regional ische-

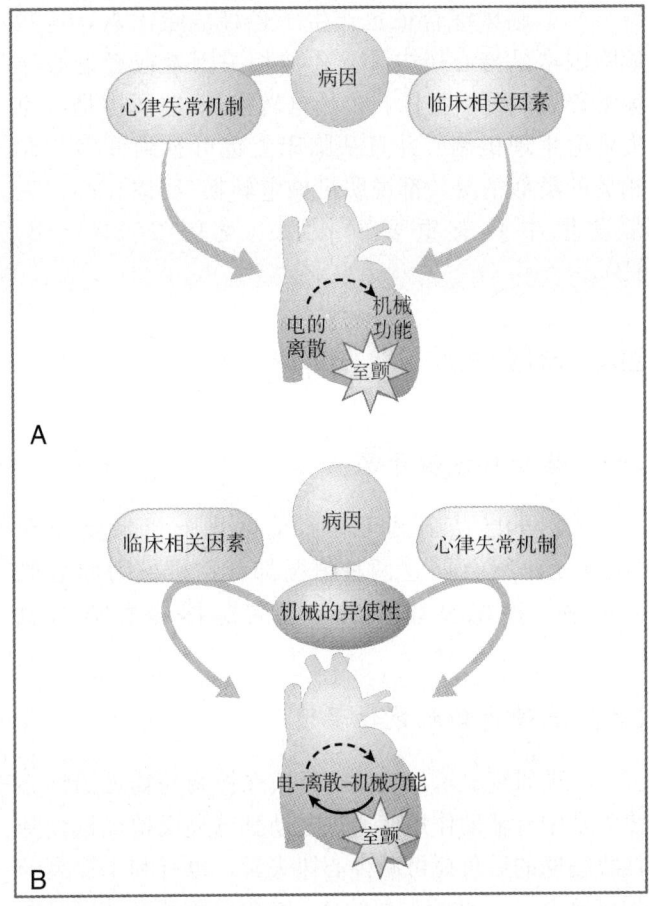

图 27-4 与机械电传导/反馈有关的病因、心律失常机制和临床相关因素　A:概况图。病因学因素（顶端中心）产生（弯曲的箭头）心律失常机制和临床相关因素,从而导致了电的离散。例如心脏的示意图中显示的那样,电改变可以影响（虚线箭头）机械功能。电的离散有利于发生室颤。B:机械电反馈通过心律失常机制和临床相关因素促发心律失常（见图27-3A和27-3B）。病因学因素产生（下连接）机械性的异质性（见图27-3A）。这就可以产生（环状箭头）心律失常机制（27-3A）和临床相关因素（27-3B）。最后,机械电反馈产生机械电的离散（mechanoelectric dispersion）,后者又组成为了机械电反馈环中的一部分（实线和虚线箭头）

mia of the pig heart,牵张心肌促进急性猪心缺血区细胞外钾离子聚集）。也就是说,对急性缺血区钾离子升高有了一个新的解释,表明牵张心肌可开放离子通道,允许钾离子漏出到细胞外,而且可能是通过K_{ATP}通道,因为该通道属于机械敏感性离子通道。

（七）本节要点

图27-4集中概括了上述这些论点。目前,大家一致公认,病因学因素产生了电生理学的心律失常机制,而后者可导致电的离散,最终发生室颤（见图

27-4A）。临床综合征也产生了各种危险因素，这些危险因素是与心律失常猝死的相关因素或者是心律失常猝死的预测指标。机械电转换/反馈同样是心律失常电生理机制，并且从临床上也可看到许多与此相关的类似情况，都说明机械电转换/反馈在心律失常发生中具有重要的作用（见图 27-3A、3B、4B）。

四、治疗方法

（一）体外机械性干预

人们早已认识到可在心前区进行机械复律和"咳嗽复律"[9,46]。这两种情况都存在机械力向心肌的传递。捶击复律常用于安装起搏器之前的急救。

（二）血管内的机械性干预

一项研究显示，机械电反馈在控制药物难治性心律失常中有辅助作用。通过主动脉球囊反搏机械性降低收缩期的后负荷可减少心律失常，也有利于提高药物疗效[44]。与此相类似的是，减少前负荷有辅助除颤的作用[48]，数学模型的研究也支持这一发现[49]。

（三）药理学

如果牵张激活通道参与牵张性心律失常，促进牵张性心律失常发展成临床心律失常，那么牵张激活通道的阻滞剂有希望成为一类新的抗心律失常药。钆，是一种实验室常用的 SAC 阻滞剂，但它不能像链霉素一样令人满意。目前正在寻找 SAC 的特异性阻滞剂，狼蛛（tarantula）的毒液很有希望[20]。因为 K_{ATP} 通道也属于牵张敏感通道，并且它可能参与"心脏震荡，commotio cordis"诱发的机械性心律失常[50]，这种通道的阻滞剂可望成为一种有效的治疗药物。不过有很多的机械感受器都能改变电信号，它们中每个都可能成为一个治疗的靶点，包括细胞骨架。

外周血管舒张剂可以减少血管壁的应力，尤其是血管紧张素转化酶抑制剂对心律失常也能产生有益的治疗作用[1,9]。血管紧张素转化酶抑制剂可以抑制心肌的重塑，减少心肌的不协调收缩。血管紧张素转化酶抑制剂还有交感活性，增加压力反射的敏感性，这些都有助于防止室性心律失常。似乎这些是与 K^+ 有关[9,14]，高钾可能是种保护因素，低钾可会造成心律紊乱。

β肾上腺素体受体拮抗剂是少数几个能有效减少心律失常性猝死的药物之一。而且，通过溴苄铵来耗竭内源性的儿茶酚胺也是有益的[42,51]。

五、理论上的深思

（一）一种整合机制

在机械反应和电生理反应之间，机械电转换（反馈）可能参与形成心肌细胞内稳定系统，后者被认为是一种整合调节系统[6]。不过它能像其他系统一样，与其他整合系统相互调节，如神经内分泌系统在不同的水平上进行调节而显示出一种自动调节的稳态吗？首先，在整合系统中，机械电反馈提供了从机械感受器到整个心脏的路径。前面的部分已经提到了这一点。第二，在不同的机械敏感性机制中存在着相互作用[14]，经常有细胞内钙和 ATP 的改变。第三，机械电反馈可以和其他的调节系统相互作用。第四，如同神经内分泌控制系统能很好的负反馈调节一样，机械电反馈顾名思义，也存在负反馈机制。最后一点，就像其他系统，当机械电反馈出现功能异常，可能会引起疾病（心血管疾病）。

（二）反馈

为什么称为机械电"反馈"，而不是机械电耦联或机械电传导？人们通常认为兴奋收缩耦联是单向的，同样也会认为机械电耦联或传导也是单向的[6]。心脏的周期性和节律性变化会引起机械电状态的变化。这些在时间和空间（解剖学）上是平行的。进一步说，在兴奋收缩耦联和电机械传导中都普遍存在着这一过程。这种单向的传递为反馈提供了基础。在心肌中，兴奋收缩耦联和机械电反馈之间的相互作用有一个精细的调节过程（见图 27-5A）。以这种方式，任何机械性的变化会影响膜的电生理和兴奋性，然后影响机械收缩功能。尽管机械电反馈缺乏严谨性，但却能反映出它的部分功能。在正常环境中，这一反馈环路使在电或机械干扰时能保持稳定，但也可能在病理条件下失去稳定。也就是，诱导心脏机械性变化的那些病理条件也会引起这种紊乱，从而产生临床综合征，而这些又在过去往往很难解释，也很难单纯从电生理的角度去治疗。

这种电和机械事件的相互作用都具有一定的范

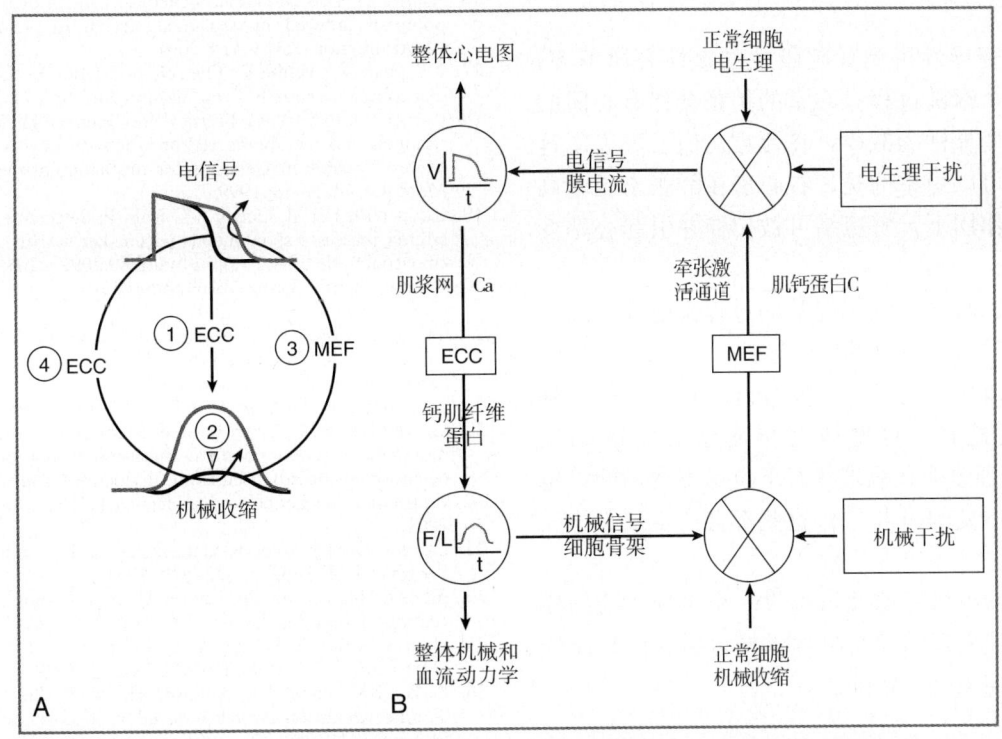

图 27-5 机械电反馈（MEF） A：简单的生物学示意图。(1) 在电信号的作用下，通过兴奋收缩耦联（ECC），图示意的动作电位会产生很强的收缩。(2) 在某种原因下，收缩减弱。(3) 通过机械电反馈的反馈使动作电位延长。(4) 这种延长会通过下一个兴奋收缩耦联增加小的机械信号。B：简单的工程学示意图：在左上是动作电位，用电压对时间（V 对 t）的曲线表示。整体表现为心电图（ECG）（上箭头）。同样，它也使肌浆网（SR）释放钙离子（下箭头）而产生兴奋收缩耦联。钙和肌纤维蛋白作用产生收缩。左下是力量或长度对时间（F/L 对 t）的曲线。这样会产生（下箭头）机械的和血流动力学的改变，如压力/容积的改变。机械信号（通过细胞骨架），包括了正常的机械收缩（底部的水平箭头），输入到了一个比较器（comparator）（右下的带叉的圆圈）。任何机械性的刺激都将进入比较器进行叠加。传出的信号（向上）通过机械电换能器诱发了机械电反馈，这些换能器包括牵张激活通道（SACs）或肌钙蛋白-C（tnc）机制。机械性激活的电流进入另一个比较器（右上带叉的圆圈），和正常的电生理信号和干扰进行叠加，从而产生一个膜电压的信号来影响动作电位（返回到了右上角）

围，这种关系的维持对于正常生理上的整体功能具有重要作用。在系统中的任何干扰都将会使系统不稳定，产生病理过程。对这种不稳定性的矫正是控制系统的一个标志。运用控制论的一个简化例子来说明电和机械事件的相互作用，可以描述为是一个反馈控制系统，它可以确保细胞的电机械关系维持在一个正常的范围内，这种关系可反映为心电图的整体表现与压力/容积负荷之间的关系。

这里控制理论的应用是有缺陷的，在图中 27-5B 中有些部分是需要区别对待的。在这样一个系统中很难去准确的定义它们，包括：具体的被调控变量，在机械电反馈环中的比较元件（即错误检测器），和传导到控制器的错误信号（控制信号和反馈信号的差别）。另外，在电压电流与机械能之间的转化功能，以及兴奋收缩耦联之间的转化功能都需要进行定义。

控制系统的破坏或正反馈将会导致生理性和病理生理性的改变。

（三）数学的方法

通过机械电反馈的实验数据得出一些方程，目前已建立起了几个数学模型[6,7,52-55]。一些模型用于验证机械电反馈诱导心律失常，以及机械性的异质性是如何成为心律失常发生基质的研究（见图 27-3A "i"）[57]。

机械电反馈作为一个反馈过程，充当了一种调节系统，使得自己成为了一种非线性的动态模型[6]。它既能接受系统的稳定，也能耐受紊乱的发生，或心律失常。它在正常生理和病理状态下的作用还有争论。

- 当出现紊乱过程导致了生理性的不适应性时，机械电反馈能稳定这一系统。

- 其他的模型也提示，在心脏的电除颤中存在一种机械性作用[49]。
- 正常心率的变异性可诱导呼吸性的窦性心律不齐，它被认为是个紊乱过程。心室的扩张会伴有心肌的衰竭和心率变异性的减少，在死亡之前已失去了这种变异性。可以想象的是，右心房在舒张末压增高和机械性的作用下，窦房结可被拉伸并引起心率变异性的减少。
- 并行心律和二联律可以用混乱的过程来解释，并且这种心律失常可以被机械性诱导。
- 对电生理的改变目前还有一些分歧，它可能是一种导致紊乱的途径，这些改变可先于心室颤动发生[44]。机械性改变在病理状态下也是不均匀的，也是一个预后不良的因素[45]。这些都会产生致心律失常的电离散。
- 超常态陡峭的电恢复曲线可提供一个再现紊乱的模型，并且这些发现与"机械性诱导可引起恢复曲线的改变"的现象是一致的。

（张幼怡　龚开政　徐　宁　译）

参 考 文 献

1. Dean JW, Lab MJ: Arrhythmia in heart failure: Role of mechanically induced changes in electrophysiology. Lancet 1:1309–1312, 1989.
2. Sideris DA: High blood pressure and ventricular arrhythmias. Eur Heart J 14:1548–1553, 1993.
3. Nazir SA, Lab MJ: Mechanoelectric feedback and atrial arrhythmias. Cardiovasc Res 32:52–61, 1996.
4. Reiter MJ: Effects of mechano-electric feedback: Potential arrhythmogenic influence in patients with congestive heart failure. Cardiovasc Res 32:44–51, 1996.
5. Taggart P, Sutton PM: Cardiac mechano-electric feedback in man: Clinical relevance. Prog Biophys Mol Biol 71:139–154, 1999.
6. Lab MJ: Mechanosensitivity as an integrative system in heart: An audit. Prog Biophys Mol Biol 71:7–27, 1999.
7. Kohl P, Hunter P, Noble D: Stretch-induced changes in heart rate and rhythm: Clinical observations, experiments and mathematical models. Prog Biophys Mol Biol 71:91–138, 1999.
8. Franz MR: Mechano-electrical feedback. Cardiovasc Res 45:263–266, 2000.
9. Reiter MJ: Contraction Excitation Feedback. In Zipes DP, Jalife J (eds): Cardiac Electrophysiology from Cell to Bedside. Philadelphia, WB Saunders, 2000.
10. Tavi P, Laine M, Weckstrom M, Ruskoaho H: Cardiac mechanotransduction: From sensing to disease and treatment. Trends Pharmacol Sci 22:254–260, 2001.
11. Guadalajara Boo JF: Mechanoelectric feedback and sudden death in heart failure. Arch Cardiol Mex 71 (Suppl 1):S69–S75, 2001.
12. Babuty D, Lab MJ: Mechanoelectric contributions to sudden cardiac death. Cardiovasc Res 50:270–279, 2001.
13. Kamkin AG, Kiseleva IS, Iarygin VN: Ion mechanisms of the mechanoelectrical feedback in myocardial cells. Usp Fiziol Nauk 32:58–87, 2001.
14. Lab MJ: Mechanoelectric feedback in heart: neurohumoral contribution and crosstalk. In Proceedings of the 3rd International Workshop on Cardiac Mechano-electric Feedback and Arrhythmias. Oxford, UK, 2003, pp 50–51.
15. Hamill OP, Martinac B: Molecular basis of mechanotransduction in living cells. Physiol Rev 81:685–740, 2001.
16. Babuty D, Lab M: Heterogeneous changes of monophasic action potential induced by sustained stretch in atrium. J Cardiovasc Electrophysiol 12:323–329, 2001.
17. Calaghan SC, White E: The role of calcium in the response of cardiac muscle to stretch. Prog Biophys Mol Biol 71:59–90, 1999.
18. Cazorla O, Pascarel C, Brette F, Le Guennec JY: Modulation of ion channels and membrane receptor activity by stretch in cardiomyocytes: Possible mechanisms for mechanosensitivity. Prog Biophys Mole Biol 71:29–58, 1999.
19. Cooper PJ, Lei M, Cheng LX, Kohl P: Selected contribution: Axial stretch increases spontaneous pacemaker activity in rabbit isolated sinoatrial node cells. J Appl Physiol 89:2099–2104, 2000.
20. Bode F, Sachs F, Franz MR: Tarantula peptide inhibits atrial fibrillation. Nature 409:35–36, 2001.
21. Takagi S, Miyazaki T, Moritani K, et al: Gadolinium suppresses stretch-induced increases in the differences in epicardial and endocardial monophasic action potential durations and ventricular arrhythmias in dogs. Jpn Circ J 63:296–302, 1999.
22. Greve G, Lab MJ, Chen R, et al: Right ventricular distension alters monophasic action potential duration during pulmonary arterial occlusion in anaesthetised lambs: Evidence for arrhythmogenic right ventricular mechanoelectrical feedback. Exp Physiol 86:651–657, 2001.
23. Lab MJ, Dean J: Myocardial mechanics and arrhythmia. J Cardiovasc Pharmacol 18 (Suppl 2):S72–S79, 1991.
24. Allessie MA, Boyden PA, Camm AJ, et al: Pathophysiology and prevention of atrial fibrillation. Circulation 103:769–777, 2001.
25. Hein S, Kostin S, Heling A, et al: The role of the cytoskeleton in heart failure. Cardiovasc Res 45:273–278, 2000.
26. Parker KK, Taylor LK, Atkinson JB, et al: The effects of tubulinbinding agents on stretch-induced ventricular arrhythmias. Eur J Pharmacol 417:131–140, 2001.
27. Tobler HG, Gornic CC, Anderson RW, Benditt DG: Electrophysiologic properties of the myocardial infarction border zone: Effects of transient aortic occlusion. Surgery 100:150–156, 1986.
28. Calkins H, Maughan WL, Kass DA, et al: Electrophysiologic properties of the myocardial infarction border zone: Effects of transient aortic occlusion. Surgery 100:150–155, 1979.
29. Calkins H, Weisman HF, Levine JH, et al: Effect of acute volume load on refractoriness and arrhythmia development in isolated chronically infarcted canine hearts. Circulation 79:687–697, 1989.
30. Zhou BY, Harrison FG, Dick DJ, et al: Ventricular arrhythmogenesis is enhanced by mechanoelectric feedback in regional ischaemic heart of the anaesthetised pig. J Physiol 473:184P, 1993.
31. Lab MJ, Zhou BY, Dick DJ, et al: Stretch-induced ventricular fibrillation in normal and globally anoxic isolated guinea pig hearts. J Physiol 473:183P, 1993.
32. Wang Z, Taylor LK, Denney WD, Hansen DE: Initiation of ventricular extrasystoles by myocardial stretch in chronically dilated and failing canine left ventricle. Circulation 90:2022–2031, 1994.
33. Horner SM, Lab MJ, Murphy CF, et al: Mechanically induced changes in action potential duration and left ventricular segment length in acute regional ischaemia in the in situ porcine heart. Cardiovasc Res 28:528–534, 1994.
34. Pye MP, Cobbe SM: Arrhythmogenesis in experimental models of heart failure: The role of increased load. Cardiovasc Res 32:248–257, 1996.
35. Kamkin A, Kiseleva I, Isenberg G: Stretch-activated currents in ventricular myocytes: Amplitude and arrhythmogenic effects increase with hypertrophy. Cardiovasc Res 48:409–420, 2000.
36. Clemo HF, Stambler BS, Baumgarten CM: Swelling-activated chloride current is persistently activated in ventricular myocytes from dogs with tachycardia-induced congestive heart failure. Circ Res 84:157–165, 1999.
37. Balke CW, Shorofsky SR: Alterations in calcium handling in cardiac hypertrophy and heart failure. Cardiovasc Res 37:290–299, 1998.
38. Siogas K, Pappas S, Graekas G, et al: Segmental wall motion abnormalities alter vulnerability to ventricular ectopic beats associated with acute increases in aortic pressure in patients with underlying coronary artery disease. Heart 79:268–273, 1998.
39. Perticone F, Ceravolo R, Maio R, et al: Mechano-electric feedback and ventricular arrhythmias in heart failure: The possible role of permanent cardiac stimulation in preventing ventricular tachycardia.

Cardiologia 38:247–252, 1993.
40. Link MS, Wang PJ, Maron BJ, Estes NA: What is commotio cordis? Cardiol Rev 7:265–269, 1999.
41. Kohl P, Nesbitt AD, Cooper PJ, Lei M: Sudden cardiac death by Commotio cordis: Role of mechano-electric feedback. Cardiovasc Res 50:280–289, 2001.
42. Garfinkel A, Kim YH, Voroshilovsky O, et al: Preventing ventricular fibrillation by flattening cardiac restitution. Proc Natl Acad Sci U S A 97:6061–6066, 2000.
43. Gatzoulis MA, Till JA, Somerville J, Redington AN: Mechanoelectrical interaction in tetralogy of Fallot: QRS prolongation relates to right ventricular size and predicts malignant ventricular arrhythmias and sudden death. Circulation 92:231–237, 1995.
44. Armoundas AA, Tomaselli GF, Esperer HD: Pathophysiological basis and clinical application of T-wave alternans. J Am Coll Cardiol 40:207–217, 2002.
45. Murphy CF, Lab MJ, Horner SM, et al: Regional electromechanical alternans in anesthetized pig hearts: Modulation by mechanoelectric feedback. Am J Physiol 267:H1726–H1735, 1994.
46. Caldwell G, Millar G, Quinn E, et al: Simple mechanical methods for cardioversion: Defence of the precordial thump. BMJ 291:627–630, 1985.
47. Fotopolous GD, Mason MJ, Jepson NS, et al: Intra-aortic balloon counterpulsation for the control of refractory ventricular arrhythmias. Circulation 94:737, 1996.
48. Strobel JS, Kay GN, Walcott GP, et al: Defibrillation efficacy with endocardial electrodes is influenced by reductions in cardiac preload. J Interv Card Electrophysiol 1:95–102, 1997.
49. Trayanova N, Ideker R, Li W, et al: Effects of mechano-electric feedback on defibrillation threshold. In Proceedings of the 3rd International Workshop on Cardiac Mechano-electric Feedback and Arrhythmias. Oxford, UK, 2003, pp 50–51.
50. Link MS, Wang PJ, VanderBrink BA, et al: Selective activation of the K(+)(ATP) channel is a mechanism by which sudden death is produced by low-energy chest-wall impact (Commotio cordis). Circulation 100:413–418, 1999.
51. Waller DG: Treatment and prevention of ventricular fibrillation: Are there better agents? Resuscitation 22:159–166, 1991.
52. Vetter FJ, McCulloch AD: Mechanoelectric feedback in a model of the passively inflated left ventricle. Ann Biomed Eng 29:414–426, 2001.
53. Knudsen Z, Holden AV, Brindley J: Qualitative modeling of mechanoelectrical feedback in a ventricular cell. Bull Math Biol 59:1155–1181, 1997.
54. Riemer TL, Sobie EA, Tung L: Stretch-induced changes in arrhythmogenesis and excitability in experimentally based heart cell models. Am J Physiol 275:H431–H442, 1998.
55. Han C, Tavi P, Weckstrom M: Modulation of action potential by [Ca2+]i in modeled rat atrial and guinea pig ventricular myocytes. Am J Physiol Heart Circ Physiol 282:H1047–H1054, 2002.
56. Rice JJ, Winslow RL, Dekanski J, McVeigh E: Model studies of the role of mechano-sensitive currents in the generation of cardiac arrhythmias. J Theor Biol 190:295–312, 1998.
57. Markhasin VS, Solovyova O, Katsnelson LB, et al: Mechano-electric interactions in heterogeneous myocardium: Development of fundamental experimental and theoretical models. Prog Biophys Mol Biol 82:207–220, 2003.

第五部分
心脏兴奋的模型

第 28 章

心脏电活动的离子机制：理论探索

Yoram Rudy

本章目录

- 心肌细胞动作电位的产生 ……………… 251
- 遗传性通道病模型 ……………………… 254
- 多细胞组织中动作电位的传播 ………… 256
- 从离子通道到心电图波形 ……………… 259
- 跋 ………………………………………… 259
- 致谢 ……………………………………… 260

心脏的兴奋是膜离子过程（电源）和多细胞组织的被动结构特点（电穴）复杂的相互作用过程。这一过程包括单个细胞的电脉冲、动作电位的产生，以及通过缝隙连接从一个细胞到另一个细胞的传导。因此，要理解兴奋性的过程，就要从单个离子通道到全细胞、到多细胞组织，从整体水平上了解其机制。

在单个心肌细胞，离子通道与膜电位、细胞的离子环境以及各种调节机制相互作用，即使在此水平上，也存在整合作用。以上都是动态过程，通过复杂的非线性相互作用，产生动作电位，并决定其形态。

在另一个整合水平上，心肌细胞通过缝隙连接实现电通讯，后者为细胞间离子流动和动作电位的传播提供了路径。因为产生动作电位的细胞与其他细胞在电学上是相互联系的，因此其膜电位可受相邻细胞离子流的影响，这一现象被称为"电负荷"（electrical loading）。反之，膜电位也影响离子通道的动力学特点和通过此通道的离子流。在多细胞组织中，动作电位的产生和传播不仅包括单细胞膜离子流的调节，还包括反映多细胞组织结构的电负荷。

研究如此复杂过程的一个有用的方法是利用数学模型和计算机模拟[1]。但应该注意的是，研究离子通道所选用的标本（如爪蛙卵母细胞）远远不同于离子通道所处的心肌细胞的生理环境[2]。数学模型是一个有用的工具，可以把离子通道"重建"到细胞相互作用的环境中，从而可以在完整的细胞上研究通道的作用。在组织水平上，电学或光学的实验标测技术并不能记录动作电位传播时的离子流。多细胞组织的理论模型能填补这一空白，提供动作电位传导的离子机制。本章就利用这样的模型来解释心脏兴奋的离子机制。在通道水平、全细胞水平和多细胞组织水平上都有这样的例子。

一、心肌细胞动作电位的产生

单细胞动作电位的产生是离子跨膜运动的结果，因此膜电容（C_m）上的电荷移动，使得膜电位（V_m）发生变化。下面的公式定量描述了这一过程：

$$dV_m/dt = -(1/C_m) \cdot I_{ion} \qquad [1]$$

I_{ion}是总跨膜电流，由细胞膜上的许多离子通道和离子交换机制所携带，dV_m/dt是V_m的变化率，与I_{ion}成正比。习惯上，负的I_{ion}代表正离子流入细胞内形成内向电流，这形成一个正的dV_m/dt，使得膜电位增加（去极化）。相反，正的I_{ion}代表正离子流出细胞外形成外向电流，形成一个负的dV_m/dt，使得膜电位减小（超极化）。总之，I_{ion}是各种内向电流和外向电流所形成的总和，其所携带的离子类型不同，相应的电流幅度、时间、对电压和离子浓度的依赖性也不同。图28-1是心室肌细胞及其电生理成分的示意图，也描述了本章中所应用的计算I_{ion}的数学模型（Luo-Rudy动态[LRd]模型）[3-5]。LRd模型的主要基础是豚鼠单细胞和离子通道的数据。该模型包括膜离子通道、参与离子跨膜转运的离子泵和交换子。也描述了钠、钾、钙等离子浓度的动态变化过程。重要的是，此模型模拟了肌浆网的钙循环和动作电位期间钙致钙释放所形成的钙瞬变。此模型的图示如图 28-1：(1) I_{Na} 的特点是快速激活和快速失活或缓慢失活[6]。(2) $I_{Ca(L)}$ 的失活是电压和钙依赖性的。钙导致的失活是一个快速过程，而电压所导致的失活是一个缓慢过程[7]。(3) 延迟整流钾电流有两个成分：快速成分 (I_{kr}) 和慢速成分 (I_{ks})[8]。(4) I_{kr}、I_{kl} 和 $I_{k(ATP)}$ 的电导与细胞外钾离子浓度 ($[K^+]_o$) 的平方根成正比。(5) 细胞内钙浓度 ($[Ca^{2+}]_i$) 增高，则 I_{ks} 也增高。(6) I_{to} 不见于豚鼠心室肌，但它在其他大多数物种的心外膜很明显[9]。

如前所述，动作电位是不同膜电流和其他细胞离子转运过程间动态地相互作用的结果。它们共同决定了细胞的整体行为、动作电位特点以及动作电位对不同生理性和病理性状态的反应。图 28-2 描述的是不同电流对动作电位的产生、形态和时程 (APD) 的影响。此图显示了动作电位、细胞内钙瞬变和动作电位期间某一离子流的时程。当细胞去极化达到其兴奋性的阈值时，快速内向钠电流 (I_{Na}) 激活并使膜以非常快的速度去极化 (dVm/dt 最快可达 393V/s)，产生动作电位的快速超射期，随后就快速失活。在动作电位的图形上，I_{Na} 表现为一个大的内向"钉样"电流。随后 $I_{Ca(L)}$ 激活（当 V_m 达到约 −25mV 时），形成一个去极化电流，与复极化的外向电流 I_{kr} 和 I_{ks} 形成动作电位的平台期。$I_{Ca(L)}$ 的特点是，动作电位期间表现为"钉样和圆顶状"[10]。它在 2.74ms 到达其第一个峰值 −4.92μA/μF，而 I_{Na} 在 1ms 到达其峰值（注意 $I_{Ca(L)}$ 的峰值比 I_{Na} 的峰值小 20%）。1ms 时，$I_{Ca(L)}$ 仍很小，只有 −0.84μA/μF，因此，$I_{Ca(L)}$ 早期的钉样成分对动作电位上升支的去极化的作用很小，它的重要生理意义是触发肌浆网的钙释放以形成钙瞬变 (calcium transient)，后者将收缩的信息传导到细胞的收缩成分，这一过程就是兴奋收缩耦联。$I_{Ca(L)}$ 的圆顶部分维持动作电位的平台期，随着 L 型钙通道的失活而逐渐减弱。同时，I_{kr} 和 I_{ks} 逐渐增强，使得外向电流占优势，膜复极化，回到静息电位。I_{NaCa} 是产电性交换子，化学当量为 $3Na^+ : 1Ca^{2+}$，在动作电位的早期，它"反向"工作，将 Na^+ 运出细胞外，产生一个相对较小的外向电流。然后，它恢复"正向"工作，排出 Ca^{2+}，产生一个明显的内向电流，延缓了动作电位晚期复极化的速度，并延长 APD。最后，I_{kl} 明显增大，与 I_{kr} 和 I_{ks} 一起，使得膜复极化，回到静息电位。需要注意的是，I_{kl} 在动作电位的终末期占优势，并在动作电位之后将膜电位保持在静息电位水平（I_{kl}

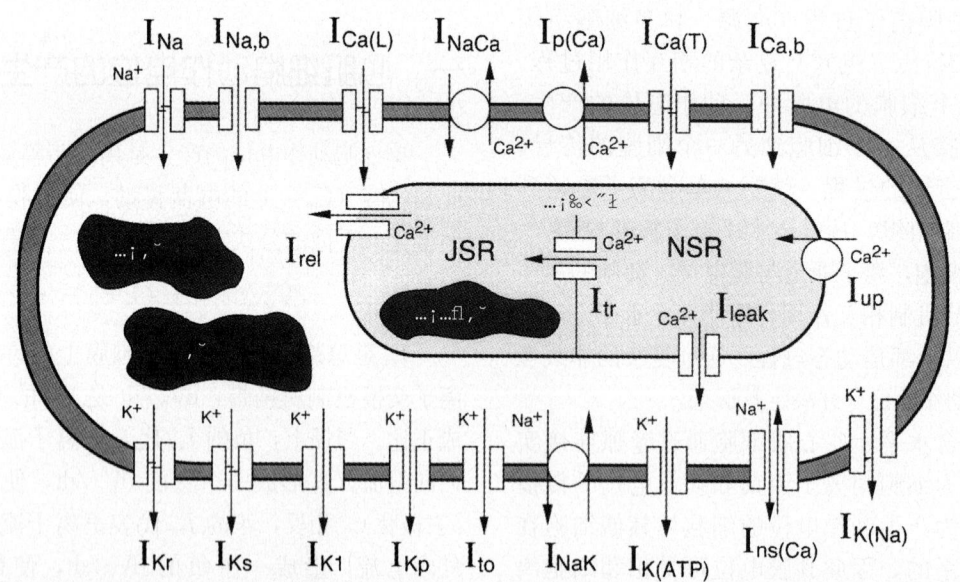

图 28-1 Luo-Rudy 动力学 (LRd) 心室细胞模型示意图 I_{Na} 快钠电流；$I_{Ca(L)}$，L 型钙通道的钙电流；$I_{Ca(T)}$，T 型钙通道的钙电流；I_{kr}，快速延迟整流钾电流；I_{ks}，缓慢延迟整流钾电流；I_{to}，瞬时外向电流；I_{k1}，内向整流钾电流；$I_{k(ATP)}$，ATP 敏感钾电流；I_{Kp}，平台期钾电流；$I_{K(Na)}$，钠激活的钾电流（在钠超载时激活），$I_{ns(Ca)}$，非特异性钙激活电流（在钙超载时激活），$I_{Na,b}$，背景钠电流，$I_{Ca,b}$ 背景钙电流；$I_{Na,K}$，钠-钾泵电流，I_{NaCa}，钠-钙交换电流；$I_{P(Ca)}$，肌膜钙泵，I_{up}，从细胞浆摄取到肌浆网 (NSR) 的钙；I_{rel}，从连接处肌浆网 (JSR) 释放的钙，I_{leak} 从 NSR 漏到胞浆的钙，I_{tr}，从 NSR 转移到 JSR 的钙。钙调蛋白和肌钙蛋白是细胞浆中的钙缓冲体。Calsequestrin 是 JSR 中的钙缓冲体。详细内容见于 www.cwru.edu/med/cBRTC（引自 Rudy Y: The cardiac ventricular action potential. In Page E, Fozzard HA, Solaro RJ [eds]: The Handbook of Physiology, section 2, vol 1: The Heart. New York, Oxford University Press, 2002, pp 531-547.）

能决定膜的兴奋性,这一点由 Hund 和 Rudy 已经讨论过)。在动作电位的平台期,I_{NaK} 也增加(化学当量为 $3Na^+:2K^+$),它能排出动作电位期间进入细胞的 Na^+。

豚鼠心室肌没有瞬时外向钾电流 I_{to},此电流见于其他种属的心外膜和心肌中层,而不见于心内膜。图 28-2 对应于豚鼠心肌,没有 I_{to},上升支之后,动作电位向着静息电位复极化。如果图中包括了 I_{to}(此图未显示,见 Rudy[3] 所著图 13-9),则上升支之后跟随一个快速早期复极期,在平台期的起始部分形成一个明显的切迹,使得动作电位呈现"尖峰和圆顶"状。

在形成动作电位各个时期的离子机制中有一个重要原则。即在正常心室肌细胞,动作电位的上升支是一个"全或无"的过程,主要由一种大的离子流 I_{Na} 所形成。相反,平台期和复极期是多种较小的内向和外向离子流精确平衡的结果。这与其生理功能相一致。上升支需要迅速、安全范围广,以保证动作电位的产生和其兴奋。而平台期和复极期则需要严密控制下的可变性和适应性。这些特点对于动作电位能适应心率的生理性变化是非常重要的。心率增快时,APD 缩短以适应新的更短的兴奋周期。APD 对各种相反过

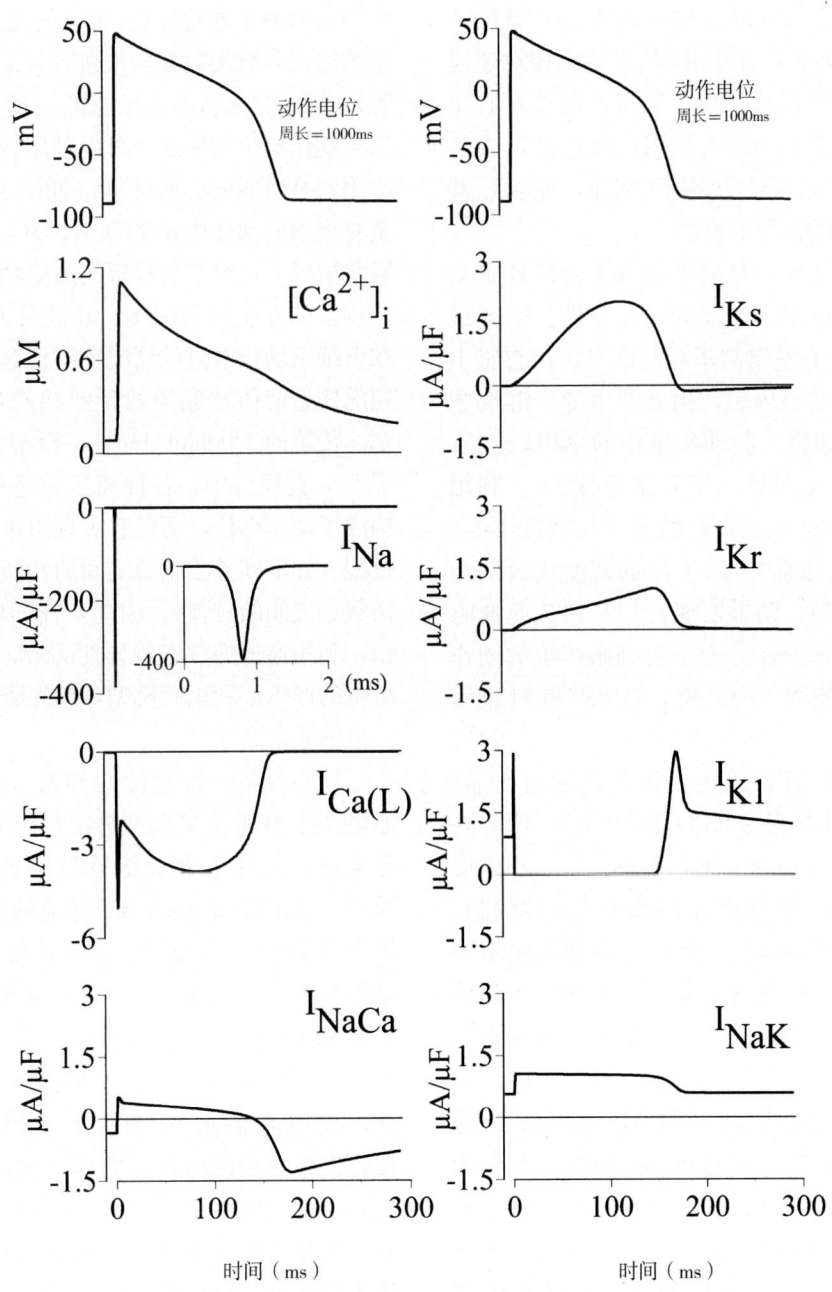

图 28-2 决定动作电位形态部分离子流 图示动作电位(AP)、钙瞬变(动作电位期间细胞内的游离钙,$[Ca^{2+}]_i$)和决定动作电位形态的部分膜离子流中 I_{Na} 的标尺增宽,所有电流都用 LRd 模型模拟。细胞以 1000ms 的周长起搏,已经达到稳定状态(引自 Rudy Y: The cardiac ventricular action potential. In Page E, Fozzard HA, Solaro RJ [eds]: The Handbook of Physiology, section 2, vol 1, The Heart. New York, Oxford University Press, 2002, pp 531-547.)

程（内向和外向电流）的依赖性，以及其间的精确平衡，产生了"控制点"，其对于最佳控制具有高度敏感性（某一电流的微小变化就可引起 APD 明显变化）和多样性。图 28-2 的模型中，当起搏周长从 1000ms 缩短到 200ms 时，APD 从其稳态的 190ms 减少了大约 50%（未显示）。

APD 随心率增加而缩短的过程包括了多个离子流，最重要的是，I_{ks} 在快速心率时增加。因为此电流失活缓慢，当动作电位期间的舒张期缩短时，此电流失活不完全而增加。心率增快时 $[Na^+]_i$ 积聚增加，所以平台期的外向 I_{NaCa} 增加，这也参与适应过程（详细请参照 Rudy[3] 所著图 13-5 和 13-6）。应该注意，APD 适应性的离子机制与种属有关。如犬，其 I_{kr} 和 I_{ks} 失活的相对速度就与豚鼠相反。豚鼠的 I_{ks} 失活慢，使得此电流对心率变化敏感，对 APD 适应性有重要作用。而犬的 I_{ks} 失活比 I_{kr} 快，因此对 APD 适应性的作用不明显，提示 I_{kr} 甚至是 $I_{Ca(L)}$ 在此过程中的作用更重要。

心室肌的一个重要特点是离子通道的表达具有空间可变性，从而导致电生理功能的不均一性。研究最多的一个例子是 I_{ks} 在心室壁的不均一性[9]，在心肌中层的密度低于心外膜或心内膜，由此产生的一群细胞（心肌中层细胞，M 细胞）其动作电位的 APD 较长，APD 对心率的依赖性更明显（APD 适应性大）。利用图 28-1 的模型模拟不同 I_{ks} 密度的情况（I_{kr} 密度不变，心外膜、心内膜和 M 细胞中 I_{ks}：I_{kr} 的密度比分别为 23:1、15:1 和 7:1），结果发现：(1) 快速起搏时（心动周期 [CL] 为 300ms)，这三种细胞产生的动作电位时程相似，都比较短（心外膜、心内膜和 M 细胞的 APD 分别为 105ms、113ms 和 135 ms）。(2) 起搏频率变慢时，M 细胞 APD 的延长比其他细胞明显。CL 为 2000 ms 时，M 细胞的 APD 为 240 ms，而心外膜和心内膜细胞分别为 168ms 和 188 ms。(3) 心率慢时，整个动作电位期间 M 细胞的 I_{ks} 都小于其他细胞。(4) 由于 M 细胞的 APD 较长，因此当心动周期缩短时，在心跳的间歇，I_{ks} 的失活时间短，从而导致其残留 I_{ks} 激活增加，I_{ks} 相对增强。当 CL 从 2000 ms 缩短到 300 ms 时，M 细胞的 I_{ks} 增加了 128%，而在心外膜仅仅增加了 33%，这就是 M 细胞 APD 适应性大的离子机制。(5) I_{NaCa} 也参与 M 细胞的适应性。因为 M 细胞的 I_{ks} 小（导致总的复极化电流也小），所以心率快时，$[Na^+]_i$ 增加，外向 I_{NaCa} 增加，使得总复极化电流相对变化较大，I_{NaCa} 在缩短 APD 方面的作用增强。需要指出的是，M 细胞的一个标志就是，对各种影响复极化离子流的因素反应敏感。在总的复极化电流相对较小的背景下，任何一个电流的明显变化都会对复极化和 APD 产生明显影响，如疾病状态下通道功能改变（例如遗传性长 QT 综合征）或药物改变了通道的状态（例如Ⅲ类抗心律失常药物阻断 I_{kr})。

二、遗传性通道病模型

长 QT 综合征

近年来，很多心律失常都与遗传缺陷（或突变）所导致的离子通道结构-功能的变化有关[14,15]。此类异常的绝大多数实验数据来自各表达系统（如爪蛙卵母细胞），而不是来自心肌细胞的生理性环境，其离子通道参与动作电位的形成。可以利用数学模型来把这些数据应用到有功能的心肌细胞（如图 28-1），以研究通道突变对全细胞动作电位的影响，并明确相应的细胞表型。通常情况下，突变所导致的通道功能变化都包括通道蛋白构型的变化（如关闭、开放及失活状态）。因此，要在全细胞动作电位的情况下模拟这些异常，就要求所选用的模型能体现通道的特殊结构状态及其相互作用关系。传统的 Hodgkin-Huxley 模型已经不能达到此要求了[16]，此模型中，各种离子通道形成的大的跨膜电流构成了动作电位，而没有表现出单通道状态之间的转换过程（如不同关闭状态之间的转换，或从关闭状态到失活状态之间的转换）。因此，我们建立了一个不同的模型，利用通道的状态特异性的 Markov 模型来模拟动作电位的产生。利用此模型，首先研究了与 LQTS 相关的一种钠通道突变[17]。

LQTS 是一种遗传性异常，特点是复极化异常，心电图上表现为 QT 间期延长，可导致多形性室性心律失常，尤其是尖端扭转型室速、晕厥和心源性猝死[18]。编码心脏不同离子通道的基因突变可产生不同类型的 LQTS。LQTS1 是 KvLQT1 基因（编码 I_{ks} 的基因）突变，引起 I_{ks} 功能丧失和电流减小。LQTS2 是 HERG 基因（编码 I_{kr} 的基因）突变，导致 I_{kr} 功能丧失。LQTS3 是 SCN5A 基因突变，导致 I_{Na} 功能增强，I_{Na} 电流增强。如前所述，动作电位的平台期和复极化期是各种内向和外向离子流精确平衡的结果，因此，复极化电流（LQTS1 中的 I_{ks} 或 LQTS2 中的 I_{kr}）的缺失或去极化电流（LQTS3 中的 I_{Na}）的增强都能使得动作电位复极化时间延长。

图 28-3 示 LQTS3 中，SCN5A 的一个突变（△KPQ 突变）导致钠通道功能增强[19-22]。此突变导

致Ⅲ-Ⅳ连接处的一段高度保守区域有3个氨基酸缺失，而此区与快速失活有关，这种结构的缺失使通道功能发生两种改变：（1）由于从失活状态恢复变快，所以当去极化时，通道在第一次开放后会再次开放，而正常通道只开放一次（图28-3A）。（2）通道在短期内不能失活，使通道在开放和关闭状态之间来回转换，从而使开放事件的频率增加。第一种模式，通道散发地再开放，称为背景模式或散发模式。第二种模式，通道开放频率增加，称为猝发模式。这两种模式在第一次开放后产生一个明显的电流。图28-3B示通过钠通道产生的跨膜电流。在正常通道，从维持电位－140mV去极化到－20mV，产生一个大的峰电流（峰值）300μA/μF，然后迅速衰减，提示在单通道水平没有晚期开放。相反，△KPQ突变中，散发模式和猝发模式的晚期开放效应产生一个大的电流（幅度约0.3μA/μF），即使去极化时间延长该电流仍持续存在（200ms）。这种晚期电流对动作电位的影响见图28-3C，示三种情况下模拟的动作电位和相应的I_{Na}：（Ⅰ）正常通道以CL＝400ms起搏，（Ⅱ）△KPQ突变以相同CL起搏，（Ⅲ）△KPQ突变以CL＝600ms起搏。△KPQ突变的实验数据见Ⅳ，可见其所测量的I_{Na}与Ⅱ中所模拟的非常相似。在CL＝400ms时，突变细胞的APD比正常细胞明显延长（为62.3ms），因为其在动作电位的晚期有I_{Na}电流，尽管此电流很小（3.0μA/μF，占I_{Na}电流峰值的1%），但也足以将电流向内向方向移动，从而延长APD。当起搏频率下降，CL＝600ms时，动作电位平台期的晚期就产生再次去极化。这种后去极化被归类于早后去极化（EAD）[23]，因为它发生于动作电位期间，在动作电位完全复极化之前。EAD形成的局部复极化延长可导致膜兴奋性的空间不均一性，利于形成单向传导阻滞和折返性心律失常。而且，在一定条件下，EAD能在周围组织产生兴奋性反应，从而触发心律失常。

在平台期去极化形成的EAD（如图28-3C所示）称为平台期EAD[24]。图28-4模拟了其发生的离子机制。其EAD的发生是由于I_{kr}功能缺失而形成的（LQT2）。图28-4显示40个连续刺激（CL＝500ms）的最后一个心跳的动作电位和相应的$I_{Ca(L)}$，以及1500ms的停搏后的另一个心跳（临床上，LQTS的心律失常发作前常常有一段停搏）。同时显示了停搏前和停搏后的数据以利于比较。停搏后的动作电位有3个平台期EAD（图28-4A），每一个EAD的上升支对应于内向$I_{Ca(L)}$的增高（图28-4B）。在停搏前动作电位中，$I_{Ca(L)}$回落到0点，因此没有形成EAD。如果把停搏后动作电位中的$I_{Ca(L)}$钳制在停搏前的水平，EAD就不会发生。很显然，$I_{Ca(L)}$是产生EAD上升支的去极化电流，是平台期EAD产生的主要机制。产生图28-4中的EAD是由于：停搏时I_{kr}降低（突变所致）和I_{ks}的失活，使得停搏后动作电位的复极化电流减少，平台期延长。而且，停搏后钙瞬变增加，使前向I_{NaCa}（内向电流）增强，也有助于延长APD。平台期的延长有助于L型钙通道从失活状态恢复并再次激活。再次激活产生的$I_{Ca(L)}$使膜去极化而形成EAD。

需要注意：（1）图28-3中，相对较短的CL（600ms）就产生了EAD，而先天性LQTS3，心律失常通常发生在睡眠或休息状态心率较慢时[18]。图28-3模拟的是所有钠通道都是△KPQ突变通道的情况，而病人一般都是LQT3杂合子，因此又模拟了50%是△KPQ、50%是野生型钠通道的情况，结果发现，当起搏心率降到CL＝1200ms时，即典型的临床心动过缓时，才发生EAD。（2）如果平台期延长到足够长时，其电压也适于$I_{Ca(L)}$的激活，就发生平台期$I_{Ca(L)}$的再激活，从而产生平台期EAD。（3）各种非特异性情况均能延长动作电位的平台期，而产生EAD。这些情况可能是钙依赖性的（如β肾上腺能刺激或停搏后，I_{NaCa}增加），也可能是非钙依赖性的（如图28-3中LQT3的晚期I_{Na}）。（4）图28-3和28-4的LQTS示例中，突变的缺陷通道不能产生导致心律失常的EAD，而是通过延长平台期，使得$I_{Ca(L)}$形成EAD。$I_{Ca(L)}$完全是一个"无辜旁观者"，完全正常，不受突变的影响。在单个心肌细胞中的这种复杂的相互关系也决定了其电生理反应。（5）EAD产生的$I_{Ca(L)}$机制不仅仅局限于平台期EAD。在动作电位的复极化晚期，复极化电位也可产生EAD。钙从肌浆网自发释放后，前向I_{NaCa}增强以排出钙离子，从而产生EAD。动作电位完全复极化之后，产生的迟后去极化也是同样机制[24]。（6）LQT2模型显示，突变的I_{kr}对动作电位的影响明显取决于其时程[26]。在动作电位早期影响I_{kr}的突变对APD影响很小，而在动作电位晚期影响I_{kr}的突变则明显延长APD。因此，把一个突变仅仅归类于"功能缺失"并不足以预测其表型特点。（7）模拟显示，通过与心肌的不同电生理介质相互作用，同一种突变可产生"双表型"[27]。例如，一种钠通道的突变（1795insD：在C端插入一个天冬氨酸）可产生两种表型，临床可观察到：一种是长QT综合征，一种是Brugada综合征[27-29]。

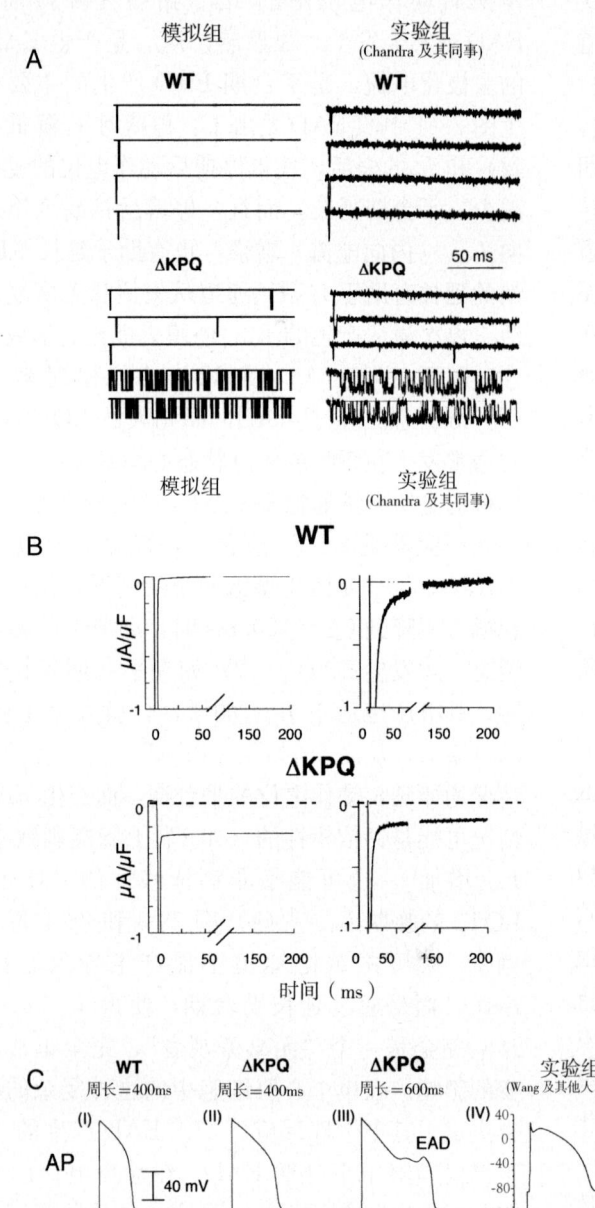

图 28-3 LQT3 患者 I_{Na} 功能增强形成早后除极（EAD） A，模拟的通道与相应实验的单通道门控。上，野生型通道门控显示只有一种开放状态。下，ΔKPQ 突变通道的门控表现为散发型（上面三条线）和簇发型（下面二条线）。B，从 -140mV 逐步去极化到 -20mV，得到的野生型和突变的 I_{Na}。上，野生型通道，I_{Na} 失活并回到零线。下，ΔKPQ 突变通道，I_{Na} 存在一个晚发（持续性）成分。模型（左）与 Bennett 等人的实验数据（右，已标准化）进行比较。I_{Na} 的标尺从 0 到 $-1\ \mu A/\mu F$ 以强调晚发电流（绝大部分早期 I_{Na} 超出此范围，图中未显示）。与模型相比，此实验中 I_{Na} 的衰减更缓慢，反映了温度的差异（模型中为 37℃，实验中为 22℃）。C，ΔKPQ 突变为全细胞动作电位的影响（上面的线条）。突变的 I_{Na} 在平台期持续存在，导致动作电位时程延长（Ⅱ，Ⅰ为野生型的动作电位时程），并且在较低起搏心率下，形成了 EAD（Ⅲ）。注意模型（Ⅱ）和实验（Ⅳ）中 I_{Na} 的密切相关性（引自 Clancy CE, Rudy Y: Linking a genetic defect to its cellular phenotype in a cardiac arrhythmia. Nature 400：566-569，1999.）

三、多细胞组织中动作电位的传播

前面部分讲述的是单个细胞动作电位的产生，不涉及电流的空间扩散。在这种情况下，全部 I_{ion} 用于对局部膜电容放电，见公式 1。而在多细胞组织中，细胞去极化所产生的 I_{ion} 分为两部分，一部分对局部膜电容放电，另一部分通过细胞间电流的流动使得邻近细胞去极化。换言之，组织中的细胞是"电负载的"。动作电位传播时，一个兴奋细胞必须为相邻的未兴奋细胞提供足够的电荷以使其膜达到兴奋阈值。

很明显，电荷的需求和电荷供给之间的平衡决定了动作电位能否传播。动作电位传播强度的一个有用的指标是传导安全系数（SF）。SF 的定义是：组织细胞的一个兴奋性循环中，产生电荷与消耗电荷的比值，可用以下公式计算[30-32]：

$$SF = \frac{\int_A I_c \cdot dt + \int_A I_{out} \cdot dt}{\int_A I_{in} \cdot dt} = \frac{Q_c + Q_{out}}{Q_{in}} \quad [2]$$

I_c 是细胞的电容电流，I_{in} 和 I_{out} 分别是流入和流出细胞的电流。将电流对时间进行积分可以计算出细胞兴奋周期中的电荷 Q（详细见 Shaw 和 Rudy[30]，

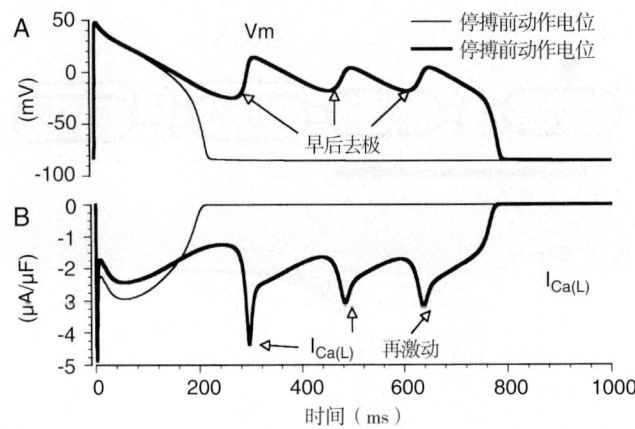

图 28-4 LQT2 中 I_{kr} 功能的缺失形成了早后除极 I_{kr} 减少的 LRd，模型细胞以 500ms 的周期起搏 40 次，经过 1500ms 停搏后，给予一个额外刺激。A，停搏前最后一个 AP（细线）和停搏后 AP 形成平台期 EAD（粗线），B，相应的 $I_{Ca(L)}$。箭头示 $I_{Ca(L)}$ 重新激活，形成 EAD（引自 Viswanathan PC，Rudy Y：Pause induced early afterdepolarizations in the long QT syndrome：A simulation study. Cardiovasc Res 42：530-542，1999.）

Wang 和 Rudy[31] 的著作）。公式 2 中的分子是使自身膜去极化（Q_c）和使相邻未兴奋细胞去极化所需要产生的电流（Q_{out}）。分母 Q_{in} 是细胞从相邻去极化细胞中所接受的电荷。SF 为 1 是个重要值，指细胞传给组织和从组织得到的电荷恰恰相等。SF 小于 1，细胞产生的电荷小于得到的电荷，不能满足对电荷的需求，传导失败。SF 大于 1 提示传导能力强（产生的电荷多于成功传导所需要的电荷），能安全传导。

前面我们讨论了心脏组织中离子通道表达的空间不均一性、其在动作电位特点中的作用及其离子机制。心脏组织的结构也存在不均一性。正常心肌结构的不均一性（如浦肯野-肌肉连接处、纤维的分支、结缔组织分隔、血管）随年龄增加和病理状态而进一步增加。例如，心肌梗死后，存活心肌组织岛与狭长的心肌带相联系。心脏的兴奋是膜的过程（离子通道和转运体的离子流）与组织的结构特点相互作用的结果。因此，检测结构不均一性的心脏的兴奋特点及其离子机制就尤为重要。

图 28-5 中，我们模拟动作电位在一个结构不均一区域的传播。在此模型中[31]，结构的不均一性是指组织通过分支形成膨胀点。此模型是由 LRd 细胞通过缝隙连接而形成的多细胞纤维。组织的传播从细胞 80 开始，有多个细胞间连接，而细胞大小（长 110μm，半径 11μm）不变。这代表了心脏组织中的传播（即一个狭长的心肌带插入梗死的存活心肌岛中），只是后者的细胞数目更多，但心肌细胞大小不变。

图 28-5 中，刺激从细胞 0 开始，从左向右传播，传入分支纤维。细胞 79 和细胞 80 之间的转换部位有一个很长的传导延迟，因为在此部位，一个小的电源（单个纤维）要为一个大的电负荷（分支纤维）提供电流。分支纤维后的膜面积大，因此膜电容也大，达到兴奋性阈值所需要的去极化电荷也大。因为分支点近端的纤维所产生的去极化电流受纤维大小的限制，所以产生足够电流的时间就延长（见公式 2），从而产生局部传导的延迟。注意，在整个延迟中，细胞 79 的平台期被"拉下"来了，反映它被转换部位后的分支纤维加载电荷。一旦分支纤维兴奋，其电负荷被移除，细胞 79 就重新获得了充分去极化（正常）的平台期电势。紧邻膨胀点远端的细胞有一个持续时间长、幅度高的尾电势，位于局部兴奋之前，它反映的是，在跨分支区域，需要很长的去极化时间才能达到兴奋阈值。

图 28-5B 显示的是不同部位纤维的 SF，以及局部 I_{Na} 和 $I_{Ca(L)}$ 的电荷（Q_{Na} 和 $Q_{Ca(L)}$）对动作电位传播的作用。当动作电位到达分支点时，SF 突然下降，提示此点是传播的关键点。在分支点以外，纤维均匀部位，I_{Na} 对传导起主要作用。相反，在分支区，$I_{Ca(L)}$ 是一个重要的去极化电流，提供的去极化电荷比 I_{Na} 多。事实上，图 28-5 中，阻断 15% 的 $I_{Ca(L)}$ 就使得兴奋不能从分支点处传入分支纤维。在包含分支的培养组织中，用尼非地平阻断 $I_{Ca(L)}$ 时，可以观察到相似的实验结果[33]。

膨胀点处 $I_{Ca(L)}$ 对电荷的作用大，是因为此处的局部传导延迟很长。在绝大多数延迟中，由于其失活动力学很快，I_{Na} 很快就失活，1ms 之后几乎可以忽略不计，因此，在膨胀区近端的细胞，其去极化电荷的唯一来源就是 $I_{Ca(L)}$。而正常传导区，没有长的局部传导延迟，I_{Na} 是主要的去极化电流。有趣的是，在传导最需要 $I_{Ca(L)}$ 的区域，$I_{Ca(L)}$ 大大增强了（峰值从 $-11\mu A/\mu F$ 增加到 $-34\mu A/\mu F$）（见图 28-5C）。相反，在分支点远端，I_{Na} 减少了。$I_{Ca(L)}$ 增强是由于局部平台期电势减少，增加了 $I_{Ca(L)}$ 的驱动电位，从而增加此电流。I_{Na} 减少是因为在去极化电势延长的末端，随着对跨分支点的细胞进行缓慢充电，钠通道失活了。

在大的组织膨胀点处，从 I_{Na} 依赖性传导转变到 $I_{Ca(L)}$ 依赖性传导，这是一个重要规律。它明确指出，在动作电位传播过程中，心肌结构与兴奋性膜电流之间有密切的联系。在这一点上,多细胞组织的结构特点决定了单个细胞上离子通道的作用。组织结构(电荷)对细胞电流(电源)的作用形成了一个反馈,来调节传导的离子机制。在需要的地方(膨胀点近端,此处 $Q_{Ca} \geq Q_{Na}$),$I_{Ca(L)}$ 增加,这形成了另外一个反馈代偿机制。结构不均一性决定了局部传导依赖于 $I_{Ca(L)}$,并通过增强此电流决定了细胞膜的反应。在细胞对的实验中可观察到 $I_{Ca(L)}$ 增加,即动作电位传导过程中,可见主导细胞的 $I_{Ca(L)}$ 强于随后的细胞[34]。需要注意的是,膨胀点效应是非对称性的(具有方向依赖性)。图 28-5 中,如果刺激细胞 159,则传播方向是从右到左,从多个分支到单一纤维。与膨胀不同,纤维的集中导致电负荷的减少,因此,这个方向上的传导连续、牢固,纤维上任何一处的 SF 都很高。此方向上的传导是由 I_{Na} 单独完成的,$I_{Ca(L)}$ 的作用可以忽略。这种组织结构的不对称性对心律失常的发生有重要意义,因为单向阻滞是折返性心律失常的必要条件之一。在结构高度复杂的组织,传导依赖于 $I_{Ca(L)}$,而在正常组织则否,这对心律失常的药物治疗来说有重要意义。它提示:作用于 $I_{Ca(L)}$ 的药物可以选择性地改变异常病理组织的传导,从而使得依赖于心肌病理状态的"功能性药物靶向作用"成为可能。

图 28-5 所示的例子可普遍应用于其他情况,即动作电位传入电荷增加的区域。例如细胞间的缝隙连接处,其局部电荷增加[31]。连接良好的区域形成一个大的电负荷,而连接差的区域,其高阻抗的缝隙连接限制了其提供去极化电流的能力。对这种情况的模拟表明[31],其表现同图 28-5 中组织膨胀处相同,在分支点处局部 SF 降低,有很长的传导延迟,传导依赖于 $I_{Ca(L)}$,而且此电流增强。需要说明的是,局部电负荷增加并不一定有解剖结构的改变,可以是功能的改变。例如,折返时旋转波的波锋沿支点转动时有一个很大的曲率[35-37]。这些情况下,波锋的一小部分为很大区域的组织提供去极化电流("扇面"效应)。螺旋波尖端也有同样的扩散效应。这些情况与图 28-5 中的组织膨胀处的传导一样,都存在电源-电负荷的不匹配。模型也提示,在大的波锋曲率处,$I_{Ca(L)}$ 可能起重要作用。缝隙连接显著减少时,在细胞水平也可产生不连续传导[30]。与图 28-5 所示的大体水平相同,细胞水平的不连续传播的特点也是局部延迟很长(发生于缝隙连接处),依赖于 $I_{Ca(L)}$[30]。

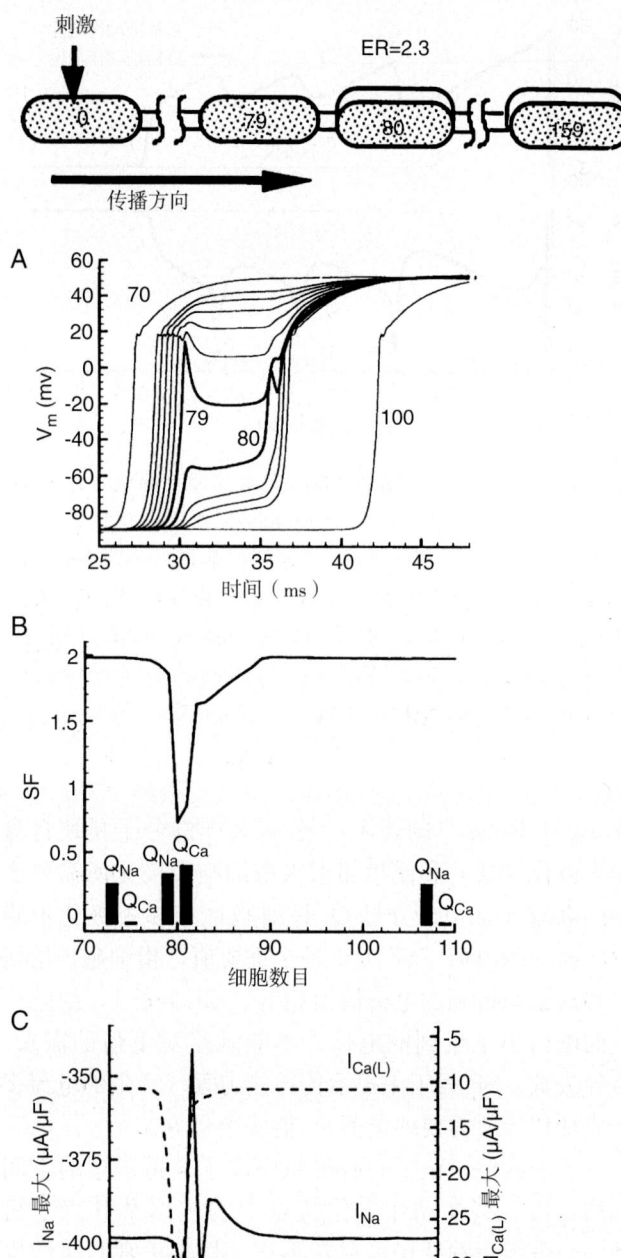

图 28-5 在组织膨大部位的扩散 上,在细胞 80 处纤维膨大,并以 2.3 的膨大系数重复了两次。A,动作电位,数字表示所选择的细胞编号。B,线指的是沿纤维传导的安全系数。竖条指的是局部 I_{Na}(Q_{Na})和 $I_{Ca(L)}$(Q_{Ca})对电荷的影响。C,沿纤维方向的 $I_{Na,max}$(实线)和 $I_{Ca(L),max}$(虚线)(引自 Wang Y, Rudy Y: Action potential propagation in inhomogeneous cardiac tissue: Safety factor considerations and ionic mechanism. Am J Physiol 278: H1019-1029, 2000.)

四、从离子通道到心电图波形

前面部分，我们利用数学模型研究了心肌组织动作电位产生和传播的离子机制。一个有临床意义的问题是，这些细胞电生理过程能否反映在体表或心脏表面记录的心电图上。鉴于我们对心律失常的分子和离子机制的进一步理解，在这些细胞过程和心电图之间建立联系，将有助于我们对心脏电生理异常的心电图表现作出诊断。本节我们简述特异性膜离子流、动作电位形态和心电图波形之间的关系[38]。

模型采用的是LRd细胞束，包括心内膜、心肌中膜（M）和心外膜，I_{ks}和I_{to}的表达具有不均一性[38]。模拟正常心室激动时，平面波从心内膜向心外膜传播，它对应于心电图波形实验中广泛应用的跨壁梯度模型。利用以下公式计算跨膜电势[41]：

$$ECG=\frac{a^2\sigma_i}{4\sigma_e}\int(-\nabla V_m)\cdot\left[\nabla\frac{1}{r}\right]dx \quad [3]$$

式中，a是纤维的半径，σ_i和σ_e是细胞内外的电导，r是从纤维的电源点到心电图记录点之间的距离（在纤维轴方向上距心外膜2.0cm）。模拟的心电图体现的是靠近心外膜的心肌所产生的电势，受心脏其他部位电活动的影响很少。注意，公式3中，心电图电势的来源是$-\nabla V_m$，即V_m的空间梯度，而不是V_m本身。因此心电图反映的是心室壁的跨膜电势梯度，及离子流和缝隙连接对它的影响。

图28-6模拟显示的是正常生理状态下跨壁动作电位的不均一性及其离子流与心电图波形的关系。正常心肌，M区的I_{ks}密度低，而从心外膜到心内膜，I_{to}密度逐渐降低。图28-6中，M细胞的I_{ks}使得APD延长，而I_{to}在心外膜和M细胞的动作电位上形成了一个早期切迹。T波的峰值对应于心外膜的完全复极化，而T波的终点由M区的完全复极化决定。尽管去极化和复极化的方向相反，但QRS和T波都是正向的。这是因为，APD的差异远远大于跨心室壁的传导时间，因此$-\nabla V_m$是由APD的不均一性决定的，而受激动顺序的影响较少。心外膜区最晚去极化，但最早复极化，在去极化期间保持$-\nabla V_m$的方向（指向心外膜）不变。如果减少缝隙连接，显著延长跨壁传导时间，则激动顺序，而不是APD的不均一性决定了复极化顺序。这时，$-\nabla V_m$与对照相反，T波倒置（见Gima和Rudy所著图2）。因为跨壁APD的不均一性主要是由I_{ks}表达的不均一性决定的，我们模拟了I_{ks}在整个纤维均匀分布时的心电图（见图28-6，中）。如我们所料，如果没有这种不均一性，则复极化的顺序与去极化相同，心外膜最后复极化。复极化时这种与去极化相反的$-\nabla V_m$，使得T波倒置。

J波（Osborn波）位于QRS波群后，其产生的离子机制见图28-6（右）。在模拟的对照情况下可见J波，并与心外膜动作电位上的切迹相对应。如果阻断I_{to}（产生动作电位的切迹），则动作电位的切迹和J波都消失，证明I_{to}是产生J波的离子基础。

图28-6有助于在离子流、动作电位和心电图图形之间建立直接和特定的联系。它仅限于正常情况，表明T波形态主要由I_{ks}的不均一性决定的，而心外膜的I_{to}产生了J波。疾病状态下，也可用此模型来解释离子通道功能变化与心电图图形的关系。Gima和Rudy[38]的研究中包括以下情况：（1）细胞外钾（高钾血症和低钾血症）对T波形态的影响。（2）三种LQTS（LQT1、LQT2、LQT3）引起的心电图改变：LQT2和LQT3延长QT间期，使T波增宽，反映复极化的离散度增加，而LQT1延长QT间期，不影响复极化的离散度，不使T波增宽。（3）Brugada综合征的ST段抬高。通过不同程度地加快I_{Na}的失活，可以引起ST段抬高，可模拟Brugada综合征[42]。随严重程度的增加，心电图图形从"马鞍形"变为"穹隆形"直至"三角形"。（4）急性心肌缺血的ST段抬高，表明ATP敏感的钾通道开放，引起ST段抬高。

五、跋

本章通过计算机模型，试图阐述心肌细胞动作电位产生和多细胞组织中动作电位传播的离子机制，以及这些过程在心电图图形上的反映。重点是各个水平（单细胞水平和多细胞组织水平）上高度复杂和非线性的相互作用，决定了其电生理反应。在单细胞水平，多个离子通道和转运子相互作用，产生了动作电位，并决定了其特点。在组织水平，细胞间通过缝隙连接相互作用，以及组织的结构特点是动作电位传播的主要决定因素。重要的是，模型提示，在不同水平间会产生相互作用，例如，动作电位传播过程中，组织结构可以调控离子通道的功能。对心电图波形作出诊断性分析时，以及治疗心律失常时，必须考虑到这些复杂的相互作用及其电生理结果。

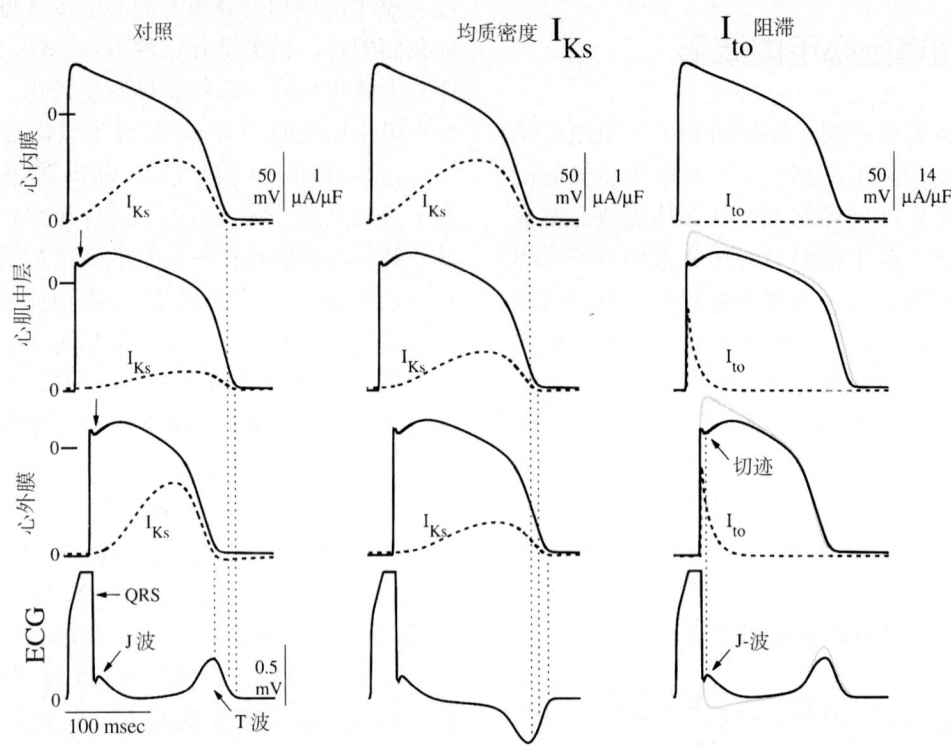

图 28-6　离子流与心电图波形之间的关系　对照组（左），相同性跨壁 I_{ks} 密度（中）和 I_{to} 缺失（右）时心内膜细胞、心肌中层细胞和心外膜细胞的模拟动作电位和相应的计算机化心电图。左，心室壁 I_{ks} 的不同密度形成了跨壁的电压梯度，产生了 T 波。心外膜和心肌中层的完全复极化分别与 T 波的顶点和终末部分相对应（竖点线）。箭头指的是心外膜和心肌中层细胞中由 I_{to} 形成的切迹。I_{to} 不均一性导致的跨壁梯度产生了心电图上的 J 波（Osborn 波）。中，去除内在的 I_{to} 不均一性后，改变了复极顺序，随之改变了激动顺序，心电图上出现 T 波倒置。右，阻断 I_{to}（灰线，对照为黑线）导致切迹和 J 波变线（引自 Gima K，Rudy Y：Ionic current basis of electrocardiographic waveforms：A model study. Circ Res 90：889-896，2002.）

资助，项目号 R37-HL33343 和 R01-HL49054。

（李　春译）

六、致　谢

本章的研究由国立医学研究院心肺血管研究所

参 考 文 献

1. Noble D, Rudy Y: Models of cardiac ventricular action potentials: iterative interaction between experiment and simulation. Phil Trans Roy Soc (Lond) 359:1127–1142, 2001.
2. Morad M, Ebashi S, Trautwein W, Kurachi Y: Molecular Physiology and Pharmacology of Cardiac Ion Channels and Transporters. Dordrecht, Kluwer, 1996.
3. Rudy Y: The cardiac ventricular action potential. In Page E, Fozzard HA, Solaro RJ (eds): The Handbook of Physiology, section 2, vol 1, The Heart. New York, Oxford University Press, 2002, pp 531–547.
4. Faber GM, Rudy Y: Action potential and contractility changes in $[Na^+]_i$ overloaded cardiac myocytes: a simulation study. Biophys J 78:2392–2404, 2000.
5. Hund TJ, Kucera JP, Otani NF, Rudy Y: Ionic charge conservation and long-term steady state in the Luo-Rudy dynamic cell model. Biophys J 81:3324–3331, 2001.
6. Fozzard HA, Hanck DA: Structure and function of voltage-dependent sodium channels: Comparison of brain II and cardiac isoforms. Physiol Rev 76:887–926, 1996.
7. Sipido KR, Callewaert G, Carmeliet E: Inhibition and rapid recovery of Ca^{2+} current during release from sarcoplasmic reticulum in guinea pig ventricular myocytes. Circ Res 76:102–109, 1995.
8. Zeng J, Laurita KR, Rosenbaum DS, Rudy Y: Two components of the delayed rectifier K^+ current in ventricular myocytes of the guinea pig type: Theoretical formulation and their role in repolarization. Circ Res 77:1–13, 1995.
9. Antzelevitch C, Dumaine R: Electrical heterogeneity in the heart: Physiological, pharmacological and clinical implications. In Page E, Fozzard HA, Solaro RJ (eds): The Handbook of Physiology, section 2, vol 1, The Heart. New York: Oxford University Press, 2001, pp 654–692.
10. Linz KW, Meyer R: Profile and kinetics of L-type calcium current during the cardiac ventricular action potential compared in guinea-pigs, rats and rabbits. Pflugers Arch 439:588–599, 2000.
11. Blaustein MP, Lederer WJ: Sodium/calcium exchange: its physiological implications. Physiol Rev 79:763–854, 1999.
12. Hund TJ, Rudy Y: Determinants of excitability in cardiac myocytes: Mechanistic investigation of memory effect. Biophys J 79:3095–3104, 2000.
13. Viswanathan PC, Shaw RM, Rudy Y: Effects of I_{Kr} and I_{Ks} heterogeneity on action potential duration and its rate-dependence: A simulation study. Circulation 99:2466–2474, 1999.
14. Keating MT, Sanguinetti MC: Molecular and cellular mechanisms of cardiac arrhythmias. Cell 104:569–580, 2001.
15. Marban E: Cardiac channelopathies. Nature 415:213–218, 2002.
16. Hodgkin A, Huxley A: A quantitative description of membrane current and its application to excitation and conduction in nerve. J Physiol (Lond) 117:500–544, 1952.

17. Clancy CE, Rudy Y: Linking a genetic defect to its cellular phenotype in a cardiac arrhythmia. Nature 400:566–569, 1999.
18. Schwartz PJ, Priori SG, Napolitano C: Long QT syndrome. In Zipes DP, Jalife J (eds): Cardiac Electrophysiology: From Cell to Bedside, 3rd ed. Philadelphia, WB Saunders, 1999, pp 788–810.
19. Bennett PB, Yazawa K, Makita N, George AL Jr: Molecular mechanism for an inherited cardiac arrhythmia. Nature 376:683–685, 1995.
20. Chandra R, Starmer CE, Grant AO: Multiple effects of the KPQ deletion on gating of human cardiac Na^+ channels expressed in mammalian cells. Am J Physiol 274:H1643–H1654, 1998.
21. Wang DW, Yazawa K, Makita N, et al: Pharmacological targeting of long QT mutant sodium channels. J Clin Invest 99:1714–1720, 1997.
22. Dumaine R, Wang Q, Keating MT, et al: Multiple mechanisms of Na^+ channel-linked long QT syndrome. Circ Res 78:916–924, 1996.
23. Vos MA, Lerman BB: Automaticity and triggered activity. In Spooner PM, Rosen MR (eds): Foundations of Cardiac Arrhythmias. New York, Marcel Dekker, pp 425–447, 2001.
24. Zeng J, Rudy Y: Early afterdepolarizations in cardiac myocytes: mechanism and rate dependence. Biophys J 63:949–964, 1995.
25. Viswanathan PC, Rudy Y: Pause induced early afterdepolarizations in the long QT syndrome: A simulation study. Cardiovasc Res 42:530–542, 1999.
26. Clancy CE, Rudy Y: Cellular consequences of HERG mutations in the long QT syndrome: Precursors to sudden cardiac death. Cardiovasc Res 50:301–313, 2001.
27. Clancy CE, Rudy Y: A Na^+ channel mutation that causes both Brugada and long QT syndrome phenotypes: A simulation study of mechanism. Circulation 105:1208–1213, 2002.
28. Bezzina C, Veldkamp MW, van den Berg MP, et al: A single Na(+) channel mutation causing both long-QT and Brugada syndromes. Circ Res 85:1206–1213, 1999.
29. Veldkamp MW, Viswanathan PC, Bezzina C, et al: Two distinct congenital arrhythmias evoked by a multidysfunctional Na(+) channel. Circ Res 86:E91–E97, 2000.
30. Shaw RM, Rudy Y: Ionic mechanisms of propagation in cardiac tissue. Roles of the sodium and L-type calcium currents during reduced excitability and decreased gap junction coupling. Circ Res 81:727–741, 1997.
31. Wang Y, Rudy Y: Action potential propagation in inhomogeneous cardiac tissue: Safety factor considerations and ionic mechanism. Am J Physiol 278:H1019–1029, 2000.
32. Kucera JP, Rudy Y: Mechanistic insights into very slow conduction in branching cardiac tissue: a model study. Circ Res 82:799–806, 2001.
33. Rohr S, Kucera J: Involvement of the calcium inward current in cardiac impulse propagation: Induction of unidirectional conduction block by nifedipine and reversal by Bay K 8644. Biophys J 72:754–766, 1997.
34. Kumar R, Joyner RW: Calcium currents of ventricular cell pairs during action potential conduction. Am J Physiol 268:H2476–H2486, 1995.
35. Girouard SD, Pastore JM, Laurita KR, et al: Optical mapping in a new Guinea pig model of ventricular tachycardia reveals mechanisms for multiple wavelengths in a single reentrant circuit. Circulation 93:603–613, 1996.
36. Fast VG, Kléber AG: Role of wavefront curvature in propagation of cardiac impulse. Cardiovasc Res 33:258–271, 1996.
37. Kléber AG, Janse MJ, Fast VG: Normal and abnormal conduction in the heart. In Page E, Fozzard HA, Solaro RJ (eds): The Handbook of Physiology, section 2, vol 1, The Heart. New York, Oxford University Press, 2002, pp 455–530.
38. Gima K, Rudy Y: Ionic current basis of electrocardiographic waveforms: A model study. Circ Res 90:889–896, 2002.
39. Yan GX, Antzelevitch C: Cellular basis for the normal T wave and the electrocardiographic manifestations of the long-QT syndrome. Circulation 98:1928–1936, 1998.
40. Shimizu W, Antzelevitch C: Cellular basis for long-QT, transmural dispersion of repolarization, and torsade de pointes in the long-QT syndrome. J Electrocardiol 32(suppl):177–184, 1999.
41. Plonsey R, Barr RC: Bioelectricity: A Quantitative Approach, 2nd ed. New York, Kluwer Academic/Plenum Publishers, 2000, pp 217–243.
42. Dumaine R, Towbin JA, Brugada P, et al: Ionic mechanisms responsible for the electrocardiographic phenotype of the Brugada syndrome are temperature dependent. Circ Res 83:803–809, 1999.

第 29 章

心肌中电激动的二维传导

Bradley J. Roth

本章目录

- 反应-弥散模型 262
- 三种波锋 263
- 螺旋波蜿蜒 264
- 螺旋波碎裂 266
- 结论 266

心肌组织中的每个细胞都能产生动作电位,但是,心肌细胞不是孤立的,细胞间通道把细胞相互联系起来,使心肌组织在功能上成为一个合胞体(syncytium)。而且,在平行于和垂直于细胞长轴(纤维)的方向上,细胞间的连接是不同的,因此,组织具有各向异性。

可以利用各种二维组织切面的方法来研究波锋在各向异性合胞体中的传播。在本书的第三版中,我讨论了与激动传播相关的三个方面:波锋速度如何决定于激动波传播方向,波锋曲率如何影响速度以及螺旋波如何蜿蜒[1](35章到38章详细介绍了螺旋波)。在本书第四版中,我更新了以上内容,然而最近5年来,Chaos杂志发行了两期"焦点问题"以利于进一步了解心脏的电活动[2,3]。而且,物理学文献中也发表了很多新的结果(如 *Physical Review E Physica D*)。本章旨在对这些结果做一个简述,并介绍这方面的最新进展。

本章着重于连续、二维组织切面的数字模型,不包括细胞自动控制以及其他空间离散效应、三维行为(见30章)、心肌组织的电刺激[11-13](见31章)及数字预测的实验检验。

一、反应-弥散模型

研究者通常用连续、二维的反应-弥散模型来描述心肌组织中波锋的传播。图29-1显示一个近似此模型的电阻网络。兴奋性模型阐述了每一片膜的特点(图29-1左中,膜盒子)。电阻格反映的是细胞内空间,并把每一片膜与其周围的膜相联系(图29-1,左下)。这些电阻考虑到了每一个细胞内电阻和细胞间通道的电阻。与细胞内空间相比,细胞外空间可以忽略不记。细胞内空间、膜、细胞外空间共同形成了二维反应-弥散模型(图29-1,右)。

在连续组织中,此电阻网络中每一个结点之间的距离都很小。其反应-弥散模型可用以下公式描述:

$$g_{ix}\frac{\partial^2 V}{\partial x^2} + g_{iy}\frac{\partial^2 V}{\partial y^2} = \beta\left[C_m\frac{\partial V}{\partial t} + J_{ion}\right] \quad [1]$$

此公式基于电路分析的两个基本概念:欧姆定律和电流的连续性。当细胞外电位为0时,跨膜电位 V 等于细胞内电位。β 是膜表面积与体积的比值,C_m 是单位面积的膜电容,J_{ion} 是膜电流密度,可以从不同离子通道的动力学模型中计算出来。

参数 g_{ix} 和 g_{iy} 是细胞内电导。因为各向异性组织中,细胞内电导依赖于两个方向,所以有两个参数:x 是平行于心肌纤维的方向,y 是垂直于纤维的方向。公式1的一个特点是:用于测量距离的标尺的变化可以改变各向异性效应。如果坐标从 (x, y) 变为 (X, Y),X=x,Y=aa,则在 X,Y 坐标系中,组织就是各向同性的。因此,将各向同性组织中计算的结果在某一方向上"伸展",就能得到各向异性组织中的行

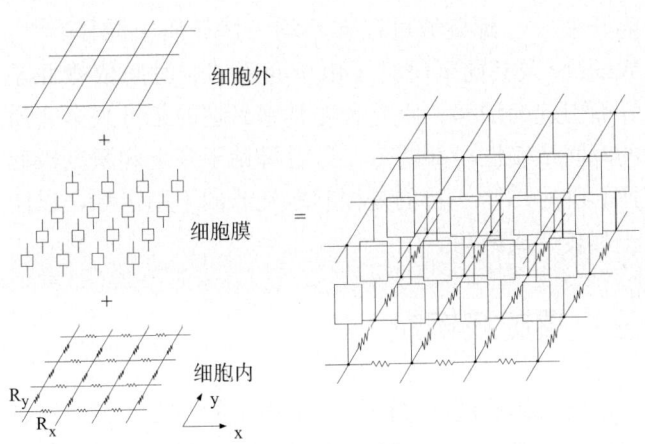

图 29-1 电阻-格栅近似于二维反应-扩散模型 下层电阻为格栅反映了细胞内空间的电特性。由于各向异性，x 方向（平行于纤维方向）的电阻小于 y 方向（垂直于纤维方向），$R_x < R_y$。膜单元反映的是膜电容，后者与离子通道的电导相关。细胞外空间已接地

为特点。同样，在各向异性组织中得到的结果在某一方向进行"压缩"，就能得到各向同性的结果。当然，只有当整个组织中的传导都是均匀的时候（均匀的心肌组织，且不弯曲），这一特点才是正确的。

二、三种波锋

公式 1 可以产生 3 种波锋。首先，如果沿着二维切面的边缘兴奋，就会产生一个跨过组织的平面波（图 29-2A）。其速度决定于传播方向与纤维方向之间的夹角 θ

$$V(\theta) = V_L \sqrt{\cos^2\theta + \frac{g_{iT}}{g_{iL}}\sin^2\theta}, \quad [2]$$

V_L 是平行于纤维方向的速度。典型的是，平行于纤维方向的速度大约是垂直于纤维方向速度的 2～2.5 倍。

如果切面内的某一点兴奋，则第二种波——环形波就向外传播（图 29-2B，如果组织是各向异性的，则波形就是椭圆形的），环形波的速度受波锋曲率的影响[14]。各向同性组织中，环形波的速度 $V_{circular}$ 与平面波的速度 V_{planar} 相关，

$$V_{circular} = V_{planar} - D/r \quad [3]$$

r 是环形波的半径。D 是"弥散常数"[15]，等于 $g_i/(\beta C_m)$，g_i 是各向同性细胞间的电导。公式 3 不仅适用于环形波，也适用于曲率随位置变化的波。它提示，沿着波锋、凸曲率大的点（因为 r 值小且为负值）

传播速度相对较慢，而凹曲率大的点（r 值小，为正值）的传播速度相对较快。如果公式 3 可被推论用于很大的曲率（此推论可能不十分恰当），则半径的临界值 $r_{critical}$ 将使得 $V_{circular}$ 等于零。半径小于 $r_{critical}$ 的波锋不能传播。$r_{critical}$ 的估计值为 100～200μm。当波锋从组织的一条窄带传入一个大的相邻区域时，或通过分隔两个较大区域的峡部时，曲率就显得非常重要了。波锋能传播的最小峡部宽度为 150μm。峡部再窄时，波锋就不能传播了，因为远端波锋的曲率很大。通过一个依赖于波锋曲率的机制，边缘锐利的非兴奋性障碍物能形成螺旋波[16,17]（图 29-3，左）。如果障碍物足够小，则很高的曲率和频率使得波锋不能围绕此障碍物，解剖折返（围绕环形障碍物的传播）就变成了功能折返（螺旋波传播甚至是螺旋波破裂）[18,19]。各向异性组织中的速度和曲率之间的关系是很微妙的[15]。Morozov 及其同事对公式 3 作出了修正，以适

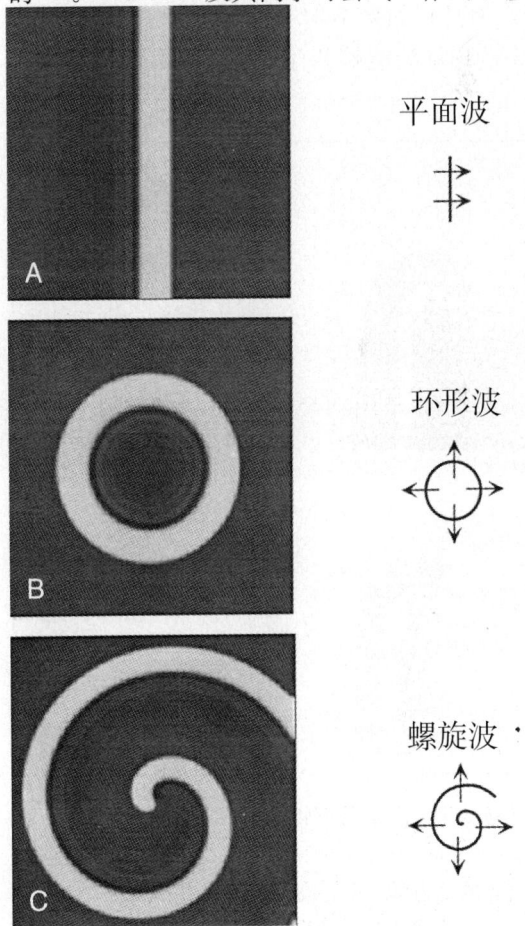

图 29-2 三种波锋：平面波（A）、环形波（B）和螺旋波在某一瞬间，在 x（水平）和 y（竖直）方向的跨膜电势 白色为去极化，黑色为静息状态。应用二维反应-扩散模型进行计算，利用 FitzHugh-Nagumo 模型表示膜兴奋性

用于各向异性的情况。

第三种波锋是螺旋波或旋转波（图 29-2C）。螺旋波有很多独特的特点。与平面波和环形波不同，螺旋波是自我维持的：一旦形成，它们就能永久存在。在螺旋波的中心或顶端，具有"时相单一性（phase singularity）"。平面波和环形波，其主导相（从静息快速去极化）和尾随相（与复极化和不应期有关）的区别是明确的。而螺旋波的主导相和尾随相在尖端附近融合，此处波锋的时相不能被分为主导相或尾随相。螺旋波尖端的曲率很大。如前所述，曲率大的波锋传导相对较慢，因此尖端附近的传播非常慢。螺旋波不必绕解剖障碍物旋转，它们能在均匀组织中绕任何一点旋转。起始的情况决定了其方向。

如果在不均一性介质中同时存在两个或更多稳定的螺旋波，其相互作用决定于不均一性的程度。某些情况下，低频率的螺旋波能被邻近高频率的螺旋波"清除"[21]。但是，如果不均一性超过了一个临界值，则不同频率的螺旋波能够共存，一个混乱区把它们分隔开来[22]。螺旋波可以在不均一性介质中漂移[23-28]。Wellner 及其同事研究了由于介质的非时间依赖性差异而引起的漂移。研究者尤其感兴趣的是可兴奋介质的时间依赖性局部调节，后者可见于多个刺激电极起搏心脏时[27,28]。目的是控制螺旋波的不稳定性，以防止其转变成颤动。

三、螺旋波蜿蜒

有时螺旋波严格围绕一个固定的中心旋转。这种情况下，螺旋波的尖端固定，或在一个环形轨道上旋转（图 29-4A）。但其他情况下，螺旋波尖端的运动很复杂，被称为"蜿蜒（meandering）"。尖端的路径像是一个多瓣的"花"。通常，这些花像是内摆线（图 29-4D），但也有其他变化（图 29-4B 和 4C），如近似线性轨道（图 29-4F），这取决于膜离子模型的具体情况。典型的蜿蜒运动包括两种频率（准周期性）：螺旋波旋转的频率和尖端蜿蜒的频率。如果这两种频率的比值等于两个整数的比值，则轨道本身就关闭了。研究者对蜿蜒的机制进行了大量的探索[29-33]。如果兴奋性很微弱，螺旋波围绕一个大的非兴奋性核心旋转，其机制已经被 Hakim 和 Karma 阐明[34,35]。Starobin 和 Starmer 发现，蜿蜒的发生与波锋从障碍物处分裂有关[17]（图 29-3）。某些情况下，"超蜿蜒"可使得螺旋波的尖端形成一个复杂的布朗（Brownian）样运动[36,37]（图 29-4E）。其他情况下，尖端可以向外盘旋[38]。

各向异性可以影响螺旋波的蜿蜒。为说明这一点，需要把细胞外空间的电阻系数引入心肌组织模型中。在公式 1 阐述的反应-弥散模型中，细胞外空间被视为 0。双域模型是对这一个模型的扩展，加入了细胞外空间的各向异性阻抗。这种细胞外阻抗产生了什么差别呢？差别是显著的，原因就是各向异性的特点。在反应-弥散模型中，坐标的一个简单变化就去掉了各向异性的作用，而在双域模型中则不是，坐标的变化去掉了细胞内各向异性后，可使得细胞外空间变成各向异性。总之，仅仅改变坐标并不能去掉各向异性的影响。各向异性对组织电学特点有着更深刻、更复杂的影响。只有细胞内和细胞外空间的各向异性程度相等时（各向异性比率相等），等比例的变化才能去除各向异性的影响。心室肌细胞内空间的各向异性远远大于细胞外空间（各向异性比率不等）。

双域模型中，各向异性比率不等明显影响螺旋波尖端的路径[39-42]。旋转和蜿蜒的频率为 2 : 1 时，蜿

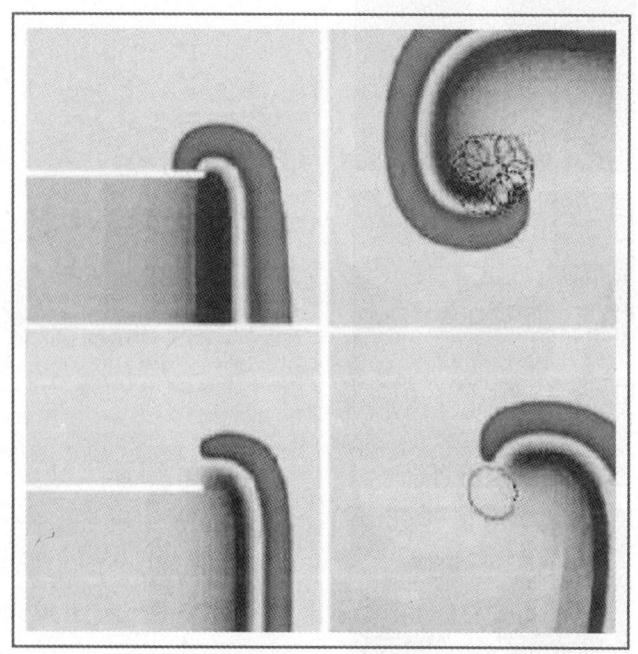

图 29-3　蜿蜒变化与波锋-障碍物阻隔-相连边缘相一致　利用 FitzHugh-Nagumo 模型来计算一个二维组织中的跨膜电势，以研究膜的动力学。上，高度可兴奋组织，下，微兴奋性组织。左，波锋与非兴奋性边缘相互作用，右，螺旋波顶端的抛物线（引自 Starobin JM, Starmer CF: Common mechanism links spiral wave meandering and wavefront-obstacle separation. Phys Rev E 55: 1193-1196, 1997.）

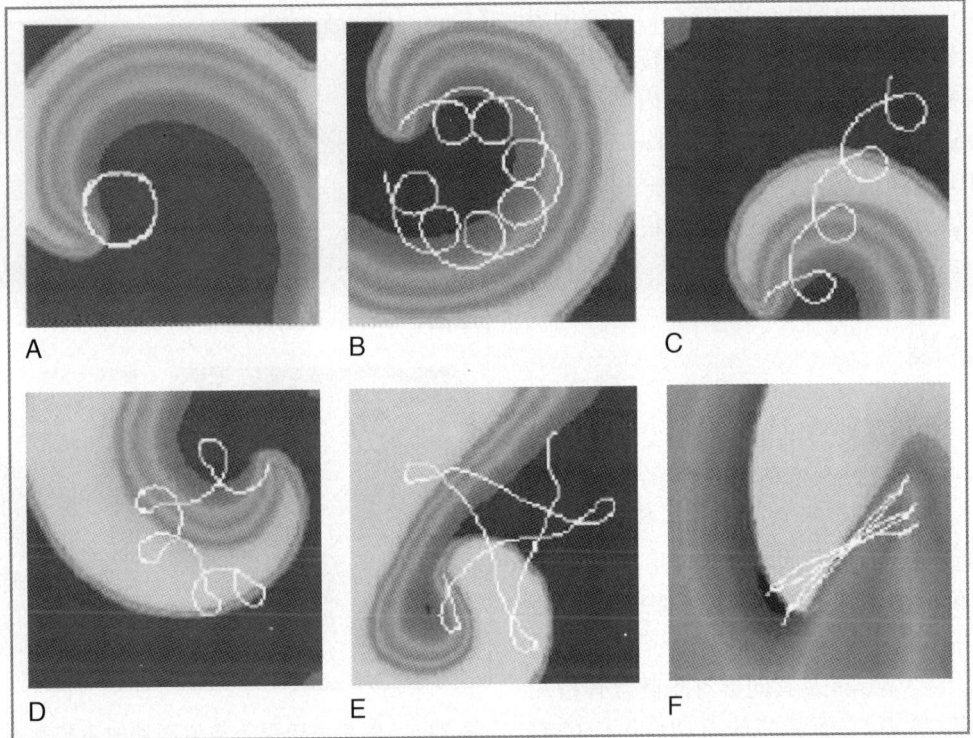

图 29-4　螺旋顶端的各种轨迹　可见环行（A）、摆线形（B）、摆线形（C）、内摆线形（D）、高度蜿蜒形（E）和线形（F）轨迹（引自 Fenton FH，Cherry EM，Hastings HM，Evans SJ：Multiple mechanisms of spiral wave breakup in a model of cardiac electrical ativity. Chaos 12：852-892，2002.）

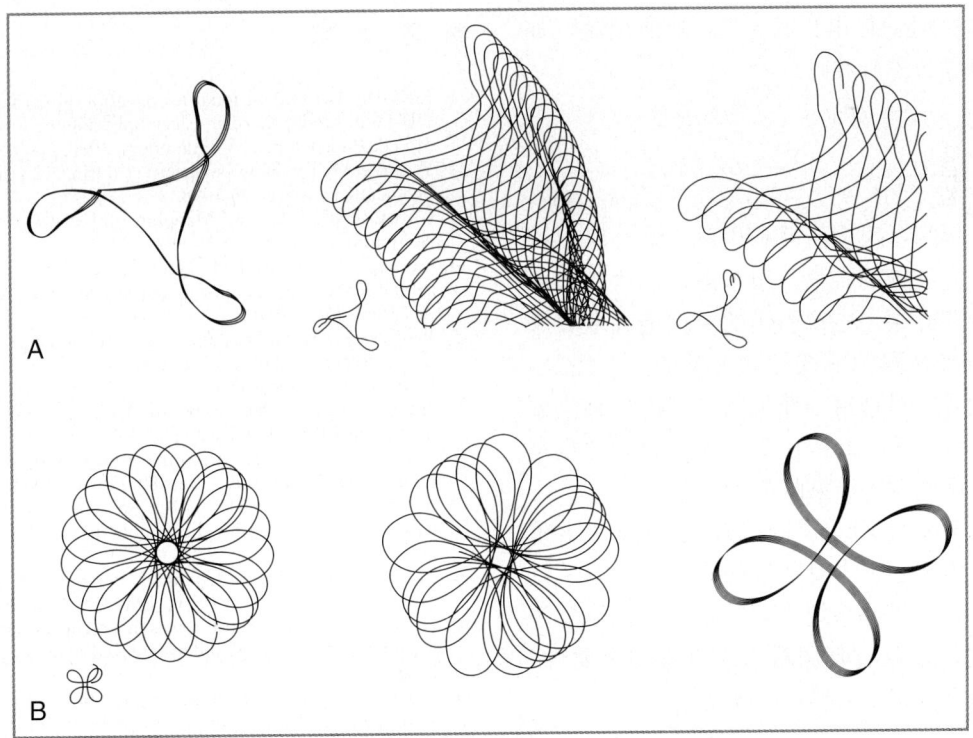

图 29-5　利用双域模型计算得到的螺旋波顶端的轨迹　A，频率比为 2：1，图形为三足内摆线形。B，频率比为 3：1，图形为四足内摆线形。左侧为各向同性的心肌组织，中间为正常心肌组织，右侧为极度各向异性的例子

蜓的路径近似一个三足的内摆线（图 29-5A）；各向异性引起一种线性漂移的蜿蜒形式。如果旋转和蜿蜒的频率为 3：1，蜿蜒的路径近似一个四足的内摆线（图 29-5B）：蜿蜒和旋转的频率被捕捉。LeBlanc 利用一个分析模型来阐明哪种情况下会导致频率捕捉，哪种情况下会导致漂移。他的分析结果与我的很多模拟结果一致。

四、螺旋波碎裂

某些情况下，螺旋波变得不稳定，衰变为一种无序状态（图 29-6）。对这种衰变的研究很多，因为它可以作为室性心动过速转变为心室颤动的模型[31,33,43-46]。最近 Fenton 及其同事发表了有关螺旋波碎裂机制的很有价值的文章。针对其中一种机制：心脏重建，Alan Garfinkel 及其同事也发表了一系列的研究结果[31,44,45,47-49]（Weiss 及其同事对此概念有精彩的解释，也参见第 36 章）。重建意味着动作电位的时程决定于前面的舒张间期：舒张间期短，则动作电位时程也短。动作电位重建曲线的斜率大于 1，则会促进变化和螺旋波碎裂。有意思的是，如果重建曲线斜率的绝对值大于 1，则"负性重建"也有利于螺旋波碎裂（舒张间期短但动作电位长）[50]。其他机制，如记忆效应，也可导致螺旋波碎裂[33,43]。

五、结 论

在过去的 5 年间，很多研究利用对二维心肌组织的数字模拟来研究波锋的传播。很多最近的研究集中于螺旋波的蜿蜒和碎裂。本章引用的文献绝大多数来自物理学杂志，来自熟悉非线性动力学的人。但是，这些看似抽象的研究对理解心律失常及其治疗有重要意义。引用 Christini 和 Glass 在 2002 年 Chaos "重点问题"中的介绍性文章来结束此章：

今天，动力学家对于临床治疗方法还没有产生重大影响，但是，鉴于心脏本身明显的非线性动力学特点及其与研究明确的物理系统之间的相似性，很多领域的创新性研究，以及心脏病对人类健康的重要性，在未来几年中一定会有令人振奋的发展。

（李　春译）

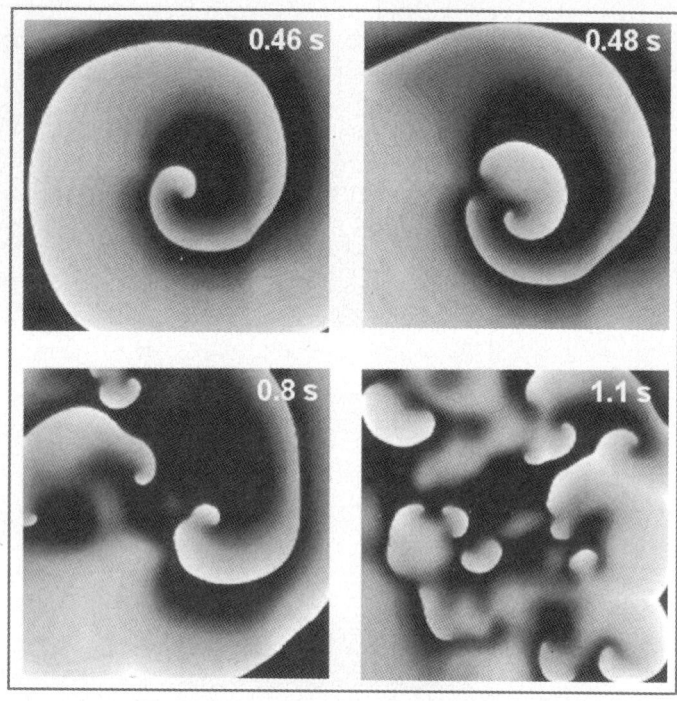

图 29-6　螺旋波碎裂为类似颤动的不规则形式（引自 Weiss JN，Garfinkel A，Karagueuzian HS，et al：Chaos and the transition to ventricular fibrillation：A new approach to antiarrhythmic drug eveluation. Circulation 99：2819-2826，1999.）

参 考 文 献

1. Roth BJ: Two-dimensional propagation in cardiac muscle. In Zipes DP, Jalife J (eds): Cardiac Electrophysiology, From Cell to Bedside, 3rd ed. Philadelphia, WB Saunders, 2000, pp 265–270.
2. Winfree AT: Evolving perspectives during 12 years of electrical turbulence. Chaos 8:1–19, 1998.
3. Christini DJ, Glass L: Mapping and control of complex cardiac arrhythmias. Chaos 12:893–902, 2002.
4. Gerhardt M, Schuster H, Tyson JJ: A cellular automaton model of excitable media including curvature and dispersion. Science 247:1563–1566, 1990.
5. Panfilov AV: Spiral breakup in an array of coupled cells: The role of the intercellular conductance. Phys Rev Lett 88:118101, 2002.
6. Feldman AB, Chernyak YB, Cohen RJ: Spiral waves are stable in discrete element models of two-dimensional homogeneous excitable media. Int J Bifurcat Chaos 8:1153–1161, 1998.
7. Bub G, Shrier A, Glass L: Spiral wave generation in heterogeneous excitable media. Phys Rev Lett 88:058101, 2002.
8. Margerit D, Barkley D: Large-excitability asymptotics for scroll waves in three-dimensional excitable media. Phys Rev E 66:036214, 2002.
9. Berenfeld O, Wellner M, Jalife J, Pertsov AM: Shaping of a scroll wave filament by cardiac fibers. Phys Rev E 63:061901, 2001.
10. Henry H, Hakim V: Scroll waves in isotropic excitable media: Linear instabilities, bifurcations, and restabilized states. Phys Rev E 65:046235, 2002.
11. Eason J, Trayanova N: Phase singularities and termination of spiral wave reentry. J Cardiovasc Electrophysiol 13:672–679, 2002.
12. Winfree AT: Various ways to make phase singularites by electric shock. J Cardiovasc Electrophysiol 11:286–289, 2000.
13. Roth BJ, Krassowska W: The induction of reentry in cardiac tissue. The missing link: How electric fields alter transmembrane potential. Chaos 8:204–220, 1998.
14. Wellner M, Jalife J, Pertsov AM: Waves in excitable media: Effects of wave geometry. Int J Bifurcat Chaos 12:1939–1951, 2002.

15. Winfree AT: A spatial scale factor for electrophysiological models of myocardium. Prog Biophys Mol Biol 69:185–203, 1998.
16. Azene EM, Trayanova NA, Warman E: Wave front-obstacle interaction in cardiac tissue: A computational study. Ann Biomed Eng 29:35–46, 2001.
17. Starobin JM, Starmer CF: Common mechanism links spiral wave meandering and wave-front-obstacle separation. Phys Rev E 55:1193–1196, 1997.
18. Xie F, Qu Z, Garfinkel A: Dynamics of reentry around a circular obstacle in cardiac tissue. Phys Rev E 58:6355–6358, 1998.
19. Comtois P, Vinet A: Curvature effects on activation speed and repolarization in an ionic model of cardiac myocytes. Phys Rev E 60:1619–1628, 1999.
20. Morozov VG, Davydov NV, Davydov VA: Propagation of curved activation fronts in anisotropic excitable media. J Biological Physics 25:87–100, 1999.
21. Xie F, Qu Z, Weiss JN, Garfinkel A: Interactions between stable spiral waves with different frequencies in cardiac tissue. Phys Rev E 59:2203–2205, 1999.
22. Xie F, Qu Z, Weiss JN, Garfinkel A: Coexistence of multiple spiral waves with independent frequencies in a heterogeneous excitable medium. Phys Rev E 63:031905, 2001.
23. Elkin YE, Biktashev VN: Drift of large-core spiral waves in inhomogeneous excitable media. J Biological Physics 25:129–147, 1999.
24. LeBlanc VG, Wulff C: Translational symmetry-breaking for spiral waves. Nonlinear Science 10:569–601, 2000.
25. Sandstede B, Scheel A: Superspiral structures of meandering and drifting spiral waves. Phys Rev Lett 86:171–174, 2001.
26. Wellner M, Pertsov AM, Jalife J: Spiral drift and core properties. Phys Rev E 59:5192–5204, 1999.
27. Rappel W-J, Fenton F, Karma A: Spatiotemporal control of wave instabilities in cardiac tissue. Phys Rev Lett 83:456–459, 1999.
28. Hwang S-M, Choe WG, Lee KJ: Complex dynamics of a spiral tip in the presence of an extrinsic local modulation. Phys Rev E 62:4799–4803, 2000.
29. Otani NF: A primary mechanism for spiral wave meandering. Chaos 12:829–842, 2002.
30. Kremmydas GP, Holden AV: Spiral-wave meandering in reaction-diffusion models of ventricular muscle. Chaos Solitons Fractals 13:1659–1669, 2002.
31. Qu Z, Xie F, Garfinkel A, Weiss JN: Origins of spiral wave meander and breakup in a two-dimensional cardiac tissue model. Ann Biomed Eng 28:755–771, 2000.
32. Kessler DA, Kupferman R: Spirals in excitable media. II. Meandering transition in the diffusive free-boundary limit. Physica D 105:207–225, 1997.
33. Fenton FH, Cherry EM, Hastings HM, Evans SJ: Multiple mechanisms of spiral wave breakup in a model of cardiac electrical activity. Chaos 12:852–892, 2002.
34. Hakim V, Karma A: Theory of spiral wave dynamics in weakly excitable media: Asymptotic reduction to a kinematic model and applications. Phys Rev E 60:5073–5105, 1999.
35. Hakim V, Karma A: Spiral wave meander in excitable media: The large core limit. Phys Rev Lett 79:665–668, 1997.
36. Ashwin P, Melbourne I, Nicol M: Hypermeander of spirals: Local bifurcations and statistical properties. Physica D 156:364–382, 2001.
37. Biktashev VN, Holden AV: Deterministic brownian motion in the hypermeander of spiral waves. Physica D 116:342–354, 1998.
38. Sabbagh H: Observation of spiral core expansion in an excitable medium. Phys Lett A 299:207–211, 2002.
39. LeBlanc VG: Rotational symmetry breaking for spiral waves. Nonlinearity 15:1179–1203, 2002.
40. LeBlanc VG, Roth BJ: Meandering of spiral waves in anisotropic tissue. Dynamics of Continuous, Discrete and Impulsive Systems, Series B 10:29–41, 2003.
41. Roth BJ: Frequency locking of meandering spiral waves in cardiac tissue. Phys Rev E 57:R3735–3738, 1998.
42. Roth BJ: Meandering of spiral waves in anisotropic cardiac tissue. Physica D 150:127–136, 2001.
43. Fenton FH, Evans SJ, Hastings HM: Memory in an excitable medium: A mechanism for spiral wave breakup in the low-excitability limit. Phys Rev Lett 83:3964–3967, 1999.
44. Qu Z, Weiss JN, Garfinkel A: Cardiac electrical restitution properties and stability of reentrant spiral waves: A simulation study. Am J Physiol 276:H269–H283, 1999.
45. Qu Z, Weiss JN, Garfinkel A: From local to global spatiotemporal chaos in a cardiac tissue model. Phys Rev E 61:727–732, 2000.
46. Weiss JN, Garfinkel A, Karagueuzian HS, et al: Chaos and the transition to ventricular fibrillation: A new approach to antiarrhythmic drug evaluation. Circulation 99:2819–2826, 1999.
47. Hastings HM, Fenton FH, Evans SJ, et al: Alternans and the onset of ventricular fibrillation. Phys Rev E 62:4043–4048, 2000.
48. Xie FG, Qu ZL, Garfinkel A, Weiss JN: Electrical refractory period restitution and spiral wave reentry in simulated cardiac tissue. Am J Physiol 283:H448–H460, 2002.
49. Qu Z, Garfinkel A, Chen P-S, Weiss JN: Mechanisms of discordant alternans and induction of reentry in simulated cardiac tissue. Circulation 102:1664–1670, 2000.
50. Zemlin CW, Panfilov AV: Spiral waves in excitable media with negative restitution. Phys Rev E 63:041912, 2001.

第 30 章

数学模型中电激动的三维传导

Craig S. Henriquez, Joseph V. Tranquillo, David Weinstein,
Edward W. Hsu, Christopher R. Johnson

本章目录
- 研究方法 ………………………… 269
- 研究结果 ………………………… 271
- 讨论 ……………………………… 273

自20世纪70年代末，计算机数学模型已经用于心脏电传导功能的研究[1]。当时由于计算机技术限制，研究主要局限于单根纤维传导束和单层心肌细胞电生理功能的研究。随着计算机技术的发展，目前心脏计算机数学模型的研究已经进入三维立体的研究，所建立的模型也更接近真实的心脏[2-4]，从而能够对心脏的生物物理学参数与电势分布和离子通道电流的基本联系进行更广泛的研究。

尽管已取得令人注目的进展，目前仍只有极少的研究能够将心脏离子通道电流的数据与心脏器官水平的参数进行整合。原因之一是，如果以单个心肌细胞的电活动作为最小计算单元，全心脏一次兴奋的波阵面传播所得的数据就已经超过目前计算机的能力。我们对以单个心肌细胞为计算单元，成人心脏1次跳动的计算机数学建模所需的数据进行估计[5]。成人心肌的总体积约为225cm³，为了模拟离子通道电流，我们首先将全心脏分解成计算机建模所需的体积大体一致的单元。每一单元的体积约为 0.1 cm³，共计 225×10^6 个计算单元。为了描述每一单元局部的电导张量，必须对其离子通道的电流的数据和校正参数进行指定。描述每一单元所需的参数约为 50 个，每个参数为 4 比特字节，全心脏数学模型的建立则需要 $50 \times 4 \times 225 \times 10^6$ 比特，即约 45GB 字节的数据。同样，如果以 $10\mu s$ 为最小研究单元，为了模拟一阵持续时间仅 10s 的心律失常，则需要大约 10×10^{10} 个参数。因此，如果以单个心肌细胞作为研究单元，目前建立人体全心脏电生理功能的计算机数学模型并不现实。这也促使研究者选用体积较小的动物心脏[2,3]，如小鼠心脏进行计算机数学模型研究。而且，目前也已经有大量心脏解剖结构和离子通道电流的数据支持体外构建小动物心脏电生理功能的计算机数学模型。

值得注意的是，小动物心脏的动作电位和兴奋波阵面的传播特征与人类心脏存在明显差异。其中部分是由于两者在心脏大小、室壁厚度、离子通道的表型和分布差异所造成的。另外，这种差异有可能影响到对某些电生理异质性的空间定位，而这些电生理异质性可导致有临床意义的心律失常的发生。

由于目前越来越多地使用小鼠作为模型研究心血管疾病，因此如何有效地将在小鼠心脏上观察到的现象与大动物、甚至人体心脏上观察到的现象紧密联系起来，也是非常重要的问题。小鼠的基因操作技术相对简单，从而导致更多的小鼠心血管疾病模型的出现，包括长 QT 综合征[6,7]、心肌肥厚[8,9]、心肌缺血[10]等疾病[11,12]。在人体心脏上的研究表明，心脏组织结构和离子通道表达的异质性增加可以诱发新的心律失常。由于小鼠心脏和人体心脏在几何形状和细胞膜动力学上的巨大差异，计算机数学模型被用来寻找两者比较的原则及心脏电生理功能上的联系。

基于上述目的，首要的步骤是建立小鼠心脏兴奋时电冲动传导的计算机模型，并且所得到的数据能够与其他实验室和临床电生理检测的数据相比较。这些检测技术包括心脏表面或跨壁电位图、心肌细胞动作电位记录和体表心电图。为达到这一目标，小鼠心脏的计算机模型应能够描述心房和心室的几何形状、传导系统纤维束的走行、细胞内和细胞外物质的特点以及离子通道的分布和激活动力学特征。并且心脏模型的特征能够随病理状态发生改变，解释实验室的结果则更加理想。

本章的主要内容是介绍一种小鼠心脏的计算机数学模型，这一模型既能对心脏离子通道的激活动力学进行详细的描述，也能逼真描述心室的几何形状和传导系统纤维束的走行。此外，本章还提供了小鼠心脏计算机快速建模，反映心脏电传导功能的范例。它通过核磁共振技术获得心脏断面解剖数据来重建心脏的几何形状和传导纤维的走行，并且通过先进的计算方法来揭示心脏电活动反应-扩散方程。我们证实通过这种方法建立的反映心脏电生理功能的计算机数学模型能够与心脏光学和电学标测的结果相联系。这些结果表明小鼠心脏电生理功能的计算机数学模型能够成为研究大动物、甚至人体心脏基本电生理现象的实验平台。

一、研究方法

(一) 核磁共振弥散张量成像

建立全心脏模型的第一步必须获得足够描述心脏几何形状和传导系统纤维走行的数据。组织切片方法是获得心脏解剖结构特征的标准方法。LeGrice 等研究者通过组织切片方法建立了狗心室的有限网格模型[13]。Vetter 和 McCulloch 用类似的方法建立兔的数学模型[2]。但是，这种依靠组织连续切片获得心脏解剖结构信息建模的方法存在明显的局限。首先，它非常耗时，并且只能获得全心脏少量的数据信息。

替代的方法是通过核磁共振成像（MRI）和弥散张量成像（DTI）技术[14]获取反映心脏解剖结构和传导纤维束走行的数据。DTI 技术通过观察组织微环境中水分子的位移情况显示心脏传导纤维的组织结构特征。组织中水分子的弥散过程能够导致核磁共振信号的衰减。心脏核磁共振信号的衰减可以用以下公式表示：

$$A(TE) = \exp[-(v^T \Sigma v)\lambda^2 \int_0^{TE}(\int_0^t G(\tau)d\tau)^2 d\tau] \quad [1]$$

其中 $t=TE$ 表示回波的时间，G 为磁场梯度向量的时间变化，λ 为螺旋磁场自旋常数。此外：

$$v^T = [g_\xi g_\eta g_\zeta] \quad \Sigma = \begin{bmatrix} D_\xi & 0 & 0 \\ 0 & D_\eta & 0 \\ 0 & 0 & D_\zeta \end{bmatrix} \quad [2]$$

$\lambda^2 \int_0^{TE}(\int_0^t G(\tau)d\tau)^2 dt$ 是已知的反映回波序列的参数。标量 $v^T \Sigma v$ 等于表现弥散系数（ADC），而 ADC 值是参考各实验室的数据确定。线性变换公式 $v=Ug$（U 为正交矩阵）将 V 转换成球面坐标系统。

$$ADC = g^T \cdot U^T \Sigma U \cdot g \quad [3]$$

通过 ADC 值，本征值（Σ）和本征向量（U）就可以通过公式 $D=U^T \Sigma U$ 计算。最大本征值对应的本征向量即是主要纤维的走行方向。而较小本征值对应的本征向量则对应于次要纤维的走行方向。

不同于以往采用的组织切片方法，本研究组首次运用核磁弥散成像（DTI）技术定量显示小鼠心脏纤维的分布和走行[15]。Scollan 等同样运用核磁弥散成像技术构建兔心脏的三维计算机数学模型，结果发现与心脏组织学的特征有良好相关性[16]。与经典组织学方法比较，核磁共振弥散张量成像技术容易获得心脏组织结构的信息，在心脏干预治疗时进行形态测定更具有优势。

(二) 反应-扩散模型

当获取到足够的关于心脏形状和纤维走行的信息后，下一步是运用数学方法建立包含上述信息的刚度矩阵。心脏组织可以近似看成由心肌细胞、胶原和血管相互交织形成的网络结构。其中心肌细胞通过胞内可传导空间相互耦联，并被细胞外间质包绕。我们用双区域模型（bidomain model）将心脏结构模拟成功能上的合胞体。在这个双区域模型中，细胞内间隙和细胞外间隙被看成是均匀连续的。为方便起见，细胞内间隙和细胞外间隙的容积在心脏组织总容积上确定。在心脏中，电流必须跨细胞膜才能从一个区域到达另一区域。因此，在双区域模型中，跨膜电流的数据经体积平均后，分配到各计算节点[18]。以下为双区域模型的方程：

$$\Delta \cdot (D_i + D_e)\phi_e = -\nabla \cdot (D_i \Delta V_m) \quad [4]$$

$$\nabla \cdot (D_i V_m) + \nabla \cdot (D_i \nabla \phi_e) = -\beta I_m \quad [5]$$

在方程中，V_m 和 ϕ_e 分别为细胞跨膜电压和细胞外电压，其中，$\beta = \dfrac{2\pi\alpha}{\pi\alpha^2/f_i} = \dfrac{2f_i}{\alpha}$ 是表面与容积的比值。f_i 是细胞内空间的分数，而 α 是细胞的内径。细胞跨膜电流的密度，即 I_m，则是根据膜电容和离子通道电流计算出来的，计算公式为：

$$I_m = C_m \frac{dV_m}{dt} + I_{ion} \quad [6]$$

由于在通常情况下，心脏传导纤维的走行方向并非完全固定不变的，因此将 $D_{i,e}$ 定义为位置函数，指定到细胞内结构区和细胞外结构区的任一点中[19]。

双域模型还可以用来模拟血液的分流效应和其他可传导介质，只要这种相邻结构中的电压变化和电流的传导符合拉普拉斯方程。在细胞内和细胞外结构中的组织-气体界面和液体-气体界面中，并非电流的传导。在组织-液体界面，细胞内结构是近乎密闭的，而细胞外结构中存在电位的变化和电流的移动[20]。因而，为解决这个问题，我们把细胞外空间的某些点的电压设定为 0V。

（三）扩散矩阵的数学离散化

在大多数情况下，对双域模型方程的分析和求解是困难的。因此，为了更多应用该模型解决现实中的问题，需要借助有关的数学方法。其中，最常用的数学方法是有限差分法。尽管有限元法更适合于解决复杂几何形状的问题，但它不如有限差分法直观。一种替代有限元法的数学方法是顶点中心有限容积法[21]。运用这种数学方法，结构区局部的电流是守恒的，计算机网格可以用相互连接的电阻来进行解释。另外由于这种方法本身排除了流量界面的因素，对于不规则几何形状和各向异性的物体比有限差分法更加有效。Penland 等对应用有限容积法对各向异性的心脏三维结构进行了详细的描述[22]。

（四）离子通道电流

公式 6 中的离子通道电流是指通过细胞膜的单个通道电流的总和。

$$I_{ion} = \sum_{x=1}^{n} I_x \quad [7]$$

通常，I_x 既可以表示跨膜电压的函数，又可以是反映离子通道门控特征的多个变量的非线性函数。如下所示：

$$I_x = G_x \left(\prod_{p=1}^{m} z_p^q \right) (V_m - E_x) \quad [8]$$

在这，Z_p 表示某特定离子通道的平均量（关闭=$0 \leq Z \leq 1$=开放），q 通常为整数。而 E_x 为 I_x 的反转电位。

同时，离子通道本身的特征也可用下列方程式表示：

$$\frac{dz}{dt} = \alpha_z (V_m)(1-z) + \beta_z (V_m) z \quad [9]$$

公式中，α_z 和 β_z 为依存于 V_m 的比例常数。另外，我们也可以用 Markov 模型对离子通道门控特征进行更详细的描述，甚至可以对基因变异所致通道异常加以研究[23]。

通道电流和动作电位形态的差异性是由于离子通道的种属差异和心脏区域性分布造成的。例如在小鼠心脏，影响心肌细胞动作电位复极过程的主要电流为瞬时外向钾电流（I_{to}），而在较大的哺乳动物心脏，快成分（I_{kr}）和慢成分（I_{ks}）复极钾电流是影响心肌细胞动作电位复极相的主要电流[24]。同样，不同离子通道在心脏不同区域的分布也会导致动作电位形态和时程的变化[25]。正是由于小鼠心肌细胞动作电位时程和人类心肌细胞动作电位时程存在明显差异，一些研究者对使用小鼠心脏作为模型研究人类心脏的电生理功能提出了质疑。

尽管目前尚无小鼠心肌细胞膜兴奋的模型，Pandit 等研究者近期发表了大鼠心肌细胞动作电位的详细数学模型[26]。我们在 Pandit 的模型基础上，进行适当的修改，主要是增加了动作电位上升支的速率（通过增加钠通道的最大电导至 1.5ms/cm）以便更接近于小鼠实验的数据[25]。

（五）模型构建

完整的小鼠心脏（C57BL/6J 品系，来自 Jackson 实验室）甲醛固定后，用环距为 1cm 的螺旋线圈组成的 7.1T 的核磁共振显微镜沿心脏短轴进行扫描。为了减少心脏位移导致的误差，小鼠心脏被放置在离心管内，因而可能导致心脏轻微变形。通过标准的、立体的、自旋回波序列和扩散加权成像方式获取小鼠心脏的图像。所获得的图像数据包括 1 幅全编码的非弥散加权图像（128×128×128 矩阵大小）和 12 幅通过弥散成像方式获得的精简图像（128×64×64 矩阵大小）[5]，而这些弥散成像的图像数据可以通过改进的定位方法重新构建成完整的小鼠心脏图像。为了减少噪声，对所获得图像数据进行自适应过滤处理。

因为在图像数据中，既包括心脏组织，也包括非心脏组织。因此必须将两者区分开来。所有图像数据用非线性的最小方差法[5]转换为线性张量数据。非心脏组织（包括脊柱和血池）的低弥散信号用最小方差法转换时排除在外。用标准的特征分解的方法将心脏组织的三维像素逐步解析成反映心脏传导纤维的走行的数据。将这些数据输入到电脑，用 BioPSE 软件系统分析处理，从而得到反映心脏有限体积的网格数据和刚度矩阵[27]。

为了建立计算机网格，首先在心脏中已知的一点放置随机计算种子，然后用填充运算的方法建立心脏其他部位的网格数据。通过类似的方法，也可以建立心脏左右心室腔的计算机网格数据。对不能用填充运算的点则排除在外，这可以导致数据的不完整。将这些点排除后，其他的点则重新计算。

（六）组织特征

心脏组织包括心脏传导纤维是各向异性的，我们假定传导纤维在层间即横断面上是各向同性的。用以下的双域电导率描述纤维纵向走行的电传导：$g_{il}=5.0\text{ms/cm}$，$g_{el}=4.0\text{ms/cm}$；而用下列公式表示纤维横向交叉的电传导：$g_{it}=0.5\text{ ms/cm}$，$g_{et}=1.33\text{ms/cm}$。根据细胞的半径为 $8.4\mu m$，计算出表面积与体积的比值为 1666 cm^{-1}。

（七）数学方法

公式 4 和 5 的计算求解是用 Grank-Nicholson 方法进行的。公式 6 中反映离子电流的状态变量是用 Euler 方法计算所得。固定的时间间期为 $2.0\mu s$。通过 Cuthill-Mckee 运算法则使计算矩阵的带宽最小化。上述公式计算结果的输出根据 GMRES 方法进行，其容差为 10^{-4}mV。所有的计算机模拟都由本研究室开发的 CRDIOWAVE 软件[28]进行。这种模块化软件系统是被设计在多处理器上运行。因此，计算机模拟是在北加利福尼亚超级计算机中心的 IBM SP Power 3 电脑系统上进行。心脏 100ms 的电活动的模拟需要 11 个处理器进行 6 小时的运算。

二、研究结果

当使用弥散张量成像扫描时，一幅非扩散加权图像通常用来获得心脏的几何形状，以利于后续的计算机模拟。图 30-1A 所示为用于建立计算机网格的、经甲醛固定的小鼠心脏形态。图 30-1B 所示为用弥散张量成像的数据构建的心脏计算机模型。构成模型的像素大小为 $75\times75\times75\mu m$，按照这样的分辨率，整个心脏由 225 236 个计算节点组成。同样心室腔也是由 793 个计算节点组成，因而双结构区计算模型中也包括血池部分。弥散张量成像中，每一像素对应一个张量。最大本征向量代表心脏传导纤维走行的方向。图 30-1B 中所示心脏传导系统纤维的走行用白色短线表示。在左心室游离壁的表面，传导纤维是从心尖斜行走向基底部，离开间隔后，环绕整个心脏。而在心内膜面，从心尖到基底部传导纤维的走行更垂直。与 LeGrice 研究组[13]、Vetter 和 McCulloch 研究组[2]所建立的数学模型不同的是，传导纤维的分布有明显的局部差异。其中部分是生理性原因，另外也可能是心

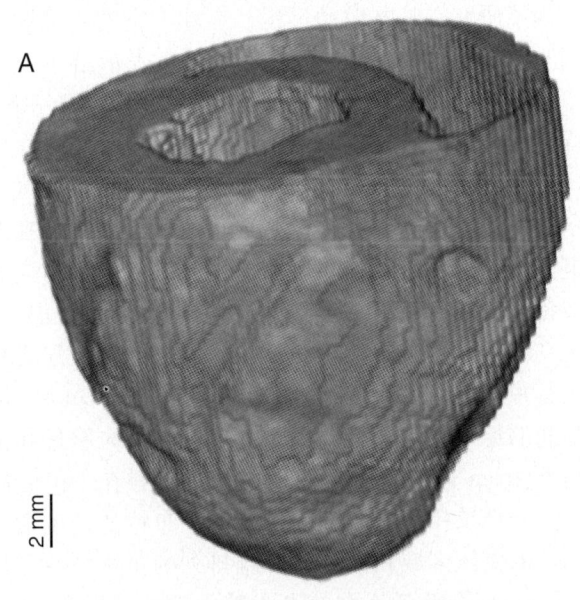

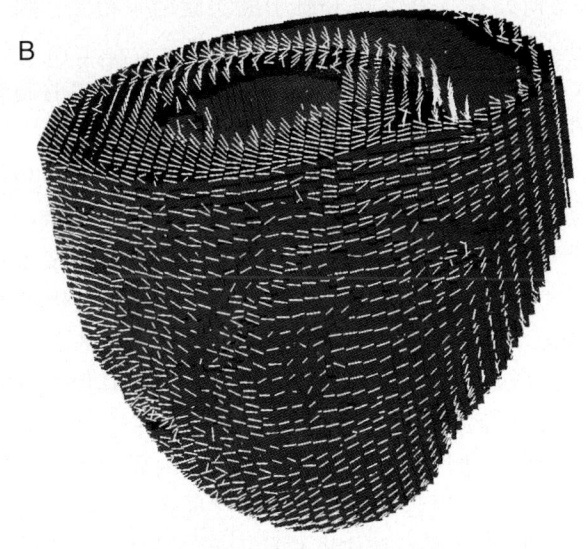

图 30-1 用核磁共振成像技术构建小鼠心脏传导的数学模型 A：核磁共振成像技术获取的小鼠部分心室图像。B：根据核磁共振断层图像构建的非连续、节段性心室模型。其中，通过弥散张量成像技术获取的表面纤维的走行用白色短线表示。

脏固定和成像时位置移动造成的。令人惊异的是，小鼠心脏中部分传导纤维呈平滑的旋绕走行，这与大动物心脏中的表现一致。旋绕的角度大约为80°～90°，而在大动物心脏，传导纤维旋绕的角度约为110°～130°。尽管在小鼠心脏中，由于左心室壁的平均厚度只有1.5mm，右心室壁的厚度只有0.6mm，纤维旋绕的程度比大动物心脏明显。从左心室和右心室均匀取样，传导纤维的三维投影在图30-2中用两幅独立的图表示。

为了研究心脏电激动过程，在左心室的心外膜给予刺激，造成心室异位搏动。图30-3表示给予刺激后，左心室表面四个不同时间点（0.5ms，6.5ms，8.5ms和10.5ms）跨膜和细胞外电势扩布图。在图中，较亮的区域表示膜去极化或正电压，而较暗区域表示膜超极化或负电压。在0.5ms时，激动部位在跨膜电势图上如同虚拟的阴极，呈去极化状态，两侧为超极化状态的区域[29]，尽管所使用的刺激强度很小，小于0.5mV。随后，心脏的激动波以椭圆形方式扩布。其中，沿纤维走行方向传导的速度为68cm/s，而纤维间的传导速度为34cm/s。激动扩布的形式和速度与Nygren等研究者[30]用电压敏感染料在小鼠心脏中的实验结果相符合。细胞外电压扩布特征是包括中心部位的负压区域和沿表面纤维排列的正压区域。这与Taccardi等研究者[31]在犬心脏中实验结果和Macchi等研究者[32]在大鼠心脏中的实验结果相似。因为小鼠心脏的左心室室壁厚度小于犬左心室的室壁厚度，因此在小鼠心脏中，室壁跨膜激动扩布中的旋绕要少于犬心脏[33]。

图30-4A是通过跟踪任一点去极化达到-60mV时所得到的心脏电激动图。在固定位置起搏刺激，心脏激动的全部时间约为24ms。图30-4B是跟踪复极化达到-60mV时所得到的心脏复极图。心脏复极图与心脏激动扩布时的靶心图相似。复极过程是由外向内，刺激部位是最后复极的部位[34]。心脏其他部分的复极方向与激动扩布方向相似。与心脏电激动图比较，心脏复极图的范围更广，而且各向异性更小，这主要是复极的时程较长所致。最终导致心脏兴奋与复极图差异的因素是动作电位的时程（APD）。动作电位时程的范围在43.2～63.9ms，刺激模型中其刺激部位的动作电位时程是最长的。值得注意的是，上述模型中的结果是在我们假定跨膜电传导特性是均一的情况下观察到的。

数学模型的一个优点是能将电描记图的数据与离

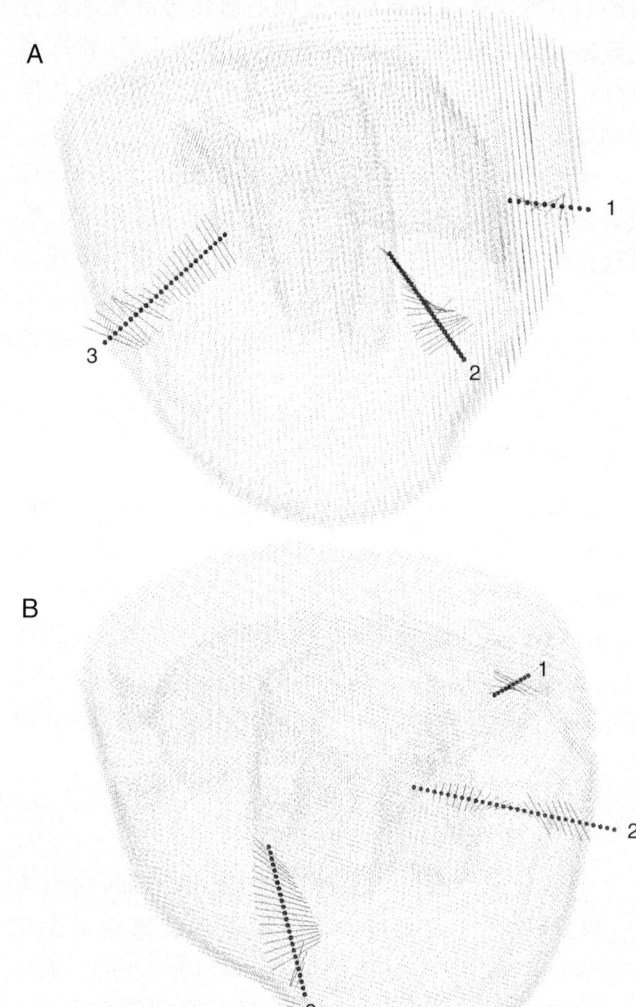

图30-2 弥散张量成像（DTI）图中所示传导纤维在小鼠心脏室壁中平滑旋绕走行

子电流的数据整合到一起。图30-5所示为具有代表性的心脏表面沿纤维走行记录到电描记图和与纤维交叉方向记录到的电描记图。在既往大动物心脏的研究中，与纤维交叉方向记录到的电压图的电压幅度更低，且形状更不对称。两种电描记图都具有显著的J波和微小的T波。数学模型的另一个优点是所获得心脏激动数据是三维立体的。图30-6所示为刺激部位附近5个部位的跨膜电压和电描记图。电描记图上最大的负向偏移与电压图上最大的去极化速度是一致的。而且在激动由心外膜向心内膜扩布时，出现轻微的向右偏移。值得注意的是，在心脏某些部位，由于激动波曲率的下降可以导致电压幅度的增加。

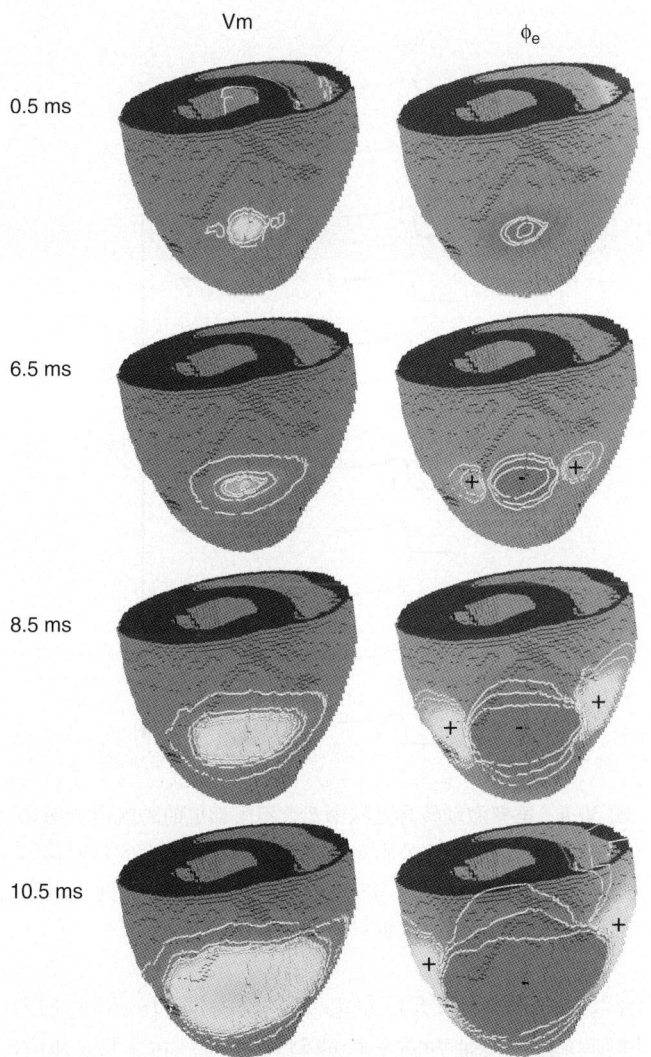

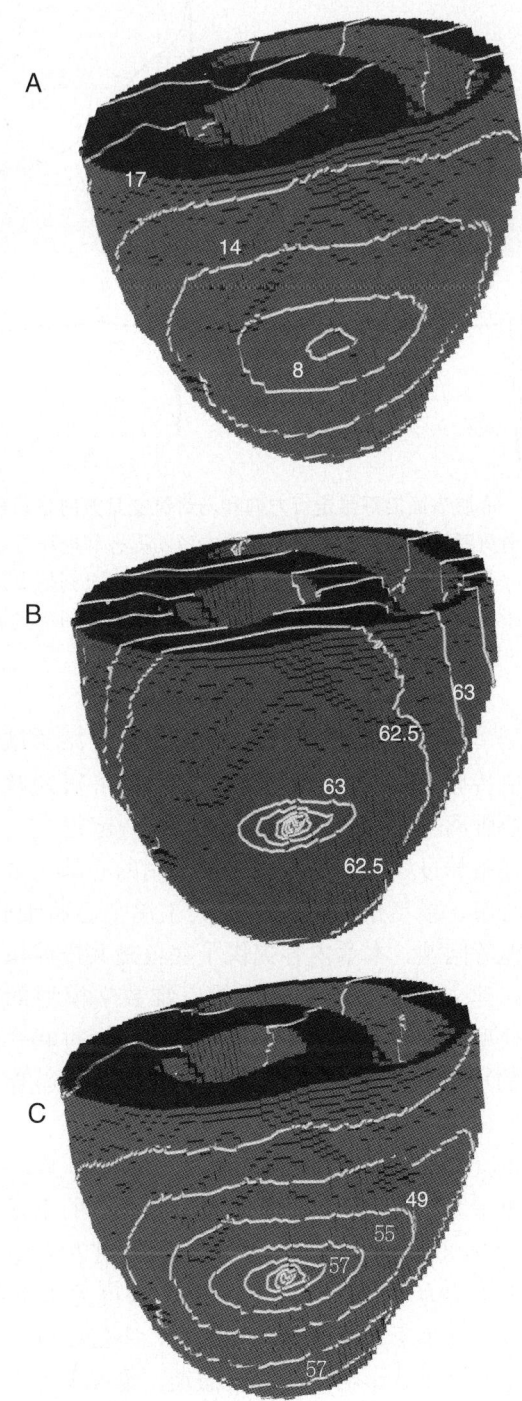

图 30-3 心外膜给予刺激，4 个时间点跨膜和细胞外电势扩布图 刺激时（最上一行图），激动部位在跨膜电势图上如虚拟阴极，呈去极化状态，邻近两侧为超极化状态的区域。下三行图表示刺激后，激动波以椭圆形方式扩布。其中，沿纤维走行方向传导的速度为 68cm/s，而纤维间的传导速度为 34cm/s。细胞外电势图的特征是中心为椭圆形的负电压区，两侧为沿纤维走行方向形成的正电压区。

三、讨论

很久以前，研究者们已经认识到，完整心脏的正常激动传导过程和许多折返性心律失常不能在小片心脏组织中复制出来，因此需要建立心脏传导的三维数学模型。早期的数学模型是在假定心脏组织各向同性的运算规则上建立的[35,36]。后期的数学模型结合了心脏及传导纤维的解剖数据，但仍然依赖于简化的 FitzHugh-Nagumo 动力学公式和自动化计算技术建立

图 30-4 激动时间（A）、复极时间（B）和动作电位时程（C）的等高线图 激动时间（A）为心脏任一点去极化达到 −60mV 的时间，而复极时间（B）是指心脏复极达到 −60mV 时的时间。激动等时线从刺激部位向外周移动，而复极的等时线与激动等时线类似，不同的是它的方向是从外周向中心移动。刺激部位是最后复极的部位。动作电位时程（APD）等高线图提示最长的动作电位时程位于刺激部位附近

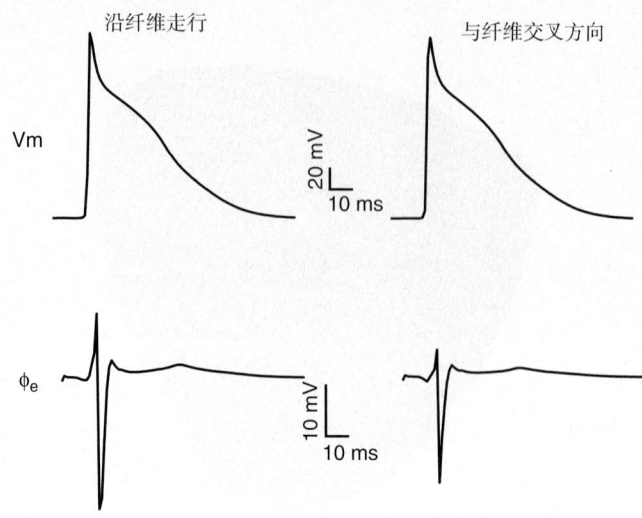

图 30-5 心脏表面沿纤维走行方向和与纤维交叉方向记录到的跨膜电势图和细胞外电势图 动作电位的形态和电压幅度与记录的方向无明显相关性，与纤维交叉方向记录到的电压图的电压幅度更低，且形状更不对称。两种电描记图都具有显著的 J 波和微小的 T 波

数学模型[37-39]。直到最近几年，研究人员开始尝试建立心脏电传导的三维数学模型。它能够将心脏的解剖数据和心脏离子通道电流的数据整合到一起[3,4,40]。但是，在建模的过程中，也存在包括采用的心脏通常小于人体心脏、模型的空间分辨力大于单个心肌细胞，计算误差等问题。本章内容提供了在核磁共振成像的基础上，建立小鼠心脏电传导的三维数学模型的方法，该模型的空间分辨力接近单个细胞。通过联合运用先进的成像技术和分析工具，以及高效的运算方法，这种建模方法也可以扩展到人体心脏。

小鼠心脏和人体心脏的差异是巨大的。正常小鼠的心脏重量为 150～175mg[12]。而人体心脏的重量可以达到 280000mg。在本研究中，小鼠心脏左心室的室壁厚度平均为 1.5ms，右心室的室壁厚度为 0.6ms。这些数据均远小于人体心脏。事实上，小鼠心脏右心室的室壁厚度显著影响室壁跨膜激动。也许更令人瞩目的是，小鼠心脏细胞的数量(10×10^6)的范围可以用来构建较大心脏的数学模型[41]。因此，借助最新的电脑技术，在小鼠心脏上，可以建立单个细胞分辨力水平、10 次心跳、接近生理情况的心脏电传导的数学模型。

尽管已经有通过组织连续切片研究心肌纤维结构的方法，但本研究首次通过无创性的核磁共振弥散张量成像技术获得心肌纤维的解剖数据。Mclean 和 Prothero 曾经报道[42]，心室壁的结构就像一块"三明

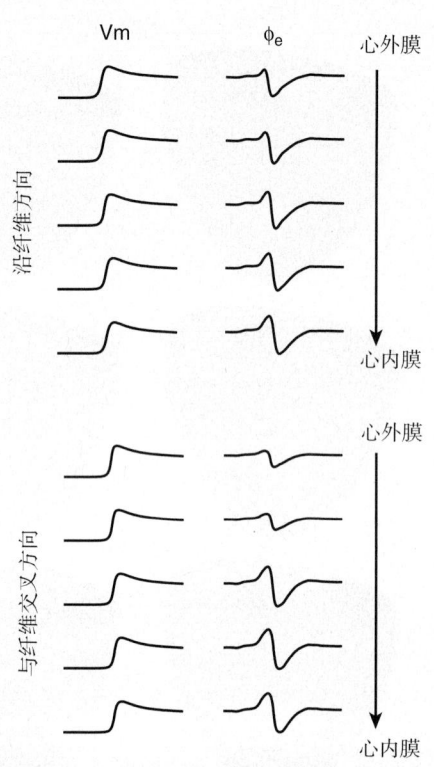

图 30-6 室壁激动传导过程中 5 个不同部位的跨膜电势图和电描记图 激动由心外膜向心内膜传导时，最大的负向偏移与电势图上最大的去极化速度是一致的，除了时间上的偏移，细胞外电势的幅度也有轻微的上升

治"，中层的肌纤维环绕心室，而内层和外层的肌纤维则与心室长轴方向平行或斜行排列，在不同心脏存在变异。在本研究中，通过弥散张量成像技术获得的纤维走行方向（尽管只是在单个心脏上）与上述报道结果相似。但纤维在层间旋绕的程度小于组织学研究的报道。这种差异与采用的方法和心脏的差异（年龄、动物品系和其他）有关。可能需要更多的研究数据支持这一差异。

另外，在本研究中采用经甲醛固定的心脏，尽管心脏的外形可能会受到一定的影响，但是与在体心脏比较，经甲醛固定的心脏可以进行长时间的成像，分辨力和信噪比更好。同时，也可以防止心脏灌注时可能导致的数据丢失，并且不会影响心脏纤维的走行[43]。尽管在本研究弥散张量成像是沿心脏长轴方向获取心脏纤维走行的数据，也有证据表明，在组织学研究的基础上，这种方法也可以研究心肌的层间结构。在本研究建立的数学模型中，心脏传导纤维小样本的研究数据并没有包括在内，传导纤维的数据主要来源于弥散张量成像获得。由于研究中采用小鼠的心

脏进行扫描，心脏轻微的位移或者心脏形状的改变都可以在心肌的边缘产生人工伪差。在对张量进行评估和删除传导纤维在各向异性比例以下的估计量之前，将获取的图像进行寄存有助于减少部分人工伪差。这些方案目前被用于改进心脏数学模型的构建。

通过具有精细空间分辨力的磁共振成像可以建立计算机网格，但由于心脏的体积较小，网格的边缘并不平滑。与边界拟合网格比较，本研究采用阶梯步骤建立的计算机网格具有速度快的优势，并且能够避免不同大小的邻近像素带来的数学问题。通过FV方案，可以直接使用核磁共振的像素作为构建模型的元素。这种方法使建立预加工的特定心脏的数学模型成为可能，并且有助于解释不同体积心脏之间电生理活动的差异。

由于心脏体积较小，使我们能够首次用双域建模方法构建了1个完整心脏电生理活动的数学模型。在这个模型中，心脏整个电传导过程，包括跨壁电压和细胞外电压均能通过模型计算。尽管模型与实验室的数据并非完全吻合，但与 Nygren 等研究者[30]在小鼠心脏用光学标测的跨室壁电压的结果比较，还是非常接近的。细胞外电压的数据也与 Mooch 等在大鼠心脏上的研究结果相似[31]。更重要的是，我们所建立的小鼠心脏模型结果与实验室在较大心脏上的结果接近，提示小鼠心脏和心脏的计算机模型可以用来研究不同条件下（包括基因水平的调节）心脏的激动波传导的过程[32]。

通过基因水平的操作，可以使小鼠心脏成为研究某些电生理异常疾病的良好实验工具。目前研究表明，某些心脏电生理功能异常不仅与特定基因或基因编码的蛋白质异常相关，而且在信号通路中蛋白质相互作用的异常也可以成为发生心脏激动传导障碍的基质。这些异常的电生理基质不仅包括细胞结构上的异常（细胞连接）[44]，也包括心肌细胞离子通道分布和动力学特征的异常[45,46]。通过小鼠心脏的数学模型，可以首先在完整心脏上对某些蛋白质的相互作用过程进行计算，然后提出假说，设计实验方案，包括对小鼠进行转基因操作，用于临床心律失常疾病的研究。

正如前面提到的，小鼠心脏数学模型目前遇到的最大的挑战是如何将小鼠心脏模型中观察到的结果推广到大动物，特别是人类心脏上。尽管如此，小鼠心脏的计算机模型仍然能够在研究心脏电生理功能上发挥重要的作用。研究人员需要将模型的复杂程度控制在合适的水平，以利于某些心脏电生理现象的研究，并且作为进一步实验室研究的基础。本研究证实，心脏数学模型上获得的结果有的能够与实验室结果相互印证，有的则不能，例如，心脏多个部位的电势图和荧光染料指示的跨膜电压图结果可以通过模型计算，但对单一离子通道的电流则不能通过模型计算。将两者的优势结合起来，将有助于从分子水平解释心律失常发生的机制。通过核磁共振成像技术和电激动光学标测技术能够快速在心脏三维数学模型上标测出基因表达情况，并进一步将其导入到转基因小鼠心脏的数学模型中[47,48]。这对于研究蛋白质相互作用异常导致的心律失常的机制是非常重要的。最后，如果将全部离子通道电流动力学特征的数据纳入到心脏三维数学模型中，将可能对心脏的体表心电图进行模拟计算，使其在心脏电生理研究中的应用从蛋白质水平上升到临床应用水平。

（李继文　译）

参 考 文 献

1. Henriquez CS, Papazoglou AA: Using computer models to understand the roles of tissue structure and membrane dynamics in arrhythmogenesis. Proc IEEE 84:334–354, 1996.
2. Vetter FJ, McCulloch AD: Three-dimensional analysis of regional cardiac function: A model of rabbit ventricular anatomy. Prog Biophys Mol Biol 69:157–183, 1998.
3. Trayanova N, Eason J, Aguel F: Computer simulations of cardiac defibrillation: A look inside the heart. Comput Visual Sci 4:259–270, 2002.
4. Harrild DM, Henriquez CS: A computer model of normal conduction in the human atria. Circ Res 87:E25–E36, 2000.
5. Cherry EM, Greenside HS, Henriquez CS: A space-time adaptive method for simulating complex cardiac dynamics. Phys Rev Lett 84:1343–1346, 2000.
6. London B, Jeron A, Zhou J, et al: Long QT and ventricular arrhythmias in transgenic mice expressing the N terminus and first transmembrane segment of a voltage-gated potassium channel. Proc Natl Acad Sci USA 95:2926–2931, 1998.
7. Mitchell GF, Jeron A, Koren G: Measurement of heart rate and QT interval in the conscious mouse. Am J Physiol 274(3 Pt 2):H747–H751, 1998.
8. Gottshall KR, Hunter JJ, Tanaka N, et al: Ras-dependent pathways induce obstructive hypertrophy in echo-selected transgenic mice. Proc Natl Acad Sci USA 94:4710–4715, 1997.
9. Johnatty SE, Dyck JR, Michael LH, et al: Identification of genes regulated during mechanical load-induced cardiac hypertrophy. J Mol Cell Cardiol 32:805–815, 2000.
10. Nossuli TO, Lakshminarayanan V, Baumgarten G, et al: A chronic mouse model of myocardial ischemia-reperfusion: Essential in cytokine studies. Am J Physiol Heart Circ Physiol 278:H1049–H1055, 2000.
11. London B: Cardiac arrhythmias: from (transgenic) mice to men. J Cardiovasc Electrophysiol 12:1089–1091, 2001.
12. Doevendans PA, Daemen MJ, de Muinck ED, Smits JF: Cardiovascular phenotyping in mice. Cardiovas Res 39:34–49, 1998.
13. LeGrice IJ, Smaill BH, Chai LZ, et al: Laminar structure of the heart: Ventricular myocyte arrangement and connective tissue architecture in the dog. Am J Physiol 269(2 Pt 2):H571–H582, 1995.
14. Basser PJ, Mattiello J, Bihan DL: MR diffusion tensor spectroscopy and imaging. Biophys J 66:259–267, 1994.
15. Hsu EW, Muzikant AL, Matulevicius SA, et al: Magnetic resonance myocardial fiber-orientation mapping with direct histological corre-

lation. Am J Physiol 274(2 Pt 2):H1627–H1634, 1998.
16. Scollan DF, Holmes A, Winslow R, Forder J: Histological validation of reconstructed myocardial microstructure obtained from diffusion tensor magnetic resonance imaging. Am J Physiol 275(6 Pt 2):H2308–H2318, 1998.
17. Tung L: A bidomain model for describing ischemic myocardial D.C. potentials [thesis]. Cambridge, MA: Massachusetts Institute of Technology, 1978.
18. Henriquez CS: Simulating the electrical behavior of cardiac tissue using the bidomain model. Crit Rev Biomed Eng 21:1–77, 1993.
19. Colli Franzone P, Guerri L, Taccardi B: Spread of excitation in a myocardial volume: Simulation studies in a model of anisotropic ventricular muscle activated by point stimulation. J Cardiovasc Electrophys 4:144–160, 1993.
20. Henriquez CS, Muzikant AL, Smoak CK: Anisotropy, fiber curvature and bath loading effects on activation in thin and thick cardiac tissue preparations: Simulations in a three dimensional bidomain model. J Cardiovasc Electrophys 7:424–444, 1996.
21. Harrild DM, Penland RC, Henriquez CS: A flexible method for simulating cardiac conduction in three-dimensional complex geometries. J Electrocardiol 33:241–251, 2000.
22. Penland RC, Harrild DM, Henriquez CS: Modeling impulse propagation and extracellular potential distributions in anisotropic cardiac tissue using a finite volume element discretization. Comput Visual Sci 4:215–226, 2002.
23. Clancy C, Rudy Y: Linking a genetic defect to its cellular phenotype in a cardiac arrhythmia. Nature 400:566–569 1999.
24. Nerbonne JM, Nichols CG, Schwarz TL, Escande D: Genetic manipulation of cardiac K(+) channel function in mice: What have we learned, and where do we go from here? Circ Res 89:944–956, 2001.
25. Knollmann BC, Katchman AN, Franz MR: Monophasic action potential recordings from intact mouse heart: Validation, regional heterogeneity, and relation to refractoriness. J Cardiovasc Electrophys 12:1286–1294, 2001.
26. Pandit SV, Clark RB, Giles WR, Demir SS: A mathematical model of action potential heterogeneity in adult rat left ventricular myocytes. Biophys J 81:3029–3051, 2001.
27. Johnson C, Parker S, Weinstein D, Heffernan S: Component-based, problem-solving environments for large-scale scientific computing. Concurrency and Computation: Practice and Experience 14:1337–1349, 2002.
28. Pormann J: A modular simulation system for the bidomain equations (thesis). Durham, NC, Duke University, 1999.
29. Wikswo JP Jr, Lin SF, Abbas RA: Virtual electrodes in cardiac tissue: A common mechanism for anodal and cathodal stimulation. Biophys J 69:2195–2210, 1995.
30. Nygren A, Clark RB, Belke DD, et al: Voltage-sensitive dye mapping of activation and conduction in adult mouse hearts. Ann Biomed Eng 28:958–967, 2000.
31. Macchi E, Cavalieri M, Stilli D, et al: High-density epicardial mapping during current injection and ventricular activation in rat hearts. Am J Physiol 275(5 Pt 2):H1886–H1897, 1998.
32. Taccardi B, Macchi E, Lux RL, et al: Effect of myocardial fiber direction on epicardial potentials. Circulation 90:3076–3090, 1995.
33. Muzikant AL, Hsu E, Wolf PD, Henriquez CS: Region specific modeling of cardiac muscle: Comparison of simulated and experimental potentials. Ann Biomed Eng 30:867–883, 2002.
34. Sampson KJ, Henriquez CS: Simulation and prediction of functional block in the presence of structural and ionic heterogeneity. Am J Physiol Heart Circ Physiol 281:H2597–H2603, 2001.
35. Lorange M, Gulrajani RM: A computer heart model incorporating anisotropic propagation. I. Model construction and simulation of normal activation. J Electrocardiol 26:245–261, 1993.
36. Miller WT, Geselowitz DB: Simulation studies of the electrocardiogram. I. The normal heart. Circ Res 43:301–315, 1978.
37. Berenfield O, Jalife J: Purkinje-muscle reentry as a mechanism of polymorphic ventricular arrhythmias in a 3-dimensional model of the ventricles. Circ Res 82:1063–1077, 1998.
38. Hren R, Nenonen J, Horacek BM: Simulated epicardial potential maps during paced activation reflect myocardial fibrous structure. Ann Biomed Eng 26:1022–1035, 1998.
39. Panfilov AV: Three dimensional wave propagation in mathematical models of ventricular fibrillation. In Zipes DP, Jalife J (eds): Cardiac Electrophysiology: From Cell to Bedside, 3rd ed. Philadelphia, WB Saunders, 1999, pp 271–276.
40. Vigmond EJ, Ruckdeschel R, Trayanova N: Reentry in a morphologically realistic atrial model. J Cardiovasc Electrophys 12:1046–1054, 2001.
41. Fenton F, Karma A: Vortex dynamics. In 3D continuous myocardium with fiber rotation: Filament instability and fibrillation. CHAOS 8:20–65, 1998.
42. McLean M, Prothero J: Myofiber orientation in the weanling mouse heart. Am J Anat 192:425–441, 1991.
43. Holmes AA, Scollan DF, Winslow RL: Direct histological validation of diffusion tensor MRI in formaldehyde-fixed myocardium. Magn Reson Med 44(1):157–161, 2000.
44. Scollan DF, Holmes A, Zhang J, Winslow RL: Reconstruction of cardiac ventricular geometry and fiber orientation using magnetic resonance imaging. Ann Biomed Eng 28:934–944, 2000.
45. Noble D: Modeling the heart—from genes to cells to the whole organ. Science 295:1678–1682, 2002.
46. Jalife J, Morley GE, Vaidya D: Connexins and impulse propagation in the mouse heart. J Cardiovas Electrophys 10:1649–1663, 1999.
47. Anumonwo JMB, Tallini YN, Vetter FJ, Jalife J: Action potential characteristics and arrhythmogenic properties of the cardiac conduction system in the murine heart. Circ Res 89:329–335, 2001.
48. Mahmood U, Tung CH, Tang Y, Weissleder R: Feasibility of in vivo multichannel optical imaging of gene expression: Experimental study in mice. Radiology 224:446–451, 2002.

第 31 章

心脏除颤模型

Natalia Trayanova, *Felipe Aguel*, *Claire Larson*, *Carlos Haro*

本章目录

- 方法 278
- 结果 278
- 讨论 282
- 结论 283

尽管已经有大量关于心脏除颤的研究，但用强电流终止致命性室性心律失常发作的机制目前仍然存在争论。实验室的资料提示，电击可以导致局部心脏跨膜电压变负或变正的改变，并称之为模拟电极极化[1-5]。而心脏除颤的数学模型研究也支持这一结果[6-11]。模拟电极极化是非均一的，并且依赖于心脏组织结构[3,12,13]。实验表明，遭受电击的心肌跨壁电压的改变以非线性方式快速改变了心肌细胞动作电位的形成过程。累积单个细胞电生理特性的变化可使整个心肌的电生理特性也会发生改变，当部分心肌仍处于不应期时，其他心肌的兴奋性已经部分甚至完全恢复。电击的结果不仅取决于电击后跨膜电压的分布，更取决于它们在空间上的相互作用，以及由此引发的新的波阵面。

上述新发现改变了心室除颤的传统观点，但仍然存在需要深入研究的问题。例如研究深层心肌电击后电活动的改变，用目前的实验记录方法是难以达到的。另外特别令人感兴趣的问题还包括电击后肌纤维电生理变化、折返活动的形成[14]，而折返的形成与电击失败、室颤再次发生有关。

肌纤维电生理改变的研究试图解释室性心动过速蜕变为室颤的机制，特别是单一折返波被分裂成多个折返波的原因[15-18]。尽管近年来某些光学记录技术包括透照技术[19]和光纤技术[20]已经初步应用于跨室壁肌纤维的研究，但距离在心脏立体结构中辨别肌纤维仍比较遥远。计算机模拟技术，对从三维结构上研究心律失常发生的电生理基质具有重要的作用（见 Fenton 等人的综述[21]）。这些研究发展了折返形成的理论，特别是折返的形成、演变及分裂为多个子波的机制，这在二维平面研究上是难以实现的。

尽管折返波的分裂机制在心肌电击后的电生理活动中起着重要的作用，但对于电击后即刻形成的折返只能部分解释。原因在于模拟电极极化机制[2]，电击本身就可以出现相位奇点。这些相位奇点在电击后不应期变化的心肌区域内演变[22]。本研究组对二维平面和 1mm 层厚犬心脏组织中进行的室性心动过速电转复的计算机模拟研究表明，电击后可以产生大量的相位奇点，其中大部分在折返形成前消失。但是，目前仍缺乏室颤电转复中自旋波条纹的动态变化以及用计算机技术进行三维模拟的研究。

本研究的目的是运用计算机技术，建立反映成功或不成功的室颤电转复中肌纤维电生理特征的动态变化的三维立体高分辨力的双域数学模型。此模型中，既包含反映心脏的几何形状、纤维走行、离子通道电流的数据，也包含通过猝发刺激诱发的室颤和电击有害效应（如细胞电穿孔）的数据。本研究组不仅建立了室颤电转复的数学模型，而且在心脏三维立体结构上，对电击后心律失常发生的电生理基质进行了研究，目前用其他的方法是难以做到的。

一、方法

有限元方法建立的兔心室和纤维走行的数学模型[23]被用来模拟心室颤动和电转复后心肌电生理改变，具体模型建立的方法见既往报道[24]。简要如下：用 MSC Patran 软件系统建立反映心室几何形状的计算机有限元网格。首先用三角测量方法确定兔心室表面 36 个六面体结构[23]；将六面体结构的数据导入 Patran 系统，并对其进行分析和适当调整；然后用三角测量的方法使分辨力达到 350μm；最终建立包含四面体计算网格数据、分辨力达到 350μm 的兔心室数学模型。用类似的方法建立心室腔的数学模型，其像素密度为 1mm。当所有的计算机网格数据获得后，在每个四面体的图心位置找到肌纤维的走行方向，并用数据指定局部的组织特征。图 31-1（左图）描述了兔心室的几何特征。图 31-1（中图和右图）所示为兔心室和肌纤维的后面观和前面观。其中，白线表示心外膜中纤维的走行，而心内膜纤维的走行用黑线表示。心室腔用等体积的均匀导体表示，导体的特征与血池接近。心外膜表面并非绝缘体，因此心外膜表面数据被用来模拟 Lengendorff 灌流的心室中的气体[3,25]。

心肌的电生理特征用双域数学模型表示。修改后的 Luo-Rudy 方法建立的心室肌动作电位模型被用来模拟细胞膜的兴奋性[26]。电转复后膜结构的变化（如电穿孔）用 DeBruim 和 Krassowska 模型表示[27,28]，用既往报道的双域模型线性四面体有限元求解方法[24]和 Vigmond 等提出的新运算法则来计算心肌组织和血池中的电压[29]。兔心室的三维数学模型在我们的前期研究结果中已经证实。

在本研究中，我们使用 Kwaku、Dillon[25] 和 Knisley 的研究[3]中类似的套囊电极，通过猝发刺激的方法诱发心室颤动，并进行电转复。以基底部的电极作为地线，通过心尖部的电极发放刺激脉冲。具体方法是发放 17 个成串的刺激，刺激的周长为 50ms，刺激脉宽为 4ms。室颤诱发后 600ms 进行电转复。

转复电流为持续 9ms 的单相波，分别采用 8 个逐级递增的电流强度进行转复，以寻找合适的除颤阈值。电流的强度为 25.69～128.43mA 之间。电转复后 300ms 是心肌电生理活动的观察期。

对电转复后心肌电生理表现的观察主要是确认自旋波（涡旋）条纹，包括它们的持续时间，在左右心室和室间隔的部位。此外对它们的类型加以确定。I

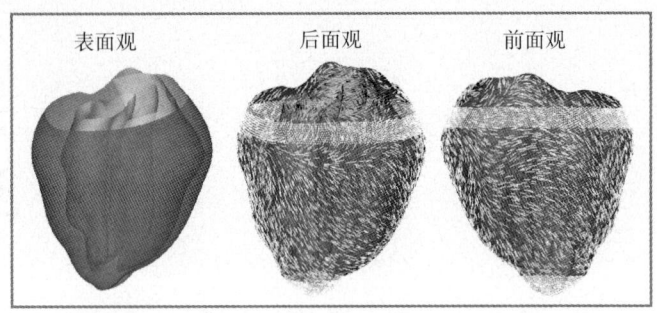

图 31-1　兔心室模型　左图为心室模型的内膜面和外膜面（表面观）；中图和右图为兔心室和肌纤维的后面观和前面观，白线表示心外膜中纤维的走行，而心内膜纤维的走行用黑线表示

型是指其末端分别与左右心室的内膜面和外膜面相接触。而 U 型是指其两端与心室内膜或外膜的同一部相位接触。O 型指呈环状。而不符合上述分类的也计算在内。

确定自旋波的运算方法来源于二维平面计算相位奇点的方法（后者在我们前期的研究报道中已经详细描述[24]）。简而言之，通过用 Gray 等[14]的方法将跨膜电图转换为相位角度图，并采用接近心肌兴奋阈值的"中心电压"和 2ms 延迟时间。然后通过将构成网格的四面体的每一面上包围三个节点的相位进行线性积分，使二维平面的计算方法[11,14]拓展到三维不规则模型。如果在四面体至少一个面上计算得到的积分为 ±2π，则认为该四面体中有自旋波条纹通过。对四面体的连接进行计算处理后，将包含自旋波条纹的四面体的中心连接起来，用绘制的球体将其包含在内。

二、结果

图 31-2 所示为通过猝发刺激诱发室颤时的兔心室基底部和正后壁电压图，包含大量激动波和可激动间隙。底部图对应的时间为诱发室颤的刺激开始发放后 1400ms，图中可以看到与心室颤动重叠的自旋波条纹，共有 9 个条纹。条纹的长度都比较短。1400ms 时间点的自旋波条纹和电压图代表心室颤动电转复前的电生理状态，而由于模拟电极极化作用，随后的电转复将以非线性方式改变上述表现。

对室颤 8 次电转复进行数学模拟后，结果表明心室颤动的除颤阈值为 106.35mA（成功转复的最小电流强度）。在 8 次电转复中，4 次成功，4 次失败。电转复时的电流强度的具体数值见图 31-3。所有的电击除颤均能在心室表面和心室内发生模拟电极极化作用。电极极化作用与我们前期的研究报道结果相一致[24]。

在本章中，对于电击后心脏电生理基质的变化，我们用自旋波条纹的演变进行定量的描述。图31-3表示电击除颤的不同时间点、自旋波条纹的数量。从图中可以看到，在除颤初期，自旋波条纹的数量是最多的。在电除颤后30ms，成功转复组中自旋波条纹的数量略多于转复失败组，分别为19.8和17.5。在电除颤100ms内，自旋波条纹的数量明显下降。特别是50ms时，下降最明显。例外情况是用最小电流25.69mA除颤后30ms，只有6个自旋波条纹，其中5个在右心室，1个在室间隔。

图31-3的结果也证实，在电除颤100ms到200～250ms时间段，心室的电活动处于调整的状态，表现为自旋波条纹数量少，而且保持稳定。事实上，在成功转复组中，电除颤100ms时，只有2个自旋波条纹。而且在200～250ms时间段，自旋波条纹消失。而电转复失败组中，电击后100ms，自旋波条纹的数量仍较多，平均数量为5.25。200ms后，自旋波条纹的数目上升，提示心室的电活动处于更加无序的状态。

图31-4和图31-5示通过心室模型中自旋波条纹的分布证实了图31-3的结果。图31-4所示为

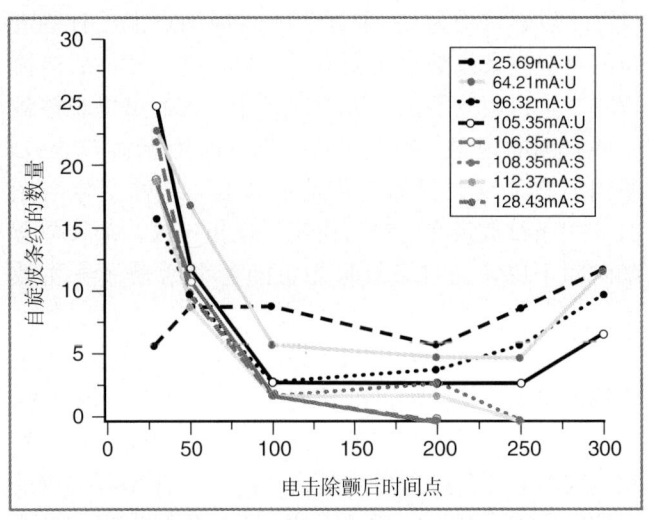

图 31-3　电击除颤的不同时间点，兔心室数学模型中自旋波条纹的数量　图例中为电流强度和相应的线条颜色，S：成功电转复，U：电转复失败。

64.21mA的电流电转复后三个时间点，心室基底部和后壁自旋波条纹的分布。这种对自旋波条纹的直观描述与图31-2不同。图31-5用灰阶的方式描述了心室跨膜电压分布情况（最深的颜色对应于-80mV，最浅的颜色对应于-30mV），用颜色将自旋波条纹区分开来。从图中可以明显看出，电除颤后30ms，条纹数目是最多的，100ms时，条纹数目明显下降，而当200ms时，条纹数目又重新上升。图31-5按电流强度顺序排列，表示电击除颤后30ms，自旋波条纹的数量和分布。左侧为心室前壁，右侧为心室后壁。图中，自旋波条纹用橘黄色或黄色表示。用其他的颜色着重表示心室外膜面和内膜面自旋波条纹的终点，条纹终点与心室的内膜面相连用红色表示，而条纹终点与外膜面相连则用紫蓝色表示。从图中可以直观地看到自旋波条纹的碎裂。另外一个有趣的发现是，当用较小的电流转复时形成较长的自旋波条纹，随着电流强度的增加，这些长条纹可以碎裂为较短的条纹，但条纹的位置和性状似乎保持不变。例如在右图中，用箭头表示的条纹，在电流从106.35mA增加到128.43mA的情况下，分裂成两条，在图中分别用黑色和灰色箭头表示。这也可以部分解释成功转复组早期自旋波条纹的数量多于转复失败组。

图31-6则描述了心室模型中自旋波条纹的形态和部位。图A、B、C分别表示左心室、右心室和室间隔。采用的时间点为电击后30ms、100ms和300ms。每一个直方图描述了不同形态自旋波条纹的数量。在成功转复组中，心室上述部位在300ms时间点上，自

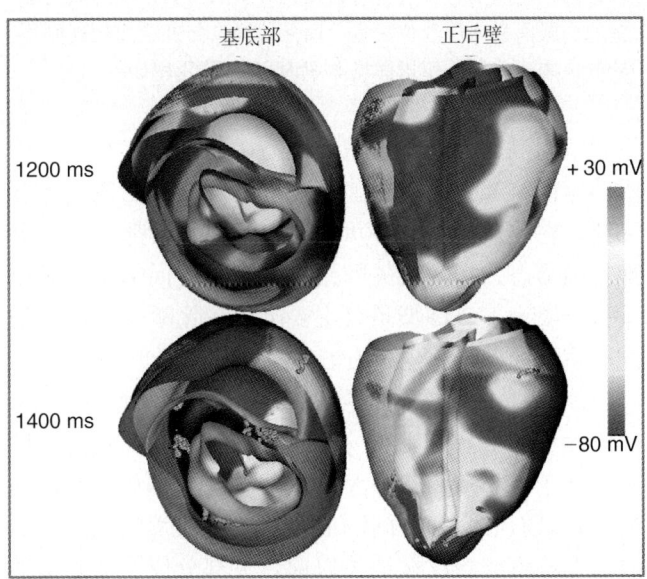

图 31-2　猝发刺激诱发室颤时，兔心室模型基底部和正后壁在两个不同时间点跨膜电压图　底部图对应的时间为诱发室颤的刺激开始发放后1400ms，图中可以看到兔心室三维数学模型中的自旋波条纹。（彩图57）

旋波条纹数目均为 0；而在 100ms 时间点上，有些部位的自旋波条纹数目也是 0。在左心室，最小的电流没有产生自旋波条纹。从图 31-6 中，我们可以观察到一些有趣的现象。在电击后早期（时间点为 30ms），不同类型条纹数目的变化是很大的。这种变化与图 31-3 中条纹数量在电击后快速下降相一致。条纹数量随时间下降，而且条纹形态也随着电活动而发生改变。

大部分 O 型条纹（最不稳定的形态）形成于电击除颤的早期。从图中可以看出，在时间点为 30ms 时，O 型条纹的数量是最多的，特别是在室间隔部位。相反，在右心室，O 型条纹是最少的。尽管在电除颤的晚期，仍然有少量的 O 型条纹，但它们只出现在左心

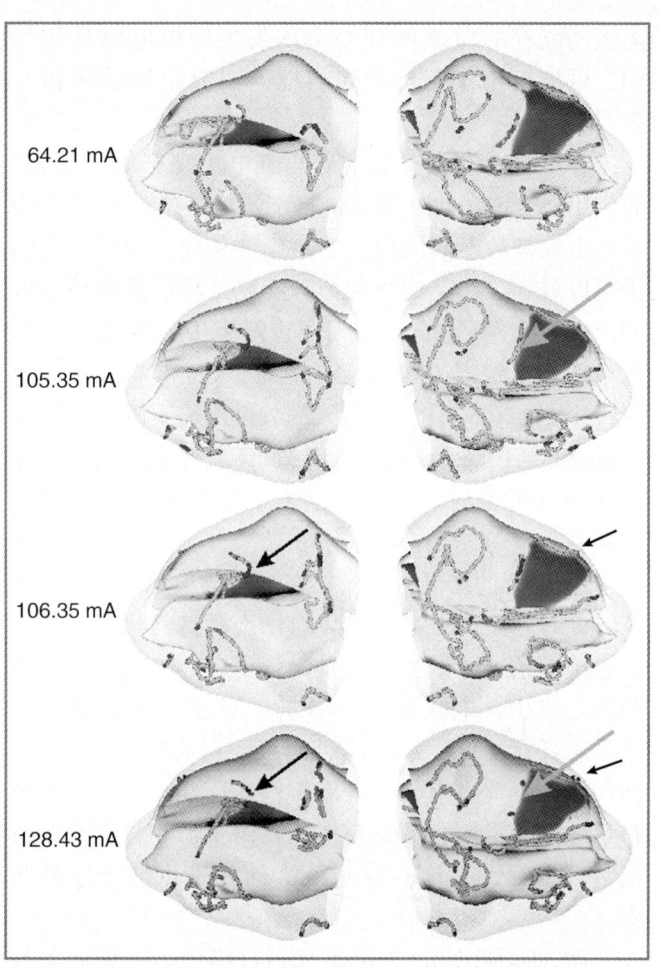

图 31-5 电击除颤后 30ms，心室模型中自旋波条纹的数量和分布　左图为心室前壁，右图为心室后壁。条纹终点与心室的内膜面相连用红色表示，而条纹终点与外膜面相连则用紫蓝色表示，箭头所指详见本章内容。（见彩图 58）

室和室间隔，可能与室壁厚度有关。另外，在电击除颤的早期（30ms），I 型条纹只出现在右心室。尽管如此，在除颤 200～300ms 时，I 型条纹都是占主导地位的形态。在转复失败组中，形式不同部位都是以 I 型条纹为主。U 型条纹主要出现在除颤后 100ms 的左心室，同样，它也是右心室早期的主要形态。

图 31-6 的结果还证实在成功除颤后 100～200ms 时间段（恰好在自旋波条纹消失之前），自旋波条纹只存在于左心室，其中大部分为 U 型。因此，在成功转复组，右心室和室间隔的自旋波条纹消失更早。而且，左心室的条纹在消失以前，大部分位于左心室的表面。而转复失败组中，同一时间段，则仍然存在较多的自旋波条纹，这与图 31-3 中的结果相一致。

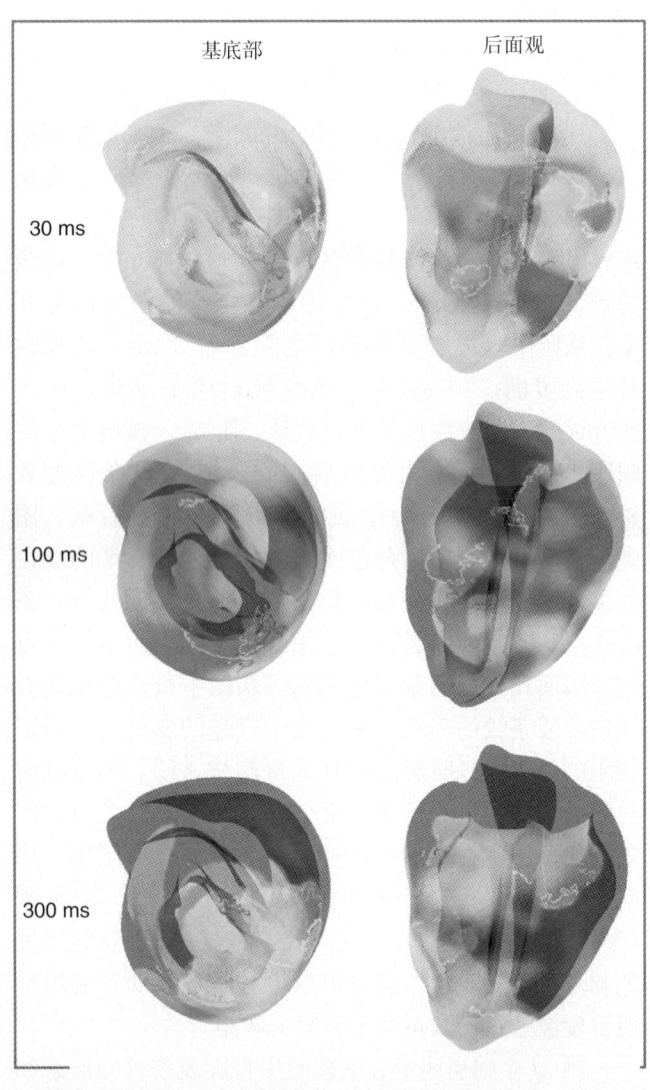

图 31-4　用 64.21mA 的电流电转复后三个时间点（30ms、100ms 和 300ms），心室基底部和后壁自旋波条纹的分布　心室模型中的阴影用来辨别自旋波条纹。

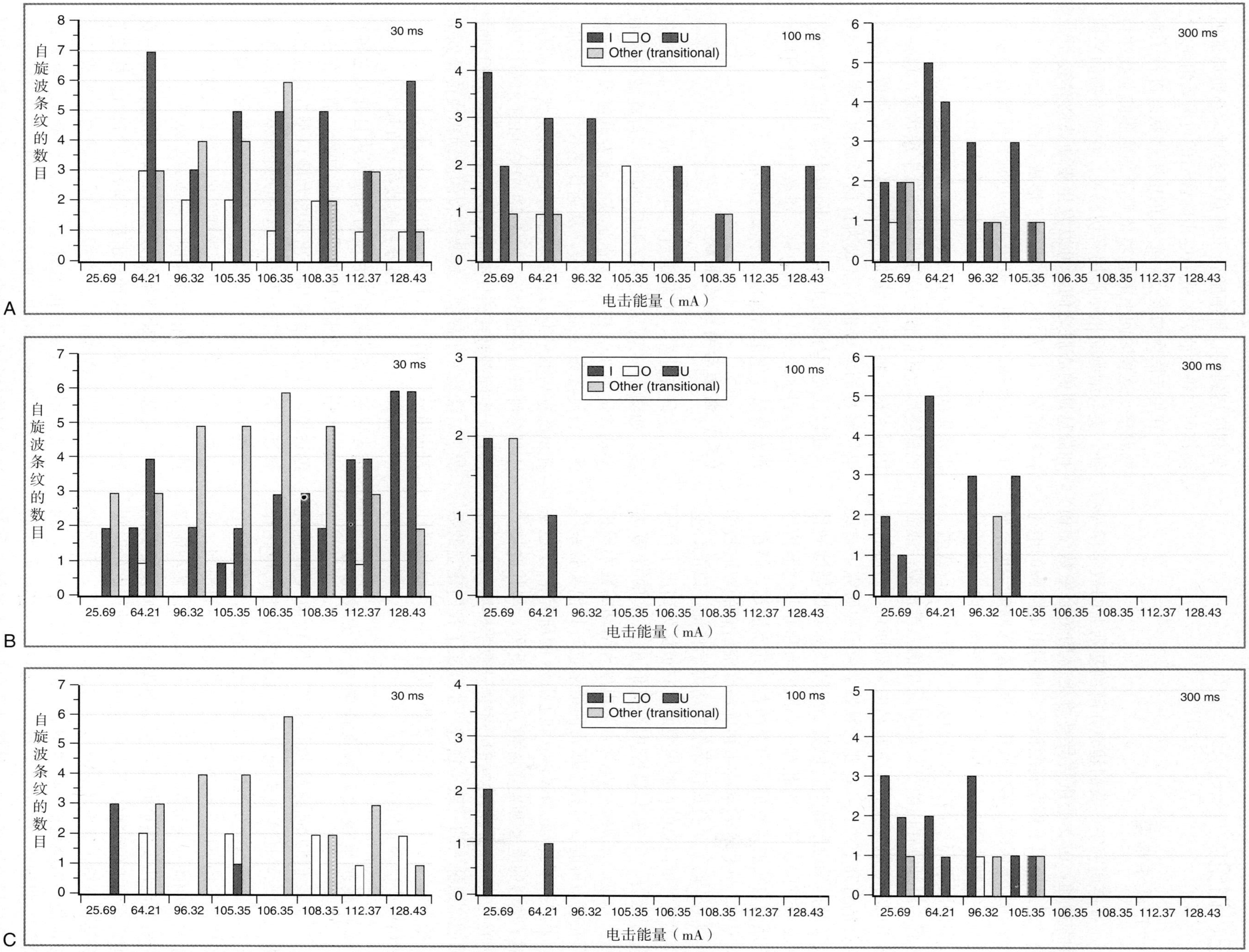

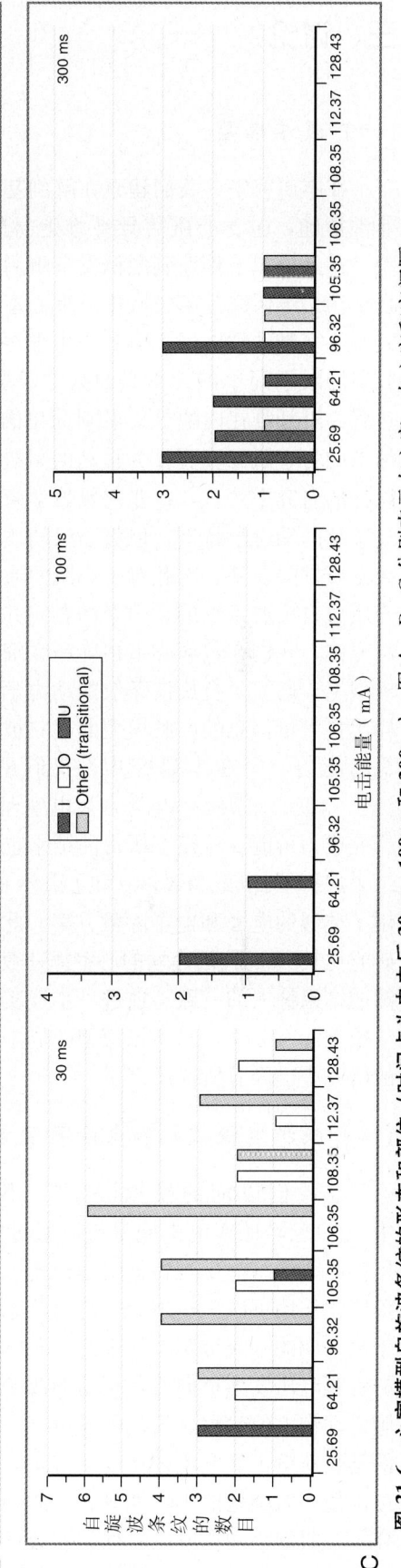

图 31-6 心室模型自旋波条纹的形态和部位（时间点为电击后 30ms、100ms 和 300ms） 图 A、B、C 分别表示左心室、右心室和室间隔。

三、讨论

（一）数学模型

在本研究中，我们建立在解剖基础上的数学模型非常精确，包含心脏传导纤维走行的兔心室数学模型，并且模拟了猝发刺激诱发室颤后电击除颤的电生理活动。本研究是第一次用三维心室双域数学模型研究了心室颤动后电击除颤的电生理过程。而以往的研究多局限于简单的二维平面数学模型[8,31-33]；或者不包含心脏纤维在内的[34]、相对简单的三维模型；或者简单的将心肌细胞膜作为被动的阻抗回路[5]。尽管在以往的研究中[16-18]，在非双域数学模型中研究了自旋波条纹的动力学特征，但将心肌间质和心肌周围的传导介质排除在外。因此对于心肌间质和心肌周围传导介质对自旋波条纹的动力学的影响并不清楚。但在本研究中，我们在包含心室精确和详细信息的双域数学模型上，研究了自旋波条纹的动力学特征。以前，这样包含大量信息的心脏模型的建立被认为超出了计算机的能力，而在本研究中，我们用高效的计算方法[29]，使心室颤动和电除颤后电生理活动的数学模拟研究成为可能。该模型所得的结果也与其他实验室的结果进行了比较。Kwaku 和 Dillon 的研究中[25]也采用了类似的电极和电击除颤方案。此外，与其他技术研究比较[30]，我们建立的心室颤动数学模型与光学标测的结果惊人的一致。这进一步证实了我们建立的数学模型的有效性。对于该模型的局限性，我们在以往的研究中已经有所描述[24]。

（二）模拟电极极化和电除颤后电生理活动

在我们以前的模拟研究[8-11]和其他大量研究中[1-5]，已经证实电击能量可以通过模拟电极极化作用使心肌细胞电生理特征发生改变。首先，电击时电极极化作用可以兴奋本处于静息状态的心肌细胞，对于兴奋期的心肌细胞，外来的微弱电流可以使细胞膜的跨膜电压发生负向或者正向的改变，从而使心肌细胞的动作电位时程延长或者缩短[22,36]。动作电位时程的延长对电击后电生理活动具有重要的意义，因为它可以使心肌细胞的不应期延长，激动的传导延迟。同样，心肌细胞动作电位时程的缩短可以使部分心肌的兴奋性提前恢复，从而使激动顺电压差传导到未兴奋组织的几率增加[37]。增加电击的能量可以导致上述动作电位时程的改变更加明显。当电击导致的电生理改变程度达到使心肌细胞处于静息状态时，心肌局部的动作电位将会消失，成为电击除颤后的可激动组织。

在电击除颤的终点，心肌的电生理状态进行了新的调整。这种时间上的调整依赖于细胞膜的非线性特征，更与细胞间相互作用密切相关。在兴奋期的心肌和静息期的心肌之间，可以发生激动波的碎裂[6,38]。这种情况一旦发生，就具备了形成折返活动的"种子"，去极化的心肌、复极期的心肌和可兴奋心肌可立即构成了折返环的组成部分。在 Efimov 等[2]对电击诱发的相位奇点研究中就已经认识到这一点。折返的最终形成还依赖于周围组织的电生理状态，包括周围可兴奋心肌和处于复极期的心肌。与之类似，动作电位时程的缩短也可以成为折返形成的"种子"[37]，这在以往光学标测的研究[39,40]和我们数学模型的研究中已经得到证实[41]。在心室三维数学模型中，同样的机制导致了电击后自旋波条纹的形成。

（三）电击后自旋波条纹

本研究证实，电除颤后，可以形成大量自旋波条纹。如图 31-3 所示，电除颤后 30ms，自旋波条纹的平均数量为 30。图 31-5 也证实，随着电流强度的加大，自旋波条纹发生碎裂，从而使条纹的数量增加。在电除颤后的早期，心室大部分处于极化状态，只有小部分维持可兴奋状态（比较图 31-3 和图 31-5），原因在于电除颤时或稍后时间内，在电极极化的相对边界上，激动发生碎裂，这些碎裂的激动很快传导到未兴奋组织，使组织去极化，如图 31-5 所示。

在图 31-3 中，大部分自旋波条纹在除颤后 50ms 消失，这种变化的原因在于有限空间内自旋波之间的相互作用，经过相互增加或抵消的过程，消失在心室的边界。另外，在除颤后出现的大量 O 型自旋波条纹被证实是最不稳定的形态，这种涡旋波缩小的速度与它的半径成反比[42,43]。与 Winfree 的预测相一致[44]，这种 O 型自旋波是"左右摇摆"的，当它接触到边界或与其他自旋波相互作用时，便会发生碎裂。

电除颤后自旋波条纹数量的下降是持续的，一直到电击后 100ms。这种电击后 100ms 时间内自旋波条纹的显著下降提示，只有很少的自旋波可以形成折返活动，绝大部分在折返发生前就已经消失。有趣的是，在成功转复组中，电击后 100ms 时，自旋波条纹的数量比转复失败组少（2 比 5.2）。这一结果是本研究组既往在二维空间上模拟终止室性心动过速[11]和在狗心脏组织条上[10]的研究结果的进一步拓展。在既往研究中，我们发现电击可以产生大量相位奇点，并且随时间快速下降。大部分相位奇点持续的时间相当于螺旋波的一半或更短。

经过电击后自旋波条纹数量快速下降的时期后，在电击后100～200ms时，进入了一段电生理活动调整期。在这期间，最明显的发现是，在成功转复组中，只有左心室存在自旋波条纹，而右心室和室间隔的条纹已经消失（见图31-6）。因而提示成功电转复后，折返只可能发生在左心室，而不是在心室的所有部位都能形成折返活动的"种子"。左心室中的折返活动在电击后200～250ms便会自行消失，如果电击的能量更大，自旋波条纹消失的时间更早。

在同一时期（200～250ms），转复失败组心室中自旋波条纹的数量增加，导致室颤的再次发生。再次发生的室颤的维持依靠自旋波条纹的形成，其中主导形态是Ⅰ型条纹，在心室的各个部分均是如此。在右心室则几乎全部是Ⅰ型条纹，而且这种电生理特点与电击后的初期情况一致（左心室和室间隔的情况不同）。原因可能与左心室和室间隔比较，右心室的室壁较薄。既往研究报道，室壁的厚度与自旋波条纹的稳定性有密切关系[45]。事实上，在Zipes等的研究结果中，室颤只来源于较厚的左心室壁，并且可以演变为稳定的室性心动过速[46]。类似的结果也可见于心脏内膜冰冻[47]或去除部分心室[48]的研究报道（具体见Fenton等最近发表的综述[21]）。因为Ⅰ型自旋波条纹是最稳定的[44]，因而似乎支持其可以在室壁较薄的右心室发生。在我们的研究中，Ⅰ型条纹的形状很少是固定的，大部分存在一定程度的弯曲。在Jlife的研究[49]和其他研究组的报告中也有类似的发现[47,50]。

四、结 论

从本研究组对兔心室除颤的三维数学模型的研究结果，我们得出以下的结论：

1. 电除颤导致的自旋波条纹在电击时是最多的，在电除颤后100ms，自旋波条纹的数量明显减少。在成功的电转复中，自旋波条纹在电击后250ms完全消失。电转复失败后，自旋波条纹的数量在电击后200～250ms又重新增加。

2. 电除颤成功后，折返活动只发生于左心室，尽管在心室三维数学模型中，可以见到一过性的折返形成的"种子"。

3. 电除颤时形成的自旋波条纹有三种形态：Ⅰ型、U型和O型。自旋波形态的演变多发生于电击后的早期。电除颤时，Ⅰ型自旋波条纹只发生于右心室，左心室主要为U型，而室间隔是以O型条纹为主。在电极后的晚期，涡旋的发生并不常见，即使是室壁较厚的左心室也是如此。在电击后200ms，主要是Ⅰ型自旋波条纹，尤其是在右心室。

（李继文 译）

参 考 文 献

1. Wikswo Jr JP, Lin SF, Abbas RA: Virtual electrodes in cardiac tissue: A common mechanism for anodal and cathodal stimulation. Biophys J 69:2195–2210, 1995.
2. Efimov IR, Cheng YN, Van Wagoner DR, et al: Virtual electrode-induced phase singularity: A basic mechanism of defibrillation failure. Circ Res 82:918–925, 1998.
3. Knisley SB, Trayanova NA, Aguel F: Roles of electric field and fiber structure in cardiac electric stimulation. Biophys J 77:1404–1417, 1999.
4. Efimov IR, Cheng YN, Yamanouchi Y, Tchou PJ: Direct evidence of the role of virtual electrode-induced phase singularity in success and failure of defibrillation. J Cardiovasc Electrophysiol 11:861–868, 2000.
5. Efimov IR, Aguel F, Cheng YN, et al: Virtual electrode polarization in the far field: Implications for external defibrillation. Am J Physiol 279:H1055–H1070, 2000.
6. Roth BJ: Strength-interval curves for cardiac tissue predicted using the bidomain model. J Cardiovasc Electrophysiol 7:722–737, 1996.
7. Roth BJ: Nonsustained reentry following successive stimulation of cardiac tissue through a unipolar electrode. J Cardiovasc Electrophysiol 8:768–778, 1997.
8. Skouibine K, Trayanova NA, Moore P: Success and failure of the defibrillation shock: Insights from a simulation study. J Cardiovasc Electrophysiol 11:785–796, 2000.
9. Lindblom AE, Roth BJ, Trayanova NA: Role of virtual electrodes in arrhythmogenesis: Pinwheel experiment revisited. J Cardiovasc Electrophysiol 11:274–285, 2000.
10. Trayanova NA, Eason J: Shock-induced arrhythmogenesis in the myocardium. Chaos 359:1327–1337, 2002.
11. Eason JC, Trayanova NA: Phase singularities and termination of spiral wave reentry. J Cardiovasc Electrophysiol 13:672–679, 2002.
12. Trayanova NA, Skouibine K, Aguel F: The role of cardiac tissue structure in defibrillation. Chaos 8:221–233, 1998.
13. Fast VG, Cheek ER: Optical mapping of arrhythmias induced by strong electrical shocks in myocyte cultures. Circ Res 90:664–670, 2002.
14. Gray RA, Pertsov A, Jalife J: Spatial and temporal organization during cardiac fibrillation. Nature 392:675–678, 1998.
15. Paniflov A, Hogeweg P: Spiral break-up in a modified fitzhugh-nagumo model. Phys Lett A 176:295–299, 1993.
16. Fenton FH, Karma A: Vortex dynamics in three-dimensional continuous myocardium with fiber rotation: Filament instability and fibrillation. Chaos 8:20–47, 1998.
17. Garfinkel A, Chen PS, Walter DO, et al: Quasiperiodicity and chaos in cardiac fibrillation. J Clin Invest 99:305–314, 1997.
18. Qu Z, Kil J, Xie F, et al: Scroll wave dynamics in a three-dimensional cardiac tissue model: Roles of restitution, thickness, and fiber rotation. Biophys J 78:2761–2775, 2000.
19. Baxter W, Mironov S, Zaitsev A, et al: Visualizing excitation waves inside cardiac muscle using transillumination. Biophys J 80:516–530, 2001.
20. Hooks DA, LeGrice IJ, Harvey JD, Smaill BH: Intramural multisite recording of transmembrane potential in the heart. Biophys J 81:2671–2680, 2001.
21. Fenton FH, Cherry EM, Hastings HM, Evans SJ: Multiple mechanisms of spiral wave breakup in a model of cardiac electrical activity. Chaos 12:852–892, 2002.
22. Trayanova NA: Concepts of defibrillation. Phil Trans Roy Soc Lond A 359:1327–1337, 2001.
23. Vetter FJ, McCulloch AD: Three-dimensional analysis of regional cardiac function: A model of rabbit ventricular anatomy. Prog

Biophys Mol Biol 69:157–183, 1998.
24. Trayanova NA, Eason JC, Aguel F: Computer simulations of cardiac defibrillation: A look inside the heart. Comput Visual Sci 4:259–270, 2002.
25. Kwaku KF, Dillon SM: Shock-induced depolarization of refractory myocardium prevents wave-front propagation in defibrillation. Circ Res 79:957–973, 1996.
26. Skouibine K, Trayanova NA, Moore PK: A numerically efficient model for simulation of defibrillation in an active bidomain sheet of myocardium. Math Biosci 166:85–100, 2000.
27. DeBruin KA, Krassowska W: Electroporation and shock-induced transmembrane potential in a cardiac fiber during fibrillation strength shocks. Ann Biomed Eng 26:584–596, 1998.
28. DeBruin KA, Krassowska W: Modeling electroporation in a single cell: I. Effects of field strength and rest potential. Biophys J 77:1213–1224, 1999.
29. Vigmond E, Aguel F, Trayanova NA: Computational techniques for solving the bidomain equations in three dimensions. IEEE Trans Biomed Eng 49:1260–1270, 2001.
30. Rodriguez B, Campbell C, Li L, et al: Effect of electrode polarity on shock-induced arrhythmogenesis [abstract]. PACE 26:978, 2003.
31. Roth BJ, Wikswo Jr JP: The effect of externally applied electrical fields on myocardial tissue. Proc IEEE 84:379–391, 1996.
32. Skouibine K, Trayanova NA, Moore PK: Anode/cathode make and break phenomena in a model of defibrillation. IEEE Trans Biomed Eng 46:769–777, 1999.
33. Anderson C, Trayanova NA, Skouibine K: Termination of spiral waves with biphasic shocks: The role of virtual electrode polarization. J Cardiovasc Electrophysiol 11:1386–1396, 2000.
34. Henriquez CS, Muzikant AL, Smoak C: Anisotropy, fiber curvature, and bath loading effects on activation in thin and thick slabs of cardiac tissue: Simulation in a three-dimensional bidomain model. J Cardiovasc Electrophysiol 7:424–445, 1996.
35. Aguel F, Eason J, Trayanova NA: Advances in modeling cardiac defibrillation. Int J Bifurcat Chaos 13, 2002.
36. Efimov IR, Gray RA, Roth BJ: Virtual electrodes and deexcitation: New insights into fibrillation induction and defibrillation. J Cardiovasc Electophysiol 11:339–353, 2000.
37. Bourn DW, Trayanova NA, Gray RA: Shock-induced arrhythmogenesis and isoelectric window. Pacing Clin Electrophysiol 25(pt 2):604, 2002.
38. Roth BJ: A mathematical model of make and break electrical stimulation of cardiac tissue by a unipolar anode or cathode. IEEE Trans Biomed Eng 42:1174–1184, 1995.
39. Wang NC, Lee MH, Ohara TO, et al: Optical mapping of ventricular defibrillation in isolated swine right ventricles: Demonstration of a postshock isoelectric window after near-threshold defibrillation shocks. Circulation 104:227–233, 2002.
40. Karagueuzian HS, Chen PS: Cellular mechanism of reentry induced by a strong electrical stimulus: Implications for fibrillation and defibrillation. Cardiovasc Res 50:251–262, 2001.
41. Eason J, Hillebrenner M, Campbell C, Trayanova NA: Assessing shock efficacy as a function of arrhythmia complexity in a slab of the canine heart. In Proceedings of the 24th Annual IEEE EMBS Conference [CD-ROM], 2002.
42. Panfilov AV, Rudenko AN: Two regimes of the scroll ring drift in the three-dimensional active media. Physica D 28:215–218, 1987.
43. Panfilov AV, Holden AV: Computer simulation of re-entry sources in myocardium in two and three dimensions. J Theor Biol 161:271–285, 1993.
44. Winfree AT: Rotors, fibrillation, and dimensionality. In Panfilov AV, Holden AV (eds): Computational Biology of the Heart. Chichester, UK, Wiley, 1997, pp 101–135.
45. Winfree AT: Electrical turbulence in three-dimensional heart muscle. Science 266:1003–1006, 1994.
46. Zipes DP, Fisher J, King RM, et al: Termination of ventricular fibrillation in dogs by depolarizing a critical amount of myocardium. Am J Cardiol 36:37–44, 1975.
47. Schalij MJ, Lammers WJ, Rensma PL, Allessie MA: Anisotropic conduction and reentry in perfused epicardium of rabbit left ventricles. Am J Physiol 263:H1466–H1478, 1992.
48. Dillon SM, Allessie MA, Ursell PC, Wit AL: Influence of anisotropic tissue structure on reentrant circuits in the epicardial border zone of subacute canine infarcts. Circ Res 63:182–206, 1988.
49. Gray RA, Jalife J, Panfilov A, et al: Mechanisms of cardiac fibrillation. Science 270:1222–1225, 1995.
50. Chen PS, Wolf PD, Dixon EG, et al: Mechanism of ventricular vulnerability to single premature stimuli on open chest dogs. Circ Res 62:1191–1209, 1988.

第六部分 心脏电活动的中枢调节

第 32 章

β 和 α 肾上腺素受体调节心脏节律的分子和细胞基础

Susan F. Steinberg, Richard B. Robinson, Michael R. Rosen

本章目录

- 心肌 β 肾上腺素受体 …………………… 285
- β 肾上腺素受体亚型信号转导的局域化 …………………… 286
- α₁ 肾上腺素受体的信号转导机制 …… 287
- β 肾上腺素受体激动对心脏动作电位和离子通道的影响 …………………… 288
- α 肾上腺素受体激动对心脏动作电位和离子通道的影响 …………………… 289
- β 和 α 肾上腺素受体在临床心律失常中的作用 …………………… 290
- 致谢 …………………… 290

儿茶酚胺可以引起心脏收缩中电和机械力的急剧变化，也可以引起心室结构、电和机械的慢性重构。关于肾上腺素受体（adrenergic receptor，AR）的调节、信号转导途径和调控离子通道等都涉及细胞生物学和分子遗传学。最近的一些研究改变了我们以往对心脏 β-和 α-AR 效应的分子和细胞机制的认识，本章简要综述这些最新研究进展。

一、心肌 β 肾上腺素受体

已有三种 β-AR 被克隆，它们都可以不同程度地被神经递质去甲肾上腺素和肾上腺分泌的激素肾上腺素激动[1,2]。人心脏组织（如同大多数哺乳动物）以 $β_1$-AR 亚型为主，约占总 β-AR 的 75%~85%。在正常生理状态，儿茶酚胺引起的正性变力、变时和舒张 (lusitropic) 效应主要由 $β_1$-AR 介导。$β_1$-AR 与刺激型三磷酸鸟苷酸（guanosine triphospahate，GTP）调节蛋白（Gs）耦联，激活腺苷酸环化酶（adenylyl caylase，AC），进而使环磷酸腺苷（cyclic adenosine monophosphate，cAMP）蓄积和 cAMP-依赖蛋白激酶（protein kinase A，PKA）激活，激活的 PKA 可使重要靶蛋白磷酸化，其中包括 L-型钙通道、受磷蛋白和肌钙蛋白 I（troponin I）。然而，心肌组织也表达 $β_2$-AR。$β_2$-AR 在介导心脏收缩中也起重要作用，特别是心衰和老年心脏由于 $β_1$-AR 选择性下调，$β_2$-AR 则在介导正性变力效应中发挥作用，因而此时 $β_2$-AR 的作用变得更重要了[3]。$β_3$-AR（在脂肪组织和消化道中具有调节生理功能作用，因而成为了减肥和抗糖尿病药物的靶受体）也在人心肌组织有表达。与 $β_1$-AR 和 $β_2$-AR 作用相反，$β_3$-AR 能抑制心脏收缩[4]。

β-AR 是典型的 G 蛋白耦联受体（G protein-coupled receptors，GPCRs）。$β_1$-AR 效应主要是通过 G_s 介导的。相反，$β_2$-AR 可以耦联几种 G 蛋白（G_s、G_i、G_{12}）和多种信号分子，比如 AC、丝裂原活化蛋白激酶（mitogen-activated protein kinase，MAPK）系统中的细胞外信号调节蛋白激酶（extracellualr signal-regulated protein kinase，ERK）和 p38-MAPK，磷酸激醇 3-激酶（phosphoinositide 3-kinase，PI3-K）以及蛋白激酶（protein kinase B/AKT）。从下面总结的 $β_2$-AR 激活 ERK 途径的多种机制可以看出 $β_2$-AR 信号途径的多面性和复杂性（引自 Luffrell 及其同事的综述[5]）。

1. $β_2$-AR 通过百日咳毒素（pertussis toxin，PTX）敏感 G 蛋白激活 ERK。PTX 敏感 G 蛋白激活

导致 PKA 依赖的 $β_2$-AR 磷酸化。$β_2$-AR 磷酸化后与 G_s（和 AC）的耦联能力降低，而与 G_i 耦联能力增强。G_i 是 βγ 亚单位二聚体的主要来源，βγ 亚单位激活 Src 激酶，进而启动 ERK 信号途径的激活[6]。

2. $β_2$-AR 通过 G 蛋白的 βγ 亚单位或 Src 激酶，转位激活表皮生长因子受体（epithelial growth factor receptors，EGFRs）来激活 ERK 途径。最近的研究证实 EGFRs、激活状态 $β_2$-AR 和催化激活的 Scr 三者稳定而直接结合在一起。这种多信号蛋白复合体也可能还含有其他接头蛋白（adapter）/信号蛋白，它们与胞浆内的信号分子相互作用，激活 ERK（可能也激活其他分子，如 p38-MAPK 和 AKT[7]）。

3. 激动剂与 β-AR 结合后，被 G 蛋白耦联受体激酶（G protein-coupled receptor kinase，GRK）磷酸化。β-AR 的磷酸化作为部分机制，终止了 cAMP 途径的信号转导。$β_2$-AR 的 GRK-依赖的磷酸化增加了 $β_2$-AR 对 β-arrestin 的亲和性，β-arrestin 从空间上阻碍了 β-AR 与 G_s 之间的相互作用。β-AR-β-arrestin 复合物为 Src 的停泊和其他信号分子的聚集提供了平台；β-AR-β-arrestin-Src 复合体被聚集到 clathrin-包被的小体（vesicle），在小体内，对 ERK 途径启动"第二次信号传递（second-wave）"。

4. 直接激活（cAMP-非依赖）Src 家族的酪氨酸激酶。β-AR 与 G_s 耦联，激活的 $Gα_s$ 亚单位[8]和 PKA 依赖的 Src 的 S^{17} 都可以进一步启动 ERK 途径的激活；最近的研究证实，Rap1 和 B-Raf 途径与 PKA-Src-ERK 激活途径有关[9]。

5. 当 $β_2$-AR 处在被激动状态时，$β_2$-AR C 末端的酪氨酸（Y^{350}）磷酸化会产生一个 SH2-结合域，SH2 可以聚集 PI3-K 的 p85 调节亚单位和 Src[10]。

值得提到的是，这些激活 ERK 的不同途径都是在不同的表达系统和表达 $β_2$-AR 的未分化细胞株中研究发现的。由于 $β_2$-AR 信号转导受很多因素的影响，在不同的细胞之间有很大差异，因此这些发现也只是为心脏 β-AR 的信号转导描绘了很好的框架图，儿茶酚胺在心脏的作用仍有很大的研究空间。

二、β 肾上腺素受体亚型信号转导的局域化

心肌细胞 $β_1$-AR 介导的 cAMP 蓄积效应与收缩力的关系非常密切。相反，许多研究表明，$β_2$-AR 介导的 cAMP 蓄积与正性变力效应关系就很弱。通过比较前列腺素 E_2（prostaglandin E_2，PGE_2）和异丙肾上腺素的作用，提示在心肌细胞中，cAMP/PKA 可被局限在某些区域中，这种局域化效应在不同的 GPCRs 表现不同。PGE_2 和异丙肾上腺素都可以增加细胞中 cAMP 水平，但是只有异丙肾上腺素可以激活 PKA，增强心脏收缩，而 PGE2 却不能[11]。β-AR 的信号空间调节概念的进一步证据来自于 Fischmeister 实验室的研究，其研究结果表明 β-AR 可引起邻近细胞膜的 cAMP 局部升高，进而导致邻近的 L-型钙通道激活[12]。这些结果为阐述传统的 GPCR 信号分子"随机碰撞"（random collision）模式不能解释的组织特异的信号空间和时间特征的机制提供了最初的线索。"随机碰撞"模式是指受体后的信号产生于游离的信号蛋白分子在细胞内的随机相互作用。

心肌细胞 $β_2$-AR 信号转导局域化概念源自于三个意外发现，这些发现不能被 GPCRs 信号转导的随机碰撞模式所解释。

1. 在成年大鼠心室肌细胞，$β_1$-AR 可以引起高于 ～20 倍的 cAMP 蓄积。$β_1$-AR 依赖的 cAMP 增加是快速的，在细胞内播散的。相反，$β_2$-AR（$β_2$-AR 和 $β_1$-AR 共同表达于成年心肌细胞表面）介导的正性变力效应，仅伴有轻微的 cAMP 蓄积增加[13]。在成年大鼠心肌细胞，$β_2$-AR 介导正性变力效应的机制（伴有很少或不伴有 cAMP 升高）是有争议的。肖及其同事[13a]提出了一个有序模式，即 $β_2$-AR 先耦联 G_s，随后与 G_i 耦联，G_i 的磷酸化使得 cAMP 限制在浆膜的某个局部。然而，也有证据表明 $β_2$-AR 有 cAMP 非依赖途径。信号使细胞内碱化，增加肌小节收缩蛋白的钙敏感性，进而增强心肌收缩力[2,13,14]。目前仍有几个实验室在致力于研究成年大鼠心肌细胞 $β_2$-AR 介导的 cAMP 蓄积作用和其他因子作用的异同。然而，更重要的问题是成年动物心脏上 $β_1$-和 $β_2$-AR 信号转导的异同（$β_1$-和 $β_2$-AR 共表达在一个心肌细胞上），这些问题目前仍不清楚。

2. $β_1$-和 $β_2$-AR 在大鼠乳鼠心肌细胞上都可以引起 cAMP 蓄积，根据这一结果，我们预期在培养的大鼠乳鼠心肌细胞上 $β_1$-和 $β_2$-AR 具有相似的 cAMP 依赖性信号转导途径。但是，我们早期的研究表明，大鼠乳鼠心室肌细胞 $β_1$-AR 介导的 cAMP 增加可以被乙酰胆碱 M 受体激动剂 carbachol 抑制，这种现象传统称之为增强拮抗（accentuated antagonism），而 $β_2$-AR 介导的 cAMP 增加则不能被 carbacol 抑制[15]。但用传统的受体和信号分子在细胞内均匀游离漂浮的模式不能解释这种受体对 β-AR 不同亚型的不同作用，这些

结果提示可能有更高层次的空间调节。

3. Ostrom 及其同事[16]报告了在心肌细胞过表达Ⅵ型腺苷酸环化酶可选择性增加 β-AR 激动剂和 forskolin 引起的 cAMP 蓄积增加，而对 PGE_2 通过其受体引起的 cAMP 蓄积无影响。同样，受体、G 蛋白和效应因子在胞浆自由移动的随机碰撞理论也不能解释这一现象。相反，这些研究结果支持了膜亚区域局域化理论。例如脂筏（lipid raft）或者小凹（cavedae）揭示了心肌细胞 β-AR 更高层次的空间调节[13]。

脂筏是哺乳动物细胞特有的现象。脂筏很小，分布在整个细胞表面，也可以是小凹。小凹由细胞内某些特殊蛋白构成，如小凹蛋白（caveolin）[一个多成员家族，至少有三个不同免疫特性 21～24KD 的同源体（isoform）]。在小凹蛋白和小凹缺失的细胞上表达小凹蛋白-1 和小凹蛋白-3 可以形成异源二聚体，这个异源二聚体形成具有小凹拓扑特征的表面小凹（pifs）[17]。信号蛋白通过以下方式定位于脂筏：（1）脂质修饰的信号蛋白分子和"流体状态"（liquid-ordered）的脂筏之间的脂质－脂质相互作用；（2）在小凹蛋白-1 或小凹蛋白-3 胞膜内侧区［称之为"小凹蛋白锚定域"（caveolin-scaffolding domain）和小凹蛋白-结合域（caveolin-binding motif）］，与结构模式为 xΦxxxxxΦ 或者 ΦxxxxΦxxΦ 区域，相互作用 Φ 指芳香族氨基酸位点。许多信号分子（Gα 亚单位和 AC 的催化亚单位、GRK2、PKA 等）都有这种特性[13]。

另一方面，小凹蛋白作为"锚钉（scaffold）"预组装成膜结合的寡聚复合物，促进高效、快速传递信号。心肌细胞对交感神经的反应速度是毫秒级的，但是 β-AR 对 AC 的调节是缓慢的，因为 AC 的表达量有限，β-AR 靠 AC 表达增加来传递交感神经的调节是不可能的。因此小凹蛋白的这一功能对交感神经系统调节心肌细胞收缩是非常重要的。此外，这些信号酶激酶的激活与抑制在一个循环完成以后，信号分子与小凹蛋白的相互作用可使 Gα 亚单位返回到二磷酸鸟苷酸的失活状态，直到下一个刺激再发生，这个循环又重新开始。

最近的研究显示多种 GPCRs，或以稳定状态，或以配体介导的激活状态存在于小凹中，可参阅 Steinberg 和 Brufon[13]、Razani 及其合作者[17]的综述。有几项研究证实在异源表达系统和心肌细胞，β-AR 存在于小凹蛋白丰富的小囊（vesicles）中[16,18,19]。我们实验室的研究[18]证实了在培养的大鼠乳鼠心肌细胞 $β_1$-和 $β_2$-AR 的调节是有差别的，后又被其他实验室证实[16,19]。从心肌细胞小凹组分中分离出了 $β_2$-AR；$β_2$-AR 激动后就离开小凹（推测是 $β_2$-AR 瞬时存在于 clathrin 包被的小囊）。相反，在大鼠乳鼠心肌细胞的小凹中很少检测到 $β_1$-AR，也检测不到 $β_1$-AR 激动后的转运。这些研究表明，$β_1$-和 $β_2$-AR 定位是有区域特异性的（在小凹中含有大量 $β_2$-AR 和极少量 $β_1$-AR，而在剩余的浆膜部分，含有大量 $β_1$-AR 而没有 $β_2$-AR）。因为 AC 富集于心肌细胞膜的小凹，这一结果可以解释长期以来观察到的 $β_2$-AR 耦联 AC 比 $β_1$-AR 更高效。

我们在小凹中检测到了 β-AR 信号转导的下游分子（包括 Gα 亚单位、AC、L-型钙通道 α 单位、PKA 的 RII 亚基和催化亚单位），支持了小凹的功能是信号转导的核心平台这一概念。$β_2$-AR 和与它结合的信号分子定位于小凹，至少从理论上解释了 $β_2$-AR 的信号转导在心肌细胞和未分化细胞株的差别。小凹大量存在于分化好的细胞（如心肌细胞），而在相对增殖较快的细胞株，小凹蛋白表达水平则比较低，在膜上小凹形成的也比较少。

有研究显示小凹蛋白-3 在心力衰竭的心脏上有表达，且受 β-AR 信号调节，这一重要发现提示在小凹蛋白-3 和 β-AR 信号之间存在调节。此外，在心衰心脏，小凹蛋白-3 的表达或许改变了心衰时自主神经对心脏收缩的调节，影响了心衰的自然病程。对不表达小凹蛋白-3 小鼠心脏结构和功能的研究支持了这一理论[20,21]。

三、$α_1$ 肾上腺素受体的信号转导机制

儿茶酚胺作用于 $α_1$-AR，引起的短期效应是调节心率、心律和心肌细胞收缩力；而长期效应引起的是一系列心肌肥厚的标志性表型和分子改变[22,23]。心肌细胞 $α_1$-AR 的信号转导途径及其对肥厚信号转导途径的作用已经被几个实验室证实。总而言之，对 $α_1$-AR 介导的动作电位和收缩的生物化学和离子机制的研究进展比较慢，至少部分原因是由于 $α_1$-AR 介导的调控作用及其信号转导途径比较复杂。$α_1$-AR 介导的收缩功能随动物的种属和年龄不同而不同，甚至因实验条件不同（如细胞外钙浓度、刺激频率）而不同。关于 $α_1$-AR 对心脏收缩的调节作用，已经明确 $α_1$-AR 激动 15～20 分钟后收缩力稳定增加，特别是在大鼠的肌小梁。有研究显示，$α_1$-AR

介导的心肌细胞收缩呈现复杂的三时相调节，在第一时相收缩幅度短暂迅速增加，在第二时相瞬时减弱，第三时相则持续增高。而人们往往忽略了α_1-AR调节的早期时相的机制。

在小鼠心脏，α_1-AR介导的收缩效应不同，在第一时相介导瞬时的收缩力增加，继而出现短暂的、明确的收缩力减弱，而在第三时相虽然收缩力增加，但是达不到第一时相水平[24]。这一结果与目前已公认的α_1-AR对心脏收缩的调节作用不同，原因在于以往的结果来自于大鼠，而大鼠心脏的α_1-AR表达量较高，α_1-AR介导磷脂酶C激活和进而引起收缩/肥厚反应。小鼠心脏的α_1-AR表达水平比较低，大鼠的研究结果可能并不适于小鼠和人，因此，小鼠和人的心脏α_1-AR的功能和分子机制尚需进一步研究[25]。

α_1-AR调控心脏起搏细胞的冲动和心肌细胞的收缩频率。α_1-AR促进乳鼠心脏起博细胞电脉冲的产生，而抑制成鼠心脏起搏细胞的电脉冲[26,27]。成年心脏的α_1-AR依赖的负性变时效应是由百日咳毒素敏感的G蛋白调节，而乳鼠的正性变时效应则不是由α_1-AR调节。早期的证据表明，α_1-AR信号转导途径与上游脱离，至少在G蛋白水平分离[26]。

根据α_1-AR对选择性配体的亲和性和其下游信号转导途径的不同，α_1-AR被分为三种亚型。最早的药理学分类，α_1-AR分为两种亚型。根据受体对WB-4101的高亲和性和对烷化剂chloroethylclonidine（CEC）的不敏感性，α_1-AR分为α_{1A}亚型和α_{1B}亚型，而α_{1B}则对WB-4101低亲和性，可被CEC完全失活，并启动磷酸肌醇水解。这也是细胞内钙池动员的机制[28]。这种分类源于对培养的乳鼠心肌细胞α_1-AR信号转导的研究。在乳鼠心肌细胞，去甲肾上腺素引起磷酸肌醇水解是由WB-4101敏感（CEC-不敏感）的α_1-AR介导的，而CEC-敏感的α_{1B}-AR不介导磷酸肌醇水解（尽管放射配基结合试验表明CEC-敏感的α_{1B}-AR占总α_1-AR的25%）[28]。

继而，α_1-AR三种亚型的基因被克隆，在不同表达体系中对其药理学特性进行了研究。最初的命名和分类有些混乱，由于使用了不恰当的命名法，造成在表达系统中的α_1-AR的特性和按药理学特性定义的自然组织中的α_1-AR亚型的特性不一致甚至矛盾，并且人们也意识到α_1-AR对许多配体的亚型选择性是很有限的，并不像人们原来所认为的那样。最近对α_1-AR亚型的再分类，明确定义克隆的α_{1C}-AR就是药理学的α_{1A}-AR（因此也称之为$\alpha_{1A/C}$-AR），克隆的α_{1b}-AR就是药理学的α_{1B}-AR，第三个克隆受体最初命名为α_{1a}-AR，再分类时定义为α_{1D}-AR。

啮齿动物的心肌细胞有α_1-AR三种亚型的mRNA表达，为研究心脏α_1-AR亚型的功能提供了很好的模型[29]。最初的研究应用了药理学手段，表明α_{1A}亚型（低浓度WB-4101可抑制，不与百日咳毒素敏感G蛋白耦联）在动物新生期介导心脏正性变时效应[27]。药理学上的α_{1B}亚型可以被CEC抑制（与百日咳毒素敏感G蛋白耦联），在成年心肌细胞α_{1B}介导负性变时效应。应用相同的药理学方法，Gambassi和他的同事[30]揭示了在成年大鼠心脏相反的变力效应：WB-4101-敏感的α_{1A}亚型增加钙瞬时振幅和细胞内pH值，导致正性变力效应，而CEC敏感的α_{1B}亚型降低钙瞬时振幅和细胞内pH值，引起负性变力效应。然而，这种在大鼠心脏的α_{1A}和α_{1B}之间的功能性拮抗作用，在小鼠心脏则并非如此。在小鼠心脏收缩的第三时相，α_{1A}-AR和α_{1B}-AR都介导负性变力效应，而且效应相加[24]。总之，这些研究揭示了α_1-AR的信号转导和效应的高度可塑性。

四、β肾上腺素受体激动对心脏动作电位和离子通道的影响

在成年和新生犬心脏的浦肯野纤维，高浓度β_2-AR激动剂salbutamol对心脏动作电位的特性和自律性的作用与β_1和β_2非选择性激动剂异丙肾上腺素的作用相似[31]。然而，异丙肾上腺素和salbutamol所引起的跨膜电位的变化都可以被β_1-AR拮抗剂CGP20712A所拮抗，而不能被β_2-AR拮抗剂ICI118551所拮抗。这些结果提示在成年和新生犬的心脏浦肯野纤维，β-AR调节的跨膜电位和自律性是由β_1-AR介导的。

但是，羊浦肯野纤维则与犬浦肯野纤维截然不同[32]。在羊浦肯野纤维，异丙肾上腺素引起动作电位的时程缩短，而不是起搏电流的增加，而且这一作用主要是β_2-AR介导的。β_2-AR在兔浦肯野纤维、乳头肌和窦房结也介导缩短动作电位效应[33]。

在羊的心室肌[34]，β_2-AR占总β-AR的30%，参与异丙肾上腺素引起的正性变力效应，与浦肯野纤维相反，不参与心肌动作电位的缩短，提示在这些种属中，心脏的不同类型细胞的β_1-和β_2-AR生物功能可以完全不同（如羊的浦肯野细胞和心肌细胞）。这也

可以解释为什么犬浦肯野纤维上β-AR的作用不同于犬心脏的其他细胞，例如，$β_2$-AR激动时增加犬窦性心率、房室传导速度和心房收缩力，以及缩短心房不应期[35-37]。值得注意的是，$β_2$-AR的这些作用都发生在犬的心室组织。在犬心室，尽管$β_2$-AR占总β-AR的15%～20%[38,39]，但$β_2$-AR不能缩短不应期[37]，仅轻度增加收缩力[35]。因此，如果细胞电生理活动中没有$β_2$-AR的功能性效应，并不意味着没有$β_2$-AR的表达。

由上述结果而产生了两个问题：（1）$β_2$-AR介导的复极在不同发育阶段有无变化；（2）如果有变化，这些变化是否与延迟整流钾电流（I_K）有关？在所有年龄段的犬心外膜，β-AR激动都增加平台期，但仅在成年期β-AR激动可以缩短动作电位时程[40]。平台期幅度增加可以用增加了L-型钙通道的钙电流强度（$I_{Ca,L}$）来解释。此外，在幼年兔心室β-AR也可以增强钙电流，尽管这种作用弱于成年兔。

因为在成年心肌细胞β-AR激动可以增强I_K，特别是I_{Ks}，我们假设心肌细胞复极的年龄差别是由于在幼年期异丙肾上腺素不能引起I_K增加所致[40]。异丙肾上腺素可使成年心肌细胞I_K增强，并在其他标本也证实了这一结果，但是异丙肾上腺素却不能增加幼年心肌细胞的I_K。这种β-AR介导I_k的年龄差异至少可以部分地解释为什么在幼年犬异丙肾上腺素不能介导动作电位缩短。但是，异丙肾上腺素可以使幼年犬心室肌细胞平台期升高和$I_{Ca,L}$增强，说明在幼年期并没有β-AR信号途径的缺失和损害。最近的研究表明β-AR介导I_{Ks}是依赖于信号分子复合物的形成，其复合物由离子通道形成小孔的亚单位C-末端、PKA、蛋白磷脂酶和靶蛋白构成[41]。在新生期，I_K对β-AR刺激不敏感可能与信号途径中的靶分子和局域化功能尚未发育成熟有关。

大多数β-AR调控I_K的单细胞数据来源于成年豚鼠心室肌。在成年豚鼠心室肌，PKA的激活是有明显的电位依赖性的，如接近域值的电压可引起更大的激活效应。在犬心肌细胞则没有这种电压依赖特性。此外，在成年狗和豚鼠的心室肌细胞，I_K的动力学和药理学特性也有不同[45]。Huang及其同事[46]将大鼠心房的延迟整流钾通道表达在蛙卵细胞，观察到非异丙肾上腺素和PKA依赖的钾电流增加。甚至在豚鼠，有人观察到了电压非依赖的和依赖的钾电流增加，是否电压依赖取决于通道被蛋白激酶C（protein kinase C，PKC）还是PKA磷酸化[43]。总之，电压依赖程度是有种属特异性的，可能与在不同组织中离子通道磷酸化的位点不同有关。

五、α肾上腺素受体激动对心脏动作电位和离子通道的影响

α-AR激动对心脏动作电位有不同的影响。最有趣的是$α_1$-AR可使去极化的第四相斜率增加，导致自律性增加；或者使其斜率降低，抑制自律性[27,48]。$α_1$-AR对动作电位调节的研究大多数都是观察的犬浦肯野纤维。$α_1$-AR激动引起自律性增加是$α_1$-AR通过介导磷酸肌醇代谢增强，进而增加细胞内钙离子浓度来实现的[48,49]。这种作用在新生犬心脏表现明显[27,47]，在新生大鼠心室也可以见到此效应[50]。随着犬心脏的生长发育和培养的新生大鼠心肌细胞去除交感神经支配，$α_1$-AR对自律性的作用也由增强变为抑制[27,50]。交感神经末梢释放的神经肽Y（neuropeptide Y）是产生这个变化的原因[51]；自律性降低是由于Na/K泵的激活[52,53]。随后的传导与一种PTX敏感的GTP调节蛋白有关[26]。根据药理学特性的分类，增加自律性的是$α_{1A/D}$受体亚型；抑制自律性的是$α_{1B}$亚型[28]。有趣的是，在窦房结表现出了明显的种属特异性，可参阅Terzic及其同事的综述[54]。

$α_1$-AR激动剂对复极的作用因组织和种属不同而不同。总体来说，在犬浦肯野纤维和犬、大鼠、兔心室肌，$α_1$-AR激动剂的作用是延长复极[33,47,55]。$α_{1A/D}$-AR部分抑制瞬时外向钾电流I_{to}[55,56]和部分阻断延迟整流钾电流[52,57]。然而，在个别的实验中，Na/K泵激活的数量很大，产生的外向电流可能限制了动作电位的延长。在豚鼠心肌，$α_1$-AR激动可缩短动作电位的持续时间[58]，这也许是Na/K泵激活所致。值得注意的是，$α_1$-AR（和β-AR）对Na/K泵的激活作用是随年龄和种属不同而不同的。在不同种属和不同发育阶段，Na/K泵亚单位的表达量各不相同，所有β-AR都是通过Na/K泵的$α_1$亚单位来调节泵的活性的，而$α_1$-AR则是通过$α_2$亚单位，两者更精确的调节还依赖于细胞内钙的水平[59]。

在心肌缺血模型，$α_1$-AR介导正性变时效应，其机制与前面所讲的正常心肌纤维的机制不同，药理学研究提示是$α_{1A}$亚型介导[60]。自律性增强是抑制钾（K^+）传导造成的，可能是通过内向整流钾电流I_{K1}实现的[52]。这一钾电流的变化可能也与动作电位第三

相终末段的延长有关。

六、β和α肾上腺素受体在临床心律失常中的作用

简单而言，我们早已知道β-AR激动可以加速心率和促进房室传导。但是，儿茶酚胺对心脏电生理过程具有多样的效应，其效应的多样性我们无法在本章中全面综述。不过，已有人在其他文章中综述过（Wit and Rosen[62]）。例如，心梗后，β-AR激动不仅增加正常起搏细胞的冲动频率，而且导致异位起搏和去极化后诱导的触发活性，所有这些都是由于β-AR激动导致细胞钙超载所致。

临床检查使我们有机会来研究β-AR介导细胞钙超载与心律失常的关系。对于年轻患者（没有心脏病），儿茶酚胺诱导的和运动引起的心动过速就是典型的例子[63,64]。然而，造成心动过速的原因不是受体本身，而是内质网Ca^{2+}释放通道[65]。已有研究报道了很多钙通道基因点突变，这些患者在儿茶酚胺增高时易发室速[65,66]。至少有部分实验结果提示内质网钙释放通道的高度磷酸化可导致病理性心动过速[76]。

对德国牧羊犬遗传性室速模型的研究提供了有关室性心动过速发生机制的证据。这种血统的德国牧羊犬有心律失常病史和心律失常致死性[68,69]。这种患病犬的心脏上有解剖结构的改变及左室前间壁交感神经分布减少[70]。

心律失常有两种发生机制。一是β-AR在触发室性心动过速中起重要作用。这种犬左室前间壁交感神经刺激信号减少，异丙肾上腺素激动β-AR时产生异常效应——延长动作电位而不是缩短动作电位[71,72]。与正常犬相比，异丙肾上腺素增加延迟整流电流I_{Ks}的作用明显减弱[73]，这就是β-AR延长动作电位的机制。在左室前间壁β-AR密度和AC活性都增加[71,72,74]。心律失常发生机制中是$β_1$-AR而不是$β_2$-AR，通过cAMP依赖途径导致Ca^{2+}信号异常[72,74]。在心室前间壁，由于交感神经分布减少，β-AR激动引起的迟后除极被认为是触发心动过速的原因[71]。此外，与正常德国牧羊犬相比，心动过速牧羊犬有明显的心肌复极透壁传导，这是心律失常的病理基础[71,72]。

心律失常遗传学的临床研究结果对$α_1$-AR的作用不像对β-AR作用那么确定。在1960年代，几项小规模的比较研究显示，在冠心病重症监护病房，非选择性α-AR拮抗剂酚妥拉明有抑制心律失常的作用。然而，这种抑制心律失常的作用是通过阻断α-AR直接引起复极延长，还是药物引起的血流动力学改变所致一直没有明确答案。从那时起，尽管各种缺血致心律失常的动物模型显示α-AR拮抗剂可以减轻心律失常[55-57]，但是还没有明确的证据确证在病人$α_1$-AR拮抗剂可以抑制心律失常。卡维地洛成功地降低了心衰病人的猝死率，是否与直接阻断α-AR有关（同时主要具有β-AR阻滞作用）尚未定论。

$α_1$-AR激动引起心律失常最有说服力的例子是早期报道的德国牧羊犬心律失常猝死模型[68,69]。$α_1$-AR激动剂可以增加先天性心律失常的德国牧羊犬的心肌动作电位时程，增强早后除极和触发活性[78]，这些病理改变是这种动物猝死的原因。除这些证据以及其他实验动物模型的研究发现外，$α_1$-AR激动引起人猝死和心律失常的机制尚不确定。

七、致　谢

在此对Eileen Franey女士在本文书写过程中的关心表示感谢。

（张幼怡　译）

参 考 文 献

1. Steinberg SF: The molecular basis for distinct β-adrenergic receptor subtype actions in cardiomyocytes. Circ Res 85:1101–1111, 1999.
2. Xiao RP: β-Adrenergic signaling in the heart: Dual coupling of the $β_2$-adrenergic receptor to G_s and G_i proteins. Sci STKE 2001:RE15, 2001.
3. Bristow MR, Ginsburg R, Umans V, et al: $β_1$- and $β_2$-adrenergic receptor subpopulations in nonfailing and failing human ventricular myocardium: Coupling of both receptor subtypes to muscle contraction and selective $β_1$-receptor down-regulation in heart failure. Circ Res 59:297–309, 1986.
4. Gauthier C, Leblais V, Kobzik L, et al: The negative inotropic effect of $β_3$-adrenoceptor stimulation is mediated by activation of a nitric oxide synthase pathway in human ventricle. J Clin Invest 102:1377–1384, 1998.
5. Luttrell LM, Daaka Y, Lefkowitz RJ: Regulation of tyrosine kinase cascades by G-protein-coupled receptors. Curr Opin Cell Biol 11:177–183, 1999.
6. Zamah AM, Delahunty M, Luttrell LM, Lefkowitz RJ: Protein kinase A-mediated phosphorylation of the β-adrenergic receptor regulates its coupling to G_s and G_i. Demonstration in a reconstituted system. J Biol Chem 277:31249–31256, 2002.
7. Maudsley S, Pierce KL, Zamah AM, et al: The $β_2$-adrenergic receptor mediates extracellular signal-regulated kinase activation via assembly of a multi-receptor complex with the epidermal growth factor receptor. J Biol Chem 275:9572–9580, 2000.
8. Ma YC, Huang J, Ali S, et al: Src tyrosine kinase is a novel direct effector of G proteins. Cell 102:635–646, 2000.
9. Schmitt JM, Stork PJ: Gα and Gβ σ require distinct Src-dependent pathways to activate Rap1 and Ras. J Biol Chem 277:43024–43032, 2002.
10. Fan G, Shumay E, Malbon CC, Wang H: c-Src tyrosine kinase binds the $β_2$-adrenergic receptor via phospho-Tyr-350, phosphorylates G-

protein-linked receptor kinase 2, and mediates agonist-induced receptor desensitization. J Biol Chem 276:13240–13247, 2001.
11. Buxton ILO, Brunton LL: Compartments of cyclic AMP and protein kinase in mammalian cardiomyocytes. J Biol Chem 258:10233–10239, 1983.
12. Jurevicius J, Fischmeister R: cAMP compartmentation is responsible for a local activation of cardiac Ca^{2+} channels by β-adrenergic agonists. Proc Natl Acad Sci USA 93:295–299, 1996.
13. Steinberg SF, Brunton LL: Compartmentalization of G-protein-mediated signal transduction components in the heart. Ann Rev Pharm Toxicol 41:751–773, 2001.
13a. Xiao RP, Avdonin P, Zhou YY, et al: Coupling of beta2-adrenoceptor to Gi protein and its psychological relevance in murine cardiac myocytes. Circ Res 84:43–52, 1999.
14. Jiang T, Steinberg SF: $β_2$-Adrenergic receptors enhance contractility by stimulating HCO_3—dependent intracellular alkalinization. Am J Physiol 273:H1044–H1047, 1997.
15. Aprigliano O, Rybin VO, Pak E, et al: $β_1$- and $β_2$-adrenergic receptors exhibit differing susceptibility to muscarinic accentuated antagonism. Am J Physiol 272:H2726–H2735, 1997.
16. Ostrom RS, Gregorian C, Drenan RM, et al: Receptor number and caveolar co-localization determine receptor coupling efficiency to adenylyl cyclase. J Biol Chem 276:42063–42069, 2001.
17. Razani B, Woodman SE, Lisanti MP: Caveolae: From cell biology to animal physiology. Pharmacol Rev 54:431–467, 2002.
18. Rybin VO, Xu X, Lisanti MP, Steinberg SF: Differential targeting of β-adrenergic receptor subtypes and adenylyl cyclase to cardiomyocyte caveolae: A mechanism to functionally regulate the cAMP signaling pathway. J Biol Chem 275:41447–41457, 2000.
19. Xiang Y, Rybin VO, Steinberg SF, Kobilka B: Caveolar localization dictates physiologic signaling of $β_2$-adrenoceptors in neonatal cardiac myocytes. J Biol Chem 277:34280–34286, 2002.
20. Yamamoto M, Okumura S, Oka N, et al: Downregulation of caveolin expression by cAMP signal. Life Sci 64:1349–1357, 1999.
21. Hare JM, Lofthouse RA, Juang GJ, et al: Contribution of caveolin protein abundance to augmented nitric oxide signaling in conscious dogs with pacing-induced heart failure. Circ Res 86:1085–1092, 2000.
22. Piascik MT, Perez DM: $α_1$-adrenergic receptors: new insights and directions. J Pharmacol Exp Ther 298:403–410, 2001.
23. Graham RM, Perez DM, Hwa J, Piascik MT: $α_1$-adrenergic receptor subtypes: Molecular structure, function and signaling. Circ Res 78:737–749, 1996.
24. McCloskey DT, Rokosh DG, O'Connell TD, et al: $α_1$-Adrenoceptor subtypes mediate negative inotropy in myocardium from $α_{1A/c}$-knockout and wild type mice. J Mol Cell Cardiol 34:1007–1017, 2002.
25. Michelotti GA, Price DT, Schwinn DA: $α_1$-adrenergic receptor regulation: Basic science and clinical implications. Pharmacol Ther 88:281–309, 2000.
26. Steinberg SF, Drugge ED, Bilezikian JP, Robinson RB: Innervated cardiac myocytes acquire a pertussis toxin specific regulatory protein functionally linked to the $α_1$-receptor. Science 230:186–188, 1985.
27. del Balzo U, Rosen MR, Malfatto G, et al: Specific $α_1$-adrenergic receptor subtypes modulate catecholamine induced increases and decreases in ventricular automaticity. Circ Res 67:1535–1551, 1990.
28. Minneman KP: $α_1$-adrenergic receptor subtypes, inositol phosphates, and sources of cell Ca^{2+}. Pharm Rev 40:87–119, 1998.
29. Rokosh DG, Stewart AFR, Chang KC, et al: $α_1$-adrenergic receptor subtype mRNAs are differentially regulated by $α_1$-adrenergic and other hypertrophic stimuli in cardiac myocytes in culture and in vivo; repression of $α_{1B}$ and $α_{1D}$ but induction of $α_{1C}$. J Biol Chem 271:5839–5843, 1996.
30. Gambassi G, Spurgeon HA, Ziman BD, et al: Opposing effects of $α_1$-adrenergic receptor subtypes on Ca^{2+} and pH homeostasis in rat cardiac myocytes. Am J Physiol 274:H1152–H1162, 1998.
31. Charpentier F, Rosen MR: β-adrenergic regulation of action potentials and automaticity in young and adult canine Purkinje fibers. Am J Physiol 266 (Heart Circ Physiol 35):H2310–H2319, 1994.
32. Cerbai E, Masini I, Mugelli A: Electrophysiological characterization of cardiac $β_2$-adrenoceptors in sheep Purkinje fibers. J Mol Cell Cardiol 22:859–870, 1990.
33. Dukes ID, Vaughan-Williams EM: Effects of selective $α_1$-, $α_2$-, $β_1$- and $β_2$-adrenoceptor stimulation on potentials and contractions in the rabbit heart. J Physiol Lond 355:523–546, 1984.
34. Borea PA, Amerini S, Masini I, et al: $β_1$- and $β_2$-adrenoceptor in sheep cardiac ventricular muscle. J Mol Cell Cardiol 24:753–764, 1992.
35. Akahane K, Furukawa Y, Ogiwara Y, et al: $β_2$-adrenoceptor-mediated effects on sinus rate and atrial and ventricular contractility on isolated, blood-perfused dog heart preparations. J Pharmacol Exp Ther 248:1276–1282, 1989.
36. Motomura S, Hashimoto K: Beta$_2$-adrenoceptor-mediated positive dromotropic effects on atrioventricular node of dogs. Am J Physiol 262 (Heart Circ Physiol 31):H123–H129, 1992.
37. Takei M, Furukawa Y, Narita M, et al: Cardiac electrical responses to catecholamines are differentially mediated by $β_2$-adrenoceptors in anesthetized dogs. Eur J Pharmacol 219:15–21, 1992.
38. Manalan AS, Besch HR, Watanabe AM: Characterization of [^{3}H] (±) Carazolol binding to β-adrenergic receptors. Application to study of β-adrenergic receptor subtypes in canine ventricular myocardium and lung. Circ Res 49:326–336, 1981.
39. Muntz KH: Autoradiographic characterization of β-adrenergic receptor subtype in the canine conduction system. Circ Res 1:51–57, 1992.
40. Charpentier F, Liu Q-Y, Rosen MR, Robinson RB: Age-related differences in β-adrenergic regulation of repolarization in canine epicardial myocytes. Am J Physiol 271:H1174–H1181, 1996.
41. Osaka T, Joyner RW: Developmental changes in the β-adrenergic modulation of calcium currents in rabbit ventricular cells. Circ Res 70:104–115, 1992.
42. Bennett PB, Begenisich TB: Catecholamines modulate the delayed rectifying potassium current (I_K) in guinea pig ventricular myocytes. Pflugers Arch 410:217–219, 1987.
43. Walsh KB, Kass RS: Distinct voltage-dependent regulation of a heart-delayed I_K by protein kinases A and C. Am J Physiol 261(Cell Physiol 30):C1081–C1090, 1991.
44. Marx SO, Kurokawa J, Reiken S, et al: Requirement of a macromolecular signaling complex for β-adrenergic receptor modulation of the KCNQ1-KCNE1 potassium channel. Science 295(5554):496–499, 2002.
45. Gintant G: Two components of delayed rectifier current in canine atrium and ventricle. Circ Res 78:26–37, 1996.
46. Huang X-Y, Morielli AD, Peralta EG: Molecular basis of cardiac potassium channel stimulation by protein kinase A. Proc Natl Acad Sci USA 91:624–628, 1994.
47. Rosen MR, Hordof AJ, Ilvento J, Danilo P: Effects of adrenergic amines on electrophysiologic properties and automaticity of neonatal and adult canine cardiac Purkinje fibers. Circ Res 40:390–400, 1977.
48. Molina-Viamonte V, Steinberg SF, Chow YK, et al: Phospholipase C modulates automaticity of canine cardiac Purkinje fibers. J Pharmacol Exp Ther 252:886–893, 1990.
49. Steinberg SF, Kaplan LM, Inouye T, et al: $α_1$-adrenergic stimulation of 1,4,5-inositol triphosphate formation in ventricular myocytes. J Pharmacol Exp Ther 250:1141–1148, 1989.
50. Drugge E, Rosen MR, Robinson R: Neuronal regulation of the development of the α adrenergic chronotropic response in the rat heart. Circ Res 57:415–423, 1985.
51. Sun LS, Ursell PC, Robinson RB: Chronic exposure to neuropeptide Y determines cardiac $α_1$-adrenergic responsiveness. Am J Physiol 261:H969–H973, 1991.
52. Shah A, Cohen IS, Rosen MR: Stimulation of cardiac α receptors increases Na/K pump current and decreases g_K via a pertussis toxin-sensitive pathway. Biophys J 54:219–225, 1988.
53. Zaza A, Kline R, Rosen M: Effects of α-adrenergic stimulation on intracellular sodium activity and automaticity in canine Purkinje fibers. Circ Res 66:416–426, 1990.
54. Terzic A, Puceat M, Vassort G, Vogel SM: Cardiac $α_1$-adrenoceptors: An overview. Pharmacol Rev 45(2):147–175, 1993.
55. Apkon M, Nerbonne JM: $α_1$-Adrenergic agonists selectively suppress voltage-dependent K$^+$ current in rat ventricular myocytes. Proc Natl Acad Sci USA 85(22):8756–8760, 1988.
56. Giles WR, Imaizumi Y: Comparison of potassium currents in rabbit atrial and ventricular cells. J Physiol 405:123–145, 1988.
57. Lee JH, Rosen MR: $α_1$-Adrenergic receptor modulation of repolarization in canine Purkinje fibers. J Cardiovasc Electrophysiol 5:232–240, 1994.
58. Dirksen RT, Sheu SS: Modulation of ventricular action potential by $α_1$-adrenoceptors and protein kinase C. Am J Physiol 258:H907–H911, 1990.
59. Mathias RT, Cohen IS, Gao J, Wang Y: Isoform-specific regulation

of the Na(+)-K(+) pump in heart. News Physiol Sci 15:176–180, 2000.
60. Anyukhovsky EP, Guo S-D, Danilo P Jr, Rosen MR: Responses to norepinephrine of normal and "ischemic" canine Purkinje fibers are consistent with activation of different α_1-receptor subtypes. J Cardiovasc Electrophysiol 8:658–666, 1997.
61. Anyukhovsky EP, Steinberg SF, Cohen IS, Rosen MR: Receptor-effector coupling pathway for α_1-adrenergic modulation of abnormal automaticity in 'ischemic' canine Purkinje fibers. Circ Res 74:937–944, 1994.
62. Wit AL, Rosen MR: Afterdepolarizations and triggered activity: Distinction from automaticity as an arrhythmogenic mechanism. In Fozzard HA, Haber E, Jennings RB, Katz AM, Morgan HE (eds): The Heart and Cardiovascular System, vol 2, 2nd ed. New York, Raven Press, 1992, pp 2113–2163.
63. Coumel P, Fidelle J, Lucet V, et al: Catecholamine-induced severe ventricular arrhythmias with Adams-Stokes syndrome in children: Report of four cases. Br Heart J 40(suppl):28–37, 1978.
64. Leenhardt A, Lucet V, Denjoy I, et al: Catecholaminergic polymorphic ventricular tachycardia in children. A 7-year follow-up of 21 patients. Circulation 91:1512–1519, 1995.
65. Priori SG, Napolitano C, Tiso N, et al: Mutations in the cardiac ryanodine receptor gene (hRyR2) underlie catecholaminergic polymorphic ventricular tachycardia. Circulation 103(2):196–200, 2001.
66. Swan H, Piippo K, Viitasalo M, et al: Arrhythmic disorder mapped to chromosome 1q42. J Am Coll Cardiol 34:2035–2042, 1999.
67. Marx SO, Reiken S, Hisamatsu Y, et al: PKA phosphorylation dissociates FKBP 12.6 from the calcium release channel (ryanodine receptor): Defective regulation in failing hearts. Cell 101:365–376, 2000.
68. Möise NS, Gilmour RF, Ricco ML: An animal model of spontaneous arrhythmic death. J Cardiovasc Electrophysiol 8:98–103, 1997.
69. Möise NS, Meyers-Wellen V, Flahive WJ, et al: Inherited ventricular arrhythmias and sudden death in German shepherd dogs. J Am Coll Cardiol 24:233–243, 1994.
70. Dae MW, Lee RJ, Ursell PC, et al: Heterogeneous sympathetic innervation in German shepherd dogs with inherited ventricular arrhythmia and sudden cardiac death. Circulation 96:1337–1342, 1997.
71. Sosunov EA, Anyukhovsky EP, Shvilkin A, et al: Abnormal cardiac repolarization and impulse initiation in German shepherd dogs with inherited ventricular arrhythmias and sudden death. Cardiovasc Res 42:65–79, 1999.
72. Sosunov EA, Gainullin RZ, Möise NS, et al: β_1- and β_2-adrenergic receptor subtype effects in German shepherd dogs with inherited lethal ventricular arrhythmias. Cardiovasc Res 48:211–219, 2000.
73. Obreztchikova MN, Sosunov EA, Anyukhovsky EP, et al: Heterologous ventricular repolarization provides a substrate for arrhythmias in a German shepard model of spontaneous arrhythmic death. Circulation 108:1389–1394, 2003.
74. Steinberg SF, Alcott S, Pak E, et al: β_1-receptors increase cAMP and induce abnormal Ca_i cycling in the German shepherd sudden death model. Am J Physiol Heart Circ Physiol 282:H1181–H1188, 2002.
75. Corr PB, Shayman JA, Kramer JB, Kipnis RJ: Increased α-adrenergic receptors in ischemic cat myocardium: A potential mediator of electrophysiological derangements. J Clin Invest 67:1232–1236, 1981.
76. Bolli R, Fisher DJ, Taylor AA, et al: Effect of α-adrenergic blockade on arrhythmias induced by acute myocardial ischemia and reperfusion. J Mol Cell Cardiol 16:1101–1117, 1984.
77. Benfey BG, Elfellah MS, Ogilvie RI, Varma DR: Antiarrhythmic effects of prazosin and propranolol during coronary occlusion and reperfusion in dogs and pigs. Br J Pharmacol 82:717–725, 1984.
78. Gilmour RF, Möise NS: Triggered activity as a mechanism for inherited ventricular arrhythmias in German shepherd dogs. J Am Coll Cardiol 27:1526–1533, 1996.

第 33 章

神经的新生与心律失常

Lan S. Chen and Peng-Sheng Chen

本章目录

- 心脏的神经支配 ………………… 293
- 心肌受损后交感神经的变性与再生 ………………… 294
- 交感神经支配的更替与心律失常 …… 294
- 交感神经的新生（神经重塑）与心律失常 ………………… 296
- 心肌梗死后由交感神经新生所致的心律失常发生机制 ………………… 296
- 交感神经高支配在功能上的不对称性 ………………… 297
- 结论 ………………… 298
- 致谢 ………………… 298

外周神经在切断、压碎、血供受阻或其他方式损伤的情况下，可发生瓦氏变性（Wallerian degeneration）和轴突的再生。这种再生过程称之为神经新生（Nerve sprouting），在中枢神经系统及外周神经系统常可见到这种现象。如果能形成许多突触，这将引起局部神经支配的永久性变化，从而导致相应的功能改变。心肌梗死可引起神经损伤和区域性的交感神经变性，随后即可发生神经的新生并导致心肌局部区域性的交感神经高支配（hyperinnervation）[1]。虽然神经新生的程度在个体间有很大差异，但神经新生造成的局部交感神经分布的密集程度与室性心律失常的发生有着密切关系[2,3]。在这一章节里，我们将对交感神经新生与心律失常的关系进行评述。

一、心脏的神经支配

支配心脏的节前交感神经发自于脊髓的胸 4 或 5 段，穿过白交通支进入交感神经干，终止于颈上神经节、颈中神经节（若存在时）和星形神经节。这些神经节发出心脏神经与迷走神经的心脏支一起组成了心脏神经丛，接着再发出分支进入心脏内部。交感神经广泛分布于表层心外膜，并伴随冠状动脉进入心肌内部。交感神经主要位于血管周围及心肌细胞之间。这些神经纤维沿心肌细胞的长轴定向分布。支配心脏的副交感神经来自于迷走神经，其心脏支是节前神经纤维，在心脏神经丛或心内神经结内能与神经节细胞形成突触连接。

通过免疫组织化学技术标记神经特异性的标记物，如 S100 蛋白（雪旺氏细胞的标记物）、神经丝、突触素、蛋白基因产物 9.5 以及各种神经调节肽（如神经肽 Y），心脏神经便可显示出来[4,5]。而分别对酪氨酸羟化酶和乙酰胆碱酯酶进行免疫标记可区分出交感神经和副交感神经。像其他外周神经一样，心脏神经包括有髓鞘神经纤维和无髓鞘神经纤维，其中前者可通过对髓鞘的标记物如碱性髓磷脂蛋白的免疫染色进行识别。应用免疫组织化学和共聚焦显微镜技术对全心脏组织标本进行观察，Marron 及其同事[6]证明，所有分布于心外膜的神经末梢均可与酪氨酸羟化酶（针对交感神经的标记物）发生免疫反应，而心内膜则主要由有髓的交感神经来支配，分布于心外膜的神经末梢却不能与乙酰胆碱酯酶发生免疫反应，在心内膜也少于 5%。然而，副交感神经主要支配于心脏的传导系统，如在窦房结与房室结组织以及房室束的分布可分别占60%和70%。资料显示，在人类心脏，交感神经的分布远比副交感神经广泛[4,7]。

二、心肌受损后交感神经的变性与再生

在外周神经损伤后，邻近损伤的部位可发生轴突的新生，而远离损伤的部位却发生瓦氏变性（见图33-1）。轴突的再生可分出许多细带而延伸到变性的神经残干的雪旺氏管。其中一些再生的轴突芽可完全被雪旺氏细胞的质膜包绕，许多轴突芽只在再生的早期存在。然而，只有那些与受体和效应器末梢发生突触联系的轴突芽能够保留下来。冗余无功能的轴突芽需要相当长的时间才能消失。

轴突再生最初是很慢的，但可逐渐加速，直到损伤后的第3天变成了恒速[8]。轴突再生速度可因损伤的类型、年龄及种属的不同而有所差别。速度差异大概是1~3 mm/d[8]。例如大鼠坐骨神经的轴突再生速度可达到3.2 mm/d。轴突再生机制目前尚不完全清楚，神经损伤部位周围的非神经组织中神经营养因子的上调是启动轴突新生的重要机制之一。这个机制也可能参与启动邻近部位未受损神经纤维侧支神经的新生。

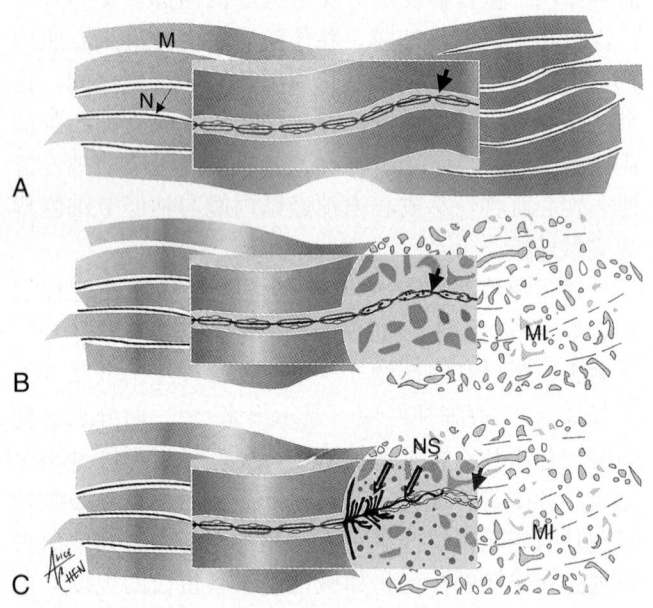

图33-1 心肌梗死后的神经新生 A：分布于血管周围及心肌细胞之间的交感神经，神经纤维沿着心肌细胞的长轴定向分布（实心箭头所示）。B：心肌梗死后梗死部位的神经纤维受到损伤。远端的残干发生了瓦氏变性（图B和C中的实心箭头所示）。C：邻近损伤的地方有神经纤维的轴突新生（空心箭头所示）。M：心肌细胞；N：神经纤维；MI：心肌梗死；NS：神经芽（见彩图6）

由于心肌梗死时心室内的神经纤维也会受到损伤，缺血损伤后便可能发生神经的新生（见图33-1）。在体心脏的交感神经可通过^{131}I间碘苄胍（Meta-[^{131}I]iodobenzylguanidine，MIBG）扫描来显示，后者是一种可被交感神经末梢摄取的去甲肾上腺素类似物。在心肌梗死后的心室可出现局部MIBG摄取的缺损（去神经支配）。这种现象可一直持续30个月[9,10]。然而，有报道在梗死后3~12个月之间可观察到梗死周围带MIBG摄取的增加，提示有神经再支配存在[11]。另外在那些没有心肌梗死的冠心病患者中也观察到有MIBG摄取的缺损，而且这种摄取缺损所占的面积与冠状动脉的狭窄程度相关[12]。冠状动脉痉挛性心绞痛患者也有MIBG的摄取缺损，但其中85%的患者摄取缺损可持续2个月，有32%的患者可持续6个月[13]。在对犬进行短暂冠状动脉闭塞的模型中可观察到慢性的去交感神经支配现象[14]。这些资料提示，心脏交感神经极易受缺血损伤，梗死心肌可出现持续的交感神经去神经支配，同时在梗死周围也可发生神经再支配。

通过对梗死心肌成像的组织学研究已经证实了交感神经的去神经支配和再支配现象。心肌损伤后神经纤维的分布可发生变化。Cao等[2]对因冠心病或特发性扩张型心肌病行心脏移植患者的心脏取材观察，结果显示患者心室肌内神经纤维的分布并不均匀。在坏死区周围或血管周围分布着大量能与S100蛋白或酪氨酸羟化酶发生免疫反应的神经纤维（见图33-2）。相比之下，梗死中心区以及纤维组织密集区却无神经分布。对比无心脏病史的心肌活检组织，移植心脏心肌组织内能与S100蛋白发生免疫反应的神经纤维的密度增加了两倍（见表33-1）。心脏内交感神经纤维远远比副交感神经纤维丰富，酪氨酸羟化酶和S100蛋白在大多数神经纤维是共存的，这些资料反映出受损心肌存在交感神经支配的增加，提示在人类心脏有交感神经的新生。

对人类心脏进行MIBG或组织学研究的资料显示，心肌损伤可引起去神经支配诱发神经重塑，即心肌的交感神经新生。心肌损伤后的神经重塑可导致交感神经的不均匀分布，出现受损部位区域性的去神经支配及邻近部位的神经高支配。

三、交感神经支配的更替与心律失常

许多研究显示，在心律失常的患者，包括特发性

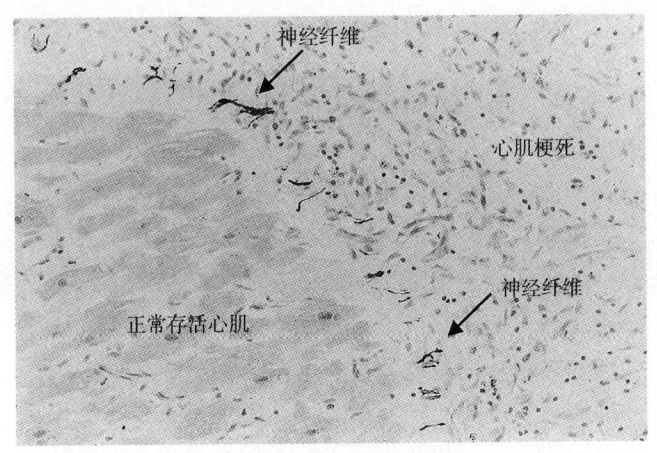

图33-2 心肌梗死后区域性的神经高支配 神经纤维（箭头）在梗死外围最丰富。相比之下，梗死的坏死区及纤维化区无神经纤维。心肌梗死后的去神经支配及神经新生可导致心脏交感神经的不均匀性分布（引自Chen P-S et al. Sympathetic nerve sprouting, electrical remodeling and the mechanisms of sudden cardiac death.*Cardiovasc Res* 2001；50：409-416.）（见彩图7）

室性心动过速（Ventricular tachycardia, VT, 简称为室速）、致心律失常性右室心肌病、右室流出道室速以及Brugada综合征，都存在区域性的MIBG摄取缺损。这些患者中交感神经去神经支配的发生率为33%~88%。Moise等[15]报道了对有较高自发性室速和心脏性猝死发生率的德国牧羊犬的研究结果，他们分析了这种德国牧羊犬在异相睡眠和锻炼后心律失常的发生趋势，揭示了交感活性在心律失常发生中的作用，同时也观察到这种犬的心脏有MIBG摄取的不均匀分布[16]。根据心电图是否有室速进行分组，室速组（n=6）比无室速组（n=5）去神经支配区域面积更大（35±16.5% 比 12±5.6%；$P < 0.02$）。MIBG摄取减少与组织学证实的交感神经分布贫乏有关。上述资料提示，区域性的交感神经去神经支配很可能与室速的发生有因果关系。去神经超敏反应可能是去神经支配诱导的心律失常的发生机制。给予无交感神经支配的心肌交感神经刺激或去甲肾上腺素输注，可表现出有效不应期的显著缩短。

Cao等[2]根据患者病史对接受心脏移植患者体内取出的心脏组织进行了分类：有持续室速、短阵室速或心脏性猝死患者的心脏组织为第1组，无心律失常病史的为第2组。结果发现，S100蛋白阳性的神经纤维密度在缺血性心肌病和非缺血性心肌病之间并无差别。然而，第1组心室神经密度明显高于第2组，揭示了心室交感神经密度与室速或心脏性猝死之间的联系（见表33-1）。室速患者的心肌组织纤维化与正常心肌细胞混合存在，同时伴有大量的神经纤维分布（见表33-2）。这些临床和组织学研究资料提示，在人类，心肌梗死后区域性的交感神经高支配与室速或心脏性猝死的发生有关。

MIBG研究结果和组织学观察资料对于解释交感神经支配的变化是如何引起室性心律失常，也就是区域性去神经支配与区域性神经高支配作为一种致心律失常发生机制产生了相反的假说。然而，这些假说并不相互排斥。MIBG区域性的摄取降低并没排除有交感神经再生的存在。Cao等[2]研究显示，邻近梗死带心肌内分布的神经末梢增加了两倍很可能是与MIBG检测灵敏度低有关。事实上，这种MIBG摄取面积的减小通常与洗脱的增加有关，提示去神经支配区有儿茶酚胺的循环增加，或者是有可能存在交感活性的增

表33-1 临床特征及心室神经密度

组别*	正常	冠心病	特发性扩张型心肌病	年龄（岁）	射血分数	每mm² 神经纤维总数
1A	30	14	16	56.7±12.1	0.22±0.07	19.6±11.21†
1B	23	11	12	56.7±12.9	0.21±0.07	13.5±6.1
2	5	—	—	60.0±9.7	未测	6.8±2.4§
3	7	7	0	63.7±8.9	未测	未测

*1A组：心律失常患者；1B组，无心律失常患者；2组：非心脏性死亡患者的尸检心肌组织；3组：经外科手术消融治疗后的室速患者的心肌组织。
†1A组与1B组比较：$P < 0.05$。
§2组与1A组比较：$P < 0.01$。
引自Cao J-M, Fishbein MC, Han JB, et al：Relationship between regional cardiac hyperinnervation and ventricular arrhythmia. *Circulation* 2000；101：1960-1969.

加。去神经支配后诱导的肾上腺素能超敏（supersensitivity）以及交感神经的高支配，二者都可能对受损心肌的电生理特性产生协同作用。而且，分散的神经高支配的存在可增加心肌受损部位交感神经分布的不均匀性。这种交感神经支配的不均匀性在室速或心源性猝死的发生中可能具有重要的作用。

四、交感神经的新生（神经重塑）与心律失常

为了进一步阐明梗死心肌区域性交感神经高支配的致心律失常作用，Cao及其同事[3]对完全性左束支传导阻滞[17,18]和心肌梗死犬进行左侧星状神经节注射神经生长因子，从而诱导出交感神经的新生。神经生长因子注射可很快增加交感神经的新生，并促进受损心肌的交感神经高支配。我们的实验证实，对3条正常犬的左侧星状神经节进行神经生长因子注射2周，也可引起心肌组织内神经的新生。我们进一步采用射频消融法以及在第一对角支下方进行的冠状动脉结扎术复制了伴完全性房室传导阻滞的心肌梗死犬模型，同时采用一台植入式心律转复除颤仪来检测室速和室颤的发生，实验组采用渗透泵对9条完全性房室传导阻滞和心肌梗死的犬进行了左侧星状神经节的神经生长因子注射，6条没有注射神经生长因子的犬作为对照组，免疫组织化学染色显示，实验组的交感神经分布密度明显高于对照组（33.2±2.1根/mm² 与 16.1±5.36根/mm²）。

所有心肌梗死的犬在第1周都出现了自发性室速（1相室速），又在术后平均13.1±6.0天可再次出现自发性室速（2相室速）。实验组中2相室速的发生率明显高于对照组，而且其发生显示出明显的昼间变异（$P<0.05$），从清晨到午后这段时间为高峰期。实验组中有4条犬因自发性室速而猝死，但对照组没有1例发生猝死。同时在另外6条无房室传导阻滞并未进行神经生长因子注射的心肌梗死犬，于术后48±5.0天可在心肌组织里观察到交感神经的新生，而且它们也没有发生心脏性猝死。

有趣的是，部分室性心律失常患者的心肌组织神经密度（19.6±11.2根/mm²）与心脏性猝死犬模型实验组心肌组织的交感神经密度（33.2±12.1根/mm²）相近[2,3]。而交感神经新生在无房室传导阻滞及未给予神经生长因子注射的6条心肌梗死犬的心肌组织中很明显。这些结果与临床研究资料相一致，即：（1）在没有外源性神经生长因子的情况下，心肌梗死后也可能发生心脏神经的新生；（2）交感神经新生，在犬模型中可采用神经生长因子注射来增强，且与室速和心脏性猝死的高发生率有着因果关系。因此，区域性交感神经的高支配是心肌梗死后致室性心律失常发生的重要机制。

最近一项采用电生理刺激左侧星状神经节诱导交感神经新生的研究报道，其结果进一步支持了交感神经的高支配在促心律失常发生中的作用。另外，对6条有心肌梗死和完全性房室传导阻滞的犬，连续电刺激（5 Hz）左侧星状神经节极易诱发室速和心脏性猝死（4条）。此外，交感神经高支配也在心房颤动的发生中具有重要的作用。长期快速的右心房起搏可诱导犬的持续性心房颤动。Chang等[19]证实，心房颤动犬其心房组织的交感神经密度可增加3~5倍。通过采用同样的模型，Jayachandran等[20]也证实了心房内交感神经支配有不均匀性的增加。

五、心肌梗死后由交感神经新生所致的心律失常发生机制

多数心脏性猝死患者都有冠心病或心肌梗死病史。心肌梗死造成的电重塑及解剖重塑在室速及心脏性猝死的发生中都是非常重要的因素。我们认为这种神经重塑及电重塑的相互作用是心肌梗死后致室性心律失常的发生机制。交感神经新生所致的神经重塑很可能是触发心律失常的扳机，而电重塑在诱发室速及心脏性猝死中却充当了基质的作用。

（一）心肌梗死后的电重塑

在实验模型中，持续结扎冠状动脉的左前降支可导致前间隔的透壁梗死。在透壁梗死的心外膜中存活下来的心肌纤维（少到几百个心肌细胞那么厚）构成了心外膜边缘带（epicardial border zone，EBZ）。EBZ已被证实是左前降支闭塞后1周（心肌梗死的治疗期）诱发性室速/室颤发生的起源点。在左前降支闭塞后1周，心肌重塑主要表现为心外膜结缔组织的增加和水肿，这将导致心肌组织局部不均匀的各向异性。EBZ的膜特性也将发生改变。EBZ区心肌细胞的L型内向钙电流峰值可发生降低[21]，且快速内向钠电流的恢复也出现延迟[22]。这种膜特性的变化改变了EBZ区心肌细胞的电兴奋性及复极后的不应性，这在早搏刺激或快速起搏时将有助于传导阻滞和折返的形

成[22]。电重塑也并不仅仅只发生在EBZ区，这种变化也可发生在非梗死区心肌。Qin等[23]证实，心肌梗死很可能导致动作电位时程（action potential duration, APD）的延长以及非梗死区心肌复极的不均匀性，这些变化可通过短暂外向钾电流的减少来解释。Aimond等[24]对幼年大鼠进行了冠状动脉结扎，4～6个月后分离心室肌细胞，结果发现长期的冠状动脉结扎导致L型钙电流的显著变化，包括峰值的降低以及缓慢失活，同时观察到心肌梗死后心肌细胞钾电流的变化。这些发现提示心肌梗死可导致EBZ及非梗死心肌明显的电重塑[25]。

（二）交感神经新生与电重塑之间的相互作用

众所周知，β肾上腺素受体激动可通过L型钙电流（I_{Ca}）、钾通道（I_{Ks}）以及氯离子通道（$I_{Cl(Ca)}$和$I_{Cl-cAMP}$）来增加离子电流。I_{Ks}的增加可缩短APD，然而I_{Ca}的增加可延长APD。在体条件下，对正常犬心室给予交感神经刺激将导致APD的缩短并降低不应性的离散度[26]，提示外向除极电流（I_{Ks}和I_{Cl}）与内向电流I_{Ca}综合结果可能有净增加。然而，当I_{Ks}被抑制或心肌梗死后发生下调，却不会出现上述变化[27]。在灌注的犬心脏，色原烷醇293B（Chromanol 293B，一个特异性的I_{Ks}阻滞剂）可延长QT间期以及心肌细胞动作电位复极90%的时程（APD_{90}），但不会使T波变宽或诱导尖端扭转型室速（Torsde de Pointes，TdP）。在持续有色原烷醇293B作用的情况下，异丙肾上腺素可缩短心外膜和心内膜细胞（而不是M细胞）的APD_{90}，促进了T波的增宽以及复极离散度的显著增强。只有在给予I_{Ks}阻滞剂以及异丙肾上腺素才能观察到自发的TdP或是程序刺激诱发的TdP。在Ⅰ型先天型QT延长综合征患者中也存在I_{Ks}的异常[28,29]。在运动实验中，这些患者可减少变时效应以及出现反常的QT间期延长[30]。肾上腺素也可诱导TdP，然而β受体拮抗剂治疗以及交感神经切除术对这些患者具有抗心律失常的作用。这些资料提示，假若存在I_{Ks}的先天异常（如Ⅰ型先天型QT间期延长综合征），药物抑制或者是受体发生下调（如心肌梗死）等情况下，交感神经的刺激具有促心律失常作用。对这些心室的交感神经刺激也可能增加复极的离散度以及诱导TdP。这个机制最可能与心外膜及心内膜细胞残余I_{Ks}的显著增强有关，但不是M细胞，因为后者的I_{Ks}本身就比较弱[27]。

假如这种交感神经刺激与I_{Ks}减少的相互作用对于心律失常以及心脏性猝死的发生具有重要的作用，那么左侧星状神经节切除术（切除或减少心脏支配）将可有效的用于预防心律失常。与这个假说相一致的是，左侧星状神经节切除术通常都显示出抗心律失常作用。在由于电重塑而导致的获得性钾离子通道异常的人或动物，左侧星状神经节切除术均可有效预防心肌梗死后心脏性猝死的发生。在Ⅰ型先天型QT间期延长综合征患者，钾离子通道的活性异常是先天的而不是获得性的，左侧星状神经节切除术虽然不是100%有效，但在预防心律失常的再发也是有效的。总之，异常的电生理基质与交感神经刺激之间的相互作用对于心律失常的发生是很重要的。

在我们的心脏性猝死犬模型中观察到一个有趣的现象，给正常犬的左侧星状神经节注射神经生长因子可引起神经的新生，但不会导致室性心律失常或心脏性猝死。在对照组，由心肌梗死和完全性房室传导阻滞诱导的电重塑也不会增加心脏性猝死。看来这种神经新生（神经重塑）以及电重塑的相互作用对引起室速、室颤或心脏性猝死的高发是必需的。

另一个遗传性室性心律失常的德国牧羊犬的心脏性猝死模型，表现为可出现自发性室颤[15]。在这个模型中，交感神经支配的不均匀性是恒定存在的[16]。而且，β肾上腺素受体密度也存在异质性的增加。对犬心脏前间隔分离的M细胞标本采用微电极检测显示，异丙肾上腺素注射可引起APD异常的延长而不是缩短[31]。这些结果提示在这种模型中，猝死的机制可能同交感神经不均匀性支配与异常的电生理基质之间的相互作用有关，其中，很可能是由于在这种模型中有钾离子通道的异常所致[32]。

六、交感神经高支配在功能上的不对称性

Zhou等[33]证实了交感神经高支配对QTc间期的不同作用。当给予心肌梗死伴完全性房室传导阻滞犬的右侧星状神经节注射神经生长因子后，交感神经的新生主要发生在右室心肌。而QTc间期的显著减少可持续2～7周。术后2相室速的发生率与单纯心肌梗死和完全性房室传导阻滞的对照组犬相比是降低的。相比之下，通过对左侧星状神经节注射神经生长因子诱导的左室交感神经高支配可伴随有QTc间期的增加以及2相室速和心脏性猝死的高发。这些发现与早期观察到的结果一致，即对左侧星状神经节刺激或右侧星

状神经节切除可导致 QTc 间期的延长，然而，左侧星状神经节切除或右侧星状神经节刺激可产生相反的结果。一个可能的机制是，来自右侧星状神经节的传入交感神经对来自左侧星状神经节的交感神经有相互抑制作用。另外一个机制是，右室选择性交感神经高支配很可能通过 I_{Ca} 增加了离子流，因此延长了右室的 APD 并减少了左室电生理的异质性。

七、结 论

许多物种（但不是所有）的心肌损伤后都可发生交感神经的新生。心肌交感神经密度和室性心律失常之间存在着一定的联系。通过对慢性心肌梗死及完全性房室传导阻滞的犬进行左侧星状神经节神经生长因子的注射，可增加交感神经的新生，并导致自发性室速、室颤及心脏性猝死的高发。交感神经新生的程度可能成为了慢性心肌梗死后室速或心脏性死亡的重要决定因素。因此，我们提出了心脏性猝死的神经新生假说，即在心肌梗死后发生由交感神经新生所致的神经重塑，它是已发生电生理重塑的心肌诱发室速或室颤的一个重要因素。（见表 33-1）

这个神经新生假说解释了 β 肾上腺素受体拮抗剂用于预防心肌梗死后心脏性猝死的作用[34]。它也可用于解释许多临床试验的结果。例如，索他洛尔（Sotalol）是 β 肾上腺素受体拮抗剂，广泛用于预防慢性心肌梗死患者室性心律失常的发生。假若失去了 β 肾上腺素受体拮抗剂的作用（如 D-索他洛尔），那么这个药物将增加心肌梗死患者的死亡率[35]。众所周知，左侧星状神经节切除术在预防人及动物心肌梗死后的心脏性猝死都是有效的。所有上述这些结果都与心脏性猝死的神经新生假说相一致。

八、致 谢

这项研究由 Pauline 和 Harold 奖，NIH R01 HL66389，NIH HL71140 以及 P50 HL52319 基金资助。我们感谢 Rita Cholakian，Elaine Lebowitz 以及 Nina Wang 的帮助。我们也感激 Alice Chen 为本文做的制图工作。

（张幼怡 龚开政 译）

参 考 文 献

1. Chen P-S, Chen LS, Cao JM, et al: Sympathetic nerve sprouting, electrical remodeling and the mechanisms of sudden cardiac death. Cardiovasc Res 50:409–416, 2001.
2. Cao J-M, Fishbein MC, Han JB, et al: Relationship between regional cardiac hyperinnervation and ventricular arrhythmia. Circulation 101:1960–1969, 2000.
3. Cao J-M, Chen LS, KenKnight BH, et al: Nerve sprouting and sudden cardiac death. Circ Res 86:816–821, 2000.
4. Marron K, Wharton J, Sheppard MN, et al: Distribution, morphology, and neurochemistry of endocardial and epicardial nerve terminal arborizations in the human heart. Circulation 92:2343–2351, 1995.
5. Chow LT, Chow WH, Lee JC, et al: Postmortem changes in the immunohistochemical demonstration of nerves in human ventricular myocardium. J Anat 192(Pt 1):73–80, 1998.
6. Crick SJ, Sheppard MN, Ho SY, Anderson RH: Localisation and quantitation of autonomic innervation in the porcine heart. I: Conduction system. J Anat 195(Pt 3):341–357, 1999.
7. Chow LT, Chow SS, Anderson RH, Gosling JA: The innervation of the human myocardium at birth. J Anat 187(Pt 1):107–114, 1995.
8. Fu SY, Gordon T: The cellular and molecular basis of peripheral nerve regeneration. Mol Neurobiol 14:67–116, 1997.
9. Bengel FM, Barthel P, Matsunari I, et al: Kinetics of ^{123}I-MIBG after acute myocardial infarction and reperfusion therapy. J Nucl Med 40:904–910, 1999.
10. Podio V, Spinnler MT, Spandonari T, et al: Regional sympathetic denervation after myocardial infarction: a follow-up study using [123I]MIBG. Q J Nucl Med 39:40–43, 1995.
11. Hartikainen J, Kuikka J, Mantysaari M, et al: Sympathetic reinnervation after acute myocardial infarction. Am J Cardiol 77:5–9, 1996.
12. Hartikainen J, Mustonen J, Kuikka J, et al: Cardiac sympathetic denervation in patients with coronary artery disease without previous myocardial infarction. Am J Cardiol 80:273–277, 1997.
13. Inobe Y, Kugiyama K, Miyagi H, et al: Long-lasting abnormalities in cardiac sympathetic nervous system in patients with coronary spastic angina: quantitative analysis with iodine 123 metaiodobenzylguanidine myocardial scintigraphy. Am Heart J 134:112–118, 1997.
14. Dae MW, O'Connell JW, Botvinick EH, Chin MC: Acute and chronic effects of transient myocardial ischemia on sympathetic nerve activity, density, and norepinephrine content. Cardiovasc Res 30:270–80, 1995.
15. Moise NS, Gilmour RF Jr, Riccio ML: An animal model of spontaneous arrhythmic death. J Cardiovasc Electrophysiol 8:98–103, 1997.
16. Dae MW, Lee RJ, Ursell PC, et al: Heterogeneous sympathetic innervation in german shepherd dogs with inherited ventricular arrhythmia and sudden cardia death. Circulation 96:1337–1342, 1997.
17. Volders PG, Sipido KR, Vos MA, et al: Cellular basis of biventricular hypertrophy and arrhythmogenesis in dogs with chronic complete atrioventricular block and acquired torsade de pointes. Circulation 98:1136–1147, 1998.
18. Vos MA, de Groot SH, Verduyn SC, et al: Enhanced susceptibility for acquired torsade de pointes arrhythmias in the dog with chronic, complete AV block is related to cardiac hypertrophy and electrical remodeling. Circulation 98:1125–1135, 1998.
19. Chang C-M, Wu T-J, Zhou S-M, et al: Nerve sprouting and sympathetic hyperinnervation in a canine model of atrial fibrillation produced by prolonged right atrial pacing. Circulation 103:22–25, 2001.
20. Jayachandran JV, Sih HJ, Winkle W, et al: Atrial fibrillation produced by prolonged rapid atrial pacing is associated with heterogeneous changes in atrial sympathetic innervation. Circulation 101:1185–1191, 2000.
21. Aggarwal R, Boyden PA: Diminished Ca^{2+} and Ba^{2+} currents in myocytes surviving in the epicardial border zone of the 5-day infarcted canine heart. Circ Res 77:1180–1191, 1995.
22. Pu J, Boyden PA: Alterations of Na^+ currents in myocytes from epicardial border zone of the infarcted heart. A possible ionic mechanism for reduced excitability and postrepolarization refractoriness. Circ Res 81:110–119, 1997.
23. Qin D, Zhang ZH, Caref EB, et al: Cellular and ionic basis of arrhythmias in postinfaction remodeled ventricular myocardium. Circ Res 79:461–473, 1996.
24. Aimond F, Alvarez JL, Rauzier JM, et al: Ionic basis of ventricular arrhythmias in remodeled rat heart during long-term myocardial

infarction. Cardiovasc Res 42:402–415, 1999.

25. Pinto JM, Boyden PA: Electrical remodeling in ischemia and infarction. Cardiovasc Res 42:284–297, 1999.
26. Takei M, Sasaki Y, Yonezawa T, et al: The autonomic control of the transmural dispersion of ventricular repolarization in anesthetized dogs. J Cardiovasc Electrophysiol 10:981–989, 1999.
27. Shimizu W, Antzelevitch C: Cellular basis for the ECG features of the LQT1 form of the long-QT syndrome: Effects of β-adrenergic agonists and antagonists and sodium channel blockers on transmural dispersion of repolarization and torsade de pointes. Circulation 98:2314–2322, 1998.
28. Sanguinetti MC, Curran ME, Zou A, et al: Coassembly of K(V)LQT1 and minK (IsK) proteins to form cardiac I(Ks) potassium channel. Nature 384:80–83, 1996.
29. Barhanin J, Lesage F, Guillemare E, Fink M, Lazdunski M, Romey G: K(V)LQT1 and lsK (minK) proteins associate to form the I(Ks) cardiac potassium current. Nature 384:78–80, 1996.
30. Swan H, Viitasalo M, Piippo K, et al: Sinus node function and ventricular repolarization during exercise stress test in long QT syndrome patients with KvLQT1 and HERG potassium channel defects. J Am Coll Cardiol 34:823–829, 1999.
31. Wu CC, Karten HJ: The thalamo-hyperstriatal system is established by the time of hatching in chicks (*Gallus gallus*): A cholera toxin B subunit study. Vis Neurosci 15:349–358, 1998.
32. Germani E, Lesma E, Di Giulio AM, Gorio A: Progressive and selective changes in neurotrophic factor expression and substance P axonal transport induced by perinatal diabetes: Protective action of antioxidant treatment. J Neurosci Res 57:521–528, 1999.
33. Zhou S, Cao JM, Tebb ZD, et al: Modulation of QT interval by cardiac sympathetic nerve sprouting and the mechanisms of ventricular arrhythmia in a canine model of sudden cardiac death. J Cardiovasc Electrophysiol 12:1068–1073, 2001.
34. Rarnaot M: Nicotine patches may not be safe. BMJ 310:663–664, 1995.
35. Waldo AL, Camm AJ, deRuyter H, et al: Effect of *d*-sotalol on mortality in patients with left ventricular dysfunction after recent and remote myocardial infarction. The SWORD Investigators (Survival With Oral *d*-Sotalol) [see comments] [published erratum appears in Lancet 348(9024):416, 1996]. Lancet 348:7–12, 1996.

第 34 章

胆碱能性心房颤动

Leonid V. Rosenshtraukh，Vadim V. Fedorov，Oleg F. Sharifov

本章目录

- 犬心房的自发胆碱能性房性心动过速 300
- 初级和次级起搏区在兔右心房自发性胆碱能性心动过速中的作用 306
- 结论 309
- 致谢 310

一个世纪以来，心房纤维颤动（简称为房颤）一直是实验及临床研究的热点。然而，尽管作为一种最常见的持续性心律失常[1]，它对于临床及基础电生理学家仍是一个神秘的难题。房颤的启动和维持的电生理基础一直未被阐明。虽然在房颤的实验研究中，可采用电刺激心房来诱发房颤，但在现实中真正启动房颤发作的机制尚不清楚。目前普遍认为神经机制在房性心动过速（简称为房速）和房颤的启动及维持中发挥着重要的作用[2,3]。大量的实验资料提示自主神经系统可促进房颤的发生，然而，迷走神经的作用要明显强于交感神经[4,5]。迷走神经刺激可通过降低心房不应期以及增加心房不应性的不均一性而有助于房颤的维持[5,6]。给犬迷走神经刺激或是持续注射乙酰胆碱均可维持电诱导的房颤，动物实验也证实这些方法在没有给心房电刺激的情况下也可诱发房颤发作[9-11]。本章将对近年来胆碱能性房颤（cholinergic atrial fibrillation）的自发启动机制的研究进展进行综述。

一、犬心房的自发胆碱能性房性心动过速

（一）迷走神经介导的胆碱能频率依赖性

虽然有学者已注意到强烈的迷走神经刺激可诱发房速和房颤[2,10,12]，但一直没有对此进行过系统的研究。我们采用5秒一串（5-second trains）的强刺激对犬迷走神经进行刺激，从而系统地研究不同胆碱能性房速及房颤的发生率[13]。我们的定义是，出现联律间期小于200ms、2次以上配对的心房激动为房速。给予犬心得安后，以10~50Hz的频率刺激右侧迷走神经，可导致房速频率进行性增加，但起始就给予40 Hz的频率刺激时，房速频率增加不会超过50%。当没有房速发作时，相对弱一点的迷走神经刺激可减慢窦性心律，稍强一点的迷走神经刺激便可产生窦性静止，继而恢复为窦性心律（见图34-1 A）。窦性静止可被一个逸搏所打断。每次房速的发作都与许多类型的迷走神经刺激诱导的缓慢性心律失常有关。这些缓慢性心律失常以及房速的发作也与迷走神经刺激的强度呈线形相关。有趣的是，在半数以上房速的发作中都伴有房颤发作。然而，有研究提示，在恰当的时候给予单次迷走神经刺激便可影响窦性节律[14]，并引起一个心房异位起搏点发生逸搏[15]。研究中并未观察到在心动周期中，强迷走神经刺激的时限对不同的迷走反应及房速频率有明显的作用。值得注意的是，尽管迷走神经刺激对窦性节律有显著的作用，但在10只犬中只有8只可诱发出房速。当同时满足以下两个条件时便可出现房颤：（1）在恰当的时间点引入一个

房性早搏（atrial premature depolarization）而触发折返激动；(2) 维持折返的心房肌发生了功能性改变。我们的研究结果表明，不同的迷走神经刺激强度（频率）触发房颤的机制可能不同。

（二）胆碱能介导的房性早搏的正常位置与异常位置

近年来，随着经导管射频消融术（radiofrequency current catheter ablation，RFCA）的发展，已将它用于房颤的临床治疗[16,17]。对犬进行迷走神经刺激诱发房颤是目前用来探讨 RFCA 治疗房颤新方法最常用的动物模型[7,18]。因此，了解胆碱能诱导的房性早搏是如何触发房颤以及它们所发生的部位，对开发新的治疗策略是非常重要的。

有资料显示，给犬的窦房结动脉注射乙酰胆碱可诱发房颤，而窦房结本身在胆碱能性房颤中的作用日益受到关注[19,20]。对游离的犬右心房进行乙酰胆碱诱发房颤的研究证实，来自不同位点的局灶性房性早搏可触发折返性房速[11,21]。这些局灶点（focal sites）沿界嵴的分布最为密集。Boineau 及其同事[22]提出假说认为，心脏存在一个分布相似的起搏系统，即起搏点复合体（pacemaker complex）。由此可见，起始的房性早搏是由多个右心房起搏点不同步激动共同形成的。这种胆碱能性房性早搏的机制与生理性心房起搏点的功能异常有关。看来有必要对离体和在体胆碱能性房性早搏进行局部解剖学上的比较研究。通过使用间距为 3～6 mm 的 256 个电极对整个心外膜进行精确的标测，我们集中观测作为启动房颤发作的第一个紧密配对电冲动（A1 和 A2）局灶位点的空间分布情况[13,23]，并采用了不同剂量的乙酰胆碱（静脉注射 10 mM 的乙酰胆碱 5～10 ml 或窦房结注射 1 μM 的乙酰胆碱 1ml）以及不同的颈迷走神经刺激强度（10～50 Hz）来诱发自发性房速及房颤的发作。为了分析，标测区被划分为 5 个区（见图 34-1 B）。在作为对照的房颤发作期，观察到所有的局灶位点都位于 CAVAL 区，它涵盖了 1cm 的腔静脉及腔静脉间带，这个区域被认为是"正常位置（normotopic）"，因为它正好与心房起搏点复合体的分布位置一致。除此之外，其他区都认为是"异位的（ectopic）"。

全身给予乙酰胆碱可引起广泛分布的房性早搏灶，这与离体右心房实验观察到的明显不同。然而，大多数 A1 局灶点都发自心房起搏复合体[22]，这与离

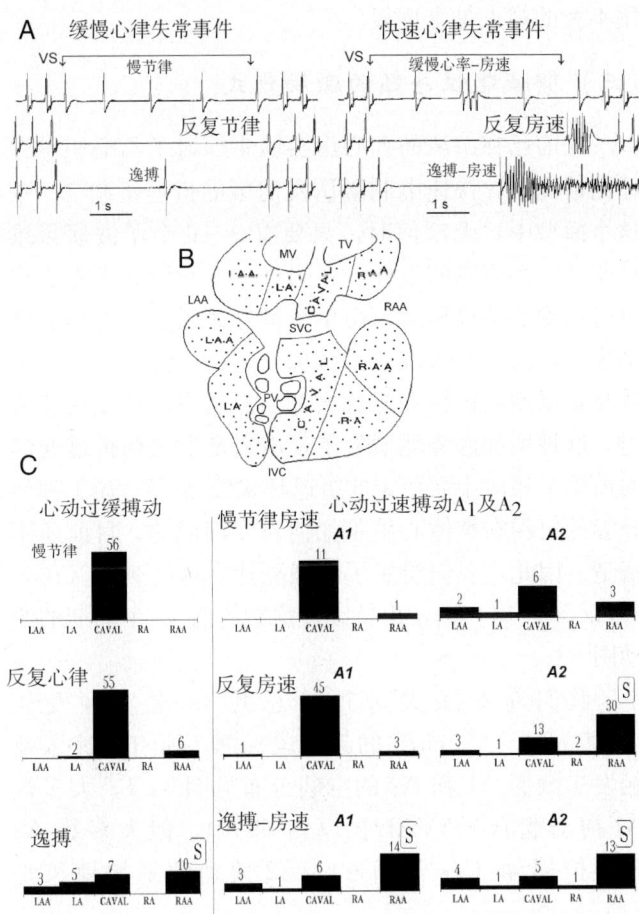

图 34-1 A：对迷走神经刺激（VS）诱发的缓慢性心律失常及心动过速的跟踪记录。每条心房电图记录代表一次心律失常。B：在主要解剖标志点上电极排列图（上腔静脉，SVC；下腔静脉，IVC；肺静脉，PV；右心耳，RAA；左心耳，LAA；二尖瓣，MV；三尖瓣，TV）。为了分析，标测区被划分为 5 个区：CAVAL，RAA，RA，LAA 及 LA。C：在迷走神经刺激下诱发不同缓慢性心律失常发作时的最早激动点以及心动过速时最早的两个搏动（A1 和 A2）空间分布的直方图。在迷走刺激前作为对照激动时，所有的最早激动点都位于 CAVAL 区（即正常位置区）。方块显示的是发自预定区的电冲动总数。虽然多数慢节律（slowed rhythm）、反复房速（return-atrial tachycardia）以及缓慢的反复心律（slowed and return rhythms）的 A1 电冲动都起源于 CAVAL 区，而它们的 A2 电冲动更多是异位的。逸搏-房速（escape-AT）以及逸搏（escape beat）的 A1 和 A2 局灶点却广泛分布于两侧高位心房，在右心耳有一个高密集（S）区（引自 Sharifov OF, Zaitsev AV, Rosenshtraukh LV, et al: Spatial distribution and frequency-dependence of arrhythmogenic vagal effects in canine atria. J Cardiovasc Electrophysiol 2000；11：1029-1042.）

体组织实验的结果类似[11]，而A2搏动更多是"异位的"，常发自右心耳，但有时也可发自右心房、左房游离壁以及左心耳。也可观察到多个灶点起源的特殊形式，提示这些房性早搏来自间隔部。有时也可观察到房性早搏起始于不同的心房区，如同时来自于左、右心耳。在给予强烈的迷走神经刺激时也可观察到，发生房性早搏的局灶兴奋点有相同的空间分布，同时伴有心房上部传播的异位搏动[13,23]。

图34-1 C显示在迷走神经刺激下，缓慢性心律失常及心动过速发作时发生了激动起源点从正常位点向异位（即CAVAL区以外）的转变。心动过缓越重，异位冲动就越多，如缓慢心律时异位冲动为零，而反复心律（return rhythm）时异位冲动为13%，逸搏时为72%。在心动过速时，A1搏动的空间分布从性质上与那些单纯的缓慢性心律失常发作时类似。A2搏动的异位起源概率较高：慢房速时为50%，反复房速时（return AT）为64%，而逸搏房速时（escape-AT）为79%。在图34-1 C中显示的所有分布模式可分为两类：一类以正常位置为主的，如对照组、缓慢性回返心律（slowed and return rhythms）以及反复心律；另一类以异位为主的，如单个逸搏，异搏房速为A1以及所有房速为A2。

窦房结注射乙酰胆碱诱发房性早搏的空间分布与离体右心房实验有相似的模式。这些局灶性房性早搏主要限于窦房结动脉支配区。因此，这些房性早搏主要起自界嵴、右肺静脉毗邻处以及房间隔。另外，这种房性早搏很少发生于右心房的游离壁以及右心耳，但从来不会在左房出现[23]。

对比在体与离体胆碱能性房性早搏局部解剖学上的差异，得到的提示是：①这种偏差可能是由于标本实际大小以及对乙酰胆碱的趋近性（accessibiliy）不同所致。②乙酰胆碱的直接作用看来是迷走神经介导的房性早搏发生的关键因素。③上述在体原位的研究中，大多数乙酰胆碱及迷走神经刺激的房性早搏与"正常位置"起搏点无关。我们设想，那些广泛分布于左右心房及房间隔的潜在起搏点能参与胆碱诱导的房性早搏及房颤的启动（见后面所述）。

汇总最近几年的临床研究结果，多数认为肺静脉是诱发房颤发生异位激动点的主要来源[16,17]。我们的研究结果显示，神经介导的房性早搏的起搏点可能位于双侧心房的静脉外区。近来对人双心房多位点标测显示，诱发房颤发作的异位启动位点47%是在双心房肺静脉外面。房颤患者中有27%为双起源[24]。这些资料对当前认为肺静脉以外的起搏点在房颤启动中作用不大的观点是个挑战。

（三）胆碱能性房颤的激动模式

先前已在游离的犬心房实验中探讨了乙酰胆碱存在的情况下，快速电刺激诱发房颤的折返机制[8]。在这个模型中，无论何时，只要有3~6个子波便可维持胆碱能性房颤的发作。在另外一次对游离犬右心房进行标测的结果显示，由单个额外刺激诱发房颤的激动模式取决于乙酰胆碱的浓度。起初，折返环和子波的数量以剂量依赖的方式增加。然而当房速变成持续时，这种增加趋势就消失了，由兴奋形成的折返便趋向由单个相对小而稳定的折返环来控制[25]。迷走神经介导的房颤在整体心脏是如何自发形成的，目前还不清楚。因此，我们绘制了由强烈迷走神经刺激（10~50Hz 5s一串）诱发出持续性房颤的前10个周期的激动图[13]。

我们对8条犬进行了总共49次房颤发作（持续30 s~15 min）的起始段标测。所有房速以及触发房颤的A1和A2的空间分布见图34-1。大多数A1搏动起自CAVAL区（占69%），但大多数A2是异位搏动（占73.5%）。A2搏动的平均周长是118±25 ms。

激动标测显示，多数房颤发作都有单个稳定的、主导的致心律失常源，并且它参与激动心房的余部（图34-2A）。任何一次运行的子波数量可根据房颤激动复杂程度的不同在3.9±1到13±2之间变化。在开始的10个周期中，所有房颤都有较高的频率（见图34-2B）。这种激动模式依赖于基本的致心律失常源的类型。所有动物至少都有两种类型的激动模式。

当从心外膜很好的标测到A2（n=15）或A3（n=2)搏动的兴奋波沿着部分不应性组织传播形成一个折返时便可记录为显性折返。折返环在不同的区域可演化，可伴有前几个周期的不稳定，到第10个周期时才变得稳定。图34-3说明折返是通过来自左心耳的单个房性早搏而触发的。在图34-3中显示的那个"8"字型折返看来在右心房或是肺静脉附近，并且不太稳定。有时也观察到通过A2搏动可同时形成两个折返环，但只有一个是稳定的。在显性折返型房颤中，那个稳定的折返环决定了房颤的频率，同时也可伴随有一个或多个额外的不稳定折返环。所有折返环都是有功能的，但可以没有解剖结构基础。图34-2 B

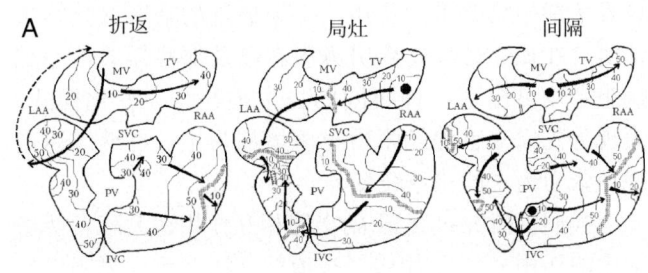

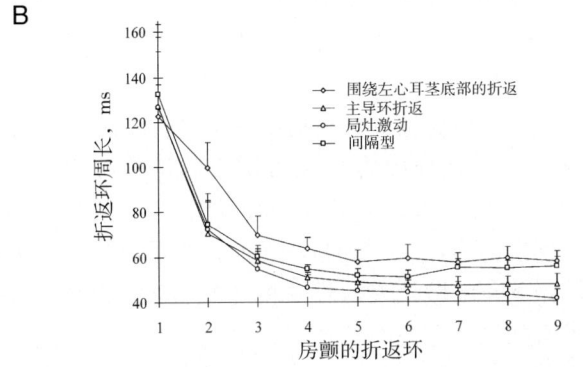

图 34-2 A：在犬模型中，房颤的一个周期里存在着不同的致心律失常起源点。Reentry 型：折返型，是指围绕在左心耳底部的折返环。子波激动左右心房而不产生任何冲突。Focal 型：局灶型，是指来自心耳局灶点的激动，在左房，两个宽子波相互碰撞引起激动的紊乱。Septal 型：间隔型，是由于在上腔静脉附近和右侧肺静脉底部同时出现两个突破点（breakthrough）。新发和先前周期中兴奋波的前部分别采用阴影线和箭头来标记。缩写的注释见图 34-1。B：在不同房颤类型中前 10 个周期里稳定的致心律失常源的周长曲线图。虽然有四条曲线显示出越跳越快的相似模式，但它们的基线明显不同。除"主环"型折返与间隔型折返的比较外，其他所有比较，P 均小于 0.05（Kolmogorov - Sharifov 双侧检验）（引自 Sharifov OF，Zaitsev AV，Rosenstraukh LV，et al：Spatial distribution and frequency-dependence of arrhythmogenic vagal effects in canine atria. *J Cardiovasc Electrophysiol* 2000；11：1029-1042.）

（左图）显示环绕左心耳的稳定折返环的一个循环。这个折返环很大，而且周长有周期性的波动。它还显示了不同的稳定性致心律失常源前 9 个周期中周长的平均曲线（A1-A2，A2-A3⋯A9-A10）。环绕左心耳的折返可表现出周长的一次缓慢、逐步的初始缩短，接着在大约 60ms 时形成了周期性波动。另外一次稳定的折返变异产生于右心房游离壁和右心耳的"主环"，在这个折返里，折返环的周长经过一次平稳快速的缩短后出现逐步稳定（见图 34-2B）。

在局灶型房颤发作中（n=12），多数激动发生在上腔静脉的靠前方（Bachmann's bundle），并且最早激动的范围涉及的区域较广。在更强的迷走神经刺激下，比其他类型房颤发作时更容易看到在左右心耳、靠近右肺静脉和左房内的局灶激动。在局灶型房颤中，不排除有微折返存在的可能。但从未观察到有两个同时发生的局灶点激动以及激动部位发生改变的现象。图 34-2 A（中图）显示起源于右心耳的局灶激动引起的心房激动顺序图，虽然稍快一些，但局灶型房颤周长的时程与"主环"折返型房颤十分相似（见图 34-2 B）。

在许多房颤病例中（n=11），间隔型激动模式可导致心房的心外膜激动（见图 34-2A，右图）。在上腔静脉基底部、下腔静脉以及右肺静脉可形成特殊的心外膜多个局灶点同时激动的现象是间隔型的特点。我们在对心房心外膜以及间隔同时标测时观察到，在不同的间隔点刺激以及在迷走神经刺激诱导间隔部的房性早搏时，都可显示出这种激动模式[27]。这是因为单独心外膜标测不能够确定这种多个局灶点同时激动的起源，而后者可引起折返性兴奋或间隔的局灶激动。另外，许多来自于右肺静脉的激动从理论上也可产生这种模式。然而，在早期的临床研究中也观察到有间隔型房颤的存在[28]。在间隔型房颤发作时，那种

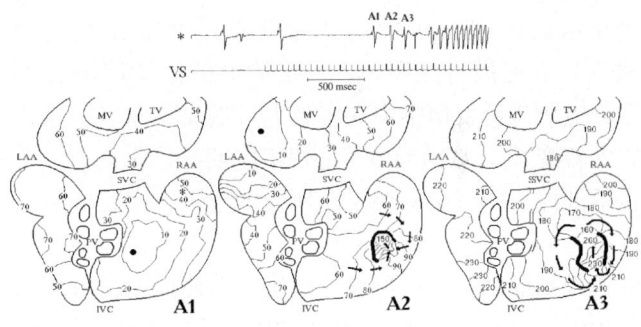

图 34-3 以 20 Hz 的迷走神经刺激强度诱发一次房性早搏触发折返的实例 来自心耳的电极（星号）显示右侧迷走神经刺激后 1s 内房颤便开始发作，但同时出现窦性静止。A1 起源于 CAVAL 区的中部。A2 以 134ms 的配对间期开始于左心耳，并通过 Bachmann 束进入右心房及房间隔。在右心房，激动沿着一个阻滞区以"8"字形顺时针或是逆时针方向旋转。激动缓慢传播 50ms 并于大约 90ms 内重返初始阻滞的近点。接着初始阻滞的远点发生逆向激动，重返初始阻滞的近点。对 A2 和 A3 采用了连续的计时标测。粗线显示的是传导阻滞，星号指示的是激动传播的方向。缩写的注释见图34-1。（引自 Sharifov OF，Zaitsev AV，Rosenstraukh LV，et al：Spatial distribution and frequency-dependence of arrhythmogenic vagal effects in canine atria. *J Cardiovasc Electrophysiol* 2000；11：1029-1042.）

多个突破点同时出现的模式经常伴随有规律的心外膜激动。没有观察到朝向房间隔前方有逆行的心外膜激动波。间隔型房颤的周长以及时程同其他类型的房颤也很相似（见图34-2B）。另外，因为有致心律失常的起源点发生转移或同时存在两到三个起源点，有9次房颤发作被认为是中间型。

Sharifov及其同事[13]证实大多数房颤发作时，在2/3搏动周期之后，或者是在一些不稳定的致心律失常起源点的事先干预之后，可逐步形成单个稳定的、主导的兴奋源。先前在对游离犬右心房的研究中观察到，持续性胆碱能性房颤与单个稳定的折返源有关[25]。另外，这种引起房颤的单个折返在对整体犬以及临床研究中也被证实[28]。当折返环周长足够短时，心房的余部就不可能产生1:1的激动，从而导致房颤。然而，在我们的研究中经常观察到，许多房颤发作都有主要致心律失常起源点的变换以及心房激动顺序由规则向不规则的改变。尽管存在周长曲线上的个体差异，尤其在它们的基线部，但各型房颤的时程及周长均相似（见图34-2B）。我们曾假设，在不同的心外膜标测中所标测到的兴奋源在起源上可能都是折返性的。早期研究已证实，在游离犬右心房，乙酰胆碱介导的折返在心外膜及心内膜表面都是三维的，可分别显示出同时发生的局灶激动模式及折返激动模式[21]。在相似的模型中，一定浓度的乙酰胆碱存在下，电刺激诱发房颤中观察到大折返模式向微折返模式的转变[25]，从而导致了心房不应期的显著缩短以及折返环减小到超出标测系统所及的范围。在我们的研究中，局灶型房颤的速度更快一些，而且在更强一点的迷走神经刺激下就可诱导出来，因此提示这可能与微折返兴奋有关。在一项对游离羊心脏的光学标测研究中，也证实了这种稳定的微折返源是诱导性胆碱能性房颤的电生理机制[29]。

（四）β肾上腺素受体对胆碱能性房颤自发启动的影响

在临床实践中，通常基于发作前自主神经张力的变化可将阵发性房颤分为两种：迷走神经诱发型和交感神经诱发型[2]。为了阐述伴有自主神经张力变化的房颤启动机制，除临床病史以外，对阵发性房颤发作前心率的变化模式也进行了分析。通常认为迷走神经诱发的房颤多为折返，而肾上腺素诱发的房颤多为自律性异常和触发激动[2,3]。然而，两种类型的阵发性房颤的根本机制目前尚未完全明了。例如Hashimoto及其同事[9]曾提出，β肾上腺素受体激动在乙酰胆碱诱发房颤中具有重要作用。一项最近的临床试验结果证实，在孤立性阵发性房颤患者以及那些器质性心脏病患者均可出现一种相同的自主神经张力变化模式，表现为先以交感神经张力显著增加为主，再继以迷走神经张力为主的快速转变[30]。

我们曾研究过交感-副交感相互作用在犬阵发性房颤中的作用[31]。采用曾经报道的方法[19,23]，复制出自发性神经诱发房颤模型，即对20条开胸的麻醉犬在没有电刺激心房的情况下，分别采用含儿茶酚胺（$1\mu M$、$10\mu M$和$100\mu M$）、乙酰胆碱或二者混合的台氏液（改良林格氏液）对窦房结动脉进行灌注。14条犬中有3条出现异丙肾上腺素诱发的房颤发作（$10\mu M$，2只；$100\mu M$，1只），6只犬中有1条出现肾上腺素诱发的房颤（$10\mu M$），然而，给予阿托品后可显著降低儿茶酚胺诱发房性早搏的发生率。而且，尽管与没有阿托品存在时相比，肾上腺素及异丙肾上腺素能引起心率显著增加，但均不能诱发房颤。由于两侧迷走神经均已被隔离开来，这些结果提示有两种可能存在，一是一定的胆碱能张力有助于促进高浓度儿茶酚胺的致心律失常作用，其次是窦房结动脉灌注儿茶酚胺可引起心脏固有神经系统激动。

在20条由乙酰胆碱灌注诱发房颤的犬模型中，我们对其中12条进行了系统的研究，即肾上腺素受体激动是如何影响乙酰胆碱诱导房颤的启动及维持的？同时给予乙酰胆碱及两种浓度的异丙肾上腺素灌注（$1\sim2\mu M$及$10\mu M$），可明显促进乙酰胆碱诱导房颤的启动，降低了乙酰胆碱诱导房颤的浓度阈值（从$3\pm1\mu M$分别降到$0.5\pm0.3\mu M$及$0.4\pm0.3\mu M$，$P<0.05$)，并延长了阵发性房颤的发作时间，从$25\pm7s$分别延长到$141\pm56s$及$233\pm54s$，$P<0.05$)。图34-4显示其中一条犬的两次房颤发作情况，在异丙肾上腺素的存在下，无论心率快慢，乙酰胆碱诱导的房颤发作都多于灌注前。相比之下，给予心得安可导致发作前心率明显减慢，需要更高浓度的乙酰胆碱才能诱发房颤。因此在这个模型中，心率依赖于β肾上腺素受体激动，在心率变慢或加快的过程中发生乙酰胆碱诱导的房颤发作。我们这些研究资料提示：(1)基础的胆碱能或交感神经张力可分别调节β肾上腺素受体或胆碱受体激动对房颤的诱导作用。(2)在这个模型中，看起来胆碱受体激动是房颤启动的必要条件。

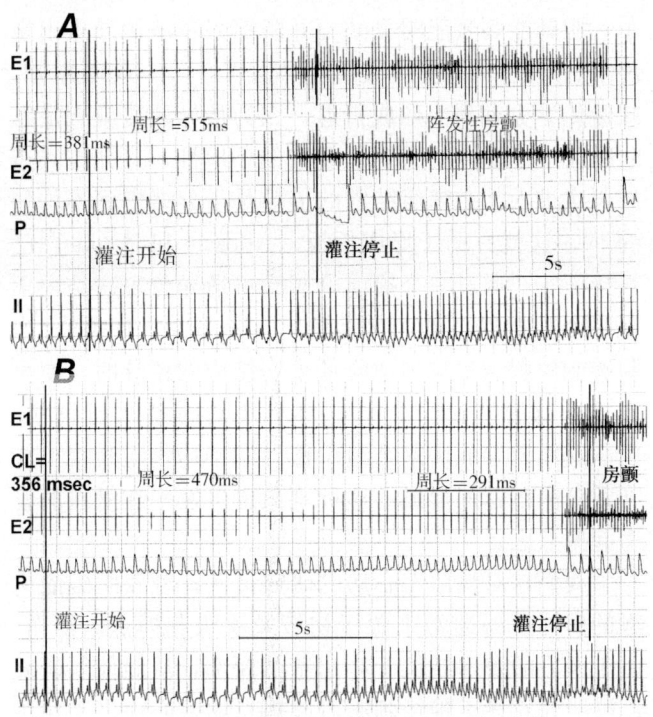

图 34-4 给犬窦房结动脉灌注含 1μM 的乙酰胆碱（A），0.1μM 的乙酰胆碱以及 2μM 的异丙肾上腺素（B）的台氏液所诱发的房颤　在对照组（A），诱导犬房颤反复发作的乙酰胆碱阈值或最低致心律失常浓度是 1μM。在另外一条犬，灌注乙酰胆碱并窦性心率减慢。当灌注 7s 之后，一个紧密配对的房性早搏触发了房颤。在立即停止灌注后发作还可持续 12s。用这个例子主要是为了强调单独乙酰胆碱灌注诱导发作前以及同时采用乙酰胆碱和异丙肾上腺素（B）灌注诱导发作前，对比两者窦性心率变化的差异。在联合灌注时，窦性心率的初始减慢比对照少，而发作时可达到一个比对照更为稳快的心率。值得注意的是，当异丙肾上腺素与乙酰胆碱同时存在时，诱发房颤的乙酰胆碱浓度比单独使用乙酰胆碱低了 10 倍。发作有些延迟但持续了 90 s（没有显示）。E1 和 E2 为心房的双极心电记录图。P2 为心房内的血压记录。Ⅱ为标准的Ⅱ肢体导联［引自 Sharifov OF, Fedorov VV, Beloshapko GG, et al: Spontaneous AF induced by sympathetic and cholinergic stimulation in dogs.（投稿中）］

（五）触发胆碱能性房颤的房性早搏的细胞机制

对触发阵发性房颤的自发性房性早搏的机制至今仍不清楚，一直是研究的热点[11-13,15-17,20-24,27,31-41]。目前提出的房性早搏的几种机制包括：触发激动、自律性异常、不同步的起搏点激动以及局部微折返。

在近来的临床研究中，主要来自肺静脉底部的触发性激动或者是自律性异常都被认为是阵发性房颤的

机制[16,17]。对整体犬心脏的实验研究已证实，高频率电刺激可诱导肺静脉及上腔静脉处的快速异位搏动，从而诱发房颤。基于对肺静脉内许多心房肌细胞存在早后除极的观察，推测在这个模型中，触发性激动有助于促进房性早搏及房颤的发生，阿托品可以完全消除快速的异位局灶点激动和房颤，而β肾上腺素受体拮抗剂则仅仅增加了高频电刺激诱发房速所需的电压水平[32]。Scherlag 及其同事[33]发现，当对原位的犬心给予刺激左肺动脉内的自主神经时，也可得到上述类似的结果。这些研究均支持副交感神经对房颤诱发的作用[32,33]。然而，触发性激动或自律性异常都不是胆碱能性房性早搏的机制，因为乙酰胆碱已被证实可抑制这种自律性[41,42]。而从理论上讲，乙酰胆碱可增加毒蕈碱样的 K^+ 外向电流（I_{KACh}），所以应该能抑制所有类型的自律性[43]。

基于撤药后兴奋，近来又提出了另外一个胆碱能诱导房性早搏的启动机制。Wang 及其同事[34]证实，从游离的猫心房肌细胞快速撤去乙酰胆碱可导致细胞内 Ca^{2+} 超载，从而引起迟后除极。他们推测这种机制可能参与了去迷走神经引起的房性早搏。然而这个机制无法解释在乙酰胆碱刺激的情况下，为什么会发生房性早搏。在我们的研究中，多数房颤发作出现在乙酰胆碱灌注或迷走神经刺激过程中，而不是恢复期。然而，我们在胆碱能性房颤的犬模型中测试了一个特异性的肌浆网钙释放通道的阻滞剂——兰尼碱的作用[35]。研究显示，全身给予兰尼碱（5μg/kg 静脉内注射）对乙酰胆碱诱导房颤的自发启动并无影响。在另外一项研究中，Fedorov 及其同事[36]研究证实，钙离子拮抗剂维拉帕米（0.2 mg/kg）静脉注射对窦房结动脉灌注乙酰胆碱诱导的房颤也无作用。这些资料提示在乙酰胆碱灌注期，房颤的自发启动很可能与细胞内钙超载所诱导的触发激动无关。

另外一个解释胆碱能性房性早搏发生的可能机制是不同步的起搏点激动[11]。在对游离右心房的实验显示，乙酰胆碱诱导的房速的前 2~3 个搏动以单灶点或多灶点的形式起源于界嵴，并可触发折返性房颤。有人认为，乙酰胆碱诱导的传入阻滞可使多个心房起搏点在不同步激动中相互保护，从而触发了房性早搏。Rozanski[15]也证实了这种阻滞的存在。在这项研究中，适时给予同步相的迷走神经刺激可诱导出副瓣叶起搏点的迟发早搏，但由于受主导房性节律的影响而表现出短暂的不应性。我们对整体犬心的研究结果

显示，乙酰胆碱及迷走神经诱导的局灶性房性早搏多为异位，广泛分布于心房的上部[13,23,27]。因此，为了将这个起搏假说应用于胆碱能性房颤的启动机制，必须假设整个心房内广泛分布着潜在的起搏点。在对犬和人的研究已证实，心房确实存在多个起搏点[12]。这些起搏点的节律以及对神经递质的反应性是不同的。值得注意的是，许多资料都提示，在肺静脉区存在着潜在的起搏点，因此，肺静脉内的房性早搏也被纳入到致心律失常的起搏点里。假如潜在的起搏点对迷走抑制的敏感性弱于生理性起搏点，那么胆碱性刺激通过抑制主节律可把它们显露出来，从而参与缓慢型及快速型心律失常的发作。均匀分布于心房上部（60%在右心房，40%在左房）的逸搏性局灶激动很可能就源于这种机制，它们在窦性静止后可以被显示出来[13]。这些细胞在窦性静止时可发生除极，从而在经迷走神经刺激导致的单向阻滞后的整齐节律期，可能引起房性早搏。因此，这种稳定或不稳定、生理或非生理性的起搏点阻滞可能就是胆碱能性或迷走性心律失常发生的一个普遍机制。

基于在兔的窦房结内以及潜在的起搏点区域存在迷走诱导的局部短暂无反应性现象（详见后述）[38-40]，提出了另外一个关于胆碱能性房性早搏及房颤的假说——局部微折返。

二、初级和次级起搏区在兔右心房自发性胆碱能性心动过速中的作用

（一）在初级和次级起搏区乙酰胆碱诱导的局部无反应性

先前，Roseenshraukh 及其同事[37]在对游离的青蛙标本研究中显示，在迷走神经刺激期，起始于窦静脉的一个单波可下传进入到迷走神经刺激产生的一个短暂无反应性心房区，这种激动波在这些区域发生前向阻滞，接着消失，或者围着阻滞区环形传播。在这项研究中，形成折返需要没有提前成对的除极。在青蛙心脏模型中的这种环形运动完全依赖于迷走刺激引起的心房传导的短暂、不均匀的阻滞，且很可能并不依赖于不应性。然而，不像在两栖动物上的研究，对游离的和在体的犬右心房，胆碱能刺激并不会在长配对间期（>200 ms）出现阻滞区。

虽然还没有证实在哺乳动物组织中存在迷走神经刺激或乙酰胆碱灌注诱导的不应性，但许多研究已显示，胆碱能刺激能明显减少并阻滞兴奋波传导进出窦房结、房室结以及次级起搏点[11,12,44,45]。众所周知，减慢传导更有利于形成折返，因为传导减慢就有足够时间让这个环内的组织恢复它的不应性，并允许兴奋波再次进入。在窦房结内的传导是十分缓慢而不均匀的[44]，这就有助于形成折返。Allessie 和 Bonke[46]已直接证实，通过一个提前电刺激可诱导兔窦房结内出现一个微折返环的一次运行（echo beat，回波）。当胆碱能性刺激不均匀地降低窦房结内的传导时，便可促进折返的形成[44]。Mazgalev 及其同事[45]已证实，由胆碱能诱导的房室结组织传导的不均匀阻滞很可能导致结内折返的形成。这种现象也可发生在潜在的心房起搏点区。

我们在对整体犬心房的研究证实，触发胆碱能房颤的房性早搏通常来源于初级及次级起搏点。然而，由于犬心的窦房结位于心房壁的深部，从而使得研究乙酰胆碱及迷走神经刺激对起搏点的致心律失常作用的细胞机制变得很困难。与犬的窦房结相比，兔右心房的下腔静脉区较薄，有窦房结和次级起搏点，在那里窦房结可从心内膜贯穿到心外膜[47]。近来，我们对游离兔右心房的房速发作期以及自发的胆碱能性房速发作期进行心外膜标测，并对一级及潜在起搏点进行了微电极记录[38-40]。

我们的研究结果显示，乙酰胆碱表面灌流或者神经节后的迷走神经刺激，都可使窦房结内初级起搏区的细胞超极化并显著降低动作电位幅度，降低到对照组的 40% 以下[39]。初级起搏细胞可保持不兴奋，并且只要胆碱能刺激得以维持，窦房阻滞就很容易出现。相比之下，来自次级起搏区周围以及心房的细胞可保持很好的兴奋性。图 34-5 显示的是乙酰胆碱对来自窦房结内初级起搏区及次级起搏区细胞的动作电位的作用。初级起搏区细胞在界嵴前激动 30ms，而界嵴前的次级起搏区细胞才激动 15ms（见图 34-5A）。乙酰胆碱表面灌流可进行性降低备用率大约为 50%。在初级起搏区细胞的动作电位逐渐降低直至消失的同时，次级起搏区细胞开始发放脉冲，其脉冲幅度仅有轻度的降低（见图 34-5B）。可使用一种慢速显示器来显示乙酰胆碱对初级起搏区细胞及次级起搏区细胞电激动的不同作用（见图 34-5 C）。经过 15min 的洗脱期，这种乙酰胆碱对同种细胞的作用可再次被诱导出来。

已观察到，乙酰胆碱刺激产生的动作电位抑制是一种可预测的现象，因为这种抑制程度与动作电位上

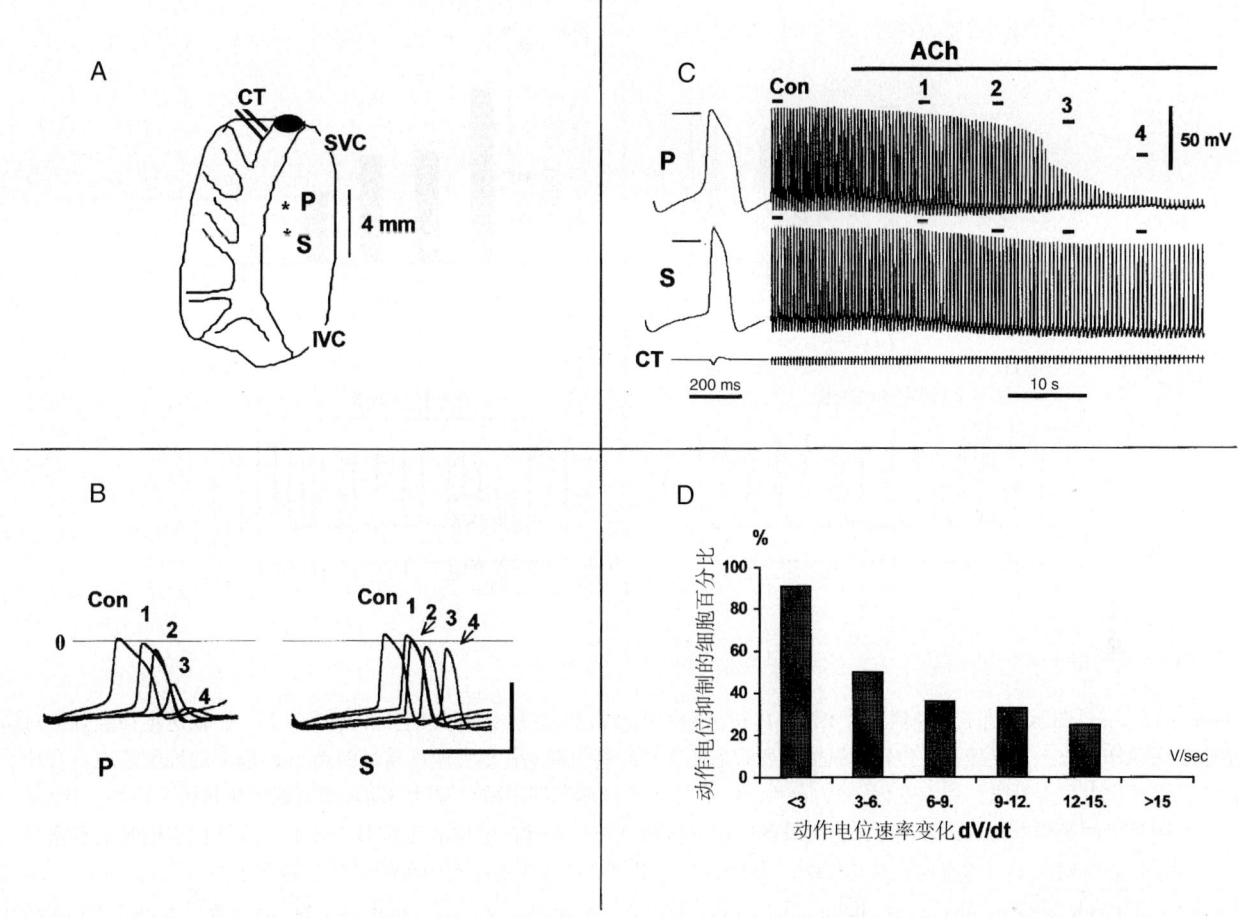

图 34-5 A：对游离兔右心房标本以及经筛选的类似记录的一个示意图，用于说明乙酰胆碱（0.1 mM）表面灌流对初级起搏区及次级起搏区细胞的作用。IVC，下腔静脉；SVC，上腔静脉；CT 代表的是采用双极电极记录到的界嵴；P 和 S 是同时发生的窦房结膜电位记录的相对位置。B：乙酰胆碱对初级起搏区及次级起搏区记录到的动作电位作用的比较。B（右侧）以一种标准的扫描基线显示，P 是来自初级起搏区细胞一个膜电位记录；S 是来自偏外周的次级起搏点的一个记录；CT 是采用双极电极记录到的界嵴。在 B（左）是部分对照记录的放大。C：取自 B 中五个点的放大图，并以 Con（对照）以及 1，2，3，4 代表在加入乙酰胆碱后 10、20、30、40 s 后获得的记录。乙酰胆碱表面灌流可抑制初级起搏区细胞的动作电位幅度，达到小于对照组的 40%，并且膜电位固定在一个接近对照最大舒张期电位的值。在次级起搏点，乙酰胆碱缩短了动作电位的时间并引起超极化。在动作电位描记图上的虚线显示的临界水平。图中比例尺代表的是 200 ms（水平），50 mV。D：乙酰胆碱对具有不同动作电位上升支速率的窦房细胞作用的比较。纵轴代表出现动作电位抑制的细胞百分比，横轴代表动作电位的速率变化（dV/dt）（引自 Vinogradova TM, Fedorov VV, Yuzyuk TN, et al: Local cholinergic suppression of pacemaker activity in the rabbit sinoatrial node. *J Cardiovasc Pharmacol* 1998；32：413-424.）

升肢的最大速率有关（见图 34-5D）。这些动作电位来自窦房结不同区的细胞，范围包括从窦房结中心的典型起搏细胞到窦房结外周典型的心房肌细胞[47]。在那些动作电位上升支速率变化超过 15V/s 的细胞不会发生无反应性。该实验取自 20 个游离右心房标本，动作电位上升支的速率低于 15V/s 的细胞（n=66），按它们的速率进行分组，在那些动作电位上升支速率小于 3V/s 的细胞中，动作电位降低的细胞共 35 个（91%），对这些细胞进行乙酰胆碱表面灌流使动作电位的抑制达到对照组的 40% 以下。

图 34-6 A 和 B 显示了短暂的神经节后迷走神经刺激对来自初级起搏区细胞及次级起搏区细胞电兴奋的作用。在心得安作用下，在窦房结有自发动作电位时给予一串持续 400ms、频率为 100Hz 的刺激。在图 34-6 A 中，初级起搏区细胞在界嵴前兴奋 30ms，迷

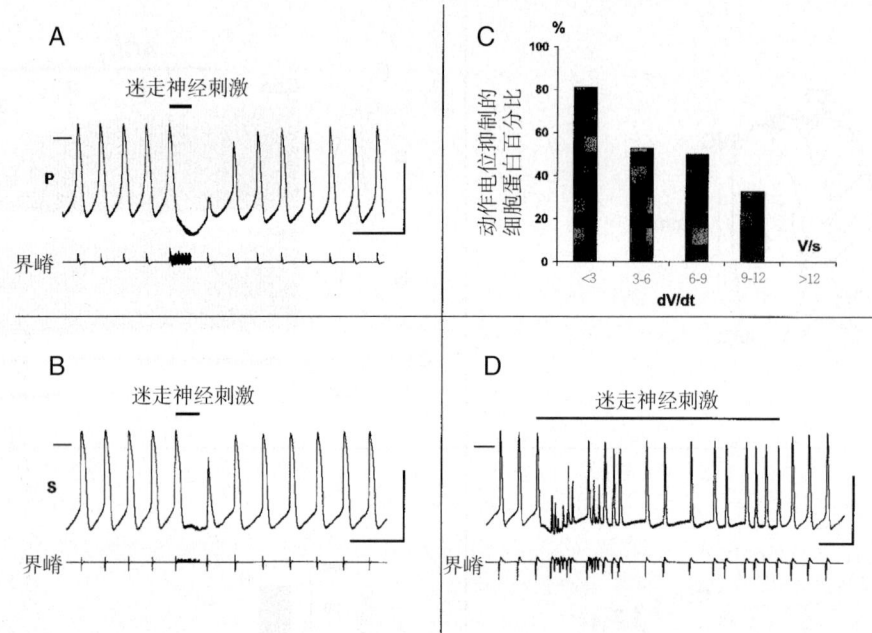

图34-6 A, B: 图示是迷走神经刺激对窦房结内初级起搏区及次级起搏区细胞膜电位的作用。C: 比较迷走神经刺激对窦房结细胞不同动作电位上升支速率的作用。纵轴代表的是迷走神经刺激期动作电位幅度被抑制到40%以下的细胞所占百分比，横轴代表的是动作电位上升支的速率变化（dV/dt）。D: 在迷走神经刺激期跟随自发性心动过速出现的短暂无反应性。A、B、D，上方一组图显示的是膜电位，下方图是来自界嵴的心房电极图。在显示动作电位前面的那一段水平线条代表的是临界水平。图左的比例尺代表时间为1s（水平向）及动作电位为50mV，用它可进行迷走神经刺激的时间定量（引自 Vinogradova TM, Fedorov VV, Yuzyuk TN, et al: Local cholinergic suppression of pacemaker activity in the rabbit sinoatrial node. *J Cardiovasc Pharmacol* 1998; 32: 413-424.）

走神经刺激可导致初级起搏区细胞膜13mV的超极化，并降低储备率达60%。结果只记录到一个亚阈值除极，而没有记录到起搏点的动作电位。这种亚阈值的除极在界嵴兴奋之后5s消失。反复的迷走神经刺激均可抑制初级起搏区细胞的兴奋。在图34-6 B中，迷走神经刺激可导致次级起搏区细胞自发激动的减慢，同时伴随有轻度的超极化（-2mV）以及动作电位幅度的降低。

在取材于20个游离右心房标本的63个细胞中，均记录到迷走神经刺激导致动作电位幅度的抑制达到了小于对照组的40%。在那些动作电位上升支速率小于3V/s的细胞中，无兴奋性发生率最高（81%）（见图34-6 C）。随着上升支速率的增加，无兴奋性的发生率降低。这种无兴奋性不会发生在速率大于3 V/s的细胞。在我们的实验中，没有观察到迷走神经刺激和乙酰胆碱表面灌流效应的不同。给予1μM的阿托品预处理可以完全阻断乙酰胆碱能的作用。在这项研究中，证实了乙酰胆碱以及迷走神经刺激均能使窦房结的局部位点不再有电活动，而窦房结的其他部分以及心房组织仍可继续产生动作电位。认为对动作电位的抑制是来自乙酰胆碱的直接作用。在同样的细胞，迷走神经刺激和乙酰胆碱灌注对动作电位的抑制作用相同。

（二）胆碱能性抑制起搏点动作电位的离子基础

对兔窦房结组织的电生理及形态学研究显示，起搏点细胞动作电位上升支的速率及细胞体积从位于窦房结中心的初级起搏点到窦房结外周逐步增加[47,48]。虽然窦房结起搏的离子机制一直处于探讨中，近来的研究证实，兔窦房结是由多种具有电生理异质性的起搏细胞组成，这些细胞的细胞膜具有不同的电学特性[48]。基于此，有人认为乙酰胆碱对窦房结中部及外周的细胞具有不同的作用[49]。已观察到在乙酰胆碱刺激过程中，窦房结的初级起搏细胞与次级起搏细胞相比，在兴奋性上有显著的不同[39]。先前的研究曾证实，透壁的迷走神经刺激通过降低总的膜阻力可降低细胞间的耦联[50]。乙酰胆碱的作用减少了窦房结细胞相互间的电影响，因此可导致附近的起搏细胞在电激动上产生明显的局部差异。

已证实，L型Ca^{2+}电流（$I_{Ca,L}$）在窦房结中心细胞的动作电位上升支中具有重要的作用，而钠离子电流（I_{Na}）在窦房结外周细胞动作电位的上升支中起重要作用[48]。迷走神经刺激或者加入乙酰胆碱都可激活窦房结细胞毒蕈碱样K^+电流$I_{K,Ach}$[43]。$I_{K,Ach}$的激活可导致细胞超极化，增加周长，缩短窦房结细胞动作电位[49]。众所周知，乙酰胆碱在游离兔窦房结心肌细胞可抑制基础的$I_{Ca,L}$。在我们的定量研究中也观察到，对典型起搏细胞的动作电位幅度的抑制可达到60%以上，与Petit-Jacques及其同事[51]报道的乙酰胆碱（10μM）对$I_{Ca,L}$的抑制作用（大约56%）相近。乙酰胆碱很可能是通过抑制基础水平的腺苷酸环化酶活性，导致了环磷酸腺苷依赖的蛋白激酶活性降低，使得钙通道（$I_{Ca,L}$）发生去磷酸化，通道活性抑制。我们认为对上升支速率小于3V/s的起搏细胞，动作电位幅度的抑制很可能是乙酰胆碱对$I_{Ca,L}$的抑制结果。

（三）游离兔心脏标测胆碱能性房性心动过速

我们的研究结果显示，迷走神经刺激以及乙酰胆碱均可抑制80%以上典型起搏细胞的兴奋[39]。众所周知，那些dV/dt最低值小于3V/s的细胞在窦房结中部占据了一个很大的区域，大约$1\times2\ mm^2$[47]。因此，在我们进行胆碱能性刺激时便可观察到，传导一旦进入该区就完全被阻滞了。因此，很可能是胆碱能诱导了无反应细胞产生了不兴奋区，这就很可能形成折返性心动过速的一个障碍或单向阻滞，从而有助于形成折返。我们观察到，迷走神经刺激以及乙酰胆碱介导的起搏点不兴奋有时可伴随自发的房速（见图34-6 D）[39]。这些房速很可能起因于窦房结内围绕不兴奋区的局部折返。

为了评价自发的胆碱能性房速的起始激动模式，我们采用64个双极电极对游离兔右心房的上下腔静脉间进行了心外膜标测，电极中心点间距在平行界嵴的方向上是1mm，垂直方向为2mm[40]。在乙酰胆碱灌注（0.1mM）下，56次灌注中有32次记录到自发性房速（57%）。通常来讲，房速常在乙酰胆碱灌注开始诱导出由数千个周长为40～200ms的搏动组成的

缓慢性心律失常中出现。激动模式显示了这些房速由于产生数次房内折返而有局部发作的特点。虽然在一定条件下，窦房结区可出现稳定的自发节律，但所有的房性早搏都是来自上下两个独立的区域，上方区域（占37%）与窦房结有关，而下方区域（占63%）位于下腔静脉与右心房下壁（也是一个潜在的起搏点区）的联合部。这些研究提示，起搏点的结构与自发性胆碱能性房速的触发和维持有关。

Vingradova及其同事[38]先前曾证实，乙酰胆碱可增加来自邻近下腔静脉的潜在起搏点区细胞动作电位时程的不均匀性，而且可抑制动作电位的幅度，这与对窦房结初级起搏细胞的作用方式相同。例如，已显示在下腔静脉区，82%的动作电位升肢速率小于3V/s的细胞在乙酰胆碱灌注时可产生动作电位幅度下降超过40%的现象。这些资料提示，在窦房结中心，也可能在靠近下腔静脉的潜在起搏区，这里短暂无反应细胞组成了一个功能阻滞区，从而形成微折返[38-40]，这类似于在青蛙心房内观察到的折返[37]。而一个激动波与这些阻滞区发生碰撞后很可能发生碎裂并导致了自发性折返性心动过速或房颤，或二者兼之。

就如在对犬[13,23,31]和兔模型[38-40]中观察到的那样，那些局灶激动是起搏点围绕不兴奋带微折返的一种反应，还是由于电标测的空间分辨率所限导致的异常，直到目前仍不清楚。实际上，在兔窦房结中经电刺激诱导的微折返环的直径大约是1～2mm[46]。另外，胆碱能刺激可降低兔窦房结细胞间的耦联[50]以及$I_{Ca,L}$[51]，从而进一步降低传导率及折返环的大小（对照"主环模型"[26]）。因此在胆碱能刺激时，窦房结内环的大小就可能小于1mm。与我们的研究相比[40]，对这些区域进行微折返的标测需要电极的密度增加至少10倍。要在这个研究领域取得进展，就需要采用高分辨率的光学标测技术对哺乳动物的上下腔静脉间区域的兴奋传播模式以及动作电位的动力学进行标测研究。对这种标测技术空间分辨率的要求是能够准确测量出引起折返启动的兴奋波传播参数的变化。

三、结 论

对在体犬心以及离体兔心的研究表明，同时给予乙酰胆碱或强烈的迷走神经刺激均可反复诱发房速和房颤。随着迷走神经刺激强度的增加可直接增加犬房速及房颤的发生率。对每次房速发作时前两个紧密配

对搏动进行最早激动位点的标测显示，A1 的起源位置多为"正常位置"，而 A2（第一个房性早搏）通常为异位起源。单个房性早搏大多数情况下足以触发折返型房颤。尽管迷走神经刺激诱导房颤具有较高的发生率，且还可以通过单个稳定的折返环使房颤得于维持，但胆碱能性刺激诱导房颤的发作受交感张力的调节，反之亦然。胆碱能刺激对整体犬房颤的自发启动是必需的。

对兔体外研究显示，迷走神经刺激以及乙酰胆碱可增加位于窦房结及下腔静脉区起搏点细胞动作电位时程的不均匀性，并诱导短暂的无反应性。我们提出的假说认为，胆碱能刺激可在初级起搏区（窦房结）及次级起搏区（下腔静脉及其他区）产生不兴奋区，从而成为单向阻滞或者微折返以及两者兼有的病理基础。胆碱能性（迷走性）介导的局部短暂不兴奋性也是对生理性和非生理性起搏点的一种保护，可使它们从主节律的重整中逃逸并引起房性早搏。

然而，为了阐明在心房起搏组织迷走神经诱导传导阻滞及不兴奋性的机制，还需进一步研究。理论上，乙酰胆碱抑制传导至少有以下三个机制：（1）抑制 $I_{Ca,L}$；（2）由于显著增加了 $I_{K,Ach}$ 而降低了膜阻抗；（3）降低细胞与细胞间的耦联。乙酰胆碱的这些作用在许多病理性传导中很可能被进一步放大，尤其是病理因素本身就可导致细胞间脱耦联或者兴奋性降低时更加明显。在临床实践中副交感神经对房颤的影响比我们实验中观察到的要小，但是我们可观察到相似的房颤启动模式。因此，研究这些实验结果，为阐述心房电现象提供了可能的模式（包括迷走神经张力增加引起的房颤）。

四、致　谢

这项工作受俄罗斯基础研究基金（02-04-4830，02-04-06103 以及 00-15-97788）的支持。本章采用的资料来源于近来发表的论文以及我们尚未发表的论文。我们非常感谢以下同事对本文所做出的努力：Alexey Zaitsev, Tatinna Vinogradova, Tatjana Yuzyuk, Alexandr Kaliadin, Galina Beloshapka 以及 Anna Yushmanova。

（张幼怡　龚开政　译）

参 考 文 献

1. Feinberg WM, Blackshear JL, Laupacis A, et al: Prevalence, age distribution, and gender of patients with atrial fibrillation. Analysis and implications. Arch Intern Med 155:469–473, 1995.
2. Coumel P: Autonomic influences in atrial tachyarrhythmias. J Cardiovasc Electrophysiol 7:999–1007, 1996.
3. Tai CT, Chiou CW, Chen SA: Interaction between the autonomic nervous system and atrial tachyarrhythmias. J Cardiovasc Electrophysiol 13:83–87, 2002.
4. Zipes DP, Mihalick MJ, Robbins GT: Effects of selective vagal and stellate ganglion stimulation on atrial refractoriness. Cardiovasc Res 8:647–655, 1974.
5. Liu L, Nattel S: Differing sympathetic and vagal effects on atrial fibrillation in dogs: Role of refractoriness heterogeneity. Am J Physiol 273(2 Pt 2):H805–H816, 1997.
6. Allessie R, Nusynowitz M, Abildskov JA, Moe GK: Nonuniform distribution of vagal effects on the atrial refractory period. Am J Physiol 194:406–410, 1958.
7. Schauerte P, Scherlag BJ, Pitha J, et al: Catheter ablation of cardiac autonomic nerves for prevention of vagal atrial fibrillation. Circulation 102:2774–2780, 2000.
8. Allessie MA, Lammers WJEP, Bonke FIM, Hollen J: Experimental evaluation of Moe's multiple wavelet hypothesis of atrial fibrillation. In Zipes DP, Jalife J (eds): Cardiac Electrophysiology and Arrhythmias. Orlando, FL, Grune & Stratton, 1985, p 265.
9. Hashimoto K, Chiba S, Tanaka S, et al: Adrenergic mechanism participating in induction of atrial fibrillation by ACh. Am J Physiol 215:1183–1191, 1968.
10. Randall WC, Armour JA: Gross and microscopic anatomy of the cardiac innervation. In Randall WC (ed): Neural Regulation of the Heart. New York, Oxford University Press, 1977, p 20.
11. Schuessler RB, Rosenshtraukh LV, Boineau JP, et al: Spontaneous tachyarrhythmias after cholinergic suppression in the isolated perfused canine right atrium. Circ Res 69:1075–1087, 1991.
12. Schuessler RB, Boineau JP, Bromberg BI, et al: Normal and abnormal activation of atrium. In Zipes DP, Jalife J (eds): Cardiac Electrophysiology: From Cell to Bedside, 2nd ed. Philadelphia, WB Saunders, 1995, pp 543–562.
13. Sharifov OF, Zaitsev AV, Rosenshtraukh LV, et al: Spatial distribution and frequency-dependence of arrhythmogenic vagal effects in canine atria. J Cardiovasc Electrophysiol 11:1029–1042, 2000.
14. Jalife J, Slenter VA, Salata JJ, Michaels DC: Dynamic vagal control of pacemaker activity in the mammalian sinoatrial node. Circ Res 52:642–656, 1983.
15. Rozanski GJ: Atrial ectopic pacemaker escape mediated by phasic vagal nerve activity. Am J Physiol (Heart Circ Physiol) 29:H1507–H1514, 1991.
16. Haissaguerre M, Jais P, Shah DC, et al: Spontaneous initiation of atrial fibrillation by ectopic beats originating in the pulmonary vein. N Engl J Med 339:659–666, 1998.
17. Chen SA, Hsieh MH, Tai CT, et al: Initiation of atrial fibrillation by ectopic beats originating from the pulmonary vein: Electrophysiological characteristics, pharmacological responses, and effects of radiofrequency ablation. Circulation 100:1879–1886, 1999.
18. Chevalier P, Obadia JF, Timour Q, et al: Thoracoscopic epicardial radiofrequency ablation for vagal atrial fibrillation in dogs. Pacing Clin Electrophysiol 22(6 Pt 1):880–886, 1999.
19. James TN, Nadeau RA: Direct perfusion of the sinus node: An experimental model for pharmacological and electrophysiologic studies of the heart. Henry Ford Hosp Med Bull 10:21–29, 1962.
20. Nadeau RA, Roberge FA, Billette J: Role of the sinus node in the mechanism of cholinergic atrial fibrillation. Circ Res 27:129–138, 1970.
21. Zaitsev AV, Rosenshtraukh LV, Fast VG, et al: Study of spontaneous acetylcholine-dependent tachyarrhythmias using isolated specimens of the right canine atrium by bilateral mapping of the spread of excitation [in Russian]. Kardiologiia 29:80–85, 1989.
22. Boineau JP, Schuessler RB, Hackel DB, et al: Widespread distribution and rate differentiation of the atrial pacemaker complex. Am J Physiol 8:H406–H415, 1980.
23. Sharifov OF, Rozenshtraukh LV, Zaitsev AV, et al: Comparison of atrial premature depolarization topography during vagal stimulation and humoral acetylcholine administration [in Russian]. Ross Fiziol

Zh Im I M Sechenova 84(11):1174–1190, 1998.
24. Schmitt C, Ndrepera G, Weber S, et al: Biatrial multisite mapping of atrial premature complexes triggering onset of atrial fibrillation. Am J Cardiol 89:1381–1387, 2002.
25. Schuessler RB, Grayson TM, Bromberg BI, et al: Cholinergically mediated tachyarrhythmias induced by a single extrastimulus in the isolated canine right atrium. Circ Res 71:1254–1267, 1992.
26. Allessie MA, Bonke IM, Schopman FJ: Circus movement in rabbit atrial muscle as a mechanism of tachycardia. III. The "leading circle" concept: A new model of circus movement in cardiac tissue without the involvement of an anatomical obstacle. Circ Res 41:9–18, 1977.
27. Sharifov OF, Rozenshtraukh LV, Beloshapko GG, et al: The role of the interatrial septum in development of supraventricular tachyarrhythmias of vagal origin in dogs [in Russian]. Ross Fiziol Zh Im I M Sechenova 84:561–588, 1998.
28. Cox JL, Canavan TE, Schuessler RB, et al: The surgical treatment of atrial fibrillation. II. Intraoperative electrophysiologic basis of atrial flutter and atrial fibrillation. J Thoracic Cardiovasc Surg 101:406–426, 1991.
29. Mandapati R, Skanes A, Chen J, et al: Stable microreentrant sources as a mechanism of AF in the isolated sheep heart. Circulation 101:194–199, 2000.
30. Bettoni M, Zimmermann M: Autonomic tone variations before the onset of paroxysmal atrial fibrillation. Circulation 105:2753–2759, 2002.
31. Sharifov OF, Fedorov VV, Beloshapko GG, et al: "Roles of Adrenergic and Cholinergic Stimulation in Spontaneous Atrial Fibrillation in Dogs", JACC 43:483-490,2004.
32. Schauerte P, Scherlag BJ, Patterson E, et al: Focal atrial fibrillation: Experimental evidence for a pathophysiologic role of the autonomic nervous system. J Cardiovasc Electrophysiol 12:592–599, 2001.
33. Scherlag BJ, Yamanashi WS, Schauerte P, et al: Endovascular stimulation within the left pulmonary artery to induce slowing of heart rate and paroxysmal atrial fibrillation. Cardiovasc Res 54:470–475, 2002.
34. Wang YG, Huser J, Blutter LA, Lipsius SL: Withdrawal of acetylcholine elicits Ca2+-induced delayed afterdepolarizations in cat atrial myocytes. Circulation 96:1275–1281, 1997.
35. Fedorov VV, Beloshapko GG, Yushmanova AV, et al: Effects of ryanodine on atrial fibrillation induced by cholinergic stimulation in the intact canine heart [abstract]. Eur Heart J 22(suppl):334, 2001.
36. Fedorov VV, Glukhov AV, Sharifov OF, et al: Effects of verapamil on atrial fibrillation spontaneous initiation in the intact canine heart [in Russian]. Kardiologiia 41:55–70, 2003.
37. Rosenshtraukh LV, Zaitsev AV, Fast VG, et al: Vagally induced block and delayed conduction as a mechanism for circus movement tachycardia in frog atria. Circ Res 64:213–226, 1989.
38. Vinogradova TM, Yuzyuk TN, Zaitsev AV, Rosenshtraukh LV: Acetylcholine induces local inexcitability in the cells with diastolic depolarization in the intercaval region of the rabbit right atrium [in Russian]. Sechenov Zh Physiol 82:1–19, 1996.
39. Vinogradova TM, Fedorov VV, Yuzyuk TN, et al: Local cholinergic suppression of pacemaker activity in the rabbit sinoatrial node. J Cardiovasc Pharmacol 32:413–424, 1998.
40. Vinogradova TM, Sharifov OF, Yuzyuk TN, et al: Spontaneous cholinergic tachyarrhythmias in the rabbit right atrium. Role of primary and subsidiary pacemaker areas. (Submitted).
41. Chen YJ, Chen SA, Chang MS, Lin CI: Arrhythmogenic activity of cardiac muscle in pulmonary veins of the dog: Implication for the genesis of atrial fibrillation. Cardiovasc Res 48:265–273, 2000.
42. Wit AL, Cranefield PF: Triggered and automatic activity in the canine coronary sinus. Circ Res 41:435–445, 1977.
43. Sakmann B, Noma A, Trautwein W: Acetylcholine activation of single muscarinic K+ channels in isolated pacemaker cells of the mammalian heart. Nature (Lond) 303:250–253, 1983.
44. Bonke FI, Allessie MA, Kirchhof CJ, Roos AG: Investigation of the conduction properties of the sinus node. In Zipes DP, Jalife J (eds): Cardiac Electrophysiology and Arrhythmias. Orlando, FL, Grune & Stratton, 1985, pp 73–79.
45. Mazgalev T, Dreifus LS, Michelson EL, Pelleg AP: Effect of postganglionic vagal stimulation on the organization of atrioventricular nodal conduction in isolated rabbit heart tissue. Circulation 74:869–880, 1986.
46. Allessie MA, Bonke FIM: Direct demonstration of sinus node reentry in the rabbit heart. Circ Res 44:557–568, 1979.
47. Bleeker WK, Mackaay AJ, Masson-Pevet M, et al: Functional and morphological organization of the rabbit sinus node. Circ Res 46:11–22, 1980.
48. Boyett MR, Honjo H, Kodama I: The sinoatrial node, a heterogeneous pacemaker structure. Cardiovasc Res 47:658–687, 2000.
49. Zhang H, Holden AV, Noble D, Boyett MR: Analysis of the chronotropic effect of acetylcholine on sinoatrial node cells. J Cardiovasc Electrophysiol 13:465–474, 2002.
50. Duivenvoorden JJ, Bouman LN, Opthof T, et al: Effect of transmural vagal stimulation on electrotonic current spread in the rabbit sinoatrial node. Cardiovasc Res 26:678–686, 1992.
51. Petit-Jacques J, Bois P, Bescond J, Lenfant J: Mechanism of muscarinic control of the high-threshold calcium current in rabbit sinoatrial node myocytes. Pflugers Arch 423:21–27, 1993.

第七部分
非线性动力学、螺旋波和心脏节律

第 35 章

折返理论

Marcel Wellner, Omer Berenfeld

本章目录

- 简介 313
- 零空间维度 314
- 一维空间 315
- 二维空间 315
- 三维空间 320

除了理论创立者本人，没有人相信理论；
除了实验者本人，任何人都相信实验。

Albert Einstein

一、简介

兴奋波沿一个闭合路径反复传播称为"折返"。通常，路径并不只是一个窄路，其几何学特性是本章和其他章的重点内容。医学上，心脏电激动的折返是一种危险的病理状态。从时间上看，折返是一种周期现象，其频率远远超过窦性心率。正常的电激动并不能折返，因为其路径有始（窦房结）有终（心室底部）。

折返的频率很快，并在一个相对心脏而言很小的地方发生单向阻滞。人心脏中，电激动沿心肌的传播速度大约 1m/s，垂直于心肌纤维的传播速度是 0.3m/s。我们发现，在一个闭合路径中，心肌的传播速度大约 0.5m/s，折返周期大约为 0.1s，折返周长长度大约为 0.05m，相当于直径为 2cm 的环路。

我们对于折返理论的理解还远远不够。然而，其基本特点之一，兴奋波的传播已经明确：它们是非线性现象，即两个可识别的不同的波，不能精确地预测可产生另外一种可识别的波。非线性系统的一个明显的特点是，它对于刺激的反应并不总是与刺激成比例。如刺激心肌或其他类似的可兴奋组织，只有刺激强度达到一个阈值时才能引起组织兴奋。非线性一方面使得人们很难得出总体的分析预测，另一方面，使得这些波的特点多变，常常令人惊讶。那么，非线性源自何处？

要回答这个问题，我们首先要列出影响波行为的因素：（1）边界和接触面的几何形状；（2）在每一个空间点上，每一个边缘点的变量值，此变量被称为扩散率张量，或结合张量，它决定了波如何从一点传播到另一点；（3）在每一点上，各个变量之间相互作用的定律（反应条件或膜动力学）。在微观上，此反应起源于膜离子流；（4）起始条件，即在一个我们认为是开始的时间点，对所有空间点的变量的简单描述。实验中或临床上，通过点电源或除颤器，给予一个外来刺激，实际上已经指明了起始条件。此刺激被称为外源电流。

通常，只有第三点（即介质的反应性，已经在前面讨论过）与其非线性有关。在非反应性介质中，兴奋在空间上扩散，还没有形成波就消失了。相应的，如果没有反应条件（没有传播，见于单个理想细胞），非线性就会存在，并增加了自发震荡的细胞变量，心脏起搏细胞就是如此。兴奋性介质常被称为反应-弥散系统。

除了非线性，在分析兴奋波时，数学家们还面临另一个困难。在处理许多物理系统，如电荷、概率、能量等时，我们应用了局部（微分）守恒（conservation)的特点。这些定律是有用的定性指标，并能为理论公式提供有力的工具。相反，兴奋性介质作为空间分布源（spatially distributed sources）或能量穴（sink of energy）。因此，局部守恒定律并不适用，不能用它来进行分析。电荷守恒尽管本身正确，但在此模型中并不适用，因此不能直接应用。

最后，我们必须提到心脏模型的另一个重要的数学特点，某些情况下，它是有用的，但在某些情况下，则使问题更加复杂。动作电位包括不同时相。上升相持续不到1ms，总的动作电位时程约200ms，两者的比率约为1：200。反映此种不均衡性的数学模型是"不灵活的（stiff）"，需要进行大量运算才能产生可信的预测结果。另一方面，如果利用一个薄层，忽略其中的慢成分，则可对陡峭的上升相进行分析。

人们利用上述工具和方法，来得到经很短时间传播的变量（如跨膜电位）的所有值，对时间积分就能得到人们想要的东西。这是在连续介质中"完全"理论模型所能预期的。

本章内容就是按照这种抽象性安排的。我们按照空间维度的增加来安排题目。尽管心肌细胞是三维的，理论家们还是从模型中的零维度开始依次上升达到现实状态。

二、零空间维度

如果细胞的内部空间结构毫无意义的话，单个分离的起搏细胞极少在零纬度折返中被提到。图35-1A示在这样一个细胞中观察到的电位（细胞来源于窦房结）。同时显示其不远处的一个心房肌细胞的同步活动以利于比较，窦房结细胞起搏并激动心房肌。

研究这些细胞使我们有机会了解其简单动力学原理。在一个典型的传播模型中，我们通过一套变量对心脏某一部位任何一个时间点的状态进行了详细描述。今天的模型可能列出8个或更多这样的变量，包括跨膜电位u以及一系列离子流v1、v2等。在图35-1B的起搏模型中，我们仅仅考虑两个变量：u和v，决定其状态。轨道反映了在此平面上u和v随时间的变化，并未显示时间这一共变量。不同起始状态常常导致不同的结果。我们把轨道看成是携带时相点（u，v）的流体，就像河流携带一个流动的软木塞一样。图35-1B示一个起搏细胞样的自发收缩状态。细胞的一个状态，固定点（FP），理论上在时间上是静止的，但在实际中并不存在，因为它不稳定：很轻微的波动，比如噪声，就能使得时相点变成流动性的，可能到达P2，最后发展为稳态震荡。最后的行为可用有限闭合曲线来表示。有限周期（limited cycle，LC）的时间特点是图35-1A的上一条曲线。同样，从LC外的某一点P1开始，细胞进入同样的稳态震荡。如果心脏功能正常，上述自动行为仅仅见于窦房结。但是，在一定条件下，许多其他心肌细胞能够以低频率自发活动。

反之，我们在图35-1C中显示的是一个更加典型的心肌细胞的时相平面，此细胞可以接受刺激产生兴奋，但通常并不产生自发收缩。也有固定点，但它是稳定的。从这一状态开始，我们从外部给予刺激，使得电位中等程度地增加（部分去极化），时相点从固定点到达一个新的起始点P1，则u就会自动降低，直到重新回到静息状态。另一方面，如果去极化足够强，在P2产生一个新的起始点，则u就在降低前自动增加，产生一个动作电位。这两种状态的区分点就是细胞的兴奋阈值。兴奋性的一个定义就是：最大电位/阈值电位的比值。

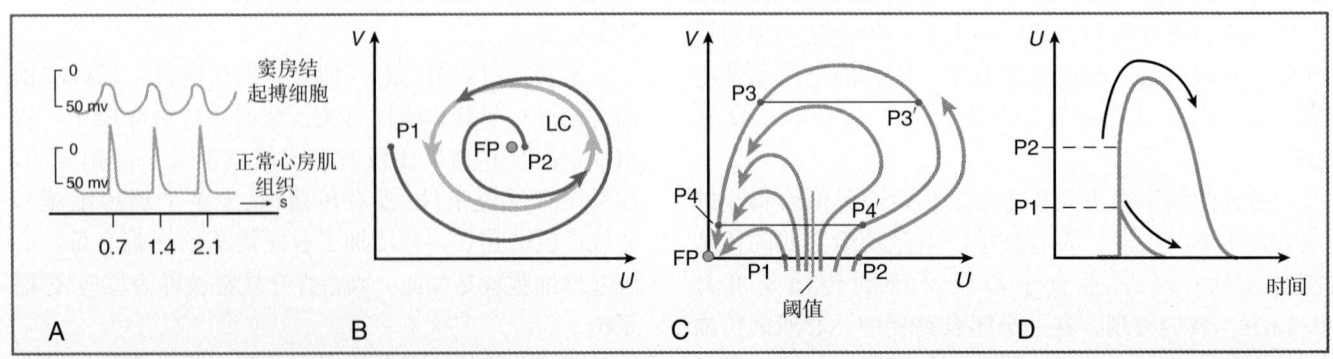

图35-1 A，窦房结起搏细胞（上）和心房细胞（下）的动作电位。B，起搏细胞的相点轨迹。固定点（FP）不稳定，且有一个限制环（LC）。C，模拟细胞的轨迹，FP稳定，且不存在LC，P1和P2代表阈下刺激和阈上刺激。D，阈上刺激P1和阈下刺激P2产生的电势的时间依赖性。

兴奋细胞的另一个特点是具有不应性,也可在图35-1C中看出来。假设在动作电位过程中,时相点位于P3,从P3到P3′,进一步去极化永远不会产生一个新的动作电位(一个已经产生的动作电位的大部分时间都处于不应期)。另一方面,从P4到P4′去极化就会产生一个新的动作电位(在动作电位的末期细胞具有兴奋性),但需要刺激很大,超过从固定点去极化的阈值。图35-1D显示其随时间变化的特点。功能正常的细胞,触发动作电位的刺激来自相邻细胞。我们认为起搏细胞和其他心肌细胞的动力学非常相似。一个足够强的刺激,如果其频率超过起搏细胞正常频率,就能以相同方式兴奋这两种细胞。

三、一维空间

实验中,在可兴奋性心肌组织环中能建立折返[2,3]。如果环很细,其细胞长轴平行于环的圆周,则我们就有一个表,可以比较精确地计算这个周期性运动波的特点,如传播速度。

对上述闭合环路的计算机模拟能提供很多信息[4]。沿环路运动的单个动作电位与沿无穷轨道运动的周期波的周长是相等的。在典型心肌模型中,如果环的周长很大时,激动将达到其最大速度,相反,如果周长减少时,速度和周期都变小。这可用离差曲线来表示(需要指出的是,尽管模型不等同于生理情况,但也随非线性离差曲线而变化)。最后,环的周长变得更小,波开始不稳定,最终电活动终止。在这个过程中,影响激动速度和形状的额外刺激,以及在原来激动周期上产生一个完全不同周期的额外刺激(两种周期并存,形成一个准周期性兴奋),都预示着折返的终止。

如果许多动作电位在同一个环中传播,它们的传播方向必须一致:两个方向相反的波碰撞后就会消失。许多波沿同一方向传播,有很多值得注意的特点。举一个数字模拟的例子,假设一对动作电位在逐渐缩小的环中传播,它们会相互挤压,波的频率就会增加。最后,环只能容下一个动作电位,因此,两个动作电位里有一个必须消失,这就是2:1阻滞。在挤压过程中,两个动作电位受到的影响是不同的,其中之一发生在另一个完全复极化之前,这个提前的动作电位时程缩短,我们就会看到长短动作电位时程交替的现象。

怎样引发或终止一个环路的折返呢?利用计算机模拟,我们可以断开或重新连接回路。由解剖环路引起的房性心动过速可以通过消融,永久切断环路而使心动过速终止。另一方面,模拟的实验电极能否引起折返?存在以下问题:环路上某一点的激动产生顺时针和逆时针方向的波,它们会在环路远端的某一点碰撞并消失(图35-2A)。单向阻滞是必须的,即环路功能上的左右对称必须被打破。这可以用不同点和不同时间的两个激动来模拟(图35-2B)。一旦折返终止,对称性就被打破,因此一个刺激位点就足够了(图35-2C和35-2D)。实际心肌组织中,对称性并不总是起作用。比如,顺时针和逆时针折返可能有不同的速度和周期。

如果整个环路都被波的不应期占据,折返就不存在了。这个区域大体上是动作电位的空间范围,即(APD)×(速度)。由此得到不等式:环周长>(APD)×(速度)。如果我们知道不等式的右边,就能够估计最小环周长和允许折返形成的最小组织长度。我们容易得出一个长的环路中单个激动的动作电位时程和速度。但实际上,折返并不是一维的,动作电位时程常明显缩短,速度减慢。这时不等式仍然正确,但作用不大。人们在小鼠心脏观察到大小为6mm的折返,而这个长度人们以前认为不能形成折返[6]。

一度空间内的折返需要一个传导的闭合环路,这是常识。然而,实验室中也有例外。假设一个开放的线上依次有A、B、C三个片段,B由于传导受损不能传播动作电位,但能在各个方向上传播电信号。在某一个维度上,与B相邻的A点的兴奋缓慢地传导到C点。C点的兴奋又传回到A点,此时A点的兴奋性已经恢复,于是兴奋就循环往复[7]。这一方法在心脏研究中也被用于起搏。

四、二维空间

关于折返绝大多数是指二维空间概念。螺旋波是其最主要的形式,是过去20年来研究的焦点。它不仅是一个数学难题,还有助于我们了解包括房颤、室颤在内的心律失常。二维空间的实际情况如何呢?可兴奋组织的一个薄层可看作二维空间。这一层的深度可能有一个细胞的厚度,如培养的组织,心脏壁的标本也可很薄,被认为是二维的。

首先我们考虑一个闭合环路对应的二维空间,即一个窄的环面。将面临两个因素:(a)基质的各向异性和(b)边缘效应,这两个因素在一维空间中并无意义。

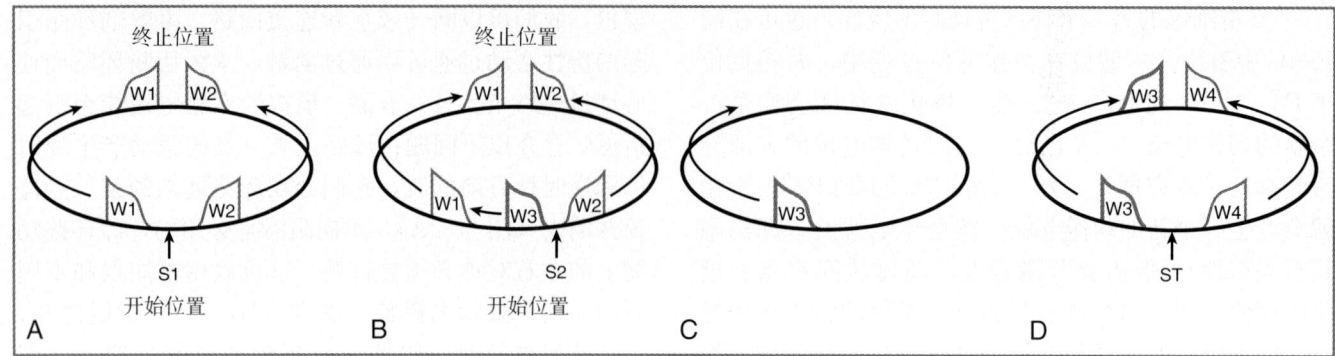

图35-2　A：一个刺激（S1）产生了两个冲动（W1和W2），它在环的远端相互湮灭；B：在W2尾端，于S1刺激后给予另一个刺激S2，只产生一个左侧的冲动（W3），右侧无冲动产生。最后，在W1和W2相互湮灭后W3继续存在；C：单个冲动，W3，有可能终止：在W3尾端给予刺激ST；D：产生单个右侧冲动，并最终与W3一同湮灭

（a）心脏的激动波沿着肌纤维方向（纵向）传播的速度是横向传播速度的3倍，因此波的形状和大小就会受影响，比如，某一点的兴奋就产生一个椭圆形波，而不是一个圆形波。理论上，如果任何一个部分的各向异性被认为在空间上是均匀分布的，则在数学上改变比例就能够将它消除。一个方法就是把速度快的方向压缩，直到两个方向上的速度相等，则椭圆波就变成圆形波。当然，改变比例会使得边缘变扭曲，圆形波变成椭圆波。此时我们认为它是各向同性的基质。（b）很自然地，人们推测在组织边缘恰当角度处的跨膜电流密度为零，既无电流状态或同质性状态，也是我们下面要讲述的问题。如果基质是各向同性的，无电流指的是包括波锋在内的等电位都在恰当角度的边缘处相逢。在一个薄环中，这种效应使得波沿环路传播，如同在一维环路中那样。

（一）转变为螺旋波

以大于内半径的尺寸扩展环的外半径，就会使得环形激动转变为环行螺旋波（图35-3A）。对于沿着解剖障碍物（如血管开口处和非兴奋性瘢痕组织）的折返而言，这种情况可能是一个合理的模型。理论上一个外半径无限远的例子很容易描述。例如某一个等电位，如半最大电位。它给出了波锋（图35-3A中的曲线f）和波尾（曲线t）的定义，并观察到以下特点：

- 激动波始终如一地旋转，其周期（周长）每一次都相等。
- 波锋和波尾在恰当角度的内环相遇（无电流状态）。
- 等电位曲线在外侧衰减，渐近地产生了平面等距离波，后者以单一速度运动，$c=c_\infty$，当从中心处测量时，c要小一些。（注意：c是依赖于定义的，如果基质是各向同性的，c就是正

常方向上波锋的速度。）
- 激动的宽度 $APD \times c$，或泛泛地讲是波锋和波尾的距离，其定义很详细：就半径而言，其半径无穷大；沿着环路测量时，它位于内环。由于APD和c都减少，后者通常要小一些。C的减少如果不是由于中心处波的曲率大而引起，至少常常伴随着中心处波的曲率大。

（二）Wiener-Rosenblueth理论（题外话）

我们为什么会得到螺旋波？作为一种定性的现象，旋转的螺旋波对于兴奋性基质来说并不特殊。它们是局部循环失衡并以有限速度传播入周围空间的产物。随着与循环中心距离的增大，传播信号的时间延迟也增大，形成螺旋周期。在均匀基质中，循环中心为周期性的，在距离中心足够远的地方，我们就认为螺旋波是阿基米得螺旋。正如在一个小圆中晃动水面就会产生旋转的螺旋波。

如前所述，环-孔位置是用Wiener和Rosenblueth于1946年发表的理论来预测的[9]，很久以后才被直接观察到。它适用于单一波锋与边缘垂直相遇，并且垂直于波锋的每一点都有共同的速度c。他们发现，波锋是圆的渐开线，在距离很远时，很难与阿基米得螺旋分辨开。螺旋周期的渐进距离为$\lambda=2\pi R$，R是孔的半径。同样，在一维环路中，$cT=2\pi R$。由于把固定常数简化，WienerRosenblueth理论错误地预测了位于孔边缘无限处波锋的曲率。就今天的知识而言，曲率大于某一有限边缘的波锋不可能传播，事实上，沿着波锋的c是变化的。

（三）转变为功能性折返

把外边缘定义为无穷远，则可把内边缘认为是逐

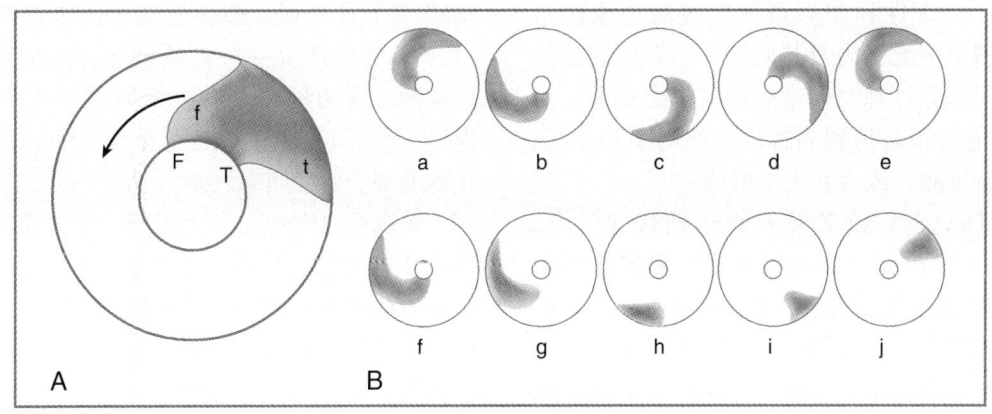

图 35-3 A：当外环增大时，波锋（f）和波尾（t）之间的冲动正形成螺旋（阴影）；B：当内环足够小时（a—e），顶端（图 35-3A 中的 F 和 T）形成了。在"孔"变得更小的过程中（f）及之后（g），出现了分离

渐缩小的[10]。在此过程中，波锋顶端（F）和波尾顶端（T）沿着圆环到达彼此的位置，最后，在环缩小为零之前，融合成为螺旋波的顶端（图 35-3A）。随着环不断缩小，顶端从圆环上脱离（图 35-3B）。在模拟情况下，有两种可能性，这取决于模型的参数，尤其是兴奋性。首先，顶端缩小直到消失。换言之，螺旋波需要一个不消失的中心孔才能存在。第二，即使在孔消失成一点之后，顶端仍以一定的比例缩小。这就是一个没有解剖障碍能自我维持的折返-功能性折返。

在上述的环缩小过程中，有两点值得注意：①在详细过程中，顶端和孔之间的距离可能有一定程度的震荡。②心脏中功能性折返的形成并不需要孔缩小机制。以下我们讨论引起人们很大兴趣的螺旋波的特点。但我们并不涉及多个螺旋波的碎裂，尽管它是一种重要的不稳定形式，一个螺旋波形成许多新的螺旋波。

稳定状态的功能性螺旋波有以下特点：
- 旋转周期 T。
- 旋转中心（固定）。
- 螺旋波的顶端，反映的是半数最大等电位。顶端是曲线最接近中心的地方，其顶端做匀速环行运动。
- 核心，即顶端轨道所在的环面。今天，在某种程度上，核心还是个谜[5]。保护它不受周围的波干扰的机制只有很少一部分被阐明。但计算机模拟可轻松产生此效应。
- 周围的平面波参数，尤其是速度 c_∞。如果某一基质能保持一个稳态螺旋波的稳定，不受小的干扰，则螺旋波就与中心坐标、旋转时相和手征性相匹配。因此，T、c_∞ 和 λ 都是基质本身的特性。
- 螺旋波可疏可密。为了表示螺旋波有多密，我们可以测量在时间或空间中，总循环中动作电位所占的比例（APD/T）。螺旋波密常常伴随兴奋性高：它们常常伴随着比环周长小的核心。

最后，讨论一下位于一个逐渐缩小的无电流的边缘内的功能性折返。螺旋波需要多大的转弯空间以避免相撞？答案是，很小[12,13]。在正方形中的模拟产生的区域比已经减小的核心本身大不了多少，折返可以在比螺旋周期小很多的区域内存在。局限区域内实际的心脏折返也有这些特征。模拟也显示：基质的兴奋性越低，核心被压缩的因素越大，波的频率增加的因素越大。

（四）理论状态

稳态螺旋波的外圈完全可以用平面波的一维理论来解释，其曲率也可用同心波理论来推理[14,15]。当曲率变大时，可精确预测速度的减少：$c = c_\infty -$（正常数）×（曲率），从平面波的模拟中可得到常数值。但人们并不知道如何把曲率-速度关系推广到重要的核心区域。因为，我们知道，周围的波被排斥在靠近顶端的区域之外，很明显，螺旋波理论必须包括核心区域才能成功。过去几年中已经有许多理论想法，在此，我们讲述三种。

- 临界曲率的引入[16]。在临界曲率时，波不再传播，因为其速度降到 0 或接近 0。顶端达到此曲率时，兴奋性波锋不再进入内侧，核心就被保护不受到影响。通过曲率-速度关系，设置 $c=0$，就可以估算曲率。临界曲率-顶端波锋的曲率由下面得到：曲率 $= c_\infty /$ 已知常数。这些由平面波数据得到的特点，在外推时有很大的不确定性。我们也注意到，临界半径（临界曲率的倒数）不能与核心半径相关，而后者是心脏病学家和数学家非常感兴趣的。
- Fife 及其他作者提出的自由边缘（free-boundary）

方法[17,18]推测有两个时间标尺,短长比 ε≪1。我们前面提到,兴奋性和非兴奋性区域的边缘区很薄,模型分别位于此区内及其两侧,交界面的溶液互相匹配。大部分计算与模型的反应参数无关。对于 ε≪1,能够很好地预测螺旋波的周期和形状。核心用一点来推测,或者其大小可调。

- Mikhailov、Davydov 和 Zykov 的运动理论[19,20]。这一方法,包括 ε≪1(尖锐波锋)和稀疏螺旋波,要求曲率-速度关系存在于整个波锋。而且,根据推测,适当条件下,顶端的任何波锋都可以增大,此点形成临界曲率。这样,顶端区域的细节就不必考虑,这比严格的自由边缘计算方法更有计算上的优势。在推测的参数范围内,可很好地预测周期和核心区的大小。

(五)螺旋波的蜿蜒和漂移

迄今为止,我们只讨论了稳态螺旋波。但是,功能性折返在解剖上并没有旋转中心,必须在相对于平移运动的中性平衡中加以考虑。可以推测,在一定的参数范围内,平移运动能够自动发生,而事实确实如此。蜿蜒[21,22]通常是不均匀的,速度慢于波速。其行为可用顶端轨道来解释,而后者的匀速环行运动提示没有蜿蜒。图 35-4A 可使人们对模拟得到的轨道的多样性有所了解。通过计算机和分析方法发现了一部分对应于不同轨道的参数空间盆地(basins in parameter space)[22-24]。对于任何支持螺旋波蜿蜒的参数值而言,后者将变为一种其平移和旋转都很独特的蜿蜒形式。其时相和空间坐标决定于起始状态的特点和时程。参数点进入蜿蜒盆地时,螺旋波(开始只有一个旋转频率)受到干扰形成第二个频率,其频率与第一个不成比例,并产生一个内摆线或外摆线样图形。如果与另一个盆地边缘交叉,就会产生超蜿蜒,一种无序状态。蜿蜒并不少见,可能是心律失常的重要特点。它可把螺旋波带到传导边缘并使之终止或带到传导"岛"并在此停留。蜿蜒过程中,多普勒效应在前向(后向)方向产生一个轻微增加(减少)的波频。人们推测,这两种频率的波相撞会产生尖端扭转型室速,一种心电图上其幅度缓慢变化的心动过速[25]。变化幅度等于两种频率之差。

蜿蜒是自发的,与之相反,漂移是对组织不均匀性或外界刺激的反应。然而,漂移与蜿蜒相同的是,是核心的平移运动。可能引起漂移的原因有:

- 边缘效应,在边缘产生漂移,漂移的方向与螺旋波相反。
- 基质的空间梯度[26]。如临床上药物分布不均匀或缺血程度不一。
- 有效的"缠绕",或局部对流[26,27],仅仅作用于电-电位变量。这是一个最常见的数学模型,在分析梯度效应时很有用。
- 外部以一定的频率对螺旋波起搏。
- 与另一个螺旋波相互作用。

在上面的列表中,梯度、起搏和螺旋波-螺旋波相互作用已经引起了人们很大的兴趣,我们做一简述。

组织的扩散率或反应功能存在空间梯度,这是局部特点。为了简化,我们来看一个各向同性组织中的梯度(如瘢痕)。我们假定一个弱的干扰,其局部空间的变化相比核心的大小要小很多。梯度本身有幅度和方向,产生的漂移也有幅度和方向,并与梯度成正比-线性关系。基质中唯一的方向是梯度的方向,因此漂移的方向与之相同或相反。但明显的是,梯度和漂移之间通常有一个角度,对其解释是:螺旋波的手性破坏了基质的左右对称性。漂移的角度和手性能相互变化。漂移角度不依赖于梯度密度,是未受影响的基质本身的特性。预测在未受影响的基质内的漂移仍需要复杂的工作。

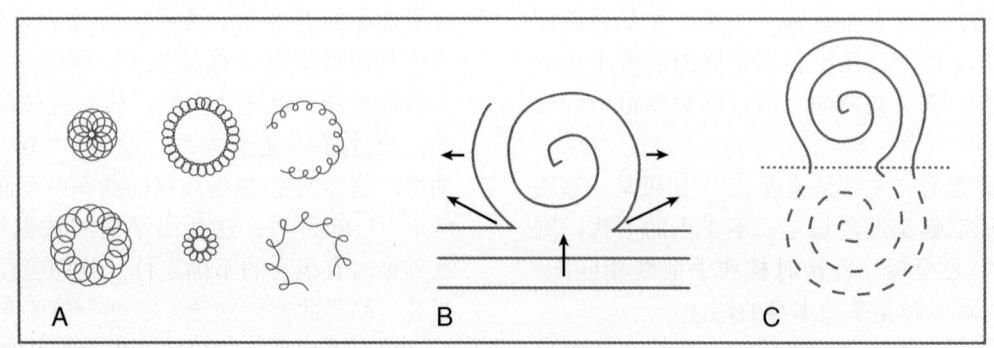

图 35-4 A:蜿蜒时顶端可能的轨道;B:平面波及螺旋波相融合;C:螺旋波与直平面相互作用(点线),加上螺旋波的几何反射(实线),实际上等同于一个"8"字形折返

重新回到均匀基质，我们讨论一下稳态螺旋波的周期 Ts 和朝向螺旋波运动的、起搏的周期性平面波的起搏周期 Tp[12,28]。来源于这两点的波锋碰撞后，各自把对方驱散开，产生一个扩展缝隙（图 35-4B）。如果 Ts 大于 Tp，则连续的碰撞将螺旋波剥得像一个洋葱，直到一个偶然的波锋到达核心。此后每一个后续的螺旋波都轻微地使核心偏移，随着时间的延长就产生了漂移。也有横向漂移。相反，如果 Ts 小于 Tp，螺旋波变得越来越紧，其核心受紧密螺旋的保护，并不漂移。用高频率把螺旋波推向边缘可终止之，但迄今为止在临床上并不可行。

一种前面所述的机制使得高频螺旋波把低频螺旋波推开。但我们知道，两种不同频率的螺旋波要共存，其核心区的组织参数必须不同，某些情况下，由此产生的空间梯度有利于产生漂移。

组织标本和计算机模拟中可产生两个受性相反的螺旋波，彼此互为镜像并持续存在[29]。这一系统被称为八面体折返，其特点等同于一个与直线无电流边缘相互作用的单个螺旋波。边缘就是产生另一个螺旋波的"镜面"（图 35-4C）。通常，单个螺旋波相对于边缘做稳定漂移，由此论证了没有任何边缘的、漂移的八面体是存在的。

漂移也可产生于起搏。干扰，可能是来源于螺旋波平面恰当角度的移动电场，覆盖了整个基质。干扰

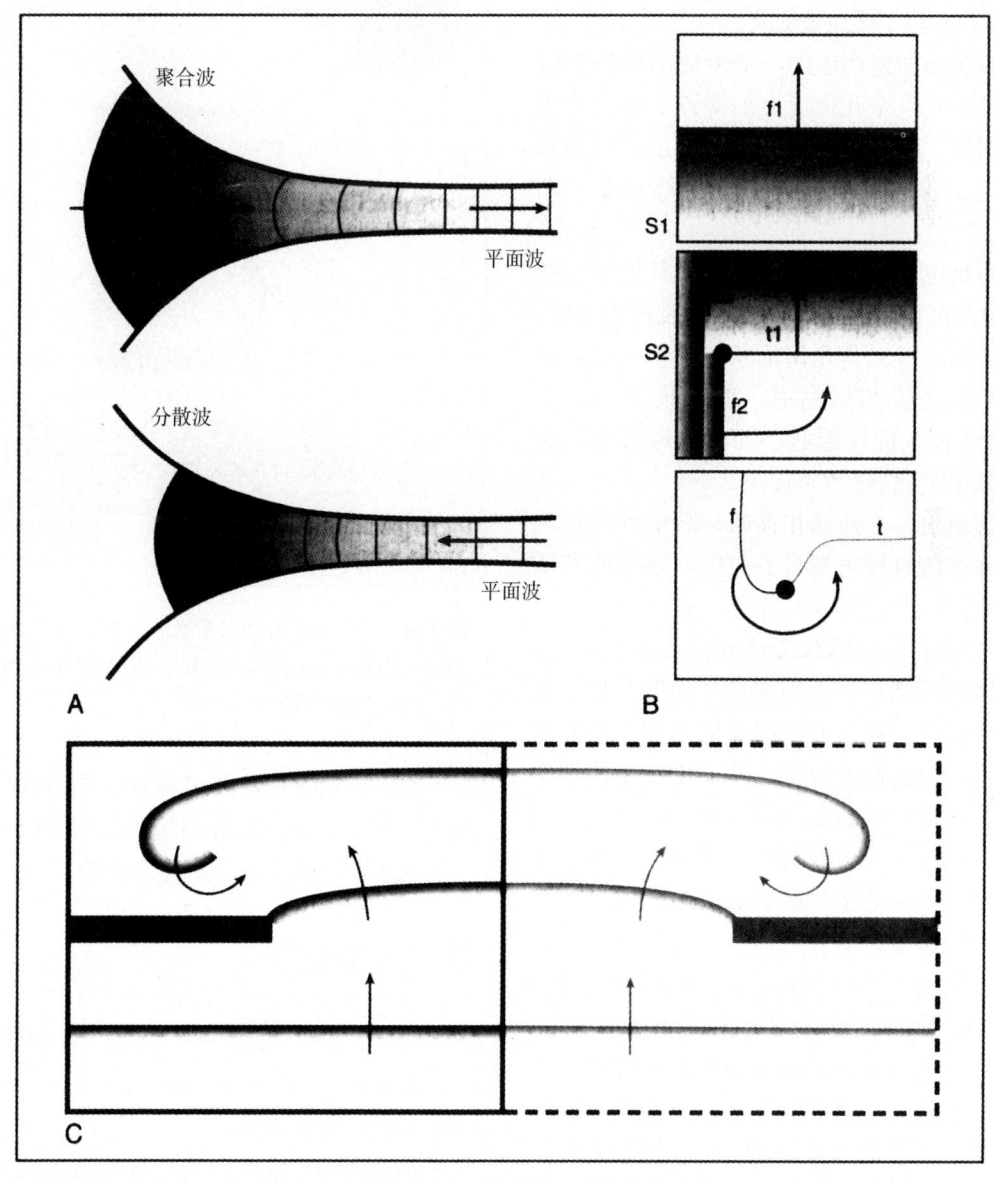

图 35-5　A，拥有无流动内壁的漏斗可以产生波的单向阻滞。如前所述，聚合波锋移动快，易于扩散，在此例中，分离波锋沿相反方向运动，到达其临界曲线并不再扩散。B，交叉部位刺激有 3 个阶段。S1 刺激产生一个向上的平面波锋（f1）（上），然后 S2 刺激产生一个向右的 f2（中），尾部（t1）上面的区域是不应期。最后，f2 成为一个螺旋波（f）（此处显示是在约 180°转身后），螺旋波的尾端（t）也显示了。C，障碍物使波破裂，从而产生一个螺旋波。与其右侧的物理学镜像一起，在障碍物之间形成沟或峡，产生了两个方向相反的螺旋波（8 字形）

和螺旋波的频率匹配时，就会产生直线漂移。如果基质存在各向异性，基质中就没有优先方向了，则漂移的方向取决于螺旋波与干扰的相对时相。如果频率匹配不完全，则漂移的轨道是圆形的。

（六）折返的起始和终止

沿着一个闭合环路的折返通常需要环路中存在单向阻滞。阻滞可以是功能性的，如图35-2中的一维例子，也可以是解剖性的，如图35-5A。在此机制中有两个原理：边缘为无电流几何体系，存在临界波锋曲率。我们注意到，高频率波可能被阻滞，而低频率波不会，就是因为上述两个原理，而且高频率时，波的速度降低。因此，即使在健康心脏，当高频率起搏时，一些潜在折返也会被激活，这在实验中已经被证实。

功能性螺旋波是如何产生的？最重要的条件是波的碎裂，即波锋存在一个几何学上的终点，能变成螺旋波的顶端。同样，这可以是功能性的，也可以是解剖上的。功能上的例子是实验中的交叉场刺激（图35-5B）。

几何学障碍物也能产生自由螺旋波，其机制与图35-5A类似，也与前面所叙述的顶端从孔脱离相类似。图35-5C是其简单示意。其几何形状有很多变化，如图35-5C，当与其镜像相粘贴时，就表现为被称为"峡部"的几何学和八面体形状。而且，螺旋波是在一个足够高的频率下偶然产生的。

当螺旋波蜿蜒与一个边缘相撞时，功能性螺旋波可自发终止。并非所有撞击都是有效的，在某些基质中，边缘把螺旋波推开或改变其漂移（被一个无电流的壁终止等同于两个八面体螺旋波相撞而消失）。如前所述，朝向边缘的漂移可由周期性平面波产生。如果药物改变了膜参数，螺旋波变得难以维持，最后也会终止。实际上，功能性折返很强壮，可在拓扑学中找到答案：波锋可被看成是曲线的一部分，必定有两个终点，一个在边缘，并沿着边缘运动，另一个在螺旋波的顶端。边缘的一个适当的刺激能够剥离波锋并使之产生第二个螺旋波，后者可能会也可能不会与第一个螺旋波共同消失。另一方面，靠近核心的刺激不会产生任何反应，因为只有顶端完全不能到达边缘，螺旋波才能终止。与一维环路的比较是很有趣的。在一维环路中，一点的刺激能够终止折返，与之对应的是二维空间中沿着螺旋的线性刺激，但在现实中并不存在。它也可在某一点上与螺旋波相遇，但很可能是错的。这样得到的碎裂波产生两个终点，即两个螺旋

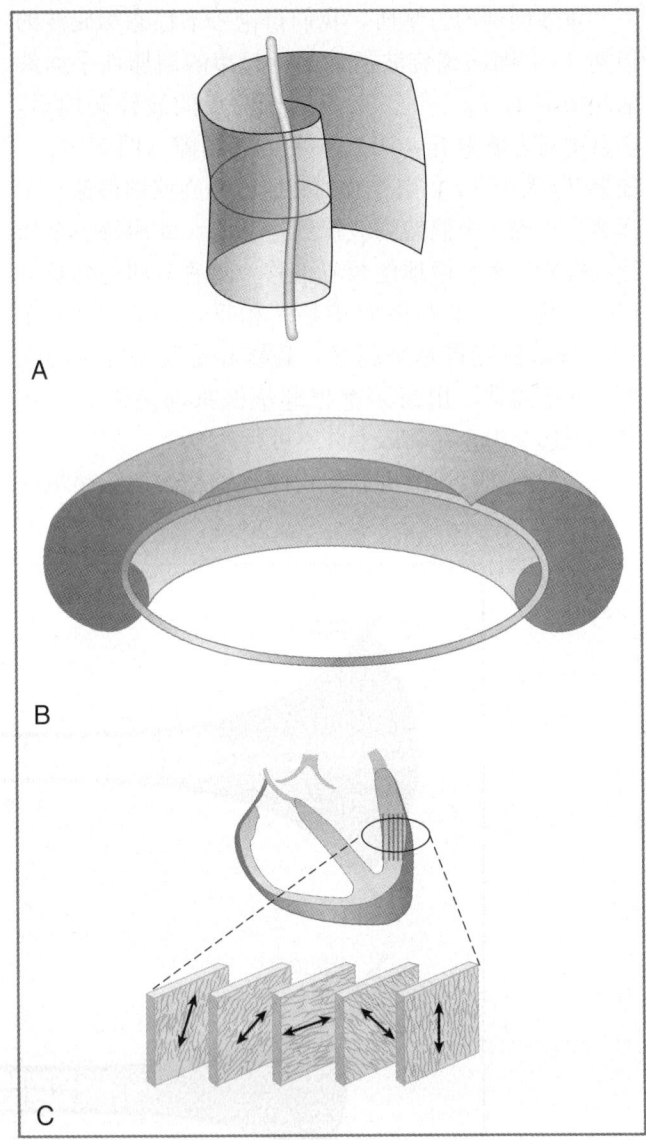

图35-6　A：卷形波是一系列螺旋波，而螺旋波围绕其旋转的轴，则是一系列核心；B：一个卷形环中的轴可以闭合。C：心肌纤维扭曲的各向异性

波。值得注意的是，许多房颤的模型就有多个螺旋波碎裂[11,30]。相反，标准的除颤就是即刻给予整个心脏一个刺激，但其机制并不完全清楚。

五、三维空间

我们在此仅仅做一个简述，详细请看第38章。人们普遍认为，卷形波（scroll）在心律失常、尤其是颤动中起了重要作用。

卷形波的三维对应物是螺旋波，其基础是一堆连续的螺旋波（图35-6A、B）。堆起来的核心所形成的静止管是卷形波的轴，卷形波围绕它旋转。如前所

述，心肌是各向异性的，在并不太大的区域内，可以认为在平行于壁表面的各层中是均匀的。在各层中纤维改变方向，但仍平行于壁表面[31]（图 35-6C）。心室壁，从心外膜到心内膜的纤维方向可旋转 120°。因此，与二维空间不同，三维空间的各向异性不能简单地利用数学方法从传播模型中去除，而且，各向异性对于卷形波的漂移运动及其轴的平衡状态有重要影响。

轴可以打开，即它有两个终点，总是位于边缘。如果纤维沿着一个无电流边缘运动，轴就会在恰当的角度与边缘相遇。轴本身可以关闭，就像在卷形波环中一样（图 35-6B）。卷形波有以下有用的特点：

- 轴的形状，包括其曲率和扭矩。
- 轴终点的位置。
- 闭合轴的拓扑学：可以是一个结，也可以与其他轴相连。
- 卷形波的即刻扭曲，这是其连续螺旋波横断面的时相沿着轴变化的速度。可见，轴是卷形波的一个重要特点，是其骨架。螺旋波横断面的其他特点见我们有关二维空间的讨论。

作为本章的总结，我们列出了以下深受人们重视的卷形波理论：

- 卷形波对心脏几何学，尤其是边缘的反应；各向异性-扭曲、弯曲或不连续性[32]；弥散或反应参数的梯度。
- 卷形波本身扭曲的机制，以及扭曲如何与轴的扭矩相互作用。
- 卷形波对起搏或其他刺激的反应；颤动理论。
- 卷形波在不同模型中不稳定性的特点；一些不稳定性是轴的漂移或瓦解，或新的轴的产生，如同多个轴碎裂一样[11,30]。
- 具有不平常拓扑结构的轴和边缘[33-35]。
- 轴末端的几何学特点[36-38]。
- 平衡轴的形状和位置[39-41]。

所有这些努力的目的就是要了解颤动和除颤，而迄今为止，这一目的还只是部分达到了。

（李 春 译）

参 考 文 献

1. Plonsey R: Electrocardiography. In Plonsey R: Bioelectric Phenomena. New York, McGraw-Hill, 1969.
2. Bernstein RC, Frame LH: Ventricular reentry around a fixed barrier: Resetting with advancement in an in vitro model. Circulation 81:267–280, 1990.
3. Fei H, Yazmajian D, Hanna MS, Frame LH: Termination of reentry by lidocaine in the tricuspid ring in vitro: Role of cycle-length oscillation, fast use-dependent kinetics, and fixed block. Circ Res 80:242–252, 1997.
4. Courtemanche M, Glass L, Keener JP: Instabilities of a propagating pulse in a ring of excitable media. Phys Rev Lett 70:2182–2185, 1993.
5. Beaumont J, Davidenko N, Davidenko JM, Jalife J: Spiral waves in two-dimensional models of ventricular muscle: Formation of a stationary core. Biophys J 75:1–14, 1998.
6. Vaidya D, Morley GE, Samie FH, Jalife J: Reentry and fibrillation in the mouse heart: A challenge to the critical mass hypothesis. Circ Res 85:174–181, 1999.
7. Jalife J, Moe GK. Excitation, conduction, and reflection of impulses in isolated bovine and canine cardiac Purkinje fibers. Circ Res 49:233–247, 1981.
8. Antzelevitch C, Bernstein MJ, Feldman HN, Moe GK: Parasystole, reentry, and tachycardia: A canine preparation of cardiac arrhythmias occurring across inexcitable segments of tissue. Circulation 68:1101–1115, 1983.
9. Wiener N, Rosenblueth A: The mathematical formulation of the problem of conduction of impulses in a network of connected excitable elements, specifically in cardiac muscle. Arch Inst Cardiol Mex 16:205–265, 1946.
10. Pertsov AM, Ermakova EA, Panfilov AV: Rotating spiral waves in a modified FitzHugh-Nagumo model. Physica D 14:117–124, 1984.
11. Panfilov AV, Pertsov AM: Ventricular fibrillation: Evolution of the multiple-wavelet hypothesis. Philos Trans R Soc Lond A 359:1315–1325, 2001.
12. Ermakova EA, Pertsov AM: Interaction of rotating spiral waves with a boundary. Biofizika 31:932–940, 1986.
13. Beaumont J, Jalife J: Rotors and Spiral Waves in Two Dimensions. In Zipes DP, Jalife J (eds): Cardiac Electrophysiology: From Cell to Bedside. Philadelphia, WB Saunders, 2000.
14. Pertsov AM, Wellner M, Jalife J: Eikonal relation in highly dispersive excitable media. Phys Rev Lett 78:2656–2659, 1997.
15. Wellner M, Pertsov AM: Generalized eikonal equation in excitable media. Phys Rev E 55:7656–7661, 1997.
16. Cabo C, Pertsov AM, Davidenko JM, Jalife J: Electrical turbulence as a result of the critical curvature for propagation in cardiac tissue. Chaos 8:116–126, 1998.
17. Fife PC: Propagator-Controller Systems and Chemical Patterns. In Vidal C, Pacault A (eds): Non-Equilibrium Dynamics in Chemical Systems. New York, Springer, 1984.
18. Margerit D, Barkley D: Cookbook asymptotics for spiral and scroll waves in excitable media. Chaos 12:636–649, 2002.
19. Mikhailov AS, Davydov VA, Zykov VS: Complex dynamics of spiral waves and motion of curves. Physica D 70:1–39, 1994.
20. Elkin YuE, Biktashev VN, Holden AV: On the movement of excitation wave breaks. Chaos Solitons Fractals 9:1597–1610, 1998.
21. Otani NF: A primary mechanism for spiral wave meandering. Chaos 12:829–842, 2002.
22. Barkley D: Spiral Meandering. In Kapral R, Showalter K (eds): Chemical Waves and Patterns. Dordrecht, Kluwer, 1995.
23. Winfree AT: Varieties of spiral-wave behavior: An experimentalist's approach to the theory of excitable media. Chaos 1:303–334, 1991.
24. Roth BJ: Meandering of spiral waves in anisotropic cardiac tissue. Physica D 150:127–136, 2001.
25. Gray RA, Jalife J, Panfilov AV, et al: Nonstationary vortexlike reentrant activity as a mechanism of polymorphic ventricular tachycardia in the isolated rabbit heart. Circulation 91:2454–2469, 1995.
26. Wellner M, Pertsov AM, Jalife J: Spiral drift and core properties. Phys Rev E 59:5192–5204, 1999.
27. Krinsky VI, Hamm E, Voignier V: Dense and sparse vortices in excitable media drift in opposite directions in electrical field. Phys Rev Lett 76:3854–3857, 1996.
28. Gottwald G, Pumir A, Krinsky VI: Spiral wave drift induced by stimulating wave trains. Chaos 11:487–494, 2001.
29. Ermakova EA, Pertsov AM, Shnol EE: On the interaction of vortices in two-dimensional active media. Physica D 40:185–195, 1989.
30. Fenton FH, Cherry EM: Multiple mechanisms of spiral wave breakup in a model of cardiac electrical activity. Chaos 12:852–892, 2002.
31. LeGrice IJ, Smaill BH, Chai LZ, et al: Laminar structure of the heart: Ventricular myocyte arrangement and connective tissue archi-

tecture in the dog. Am J Physiol 269:H571–H582, 1995.
32. Wellner M, Berenfeld O, Pertsov AM: Predicting filament drift in twisted anisotropy. Phys Rev E 61:1845–1850, 2000.
33. Winfree AT: Stable particle-like solutions to the nonlinear wave equations of three-dimensional excitable media. SIAM Rev 32:1–53, 1990.
34. Winfree AT: Persistent tangled vortex rings in generic excitable media. Nature 371:233–236, 1994.
35. Keener JP, Tyson JJ: The dynamics of scroll waves in excitable media. SIAM Rev 34:1–39, 1992.
36. Pertsov AM, Wellner M, Vinson M, Jalife J: Topological constraint on scroll wave pinning. Phys Rev Lett 84:2738–2741, 2000.
37. Pertsov AM, Vinson M: Dynamics of scroll waves in inhomogeneous excitable media. Philos Trans R Soc Lond A 347:687–701, 1994.
38. Vinson M, Pertsov AM, Jalife J: Anchoring of vortex filaments in 3D excitable media. Physica D 72:119–134, 1993.
39. Berenfeld O, Jalife J: Purkinje-muscle reentry as a mechanism of polymorphic ventricular arrhythmias in 3-dimensional model of the ventricles. Circ Res 82:1063–1077, 1998.
40. Berenfeld O, Wellner M, Jalife J, Pertsov AM: Shaping scroll wave filament by cardiac fibers. Phys Rev E 63:061901, 1–9, 2001.
41. Wellner M, Berenfeld O, Jalife J, Pertsov AM: Minimal principle for rotor filaments. Proc Natl Acad Sci U S A 99:8015–8018, 2002.

第 36 章

心肌兴奋和传导的非线性动力学

Zhilin Qu and Alan Garfinkel

本章目录

- 周期性刺激单细胞的非线性传导动力学 323
- 在一维传导线上波的传播 325
- 二维和三维组织折返的动力学：螺旋波和漩涡波的稳定性 325
- 颤动过程中转变为混乱传导的证据 329
- 基于螺旋波传导动力学的心律失常分类 330

心脏的正常收缩是由起源于窦房结的电兴奋并传遍整个心脏而引起的。心律失常时，局部心肌的兴奋，诸如异位兴奋灶或折返波病理性出现，导致心脏的同步收缩丧失。自从 Moe 和他的同事们[1]提出颤动的多子波假说以来，动物实验已证实了单个或多个功能折返波是心律失常的产生机制[2-6]。

心室颤动（ventricular fibrillation，VF）是以一种有序的方式开始的。Wiggers[7]的研究表明，室颤开始于一个更有组织的短期行为，像是心动过速的习性。特别是最近以来，Chen 及其同事[5,6]的研究已经表明，在室颤的早期，即 Wiggers I 期和 II 期，通过期前刺激可产生一个螺旋波或一对旋转方向相反的波，然后这些螺旋波变得不稳定，并且最终完全碎裂发展为颤动。产生室颤的中心问题是什么因素导致一个折返的螺旋波变得不稳定并碎裂为多个子波？

波的碎裂可由动力学不稳定[8,9]或严重的电生理不均一性[10,12]引起。心脏组织动力学不稳定的主要原因之一是陡峭的动作电位时程（action potential duration，APD）回复曲线和传导速度（conduction velocity，CV）回复曲线。动作电位时程回复曲线就是当前的动作电位时程是前一舒张期（diastolic interval，CI）的函数：

$$APD_{n+1} = f(DI_n) \quad [1]$$

对于 CV 回复曲线也相似：

$$CV_{n+1} = g(DI_n) \quad [2]$$

这两个回复特性是心脏组织的传导发生混乱和螺旋波碎裂的关键，也是从室速（ventricular achycardia，VT）转变为室颤（ventricular fibrillation，VF）的关键。图 36-1A-C 显示的是典型的回复曲线。该篇文章复习有关心脏组织发生的从规律的动力学到不规律的动力学的转变，特别是两个回复曲线的特性。

一、周期性刺激单细胞的非线性传导动力学

动物实验和计算机模拟实验都已反复证实了心脏细胞在周期性刺激时所发生的复杂的传导动力学[13-17]。心脏病学家 Nolasco 和 Dahlen[13]作了最早的研究，他们研究了剥离出的蛙心室肌在受到电刺激时，蛙心室肌的反应，研究表明，当动作电位时程回复曲线的斜率大于 1 时，周期性的刺激产生交替性的变化。Nolasco 和 Dahlen 精确地证明当动作电位时程回复曲线大于 1 时，平衡点是不稳定的。对于一个恒定的起搏频率，方程 1 可被改写为：

$$APD_{n+1} = f(DI_n) = f(CL-APD_n) \quad [3]$$

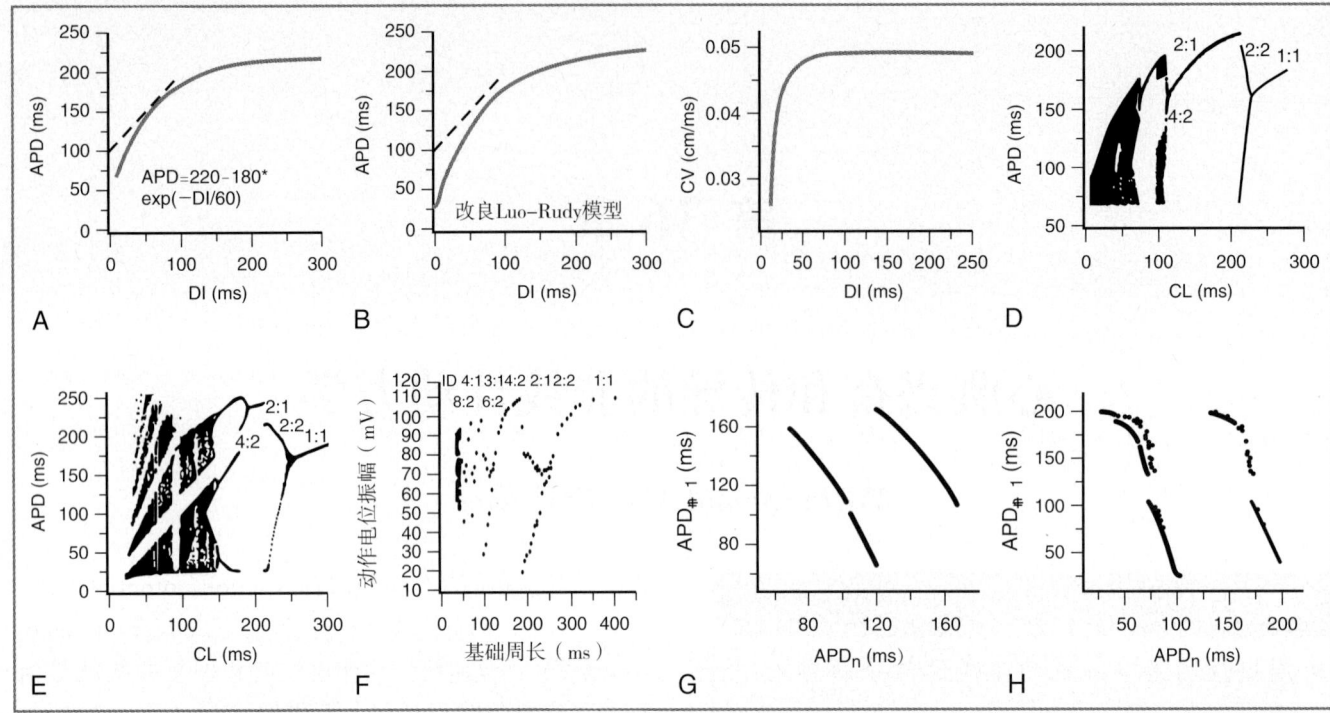

图 36-1 A：动作电位时程（APD）回复曲线；B：改良的 Luo-Rudy 模型的动作电位时程回复曲线；C：Luo-Rudy 模型的传导速度（CV）回复曲线；D：方程 3 的分叉图；E：周期性刺激 Luo-Rudy 模型出现的分叉图；F：由绵羊心脏的蒲肯野纤维获得的分叉图；G：周长（CL）=6ms 时动作电位时程从图 G 转为该图；H：Luo-Rudy 模型，当周长 CL=105ms 时，图 E 转为该图

这里 APD_n+DI_n 是起搏周期，平衡点 $[DI_0, APD_0]$ 满足方程 $APD_0=f(DI_0)=f(CL-APD_0)$。对每一个起搏周长（cycle length, CL），就有一个平衡点位于回复曲线上。现在假定这个平衡点产生了小的紊乱，即 $DI_n=DI_0+\triangle DI_n$，那么根据方程 3，可得出如下结果：

$$APD_{n+1}=f(DI_0+\triangle DI_n)=f(DI_0)+f'(DI_0)\triangle DI_n=APD_0+\triangle APD_{n+1} \quad [4]$$

或

$$\triangle APD_{n+1}=f'(DI_0)\triangle DI_n=-f'(DI_0)\triangle APD_n \quad [5]$$

而点 $f'(DI_0)=df(DI_n)/dDI_n|DI_n=DI_0$ 是平衡点在动作电位时程回复曲线的斜率。根据方程 5，我们能够看到，当 $|f'(DI_0)|<1$ 时，平衡点是稳定的，因为小的紊乱会变得越来越小。当 $|f'(DI_0)|>1$ 时，平衡点是不稳定的，因为小的紊乱变得越来越大。当平衡点变得不稳定时，动作电位时程交替和混乱振荡就会发生。

图 36-1D-F 显示的是回复功能 $f(DI)=220-180e^{-DI/60}$ 由方程 3 得出的分叉图（见图 36-1D），周期性起搏改良的 Luo-Rudy 动作电位模型[18]（见图 36-1E），和周期性起搏绵羊心脏的蒲肯野纤维（见图 36-1F）[15]。这三个例子都表明了相似的分叉结果：1∶1，2∶2，2∶1，4∶2，并且随着周长（CL）的减小，会有更复杂的反应。其中一个重要的观察结果就是传导紊乱仅发生于传导阻滞之后。在这 3 个系统图中，传导紊乱的机制与在转换图谱中紊乱的机制是一致的，这种转换图谱在非线性动力学中有着很好的研究[19]，当传导阻滞发生时，方程 3 必须改写为：

$$APD_{n+1}=f(CL-APD_n), if\ APD_n+DI_{min}<CL,$$
$$APD_{n+1}=f(2CL-APD_n), if\ CL<APD_n+DI_{min}<2CL, \quad [6]$$
$$\vdots$$
$$APD_{n+1}=f(mCL-APD_n), if\ (m-1)CL<APD_n+DI_{min}<mCL,$$

这里 DI_{min} 就是一个刺激引起动作电位的最小 DI，小于这个 DI 时，传导阻滞就会发生。方程 6 与转换图谱相似，因为一个传导阻滞导致 DI，使动作电位时程的转变，也会使 CL 增大。表 36-1G 和 H 表明在混乱状态下方程 3 和 Luo-Rudy 模型刺激的转换图，这个图形类似转换图。混乱发生的关键因素如下：（1）动作电位时程回复曲线斜率大于 1（这就放大了差异），传导阻滞使传导动力学回到较大的 DI 和较大的动作电位时程。

除了前面所述的分叉结果外，当回复曲线可变时，一个双期的分叉就会发生[20]。在这种情况下，在传导阻滞之前，混乱传导就会发生。此时混乱传导的机制与 logistic 图或在非线性动力学中引起双期路线到混乱的单峰图的机制相似[19]。然而斜率大于 1 仍然是必需的。

因为动作电位模型或真正的心脏细胞是一个多维系统，一维（ID）图形如方程 3 就不能完全描述系统的动力学。例如心脏的记忆性就是另外一个影响系统稳定性的因素。Fox 和他的同伴[21]证实在记忆存在的情况下，即使平衡点所在动作电位时程回复曲线那一点的斜率大于 1，这个平衡点仍然可能是稳定的。

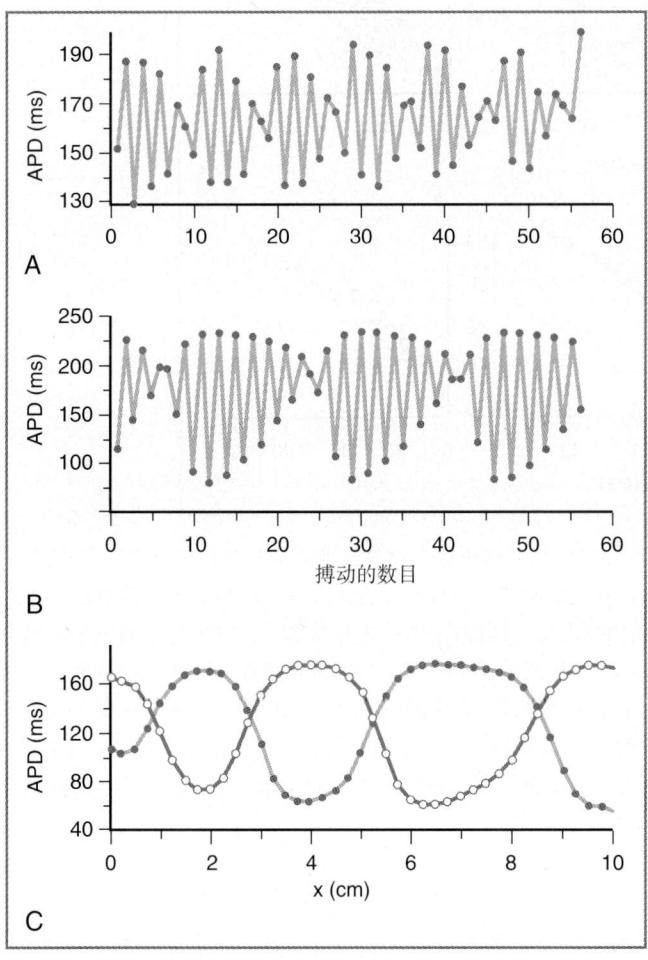

图 36-2　A：在三尖瓣口周围[23]记录到的犬心房组织的调整的动作电位时程；B：应用改良的 Luo-Rudy 动作电位模型[18]从一个相似的环路中记录到的调整的动作电位时程；C：在一个通道中两个连续心搏的动作电位时程空间分布

二、在一维传导线上波的传播

Mine[22]首先证实了在一个环路中的持续性折返。随后，Frame 和 Simon[23]描述了犬心房组织环绕三尖瓣的交替性变化。Courtemanche 和他的同伴[24]以及 Karma 和他的同伴[25]系统地分析了这种准周期的变化。Courtemanche 和他的同伴[24]应用延迟的微分方程证实要让交替性变化发生在环路中，那么在平衡点处动作电位时程回复曲线的斜率必须大于 1。除了这一点，另一种情况也是必需的，即传导速度回复曲线非零斜率的存在。如果传导速度回复曲线是完全平坦的（dCV/dDI），其分支不是 Hopf 分支并且没有准周期性的变化发生。这就说明，动作电位时程回复曲线的斜率决定着交替的发生。但 CV 回复曲线的斜率决定着交替的频率和空间的波长。图 36-2B 表明了在模拟的心肌细胞环路中应用动作电位模型满足动作电位时程和 CV 回复曲线的要求所发生的动作电位时程交替的实例。这与 Frame 和 Simson[23]在图 36-2A 所观察到的结果相似。

对于一个不变的动作电位时程回复曲线，一旦折返环变得不稳定，准周期行为在任何长度的折返环中都会发生，直到传导阻滞发生。但当动作电位时程回复曲线变化时，就会发生从准周期到混乱传导的转变[26]，而在单细胞中，同样的动作电位时程曲线就会导致双期到混乱的转变[20]。

如果动作电位时程回复曲线的斜率大于 1，那么快速起搏一个单细胞就会产生动作电位时程交替和复杂的图形摆动。如果起搏成对的心脏细胞传导线的末端，就会发生不同的动力学现象。最重要的新的现象是空间的不协调交替（见图 36-2C）。这个现象已在动物实验[27,28]和模拟实验[29,30]中证实。产生不协调交替的重要性就在于它增加了不应期的离散性，而不应期离散度的增加是产生心律失常的关键[27,28]。

三、二维和三维组织折返的动力学：螺旋波和漩涡波的稳定性

在均一介质中应用 FitzHugh-Nugh-Nagumo 模型的模拟研究表明[31,32]，当一个螺旋波蜿蜒曲折传导，它的前端形成各种各样花样图案时[31]，最简单的不稳定就会发生。已经证实，这种不稳定是通过一个二级的 Hopf 分支产生的[32]，这就会导致一个准周期的运

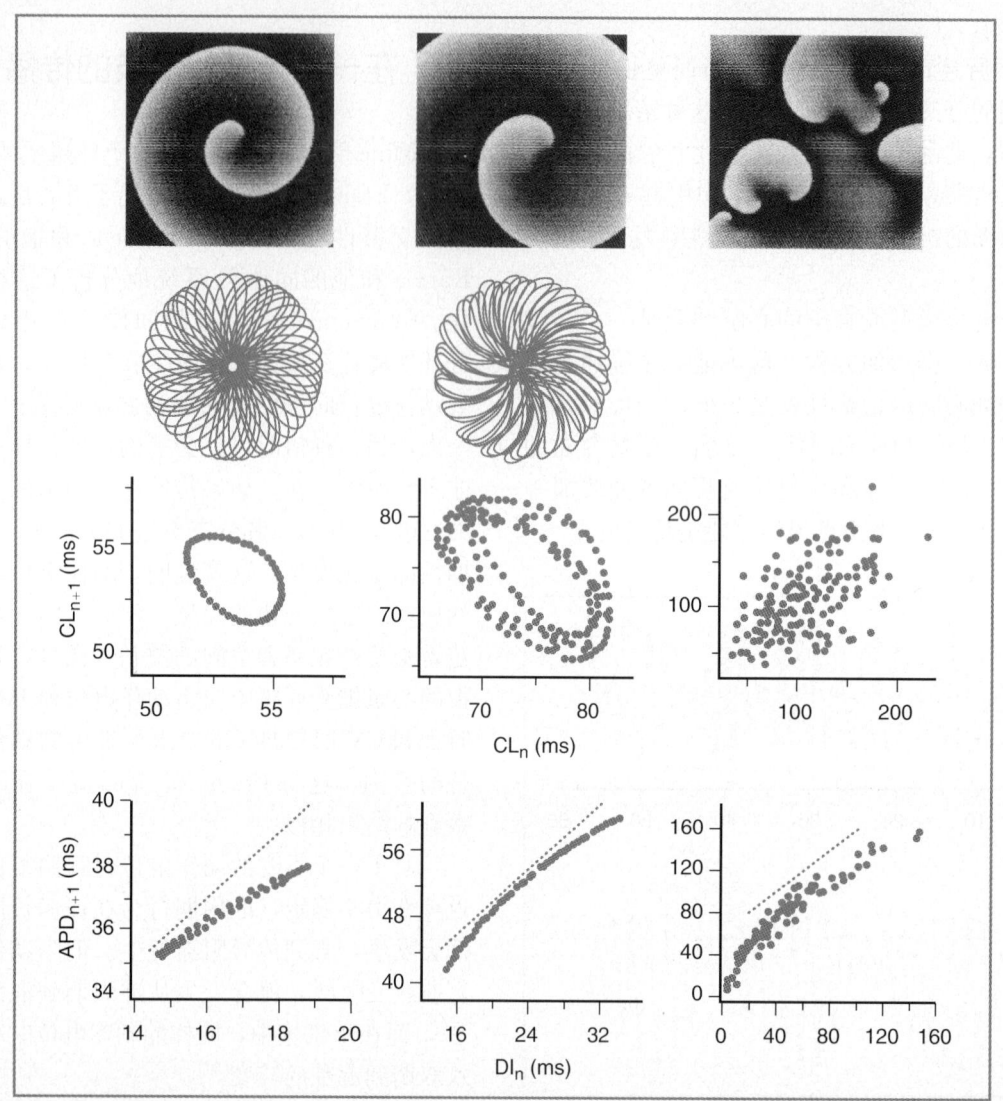

图 36-3 改良的 Luo-Rudy 动作电位模型在二维心脏组织中从曲折传导到混乱的曲折传导到螺旋波碎裂的过渡转变[18] 控制参数是最大的钙通道传导，该通道被设置以产生一个准周期性的曲折传导的螺旋波（左列）转变为混乱的曲折传导的螺旋波（中列）或螺旋波碎裂（右列）。第一行：在一个时间内电压的空间分布照相图。由白到黑的排列分布显示：白色是最高电压，黑色是最低电压。第二行：整个时间中螺旋顶的路径。第三行是空白，因为螺旋波碎裂，许多的螺旋顶被连续产生又被破坏。第三行：以前一周长（CL）为背景在一点上画出周长的 Poincare 图。左图：环形图是准周期性的诊断。中图：模糊的环提示从准周期已经发生了低维混乱。右图：当系统显示多维混乱时，在螺旋碎裂的区域环形消失。第四行：三种状况下 APD_{n+1} 对 DI_n 从二维螺旋波模拟中记录的资料。圆点线为斜率为 1 的参考线。注意在曲折传导时，任何地方的斜率都小于 1，但是在混乱的曲折传导时和碎裂时有些区域的斜率大于 1。ADP：动作电位时程；DI：舒张期

动。下一个转变就是从准周期到混乱的传导，在这个过程中，单个的螺旋波变成一种不规则型传导（这种方式也称为次级曲折传导 [bypermeander][31]，它是一种混乱传导[33]）。这种进一步的转变随即产生一种新的状态，即螺旋波碎裂，在这个过程中，许多的螺旋波不断地产生并且碎裂[34]。

在二维均一介质中用心脏动作电位模型产生的模拟实验[35-39]也表明了上述相似的转变：从曲折传导到混乱的曲折传导到螺旋波碎裂，这种转变与动作电位时程回复曲线的斜率有密切关系。图 36-3 显示了在二维组织使用改良的 Luo-Rudy 动作电位模型下的这种转变[37,39]。它表明当动作电位时程曲线斜率增加时，就会发生从准周期的曲折传导到混乱的曲折传导，然后到碎裂发生的转变。这样，波传导的动力学就会变得更加复杂，正如 CL 回复图所表示的那样（见图 36-3，第 3 排）。尽管对这种不稳定的机制是如何发生的还未作过分析性的研究，但我们基于自己的模拟实验资料试图解释其发生机制[38,39]。基本的观察结果如

下：(1) 螺旋波的固有周长取决于组织兴奋性、不应期和前波的曲率。由于曲率的改变，从螺旋波顶端到螺旋波臂的可激动间隙增加，值得注意的是周期性驱动的细胞其周长是受外部因素调控的，环中的 CL 取决于环长。(2) 假如在选定的 CL 上动作电位时程回复曲线的斜率小于 1，除了在中心部位产生 Hopt 分叉外，螺旋波不会变得不稳定（这就是为什么在一个扁平的动作电位时程回复曲线上能够看到曲折传导的原因）。如果斜率大于 1，波长的摆动就会发生，与在一个环路上波长的摆动是相似的。(3) 在一个环路中波长的摆动是纵向摆动，但对于一个螺旋波，除了不稳定的纵向摆动，不稳定的横向摆动也会发生，这就引起回波发展到"跳动传播"。这种跳动传播引起了局部传导阻滞，从而在组织中形成新的螺旋波。如果局部传导阻滞仅在区域的顶端发生，则会产生混乱的曲折传导，但不会产生新的螺旋波。假如局部传导阻滞发生在波臂，会形成新的螺旋波并发生碎裂。(4) 与在一个周期性的驱动细胞内产生混乱传导的机制相似，只要有局部传导阻滞和陡峭的动作电位时程回复能力，就会产生混乱传导。然而这种混乱传导并不像单个细胞的低维传导，而是多维空间的混乱传导。因此，我们不能用一个简单的一维方程（如图 36-1）去描述系统中发生的混乱传导。

根据动作电位时程回复曲线的形态，螺旋波碎裂可能不是混乱的。例如，对于一个 S 形动作电位时程回复曲线，通过正交场（cross-field）方法诱导一个螺旋波后，这个螺旋波碎裂成许多螺旋波，但这个碎裂过程最终停止，形成一个稳定的系统，Karma 称之为螺旋玻璃[35]。

由组织厚度引起的不稳定性也应该考虑。三维空间的折返波称为"漩涡波"。Winfree[40] 已经表明缠结在一起的漩涡波存在于三维可兴奋组织中，值得注意的是，由三维均一介质的厚度引起的螺旋波的不稳定性可通过复杂的 Ginzburg-Landau 方程[41] 和 FitzHugh-Nagumo 模型[42] 表现出来。这些研究表明，尽管在二维介质中螺旋波是稳定的，但在三维介质中可能会碎裂，导致波的时空传导的混乱，但在正常兴奋性的心脏组织中，没有观察到这种不稳定性[43]，然而在低兴奋性状态下，这种不稳定却可能发生[44]。Wu 和他的同伴们[45] 已经观察到了这种不稳定，他们演示了基线室颤转变为室速，然后室速又转变为其他类型的室速（"慢室速"），这种情况发生在用 Langendorff 灌注的兔的心脏中，当浓度达到 D600 时就会出现。D600 致

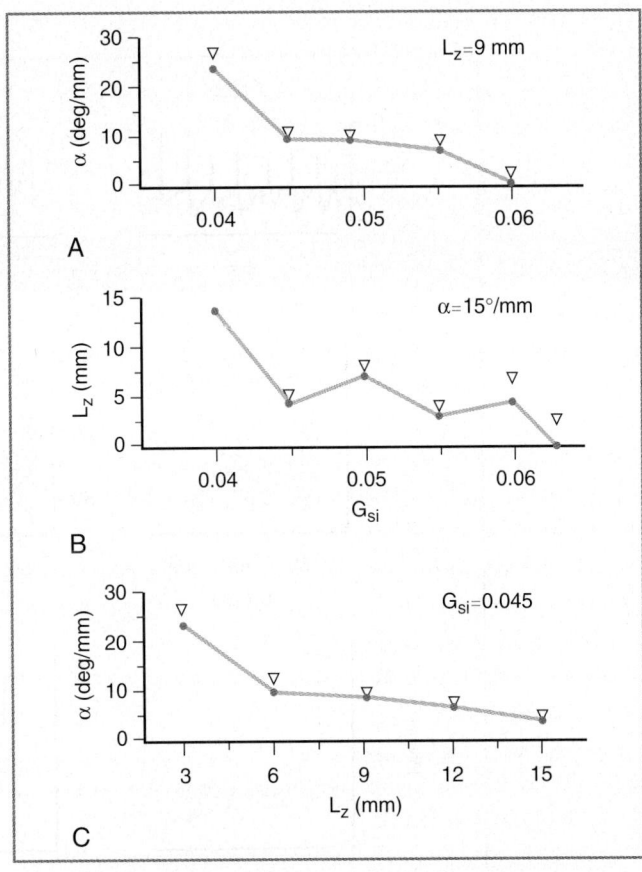

图 36-4 三维螺旋现象和 G_{si}（在 Luo-Rudy 模型中，最大 Ca^{2+} 通道传导，控制动作电位时程回复斜率）、纤维交替率 α 和组织厚度 L_z 的关系 实心圆表示没有碎裂发生，三角形表示有碎裂发生。我们将圆点用线连接起来从而区分出无碎裂区和碎裂区（线以下的为无碎裂区，线以上的为碎裂区）。A: α-G_{si} 参数空间；B: L_z-G_{si} 参数空间；C: α-L_z 参数空间。(选自 Qu Z, Kil J, Xie F, et al: Scroll wave dynamics in a three-dimensional cardiac tissue model: roles of restitution, thickness, and fiber rotation. Biophys J 78: 2761-2775, 2000.)

动作电位时程回复曲线平坦可引起第一个转变。而 D600 引起传导速度减慢（兴奋性下降）从而导致第二个转变。使用河豚毒素降低组织的兴奋性也可观察到同样的现象。

当然真正的心脏是一个不均一的组织，它有各种各样的异质性，包括结构的和电生理的异质性。除了动作电位时程回复曲线的斜率和组织的低兴奋性外，组织的不均一性在折返的不稳定方面可能起作用。在旋转的各向异性的三维模型的模拟实验中表明[43,46]，这种纤维旋转促进了由于纤维丝不稳定引起的螺旋波碎裂。我们已经证实为了螺旋波的稳定性，纤维旋转的效应必须与动作电位时程回复曲线诱导的不稳定性

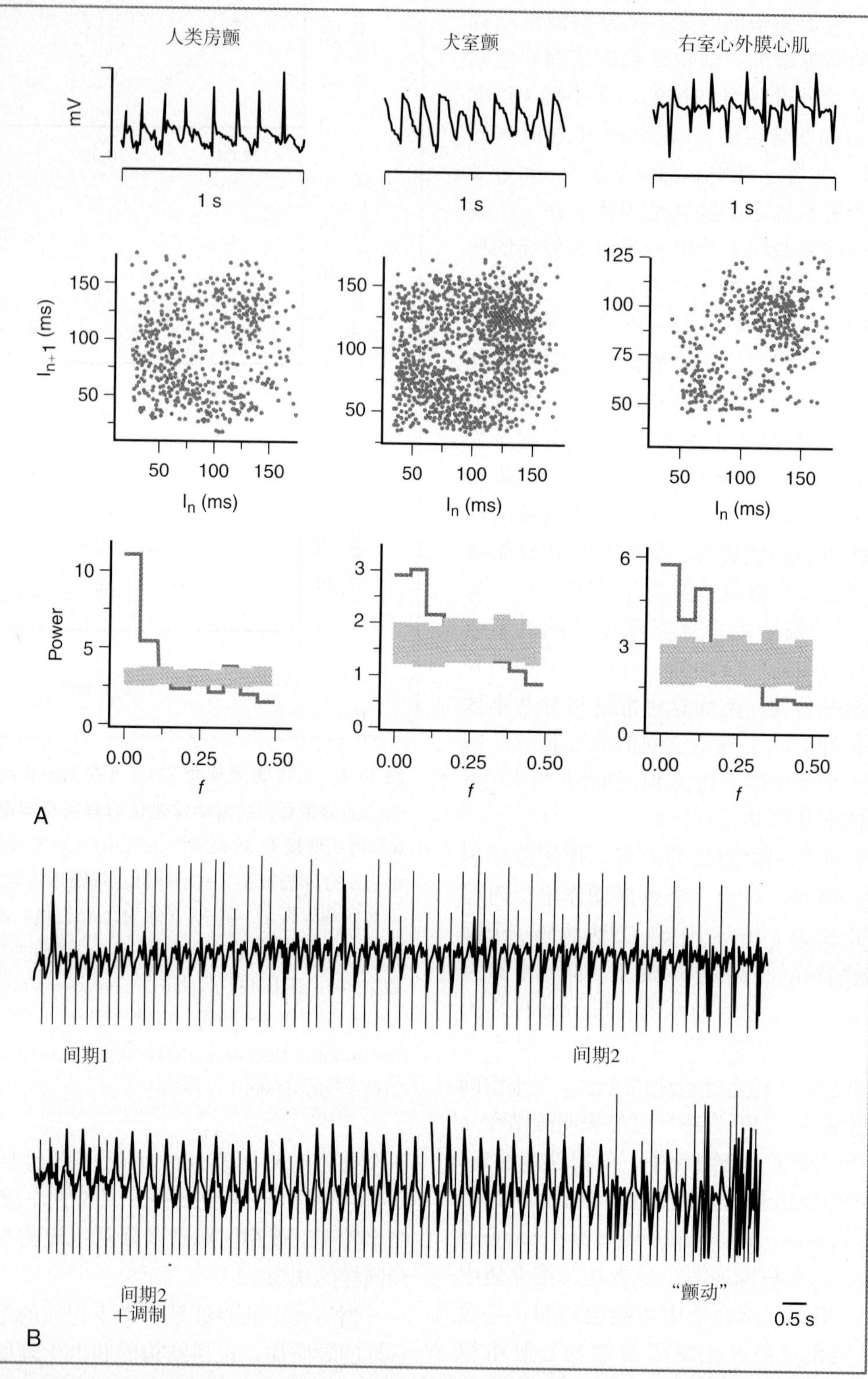

图 36-5 颤动时从准周期传导到混乱传导的证据 A：人心房颤动的心内电活动（左），犬室颤的心内电活动（中），分离的犬心室肌的类颤动（右）。第一行：简短摘录的局部的心内心电图。第二行：从第一行摘出的关于两个间期（I_{n+1} 与 I_n）完整的数据资料的 Poincare 图。第三行：连续间期的傅立叶频谱图。黑线是实际数据的频谱。灰色区域是同样间期的 99% 的可信区间〔（这样在灰色区域以外的黑线上的任何部分都是有意义的 ($P<0.01$)〕。B：颤动发生前即刻准周期的不稳定。将人右室心外膜置于 K^+ 通道开放剂 cromakalim（$10\mu M$）中，记录组织表面电图。注意在房颤开始前即刻出现调制振荡

相一致[43]。图 36-4 概括了最大的钙通道传导、纤维旋转率和促进螺旋波不稳定性的室壁厚度的关系。在 Luo-Rudy 模型中[18]，增加钙通道传导就会增加动作电位时程回复曲线的斜率，这样，传导动力学就会变得不稳定。传导动力学越不稳定，引起不稳定所需的纤维旋转和组织厚度就越小。

在均一介质中除了由陡峭的动作电位时程回复曲线引起螺旋波碎裂外，心电回复和电生理异质性或几何形状之间的相互作用，以及单一的严重的电生理异质性能够产生多个复合的螺旋波[11,12,47]，这与颤动相似。然而最近的研究表明[48,51]，在动物实验中用降低动作电位时程回复曲线斜率的药物能使室颤转变为室速，表明了动作电位时程回复曲线在控制心律失常中的重要性。

四、颤动过程中转变为混乱传导的证据

在周期性驱动的心脏细胞[14,15,20]和细胞的数学模型[16,17]中，已证实了转变为混乱状态的过程。用计算机模拟的一维环路[26]和二维螺旋波折返[38,39]，也发生转变为混乱传导的过程。尽管在急性室颤过程中，寻找混乱传导的直接证据是困难的，然而在动物实验中已取得了混乱传导的证据[52,53]。

当螺旋波曲折传导时，由于曲折传导的周期性调整了螺旋波的周期性，系统被认为是准周期的，当有几个摆动模式同时显示时，系统就是准周期性的。准周期性变化可形成多种方式，最常见的形式是在易变的涡流和螺旋波中发现的，开始是一个单一的频率，与漩涡波的传导动力学相一致。在液体中当发现对流滚动开始时或是在心脏组织当螺旋波开始折返时可见到这种情形。在螺旋波内，随着最初始的摆动波频率或振幅（或两者间有）的周期性调整，出现第二个频率的螺旋波，引起螺旋波的曲折传导。

系统的准周期性是一个重要的发现，因为它可以精确表明准周期行为趋于不稳定。一个准周期系统不能继续增加更多的摆动模式，因为多频率的准周期具

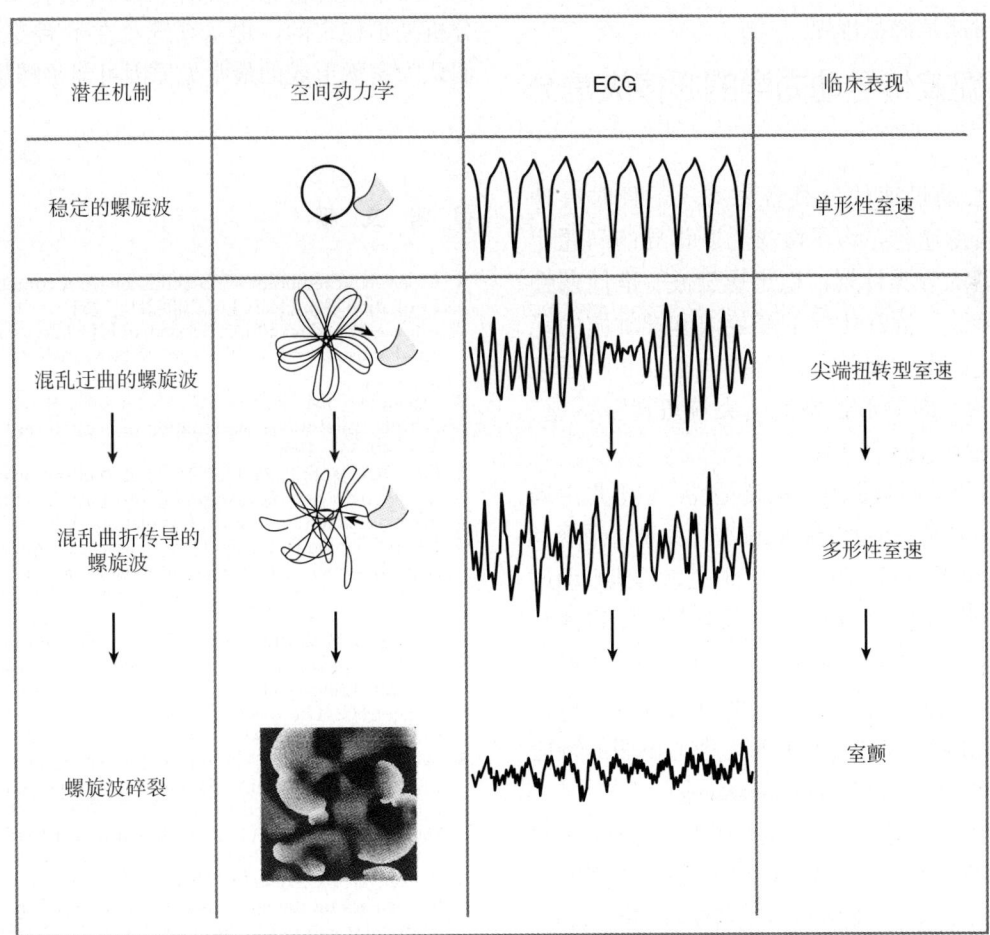

图 36-6 螺旋波表型和相应的临床表现 第一列：螺旋波表型。第二列：螺旋波以灰色表示，螺旋波顶部的路径以实线表示。螺旋波碎裂的路径没有表现出来，因为它是在不断产生和破坏的过程中。ECG：心电图

有内在的不稳定性（三个或更多的摆动模式），并且退化为混乱传导[54]。在心脏组织中，准周期曲折传导的螺旋波已有两个频率，由于回复的不稳定引起的摆动充当了额外的不稳定摆动。

我们研究小组[52,53]已经提出心脏颤动时，准周期传导已转化为混乱传导（图36-5）。简言之，证据如下：三种不同类型的颤动相互作用间期的Poincare图都表明有一个类环状的图形，它是从准周期发展而来，是混乱传导的特征（见图36-5A，第二行）。三种颤动中，相互作用间期的低频调整均有统计意义，它是混乱传导的另一个特征，源于准周期（见图36-5A，第三行）。在制备的心外膜，颤动开始前即刻能够直接观察到准周期的频率和振幅的调整（见图36-5B）。

近来的研究表明[48,49]，在心脏组织实验中，动作电位时程回复曲线斜率的改变，产生了周期性振荡到不规则振荡的转变，表明传导动力学从简单到复杂的转变，在这个过程中，极大可能产生了从周期性到时空的混乱传导的转变。室颤的快速傅立叶转换频谱分析（FFT）[12,55,56]表明有多峰的宽带频谱，提示室颤的潜在动力学可能是混乱传导。

五、基于螺旋波传导动力学的心律失常分类

目前有关心动过速的分类各家不一，且时有冲突。基于四种折返途径，为了解决心脏传导的问题应该出台一个合理的分类计划：稳定螺旋波、准周期性曲折传导的螺旋波、混乱传导的螺旋波和螺旋波的碎裂。我们认为这四个类型问题的解决与室性心动过速的解决是一致的，即单形性室速、尖端扭转型室速、多形性室速和室颤（图36-6）。

单形性室速的机制是折返（也就是说，它不是由局灶活动引起的），它是一个稳定的螺旋波，关于这个观点目前没有争议（见图36-6，第一行）。但是，其他心动过速的机制尚无一致结论。我们建议，尖端扭转型室速与准周期曲折传导螺旋波是一致的，该建议首先由Winfree[57]提出并已在实验中证实[58,59]（见图36-6第二行）。准周期的曲折传导赋予了尖端扭转型室速心电图的特征即逐渐变大和逐渐变小（waxing-and-waning）。

当曲折传导变得更混乱时，心电图图形将失去与尖端扭转有关的周期性变化，出现大小和形态更不规则的宽QRS波群，即多形性室速[4]和室颤（见图36-6，第三行）。

我们认为，充分发展的室颤与第四种螺旋波即螺旋波碎裂一致。但有关室颤形成的确切机制仍有争议。例如有些作者认为[60]，颤动是一个单一的混乱的曲折传导的螺旋波，他们认为，这样一个波在心电图上产生类似室颤的图形，近来提出了VF的"母转子波（mother rotor）"理论[10]，这个理论认为，室颤是由一个快速颤动的波称为母转子波（mother rotor）驱动的颤动传导的结果。FFT频谱分析指出，用单一的频率支配多个范围，就会产生类似室颤的伪心电图。在交替假说中[8,9]，认为是螺旋波碎裂的多重折返。在心脏模型中，螺旋波碎裂，部分螺旋波重复碎裂，形成新的螺旋波已有报道[35,39,43,46]。关键的问题是：螺旋波的碎裂对于室颤是否是必需的？第一，很多研究表明[12,45,49]：室颤过程中，有多个螺旋波。第二，因为室颤一般开始于一个单一的心动过速的螺旋波，我们能够推断有些螺旋波碎裂从单一螺旋波的心动过速产生出多个螺旋波[5,6]。第三，研究已表明在心脏组织中，螺旋波的寿命有限[12,56]，当它们遇到不应期时会自动消失，而这个不应期可由螺旋波本身或其他螺旋波产生或遇到组织结构的不应期。因为螺旋波总是在消逝，它们必须被以相同的频率连续产生，以维持室颤的稳态。最后FFT分析表明[12,55,56]，频谱分析是不稳定的，提示系统总在不断变化。因此，我们认为室颤形成的最常见原因可能是螺旋波的碎裂。

（黄织春　译）

参 考 文 献

1. Moe GK, Rheinboldt WC, Abildskov JA: A computer model of atrial fibrillation. Am Heart J 67:200–220, 1964.
2. Allessie MA, Bonke FIM, Schopman FJC: Circus movement in rabbit atrial muscle as a mechanism of tachycardia. Circ Res 33:54–77, 1973.
3. Davidenko JM, Pertsov AM, Salomonsz R, et al: Stationary and drifting spiral waves of excitation in isolated cardiac muscle. Nature 355:349–351, 1992.
4. Gray RA, Jalife J, Panfilov AV, et al: Nonstationary vortexlike reentrant activity as a mechanism of polymorphic ventricular tachycardia in the isolated rabbit heart. Circulation 91:2454–2469, 1995.
5. Lee JJ, Kamjoo K, Hough D, et al: Reentrant wave fronts in Wiggers' stage II ventricular fibrillation. Characteristics and mechanisms of termination and spontaneous regeneration. Circ Res 78:660–675, 1996.
6. Chen P-S, Wolf PD, Dixon EG, et al: Mechanism of ventricular vulnerability to single premature stimuli in open chest dogs. Circ Res 62:1191–1209, 1988.
7. Wiggers C: The mechanism and nature of ventricular fibrillation. Am Heart J 20:399–412, 1940.
8. Weiss JN, Garfinkel A, Karagueuzian HS, et al: Chaos and the transition to ventricular fibrillation: A new approach to antiarrhythmic drug evaluation. Circulation 99:2819–2826, 1999.
9. Weiss JN, Chen PS, Qu Z, et al: Ventricular fibrillation: How do we stop the waves from breaking? Circ Res 87:1103–1107, 2000.
10. Zaitsev AV, Berenfeld O, Mironov SF, et al: Distribution of excitation frequencies on the epicardial and endocardial surfaces of fibrillating ventricular wall of the sheep heart. Circ Res 86:408–417, 2000.
11. Xie F, Qu Z, Weiss JN, Garfinkel A: Coexistence of multiple spiral waves with independent frequencies in a heterogeneous excitable medium. Phys Rev E 63:031905, 2001.

12. Valderrabano M, Yang JZ, Omichi C, et al: Frequency analysis of ventricular fibrillation in swine ventricles. Circ Res 90:213–222, 2002.
13. Nolasco JB, Dahlen RW: A graphic method for the study of alternation in cardiac action potentials. J Appl Physiol 25:191–196, 1968.
14. Guevara MR, Glass L, Shrier A: Phase locking, period-doubling bifurcations, and irregular dynamics in periodically stimulated cardiac cells. Science 214:1350–1353, 1981.
15. Chialvo DR, Gilmour RF, Jalife J: Low dimensional chaos in cardiac tissue. Nature 343:653–657, 1990.
16. Vinet A, Chialvo DR, Michaels DC, Jalife J: Nonlinear dynamics of rate-dependent activation in models of single cardiac cells. Circ Res 67:1510–1524, 1990.
17. Lewis TJ, Guevara MR: Chaotic dynamics in an ionic model of the propagated cardiac action potential. J Theor Biol 146:407–432, 1990.
18. Luo CH, Rudy Y: A model of the ventricular cardiac action potential: Depolarization, repolarization, and their interaction. Circ Res 68:1501–1526, 1991.
19. Ott E: Chaos in Dynamical Systems. New York, Cambridge University Press, 1993.
20. Watanabe M, Otani NF, Gilmour RF: Biphasic restitution of action potential duration and complex dynamics in ventricular myocardium. Circ Res 76:915–921, 1995.
21. Fox JJ, Bodenschatz E, Gilmour RF: Period-doubling instability and memory in cardiac tissue. Phys Rev Lett 89(13):138101, 2002. Epub Sep 9, 2002.
22. Mines GR: On circulating excitation on heart muscles and their possible relation to tachycardia and fibrillation. Trans R Soc Can 4:43–53, 1914.
23. Frame LH, Simson MB: Oscillations of conduction, action potential duration, and refractoriness: A mechanism for spontaneous termination of reentrant tachycardias. Circulation 78:1277–1287, 1988.
24. Courtemanche M, Glass L, Keener JP: Instabilities of a propagating pulse in a ring of excitable media. Phys Rev Lett 70:2182–2185, 1993.
25. Karma A, Levine H, Zou X: Theory of pulse instability in electrophysiological models of excitable tissues. Physica D 73:113–127, 1994.
26. Qu Z, Weiss JN, Garfinkel A: Spatiotemporal chaos in a simulated ring of cardiac cells. Phys Rev Lett 78:1387–1390, 1997.
27. Pastore JM, Girouard SD, Laurita KR, et al: Mechanism linking T-wave alternans to the genesis of cardiac fibrillation. Circulation 99:1385–1394, 1999.
28. Cao JM, Qu Z, Kim YH, et al: Spatiotemporal heterogeneity in the induction of ventricular fibrillation by rapid pacing: Importance of cardiac restitution properties. Circ Res 84:1318–1331, 1999.
29. Qu Z, Garfinkel A, Chen PS, Weiss JN: Mechanisms of discordant alternans and induction of reentry in simulated cardiac tissue. Circulation 102:1664–1670, 2000.
30. Watanabe MA, Fenton FH, Evans SJ, et al: Mechanisms for discordant alternans. J Cardiovasc Electrophysiol 12:196–206, 2001.
31. Winfree AT: Varieties of spiral wave behavior: An experimentalist's approach to the theory of excitable media. Chaos 1:303–334, 1991.
32. Karma A: Meandering transition in two-dimensional excitable media. Phys Rev Lett 65:2824–2827, 1990.
33. Biktashev VN, Holden AV: Deterministic Brownian motion in the hypermeander of spiral waves. Physica D 116:342–354, 1998.
34. Panfilov AV, Hogeweg P: Spiral breakup in a modified FitzHugh-Nagumo model. Phys Lett A 176:295–299, 1993.
35. Karma A: Electrical alternans and spiral wave breakup in cardiac tissue. Chaos 4:461–472, 1994.
36. Courtemanche M: Complex spiral wave dynamics in a spatially distributed ionic model of cardiac electrical activity. Chaos 6:579–600, 1996.
37. Qu Z, Weiss JN, Garfinkel A: Cardiac electrical restitution properties and the stability of reentrant spiral waves: A simulation study. Am J Physiol 276:H269–H283, 1999.
38. Qu Z, Weiss JN, Garfinkel A: From local to global spatiotemporal chaos in a cardiac tissue model. Phys Rev E Stat Phys Plasmas Fluids Relat Interdiscip Topics 61:727–732, 2000.
39. Qu Z, Xie F, Garfinkel A, Weiss JN: Origins of spiral wave meander and breakup in a two-dimensional cardiac tissue model. Ann Biomed Eng 28:755–771, 2000.
40. Winfree AT: Persistent tangled vortex rings in generic excitable media. Nature 371:233–236, 1994.
41. Aranson IS, Bishop AR: Instability and stretching of vortex lines in the three-dimensional complex Ginburg-Landau equation. Phys Rev Lett 79:4174–4177, 1997.
42. Qu Z, Xie F, Garfinkel A: Diffusion-induced 3-dimensional vortex filament instability in excitable media. Phys Rev Lett 83:2668–2671, 1999.
43. Qu Z, Kil J, Xie F, et al: Scroll wave dynamics in a three-dimensional cardiac tissue model: roles of restitution, thickness, and fiber rotation. Biophys J 78:2761–2775, 2000.
44. Fenton FH, Cherry EM, Hastings HM, Evans SJ: Multiple mechanisms of spiral wave breakup in a model of cardiac electrical activity. Chaos 12:852–892, 2002.
45. Wu TJ, Lin SF, Weiss JN, et al: Two types of ventricular fibrillation in isolated rabbit hearts: Importance of excitability and action potential duration restitution. Circulation 106:1859–1866, 2002.
46. Fenton F, Karma A: Vortex dynamics in three-dimensional continuous myocardium with fiber rotation: Filament instability and fibrillation. Chaos 8:20–47, 1998.
47. Xie F, Qu Z, Garfinkel A, Weiss JN: Electrophysiological heterogeneity and stability of reentry in simulated cardiac tissue. Am J Physiol 280:H535–H545, 2001.
48. Riccio ML, Koller ML, Gilmour RF Jr: Electrical restitution and spatiotemporal organization during ventricular fibrillation. Circ Res 84:955–963, 1999.
49. Garfinkel A, Kim YH, Voroshilovsky O, et al: Preventing ventricular fibrillation by flattening cardiac restitution. Proc Natl Acad Sci U S A 97:6061–6066, 2000.
50. Lee MH, Lin SF, Ohara T, et al: Effects of diacetyl monoxime and cytochalasin D on ventricular fibrillation in swine right ventricles. Am J Physiol 280:H2689–H2696, 2001.
51. Banville I, Gray RA: Effect of action potential duration and conduction velocity restitution and their spatial dispersion on alternans and the stability of arrhythmias. J Cardiovasc Electrophysiol 13:1141–1149, 2002.
52. Garfinkel A, Chen PS, Walter DO, et al: Quasiperiodicity and chaos in cardiac fibrillation. J Clin Invest 99:305–314, 1997.
53. Kim YH, Garfinkel A, Ikeda T, et al: Spatiotemporal complexity of ventricular fibrillation revealed by tissue mass reduction in isolated swine right ventricle. Further evidence for the quasiperiodic route to chaos hypothesis. J Clin Invest 100:2486–2500, 1997.
54. Ruelle D, Takens F: On the nature of turbulence. Commun Math Phys 20:167–192, 1971.
55. Choi BR, Liu T, Salama G: The distribution of refractory periods influences the dynamics of ventricular fibrillation. Circ Res 88:E49–E58, 2001.
56. Choi BR, Nho W, Liu T, Salama G: Life span of ventricular fibrillation frequencies. Circ Res 91:339–345, 2002.
57. Winfree AT: Electrical instability in cardiac muscle: Phase singularities and rotors. J Theor Biol 138:353–405, 1989.
58. Asano Y, Davidenko JM, Baxter WT, et al: Optical mapping of drug-induced torsades de pointes in the isolated rabbit heart. J Am Coll Cardiol 27:24A, 1996.
59. El-Sherif N, Caref EB, Yin H, Restivo M: The electrophysiological mechanism of ventricular arrhythmias in the long QT syndrome: Tridimensional mapping of activation and recovery patterns. Circ Res 79:474–492, 1996.
60. Gray RA, Jalife J, Panfilov AV, et al: Mechanisms of cardiac fibrillation. Science 270:1222–1225, 1995.

第 37 章

二维空间的旋转子和螺旋波

Leslie Tung，*Nenad Bursac*，*Felipe Aguel*

本章目录

- 二维折返模型 ………… 332
- 二维折返的常见类型 ………… 333
- 螺旋的开始和边界的作用 ………… 336
- 加速和增殖的旋转波 ………… 336
- 多边界的旋转子 ………… 337
- 总结 ………… 339

折返机制所致的心律失常是最常见并且具有潜在致死性的心律失常。折返型心律失常可以有功能学和解剖学的基础。解剖学意义上的折返指的是环绕解剖阻滞区（指的是在任何情况下都无法兴奋的组织，占据一定的解剖区域，与周围组织有明显的分界）的环形通路。这种类型的折返通常在定义上指的是组织学上的折返环路。比如：常见的折返发生在围绕浦肯野纤维、束支、房室结以及三尖瓣环周围的肌肉等组织。另外一种折返是功能学意义上的折返。该类型折返通常并不需要环绕中央解剖阻滞区，却是许多房性和室性心律失常以及颤动的内在机制。功能性折返的机制常常被描述为大折返、螺旋波、8字形折返以及各向异性折返。所有这些折返形式都可以被认为是螺旋波的不同表现形式。这些螺旋波表现为可兴奋的、可以重复的以及可自行中止的循环扩布。在兴奋中不同的折返形式相互融合。这种不同形式的折返的相互融合取决于细胞兴奋或不应期特性的联合或融合。

以上所有这些现象是二维折返的基本特点。与三维空间的折返明显不同。实验和理论研究均是在二维空间中进行的，实验所研究的空间范围为1~2cm，刚好可以完成动态和不中断的折返环路。折返环路的边界阻止外来的螺旋波的波锋打入并干扰正在进行研究的二维系统折返波。缺少三维空间也有助于折返波的稳定。而且，在折返的数理或分析模型的构建方面，二维系统比三维系统的困难少得多，后者有更多的空间、参数以及行为模式。因而，对折返的二维系统的细致入微的以及设置有对照组的研究可以揭示折返的最基本的机制，从而对生理相关的折返系统提供更有价值的认识。

一、二维折返模型

研究螺旋波的二维计算机模型主要分为三种：细胞自动操作模型、简化模型和以离子为基础的模型。细胞自动操作模型在生理学上机制不清，常常建立在探索和假说的基础上。为了简便起见，不会深入讨论这些模型。除非在解释该模型中的复杂的行为方面如：兴奋过程的失活、扩布耦联、波锋偏离等。简化模型（又叫做FitzHugh-Nagumo模型）是两个或三个代表心脏生物物理行为的变量，在计算上简便化。该模型是通过对基本的动态行为的控制来提供有益的认识。而基本的动态行为在激动波的形成、稳定或中止中起着关键的作用。这一模型的主要缺陷在于内在的参数常常缺少生理学的认同。即便如此，简化的模型仍然对于识别和确定折返波的可能的动态行为方面颇有价值。另外，该模型也为分析和理解实验结果提供了一个平台。另一方面，在最近刚刚过去的几十年中，人们又提出了以离子通道为基础的详细的细胞模型、传输介质、缓冲介质、存储间隔以及缝隙连接等模型。虽然这些模型非常复杂，在运算上也有难度，但是这些模型进行了严谨的基础研究，解释了除极、复极和不应期的概念，而这些概念是研究折返的基础。而且，这些模型可以帮助我们理解组织对电学刺激的反应，并能确定药物或分子治疗的特异靶点。

与计算机模型相对应的是实验模型,是指二维的薄的心肌组织切片做为基质。例如:(1)在兔或犬心脏中,通过灌流分离出的心房游离壁细胞;(2)从山羊或犬心脏表面用刀片切割下来的约 0.5mm 厚的组织切片;(3)豚鼠或兔心脏内膜行冷冻消融后,存活下来的心外膜薄的组织切片;(4)从猪右室游离壁分离出的心外膜组织块;(5)心肌梗死后犬存活的心外膜组织。虽然这些组织切片为二维的,但却已经很好地帮我们理解折返波的行为(如螺旋波行为、波锋偏离、APD 变量)。晚近,光学标测的进展又提供了一种新的有价值的工具用来监测二维折返波的电波锋在时间和空间上的传导。

理想的二维组织模型指的是经过培养的心肌细胞薄层。这样的细胞网络可以在单个细胞和整个组织之间建立结构和功能的相互作用。并且可以代表在几个厘米范围内成百上千细胞的聚集的特性。该细胞网络具有特异性的细胞构成,快速的扩散途径,而没有分离组织导致的损伤区域,可以通过定向生长的方法来控制细胞层的扩展方向,可以联合控制几何形态的方法来进行一个细胞和一个细胞之间的、精确的对于二维计算模型的反应。由于该细胞层可以牢牢地粘附在培养基质的表面,因而在电刺激或光学记录的过程中的移动伪差相对于其他的组织要小得多。培养的细胞可以允许长期的研究、操作、模拟不同的条件(如药物、基因向量、伸展、或程序刺激),时间可以长达几天到几周不等。"盘子中的心脏折返的研究"能在理论上适合于离子通道作用的基因研究和分子结构-功能研究、载体研究、以及在组织层面上的折返上的缝隙连接的研究。细胞培养模型也可以允许精确的组织构建,有可能用来研究器质性心脏病的心肌电生理特性。如果计算机模型作为一种揭示和理解复杂生物系统的方法获得了广泛的接受,并且在药物治疗的区域作为筛选的工具,那么二维细胞薄层也可以作为该模型的有效的"试验床"。在目前的计算机中可以完全具备在二维空间研究离子电流、载体和室。动作电位的光学记录可以为 APD 和传导速度(折返的十分重要的参数)提供信息。而这些测量目前仅仅限于组织的表面和以下的研究,还达不到在三维空间的研究。

目前,主要有两个研究小组在应用细胞培养来研究二维细胞单层的折返。Bub 及其同事报道了在鸡胚单层细胞上的自发开始和中止的钙的旋转子波。Tung 及其同事研究了在新生鼠心室肌单层细胞上发生的折返。心室肌单层细胞由电压敏感的染色所点缀,不仅可以测量激动波的前锋,而且还有复极时间和 APD(动作电位时间)。结果显示:解剖学上的折返可以从电学上诱发和中止,与可激动间隙相关。结果还显示:功能性折返环也可以在各向同性单层细胞上诱发和中止。而且,方向性的增长方法可以用来控制单层的各向异性。

二、二维折返的常见类型

研究折返我们首先要简单谈谈一维空间系统。因为二维空间系统不仅包括了多维空间的特点,还包括了一维空间的特点。最常见的一维空间的折返环路模型是围绕着某个大的解剖阻滞区域的固定的传导通路(常常被认为菲薄的环路)。密闭的环路常常认为是没有边界的一维的环路。很多描述二维折返的概念源自于一维环路。这些包括以下几个方面的理论研究:(1)传导沿着某个方向的单向阻滞以及落在诱发带内的适时间期和位点的早搏所诱发的折返;(2)折返的诱发和稳定受到细胞的解耦联的影响;(3)细胞膜结构或组织构造上的各向异性导致了折返的容易诱发;(4)折返的波锋和波尾相互作用导致了动作电位和折返周期的变化;(5)引起折返自发中止的变量。这些变量的性质(自变量或因变量)实质上是 APD 和传导速度(CV)之间的回归曲线(恢复或频率依赖性)的形态和功能。

一维折返环中应用的两个概念目前仍然在应用于二维系统。这两个概念分别是波长(wave length,WL)和可激动间隙(exitable gap,EG)。图 37-1 表示的是通过接触性荧光视觉标测系统对折返环路的波锋的记录(折返波的内径 3mm,外径 17mm)。因为环路不单是薄薄的环路,故该环路表现为一维和二维系统的特点(二维解剖折返)。在图 37-1A 中环路长度(path length,PL)指的是围绕在阻滞区外的折返波的长度。波长(WL)指的是对外在刺激无反应的激动波的长度,它等于有效不应期和传导速度的乘积。WL 和 PL 的比值决定环路维持折返的能力。因此,折返发生的条件必须是 WL 小于 PL。可激动间隙(EG)在空间上的测量是从波锋到波尾的距离。EG 的大小决定了通过应用外界刺激在超速起搏、拖带或中止心动过速时,外界刺激打入折返环路的能力。在特定的空间上的某点,跨膜动作电位会周期性的经历环路长度、有效不应期和舒张间期的变化(见图 37-1B)。在任一瞬间,都可以看出:环路长度(PL)=波长(WL)+可激动间隙(EG),折返环间期(CL)=有效不应期(ERP)+舒张间期(DI)。在非常严格的条件下(如:在同一介质的环路中,不伴有改变的、稳定的折返环路),描述空间的三个参数(PL、WL 以及 EG)分别和描述时间的三个参数(CL、ERP 以及 DI)有直接相关性。

图 37-1A 也显示出将 PL、WL 和 EG 三个参数的定

义直接应用到二维系统中还存在一些困难。例如：常常会见到当折返波跨越的通路的不同，这些参数也会发生变化。正如以后要谈到的那样，在二维解剖折返中，明确的环路常常在围绕在阻滞区的外面。

虽然在理想的数学模型中，对于 WL 和 EG 这两个概念已经研究得十分成熟。但是生理状态下，这两个参数不可能总是保持不变。即使对于一维折返环路也是这样。下面是它们相互关系的方程式：

$$WL = ERP \times CV = k \times APD \times CV \quad [1]$$
$$APD = f_1(DI, a, t, x \cdots) \quad [2]$$
$$CV = f_2(DI, a, t, x \cdots) \quad [3]$$

方程式 1 是 WL 的传统定义。但在这里 ERP 被 APD 所代替。这也是实验人员通常所采取的近似值，因为 APD 常常容易测量。设置参数 k 的目的明确 ERP 和 APD 不同。k 值通常是 1，但是在复极后不应期的情况下，k 值可以远远大于 1。公式 2 和 3 表明 APD 和 CV 均是与许多变量的函数。回归方程提示 APD 和 CV 是舒张间期 DI 的函数。DI 是指两个参数的前面舒张间期（diastolic interval）。正因为如此，在高频状态时，由于 APD 和 CV 的下降，WL 可以缩短。所以回旋波开始形成时 WL 长于组织的直径，随着时间的推移，逐渐改变然

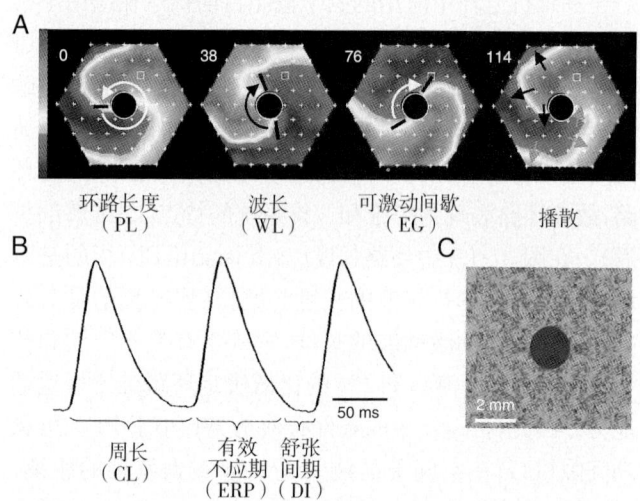

图 37-1　折返参数　A：在新生的小鼠细胞薄层切片，单次折返周期中的光学标测（中央阻滞区内径 3mm，外径为 18mm）。细胞由 RH237 染色，同时监测白色光点标记的 60 个记录部位的光学动作电位。左侧的彩条表示相对电压，蓝色代表静息细胞或完全复极化的细胞。红色代表完全除极化的细胞。数字表示时间，并以毫秒为计量单位。前三个图形表示了在障碍物的周长所测量出的环路长度（PL）、波长（WL）以及可激动间隙（EG）。在右侧的最后一个图形显示出波锋（用黑色箭头表示）和波尾（用灰色箭头表示）扩布的方向。B：在同一次折返中，对某个记录部位通过光学过滤记录到的动作电位。图中显示出了三个参数：环路长度（CL）、有效不应期（ERP）以及舒张间期（DI）。C：另外一个通过培养的显微结构的显微照片。环形解剖阻滞的直径为 2mm。细胞肌动蛋白通过荧光染色得以显现（引自 Y. Nabutovsky, N, Bursac, and L, Tung，未公开发表的资料）（见彩图 8）。

后适应了较小的组织周围路径。这一概念说明：维持回旋波所需要的组织面积可以小于回旋波开始时所需要的面积。而且，APD 和 CV 也是以下几个变量的函数关系：(1) a 角度，与肌纤维相关的波锋扩布的方向。(2) 时间参数 t，记忆效应会改变回归方程的特性，随着心动过速的持续，会出现电重构。(3) 在环路上的位置 x，该参数反映了环路在空间上的异质性。如：以细胞、结构、或功能为基础的缓慢传导区域。(4) 其他的影响因素如组织边界或离子浓度的改变、温度、代谢状态、神经内分泌入路、机械张力以及缝隙连接传导。因而，波长是个定性的概念，但是需要仔细地定义，在二维折返中具有高度的可变性。当 CV 和 APD 的基本参数是与历史相关的，并且是空间、组织结构以及其他可以调节的作用的函数关系时，需要在二维系统进行更加复杂的分析。以上的情况也同样应用于可激动间歇（EG）。

折返波的行为特性会随着障碍的大小而改变。理论研究已经证实，随着障碍区域的变化，波的行为特性也发生连续的改变。对于大的障碍以及窄的传导路径来说，波锋相对较直，且与整个环路呈垂直关系。然而，随着障碍的区域减小以及环路宽度的增加，波锋会出现弯曲，且半径越小，弯曲越大（见图 37-1A）。而且，环绕在障碍区周围的 CV 和折返间期随着障碍区的增加而减小。弯曲（边缘绝缘于中心）导致了比平坦时的波的缓慢扩布。这也是波锋激动电流前面的未兴奋的静息组织的电负荷增加所致。弯曲越大，负荷越重，心肌越难兴奋，因而传导速度越慢。当存在一个最小的弯曲半径时，扩布就不能持续（而且还会发生传导阻滞），这个最小的弯曲半径在正常的心室肌估计是非常小的，大约是 150μm[26]。波锋弯曲的另外一个后果是波锋可以获得向外侧放射的速度。因此，在二维解剖折返中，折返波除了在阻滞区周围外，不再围绕着同一区域来循环。而是逐渐离开阻滞区。折返波成为附属于阻滞区的一支。只有沿着附属于阻滞区的波锋的周长，PL 才有意义。因为在此，折返波才能循环，再次激动同一区域。波锋弯曲也会影响 APD 和 CV 回归关系，导致 EG（可激动间隙）沿着折返波的分支受到调节[27]。

解剖学上定义的障碍或其他的结构上的异质性不是折返发生的必需条件。在此种情况下，折返（功能性折返）产生一个围绕着中点（转子）的波，同时波也向离开中

---

*"旋转子"这一术语广泛应用于很多文学作品，并且有很多定义。Winfree[4]将旋转子定义为"螺旋波的自我维持"，并且为时相单一性所在。它是螺旋形状的波的组织中心。我们使用该术语包括任何一种二维功能性折返波，如：主导环或螺旋波折返。在主导环折返中，旋转子是穿越主导环的波的一部分。在螺旋波的折返中，旋转子是指时相相同一性周围的区域，该区域紧随一个或几个羊组成的折返轨道。

心的方向扩布。这与二维解剖折返的情况十分相似。功能性障碍区可以由该区域的兴奋性下降或残留的或持续的不应期产生。组织的不应性的产生与动作电位和恢复时间的延长相关,或者与主导折返环的电持续相关。在主导环折返中,沿着波的扩布方向上,存在一个大的直径(估计在兔的心肌组织该直径达到 6～8mm)的闭合环路(主导环路)。刚好 PL 等于 WL(见图 37-2A)。因而,完全没有可激动间歇。波持续性向心扩布导致了闭合环路始终处于不应期,而同时波从主导环向外放射性地扩布。理解主导环概念的一个困难是很难知道波长优先。考虑到以上所谈到的 ERP 和 CV 的可变性,波长等于局部的 ERP 和 CV 的乘积,沿着主导环路的闭合环路而变化。

另外,中央阻滞区甚至可能并不存在。螺旋波[6]是一种目前研究得比较透彻的一种功能性折返形式,该折返存在于反应-扩散动力学的非线性可激动系统[28]。数字模拟研究已经揭示了在同源介质的螺旋波的特点。虽然仅有一部分特性行为得到心肌实验研究的证实(如:螺旋波的完全反转也很少能观察到)。我们可以从数学模型上将螺旋波的尖端定义为时相同一性的点(而动作电位的不同时相可以在空间上的某一个点相遇),该点保持部分除极和部分不应期(图 37-2B)。在螺旋波的尖端的比较大的波锋弯曲不可能保证尖端向所有的方向同等的扩布。相反,尖端沿着同轴的轨道运行,轨道的外形取决于与平面 WL 轨道相关的中轴的长度[26]。转子围绕着大的中轴"核心"区域作圆形或椭圆形的旋转(头尾很少相互作用)。Z 形轨道会伴长短的中轴(头尾相互作用较强,没有 EG)。弯弯曲曲的花朵外形的轨道会伴有通常 WL 的长度[26]。当核心区域存在时,在核心的心胞可被激动,但是永远无法激动[8,29]。这一特点将螺旋波和主导环路的转子相区别开来,前者的中央阻滞区域的细胞是完全处于不应期的。而且,当螺旋波折返时,离心波向外扩布,EG 存在于核心和外周[28]。核心是几毫米宽的未激动的组织[8,11],对外层的细胞具有强烈的电学影响[21],因而降低了动作电位的幅度、时程和除极的速度,缩短了折返的 WL[6,8,21]。这些边界细胞被认为与功能性折返的维持和动态变化有关[14]。例外,在二维可激动媒介(不仅仅是心脏组织)中进行的大量研究已经揭示了螺旋波的形成[4,30,31]、弯曲和漂流行为[28,32]以及中止的机制[19,27]。螺旋波可以在不应性、兴奋性、传导速度以及纤维方向均不同的异质性组织中传导和扩布[6,26]。螺旋波的自发性碎裂或扩增为子波可能是稳定性心律失常退化为颤动的基础。其机制为核心的动态变化、APD 和 CV 回归关系的形态以及其他因素如双稳态、滞后和 Doppler 扩布[19,20]。

转子可以固定在某一处或者漂移[28]。四处飘移的

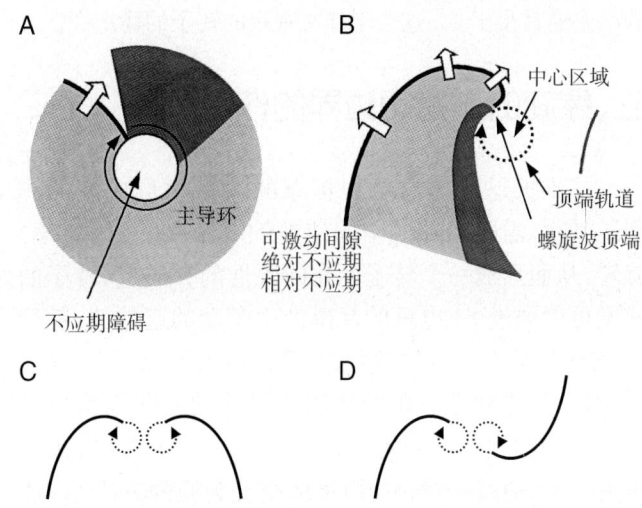

图 37-2 各种功能折返的不同形式 波锋用黑色表示,黑灰色表示相对不应期的波尾,波的绝对不应期(不能兴奋的)用浅灰表示。A:主导环路折返。波的内层沿着最小的主导环路,在该环路内波锋和波尾相遇。B:螺旋波折返。波的三个阶段相遇在一个单一的点,该点沿着核心的轨道旋转。C:两个相反折返方向的波成了 8 字折返模型。该图显示出波锋和轨道的头端。两个转子的阶段相反。D:相连的转子具有同一个手形,形成了双臂折返模型。两个转子刚好在时相上相差 180°

转子波可以产生多形性心电图[28,33]。但是也可以固定在某个最小的解剖障碍区域[6,9,10],导致单形性心电图。因而,障碍可以对于飘移的转子波有稳定作用。最小的障碍区的大小决定于弯曲的外形和弯曲的半径。小的障碍区场常常外形锐利[26,30]。一旦粘附在一起,转子旋转变慢[6,9],成为二维解剖学折返的一种形式。

心肌的各向异性的结构被认为导致在 CV 的方向上的差异,从而引起了传导上的阻滞[34]。各向异性的折返是心肌纤维不同方向上的排列的结果[2]。按照理论模型,各向异性可以导致系统在电学方面的"伸长"。而波旋转的间期不受影响[6]。在各向异性介质中的转子沿着椭圆形[6]或 Z 形的轨道做前后的摆动[13]。各向异性折返包括时间相关性的 EG,原因是在波的中轴的轨道末端传导变慢[2,22]。轴心的传导的减慢也提示在此处存在有较强烈的头尾相互作用。轨道的线性部分产生的原因是沿着相反方向旋转的波的不应期形成的。

在二维细胞单层,各向异性可以应用微磨损或微模型的方法预处理生长表面来获得[15]。图 37-3 的左侧部分为免疫荧光图像显示出不同细胞的肌动纤维的排列方向,而右侧部分是顺钟向折返的一个周期的激动时间的先后顺序[51]。沿着细胞长轴的方向转子被拉长了,在垂直方向的阻滞线的方向周围扩布。左下部分是模拟心电图(pECG),该心电图是通过计算所有记录点的跨膜电位计算出的。而额外的功能是由导联面积运算法则决定的[18]。稳态的、单个的转子的 pECG 是单形的。应当注意的是:我们发现在培养的新生的鼠细胞中,APD 回归方程

的斜率通常小于1。这会增加所观察的转子的稳定性。

三、螺旋的开始和边界的作用

二维折返首先需要在扩布的波锋中形成波的碎裂。其次,需要足够的空间使波的自由端(波的尖端)旋转,从而形成一个转子。在同源性的介质里,转子的诱发可以通过S1电极的起搏产生激动的起始波,随后S2电极发放合适的早搏刺激,刚好落入不应期内(风轮实验)[4]。这种方法曾经应用在培养的心肌细胞单层中[18]。其他的方法也可以在同源性的介质中诱发出转子来。如:通过一对相交电极的交叉刺激的方法[11],或通过起搏各向异性不同的组织来诱发,或使激动波脱离障碍区的方法(漩涡分流)[30]。因为一旦脱离,激动波就会"碎裂",碎裂的激动波就会获得一个尖端,然后以此尖端为中心旋转。前提是它有足够小的旋转半径。在异质性的媒介中,空间上的不应期和回归参数都会变化。在某个点上的快速的起搏可以导致传导阻滞、激动波的碎裂,或诱发出功能性折返[31,35]。在所有的情况下,转子的数目可能会因为形成了相反方向的转子对而增加,亦有可能保持不变,原因是拓扑限制[36]。然而,如果单个的转子漂移到媒介的边界或到达仍然处于不应期的区域,转子就会中止[37]。

图37-4 显示的是在各向异性的单细胞层中的转子的诱发[51]。各向异性比值(即在经度上的传导速度和纬度上的传导速度之比值)为2.2。显示出的两栏为左侧的电压图和右侧的相位图[38]。经过一段时间的快速起搏后,

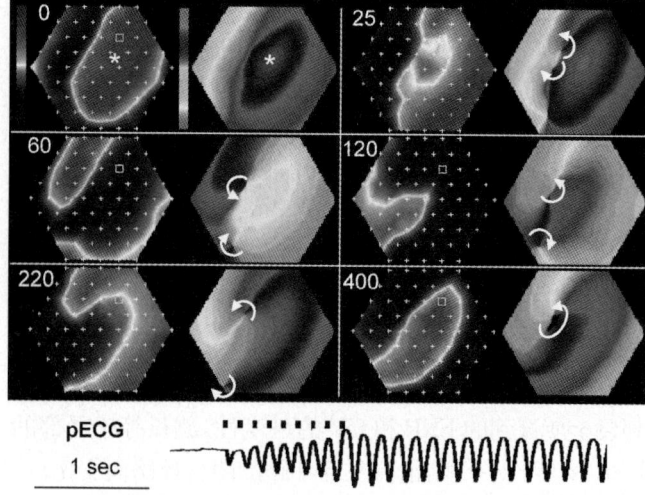

图37-4 通过单一的点电极的快速起搏所诱发的单环折返:通过开始时的电压所致的电压和相应的时相点 左图显示的电压彩条和图37-3中的相同。第一时相左侧的彩条显示从$-\pi$(0%)到$+\pi$(100%)。图形阅读从左到右,从上到下。数字显示为ms。星号显示起搏位点。箭头显示转子的方向。稳定的快速起搏导致25ms时波的碎裂(见彩图10)

形成了一对不同的相位。应用的最后的刺激显示在第一个图像中(0ms)。用星号标记出。单个相位的位置在不同相位点的相位图中很容易认出。方向性(旋转的方向)用弯箭头表示出来。额外的刺激开始诱发出了8字折返(25ms),但是其中一个相位离开单层细胞的边界(60~220ms),仅仅留下了一个相位(400ms)。余下的相位的轨道由黑色的线条来表示。线条短而成线性。在余下的转子稳定后,pECG成为稳定的单形。

在准备各向异性的心肌单层细胞时,特别要注意应用视觉检查、起搏位点的电生理的测量以及心肌细胞和非心肌细胞的免疫荧光染色来确保功能和结构的高度的一致性[15]。另外一方面,即使如此,也不能除外存在着随机分布的微观的结构上的异质性(非细胞的区域小于80μm,细胞大小和方向的局部变化,或缝隙连接耦联)。而且也不能除外存在着功能上的异质性(如:细胞膜离子电流的空间上的变化)。这些微观上的异质性导致了APD和CV回归特性的空间上的离散。从一个位点的快速的起搏常常能够成功地诱发出波的碎裂(图37-4),提示出某种程度的异质性可以促使转子的诱发。目前还不了解是否微观上、解剖上的异质性能够影响转子的稳定性。总是能够观察的某些转子的漂移以及在同一单层细胞不同位点的起搏均能诱发出转子的事实表明所观察到折返的功能的同一性。

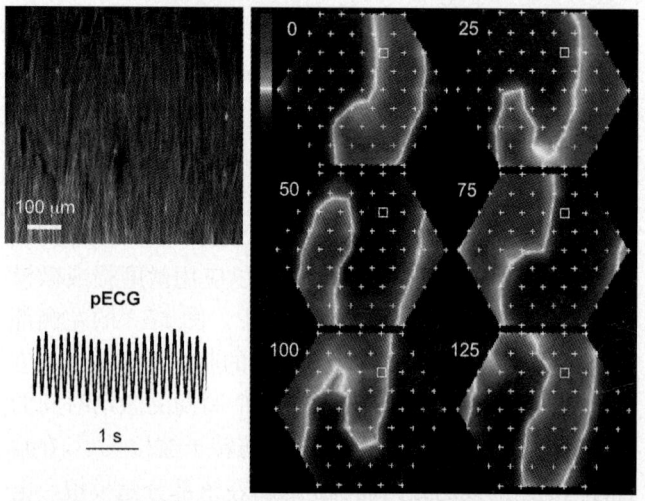

图37-3 各向异性单层构筑可通过florescinphalloids染色显示肌动蛋白纤维 右侧图显示单个顺时针方向旋转的转子。彩色棒状线表示正常电压水平;如图37-1所示,从左向右、从顶端至底部阅读该幅图,数字表示时间,单位ms。折返环长度135ms。伪心电图(pECG)在左下图显示,呈单形性(见彩图9)

四、加速和增殖的旋转波

在持续性多形性室性心动过速的复律治疗中,通常是

在单一位点以稍高于自身折返频率的起搏频率进行抗心动过速治疗[39]。这种快速起搏治疗除了有拖带和终止心动过速的作用外，还能导致心动过速频率的加速以及单形和多形的心电图形态的快速转变。但仅有少数的试验研究证实，发生频率加速的原因是由于快速起搏了解剖上的预激通路或功能上的折返路径，参见下一段所述。

起搏固定的旋转波能够影响其稳定性，导致其湮灭、核心的转移或波形的增殖[11]。心脏实验中发现，快速起搏是通过两个完全不同的模式导致旋转波的加速：(1)非增殖性：是指虽然是单一旋转波，但具有加速的动力学特性或(2)增殖性：是指单一旋转波增殖成几个稳定共存的旋转波。就解剖折返来说，通过快速起搏和由障碍区分离折返波能够得到加速的非增殖模式，接着，再回到一小障碍区或是转变成另一个功能旋转波[31]。另一方面，在解剖折返上有大的可激动间隙能够得到增殖性模式，快速起搏导致第二循环波(双波)的出现。双波是指沿着同样路径围绕着同一解剖障碍区以相同的频率和方向旋转的两个波，因而双波能够在此路径上能以同一加速频率激动每一个位点[40]。

就功能性折返而言，快速起搏通过一个支持快速旋转频率的区域(例如，一个有结构或电生理特性改变的区域)替代它而使旋转波加速。在没有增殖的情况下，即使是在同一媒介中(例如，由于核心直径的减少出现色满卡林导致的加速[41])，功能性折返也能够由药物所诱发。唯一的增殖模式的范例是通过快速起搏，或在反向旋转螺旋波予以额外刺激(例如，8字形折返的形成)[11,14,28]。加速的程度依赖于两个旋转环之间的距离[28]。

我们的研究发现，在同一各向异性的单层心肌细胞中，由于存在不同类型的增殖，快速的起搏不能终止由单环功能性折返所导致的折返加速[51,52]。不仅形成了8字形折返，而且形成了最常见的加速模式，这种模式是指包括同样手式旋转的2~3臂旋转。先前在别的激动媒介中已经形成了稳定旋转的多臂旋转波：(1)化学形式[42]或激光形式[43]在B-Z化学反应区中非激动的中心障碍区被顺次移开或(2)在阿米巴 Dictyostelium discoideum 的聚集体中发生的空间上致密的多重碎裂。这样的诱导模式并没有在心脏组织螺旋波形成的过程中发生。我们在心脏单层组织中的研究表明，对于单个转子的电刺激可以诱导出多个转子的形成。其中一个转子的方向与起始转子的方向相同[52]。

五、多边界的旋转子

在8字形折返的形成中，一对边界的旋转子(即稳

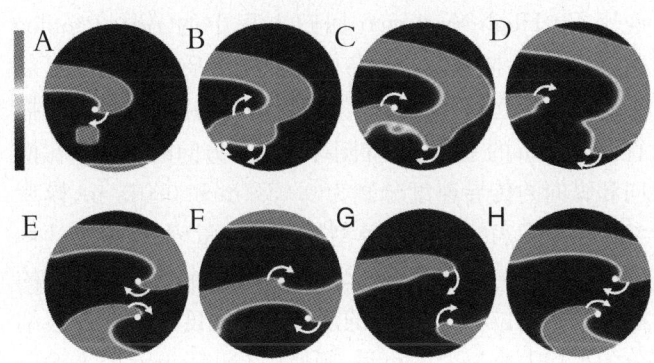

图 37-5　计算机模拟双支螺旋波的起始和维持　A 到 D，在螺旋波上发放单个 S3 刺激，导致了新的双支螺旋波。每个图形之间的间距为 50ms。白色的标记表示单相波的时相。E 到 H，完整的双支螺旋波。图形之间的间距为 100ms(见彩图 11)

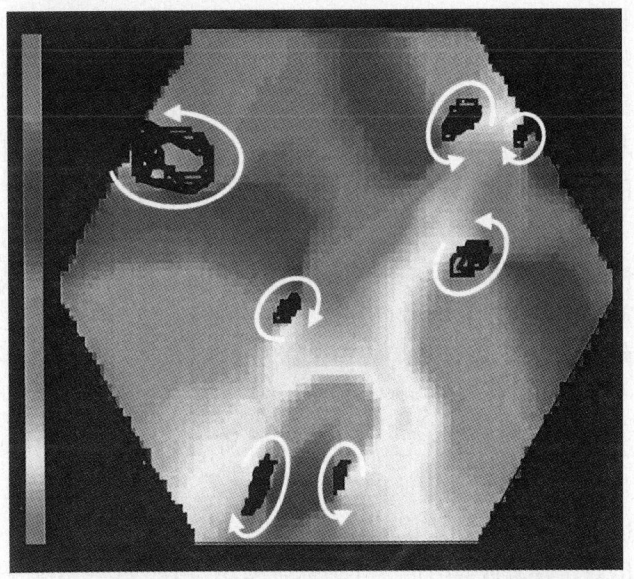

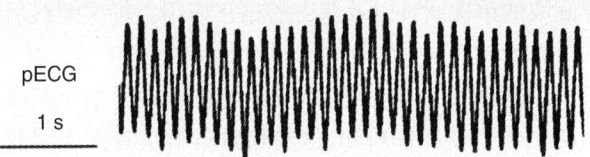

图 37-6　复杂但稳定的静态的 7 个转子组成的折返的示意图，彩条和图 37-4 相同　白色箭头表示 7 个并存的、频率和时相相同的转子的旋转方向。在 5s 的活动中，旋转轨道的尖端用黑色表示。时相心电图是单相的(参见彩图 12)

态的、紧密相连的旋转子)已为人熟知。8字形折返涉及到一对旋转方向相反的波。这两个波具有相同的波长、并且两者沿着2个功能阻滞区域为中心的具有相同的时相性(如同镜像改变)。其中一个波的时相和另一个波的时相刚好相反(此处时相指的是波锋与波尾之间的中心区域的相对的螺旋方向，参见图 37-2C)。在双支折返，刚刚形成的旋转子的起始部分以相同的方向旋转，具有相同的波长，时相固定。其中一个波的时相可以与另一个波相差大约 180°(见图 37-2D)[52]。这种折返形式在我们的单层细胞实验以及完整的兔心脏中得到证实[45]。

应用 FitzHugh-Nagnmmo 回归方程中的 Alier-Panfilov 版本，我们在同源性但是各向异性的介质中复制出了双支旋转子的起始和维持。为达到最佳的模仿效果，选择直径为 2cm 的主导环，伴随纤维水平方向的走行。在横向和纵向的传导速度分别为 0.05s/m 和 0.01s/m，模型参数与已发表的相同。模型的时间变量固定，单个动作电位的时程为 262ms，快速变量参数用来代表-80mV 的静息跨膜电位和 100mV 的动作电位幅度。主导环被细分为平均大小为 150μm 后，则使用 Galeilain 有限方法以及 Enler 分析方程 $\nabla \cdot (\sigma_m \nabla V_m) = \beta I_m$ 来分析。时相单一性通过转换电压资料为时相，然后计算出线性回归方程，以出现拓扑代数变化[38]。在应用标准的 S1S2 刺激程序引发出单一旋转子后，在旋转子启动后的几秒钟后，不同的时间点和周长发放一个或四个 S3。S3 刺激要么落入上一个螺旋波后的不应期内导致波的碎裂，要么引起螺旋波的其中的一个分支波的碎裂。正如我们所预期的那样，螺旋波碎裂为一对方向相反的新的螺旋波。对于一些时间-周期长度的联合，新产生的与初始的波方向相反的螺旋波会离开折返的组织，主要是因为新的螺旋波离组织的边界较近。余下的新的螺旋波与初始的波的方向相同，会演变为双支螺旋波。

图 37-5A 表明 S3 电极的位置，起始的螺旋波在单个 S3 期前刺激后立刻生成了双支螺旋波。图 37-5 B~D 显示诱发出的螺旋波的碎裂以及随后产生的一对螺旋波。方向和极性相反的螺旋波离开了组织的边界，余下的两个螺旋波具有同一个方向。图 37-5 E~H 表明双支螺旋波的单次回旋以及双支的相互作用。每次螺旋后的两个波锋相互碰撞，导致每半个螺旋分支转换一次（图 37-5E 和 H）。在本例中，双支螺旋持续到了整个刺激间期（20 秒）。就我们所知，这些刺激资料是首次表明双支螺旋波可以在正常可激动组织中存在，并且伴有快速上升的心脏样动作电位。从现实的角度，可以在心脏组织诱发出来。既往的大量的研究在同质性的 FitzHugh-Nagumo 计算机模型上成功地模仿和诱发出了双支螺旋波。但是这些都是在低的可激动性方面[48,49]。而且，典型的双支螺旋波可以被以下两种方式诱发：（1）随机分布快激活和慢失活变量的起始条件或（2）操控双变量以利于形成同一个转子的方向的起始条件[50]。

通常来说，在我们的实验中，不同加速阶段形成的转子的数目在 2~7 之间，尽管在相对小的介质面积上（2cm 直径环路的平均单个螺旋波的周长 WL 大约为 4cm）[52]。这些稳定的转子以同样的频率在一起旋转，表现出相对稳定的核心，导致加速的折返频率。但是大多数保持体表心电图的单形性。常常形成较短的局灶性波的碎裂，但是并不能影响强烈的时间和空间上的周期性以及体表心电图的单形性。加速的程度和多重转子的数目成正相关[52]。

图 37-6 显示在单层细胞的快速起搏所诱发的最为复杂的折返。该折返包括 7 个同时存在的、稳定的以及相对来说固定的转子，围绕着小的核心在旋转。形成的体表心电图非常快但是单形的。箭头显示，在 7 个转子中的其中 4 个为同一方向旋转，而剩余的 3 个为相反的方向旋转（见图 37-6 中箭头的方向）。不同转子的核心的不同（由旋转的时相性表示）展现出不同的形态和大小。这些不同之处可能导致了对于相邻的核心和介质边界的不同的电学影响，而且有可能导致结构或功能异质性的细微改变。我们认为异质性是潜在的，在通常的平面的扩布上表现不出来。例如：当高频刺激频率或波锋曲度（引起传导速度下降和 APD 缩短）导致 WL 逐渐减小时，微结构的异质性改变与 WL 相比变得显著，其结果是旋转子之间相互作用提高，以及有可能导致异质性的固定。

如前所述，各向异性的单层心脏组织代表了高度结构和功能同向性的可激动介质。按照计算机的模拟，如果多个功能稳定的转子以不同的频率旋转，那么它们不可能并存[46]。我们相信在二维新生鼠心肌单层细胞上的多支和多个转子模型的高度稳定性的原因为：相同频率转子的旋转（由于介质的相对同源性以及在转子之间可能的相互影响）；缺少 APD 的变化；单层的心肌组织的面积太小限制形成碎裂波以及漂移的转子消失在边界[37]。复杂的功能性折返的不同类型涉及多个、稳定的转子。可按照每个不同极性的稳定转子的数目来分类[52]。例如：单环折返（见图 37-4）是类型 1/0，表示只有 1 个某个方向的转子而相反方向的转子为 0。8 字折返（图 37-4）是类型 1/1，表示有两个转子，方向相反。双支折返是类型 2/0，四支折返是类型 2/2，图 37-6 中的折返为类型 4/3，等等。大量的研究提示类型 1/1、2/0 以及 3/0 折返在介质中稳定，具有相对低的兴奋性，形成多边界的螺旋波的"分子"[50]。

最后，在复杂的多边界转子中给予单点额外的快速起搏刺激可以引起以下几种结果：（1）旋转的频率无变化，（2）加速和增殖为更加复杂的类型（转子的数目增加）或（3）减速和简化为不太复杂的类型（转子的数目减少）。实际上在所有的情况下，复杂的折返最终都能够被不同间期和频率的起搏所中止。要么是转子漂移和消失在单层组织的边界，要么是消除了转子的可激动间隙，使转子遇到了组织的不应期。

六、总结

我们对心脏组织中的折返活动的理解大多数来源于对二维螺旋和折返波的实验研究和数学模型。如同数学模型一样，单层面的细胞代表了理想的二维系统。新的实验证据表明对单一折返环的电刺激可能导致了多个子波或多个界面的折返环路。在心脏组织中的快速起搏能够对复杂类型的折返产生加速现象或中止，对这一现象的深入理解可能对临床和 ICD 的起搏策略提供帮助。

（赵战勇 译）

参 考 文 献

1. Rudy Y: Reentry: Insights from theoretical simulations in a fixed pathway. J Cardiovasc Electrophysiol 6(4):294–312, 1995.
2. Wit AL, Dillon SM, Coromilas J: Anisotropic reentry as a cause of ventricular tachyarrhythmias in myocardial infarction. In Zipes DP, Jalife J: Cardiac Electrophysiology: From Cell to Bedside, 3rd ed. Philadelphia, WB Saunders, 1995, pp 511–526.
3. El-Sherif N: Reentrant mechanisms in ventricular arrhythmias. In Zipes DP, Jalife J: Cardiac Electrophysiology: From Cell to Bedside, 2nd ed. Philadelphia, WB Saunders, 1995, pp 567–582.
4. Winfree AT: The Geometry of Biological Time, 2nd ed. New York, Springer-Verlag, 2001.
5. Feldman AB, Chernyak YB, Cohen RJ: Cellular automata model of cardiac excitation waves. Herzschr Elektrophys 10:92–104, 1999.
6. Pertsov AM, Davidenko JM, Salomonsz R, et al: Spiral waves of excitation underlie reentrant activity in isolated cardiac muscle. Circ Res 72(3):631–650, 1993.
7. Allessie AM, Bonke FI, Schopman FJ: Circus movement in rabbit atrial muscle as a mechanism of tachycardia. III. The "leading circle" concept: A new model of circus movement in cardiac tissue without the involvement of an anatomical obstacle. Circ Res 41(1):9–18, 1977.
8. Athill CA, Ikeda T, Kim YH, et al: Transmembrane potential properties at the core of functional reentrant wave fronts in isolated canine right atria. Circulation 98(15):1556–1567, 1998.
9. Ikeda T, Yashima M, Uchida T, et al: Attachment of meandering reentrant wave fronts to anatomic obstacles in the atrium. Role of the obstacle size. Circ Res 81(5):753–764, 1997.
10. Davidenko JM, Pertsov AV, Salomonsz R, et al: Stationary and drifting spiral waves of excitation in isolated cardiac muscle. Nature 355(6358):349–351, 1992.
11. Davidenko JM, Salomonsz R, Pertsov AM, et al: Effects of pacing on stationary reentrant activity. Theoretical and experimental study. Circ Res 77(6):1166–79, 1995.
12. Girouard SD, Rosenbaum DS: Role of wavelength adaptation in the initiation, maintenance, and pharmacologic suppression of reentry. J Cardiovasc Electrophysiol 12(6):697–707, 2001.
13. Schalij MJ, Boersma L, Huijberts M, Allessie MA: Anisotropic reentry in a perfused 2-dimensional layer of rabbit ventricular myocardium. Circulation 102(21):2650–2658, 2000.
14. Kamjoo K, Uchida T, Ikeda T, et al: Importance of location and timing of electrical stimuli in terminating sustained functional reentry in isolated swine ventricular tissues: evidence in support of a small reentrant circuit. Circulation 96(6):2048–2060, 1997.
15. Bursac N, Parker KK, Iravanian S, Tung L: Cardiomyocyte cultures with controlled macroscopic anisotropy. A model for functional electrophysiological studies of cardiac muscle. Circ Res 91:e45–e54, 2002.
16. Bub G, Glass L, Publicover NG, Shrier A: Bursting calcium rotors in cultured cardiac myocyte monolayers. Proc Natl Acad Sci U S A 95(17):10283–10287, 1998.
17. Entcheva E, Lu SN, Troppman RH, et al: Contact fluorescence imaging of reentry in monolayers of cultured neonatal rat ventricular myocytes. J Cardiovasc Electrophysiol 11(6):665–676, 2000.
18. Iravanian S, Nabutovsky Y, Kong C-R, et al: Functional reentry in cultured monolayers of neonatal rat cardiac cells. Am J Physiol 285:H449–H456, 2003.
19. Fenton FH, Cherry EM: Multiple mechanisms of spiral wave breakup in a model of cardiac electrical activity. Chaos 12:852–892, 2002.
20. Xie F, Qu Z, Garfinkel A, Weiss JN: Electrical refractory period restitution and spiral wave reentry in simulated cardiac tissue. Am J Physiol Heart Circ Physiol 283(1):H448–H460, 2002.
21. Beaumont J, Davidenko N, Davidenko JM, Jalife J: Spiral waves in two-dimensional models of ventricular muscle: formation of a stationary core. Biophys J 75(1):1–14, 1998.
22. Peters NS, Coromilas J, Hanna MS, et al: Characteristics of the temporal and spatial excitable gap in anisotropic reentrant circuits causing sustained ventricular tachycardia. Circ Res 82(2):279–293, 1998.
23. Gray RA, Jalife J: Ventricular fibrillation and atrial fibrillation are two different beasts. Chaos 8(1):65–78, 1998.
24. Xie F, Qu Z, Garfinkel A: Dynamics of reentry around a circular obstacle in cardiac tissue. Phys Rev E 58(5):6355–6358, 1998.
25. Comtois P, Vinet A: Curvature effects on activation speed and repolarization in an ionic model of cardiac myocytes. Phys Rev E 60(4 Pt B):4619–4628, 1999.
26. Fast VG, Kleber AG: Role of wavefront curvature in propagation of cardiac impulse. Cardiovasc Res 33(2):258–271, 1997.
27. Qu Z, Xie F, Garfinkel A, Weiss JN: Origins of spiral wave meander and breakup in a two-dimensional cardiac tissue model. Ann Biomed Eng 28(7):755–771, 2000.
28. Davidenko JM: Spiral waves in the heart: experimental demonstration of a theory. In Zipes DP, Jalife J: Cardiac Electrophysiology: From Cell to Bedside, 2nd ed. Philadelphia, WB Saunders, 1995, pp 478–488.
29. Beaumont J, Jalife J: Rotors and spiral waves in two dimensions. In Zipes DP, Jalife J: Cardiac Electrophysiology: From Cell to Bedside, 3rd ed. Philadelphia, WB Saunders, 2000, pp 327–335.
30. Cabo C, Pertsov AM, Davidenko JM, Jalife J: Electrical turbulence as a result of the critical curvature for propagation in cardiac tissue. Chaos 8:116–126, 1998.
31. Krinsky V: Qualitative theory of reentry. In Zipes DP, Jalife J: Cardiac Electrophysiology: From Cell to Bedside, 3rd ed. Philadelphia, WB Saunders, 2000, pp 320–327.
32. Chernyak YB, Starobin JM: Characteristic and critical excitation length scales in 1D and 2D simulations of reentrant cardiac arrhythmias using simple two-variable models. Crit Rev Biomed Eng 27(3–5):359–414, 1999.
33. Boersma L, Zetelaki Z, Brugada J, Allessie M: Polymorphic reentrant ventricular tachycardia in the isolated rabbit heart studied by high-density mapping. Circulation 105(25):3053–3061, 2002.
34. Spach MS, Josephson ME: Initiating reentry: the role of nonuniform anisotropy in small circuits. J Cardiovasc Electrophysiol 5(2):182–209, 1994.
35. Qu Z, Garfinkel A, Chen PS, Weiss JN: Mechanisms of discordant alternans and induction of reentry in simulated cardiac tissue. Circulation 102(14):1664–1670, 2000.
36. Huyet G, Dupont C, Corriol T, Krinsky V: Unpinning of a vortex in a chemical excitable medium. Int J Bifurc Chaos 8:1315–1323, 1998.
37. Aslanidi OV, Bailey A, Biktashev VN, et al: Enhanced self-termination of re-entrant arrhythmias as a pharmacological strategy for antiarrhythmic action. Chaos 12(3):843–851, 2002.
38. Iyer AN, Gray RA: An experimentalist's approach to accurate localization of phase singularities during reentry. Ann Biomed Eng 29(1):47–59, 2001.
39. Block M, Breithardt G: Implantable cardioverter-defibrillators: Clinical aspects. In Zipes DP, Jalife J: Cardiac Electrophysiology: From Cell to Bedside, 3rd ed. Philadelphia, WB Saunders, 2000, pp 958–970.
40. Cheng J, Scheinman MM: Acceleration of typical atrial flutter due to double-wave reentry induced by programmed electrical stimulation. Circulation 97(16):1589–1596, 1998.
41. Uchida T, Yashima M, Gotoh M, et al: Mechanism of acceleration of functional reentry in the ventricle: effects of ATP-sensitive potassium channel opener. Circulation 99(5):704–712, 1999.
42. Agladze KI, Krinsky VI: Multi-armed vortices in an active chemical medium. Nature 296:424–426, 1982.
43. Steinbock O, Muller SC: Multi-armed spirals in a light-controlled excitation reaction. Int J Bifur Chaos 3(2):437–443, 1993.
44. Rietdorf J, Siegert F, Weijer C: Analysis of optical density wave propagation and cell movement during mound formation in *Dictyostelium discoideum*. Dev Biol 177(2):427–438, 1996.
45. Wu TJ, Bray MA, Ting CT, Lin SF: Stable bound pair of spiral waves in rabbit ventricles. J Cardiovasc Electrophysiol 13(4):414, 2002.
46. Xie F, Qu Z, Weiss JN, Garfinkel A: Interactions between stable spiral waves with different frequencies in cardiac tissue. Phys Rev E 59(2):2203–2205, 1999.
47. Aliev RR, Panfilov AV: A simple two-variable model of cardiac excitation. Chaos Solitons Fractals 7(3):293–301, 1996.
48. Vasiev B, Siegert F, Weijer C: Multiarmed spirals in excitable media. Phys Rev Lett 78(12):2489–2492, 1997.
49. Zaritski RM, Pertsov AM: Stable spiral structures and their interaction in 2D excitable media. Phys Rev E 66(6 Pt 2):066120, 2002.
50. Lin SF, Roth BJ, Wikswo JP Jr: Quatrefoil reentry in myocardium: An optical imaging study of the induction mechanism. J Cardiovasc Electrophysiol 10(4):574–586, 1999.
51. Bursac N, Iravanian S, Parker KK, Tung L: Anisotropic reentry in cultured cardiac myocytes (abstr). PACE 25(4, Part 2):578, 2002.
52. Bursac N, Tung L: Novel stable functional reentry patterns induced by rapid pacing in uniformly anisotropic cardiomyocyte cultures (abstr). Circ 106(19, Suppl II): II–304, 2002.
53. Nabutovsky Y, Iravanian S, Bursac N, et al: Resetting and termination of reentrant activity in circular annuli of cultured ventricular cell monolayers by single electrical field pulses (abstr). PACE 25(4, Part II):604, 2002.
54. Winfree AT: Spiral waves of chemical acitvity. Science 175:634–636, 1972.
55. Vigmond EJ, Aguel F, Trayanova NA: Computational techniques for solving the bidomain equations in three dimensions. IEEE Trans Biomed Eng 49:1260–1269, 2002.

第 38 章

三维空间的回旋波

Arkady M. Pertsov

本章目录

- 回旋波 340
- 回旋波的发生 343
- 回旋波的动力学 343
- 轴丝的不稳定导致了心动过速向颤动的转变 346
- 回旋波成像 347
- 致谢 349

为了理解多形性室性心动过速和心室颤动的发生机制,研究三维结构中(three-dimension,3D)心肌的空间结构和折返激动的动力学特性很重要。由于三维标测存在技术上的问题,因此积累的有关心脏三维折返传播的经验有限,但目前在三维折返理论和计算机模型方面已取得了重要的进展。本章节回顾了一些研究成果,其中包括了本书原版本中未提到的最新进展[1,2],特别是有关心肌结构在三维折返的形成、动力学以及形态学中的重要性,这些内容在过去三年已有所阐述。另外,本书也对心肌内部三维折返成像的方法做了简洁的描述。与本书原版本一样,我们尽量简化技术细节,使更多的读者(包括基础和临床心脏电生理学家)能够理解,同时我们尽量保持原文的释义,使理论学家能够接受。特别需要指出的是,有关三维折返和其结构中心我们一直使用回旋波(scroll wave)和轴丝(filament)这两个术语。我们深信,这些术语正逐渐被大家熟悉、接受,使我们能用更深层次的视角洞悉其原理,以及在生物化学激动系统中领悟大量实验文献所提到的"类折返"(reentry-like)现象。我们设想读者也熟悉螺旋波折返(spiral wave reentry)这一概念[3,4](注解见第35~37章)。

一、回旋波

(一) 单一回旋波

在室性心动过速和心室颤动的动物模型[5]和人[6]的试验中,有许多关于在心外膜和心内膜观察到螺旋波的报道,显而易见,这提出了一个问题:当心肌表面出现螺旋波时,在其内部又发生了怎样的变化呢?尽管这个问题的答案带有明显的经验性,但计算机模型给出了一个能够预测三维激动模式的很好的思路。

图 38-1A 显示的是解释心肌表面螺旋波激动的最简单的三维回旋波模型。根据其形状命名为"回旋波"(scroll wave)[7]。回旋波跨越所有的心肌,围绕着中线(f-f′)旋转,因此称中线为轴丝(filament)(Pertsov 及其合作者给出了更确切的定义[8])。在回旋波与轴丝垂直的部分,研究者也能看见同样旋转的螺旋波(spiral wave)。左图显示的是距离轴丝不同距离时所记录的跨膜电位。围绕着轴丝的细胞与二维螺旋波核心的细胞相类似[3,9],虽然激动波幅较小,但功能正常,当轴丝向不同方向移动时能表现正常的动作电位,在试验研究中使用接近中心的低振幅波是为了定位轴丝[10,11]。由于回旋波的轴丝跨越了所有的心肌,所以常常称之为"透壁回旋波"(transmural scroll wave)。

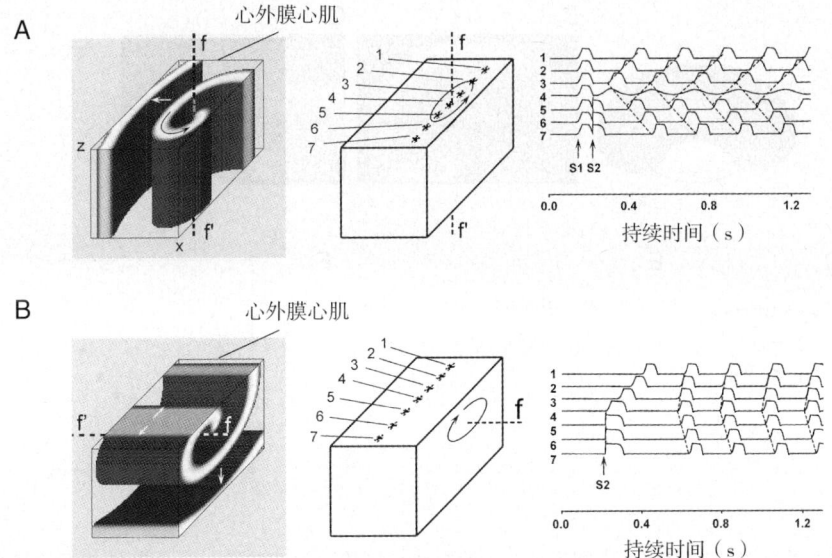

图 38-1 回旋波折返 A：计算机模拟研究中利用 FHN（FitzHugh-Nagumo）模型得出的三维回旋波[16]。模型由 48×48×48 兴奋元素的阵列组成，元素之间互相通过扩散相连接。该阵列呈各向异性，因为沿着 y 轴的元素大小是 X 轴和 Z 轴大小的两倍。左图：逆时针旋转的回旋波相片。非兴奋区是透明的，f（轴丝）以折线表示，白色箭头表示传播方向，利用正交场刺激激发出回旋波；基础刺激（S_1）和期前刺激（S_2）分别来自前方和左侧（图中未标出）。右图：距轴丝不同距离的立方形上方所记录到的动作电位，数字表示的是插入记录区的位置，迹线下方的箭头表示刺激的时间。B：轴丝平行于心外膜表面的单一回旋波。尽管其折返特性肉眼可见，但心外膜标测仍不能揭示其折返激动机制，仅能观察到一些大的突破区

需要注意的是，就心肌表面而言，相同的回旋波由于轴丝的方向不同而有完全不同的表面现象。图 38-1B 显示的是回旋波的轴丝不是跨越心室壁，而是平行于心肌表面的方向，因此称这一类回旋波为"壁内（intransmural）回旋波"，以区别于图 38-1A 中的"透壁（transmural）回旋波"。壁内回旋波不是作为螺旋波出现在心内膜和心外膜表面，而是产生大量的突破区（breakthrough area）。尽管试验显示，发现壁内回旋波要比发现跨壁回旋波难，但根据上述原理，壁内回旋波可能更普遍存在。事实上，近年的计算机成像模式已经发现回旋波轴丝有和心肌纤维平行排列的趋势[12-14]。假使心肌纤维多与心肌表面平行排列，这就进一步提示，轴丝将有助于壁内回旋波的定位。

与其他轴丝方向的回旋波相比，其轴丝方向与心肌纤维平行排列的壁内回旋波有以下优势：有尽可能小的波长 λ（波长＝不应期×传导速度）。在特定的方向，回旋波总是穿过心肌纤维传播，传导速度最小，因此 λ 值最小。相反，透壁回旋波则需要相当大的空间来稳定其旋转方向，它沿着心肌纤维传导的速度至少是旋转周期的一半，因此 λ 值较大。试验证据表明，心肌组织中很少存在单一回旋波。然而，有关透壁和壁内回旋波的文献报道却有许多[15-17]，这些数据将在下文有更详尽的讨论。

（二）环状回旋波

在前面两个示例中我们讨论的是有直线轴丝的回旋波。但是，回旋波的轴丝不全都是直的，它可弯曲、缠绕，甚至可以是一个闭合的环。轴丝呈闭合环形的回旋波称为环状回旋波（Scroll Ring）。环状回旋波是个三维的类似体，即心脏电生理学家所说的 8 字形折返（figure-of-eight reentry）。图 38-2A 显示的是在空间各向同性可激动媒质中，"理想"的环状回旋波的相片。折返激动是围绕环形轴丝（位于图片挖剪部分的实线）而构建的。波前部沿着轴丝缠绕，形成一个圈饼样的形状。交叉部分的前面与 8 字形折返一样，是一对相互旋转的螺旋。螺旋中心的空间大小决定了三维 8 字形的峡部。峡部的宽度与环的直径相同。

环状回旋波的结构不稳定，常常在一定数量的旋转后湮灭（collapse）[18,19]；环的直径随着时间延长而逐渐变小，直到峡部消失。然而，如果最初环的直径很大，可能在环湮灭前发生了几百次的旋转周期。因此，环状回旋波只有在非持续性心动过速时才可以计数，这一点将三维 8 字形与其二维形态区别开来，因为后者通常是稳定的。

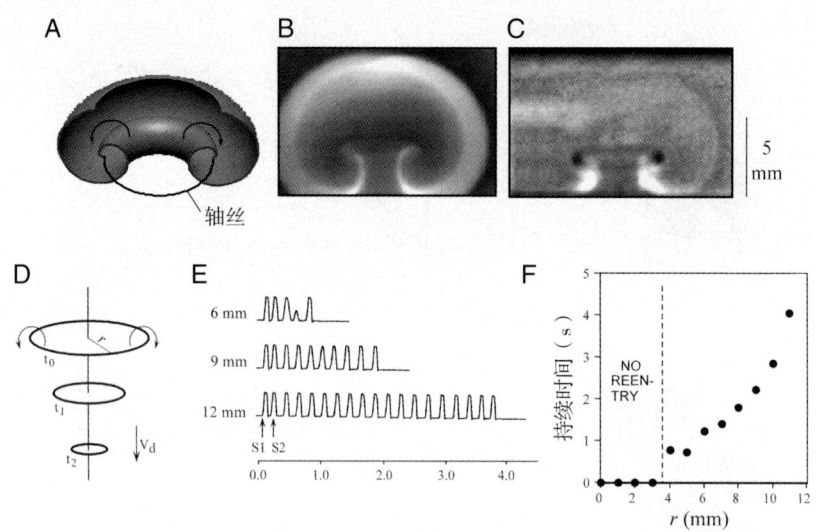

图 38-2　环状回旋波　A：交叉部分的原理。中间半径为 r 的黑环是环状回旋波的轴丝，回旋波围绕着轴丝旋转。箭头表示其旋转方向。B：凝胶固定发生 B-Z（Belousov-Zhabotinsky）反应的倾斜的环状回旋波侧面投射的相片，兴奋区（氧化区）着色浅，环的平面和垂直轴的夹角为 11°。C：同样角度投射的轴丝相片。轴丝呈一模糊的环，由于投照角度的原因，看起来更像椭圆形（引自 Vinson M，Mironov S，Mulvey S，Pertsov AM：Control of spatial orientation and lifetime of scroll rings in excitable media. Nature 386：477-480，1997. Copyright 1997，MacMillian Magazines Ltd.）D：轴丝的动力学（原理）。三幅连续的相片：轴丝逐渐收缩，同时沿着垂直于平面环的轴漂移。E：不同大小的环状回旋波导致的心动过速（激发环的大小分别为 6、9、12mm），FHN 模型。F：激发环的大小与心动过速时程的函数关系

图 38-2D 显示的是一个湮灭环状回旋波轴丝的连续相片。除了收缩运动，环也沿着其轴丝漂移[18]。当轴丝半径逐渐变小时其收缩和漂移的速度加快[18,19]。环状回旋波维持的寿命与轴丝的面积成比例——环越大，其维持时间越长[18]。图 38-2E 显示的是环状回旋波在不同的激发半径破碎时引起的三次非持续性心动过速事件。图 38-2F 显示了激发环的大小与心动过速时程的函数关系曲线。

环状回旋波和单一回旋波的旋转周期大致相同。与漂移的螺旋波相似，由于涡形运动产生的多普勒效应[20]而偏离了主频率。需要注意的是在回旋波湮灭前应激期的变化（见图 38-2D）。

环状回旋波的发现提出了一个具有挑战性的任务。目前，只有间接的证据表明在心肌组织中存在环状回旋波[21]，与单一回旋波相比，环状回旋波难以被发现的原因主要有两个。首先，与单一回旋波不同，在心肌表面不能证明环状回旋波的折返激动，即使利用表面标测技术也不能明确之。其次，折返环发生的重要部分位于峡部，由于室壁内标测的空间分辨力有限，峡部很容易被忽略。然而，随着视频图像和传统的心电图标测技术的快速发展，这些难点将来逐步会一一克服的。

在三维化学激动系统中，扩散波的可视化已经不是一个技术问题（肉眼即能看见扩散波）。回旋波的发现已经有 20 多年了[7,22]，并且已在重要的细节上研究了其性能[11]。图 38-2B 和 C 显示了用凝胶固定发生 B-Z 反应的环状回旋波侧面和轴丝影像，化学激动系统也支持浓集波在性能上与心肌动作电相位似。

（三）U 型和 L 型回旋波

如果把在心肌组织中可能观察到的回旋波的构型完全罗列出来，还需要讨论有 U 型和 L 型轴丝的回旋波[1]，特别是作用在心肌表面的、在强烈的电刺激下形成的 U 型轴丝[23]。U 型和 L 型回旋波的动力学改变与环状回旋波的动力学改变是一致的。解剖学上，它们可能是组成环状回旋波的一部分：分别是 1/2 和 1/4。正常激动时，U 型和 L 型回旋波都在几次旋转后湮灭，因而仅能解释非持续性心动过速的发生。而在某些情况下，仅利用心外膜和心内膜激动标测技术就能发现 U 型和 L 型回旋波，这一特殊表现使我们能将 U 型、L 型回旋波与有其他构型的回旋波区分开来，原因是这一表现说明折返激动仅仅是发生在心肌表面的一个现象[1]。相比而言，单一回旋波是发生在心肌两面，突破区也位于两面（见图 38-1）。

二、回旋波的发生

回旋波发生的机制源自于著名的二维螺旋波发生的机制。第一个例子[21]是基于著名的由不应期各向异性引起的8字形折返的发生机制。事实上,已知的二维机制能够扩展到三维中去。近来提出了另一个有关回旋波发生的可能机制,即所谓的回旋波发射效应(vortex-shedding effect)。第一次描述回旋波发射效应的是在激动媒质的二维计算机模式中[20],之后在一系列试验中(在薄层心肌组织中减少激动次数、提高起搏频率、或者二种方法均采用)也得到了证实[25]。

图38-3A通过羊的心外膜切片显示了二维螺旋波的发生是由于回旋波发射机制引起的。随着波阵面(wave front)逐渐从功能障碍区边缘(等时线,16～48ms)分开,螺旋也逐渐开始形成。当松散的波阵面末端(即波破碎处)逐渐远离功能障碍区时,它逐渐卷绕起来,形成了螺旋的核心。有关回旋波发射机制的三维模型的假说如图38-3B中的图示,一个矩形的非兴奋的功能障碍区附近的平面波逐渐从障碍区边缘分开,形成一个单一回旋波(与图38-1B所示类似)。在显现出的回旋波前方的投照部分,激动模式与图38-3A所示的二维等时图相同。

回旋波的发生中,结构的各向异性不是必要条件。即使在一个理想的、完全不同的激动媒质中,利用垂直于扩散波尾部的强电场也能刺激产生回旋波[26]。这个方法,即通常所说的"正交场刺激"(cross-field stimulation),已经作为激发螺旋波和回旋波的发生而在动物模型中广泛应用[15,27]。

近来也有利用心肌组织壁内、壁外区各向异性的差异,通过电刺激来描述回旋波的发生机制(见Efimov等的综述,也见本书第29、31章节所述),此机制也是二维机制的扩展[28]。在强烈的电刺激下,壁内、壁外区各向异性差异产生的心肌极化的非一致性能够引起折返激动[29]。

三、回旋波的动力学

(一) 轴丝形状的作用

在同一媒质中,螺旋波的动力学完全由激动媒质的性能所决定,而回旋波不是这种情形。三维结构中影响折返动力学和寿命的一个主要因素是轴丝的形状。在同一媒质中,轴丝形状不同的螺旋波可以有完全不同的动力学。典型的例子就是单一回旋波和环状回旋波动力学的差异:单一回旋波的媒质是稳定的,而环状回旋波则能自发的湮灭(见图38-2)。

将回旋波三维动力学与其轴丝的形状联系起来的理论正得到蓬勃发展[30,31],有关这一理论在此未做定量方面的讨论。然而,了解一些常规的法则对理解回旋波的全部动力学表现也很重要,这些已经简短讨论过了。其中一条法则如下所示:正常激动时,回旋波的轴丝长度上趋向最小化。值得注意的是,环状回旋波的湮灭完全合乎于该法则。简言之,单一回旋波的稳定性也遵从该法则:由于直线距离最小,轴丝的末端不能从表面分离。这后一特性与其局部解剖有关,其解剖特点使得轴丝在激动媒质内部没有松散的末端[8]。

在心肌组织中应用"最小长度"(minimal length)法则可以作出如下有趣的预测:轴丝跨越心外膜到心内膜的单一回旋波能够漂移到最薄的区域,使得长度最小化。正常心肌组织中,接近心尖部厚度很小。因此,不论其激动部位,单一回旋波将向心尖部漂移。然而,透壁梗死时情况就会改变。在透壁梗死时,可

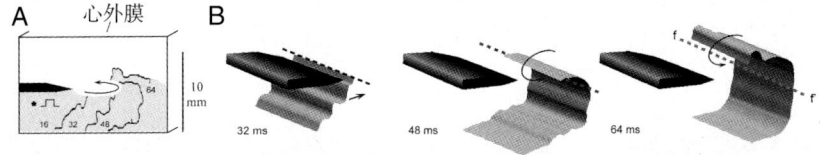

图 38-3 螺旋发射机制引起单一回旋波　A:羊心外膜切片的等时标测图显示出由螺旋发射机制导致的螺旋波发生。增加15mM河豚毒素(tetrodotoxin)其兴奋性受到抑制,刺激点(星号所示)位于非兴奋功能障碍区(左侧的黑色楔形标记)的下面。接近等时区的数字显示的是时间,以毫秒(ms)表示(引自Davidenko JM, Cabo C, Jalife J: Wavefront curvature leads to slow conduction and block in two-dimensional cardiac muscle. In Spooner PM, Joyner RW, Jalife J [eds]: Discontinuous Conduction in the Heart. Armonk, NY, Futura Publishing. 1997.) B:螺旋发射机制在三维中的扩展。以16ms的间隔的波阵面连续快照,由于图像模糊,功能障碍区和波阵面的形状在A图中显示的要清楚。折线表示回旋波的轴丝

激动组织的最薄处位于存活心肌的心外膜边缘。因此，单一回旋波将向该部位漂移[32]。尽管没有直接的证据表明真正的回旋波是向心肌最薄区域移动，但在文献中有报道：正常心肌中可以观察到回旋波趋于接近心尖部[6,33]，而在梗死心肌中正相反，它常常定位于存活的心外膜边缘[32]。

近来已表明，"最小长度"法则能扩展到心肌组织各向异性的非一致性中[34]。值得注意的是，在各向异性的表现中，最小长度不总是直线，有时是一些特殊的曲线，即所谓的短程线（geodesic），也具有最小距离的特征[34]。因此，心肌纤维在回旋波轴丝的形成中发挥了重要的作用。

（二）各向异性的作用

迄今为止，我们关注的是回旋波在同质激动系统中的内在动力学。然而，心脏组织即使在正常情况下也具有较高的各向异性（heterogeneous）。那么各向异性是如何影响回旋波的动力学呢？结合其对动力学的影响，可以将各向异性分成两种不同的类型：平滑/梯度（smooth/gradients）和局部/缺损（localized/defects）。

正常心肌组织中，平滑各向异性的典型例子是透壁[35]和心外膜[36]动作电位时程的梯度。另一个与心肌组织中自发出现梯度的例子是电偶（electrical coupling）梯度[12]。以上梯度源自于心肌纤维在深度方面的逐渐变化，这已在传感器的组成中得到证实，并已用于描述心肌细胞之间的电偶[12,13]。这一点都知道，急性心肌缺血时，正常区域和灌注不良区域的交界处会形成显著的梯度差异[37]。

另一个有关各向异性的类型——局部缺损，同样也有许多示例。其中具有代表性的例子是冠状动脉血管和非兴奋纤维碎片（inexcitable fibrotic patches）。为限定局部缺损，碎片不要求一定是非兴奋的，因性能显著不同于其余组织的小片的激动组织碎片也提示局部缺损。

在轴丝动力学方面，梯度和局部缺损具有相反的作用。平滑梯度引起漂移和轴丝的缠绕，最终导致轴丝破碎（breakup）；局部缺损则有稳定轴丝的趋势，即锚定（anchor）。

（三）梯度诱发的漂移

轴丝动力学梯度的主要作用是导致轴丝的漂移。当梯度垂直于轴丝有一投照时能够观察到漂移现象[16,38]。图 38-4 示由于壁内纤维的旋转，电偶梯度引起了穿越心肌组织的回旋波轴丝的漂移[12]。纤维方向在深度上（见图 38-4，点线）的变化影响了扩散张量（diffusivity tensor）的成分 D_{xx}，这对漂移有一定的作用。本例中漂移的速度通过分析能够预测[13]。只有当轴丝到达梯度缺如层时才发生漂移（见图 38-4 中右图），达到这一层时，轴丝趋于稳定。需要注意的是，如此稳定的状态是与轴丝平行于心肌纤维层面时相对应的。

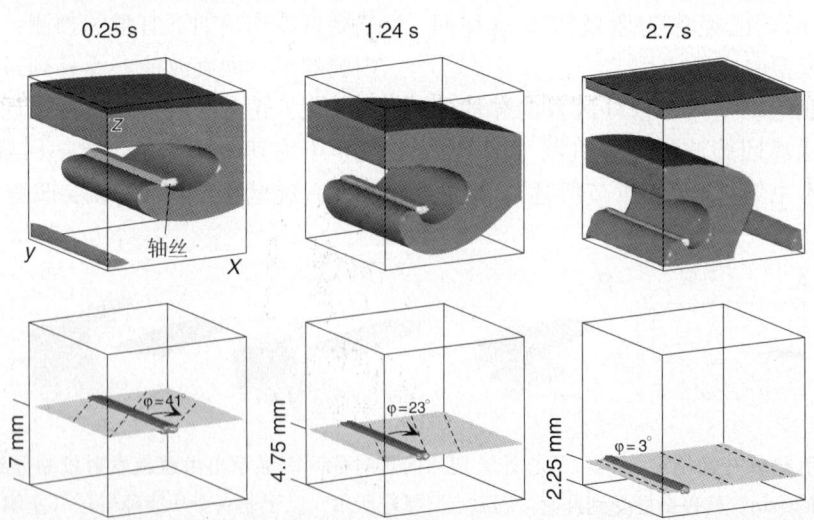

图 38-4 纤维方向变化引起壁内回旋波的漂移 上部和底部箭头分别表示回旋波和轴丝相继的位置。虚线表示轴丝附近纤维的方向。随着时间的增加（见上图所标数字），在轴丝和纤维（轴丝附近的纤维）之间逐渐缩小的角度 φ（引自 Berenfeld O, Pertsov A：Dynamics of intramural scroll waves in three-dimensional continuous myocardium with rotational anisotropy. J Theor Biol 199：383-394，1999.）

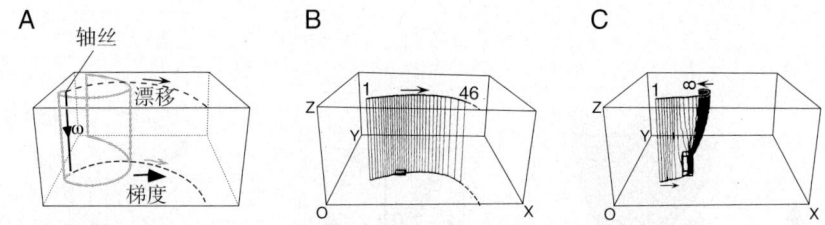

图 38-5 异质媒质中单一回旋波的动力学　A：单一回旋波在垂直于轴丝的参数梯度中的漂移。此为回旋波示意图，黑线表示轴丝，灰色曲线为波阵面，梯度方向在右侧。B：漂移轴丝的连续快照。小范围的局部缺损（底部小的立方形）不影响轴丝的运动。C：轴丝锚定到大的缺损处（引自 Vinson M Pertsov AM，Jalife J：Anchoring of vortex filaments in 3D excitable media. Physica D 72：119-134，1993.）

有趣的是，漂移常常发生在梯度的角部，角度的变化显著依赖于梯度的特性和回旋波旋转的方向。计算机模式显示出轴丝能够垂直于梯度漂移，有时方向甚至与梯度相反。不过，梯度诱发漂移的原理仍在探讨中。

梯度诱发的漂移通过将轴丝带到其消退的边缘而使回旋波消除。图 38-5A 和 B 显示的是梯度诱发回旋波消除的例子。本例中，回旋波具有透壁方向。当梯度达到激动阈值时，即沿着 X 轴呈线性增加[3,9]。计算机模式也显示出，如同前面示例所见，轴丝未发生变形，而是平行于自身漂移，虽有微小的干扰，但很稳定[38]。最终，轴丝和媒质边缘发生碰撞而消退（annihilates）[3]。

梯度诱发的漂移也能引起以反方向旋转的回旋波（或螺旋波）的碰撞和消退[39,40]。根据这一理论，垂直于梯度的漂移部分可以引起碰撞，这些部分使反向回旋波彼此接近，直至相互消退。反向旋转回旋波之间发生的漂移基于如下的事实：漂移速度的正交成分对不同手性的回旋波有相反的征象。应用相对较小的外部梯度有可能消除回旋波，这一可能性使得研究控制漂移速度参数的兴趣点发生了转移，从其作为实际观点而转移到可能作为终止心律失常的一部分。

（四）锚定

与梯度相反，局部缺陷能使回旋波稳定。二维结构中显示，当奇数轨道带着回旋波接近缺损时，是面对缺损发生移动的，直至与缺损互相接触[3,9,38,41,42]。一旦锚定，回旋波能够维持。当奇数轨道距离功能障碍区太远时，而该功能障碍区在其吸引下没有下落时，螺旋波漂移而没有被锚定。

三维结构中也能发生回旋波的锚定，但与上述有明显差别[38]。三维结构中，只有部分轴丝吸引到缺损处；而没有吸引到缺损的那部分轴丝继续进展。因此，在轴丝结束和未结束的锚定之间发生了竞争。在三维结构中，这种竞争产生了不同性质的动力学（见图 38-5C 所示）。图中可见，缺损高度是媒质高度的 1/4，轴丝通过缺损部位的轨道是竞争发生的条件。如二维示例所示，轴丝下部被吸引并锚定到缺损处，而上部持续漂移。顶端轨道开始卷曲环绕，围绕缺损旋转（轴丝底部已被锚定），直到在接近 60 个旋转周期后达到平衡。三维空间的平衡慢于二维空间，后者中，当漂移的螺旋遇见功能障碍区时，于 2~3 个旋转周期后即迅速锚定它[3,38,40]。当缺损高度增加时，这两种情况的差别变小，大的功能障碍区吸引了更多的轴丝，使剩余的部分能更快达到平衡。

（五）缠绕

与早先所讨论的关于平行于轴丝的梯度不引起轴丝移动的情况正相反，由于沿着轴丝不同点的差别引起了轴丝的缠绕，也就产生了旋转的内在频率（natural frequency）[43,44]。考虑到有轴丝局部的内在旋转频率 ω_1 和 ω_2，人们期望这两点间最初的时相不同，而在时间上呈线性增长，$\Delta\Psi=(\omega_1-\omega_2)t$，这些不同的旋转即引起了缠绕的发生。缠绕的回旋波已经从 Winfree 和 Strogatz[45] 的拓扑分析中得到了预测，也可在 Pertsov 及其同事试验的 BZ 反应中观察到[43]。

图 38-6 显示出缠绕的回旋波是从一个最初平行于轴丝方向的梯度开始的。尽管波阵面的出现很复杂，但它只是一个有着直线轴丝的简单缠绕的回旋波。事实上，如图 38-6B 所示，垂直于轴丝的交叉部分包含有简单的螺旋波。当轴丝从顶部横穿到底部时，螺旋的时相发生了移动。图 38-6B 显示了三个这样的交叉部分，中部相对于上部有一个时相的漂移 $\Delta\Psi=\pi$，底部切片漂移的更远。如图 38-6A（右侧）所示，包含轴丝的波阵面交叉部分具有树枝模式的特征。

由梯度而发生的缠绕能够明确的发展；如果梯度

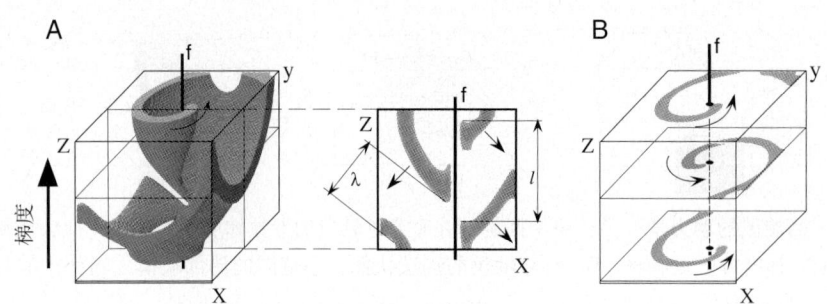

图 38-6 平行于轴丝的参数梯度中的缠绕回旋波 A：FHN 计算机模式下的均衡缠绕的回旋波，其典型的结构是圆锥形。插图（右侧）显示的是通过轴丝的垂直于缠绕波的交叉部分，其中特定的分支结构指的是缠绕。箭头指示传播方向，中间的垂线表示轴丝，跟随波阵面的是分支线。λ 表示回旋波波长，l 表示时相移动为 2π 的距离。B：回旋波在 A 图中的三个水平部分，显示出其螺旋结构，轴丝以灰线表示（引自 Pertsov AM，Vinson M：Dynamics of scroll waves in inhomogeneous excitable media. Phil Trans R Soc Lond A 347：687-701，1994.）

不是太大，缠绕可以达到一个平衡值。梯度越大，平衡缠绕就越大。平衡机制包括了轴丝慢部分的加速，这一机制能导致稳定的缠绕波快速旋转[44,46]，因此，缠绕能够明显增加旋转的频率。

如果梯度超过临界值，缠绕就不能达到平衡。过大的梯度难以避免地会引起回旋波的破碎，形成了类似于颤动的、复杂的、湍流样的状态。这种现象将在下一章节作更深入的探讨。

四、轴丝的不稳定导致了心动过速向颤动的转变

本章节讨论的是轴丝不稳定能产生复杂的颤动样动力学。上文已经提到了有关不稳定的几个机制，尽管在这些机制中有一部分已经得到关注，但其余的却很少被人所知，即使在有关心脏电生理的文献中也常常忽视了。本章节集中讨论了三维不稳定性。这些不稳定性仅在三维中发展，不在二维或一维中发生。我们是在均匀激动媒质中从低兴奋性发生的内在不稳定性开始讨论的，由于其负性的轴丝张力（filament tension），所以通常认为它是不稳定的[31]。这种不稳定不能与发生在正常兴奋性的螺旋波破碎机制相混淆（可参照 37 章详细的讨论）。

（一）负性轴丝张力导致的不稳定

缺血心肌中通常可见低兴奋性所导致的轴丝动力学的动态变化。兴奋性减低时，回旋波的轴丝长度不是缩短，而是增加，因而违反了"最小长度"法则，我们把这种特点称为"负性张力"（negative tension），与引起轴丝收缩的正性张力相反，它使回旋波内部发生不稳定，从而使环状回旋波不是收缩而是扩展。稳定的单一回旋波常常发生自发的不稳定[31]，这种不稳定是自发的、在轴丝内部发生的混乱，这种混乱迅速蔓延，最终接触到边缘。在接触区，轴丝破碎成两个独立的轴丝（回旋波），而新形成的轴丝不断增长扩散，出现复杂的、不断变化的激动模式。目前，已经形成了这样的假说：这种不稳定在病损心肌中可能更有利于心动过速向颤动的转变。

（二）缠绕各向异性引起的不稳定

心肌组织中，由于纤维方向一层一层的逐渐变化，导致了传播速度的缠绕各向异性，实验模型研究预测了这些各向异性可能是回旋波不稳定的原因[47,48]。与前面所讨论的内在不稳定性相似，这些不稳定性也可导致轴丝长度的增加、数目的增长和颤动样激动模式的复杂化。根据 Fenton 和 Karma 所报道的结果[48]，当兴奋性下降时，心肌纤维旋转引起的不稳定性会消失。这将后一种不稳定性与负性张力引起的不稳定性区分开了，负性张力引起的不稳定在兴奋性增加时反而消失。缠绕各向异性仅在特定的轴丝方向引起不稳定，这一点仅在跨越心肌壁的轴丝（其方向垂直于纤维）中得到证实。当轴丝平行于心肌表面时，旋转各向异性引起轴丝的移动但不减小稳定性。这种由旋转各向异性引起的不稳定机制目前尚不完全清楚。

（三）梯度导致的不稳定

沿着回旋波轴丝的梯度能引起复杂的不稳定性改

了回旋波发生缠绕，见侧面投射的圆锥模型所示（t=25min），t=52min 时，回旋波破碎，在接近其末端形成复杂的、混乱样状态（见图 38-7A，下方）。以 a、b、c 标记的可视密度记录（见图 38-7B）显示了沿着垂线的最初时相是恒定的，这与预期的未缠绕的垂直回旋波是一致的。在随后的 30min 内，如图所示，随着三次系列中时相差别的增加，缠绕也在逐渐增加。30min 之后，b、c 点的模式变得复杂，没有周期性，提示发生了混乱状态。需要注意，在多形性心动过速时所记录的这些心电图波形形态之间的类同之处。

心律失常中缠绕回旋波发生的缠绕（twisting）和崩溃（breakdown）可能也很重要。心肌组织通过厚的心壁时有平滑的各向异性[35]。急性缺血时，心肌正常区域与灌注不良区域的边缘带会出现显著的梯度变化[37]，边缘带即通常我们所说的心律失常"源"（arrhythmogenic），在这些区域形成的回旋波将会发生缠绕，这一点在前文已有所讨论。如果各向异性足够大，缠绕终将超过临界值，于是回旋波发生破碎，这与在 B-Z 反应中所见的一样。如果是发生在心肌中的各向异性，回旋波会破碎成多形的、无结构的漩涡，而发生类似于颤动的现象。

五、回旋波成像

近年来，在心肌中研究三维激动传播的唯一可行的方法是多电极标测（multiple electrode mapping）。在多电极标测中，针电极（plunge-needle electrodes）插入到心肌中，每个插入针电极都有几个平行的沿着针轴的双极电极对组成。目前，许多先进的系统包括了几百个针，可记录到多达 1000 个记录位点。利用这项技术得到的实验数据首先提出了跨膜回旋波的存在[15]（由这些数据得到的回旋波的重建见前文图 39-2 所述[2]）。

尽管多电极标测技术很有用，但其空间分辨力常常不足以精确地标测复杂的激动传播的三维模式，特别是在室性快速性心律失常时。这项技术最主要的缺点是穿刺针电极所引起的心肌组织的损伤，当穿刺部相位互之间距离太近时，显著影响了激动的传播，甚至可以引起传播的阻滞。

多电极标测的内在局限性提出了需要发展一个可替代的、侵入性伤害小的技术，三维技术的高空间分辨力和瞬时清晰度能够弥补传统多电极标测的不足。近来的研究指出，利用电压敏感染色（voltage-sensi-

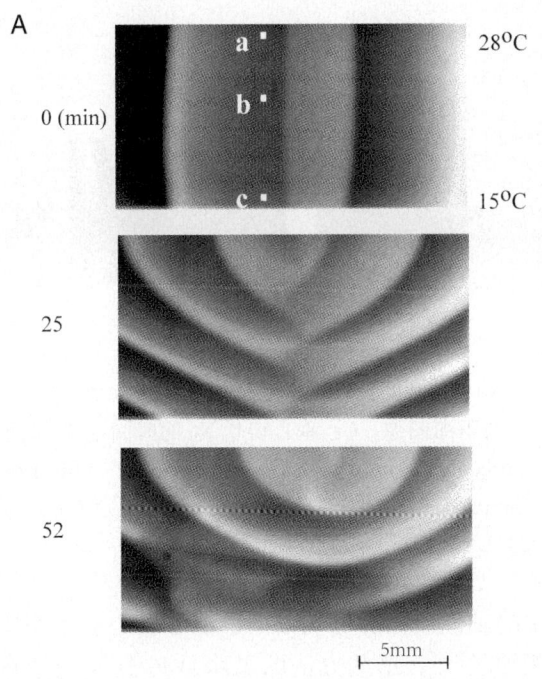

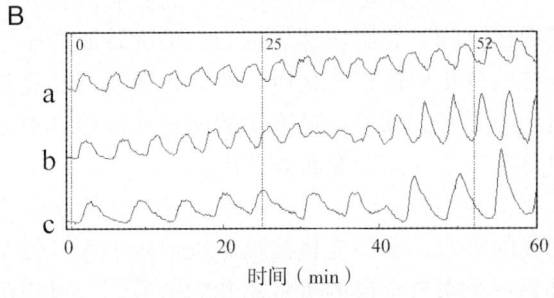

图 38-7 B-Z 反应中由于温度梯度导致单一回旋波的不稳定

A：三个不同时间的侧面投影相片。t=0min（梯度刚出现的时刻）时回旋波未发生缠绕；t=25min（中图）时波群开始缠绕，但没有结构的紊乱；t=52min（下图）时回旋波不再是明确可辨的模式。B：A 中最上方图中的 a 到 c 的时间序列，垂直的虚线表示 A 图拍照的时间（引自 Mironov S, Vinson M, Mulvey S, Pertsov A：Destabilization of three-dimensional rotating chemical waves in an inhomogeneous BZ reaction. J Phys Chem 100：1975-1983，1996. Copyright American Chemical Society.）

变，表明室性心动过速有向心室颤动转变的可能。通常，沿着轴丝的梯度仅产生缠绕（见前文）。然而，在梯度足够大时，所诱发的缠绕不能维持平衡，回旋波破碎，形成了复杂的、混乱样的状态[10,43]。图 38-7 显示了在 B-Z 反应中梯度所诱发的单一回旋波的不稳定性改变。将回旋波放置在平行于轴丝的常温梯度中，在早期，回旋波没有发生缠绕（见图 38-7A，t=0min）。之后，由温度梯度引起的旋转周期的差别导致

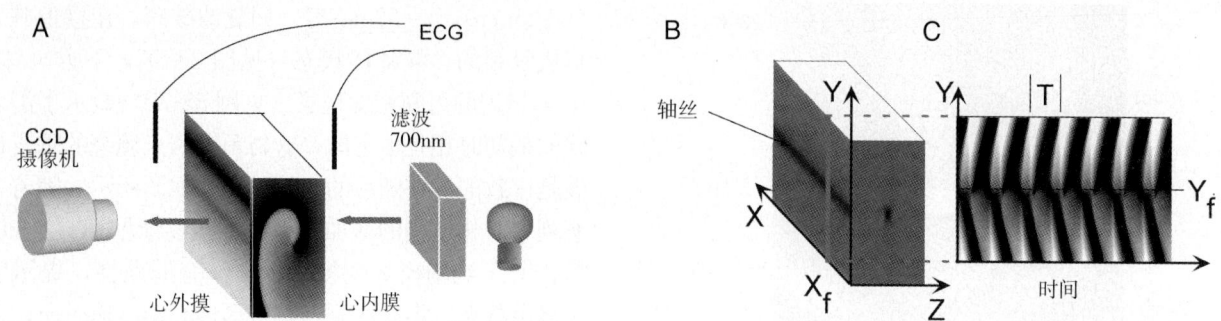

图 38-8　利用 X 线透视技术（计算机模式）观察到的轴丝　A：中间的三维阻滞表示的是有旋转回旋波的心肌组织的切片。灰色部分表示计算出的光强度。B：通过时间-叠加序列框架得出的轴丝投影的阻滞图像。C：垂直切片 X_l 的时间-空间曲线图（Y，T），呈之字形排列，表示了切片中轴丝的位置（引自 Pertsov AM：Three-dimensional organization of reentry in fibrillating ventricular wall. In Virag N，Blanc O，Kappenberger L [eds]：Computer Simulation and Experimental Assessment of Cardiac Electrophysiology．Lausanne，Switzerland，Futura Publishing，pp63-68，2001.）

tive dyes）的可视图像能够成为取代它的产品。染色剂能够通过冠脉血流而不引起明显的组织损害。另外，利用光电二极管阵列和电荷耦合器件（charge-coupled device，CCD）相机能明显简化所记录和解释的数据，能提供优质的空间分辨力。尽管目前所使用的电压敏感阵列最初是应用于成像表面活性的二维模式中，但已有许多迹象表明，这项技术在三维模式的应用中也会有很大的潜力。近来，几个实验室已经报道了在心肌表面记录的传统的荧光图像是源自于心肌的深层[16,17]。尤其在利用了传统的可视图像后，Efimov 及其同事[17]能够观察到在强电流刺激下心外膜下回旋波内部的构型。Baxter 及其同事[16]利用 X 线透视技术进一步扩展了回旋波可视图像的能力。利用这项技术，他们能够发现隐藏在心肌深部的壁内回旋波。

轴丝的显像

近来的研究提示，早期所用在化学凝胶固定激动系统中的轴丝监测的可视方法也能够在心肌组织中用于监测轴丝[50]，这些方法的思路是基于 X 线透视技术的应用。将电压敏感染色后着色的心肌放置在光源与摄影机之间，心肌内部兴奋的三维旋转波产生了跨膜电压的变化，这些变化所导致的光强度的变化被摄像机记录下来。轴丝，更确切的说是其投照，通过计算机分析所记录的图像而被重建。

兴奋的旋转波产生的跨膜电压的变化影响了染色剂的光的吸收，这些变化被摄影机记录下来。每个图像都是一个来自全层的重量总和的信号，与可视的 X 线断层投射相似，用比旋转频率大的速度来拍摄一系列这样的图像，能够得到多个同样旋转波的投射。利用 Mironov 及其同事所描述的运算法则[10]，通过运算包含有这些投射的信息能够依次看见轴丝。

图 38-8 是运用时间叠加法（time averaging

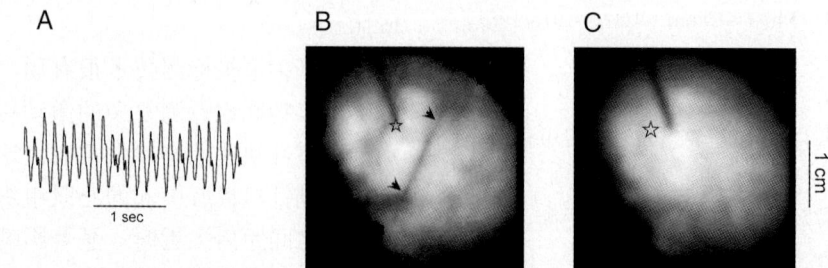

图 38-9　右心室除颤时的回旋波轴丝　A：心室颤动时记录的心电图。B：X 线透视下的时间-叠加显像，箭头指示轴丝位置。C：电复律后的图像（引自 Pertsov AM：Three-dimensional organization of reentry in fibrillating ventricular wall．In Virag N，Blanc O，Kappenberger L [eds]：Computer Simulation and Experimental Assessment of Cardiac Electrophysiology．Lausanne，Switzerland，Futura Pub-lishing，2001，pp63-68.）

method) 在 X 线透视中轴丝的重构[51]。这种方法是利用轴丝的附近没有被循环兴奋波所激动这一现象。图 38-8A 显示了回旋波方向平行于表面的心肌组织阻滞的三维模式。在这一模式中，利用 Luo-Rudy 公式描述了兴奋细胞的电特性，采用壁内光强度指数式衰减的方法可以计算出透视信号。图 38-8A 中，在阻滞边缘区可以看见螺旋和轴丝的末端，在一个或多个旋转周期的连续框架中显示出一个黑的阴影，这个阴影是轴丝在标本表面的投影，阴影的位置（见图 38-8B，中部）是轴丝真正的位置。图 38-8C 显示了基于时间-空间曲线分析重构轴丝的另一个方法[51]。这两种方法都得出了同样的结果。

用同样的方法在真正的心肌组织中也可以看见轴丝。图 38-9 显示的是羊的右心室壁在发生多形性室性心动过速时，通过 X 线透视可以发现回旋波轴丝（心外膜投照）。利用 RH-155 吸收电压敏感染色后标本可以着色，使用高速数字式 CCD 摄影机，计算以 700nm 光速穿过组织的能见度时能够发现跨膜电压的变化。光源和摄像机分别放置在标本的心内膜和心外膜的两侧。图 38-9B 显示的是利用时间-叠加方法所得到的轴丝的图像。黑色阴影部分是轴丝（见图 38-9B，箭头所示），在心动过速发生之前和终止之后都没有这些阴影（见图 38-9C），而当心律失常终止后，从刺激电极处来的阴影一直都有（见图 38-9C，星号所示）。

六、致谢

本研究得到美国心脏和血管协会 HL39707 基金的支持。作者衷心感谢 Drs. Christopher Hyatt, Sergey Mironov 和 Marcel Wellner 细心审阅刊物，提出有益意见。衷心感谢技术助手 Stephen Simons 热心准备相关的图片。

（马建新 译）

参 考 文 献

1. Pertsov AM, Jalife J: Three-dimensional vortex-like reentry. In Zipes DP, Jalife J (eds): Cardiac Electrophysiology: From Cell to Bedside. Philadelphia, WB Saunders, 1995, pp 403–410.
2. Pertsov AM, Jalife J: Scroll waves in three-dimensional cardiac muscle. In Zipes DP, Jalife J (eds): Cardiac Electrophysiology: From Cell to Bedside. Philadelphia, WB Saunders, 2000, pp 336–344.
3. Pertsov AM, Davidenko JM, Salomonsz R, et al: Spiral waves of excitation underlie reentrant activity in isolated cardiac muscle. Circ Res 72:631–650, 1993.
4. Krinsky VI: Mathematical models of cardiac arrhythmias (spiral waves). Pharmacol Ther [B] 3:539–555, 1978.
5. Gray RA, Jalife J, Panfilov AV, et al: Mechanisms of cardiac fibrillation. Science 270:1222–1223; discussion 1224–1225, 1995.
6. Downar E, Harris L, Kimber S, et al: Ventricular tachycardia after surgical repair of tetralogy of Fallot: Results of intraoperative mapping studies. J Am Coll Cardiol 20:648–655, 1992.
7. Winfree AT: Scroll-shaped waves of chemical activity in three dimensions. Science 181:937–939, 1973.
8. Pertsov AM, Wellner M, Vinson M, Jalife J: Topological constraint on scroll wave pinning. Phys Rev Lett 84:2738–2741, 2000.
9. Davidenko JM, Pertsov AV, Salomonsz R, et al: Stationary and drifting spiral waves of excitation in isolated cardiac muscle. Nature 355:349–351, 1992.
10. Mironov S, Vinson M, Mulvey S, Pertsov A: Destabilization of three-dimensional rotating chemical waves in an inhomogeneous BZ reaction. J Phys Chem 100:1975–1983, 1996.
11. Vinson M, Mironov S, Mulvey S, Pertsov A: Control of spatial orientation and lifetime of scroll rings in excitable media. Nature 386:477–480, 1997.
12. Berenfeld O, Pertsov AM: Dynamics of intramural scroll waves in three-dimensional continuous myocardium with rotational anisotropy. J Theor Biol 199:383–394, 1999.
13. Wellner M, Berenfeld O, Pertsov AM: Predicting filament drift in twisted anisotropy. Phys Rev E Stat Phys Plasmas Fluids Relat Interdiscip Topics 61:1845–1850, 2000.
14. Berenfeld O, Wellner M, Jalife J, Pertsov AM: Shaping of a scroll wave filament by cardiac fibers. Phys Rev E Stat Nonlin Soft Matter Phys 63:061901, 2001.
15. Frazier DW, Wolf PD, Wharton JM, et al: Stimulus-induced critical point. Mechanism for electrical initiation of reentry in normal canine myocardium. J Clin Invest 83:1039–1052, 1989.
16. Baxter WT, Mironov SF, Zaitsev AV, et al: Visualizing excitation waves inside cardiac muscle using transillumination. Biophys J 80:516–530, 2001.
17. Efimov IR, Sidorov V, Cheng Y, Wollenzier B: Evidence of three-dimensional scroll waves with ribbon-shaped filament as a mechanism of ventricular tachycardia in the isolated rabbit heart. J Cardiovasc Electrophysiol 10:1452–1462, 1999.
18. Panfilov AV, Pertsov AM: Vortex rings in a three-dimensional medium described by reaction-diffusion equations. Doklady Biophysics 274:58–60, 1984.
19. Jahnke W, Hanze C, Winfree A: Chemical vortex dynamics in three-dimensional excitable media. Nature 336:662–665, 1998.
20. Wellner M, Pertsov AM, Jalife J: Spatial Doppler anomaly in an excitable medium. Phys Rev E Stat Phys Plasmas Fluids Relat Interdiscip Topics 54:1120–1125, 1996.
21. Medvinsky AB, Panfilov AV, Pertsov AM: Properties of rotating waves in 3 dimensions: Scroll rings in myocardium. In Krinsky VI (ed): Self-Organization: Autowaves and Structures Far from Equilibrium. New York, Springer-Verlag, 1984, pp 195–199.
22. Welsh B, Gomatam S, Burgess A: Three-dimensional chemical waves in the Belousov-Zhabotinsky reaction. Nature 304:611–614, 1983.
23. Efimov IR, Gray RA, Roth BJ: Virtual electrodes and deexcitation: New insights into fibrillation induction and defibrillation. J Cardiovasc Electrophysiol 11:339–353, 2000.
24. Panfilov A, Pertsov AM: Mechanism of spiral wave initiation in active media connected with critical curvature phenomenon. Biofizica 27:868–888, 1982.
25. Cabo C, Pertsov AM, Davidenko JM, et al: Vortex shedding as a precursor of turbulent electrical activity in cardiac muscle. Biophys J 70:1105–1111, 1996.
26. Winfree AT: Electrical instability in cardiac muscle: Phase singularities and rotors. J Theor Biol 138:353–405, 1989.
27. Davidenko JM, Kent P, Jalife J: Spiral waves in normal isolated ventricular muscle. Physica D 49:182–197, 1991.
28. Lindblom AE, Roth BJ, Trayanova NA: Role of virtual electrodes in arrhythmogenesis: Pinwheel experiment revisited. J Cardiovasc Electrophysiol 11:274–285, 2000.
29. Lin SF, Roth BJ, Wikswo JP Jr: Quatrefoil reentry in myocardium: An optical imaging study of the induction mechanism. J Cardiovasc Electrophysiol 10:574–586, 1999.
30. Keener JP, Tyson JJ: The dynamics of scroll waves in excitable media. SIAM Rev 34:1–39, 1992.
31. Biktashev VN, Holden A, Zhang H: Tension of organizing filaments of scroll waves. Philos Trans R Soc Lond A 347:611–630, 1994.

32. Wit AL, Dillon SM, Coromilas J, et al: Anisotropic reentry in the epicardial border zone of myocardial infarcts. Ann NY Acad Sci 591:86–108, 1990.
33. Downar E, Harris L, Mickleborough LL, et al: Endocardial mapping of ventricular tachycardia in the intact human ventricle: Evidence for reentrant mechanisms. J Am Coll Cardiol 11:783–791, 1988.
34. Wellner M, Berenfeld O, Jalife J, Pertsov AM: Minimal principle for rotor filaments. Proc Natl Acad Sci U S A 99:8015–8018, 2002.
35. Antzelevitch C, Sicouri S, Litovsky SH, et al: Heterogeneity within the ventricular wall: Electrophysiology and pharmacology of epicardial, endocardial and M cells. Circ Res 69:1427–1449, 1991.
36. Rosenbaum DS, Kaplan DT, Kanai A, et al: Depolarization inhomogeneities in ventricular myocarium change dramatically with abrupt cycle length shortening. Circulation 84:1333–1345, 1991.
37. Coronel R, Wilms-Schopman FJ, Opthof T, et al: Injury current and gradients of diastolic stimulation threshold, TQ potential, and extracellular potassium concentration during acute regional ischemia in the isolated perfused pig heart. Circ Res 68:1241–1249, 1991.
38. Vinson M, Pertsov AM, Jalife J: Anchoring of vortex filaments in 3D excitable media. Physica D 72:119–134, 1993.
39. Rudenko AN, Panfilov AV: Drift and interaction of vortices in two-dimensional heterogeneous active medium. Stud Biophys 98:183–188, 1983.
40. Steinbock O, Schutze J, Muller SC: Electric-field-induced drift and deformation of spiral waves in an excitable medium. Phys Rev Lett 68:248–251, 1992.
41. Zou X, Levine H, Kessler DA: Interaction between a drifting spiral and defects. Phys Rev E Stat Phys Plasmas Fluids Relat Interdiscip Topics 47:R800–R803, 1993.
42. Ikeda T, Yashima M, Uchida T, et al: Attachment of meandering reentrant wave fronts to anatomic obstacles in the atrium. Role of the obstacle size. Circ Res 81:753–764, 1997.
43. Pertsov AM, Aliev RR, Krinsky VI: Three-dimensional twisted vortices in an excitable chemical medium. Nature 345:419–421, 1990.
44. Panfilov AV, Rudenko AN, Pertsov AM: Twisted scroll waves in three-dimensional active media. In Krinsky VI (ed): Self-Organization: Autowaves and Structures Far from Equilibrium. Berlin, Springer-Verlag, 1984, pp 103–105.
45. Winfree AT, Strogatz SH: Organizing centers of three-dimensional chemical waves. Chaos 311:611–615, 1984.
46. Mikhailov AS, Panfilov AV, Rudenko AN: Twisted scroll waves in active three-dimensional media. Phys Lett A 109:246–249, 1985.
47. Panfilov AV, Keener JP: Re-entry in three-dimensional FitzHugh-Nagumo medium with rotational anisotropy. Physica D 84:545–552, 1995.
48. Fenton F, Karma A: Vortex dynamics in three-dumensional continuous myocardium with fiber rotation: Filament instability and fibrillation. Chaos 8:20–47, 1998.
49. Zhang S, Skinner JL, Sims AL, et al: Three-dimensional mapping of spontaneous ventricular arrhythmias in a canine thrombotic coronary occlusion model. J Cardiovasc Electrophysiol 11:762–772, 2000.
50. Pertsov AM, Mironov SF, Zaitsev AV, Jalife J: Visualization of stable intramural reentry during fibrillatory activity in perfused sheep right ventricle [abstract]. Circulation(suppl 1)1999;100:I-872.
51. Pertsov AM: Three-dimensional organization of reentry in fibrillating ventricular wall. In Virag N, Blanc O, Kappenberger L (eds): Computer Simulation and Experimental Assessment of Cardiac Electrophy. Armonk, NY, Futura, pp 63–68.

第八部分
心律失常发生的机制

第 39 章

肺静脉的电生理特性：房颤发生的机制

Jeffrey E. Olgin

本章目录

- 局灶性房颤 ………………………… 351
- 肺静脉的电生理特性 ……………… 352
- 肺静脉的解剖和组织学 …………… 353
- 局灶性房颤的发生机制 …………… 354
- 结论 ………………………………… 356

早在 1876 年[1]，Brunton 和 Fayrer 首次描述肺静脉内存在自发的、独立的电激动。他们在文中写道"在生理学家和临床医生注意到肺静脉激动之前，肺静脉的现象就已被提出，但长期未受到重视……。"最近，这种"肺静脉激动"引起了电生理医生的注意，将肺静脉内的触发活动作为房颤的起源点，最早是由 Haissaguerre 等于 1998 年报道的[2]。

尽管早在一个世纪前就已对肺静脉收缩功能进行了描述，但并不了解它的电生理特性和致心律失常的特殊机制。不同的种属其心房的肌性结构延展到肺静脉内的程度不同[3-7]。早期的研究显示激动沿着这些肌纤维从心房传播[8,9]，这些肌纤维具有与心房肌相似的动作电位和电传导特性，提示这些肌纤维起源于心房[3,8,9]。

现在已清楚肺静脉是房性心动过速常见的局灶性起源[10,11]。另外，由于外科迷宫手术就是切割和隔离肺静脉，有助于了解肺静脉在房颤发生中的重要性[12]。临床研究已经显示最常见的阵发性房颤的触发因素是起源于肺静脉的早搏[2,13]。然而，肺静脉内局灶性激动的机制，以及什么使肺静脉内产生了局灶性激动仍不清楚。

一、局灶性房颤

多子波假说作为大多数房颤维持的机制已被普遍接受，局灶性房颤是在 90 年代后期作为临床相关概念再度出现的，因为肺静脉是房颤射频消融治愈的靶点（参照 112 章和 113 章）。1947 年 Scherf[14] 描述了实验条件下的局灶性房颤，将乌头碱（可引起局灶性后除极和局灶性心动过速）注射到右心耳处制做房颤的模型，心动过速频率加快后，就可能发展为房颤。当将右心耳从心房分离后，房颤就终止。Haissaguerre 等[2]在阵发性房颤的病人中报道了相似的机制，在这项研究中，45 例局灶性房颤的患者中 41 例的局灶起源在肺静脉，大多数病例（31 例）的局灶性激动起源于左上肺静脉，其次是右上肺静脉（17 例），余下的起源左下肺静脉（11 例）和右下肺静脉（6 例）。在另外一项 97 例病人的研究中，90％局灶性房颤的激动起源于肺静脉[13]。重要的是这两项研究均证明了局灶性消融可以消除房颤。

临床上，局灶性房颤可以分为两种类型：局灶性触发和局灶性驱动。局灶性触发的因子就是房早（或几个房早，或一串快速房速），它们能够触发多子波折返和导致自发的持续性房颤（图 39-1）。房颤的维持并不需要连续的局灶性激动，局灶消融也不能终止房颤，但是可以防止房颤再复发。局灶性驱动是由连续性局灶性激动产生的，它对于延续和维持房颤是必要的（图 39-2A）。局灶性驱动的消融可以终止房颤（图 39-2B）。这两种机制的证据在病人中均存在。

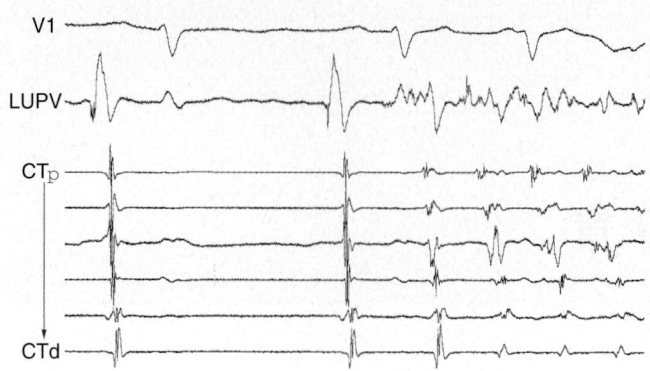

图 39-1 左上肺静脉的触发灶诱发的自发性房颤 一个左上肺静脉内的早搏触发了多子波折返,产生持续性房颤。该患者的这一现象反复发生,在 2 小时的电生理检查中,复律后反复发作了 25 次。在左上肺静脉的消融没有终止房颤,但在消融后行电复律,则房颤不再被诱发。CT:界嵴;d:远端;p:近端

二、肺静脉的电生理特性

尽管已清楚大多数病人中,局灶性房颤起源于肺静脉内或肺静脉周边,但还不清楚为什么这些部位在致心律失常中是易感区。在电生理实验室中,可以获得一种离散的、高频的细胞外电位(被称作肺静脉电位),一般存在于肺静脉口到其远端 4cm 处,而下肺静脉则短一些[8]。这些电活动代表的是从左房深入肺静脉的肌袖的电位,肌袖深入到肺静脉的深度在种属与种属之间存在差异,在哺乳类动物,肌袖主要局限在肺静脉外;在啮齿类动物[15],肌袖延展至肺静脉内。1972 年 Spach 和其他人[8]首先研究了肺静脉内的激动,他们观察了 2 名进行心外科手术的患者(无房颤)和犬,在距肺静脉口 1~4cm 处可记录到激动及其传导现象。左上肺静脉内激动传导的距离最长。单极记录特别是右上肺静脉内可记录到双电位,这些分别是远场的心房信号和局部肺静脉内心肌激动。

在电生理实验室,从肺静脉内记录到的电位通常与来自左房的、远场的、低频的信号分开的,并且紧随其后(图 39-3)。这种情况既可在正常人中见到,也可在房颤患者中见到,反映的是来自左房的激动进入肺静脉后的正常传导顺序。然而,作为心律失常的致病区,肺静脉内这些电位的激动顺序可以颠倒,例如在房性早搏时,可见肺静脉电位领先于远场电位(图 39-3)。这些信号分开的距离,特别是起自致心律失常肺静脉的早搏时,两种电位的间距可达 160ms 以上[16]。有趣的是,窦性心律下,在肺静脉近端,电位

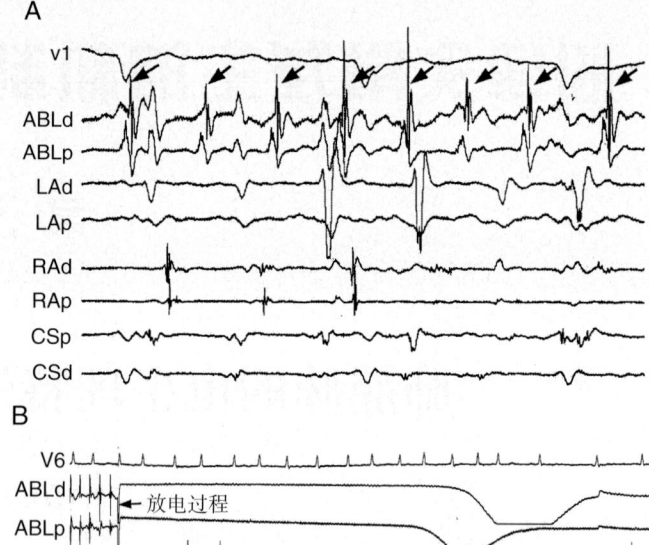

图 39-2 右上肺静脉起源的局灶性驱动的房颤 A. 在右上肺静脉用消融导管记录的局部心内电图,房颤发生时记录到规则的尖锋电位(箭头标示),周期 160ms,从肺静脉到左房存在不规则性传导。B. 在该部位放电时,房颤 7s 内终止,如箭头所示。ABL:消融;CS:冠状窦;d:远端;p:近端;LA:左房;RA:右房

和左房远场电位不明显分开。从心房的不同部位起搏,可将局部肺静脉电位与左心房电位分开。例如在冠状窦远端起搏,可以将左上肺静脉内的电位分开。另外,应用快频率起搏或期前刺激,均可将这些电位分开[17]。局部记录中所见的电位分开的基础尚不清楚。尽管如此,有证据证实在肺静脉近端存在着缓慢传导。在肺静脉内可记录到碎裂电位,通常位于环绕左房和肺静脉连接处[18]。这些电位碎裂的程度不同,依赖于起搏部位。

Arora[19]等应用高分辨光学标测技术观察了灌流下完整心房的电活动。在这项研究中,可见肺静脉近端是一个具有缓慢传导碎裂区域(图 39-4),缓慢传导区域的传导速度为 31.3±4.47cm/s,而心房内的传导速度为 90.2±20.7cm/s。Hocini[20]等应用高密度片状电极标测灌流的犬心脏时,也有类似发现。缓慢传导区域就是那些肌细胞纤维的排列方向突然改变的部位[20,21]。

为什么在心房不同部位起搏会导致左房电位和肺静脉电位分离的程度不同,或增加碎裂电位,这一机制尚不清楚。有一个假说,就是进入肺静脉的激动具

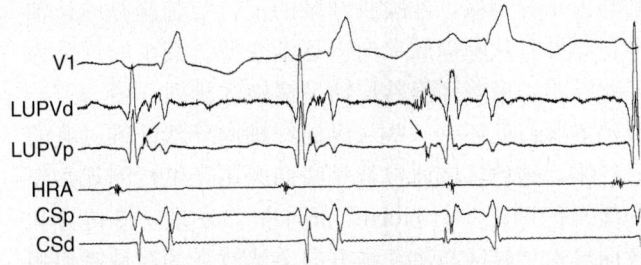

图39-3 位于左上肺静脉导管记录到心房期前收缩时的"肺静脉电位" 窦性心律时,箭头所指的尖锐的局部电位,代表的就是肺静脉肌袖的局部电活动。肺静脉电位落在左房电位之后,且为低频信号,它与冠状窦的心房信号同步。从左侧数第三跳,发生了一次房早,并且肺静脉电位领先左房电位,在左上肺静脉导管的远端,可记录到局部碎裂电位。CS:冠状窦;d:远端;p:近端;HRA:高右房

有高度各向异性,因此,在肺静脉口会有很多条路径进入肺静脉[18]。

另外,在肺静脉近端缓慢传导离散电位区,具有递减传导特性[17,19,22,23],这种递减传导在人和犬中均可以见到,这种递减传导更多见于有阵发性房颤病史的患者[17]。有趣的是,这种递减现象出现在肺静脉近端缓慢传导的离散区[19]。有些病人中,在较长的心动周期中,递减传导可表现为2:1传导或文氏传导(图39-5)。这些传导形式有时使左右心房的激动表现为不规则的,而肺静脉内的激动却是规则的(图39-2A)。另外,来自肺静脉内联律间期较短的早搏,可能会被这种传导阻滞掉,形成一个隐匿性房早。

正常人中,肺静脉内心肌的有效不应期长于邻近的心房肌(282 ± 45ms vs 253 ± 41ms, $p=0.009$)[17]。与此相似的情况在犬模型中也可以见到,应用光学标测技术,在以80%除极动作电位时限(APD_{80})计算,肺静脉内长于左房(187 ± 15ms vs 125.1 ± 16.5ms, $p<0.001$)[19]。在正常的犬模型中,应用光学标测可以见到肺静脉内除极的各向异性是增加的[19]。Cheung[24]研究了豚鼠的肺静脉。应用微电极记录,他发现肺静脉远端静息膜电位是~66mV,近端为~71mV,肺静脉近端的动作电位与心房非常相似,肺静脉近端的动作电位较远端长。Hocini和同事[20]在离体灌流犬心脏中也有相似的发现,他们应用微电极在肺静脉近端心房肌记录到相似的动作电位,而在肺静脉远端记录的动作电位缺乏平台期,动作电位时限短,超射速度较慢(图39-6)。

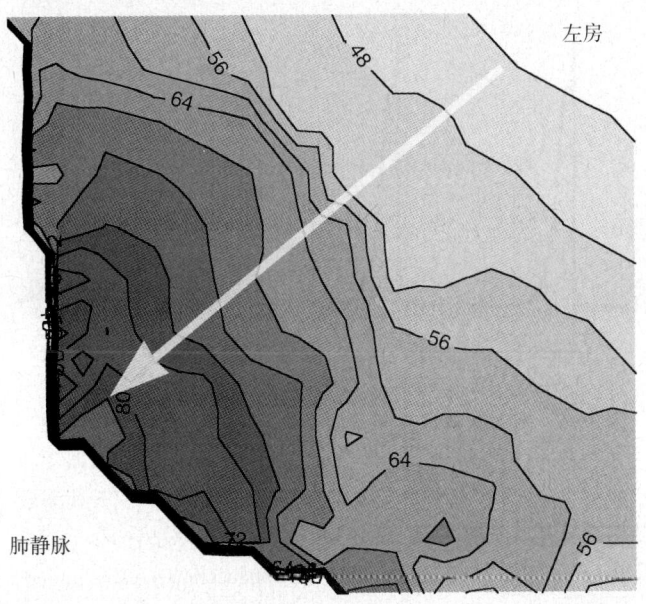

图39-4 利用光学标测技术,在一只正常犬的肺静脉近端$4cm^2$的区域进行了等时标测 从左房起搏产生的激动沿着箭头标记的方向传导,左房和肺静脉远端已标记,在肺静脉的近端有明显的缓慢传导,等时线的间距较拥挤,等时标记线的数字单位是ms

三、肺静脉的解剖和组织学

有关肺静脉肌袖的解剖结构和组织学特征在人和犬中均已有研究,典型的情况下,人有4根肺静脉分别开口,而这些肺静脉的位置有很大的差异,HO和他的同事从正常人的尸检研究中发现,25%的尸检可见常规的左、右静脉开口,40%的尸检标本中上下肺静脉开口距离小于3mm,他们还发现最长的肺静肌袖位于上肺静脉内,可达2.5mm长;靠近肺静脉口

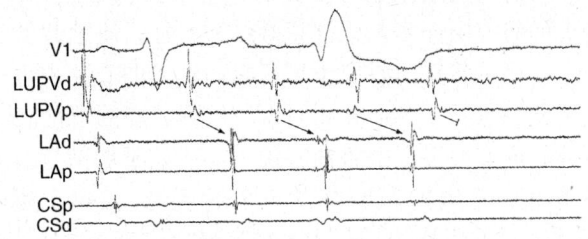

图39-5 左上肺静脉内记录的局灶性房性早搏 在第1跳窦性心律之后紧随4个房性早搏,最早激动点位于左上肺静脉内,当把左房电极导管放置在左上肺静脉内时显示出起源于左上肺静脉的局灶房早向心房传导呈逐渐延长,直至向左房传导发生阻滞,表现为文氏现象。CS:冠状窦;d:远端;p:近端。

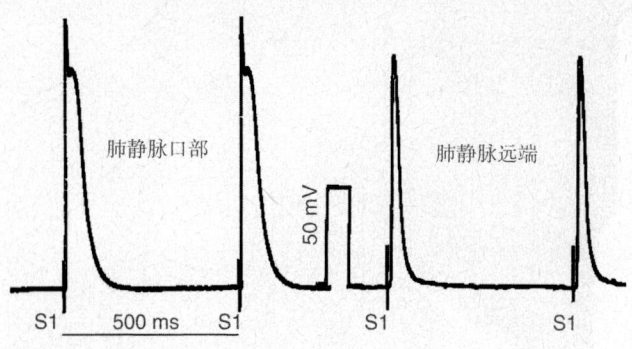

图 39-6 利用微电极在灌流的犬肺静脉内记录的动作电位

肺静脉近端的动作电位（左侧）的形态和特征与心房肌动作电位非常近似。肺静脉远端的动作电位（右侧）上升速率较慢，缺乏平台期，时限较短。S₁：短阵刺激（引自 Hocini M, Ho SY, Kawara T et al. Electrical conduaction in caine pulmonary veins: Electrophysiological and anatomic correlation. Circulation 105：2442-2448, 2002.）

处的肌袖最厚，其次是上肺静脉靠下的部位，其比下肺静脉上部的肌袖厚，这些部位肌袖厚度范围约0.5～1.98mm。肌袖的厚度从肺静脉左房开口向内逐渐变薄。组织学检查证实肌袖结构呈环形纤维（沿着肺静脉的长轴呈螺旋样结构），也还有一些纵向纤维（沿肺静脉长轴排列），这些纤维通常紧靠着环形纤维走行，也是在肺静脉口处较厚，进入肺静脉远端逐渐变薄。环形纤维区域之间有明显的连接，有些区域也缺乏连接，被结缔组织分割。肺静脉的远端，结缔组织形成的分割较多，心肌组织可以被纤维组织环绕分割（图 39-7）[26]。在那些有或没有房颤史患者尸检的研究中，Saito 等[26]发现在这些人群中，肌袖的形态、长度、微结构或纤维走向无明显差异。另外，该研究发现在肺静脉肌袖内没有特异性传导和结样组织。

目前认为肌袖起源于左房，Spach 和同事[8]在人和犬的研究中证实，根据超微结构特征，肌袖起源于心房，可见特殊的心房小体。我们在犬的心脏中也证实了这一点[21]。Spach 和同事[8]进行了胚胎学的相关研究，证实在发育中肌袖起源于心房的延展部分，而不是由中胚层的原腔静脉壁分化而来。Blom 和同事[27]发现在发育的过程中，肺静脉内含有 HNK-1 抗原，它是房室特殊传导系统发育的标志物。这些资料提示：至少肺静脉周围的心肌发育来自原始的房室结组织。然而，有关成人和犬的起搏细胞的来源尚缺乏证据[10,20,21,25]。

我们进一步研究了肺静脉肌袖的解剖学、组织学、超微结构和缝隙连接的分布[21]。发现犬肺静脉肌袖与人十分相似，外膜肌纤维的走行与肺静脉的长轴平行，并且从肺静脉口向内逐渐变薄。其余的纤维为环状纤维，沿着肺静脉长轴呈螺旋样排列（图 39-7）。在肺静脉口处还有一些从纵向纤维向环状纤维过渡的肌纤维，这种区域通常就是我们应用光学标测观察到的缓慢传导区[19]。Hocini 和同事[20]发现，慢传导和各向异性传导区与肌纤维方向突然改变的区域密切相关，连接蛋白 43 在肺静脉的分布与左房中没有明显差异[21]。然而，与左房相比，肺静脉内连接蛋白 40 是缺乏的。

有或没有房性心律失常的人肺静脉组织切片三维结构显示肺静脉纤维方向较复杂[25,26]，这种结构就会导致不均一的各向异性[28]。当发生纤维化导致细胞之间具有不连续性时，不均一的各向异性就会加重，这是折返形成的基质。我们和其他研究者都证实了在肺静脉口存在缓慢传导、递减传导和传导阻滞区[19,20]。我们还证明了在正常犬肺静脉内可以发生折返。这些区域的失耦联可能是由于连接蛋白 40 的减少，可以影响异位灶的传导。计算机模型提示某种程度的失耦联可以抑制异位灶激动的传导[29]。因而，这些部位的解剖结构特征使其易发生折返和异位搏动。

四、局灶性房颤的发生机制

肺静脉起源的局灶性房颤发生的机制目前尚不十分清楚，有可能与自律性升高、触发活动和折返相关。在豚鼠的肺静脉内，Cheung[24]等研究表明肺静脉内的平滑肌细胞具有稳定的静息膜电位，但刺激不能产生动作电位。另外，平滑肌细胞与肌袖之间被一层纤维组织分开，应用电镜和缝隙连接染色都未见在这两者之间存在连接，因而，这些平滑肌细胞应该不会产生异位激动。Masani[15]通过电镜研究细胞的超微结构确认在肺静脉内存在结样细胞。在该研究中可观察到清晰的细胞结构，其具有结样结构，但并没有研究这些细胞的电生理特性。在人和正常犬的肺静脉内也可以观察到非特异性结样细胞[26]。在逆向灌流分离的兔肺静脉细胞中，可以看到具有心房细胞和起搏细胞两种特征的混合型细胞（慢的动作电位超射和自动的 4 相除极）[30]。在豚鼠的肺静脉远端可记录到具有自动舒张期除极的起搏细胞的电位。该研究完整地分离出豚鼠肺静脉细胞，并应用微电极记录电位。在分离的 17 个静脉中有 7 个静脉具有自发的肺静脉节律。在肺静脉的远端，通过微电极记录可以观察到自动的

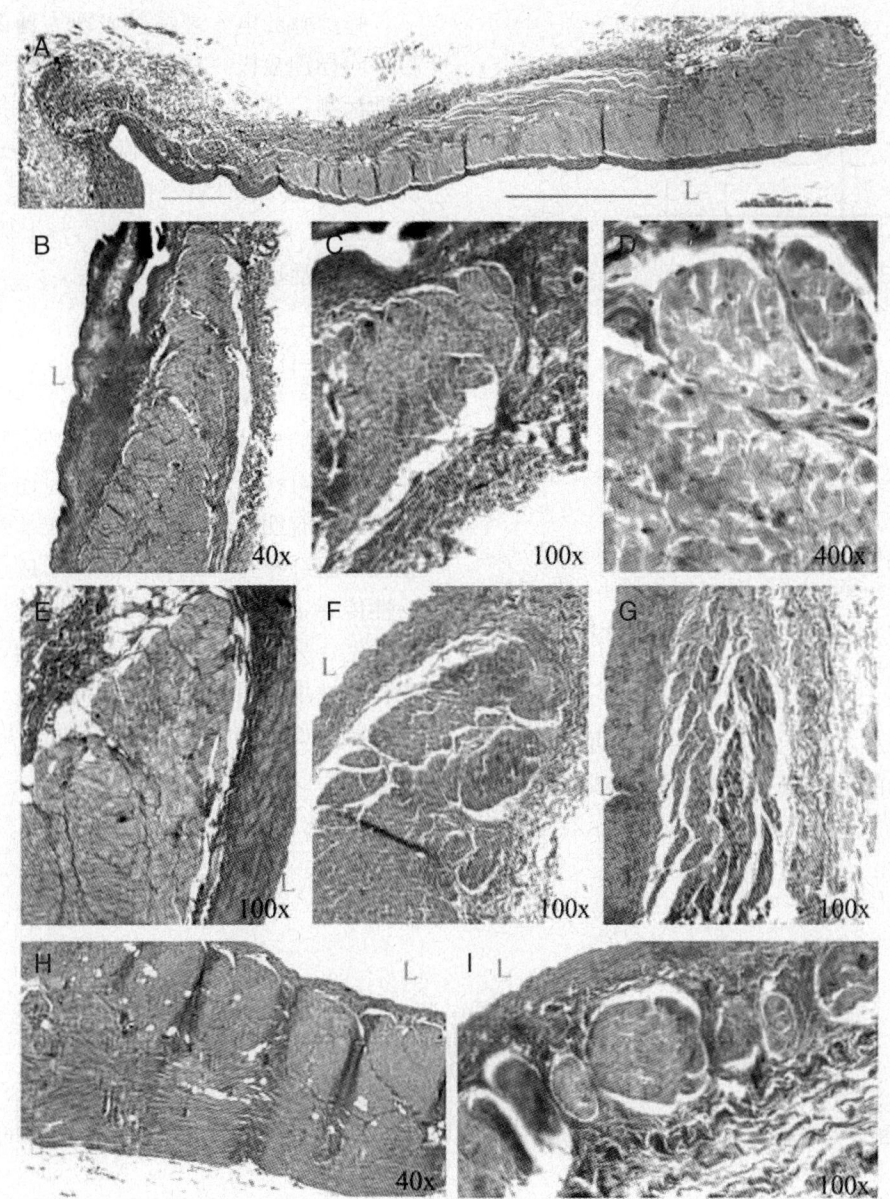

图 39-7 正常犬肌袖组织学横向切片 A、B 和 C 是右下肺静脉的切片，靠近肌袖的顶端。A 和 B 图取自同一切片的相对侧，C 图是对 B 图的放大，D 图和 E 图是肌袖中部的横向切片，图示为血管内的环状纤维，F 图和 G 图是靠近静脉口的横向切片，H 图是取自肺静脉近端靠内膜的环状纤维和靠近外膜的纵向纤维的低倍视野。I 图是肺静脉远端孤立的肌纤维（引自 Verheule S, Wilson EE, Arora R, Engle SK, Scott LR, Olgin JE: Tissue structure and connexin expression of canine pulmonary veins. Cardiovasc Res 55：727-738，2002.）

4 相除极。有趣的是，去甲肾上腺素和血管周围神经元的直接刺激可以通过增加自动除极的频率抑制自发电活动，与窦房结的反应相似[24]。在表面灌流的正常犬肺静脉细胞，可以观察到自动 4 相除极（图 39-8）[31]，这种自发活动的频率较低（1000ms）。另外，在完整的犬肺静脉没有看到自动除极现象。

肺静脉内也存在触发活动，Cheung[32] 观察到豚鼠肺静脉远端存在洋地黄诱发的电活动的起源点。在有些分离的兔肺静脉肌细胞中存在早后除极和晚后除极[30]，在分离的犬肺静脉标本中，持续快速起搏刺激几周，可见自发性节律。在该研究中，正常犬和持续 6~8 周的快速心房起搏的犬均可见到肺静脉内存在高频电活动，并伴有早后除极（图 39-9）[31]，但快速起搏组明显高于对照组（93% vs 41%），异丙肾上腺素和电刺激可增加其发生率，而心得安、钙拮抗剂、乙酰胆碱则可抑制高频电活动的发生[31]。然而，现在还不清楚缺血会起什么样的作用。Arora 等[33] 在用二尖瓣反流制作的左房增大的模型上经冠状动脉进行灌

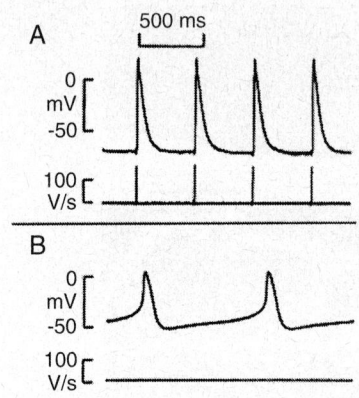

图 39-8 表面灌流犬肺静脉的微电极记录 A. 为 2Hz 的频率起搏时的正常动作电位,伴快速 0 相除极。B. 为自发活动和 4 相除极(引自 Chen YJ, Chen SA, Chang MS, Lin CI: Arrhytnmogenic activity of cardiac muscle in pulmonary veins of the dog: implication for the genesis of atrial fibrillation. Cardiovasc Res 48: 265-273, 2000.)

流,利用光学标测技术标记电活动情况,可见到局部电活动增加,这样的节律可见于起搏后,或起搏后可使自发活动频率增加。光学标测的数据显示有关触发活动的资料较少。

肺静脉的电生理特性表现为局部存在缓慢性传导和各向异性复极,这是折返发生的基质。应用高分辨光学标测,我们看到在犬的肺静脉内存在折返(图 39-10)[19]。在近 50% 的肺静脉中折返可以被期前刺激诱发,折返环的大小约 1～2cm,其典型的周长为 150～180ms。在本研究中,异丙肾上腺素灌注可产生持续性折返活动。

五、结 论

房颤的触发灶起源于从左房延展至肺静脉的肌袖,尽管有些资料相互矛盾,但还是提示肺静脉的心房肌内没有明显的结样组织,在从左房至肺静脉的交界区,肌纤维排列的各向异性形成了这一区域的不均一性传导,肺静脉内的缓慢和递减性传导促进了折返的发生。另一机制,尚缺乏有力的证据,即触发活动或自律性增加可以促进房颤的发生。目前尚不清楚肺静脉肌袖如何作为房颤的机制促进房颤发生的。

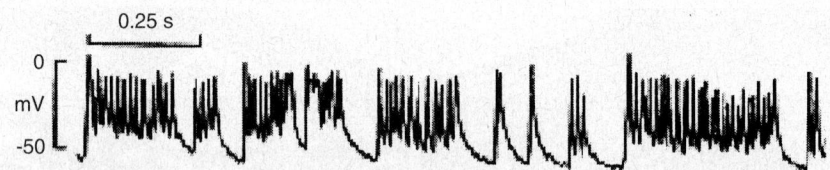

图 39-9 微电极记录的表面灌流犬肺静脉自发性电活动在 3 相复极中存在早后除极 这些后除极随着起搏和异丙肾上腺素灌流增加,可被心得安、尼非地平和乙酰胆碱抑制(引自 Chen YJ, Chen SA, Chang MS, Lin CI: Arrhytnmogenic activity of cardiac muscle in pulmonary veins of the dog: implication for the genesis of atrial fibrillation. Cardiovasc Res 48: 265-273, 2000)

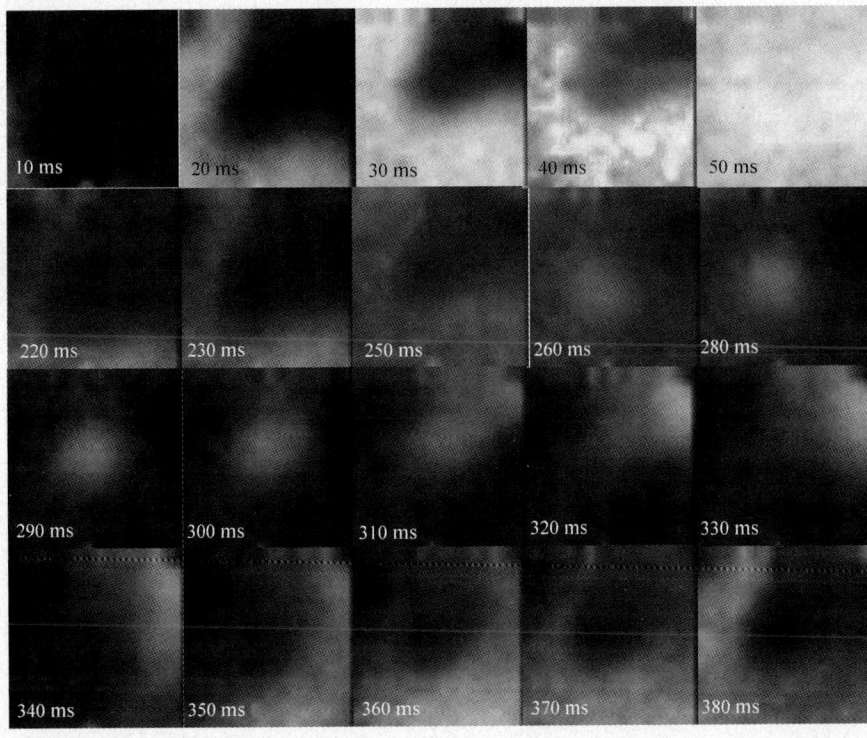

图 39-10　应用光学标测肺静脉折返活动激动的时间顺序　在冠状动脉灌流的犬肺静脉 $2×2cm^2$ 的区域中，用 256 个通道的光敏二极管阵列记录电活动，通过 Di-4-ANEPS 荧光信号可以记录到动作电位，亮颜色是高密度荧光，代表的是除极状态，第一排 S_1 起搏后传导状态，后三排是 S_2 形成的传导，有一个缓慢传导的中心带，S_1 激动被阻滞在 250ms 框的右下角。激动跨过缓慢传导区（260～320ms 框），形成折返（引自 Arora R，Verheule S，Scott L et al：Arrhythmogenic substrate of the pulmonary veins assessed by high-resolution optical mapping。Circulation 107：1816-1821，2003.）

（张　萍　译）

参 考 文 献

1. Brunton TL, Fayrer J: Note on independent pulsation of the pulmonary veins and vena cava. Proc Royal Soc Lond 25:174–176, 1876.
2. Haissaguerre M, Jais P, Shah DC, et al: Spontaneous initiation of atrial fibrillation by ectopic beats originating in the pulmonary veins. N Engl J Med 339:659–666, 1998.
3. Paes de Almeida O, Bohm CM, et al: The cardiac muscle in the pulmonary vein of the rat: A morphological and electrophysiological study. J Morphol 145:409–433, 1975.
4. Karrer HE, Cox J: The striated musculature of blood vessels. J Biophys Biochem Cytol 6:383–390, 1959.
5. Nathan H, Eliakim M: The junction between the left atrium and the pulmonary veins. An anatomic study of human hearts. Circulation 34:412–422, 1966.
6. Carrow R, Calhoun ML: The extent of cardiac muscle in the great veins of the dog. Anat Rec 150:249–256, 1964.
7. Eliakim M, Stern S, Nathan H: Site of action of hypertonic saline in the pulmonary circulation. Circ Res 9:327–332, 1961.
8. Spach MS, Barr RC, Jewett PH: Spread of excitation from the atrium into thoracic veins in human beings and dogs. Am J Cardiol 30:844–854, 1972.
9. Zipes DP, Knope RF: Electrical properties of the thoracic veins. Am J Cardiol 29:372–376, 1972.
10. Anderson KP, Stinson EB, Mason JW: Surgical exclusion of focal paroxysmal atrial tachycardia. Am J Cardiol 49:869–474, 1982.
11. Lesh MD, Van Hare GF, Epstein LM, et al: Radiofrequency catheter ablation of atrial arrhythmias. Results and mechanisms. Circulation 89:1074–1089, 1994.
12. Cox JL, Schuessler RB, Lappas DG, Boineau JP: An 8?-year clinical experience with surgery for atrial fibrillation. Ann Surg 224:267–273, 1996; discussion 273–275.
    logical characteristics, pharmacological responses, and effects of radiofrequency ablation. Circulation 100:1879–1886, 1999.
14. Scherf D: Studies on auricular tachycardia caused by aconitine administration. Proc Soc Exp Biol NY 64:233–239, 1947.
15. Masani F: Node-like cells in the myocardial layer of the pulmonary vein of rats: An ultrastructural study. J Anat 145:133–142, 1986.
16. Hocini M, Haissaguerre M, Shah D, et al: Multiple sources initiating atrial fibrillation from a single pulmonary vein identified by a circumferential catheter. Pacing Clin Electrophysiol 23:1828–1831, 2000.
17. Jais P, Hocini M, Macle L, et al: Distinctive electrophysiological properties of pulmonary veins in patients with atrial fibrillation. Circulation 106:2479–2485, 2002.
18. Chen YJ, Tai CT, Hsieh MH, et al: Dependence of electrogram duration in right posteroseptal atrium and atrium-pulmonary vein junction on pacing site: Mechanism and implications regarding atrioventricular nodal reentrant tachycardia and paroxysmal atrial fibrillation. J Cardiovasc Electrophysiol 11:506–515, 2000.
19. Arora R, Verheule S, Scott LR, et al: Arrhythmogenic substrate of the pulmonary veins assessed by high-resolution optical mapping. Circulation 107:1816–1821, 2003.
20. Hocini M, Ho SY, Kawara T, et al: Electrical conduction in canine pulmonary veins: Electrophysiological and anatomic correlation. Circulation 105:2442–2248, 2002.
21. Verheule S, Wilson EE, Arora R, et al: Tissue structure and connexin expression of canine pulmonary veins. Cardiovasc Res 55:727–738, 2002.

22. Tada H, Oral H, Ozaydin M, et al: Response of pulmonary vein potentials to premature stimulation. J Cardiovasc Electrophysiol 13:33–37, 2002.
23. Haissaguerre M, Shah DC, Jais P, et al: Mapping-guided ablation of pulmonary veins to cure atrial fibrillation. Am J Cardiol 86:K9–K19, 2000.
24. Cheung DW: Electrical activity of the pulmonary vein and its interaction with the right atrium in the guinea-pig. J Physiol 314:445–456, 1981.
25. Ho SY, Cabrera JA, Tran VH, et al: Architecture of the pulmonary veins: relevance to radiofrequency ablation. Heart 86:265–270, 2001.
26. Saito T, Waki K, Becker AE: Left atrial myocardial extension onto pulmonary veins in humans: Anatomic observations relevant for atrial arrhythmias. J Cardiovasc Electrophysiol 11:888–894, 2000.
27. Blom NA, Gittenberger-de Groot AC, DeRuiter MC, et al: Development of the cardiac conduction tissue in human embryos using HNK-1 antigen expression: Possible relevance for understanding of abnormal atrial automaticity. Circulation 99:800–806, 1999.
28. Spach MS, Josephson ME: Initiating reentry: The role of nonuniform anisotropy in small circuits. J Cardiovasc Electrophysiol 5:182–209, 1994.
29. Wilders R, Wagner MB, Golod DA, et al: Effects of anisotropy on the development of cardiac arrhythmias associated with focal activity. Pflugers Arch 441:301–312, 2000.
30. Chen YJ, Chen SA, Chen YC, et al: Electrophysiology of single cardiomyocytes isolated from rabbit pulmonary veins: Implication in initiation of focal atrial fibrillation. Basic Res Cardiol 97:26–34, 2002.
31. Chen YJ, Chen SA, Chang MS, Lin CI: Arrhythmogenic activity of cardiac muscle in pulmonary veins of the dog: Implication for the genesis of atrial fibrillation. Cardiovasc Res 48:265–273, 2000.
32. Cheung DW: Pulmonary vein as an ectopic focus in digitalis-induced arrhythmia. Nature 294:582–584, 1981.
33. Arora R, Verheule S, Everett T, Olgin JE: Effect of chronic left atrial dilatation from mitral regurgitation on electrophysiology of the pulmonary vein. Circulation 106:II-179, 2002.

第 40 章

心房颤动的维持机制

Omer Berenfeld

本章目录

- 心房颤动的时空特点 ········· 359
- 心房颤动的维持来源于折返活动 ········· 360
- 折返活动的产生 ········· 362
- 左右心房内（电）活动的关系 ········· 364
- 波动崩溃为碎裂传导 ········· 364
- 起源频率和传导一致性 ········· 368
- 总结 ········· 368

目前在美国有超过两百万人患有心房颤动（AF），这是最常见的持续性心律失常。随着人口老龄化预测将会增加更多病例[1]。尽管一个多世纪来对心房颤动进行了广泛的研究，但是仍没有完全澄清它的确切机制。心房的解剖结构是具有不同大小的肌束和开口的复杂的三维结构。另外，当考虑到心房的许多离子机制还不清楚以及多种心脏疾病可改变心脏激动基质使房颤更易发生，就不难理解为什么房颤对那些研究房颤发生和维持机制的科学家们来讲一直是巨大挑战了[2,3]。分析房颤时激动波传播的时空特性可以为阐明它的潜在机制提供重要线索。折返被越来越广泛地认为是多种室颤和房颤的主要起源；然而，目前对这些折返的确切实质还有争议。房颤可能是由多个环行运动、随机传播的微环碎裂而成；也可能是由个别不连续且行环行运动的激动波遇到固定的异质性部位，从而使环形运动破坏而造成。这两种不同机制会表现为颤动的不同动力学特征：后者的传播更加规则和稳定。

本章将要讨论近来我们实验室的一些资料。这些资料支持发生在结构正常的绵羊心脏的急性房颤不是完全随机现象的假说[6-11]。如下所述，传播的结构模式提示急性房颤的维持依赖于左房局部的折返源和右房的碎裂传播。这里所说的研究是在台氏液冠脉灌流完整的或切开的正常绵羊心脏进行的。台氏液里含停跳心肌的不同浓度的甲氧维拉帕米（D600）和用来调节房颤心率的乙酰胆碱（ACh）。为了研究心房激动模式的特征，我们联合应用高分辨率视频成像和双极电图记录（EGs）技术[12]。本章集中描述心房激动的时空特点，利用能谱和相位分析以客观、可靠地量化房颤的复杂传播模式[8,13]。

一、心房颤动的时空特点

因为传统观点认为房颤是一系列复杂的顺序激动所致，所以我们用高分辨率光学标测直接揭示其形态特点[6]。图 40-1 是 Langendorff 灌流下绵羊心脏发生房颤时的活动特点。在灌流液里加 $2\mu M$ D600 停跳心肌，另加 $0.1\sim0.5\mu M$ ACh。在 6 次实验的 20 阵房颤发作中，波动形态是复杂的，包括各种类型折返活动、心外膜穿透模式、波动中断和碰撞[6]。图 40-1A 是房颤发作时的双极电图，显示了房颤时的不规则电活动。能谱是通过快速傅立叶转换获取的，显示有多个分离的窄锋。在 8.3 Hz 处有一明显窄锋，它的谐波位于 16.7 Hz 处。也能看到其他小幅窄锋，包括发作中的室颤在 13.9 Hz 处引起的窄锋。在所有房颤发作中，双极电图频谱分析显示有多个窄锋，其中有一个主锋，也就是主频（DF）。6 次实验中双极电图的主频从 $6.4\sim16.7Hz$ 不等（均值±STD：9.4±2.6 Hz)。

为了研究房颤时整体测量中得出的各种锋的起源，还对拟心电图进行了能谱分析。这种拟心电图（pseudo-ECG）是通过整合光标测像素到个体心房整体标测图而构建的。从图40-1B可见左房拟心电图与双极电图（见图40-1A）和右房拟心电图相比（见图40-1C）看上去更规则。左房拟心电图能谱分析显示在8.2 Hz处有一分离的窄的主锋。这与双极能谱电图中8.3 Hz处的主锋相对应。右房拟心电图的特点是形态规则，激活较慢。这被有6.3 Hz和4.0 Hz主锋的宽的带状能谱所确证。总体双极电图的能谱也可见此种主锋。

在确定了左右房光标测能谱图的主锋后，我们进一步研究在这些频率处激动起源的本质特点。图40-1D示在490ms时间（见图40-1B的水平条）内从左房记录的四幅连续的彩色激动等时线图。从这些图明显可见在这段时间左房的游离壁和心耳被来自标测图右下的同一位置的波锋反复激动。波锋在整个3s的记录时间内是周期性的（如图40-1B中左房拟心电图所示的规整周期）。激动的周长是120ms（8.3Hz），与左房拟心电图和双极电图的主锋对应。然而，仔细观察这四幅连续的左房等时图（图40-1D）会发现相邻图间波锋的传播有一定的变异。这也许导致了左房拟心电图形某种程度的变异（见图40-1C），也可能使主锋变宽，从而产生能谱中相应的附加小锋（见图40-1B和D）。图40-1 E示三幅右房8.3ms彩色等时图，在时间上和图40-1D相对应。与左房中的时空周期性不同，右房里没有这种周期特点。正如别处报道[12]，右房等时图表现为不完整折返，突破样式和整个标测区千变万化的传导阻断。很明显，这种复杂的激动模式导致右房拟心电图的显著变异，是双极电图不规则活动的重要因素。传播的复杂模式直接引起右房拟心电图能谱锋的增宽。值得注意的是，为了将来参考，右房能谱主锋与左房的相比在更低的频段处。图40-1的数据代表了起源于左房的19阵房颤发作的时空周期特点。的确，分析所有房颤发作后发现左房的周期性时空活动更常见；左房的19次都有时空周期而20次右房记录中只有12次（60%）有此特点。此外，在同一次房颤发作中双房都有时空周期的记录中，左房来源的周期活动的频率高于或等于右房来源者。

房颤时激动的传播模式已被广泛研究。最初Moe及同事们[4]提出了房颤的多子波假说，并被Allessie等[5]的实验证实，认为（房颤时）心房是由多个随机运动的分离的波激动的，这些波互生互灭。然而，最近更多人体研究的统计数据揭示了房颤的潜在规律[14,15]。Botteron和Smith[14]关于人体房颤的双极记录表明，6cm内的记录是交叉相关的。Gerstenfeld及其同事们也发现在人一分钟的房颤发作中的非随机的瞬时联系，表现为相继的图形数目为6～14，变异小于30°（也就是有相关）。此外，近来应用多电极记录的外科记录[16,17]提示在单纯二尖瓣疾患病人的房颤发作时左房有规则的重复活动。总之，这些研究强烈支持房颤不是完全随机的现象。

二、心房颤动的维持来源于折返活动

因为房颤时主频（DFs）是规整的，而且局部活动率可以用来判断整体记录能谱[6]，我们着手联合应用光标测和频率分析寻找房颤的维持机制。我们假设在乙酰胆碱存在条件下，Langendorff灌流绵羊心脏的房颤来自于一个或者少数几个分离的稳定的来源，这些来源就位于那些活动最快最稳定的地方，也就是左房。正如最近的研究所述，反复激动可起自房间隔或肺静脉[18,19]。我们承认，正如体表心电图所见，当来自上述起源的快速连续的波锋在双房传播遇到解剖或功能障碍时会导致碎裂波形成[20]。图40-2示房颤发作时高频周期活动的局部起源[7]。这次房颤的发作机制基于对左房光标测电影的研究。在图40-2A，左房光标测的等时图显示一个以67ms（约14.7 Hz）为周期的顺时针旋转的漩涡，旋转持续了整个发作时间（25min）。起源频率等于在所有位置记录到（光学或电学记录，见Mandapati等[7]）的最快最窄的主频（最规则的信号），这提供了这次房颤发作维持的折返机制的直接证据[20]。实际上，视野中活动（图40-2B左房拟心电图）的总和表明整个左房在14.7 Hz被激动。为了评价折返活动在判断一次发作的总体主频中的作用，我们收集了14个仅在左房中的折返环完整的漩涡运动。图40-2C示漩涡旋转周期与从相应左房拟心电图的能谱获得的总体主频倒数的关系。直线斜率是0.93（R=0.91），强烈提示相关螺旋波的周期是光标测区域主频的主要影响因素。对不同情况下房颤的不完全折返和不稳定多折返环已有描述[5,12,18,21,22]。然而，自从Allessie等第一次验证多环假说，少有研究涉及Lewis[23]和Scherf[24]相继提出的单一高频稳定折返维持房颤的假说。然而Schuessler和同事[25]发现在分离的犬右房增加乙酰胆碱浓度使多

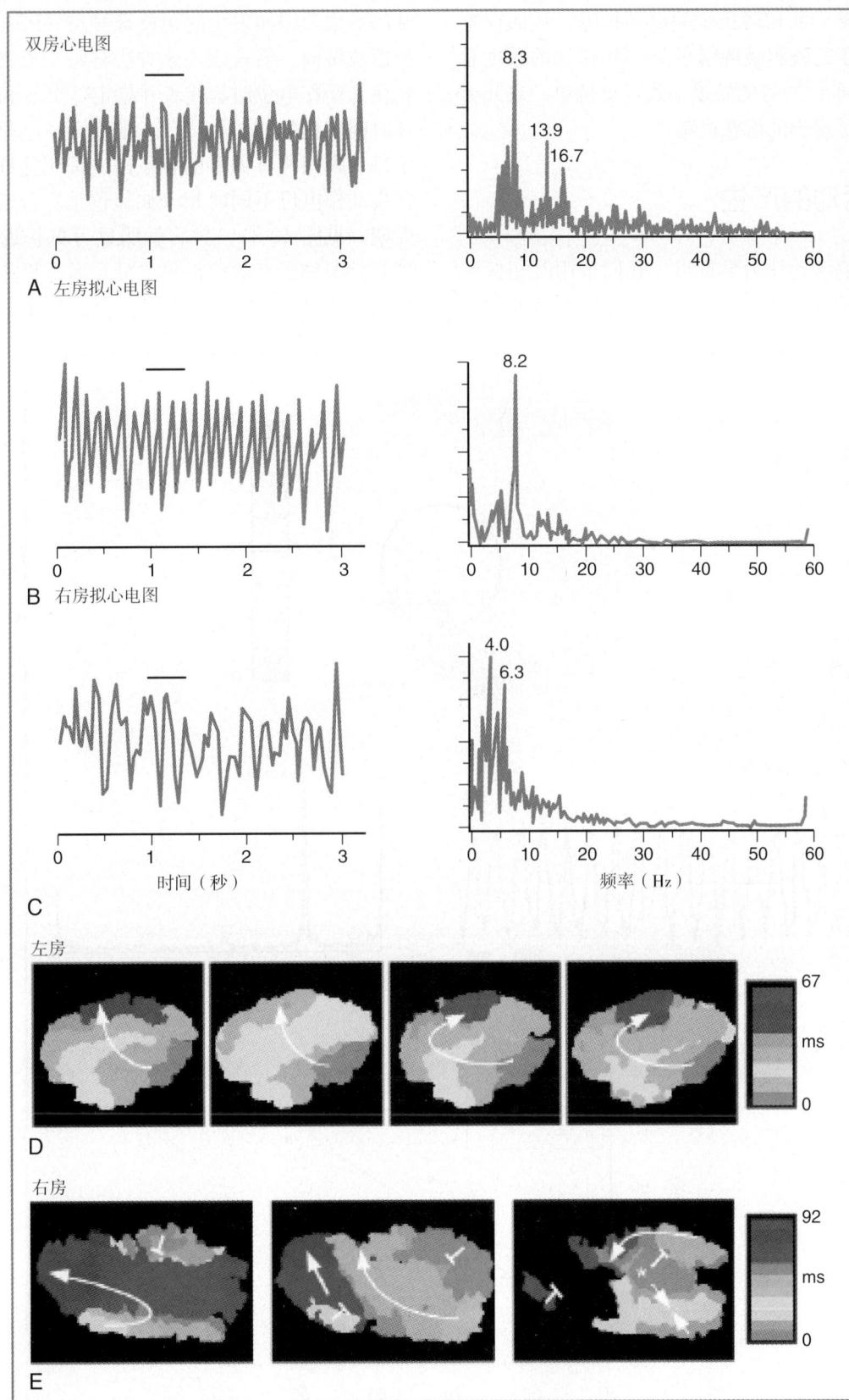

图 40-1 一次房颤发作的频谱和等时图 A：双房整体活动的双极电图记录及相应能谱。B 和 C：左房和右房及相应能谱。连续左房（D）和右房（E）同步记录等时图。等时图时间由水平标尺指示（改自 Skanes A，Mandapati R，Berenfekl O，等：Spatiotemporal periodicity during atrial fibrillation in the isolated sheep heart. Circulation 98：1236-1248，1998.）（见彩图 13）

折返环转变为单一的相对稳定的高频折返,从而产生碎裂传导。由于乙酰胆碱持续存在,图 40-2 的数据看起来同 Schuessler[25]等的结果一致,支持单一或几个稳定折返活动是房颤的潜在机制。

三、折返活动的产生

为量化折返活动动力学特点,我们采用时相标测技术。这是一种刚建立的方法,它可有效显示波的中断的形成及因而发生的相位奇异点(PSs),在这些点折返波转向。简言之,该方法将每个象素的跨膜信号转化为动作电位时程代表并指定一个 p 和-p 弧度间的随时间变化的相位值[9,13]。相位值经色彩编码就形成了每一瞬间所有象素的相位图。按照这种转换,颜色代表动作电位不同时相(如蓝色是平台期,红色是不应期,见图 40-3)。然后就明显可见折返活动的转向处就是那些所有颜色汇集之处,而这里相位没有确定(也就是相位奇异点)。在所分析的房颤发作中表现为

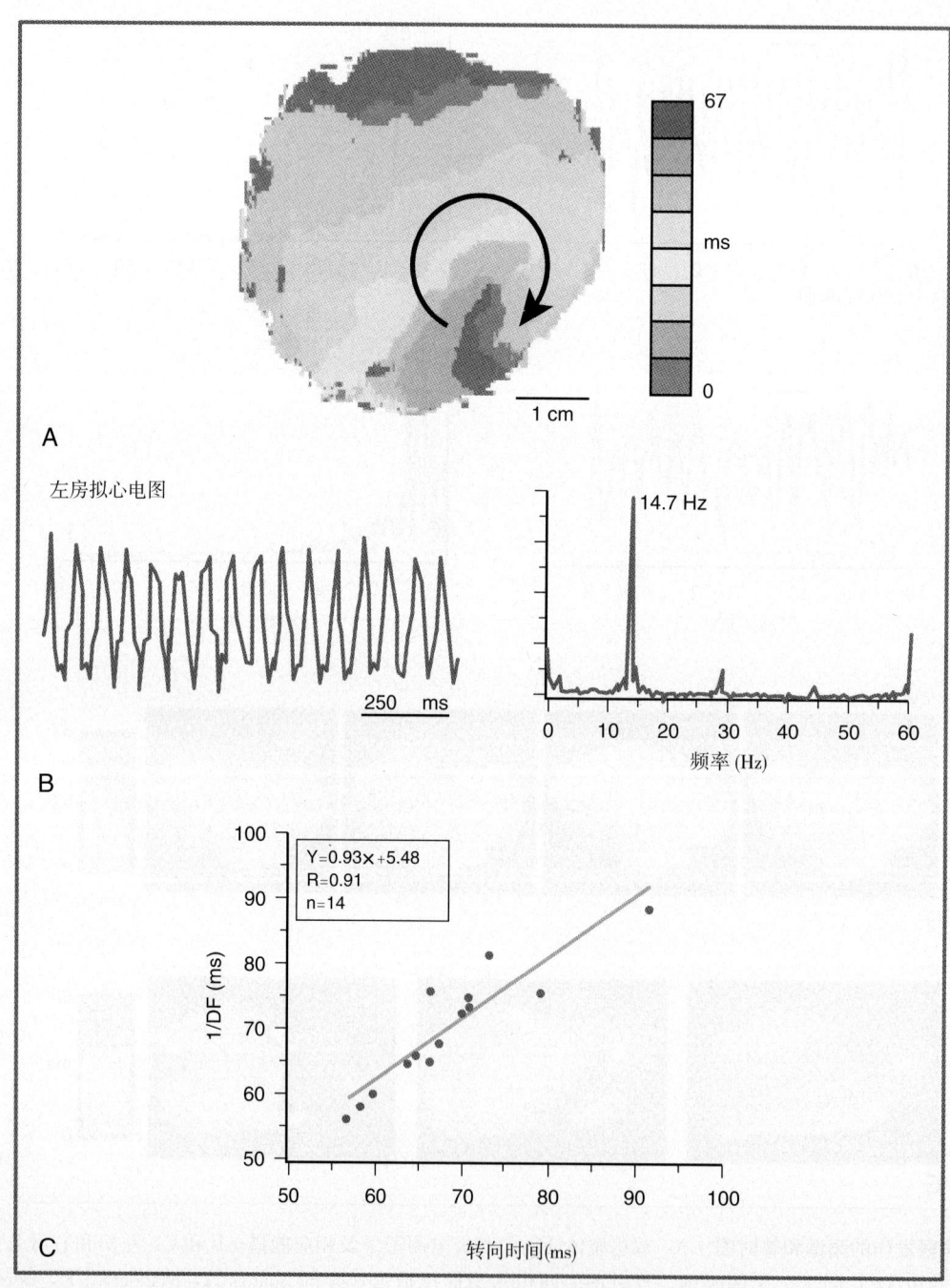

图 40-2 房颤的折返源 A:持续房颤时左房游离壁的光标测等时图,示顺时针折返。B:同次发作的左房拟心电图及相应能谱。C:全部视频记录拟心电图的主频倒数同房颤折返周期的相关性(改自 Mandapati R, Skanes A, Chen J, et al: Stable microreentrant sources as a mechanism of atrial fibrillation in the isolated sheep heart. Circulation 101:194-199,2000.)(见彩图 14)

相位奇异点的波动中断经常发生。每 400ms 记录（50 幅）[9]中相位奇异点平均总数为 70±40（23～154）。当追踪相位奇异点的轨迹时发现虽然相位奇异点迂回漂移，但是还是倾向于在特定的标测区域聚集，空间分布并不是随机的。多数情况下，相位奇异点的持续时间特别短，平均为 19.5±18.3ms，从 8.33（1 幅）到 200ms 不等。我们的实验中约 98%的相位奇异点持续时间短于一个螺旋周期（~85ms）；在持续房颤的 556 个相位奇异点中只有 10 个持续时间大于或等于一个螺旋周期[9]。

图 40-3 是对波动中断起始机制理论预测的深入实验验证，继发于房颤时波锋与功能性阻滞的相互作用（涡旋脱落）[26,27]。图 40-3A 示左房心外膜碎裂波断端[9]一对相位奇异点的产生，并导致相对较长时间的"8"字折返（约 3 圈）。在 0s 有两个除极波锋（绿/黄）。视野上缘的波向下传播过程中遇到视野中央不应期组织（红）而湮灭。如 16ms 那幅图所示，标测区域下缘的波向上传播，遇到功能性障碍（红）而被打碎形成具有相反手性的两相位奇异点（"+"和"-"）。在 32ms 两个逆向旋转的子波开始绕两个相位奇异点传播。在 56ms，两个子波的游离端融合开始在相位奇异点间传播。这时奇位异点间距是 6.8 mm。80ms 时的图示成功通过功能性峡部，完成一个完整"8"字折返后的波锋。在我们的研究中，也发现奇异点间功能性峡部宽度不足以传播的案例。图 40-3B 示房颤的相位图。这里有两个碎裂后形成的逆向旋转的子波。不能完成一圈旋转。0ms 时，可见黄绿色波锋传进异质性区域，导致两个碎裂波：中央红色不应期区域两侧一边一个。8ms 时，每一个新形成的相位奇异点的手性以"+"和"-"表示。16ms 时，两个逆向旋转的子波前缘出现在旋转环的中间，包绕那两个相位奇异点。在 24ms 时，子波融合试图在两个相位奇异点间传播，相位奇异点间距是 3.3 mm。32ms 的图示这两个逆向旋转的子波相互消减，没有完成折返（子波围绕相应相位奇异点旋转，但是完成折返前就消失）。在我们的试验中，测量了 15 例完全的和 25 例不完全的"8"字折返的相位奇异点间距。我们发现两组的相位奇异点间距均匀分布但是范围不同；所有不完全折返的相位奇异点间距小于～4mm，然而所有完全折返的相位奇异点间距要大一些（$P<0.001$）。从而我们建立了左房"8"字折返的最小相位奇异点间距，在我们模型中大约是 4mm。这一结论证实了 Cabo 等[27]的观察，他们在心室组织估测了阻断传播的临界峡部是 2.5～3.5mm，这依赖于刺激频

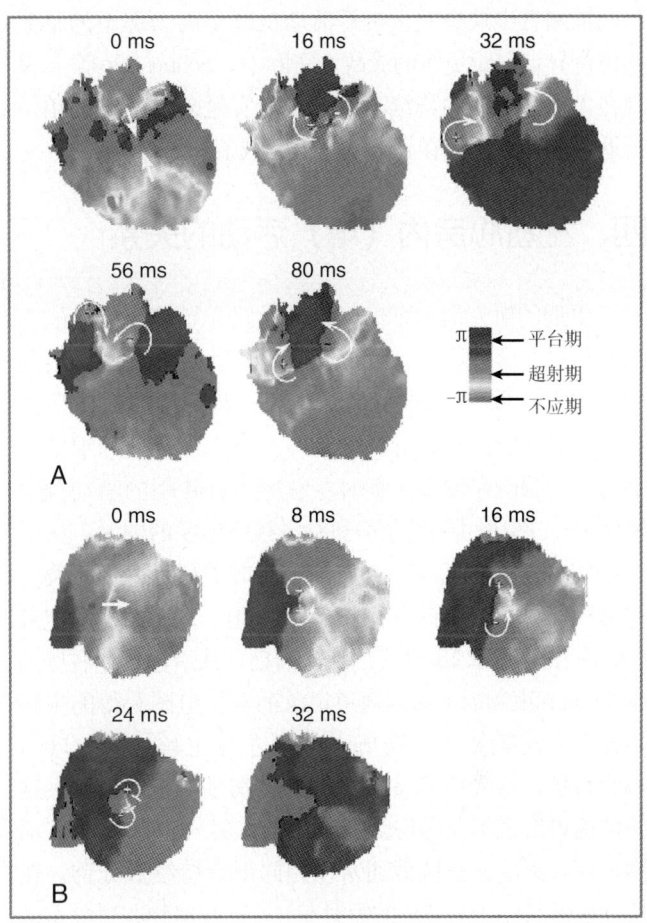

图 40-3 波动碎裂和折返形成时相图示 A："8"字折返的序列时相图。在 0ms，两个波锋（绿/黄）以相反方向移动。向下的波遇到不应期组织（红）而湮灭。16ms，向上的波在 0ms 遇到不应期碎裂形成两个相位奇异点（"+"and"-"示它们相应手性）。32ms，两波锋绕相位奇异点旋转。56ms，波锋融合开始在两个相位奇异点间扩布（相位奇异点间距 6.8mm）。80ms，折返完成一次"8"字折返。B：折返形成失败的时相图。0ms，波锋（绿/黄）左向右扩布。8ms，遇到不应期碎裂形成两个相位奇异点（"+"and"-"）。16ms，两波锋绕相位奇异点旋转。24ms，波锋融合试图在两个相位奇异点间扩布（相位奇异点间距 3.3 mm）。32ms 时，折返失败。彩条示时相值的弧度（改自 Chan J, Mandapati R, Berenfeld O, et al: Dynamics of wavelets and their role in atrial fibrillation in the isolated sheep heart. Cardiovasc Res 48：220-232，2000.）（见彩图 15）

率和肌纤维定向。因此，例证了房颤折返源的产生可能是波锋与功能性屏障的碰撞。相位奇异点倾向与在某一区域聚集提示组织的潜在结构和其他固有特性，也与屏障的产生有关。图 40-2 的折返在标测区没有可见的如图 40-3A 所示的逆向传导活动来完成"8"字折返。然而我们不能排除在其他地方有此活动，也不认为单一折返可以以相同机制产生（见第 35 章）。基于这些发现，

我们推测右房缺少完全折返活动也许是因为那里的临界相位奇异点间距更大的缘故。实际上，Schuessler等[25]发现在犬孤立右房的持续心律失常确实是来自稳定的单一折返，这种折返仅在高浓度乙酰胆碱条件下可见。

四、左右心房内（电）活动的关系

更近的研究揭示了房间传导通路介导碎裂传导的方式以及左右房间频率梯度的建立，显著扩展了房颤的前期工作[10]。Bachmann束（BB）和冠状窦下的后下房间通道是房间电活动传导通道[28,29]。我们在分离的绵羊心脏的光标测研究发现房颤时左右房间有陡峭的激动频率梯度[6-8]。图40-4A是左房到右房频率梯度的图示，显示3s的房颤发作（见Mansour等[10]）时光信号的主频及左右房和Bachmann束左右侧的双极电图。左房的光学记录（图40-4A）显示18.8Hz的快速活动。从沿连接左右房的Bachmann束和后下房间通道记录的双极电图获得的主频重叠在心房轮廓上。Bachmann束左端主频是18.7Hz，随着右移，右端是14.5Hz，最后右房主频是9.8Hz。这些数据再次说明左房房颤频率高于右房[6,7,10]。在所有动物，主频离散分布区域通常以相同形态持续数分钟，在持续房颤有小于～20%的短时变异[8]。左房和右房分布区域的平均面积[8]分别是2.99 ± 1.49和1.17 ± 1.57 cm^2。主频稳定的空间构型，同时左房既快又规整强烈提示左房的电生理结构比右房支持更高的激动频率。此外，左右房间最大的频率衰减发生在Bachmann束和右房之间，提示梳状肌的内在结构是右房游离壁碎裂扩布的基质[10,12]。

检测至少三个连续电极所覆盖距离，沿Bachmann束和后下通路的传导方向——也就是2cm Bachmann束和2.6cm的后下通路，提供了对上述假设的更进一步支持[10]。图40-4B示一阵3s的房颤发作时沿Bachmann束由左向右扩布的情况，该房颤具有从左向右主频递减的特点。定量研究表明沿Bachmann束和后下通路分别有81%和80%所分析的波可以左向右扩布。相反，仅有很少的右向左扩布。

我们已经阐述折返可以是时空周期活动的基础，以至于左房来源的周期决定了我们的实验性房颤模型频谱的主峰（图40-1到40-3）[6,7,9]。这些资料加上图40-4A和B中的数据提示在我们的模型中房颤起源于左房高频冲动。这些冲动沿房间通道扩布以复杂的空间方式激动右房。由于这种情况被认为是碎裂扩布，所以常常会以为存在左右房频率梯度，这种梯度与来源频率（房颤时最大局部频率）直接相关，频率越快间断阻滞的程度越大。为此，我们用D600减慢频率（n=4）。维拉帕米类似物可以增加室颤规整度，伴随室颤主频的降低[30]。在另一组实验，我们增加乙酰胆碱浓度以增加房颤频率（n=4）。如图40-4C，D600使最快的左房频率从19.7 ± 4.4减到16.2 ± 3.9 Hz（$P<0.01$），奇怪的是却使右房主频从8.6 ± 2.0增加到10.7 ± 1.8 Hz（$P<0.05$）。相反，把乙酰胆碱浓度从0.2 μM增加到使左右房频率梯度从4.9 ± 1.8增加到8.9 ± 1.8 Hz（$P=0.02$），如图40-4D所示。因此很明显左右房频率梯度和右房频率是由左房频率决定的。这一结论同独立右房的多环折返假说矛盾，只能用左房来源的激动碎裂扩布离开左房时的频率依赖性的变化来解释，允许大量波可以到达低频区域。实际上，由于房间传导通道和右房成分的电穴-电源不匹配，更高的起源频率会导致间断阻滞。当起源频率降低时，右房主频增加（仍比左房主频低），这意味着低频区不匹配度降低，可以解释D600的实验结果。此外，乙酰胆碱引起的左房主频升高也提示，不管我们的模型中有无局部活动，持续房颤的机制也不可能是节律点或触发机制。

五、波动崩溃为碎裂传导

至少在某些情况下，房颤是由左房相对稳定的高频活动向右房传播引起的。我们通过在Bachmann束右端直接起搏细致研究右房对左房高频激动的反应。为此我们用分离的、冠脉灌流的右房标本，这可以为定量来自Bachmann束进入右房的波锋扩布的频率依赖特性及碎裂传导的基础提供真实可控的条件。在我们的完整绵羊心脏模型的实验性房颤中，左房稳定的折返源通常产生高于7Hz的激动[6-8]。然而，房颤发作时右房一般在更低的频率激动，提示一定有一个左房右房1:1输入输出临界频率。因此我们推测正常右房由梳状肌构成的复杂束状结构是传导频率依赖性延迟和阻滞（碎裂传导的标志）的基质。如图40-5A主频图（Berenfeld等[11]）所示，对Bachmann束的5.0Hz节律刺激导致整个右房输出频率也是5.0Hz的1:1激动。然而，在7.7Hz时激动不在是1:1。取而代之的是心内膜和心外膜异质性分布的主频域，频率在3.5～7.7Hz。图40-5B综合了5次实验结果。心内膜测得的主频标绘为起搏频率的功能。很明显，在6.7 Hz以下反应主频在所有实验中都没有离散，意味着所有区域的激动是1:1的。超过6.7Hz的"崩溃频率"，就会有严重的主频离散，表现为多个频率小

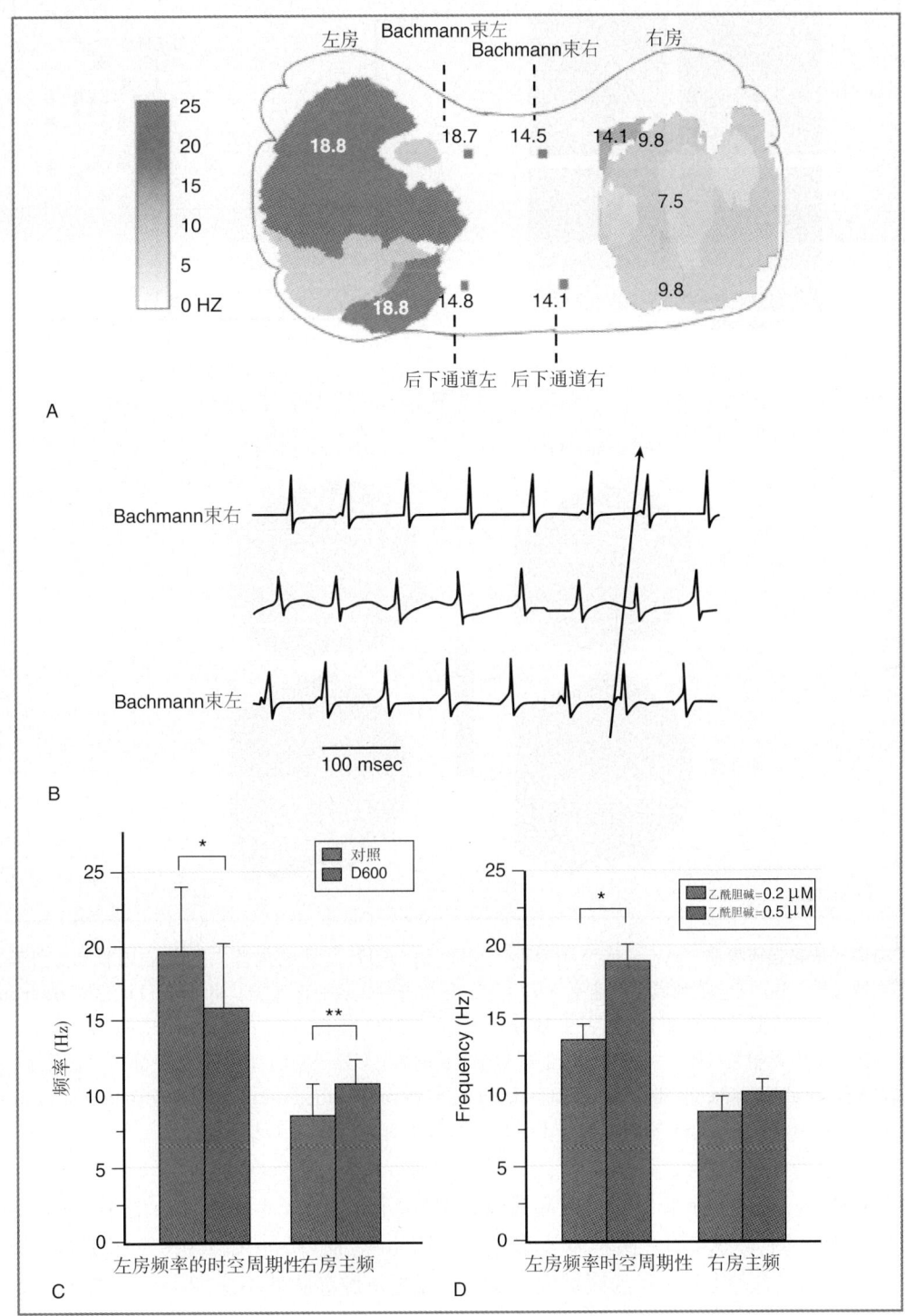

图 40-4 左右房之间激动的关系 A：左房-右房主频梯度。左右房心外膜主频图，及沿 Bachmann 束和后下通道的主频。单位是赫兹。频率图面积示光标测区域。B：激动扩布左-右方向性。记录来自沿 Bachmann 束的三个电极。下图的记录来自最左边电极的电图。D600（C）、乙酰胆碱（D）对左右房频率的影响。（改自 Mansour M, Mandapati R, Berenfeld O, et al: Left-to-right gradient of atrial frequencies during acute atrial fibrillation in the isolated sheep heart. Circulation 103：2631-2636，2001.）

于等于起搏频率的频域。

图 40-5A 和 B 所示的主频空间离散可能是因为分支处或附近电穴-电源不匹配造成的。分支束电穴-电

源效应使几位研究者转向房颤时心房心内膜下解剖结构的作用[12,25,32-34]。然而，传导途径上不应期的内在异质性也会起作用[35,36]。因此我们决定检测慢速起搏

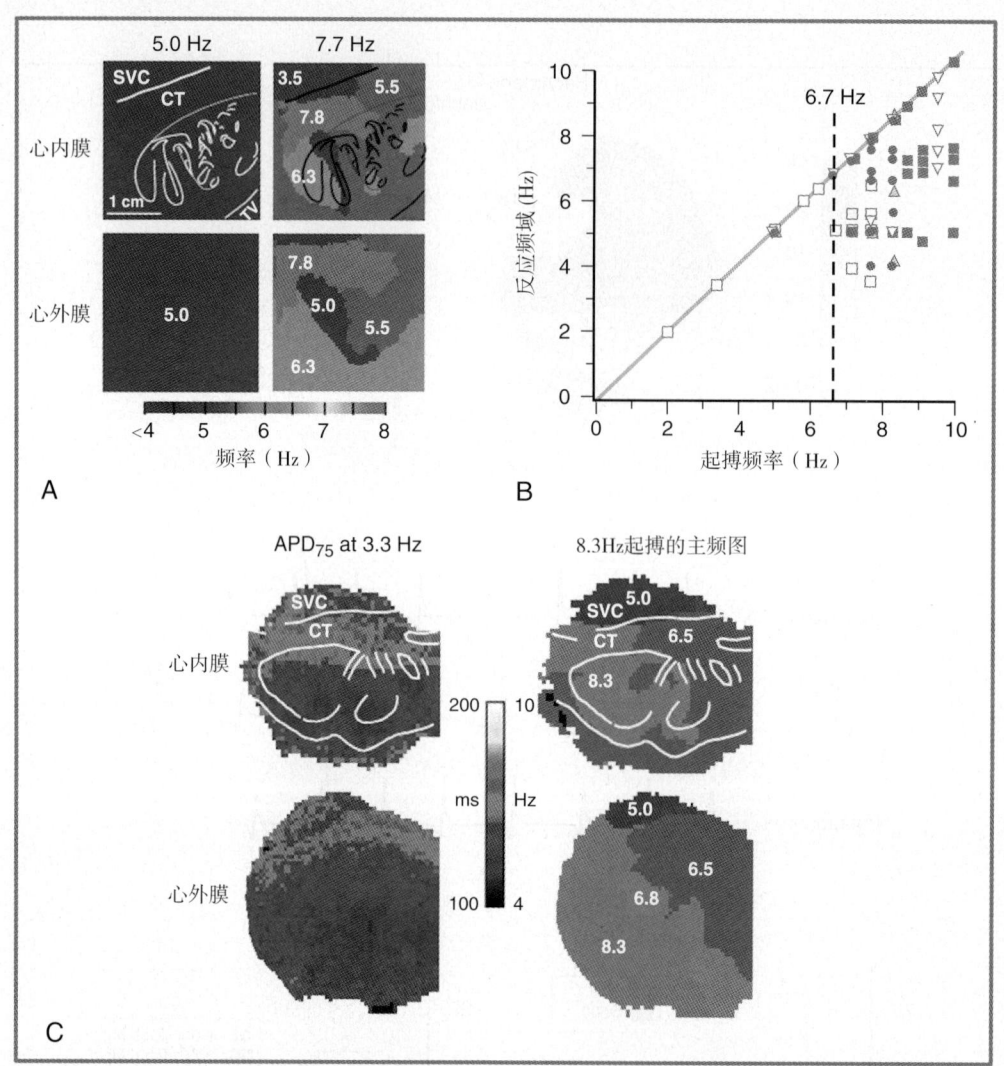

图40-5 右房扩布模式依赖起搏频率 A："崩溃频率"。5.0Hz 和 7.7Hz 起搏的离体右房的心内膜和心外膜主频图。注意 7.7Hz 时出现主频域异质。B：反应主频域起搏速率（n = 5）。每个符号代表一次实验。低于 6.7Hz 起搏 Bachmnnn 束产生 1：1 激动。在更高频率频域增加但是主频下降。C：主频分布不依赖 APD 离散。左，3.3Hz 起搏的 APD_{75} 图；右，同一标本 8.3Hz 起搏的主频图。两图无相关（$R^2 = 0.05$）。APD：动作电位时程；CT：界嵴；SVC：上腔静脉（改自 Berenfeld O, Zaitsev AV, Mironov AF, et al: Frequency-dependent breakdown of wave propagation into fibrillafory conduction across the pectinate muscle network in the isolated sheep right atrium. Circ Res 90：1173-1180，2002.）（见彩图 16.）

时动作电位时程（APD）的空间分布[37]与快速起搏时主频（DF）分布比较。图 40-5C 示一次样本实验的 APD（左）和主频（右）。注意长 APD 的区域同时有最大主频，同不应期离散决定主频的预期相反。实际上，有五个心脏 APD 和主频分布无明显相关性（$R^2 < 0.05$；0.018 ± 0.021，n = 5），说明 3.3Hz 处 APD 离散是主频很差的预测因素，不应期离散并不是房颤主频异质性的原因。

低频刺激的不应期和 APD 空间离散常被用来解释房颤波的复杂传播[38]。Wang 等[35]发现在罹患持续性房颤的狗用 250ms 的周期刺激时，右房心外膜不应期离散是 19±3ms，最长的不应期在游离壁，长约 120ms，而 Satoh 和 Zipes[39]报道的结果是在界嵴下部靠近下腔静脉处不应期最短。然而，这些表面上矛盾的研究没有测量梳状肌区的不应期，因此这些数据也很难跟我们的结果比较。我们以 300ms（3.3Hz；见图 40-5C）周期建立了高分辨 APD 图来间接评价不应期离散的程度[37]。与 Feng 等[40]的结果类似的是，我们的结果也提示在低频（3.3Hz）起搏时界嵴有最长的 APD。Spach 等[41]也报道在 1.7Hz 低频起搏下界嵴的 APD 比梳状肌 APD 长。Yamashita 等[42]报道在单细胞 1Hz 起搏时兔界嵴 APD 比梳状肌长。然而，

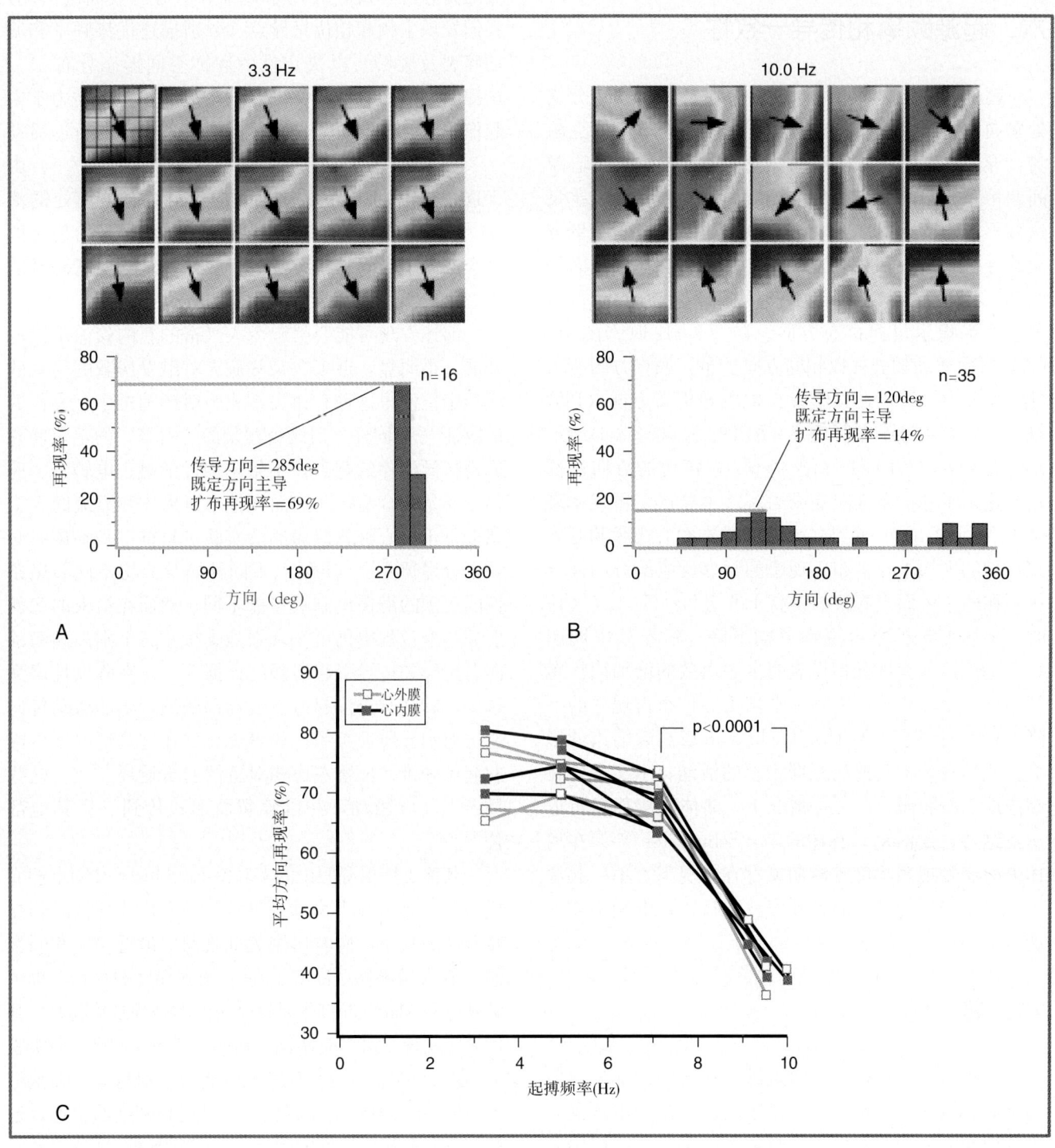

图 40-6 优势传导方向（PD）的频率依赖 上图，心内膜同一位置 3.3Hz（A）和 10Hz（B）起搏的 15 幅连续的等时图。两图的色价以红比蓝标准化。下图，既定方向主导扩布再现率（RPD）的直方图。C，5 次实验中心内膜（Endo）和心外膜（Epi）平均 RPD 的起搏频率依赖。注意超过 6.7Hz 起搏时 RPD 突然下降（改自 Berenfeld O, Zaitsev AV, Mironov AF, et al: Frequency-dependent breakdown of wave propagation into fibrillatory conduction across the pectinate muscle network in the isolated sheep right atrium. Circ Res 90：1173-1180，2002.）（见彩图 17）

在我们的实验里以与房颤时左房激动可比的频率（>7 Hz）起搏 Bachmann 束时，界嵴一直具有最大主频。因而，APD 分布看来不同于主频分布，这使我们推测从正常频率的不应期离散很难预测房颤间断阻滞模式的空间分布。

六、起源频率和传导一致性

超高频起搏 Bachmann 束会导致右房束主要分支处单向阻滞[11]。因此自然会发生不同步的多位点阻滞，导致高度不均一的激动。我们通过检测每个心跳间期扩布方向的改变并与主频结构改变相联系来定量这种不均一度（图 40-5）。图 40-6A 和 B 显示一例方向性分析。最上栏是梳状肌区以 25 像素（记录面积约 $2.5 \times 2.5 \text{ mm}^2$）记录的 15 次连续搏动的等时图，黑色箭头指示每搏扩布方向。在 3.3 Hz 时（图 40-6A）每次波动的波锋以相同方向扩布。如直方图所示（图 40-44 左下），在该组像素中主导扩布方向（PD）是 285°，其主导扩布再现率（RPD）为 69%（Berenfeld 等[11]）。在 10 Hz（图 40-6B），每搏的方向性都在变化，主导扩布方向变成 120°，主导扩布再现率降到 14%。图 40-6C 总结了对五个样本的心内膜和心外膜标测的平均主导扩布再现率的频率反应的方向性分析。在两个表面当起搏频率高于 6.7 Hz（$P < 0.01$）时，平均主导扩布再现率急剧下降。临界频率同图 40-5 的崩溃频率的相似性表明主频离散的增加同扩布复杂程度增加相关，表现为平均主导扩布再现率的下降[11]。由于我们主要研究 Bachmann 束高频输入的影响，我们只分析起搏后立即中止的活动。事实上，在高浓度乙酰胆碱[25,43,44]等情况下，离体右房能以折返形式维持自发活动。有趣的是，Schuessler 等[25]在离体犬右房发现高浓度乙酰胆碱存在情况下，单一起源就可产生碎裂传导，而且碎裂波数目同折返频率成比例。

七、总 结

对折返波决定持续性房颤激动模式的论证为理解房颤的机制提供了新视野，使单起源维持房颤的概念重新引起人们的注意[23,24]。自从 Moe 及同事[4]提出多子波假说，并被 Allessie 及同事[5]实验证实以来，房颤一直被认为是由心房内互生互灭连续扩布的颤动波维持的。然而，更近的研究发现心房局部活动的频率并不是随机分布的，越来越多的人体和动物模型资料提示左房标志性频率可能比右房高[16,17,45]。离体绵羊心脏持续房颤时高分辨视频成像技术的应用不仅能显示左房激动快于右房，而且证实左房具有空间稳定的周期性的波的特点，这是右房所没有的[6,7]。光学标测的高分辨率使它可用来详细分析心房表面的活动，我们发现主频和相位奇异点（分别描述优势频率和波动碎裂及旋转）以决定性的簇样空间形态分布[8-10]。这提示心房固有结构特点在波动形成和扩布动力学中起作用。此外的研究直接显示了左房表面的折返活动[7,9]，发现折返时心房表面最快最规整的活动[6,7]。由于这些位于左房游离壁活动被证明决定了别处的活动[7,10]，强烈提示至少在某些情况下房颤是由稳定的一个或几个高频来源驱动的。我们发现右房所表现的碎裂传导实际上是左房高频周期活动的结果[11]。

前述发现可能会引起令人兴奋的新的诊治手段的开展。很明显，近来在某些病人对触发房颤的局灶的成功定位使得这种心律失常成为射频消融中止发作的适应证[19]。同样，对维持房颤的"引擎"的定位使它成为特异治疗的靶点，不管是通过消融、电转复、药物、还是联合治疗。然而在把来自离体和灌流的人工条件下正常心脏急性房颤的实验资料推广到临床时必须十分谨慎[6-11]。实际上不同种属及心房不同易患条件的房颤的潜在机制很可能不同。然而在给人的房颤射频消融过程中仍可发现强烈支持左房个别高频激动向右房碎裂传导引起房颤的证据[46,47]。在阵发性房颤病人，肺静脉异位起搏点或局部触发产生的激动传向左房遇到异质性组织。很容易想到在这些情况下房颤的起始和维持依赖左房相对持续的折返环[6,7,9]，这些环产生高频激动，并以碎裂波形式传到心房其他部位[10,11,20]。

其他支持单源假说的实验是 Roithinger 及同事们完成的[48]，他们在犬房颤模型选择性左房线性消融明显减慢房颤频率，而右房则无此现象。最近 Wu 和同事们[49]在犬房颤模型证实了左-右频率梯度的存在，提示肺静脉和 Marshall 韧带是维持房颤的高频激动起源。其他研究发现左房不应期比右房短。最近 Li 等[50]的实验强烈提示低频时左房-右房不应期的差别与双房细胞记录到的 APD 内在差异相关。左房更高密度的快速延迟整流电流看起来与低频起搏时心腔特异的 APD 差异一致[50]。这些差别能否解释左房以 18 Hz 激动的能力、左房-右房频率梯度和房颤时右房[11]波碎裂还有待确定。据我们所知，决定左房和肺静脉具有最高频率倾向的分子、细胞和病理生理机制仍是个谜。也许需要综合从分子水平到膜通道、细胞和组织，到整体水平的研究来回答这一重要的临床问题。

（张 萍 译）

参 考 文 献

1. Feinberg WM, Blackshear JL, Laupacis A, et al: Prevalence, age distribution, and gender of patients with atrial fibrillation. Arch Intern Med 155:469–473, 1995.
2. Nattel S: New ideas about atrial fibrillation 50 years on. Nature 415:219–226, 2002.
3. Jalife J, Berenfeld O, Mansour M: Mother rotors and fibrillatory conduction: A mechanism of atrial fibrillation. Cardiovasc Res 54:204–216, 2002.
4. Moe GK, Rheinboldt WC, Abildskov JA: A computer model of atrial fibrillation. Am Heart J 67:200–220, 1964.
5. Allessie MA, Lammers WJEP, Bonke FIM, Hollen J: Experimental evaluation of Moe's wavelet hypothesis of atrial fibrillation. In Zipes DP, Jalife J (eds): Cardiac Electrophysiology and Arrhythmias. Orlando, Fla, Grune & Stratton, 1985.
6. Skanes AC, Mandapati R, Berenfeld O, et al: Spatiotemporal periodicity during atrial fibrillation in the isolated sheep heart. Circulation 98:1236–1248, 1998.
7. Mandapati R, Skanes A, Chen J, et al: Stable microreentrant sources as a mechanism of atrial fibrillation in the isolated sheep heart. Circulation 101:194–199, 2000.
8. Berenfeld O, Mandapati R, Dixit S, et al: Spatially distributed dominant excitation frequencies reveal hidden organization in atrial fibrillation in the Langendorff-perfused sheep heart. J Cardiovasc Electrophysiol 11:869–879, 2000.
9. Chen J, Mandapati R, Berenfeld O, et al: Dynamics of wavelets and their role in atrial fibrillation in the isolated sheep heart. Cardiovasc Res 48:220–232, 2000.
10. Mansour M, Mandapati R, Berenfeld O, et al: Left-to-right gradient of atrial frequencies during acute atrial fibrillation in the isolated sheep heart. Circulation 103:2631–2636, 2001.
11. Berenfeld O, Zaitsev AV, Mironov SF, et al: Frequency-dependent breakdown of wave propagation into fibrillatory conduction across the pectinate muscle network in the isolated sheep right atrium. Circ Res 90:1173–1180, 2002.
12. Gray RA, Pertsov AM, Jalife J: Incomplete reentry and epicardial breakthrough patterns during atrial fibrillation in the sheep heart. Circulation 94:2649–2661, 1996.
13. Gray RA, Pertsov AM, Jalife J: Spatial and temporal organization during cardiac fibrillation. Nature 392:75–78, 1998.
14. Botteron GW, Smith JM: Quantitative assessment of the spatial organization of atrial fibrillation in the intact human heart. Circulation 93:513–518, 1996.
15. Gerstenfeld EP, Sahakian AV, Swiryn S: Evidence for transient linking of atrial excitation during atrial fibrillation in humans. Circulation 86:375–382, 1992.
16. Harada A, Sasaki K, Fukushima T, et al: Atrial activation during chronic atrial fibrillation in patients with isolated mitral valve disease. Ann Thorac Surg 61:104–112, 1996.
17. Sueda T, Nagata H, Shikata H, et al: Simple left atrial procedure for chronic atrial fibrillation associated with mitral valve disease. Ann Thorac Surg 62:1796–1800, 1996.
18. Kumagai K, Khrestian C, Waldo AL: Simultaneous multisite mapping studies during induced atrial fibrillation in the sterile pericarditis model. Insights into the mechanisms of its maintenance. Circulation 95:511–521, 1997.
19. Haissaguerre M, Jais P, Shah DC, et al: Spontaneous initiation of atrial fibrillation by ectopic beats originating in the pulmonary veins. N Engl J Med 339:659–666, 1998.
20. Jalife J, Berenfeld O, Skanes A, Mandapati R: Mechanisms of atrial fibrillation: Mother rotors or multiple daughter wavelets, or both? J Cardiovasc Electrophysiol 9:S2–S12, 1998.
21. Ortiz J, Niwano S, Abe H, et al: Mapping the conversion of atrial flutter to atrial fibrillation and atrial fibrillation to atrial flutter. Insights into mechanisms. Circ Res 74:882–894, 1994.
22. Ikeda T, Wu TJ, Uchida T, et al: Meandering and unstable reentrant wave fronts induced by acetylcholine in isolated canine right atrium. Am J Physiol 273:H356–H370, 1997.
23. Lewis T: The mechanism and graphic registration of the heart beat. London, Shaw & Sons, 1925.
24. Scherf D: Studies on auricular tachycardia caused by aconitine administration. Proc Soc Exp Biol Med 64:233–239, 1947.
25. Schuessler RB, Grayson TM, Bromberg BI, et al: Cholinergically mediated tachyarrhythmias induced by a single extrastimulus in the isolated canine right atrium. Circ Res 71:1254–1267, 1992.
26. Starobin JM, Zilberter YI, Rusnak EM, Starmer CF: Wavelet formation in excitable cardiac tissue: The role of wavefront-obstacle interactions in initiating high-frequency fibrillatory-like arrhythmias. Biophys J 70:581–594, 1996.
27. Cabo C, Pertsov AM, Davidenko JM, et al: Vortex shedding as a precursor of turbulent electrical activity in cardiac muscle. Biophys J 70:1105–1111, 1996.
28. Antz M, Otomo K, Arruda M, et al: Electrical connections between the right atrium and the left atrium via the musculature of the coronary sinus. Circulation 98:1790–1795, 1998.
29. Dolber PC, Spach MS: Structure of the canine Bachmann's bundle related to propagation of excitation. Am J Physiol 257:H1446–H1457, 1989.
30. Samie FH, Mandapati R, Gray RA, et al: A mechanism of transition from ventricular fibrillation to tachycardia: Effect of calcium channel blockade on the dynamics of rotating waves. Circ Res 86:684–691, 2000.
31. Kucera JP, Kleber AG, Rohr S: Slow conduction in cardiac tissue. II: Effects of branching tissue geometry. Circ Res 83:795–805, 1998.
32. Spach MS, Dolber PC, Heidlage JF: Interaction of inhomogeneities of repolarization with anisotropic propagation in dog atria. A mechanism for both preventing and initiating reentry. Circ Res 65:1612–1631, 1989.
33. Olgin JE, Kalman JM, Fitzpatrick AP, Lesh MD: Role of right atrial endocardial structure as barriers to conduction during human type I atrial flutter. Activation and entrainment guided by intracardiac echocardiography. Circulation 92:1839–1848, 1995.
34. Ikeda T, Yashima M, Uchida T, et al: Attachment of meandering reentrant wave fronts to anatomic obstacles in the atrium. Role of the obstacle size. Circ Res 81:753–764, 1997.
35. Wang Z, Feng J, Nattel S: Idiopathic atrial fibrillation in dogs: Electrophysiologic determinants and mechanisms of antiarrhythmic action of flecainide. J Am Coll Cardiol 26:277–286, 1995.
36. Kim KB, Rodefeld MD, Schuessler RB, et al: Relationship between local atrial fibrillation interval and refractory period in the isolated canine atrium. Circulation 94:2961–2967, 1996.
37. Efimov IR, Huang DT, Rendt JM, Salama G: Optical mapping of repolarization and refractoriness from intact hearts. Circulation 90:1469–1480, 1994.
38. Roithinger FX, Karch MR, Steiner PR, et al: The spatial dispersion of atrial refractoriness and atrial fibrillation vulnerability. J Interv Card Electrophysiol 3:311–319, 1999.
39. Satoh T, Zipes DP: Unequal atrial stretch in dogs increases dispersion of refractoriness conductive to developing atrial fibrillation. J Cardiovasc Electrophysiol 7:833–842, 1996.
40. Feng J, Yue L, Wang Z, Nattel S: Ionic mechanisms of regional action potential heterogeneity in the canine right atrium. Circ Res 83:541–551, 1998.
41. Spach MS, Dolber PC, Anderson PAW: Multiple regional differences in cellular properties that regulate repolarization and contraction in the right atrium of adult and newborn dogs. Circ Res 65:1594–1611, 1989.
42. Yamashita T, Nakajima T, Hazama H, et al: Regional differences in transient outward current density and inhomogeneities of repolarization in rabbit right atrium. Circulation 92:3061–3069, 1995.
43. Wu TJ, Yashima M, Xie F, et al: Role of pectinate muscle bundles in the generation and maintenance of intra-atrial reentry: Potential implications for the mechanism of conversion between atrial fibrillation and atrial flutter. Circ Res 83:448–462, 1998.
44. Gray RA, Takkellapati K, Jalife J: Dynamics and anatomical correlates of atrial flutter and fibrillation. In Zipes DP, Jalife J (eds): Cardiac Electrophysiology: From Cell to Bedside. Philadelphia, WB Saunders, 2000.
45. Morillo CA, Klein GJ, Jones DL, Guiraudon CM: Chronic rapid atrial pacing: Structural, functional, and electrophysiological characteristics of a new model of sustained atrial fibrillation. Circulation 91:1588–1595, 1995.
46. Jais P, Haissaguerre M, Shah DC, et al: A focal source of atrial fibrillation treated by discrete radiofrequency ablation. Circulation 95:572–576, 1997.
47. Lu TM, Tai CT, Hsieh MH, et al: Electrophysiologic characteristics in initiation of paroxysmal atrial fibrillation from a focal area. J Am Coll Cardiol 37:1658–1664, 2001.

48. Roithinger FX, Steiner PR, Goseki Y, et al: Electrophysiological effects of selective right versus left atrial linear lesions in a canine model of chronic atrial fibrillation. J Cardiovasc Electrophysiol 10:1564–1574, 1999.
49. Wu TJ, Ong JJC, Chang CM, et al: Pulmonary veins and ligament of Marshall as sources of rapid activations in a canine model of sustained atrial fibrillation. Circulation 103:1157–1163, 2001.
50. Li D, Zhang L, Kneller J, Nattel S: Potential ionic mechanism for repolarization differences between canine right and left atrium. Circ Res 88:1168–1175, 2001.

第 41 章

电重构与慢性心房颤动

David R. Van Wagoner

本章目录

- 心房电重构发生较快而且早期可逆转 371
- 心房电重构的分子基础 371
- 心房电重构的发生机制 374
- 未来的发展方向 374
- 致谢 374

心房颤动（房颤）多见于老年患者，其临床病程常呈进行性进展。虽然房颤的早期常呈阵发性发作和自限性，但是随着病程的延长，房颤发作的持续时间逐渐延长，有时变成持续性房颤。房颤从阵发性到持续性再发展成持久性的整个病程中，心房将发生结构的重构改变，如扩张、肌小梁增多、纤维化、脂肪浸润等，以及心房肌细胞发生的生化改变，如心肌细胞肥大和离子通道密度及分布异常。心房这种对房颤的病理生理适应性改变从广义上讲称为重构。更确切地说，这些改变主要影响心房肌细胞的兴奋性和电激动过程，称为电生理重构。心房扩张改变、胶原沉积和大体组织学改变称为结构重构。本章主要讨论近年来关于人体心房肌电重构的证据以及与动物实验的相关性，同时讨论人类房颤的这些变化以及引起这些变化的分子学机制。房颤时电重构的组织学改变将在近期述评中讨论[1,2]。

一、心房电重构发生较快而且早期可逆转

Wijffels 和同事[3]的基础研究表明，猝发式起搏建立的山羊持续性房颤模型能引起心房重构，而且在持续性房颤情况下，心房有效不应期发生改变，特点是心房有效不应期快速缩短，最明显的改变发生在房颤发生后 24h 内。有效不应期的缩短能在快速起搏后 1 周内发生。随访研究显示，心房的这种电生理重构的逆转随着时间的延长又可回到最初水平，房颤持续 5 天内，心房的电重构容易逆转，且房颤持续 2 天之内完全可以逆转[4]。图 41-1 显示，心房电重构过程可以反复几次，但有效不应期并没有明显的累加变化。临床研究表明，甚至极短暂的猝发式快速起搏（几分钟）就能引起心房有效不应期的可逆性缩短[5]。临床观察还发现，有效不应期无累加改变，持续性房颤形成的过程比心房电重构要慢，提示有其他因素（结构重构）也可能在房颤发生中起十分重要的作用。这些因素将在本章有关房颤发生机制中作简要讨论。

二、心房电重构的分子基础

心房肌细胞的动作电位与其他可兴奋细胞一样，反映了细胞膜上所有离子通道的完全激活及细胞膜上离子泵的分布情况，并影响细胞膜电位。图 41-2 显示健康人和房颤患者的心房肌细胞的动作电位（上图），这些离子通道中有数个相关的分子相同（右栏注解），而且离子通道电流密度的相应改变与慢性房颤的发生有关（左栏注解）。这些离子流和离子通道亚单位在

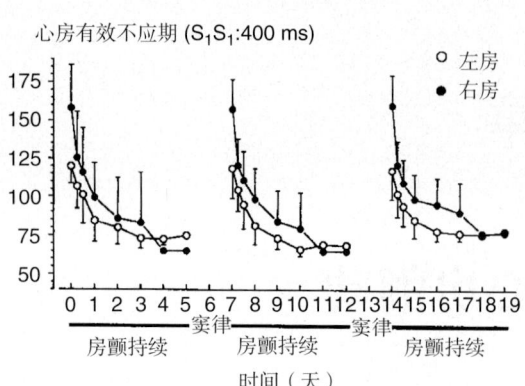

图 41-1 心房电重构发生较快，而且早期可以逆转 本图显示，在持续性房颤时，心房有效不应期的变化比较快。这种变化在左右心房之间相似。在房颤发作5天期间中，最初2天内可以逆转的，且2天后心房有效不应期也无累加改变（引自 Garratt CJ, Duytschaever M, Killian M, et al. J Cardiovasc Electrophysiol, 1999; 10: 1101-1108)

持续性房颤患者的心房肌细胞中的表达变化将在下文讨论。

（一）内向整流 K^+ 电流

1. I_{K1}

心房肌细胞的静息电位主要由内向整流 K^+ 电流（I_{K1}）形成[6]。I_{K1} 电流在心房肌细胞比心室肌细胞少得多，但在正电位时外向电流通常较小。最新研究表明，内向整流钾通道的亚单位 Kir2.1 和 Kir2.3 的不同表达是各个房室之间 I_{K1} 电流密度不同所致[7]。有趣的是，房颤患者的 I_{K1} 电流密度是增加的[8-10]，这可能是频繁除极时的代偿机制。

2. I_{KACh}

心房肌细胞存在乙酰胆碱 K^+ 电流（I_{KACh}），但心室肌细胞没有，它由迷走神经兴奋或循环中的腺苷来激活，对心房肌细胞和窦房结细胞的静息电位和兴奋性也有很强的调节作用。最新研究表明，慢性房颤时 I_{KACh} 减少而 I_{K1} 增加[10]，而且 GIRK4 mRNA 的表达也减少[11]。房颤患者的心房肌 I_{K1} 分布的各向异性变化与以前报告的除极组织的面积增加有关。

（二）外向 K^+ 电流

1. I_{kur}

与心室肌相比，心房肌的复极钾电流的密度及各向异性较大。心房肌细胞的这些电流密度的增加可以解释心房肌细胞动作电位呈"三角"形而心室肌细胞呈"直角"形的机制。心房肌细胞特异钾电流之一是超速延迟整流钾电流（I_{kur}），其分子基础与 $K_V1.5$ 亚单位的表达有关[21,22]。在人类房颤相关的钾电流变化的早期研究表明，房颤对持续性外向钾电流（I_{kur}）有明显影响[8]。I_{kur} 与已报道的 I_{TO} 电流是同义词，无论是左心房还是右心房，其电流均降低 50%。I_{kur} 包括两种成分，其一是 I_{kur}，是主要成分；其二是其他延迟整流钾电流。蛋白印迹杂交对 K_{Va} 亚单位表达的特异抗体的分析显示，房颤患者的心房肌细胞膜 $K_V1.5$ 蛋白的表达明显降低[8]，而另一种电压依赖性钾通道 a 亚单位 Kv2.1 的表达明显增加，且不受房颤的影响[8]。但另有研究表明，房颤的心房肌细胞的 I_{kur} 电流和 $K_V1.5$ 电流的表达有同样改变[15]。

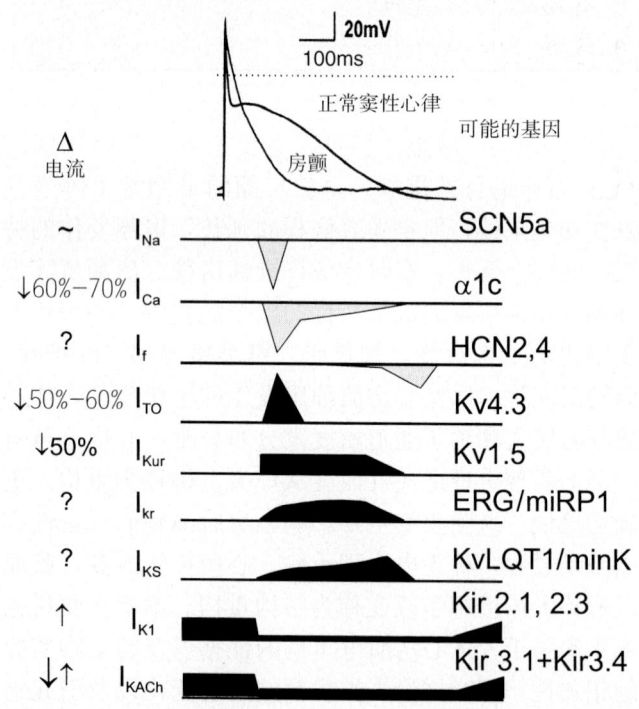

图 41-2 心房颤动对人体心房肌细胞动作电位和离子流的影响 图示1例26岁健康男患正常窦性心律时的动作电位；以及1例73岁持续性房颤3年后的动作电位。参与人体心房动作电位的电流用图解法描述，以及相关的功能电流变化（左侧）和基因异常（右侧）

2. I_{TO}

暂时外向钾电流（I_{TO}）是人类心房和心室肌细胞动作电位的快速复极早期（1相）的主要电流[12-14]。在人类，心房肌细胞的 I_{TO} 密度明显高于心室肌细胞，机制可能是心房肌细胞的动作电位时程较短。Kv4.3 蛋白是形成 I_{TO} 的主要亚单位。这种亚单位的激活可能由几个辅助亚单位调节（β亚单位和 KChIPs）。对正常人的心房，辅助亚单位表达区域的分布尚未进行过研究。已完成的几项研究是对心肌细胞的外向钾电流的密度及分子组成的变化进行了评估，其分离的心房肌细胞来自心房颤动患者的心房。最早的报告显示，I_{TO} 的电流密度明显降低（≈60%），但随后对房颤患者与非房颤外科手术患者（对照组）进行了比较，左、右心房肌细胞的 I_{TO} 是相同的[8]。左心房与右心房相比较，二尖瓣疾病最易影响左心房，其主要影响因素是房颤而不是瓣膜病，因房颤能使 I_{TO} 减少。对于有折返性房颤病史的患者，外科手术时常呈窦性心律，心房肌的 I_{TO} 电流和正常对照组患者间没有区别[8]。其他几项研究也有相同的观察结果，人体房颤时 I_{TO} 电流明显降低[9,15]。有趣的是，在扩张型心肌病患者，虽无心房颤动，但心肌细胞的 I_{TO} 表达也发生下降[16]。通过对快速起搏犬模型的实验研究证实，I_{TO} 表达减少[17]。还有几项研究也对 I_{TO} 减少的分子机制做了评估，发现 Kv4.3 mRNA 的表达变化与 I_{TO} 电流的减少有关[18,19]。除此，在快速起搏的犬模型，对蛋白表达的分析也显示，Kv4.3 的表达变化与该电流功能的降低相一致[20]。而其他亚单位可能修饰 I_{TO} 通道的功能特性，但尚无关于房颤相关的这些亚单位表达变化方面的研究报告。

3. I_{Kr} 和 I_{Ks}

I_{Kr} 和 I_{Ks} 是短效抗心律失常药物的主要靶点，对 I_{Kr} 电流选择性阻滞的药物有得菲利特（dofetilide）和 D-索他洛尔，并可由多种药物进行间接调节，但对 I_{Kr} 通道的兴奋呈弱的抑制作用[24,25]。I_{Ks} 可由 azimilide 和其他（正在研制中）药物来阻滞[26]。这些延迟整流钾通道存在人的心房肌细胞，而且在心房复极过程中具有重要作用[27]。因此，充分了解房颤对这些电流分布的影响倍受关注。值得注意的是，至少认为 I_{Ks} 阻滞剂的疗效在房颤和房扑早期更为明显，对持续性房颤和房扑的疗效较差[28]。这可以根据动作电位的形态反映心房电重构的过程，并根据心律失常的复杂性反映离子通道结构的改变。

由于很难解释人体的游离心房肌细胞 HERG 基因相关的离子通道改变所产生的电流，所以根本不可能决定房颤对离子通道功能激活的作用。迄今为止，还几乎没有几篇关于 HERG（I_{Kr}）亚单位表达变化的报告，他们报告的结果是 HERG 蛋白的表达下调[29]，但没有 HERG mRNA 的表达改变[23]。

需要强调，对 KCNQ1（KvLQT1）功能突变的分析表明，房颤的最初基因型可能与 I_{KS} 电流表达的增加有关[30]。从理论上讲，KCNQ1 功能改变能够引起心房动作电位时程的缩短，从而使传导波长缩短及多重子波折返环得以维持。

（三）内向电流

1. $I_{Ca,L}$

L 型二氢吡啶敏感性钙电流（$I_{Ca,L}$）也是在细胞膜除极时被激动，并形成心房动作电位的平台期[31]。由于房颤时钾电流的密度减小以及慢性房颤时心房组织的动作电位和有效不应期缩短，因而有证据提示，心房肌有效不应期和动作电位时程缩短的同时有 $I_{Ca,L}$ 密度的降低[32]。快速心房起搏犬模型令人信服地说明，$I_{Ca,L}$ 减小使动作电位的平台期消失。除此，还有一系列有关人体心房肌细胞的实验研究来验证这个假说，通过与正常窦性心律对照组患者在外科手术中获取的心房肌细胞进行比较，表明慢性房颤患者心房肌细胞的 $I_{Ca,L}$ 密度明显降低（约为 2/3）[9,33]。且在持久性房颤时 $I_{Ca,L}$ 的密度较低，但有趣的是，这仅仅是这些研究的结果之一[33]，而对照组的 $I_{Ca,L}$ 的密度更低，其更可能是手术后发生房性心律失常的机制。据研究报告，$I_{Ca,L}$ 的密度改变能引起心律失常，其机制与持续性快速激动的代偿适应机制显著不同[33]。除此，还应强调钙超载在房性异位电激动中的介导作用[34]。

2. I_{Na}

心脏的传导功能主要取决于电压依赖性钠电流（I_{Na}）的激活，而且 I_{Na} 是动作电位上升支（除极 0 相）的主要离子流[35]。尽管 I_{Na} 十分重要，但几乎没有关于房颤时 I_{Na} 的研究报告。一项关于持续性房颤患者的心房肌细胞的研究中，Bosch 和同事[9]报告慢性房颤患者的心肌细胞上 I_{Na} 密度没有明显降低。然而有趣的是，电压依赖性 I_{Na} 失活改变（≈10mV）在房颤患者的心肌细胞趋向于更大正电位（b∞）[9]。这是房颤时离子流的电压依赖性生物物理变化（而不是密度）的首要证据。对于持续性房颤患者，房颤没有对I_{Na}密度影响与心房传导速度没有减小呈一致结果。但是，这项研究结果与心房快速起搏的犬模型观察到的结果不同，即随着心房快速起搏时间的延长其I_{Na}密度呈明显的进行性降低[36]。

三、心房电重构的发生机制

虽然钙超载可能是房颤的始动因素，但钙超载引起心房电重构的亚细胞机制尚不清楚。可能的机制包括细胞蛋白激酶的激活（如 calpains[37,38]）、钙依赖性激酶和磷酸酶激活和细胞内氧化张力增加[39]，这些可能由线粒体功能改变或炎性机制所致[40]。所有这些机制和更多的其他机制参与了心房电重构过程。然而，最新的研究中，我们主要关注氧化信号和损伤相关的通路。我们的最近研究证实，持久性房颤患者的心房组织中蛋白酪氨酸硝酸盐增加，明显提示过氧硝酸盐形成[39]。蛋白硝酸盐增加的程度与肌酸激酶的激活（可提供给心肌纤维三磷酸腺苷）和肌球蛋白异构重整的转化有关[39]。

为验证这个假说，即在心房电重构过程中氧化物的形成十分重要，我们做了一系列快速起搏犬模型的实验研究。预治疗及每日给犬补充维生素 C（抗氧化剂）能使快速心房起搏 24～48h 后的有效不应期无明显改变[41]。从这些动物模型所取的组织显示，随着起搏时间的延长蛋白硝酸盐逐渐增加，而维生素 C 能阻止这种变化[41]。因而，起搏可能是很强的致氧化刺激剂。最近，研究人员在快速起搏心室所致的心力衰竭领域的研究中得到同样的结论[42,43]。因而在临床应用抗氧化治疗减小心房快速激动的影响方面具有重要意义。

心房的血管紧张素受体表达的明显变化已在房颤患者得到证实[44]。血管紧张素Ⅱ能调节多种细胞内通路，特别是控制细胞内基质成分的形成和降解方面（纤维化）[45]。纤维化的程度与房颤的诱发和维持有关[40]。

四、未来的发展方向

心房颤动是一种复杂的多因素疾病。其病因在不同的患者亚群体中不同。但电重构是常见的，其可能是房颤持续的重要因素。除电重构外，结构重构（无论在亚细胞水平还是组织水平）也常存在，而且与促使房颤维持的组织基质改变有关[47]。但实验研究的结果表明，电生理改变是可逆的，但结构重构是很慢的及难修复的[48]。

上述研究结果提示，对于房颤患者，长期减少$I_{Ca,L}$是心房有效不应期和兴奋性改变的重要因素[32]。钙电流能触发心肌的兴奋-收缩耦联的反应，因此它是心房收缩的调节因子。因而钙电流的减小能引起心房收缩性的降低[49]。有趣的是，慢性房颤引起的改变与无房颤只有心房扩张（$I_{Ca,L}$和I_{TO}减小）的改变极为相似[16]。

最新研究表明，心房电重构过程涉及到不同的病理机制，而且需要进一步进行实验研究来评价心房重构过程中这些机制的相对权重。虽然离子通道阻滞剂在治疗房颤方面的疗效有限，但各种以新的机制为基础的通道阻滞剂正在研发，而且在药物治疗房颤方面的进展在不远的未来有望得到突破。

五、致　谢

本工作得到国家卫生机构的资助，编号为 R01 HL-65412。

（刘元生　译）

参 考 文 献

1. Waldo AL, Van Wagoner DR: Atrial Fibrillation. In Spooner PM, Rosen MR (eds): Foundations of Cardiac Arrhythmias, New York, Marcel Dekker, 1999.
2. Allessie MA: Atrial electrophysiologic remodeling: another vicious circle? J Cardiovasc Electrophysiol 9:1378–1393, 1998.
3. Wijffels MC, Kirchhof CJ, Dorland R, Allessie MA: Atrial fibrillation begets atrial fibrillation. A study in awake chronically instrumented goats. Circulation 92:1954–1968, 1995.
4. Garratt CJ, Duytschaever M, Killian M, et al: Repetitive electrical remodeling by paroxysms of atrial fibrillation in the goat: no cumulative effect on inducibility or stability of atrial fibrillation. J Cardiovasc Electrophysiol 10:1101–1108, 1999.
5. Daoud EG, Bogun F, Goyal R, et al: Effect of atrial fibrillation on atrial refractoriness in humans. Circulation 94:1600–1606, 1996.
6. Koumi S, Backer CL, Arentzen CE: Characterization of inwardly rectifying K+ channel in human cardiac myocytes. Alterations in channel behavior in myocytes isolated from patients with idiopathic dilated cardiomyopathy. Circulation 92:164–174, 1995.
7. Melnyk P, Zhang L, Shrier A, Nattel S: Differential distribution of Kir2.1 and Kir2.3 subunits in canine atrium and ventricle. Am J Physiol Heart Circ Physiol 283:H1123–H1133, 2002.
8. Van Wagoner DR, Pond AL, McCarthy PM, et al: Outward K+ current densities and Kv1.5 expression are reduced in chronic human atrial fibrillation. Circ Res 80:772–781, 1997.
9. Bosch RF, Zeng X, Grammer JB, et al: Ionic mechanisms of electrical remodeling in human atrial fibrillation. Cardiovasc Res 44:121–131, 1999.
10. Dobrev D, Wettwer E, Kortner A, et al: Human inward rectifier potassium channels in chronic and postoperative atrial fibrillation. Cardiovasc Res 54:397–404, 2002.

11. Dobrev D, Graf E, Wettwer E, et al: Molecular basis of downregulation of G-protein-coupled inward rectifying K⁺ current ($I_{K,ACh}$ in chronic human atrial fibrillation: decrease in GIRK4 mRNA correlates with reduced $I_{K,ACh}$ and muscarinic receptor-mediated shortening of action potentials Circulation 104:2551–2557, 2001.
12. Fermini B, Wang Z, Duan D, Nattel S: Differences in rate dependence of transient outward current in rabbit and human atrium. Am J Physiol 263:H1747–H1754, 1992.
13. Wang Z, Feng J, Shi H, et al: Potential molecular basis of different physiological properties of the transient outward K⁺ current in rabbit and human atrial myocytes. Circ Res 84, 551–561, 1999.
14. Kaab S, Dixon J, Duc J, et al: Molecular basis of transient outward potassium current downregulation in human heart failure: A decrease in Kv4.3 mRNA correlates with a reduction in current density. Circulation 98:1383–1393, 1998.
15. Brandt MC, Priebe L, Bohle T, et al: The ultrarapid and the transient outward K⁺ current in human atrial fibrillation. Their possible role in postoperative atrial fibrillation. J Mol Cell Cardiol 32:1885–1896, 2000.
16. Le Grand B, Hatem S, Deroubaix E, et al: Depressed transient outward and calcium currents in dilated human atria. Cardiovasc Res 28:548–556, 1994.
17. Yue L, Feng J, Gaspo R, et al: Ionic remodeling underlying action potential changes in a canine model of atrial fibrillation. Circ Res 81:512–525, 1997.
18. Gaspo R, Bosch RF, Talajic M, Nattel S: Functional mechanisms underlying tachycardia-induced sustained atrial fibrillation in a chronic dog model. Circulation 96:4027–4035, 1997.
19. Grammer JB, Bosch RF, Kuhlkamp V, Seipel L: Molecular remodeling of Kv4.3 potassium channels in human atrial fibrillation. J Cardiovasc Electrophysiol 11:626–633, 2000
20. Yue L, Melnyk P, Gaspo R, et al: Molecular mechanisms underlying ionic remodeling in a dog model of atrial fibrillation. Circ Res 84:776–784, 1999.
21. Fedida D, Wible B, Wang Z, et al: Identity of a novel delayed rectifier current from human heart with a cloned K⁺ channel current. Circ Res 73:210–216, 1993.
22. Feng J, Wible B, Li GR, et al: Antisense oligodeoxynucleotides directed against Kv1.5 mRNA specifically inhibit ultrarapid delayed rectifier K⁺ current in cultured adult human atrial myocytes. Circ Res 80:572–579, 1997.
23. Brundel BJ, Van Gelder IC, Henning RH, et al: Alterations in potassium channel gene expression in atria of patients with persistent and paroxysmal atrial fibrillation: Differential regulation of protein and mRNA. J Am Coll Cardiol 37:926–932, 2001.
24. Cavero I, Mestre M, Guillon JM, Crumb W: Drugs that prolong QT interval as an unwanted effect: assessing their likelihood of inducing hazardous cardiac dysrhythmias. Expert Opin Pharmacother 1:947–973, 2000.
25. Nattel S: Electrophysiologic remodeling: are ion channels static players or dynamic movers? J Cardiovasc Electrophysiol 10:272–282, 1999.
26. Karam R, Marcello S, Brooks RR, et al: Azimilide dihydrochloride, a novel antiarrhythmic agent. Am J Cardiol 81:40D–46D, 1998.
27. Wang Z, Fermini B, Nattel S: Delayed rectifier outward current and repolarization in human atrial myocytes. Circ Res 73:276–285, 1993.
28. Norgaard BL, Wachtell K, Christensen PD, et al: Efficacy and safety of intravenously administered dofetilide in acute termination of atrial fibrillation and flutter: A multicenter, randomized, double-blind, placebo-controlled trial. Danish Dofetilide in Atrial Fibrillation and Flutter Study Group. Am Heart J 137:1062–1069, 1999.
29. Brundel BJ, Van Gelder IC, Henning RH, et al: Ion channel remodeling is related to intraoperative atrial effective refractory periods in patients with paroxysmal and persistent atrial fibrillation. Circulation 103:684–690, 2001.
30. Chen YH, Xu SJ, Bendahhou S, et al: KCNQ1 gain-of-function mutation in familial atrial fibrillation. Science 299:251–254, 2003.
31. Escande D, Coulombe A, Faivre JF, Coraboeuf E: Characteristics of the time-dependent slow inward current in adult human atrial single myocytes. J Mol Cell Cardiol 18:547–551, 1986.
32. Boutjdir M, Le Heuzey JY, Lavergne T, et al: Inhomogeneity of cellular refractoriness in human atrium: Factor of arrhythmia? Pacing Clin Electrophysiol 9(6 Pt 2):1095–1000, 1986.
33. Van Wagoner DR, Pond AL, Lamorgese M, et al: Atrial L-type Ca^{2+} currents and human atrial fibrillation. Circ Res 85:428–436, 1999.
34. Goette A, Honeycutt C, Langberg JJ: Electrical remodeling in atrial fibrillation. Time course and mechanisms. Circulation 94:2968–2974, 1996.
35. Sakakibara Y, Wasserstrom JA, Furukawa T, et al: Characterization of the sodium current in single human atrial myocytes. Circ Res 71:535–546, 1992.
36. Gaspo R, Bosch RF, Bou-Abboud E, Nattel S: Tachycardia-induced changes in Na⁺ current in a chronic dog model of atrial fibrillation. Circ Res 81:1045–1052, 1997.
37. Goette A, Arndt M, Rocken C, et al: Calpains and cytokines in fibrillating human atria. Am J Physiol Heart Circ Physiol 283, H264–H272, 2002.
38. Brundel BJ, Ausma J, Van Gelder IC, et al: Activation of proteolysis by calpains and structural changes in human paroxysmal and persistent atrial fibrillation. Cardiovasc Res 54:380–389, 2002.
39. Mihm MJ, Yu F, Carnes CA, Reiser PJ, et al: Impaired myofibrillar energetics and oxidative injury during human atrial fibrillation. Circulation 104:174–180, 2001.
40. Chung MK, Martin DO, Wazni O, et al: C-reactive protein elevation in patients with atrial arrhythmias: inflammatory mechanisms and persistence of atrial fibrillation. Circulation 104:2886–2991, 2001.
41. Carnes CA, Chung MK, Nakayama T, et al: Ascorbate attenuates atrial pacing-induced peroxynitrite formation and electrical remodeling and decreases the incidence of postoperative atrial fibrillation. Circ Res 89:E32–E38, 2001.
42. Ekelund UE, Harrison RW, Shokek O, et al: Intravenous allopurinol decreases myocardial oxygen consumption and increases mechanical efficiency in dogs with pacing-induced heart failure. Circ Res 85:437–445, 1999.
43. Ukai T, Cheng CP, Tachibana H, et al: Allopurinol enhances the contractile response to dobutamine and exercise in dogs with pacing-induced heart failure. Circulation 103:750–755, 2001.
44. Goette A, Arndt M, Rocken C, et al: Regulation of angiotensin II receptor subtypes during atrial fibrillation in humans. Circulation 101:2678–2681, 2000.
45. Goette A, Lendeckel U, Klein HU: Signal transduction systems and atrial fibrillation. Cardiovasc Res 54:247–258, 2002.
46. Goette A, Juenemann G, Peters B, et al: Determinants and consequences of atrial fibrosis in patients undergoing open heart surgery. Cardiovasc.Res 54:390–396, 2002.
47. Ausma J, Wijffels M, Thone F, et al: Structural changes of atrial myocardium due to sustained atrial fibrillation in the goat. Circulation 96:3157–3163, 1997.
48. Ausma J, Litjens N, Lenders MH, et al: Time course of atrial fibrillation-induced cellular structural remodeling in atria of the goat. J Mol Cell Cardiol 33:2083–2094, 2001.
49. Schotten U, Ausma J, Stellbrink C, et al: Cellular mechanisms of depressed atrial contractility in patients with chronic atrial fibrillation. Circulation 103:691–698, 2001.

第 42 章

室性快速性心律失常的发生机制

Jiashin Wu，Jianyi Wu，Douglas P. Zipes

本章目录

- 局灶性放电 ……………………………… 376
- 折返激动 ………………………………… 377
- 临床意义 ………………………………… 384
- 致谢 ……………………………………… 384

关于室性心动过速的发生机制早在20世纪初就做了大量的研究。多项研究内容包括临床观察、在体和离体的实验研究、细胞和基因水平、理论分析和许多类似的研究。绝大多数室性心动过速是由心室的一个或几个部位的自发除极引起，这些电激动能引起或促使折返形成以维持室性心动过速。虽然绝大多数室性心动过速发生在心脏病患者，如冠心病、心肌病、离子通道异常和其他疾患，但室性心动过速也可能是功能性的，发生在表面看来是正常的心脏，当条件成熟时，室性心动过速就可发作。因为室性心动过速有可能导致心脏性猝死，以及发达国家的人口呈现越来越老龄化趋势，所以处理室性心动过速是一项非常有意义而又十分重要的临床任务。其中，了解室性心动过速的发生机制是制定预防和治疗室性心动过速的临床策略的关键一步。然而，室性心动过速的发生机制尚不完全清楚，其相关内容在本章将做一简要阐述。

一、局灶性放电

快速局灶性放电是室性心动过速的发生机制之一，其可能由微折返、早后除极、迟后除极、正常或异常自律性增高引起。绝大多数心室肌细胞能在较早激动后通过动作电位的4相自动除极、2相和3相的早后除极、4相的迟后除极而产生自动放电。正常时，起源于窦房结较快的激动能抑制健康心室肌的自律性。但在病理情况下或在药物作用下如儿茶酚胺浓度过高时，心室肌的自律性加速，能引起室性早搏，进而室性早搏能够演变为心室激动的主导起源点，导致室性心动过速。这些情况时，常有一个或几个心室区自律性最高并控制了心室激动。长QT综合征(LQTS)的患者，局灶性激动可能由早搏触发，该早搏以早后除极或迟后除极的形式出现。局灶性激动也可能出现在心肌缺血和心肌梗死区的周围区域。

(一) 长QT综合征时的局灶性激动

尖端扭转型室性心动过速是多形性室性心动过速的一种类型，并可导致心脏性猝死，其机制可能是长QT综合征患者发生早后除极所致[1,2]。心肌细胞膜离子通道的遗传性基因缺陷可引起长QT综合征。约有50多种药物，包括经典的抗心律失常药物如奎尼丁，以及某些抗生素、抗精神病药物和其他药物，都能影响膜的复极离子流，结果引起心电图的QT间期延长，已被证实其与获得性长QT综合征有关[3]。实际，部分明显为获得性长QT综合征的患者仅存在轻微的先天表型，当接触了前面提到的某种药物后才出现症状。而先天性长QT综合征可以分为多个亚型，其分型的依据是受累的膜离子流（例如LQT1、LQT2和LQT3是由I_{Ks}、I_{Kr}的改变和I_{Na}失活引起，见第70章）。

心室除极之间的长间歇能使心室动作电位的时程延长[4]，增加了跨室壁的复极离散度，并增加了细胞

内 Ca^{2+} 浓度[5]。这些变化能促使浦肯野纤维[6]和室壁中层单个心室肌细胞（M 细胞）[7]的膜电位震荡的振幅增加，并引发早后除极。早后除极也可能在心外膜和心内膜心肌细胞的单向动作电位图上记录到，除此，还可在豚鼠心室肌细胞微注射内向电流后记录到，其类似于细胞间不同复极速度的缝隙连接电流[9]，提示尖端扭转型室性心动过速是由早后除极触发，因其来自于心内膜（包括浦肯野纤维网）[4,6,11,12]和室壁中层 M 细胞[7]的早后除极的振幅超过激动阈值而引起[10]。我们观察了离体动脉直接接触再灌注后发生的长 QT 综合征的犬心室楔嵌模型的跨壁表面电位（长 QT 综合征由海葵毒素 II 制备），记录了多个部位的局灶激动、折返、跨壁周长差异程度及膜震荡时限，它们能引起不同的激动通路并改变心电图 QRS 波的时相和振幅，进而引起尖端扭转型室性心动过速样室性心动过速。在海葵毒素 II 制备的离体再灌注心室楔嵌模型上，自发性局灶激动和室性心动过速在心肌缺血早期 40min 内明显增加。

（二）心肌缺血周围区的局灶性激动

急性心肌缺血时 K_{ATP} 通道开放，并引起酸中毒和低氧/缺氧。外向 K^+ 电流能增加缺血区的细胞外 K^+ 浓度（$[K^+]_o$），增加跨缺血区周围心肌的复极离散度。$[K^+]_o$ 能通过改变 K^+ 平衡电位和 K^+ 传导特性调节心肌的自律性、兴奋性和不应期。$[K^+]_o$ 的少量增加（如从 5.4～7.0mM）对激动阈值和动作电位的最大速率（V_{max}）的影响也较小，但能增加静息膜电位和组织的兴奋性。当 $[K^+]_o$ 进一步增加时能使静息膜电位降低至很低水平，从而降低 V_{max} 和组织的兴奋性。因此，急性心肌缺血能引起心肌组织的兴奋性在缺血早期 1～3min 增加和随后的降低[13]。在原位猪心实验中，心肌缺血过程中 $[K^+]_o$ 增加，其与心率 90～150 次/分之间的变化[14]及周围心肌细胞外的 pH 值无关[15]。缺血周围心肌的动作电位离散度能产生缺血细胞和正常细胞间的损伤电流，能引起周围心肌附近的正常组织的兴奋性增加，从而导致浦肯野纤维的自发性除极并触发室性心动过速。事实上，在急性心肌缺血时，局灶性激动能引起缺血周围心肌心律失常中的 75%。在心肌缺血再灌注早期，组织兴奋性的各向异性的快速改善能产生局灶激动，进而引起室性心动过速[16]。

二、折返激动

室性心动过速是由心室肌的快速反复激动引起的。除了持续性快速局灶性激动外，室性心动过速的快速激动也可能由触发事件（例如期前激动、外来的电或机械刺激）引起的折返所致。折返激动的形成需要两个基本条件：传导的单向阻滞（在一个方向上能成功传导，但在相反方向上不能传导）引起反复的折返运动，折返环周长长于折返环路径心肌组织的最长不应期，从而使激动反复发生[17]。这两个基本条件是发生折返的必需条件，其可能由解剖学异常（被动过程）、膜离子流异常（主动过程）以及兴奋波、组织不应性和心室肌之间的动态相互作用而形成。折返激动的最简单形式是折返波沿着稳定周长的固定环路进行反复运动时，产生单形性室性心动过速。当折返波围绕一个核心运动时，而这个核心是不能被兴奋或兴奋性极低时（如主要动脉、梗死区或其他基质），也会形成折返激动。而当组织不应性和非解剖学各向异性产生的新的激动波之间在瞬时内相互作用时，就能产生功能性折返激动。心室颤动通常由复杂的折返波引起，若多个折返波同时运动、相互碰撞、相互融合及沿着稳定变化的路径呈分叉运行时就能引起心室颤动。在折返性心室颤动中，心室的多个区域同时收缩和同时舒张。这种非同步的区域性心室收缩使心室的输出量几乎为零，成为心脏性猝死的最常见原因。

（一）单向传导阻滞

折返形成的基本条件之一就是传导的单向阻滞，其可能是基质（包括组织的局部特征和几何形状）或瞬时事件（多个碰撞波的波锋和波尾的位置和方向）的非对称性所致，或由于在组织解剖、传导速度及动作电位的波形方面的各向异性（方向依赖性）所致，或由于心室肌的非连续性所致。心室肌不同区域的膜离子流密度的差异能形成心室肌兴奋性和动作电位时程在不同区域间的离散性。

1. 不应期离散引起的单向阻滞

心室肌的动作电位存在着各向异性[18]。动作电位的时程在心底部心肌要比心尖部心肌长，而且心内膜下心肌要比心外膜下心肌长。室壁中层心肌细胞与心内膜下和心外膜下心肌相比其动作电位时程最长。心外膜下心肌细胞的短暂外向电流（I_{TO}）比心内膜下心肌要大，且缺血诱导较强的 K_{ATP} 电流可被 glibenclamide 阻断，动作电位的形态呈较大的尖锋和穹隆状，有明显的频率依赖性，缺血诱导的动作电位时程的缩短，对缺血更为敏感，以及 I_{NaCa} 交换电流增强[19]。心内膜下浦肯野纤维网与跨壁动作电位离散度和组织兴奋性有关。病理情况下（例如缺血、LQTS）可进一步增加组织的兴奋性和不应期的离散度，促使发生单向传导阻滞。

不应期离散度的增加常能引起折返激动和室性心动过速[20]。复极离散度的增加能引起临床心律失常性猝死，并在离体 LQT2 兔心脏模型上诱发出尖端扭转型室性心动过速[10]。若减小复极离散度能减少室性心动过速的发作频率[21]。并已在计算机模拟研究的结果显示，单向传导阻滞可在期前刺激的不应期各向异性基质的中心产生[22]。期前刺激产生的激动可以向不同不应期层次的区域扩布，该区域的组织兴奋性已经恢复，而相反方向的传导因该区域仍处在不应期而发生阻滞。正常组织在动作电位复极期的易损期很窄，期前刺激能引起单向传导阻滞[49]。膜兴奋性的各向异性的减小能明显增加单向传导阻滞的可能性。

心肌缺血能增加不应期的离散度。而缺血后期则能延长动作电位的不应期。缺血引起 $[K^+]_o$ 增加能引起膜电位的部分除极，使 Na^+ 通道恢复可激动性的速度减慢，从而引起复极后的不应期延长[13]。在非缺血的心室肌，不应期与动作电位时程密切相关。但在人体心肌缺血 1min 后不应期与动作电位时程间的相关性就已消失[50]。然而，由于缺血周围区的离子不同，缺血区之间的部位与正常区相比，其不应期缩短，而缺血中心区的不应期延长。缺血周围区的 $[K^+]_o$ 的各向异性最大[15]。在急性心肌缺血时，缺血区域的 $[K^+]_o$ 各向异性、细胞间失耦联和非一致性都能产生单向阻滞和随后的室性心律失常[51]。应用 glibenclamide 阻滞 K_{ATP} 通道时能降低心肌缺血时的 $[K^+]_o$ 的聚集速率[13]，减小缺血周围区的动作电位时程的离散度，并降低心肌缺血和再灌注性心律失常的发生率[52]。

2. 各向异性基质区内的单向阻滞

虽然心肌组织的各向异性能引起单向传导阻滞，但各向异性并不是必需条件。单向传导阻滞和折返激动可以发生在各向异质区，由多个传导波的头尾短暂相互作用所致。在各向异性基质区刺激两个局部非对称位点，分别为 S_1 和 S_2，若在较早 S_1 刺激波的波尾给予 S_2 刺激时，S_2 激动波能够扩布至 S_1 激动波的不应期后，但不能沿相反方向扩布至不应区。然后，S_2 激动波传导至 S_1 激动波的波尾后的不应期区，还能再回到局部不应期后的 S_2 刺激位点。这种传导的单向阻滞能够在各向异性基质区引起螺旋波折返。

3. 动作电位时程改变引起的单向阻滞

当心率足够快时，短周期不能使心室动作电位完全复极，则引起动作电位时程呈短长序列变化。动作电位时程改变能引起心电图 T 波的振幅和形状发生逐波变化。随着激动频率的进一步增加，动作电位复极的区域同步性能够消失，引起动作电位时程在邻近区之间出现反向改变，进而引起心室内动作电位时程的显著空间差异和离散度。动作电位的这种不协调改变能引起单向传导阻滞，并引起折返激动和心室颤动[53]。有明显复极离散的 LQT3 模型上，当起搏周长突然缩短时 T 波的改变能引起尖端扭转型室性心动过速[23,24]。

动作电位的特性决定动作电位时程的改变。动作电位形成的曲线是对前一舒张间期的动作电位时程描绘出来的曲线，并能表明前一舒张间期的干扰（如期前激动）如何影响下一次激动的动作电位时程，从而改变下一次舒张间期。如果动作电位曲线的上升支比 1 相缓慢，则可通过单次期前激动干扰的放大作用，使随后激动的动作电位时程发生改变，并导致单向传导阻滞和心室颤动。

4. 单向阻滞与有效电极

绝大多数心室肌细胞的形态近似长圆柱形，其长度约 $30\sim130\mu m$，直径约 $8\sim20\mu m$，这种长圆柱形心肌细胞能使细胞内出现各向异性。如果认为细胞内阻抗主要集中在缝隙连接处，那么会把 r_n 定义为两个邻近心肌细胞之间的连接阻抗，把 k 定义为心肌细胞的长径与宽径的几何比率。对于侧侧平行的心肌细胞，其侧面长度等于心肌细胞的长度，沿着心肌细胞的长径是 1 个心肌细胞和横向跨度方向的 k 心肌细胞。在纵向方向上，k 心肌细胞是平行的，所以纵向阻抗是 r_n/k。沿着横向跨度，有一系列 k 心肌细胞。因此横向跨度阻抗是 kr_n。因此，横跨方向阻抗的各向异性比率减去纵向方向阻抗的各向异性比率等于 k^2，而且横跨方向的阻抗比纵向方向的阻抗大得多[25]。但是，细胞外阻抗比细胞内阻抗低得多。除了细胞形成闰盘外，心肌细胞占据的空间更大，接触的细胞外间隙等于或大于 $1\mu m$。此外，细胞外间隙的电流比细胞内腔小得多。

对心外膜通过真正电极的强刺激能引起折返激动。由于细胞内和细胞外组织阻抗各向异性的比率不同，定点刺激电流能产生细胞内和细胞外间隙不同的各向异性电位反应。跨膜电位在细胞内电位和细胞外电位之间不同，可能在邻近区发生除极和过度极化[54]。细胞外给予强的阴极刺激能够产生早期激动的犬骨形区（dog bone-shaped region），该区定位于刺激部位两侧的肌纤维，也能暂时形成两个超极化区，其离肌纤维轴的刺激部位约几毫米。有效的电极刺激能引起单向传导阻滞和折返激动。有效的阳极刺激能够延迟，甚至短暂阻滞从刺激部位的外向传导，而波锋是从有效阴极部位进行扩布，当波锋到达足够晚时，该波锋能激动同一区域。实验研究也证实了这种有效的电极现象[26,54]。

5. 单向阻滞和各向异性

实验观察 动作电位的传导速度和形态在心室肌呈各向异性。虽然动作电位的波锋在各个细胞间明显不同，但在组织水平存在明显的方向差异[27]。与从直角向心肌纤维的传导相比，沿肌纤维长轴的传导速度较快，而且在期前刺激时更易被阻滞，细胞外动作电位的幅度更大，细胞内的动作电位的除极最大速率（V_{max}）降低，上升支的脚时间常数（T_{foot}）较大，波锋振幅（Vi^{peak}）降低[27,28]。传导的各向异性能引起单向传导阻滞及诱发折返激动。Spach 及同事[27,28]对犬心肌的研究发现，期前激动不能沿肌纤维的长轴传导，而完全能横跨肌纤维传导，再进入纵向传导部位。动作电位和传导阻滞的各向异性与经典的一维光缆理论（one-dimensional cable theory）的预测值相反，该理论是 1855 年 Lord Kelvin 为跨大西洋光缆而提出的概念，并已经广泛应用于许多传导现象，包括物理学、工程学和生物学。该一维光缆理论认为，动作电位的波形和传导阻滞与轴阻抗无关，而且传导速度 θ 增加，由离子流增加引起，引起动作电位的 V_{max} 增大、T_{foot} 减小和 Vi^{peak} 增大，其结论与以前讨论的实验结果相矛盾[25,27,29]。

拟一维光缆理论（quasi-one-dimensional theory）**和实验研究** 最近提出的拟一维光缆理论用于可兴奋基质在紊乱情况下的传导扩布解释[25,29]，并能提供所观察的动作电位各向异性的理论基础，还能解决在经典的一维光缆理论和实验观察结果之间存在的矛盾。拟一维光缆理论包括细胞外间隙的激动电流影响的简要论述和心肌表面与深层之间的阻抗耦联。拟一维光缆理论的公式：

$$\frac{a}{2(R_i+\gamma R_e)\theta_x^2}\frac{d^2V_m(x,t)}{dt^2}=C_{app}\frac{dV_m(x,t)}{dt}+I_{app}(x,t)$$

也同样称为一维光缆理论。因此，在一维光缆理论中，膜容积和离子流可用表观膜容积（apparent membrane capacitance）替代，$C_{app}=C_m+C_{vir}$，以及表观膜离子流（apparent membrane ionic current），是有效膜容积和有效膜离子流，

$$I_{app}(x,t)=I_{ion}(x,t)+I_{vir}(x,t)$$ 这里 $C_{vir}=\frac{1}{\pi R_i^z\theta_z}$

$$I_{vir}(x,t)=-\frac{\gamma R_e}{R_d(R_i+\gamma R_e)}V_e(x,t)+\frac{1}{\pi R_i^z\theta_z}\frac{dV_e(x,t)}{dt}$$

代表心肌纤维表面和深层之间的耦联电流效应，以及离开组织表面进入液体容器颈部（bulk of the bath）的细胞外电流。a 代表心肌纤维的半径（cm）；R_i 和 R_e 各自代表心肌纤维的细胞内和细胞外轴阻抗（kΩcm）；γ 代表从细胞内到细胞外的等价横切面面积的比值；$V_m(\chi, t)$ 和 (x, t) 代表细胞膜表面的跨膜电位和细胞外电位（mV），其中 x 代表心肌纤维长轴上的位点，t 代表时间（ms）；z 与心肌纤维表面呈垂直方向；C_m 代表每单位面积细胞膜的特定膜容积（$\mu F/cm^2$）；$I_{ion}(x, t)$ 表示跨膜离子流的密度（$\mu A/cm^2$）；θ_χ 和 θ_z 代表稳定的 $V_m(x, t)$ 沿 x 轴和 z 轴扩布的速度（cm/ms）。R_i^z 表示沿 z 轴的细胞内耦联电阻（kΩcm），R_d 代表膜表面沿 z 轴的细胞外电流成分的等价深度阻抗（kΩcm²）。依据经典的一维理论，拟一维理论揭示了动作电位波形的各向异性，其原因是有效膜离子流和有效膜容积的改变。该理论也表明，电激动是在纵向传导而不是在横向传导，其可用经典的一维电缆理论解释。最近，该理论还表明，间质毛细血管也是有效容积成分，能使局部环路改变 C_{app}，并影响 T_{foot}[30]。因此，心肌纤维的表面和深层之间及心肌纤维和毛细血管之间的耦联引起心肌动作电位的波形存在着各向异性。

拟一维理论已得到进一步发展，并在乌贼的巨大神经轴突和刺激模型得到证实（图 42-1）[29]。拟一维光缆理论预言，就像实验研究证实的那样，细胞内和细胞外动作电位的形态与细胞外间隙的阻抗有关。在不同阻抗的细胞外间隙中的巨大轴突的细胞内动作电位和细胞外动作电位形态间的相关性与心肌动作电位的各向异性相似。由于乌贼轴突的动作电位波形发生改变，无论是三维结构还是非连续性，两者常常都与心肌的各向异性传导无关，这是动作电位波形发生改变必需的条件。虽然两者都不需要，但三维结构和非连续性实际上都与心肌各向异性的传导扩布有关[30]。

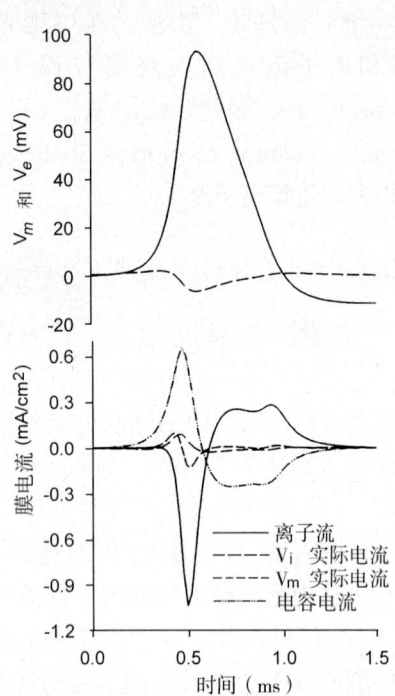

图 42-1 膜离子流、有效膜电流 V_i 和 V_m（下图）和 V_m 和 V_e 的优化时间（上图） 乌贼的巨大神经轴突在液体容器中的阻抗 653Ω（引自 Wu J, Wikswo JP Jr. Effects of bath resistance on action potentials in the squid giant axon: myocardial implication. Biophys J, 1997; 73: 2347-2358）

6. 单向阻滞和组织的几何形态、非连续性及电荷

心室肌由各个细胞的耦联束（直径<500μm）构成。在这些耦联束内，各个细胞相互之间在某种程度上存在电的连接，以致该束能作为单条纤维发挥效应[31]。相反，这种耦联束在侧方方向相互间的连接不十分广泛，从而使肌束表面的横向扩布到肌束长轴的过程被中断。心室肌的非连续性能引起单向传导阻滞[32]。与年轻人心脏的心肌相比，老龄和病人心脏的心肌细胞间的连接相对好，形成大量的连接组织，而使心肌纤维的横向连接呈明显的非连续性。心肌组织的非连续性和各向异性能引起电源与电荷之间的电阻不匹配，进而引起传导速度、动作电位参数的改变和单向阻滞。通过从主要分支束电荷引导的除极电流，心肌的分支束能使传导减慢，并能通过再注入主要分支束的电流引起分支束的除极，并增加传导的安全性[33,34]。

由心肌的非连续性产生的复杂扩布形式与心肌的各向异性传导有关[27]。细胞的非连续性可引起各个细胞的电荷明显不同，导致不同细胞的 V_{max} 和 T_{foot} 的差异，但统计学上观察到动作电位和传导的各向异性仍然存在[27,30]。此外，还能证实阻抗的非连续性能产生相反的动作电位 T_{foot} 的变化（例如 T_{foot} 越小，传导速度越快），虽然传导速度和 V_{max} 间的关系雷同于实验观察结果[27,25,35]。这种争议能用拟一维理论（quasi-1D theory）来解释，通过引入真正的膜容积分析解释 T_{foot} 的各向异性，该膜容积来自肌纤维表面和深层之间、心肌细胞和毛细血管之间的耦联关系，还可能来自细胞外电流的空间分布变量。

当非连续性类似或大于膜空间常数时，则空间非连续性对传导的影响显得十分显著。膜空间常数是一个概念，来自于呈被动性膜的一维光缆理论，表示跨越该膜区的电位距离，蜕变为源电位的1/e。然而，心室肌细胞膜具有可激动的离子通道。因此，为可激动膜新提出的空间变量概念对心室肌的传导更适合[35]。随着膜激动时 Na^+ 通道的开放，膜的传导性 G_m (x, t) 增加，而 λ_{active} (x, t) 减小（图 42-2）。

$$\lambda_{active}(x,t) = \sqrt{\frac{\alpha}{2G_m(x,t)R_{axial}}}$$

R_{axial} 代表轴阻抗。当膜的传导达峰时，空间变量 λ_{active} (x, t) 最小。应用 Luo-Rudy 膜离子流[36]和实验室测定的组织阻抗[37]指标，完全兴奋的 Na^+ 电流可使静息膜电位的相应空间常数 428.6μm 和 158.4μm，沿着或横跨心室肌纤维传导的 λ_{active} (x, t) 降低为 88.8μm 和 32.8μm。因此，组织的非连续性能诱发出明显的非连续性行为，其来自连续性理论的预测值。动作电位形态和传导性的各向异性是由组织的非连续性引起的，能促使折返的形成。

（二）激动时充分的折返延迟

折返形成的第二个条件是，折返环路的周长值超过折返通路各组织的最长不应期。折返波的延迟与折返通路的长度成正比，而与传导速度成反比。折返通路中各组织的最长不应期能为折返的形成提供最小的折返的延迟时间。

折返只能够在一块大于"临界体积"的心室肌内发生，而"临界体积"是指能容纳最小折返环所需的周长延迟时间，其等于该折返环心肌组织的最长不应期。"临界体积"的大小取决于折返通路的传导速度和最长不应期。这在原位局部心室肌用高钾除极过程能得到证实，当可兴奋组织减少到维持颤动的临界体积以下时，心室颤动就能终止[22,38]。许多生理的、病理的、药理的因素能够改变传导速度和心肌不应期，从而影响临界体积的大小。在鼠的心脏动作电位时程

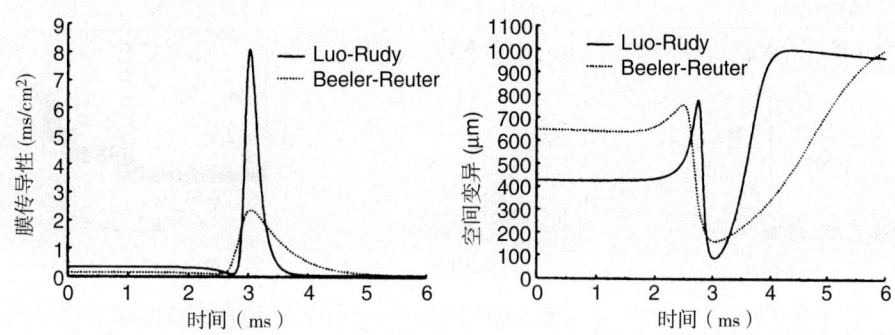

图42-2 同时有Luo-Rudy和Beeler-Reuter描述的膜离子流模型中动作电位除极过程中膜传导性（左图）和空间变异（右图）
（引自Wu J. Zipes DP. Effects of spayial segmentation in the continuous model of excitation propagation in cardiac muscle. J Cardiac Electrophysiol, 1999; 10: 965-972.）

较短，在小于$100mm^2$的面积内能发生心室颤动[2,55]。当缝隙连接失耦联而使传导速度足够慢时，折返甚至可在极小区域（$<1mm^2$）的心肌内发生[39]。

心肌缺血也能改变心室肌的传导速度和不应期。在冠状动脉闭塞后的最初2min内传导速度增加，然后降低，因为随着细胞外K^+和缝隙连接失耦联的增加使传导速度先增加后降低[13]。缺血使传导速度减慢时能促进形成跨室壁的折返[40,41]。

（三）急性全心缺血时的跨壁折返

急性心肌缺血是室性心律失常的主要原因之一。绝大多数心肌缺血引起的室性心律失常发生在心肌缺血的最初10~15min内，是因局灶性激动和跨壁折返引起[13,40-42]。在健康与缺血区之间，冠脉血流的差异及细胞对缺血反应的各向异性能引起室性心动过速。缺血区边缘的局灶性激动的发生机制已在本章前文讨论过。本部分主要讨论心肌组织对急性全心缺血反应的各向异性引起的室性心动过速的发生机制。

急性心肌缺血时，跨壁膜的动作电位和离子流的各向异性能引起透壁传导速度的不对称。急性全心缺血能抑制兴奋性和传导速度，其传导速度在心外膜比心内膜快，从而增加心肌组织的兴奋性和不应期的跨壁离散度[13]。在急性心肌缺血时，传导速度缓慢和单向传导阻滞两者都参与折返形成。急性心肌缺血和再灌注能迅速改变组织的兴奋性和传导速度的跨壁离散度并产生动态基质，使折返能够发生和维持，然后消失。

1. 急性全心缺血和再灌注时由心内膜起搏产生折返

Wu和Zipes[40]先诱导全心缺血25min，然后给予心肌再灌注，并从犬左室游离壁分离的36个动脉灌注的楔形组织块的不同跨壁层面记录电活动。他们记录了心肌缺血时由心内膜起搏引发的跨壁折返（图42-3）。缺血570±165s或更长时间（34个楔形组织块）能引起1:1、2:1和4:1组织区对心内膜起搏的反应（周长为300ms），其顺序一般是从心内膜到心外膜。心内膜起搏不能呈1:1直接下传到心外膜和室壁中层的特定区域，因为这些区域的不应期比起搏周长长，引起2:1或4:1的反应，或两者都可以，但若能以1:1比例下传到某些区域，则表明该区的不应期较短。单向传导阻滞发生在不同比例反应区之间的交界处。当局部不应期结束后，从心外膜侧进入2:1和4:1区，然后再从心外膜侧跨壁传导经过2:1或4:1区，或两者，再次进入心内膜下，在该处形成激动并形成折返。跨壁折返发生在心肌缺血的535±146s后（31个楔形组织块）。在心肌缺血的747±312s后（10个楔形组织块），缺血减慢传导能提供折返波锋所必需的折返环延迟时间，并允许恢复心内膜的可兴奋性，引起持续性折返。进一步缺血发生时能引起进行性心外膜电失活而抑制折返（24个楔形组织块）。在再灌注的最初几分钟内，组织的兴奋性和不应期的恢复不一致，心内膜下比心外膜下恢复得更快。心外膜下心肌和室壁中层心肌（在缺血25min后不能激动）进一步再激动，形成4:1和2:1传导，然后呈1:1传导或产生快速性折返激动。持续性折返和颤动与起搏刺激反应的空间离散度有关，出现在再灌注的93±49s后（8个再灌注楔形组织块中有2个）。

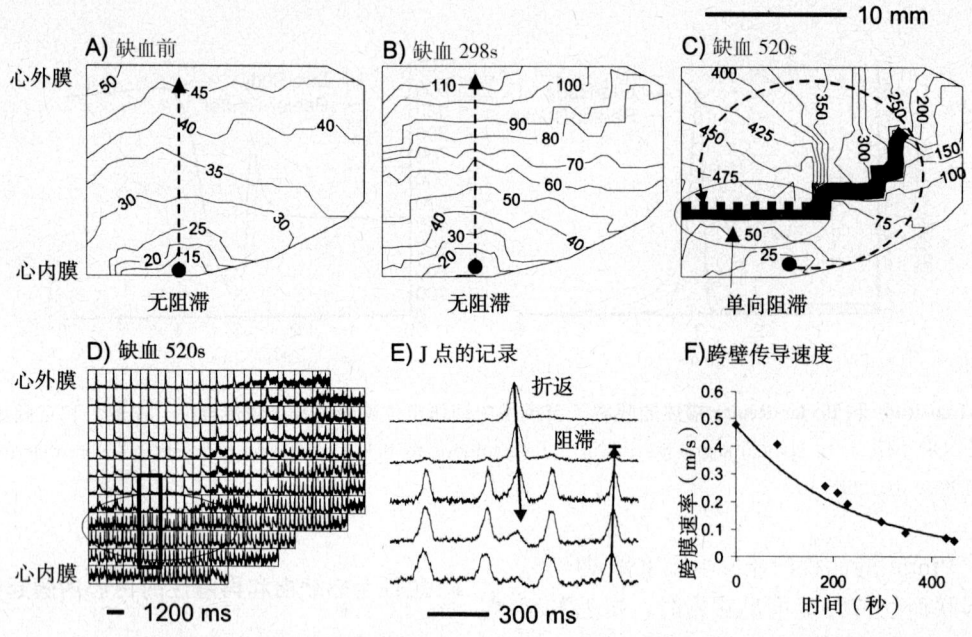

图 42-3 急性全心缺血时不应期的跨壁梯度引起心内激动的单向阻滞　在楔形离体犬左室游离壁的跨壁切面上记录的激动。急性全心缺血是由停止冠脉灌注产生的。缺血的时间由小标题标出。传导顺序（A-C）是从起搏的心内膜开始记录（点标，周长为300ms），显示在等时线上（时间点用 ms 显示），沿着细点箭头线方向移动。而在 C 图显示，粗实线、一侧点线分别表示传导的完全阻滞和单向阻滞。动作电位镶嵌栅栏隔离邻近的感受器信号。跨壁的传导速度（F）可以从两个记录位点计算，沿着跨壁线的这两个记录点的距离为11mm，通过了起搏位点。从心内膜的起搏位点跨壁传导，其周长为300mm。通过较长的不应期，在中层心肌（C-E）的传导被阻滞。因此，激动沿相反方向（指向心内膜）传导，穿透中层心肌（C-E）引起 C-E 单向阻滞，直到与另一个激动的心内膜被持续性心内膜起搏引起的有效不应期相撞（引自 Wu J, Zipes DP. Transmural reentry during global acute ischemia and reperfusion in canine ventricular muscle. Am J，Physiol Heart Circ physiol, 2001；280：H2717-H2725.）

因此，急性全心缺血和再灌注能提供折返产生的条件：单向传导阻滞，其由缺血增加不应期的跨壁差异和传导延迟引起。缺血和再灌注提供的条件是暂时的，当进一步缺血使组织不能兴奋或进一步再灌注使组织的各向异性减小时，折返则会终止。

2. 心外膜起搏诱发的折返

除了不应期跨壁梯度外，急性全心缺血还能增加组织兴奋性的跨壁梯度。Wu 和 Zipes[41] 标测了全心缺血时的跨壁传导特性，标测时，起搏位置在心外膜和心内膜之间变换，其标本来自分离的犬左室壁的 22 个再灌注楔形组织块。急性缺血能增加跨壁离散度，其中对心外膜比心内膜能更明显地抑制兴奋性和传导性。当缺血抑制了心外膜的传导并使兴奋性降低时，心内膜下仍有足够的兴奋性支持传导。在心肌缺血 $719\pm399s$ 后，18 个楔形组织块中 9 个通过心外膜刺激能诱发折返，其激动能够跨壁穿透心室壁（从心外膜起搏位点传到心内膜），但不能沿着心外膜表面向侧面传导，从而产生单向传导阻滞。穿透的激动然后沿心外膜和室壁中层心肌向侧面传导，再进入心外膜而完成折返。在上述心外膜诱发的折返前后，即刻给予心内膜刺激能产生激动，并能沿着心内膜快速传导，然后跨壁传向心外膜，但在 9 个楔形组织块并没有形成折返。因此得出结论，缺血引起的跨壁兴奋性梯度能提供心外膜刺激的折返基质（图 42-4）。

（四）螺旋波折返和三维转子

室性心动过速和心室颤动可由多个快速旋转的三维转子在心室壁内游走而产生。三维转子能在心外膜下形成多种形式的波锋（例如螺旋波折返、局灶性激动和急速移动的波锋），这些波锋取决于暴露在心外膜面的转子核心的形状和转子切面。肌纤维的壁内转子和室壁边缘可以扭转并使转子核心不稳定，引起转子核心的漂移、碎裂及增殖[22,43,44]。在心室心外膜下心肌薄层切片及在局限性面积的各向同性基质内的刺激下，螺旋波变得稳定并维持。螺旋波漂移并最后终

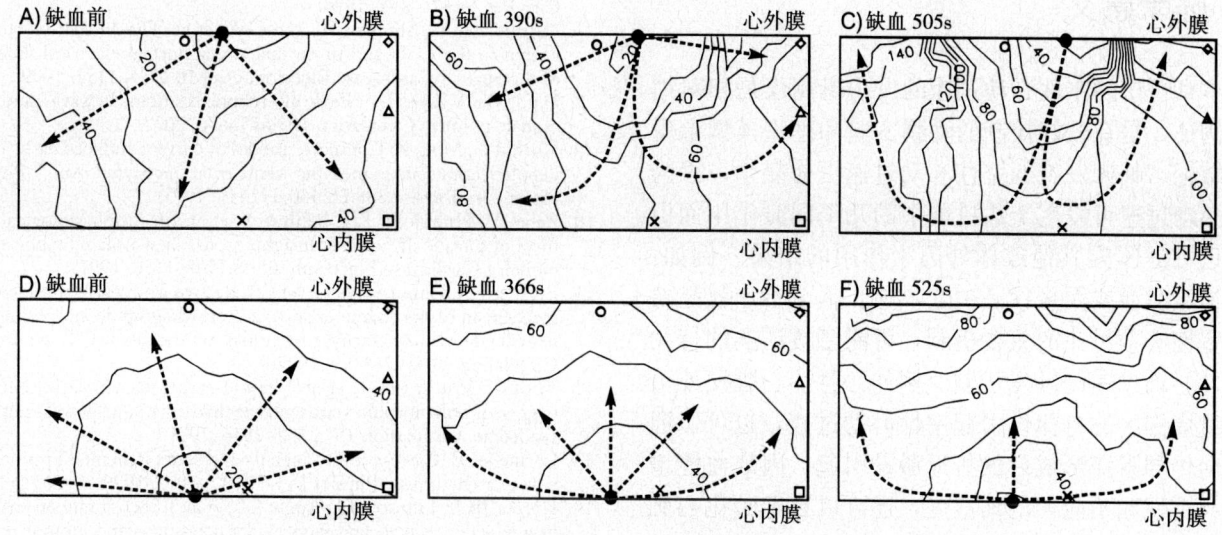

图 42-4 急性全心缺血时起源于心外膜的激动发生单向传导阻滞和跨壁的非对称性传导 离体的楔形心室肌块与图 42-3 相似。在心内膜和心外膜之间不同位点刺激楔形心室肌块,图中用点线显示。缺血能抑制组织的兴奋性,对心外膜的抑制作用比心内膜要快。在缺血 505s 时 (C),心外膜起源的激动跨壁穿透心室壁,但不能沿着心外膜向两侧传导,然后在心内膜和室壁中层向两侧传导,最后再进入心外膜。当缺血 525s 时 (F),心内膜刺激产生的激动能迅速沿心内膜扩布,然后跨壁激动心外膜而未再激动心内膜。因此,缺血诱导的跨壁兴奋梯度提供了心外膜刺激时的折返基质。记录区域跨壁深度为 10mm,而在心外膜范围是 18mm。(引自 Wu J, Zipes DP. Transmural reentry triggered by epicardial stimulation during acute ischemia in canine ventricular muscle. Am J HEART Circ Physiol,2002;H2004-H2011epicardial)

止在有兴奋梯度的基质内[22]。而且螺旋波能够锚定组织内各向异性的小面积区域并变得稳定。除此,在心室的不可激动边缘,螺旋波和三维转子能够由局灶性激动和单向传导阻滞或碎裂波而诱发。

(五) 8字形折返

"8字形折返"是指两个几乎对称的折返环在相反方向旋转,并共享环的共同通道。8字形折返可由不同的实验方案形成,例如,在极短时间内,对两个不同位点给予两个刺激时,其激动传导由期前刺激(S_2)诱发。当在不应期梯度的中心用 S_2 刺激时,而且此前已在不同位点给予了 S_1 刺激,则可引起单向阻滞[45]。S_2 刺激可引起局部不应期的延长,并在 S_1 和 S_2 刺激位点之间产生激动,因该阻滞已脱离不应期。S_2 刺激引起的激动从较早的位点(S_1 和 S_2 刺激位点之间)沿着围绕 S_2 位点(局部不应期延长)的两条通路扩布,传向 S_2 位点的相反方向,并折返回到 S_2 位点(该点局部已脱离不应期),形成8字形折返。

"8字形折返"也能见于梗死4天的犬心肌梗死的心外膜下愈合心肌的边缘区[46]。该心外膜下的边缘区,心肌梗死能引起明显的各向异性,存在明显的缝隙连接不连续性和分布的改变,并在存活心肌纤维之间形成较多扭曲的结缔组织。给予刺激产生的激动传导能遇到功能性传导阻滞区,有明显的缝隙连接中断和肌纤维间的侧侧分离,而纵向传导没有障碍。两个平行侧向功能传导的阻滞能形成8字折返型室性心动过速折返环的中心共同通路。短耦联间期的强电击也能诱发出8字形折返[47]。

(六) 围绕M细胞的折返激动

Mines[56]最早将解剖学折返定义为围绕不可兴奋的解剖结构的折返激动。最近研究证实,解剖学上的折返路径也能因功能性传导阻滞引起,该阻滞由心室中层心肌细胞不应期较长所致。而最长的动作电位时程在解剖学上位于中层心肌[7]。M细胞的动作电位时程在慢频率激动和药物诱发的 LQTS 模型上明显延长[21,24]。在离体的 D-索他洛尔诱发的 LQT2 心室肌组织,中层心肌细胞的动作电位时程较长,能产生传导阻滞区,导致室壁中层 M 细胞区的折返[48]。这种情况下,尽管折返路径是由 M 细胞的解剖部位决定的,但所有 M 细胞是可兴奋的,传导阻滞属于功能性的。

三、临床意义

本章讨论的室性心动过速的发生机制仅是相对简单的例证，是在较好控制的动物实验和理论模型上得到的结论。临床发生的室性心动过速更为复杂，因为室性心动过速可发生上述机制中的几个同时作用而引起，也可是体内其他或体外因素作用的结果。例如，自主神经激活或大量饮酒引起室速。临床治疗就是要抑制室性心动过速的主要机制，可能已被证实的持续性室性心动过速的继发机制。例如，急性心肌梗死可以通过周围区的自律性引起室性心动过速，也可以通过单向传导阻滞形成后的折返激动引起，因缺血能增加可兴奋性和不应期的离散度，还可以是老龄化心脏的各向异性和心室肌内广泛分布的连接组织的非连续传导引起。折返形成也有不同机制，其治疗策略也有区别。药物治疗和射频消融都能对室性心动过速的不同发生机制产生抑制或促进作用。例如，通过减少Na^+电流抑制组织的兴奋性而降低局灶性激动的发生，而传导速度的减慢能促进折返。射频消融能消融局灶位点和打断解剖学折返环路。但是，射频消融也能为新的折返提供不可兴奋性的核心区域。因此，证实室性心动过速的发生机制、选择适当的治疗和监测治疗反应是室性心动过速患者治疗的关键环节，这对完整心脏来说十分复杂和有一定难度。

四、致　谢

本文得到美国心脏病协会中西部分会（0256112Z）和酒精饮料医学研究基金及 Herman C. Krannert 基金、Indianapolis 和 IN 的资助。

（刘元生　译）

参 考 文 献

1. Volders PG, Vos MA, Szabo B, et al: Progress in the understanding of cardiac early afterdepolarizations and torsades de pointes: Time to revise current concepts. Cardiovasc Res 46:376–392, 2000.
2. Roden DM: Acquired long QT syndromes and the risk of proarrhythmia. J Cardiovasc Electrophysiol 11:938–940, 2000.
3. Wehrens XHT, Vos MA, Doevendans PA, Wellens HJJ: Novel insights in the congenital long QT syndrome. Ann Intern Med 137:981–992, 2002.
4. Yan GX, Antzelevitch C: Cellular basis for the normal T wave and the electrocardiographic manifestations of the Long-QT syndrome. Circulation 98:1928–1936, 1998.
5. Bouchard RA, Clark RB, Giles WR: Effects of action potential duration on excitation-contraction coupling in rat ventricular myocytes. Circ Res 76:790–801, 1995.
6. El-Sherif N, Caref EB, Yin H, Restivo M: The electrophysiological mechanism of ventricular arrhythmias in the long QT syndrome. Circ Res 69:474–492, 1996.
7. Antzelevitch C, Shimizu W, Yan G-X, et al: The M cell: Its contribution to the ECG and to normal and abnormal electrical function of the heart. J Cardiovasc Electrophysiol 10:1124–1152, 1999.
8. Wu J, Wu J, Zipes DP: Early afterdepolarizations, U waves, and torsade de pointes. Circulation 105:675–676, 2002.
9. Nordin C, Ming Z: Computer model of current-induced early afterdepolarizations in guinea pig ventricular myocytes. Am J Physiol Heart Circ Physiol 268:H2440–H2459, 1995.
10. Zabel M, Hohnloser SH, Behrens S, et al: Electrophysiological features of torsade de pointes: Insights from a new isolated rabbit heart model. J Cardiovasc Electrophysiol 8:1148–1158, 1997.
11. El-Sherif N, Chinushi M, Caref EB, Restivo M: Electrophysiological mechanism of the characteristic electrocardiographic morphology of torsade de pointes tachyarrhythmias in the long QT syndrome. Circulation 96:4392–4399, 1997.
12. Yan GX, Wu Y, Liu T, et al: Phase 2 early afterdepolarization as a trigger of polymorphic ventricular tachycardia in acquired long-QT syndrome. Circulation 103:2851–2856, 2001.
13. Carmeliet E: Cardiac ionic currents and acute ischemia: From channels to arrhythmias. Physiol Rev 79:917–1017, 1999.
14. Harper JR Jr, Johnson TA, Engle CL, et al: Effect of rate on changes in conduction velocity and extracellular potassium concentration during acute ischemia in the in situ pig heart. J Cardiovasc Electrophysiol 4:661–671, 1993.
15. Coronel RD, Wilms-Schopman FJG, Dekker LRC, Janse MJ: Heterogeneities in $[K^+]_o$ and TQ potential and the inducibility of ventricular fibrillation during acute regional ischemia in the isolated perfused porcine heart. Circulation 92:120–129, 1995.
16. Pogwizd SM, Corr PB: Reentrant and nonreentrant mechanisms contribute to arrhythmogenesis during early myocardial ischemia: Results using three-dimensional mapping. Circ Res 61:352–371, 1987.
17. Antzelevitch C: Basic mechanisms of reentrant arrhythmias. Curr Opin Cardiol 16:1–7, 2001.
18. Antzelevitch C, Fish J: Electrical heterogeneity within the ventricular wall. Basic Res Cardiol 96:517–527, 2001.
19. Zygmunt AC, Goodrow RJ, Antzelevitch C: I_{NaCa} contributes to electrical heterogeneity within the canine ventricle. Am J Physiol Heart Circ Physiol 278:H1671–H1678, 2000.
20. Robert E, Aya AGM, de la Coussaye JE, et al: Dispersion-based reentry: Mechanism of initiation of ventricular tachycardia in isolated rabbit hearts. Am J Physiol Heart Circ Physiol 276:H413–H423, 1999.
21. Shimizu W, Antzelevitch C: Sodium channel block with mexiletine is effective in reducing dispersion of repolarization and preventing torsade de points in LQT2 and LQT3 models of the long-QT syndrome. Circulation 96:2038–2047, 1997.
22. Jalife J: Ventricular fibrillation: Mechanisms of initiation and maintenance. Annu Rev Physiol 62:25–50, 2000.
23. Chinushi M, Restivo M, Caref EB, El-Sherif N: Electrophysiological basis of arrhythmogenicity of QT/T alternans in the long-QT syndrome. Circ Res 83:614–628, 1998.
24. Shimizu W, Antzelevitch C: Cellular and ionic basis for T-wave alternans under long-QT conditions. Circulation 99:1499–1507, 1999.
25. Wu J, Johnson EA, Kootsey JM: A quasi-one-dimensional theory for anisotropic propagation of excitation in cardiac muscle. Biophys J 71:2427–2439, 1996.
26. Wu J, Roden DM, Wikswo JP Jr: Delayed activation and retrograde propagation in cardiac muscle due to virtual electrode effects. Ann Biomed Eng 28:1318–1326, 2000.
27. Spach MS. Heidlage JF: The stochastic nature of cardiac propagation at a microscopic level. Electrical description of myocardial architecture and its application to conduction. Circ Res 76:366–380, 1995.
28. Spach MS: Anisotropy of cardiac tissue: A major determinant of conduction? J Cardiovasc Electrophysiol 10:887–890, 1999.
29. Wu J, Wikswo JP Jr: Effects of bath resistance on action potentials in the squid giant axon: Myocardial implications. Biophys J 73:2347–2358, 1997.
30. Spach MS, Heidlage JF, Dolber PC, Barr RC: Extracellular discontinuities in cardiac muscle: Evidence for capillary effects on the action potential foot. Circ Res 83:1144–1164, 1998.
31. Peters NS, Wit AL: Myocardial architecture and ventricular arrhythmogenesis. Circulation 97:1746–1754, 1998.

32. Spach MS, Boineau JP: Microfibrosis produces electrical load variations due to loss of side-to-side cell connections: A major mechanism of structural heart disease arrhythmias. Pacing Clin Electrophysiol 20:397–413, 1997.
33. Kucera JP, Kleber AG, Rohr S: Slow conduction in cardiac muscle, II: Effects of branching tissue geometry. Circ Res 83:795–805, 1998.
34. Kucera JP, Rudy Y: Mechanistic insights into very slow conduction in branching cardiac muscle. A model study. Circ Res 89:799–806, 2001.
35. Wu J, Zipes DP: Effects of spatial segmentation in the continuous model of excitation propagation in cardiac muscle. J Cardiovasc Electrophysiol 10:965–972, 1999.
36. Hund TJ, Kucera JP, Otani NF, Rudy Y: Ionic charge conservation and long-term steady state in the Luo-Rudy dynamic cell model. Biophys J 81:3324–3331, 2001.
37. Clerc L: Directional differences of impulse spread in trabecular muscle from mammalian heart. J Physiol (Lond) 255:335–346, 1976.
38. Kim Y-H, Garfinkel A, Ikeda T, et al: Spatiotemporal complexity of ventricular fibrillation revealed by tissue mass reduction in isolated swine right ventricle: Further evidence for the quasiperiodic route to chaos hypothesis. J Clin Invest 100:2486–2500, 1997.
39. Rohr S, Kucera JP, Kleber AG: Slow conduction in cardiac muscle, I: Effects of a reduction of excitability versus a reduction of electrical coupling on microconduction. Circ Res 83:781–794, 1998.
40. Wu J, Zipes DP: Transmural reentry during global acute ischemia and reperfusion in canine ventricular muscle. Am J Physiol Heart Circ Physiol 280:H2717–H2725, 2001.
41. Wu J, Zipes DP: Transmural reentry triggered by epicardial stimulation during acute ischemia in canine ventricular muscle. Am J Physiol Heart Circ Physiol 283:H2004–H2011, 2002.
42. Valderrábano M, Lee M-H, Ohara T, et al: Dynamics of intramural and transmural reentry during ventricular fibrillation in isolated swine ventricles. Circ Res 88:839–848, 2001.
43. Gray RA, Jalife J, Panfilov AV, et al: Mechanisms of cardiac fibrillation. Science 270:1222–1223, 1995.
44. Gray RA, Pertsov AM, Jalife J: Spatial and temporal organization during cardiac fibrillation. Nature 392:75–78, 1998.
45. Chen P-S, Wolf PD, Dixon EG, et al: Mechanism of ventricular vulnerability to single premature stimuli in open-chest dogs. Circ Res 62:1191–1209, 1988.
46. Peters NS, Coromilas J, Nicholas JS, Wit AL: Disturbed connexin43 gap junction distribution correlates with the location of reentrant circuits in the epicardial border zone of healing canine infarcts that cause ventricular tachycardia. Circulation 95:988–996, 1997.
47. Banville I, Gray RA, Ideker RE, Smith WM: Shock-induced figure-of-eight reentry in the isolated rabbit heart. Circ Res 85:742–752, 1999.
48. Akar FG, Yan G-X, Antzelevitch C, Rosenbaum DS: Unique topographical distribution of M cells underlies reentrant mechanism of torsade de pointes in the long-QT syndrome. Circulation 105:1247–1253, 2002.
49. Shaw RM, Rudy Y: The vulnerable window for unindirectional block in cardiac tissue: characterization and dependence on membrane excitability and intercellular coupling. J Cardiovasc Electrophysiol 6:115–131, 1995.
50. Sutton PM, Taggart P, Opthof T, et al: Repolarisation and refractoriness during early ischaemia in humans. Heart 84:365–369, 2000.
51. Muller-Borer BJ, Johnson TA, Gettes LS, Cascio WE: Failure of impulse propagation in a mathematically simulated ischemic border zone: influence of direction of propagation and cell-to-cell electrical coupling. J Cardiovasc Electrophysiol 6:1101–1112, 1995.
52. Picard S, Rouet R, Ducouret P, et al: K_{ATP} channel and 'border zone' arrhythmias: role of the repolarization dispersion between normal and ischaemic ventricular regions. Brit J Pharmacol 127:1687–1695, 1999.
53. Pastore JM, Rosenbaum DS: Role of structural barrierss in the mechanism of alternans-induced reentry. Circ Res 87:1157–1163, 2000.
54. Wikswo JP Jr, Lin SF, Abbas RA: Virtual electrodes in cardiac tissue: a common mechanism for anodal and cathodal stimulation. Biophys J 69:2195–2210, 1995.
55. Vaidya D, Morley GE, Samie FH, Jalife J: Reentry and fibrillation in the mouse heart: a challenge to the critical mass hypothesis. Circ Res 85:174–181, 1999.
56. Mines GR: On dynamic equilibrium in the heart. J Physiol (Lond) 43:349–383, 1913.

第 43 章

正常心脏心室颤动的动力学与分子机制

José Jalife

本章目录

- 目前的证据 ………………………………… 386
- 颤动有序 …………………………………… 387
- 稳定转子与心室颤动 ……………………… 387
- 核心对动作电位时程与转动频率的影响 ………………………………………… 387
- I_{K1} 对心室颤动动力学的作用 …………… 388
- 野生 I_{K1} 中通道蛋白 Kir2.1 的作用 ……… 388
- 左心室与右心室的背景电流 ……………… 388
- 稳态心室颤动的离子机制 ………………… 389
- 通道蛋白的 Kir 家族 ……………………… 389
- 内向整流与 Kir2.x 通道 …………………… 390
- 为什么是 Kir2.x 通道在起作用 …………… 391
- 其他内向整流通道的作用 ………………… 391
- 心室颤动时其他离子通道的作用 ………… 392
- 如何应用这些新信息 ……………………… 392

人类认识心脏颤动可致死亡已有数千年。但发现生物电并由此揭示心房和心室颤动的机理尚不足 200 年。穿越 20 世纪，许多学者在器官、细胞水平做了大量研究，为理解其复杂的机制作出了贡献。21 世纪序幕初揭，用分子生物学技术研究细胞膜离子通道的结构、功能和调节的进步，以及能够直视心脏波二维和三维扩布的动力学，这些进展共同打开了这一领域的新视窗，以便用精确方式证实启动和维持心房与心室颤动的心肌分子结构。本章我们重点关注心室颤动（简称室颤）的维持机制。尤其要复习有关内向整流通道在室颤机制中可能作用的那些令人激动的研究结果。这些新知识可能是详细理解室颤分子学基础的起步，并有希望发展新的措施以便在高危患者中预防室颤。

一、目前的证据

室颤是无序的电冲动使心室快速、非同步和不协调的方式收缩。出现时很少或无血流经心脏泵出。除非立刻提供医疗救助，否则休克、昏迷和心脏性猝死将接踵而至。在工业化国家，室颤确实是心脏性猝死的即刻和主要原因，仅在美国每年约造成 30 万人的猝死[1-3]。心电图（ECG）室颤的特点是 QRS 波群存在着形态、幅度和频率不断变化的不规则波动，以至于心脏电生理学家将室颤定义为心脏紊乱的电活动[4]。人的室颤发生时，不规则心室波群超过 500 bpm 的频率。然而，心电图对理解颤动过于间接，需要知道心脏自身的电波发生了什么以及这些波传播的细胞和分子基质。

因此，心脏电生理研究的一个主要目标是用高分辨率的记录技术观察波的二维与三维移动，并确定其动力学特点。更进一步，目前为了详细和精确理解颤动中紊乱的电活动机理，需要有从分子到器官各层面混成广阔的视野。所以，本章有三个目的：第一、复习有关波传播动力和室颤维持的最有意义的文献；第二、讨论新近发表的数据，强烈支持下列假定，即心脏钾通道表达的腔室特异化差异可部分解释结构和电生理正常的心脏发生室颤的分子机制；第三、为进一步开展研究，进而在心脏性猝死的高危患者中更好地理解和更有效地预防室颤提供一些新思路。

二、颤动有序

室颤最早的定量描述，多发小波学说认为，颤动的心肌跟从随机变化的路径同时独立存在并形成多个小波[5]。然而，新近的理论和实验已证明在室颤特征性貌似复杂的活动背后，藏有显著的有序[6-10]。另外也提出了心脏兴奋的转子是室颤维持机制的内在有序中心。一种观点认为室颤紊乱的特性由不稳定的转子维持，不稳定性因素最终导致转子的破裂[11-15]。有观察认为（复原假说[16-18]），转子的破裂由动作电位时程（action potential duration，APD）足够振幅的振荡造成转子波锋传导阻滞引发[16,17]。基于主导频率相对集中的分布特点[19]，另一些学者认为室颤中存在相对稳定的高频率周期性起源[20]。按照这一理论，室颤是由这些相对稳定的起源的颤动样传导所致[20]。

三、稳定转子与心室颤动

最近，在 Langendorff 灌注的离体豚鼠心脏，我们发现的新证据强烈支持这样的学说，即在这一动物种群，室颤的机制是一个稳定的高频率折返源伴颤动样传导[20]。通过光学记录的心室外膜电势敏感性颜料荧光图与容积传导的整体心电图的同时记录，能对每一像素的光信号作频谱分析，每一像素的主导频率（dominant frequency，DF）绘成主导频率标测图（见 Samie 和其他作者[21]），进而揭示整个心室主导频率呈明显的局限分布（图 43-1），最快的主导频率总见于左室前壁。某些实验中，左室前壁清晰可见稳定的转子，转子的转动频率与主导频率标测图的最高主导频峰一致，证明转子是室颤活动的起源。另外，光学数据显示在高、低频率的交界区发生波破裂和间断的传导阻滞，表明由转子发散的波呈颤动样传导[20]。再者，某些实验用高分辨光学与微电极的同步记录，确认激动的高度可预测性。图 43-1 示例中，彩色主导频率图显示的最大主导频率（约 26 Hz）确实位于左室前壁的表面。在此区域的单一像素证实极短的动作电位以 26.1Hz 的频率出现。随后在右室选择性分析两个不同部位，证实频率约 15Hz。因此，上述结果表明在离体豚鼠心脏左室稳定的高频率折返源是维持室颤的机制。

四、核心对动作电位时程与转动频率的影响

室颤时，激动的频率明显快于起搏活动和快速起搏可达到的频率[22,23]。在我们的实验中，转子能达到的周长几乎等于 30～40 ms，明显短于豚鼠心脏的期望值，其动作电位时程在 1Hz 接近于 200ms[24]。新近，计算机模拟结果提示转子达到的极大速度来自于其核心对复极的极量影响，使动作电位时程极大缩短。这一作用能用 1950 年代 Weidmann 发现的"全或无"复极现象解释[25]。然而，正如图 43-2 所示，随着距核心的距离增大，这一效应将大大减弱，动作电位时程增长[26]。其后果为紧邻核心的组织达到非常快的周长，而远离核心的心肌在转子的速率下不能传导，形成非均匀性（非 1∶1）传导。根据这一理论，上述作用为豚鼠心室室颤时观察到的主导频率梯度提供了基础（图 43-1）。如同别的图示一样，紧邻转子的扩布传导通常为1∶1，而距转子一定距离时，产生了间断性传导阻滞和波的碎裂，形成缓慢的主导频率区域[20]。然而，虽然此机制阐明了动作电位时程缩短

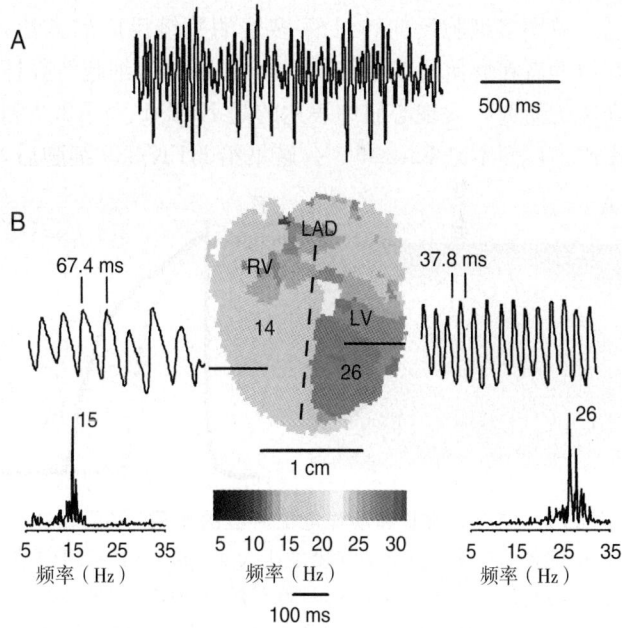

图 43-1 室颤主导频率的分析　A：心电图，B：主导频率标测图与左（右侧）、右（左侧）心室的单一像素记录和相应的功率谱（曲线的下面）。LAD，左前降支（引自 Samie FH, Berenfeld O, Anumonwo J, et al：Rectification of the background potassium current：A determinant of rotor dynamics in ventricular fibrillation. Circ Res 89：1216-1223，2001.）（见彩图 18）

和主导频率区域的形成，但不能解释最快的主导频率区域为何总位于左室前壁。

五、I_{K1}对心室颤动动力学的作用

内向整流电流[27]在心肌细胞的动作电位复极末期和静息电位中起重要的基础作用[28]。在反转电位正侧的外向电流减低，由镁（Mg^{2+}）[29,30]和多肽阻滞钾（K^+）选择性通道介导[31-33]。我们的实验结果表明背景电流的电流密度-电压关系中，外向成分在左室明显大于右室[20]。将实验数据合成实时的离子流模型时，我们观察到模拟左室内向整流钾电流（I_{K1}）存在大的外向电导，使动作电位时程大幅度缩短，足以建立稳定的高频率转子。

六、野生I_{K1}中通道蛋白Kir2.1的作用

Nakamura与同事应用反信-低聚核苷酸技术研究大鼠心室野生I_{K1}电流中Kir2.1通道蛋白的作用[34]。其结果证实Kir2.1基因编码的是一个特异的野生21-pS K^+通道蛋白，该通道在心脏I_{K1}的产生中起重要作用。应用多细胞反向转录酶-多聚酶酶链反应的方法，其他学者在豚鼠心肌细胞作Kir2亚单位的细胞特异性表达的研究，发现心肌中表达的是Kir2.1、Kir2.2和Kir2.3，而不是Kir2.4[35]。转染给HEK-239细胞后，

膜片钳分析提示豚鼠心肌细胞（23.8 pS）中的内向整流通道的断续电导与Kir2.1相对应[35]。我们对信使RNA水平的初步分析证明，左室Kir2.1的表达是右室的两倍以上，而其他通道蛋白则无显著性差异[36]。此外，在Kir2.x通道中，Kir2.1在人胚肾细胞的表达显示出最大的外向峰电流（$r=0.28\pm0.02$），提示该同构体对豚鼠心脏I_{K1}的腔室特异性差别负责（与A. S. Dhamoon的个人通信）。

再者，用整体细胞的膜片钳技术和计算机模拟，我们首次证明内向整流通道区域性分布的差别，其可能是室颤起源定位于左室，而左、右室激动频率存在一致梯度的离子机制[20]。在后续讨论中，我们将从该工作的基础上派生出许多实验研究思路，以增强我们对室颤分子机制的理解。

七、左心室与右心室的背景电流

数字模拟能够显示背景I_{K1}在建立快速和稳定折返中的重要性[26,37]。如图43-2B的动作电位重叠插图所示，预计核心对其周围紧邻组织的复极影响，导致接近电位平台范围的I_{K1}外向成分激活和提早复极；此外，I_{K1}也是维持稳定转子的基础[37]。

因此，我们决定用整体细胞电压钳技术研究左、右室背景电流的特点并将其空间分布与兴奋频率的差异相关联。图43-3A显示同一心脏左、右室两个不同细胞的背景电流的电流密度-电压关系[20]。可见左室细胞的外向电导明显大于右室细胞。从10个豚鼠离体心脏的19个左室细胞和18个右室细胞获得的结果相似。图43-3B显示这些细胞的平均电流-电压关系，表明左室的外向电导的强度明显高于右室（-50mV：右室5.3 ± 0.4 pA/pF；左室7.4 ± 0.6 pA/pF；$p=0.009$）。另外的实验在有和无1 mM钡（Ba^{2+}）的条件下，用标准的萃取技术获得Ba^{2+}敏感电流，确认左室细胞的I_{K1}外向成分的确明显大于右室细胞[38]。许多机理可解释左、右心室的I_{K1}外向成分的上述差别。基于左、右心室特异基因表达不同的两种可能性为：（1）特殊离子通道基因的不同，或者（2）直接或间接调节通道功能的蛋白基因不同。然而，我们明确发现双室的内向成分的密度基本相同（图43-3），可能原因是其他电导对心肌细胞的内向背景电流有所影响，尤其是钠背景电流。如同下文进一步讨论中所述。另一种解释是，管理I_{K1}的内向整流通道复合体实际由蛋白的同构异质多体形成，该蛋白同体由密切

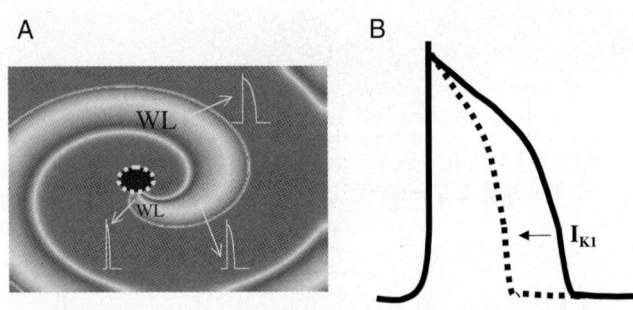

图43-2 核心对波长和动作电位时程的作用 A：在2×2 cm的各向异性（长与宽速度之比为4:1）心脏组织中的自旋波活动，遵照Luo与Rudy修正的全动作电位模型建立的方法（技术细节见Gilmour等[26]）。波锋为红色，波尾为绿色，静息组织为蓝色。注意波锋曲度沿转动中心方向增大（核心为虚线圈）。随曲度增大传导速度减慢。波长定义为兴奋状态的空间范围，从中心到周边增长。其原因是由于核心的电张作用，动作电位时程从中心到周边增长（局部波长等于传导速度×动作电位时程）。B：功能性折返中I_{K1}导致动作电位时程缩短的示意图（见彩图19）

相关的2个或更多的基因编码[39]。

八、稳态心室颤动的离子机制

正如上述,我们的初期研究强烈提示左室转子的稳定性与左、右心室细胞的 I_{K1} 密度不同有关。单通道电导和 I_{K1} 开放时间分别为 40pS 和 100 ms[40]。I_{K1} 供给膜电位在 E_k 以下的较大的内向电导,与电位刚好超过 E_k 的相对较大的外向电导一同作用,有助于使静息膜电位维持在近于 E_k 的水平。此外,I_{K1} 是正常动作电位形态和时程的重要决定因素,也有助于 I_{kr} 和 I_{ks} 结束平台期,负责快速复极的终末阶段[41]。然而,在功能性折返中,紧邻转动中心的动作电位时程明显缩短[37]。这种情况下,紧邻核心的提早复极不依赖于 I_{kr} 或 I_{ks},而是在 I_{K1} 的影响和核心提供的电张复极电流的相互作用下出现[20,26,37]。计算机模拟显示,I_{K1} 除控制动作电位时程外,还通过减小波锋-波尾的交互作用而使折返稳定[37]。如上所述,随后的实验表明左、右心室细胞的 I_{K1} 电流-电压关系中的外向成分不同(图43-3)。有了这些数据后,我们进行了更多的数字研究,以确定外向电流密度的不同对转子动力学和发散波的作用。如图43-4A所示,将这些数据拟合于心脏折返激动的二维模型,用 I_{K1} 较小的外向电导的模型,模拟右心室,由于波锋和波尾碰撞,转子尖陷落,活动终止,转子不能维持。相反,图43-4B 用 I_{K1} 较大的外向电导的模型,模拟左心室,产生动作电位时程足够的缩短,容许建立起稳定的高频转子。进而,将左、右心室模型合而二而成为一个二维组织,数字结果准确地再现了室颤的实验数据。在此情形下,左室的高频转子(中心)成为维持双室整体活动的发动机,右室(周边)生成多个短命的碎裂波,非持续折返的固有频率明显慢于左室。因此,我们的结果预计,左室心肌细胞大幅的外向电流成分,通过减低紧邻核心的动作电位时程和预防波锋与波尾的交互作用,使左室的高频转子稳定。

九、通道蛋白的 Kir 家族

最近几年克隆出许多的编码钾通道基因,就此课题已有数篇优秀的综述[41-42]。如图43-5所示,称为内向整流钾通道(Kir)的家族成员由4个亚单位构成[43-44]。然而,有关活体中这些通道是以同质还是异

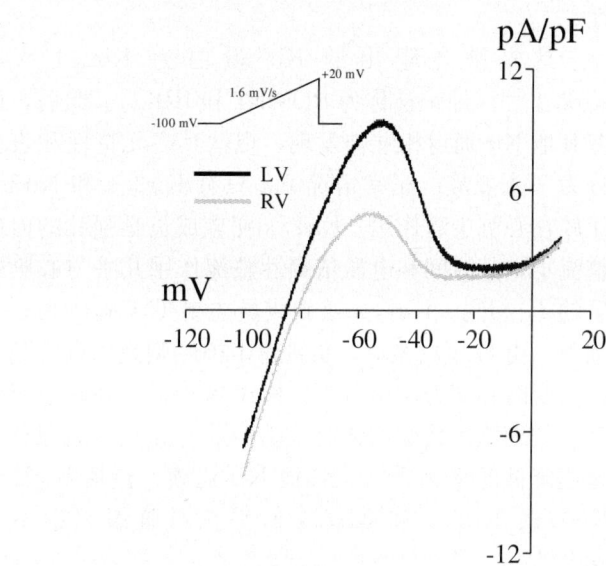

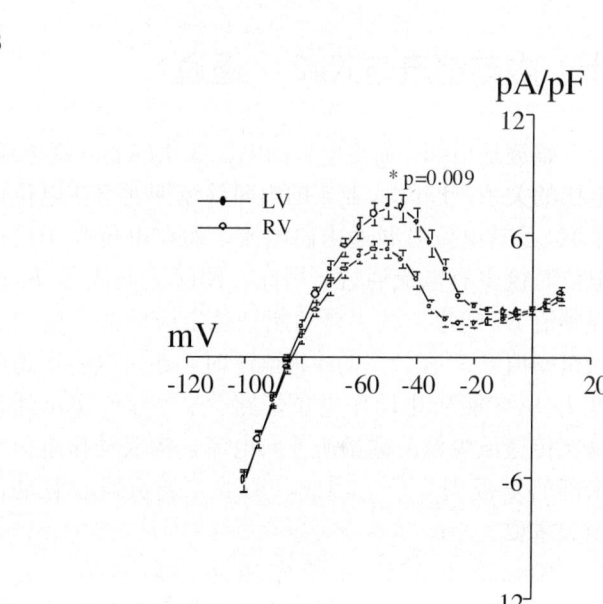

图43-3 背景电流的电流电压关系 A:同一心脏左、右心室细胞的背景电流 I_B 的电流密度-电压关系。嵌入:从-100~+20mV 的平持电位应用1.6mV/s 的斜率。B:背景电流的平均电流-电压关系(右室数18,左室数19)。电流经细胞电容校正和平均。右、左心室的平均电容分别为 165pF 和 167pF(引自 Samie FH,Berenfeld O,Anumonwo J,et al:Rectification of the background potassium current:A determinant of rotor dynamics in ventricular fibrillation Circ Res 89:1216-1223,2001)

质四聚体的形式存在,证据不一致[45-48]。如图43-5A 所示,每一亚单位有胞浆内的 N 端和 C 端与两个跨膜主体(M1 和 M2)[27]。图43-5B 示 M1 和 M2 之间的环状结构(P 或 H5)负责形成孔道[49]。P 环含有典型的 GYG/GFG 延展,决定了所有钾通道的 K^+ 选择

性[49-53]。

首先被克隆出的 Kir 蛋白为 Kir1.1[54] 和 Kir2.1[55]（原来被称为 ROMK1 和 IRK1）。此后，许多其他 Kir 通道相继被发现，现按其多元特性和表型分为 7 个亚族。正常情况下，只有 Kir2.x 和 Kir3.x 亚族在心脏中起作用。Kir2.x 亚族成员是强壮的内向整流子，其时间和电压依赖性整流作用几乎与心脏野生的 I_{K1} 相同。Kir3.x 亚族成员主要见于起搏和心房细胞，由 G 蛋白激活，负责迷走神经刺激后观察到的负向变时和变力作用[56,57]。Kir6.x 通道只在缺血时由感受到细胞内代谢增强时三磷酸腺苷和二磷酸腺苷的比值降低时激活[58,59]。其他 Kir 亚族，包括 Kir1.x、Kir4.x、Kir5.x 和 Kir7.x 似乎在心脏组织中不表达[60,61]。

十、内向整流与 Kir2.x 通道

整流是指某一通道电导随电压变化的非欧姆电流-电压的关系。Kir2.x 亚族的内向整流钾通道在电位低于 K^+ 反转电位时开通内向电流，而在电位高于反转电位时极少有电流通过。因此，Kir2.x 是携带 I_{K1} 的强整流 K^+ 通道，其主要功能是稳定膜的静息电位和兴奋阈值[27]；在较高的除极电压时，通过这些通道的低 I_{K1} 电导能防止动作电位短路[27]。然而，Kir 通道确实传递虽少但关键量的外向电流，构成动作电位终末部的复极成分[28]。因此，Kir2.x 通道对心脏功能至关重要。

Katz[62] 于 1949 年首先描述内向整流，Armstrong[63] 提议内向整流由细胞内的正电分子阻止通道的孔道所致。随后在心肌细胞的研究证明细胞内 Mg^{2+} 以电压依赖的方式阻止 Kir 通道[29,30]。20 世纪 90 年代早期，Kir 蛋白被克隆后，细胞内多肽作为整流分子在内向整流钾通道中的更为关键的作用得到确立[31,32]。与 Mg^{2+} 相比，多肽以更为陡峭的电压依赖方式阻止通过 Kir 通道的外向电流。有趣的是，虽然多肽阻止所有的 Kir 通道，但阻止的灵敏性随 Kir 亚族的不同而不同[31]。弱的内向整流子能容许更多的外向电流通过，与之相反，强的整流子容许较少的电流通过。至今尚未全面了解整流范围的特点，Kir2.x 亚族的 Mg^{2+}、多肽敏感性和电流-电压关系均限于哺乳动物的表达系统。Liu 与同事[35] 最近用单通道记录研究了豚鼠 Kir2.x 序列的电流-电压关系，但只描述了内向电流，而未研究外向电流，因此未探讨 Kir2.x

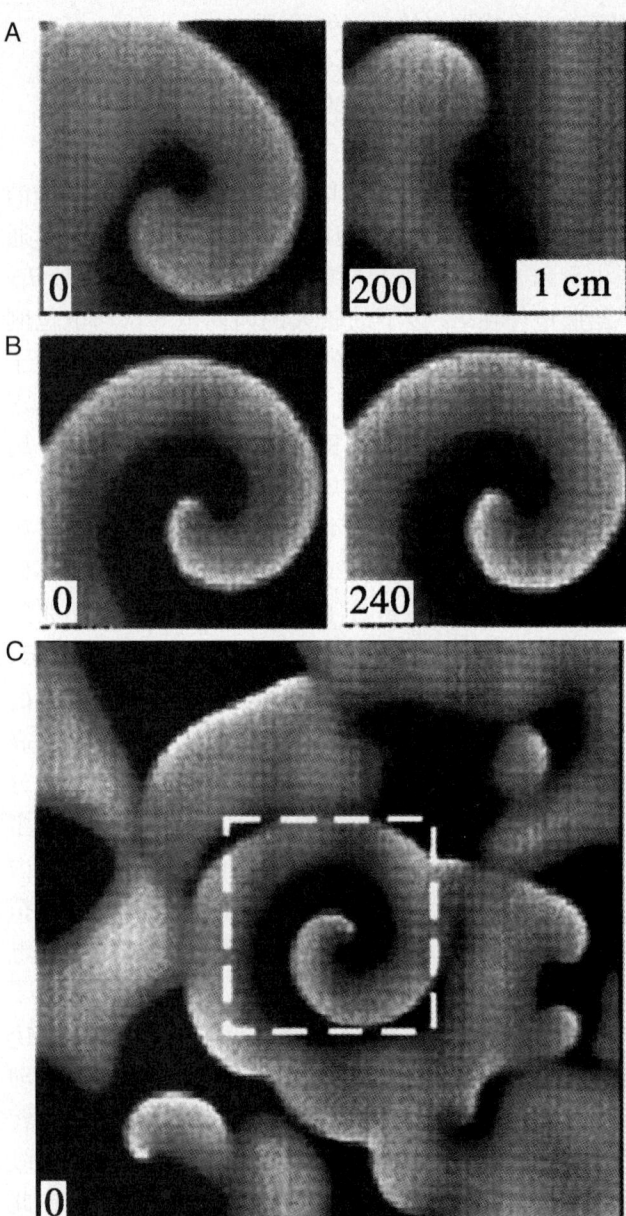

图 43-4 在 Luo 与 Rudy 修正模型，用实验获得的 I_{K1} 电流-电压关系作计算机模拟的功能性折返 模拟 A：模拟右室的 $3\times 3\ cm^2$ 组织数据的 2 张快照。B：同样大小的左室模型数据的 2 张快照（与 A 相比电位的平台范围有更大的外向电流）。C：左、右心室结合的 $6\times 6\ cm^2$ 组织模型的数据快照。各幅内的数据单位均为毫秒。C 幅中的虚线框为左室模型的周边界（面积 $2\times 2\ cm^2$）（引自 Samie FH, Berenfeld O, Anumonwo J, et al: Rectification of the background potassium current: A determinant of rotor dynamics in ventricular fibrillation Circ Res 89：1216-1223，2001）

亚族成员间整流程度的差异。同样，尽管在爪蟾卵母细胞和哺乳动物的细胞组织进行了基础电生理研究，由于不同实验室的实验槽和吸移管溶液的离子条件不

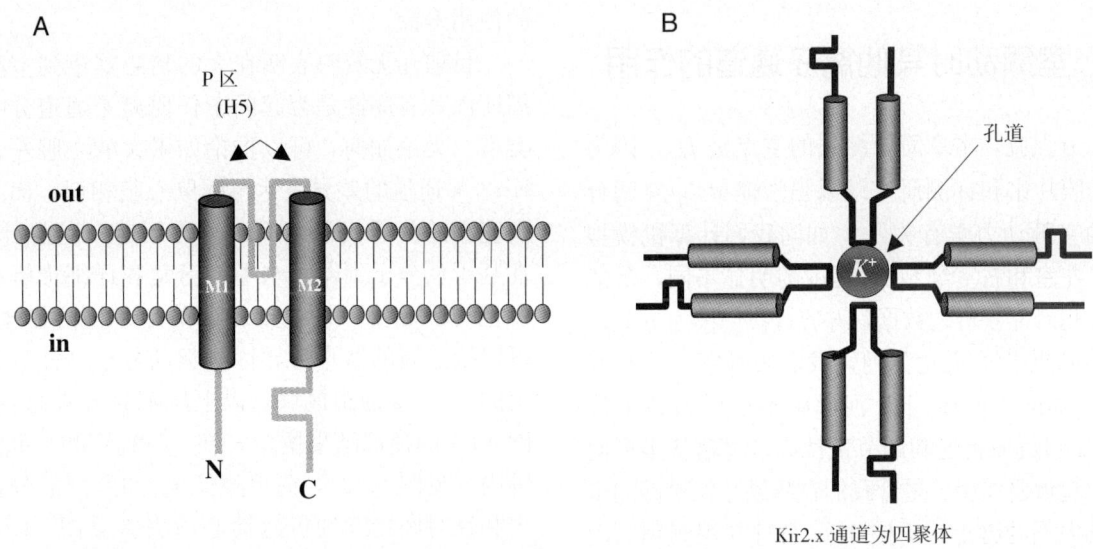

图 43-5 Kir 通道 A：Kir 通道结构的推导简图。B：Kir 通道的四个亚单位，组成 P 区孔道的衬套。Kir2.x 通道为四聚体。详见正文

同，没有一致的数据来比较所有 Kir2.x 的同构体。

目前急需研究哺乳动物细胞中 Kir2.x 的特点，确定整体细胞的 I_{K1} 不同是否取决于 Kir2.x 同构体的特性以及它们在心脏中如何表达。

十一、为什么是 Kir2.X 通道在起作用

我们的实验观察到左、右心室的整流特性不同，进而得出结论认为，Kir2.x 亚族起关键作用是出于以下考虑。第一，我们实验室的最新数据表明在豚鼠心脏中 Kir2.1 和 Kir2.3 的副本表达不同[36]，第二，它们的整流特性与镜像整体细胞 I_{K1} 非常接近，但在哺乳动物细胞表达时，克隆的 Kir2.1 和 Kir2.3 的整流外向成分明显不同[36]，第二，这些通道与 Kir3.x 和 Kir6.x 亚族不同，传递电流不需要细胞内因子（如 G 蛋白）的调节。据我们所知，没有人研究过 Kir2.x 亚族成员的个性构成，以及心脏不同区域 I_{K1} 的差别，并以此信息来理解室颤，第四，Kir2.1 功能的显性负向突变可产生 Andersen 综合征，又称 LQT7，Kir2.1 功能突变能引起畸形、周期性无力和心律失常[64]。Preisig-Muller 及同事[39]新近发表的有力证据表明负责 Andersen 综合征的 Kir2.1 等位基因突变可能与其他野生型 Kir2.1、Kir2.2 和 Kir2.3 蛋白结合，形成 Kir2.x 钾通道的非均质四聚体，引起这种病人很大的表型变异。已经确定 Andersen 综合征由 KCNJ2 突变所致，后者编码为 Kir2.1[64]。一项晚近的研究中，

Tristani-Firouzi 及同事[65]证明对于基因突变的携带者，长 QT 综合征通常是原发的心脏表现，此类病人约 64% 有心律失常。然而，该组研究的病人无一例发生心脏性猝死。在心室单细胞的数字模型中研究 Kir2.1 减少的作用，上述研究者发现动作电位终末期延长[65]。模拟细胞外 K^+ 减低时，出现 Na^+/Ca^{2+} 交换依赖型延迟后除极和自发性心律失常。虽然这些观察提示 Andersen 综合征易感心律失常的基质可能与其他遗传性长 QT 综合征不同，但为何此类病人无心脏性猝死未能提供任何见解。我们推测 Andersen 综合征患者 I_{K1} 降低引起了重要程度的保护，以免诱发折返性心律失常。如图 43-4A 计算机二维模拟结果所示，I_{K1} 的降低产生动作电位时程和波长的延长，由于波锋和波尾相互作用导致折返的自发终止，可能致使这些病人的心室不能维持稳定的转子。

十二、其他内向整流通道的作用

TWIK-1 是双孔道主导 K^+ 通道（K_{2p}）家族的一员，有可能这一弱的内向整流子也介入我们观察到的整流特性的差别。Wang 等[66]发现人类心脏有 TWIK-1 副本，并造成心房和心室内向整流性质的不同。此外，他们还研究了 Kir2.1、Kir2.2、Kir2.3 和 TWIK-1 在心房和心室间的表达差异，但同样无人研究这些通道在左、右心室间的表达。再者，尚未克隆豚鼠的 TWIK-1 通道蛋白基因，不清楚是否这一通道

对 I_{K1} 有所作用。

十三、心室颤动时其他离子通道的作用

应当十分强调，本章简要综述的重点是 I_{K1}，因为我们以前的膜片钳和标测研究结果强烈提示 I_{K1} 空间分布与豚鼠的室颤动力学有关[20]。如同我们计算机模拟结果所示，左室和右室细胞 I_{K1} 密度的明显不同，足能解释光学标测研究获得的数据，并容许我们极为近似地再现颤动的结果[37]。无论如何，我们实验室[37,67]和其他研究者[68]都证明电压门控-河豚毒素敏感型钠电流（I_{Na}）在稳定自旋波折返和调节室性心动过速从多形向单形转换中起重要作用。尽管我们在豚鼠心外膜标测未发现自旋波尖端的游走，不排除 I_{Na} 特性在观测到的动力学中发挥作用。与此类似，已发现二氢吡啶敏感型钙电流（I_{Ca}）的阻滞剂通过降低转子频率和波锋碎裂而稳定折返并使室颤转化为室速[21]。

十四、如何应用这些新信息

很明显，在小豚鼠心脏获得的结果不能用于大的种群，更别说人体，欲将上述讨论的概念泛化应用时必须十分小心。无论怎样，从豚鼠心脏获得的知识可用来部分解释为什么许多 Andersen 综合征的病人无心脏性猝死的危险。有关 Kir2.x 通道在室颤中作用的新信息也有助于理解其他通道疾病中致命性心律失常的始发和维持机制。

在 Lewis[69] 时代就存在对"母亲转子"假说解释心房和心室颤动机理是否适宜的质疑。此外，以前在许多人体和大动物的室颤标测研究中并未发现这样的转子。但是，新近的研究[70,71] 证明与豚鼠和家兔心脏类似[20,67]，大心脏的颤动激动波波锋存在优势传导方向和时间与空间的周期性。例如，Nanthakumar 与同事[70] 发现猪心左室外膜的激动并非在所有方向都呈随机扩布。相反，冲动波锋主要沿平行于房室沟的方向扩布。此外，Rogers 与同事[71] 证明在某些大心脏的颤动同样始终存在持续的心外膜折返。然而，需要更多的研究来确认这些结果不只限于猪心，也见于其他大动物的心脏，包括人体心脏。可以想象这些新的信息在预防和治疗室颤时的潜在临床意义。例如，有关室颤活动的折返源通常稳定在左室的认识，可能启发我们设计新的植入型心脏转复除颤器和导管，以便在起源部位发放有效电击而终止折返。这将有可能用更小的电击能量完成，从而延长植入型心脏转复除颤器的使用寿命。

目前还无资料表明在大的猪心观察到室颤的高度周期性和有序性是否起因于任何离子通道分布的特殊类型。无论如何，可以推论如果大的心脏左、右心室 Kir2.x 通道的差异表达与豚鼠心脏相似，而且也介入到室颤的分子机制，那么就可用这一信息作为起点，在基于从分子到器官水平上清楚和详细理解心律失常机理的基础上，设计全新的治疗和预防措施。例如，可以制造新的器官特异性抗颤动分子，针对心室中一定的 Kir2.x 通道区域，以电压依赖方式修正 I_{K1}。如图 43-4 的模拟结果所示，在 $-50mV$ 和 $-20mV$ 的范围内（见图 43-3），简单降低 I_{K1} 的外向成分，可将稳定和长时间持续的折返性心律失常（图 43-4B）转变为不稳定和短阵的心律失常（图 43-4A）。因此，可以预见在不远的将来，发展新一代安全有效的修正 Kir 的抗颤动药物，有可能用药使心脏性猝死的高危病人能完全预防室颤的发生。

（郭成军 译）

参 考 文 献

1. Myerburg RJ, Castellanos A: Cardiac arrest and sudden cardiac death. In Braunwald E (ed): Heart Disease: A Textbook of Cardiovascular Medicine. Philadelphia, PA, WB Saunders, 1997, pp 742-779.
2. Zipes DP, Wellens HJ: Sudden cardiac death. Circulation 98: 2334-2351, 1998.
3. Myerburg RJ, Spooner PM: Opportunities for sudden death prevention: directions for new clinical and basic research. Cardiovasc Res 50:177-185, 2001.
4. Wiggers CJ: The mechanism and nature of ventricular fibrillation. Am Heart J 20:399-412, 1940.
5. Moe GK, Rheinboldt WC, Abildskov JA: A computer model of atrial fibrillation. Am Heart J 67:200-220,1964.
6. Krinskii VI: Excitation propagation in nonhomogenous medium (actions analogous to heart fibrillation). Biofizika 11:676-83, 1966.
7. Winfree AT: Sudden cardiac death: a problem in topology. Sci Am 248:144-161, 1983.
8. Gray RA, Pertsov AM, Jalife J: Spatial and temporal organization during cardiac fibrillation. Nature 392:75-78, 1998.
9. Panfilov AV: Spiral breakup as a model of ventricular fibrillation. Chaos 8:57-64, 1998.
10. Karma A: Electrical alternans and spiral wave breakup in cardiac tissue. Chaos 4:461-472, 1994.
11. Fenton F, Karma A: Vortex dynamics in three-dimensional continuous myocardium with fiber rotation: Filament instability and fibrillation. Chaos 8:20-47, 1998.
12. Riccio ML, Koller ML, Gilmour RF, Jr: Electrical restitution and spatiotemporal organization during ventricular fibrillation. Circ Res 84:955-963, 1999.
13. Watanabe M, Otani NF, Gilmour RF, Jr: Biphasic restitution of action potential duration and complex dynamics in ventricular myocardium. Circ Res 76:915-921, 1995.
14. Weiss JN, Garfinkel A, Karagueuzian HS, et al: Chaos and the transition to ventricular fibrillation: a new approach to antiarrhythmic drug evaluation. Circulation 99:2819-2826, 1999.
15. Witkowski FX, Leon LJ, Penkoske PA, et al: Spatiotemporal evolution of ventricular fibrillation. Nature 392:78-82, 1998.
16. Nolasco JB, Dahlen RW: A graphic method for the study of alternation in cardiac action potentials. J of Appl Physiol 25:191, 1968.

17. Garfinkel A, Kim YH, Voroshilovsky O, et al: Preventing ventricular fibrillation by flattening cardiac restitution. Proc Natl Acad Sci U S A 97:6061–6066, 2000.
18. Gilmour RF, Jr., Otani NF, Watanabe MA: Memory and complex dynamics in cardiac Purkinje fibers. Am J Physiol 272:H1826–H1832, 1997.
19. Zaitsev AV, Berenfeld O, Mironov SF, et al: Distribution of excitation frequencies on the epicardial and endocardial surfaces of fibrillating ventricular wall of the sheep heart. Circ Res 86:408–417, 2000.
20. Samie FH, Berenfeld O, Anumonwo J, et al: Rectification of the background potassium current: a determinant of rotor dynamics in ventricular fibrillation. Circ Res 12:1216–1223, 2001.
21. Samie FH, Mandapati R, Gray RA, et al: A mechanism of transition from ventricular fibrillation to tachycardia: effect of calcium channel blockade on the dynamics of rotating waves. Circ Res 86:684–691, 2000.
22. Gray RA, Jalife J, Panfilov AV, et al: Mechanisms of cardiac fibrillation. Science 270:1222–1223, 1995.
23. Boersma L, Brugada J, Kirchhof C, Allessie M: Mapping of reset of anatomic and functional reentry in anisotropic rabbit ventricular myocardium. Circulation 89:852–862, 1994.
24. Priori SG, Napolitano C, Cantu F, et al: Differential response to Na$^+$ channel blockade, beta-adrenergic stimulation, and rapid pacing in a cellular model mimicking the SCN5A and HERG defects present in the long-QT syndrome. Circ Res 78:1009–1015, 1996.
25. Weidmann S: Effect of current flow on the membrane potential of cardiac muscle. L Physiol. 115:227–236, 1951.
26. Beaumont J, Jalife J: Rotors and spiral waves in two dimensions. In: Zipes DP, Jalife J, eds: Cardiac Electrophysiology From Cell to Bedside. Philadelphia, PA, WB Saunders, 2000, pp 327–335.
27. Nichols CG, Makhina EN, Pearson WL, et al: Inward rectification and implications for cardiac excitability. Circ Res 78:1–7, 1996.
28. Shimoni Y, Clark RB, Giles WR: Role of an inwardly rectifying potassium current in rabbit ventricular action potential. J Physiol 448:709–727, 1992.
29. Vandenberg CA: Inward rectification of a potassium channel in cardiac ventricular cells depends on internal magnesium ions. Proc Natl Acad Sci U S A 84:2560–2564, 1987.
30. Matsuda H: Effects of external and internal K$^+$ ions on magnesium block of inwardly rectifying K$^+$ channels in guinea-pig heart cells. J Physiol 435:83–99, 1991.
31. Fakler B, Brandle U, Bond C, et al: A structural determinant of differential sensitivity of cloned inward rectifier K$^+$ channels to intracellular spermine. FEBS Letters 356:199–203, 1991.
32. Lopatin AN, Makhina EN, Nichols CG: Potassium channel block by cytoplasmic polyamines as the mechanism of intrinsic rectification. Nature 372:366–369, 1994.
33. Ficker E, Taglialatela M, Wible BA, et al: Spermine and spermidine as gating molecules for inward rectifier K channels. Science 266:1068–1072, 1994.
34. Nakamura TY, Artman M, Rudy B, Coetzee WA: Inhibition of rat ventricular IK1 with antisense oligonucleotides targeted to Kir2.1 mRNA. Am J Physiol 274:H892–H900, 1998.
35. Liu GX, Derst C, Schlichthorl G, et al: Comparison of cloned Kir2 channels with native inward rectifier K$^+$ channels from guinea-pig cardiomyocytes. J Physiol 532:115–126, 2001.
36. Dhamoon AS, Bagwe S, Guha P, et al: Differential expression and whole-cell rectification profiles of guinea pig Kir2.x channels. Biophys J (Abstract) 82:587a, 2002.
37. Beaumont J, Davidenko N, Davidenko JM, Jalife J: Spiral waves in two-dimensional models of ventricular muscle: formation of a stationary core. Biophys J 75:1–14, 1998.
38. Warren M, Guha PK, Berenfeld O, et al: Blockade of the inward rectifying potassium current terminates ventricular fibrillation in the guinea pig heart. J Cardiovasc Electrophysiol. 14:621–631, 2003.
39. Preisig-Muller R, Schlichthorl G, Goerge T, et al: Heteromerization of Kir2.x potassium channels contributes to the phenotype of Andersen's syndrome. Proc Natl Acad Sci U S A 99:7774–7779, 2002.
40. Ishihara, K., and M. Hiraoka: Gating mechanism of the cloned inward rectifier potassium channel from mouse heart. J Membr Biol 142:55–64, 1994.
41. Nichols CG, Lopatin AN: Inward rectifier potassium channels. Annu Rev Physiol 59:171–191, 2003.
42. Nerbonne JM: Molecular basis of functional voltage-gated K$^+$ channel diversity in the mammalian myocardium. J Physiol 525:285–298, 2000.
43. Yang J, Jan YN, Jan LY: Determination of the subunit stoichiometry of an inwardly rectifying potassium channel. Neuron 15:1441–1447, 1995.
44. Glowatzki E, Fakler G, Brandle U, et al: Subunit-dependent assembly of inward-rectifier K$^+$ channels. Proc R Soc Lond B Biol Sci 261:2512–2561, 1995.
45. Tinker A, Jan YN, Jan LY: Regions responsible for the assembly of inwardly rectifying potassium channels. Cell 87:857–868, 1996.
46. Cohen NA, Sha Q, Makhina EN, et al: Inhibition of an inward rectifier potassium channel (Kir2.3) by G-protein betagamma subunits. J of Biol Chem 271:32301–32305, 1996.
47. Fink M, Duprat F, Heurteaux C, et al: Dominant negative chimeras provide evidence for homo and heteromultimeric assembly of inward rectifier K$^+$ channel proteins via their N-terminal end. FEBS Letters 378:64–68, 1996.
48. Kubo Y, Reuveny E, Slesinger PA, et al: Primary structure and functional expression of a rat G-protein-coupled muscarinic potassium channel. Nature 364:802–806, 1993.
49. Heginbotham L, Abramson T, MacKinnon R: A functional connection between the pores of distantly related ion channels as revealed by mutant K$^+$ channels. Science 258:1152–1155, 1992.
50. Hartmann HA, Kirsch GE, Drewe JA, et al: Exchange of conduction pathways between two related K$^+$ channels. Science 251:942–944, 1991.
51. MacKinnon R, Yellen G: Mutations affecting TEA blockade and ion permeation in voltage-activated K$^+$ channels. Science 250:276–279, 1990.
52. Yool AJ, Schwarz TL: Alteration of ionic selectivity of a K$^+$ channel by mutation of the H5 region. Nature 349:700–704, 1991.
53. Doyle DA, Morais CJ, Pfuetzner RA, et al: The structure of the potassium channel: molecular basis of K$^+$ conduction and selectivity. Science 280:69–77, 1998.
54. Ho K, Nichols CG, Lederer WJ, et al: Cloning and expression of an inwardly rectifying ATP-regulated potassium channel. Nature 362:31–38, 1993.
55. Kubo Y, Baldwin TJ, Jan YN, Jan LY: Primary structure and functional expression of a mouse inward rectifier potassium channel. Nature 362:127–133, 1993.
56. Noma A, Peper K, Trautwein W: Acetylcholine-induced potassium current fluctuations in the rabbit sinoatrial node. Pflugers Archiv Eur J Physiol 381:255–262, 1979.
57. Soejima M, Noma A: Mode of regulation of the ACh-sensitive K-channel by the muscarinic receptor in rabbit atrial cells. Pflugers Archiv Eur J Physiol 400:424–431, 1984.
58. Noma A, Takano M: The ATP-sensitive K$^+$ channel. Jpn J Physiol 41:1771–1787, 1991.
59. Fujita A, Kurachi Y: Molecular aspects of ATP-sensitive K$^+$ channels in the cardiovascular system and K$^+$ channel openers. Pharmacol Ther 85:39–53, 2000.
60. Zhou X, Wolf PD, Smith WM, et al: Effects of peroneal nerve stimulation on hypothalamic stimulation-induced ventricular arrhythmias in rabbits. Am J Physiol 267:H2032–H2041, 1994.
61. Kubo Y, Iizuka M: Identification of domains of the cardiac inward rectifying K$^+$ channel, CIR, involved in the heteromultimer formation and in the G-protein gating. Biochem Biophys Res Comm 227:240–247, 1996.
62. Katz B: Les constantes electriques de la membrane du muscle. Arch Sci Physiol 2:285–299, 1949.
63. Armstrong CM: Inactivation of the potassium conductance and related phenomena caused by quaternary ammonium ion injection in squid axons. J Gen Physiol 54:553–575, 1969.
64. Plaster NM, Tawil R, Tristani-Firouzi M, et al: Mutations in kir2.1 cause the developmental and episodic electrical phenotypes of andersen's syndrome. Cell 105:511–519, 2001.
65. Tristani-Firouzi M, Jensen JL, Donaldson MR, et al: Functional and clinical characterization of KCNJ2 mutations associated with LQT7 (Andersen syndrome). J Clin Invest 10:381–388, 2002.
66. Wang Z, Yue L, White M, et al: Differential distribution of inward rectifier potassium channel transcripts in human atrium versus ventricle. Circulation 98:2422–2428, 1998.
67. Mandapati R, Asano Y, Baxter WT, et al: Quantification of effects of global ischemia on dynamics of ventricular fibrillation in isolated rabbit heart. Circulation 98:1688–1696, 1998.

68. Starobin JM, Zilberter YI, Rusnak EM, Starmer CF: Wavelet formation in excitable cardiac tissue: The role of wavefront-obstacle interactions in initiating high-frequency fibrillatory-like arrhythmias. Biophys J 70:581–594, 1996.
69. Lewis T: The Mechanism and Graphic Registration of the Heart Beat (3rd ed.), London, Shaw, 1925, pp 319–374.
70. Nanthakumar K, Huang J, Rogers JM, et al: Regional differences in ventricular fibrillation in the open-chest porcine left ventricle. Circ Res 91:733–740, 2002.
71. Rogers JM, Huang J, Melnick SB, Ideker RE: Sustained reentry in the left ventricle of fibrillating pig hearts. Circ Res 292:539–545, 2003.

第 44 章

缺血性心室颤动的机制：谁是凶手？

Alexey V. Zaitsev

本章目录
- 引言 395
- 急性区域缺血致心律失常的时间与空间类型 395
- 高血钾 397
- 凝血酶 397
- 细胞间的去耦联 398
- 儿茶酚胺 399
- 牵张作用 399
- 排除嫌疑犯 399
- 结束语 400

一、引言

心室颤动（简称室颤）与心肌缺血在很多方面不可分割。区域性心肌缺血（阻断某支冠状动脉的血流）与室颤的发生高度相关，在动物实验中可以复制[1]。另一方面，除非人工维持正常的心肌灌注血流，任何起源的室颤均伴有整体心肌的缺血。这种继发性整体缺血反过来能引起室颤的持续[2]，影响除颤电击和颤动心脏的交互作用[3]。显然，若不理解缺血和室颤间存在的复杂关系，任何有关室颤和除颤的现代理论都不完整。

20世纪后半叶，许多研究的重点一直侧重急性心肌缺血促发心律失常的各种原因。对此的系统考证已有数篇综述[1,4,5]。然而，这些影响因素呈多样性。不完全的列出包括：三磷酸腺苷（adenosine triphosphate，ATP）的耗竭、酸中毒、细胞外钾离子堆集、细胞内钙和钠离子堆积、细胞与细胞间脱耦合、氧自由基的产生、双亲性脂肪酸水平升高、凝血酶释放、儿茶酚胺的局部和系统释放、兴奋性降低、动作电位时程（action potential duration，APD）缩短、缺血组织的机械特性改变等[4]。

尽量详尽了解这些因素不太容易，而且，为了治疗缺血性心律失常而针对如此广泛的原因治疗，几乎不可行。当然，最好的治疗选择是预防缺血性心脏病，但除非全世界数亿人口从根本上改变生活和卫生习惯，改变社会、经济状况，否则处置缺血性心律失常，尤其是室颤，仍将是全球性的挑战[6]。

这种情形下，将重点侧重于启动和维持缺血性室颤的关键因素至关重要。但是我们能否针对一或二项因素，通过对其分别控制而减低缺血室颤的发生率或增加除颤的成功率。

因此，我们依据新近文献和我们自己结果的重要线索，萃取缺血性室颤的关键因素。我们将重点讨论以下因素：钾浓度升高、凝血酶释放、儿茶酚胺的局部代谢性释放和缺血心肌的异常牵张。最后，我们将依据一项实验观察进一步缩小对关键性因素的包围圈。根据推理的原则，最终我们将能发现罪犯。

二、急性区域缺血致心律失常的时间与空间类型

我们的第一条线索是早期缺血性心律失常发生在两个明确的时间段（图44-1A）[7]。这两个时段分别称为1a和1b期，这能够区分发生在5～72小时的心律失常（Ⅱ期）和心肌梗死后慢性期的心律失常（Ⅲ

期)[1]。这种缺血早期的心律失常最早在犬模型中发现[7]，在麻醉猪中也是一样（图 44-1B）。在猪的心梗模型中大多数室颤发生在 1b 期（即冠脉阻塞后 15～40min 之间），峰值出现于 25～30min。虽然我们下文讨论重点基于这一双期模型，但应当注意这种情况在不同物种并非普遍发现。很明显，鼠和兔的模型中心律失常的发生只有一个高峰期[8]。此外，在临床心梗患者并未确定缺血性室颤的确切时间，1a 和 1b 期与临床的相关性有待研究确立。对临床病人很难确定冠脉闭塞的确切时间，使上述情形复杂化。进而，慢性缺血性心脏病患者冠脉完全闭塞前先有血流降低，后者可能影响心律失常的发生率和发生时间[9]。

双期模型的重要性在于两期内心律失常的发生机制不同，下文将详尽讨论。我们假定根据物种和病理条件的不同，实际缺血性心律失常的机理或者与 1a 期有关，或与 1b 期有关，或与两期均有关。然而，这种情形临床数据的重要性很难理解。

很多情况时，缺血性室颤的维持机制与其启动机制不同。缺血性室颤的启动常在适宜的基质存在时，需要有触发因素（室性早搏，简称室早或室性心动过速，简称室速）[1]。缺血时的许多因素可影响触发因素，基质可能对两者均有影响。室颤的基质可通过额外期前刺激测试。测试表明 1a 和 1b 期室颤的可诱发性增高[10,11]。由于自然触发因素的出现也遵循双期规律（图 44-1A），我们认为早期缺血性心律失常在两期内的室颤发生几率增加，与同时存在的触发因素和颤动基质有关。

缺血性室颤的触发因素和基质均有特殊的空间类型。已经明确在 1a 和 1b 期时缺血性室颤的触发因素多数出现在缺血区或边缘带（border zone，BZ）[12-15]。这一实验结果表明缺血和非缺血心肌的相互作用在产生触发因素中的重要性。触发因素的确切机理尚不清楚，下文将讨论可能的候选原因。

维持缺血性室颤的基质是哪些因素，为什么引起心室除极波的碎裂？Janse 与同事[12]证明 1a 期内室速向室颤的转变与缺血区内心室除极波的碎裂有关。相反，Rankovic 与同事[13]认为在室颤的维持中缺血区只起旁观者的作用，因为它不影响非缺血区激动的频率和有序性。但是，用高分辨率（<1mm）的视频成像技术仔细检查时发现，区域性缺血直到 15min，缺血的边缘区是室颤时波碎裂的主要位置（图 44-2）。波的碎裂率升高与跨缺血的边缘带不应期的显著梯度有关（图 44-2B）[16]。值得注意的是，缺血区中心部

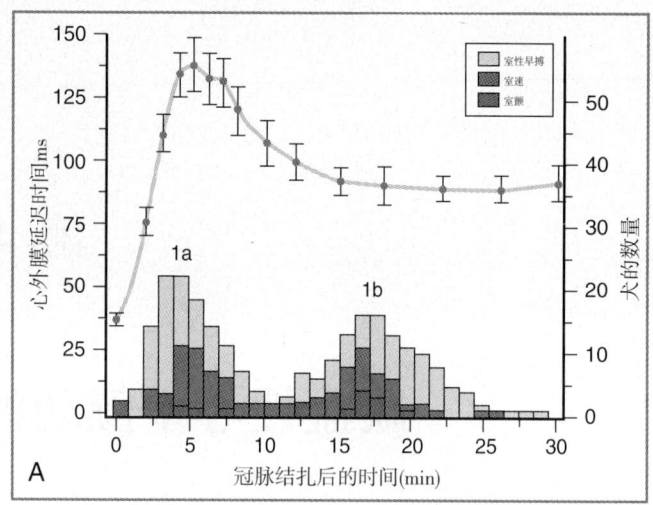

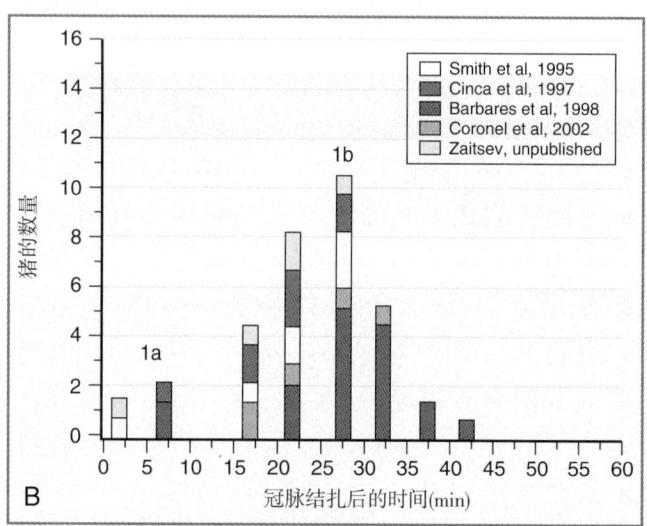

图 44-1 A：麻醉犬结扎冠状动脉后区域性心肌缺血 30min 内室性心律失常的发生率和严重度（竖条图），以及缺血区心外膜下传导延迟的动态变化（黑点）。VF，心室颤动；VPB，室性早搏。（引自 Kaplinsky E, Ogawa S, Blake CW, Dreifus LS: Two periods of early ventricular arrhythmias in the canine acute myocardial infarction model. Circulation 60：397-403，1979）。B：麻醉猪区域性心肌缺血 60min 内 VF 的发生率。注意犬和猪模型早期缺血性心律失常均有两个时期（1a 和 1b）（取自参考文献 15，44，45 和 56）

位激动波的碎裂减少（图 44-2A）。因此，在有血流灌注的离体猪心脏，区域性缺血具有致颤和抗颤的双重作用，亦即缺血在缺血的边缘带增加除极波碎裂的发生率，与此同时缺血区除极波碎裂的发生率却较低。这些作用均可用急性缺血的单一后果解释，即与高血钾有关。

三、高血钾

跨缺血边缘区细胞外钾浓度（$[K^+]_o$）的梯度可能是急性缺血的早期（1a）发生心律失常的基本因素[10]。缺血区K^+的聚集于停止灌流的15s内就已开始，常常在缺血5～15min达到平台期[17]。在缺血边缘区，出现$[K^+]_o$的恢复主要是由于钾离子从缺血边缘区的洗脱和扩散[18]。在Carmeliet精湛的综述中[4]详细讨论了缺血时细胞外K^+聚集的机理。高血钾与室颤有关的后果包括：静息膜电位的除极，备用钠通道的减低和动作电位时程的缩短。然而，有效不应期延长，并超越动作电位的复极期，称为复极后不应性[4]。Shaw和Rudy的研究表明[19]，缺血早期的三个主要因素（$[K^+]_o$升高、酸中毒、低氧）中，$[K^+]_o$升高是导致传导减慢和传导阻滞的主要决定因素，这是折返性心律失常发生的重要的条件。在缺血初期15min，$[K^+]_o$梯度[18]加大、缺血区的传导最大延迟（图44-1A）[7,14]、诱发性室颤[10]、自发性室颤[7,12,17,18]、室颤时边缘带碎裂波繁衍增加[20]等因素在时间上与其密切相关（图44-2）。

缺血区$[K^+]_o$升高导致的静息膜电位减小和延迟激动，为缺血与非缺血区之间的损伤电流的流动创造了条件[12,21]。损伤电流可能导致边缘带正常侧细胞的再度兴奋[22]或诱导自发的电活动[23]。因此，缺血的单一因素，即跨边缘带的K^+梯度，可能为1a期室颤提供触发和基质双重基础。在病人[24]和离体鼠[8]心脏低血钾增加缺血性室颤的发生几率，支持跨边缘带K^+梯度的大小、非缺血区K^+浓度的绝对值是室颤原因的观点。在离体的猪心脏，尽管存在$[K^+]_o$梯度，自发室颤却非常少见[15]。提示离体灌注的心脏缺乏一些其他因素的重要性，本章后文将进一步讨论。

虽然区域性高血钾产生的条件有利于传导阻滞、折返的发生，和边缘带反复的除极波碎裂，而整体的高血钾却抵抗室颤的发生，因为它在室颤中有稳定波锋的作用并能减低碎裂波的发生率。图44-3A所示，室颤的平均激动频率和波碎裂的奇点[25]密度随$[K^+]_o$升高而降低，直至$[K^+]_o$相当于浓度12.5mM时室颤转化为室速。整体缺血初期5min内，室颤变得更加具有周期性和有序，而且能转换为单一自旋波源驱动的单形室速（44-3B）[2]。因此，激发室颤的同一条件一旦引发室颤又阻碍颤动的进程。然而，矛盾的是随缺血发展虽然室颤的有序性增加[2]，但通常除颤阈值升高[26]。室颤后随着整体缺血除颤阈值升高最有可能是兴奋性降低的结果[27]，但双相电击波的阈值明显低于单相电击波[28]。因此应当进一步研究优化电击波的波形，以适合伴随整体缺血高血钾和兴奋性降低的条件，这对相对较长时间室颤的转复尤其重要[29]。

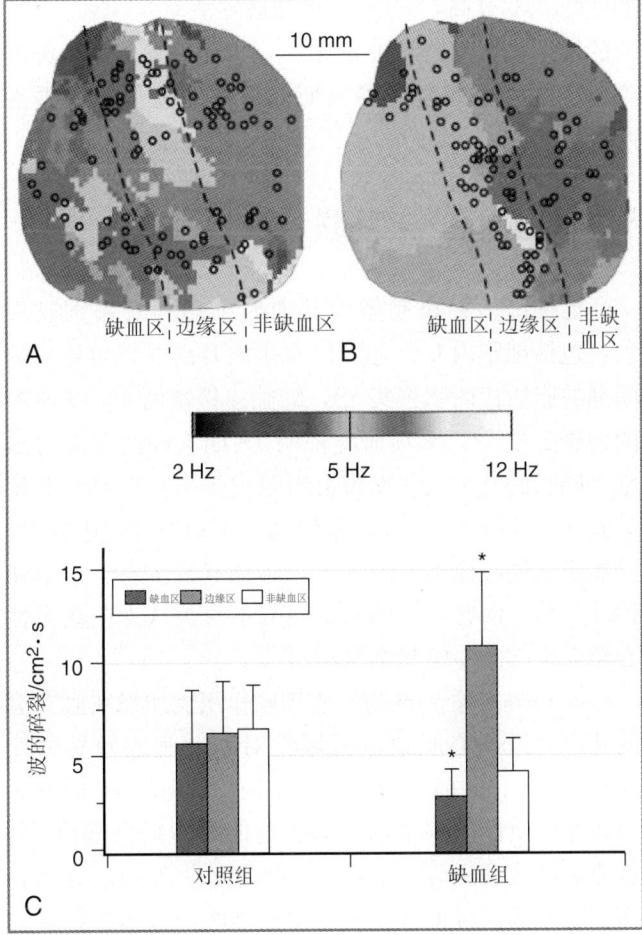

图44-2 心脏区域性缺血引发室颤时在缺血边缘带小波的形成增加 彩图代表室颤时主导兴奋频率（DF）的空间分布。DF与局部冲动的周长成反比，周长与局部不应期相关[16]。圆圈标注波的碎裂位置，导致室颤时的小波形成。A与B图中，波碎裂的分布与围缺血期室颤（A）和缺血室颤（B）的DF标测图。注意跨缺血的边缘带的不应期较大梯度区与密集的波碎裂区相连。C，6次实验缺血区（IZ）、边缘区（BZ）和非缺血区（NIZ）的平均波碎裂的密度。星号表示与对照组对应区域相比有显著性差异（引自Zaitsev AV, Sarmast F, Kolli A, et al: Wave break formation during ventricular fibrillation in the isolated, regionally ischemic pig heart. Circ Res 92：546-553，2003）（见彩图20）

四、凝血酶

病人急性心肌梗死通常由动脉硬化合并血栓所

致[30]。已经证实冠状动脉血栓性闭塞比非血栓性球囊闭塞引起室速/室颤的发生率更高[31]。血栓性闭塞引起室颤发生率的增高主要见于1a期（其他期的发生率非常低），并与激动时间明显延迟相关[14,32]，同非血栓性闭塞相比ST段的抬高更为明显[32]。血栓性闭塞的作用可能取决于完全阻塞前是否先有血流的降低[9,33]，将凝血酶注入实验性和自然发生闭塞的左前降支时，有增加室颤发生率的事实，表明这些凝血因子有直接导致心律失常的作用[32]。目前已知凝血酶至少通过三种机制发挥心脏电生理作用。第一，凝血酶激活磷脂酶 A_2[34]，后者导致心肌细胞内磷脂酸胆碱

(lisophosphatidicholines；LPC) 聚集[35]。LPCs能减慢 I_{Na} 失活的恢复速度[36]，增加细胞内 $[Na^+]_i$[37]。第二，凝血酶激活心肌纤维的 Na^+-H^+ 交换，在细胞内酸中毒时也使 $[Na^+]_i$ 增加[38]。第三，凝血酶增加 I_{Na} 峰电流，使激动-电压关系移向更负的膜电位区，使 Na^+ 窗电流大幅增加，也造成缺血时细胞内钠的聚集[39]。因此，很明显凝血酶的不同作用机制都能促进缺血时的钠负荷。由于反向的 Na^+-Ca^{2+} 交换和后继的 $[Ca^{2+}]_i$ 升高，$[Na^+]_i$ 增加触发活动[4]。Na^+ 窗电流的增加也可导致除极异常[39]，进而加强了高血钾的作用。这可解释凝血酶为何能使缺血区传导缓慢加重[32]。

五、细胞间的去耦联

已提出多种机制解释缺血时细胞间的去耦联现象，包括细胞内 Ca^{2+} 和 H^+ 水平的升高[40,41]可使去耦联剂的脂质代谢物聚集[42]，缝隙连接蛋白43（Cx43）的去磷酸化[43]。多项研究证明1b期室颤的多发与细胞去耦联的发生（表现为组织阻抗升高）在时间上相关联（图44-4）[15,44,45]。鼠缺血后Cx43的表达减少，并加速室性心律失常的发生，增加其发生率、频率和持续时间。因此，电耦联的减弱本身被认为在缺血性心律失常的发生中起重要作用[46]。

de Groot 等[11]认为，去耦联作用能加强缺血室颤的基质，增加心肌缺血区域性对期前刺激的易感性（图44-1C）。的确，缺血性心律失常发生的1b期可能存在非均质性的去耦联，为折返的发生提供基质[11]。也能促进触发活动。新近的模型研究[47]发现传导早后除极的形成区与正常区的中度去耦联，直接加强早后除极的启动和向邻近区域的扩布。在实验模型中，特定程度的去耦联可延长复极，促发早后除极的发生，并容许膜电位显著升高并促进激动向周围组织传递[47]。

虽然细胞间阻抗的升高可促进触发活动，但其本身并不产生触发活动。因此，单纯电耦联的减低不能解释1b期室颤发生率的增加。这一看法有下列事实支持：无心肌缺血时，Cx43缺陷的鼠不发生心律失常[46]。此外，尽管左前降支闭塞后细胞去耦联的时间过程一样，但离体猪心室颤的发生率几乎为零，而在体猪心室颤发生率却很高[15]。因此，细胞去耦联可能是心脏性猝死发生中重要但非必需的要素。

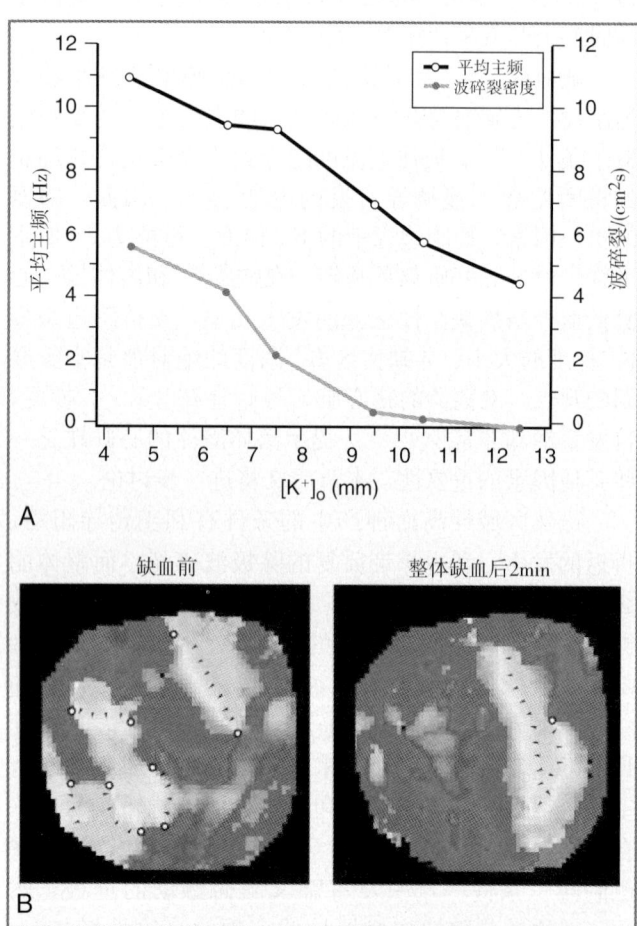

图 44-3 离体灌注猪心整体的缺血和高血钾的抗颤作用
A：室颤（VF）时平均兴奋主导频率（DF）与波碎裂（WB）的密度作为细胞外钾（K^+）的函数。随着 $[K^+]_o$ 的升高，室颤波变得更有周期性和更加有序，直至 $[K^+]_o$ 浓度相当于12.5mM时变为室速。B：室颤时心肌整体缺血前后2min时左室前壁心外膜的标测。箭头指示波锋的扩布，圆圈表示新生小波的位点。在正常灌注的心脏，标测区域最多同时存在5个小波。而整体缺血后2min，观察区仅见单一的自旋波（见彩图21）

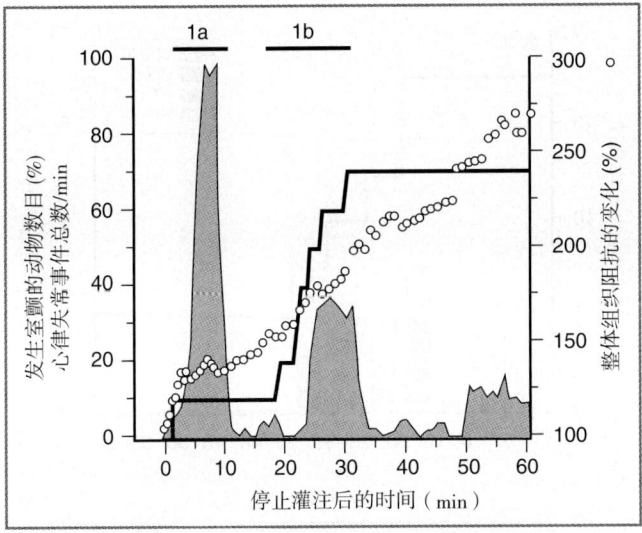

图44-4 麻醉猪区域性缺血后室颤（VF）发生比率（实线，左标尺）、心律失常事件的总数（阴影区）和整体组织的阻抗（圆圈，右标尺）之间的时间关系 实线标注出1a和1b期缺血性心律失常，注意多数室颤发生在1b期，与心肌组织阻抗的二次升高所显示的细胞间去电耦联相关（引自Smith WT, Fleet WF, Johnson TA, et al: The 1b phase of ventricular arrhythmias in ischemic in situ porcine heart is related to changes in cell-to-cell electrical coupling. Circulation 92: 3051-3060, 1995）

六、儿茶酚胺

多年来已经明确，交感神经在调节心肌缺血过程和心律失常的发生中起重要作用[48-50]。虽然中枢介导的儿茶酚胺释放能增加极早期（10min内）缺血性室颤的发生率[49]，但其在后期的作用被另一种机制掩盖，即被正常神经摄入的非细胞外物质所逆转，其不受局部和中枢神经刺激的影响[51]。作为非细胞外局部代谢性释放的后果，在体[52]或离体[51]细胞外去甲肾上腺素的浓度在缺血30min内达到正常值的100～1000倍。在缺血初期10min，去甲肾上腺素的浓度维持在生理范围，在缺血和非缺血区的增加均低于5倍[51,52]。因此，由于神经的再吸收机制能逆转导致缺血心肌组织间去甲肾上腺素的聚集，其只与缺血1b期心律失常的发生有关，而与1a期不相关。

缺血后20～30min缺血区去甲肾上腺素的升高即使对完整的心室肌细胞也能诱发早后除极、迟后除极和触发活动[51-53]。在缺血这一阶段细胞内$[Ca^{2+}]$的升高使上述机制进一步强化[4]。

七、牵张作用

牵张引起的电生理变化（机械电反馈）在心律失常发生机制中的重要性正在得到认识[54]。牵张作用在心律失常发生中发挥作用的假说认为，其介导非选择性阳离子牵张激活通道（stretch-activated channels，SACs）携带的激动电流，开启和放大自律性和触发活动[54]。新近发现了这一通道的特异性阻断剂，具有对抗心房颤动的抗心律失常作用，点燃了对该项目的兴趣[55]。然而更为重要的是，实验[56]和理论[57]研究结果支持缺血心肌发生的异常机械变化与缺血性心律失常的发生相关。在麻醉猪，发生缺血性室颤的动物比未发生室颤的动物其缺血区舒张末期节段长度异常的增加更为明显，而且经治疗和其他因素校正后，这一变化是强烈预测心律失常的因子[56]。这一结果提示机械电反馈的参与作用，然而非选择性阳离子SAC阻止剂Gd^{3+}在此模型中未能预防缺血性室颤[56]。这一显著的矛盾可用研究中的Gd^{3+}浓度不足，或存在对Gd^{3+}不敏感的SAC通道，或有不依赖SAC的其他机制参与，如自主神经反射来解释[56]。然而，Coronel与同事[15]证明牵张力在离体血流灌注的猪心导致缺血性心律失常增加，这一过程中并无自主神经的反射参与。作者证明在非工作的心室缺血1b期无心律失常发生，但在机械负荷存在时，心律失常很常见（图44-5）[15]。由于此模型中1b期室颤为主要死因（图44-1B、44-4、和44-5），因而容易看出牵张的关键作用。

八、排除嫌疑犯

令人困惑的是经Langendorff灌流的心脏自发缺血性室颤的发生几率明显低于在体心脏（图44-5A和B）。无论如何，孤立的心脏不应该比原装在机体中的心脏更健康，但是前者对缺血的挑战更有抵抗力。与Coronel和同事[15]的结果一致，我们的实验中6只麻醉猪4只有室颤（66%），而9只离体灌流的心脏仅2只发生了室颤（22%）（$P<0.05$）。究竟什么原因使离体心脏对缺血性室颤有这样的抵抗力？也许我们应该在两种实验的不同条件中寻找答案。Langendorff灌流心脏与在体模型相比缺乏以下已知的候选因素：（1）中枢神经激素的影响；（2）适宜的机械负荷。已有证据表明两种模型中其他心律失常发生因素同样存

在，如离子浓度的偏移和细胞去耦联[15]。事实上缺血1b期的缺血区和边缘带是大多数缺血性触发因素的发生部位，也是去甲肾上腺素的主要来源，但其局部代谢性释放不依赖于中枢刺激[51,52]，削弱了（但未排除）中枢神经机制的作用。而且，在离体心脏尽管去甲肾上腺素高达中毒的浓度，在无心脏负荷时并不发生明显的心律失常。灌流系统中一旦引入室壁压力，1b期室早和室速的发生率迅速达到在体心脏的水平（图44-5C）。但室颤的发生率仍旧较低。因此，离体心脏模型中还遗漏了除牵张以外的因素。一种可能性是中枢介导的儿茶酚胺释放通过选择性缩短了非缺血区的不应期[16]，促进缺血的边缘带除极波碎裂[20]（图44-2），以及有适当的触发因素时对室颤的易感性增强，这对室颤的基质具有重要的意义。还应当提及凝血酶的作用，本章前文已经讨论。然而，凝血酶似乎选择性影响1a期心律失常的发生[32]，猪模型中室颤却多数出现在1b期（图441B）。

因此，与在体的模型相比，在离体血液灌流的猪心模型中，缺血性室颤的发生率低，这容许我们排除体内和体外存在的多种候选机制。这也提示尽管缺血的几乎每项后果均有潜在促心律失常的作用[4]，但鉴别和确定关键因素为目标能够明显降低缺血性室颤的死亡率。为了鉴别缺血性室颤的关键机制，我们需要建立这样的实验模型，容许我们通过选择性引入候选因素，控制缺血性心律失常的类型和发生率。Langendorff灌流猪心脏可为此模型提供好的基础。在此模型中引入机械负荷造成非持续性心律失常但并不使室颤的发生率增加[15]。因此，必须做更多的工作以便在急性心肌缺血实验模型中获取对缺血性室颤更好的控制。

九、结束语

尽管对阻断冠脉血流后所伴发的代谢、电生理和形态结构的改变已进行了大量的研究，这些变化与缺血性室颤启动机制间的联系仍不清楚。本章推理性分析表明只有少数因素对缺血性室颤的发生机理十分关键。

在已知的因素中，用来解释离体灌流模型比在体模型缺血性室颤的发生率更高的现象时，机械牵张和中枢介导的交感刺激是首选因素，因为两种模型中其他促心律失常因素相同。在离体灌流模型引入机械负荷后可以增加室早和室速的发生率。以离体灌流模型

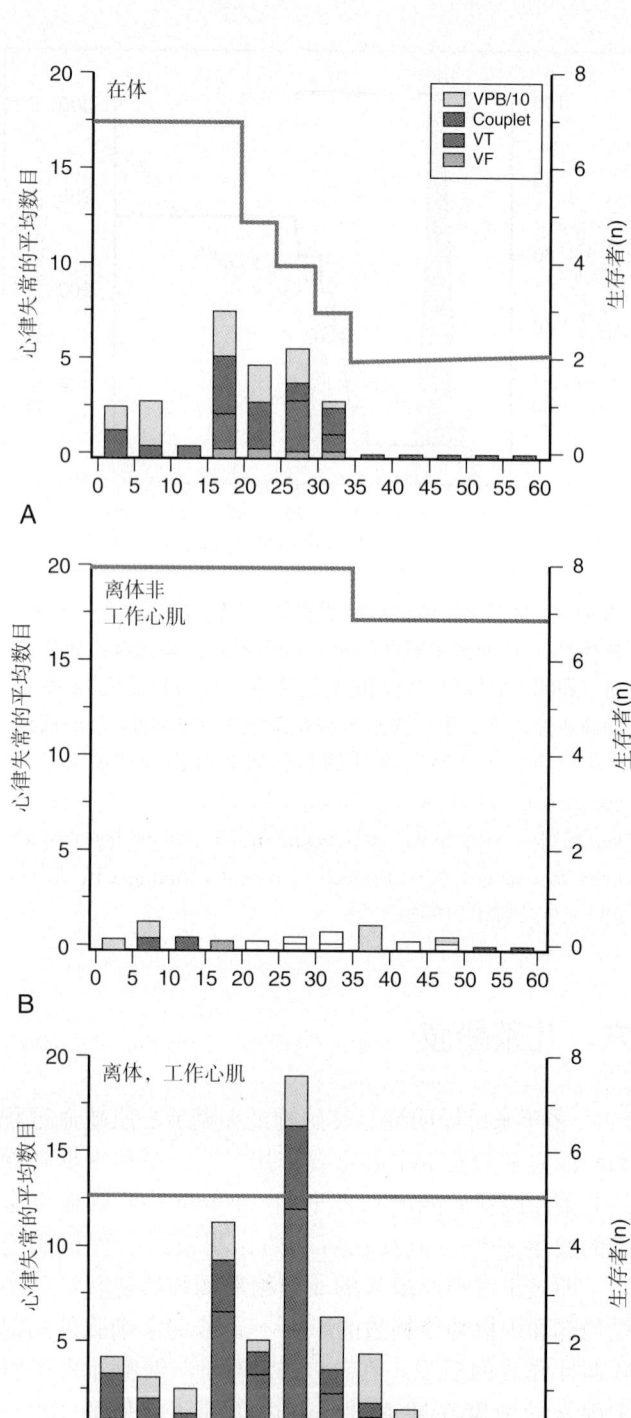

图44-5 心律失常在猪区域性缺血三种模型中的发生率 A：在体心脏；B：离体非工作心脏；C：离体工作心脏。注意与在体模型A相比，离体非工作心脏模型B的缺血性心律失常发生率极低。在离体非心脏灌流模型中引入机械负荷时，能恢复非持续性心律失常的发生率，但室颤（VF）发生率无变化（引自Coronel R, Wilms-Schopman FJG, deGroot JR: Origin of ischemia-induced phase 1b ventricular arrhythmias in pig heart. J Am Coll Cardiol 39：166-176, 2002.）

为基础，我们能选择性地引入其他候选因素，直至完全重复缺血性室颤的发生率，这样才能证明测试的因素与室颤的真正因果关系。

一旦我们在实际的实验模型中能对室颤的发生率进行控制，我们就能在电激动产生和扩布中应用已有的电生理方法全面探测缺血性室颤的电生理机制。

区域性缺血是室颤的主要原因，而整体缺血却是任何部位起源的室颤引起的后果。明显，一旦心律失常发生，激发室颤的同一条件又可降低室颤波的密度并稳定波锋。这一作用可由整体高血钾复制。在设计新的电或电药理结合的抗颤动策略中，应当考虑整体缺血时的促进和抗心律失常的双重作用。

（郭成军　译）

参 考 文 献

1. Janse MJ, Wit AL: Electrophysiological mechanisms of ventricular arrhythmias resulting from myocardial ischemia and infarction. Phys Rev 69:1049–1169, 1989.
2. Chen J, Mandapati R, Berenfeld O, et al: Spatiotemporal organization of ventricular fibrillation increases during global ischemia in the isolated rabbit heart. In Aliot E, Clementy J, Prystowsky EN (eds): Fighting Sudden Cardiac Death: A Worldwide Challenge. Armonk, NY, Futura Publishing, 2000, pp 81–98.
3. Cheng Y, Mowrey KA, Nikolski V, et al: Mechanisms of shock-induced arrhythmogenesis during acute global ischemia. Am J Physiol Heart Circ Physiol 282:H2141–H2151, 2002.
4. Carmeliet E: Cardiac ionic currents and acute ischemia: From channels to arrhythmias. Phys Rev 79:917–1017, 1999.
5. Cascio WE, Johnson TA, Gettes LS: Electrophysiologic changes in ischemic ventricular myocardium: I. Influence of ionic, metabolic and energetic changes. J Cardiovasc Electrophysiol 6:1039–1062, 1995.
6. Aliot E, Clementy J, Prystowsky EN (eds): Fighting Sudden Cardiac Death: A Worldwide Challenge. Armonk, NY, Futura Publishing, 2000.
7. Kaplinsky E, Ogawa S, Blake CW, Dreifus LS: Two periods of early ventricular arrhythmias in the canine acute myocardial infarction model. Circulation 60:397–403, 1979.
8. Curtis MJ: Characterisation, utilisation and clinical relevance of isolated perfused heart models of ischaemia-induced ventricular fibrillation. Cardiovasc Res 39:194–215, 1998.
9. Kabell G, Scherlag BJ, Hope RR, Lazzara R: Regional myocardial blood flow and ventricular arrhythmias following one-stage and two-stage coronary artery occlusion in anethesized dogs. Am Heart J 104:537–544, 1982.
10. Coronel R, Wilms-Schopman FJG, Dekker LRC, Janse MJ: Heterogeneities in $[K^+]_o$ and TQ potential and the inducibility of ventricular fibrillation during acute regional ischemia in the isolated perfused porcine heart. Circulation 92:120–129, 1995.
11. de Groot JR, Wilms-Schopman FJG, Opthof T, et al: Late ventricular arrhythmias during acute regional ischemia in the isolated blood perfused pig heart: Role of electrical cellular uncoupling. Cardiovasc Res 50:362–372, 2001.
12. Janse MJ, van Capelle FJL, Morsink H, et al: Flow of "injury" current and patterns of excitation during early ventricular arrhythmias in acute regional myocardial ischemia is isolated porcine and canine hearts: Evidence for two different arrhythmogenic mechanisms. Circ Res 47:151–165, 1980.
13. Rankovic V, Patel N, Jain S, et al: Characteristics of ischemic and peri-ischemic regions during ventricular fibrillation in the canine heart. J Cardiovasc Electrophysiol 10:1090–1100, 1999.
14. Zhang S, Skinner JL, Sims AL, et al: Three-dimensional mapping of spontaneous ventricular arrhythmias in a canine thrombotic coronary occlusion model. J Cardiovasc Electrophysiol 11:762–772, 2000.
15. Coronel R, Wilms-Schopman FJG, deGroot JR: Origin of ischemia-induced phase 1b ventricular arrhythmias in pig hearts. J Am Coll Cardiol 39:166–176, 2002.
16. Opthof T, Coronel R, Vermeulen JT, et al: Dispersion of refractoriness in normal and ischaemic canine ventricle: effects of sympathetic stimulation. Cardiovasc Res 27:1954–1960, 1993.
17. Cascio WE: Myocardial ischemia: What factors determine arrhythmogenesis? J Cardiovasc Electrophysiol 12:726–729, 2001.
18. Coronel R, Fiolet JWT, Wilms-Schopman FJG, et al: Distribution of extracellular potassium and its relation to electrophysiologic changes during acute myocardial ischemia in the isolated porcine heart. Circulation 77:1125–1138, 1988.
19. Shaw RM, Rudy Y: Electrophysiologic effects of acute myocardial ischemia: A mechanistic investigation of action potential conduction and conduction failure. Circ Res 80:124–139, 1997.
20. Zaitsev AV, Sarmast F, Kolli A, et al: Wavebreak formation during ventricular fibrillation in the isolated, regionally ischemic pig heart. Circ Res 92:546–553, 2003.
21. Coronel R, Wilms-Schopman FJ, Opthof T, et al: Injury current and gradients of diastolic stimulation threshold, TQ potential, and extracellular potassium concentration during acute regional ischemia in the isolated perfused pig heart. Circ Res 68:1241–1249, 1991.
22. Katzung BG, Hondeghem LM, Grant AO: Letter: Cardiac ventricular automaticity induced by current of injury. Pflugers Arch 360:193–197, 1975.
23. Kumar R, Joyner RW: An experimental model of the production of early after depolarizations by injury current from an ischemic region. Pflugers Arch 428:425–432, 1994.
24. Nordrehaug JE, Johanessen HA, von der Lippe G: Serum potassium concentration as a risk factor of ventricular arrhythmias early in acute myocardial infarction. Circulation 71:645–649, 1985.
25. Gray R, Pertsov AM, Jalife J: Spatial and temporal organization during cardiac fibrillation. Nature 392:75–78, 1998.
26. Jones JL, Tovar OH: Electrophysiology of ventricular fibrillation and defibrillation. Crit Care Med 28:N219–N221, 2000.
27. Ujhelyi MR, Schur M, Frede T, et al: Differential effects of lidocaine on defibrillation threshold with monophasic versus biphasic shock waveforms. Circulation 92:1644–1650, 1995.
28. Tovar OH, Jones JL: Electrophysiologic deterioration after one-minute fibrillation increases relative biphasic defibrillation efficacy. J Cardiovasc Electrophysiol 11:645–651, 2000.
29. Walcott GP, Melnick SB, Chapman FW, et al: Relative efficacy of monophasic and biphasic waveforms for transthoracic defibrillation after short and long durations of ventricular fibrillation. Circulation 98:2210–2215, 1998.
30. Libby P, Ridker PM, Maseri A: Inflammation and atherosclerosis. Circulation 105:1135–1143, 2002.
31. Goldstein JA, Butterfield MC, Ohnishi Y, et al: Arrhythmogenic influence of intracoronary thrombosis during acute myocardial ischemia. Circulation 90:139–147, 1994.
32. Coronel R, Wilms-Schopman FJG, Janse MJ: Profibrillatory effects of intracoronary thrombus in acute regional ischemia of the in situ porcine heart. Circulation 96:3985–3991, 1997.
33. Harris AS: Delayed development of ventricular ectopic rhythms following experimental coronary occlusion. Circulation 1:1318–1328, 1950.
34. McHowat J, Creer MH: Thrombin activates a membrane-associated calcium-independent PLA2 in ventricular myocytes. Am J Physiol 274:C447–C454, 1998.
35. McHowat J, Creer MH: Lysophosphatidylcholine accumulation in cardiomyocytes requires thrombin activation of Ca^{2+}-independent PLA2. Am J Physiol 272:H1972–H1980, 1997.
36. Shander GS, Undrovinas AI, Makielski JC: Rapid onset of lysophosphatidilecholine-induced modification of whole cell cardiac sodium current kinetics. J Mol Cell Cardiol 28:743–753, 1996.
37. Yan GX, Park TH, Corr PB: Activation of thrombin receptor increases intracellular Na^+ during myocardial ischemia. Am J Physiol 268:H1740–H1748, 1995.
38. Avkiran M, Haworth RS: Regulation of cardiac sarcolemmal Na^+/H^+ exchanger activity by endogenous ligands: Relevance to ischemia. Ann N Y Acad Sci 874:335–345, 1999.
39. Pinet C, Le Grand B, John GW, Coulombe A: Thrombin facilitation of voltage-gated sodium channel activation in human cardiomyocytes:

Implications for ischemic sodium loading. Circulation 106:2098–2103, 2002.
40. Burt JM: Block of intercellular communication: Interaction of intracellular H$^+$ and Ca^{2+}. Am J Physiol 352:C607–C612, 1987.
41. White RL, Doeller JE, Versellis VK, Wittenberg BA: Gap junctional conductance between pairs of ventricular myocytes is modulated synergistically by H$^+$ and Ca^{++}. J Gen Physiol 95:1061–1075, 1990.
42. Wu J, McHowat J, Saffitz JE, et al: Inhibition of gap junctional conductance by long-chain acylcarnitines and their preferential accumulation in junctional sarcolemma during hypoxia. Circ Res 72:879–889, 1993.
43. Beardslee MA, Lerner DL, Tadros PN, et al: Dephosphorylation and intracellular redistribution of ventricular connexin43 during electrical uncoupling induced by ischemia. Circ Res 87:656–662, 2000.
44. Cinca J, Warren M, Carreno A, et al: Changes in myocardial electrical impedance induced by coronary artery occlusion in pigs with and without preconditioning: Correlation with local ST-segment potential and ventricular arrhythmias. Circulation 96:3079–3086, 1997.
45. Smith WT, Fleet WF, Johnson TA, et al: The 1b phase of ventricular arrhythmias in ischemic in situ porcine heart is related to changes in cell-to-cell electrical coupling. Circulation 92:3051–3060, 1995.
46. Lerner DL, Yamada KA, Schuessler B, Saffitz JE: Accelerated onset and increased incidence of ventricular arrhythmias induced by ischemia in Cx43-deficient mice. Circulation 101:547–552, 2000.
47. Saiz, Ferrero JM Jr, Monserrat M, et al: Influence of electrical coupling on early afterdepolarizations in ventricular myocytes. IEEE Trans Biomed Eng 46:138–147, 1999.
48. Corr PB, Gillis RA: Autonomic neural influences on the disrhythmias resulting from myocardial infarction. Circ Res 43:1–9, 1978.
49. Lown B, Verrier RL: Neural activity and ventricular fibrillation. N Engl J Med 294:1165–1170, 1976.
50. Malliani A, Schwartz PJ, Zanchetti A: Neural mechanisms in life-threatening arrhythmias. Am Heart J 100:705–715, 1980.
51. Schomig A: Catecholamines in myocardial ischemia: Systemic and cardiac release. Circulation 82(Suppl 3):II13–22, 1990.
52. Lameris TW, de Zeeuw S, Alberts G, et al: Time course and mechanism of myocardial catecholamine release during transient ischemia in vivo. Circulation 101:2645–2650, 2000.
53. Priori SG, Corr PB: Mechanisms underlying early and delayed afterdepolarizations induced by catecholamines. Am J Physiol 258:H1796–H1805, 1990.
54. Sachs F: Mechanoelectric transduction. In Zipes DP, Jalife J (eds): Cardiac Electrophysiology: From Cell to Bedside. Philadelphia, WB Saunders, 2004.
55. Bode F, Sachs F, Franz MR: Tarantula peptide inhibits atrial fibrillation. Nature 409:35–36, 2001.
56. Barrabes JA, Garcia-Dorado D, Padilla F, et al: Ventricular fibrillation during acute coronary occlusion is related to the dilation of the ischemic region. Basic Res Cardiol 97:445–451, 2002.
57. Kohl P, Hunter P, Noble D: Stretch-induced changes in heart rate and rhythm: Clinical observations, experiments and mathematical models. Prog Biophys Mol Biol 71:91–138, 1999.

第 45 章

除颤的细胞机制

Vladimir G. Fast

本章目录

- 电击诱导 ΔVm 的决定因素 ············ 403
- 细胞培养中进行除颤诱导 ΔVm 的
  光学标测 ································ 404
- 组织微观结构在 ΔVm 中的作用 ······ 404
- 非线性 ΔVm 的离子机制 ··············· 406
- 完整心肌的壁内 ΔVm ··················· 408
- 结论 ··· 411

目前，终止室颤的唯一可靠方法是给心脏强大的电击。尽管这种方法在临床实践和实验中被广泛应用，但其除颤机制仍未阐明。通常认为电击通过直接使可兴奋心肌瞬间除极终止颤动[1]。刚被激动的心肌组织形成一个功能阻滞区，从而阻断了激动波的扩布并使颤动终止。此外，通过使电击时处于不应状态心肌的动作电位时程（APD）和不应期延长也有助于颤动波的终止[2]。虽然大家公认这两种作用都是细胞膜电位（Vm）发生改变的结果，但关键的问题是这种变化（ΔVm）如何产生的。首要的问题是远离组织-电极或组织-液体交界处的心肌组织其 ΔVm 如何引起？为了使除颤成功，一个重要的条件是电击必须使临界质量的心肌组织发生改变，这个临界质量约为心脏总质量的 80%～90%[3,4]。然而，根据经典的电缆模型，由均一细胞外电场产生的 ΔVm 应该局限在除颤电击部位的附近。随着距除颤电极距离的增加，ΔVm 将呈指数样衰减，从而使大面积心肌并不受电击的影响。接下来的一个重要问题是电击导致的 ΔVm 如何演变，其演变过程最终决定了 ΔVm 的大小和模式，从而决定了除颤的效果。

一、电击诱导 ΔVm 的决定因素

在静息状态的组织中，当外部电流通过细胞膜时 Vm 将发生变化。如果这种电流不是来自除颤电极或组织-液体交界面，那么它被称为继发源或虚拟电极。这两个名字也能用来区别并命名由这些电流来源造成的 ΔVm。可激动组织的理论和数学模型显示继发电流来源和由此导致的 ΔVm 可以通过两种机制引起。第一个机制认为 ΔVm 和除颤电击引起的不均一电场有关[5,6]。在该机制中，局部电流来源的强度和细胞外电场的第一空间导数成正比。第二个机制认为 ΔVm 和电阻性组织的特性不均一有关。在这种机制中，电流来源的强度和电场强度成正比。这种由电阻性不均一引起的电流来源可能由组织结构的变化而引起，而组织结构的变化又由解剖学的不连续[7]或纤维的扭转而引起[8]。

这两种继发电源的机制并不互相排斥，而是不同情况时各自分别占主导地位。非均一场理论被认为在小的电极刺激组织情况时起重要作用。在这种情况下，非均一场理论是导致除颤呈狗骨（dog bone）模式的原因，并可以解释激动的终止[9]。此外，在容易形成强大电场梯度的情况时，例如通过电极导管进行电击，非均一场也在除颤过程中起作用[10]。在电场分布更加均一的情况下，例如通过巨大的金属板电极进行经胸除颤的过程中，非均一电阻理论被认为比非均一场理论起着更重要的作用。

由于多种原因，很难明确心脏 Vm 变化的确切机

制。目前在方法学一个主要的障碍是在三维心肌中无法在空间精确地测量 Vm。即使能够获得三维 Vm 的数据，解释这些数据也存在问题。事实上，在一个细胞外间隙十分有限的组织中，Vm 的变化和细胞外电场的变化相辅相成。因此，由组织结构的非均一导致的 ΔVm 必然引起电场的非均一，从而造成类似"鸡生蛋还是蛋生鸡"的问题。由于心脏结构的复杂性使 ΔVm 很难和特定的结构联系起来，而且细胞膜的电导并不恒定，而是和 Vm 呈非线性时间依赖关系，导致 ΔVm 的解释将变得更加复杂。由于除颤-组织之间相互作用的复杂性，因此直到最近发展出计算机模型之前，有关心脏组织 Vm 变化机制的详尽研究十分有限[7,11-13]。随着新的研究手段的出现，即联合利用"patterned growth"细胞培养和高分辨率的 Vm 光学标测，这些问题才得到部分解决。

二、细胞培养中进行除颤诱导 ΔVm 的光学标测

利用细胞培养研究除颤-组织之间的相互作用有几个重要的优点。培养的细胞呈二维单层生长，避免了完整组织的三维复杂性。培养细胞的结构可以在亚细胞水平进行精确定位，并且正好能和电生理参数联系在一起，细胞外离子环境和电场分布也可以精确控制和测量。细胞培养最重要的优点是可以通过"patterned cell growth"技术对单层几何学结构按所需的方式进行改造，从而使结构和功能关系的研究成为可能。目前已经发展了许多生长技术，从而对心脏中存在的各种结构进行复制，包括细胞条、几何学扩展[14,15]、分歧[16]和各向异性模式[17,18]。细胞培养物的电生理特性，如传导速度和最大上升支的上升速度都与成体心室组织中测量的结果相同[19]。当然，细胞培养物也和成体组织存在不同之处，包括细胞较小、细胞周围的缝隙连接分布更加均一以及离子通道表达水平的不同[20]。在分析除颤效果时，这些差异都应当考虑。

通过利用 Vm 敏感性染料和光学探测器阵列，可以对细胞培养物的 Vm 反应进行多部位的监测，并且可以达到亚细胞水平和高时间分辨率。光学标测已广泛用于心脏激动研究的各个方面[21]。最近，这种方法用来对心肌细胞培养物中的除颤诱导 Vm 反应进行显微标测[16,22-26]。和电学标测不同，光学标测可以反映 Vm 的变化并且能对抗除颤伪差的干扰，因此它特别适合于这类研究。最近，在一系列研究中采用了这种方法。这些研究集中在电场-组织相互作用的以下两个方面：（1）组织微观结构在诱导性 ΔVm 中的作用；（2）离子膜特性在 ΔVm 动力学中的作用。

三、组织微观结构在 ΔVm 中的作用

在不同观察水平下，心脏是由多种具有结构非均一性的组织构成。在最微观的水平，心脏组织由单个细胞组成，这些细胞与细胞之间的边界构成电流运动的电阻屏障，从而成为形成 ΔVm 的基质。在比较宏观的水平，由于血管和结缔组织的分割，细胞之间有很多的间隙。在更宏观的水平，这些组织构成细胞束，而细胞层则稀疏地分布在细胞束之间。为了评价各种结构对诱导性 ΔVm 的作用，必须在细胞培养物中将它们分别复制出来。

（一）细胞边界的作用

细胞边界是心肌中最常见的一种不连续结构的类型。因此，最初将它们作为引起心脏除颤诱导性 ΔVm 的最可能原因毫不奇怪[7,11]。这种机制是在综合了周期性电阻屏障的一维电缆模型中发现。在这种模型中，Vm 的变化似乎呈周期性（锯齿样）震荡，即在电阻性屏障的一侧出现阴性 ΔVm，而在另一侧出现阳性 ΔVm。目前已经在培养的细胞条上采用光学标测在亚细胞水平对这种假说进行了检验[22]。

细胞边界在除颤诱导性 ΔVm 中的作用已经在窄细胞条（宽 30～60μm）中加以研究。由于细胞边缘的影响，细胞沿细胞条的轴线排列。均一的细胞外除颤电场沿着轴线作用于细胞条，同时利用分辨率为 6μm 的二极管测量 Vm 的变化。图 45-1 显示了细胞边界的除颤诱导性 ΔVm 的典型图像。继发源被认为在通过细胞边界时 ΔVm 从阳性变为阴性的变化过程中起了作用。然而，实验并没有发现这种极性的改变。在标测野的所有记录部位，细胞膜在除颤期间都处于超极化状态。并且位于相邻细胞间的局部记录也没有发现 ΔVm 强度的变化。

对继发源锯齿理论和实验结果之间差异的一个可能的解释是用于描述微观传导的"横向平均"效应[19]。锯齿理论假设轴向电流被迫穿过各细胞间隙，从而引起巨大的电压降。然而，在二维组织中，一部分轴向电流可以绕过某一间隙而从侧面的细胞连接通过。在细胞培养物中，由于细胞周围缝隙连接的分布比较均匀，因此这种平均效应可能特别明显[18]。在成

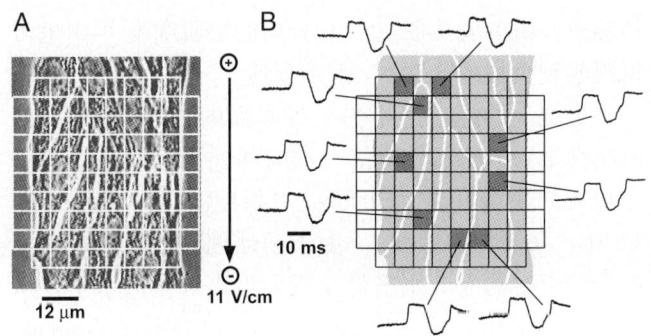

图 45-1 细胞边界在电击诱导 ΔVm 中的作用 A：采用叠加光电二极管阵列栅格制作的相位对照成像。B：对于在细胞边界测量的电击诱导 ΔVm 进行的光学标测记录。最初的正向部分代表了动作电位的上升支，而负向部分是由电击造成的（引自 Gillis AM，Fast VG，Rohr S，Kleber AG：Effects of defibrillation shocks on the spatial distribution of the transmembrane potential in strands and monolayers of cultured neonatal rat ventricular myocytes. Cir Res 79：676-690，1996）

体心肌中，细胞边界的 ΔVm 可能较大，因为细胞较大而且缝隙连接更加集中地分布在细胞端对端的连接。在分离的端对端连接的成对细胞中，检测到的 ΔVm 较小[27]。然而，在整体的三维组织中，这种效果将被众多的侧侧连接所抵消。在兔乳头肌中，利用一个放在亚细胞平台上的游动微电极对 Vm 变化的测量结果并没有发现微观继发源[28]，这进一步证实了来自细胞培养物实验的结论。

（二）细胞间隙的作用

细胞间隙是心肌中另一种常见的解剖结构不连续的类型。在数个细胞长度，即数百微米的水平这种间隙是由血管和结缔组织而造成细胞间连续性的中断。在具有各种大小的模式细胞间隙的单层细胞中，研究者对这种不连续性对 Vm 的影响进行了研究[23]。

图 45-2 显示了一次电击对大小约为 $240 \times 60 \mu m$ 的细胞间隙 Vm 的作用。在这个例子中，ΔVm 的分布和继发源理论一致。在某一除颤极性下（图 45-2A 和 B），细胞间隙一侧的细胞呈阳性极化，而另一侧细胞呈阴性极化，分别相对于电源和电穴（sinks）。当除颤极性反转时，阳性极化和阴性极化区域也随着反转（图中没有显示）。ΔVm 的大小随着间隙长度的增加而增大。据估计，引起舒张期（25mV）细胞兴奋所必需的 ΔVm 阈值可以在间隙长度为 $171 \pm 7 \mu m$ 并且除颤平均强度为 8.5V/cm 时达到。在舒张期给予这种电击时，可以直接引起间隙附近的细胞发生兴奋

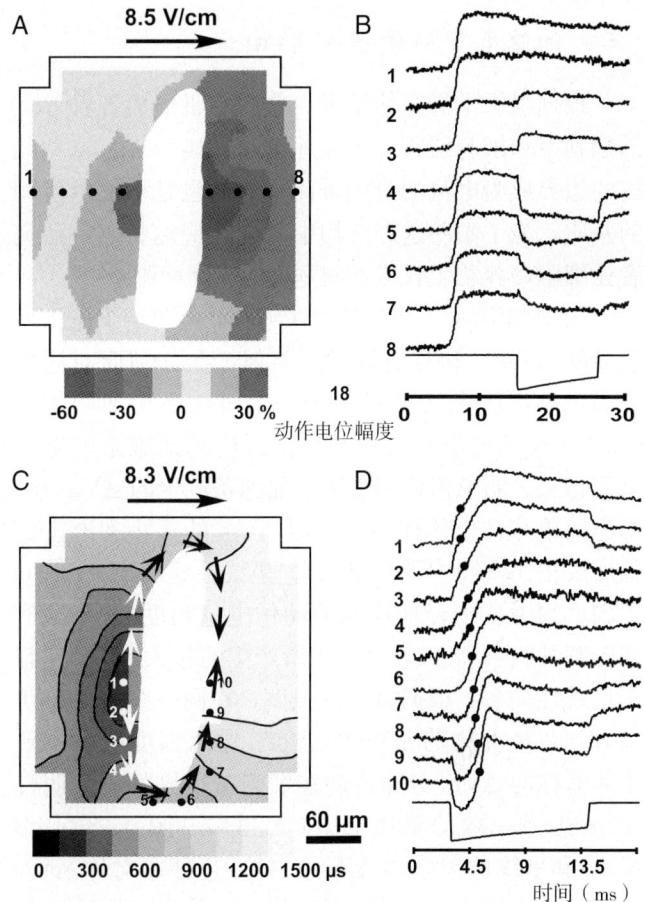

图 45-2 细胞间隙在电击诱导 ΔVm 和组织激动中的作用
A 和 B：极性相反时电击诱导 ΔVm 的等势标测。中间的白色区域表示细胞间隙。轮廓对应于光电二极管阵列的边界。C 和 D：来自舒张期电击产生继发源形成的激动扩布的等时标测。箭头提示激动扩布的方向。激动时间通过标测区域中最早激动的时间来确定（引自 Fast VG，Rohr S，Gillis AM，Kleber AG：Activation of cardiac tissue by extracellular clefts in monolayers of cultured myocytes. Cir Res 82：375-385，1998.）（见彩图 22）

（图 45-2C），而在动作电位（AP）平台期给予电击的细胞则发生阳性极化。在间隙的另一侧，电击最初使细胞超极化，然后再被扩布的激动波除极（图 45-2D）。平均强度为 8.2V/m 的电击直接导致细胞兴奋所需要的临界间隙长度在 $84 \sim 196 \mu m$ 之间，这个数字和由 AP 平台期除颤诱导性 ΔVm 的测量数值一致。几百微米直至更大尺寸的不连续性在心室肌中很常见。在人体心脏的梳状肌中，这种大小的结缔组织间隔可见于年轻人的心室组织中，而更大一些（最大 1mm）的组织间隔可见于老年人中[29]。在细胞培养物中的研究显示这种间隙可能影响到心脏的兴奋和除颤过程。

(三) 细胞条中的诱导性 ΔVm

根据组织学研究的结果，壁内心肌形成各种厚度的细胞束和细胞层并且稀疏地相互连接[30,31]。这些结构的边界成为电流通过的屏障，从而也是形成继发源的基质。为了阐明这种结构中 Vm 反应的特点，研究者让细胞培养物生长成不同宽度的线性细胞条[24]。

图 45-3 显示了细胞条中在 AP 平台期给予电击所诱导的 ΔVm。和其他继发源类似，在分别面对阴极和阳极的细胞条的相对两侧产生阳性极化和阴性极化。ΔVm 的形态和大小与电击强度和细胞条的宽度密切相关。弱电击作用于狭窄细胞条产生的 ΔVm 小，形态简单并且呈线性关系，即 ΔVm 的大小和电击的强度成正比（图中没有显示）。呈线性膜反应的 ΔVm 范围大约为从平台期算起的动作电位幅度的 ±40%。在较宽细胞条和/或较强电击所产生的较大 ΔVm 明显不呈线性关系。根据电击的强度，在同一细胞条中可以看到两种类型的非线性 ΔVm。中等强度的电击产生非对称的 ΔVm 分布，即在细胞条边界的一端阴性 ΔVm 比另一端的阳性 ΔVm 大很多（图 45-3B，细线）。和呈线性关系的 ΔVm 一样，这种非对称 ΔVm 的波形也表现为简单的形状。此外，在其他组织中包括豚鼠心脏的乳头肌[32,33]和分离的心肌细胞[34]中也可以观察到类似的非对称 ΔVm 反应。

更强大的电击产生另一种类型的 ΔVm 反应，此时阴性 ΔVm 表现为非单一的时间曲线，即在最初一个较大的超极化之后跟随一个阳性的 Vm 偏移（图 45-3B，灰线和粗黑线）。由于阳性偏移的结果，因此电击结束时的 Vm 水平低于较弱电击产生的水平，从而极大地减轻了 ΔVm 的非对称性。当阴性 ΔVm 的峰值大约超过动作电位幅度的 200% 时就能观察到这种 ΔVm 波形（图 45-3C）。这些结果提示电击期间膜电导不是恒定的，而是沿 Vm-时间曲线而变化。

四、非线性 ΔVm 的离子机制

(一) 非对称 ΔVm 的机制

非对称 ΔVm 是指阴性 ΔVm 大于阳性 ΔVm，其反映了膜电流平衡时的外向偏移。因此，可以推测 ΔVm 非对称和外向钾离子流有关，并且应用钾通道阻滞剂应该减轻 ΔVm 非对称的程度。然而，和这种推测恰好相反，应用钾通道阻滞剂氯化钡（内向整流电流）、多菲利特（延迟整流电流）和 4-氨基吡啶（短暂外向电流）并没有减轻 ΔVm 非对称性[24,35]，提示这些外向电流和 ΔVm 非对称性无关。

令人感到意外的是，应用钙通道阻滞剂可以逆转 ΔVm 的非对称性。图 45-4 显示硝苯地平在线状细胞条中对除颤诱导性 ΔVm 的效果。在对照组，最大阴性 ΔVm 平均超过最大阳性 ΔVm 的 2.52±0.5 倍（图 45-4D）。应用硝苯地平可使最大阳性 ΔVm 大大增强，而阴性 ΔVm 仅发生轻微的变化（图 45-4A 和 C）。这使平均非对称率降低到 1.62±0.2（$P<0.001$）（图 45-4D）。

硝苯地平对 ΔVm 的作用提示 ΔVm 非对称性是由除极部分细胞条的外向 I_{Ca} 引起。在生理范围的 Vm，I_{Ca} 为内向电流，而一旦 Vm 超过 I_{Ca} 反转电位时，就变成外向电流。根据膜片钳的研究结果，大鼠和家兔的 I_{Ca} 反转电位为 45~50mV[36,37]。因此，当阳性 ΔVm 幅度超过 45~50mV 时，它必然由于外向 I_{Ca} 而降低，从而解释了硝苯地平对阳性 ΔVm 的作用。

ΔVm 非对称效应在整体心脏除颤中可能具有重要的意义。在室颤时，大部分心肌处于除极化状态。因此，可以推测除颤电击对 Vm 的效果是非对称性的，即大部分心肌发生阴性而不是阳性 Vm 变化。众所周知，超极化和除极化区域的相互作用能导致波

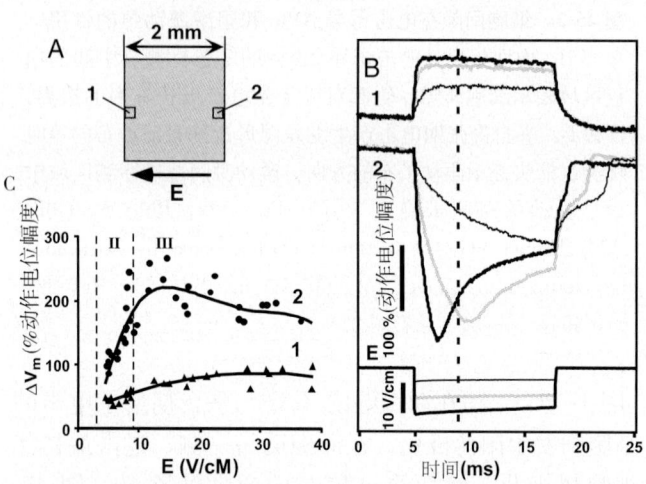

图 45-3 细胞条中电击诱导的 ΔVm A：细胞条和位于细胞条两侧的光电二极管的草图。B：不同强度的电击期间在细胞条边界处记录的 ΔVm。C：在细胞条相对两侧记录到的最大阳性和阴性 ΔVm 与电击强度的关系。垂直虚线将单纯非对称性 ΔVm（Ⅱ）和非单一 ΔVm（Ⅲ）区域分隔开来（引自 Fast VG, Rohr S, Ideker RE: Non-linear changes of transmembrane potential caused by defibrillation shocks in strands of cultured myocytes. Am J Physiol Heart Circ Physiol 278: H688-697, 2000)

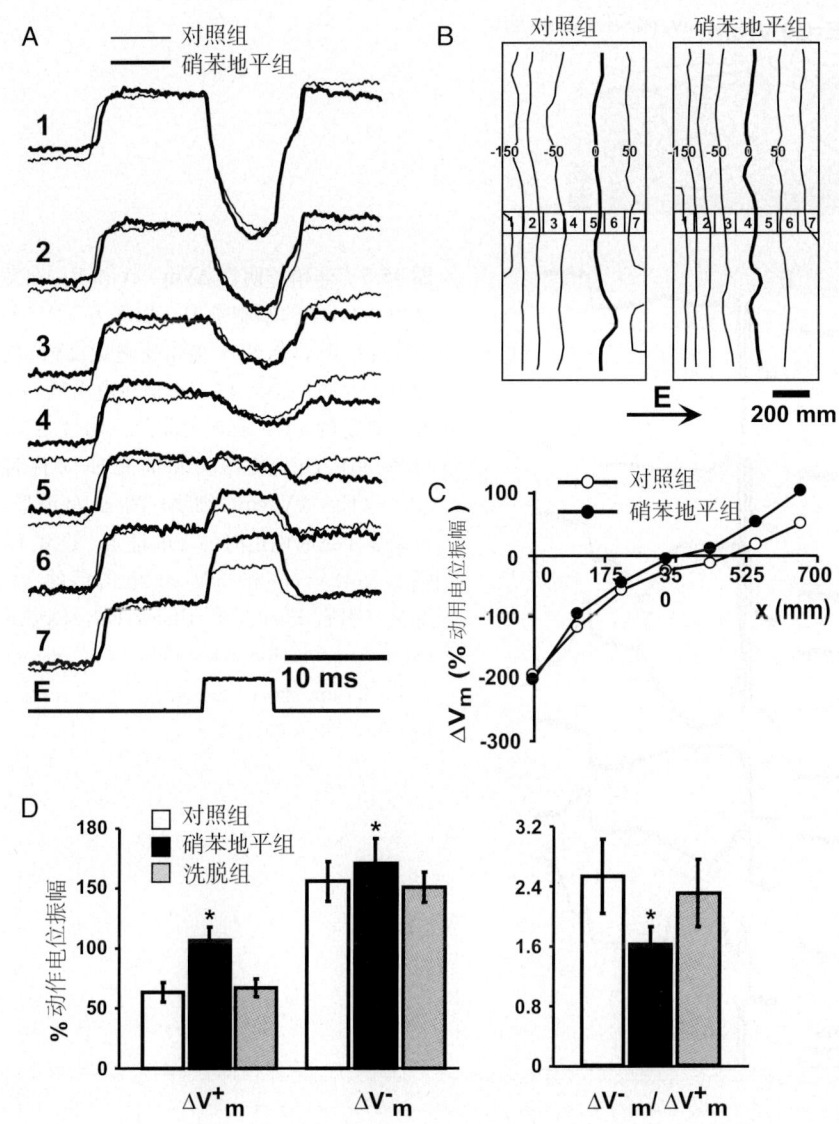

图 45-4 Ca^{2+} 电流在非对称性 ΔVm 中的作用 A：在宽度为 0.8mm 的细胞条中，来自选择性二极管和对照组以及硝苯地平组除颤波形的光学标测记录。相应的电击强度为 10.8 和 10.6V/cm。B：电击 5ms 之内 ΔVm 分布的等电位标测。粗线代表 0 等值线，它将除极化和超极化区域分隔开来。C：整个细胞条 ΔVm 的空间曲线。D：在 8 个细胞条中，当电击强度为 9.3±0.8V/cm 时硝苯地平对阳性 ΔVm、阴性 ΔVm 和非对称比率阳性 ΔVm/阴性 ΔVm 的影响（引自 Cheek ER，Ideker RE，Fast VG：Non-linear changes of transmembrane potential during defibrillation shocks：Role of Ca^{2+} current. Cir Res 87：453-459，2000.）

的碎裂和除颤失败[10]。由于 ΔVm 的非对称性决定了超极化和除极化区域的大小和形状，因此它必然影响除颤的效果。这个过程有可能应用药物进行调节，从而提高除颤效果。

（二）非单一阴性 ΔVm 的机制

以下两种原因都可以造成强大电击诱导性超极化后 Vm 的阳性偏移：(1) 激活超极化诱导性内向离子流或 (2) 膜电转导致非特异性内向电流。在巨大阴性 Vm 时存在两种内向电流：内向整流电流（I_{kl}）和超极化诱导性电流（I_f）[38]，后者在阳极碎裂中的作用在前面已经提到[39]。研究人员采用相应的通道阻滞剂对 I_f 和 I_{kl} 电流在 ΔVm 中的作用进行了观察[40]。结果发现给予 4mM 的氯化铯（I_f 阻断剂）或 0.4mM 的氯化钡（I_{kl} 阻断剂）后阴性 ΔVm 没有变化，提示这些电流和非单一阴性 Vm 反应无关。

非单一阴性 Vm 反应的另一种解释是膜的电转作用。一个观察电转的直接方法是在电击时将细胞暴露在不能通过细胞膜的荧光染料中，并且测量电击诱导细胞摄取染料的情况。最近，研究人员采用这种技术在培养的单层细胞中利用 Lucifer yellow 染料进行研究[26]。结果发现在细胞条上多次给予强度达 50V/cm 的电击后，没有检测到染料的摄取，即使这种电击产生了非常明显的非单一阴性 ΔVm。文献报道中检测膜电转的另一种方法是测量电击后舒张期 Vm[41,42]。研究人员用这种方法观察在细胞培养物中进行电击后的效果。图 45-5 比较了两种电击强度分别产生单一和非单一阴性 ΔVm 波形的效果。在较弱的电击期间（图 45-5C，细线），阴性 ΔVm 波形呈单一形态（线条 1～4），Vm 逐渐下降直至电击结束。电击后的 Vm 记

408　第八部分　心律失常发生的机制

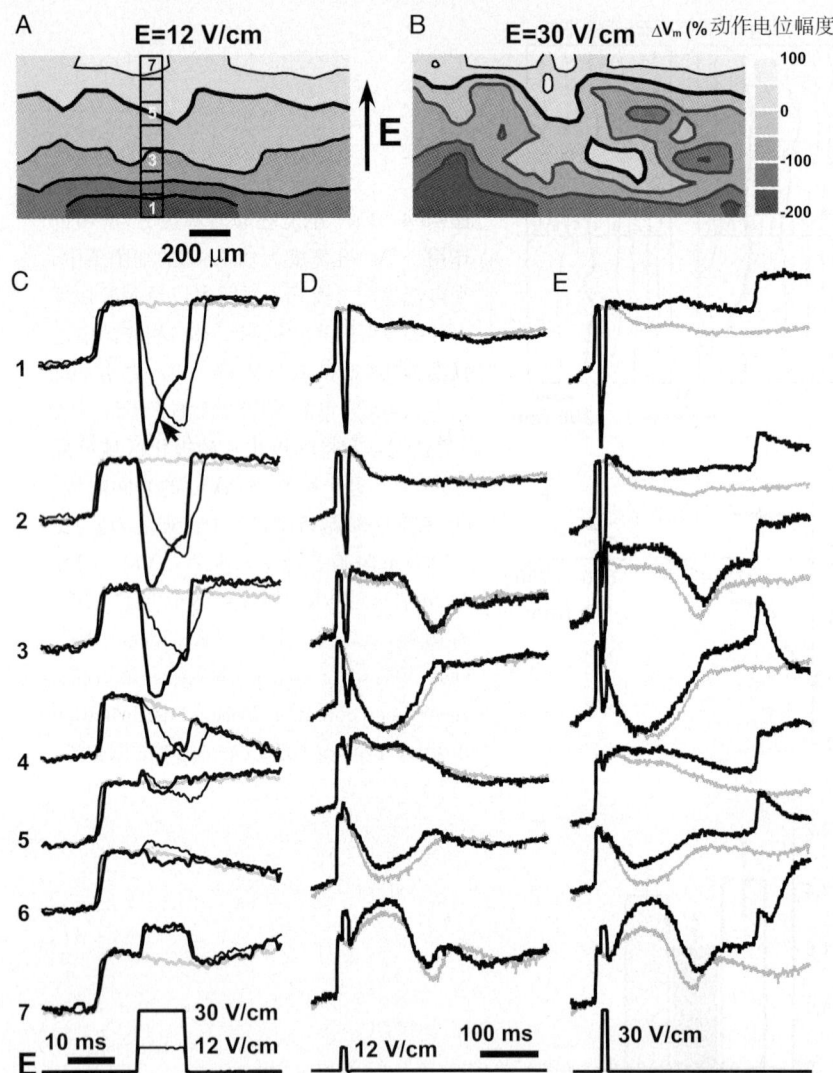

图 45-5　非单一阴性 ΔVm　A 和 B：在宽度为 0.8mm 的细胞条中，强度为 12V/cm（A）和 30V/cm（B）电击所造成 ΔVm 的等电位标测。ΔVm 的大小是在电击后 5ms 开始测量的。C：表现为非单一阴性 ΔVm（E＝30V/cm，粗线）和简单非对称性 ΔVm（E＝12V/cm，细线）的 ΔVm 波形。灰线表示没有电击时的 Vm 记录。D 和 E：强度为 12V/cm 和 30V/cm 电击后的 Vm 变化（引自 Fast VG, Cheek ER：Optical mapping of arrhythmias induced by strong defibrillation shocks in myocyte cultures. Cir Res 90：664-670，2002.）

录结果（图 45-5D）显示这种电击没有影响舒张期 Vm。相反，较强电击产生的阴性 ΔVm 波形呈非单一形态（图 45-5C，粗线）：在最初巨大的超极化（线条 1～3）之后紧接着 Vm 向更阳性的方向明显偏移（≈120％动作电位幅度）。在对电击和不电击后 Vm 的记录进行比较后（图 45-5E）提示这种电击导致舒张期 Vm 增大。除此之外，电击还能诱发一次额外收缩（图 45-5E）。

尽管关于舒张期 Vm 的数据没有根据电转或离子流调节对膜电导改变的两种机制进行区分，但是电转似乎是一种更有可能性的解释。事实上，电击后离子通道变化持续数秒钟的可能性不大，而此时却能观察到 Vm 增大。在这种情况时，染料摄取测量结果阴性可能和测量敏感度不足，以及电转时间较短从而使进入细胞的染料分子不足以被检测到有关。

五、完整心肌的壁内 ΔVm

上述细胞培养物中的研究显示电击期间 Vm 的改变可能是微观水平组织结构不连续的结果，并且 ΔVm 和非线性的模特性密切相关。一个重要的问题是如何将这些发现应用到完整心肌中，尤其是左心室的心肌。最近有一个研究对这个问题进行了探讨，研究人员测量了冠状动脉灌注的分离左心室标本的壁内 ΔVm[43]。即给予室壁不同强度的方波电击，同时采用光学标测技术从室壁表面以每个二极管 1.2mm 的分辨率标测电击诱导的 ΔVm。

这些研究结果显示了整体心肌研究和细胞培养物研究的重要相似性和明显的区别。和细胞培养物研究类似，弱电击（≈2V/cm 或更弱）产生相对简单的 ΔVm 模式，即在面向阴极的组织边缘产生阳性 ΔVm，而在面向阳极的边缘产生阴性 ΔVm。最大阳

性 ΔVm 和阴性 ΔVm 大小相似，并且通常在室壁边缘产生。在边缘之间，室壁中央的除极化基本上检测不到，而两侧 ΔVm 的大小相对逐渐移行。弱电击导致阳性 ΔVm 区域的 APD 延长，而阴性 ΔVm 区域基本不变或变化很小。

逐渐增加电击强度时出现两种类型的壁内 ΔVm，这取决于电击的强度。图 45-6A 和 B 显示了 8.8V/cm 电击的效果，和较弱电击相比有 4 方面不同：(1) 强电击在壁内产生局部 ΔVm，其极性随电击的极性而改变。其中一个这样的区域只在标测区域的左下部分的心外膜出现（图 45-6B，位置 13）。这种孤立的除极以及整体上跨壁 ΔVm 的不均一分布明确地提示存在壁内继发源。(2) 和细胞培养物研究结果类似，壁内除极模式明显呈非对称性，即阴性 ΔVm 远大于阳性 ΔVm，并且阴性 ΔVm 占据的区域远比阳性 ΔVm 所占据的区域大。(3) 和细胞培养物研究结果相反，左室壁组织中阴性 ΔVm 可以向阴极边缘延伸。(4) 电击使跨阳性 ΔVm 和阴性 ΔVm 室壁所有部位的 APD 均延长（图 45-6A）。

继续增加电击强度产生的 ΔVm，其模式更加偏离预期的行为。一次 26V/cm 电击引起整个跨壁表面均为负性的除极化（图 45-6D），并且和电击极性无关（图中没有显示结果）。此外，电击使所有部位的 APD 均延长，而无论电击极性或局部的 ΔVm 如何（图 45-6C）。

因此，这些实验提示电击事实上引起左心室壁的壁内 ΔVm，并且可以出现两种类型：极性随电击极性而变化的局部非对称性 ΔVm 和总体上呈阴性的 ΔVm。考虑到在没有组织存在的溶液中除颤场均匀分布的事实，这两种类型的除极化可以归咎于结构因素。第一种类型的外切 ΔVm 可能和宏观水平的组织结构非均一性，例如纤维扭转[13]、表面积/体积比[44]或大血管等有关。由于在某些深度的光学积分，因此表面和表浅组织的非均一性和这些 ΔVm 有关。

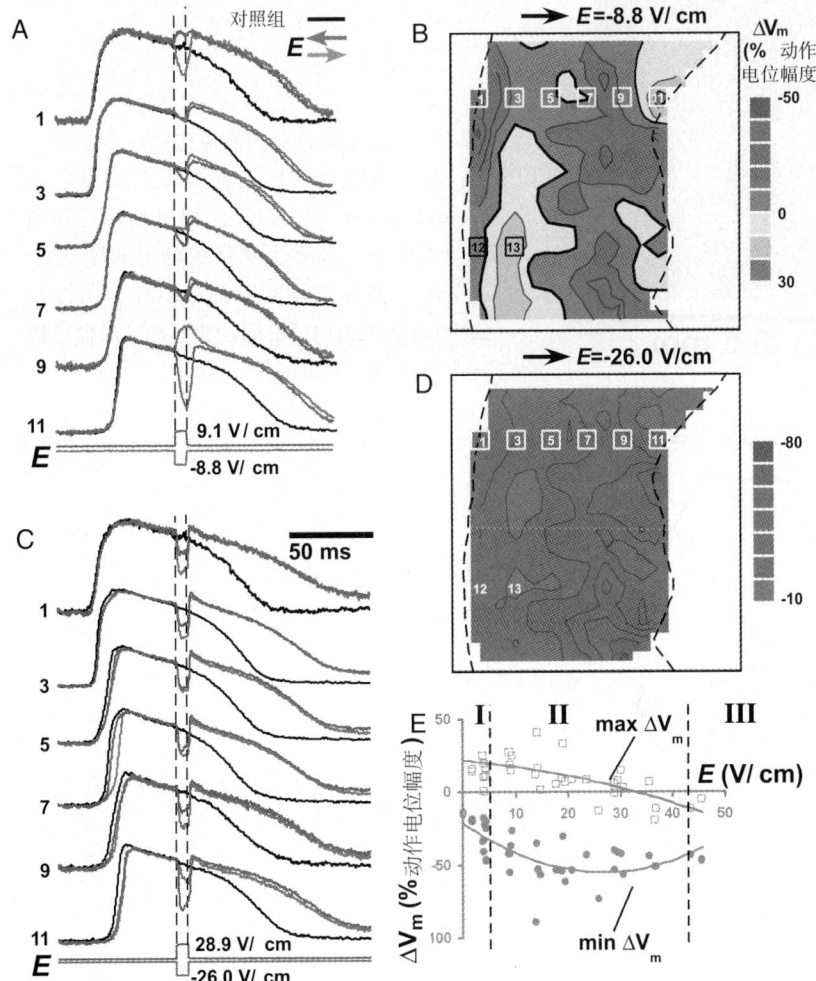

图 45-6 猪左心室壁内的虚拟电极 A 和 C：对照组（黑线）壁内 Vm 和除颤电场 (E) 和两个极性相反电击的光学标测记录。数字和 B、D 中的光电二极管相对应。B 和 D：在两个强度电击 9ms 后测定的 ΔVm 分布等电位标测。8.8V/cm 电击造成孤立性壁内 ΔVm，而 26V/cm 电击则造成总体阴性壁内 ΔVm。E：最大和最小 ΔVm 和电击强度之间的关系。虚线将 Vm 反应为几乎对称性（Ⅰ）、非对称性孤立壁内 ΔVm（Ⅱ）和总体阴性 ΔVm（Ⅲ）这三个区域分隔开来（引自 Fast VG, Sharifov OF, Cheek ER, et al: Intramural virtual electrodes during defibrillation shocks in left ventricular wall assessed by optical mapping of membrane potential. Circulation 106: 1007-1014, 2002）（彩图 23）

另一种类型的壁内 ΔVm 即总体阴性的 ΔVm 特性更难以解释。它们的存在和常规的观点相矛盾，并且细胞培养物的研究结果即电击引起两种极性的除极化反映了在某些部位有内向电流，而在另一些部位则有外向电流。对这种 ΔVm 的可能解释是微观水平组织结构非均一性造成继发源的结果。图 45-7A 描述了引起这些继发源的一个可能的解剖基质，即显示了左室壁胶原间隔的分布。例图证实壁内组织由细胞层构成，这和以往的组织学研究一致[31]。在这种结构中电击诱导的 ΔVm 可以从培养细胞条中 Vm 的反应推理而来。如上所述，在高分辨率测量时（<0.1mm），这些反应显示在细胞条的相对两侧分别出现阳性和阴性 ΔVm，而在 AP 平台期则通常呈非对称性，即阴性 ΔVm 大于阳性 ΔVm（图 45-7B，左）。然而，如果这些除极化在宏观水平进行测量时（1.2mm），即超过结构宽度的水平，那么阴性和阳性的除极化将被平均，从而产生阴性 ΔVm（图 45-6B，右）。应该指出，在三维组织中，深层细胞层的光学效应可使空间信号平均得到加强。这种光学信号可以解释强电击期间壁内 ΔVm 总体上为阴性，以及最大 ΔVm 相对较小，即从来不会超过 100% 的动作电位幅度（图 45-6E），而在细胞培养物的高分辨率测量中可以达到 300% 的动作电位幅度（图 45-3）。此外，空间平均效应也可解释为缺乏可检测的 ΔVm，发生在弱电击期间 ΔVm 更加对称时。

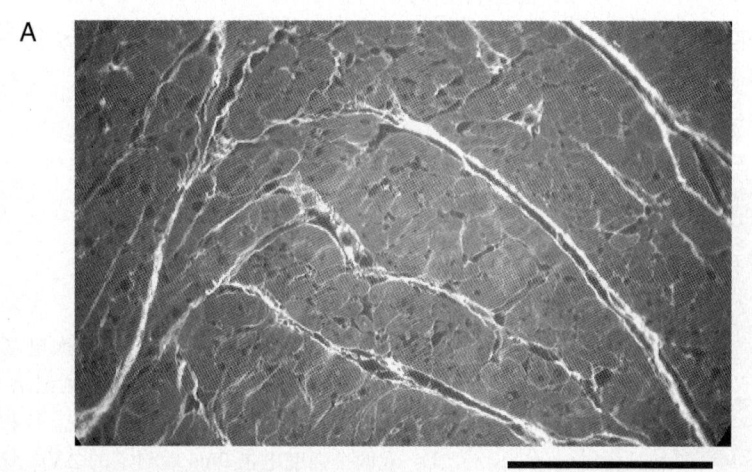

图 45-7　总体阴性壁内除极化的假定机制
A：左室跨壁切片的荧光现象，胶原采用 picrosirius red 染色。B：空间平均对跨细胞条（宽度为 0.8mm）测量的电击诱导 ΔVm 的影响。高分辨率测量提示阳性和阴性的 ΔVm 都表现为明显的阴性非对称，而低分辨率记录则提示只有阴性 ΔVm

六、结 论

在细胞培养物和整体组织中的光学标测研究结果提示微观水平组织结构在除颤过程中起到重要的作用，并且可以解释除颤电场和细胞 Vm 变化之间的关系。引起微观水平继发源最可能的解剖学基质是广泛的网状胶原间隔和血管，而单个细胞边界的作用似乎较小。这些研究还显示电击诱导的 ΔV_m 明显呈非线性。在 AP 平台期，ΔV_m 明显呈非对称，即阴性极化远远大于阳性极化。这可能和已经除极化组织的外向钙电流有关。此外，非常强大的电击产生的阴性 ΔV_m 也呈非单一性，并且已有的资料显示这种效应的机制是膜电转。这些发现可以帮助我们更好地理解在整体心脏中电击引起的细胞水平的改变。

（钟幼民 译）

参 考 文 献

1. Gurvich NL, Yuneiv GS: Restoration of regular rhythm in the mammalian fibrillating heart. Am Rev Sov Med 3:236–239, 1946.
2. Dillon SM, Kwaku KF: Progressive depolarization: A unified hypothesis for defibrillation and fibrillation induction by shocks. J Cardiovasc Electrophysiol 9:529–552, 1998.
3. Zipes DP, Fisher J, King RM, et al: Termination of ventricular fibrillation in dogs by depolarizing a critical amount of myocardium. Am J Cardiol 36:37–44, 1975.
4. Zhou XH, Daubert JP, Wolf PD, et al: Epicardial mapping of ventricular defibrillation with monophasic and biphasic shocks in dogs. Circ Res 72:145–160, 1993.
5. Sobie E, Susil R, Tung L: A generalized activating function for predicting virtual electrodes in cardiac tissue. Biophys J 73:1410–1423, 1997.
6. Muzikant A, Henriquez C: Bipolar stimulation of a three-dimensional bidomain incorporating rotational anisotropy. IEEE Trans Biomed Eng 45:449–462, 1998.
7. Plonsey R, Barr RC, Witkowski FX: One-dimensional model of cardiac defibrillation. Med Biol Eng Comput 29:465–469, 1991.
8. Trayanova N, Skouibine K, Aguel F. The role of cardiac tissue structure in defibrillation. Chaos 8:221–233, 1998.
9. Wikswo J: Tissue anisotropy, the cardiac bidomain and the virtual electrode effect. In Zipes DP, Jalife J (eds): Cardiac Electrophysiology: From Cell to Bedside, 2nd ed. Philadelphia, WB Saunders, 1995, pp 348–361.
10. Efimov IR, Cheng Y, Van Wagoner DR, et al: Virtual electrode-induced phase singularity. A basic mechanism of defibrillation failure. Circ Res 82:918–925, 1998.
11. Keener JP, Panfilov AV: A biophysical model for defibrillation of cardiac tissue. Biophys J 71:1335–1345, 1996.
12. Roth B, Krassowska W: The induction of reentry in cardiac tissue. The missing link: How electric fields alter transmembrane potential. Chaos 8:204–220, 1998.
13. Trayanova N: Concepts of ventricular defibrillation. Phil Trans R Soc Lond A 359:1327–1337, 2001.
14. Fast VG, Kléber AG: Cardiac tissue geometry as a determinant of unidirectional conduction block: Assessment of microscopic excitation spread by optical mapping in patterned cell cultures and in a computer model. Cardiovasc Res 29:697–707, 1995.
15. Rohr S, Kucera JP, Fast VG, Kléber AG: Paradoxical improvement of impulse conduction in cardiac tissue by partial cellular uncoupling. Science 275:841–844, 1997.
16. Gillis AM, Fast VG, Rohr S, Kleber AG: Mechanism of ventricular defibrillation. The role of tissue geometry in the changes in transmembrane potential in patterned myocyte cultures. Circulation 101:2438–2445, 2000.
17. Fast VG, Kléber AG: Anisotropic conduction in monolayers of neonatal rat heart cells cultured on collagen substrate. Circ Res 75:591–595, 1994.
18. Fast VG, Darrow BJ, Saffitz JE, Kléber AG: Anisotropic activation spread in heart cell monolayers assessed by high-resolution optical mapping: Role of tissue discontinuities. Circ Res 79:115–127, 1996.
19. Fast VG, Kléber AG: Microscopic conduction in cultured strands of neonatal rat heart cells measured with voltage-sensitive dyes. Circ Res 73:914–925, 1993.
20. Huynh TV, Chen F, Wetzel GT, et al: Developmental changes in membrane Ca^{2+} and K^+ currents in fetal, neonatal, and adult rabbit ventricular myocytes. Circ Res 70:508–15, 1992.
21. Rosenbaum DS, Jalife J (eds): Optical Mapping of Cardiac Excitation and Arrhythmias. Armonk, NY, Futura, 2001.
22. Gillis AM, Fast VG, Rohr S, Kléber AG: Effects of defibrillation shocks on the spatial distribution of the transmembrane potential in strands and monolayers of cultured neonatal rat ventricular myocytes. Circ Res 79:676–690, 1996.
23. Fast VG, Rohr S, Gillis AM, Kléber AG: Activation of cardiac tissue by extracellular electrical shocks: Formation of "secondary sources" at intercellular clefts in monolayers of cultured myocytes. Circ Res 82:375–385, 1998.
24. Fast VG, Rohr S, Ideker RE: Non-linear changes of transmembrane potential caused by defibrillation shocks in strands of cultured myocytes. Am J Physiol Heart Circ Physiol 278:H688–H697, 2000.
25. Tung L, Kleber AG: Virtual sources associated with linear and curved strands of cardiac cells. Am J Physiol Heart Circ Physiol 279: H1579–H1590, 2000.
26. Fast VG, Cheek ER: Optical mapping of arrhythmias induced by strong electrical shocks in myocyte cultures. Circ Res 90:664–670, 2002.
27. Sharma V, Tung L: Theoretical and experimental study of sawtooth effect in isolated cardiac cell-pairs. J Cardiovasc Electrophysiol 12:1164–1173, 2001.
28. Zhou X, Knisley SB, Smith WM, et al: Spatial changes in the transmembrane potential during extracellular electric stimulation. Circ Res 83:1003–1014, 1998.
29. Spach MS, Dolber PC: Relating extracellular potentials and their derivatives to anisotropic propagation at a microscopic level in human cardiac muscle. Evidence for electrical uncoupling of side-to-side fiber connections with increasing age. Circ Res 58:356–371, 1986.
30. Sommer JR, Scherer B: Geometry of cell and bundle appositions in cardiac muscle: Light microscopy. Am J Physiol Heart Circ Physiol 17:H792–H803, 1985.
31. Le Grice IJ, Smaill BH, Chai LZ, et al: Laminar structure of the heart: Ventricular myocyte arrangement and connective tissue architecture in the dog. Am J Physiol Heart Circ Physiol 38:H571–H582, 1995.
32. Zhou XH, Rollins DL, Smith WM, Ideker RE: Responses of the transmembrane potential of myocardial cells during a shock. J Cardiovasc Electrophysiol 6:252–263, 1995.
33. Zhou XH, Smith WM, Rollins DL, Ideker RE: Transmembrane potential changes caused by shocks in guinea pig papillary muscle. Am J Physiol Heart Circ Physiol 271:H2536–H2546, 1996.
34. Cheng DK, Tung L, Sobie EA: Nonuniform responses of transmembrane potential during electric field stimulation of single cardiac cells. Am J Physiol Heart Circ Physiol 277:H351–H362, 1999.
35. Cheek ER, Ideker RE, Fast VG: Non-linear changes of transmembrane potential during defibrillation shocks: Role of Ca^{2+} current. Circ Res 87:453–459, 2000.
36. Yuan W, Ginsburg KS, Bers DM: Comparison of sarcolemmal calcium channel current in rabbit and rat ventricular myocytes. J Physiol 493:733–746, 1996.
37. Gomez JP, Potreau D, Branka JE, Raymond G: Developmental changes in Ca^{2+} currents from newborn rat cardiomyocytes in primary culture. Pflugers Arch 428:241–249, 1994.
38. Yu H, Chang F, Cohen IS: Pacemaker current I_f in adult canine cardiac ventricular myocytes. J Physiol 485:469–483, 1995.
39. Ranjan R, Chiamvimonvat N, Thakor NV, et al: Mechanism of anode break stimulation in the heart. Biophys J 74:1850–1863, 1998.
40. Cheek ER, Fast VG: The role of membrane electroporation in non-linear V_m changes induced by defibrillation shocks in myocyte cul-

tures. Pacing Clin Electrophysiol 24:II-650, 2002.
41. Neunlist M, Tung L: Dose-dependent reduction of cardiac transmembrane potential by high-intensity electrical shocks. Am J Physiol Heart Circ Physiol 273:H2817–H2825, 1997.
42. Al-Khadra A, Nikolski V, Efimov IR: The role of electroporation in defibrillation. Circ Res 87:797–804, 2000.
43. Fast VG, Sharifov OF, Cheek ER, et al: Intramural virtual electrodes during defibrillation shocks in left ventricular wall assessed by optical mapping of membrane potential. Circulation 106:1007–1014, 2002.
44. Fishler MG: Syncytial heterogeneity as a mechanism underlying cardiac far-field stimulation during defibrillation-level shocks. J Cardiovasc Electrophysiol 9:384–394, 1998.
45. Fast VG, Cheek ER: Optical mapping of arrhythmias induced by strong defibrillation shocks in myocyte cultures. Circ Res 90:664–670, 2002.

第 46 章

除颤的总体机制

Richard A. Gray

本章目录
■ 历史 ……………………………… 413
■ 除颤诱发的跨膜变化和致心律失常性
……………………………………… 414
■ 概述 ……………………………… 414
■ 震荡电场和相位锁定 …………… 414
■ 恒定电场和稳态模式 …………… 417
■ 除颤 ……………………………… 417
■ 讨论 ……………………………… 419
■ 局限性 …………………………… 420

一、历 史

随着更多研究结果的问世和实验技术的改进，原有的除颤机制近年来已有了很大的改变。一般来说，随着认识的提高及资料的积累，相关研究将变得越来越复杂，从而使除颤机制也越来越详细，但我们对其的理解依然不完整。

1968 年，Dudel[1] 提出成功除颤的电击必须强大到足以使整个心脏麻痹。Wiggers[2] 推测为了使除颤成功，电击只需要大到能够终止颤动期间的所有激动波锋。Mower 及其同事[3] 和 Zipes 及其同事[4] 提出电击只需能够在"临界质量"的心肌中终止激动的扩布即可，这样残留的颤动波就无法维持。

有趣的是，在"易损期"给予的电除颤可以诱发颤动[5]。正如最初 Fabiato 及同事[6] 提出的那样，目前普遍认为除颤的许多机制也在除颤时诱发颤动的过程中起作用。诱颤和除颤机制相似的思想产生了一个革命性的观点，即除颤失败可能是由于颤动再次诱发的缘故，即使电击终止了所有颤动性电活动。第一个旨在解释这种再次诱发的机制是"临界点"理论，该理论认为在电击期间在临界局部场强和临界恢复期水平的交接点形成折返[7,8]。这个临界点理论包含了电击附近组织不应期延长这一重要现象[8,9]。此外，研究人员发现除颤期间整个心脏（不只是电极附近）的不应期和动作电位时程均延长，这也和除颤效率提高有关[10-13]。

尽管临界点理论解释了除颤诱发折返形成的机制[8]，但是它并不能解释电击后观察到的所有激动模式。例如，许多研究中发现，在电击后可以观察到激动的局部模式和一段时间的电静止即所谓的"等电窗"[7,14-17]。跨壁记录提示跨壁折返不是等电窗的机制[18,19]。已经有研究提示在等电窗期间可以出现难于检测到的"分级扩布反应"[20]，但是这不能解释观察到的局部激动模式。虽然已经在高电压双极刺激部位附近观察到了分级扩布反应[9]，但只是在最近才在远离除颤电极的部位观察到这种现象[21,22]。此外，在等电窗期间也可以出现检测不到的"微折返"，并且在没有紧密间隔跨壁精确记录的情况下很难排除这种可能性。最后，在等电窗期间可能没有波锋的传导，因此触发活动和电击后出现的第一次心搏有关[14,23-25]。

有助于我们理解除颤机制的第二个革命性观点是细胞外单极刺激同时使细胞膜发生除极化和超极化[26]。发生细胞膜超极化的区域称为虚拟电极。心脏组织细胞间质和细胞内传导各向异性不均的特点有重要的意义。研究人员利用心脏双区模型[27] 研究这一事实的意义[28-32]，并且实验证实了预测的除极化"狗骨"模式[33-37]。Sobie 及同事[38] 扩展了 Rattay[26] 的激动函数，把它和双区效应结合起来，推导出一个影响被动细胞膜电击诱导性跨膜变化因子的数学公式。Sobie及同事将激动函数总结如下："虚拟电极经细胞内电导加权的二次导数或经细胞内电导微商加权的细胞外电压梯度组成"。

二、除颤诱发的跨膜变化和致心律失常性

近期的实验研究已将虚拟电极除极化和电击后即刻形成的折返波联系起来[39-42]，后者被称为"虚拟电极诱发的相位奇点"或VEIPS。然而，电击期间跨膜电位的变化即虚拟电极和除颤或诱颤之间的关系尚未彻底阐明。研究人员对电极附近（近场）的虚拟电极模式有了很多的了解，并且近场折返形成的机制是发生在阳性和阴性除极化交接区附近的"碎裂"激动[39-40]。然而，对发生在远离电极（远场）的虚拟电极模式和由此产生的电击后激动模式却了解不多。研究证实心房除颤电击可以在右心房消除或引起相位奇点[42]。来自家兔心脏的光学记录发现第一次折返激动的发生部位和时间符合临界点理论，尽管引起电击后激动的精确事件有所不同[41]。晚近，Evans及其同事[43]在离体家兔心脏中通过分析跨膜电位和折返动力学研究了电击对稳定折返的影响。他们发现多种机制和折返波的消除、形成以及重整有关。例如，在相位奇点的阳性和阴性除极化期间都可以出现折返波的消除，并且临界点和VEIPS机制都可以导致即刻折返的形成[43]。

三、概 述

为了模拟临床使用的电击波形，所有用电极诱发跨膜电位变化、电击后激动以及致心律失常性的研究都采用窄脉宽（~10ms）电击。尽管研究显示在这种短暂电击期间电极附近可以出现稳定的虚拟电极[39]，但是对远场中的时间过程和虚拟电极模式并不了解。因此，我们设计了一系列研究来观察离体家兔心脏表面跨膜电位对长时程（1~2s）电场的反应。

我们采用双照相机高速充电耦联装置（CCD）系统和一种电压敏感性染料（2-4-ANEPPS）记录离体家兔心脏表面的跨膜电位。摄像系统、方法和信号处理步骤以前已经报道过[41,44]。电场来自两种不同的系统：1号电极配置是一个和右心室以及左房顶部的1cm长的螺旋电极相连接的恒流装置，而心脏浸于含有导电液体的池中（图46-4A）[41]，而2号电极配置是一个和肋网相连接的恒压装置，这样电场就和心脏长轴（垂直）平行，如图46-4B[45]。这些实验在两个不同的实验室进行，两个实验室分别用阿拉巴马（AL）和纽约（NY）来表示。

每个位置（x, y）的相位变量（θ）都按照以前方法[46]记录的跨膜激动计算而来。

$$\theta_{x,y,t} = \arctan[V_{x,y,t+\tau} - V^*, V_{x,y,t} - V^*], \quad [1]$$

t代表时间，τ代表时间延迟（此处等于16ms），而V^*是重建状态空间的原点（此处等于动作电位幅度的50%）。相位的空间离散（$\theta_{t,sd}$）按照空间标准差$\theta_{x,y,t}$进行计算。相位奇点是指某个点的相位不定，并且接闭合回路线积分接近于±2π。相位奇点通过采用一个自动程序[47]计算每个部位的拓扑充电（n_t）来确定：

$$n_t = \frac{1}{2\pi}\oint_c \nabla\theta \cdot d\vec{\ell}, \quad [2]$$

θ代表局部相位。符号n_t表示围绕其旋转波锋的手性，并且n_t数值是±1。

所有数值都以均数±均数的标准误表示。除非特别注明，否则用Student's t检验进行比较。空间模式采用线性相关系数（r）进行比较，这个系数提供了一个两种图像相似性的正态测量（范围是-1~1）[48]。曲线拟合通过最小平方法进行，尽可能减小误差，或者采用Levenberg-Marquardt方法解决非线性最小平方的问题（Origin, Microcal Software, Northhampton, MA）。P值小于0.05认为有统计学差异。

四、震荡电场和相位锁定

以往利用2号电极配置的研究结果证实无论心脏的状态如何，在给予脉宽1~2s、频率5~20Hz的正弦波刺激时，只要电场超过一个临界强度（24V），都能导致记录表面所有部位的相位锁定和不完全恢复，同时伴有周期性重复的跨膜电活动的空间模式[45]。尽管在5~20Hz的频率范围内跨膜电位的模式没有变化，但如图46-1显示跨膜电位震荡的幅度和诱发颤动的能力随着交流电（AC）的不同频率和幅度而不同。当交流电的频率低于5Hz时，各种测试幅度都能诱发室颤（VF）。图46-1（底部）显示了10Hz交流电期间锁相跨膜电位震荡和室颤（由10s的电击诱发）期

间跨膜电位震荡的相似性。此外，如图46-1（底部右侧）所示，10Hz 交流电刺激和室颤之间的重建矢量空间的轨道也类似。

这里显示了交流电刺激的致心律失常性以及相位同步的细节和持续 1s 的某一特定混乱波形。由于已经有研究证实在系统的主频附近给予假性周期性输入驱动时，可以使空间扩展非线性周期性系统同步化（在同一相位的所有部位），因此我们选择了这个特定的混乱波形[49]。当然，颤动并非严格意义上呈周期性，但是颤动期间记录的心电图显示多数种属出现中心接近 10Hz 的窄带频谱[50]。因此，某一显示接近颤动主频的强周期成分特征的特定混乱波形（由"Rossler"公式推导而来）[51]可能十分适合于使心脏活动的同步化。产生的混乱波形使得波形起始和终止时的刺激幅度为零。

如图46-2 所示，低强度（<24V）的 10Hz 刺激可诱发室颤，而更高强度（>24V）的刺激却不能诱发室颤。相图即 $\theta_{x,y}$（左侧）提示在低强度刺激结束时存在相位奇点，而高强度刺激结束时却不存在。除相图之外，另一种直观显示相位空间分布的方法是在一桢重建矢量空间中描出许多点（散点图），如图 46-2（右侧）所示。为了便于比较，图46-2A 显示了持续性室颤的相图和散点图（>200 个位置）。高强度刺激的相位均一性能通过相图颜色的变化和散点图中各点的角度进行评价。当存在相位奇点时，散点图中的点云必定围绕在原点（V^*，V^*）周围，如图 46-2A 和 B 所示。相位奇点的存在表明心脏表面的某些区域，相图上可以划出一个拓扑充电不为零的闭合环。在重建矢量空间（图 46-2A 和 B 都反映了一个顺钟向和一个逆钟向的相位奇点）中，顺钟向和逆钟向相位奇点都可以用类似的方式表现出来。如果没有奇点存在，如高强度刺激结束处（图 46-2C 和 D），则空间中没有级数为 2π 的连续环（即拓扑充电处为零）。和诱发室颤的事件相比，没有诱发室颤的事件中刺激结束处的 θ_{sd} 远小于前者（0.4 ± 0.09 和 0.67 ± 0.09 弧度，$P<0.05$）。在电击结束时，我们计算的其他参数（即超过 V^* 的心脏百分比、V 的空间均数、V 的空间标准差或 2 的空间均数）在没有室颤诱发（N 室颤 I）和诱发室颤（室颤 I）的事件之间无统计学差异。36V 正弦刺激的 $\theta_{t,sd}$ 和持续 1s，频率 10Hz 的刺激（都没有诱发室颤）的混乱波形之间的时间变异却不同。混乱波形的 $\theta_{t,sd}$ 最小值及其发生时间都明显较小（0.8 ± 0.2 vs 1.3 ± 0.1 弧度和 0.15 ± 0.02 vs $0.2 \pm$

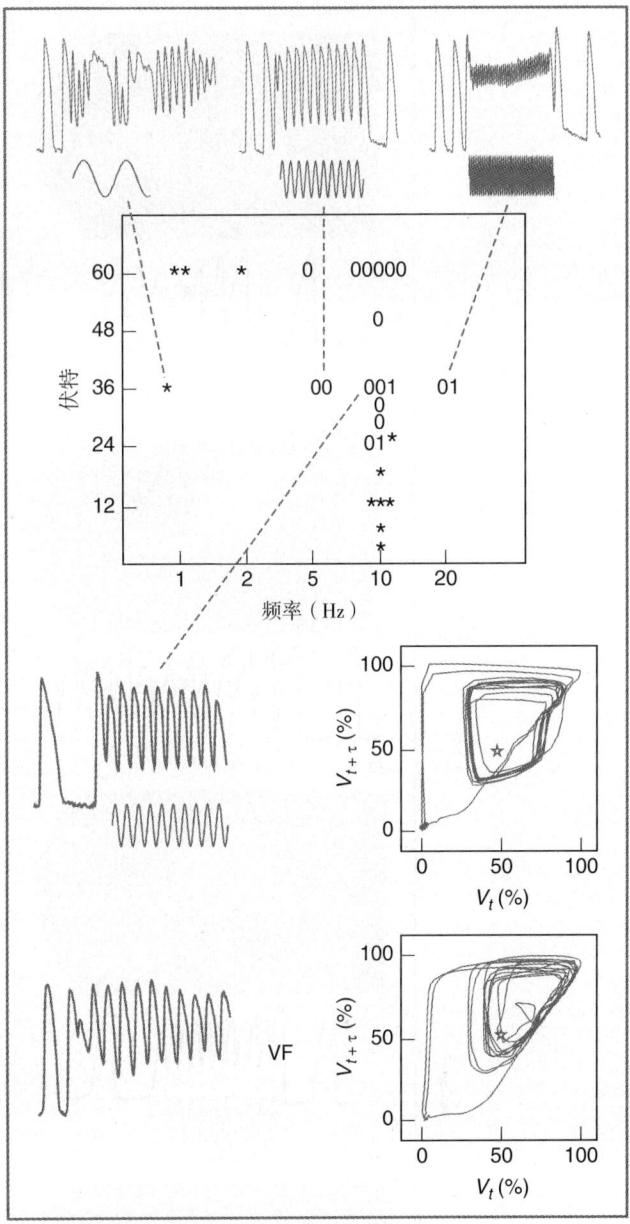

图46-1 交流电刺激和心律失常的诱发 长时程（1 或 2s）的正弦曲线波形电击的结果分为三组：0，没有期外搏动；1，一次期外搏动；*，29 个事件其期外搏动超过 1 次（NY）。低幅和低频电击诱发颤动。1、5 和 20Hz 事件（36V）的跨膜信号如图所示（顶部）。来自1Hz 电击的跨膜信号显示刺激没有造成相位锁定，而 5 和 20Hz 电击则观察到相位锁定。底部，10Hz（36V）电击和持续性室颤（VF）期间的跨膜信号如左图所示，同样的信号还在重建状态空间中加以显示（右）

0.005s）。如图46-2D，相图显示了 10Hz 混乱刺激结束处的相位的均一性。

从图 46-2 可以看到，诱发和不诱发室颤的交流电刺激其相位的空间分布不同。诱发室颤刺激期间

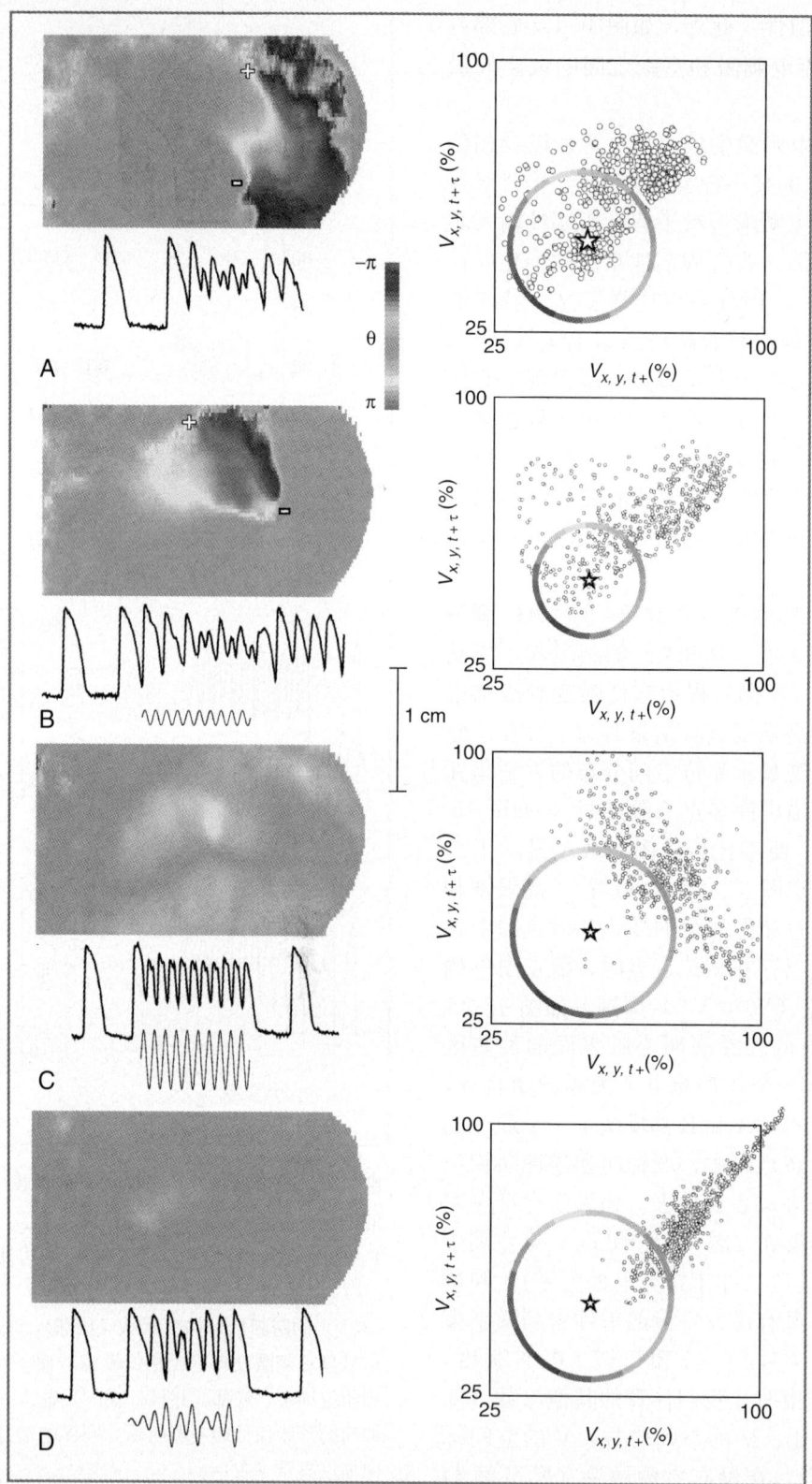

图 46-2 室颤时的相位标测和散点图 室颤（A），时限 1s，电压 12V；频率 10Hz 的正弦曲线波形电击（B），时限 1s，电压 48V；频率 10Hz 正弦曲线波形电击（C）和时限 1s，电压 36V；频率 10Hz 混乱波形电击（D）期间的相位标测和散点图。来自一个部位的跨膜信号和刺激波形都显示在每幅相位图的下方。在 12V 正弦曲线波形电击期间（B），形成一对手性相反的相位奇点（+，顺时针方向；-，逆时针方向），从而诱发颤动。☆表示状态空间中的原点（V^*，V^*）。彩色圆圈代表由公式 1 计算的相角（见彩图 24）

（图46-2B）的相位空间分布与持续性室颤期间（图46-2B）的相位空间分布与持续性室颤期间所观察到的（图46-2A）类似。然而，对于高强度刺激而言，相位的空间分布更加均一（图46-2C和D），尽管多数部位呈现和室颤期间观察到的相似的跨膜震荡，如图46-1。区别在于交流电刺激期间跨膜震荡在刺激时发生相位锁定（图46-3A）[45]。随着强度逐渐增加到24V，对10Hz的刺激发生1:1相位锁定的组织比例也逐渐增加，然后保持在强度超过24V的70%这一相对稳定的水平。发生1:2相位锁定的组织比例（即跨膜震荡的周期为50ms）在强度接近24V时开始增加，直至48V的27%这一水平。对交流电刺激发生相位锁定的组织总量（PLT）在整个强度范围内逐渐增加，并且能通过曲线很好地拟合。

$$PLT = 100 - A^* \exp(-volts/B) \quad [3]$$

其中，$A = 230 \pm 17\%$，$B = 12 \pm 0.7V$。交流电刺激（$<PS>/T_0$）期间每个阶段的平均奇点数量（PSs）随着刺激强度的增加而减少，如图46-3B所示。这种关系可以用线性回归很好地进行拟合（$P < 0.05$）。

$$<\#PS>/T_0 = C + D^* volts \quad [4]$$

其中，$C = 2.5 \pm 0.5$，$D = 0.04 \pm 0.02V^{-1}$

五、恒定电场和稳态模式

中等脉宽的电击防止波锋的传导

中等脉宽（100ms）、足够强度的矩形恒定电流波形可以防止波锋的传导，从而使整个心脏处于稳态模式（AL：n=8）。图46-4A显示了一个稳态模式。电击的强度范围0.75~3.0安培（A），数据通过电击前、中、后的片格和刺激结束处片格的线性相关系数（r）进行定量。强度超过1.5A的电击都能阻断波锋的传导，从而使跨膜电位达到稳态模式（定义为电击期间$r > 0.8$，至少持续50ms）。这个模式并不取决于电击前即刻心脏的状态（起搏或心律失常）（在每个动物中，$>1.5A$的稳态模式的所有组合的相关系数$r > 0.89$）。此外，在强度为24~60V和持续时间为100ms的恒压电击时（2号电极配置），也可以达到稳态模式。此时电击的极性在50ms后反转，从而形成电击的第一相和第二相（NY：n=4）。某个心脏在第一相结束处的模式如图46-4B。三个部位的动作电位如图46-4C所示。心脏表面的空间模式大约在15ms

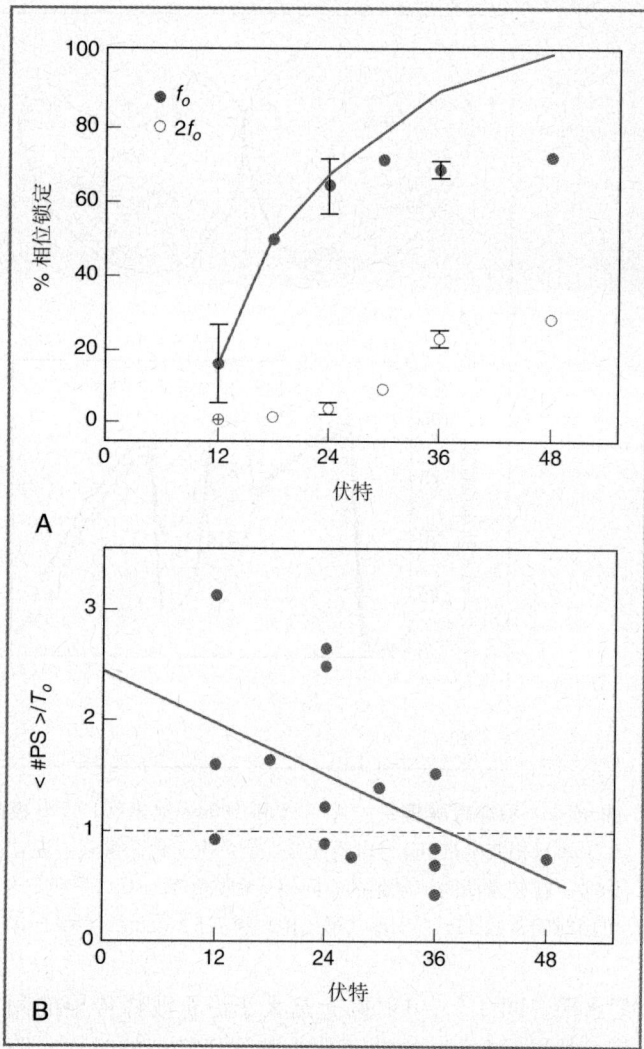

图46-3 交流电（AC）的相位锁定和AC期间的相位奇点

A：根据AC强度函数，记录到1:1锁相（实心符号，f_0）和1:2锁相（空心符号，$2f_0$）区域的百分比。实线表示所有锁相部位的百分比（包括1:1和1:2）。B：根据刺激强度函数，AC期间每个阶段$<PS/T_0>$相位奇点的平均数目。实线表示线形回归。虚线表示数值=1，由于为持续一个周期而维持折返，只需要一个相位奇点。图示代表的是平均效应，因为在AC刺激1s内相位奇点的数目有波动

内达到稳定（图46-4D），并且与电击前的状态无关。

六、除　颤

（一）短时程电击

通过8个动物中的20次电击结果（1号电极配置，AL）和Boltzmann分布（4.1 ± 0.2）进行拟合[52]，即可确定除颤阈值（即50%的除颤都能成功

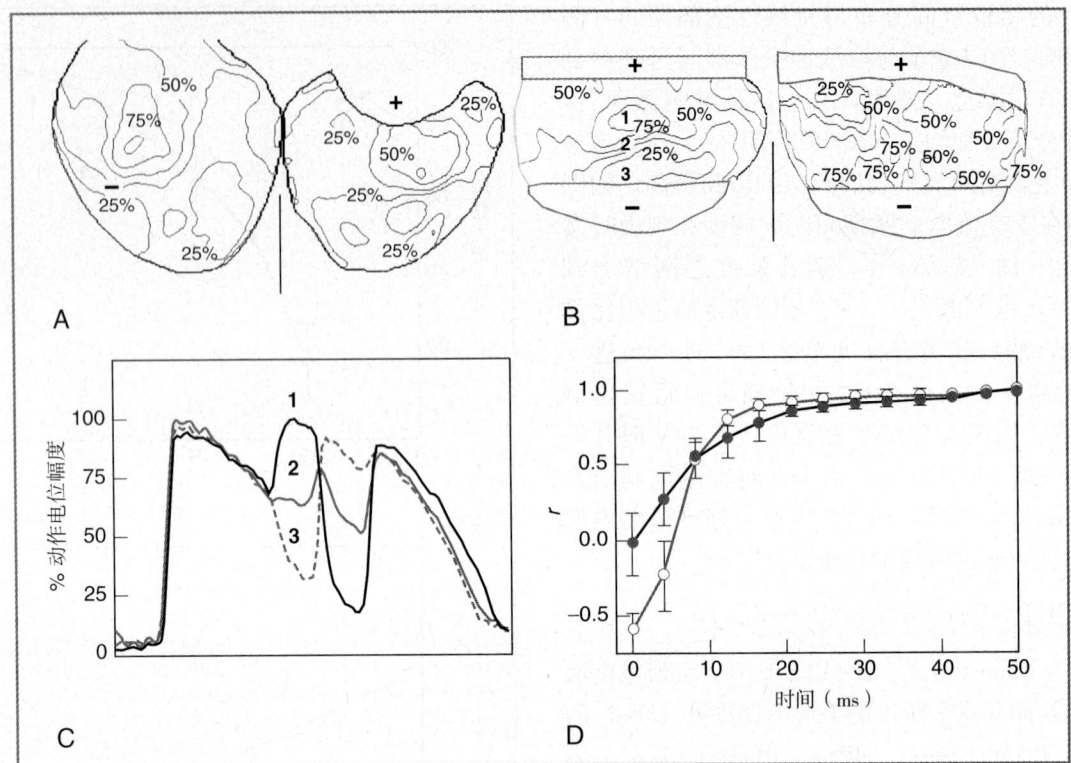

图 46-4　稳态跨膜模式　A：3A 和 100ms 电击（1 号电极配置）产生的稳态模式，左，前面观；右，后面观。B：48V 和 100ms 双相波电击（2 号电极配置）所产生的稳态模式，左，前面观；右，后面观。C：在 B、D 事件中，来自三个部位的跨膜信号。在刺激期间记录到的空间模式和除颤第一相（黑色符号）以及第二相（灰色符号）结束处观察到的模式类似。这些数据可由时间常数 11±0.4ms（第一相）和 7.5±0.8ms（第二相）的指数曲线进行很好地拟合（$P<0.001$）

的水平，DFT_{50}）。DFT_{50} 远远大于终止波锋传导的阈值，其提示 DFT_{50} 取决于使心脏到达稳态的时间，跨膜电位的稳态模式对于除颤很重要。相应之下，我们认为矩形波形电击结束时心脏的跨膜电位 $V_{x,y}$ 将由下面公式决定：

$$V_{x,y,t_+} = V_{x,y,t_\infty} + [V_{x,y,t_-} - V_{x,y,t_\infty}] * \exp\left[\frac{T_- - T_+}{\tau_s}\right] \quad [5]$$

t_+ 表示电击结束时的时间，t_- 表示电击前的时间，V_{x,y,t_∞} 是 100ms 恒定电流除颤形成的稳态模式，τ_s 代表电击时膜电位变化的时间常数。分别记录成功除颤和除颤失败期间整个离体家兔心脏表面的跨膜电活动，即 $V_{x,y,t}$（AL；n=8）。短暂（100ms）矩形恒流波形强度范围为 3～5A。我们将电击结束时跨膜电位的模式和由公式 5 预测的模式进行比较。结果发现公式 5 能够很好地预测 $V_{x,y,t}$（$r=0.74±0.04$，相似性通过线性相关系数进行评价）。τ_s（$\tau_s=8.2±1ms$）随着最大的 r 而变化。

（二）中等时程的电击

根据上述结果以及无论心脏的最初状态如何在两个阶段都可以达到相位锁定，研究人员设计了一个前瞻性研究检验正弦波形和持续 200ms、频率 10Hz 的混乱波形的除颤效果。研究在 7 只离体家兔心脏中进行，并且没有使用任何可使机械-电脱耦联的药物（NY：2 号电极配置）。结果如图 46-5 所示。在所有受试动物的心脏都可诱发室颤，并且由此产生的除颤成功曲线呈 S 形，提示在高电压电击时不会再次诱发室颤。混乱波形和 10Hz 正弦波形的结果将在下文显示。除颤成功曲线并不适合短暂（10ms）矩形单相波和双相波电击（模拟现代除颤装置中的短暂波形），因为装置在最大输出时也不能达到 100% 的成功率。因此，研究人员将这些结果和上述离体家兔心脏采用相同电极配置的短暂单相波形研究相比较[52]。由于要对不同时程的波形进行比较，因此提出三个评价除颤效果的指标：（1）峰电压；（2）平均功率（总能量除以时间）；（3）总能量：混乱波形（33.1±2.0V）和正弦波形（33.7±3.1V）的峰电压比单相波形（89.0±6.3V）

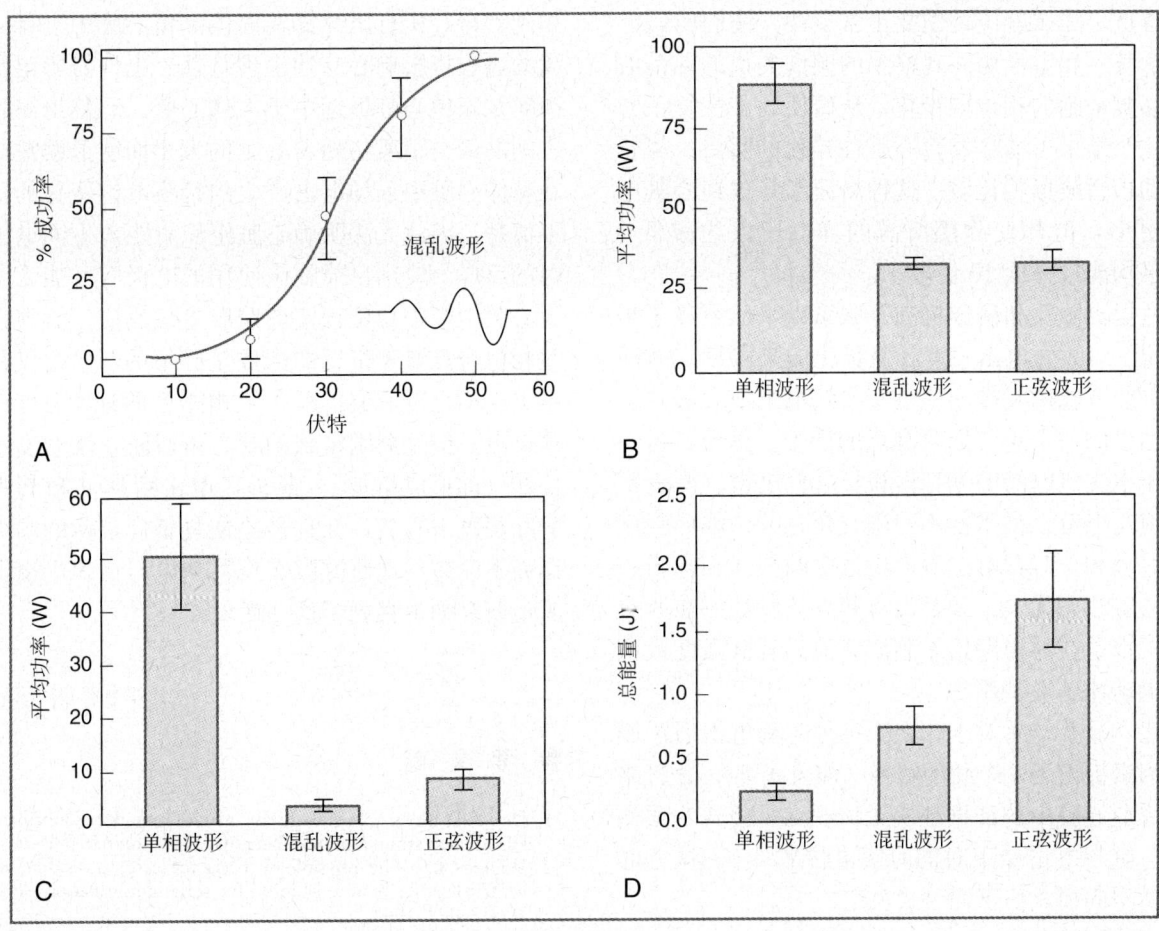

图 46-5 混乱性波形除颤 来自 200ms 混乱性波形和正弦曲线波形的结果（2 号电极配置：NY）。A：200ms 混乱性波形除颤成功率和除颤强度之间的关系。所有 50V 的电击都能成功除颤（21/21），而 10V 电击没有一次成功（0/21）。B：DFT_{50}（50% 的电击能成功除颤）的峰电压。C：DFT_{50} 的平均功率（W）。D：DFT_{50} 的总能量（J）。斜率为 58% 的截断指数单相波形的数据来自参考文献 52，并且种属和电极配置均相同（n=23）

低。和单相波形相比（78.4±11W），混乱波形释放到心脏的平均功率（3.8±0.72W）低很多，尽管混乱波形的总能量（0.76±0.14J）远大于单相波形（0.39±0.05J）。正如 Bonferroni 校正方差分析和 Student's t 检验所显示的结果，正弦波形和单相波形的数值没有不同，但是两者的三个参数都不同于单相波形（P<0.05）。

七、讨 论

这些结果证实通过整个心脏对刺激的相位锁定，超过某一强度的震荡电场可以驱动心脏产生某一特定的周期性跨膜电位模式。长时程正弦波电击的幅度和频率决定了是否诱发室颤（图 46-1）。超过某一强度的恒定电场能终止波锋的传导，并且导致离体家兔心脏表面跨膜电位稳态模式的形成。来自豚鼠乳头肌单一部位的跨膜电位微电极的记录显示，电场产生的除极化和超极化都可以阻断动作电位的传导[53]。乳头肌的结构和整个心脏的结构明显不同，因此尚不明确除颤期间整个心脏跨膜电位的改变。此处显示的模式在空间上并不均一，并且与模式有关的因素尚不明确，尽管它似乎很大程度上取决于心脏的几何构型，因为不同电极配置的模式在量上相似（图 46-4）。达到稳态模式所需要的时间大约为 10ms，并且 DFT 是终止波锋传导所需阈值的两倍。这些事实都提示长时程电击所产生的稳态模式和除颤有关。电击结束时的跨膜电位可由公式 5 推导出来，并且 10Hz 混乱波形和正弦波形可以降低除颤的峰电压和平均功率都支持这个结论（图 46-5）。

这些结果证实电击后恢复正常节律和刺激结束时相位的空间离散度（即 $θ_{sd}$）小有关。$θ_{sd}$ 的数值小和缺乏相位奇点有关，因此如果电击结束时心脏没有出现相位奇点，那么就应该恢复正常节律。我们的研究结果显示某一和室颤期间观察到的频谱类似的混乱波形可使心脏细胞的相位同步化，从而使心脏恢复正常节律。这个结果可能将改善心脏性猝死的防治。尽管和传统的短暂波形相比较，这种新波形释放到心脏中的能量更多，但却使除颤所需的峰电压大约减低 3 倍，使平均能量降低 10 倍多。

自从提出除颤和诱颤机制有联系以来已经过了半个多世纪[6]。短暂电击只有在复极化的某段特定时间（即易损期）才能诱发颤动的事实导致电击前心脏状态是决定结果的一个重要因素观点的产生。然而，这一观点对于本文研究的中等时程和长时程电击（两者都是震荡恒定电流）似乎并不正确。超过某一临界强度的中等时程和长时程电击所产生的空间模式和电击前即刻的心脏状态无关，并且没有频率依赖性。在所有情况下，都是在易损期给予刺激，但只有低强度或低频长程电击才诱发了颤动。

总之，这些结果对于什么决定短时程电击后跨膜电位的因素提出了一个新的解释（即公式 5），并且来自离体家兔心脏中的证据证实了该观点。公式 5 预测了整体心脏在电击结束时的跨膜电位 V_{x,y,t^+}。这一时刻的相位空间模式由下面公式决定：

$$\theta_{x,y,t^+} = \arctan[V_{x,y,t^+ + \tau} - V^*, V_{x,y,t^+} - V^*] \quad [6]$$

通过相位图可以发现电击结束时的相位奇点。如果心脏存在相位奇点并且变成自我维持的旋转子时，那么除颤将失败或诱发或再次启动室颤。如果电击结束时心脏不存在相位奇点，那么颤动将不再继续或形成。根据这些结果，我们认为：（1）电击前心脏的状态在决定电击后跨膜电位的模式中起到重要作用；（2）随着电击时程和能量的降低，电击前状态对电击后状态的重要性也降低；（3）心脏相位奇点将跨膜电位模式和折返联系在一起。重要的是，这些观点假定折返是除颤失败或再次诱发室颤的原因（其他可能见本章前言）。

八、局限性

了解和牢记每个研究的细节常是明智的[54]，因此在此再次指出这个研究的几个重要方面。电-机械脱耦联药物可以改变细胞膜的动力学，尽管对交流电和混乱波形的除颤研究是在没有使用脱耦联药物的情况下进行。虽然所有研究都是在正常家兔心脏上进行，因此心脏疾病和种属差异性使这些研究结果无法直接应用到临床。所有研究都在离体家兔心脏中进行，但分离的过程将影响心脏的生理特性。也许需要记住最终事实是家兔心脏远远小于人体心脏。心脏组织和电极之间的最大距离将随着心脏的大小而明显缩短。由于在整体心脏中远场电击产生的跨膜电位变化的机制尚不清楚，因此无法明确心脏组织对距离不同电极除颤时的反应。应用目前临床使用的电极有可能无法在较大心脏中产生相位锁定的跨膜电位反应。必须强调的是相位奇点对于折返的形成是必须的，但是仅具备这一点还不足以形成折返[46]。电击后即刻就可能存在相位奇点，但是周围组织的状态可以防止激动发生完全旋转（即形成折返）。此外，电击后搏动和某些失败的除颤电击有关，并且最终恢复窦性节律的动力学机制尚不清楚。本研究没有观察到电击后等电窗，但是其他研究却观察到了这一现象。

（钟幼民　译）

参 考 文 献

1. Dudel J: Elektrophysiologische grundlagen der defibrillation und künstlichen stimulation des herzens. Med Klin 63:2089–2091, 1968.
2. Wiggers CJ: The physiologic basis for cardiac resuscitation from ventricular fibrillation: Method for serial defibrillation. Am Heart J 20:413–422, 1940.
3. Mower MM, Mirowski M, Spear JF, et al: Patterns of ventricular activity during catheter defibrillation. Circulation 49:858–861, 1974.
4. Zipes DP, Fischer J, King RM, et al: Termination of ventricular fibrillation in dogs by depolarizing a critical amount of myocardium. Am J Cardiol 36:37–44, 1975.
5. Hoffa M, Ludwig C: Einige neue versuche über herzebewegung. Z Rationelle Med 9:107–144, 1850.
6. Fabiato A, Coumel P, Gourgon R, et al: Le seuil de réponse synchrone des fibres myocardiques. Application à la comparaison expérimentale de l'efficacité des différentes formes de chocs électriques de défibrillation. Arch Mal Cœur 60:527–544, 1967.
7. Shibata N, Chen P-S, Dixon EG, et al: Influence of shock strength and timing on induction of ventricular arrhythmias in dogs. Am J Physiol 255:H891–H901, 1988.
8. Frazier DW, Wolf PD, Wharton JM, et al: Stimulus-induced critical point: Mechanism for electrical initiation of reentry in normal canine myocardium. J Clin Invest 83:1039–1052, 1989.
9. Gotoh M, Uchida T, Mandel WJ, et al: Cellular graded responses and ventricular vulnerability to reentry by a premature stimulus in isolated canine ventricle. Circulation 95:2141–2154, 1997.
10. Sweeney RJ, Gill RM, Steinberg MI, et al: Ventricular refractory period extension caused by defibrillation shocks. Circulation 82:965–972, 1990.
11. Zhou X, Knisley SB, Wolf PD, et al: Prolongation of repolarization time by electric field stimulation with monophasic and biphasic shocks in open chest dogs. Circ Res 68:1761–1767, 1991.
12. Jones JL, Tovar OH: The mechanism of defibrillation and cardioversion. Proc IEEE 84:392–403, 1996.
13. Dillon SM, Kwaku KF: Progressive depolarization: A unified hypothesis for defibrillation and fibrillation induction by shocks. J Cardiovasc Electrophysiol 9:529–552, 1998.
14. Moe GK, Harris AS, Wiggers CJ: Analysis of the initiation of fibrillation by electrographic studies. Am J Physiol 134:473–492, 1941.
15. Gray RA, Jalife J: Effects of atrial defibrillation shocks on the ventricles in isolated sheep hearts. Circulation 97:1613–1622, 1998.
16. Idriss SF, Wolf PD, Smith WM, et al: Effect of pacing site on ventricular fibrillation initiation by shocks during the vulnerable period.

Am J Physiol 277(5 Pt 2):H2065–H2082, 1999.
17. Chattipakorn N, KenKnight BH, Rogers JM, et al: Locally propagated activation immediately after internal defibrillation. Circulation 97:1401–1410, 1998.
18. Chen P-S, Shibata N, Dixon EG, et al: Activation during ventricular defibrillation in open-chest dogs: Evidence of complete cessation and regeneration of ventricular fibrillation after unsuccessful shocks. J Clin Invest 77:810–823, 1986.
19. Chen P-S, Wolf PD, Melnick SD, et al: Comparison of activation during ventricular fibrillation and following unsuccessful defibrillation shocks in open chest dogs. Circ Res 66:1544–1560, 1990.
20. Chen PS, Swerdlow CD, Hwang C, et al: Current concepts of ventricular defibrillation. J Cardiovasc Electrophysiol 9:553–562, 1998.
21. Bourn DW, Trayanova NA, Gray RA: Shock-induced arrhythmogenesis and isoelectric window. PACE 25:604, 2002.
22. Evans FG, Gray RA: Shock-induced changes in transmembrane potential and arrhtyhmia induction in isolated sheep ventricles: Evidence of propagated responses, reflection, and transmural reentry. PACE 26:1111, 2003.
23. Moore EN, Spear JF: Electrophysiologic studies on the initiation, prevention, and termination of ventricular fibrillation. In Zipes DP, Jalife J (eds): Cardiac Electrophysiology and Arrhythmias. Orlando, Fla, Grune & Stratton, 1985, pp 315–322.
24. Chattipakorn N, Banville I, Gray RA, et al: Mechanism of ventricular defibrillation for near-defibrillation threshold shocks: A whole heart optical mapping study in swine. Circulation 104:1313–1319, 2001.
25. Chattipakorn N, Fotuhi PC, Chattipakorn SC, et al: Three-dimensional mapping of earliest activation after near-threshold ventricular defibrillation shocks. J Cardiovasc Electrophysiol 14:65–69, 2003.
26. Rattay F: Analysis of models for extracellular fiber stimulation. IEEE Trans Biomed Eng 36:676–682, 1989.
27. Tung L: A bidomain model for describing ischemic myocardial DC potentials [PhD thesis]. Cambridge, Mass, Massachusetts Institute of Technology, 1978.
28. Plonsey R, Barr RC: Current flow patterns in two-dimensional anisotropic bisyncytia with normal and extreme conductivities. Biophys J 45:557–571, 1984.
29. Plonsey R, Barr RC: Effect of microscopic and macroscopic discontinuities on the response of cardiac tissue to defibrillating (stimulating) currents. Med Biol Eng Comput 24:130–136, 1986.
30. Sepulveda NG, Roth BJ, Wikswo JP Jr: Current injection into a two-dimensional anisotropic bidomain. Biophys J 55:987–999, 1989.
31. Eason J, Trayanova N: The effects of fiber curvature in a bidomain tissue with irregular boundaries. Proceedings of the 15th Annual International Conference of the IEEE Engineering in Medicine and Biology Society. pp 744–745, 1993.
32. Fishler MG: Syncytial heterogeneity as a mechanism underlying cardiac far-field stimulation during defibrillation-level shocks. J Cardiovasc Electrophysiol 9:384–394, 1998.
33. Wikswo JP Jr, Wisialowski TA, Altemeier WA, et al: Virtual cathode effects during stimulation of cardiac muscle: Two-dimensional in vivo experiments. Circ Res 68:513–530, 1991.
34. Knisley SB, Hill BC, Ideker RE: Virtual electrode effects in myocardial fibers. Biophys J 66:719–728, 1994.
35. Neunlist M, Tung L: Optical recordings of ventricular excitability of frog heart by an extracellular stimulating point electrode. Pacing Clin Electrophysiol 17:1641–1654, 1994.
36. Wikswo JP Jr, Lin S-F, Abbas RA: Virtual electrodes in cardiac tissue: A common mechanism for anodal and cathodal stimulation. Biophys J 69:2195–2210, 1995.
37. Efimov IR, Cheng YN, Biermann M, et al: Transmembrane voltage changes produced by real and virtual electrodes during monophasic defibrillation shocks delivered by an implantable electrode. J Cardiovasc Electrophysiol 8:1031–1045, 1997.
38. Sobie EA, Susil RC, Tung L: A generalized activating function for predicting virtual electrodes in cardiac tissue. Biophys J 73:1410–1423, 1997.
39. Efimov IR, Cheng Y, Van Wagoner DR, et al: Virtual electrode-induced phase singularity: A basic mechanism of defibrillation failure. Circ Res 82:918–925, 1998.
40. Lin SF, Roth BJ, Wikswo JP Jr: Quatrefoil reentry in myocardium: An optical imaging study of the induction mechanism. J Cardiovasc Electrophysiol 10:574–586, 1999.
41. Banville I, Gray RA, Ideker RE, et al: Shock-induced figure-eight reentry in the isolated rabbit heart. Circ Res 85:742–752, 1999.
42. Gray RA, Jalife J: Video imaging of atrial defibrillation. In Zipes DP, Jalife J (eds): Cardiac Electrophysiology: From Cell to Bedside, 3rd ed. Philadelphia, WB Saunders, 2000, 432–439.
43. Evans FG, Ideker RE, Gray RA: Effect of shock-induced changes in transmembrane potential on reentrant waves and outcome during cardioverison of isolated rabbit hearts. J Cardiovasc Electrophysiol 13:1118–1127, 2002.
44. Gray RA, Jalife J, Panfilov AV, et al: Non-stationary vortex-like reentry as a mechanism of polymorphic ventricular tachycardia in the isolated rabbit heart. Circulation 91:2454–2469, 1995.
45. Gray RA, Mornev OA, Jalife J, et al: Standing excitation waves in the heart induced by strong alternating electric fields. Phys Rev Lett 87:168104:1–4, 2001.
46. Gray RA, Pertsov AM, Jalife J: Spatial and temporal organization during cardiac fibrillation. Nature 392:675–678, 1998.
47. Iyer AN, Gray RA: An experimentalist's approach to accurate localization of phase singularities during reentry. Ann Biomed Eng 29:47–59, 2001.
48. Press WH, Flannery BP, Teukolsky SA, et al (eds): Numerical Recipes. The Art of Scientific Computing. New York, Cambridge University Press, 1986.
49. Carroll TL, Pecora LM: Using chaos to keep period multiplied systems in phase. Phys Rev E Stat Phys Plasmas Fluids Relat Interdiscip Topics 48:2426–2436, 1993.
50. Gray RA, Jalife J, Panfilov AV, et al: Mechanisms of cardiac fibrillation: Drifting rotors as a mechanism of cardiac fibrillation. Science 270:1222–1225, 1995.
51. Rossler OE: An equation for continuous chaos. Phys Rev Lett A 57:397–398, 1976.
52. Kwaku KF, Dillon SM: Shock-induced depolarization of refractory myocardium prevents wave-front propagation in defibrillation. Circ Res 79:957–973, 1996.
53. Zhou X, Smith WM, Ideker RE: Prevention of action potentials during extracellular electrical stimulation of long duration. J Cardiovasc Electrophysiol 8:779–789, 1997.
54. Ideker RE, Chattipakorn N, Gray RA: Defibrillation mechanisms: The parable of the blind men and the elephant? J Cardiovasc Electrophysiol 11:1008–1013, 2000.
55. Gray RA, Foster E, Jalife J: Entrainment of the intact ventricles using field stimulation [abstract]. Pacing Clin Electrophysiol 19:666, 1996.
56. Gray RA, Banville I, Evans FG, et al: Long duration shocks prevent wave front propagation [abstract]. Circulation 100:I-839, 1999.

第 47 章

除颤波形

Raymond E. Ideker, Jian Huang, Gregory P. Walcott

除颤波的形状和持续时间对除颤所需的能量、峰电压和峰电流有重大的影响。它还影响到电击所造成心肌损伤和心功能不全的程度。研究人员认为除颤有益和有害作用的形成原因和电击造成的细胞外和细胞内电流通过有关，这些电流改变了跨膜电位。这种机制和小得多的电脉冲通过产生新的动作电位起搏心脏一样。因此，一些研究人员试图应用几十年前提出的将电脉冲波形和起搏阈值联系起来的数学模型，并用它们研究不同除颤波形对除颤阈值的影响。

这些模型主要有两种，它们最初都用于不同时程的方波刺激研究。第一种模型由Weiss[1]和Lapicque[2]提出，其假设波形的重要特征是它的平均电流，并且假设随着波形时程的增加起搏心肌所需要的平均电流将逐渐降低[3]。因此，这个模型并没有对方波、骤降的正弦波、截断指数波形或其他类型的下降或上升波形进行区分（图47-1）。他假设所有平均电流和时程相同的波形其起搏心肌的能力相同。第二个模型由Blair[4]提出，将波形的起搏能力归结为一个指数函数，在物理学可以由一个平行电阻-电容（RC）的电路表示。在该模型中，波形的起搏能力与通过平行RC电路产生的峰电压成正比。有些研究人员将平行RC电路转换成细胞膜的电阻和电容，这样RC电路的时间常数就和心肌细胞膜的时间常数联系起来。尽管对方波而言，Blair模型和Weiss-Lapicque模型的结果相似，但对于其他波形而言则不同，因为同一平均电流和时程的不同波形可以改变RC网络，从而产生不同的峰值。Blair模型预言对于某一给定的除颤时程，用峰电压表示的阈值以方波为最低（图47-1A），而用能量表示的阈值却是一种特定类型的上升波形为最低（图47-1D）[5]。当下降波形如截断指数的衰减波形用于植入式除颤器时（图47-1C），无论用电压或能量来表示的阈值都较高。

假定模型中除颤所需的某一最小峰电压（对于起搏而言）和用于体内除颤器模型的时间常数为2.8～4ms[6-8]，而用于体外除颤器的时间常数为5ms[9]时，这两种模型不但能很好地预测起搏阈值，还能够很好地预测除颤阈值。然而，这两个模型却无法完美地拟合实验数据。造成这种差异的原因可能有两个。第一是方波造成的跨膜电位改变不是一个只具有一个时间常数的单纯指数函数。而是在动作电位或舒张期的不同时段给予刺激时，最适合的指数时间常数不同；另外，跨膜电位除极化和超极化的最适指数时间常数不同，并且这两个数值与刺激结束后跨膜电位恢复的最佳指数时间常数也不同[10,11]。第二个原因是在舒张期起搏心脏和除颤所需的跨膜电位变化不同。这方面的证据是研究发现随着方波的时限达到无穷大，起搏电压阈值和电流阈值向渐近线靠拢；而随除颤波形时程的增加，除颤电压阈值或电流阈值先达到最小值，然后开始增加[12]。起搏和除颤之间差别的可能原因是：(1)除颤需要改变许多处于不同状态的心肌细胞的跨膜电位，此时即使有也只有少数细胞处于舒张期，而起搏时却不需要这样[13]；(2)除颤需要使全部或大部分心肌细胞的跨膜电位发生改变，而起搏只需要使起搏电极附近的少量细胞的跨膜电位发生变化；(3)除颤不仅仅是起搏，还需要延长动作电位，产生分级反应，而又不能引起再次诱发颤动的折返或触发活动[14-17]。

此外，这两种模型都已用于双相除颤波形中，后

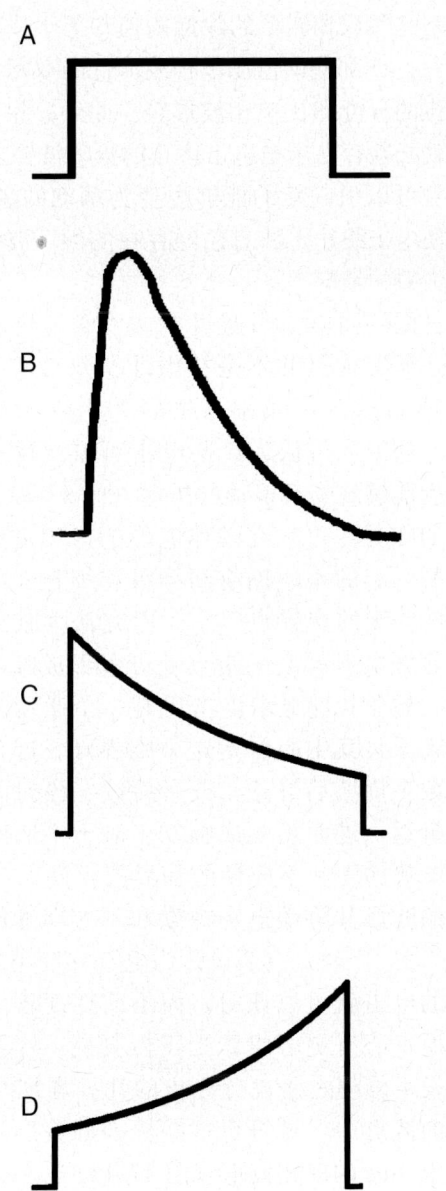

图47-1 不同的除颤波形 A：方波；B：骤降正弦波；C：截断指数下降波形；D：截断指数上升波形

者假定双相波形的第一相起搏心肌细胞并产生类似单相波形的除颤效应，而第二相能起到降低除颤阈值的辅助作用[7,18]。这些假定与第一次解释某些双相波形可以增加除颤效率的理论恰好相反，也就是第一相是准备阶段，它能够使跨膜电位超极化从而恢复兴奋性，这样第二相就可以更加容易起搏心肌并达到除颤效果[19]。然而，有些研究结果支持这些假设。这些研究结果包括那些除颤阈值最小的双相波形，其第一相充电比第二相多很多[20]，而且是第一相而不是第二相的强度-时间曲线和单相除颤波形类似[21]。这些模型发现对双相波形而言，当第一相和除颤阈值最小的单相波形相等并且其电压或电流的第二相等于或稍低于第一相起始数值时双相波形的除颤阈值最小（图47-2）[7,9,18]。

为了达到除颤效果，电击必须使整个心肌的跨膜电位发生改变，这样就可以终止颤动波的波阵面，而又不引起能够诱发颤动的新波阵面[22]。电击改变跨膜电位的方式很复杂，并且由于心肌的双域（bi-domain）结构（细胞内和细胞外结构域）涉及电击在整个心肌中产生的细胞外电势梯度、细胞外电势梯度的导数、心肌纤维的曲率和其他电阻系数改变的原因，如心肌细胞由结缔组织分隔成肌纤维束[23]。研究证实这些因素中的首要因素即电击产生的电势梯度是一个和除颤成功或失败以及电击后激动波阵的最早部位有关的重要变量[24]。为了使除颤成功，全部或大部分心肌的电击电势梯度需要达到一个最小值[25]。对于不同波形而言，这个最小电势梯度也不同。为了使除颤成功率达到大约80%，在使用10ms截断指数下降的单相波形时，所需的平均电势梯度为5.4 ± 0.8（SD）V/cm，而在使用双相截断指数下降波形并且第一相和第二相的时限均为5ms时，所需的平均电势梯度只有2.7 ± 0.3 V/cm[26]。由于对双相波形而言，强度较弱的电击就可以产生这个较低的最小电势梯度，因此双相波形的除颤阈值低于单相波形。

对于大多数除颤电极而言，随着组织到电极距离的增加其电势梯度迅速降低[24]。对于位于心脏的电极而言，电极附近最大的电势梯度比远离电极的心肌最小电势梯度大20多倍[25]。因此，为了使除颤电场最弱处的电势梯度达到5.4V/cm，单相波形在除颤电极附近产生的电势梯度必须超过100V/cm，而双相波形为了使除颤电场最弱处的电势梯度达到2.7V/cm，它在除颤电极附近产生的最大电势梯度必须超过大约50V/cm。电极附近的高电势梯度可以引起心脏损害或功能障碍[27,28]。不同波形造成的损伤或功能障碍的程度不同，在电击强度相同的情况下，双相波形的损害效应比单相波形小[29]。一次10ms单相波形电击可以造成一过性传导阻滞，此时平均电势梯度大于64 ± 4V/cm；而第一相和第二相时限均为5ms的双相波形电击并不引起传导阻滞，除非平均电势梯度超过71 ± 6V/cm[30]。因此，在电势梯度谱两端，双相波形均优于单相波形，即双相波形除颤所需的电势梯度较小，而引起功能障碍的电势梯度较大。

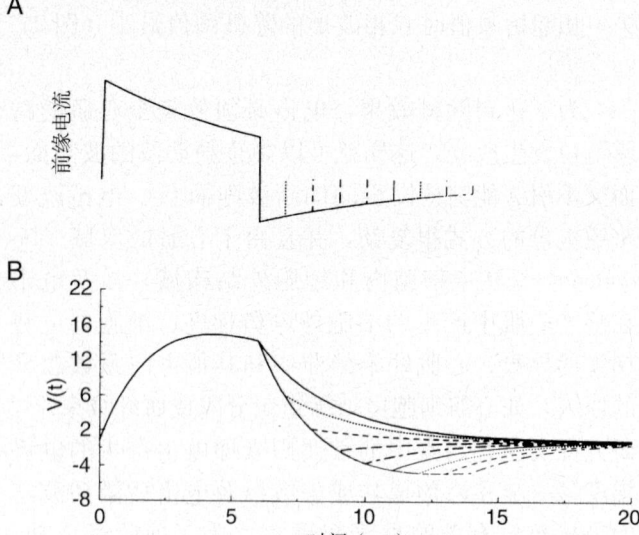

图 47-2 时间常数为 7s 的双相截断指数波形除颤反应的模型

输入波的前缘电流是 10A。A：输入波形的形状第一相的时限为 6ms。第二相的时限分别为 0、1、2、3、4、5、6、7 和 8ms，并且以不同的线条表示。B：模型反应，V（t），模型反应没有回到起始值，直到第二相时限超过 2ms 后其数值即超过起始值（引自 Walcott GP, Walker RG, Cates AW, et al: Choosing the optimal monophasic and biphasic waveforms for ventricular defibrillation. J Cardiovasc Electrophysiol 6：737-750，1995）

最近几年，研究人员提出了几种机制解释某些双相波形除颤阈值明显低于单相波形的原因。和上述假说有关（即由于双相波形第一相使组织超极化，从而使组织对第二除颤相的反应更敏感，因此双相波形起搏优于单相波形）的假说[31]是由于双相波形比单相波形更加延长动作电位（除颤诱发分级反应的结果），因此其除颤阈值较低[19,32]。这个假说的理论基础是电击造成的不应期延长使电击后颤动波锋继续存在的可能性降低，否则后者将遇到可兴奋心肌，从而继续传导并维持颤动[33,34]。根据这个论点可知，随着动作电位延长的程度和时限增加，残存颤动波锋遇到不应期组织和阻滞的机会就增加，从而使除颤成功。一个对上述假说进行改进的理论认为：为了使除颤成功，必须使电击后动作电位延长到使所有心肌同时恢复兴奋性的程度[35]。研究人员认为兴奋性同时恢复可以消除电击后不应期的离散，而后者可以通过未被电击终止的残留颤动波锋发生单向阻滞，从而引起折返形成。

研究结果似乎和这些假说相矛盾。虽然和单相波形相比某些双相波形更加明显地延长动作电位和不应期，但是这些双相波形的除颤阈值却等于或高于单相波形[36,37]。而那些阈值比单相波形低的双相波形延长动作电位的程度却比单相波形轻。此外，除颤失败也不一定就必须存在未被电击终止的颤动波锋[38]。由于电击本身可以引起新的能够蜕变为颤动的激动波锋，因此即使电击终止了所有已经存在的颤动波锋也能发生除颤失败的情况[39]。

在试图阐明电击引起再次诱发颤动机制的多数研究中，研究人员并不是在颤动期间给予电击，而是在起搏心律下在动作电位的 2 相或 3 相给予电击[40-44]。研究人员认为这些电击可以通过形成临界点而产生能够蜕变成颤动的折返（图 47-3）。其中一个类型的临界点可以在动作电位的 3 相形成，此处为电击所引起的不应期空间等级和细胞外电势梯度场的空间等级的交界点[40,45]。研究认为临界不应期和临界除颤电势梯度的交点处可以形成临界点（图 47-3A）。电学标测显示电击后有一个激动波锋形成一个旋转子，其中心就是这个临界点。这个旋转子或者在数个周期后终止，或者持续一段时间并形成继发性折返，进而蜕变成颤动。对于不同的波形而言，其电势梯度和不应期的临界值不同[46]。除颤阈值最小的波形其除颤电势梯度和不应期度的临界值也较低（图 47-4）。有假设认为电势梯度小的优势在于较小的电击就可以获得，而不应期度较小的优势在于折返中心有更多组织处于恢复期，这可能使旋转子在发生颤动之前自行终止的几率增加[46]。在所有测试的波形中，最符合这些标准的波形是每一相时限均为 4ms 的双相波形（图 47-4）。

在其他类型临界点中的重要变量是电击所造成的超极化和除极化模式，而不像第一种类型临界点中的除颤电势梯度的强度或不应期度[43,44]。光学标测显示由于心肌的双域结构，电击可造成相邻的超极化和除极化区域，即所谓的虚拟电极。在超极化区域，即使它处于动作电位的 2 相并且因此而处于有效不应期，心肌细胞也发生"去激动"，这样它的动作电位就被截断，从而恢复兴奋性。兴奋性恢复使邻近的除极化区域激动超极化组织，引起一个激动波阵并在围绕某个临界点形成旋转子，而临界点出现在相邻超极化和除极化减弱至某个点的时刻，此时电击后激动的波锋没有产生（图 47-3B）。研究人员认为虚拟电极对于终止电击时出现的颤动波锋是必需的，但是电击后在去激动区域形成的激动波锋可以导致再次发生折返，从而使除颤失败[43,44]。Efimov 及同事[44]提出双相波形

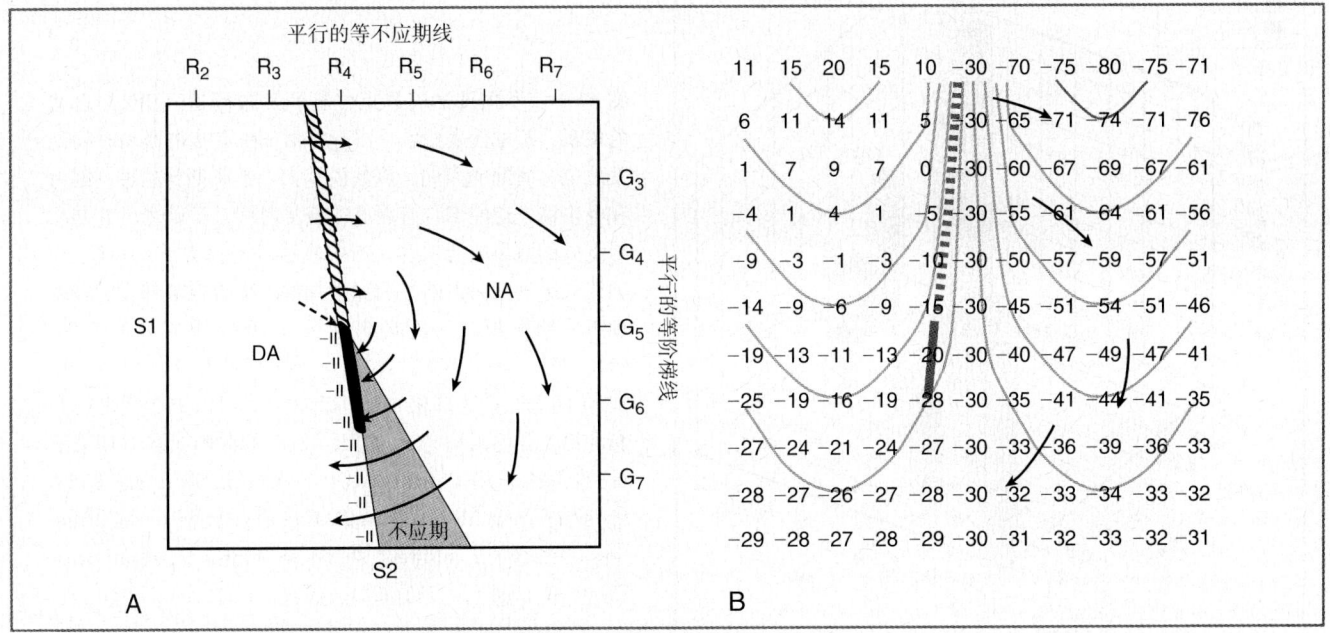

图47-3 两种类型的临界点假说 A：在临界除颤电势梯度 G_5 和临界组织不应期 R_4 交界处形成的临界点的理想模式图。S_1 起搏从左侧进行，从而造成 S_2 电击时不应期离散，即 R_2 不应期较短，而 R_7 不应期较长。从底部区域的易损期内给予 S_2 电击，此区域底部 G_7 梯度较大，而顶部 G_3 梯度较小。标记为 DA 的区域充分恢复，这样它就由梯度电场直接激动。用点标出的区域尽管暴露在更大的梯度下，但可兴奋性更差，并且发生不应期延长（RPE），因此，DA 区域的激动并不能通过这个区域传导。NA 区域的可兴奋性也很差，以至于即使在巨大梯度的作用下也不受影响。因此，扩布只能由顶部从 DA 区域向 NA 区域单向传导，围绕临界点成顺时针方向旋转并再次进入 DA 区域，从而形成折返环路。B：由除颤引发的相邻除极化和超极化跨膜电位改变的区域所形成临界点的理想模式图。数字代表电击结束时的跨膜电位，等值线起始为 −45mV，两条线之间相隔 10mV。一个具有巨大膜除极化梯度的带状区将除极化区域（左上）和超极化区域（右上）分隔开，距离狭窄的等值线表示这个带状区。带状区中的除极化组织可以激动邻近的超极化组织，从而形成可以经超极化区域扩布（箭头）的激动波锋（虚线）。下方区域，由于跨膜电位梯度较小，因此不能发生扩布。在片格和阻滞线交界处即形成临界点，而在阻滞线处扩布激动波的波锋在两个条格中都终止（引自 Chattipakorn N, Ideker RE: Mechanism of Defibrillation. In Aliot E, Clemety J, Prystowsky EN [eds]: Fighting Sudden Cardiac Death: A Worldwide Challenge. Armonk, NY, Futura, 2000, pp 593-615）

更容易除颤的原因是第二相使跨膜电位恢复到电击前的状态，从而消除了虚拟电极并防止了电击后在超极化区域产生激动波锋（图47-5）[44]。需要注意，这个理论和前面讨论的模型相符合，即除颤阈值最小的双相波形是那些模型反应能够重新恢复到电击前数值的波形（图47-2）[7,18]。4705

一个例外情况是[44]，颤动期间给予强度接近除颤阈值的电击时，心外膜和跨壁电学和光学标测并没有观察到在起搏节律给予强度接近心室颤动阈值的电击时所出现的临界点类型[47-50]。相反，激动起源于局部并且向各个方向传导，从而激动整个心肌（图47-6）。在除颤失败时，这些起源点迅速出现并重复超过三个周期之后激动波锋蜕变成颤动。如果局灶点持续一个或两个周期，则不会再次诱发颤动，除颤即告成功。

虽然对于图 47-3 所示的两种类型的临界点而言，最早激动几乎在电击后即刻就出现，但是在电击后大约 50~70ms 内并没有观察到第一个电击后局灶点（图47-6）。这个局灶点有可能来自扩布的分级反应，或者来自触发激动。考虑到从电击到观察到第一个局灶活动的时间较长，因此有假设认为这种触发激动是迟后除极。[50] 此外，最近的研究表明迟后除极抑制剂 flunarizine 可使猪的除颤阈值大约降低 40%[51]。然而，在撰写本章时，尚无标测研究提示迟后除极抑制剂是否可以消除电击后局灶活动的文章发表，这类文章可以提供局灶活动来自触发活动的证据。此外，还有一些研究提示这些延迟局灶来自缓慢扩布的分级反应[52,53]。然而，如果这些局灶确实来自迟后除极，那么双相波形除颤阈值低于单相波形的机制可能在于双相波形引起电击后动作电位延长的程度较轻，因为动作电位时程延长能增加迟后除极的发生几率[54]。

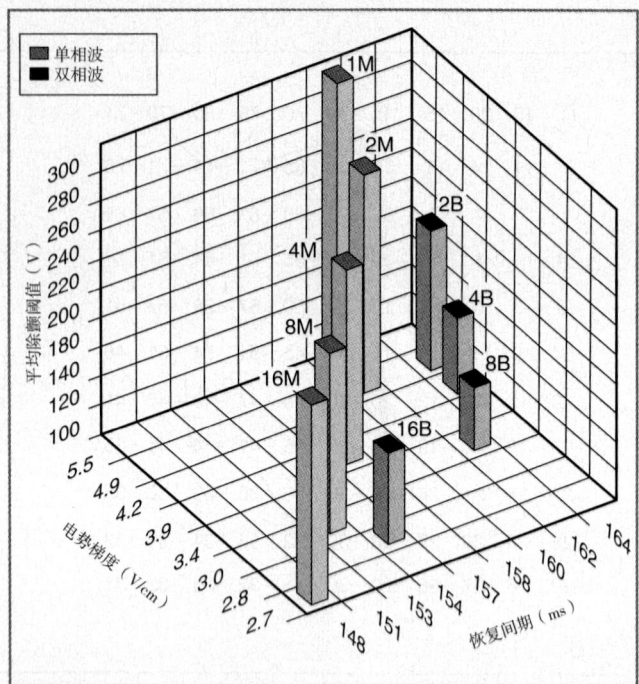

图 47-4 不同波形临界点位置和除颤阈值（DFT）之间的关系 X轴代表最后一次起搏形成临界点的激动时间到发放电击时间的间期。该数值越大，不应期就越短，因为在电击前，这些部位有更多的恢复时间。Y轴表示的是临界点处的除颤电势梯度。图中显示了6只犬的平均值。Z轴代表另外8只犬的平均除颤阈值。随着电势梯度的降低和不应期缩短（恢复间期延长），除颤阈值显著下降。1M、2M、4M、8M、16M代表时限为1、2、4、8、16ms的截断指数单相波形。2B、4B、8B、16B代表第一相和第二相时限均为1、2、4、8ms的截断指数双相波形（引自 Ideker RE，Alferness C，Melnick S，et al：Reentry site during fibrillation induction in relation to defibrillation efficacy for different shock waveforms. J Cardiovasc Electrophysiol 12：581-591，2001.）

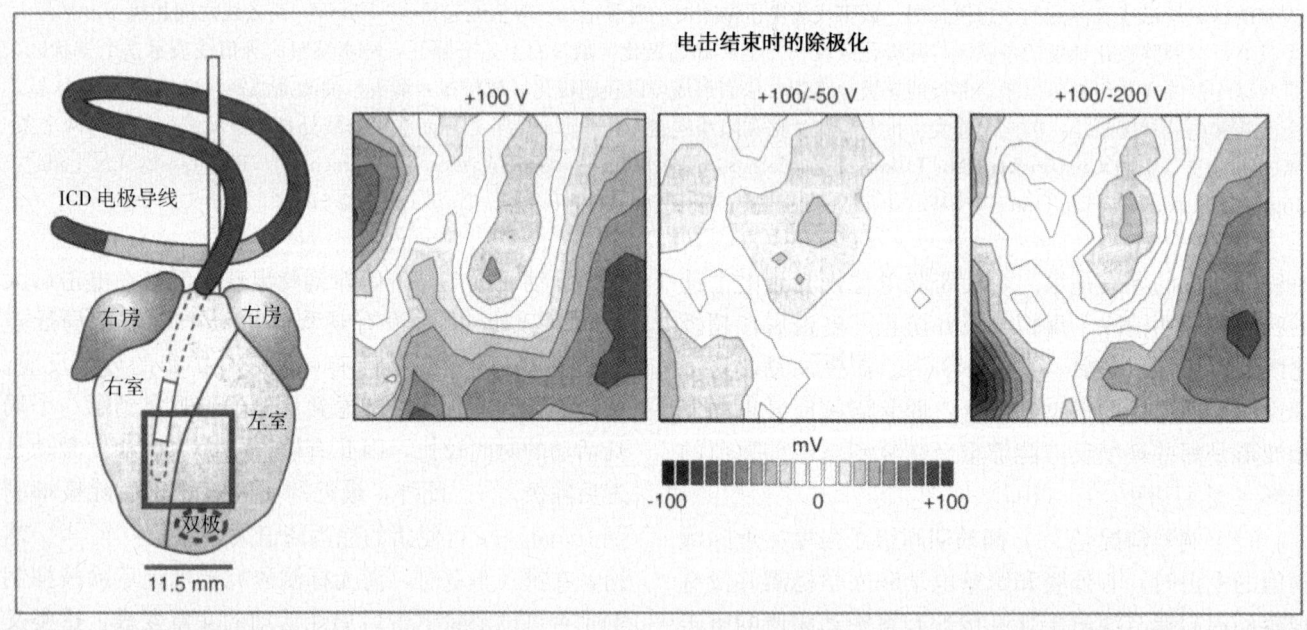

图 47-5 单相波除颤（+100V，8ms电击的第7ms）、第一相比第二相充电更多的优化双相除颤（+100V/-50V，16ms电击的第15ms）和第一相比第二相充电更少的非优化双相除颤（+100V/-200V，16ms电击的第15ms）结束处的除极化空间模式 心脏图例中的方框代表光学记录的部位。图例显示了除极化数值和电击前跨膜电压的关系，阳性和阴性除极化分别以不同的灰度水平表示，而白色表示没有发生除极化的区域（引自 Efimov IR，Cheng Y，Van Wagoner DR，et al：Virtual electrode-induced phase singularity：a basic mechanism of defibrillation failure. Cir Res 82：918-925，1998.）

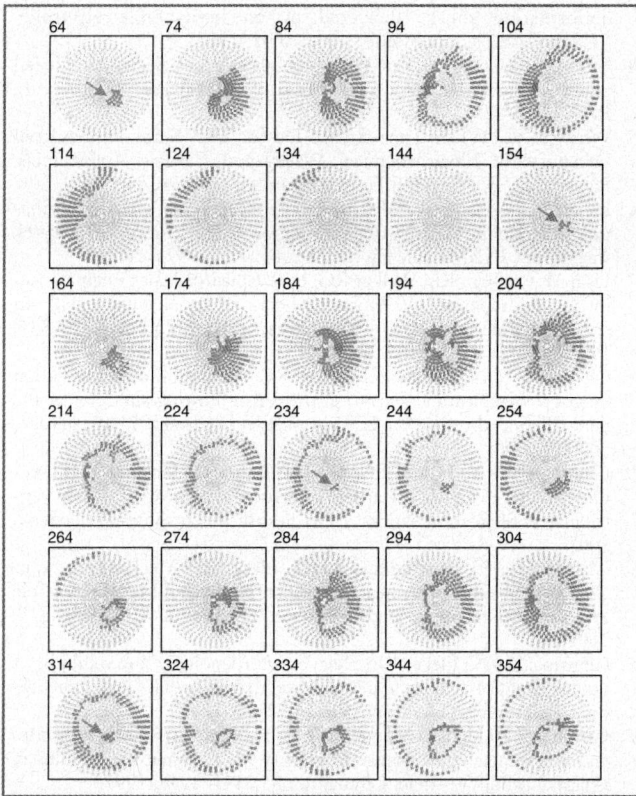

图 47-6　从右心室心尖部和上腔静脉电极给予强度接近除颤阈值的电击而除颤失败后的周期示例　通过分布在猪的心外膜 504 个电极同时记录。在极性投射中，房室沟位于周边，而左室心尖位于中央，灰线表示电极的位置。图像的底部代表前，右侧代表左心室。每一幅图都以黑色表示在 10ms 期间任何时刻 dV/dt=-0.5V/s 的电极位置。每一幅图上方的数字表示相对于电击开始的每个间期（单位 ms）。箭头表示每个周期中最早记录到激动的位置。第一个周期出现在电击后 64ms 前左心室心外膜上。第二个周期（154ms）出现在心外膜和第一个周期相同的部位，并且以局灶方式向外传导。第三个（235ms）和第四个（315ms）周期出现在前一个周期消失处（引自 Chattipakorn N，Fotuhi PC，Ideker RE：Prediction of defibrillation outcome by epicardial activation patterns following shocks near the defibrillation threshold. J Cardiovasc Electrophysiol 11：1014-1021，2000.）

（钟幼民　译）

参 考 文 献

1. Weiss G: Sur la possibilite de rendre comparables entre eux les apareils servant a l'excitation. Arch Ital de Biol 35:413–446, 1901.
2. Lapicque L: Sur l'excitation électrique de nerfs traitée comme une polarisation. J Physiol Pathol Gen 49:620–635, 1907.
3. Irnich W: The fundamental law of electrostimulation and its application to defibrillation. Pacing Clin Electrophysiol 13:1433–1447, 1990.
4. Blair HA: On the intensity-time relations for stimulation by electric currents. II. J Gen Physiol 15:731–755, 1932.
5. Fishler MG: Theoretical predictions of the optimal monophasic and biphasic defibrillation waveshapes. IEEE Trans Biomed Eng 47:59–67, 2000.
6. Kroll MW: A minimal model of the monophasic defibrillation pulse. Pacing Clin Electrophysiol 16:769–777, 1993.
7. Walcott GP, Walker RG, Cates AW, et al: Choosing the optimal monophasic and biphasic waveforms for ventricular defibrillation. J Cardiovasc Electrophysiol 6:737–750, 1995.
8. Swerdlow CD, Brewer JE, Kass RM, Kroll MW: Application of models of defibrillation to human defibrillation data: Implications for optimizing implantable defibrillator capacitance. Circulation 96:2813–2822, 1997.
9. White JB, Walcott GP, Wayland JL, et al: Predicting the relative efficacy of shock waveforms for transthoracic defibrillation in dogs. Ann Emer Med 34:309–320, 1999.
10. Zhou X, Rollins DL, Smith WM, Ideker RE: Responses of the transmembrane potential of myocardial cells during a shock. J Cardiovasc Electrophysiol 6:252–263, 1995.
11. Mowrey KA, Cheng Y, Tchou PJ, Efimov R: Kinetics of defibrillation shock-induced response: Design implications for the optimal defibrillation waveform. Europace 4:27–39, 2002.
12. Schuder JC, Stoeckle H, Dolan AM: Transthoracic ventricular defibrillation with square-wave stimuli: One-half cycle, one cycle, and multicycle waveforms. Circ Res 15:258–264, 1964.
13. Swartz JF, Jones JL, Fletcher RD: Characterization of ventricular fibrillation based on monophasic action potential morphology in the human heart. Circulation 87:1907–1914, 1993.
14. Tovar OH, Jones JL: Relationship between "extension of refractoriness" and probability of successful defibrillation. Am J Physiol Heart Circ Physiol 272:H1011–H1019, 1997.
15. Knisley SB, Smith WM, Ideker RE: Effect of field stimulation on cellular repolarization in rabbit myocardium: Implications for reentry induction. Circ Res 70:707–715, 1992.
16. Sweeney RJ, Gill RM, Steinberg MI, Reid PR: Ventricular refractory period extension caused by defibrillation shocks. Circulation 82:965–972, 1990.
17. Kao CY, Hoffman BF: Graded and decremental response in heart muscle fibers. Am J Physiol 194:187–196, 1958.
18. Kroll MW: A minimal model of the single capacitor biphasic defibrillation waveform. Pacing Clin Electrophysiol 17:1782–1792, 1994.
19. Swartz JF, Jones JL, Jones RE, Fletcher R: Conditioning prepulse of biphasic defibrillator waveforms enhances refractoriness to fibrillation wavefronts. Circ Res 68:438–449, 1991.
20. Dixon EG, Tang ASL, Wolf PD, et al: Improved defibrillation thresholds with large contoured epicardial electrodes and biphasic waveforms. Circulation 76:1176–1184, 1987.
21. Hillsley RE, Walker RG, Swanson DK, et al: Is the second phase of a biphasic defibrillation waveform the defibrillating phase? Pacing Clin Electrophysiol 16:1401–1411, 1993.
22. Ideker RE, Chattipakorn N, Walcott G, Fast VG: Electrophysiology of defibrillation. In Santini M (ed): Sudden Death: Non-Pharmacological Treatment. Casalecchio, Italy, Arianna Edtrice, 95–118, 2003.
23. Newton JC, Knisley SB, Zhou X, et al: Review of mechanisms by which electrical stimulation alters the transmembrane potential. J Cardiovasc Electrophysiol 10:234–243, 1999.
24. Chen P-S, Wolf PD, Claydon FJ III, et al: The potential gradient field created by epicardial defibrillation electrodes in dogs. Circulation 74:626–636, 1986.
25. Wharton JM, Wolf PD, Smith WM, et al: Cardiac potential and potential gradient fields generated by single, combined, and sequential shocks during ventricular defibrillation. Circulation 85:1510–1523, 1992.
26. Zhou X, Daubert JP, Wolf PD, et al: Epicardial mapping of ventricular defibrillation with monophasic and biphasic shocks in dogs. Circ Res 72:145–160, 1993.
27. Van Fleet JF, Tacker WA: Cardiac damage from transchest and ICD defibrillator shocks. In Tacker WA Jr (ed): Defibrillation of the Heart: ICDs, AEDs, and Manual. St Louis, Mosby-Year Book, 1994, pp 259–298.
28. Tacker WA: Defibrillation of the Heart: ICDs, AEDs, and Manual. St Louis, Mosby-Year Book, 1994, p 382.
29. Osswald S, Trouton TG, O'Nunain SS, et al: Relation between shock-related myocardial injury and defibrillation efficacy of monophasic and biphasic shocks in a canine model. Circulation 90:2501–2509, 1994.
30. Yabe S, Smith WM, Daubert JP, et al: Conduction disturbances

caused by high current density electric fields. Circ Res 66:1190–1203, 1990.
31. Jones JL, Jones RE: Improved defibrillator waveform safety factor with biphasic waveforms. Am J Physiol Heart Cell Physiol 245: H60–H65, 1983.
32. Fishler MG, Sobie EA, Tung L, Thakor NV: Modeling the interaction between propagating cardiac waves and monophasic and biphasic field stimuli: The importance of the induced spatial excitatory response. J Cardiovasc Electrophysiol 7:1183–1196, 1996.
33. Dillon SM, Kwaku KF: Progressive depolarization: A unified hypothesis for defibrillation and fibrillation induction by shocks. J Cardiovasc Electrophysiol 9:529–52, 1998.
34. Tovar OH, Jones JL: Biphasic defibrillation waveforms reduce shock-induced response duration dispersion between low and high shock intensities. Circ Res 77:430–438, 1995.
35. Dillon SM: Synchronized repolarization after defibrillation shocks: A possible component of the defibrillation process demonstrated by optical recordings in rabbit heart. Circulation 85:1865–1878, 1992.
36. Daubert JP, Frazier DW, Wolf PD, et al: Response of relatively refractory canine myocardium to monophasic and biphasic shocks. Circulation 84:2522–2538, 1991.
37. Zhou X, Knisley SB, Wolf PD, et al: Prolongation of repolarization time by electric field stimulation with monophasic and biphasic shocks in open chest dogs. Circ Res 68:1761–1767, 1991.
38. Chen P-S, Shibata N, Dixon EG, et al: Activation during ventricular defibrillation in open-chest dogs: Evidence of complete cessation and regeneration of ventricular fibrillation after unsuccessful shocks. J Clin Invest 77:810–823, 1986.
39. Shibata N, Chen P-S, Dixon EG, et al: Epicardial activation following unsuccessful defibrillation shocks in dogs. Am J Physiol Heart Circ Physiol 255:H902–H909, 1988.
40. Frazier DW, Wolf PD, Wharton JM, et al: Stimulus-induced critical point: Mechanism for electrical initiation of reentry in normal canine myocardium. J Clin Invest 83:1039–1052, 1989.
41. Idriss SF, Wolf PD, Smith WM, Ideker RE: Effect of pacing site on ventricular fibrillation initiation by shocks during the vulnerable period. Am J Physiol Heart Circ Physiol 277:H2065–H2082, 1999.
42. Chattipakorn N, Rogers JM, Ideker RE: Influence of postshock epicardial activation patterns on initiation of ventricular fibrillation by upper limit of vulnerability shocks. Circulation 101:1329–1336, 2000.
43. Efimov IR, Cheng YN, Biermann M, et al: Transmembrane voltage changes produced by real and virtual electrodes during monophasic defibrillation shocks delivered by an implantable electrode. J Cardiovasc Electrophysiol 8:1031–1045, 1997.
44. Efimov IR, Cheng Y, Van Wagoner DR: Virtual electrode-induced phase singularity: A basic mechanism of defibrillation failure. Circ Res 82:918–925, 1998.
45. Winfree AT: When Time Breaks Down: The Three-Dimensional Dynamics of Electrochemical Waves and Cardiac Arrhythmias. Princeton, NJ, Princeton University Press, 1987, p 153.
46. Ideker RE, Alferness C, Melnick S, et al: Reentry site during fibrillation induction in relation to defibrillation efficacy for different shock waveforms. J Cardiovasc Electrophysiol 12:581–591, 2001.
47. Usui M, Callihan RL, Walker RG, et al: Epicardial sock mapping following monophasic and biphasic shocks of equal voltage with an endocardial lead system. J Cardiovasc Electrophysiol 7:322–334, 1996.
48. Chattipakorn N, Fotuhi PC, Ideker RE: Prediction of defibrillation outcome by epicardial activation patterns following shocks near the defibrillation threshold. J Cardiovasc Electrophysiol 11:1014–1021, 2000.
49. Chattipakorn N, Fotuhi PC, Chattipakorn SC, Ideker RE: Three-dimensional mapping of earliest activation after near-threshold ventricular defibrillation shocks. J Cardiovasc Electrophysiol 14:65–69, 2003.
50. Chattipakorn N, Banville I, Gray RA, Ideker RE: Mechanism of ventricular defibrillation for near-defibrillation threshold shocks: A whole heart optical mapping study in swine. Circulation 104:1313–1319, 2001.
51. Chattipakorn N, Ideker RE: Delayed afterdepolarization inhibitor: A potential pharmacological intervention to improve defibrillation efficacy. J Cardiovasc Electrophysiol 14:72–75, 2003.
52. Gotoh M, Uchida T, Mandel WJ, et al: Cellular graded responses and ventricular vulnerability to reentry by a premature stimulus in isolated canine ventricle. Circulation 95:2141–2154, 1997.
53. Eason J, Hillebrenner M, Campbell C, Trayanova N: Assessing shock efficacy as a function of arrhythmia complexity in a slab of the canine heart. In Proceedings of the Second Joint EMBS/BMES Conference, Houston, TX, 2002, pp 1413–1414.
54. Henning B, Wit AL: The time course of action potential repolarization affects delayed afterdepolarization amplitude in atrial fibers of the canine coronary sinus. Circ Res 55:110–115, 1984.
55. Chattipakorn N, Ideker RE: Mechanism of Defibrillation. In Aliot E, Clémenty J, Prystowsky EN (eds): Fighting Sudden Cardiac Death: A Worldwide Challenge. Armonk, NY, Futura, 2000, pp 593–615.

第九部分
分子遗传学和药物基因组学

第 48 章

心律失常的小鼠模型

Barry London

本章目录

- 构建转基因小鼠和基因打靶小鼠的方法 429
- 研究转基因小鼠和基因敲除小鼠的方法 431
- 小鼠的心律失常模型 435
- 总结 437

哺乳动物心脏的发育和功能发挥需要许多基因及其产物的参与。在人类，这些基因的天然突变可导致许多先天性疾病，由此我们也得知了这些基因的重要性[1,2]。自从20世纪下半叶以来，人们越来越清楚地知道突变在小鼠身上很容易实现。心脏基因可以被添加、删除或者修饰，而这些变化所引起的心脏生理学表型也可以被量化[3]。因此，转基因和基因打靶小鼠在现代心血管研究中充当着重要的角色。

小鼠心脏与人类心脏在电生理上有比较大的差异。尽管如此，利用基因工程小鼠来复制心律失常模型还是越来越被研究者们所接受。本章将具体阐述如何构建基因工程小鼠以及研究其电生理功能的方法，并将探讨现有的遗传学模型。同时，也将讨论小鼠作为心律失常模型的优缺点。

一、构建转基因小鼠和基因打靶小鼠的方法

（一）转基因的过表达

通过转基因小鼠我们可以在心脏上表达某个基因并研究其效应（见图48-1）。一个转基因构建体由一个心脏特异性的启动子、待表达的目的基因以及用于稳定核糖核酸（RNA）的多聚腺苷尾巴构成。最常用的启动子来自于大鼠或小鼠的α-肌球蛋白重链基因。因为这种启动子在接近出生时才会有活性（可避免胚胎期死亡），可将所转基因特异性地表达于成年小鼠的心房和心室[3]。转基因构建体直接注入小鼠的受精卵原核，然后将该受精卵植入假孕的母鼠。通过对存活下来后代的尾部进行取材活检，提取脱氧核糖核酸（DNA），进而通过聚合酶链反应（polymerase chain reaction，PCR）或基因组 Southern 印迹分析可筛选获得 F_0 代。F_0 代与野生小鼠交配将产生杂合子的 F_1 代。F_1 的小鼠用于检测转基因的表达。因此，研究只需要两代小鼠，一年内即可完成。同时，同窝的对照也很容易从 F_1 代中获得。

显性负相（dominant negative）转基因策略可用于在心脏中减少某种基因的表达[4]。例如，利用有功能的钾离子（K^+）通道的形成需要四个相关的α亚单位共组装的特点，可将含有点突变或序列缺失的亚单位与野生型亚单位一起共组装。假设一个单独的突变亚单位就足以阻止功能性的通道形成，并且天然的亚单位和突变的亚单位可以随机地进行共组装，那么大量表达突变的转基因将有效地减少野生型通道的功

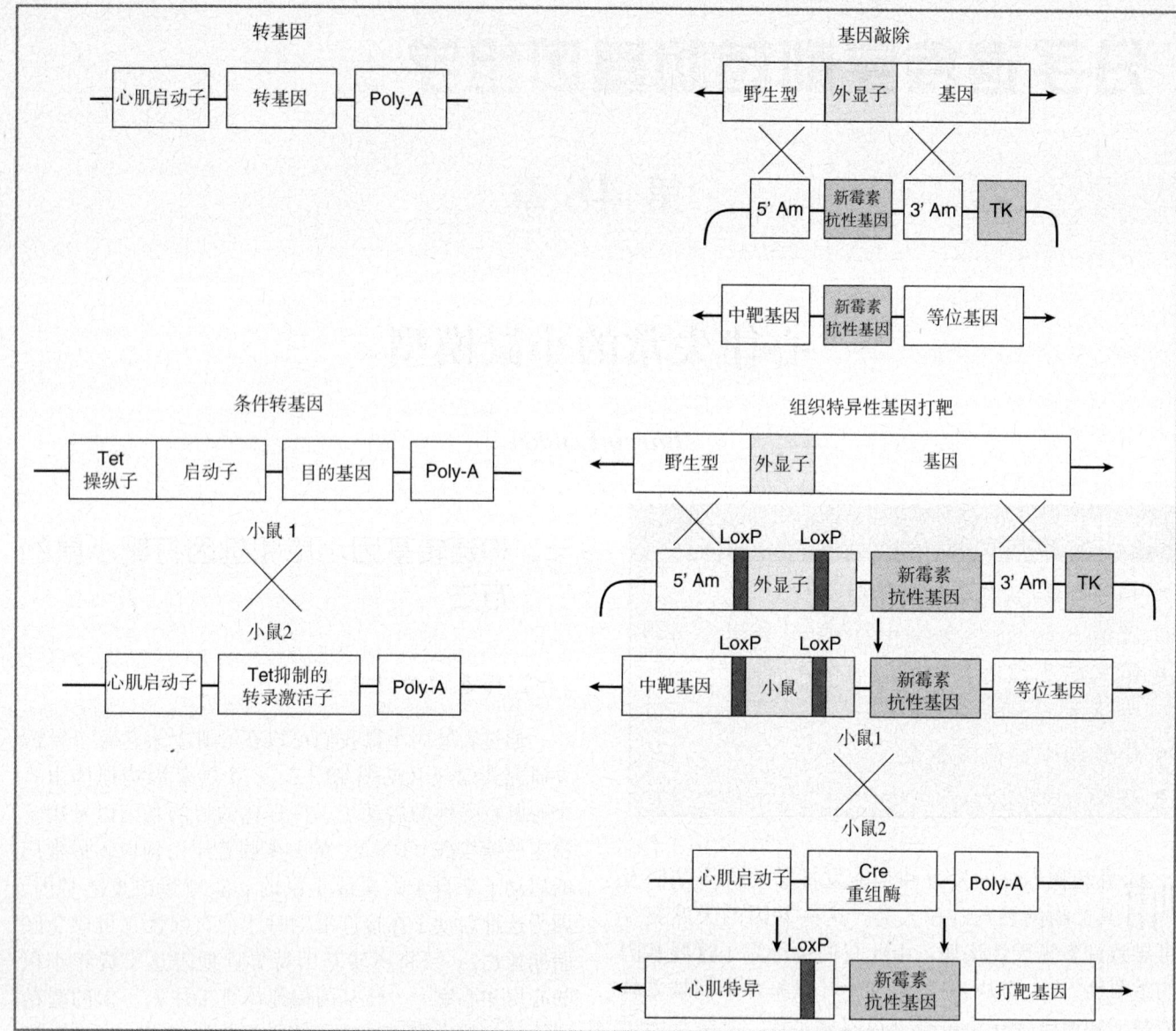

图 48-1 对用于基因工程转基因的（上左）、条件转基因（下左）、基因打靶的（上右）和组织特异性基因打靶小鼠（下右）的技术比较　　转基因的构建体随机插入小鼠染色体。而基因打靶要求在胚胎干细胞中同源重组进而产生小鼠。条件转基因和组织特异性基因打靶都要求将两个遗传学修饰的小鼠进行交配以获得想要的特性。poly-A：多聚腺苷尾巴；LoxP：34 个碱基对的元件，在 cre 重组酶存在的情况下可以内部重组；NeoR：新霉素抗性基因；Tet：四环素；TK：胸腺嘧啶激酶基因

能。另外，一种转基因还可能同时影响几种通道亚单位。这一点是很有优势的，它使我们可以迅速检测心脏中某一类离子通道的功能。然而，这也使我们有时很难确定实际上究竟是哪一种通道受到了转基因的干扰。

理想情况下，目的基因在心脏表达应可以被随意开关。研究者因此开发了多种系统，其中许多采用四环素反应启动子元件（见图 48-1）[5]。但迄今为止，有限的成功率以及转基因的组织特异性的变化限制了这项技术的广泛应用。

将目的基因随机参入小鼠染色体可能干扰插入位点的天然基因的功能。通常需要研究两种以上独立品系的转基因小鼠，才能确定观测的表型是否是转基因表达的直接结果。同时我们还可以对表达不同量突变亚单位的不同品系进行检测。通过两个杂合子小鼠交配可获得纯合子的转基因小鼠，由此可进一步提高转基因的表达水平。纯合子的品系更容易产生来自于位点插入的表型改变。

转基因小鼠的潜在问题在于突变蛋白的大量过表达。突变蛋白可能逐步中和细胞中的重要因子，比如

β亚单位，或者对心肌细胞产生直接的毒性作用。例如在心脏中过表达一种绿色荧光蛋白就可导致扩张性心肌病[6]。

（二）基因打靶

胚胎干细胞（embryonic stem，ES）同源重组技术可以使小鼠的单个基因失活（基因敲除）或被修饰（基因敲入，靶向突变），见图48-1[7]。这些ES细胞具有全能性，因为它们保持着分化成包括生殖细胞在内的所有细胞的能力。

胚胎干细胞来自动物囊胚的内细胞团，并可在体外加以扩增。最常用的细胞取自SV19小鼠，SV19含有纯合的编码灰色被毛的显性基因。人们先克隆出感兴趣基因的DNA，进而利用基因工程的方法构建打靶的构建体。该构建体包括一个在待修饰区域5'端数千个碱基对（basepair，bp）的片段上接一个用作正性筛选的抗生素抗性基因，通常为新霉素抗性基因（neomycin resistance gene，NeoR），同时在待修饰区域3'端接上一个作为负性筛选的胸腺嘧啶核苷激酶（thymidine kinase，TK）基因。用电穿孔的办法（电休克法）将这个线性构建体导入ES细胞，其中有一小部分ES细胞可发生同源重组。在这种情况下，发生了两个交换事件，即带有NeoR的打靶构建体替换了目的基因在对应于打靶构建体的两个同源臂之间的部分。因而造成一小部分ES细胞在打靶的等位基因表现为杂合型。

杂合型中靶的ES细胞可在氨基糖苷类抗生素G418存在的情况下存活（因为他们拥有NeoR基因）和甘昔洛韦（或它的类似物，FIAU）存在的情况下存活（因为他们没有TK基因）。用甘昔洛韦或FIAU做二重筛选可以消除打靶构建体随机插入染色体的克隆。这些克隆具有功能性的TK基因，上述试剂可将其致死。双阳性的克隆将经由PCR或基因组Southern印迹分析的方法筛选，进而扩增并注射入黑色被毛的C57BL/6小鼠的囊胚，然后再植入假孕的母鼠。

嵌合体后代的细胞部分来自ES细胞，部分来自供体囊胚细胞。故可从其灰黑相间的被毛颜色而确认。将雄性嵌合体与雌性的C57BL/6小鼠交配。如果后代为灰毛的，说明ES细胞来源的精子在生殖过程中被传递下来。这些灰毛小鼠后代的半数携带一个拷贝的中靶等位基因。两个杂合子的雌雄交配可获得纯合子基因打靶小鼠。

这种形式的基因操纵有几个重要的缺陷。重组的等位基因存在于该基因所表达的所有细胞类型。因此，任何表型的改变不仅反映了该基因在心脏中的缺失，也反映了该基因在神经系统和其他组织的缺失。另外，重组的等位基因存在于整个胚胎发育过程。因此，成年小鼠的表型改变可能被其他基因的长期代偿作用而得以修饰。而胚胎性死亡则无法研究某些基因在成年鼠中的作用。

利用cre/lox系统（见图48-1）人们可以实现基因的时间限制性和组织限制性敲除。该系统中，待敲除的基因被两个由34个碱基对构成的元件所包围。将纯合子基因打靶小鼠以组织特异性或时间特异性的方式与表达cre重组酶的转基因鼠交配。由于cre重组酶蛋白的表达，基因在两个元件之间的部分被去除，因而实现了条件性的组织特异性基因敲除。

小鼠的品系也会影响基因操纵的表型。如按上述操作得到的基因打靶小鼠是一个混合遗传背景的（50%SV129；50%C57BL/6）。纯SV129背景的小鼠可通过将雄性的生殖系嵌合体与SV129的雌鼠交配获得。绝大部分为C57BL/6背景的小鼠可通过混合背景的杂合子小鼠与野生型C57BL/6小鼠回交获得。经过5~10代，大部分等位基因将与C57BL16系小鼠相匹配，同时去除了和打靶基因的等位基因连锁的基因，使得与等位基因共分离。

二、研究转基因小鼠和基因敲除小鼠的方法

（一）分子水平的研究

需要对修饰基因的RNA和蛋白水平的表达情况进行检测。量化以及定位RNA的标准方法有Northern印迹、核酸酶保护实验（ribonuclease protection assay，RPA）、反转录PCR（包括定量技术，如实时PCR）和原位杂交。定量及定位蛋白质的技术包括Western印迹、酶联免疫吸附实验、免疫荧光以及免疫组织化学方法。

对于基因敲除模型，天然的基因产物通常在杂合子中明显减少而在纯合子中不存在。但在某些情况下，代偿机制可以使杂合子表现出正常的蛋白质水平。当基因打靶应用于突变或替换某个基因，人们希望获得与天然基因相似的表达水平和组织特异性。对

于转基因模型，转基因的 RNA 和蛋白质是存在的，其组织定位取决于启动子。

接下来需要研究与心脏电生理相关的其他基因的 RNA 和蛋白质水平的表达，这些基因通常包括离子通道蛋白和连接蛋白。某个基因的缺失可能导致相关基因的代偿性上调。例如，Kv1.5 基因打靶小鼠缺失心脏 $I_{K,slow}$ 的 4 氨基吡啶敏感成分[8]，而编码 4 氨基吡啶不敏感 $I_{K,slow}$ 成分的基因 Kv2.1 则出现蛋白水平的上调。这种代偿性上调使得总的 $I_{K,slow}$ 或总的钾外流保持不变。

（二）细胞电生理学

在 Langendorff 灌流装置上，用胶原酶经主动脉逆行灌流小鼠心脏可以分离到单个的成年小鼠心肌细胞[9]。采用类似于大鼠的胰酶消化方案可以分离新生小鼠的心肌细胞。利用穿膜膜片钳（perforated patch）或全细胞透析技术，动作电位（action potentials，APs）和离子流可分别以电流钳和电压钳模式放大并加以记录。小鼠的动作电位极短，类似三角形没有平台期（图 48-2）。动作电位时程（action potential duration，APD）$_{75}$ 将近 15ms，（APD）$_{90}$ 将近 40ms[9]。

小鼠心脏的离子通道与稍大一些哺乳动物的非常相似[10]。事实上，大多数小鼠和人的离子通道在蛋白质水平上至少 95％是相同的，并且具有相似的电生理学和药理学特性。在两个种属中，都是主要由 SCN5A 编码的钠离子（Na^+）电流（I_{Na}）来起始动作电位，而由 $K_{ir}2.1$ 编码的内向整流（I_{K1}）作用在于维持静息的膜电位。

然而，关于钾通道基因的含量和它在心肌复极中的作用，在小鼠和人的心脏中显著不同（见图 48-2）[11]。其实考虑到小鼠的心率快（＞600 bpm）和 AP 短，这也就不足为奇了。在人的心脏中主要的复极电流：KvLQT1 编码的延迟整流的缓慢激活成分（I_{Ks}）和它的 β 亚单位微小钾通道蛋白（minK），人的 ether-a-go-go-related 基因（HERG）编码的延迟整流的快速成分（I_{Kr}）以及可能的 β 亚单位 MiRP1。这些基因的突变会导致常染色体显性和隐性长 QT 综合征（Long QT syndrome，LQTS）。Kv4.3 和 Kv1.4 编码的瞬时外向离子流（I_{to}）的重要性尚不

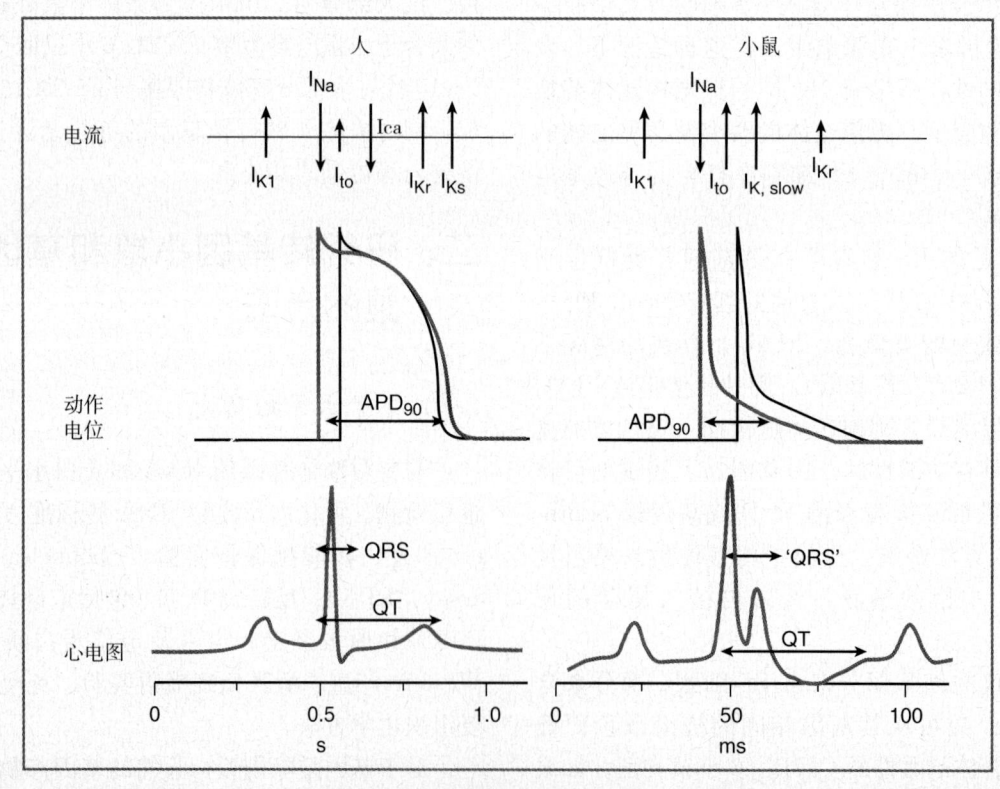

图 48-2　比较人（左侧）和小鼠（右侧）心脏离子通道、动作电位和心电图　每个电流的箭头大小大致上与他们的强度成比例。指示外向电流的箭头朝上。每次心脏搏动，最先除极细胞的 APs 用实线表示，最后除极的用虚线表示。动作电位时程（APD）$_{90}$ 即 AP 达到 90％复极的时间。小鼠的心电图是五个连续的搏动的平均信号。人的心电图是模拟的。注意，在小鼠表现出的 "QRS" 时程对应于除极和早期复极

十分清楚。Kv1.5 和/或 Kv2.1 编码超快激活缓慢失活电流（I_{Kur}，$I_{K,slow}$）则局限于心房表达。在小鼠的心室，主要的复极电流是 Kv4.3 和 Kv4.2 编码的 I_{to} 的快速成分（$I_{to,f}$）、Kv1.4 编码的 I_{to} 的缓慢成分（$I_{to,s}$）以及 Kv1.5 和 Kv2.1 编码的 $I_{K,slow}$。还存在某些 Merg1 编码的 I_{Kr}（小鼠 HERG 类似物）。尽管有人认为有 KvLQT1 的存在，但在成年小鼠心室肌细胞是否有 I_{Ks} 尚无定论，可能是 minK 表达不够广泛的缘故[12]。

（三）整体心脏的电生理

单相动作电位（monophasic action potenitials, MAPs）使得细胞外吸附电极测量 AP 形状和 APD 成为可能。这些技术已被成功地用于小鼠心脏的研究。尽管该项技术的优点尚不十分清楚[13]。

小鼠心脏外表面的激活和复极可以通过电极芯片进行标测。但是小鼠心脏的体积较小，加之电极芯片空间分辨率的限制，因而光学标测技术已经取代了电极标测[14]。

光学标测依赖于一些细胞内染料。这些染料可以随着电压的变化而改变其荧光特性[15,16]。人们将小鼠心脏固定在 Langendorff 灌流装置上，并从冠状动脉灌入染料（通常为 di-4-ANNEPS），接着用激发光照射心脏，相对较长波长的发射光被滤过并投射到光电二极管芯片或一个电荷耦联的装置（charge-coupled device，CCD）相机（见图 48-3）。这就可对每分钟跳动 600 次的小心脏以高时间分辨率和高空间分辨率持续测定 AP。同时可以测定 APD、传导速度和复极特性。程序刺激（早搏，短阵快速起搏）可用来诱发室性或房性的心率失常（见图 48-3 B 和 C）。该技术的局限性是：（1）对心室壁的测量深度不够；（2）人为造成的移动，尤其是应用二乙酰单氧化物（diacetyl monoxide）和 cytochalasin-D（细胞松弛素 D）等兴奋收缩脱耦联剂时可能引起 AP 波形较大的改变[16]。

钙敏感的染料可用以描记小鼠心脏的钙瞬变[17]。光学标测技术也可用于研究成年小鼠的传导系统以及胚胎鼠和新生鼠的发育变化[18,19]。

（四）心电图记录和无线遥测技术

心电图（electrocardiogram，ECG）也可用于小鼠研究。需要考虑的技术问题是导联的设置（通常为皮下或足垫）、导联的放置以及麻醉的应用。麻醉可能会改变心率或 AP 的特性。另外，为了精确地量化 ECG 信号，需采用很高的采样频率（>400 Hz）并对信号进行适当的滤过。

人的心电图由一个 P 波（心房除极）、一个 QRS 波群（心室除极）、一个等电线的 ST 段（当整个心脏除极后形成的 AP 的平台期）以及一个 T 波（心室复极）构成。双侧心室的心内表面几乎同时兴奋，QRS 波群的延长表明有传导系统的疾病。而 QT 间期则反映了 APD 时程，APD 延长或 APD 弥散增强可造成 QT 间期的延长。

小鼠的 ECG 由一个 P 波、一个 QRS 波群、一个低幅的 ST 段以及 T 波（仅见于部分导联）构成（见图 48-2）。小鼠 ECG 的解释很复杂，因为鼠的心脏传导迅速、心室 AP 较短缺乏平台期。一部分心脏的去极与另一部分的复极同时发生。鼠 ECG 高振幅的"QRS"波群不仅代表去极沿着心室扩散，也代表复极的早期相。同时，低幅的 ST 段和 T 波则对应于复极的晚期相（AP 的低幅尾部）。因此，QRS 波群的延长可能提示传导系统的异常或者复极的延迟。另外，QT 间期需用取自小鼠并经小鼠检测的公式加以校正[9]。由于人和小鼠 ECG 的差异造成了文献数据的混乱。

皮下植入式无线电遥感 ECG 装置通常用于记录心脏的长期节律，包括猝死时的心脏节律（图 48-4 A）。奇怪的是大部分的转基因小鼠模型在死亡时均表现为缓慢性心律失常[20]。应用遥感检测还可以测定清醒状态下走动的小鼠对药物的反应以及心率变异指数[21,22]。不过，对小鼠心率变异的解释还很困难。

小鼠心脏节律解释起来也很困难。比如宽大的室性节律波群在心率 500 bpm 的转基因小鼠中可能被称为室性心动过速，但在一个心率超过 600 bpm 的自然动物却可能代表加速性室性逸搏心律。与此类似的例子，某些野生型小鼠天然状态下也可以偶发一些高度的心脏传导阻滞（见图 48-4A）。

（五）程序刺激

采用多极导管实施程序刺激的临床电生理检查也被应用于小鼠的研究[23]。方法有开胸小鼠的心外刺激以及经颈内静脉至左房和左室的心内刺激。也可以描记希氏束电图（见图 48-4B）[24]。

到目前为止，在实验中对一只小鼠只能进行一次程序刺激。人们正在发展可以重复刺激的技术。另外

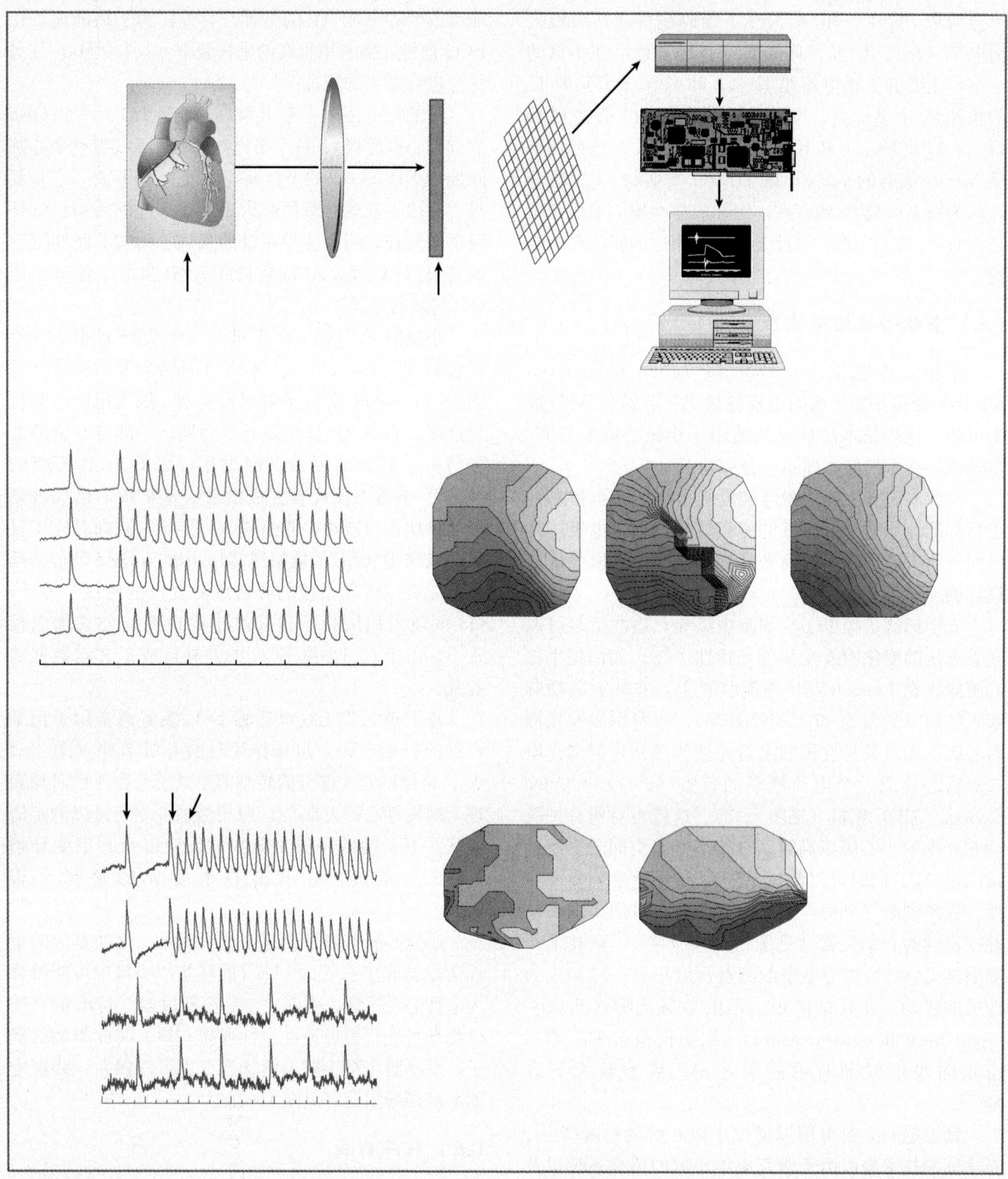

图 48-3　小鼠动作电位（APs）的光学标测　A：应用小鼠进行光学标测的简图[16]。B：采自四个光电二极管的光学信号显示在过表达肿瘤坏死因子（TNF）α的心力衰竭小鼠，单个额外刺激诱导出单形性室性心动过速。左侧显示的是基础搏动（S1）、早搏（S2）和室性心动过速的第四个搏动的同时激动图。C：用一个单独的房性早搏诱导房扑（频率约 1400 bpm）。顶端的两个通道记录的是房性的 APs，而底端的两个通道记录的是间断的室性激动

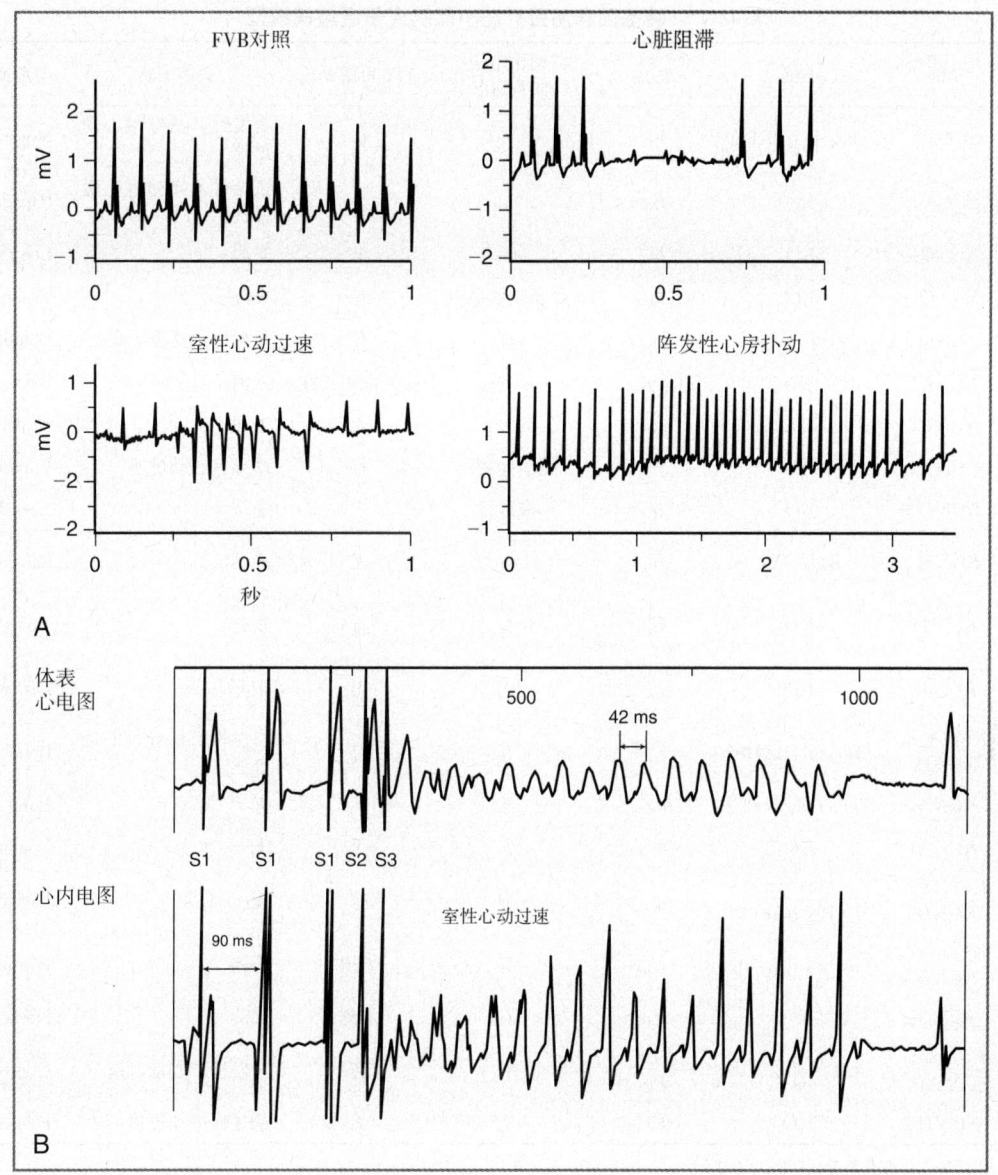

图 48-4 A：FVB 对照和肿瘤坏死因子（tumor necrosis factor，TNF）α 转基因心力衰竭小鼠的体表心电图。对照小鼠有高度的传导阻滞。TNFα 小鼠有室颤和房扑发作。B：在一只对照小鼠，经颈内静脉放置多极导管，用两个右室额外刺激诱导出了多形性非持续性室性心动过速。（本图由 Pittsburgh 大学的 Samir Saba 提供）

一个较大的问题在于对研究结果的解释。实施人为程序刺激时，大量过激的刺激可在非病理变化的心脏上也探测到心律失常。对于异常小鼠心电生理，目前尚没有明确的定义。另外，小鼠的种系和性别差异使得其心电生理学研究的解释更为复杂[22,25]。

三、小鼠的心律失常模型

（一）离子通道病

常染色体显性和隐性 LQTS 是由于心脏钾离子通道基因突变导致外向电流减少和钠离子通道基因突变导致钠离子通道不能完全失活[2]。心脏钠离子通道的功能丢失性突变可导致 Brugada 综合征。这些基因是小鼠基因突变的天然靶点，可不同程度地反映出人类某些疾病的特点（见表 48-1）。

携带 SCN5A ΔKPQ 突变的基因打靶小鼠表现为 APD 和 QT 间期延长，并伴有可诱发性心律失常[26]。这些小鼠最令人惊讶的特征是在心率突然增加或早搏之后，出现非常显著的 APD 延长以及早期后除极（early afterdepolarizations，EADs）。需要明确的是人类的这种 LQT3 突变是否具有相似的变化，以及这

表 48-1 转基因和基因打靶小鼠的离子通道病模型

通道	基因	小鼠	电流	动作电位时程延长	QTc 间期延长	心律失常	参考文献
$Na_v1.5$	SCN5A	Targeted△KPQ	I_{Na}	有	有	自发性，诱导性心动过速	Nuyens et al. 2001
$Na_v1.5$	SCN5A	KO	I_{Na}	无	无	诱导性心动过速；缓慢性？	Papadatos et al. 2002
KvLQT1	KCNQ1	KO	I_{Ks}	无	无	未测	Lee et al. 2000
KvLQT1	KCNQ1	KO	I_{Ks}	单相动作电位	有	未测	Casiimiro et al. 2000
KvLQT1	KCNQ1	TG：DN	I_{Ks}	有	有	缓慢性：莫氏1型	Demolombe et al. 2001
MinK/IsK	KCNE1	KO	I_{Ks}	未进行	有频率相关性	未测	Drici et al. 1998
MinK/IsK	KCNE1	Targeted：LacZ	I_{Ks}	无	无	未测	Kupershmidt et al. 1999
Merg1	KCNH2	Merg1$^{+/-}$	I_{Kr}	光学标测到	有	诱导性心动过速	London et al. 1998a
Merg1b	KCNH2	KO	I_{Kr}	未进行	无	窦缓	Lees-Miller et al. 2003
Merg1	KCNH2	TG：DN	I_{Kr}	有	无	未测	Babij et al. 1998
$K_{ir}2.1$/IRK1	KCNJ1	KO	I_{K1}	有	有	未测	Zaritsky et al. 2002
$K_{ir}2.2$/IRK2	KCNJ2	KO	I_{K1}	无	无	未测	Zaritsky et al. 2002
Kv1.4 & Kv1.5	KCNA4 & KCND5	TG：Kv1.1DN	I_{Kslow} & $I_{to,s}$	有	有	自发性，诱导性心动过速	London et al. 1998
Kv1.5	KCNA5	Targeted：Kv1.1	I_{Kslow}	无	无	无	London et al. 2001
Kv1.4	KCNA4	KO	$I_{to,s}$	无	无	无	London et al. 1998b
Kv4.2 & Kv4.3	KCND2 & KCND3	TG：DN pore	$I_{to,f}$	有	有	无	Barry et al. 1998
Kv4.2 & Kv4.3	KCND2 & KCND3	TG：DN truncation	$I_{to,f}$	有	未测	未测	Wichenden et al. 1998
Kv4.2	KCND2	KO	$I_{to,f}$	有	未测	未测	Nerbonne et al. 2001
Kv1.4 & Kv4.2, 3	KCNA4 & KCND2, 3	Kv1.4 KO	$I_{to,f}$ & $I_{to,s}$	有	有	自发性，心动过速	Guo et al. 2000
KChIP2	KCNIP2	KO	$I_{to,f}$	有	无	诱导性心动过速	Kuo et al. 2001

注：DN，显相负性；KO，基因敲除；TG，转基因
见参考文献 9，11，12，20，26-31，33-35，37~39，41~43

种机制是否与缓慢依赖性心律失常相关。SCN5A 的杂合子基因打靶小鼠表现出体表 ECG 的 PR 间期延长[27]。离体灌流的 SCN5A$^{+/-}$ 心脏表现出房室结和心室不应期的明显异常，并伴有可诱发的室性心动过速。

基因打靶和显性负相技术也被用于对 KvLQT1 和 minK 基因的操纵，它们在大型哺乳动物心脏中参与编码 I_{Ks} 的基因[12,28-31]。Lee 和其同事在 KLQT1 第一个外显子双敲除（KvLQT1$^{-/-}$）的小鼠上没有观察到 ECG 的异常[28]。然而 Casimiro 和他的同事[29]则报道了该模型小鼠的 QT 间期延长，但在离体心脏没有观察到这种现象。一种 KvLQT1 的显性负相小鼠表现为 QT 间期延长和心动过缓，伴有 I_{K1} 和 I_{to} 的减低。MinK 基因敲除小鼠的心血管表型也很有争议。一个研究小组报道，MinK 基因敲除可引起心率相关的异常 QT 反应[12,31]。麻醉的差异也许可以用来解释一些分歧。通过 lacZ 基因靶向替换 minK 基因可帮助我们在小鼠传导系统上定位 minK 的表达[12]。因此，目前还不清楚，在这些小鼠模型中与 I_{Ks} 缺失相关的表型是作为一种对变化的代偿性矫正呢，还是一种基因缺失的非心脏效应。值得注意的是，minK 在小鼠心脏的过表达便于对 minK/KvLQT1 复合体进行生化研究[32]。

过表达一种 HERG-显性负相构建体的小鼠虽然没有心律失常，但可表现出有一种小的 I_{Kr} 电流[33]。靶向干预 Merg1 的纯合子小鼠，胚胎期即发生死亡。而 Merg1 杂合子（Merg1$^{+/-}$）具有轻微的 QT 间期延

长，经α-肾上腺素受体激动剂处理后可发生心律失常[34]。靶向干预 Merg1b 亚型可以减少成年小鼠的 I_{Kr}[35]。这些 Merg1b-/- 小鼠更容易发生缓慢性心律失常，不过这些发现与 I_{Kr} 减低的关系尚不明确。

Kir2.1 的突变减少了内向整流 I_{K1} 并可致 Andersen 综合征[36]。靶向缺失 Kir2.1 基因的小鼠生后即因腭裂死亡[37]。虽然这些新生小鼠有 APD 延长，但是并没有观察到心律失常。靶向缺失 Kir2.2 基因可导致小鼠 I_{K1} 减低 50%[37]。

目前认为 I_{to} 和 $I_{K,slow}$ 对于小鼠心脏的复极最为重要。因此低水平表达这些电流的离子通道编码基因的转基因小鼠被广泛用于研究（见表 48-1）。表达 Kv1.1（缺失 $I_{K,slow}$ 的 4-氨基吡啶敏感成分）的一个 N 端片段的显性负相小鼠可表现为 APD 和 QT 的延长，并具有自发性和可诱导性心律失常[9]。有趣的是，主要的心律失常为单形的室性心动过速。与人类的 LQTS 中多形的室性心动过速以及尖端扭转型室速相反。光学标测可以研究心律失常易感性增强的机制，人们发现从心尖到基底部的复极和不应期的弥散增大了[16]，小鼠不会死于快速心律失常，这是在长 QT 小鼠模型可以经常看到的现象。

基因打靶也用于将 Kv1.5 替换为 Kv1.1[8]。这些小鼠也缺乏 $I_{K,slow}$ 的 4-氨基吡啶敏感成分。然而由于 Kv2.1 的上调可使 APD 或 QT 间期并不延长。事实上，这些小鼠在药物诱导的 QT 间期延长中是被 4-氨基吡啶保护的。而且小鼠并没有自发性心律失常。缺乏 Kv1.4 的基因打靶小鼠（Kv1.4-/-）也没有 APD 延长、QT 间期延长和心律失常[38,39]。缺乏 Kv2.1 基因的显性负相小鼠确实表现为 APD 和 QT 间期延长，但没有自发性心律失常[40]。

过表达 Kv4.2 小孔突变体的显性负相转基因小鼠，由于缺乏 $I_{to,f}$，故而导致 APD 和 QT 间期延长[41]。这种 Kv4.2DN 小鼠具有 Kv1.4 和 $I_{to,s}$ 代偿性的上调，所以没有复极的弥散增加和心律失常。将 Kv4.2DN 小鼠与 Kv1.4-/- 小鼠交配获得的小鼠完全缺乏 I_{to}，表现为明显的 QT 间期延长和心律失常[39]。在这种小鼠的心肌细胞可以检测到 APD 延长和 EADs 的增加。最近有报道认为靶向的干预 Kv1.4 会减少 $I_{to,f}$[11]。

应用显性负相技术过表达一种序列缺失的 Kv4.2 可以实现对 I_{to} 的干预。这种小鼠会发生进行性的心肌病[42]。但是单纯 I_{to} 缺失不足以解释这种心肌病表型。这一研究也强调了在对转基因和基因敲除小鼠的表型进行解释时需要谨慎。

对小鼠 KChIP2 基因的靶向干预（Kv4.x 家族的一个辅助性亚单位）可引起 I_{to} 的缺失、APD 和 QT 间期延长以及心律失常[43]。这些小鼠模型中电流的改变、心律失常以及死亡率的关系有待进一步明确。这些研究充分展示了利用基因打靶小鼠来证实基因产物对正常心电生理功能影响的重要性。

（二）传导紊乱

敲除缝隙连接蛋白 43（connexin43）的纯合子小鼠都死于围产期[44]。光学标测研究表明，这些小鼠在胚胎和新生时即发生慢传导和心律失常[44]。特异性敲除心脏缝隙连接蛋白 43 的小鼠表现为传导缓慢并死于心室纤颤[45]。这是小鼠明确的死于快速性心律失常少有的几个例子之一，揭示了细胞间耦联在防止致死性心律失常中的重要性。

缝隙连接蛋白 40 可表达于特殊传导系统。敲除缝隙连接蛋白 40-/- 的纯合子小鼠将发生传导减慢、束支阻滞和心房的缓慢性心律失常[18,24,46]。

心脏的传导异常在越来越多的其他转基因和基因打靶小鼠中得以明确。例如，缺乏转录因子 HF-1b 的小鼠发展为房室阻滞和室性心律失常[47]。过表达钙网织蛋白（calreticulin）的小鼠表现为慢传导和心脏传导阻滞。这可能是缝隙连接蛋白 43 和缝隙连接蛋白 40 减少的缘故[48]。类似的这些研究可望有助于从分子水平更好地理解心脏传导系统的调节。需要注意的是，病变小鼠由于代谢的干扰（缺氧、酸中毒、低温）也可通过一些非特异机制导致心动过缓和心脏传导阻滞。

（三）心肌病

异常收缩蛋白在心脏的异位表达被用于复制肥厚性心肌病的转基因和基因打靶小鼠模型[1]。心律失常可能出现于许多这些肥厚性心肌病小鼠模型[49]。其他先天性心肌病的小鼠模型如强直性肌萎缩也会发生心律失常，然而其与猝死的关系在人类尚不明确。

过表达炎性细胞因子肿瘤坏死因子-α（TNFα）的小鼠表型是扩张性心肌病。这种心肌病表现有室性快速心律失常以及房扑或房颤。在这个模型中，电压以及钙调节的异常似乎是心律失常发生的原因。

四、总 结

转基因和基因打靶技术使人们可以确定离子通道

基因承担着小鼠心脏的复极和细胞间传导的作用。在更高等的哺乳动物这两者也有很明确的相关性。

利用小鼠作为研究人的心律失常和猝死的模型，其价值尚不十分肯定。小鼠模型有很大的局限性，小鼠心率比人类的快近十倍，其心脏离子通道亦与人类不同。由于个体较小，小鼠心脏电生理比人的更稳定，室性心律失常很少引起猝死，但是所有小鼠临终时都有异常的心脏节律。心室异位搏动与可诱导性室性心律失常的相关性尚不清楚，这种因果关系不可臆测。

用转基因小鼠研究心律失常还不到一个世纪。我们必须慎重地解释这些发现。进一步繁殖扩增心律失常小鼠是必要的，如果能合理地利用这些基因工程小鼠，可望对基因产物以及基因突变与心律失常发生机制的关系有更多的了解。

(张幼怡　张　惠　龚开政　译)

参 考 文 献

1. Seidman JG, Seidman C: The genetic basis for cardiomyopathy: From mutation identification to mechanistic paradigms. Cell 104:557-567, 2001.
2. Keating MT, Sanguinetti MC: Molecular and cellular mechanisms of cardiac arrhythmias. Cell 104:569-580, 2001.
3. Izumo S, Shioi T: Cardiac transgenic and gene-targeted mice as models of cardiac hypertrophy and failure: A problem of (new) riches. J Card Fail 4:349-361, 1998.
4. London B: Use of Transgenic and Gene-Targeted Mice to Study K+ Channel Function in the Cardiovascular System. In Archer SA, Rusch JF (eds): Potassium Channels in Cardiovascular Biology. New York, Plenum, 2001.
5. Fishman GI: Timing is everything in life: Conditional transgene expression in the cardiovascular system. Circ Res 82:837-844, 1998.
6. Huang WY, Aramburu J, Douglas PS, Izumo S: Transgenic expression of green fluorescence protein can cause dilated cardiomyopathy. Nat Med 6:482-483, 2000.
7. Van der Weyden L, Adams DJ, Bradley A: Tools for targeted manipulation of the mouse genome. Physiol Genomics 11:133-164, 2002.
8. London B, Guo W, Pan XH, et al: Targeted replacement of Kv1.5 in the mouse leads to loss of the 4-aminopyridine-sensitive component of I(K,slow) and resistance to drug-induced qt prolongation. Circ Res 88:940-946, 2001.
9. London B, Jeron A, Zhou J, et al: Long QT and ventricular arrhythmias in transgenic mice expressing the N-terminus and first transmembrane segment of a voltage-gated potassium channel. Proc Natl Acad Sci U S A 95:2926-2931, 1998.
10. Wang L, Duff HJ: Developmental changes in transient outward current in mouse ventricle. Circ Res 81:120-127, 1997.
11. Nerbonne JM, Nichols CG, Schwarz TL, Escande D: Genetic manipulation of cardiac K+ channel function in mice: What have we learned, and where do we go from here? Circ Res 89:944-956, 2001.
12. Kupershmidt S, Yang T, Anderson ME, et al: Replacement by homologous recombination of the minK gene with lacZ reveals restriction of minK expression to the mouse cardiac conduction system. Circ Res 84:146-152, 1999.
13. Knollmann BC, Katchman AN, Franz MR: Monophasic action potential recordings from intact mouse heart: Validation, regional heterogeneity, and relation to refractoriness. J Cardiovasc Electrophysiol 12:1286-1294, 2001.
14. Guerrero PA, Schuessler RB, Davis LM, et al: Slow ventricular conduction in mice heterozygous for a connexin43 null mutation. J Clin Invest 99:1991-1998, 1997.
15. Morley GE, Vaidya D, Samie FH, et al: Characterization of conduction in the ventricles of normal and heterozygous connexin43 knockout mice using optical mapping. J Cardiovasc Electrophysiol 10:1361-1375, 1999.
16. Baker LC, London B, Choi BR, et al: Enhanced dispersion of repolarization and refractoriness in transgenic mouse hearts promotes reentrant ventricular tachycardia. Circ Res 86:396-407, 2000.
17. London B, Baker LC, Lee JS, et al: Calcium-dependent arrhythmias in transgenic mice with heart failure. Am J Physiol Heart Circ Physiol 284:H431-441, 2003.
18. Tamaddon HS, Vaidya D, Simon AM, et al: High-resolution optical mapping of the right bundle branch in connexin40 knockout mice reveals slow conduction in the specialized conduction system. Circ Res 87:929-936, 2000.
19. Rentschler S, Vaidya DM, Tamaddon H, et al: Visualization and functional characterization of the developing murine cardiac conduction system. Development 128:1785-1792, 2001.
20. London B. Cardiac arrhythmias: From (transgenic) mice to men. J Cardiovasc Electrophysiol 12:1089-1091, 2001a.
21. Gehrmann J, Hammer PE, Maguire CT, et al: Phenotypic screening for heart rate variability in the mouse. Am J Physiol Heart Circ Physiol 279:H733-H740, 2000.
22. Shusterman V, Usiene I, Harrigal C, et al: Strain-specific patterns of cardiac rhythm and autonomic nervous system activity in mice. Am J Physiol 282:H2076-2083, 2002.
23. Berul CI, Aronovitz MJ, Wang PJ, Mendelsohn ME: In vivo cardiac electrophysiology studies in the mouse. Circulation 94:2461-2468, 1996.
24. VanderBrink BA, Sellitto C, Saba S, et al: Connexin40-deficient mice exhibit atrioventricular nodal and infra-Hisian conduction abnormalities. J Cardiovasc Electrophysiol 11:1270-1276, 2000.
25. Trepanier-Boulay V, St-Michel C, Tremblay A, Fiset C: Gender-based differences in cardiac repolarization in mouse ventricle. Circ Res 89:437-444, 2001.
26. Nuyens D, Stengl M, Dugarmaa S, et al: Abrupt rate accelerations or premature beats cause life-threatening arrhythmias in mice with long-QT3 syndrome. Nat Med 7:1021-1027, 2001.
27. Papadatos GA, Wallerstein PM, Head CE, et al: Slowed conduction and ventricular tachycardia after targeted disruption of the cardiac sodium channel gene Scn5a. Proc Natl Acad Sci U S A 99:6210-6215, 2002.
28. Lee MP, Ravenel JD, Hu RJ, et al: Targeted disruption of the KvLQT1 gene causes deafness and gastric hyperplasia in mice. J Clin Invest 106:1447-1455, 2000.
29. Casimiro MC, Knollmann BC, Ebert SN, et al: Targeted disruption of the Kcnq1 gene produces a mouse model of Jervell and Lange-Nielsen syndrome. Proc Natl Acad Sci U S A 98:2526-2531, 2001.
30. Demolombe S, Lande G, Charpentier F, et al: Transgenic mice overexpressing human KvLQT1 dominant-negative isoform, part I: Phenotypic characterization. Cardiovasc Res 50:314-327, 2001.
31. Drici MD, Arrighi I, Chouabe C, et al: Involvement of IsK-associated K+ channel in heart rate control of repolarization in a murine engineered model of Jervell and Lange-Nielsen syndrome. Circ Res 83:95-102, 1998.
32. Marx SO, Kurokawa J, Reiken S, et al: Requirement of a macromolecular signaling complex for beta adrenergic receptor modulation of the KCNQ1-KCNE1 potassium channel. Science 295:496-499, 2002.
33. Babij P, Askew GR, Nieuwenhuijsen B, et al: Inhibition of cardiac delayed rectifier K+ current by overexpression of the long-QT syndrome HERG G628S mutation in transgenic mice. Circ Res 83:668-678, 1998.
34. London B, Pan XH, Lewarchik CM, Lee JS: QT interval prolongation and arrhythmias in heterozygous Merg1-targeted mice [abstract]. Circulation 98:I-56, 1998a.
35. Lees-Miller JP, Guo J, Somers JR, et al: Selective knockout of mouse ERG1B potassium channel eliminates I(Kr) in adult ventricular myocytes and elicits episodes of abrupt sinus bradycardia. Mol Cell Biol 23:1856-1862, 2003.
36. Tristani-Firouzi M, Jensen JL, Donaldson MR, et al: Functional and clinical characterization of KCNJ2 mutations associated with LQT7 (Andersen syndrome). J Clin Invest 110:381-388, 2002.
37. Zaritsky JJ, Redell JB, Tempel BL, Schwarz TL: The consequences of disrupting cardiac inwardly rectifying K+ current (I(K1)) as revealed by the targeted deletion of the murine Kir2.1 and Kir2.2

genes. J Physiol 533:697–710, 2001.
38. London B, Wang DW, Hill JA, Bennett PB: The transient outward current in mice lacking the potassium channel gene Kv1.4. J Physiol 509:171–182, 1998b.
39. Guo J, Li H, London B, Nerbonne JM: Functional consequences of elimination of i(to,f) and i(to,s): Early afterdepolarizations, atrioventricular block and ventricular arrhythmias in mice lacking Kv1.4 and expressing a dominant-negative Kv4 α subunit. Circ Res 87:73–79, 2000.
40. Xu H, Barry DM, Li H, et al: Attenuation of the slow component of delayed rectification, action potential prolongation, and triggered activity in mice expressing a dominant-negative Kv2 α subunit. Circ Res 85:623–633, 1999.
41. Barry DM, Xu H, Schuessler RB, Nerbonne JM: Functional knockout of the transient outward current, long-QT syndrome, and cardiac remodeling in mice expressing a dominant-negative Kv4 α subunit. Circ Res 83:560–567, 1998.
42. Wickenden AD, Lee P, Sah R, et al: Targeted expression of a dominant negative Kv4.2 K+ channel subunit in mouse heart. Circ Res 85:1067–1076, 1999.
43. Kuo HC, Cheng CF, Clark RB, et al: A defect in the Kv channel-interacting protein 2 (KchIP2) gene leads to a complete loss of I(to) and confers susceptibility to ventricular tachycardia. Cell 107:801–813, 2001.
44. Vaidya D, Tamaddon HS, Lo CW, et al: Null mutation of connexin43 causes slow propagation of ventricular activation in the late stages of mouse embryonic development. Circ Res 88:1196–1202, 2001.
45. Gutstein DE, Morley GE, Tamaddon H, et al: Conduction slowing and sudden arrhythmic death in mice with cardiac-restricted inactivation of connexin43. Circ Res 88:333–339, 2001.
46. Kirchhoff S, Nelles E, Hagendorff A, et al: Reduced cardiac conduction velocity and predisposition to arrhythmias in connexin40-deficient mice. Curr Biol 8:299–302, 1998.
47. Nguyen-Tran VT, Kubalak SW, Minamisawa S, et al: A novel genetic pathway for sudden cardiac death via defects in the transition between ventricular and conduction system cell lineages. Cell 102:671–682, 2000.
48. Nakamura K, Robertson M, Liu G, et al: Complete heart block and sudden death in mice overexpressing calreticulin. J Clin Invest 107: 1245–1253, 2001.
49. Berul CI, Christe ME, Aronovitz MJ, et al: Electrophysiological abnormalities and arrhythmias in alpha MHC mutant familial hypertrophic cardiomyopathy mice. J Clin Invest 99:570–576, 1997.
50. Berul CI, Maguire CT, Gehrmann J, Reddy S: Progressive atrioventricular conduction block in a mouse myotonic dystrophy model. J Interv Card Electrophysiol 4:351–358, 2000.

第 49 章

人类分子遗传学与心脏

Jeffrey A. Towbin，*Neil E. Bowles*

本章目录

- 遗传学基础 ············ 440
- 遗传性疾病的起源 ········ 441
- 单基因遗传病 ·········· 441
- 已知致病基因的分析与确定 ·· 444
- 与心肌病有关的快速性心律失常 ······ 446
- 总结 ················ 456

在许多心血管疾病的发病机理中，遗传因素起重要作用。先天性心脏病和血管畸形在婴儿中发生率约1%，在死产婴儿中的发生率估计要高出10倍[1]。细胞遗传学主要研究染色体及其异常，它与分子遗传学的联合应用将有助于我们破译心血管疾病的遗传基础。基因诊断和基因异常的筛选即将被纳入到临床实践中[2]。"人类基因组计划"的目标是在2001年前明确所有的基因，这个目标已基本实现[3-4]。临床心血管病学专家和实验心血管病学专家所面临的挑战是将这些基因和它们特异的生理和病理生理功能联系起来。心血管病专家们要想更好地从医学、伦理和道德的角度来认识这些遗传性疾病，那么了解这些遗传性疾病的基础是非常必要的[5]。

一、遗传学基础

所有的遗传信息都是通过DNA来传递的，DNA是一种由嘌呤（鸟嘌呤和腺嘌呤）和嘧啶（胞嘧啶和胸腺嘧啶）碱基组成的双链结构[6]。遗传的基本单位是基因，它是由负责编码特异多肽（蛋白质）的不同DNA片段组成的。尽管全部DNA足够编码几十万个基因，但事实上估计只有大约100 000个基因。而且，只有不到5%的DNA用于编码基因。每个个体都有一个基因的两个拷贝，将其称为等位基因。基因位于23对染色体（从父母双方获得，外形为棒状）的线性序列上。父母双方各提供每对染色体中的一个染色体（成对的染色体称作同源染色体）和一份拷贝的基因。基因在特异的染色体上所占的位置称为基因位点。特定的基因往往位于特定染色体的相同基因位点，所以染色体上的基因位点是相同的，但位于这些基因位点上的等位基因可以是相同或不同的。如果两个同源染色体的相同基因位点上有相同等位基因，该个体的这个等位基因为纯合；如果两个基因不同，即基因位点上的两个等位基因不同，该个体的这个等位基因即为杂合。每个个体都可表现出在一些基因位点上为纯合，而在其他基因位点上为杂合，而且基于目前所知，至少有三分之一的人具有基因的多态性。通过精子和卵子的结合，基因在传给后代的同时，也将遗传信息传递给了后代（基因型），以此通过合成相应蛋白质来决定个体的表观特性（表型）[6]。DNA所携带的每个基因的遗传信息都是由四种碱基来编码。通过信使核苷酸（messenger ribonucleic acid，mRNA）传递遗传密码，遗传信息翻译为蛋白质，每个特异的氨基酸由三个碱基编码，称之为密码子[6]。由基因转录而来的mRNA，其作为模板决定了所合成的多肽包含哪些氨基酸，以及氨基酸的序列。一个基因编码一个特定的蛋白质，但我们更倾向于一个基因编码一个多肽的说法，因为尽管有很多蛋白质是一个多肽，但也有很多蛋白质包含多个多肽，其可由一个或几个基因来编码。人的 23 对染色体包括了 22 对常染色体（1～22 号）和 1 对性染色体（X 和 Y）。女性为两条 X 染色体，男性为一个 X 和一个 Y。在常染色体，等位基因的每一方的 DNA 序列都有可能活化而决定 RNA 拷贝，但每个基因是否表达取决于细胞类型、发育阶段以及调节分子，其中调节分子可与启动子序列及增强子序列相互作用，控制基因转录。在含有两条 X 染色体的细胞里，无论是正常个体，还是含有 XXY 的 Klinefelter 综合征（先天性睾丸发育不全）患者，在胚胎发育早期只有一个 X 染色体有活性。

二、遗传性疾病的起源

遗传性疾病包括三大类：染色体病、单基因病、多基因病[6]。故遗传性疾病和先天性疾病可归于染色体异常或单基因突变或多基因突变。突变是在 DNA 上出现稳定的、遗传性的改变。可由多种原因，如环境因素（比如辐射、化学药物、病毒）引起基因传递过程中序列的精确度发生了改变而导致。因为子代与亲代相似，故认为 DNA 核苷酸序列是稳定的。但是碱基序列确实会发生改变。发生这些改变的机制也各不相同，突变可以是发生于染色体水平的显性改变，如染色体部分缺失或移位，可导致相应的一些基因缺失或改变[6]。染色体数目改变，尤其是出现整倍性（euploidy）的变化，在人类的发育中是很常见的。每一个密码子序列决定一个氨基酸，mRNA 的线性密码子序列决定蛋白质的氨基酸序列。如果一个对蛋白质的功能起关键作用的氨基酸发生改变，将会导致蛋白质的功能改变或缺失，同时可伴随表型的改变。蛋白质是基因功能的执行分子，无论这个蛋白质是酶、调节蛋白或结构蛋白，基因突变都是通过蛋白质结构改变来表现其有害作用的。一般来讲，每 106 次细胞分裂就会产生一次突变，只有发生于配子的突变才被传递下去[6]。一般来讲，一个基因每 200 000 年经历一次突变。

三、单基因遗传病

由单个基因异常引起的遗传病遗传至后代时，其表型常可预测，这被称之为孟德尔遗传[6]。这些遗传方式所产生的遗传表型遵循孟德尔遗传定律。如前所述，每个基因有分别从父方和母方得到的两份拷贝（指等位基因）。孟德尔第一定律指出，一对等位基因中的每一个基因，位于相互分离的两条染色体，在子代的形成过程中独立地、毫不改变地传于不同的配子[6]。因而，得到母方或父方等位基因的几率是随机的，或者说各占 50%。孟德尔第二定律指出，同一染色体上的基因在染色体交换过程中独立分配。两个基因位点相距越远，遗传过程中它们就越易被分开[6]。突变的异常基因可以位于 22 对常染色体和两条性染色体的任何一个，遗传按其产生的表型可分为：常染色体遗传（显性遗传和隐性遗传）和 X 连锁遗传[7]。如果不同的基因产生相同的表型，称为遗传异质性（或不均一性），许多人类疾病都显示出遗传异质性[7]。同一种疾病可能源于同一个基因的多个突变（等位基因的异质性），或源于两个或两个以上基因的一个或多个突变（基因位点的异质性）。然而，在同一家族内致病基因和突变是相同的，仅在少数情况下两个基因导致同一疾病。家族性长 QT 综合征（familial long QT syndrome，LQTS）就是一个很好的例子，可导致这种疾病的基因已发现了七个，每一个基因均可有多个位点突变（参见第 50 章）[8,9]。遗传异质性须与多基因遗传病相鉴别，例如动脉粥样硬化，它由几个基因相互作用而致。如前所述，突变包括光镜下可见的改变，例如部分染色体的缺失或移位，也包括一个密码子 DNA 序列上一个嘌呤或一个嘧啶碱基的微小改变。仅为一个核苷酸的突变称为点突变，成年单基因疾病中有 70% 以上为点突变所致。点突变是一个核苷酸被另一个核苷酸置换，导致编码为另一种氨基酸（missense mutation，错义突变）或者是变为终止密码子，使蛋白质合成截止（truncate mutation，截断突变），有时也可改变终止密码子而使肽链继续延伸（elongated mutation，延伸突变）。还有，一个核苷酸可以被删除或添加，导致移码而使整个基因编码完全不同（nonsense mutation，无义突变），最终合成一个无功能的蛋白质。如果一个嘌呤碱基被一个嘧啶碱基置换，这种突变称为颠换（transversion）；如果嘧啶被另一种嘧啶置换或嘌呤被另一种嘌呤置换则被称为转换（transition）。其他突变可由几个核苷酸的缺失或添加引起。由核苷酸添加导致疾病的一个例子就是强直性肌营养不良，它是几千个核苷酸长度的三次重复序列添加到基因的 3' 端[10]。另一种突变叫做基因转换（gene conversion），两个基因相互作用，一个基因的部分核苷酸序列参入到另外一个基因中。基因突变通过使酶、调节蛋白以及结构蛋白发生结构上的改变来产生其不利作用。显性遗传（dominant inheritance）和隐性遗传（recessive inheritance）是指表型特征，不是指基因本身的特征[7]。显性遗传指当一个个体具有一份拷贝的突变等位基因和一份拷贝的正常等位基因，就表现为突变等位基因的表型；相反，隐性遗传指两个等位基因均为突变基因时才表现突变表型。这种情况常发生于患者双亲之间具有血缘关系，且每人均携带突变的等位基因，或者突变基因在人群中常见，例如镰状细胞贫血。

（一）遗传的外显率和表现度

携带致病基因的个体中，表现出疾病特征（一个或多个）的个体所占的比例称为外显率[6]。外显是全或无的，只要个体出现出疾病的特征，无论多么微小的表现，都表明这个基因在这个个体为完全外显。不外显是指不具有任何可观察到的表型。这种特性要和表现度相鉴别，表现度（expressivity）是指个体在疾病所有的临床特点中的表现程度。因而可以确切地讲，只要存在表现度，那么这个特性在这个个体肯定是外显的。许多遗传因素和环境因素都可影响基因表达，因此想要确定哪个因素对于某个特定的个体或特定的疾病最重要几乎是不可能的。这些因素包括：（1）遗传背景；（2）年龄依赖性；（3）性别影响和性别局限；（4）外源性因素；（5）母系的影响；（6）基因位点修饰；（7）基因突变。

（二）遗传的类型

1. 常染色体显性遗传

显性遗传是指在杂合子个体表现出疾病表型，而杂合子是指仅携带一个异常等位基因，位于同源染色体上的另一个等位基因正常。因为在减数分裂中等位基因独立分配，每一个杂合子后代都有50%的机会得到突变的等位基因，常染色体显性疾病男女均可患。然而，并非所有患病个体其父母都会有一方受累，因为有相当数量患病为新产生的突变所致（如散发病例）。因为突变仅累及一个配子细胞，故配子中含有新发突变的个体临床表现虽正常，但却会将致病的等位基因传递给一半的子女。如果父母携带突变的等位基因而表型正常，或者为婚外生子，常染色体显性遗传疾病常被误诊为散发病例。以下为常染色体显性遗传的特点（可见图49-1）：（1）除非是疾病源于新发突变，或杂合子父母呈低表现度，每一个患病个体均有一个患病的亲本（父或母）；（2）从统计学上来讲，子代正常或患病的概率均等（即各占50%）；（3）患者的正常子女，其子代均正常；（4）男女患病概率均等；（5）父方和母方有均等机会将异常等位基因传给儿子或女儿，可以有"男传男"（父亲传给儿子）；（6）可有连续数代垂直传递。常染色体显性遗传疾病区别于常染色体隐性遗传疾病的另外两个特征是：发病年龄延迟和临床表现多变。如家族性肥厚型心肌病（hypertrophic cardiomyopathy，HCM）发病年龄较晚[11,12]，而长QT综合征患者临床表现多样，常有异常QT间期或异常T波或二者同时兼有。常染色体显性遗传的原发性心脏疾病包括HCM和Romano-Ward LQTS。

2. 常染色体隐性遗传

当疾病所对应的基因位点上两个等位基因均为突变基因时（即纯合），患者有常染色体隐性表型的临床表现。因致病基因位于22对常染色体上，故男女患病的概率均等。临床表现一致且典型，多为早期发病。与显性遗传疾病相比，隐性遗传疾病常于童年即可诊断。仅四分之一（平均25%）子代患病。以下为常染色体隐性遗传疾病的特点，可见图49-1：（1）父母是临床正常的杂合子；（2）隔代发病，无垂直传递；（3）男女患病的几率均等；（4）每一个子代个体都有25%的患病概率，50%的概率为未患病携带者，25%的概率为正常等位基因。累及心脏的常染色体隐性疾病有Jervell-Lange-Nielsen长QT/耳聋综合征[13]。

3. X-连锁遗传

X-连锁遗传疾病是由位于X染色体的基因所致，因此疾病的临床患病风险和严重程度因性别而异[14]。女性有两条X染色体，因其可携带一个突变等位基因（杂合子），也可携带一对突变等位基因（纯合子），故可有显性或隐性表现特征。男性只有一个X染色体和一个Y染色体，故无论其母亲（携带有异常等位基因）为临床显性还是临床隐性，只要他从母方遗传到异常等位基因，就可有临床表现。因此，X-连锁显性和X-连锁隐性这两个名词也就只适用于女性。男性亲本虽然必定将其Y染色体传给其每一个男性子代，但不能将其突变的X染色体等位基因传给儿子，因而X-连锁疾病不存在"男传男"的现象。另一方面，男性必须将其X染色体传给女儿。所有接收到突变X染色

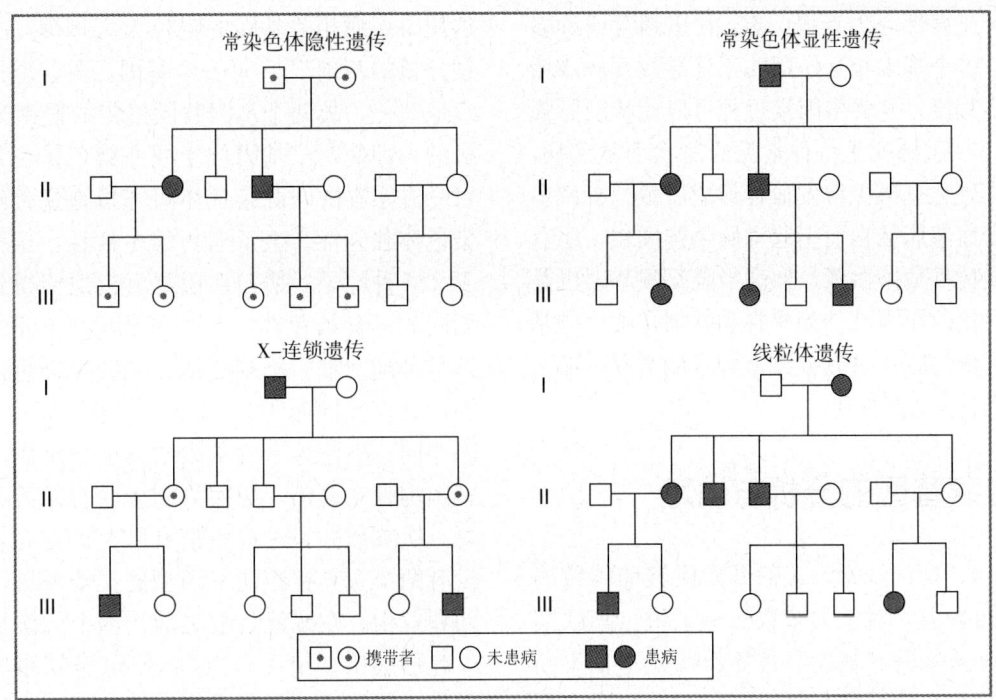

图 49-1 遗传方式 例举人类疾病的遗传方式。上排图为常染色体遗传方式；上左为常染色体隐性遗传，两个非患病的携带者双亲提供亲本的异常基因拷贝给患病子代（25%患病，50%为携带者，25%为正常）；上右为常染色体显性遗传，患病的杂合子亲本将致病基因遗传给50%的子代。下排左图为X-连锁遗传：无"男传男"，因此患病男性将致病基因遗传给女儿（携带者），女儿又可将致病基因传给她的女儿（携带者）或儿子（患者）。下排右图为线粒体遗传：为母系遗传，两种性别均可患病，但只有女性可将疾病传给子代

体的女性均表现为携带者，具有临床表现的女性称为显性女性携带者。X-连锁遗传的特点可见图 49-1，包括：(1) 无"男传男"现象；(2) 男性患者的所有女儿均为携带者；(3) 女性携带者，其儿子有50%的概率患病，其女儿有50%的概率成为携带者；(4) 只有男性患者和女性携带者所生子女才有可能出现患病的女性纯合子；(5) X-连锁隐性遗传家系出现倾斜，表现为正常的携带者的儿子和男性患者姐妹的儿子患病（即：叔叔和侄子患病）。X-连锁隐性遗传心脏疾病包括 X-连锁心肌病[14,15]，X-连锁心肌骨骼肌样变（即 Barth 综合征）[16]；累及心脏的 X-连锁疾病例如有肌营养不良（即 Duchenne/Becker 肌营养不良和 Emery-Dreifuss 肌营养不良）[17]。

4. 线粒体遗传

另一种遗传疾病是因为线粒体基因组的先天缺陷[18-20]。能量生成依赖于线粒体内的氧化磷酸化过程。多数线粒体内含有单个的染色体，它编码众多氧化磷酸化所需的酶（即 69 种蛋白质中 13 种氧化代谢所需），以及转运 RNA 和核糖体 RNA。氧化磷酸化过程所需的其他酶类由核染色体的基因编码，所合成的蛋白质运送到线粒体。因此，氧化磷酸化的基因缺陷可以源于 X 染色体或常染色体（即核染色体）的基因突变，所致疾病遵循孟德尔隐性遗传规律；也可源于线粒体基因组缺陷，所致疾病具有非孟德尔式遗传特征。其差别可以用受孕来解释，因为精子细胞提供极少甚至不提供线粒体给受精卵，胎儿的线粒体成分几乎全部来自卵母细胞胞浆。而且，线粒体突变也证明线粒体遗传为母系遗传。线粒体遗传病的特点有（见图 49-1）：(1) 男女患病几率和患病严重程度概率相同；(2) 仅通过母系遗传，男性患者的后代均不患病；(3) 女性患者的所有子代均患病；(4) 一个家族内的患病表现可能差异极大（可能包括表型上不外显）；(5) 表型具有年龄依赖性；(6) 器官镶嵌现象常见。线粒体遗传心脏病的一个例子就是传导系统疾病和 Kearns-Sayre 综合征心肌病[21]。

5. 心脏疾病的多基因遗传

高血压和缺血性心脏病是多个基因均发生突变的多基因疾病。多基因遗传病的致病基因难于定位，因为用于描述这种遗传方式的计算方法还未研究成功[22]。在过去的 20 年，发现这种遗传方式存在于很多种疾病，包括

冠状动脉疾病、充血性心力衰竭，等。在多因素或称多基因遗传病中，多个基因相互作用并累计导致发病或增加了患病的风险程度，这种多因素过程可以冠状动脉疾病为例来说明。心肌梗死是一种常见的冠状动脉疾病，它是在动脉粥样硬化基础上继发血栓形成所致。有许多单基因病可改变血浆脂蛋白而引起动脉粥样硬化，还有其他已明确的遗传性危险因素，如高半胱氨酸基因也是造成动脉粥样硬化的原因[23]。如果在动脉粥样硬化的基础上又存在纤维蛋白原[24]或其他凝血因子的突变，那么这个人就易于患急性心肌梗死。

四、已知致病基因的分析与确定

从20世纪80年代开始，人们开始能够证实致病基因，明确未知蛋白。对于大多数疾病来讲，其缺陷基因和蛋白都是未知的。辅助染色体作图技术在不断的进步，包括：（1）计算机连锁分析[25]，（2）建立高信息量的DNA标记物[26,27]，（3）利用聚合酶链反应（polymerase chain reaction，PCR）检测遗传标记[6]。人类基因组的46个染色体包含了30亿碱基对（bp）。为了确定某个特定基因的位置，首先要确定其染色体的位置和其相对位置，这需要对染色体进行标记。如果我们感兴趣的疾病相关基因与这些标记之一位于同一染色体且距离上很靠近，那么我们就有可能确定这个致病的等位基因，常用的方法为基因连锁分析[6]。这项技术需要这种疾病连续遗传两到三代的一个家族，这个家族最好至少有十个成员发病。根据家庭的结构，有时有六、七名患病个体也可以[7]。遗传标记是指DNA或染色体标记，它是一段多态性DNA序列，其在染色体上的位置是已知的，可通过个体的DNA分析来鉴定其存在。在过去十年的研究中，最大的局限就是缺乏平衡分布于每一个染色体的遗传标记。在所有染色体中，至少每一百万碱基对就要有一个标记才能保证有效利用[28,29]。基因图距以厘摩（cM）为单位，该单位是以遗传学家T. H. Morgan命名的，1cM大约1 000 000碱基对左右。遗传标记与基因一样，也是一对等位基因，其遗传也遵循孟德尔定律，也可分为遗传标记的纯合体和杂合体。如果某标记为纯合，该标记不能为基因连锁提供信息。所以，在同一区带上的几个标记需要加以分析，找出在该个体的杂合标记。在每一个染色体上定位所有的标记，并估计他们之间的基因图距称之为基因作图。目前已建立了包含超过5 000个高信息量标记的基因图，

这使得疾病相关基因的定位大大加速，奠定了基因连锁分析的基础[29]。每一个基因、等位基因和标记均独立地遗传，故两个基因共同遗传的概率为50%，是随机的，即使两个基因位于同一染色体也是如此。来自每一方亲本的同源染色体可随机地遗传给后代。同源染色体独立性产生了遗传的多样性，这种多样性产生了223种配子。换句话说，后代遗传得到与亲本完全相同的一套染色体，其概率为1/8 388 608[30]。如果这是分配的唯一机制的话，某特定染色体上的所有基因还有可能同时遗传到另一子代，但这不可能发生。除非同一染色体上的基因之间的物理距离极近，否则基因均独立遗传。交换机制使一对同源染色体之间在每一次减数分裂过程中都有频繁的混合，这也是为何没有两个人具有相同基因型的主要原因，除非他们是同卵双生。在减数分裂之前，两个同源染色体聚集到一起形成桥（交叉），它们等同部分的片段发生相互交换，使不同的基因之间发生交换。交换不会造成任何染色体成分或基因的丢失，但会使染色体之间频繁混合，以至于任何两个子代都不会完全相同。交换只发生在同源染色体之间。基因位点在一个同源染色体上的位置通常与在结合交换前它在另一个同源染色体上的位置相同。一般来讲，一次减数分裂要发生33次交换[30]。这种交换在遗传学上称为重组。

（一）遗传连锁分析的概念

尽管染色体和基因独立分配，两个或更多基因位点上的（等位）基因常会发生共同遗传，如果它们距离很近的话，在它们之间形成交叉桥的几率就较低，就不会发生染色体断裂和重组，发生共同遗传的几率就比单纯随机发生要高得多；明确地讲，这就意味着两个基因位点连锁遗传。任何两个基因位点共同遗传概率超过50%就成为遗传连锁。为定位疾病相关基因在染色体上的位置，我们利用平衡分布于染色体的DNA标记，收集一个家族中所有成员（包括正常和患者）的DNA来分析这些标记。如果一个或多个DNA标记在一半以上患者中存在共同遗传，那么就意味着这个标记所在的基因位点与疾病相关基因所在的基因位点位于同一染色体上，而且二者物理距离很近，称为疾病相关基因与标记遗传连锁。如果疾病与一个已知染色体基因位点的标记连锁，那么该疾病基因的基因位点与标记的基因位点也位于同一染色体，且二者距离很近。证实致病基因与标记之间存在遗传连锁非常必要，其计算很复杂，需要先进的计算机程序。有、无连锁的几率均需要计算，支持

存在连锁的几率最低为1000∶1才认为连锁存在。这种几率的表示方法比较繁琐（1000∶1），故用10的对数来表示，则1000∶1这个几率的对数（LOD）值就是3。如果LOD值为-2，即10^{-2}或无连锁的几率为100∶1，就可除外存在连锁。如果两个基因之间的距离增大，那么在重组过程中被分开的可能性也随着增加。发生连锁时，标记和致病基因之间的距离变化很大，可在1000至50 000千碱基对之间，但通常是在1000至10 000碱基对之间[6]。如果遗传连锁分析的结果在1000碱基对则更好。如果估计多个标记之间的距离都在几个厘摩之间，那么仅依靠连锁分析就能够构建出所有标记的染色体图。这是对多个标记在减数分裂中重组数量进行复杂计算后的结果。发生在两个标记、两个基因或一个基因和一个标记之间的重组频率是指交换次数和减数分裂次数之比。在标记和疾病相关基因位点之间的重组频率越低，二者在染色体上的物理距离越近。即使标记和疾病相关基因的基因位点足够近以至于可发生遗传连锁，重组仍有可能发生，对于已发生了重组的情况，则说明它（组合频率）仅代表了两个基因位点之间大概的物理距离。重组因子（θ）用于估计两个连锁遗传的基因位点之间的图距（cM）。如果两个基因位点（无论是两个基因或一个基因和一个标记的基因位点）的重组（或交换）频率为1%，那么它们之间的物理距离大概是一百万碱基对（1cM）[16]。一个标记和一个基因相距1cM意味着它们在减数分裂过程中发生交换的频率仅为1%，因而二者共同遗传的几率为99%。但这是从遗传作图中计算得来的结果，这个距离只是大概值。交换频率和以碱基对估计的物理距离，二者之间的相关性因不同的染色体、不同的区带而不同，甚至在同一染色体上也是如此。例如，交换频率在末端着丝粒染色体就比在着丝粒处的染色体要高，在女性要更高一些。如果标记和疾病相关基因的基因位点相距很近，比如5~10 cM，单交换和双交换均不多见。但如果距离在20~40 cM之间，可能出现双交换，这使得两个基因位点均与另一同源染色体发生重组并导致二者共同遗传（两个基因位点连锁）。在这种情况，基因图距将出现误差，低估了两个基因位点的真实物理距离。

（二）候选基因筛查和突变分析

在心血管疾病中，特别是容易发生猝死的疾病，可用于连锁分析的大家系相对少见。而且，由于人类基因组计划已经明确了大部分基因及其在染色体上的位置，筛查这些基因的突变成为明确致病基因的好方法。明确心血管疾病的生理基础使我们可直观地选择可能导致临床表型的基因，目前已有很规范的快速筛选基因的方法。常用方法有：直接DNA测序、单链构象多态性（single-strand conformational polymorphism，SSCP）检测、变性高效液相色谱（denaturing high-performance liquid chromatography，DHPLC），详述如下：

1. 直接DNA测序

可用一种叫做循环测序的DNA测序程序对备选基因进行突变筛查[31]。这种方法是将患病个体的基因组DNA进行PCR，扩增备选基因片段，然后使用PCR循环仪，在不同脱氧核苷酸和放射性标记的引物中加入耐热DNA聚合酶，将PCR产物多重循环进一步扩增。所得到的放射性标记的反应产物在聚丙烯酰胺凝胶上分离，利用放射自显影使之显影，这样异常序列就可以明确了。更快速的方法是利用自动DNA测序仪，短时间内就可直接测得大量序列。

2. 单链构象多态性

这个方法利用了DNA序列上单核苷酸的改变会使单链DNA在非变性凝胶上的迁移发生改变这一特性[32]。这个方法是在变性缓冲液中通过加热将DNA解链为单链，扩增我们感兴趣的基因条带。分离的单链在可区分出两个分子间一个核苷酸差异的条件下进行聚丙烯酰胺凝胶电泳分离。链内相互作用的改变会导致结构改变，故利用这种方法可鉴别序列差异。这种方法的最大缺陷在于检测不到真正的碱基突变。任何异常条带（构象异构体）均需要DNA测序方能明确基因突变。

3. 变性高效液相色谱

在100~1500碱基对的DNA片段中，单个碱基的置换、缺失和添加均可在反相柱上用分离异源双链体的方法检测[33,34]。可被PCR扩增的所有基因组DNA单拷贝片段，均可被快速自动检测。杂合子个体的DNA经过PCR扩增得到的是野生型和突变型双链DNA的混合物（见图49-2）。PCR变性和复性产生异源双链DNA和同源双链DNA。异源双链DNA与完全互补的同源双链DNA的熔点不同，变性高效液相色谱分析就是利用了在部分热变性条件下同源和异源双链分子的存留量差异（见图49-2）。变性高效液相色谱仪自动显示异常峰，然后进行DNA测序（见图49-2），可快速灵敏地检出突变。

(三) 心律失常疾病的遗传病图

在过去十年里，已揭示了一些心律失常疾病的遗传学基础。如第 50 章里 Priori 等所述，心律失常疾病最初是在研究 LQTS（Romano-Ward 综合征和 Lange-Nielsen 综合征）时发现了编码离子通道致病基因存在遗传异质性[35]。LQTS 为复极化疾病，起因是钾通道（KCNQ1、HERG、KCNE1 和 KCNE2）改变而功能减退，钠通道（SCN5A）改变而功能增强[35]。近来 Andersen 综合征钾通道基因 $Kir2.1$ 的发现进一步说明 LQTS 是一种离子通道病[36]。而且，LQT4 的临床表型（心动过缓和房颤）与其他型不同，编码锚蛋白 B 的 LQT4 基因又为这一观念增加了复杂性[37]（可参阅第 50 章）。

随着 LQTS 致病基因的明确，对其他心律失常综合征的研究热度也随之增加，近来报道了 Brugada 综合征和多形性室速/儿茶酚胺性室速的致病基因。如第 50 章所述，我们已明确了 Brugada 综合征的致病基因是 SCN5A[38]，LQT3 的致病基因是心脏钠离子通道基因，多形性室速是因为兰尼定（ryanodine）受体和肌集钙蛋白（这二者对钙稳态有重要意义）的基因突变[39,40]。故而，许多快速型心律失常疾病的遗传学基础已经阐明。而且，伴有心动过速的疾病例如心肌病也有研究，我们将在本章随后详述。

另外，对缓慢性心律失常也有所研究。近来发现，孤立的房室阻滞以及与纤维化有关的（如 Lev-Lenegre 综合征）房室阻滞也因 SCN5A 突变所致[41]。房室阻滞的其他原因多与心肌病有关，将在本章随后一并详述。

五、与心肌病有关的快速性心律失常

(一) 肥厚型心肌病（HCM）

肥厚型心肌病（HCM）以心肌肥厚伴多种症状为特征，包括呼吸困难、胸痛和晕厥[11]，1 年死亡率在早期报道中可达 2%～4%，主要死因是无症状性猝死，但现在公认的死亡率为每年 0.1%。该病可引起年轻患者和运动员猝死[11]。家族性肥厚型心肌病年轻患者的 1 年死亡率要高于年长患者。该病诊断基于典型临床特点和二维超声心动图证实存在无法解释的左室、右室或双室肥厚。患者常有不对称的左室肥厚，多局限于室间隔，也可是累及整个左室的向心性肥厚（见图 49-3）。单纯右室肥厚患者仅占不到 5%。单纯心尖肥厚除日本之外极少见，据报道在日本可占

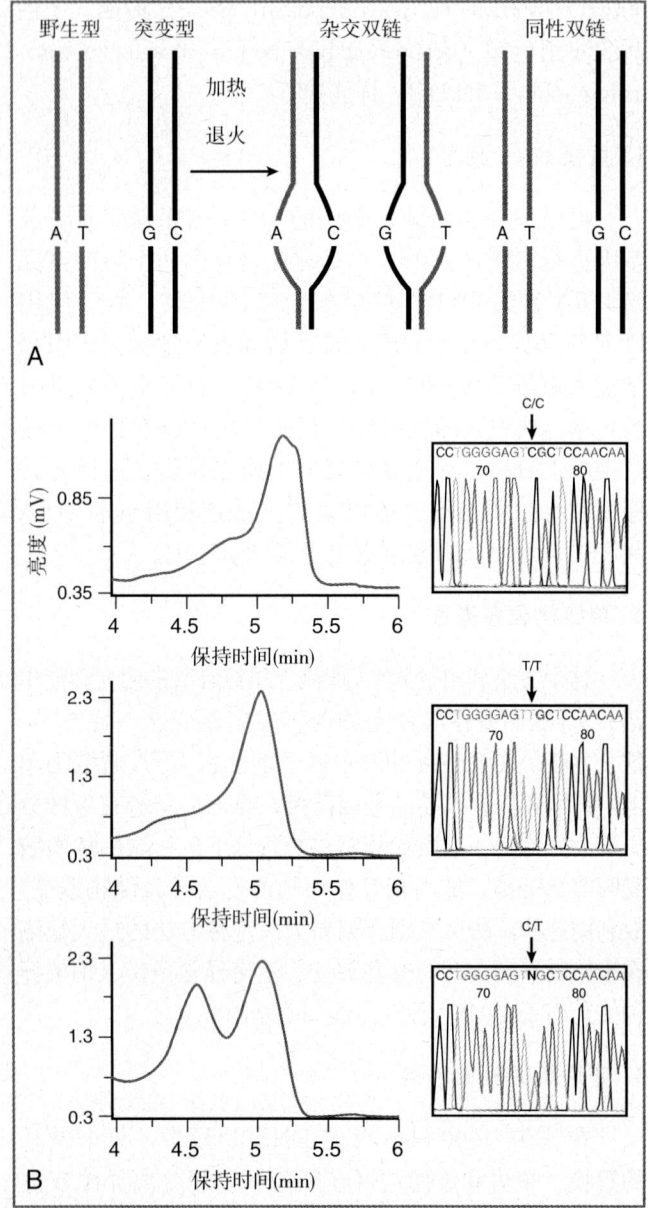

图 49-2 变性高效液相色谱检测 DNA 突变 A：对于常染色体显性遗传疾病，所有的突变都在一条染色体上，因此，PCR 对突变基因的扩增包含了野生型和突变型 DNA 序列的混合双链。在加热变性与退火复性的过程中形成了 DNA 杂交双链（heteroduplexe）以及 DNA 同性双链（homooduplexe）。B：左边显示的是变性高效液相色谱分析图，右边是对一些 C 纯合型（顶）、T 纯合型（中）以及 T 和 C 杂合型（底）个体基因多肽性分析的 DNA 序列图。值得注意的是，纯合型序列分析结构与变性高效液相色谱分析结果相似，而杂合型的可出现一个额外的高峰，这是因为杂交双链在变性高效液相色谱柱里停留时间较短

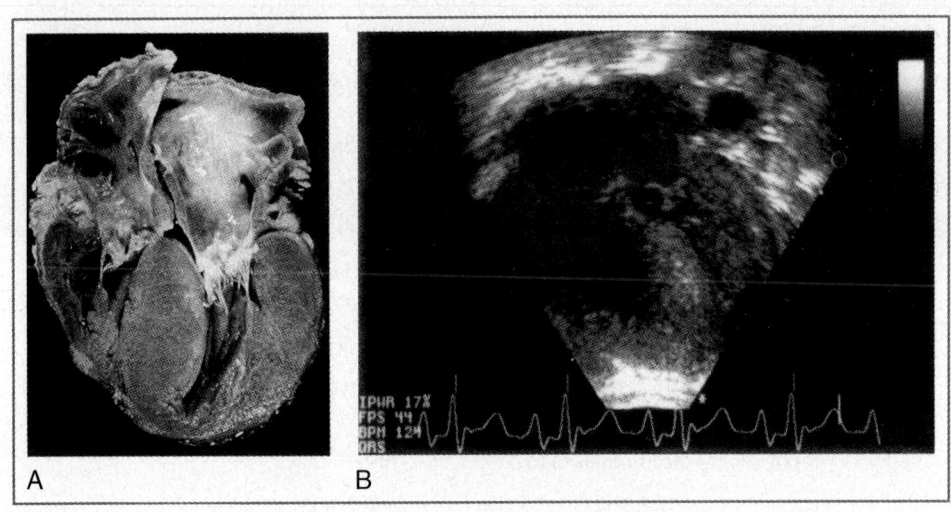

图 49-3 肥厚型心肌病 A：大体解剖标本，显示室间隔明显肥厚，左室腔呈裂缝样，左室后壁增厚以及左房扩张。B：超声心动图的四腔图也反映出相同的病变

20%～30%，或见于年长患者。患者伴心律失常比较常见，特别是室性心动过速和心室颤动，部分患者可见房颤和室上速。一小部分患者可并发 Wolff-Parkinson-White（WPW）预激综合征，还有患者可见 QT 间期延长。30% 患者会发生流出道梗阻。组织学上，心肌肥厚包括心肌细胞肥大、细胞和肌纤维紊乱和心肌纤维化，家族性肥厚型心肌病最明显的标志就是心肌纤维排列紊乱[11]。

1. 家族性肥厚型心肌病的基因定位

利用基因组连锁分析，家族性肥厚型心肌病的第一个基因定位于 14 号染色体 14q11.2-q12，后来又有关于家族性肥厚型心肌病基因位点异质性的报导[42]，将家族性肥厚型心肌病的第二个基因位点定位于 1 号染色体 1q3，第三个基因位点定位于 15 号染色体 15q2（表 49-1）。第 4 号基因位点位于 11p11.2（图 49-4）。其后报道的 5 个基因位点分别定位于：7q3、3q21.2-3p21.3、12q23-q24.3、15q14 和 2q31[42,43]。

2. 家族性肥厚型心肌病的基因鉴定

纯肥厚型心肌病的所有致病基因均编码肌小节（即肌丝）蛋白质，肌小节是一个具有精确化学计量学（stoichiometry）的复杂结构，含有多个蛋白质-蛋白质相互作用的位点[42]。所编码的蛋白（图 49-5）包括三种肌丝蛋白：β-肌球蛋白重链（β-myosin heavy chain，β-MyHC），心室肌球蛋白轻链 1（myosin essential light chain 1，MLC-1s/v）和心室肌球蛋白调节重链 2（MLC-2s/v）；四个细肌丝蛋白：心肌动蛋白，心肌钙蛋白 T（cardiac troponin T，cTnT），心肌钙蛋白 I（cardiac troponin I，cTnI）和 α-原肌球蛋白（α-tropomyosin，α-TM）；还有一种肌球蛋白结合蛋白 C（cardiac myosin-binding protein，cMyBP-C）。肌联蛋白突变最近也有报导。这些蛋白每一个都由多基因家族编码，因而表现为组织特异性的、不同发育阶段的和生理性调节的表达方式[43]。

3. 肥厚型心肌病和肌球蛋白亚单位

肌球蛋白是转换能量的分子马达，它将三磷酸腺苷水解产生的能量转换为直接的运动，在此过程中，使肌小节变短、肌肉收缩。心肌球蛋白包括两条重链（myosin heavy chain，MyHC）和两对轻链（myosin light chain，MLC），两对轻链分别为必需（或称碱性）轻链（MLC-1）和调节（或称磷酸化）轻链（MLC-2）[44]。肌球蛋白分子高度不对称，包含了两个球形头部和一个杆状尾部。轻链以头尾相连形式串联。目前对它们的功能还不完全明确。任何一种轻链都不是肌球蛋白头部 ATP 酶活化所必需的成分，但它们可能参与肌动蛋白的调节、与颈部（有人提出假说颈部具有杠杆臂的功能）的硬度有关。在重链和两种轻链上均已发现了基因突变。

肌球蛋白结合蛋白 C（cMyBP-C）也是肌小节粗肌丝的一部分，位于肌小节 A 带横纹区[42]。其功能尚不清楚。但通常认为它参与肌小节的构成和调节，包括钙敏感性。另外，cMyBP-C 磷酸化可改变自然状

表 49-1 已知的心肌病病因

表型	遗传特性	基因座	基因	蛋白	骨骼肌
扩张型心肌病	X-连锁	Xp21	Dystrophin (DYS)	Dystrophin	Duchenne 肌营养不良/Becker 肌营养不良
	X-连锁	Xq28	G4.5 (TNZ)	Tafazin	Barth 综合征
	常染色体显性	15q14	肌动蛋白 (ACTC)	肌动蛋白	Namaline 肌病
		2q35	结蛋白 (DES)	结蛋白	结蛋白肌病
		5q33	δ-Sarcoglycan (SGCD)	δ-Sarcoglycan	LGMD2F
		1q32	肌钙蛋白 T (TNNT2)	肌钙蛋白 T	?
		14q11	β-肌浆球蛋白重链 (MYH7)	β-肌浆球蛋白重链	?
		10q22	Metavinculin (VCL)	Metavinculin	?
		15q2	α-原肌球蛋白 (TPM1)	α-原肌球蛋白	Namaline 肌病
		2q31	肌联蛋白 (TTN)	肌联蛋白	Tibial 肌营养不良
	线粒体	4q21	β-Sarcoglycan (SGCB)	β-Sarcoglycan	LGMD2E
		mtDNA	mtDNA	线粒体呼吸链	线粒体肌病
伴扩张型心肌病的传导性疾病	X-连锁	Xq28	Emetin	Emetin	Emery-Dreifuss 肌营养不良
	常染色体	1q21	Lamin A/C (LMNA)	Lamin A/C	Emery-Dreifuss 肌营养不良
肥厚型心肌病	常染色体显性	14q11	β-肌浆球蛋白重链 (MYH7)	β-肌浆球蛋白重链	?
		1q32	肌钙蛋白 T (TNNT2)	肌钙蛋白 T	?
		12q23	肌钙蛋白 I (TNNI)	肌钙蛋白 I	?
		15q2	α-原肌球蛋白 (TPM1)	α-原肌球蛋白	Namaline 肌病
		11p11	肌球蛋白结合蛋白 C (MYBPC3)	肌球蛋白结合蛋白 C	?
		3q21	肌球蛋白必需轻链 (MELC)	肌球蛋白必需轻链	?
		3q21	肌球蛋白调节轻链 (MRLC)	肌球蛋白调节轻链	?
		2q31	肌联蛋白	肌联蛋白	?
肥厚型心肌病/WPW		7q3	AMPK	AMPK	?
		mtDNA	mtDNA	线粒体呼吸链	线粒体肌病
致心律失常右室发育不良/心肌病	常染色体显性	1q42	兰尼定受体 (RyR2)	兰尼定	?
	AR (Naxos)	6p24	Desmoplakin (DES)	Desmoplakin	
		17q21	盘状球蛋白 (PLAK)	盘状球蛋白	
	Carvajal	6p24	Desmoplakin (DES)	Desmoplakin	?
左室壁松散	X-连锁常染色体显性	Xq28	G4.5	Tafazzin	Barth 综合征
		18q12	α-Dystrobrevin	α-Dystrobrevin	肌营养不良

注释：AMPK，AMP 活化的蛋白激酶；LGMD，肢带肌营养不良；左室壁松散（Left ventricular noncompaction）；WPW，Wolff-Parkinson-White 综合征。

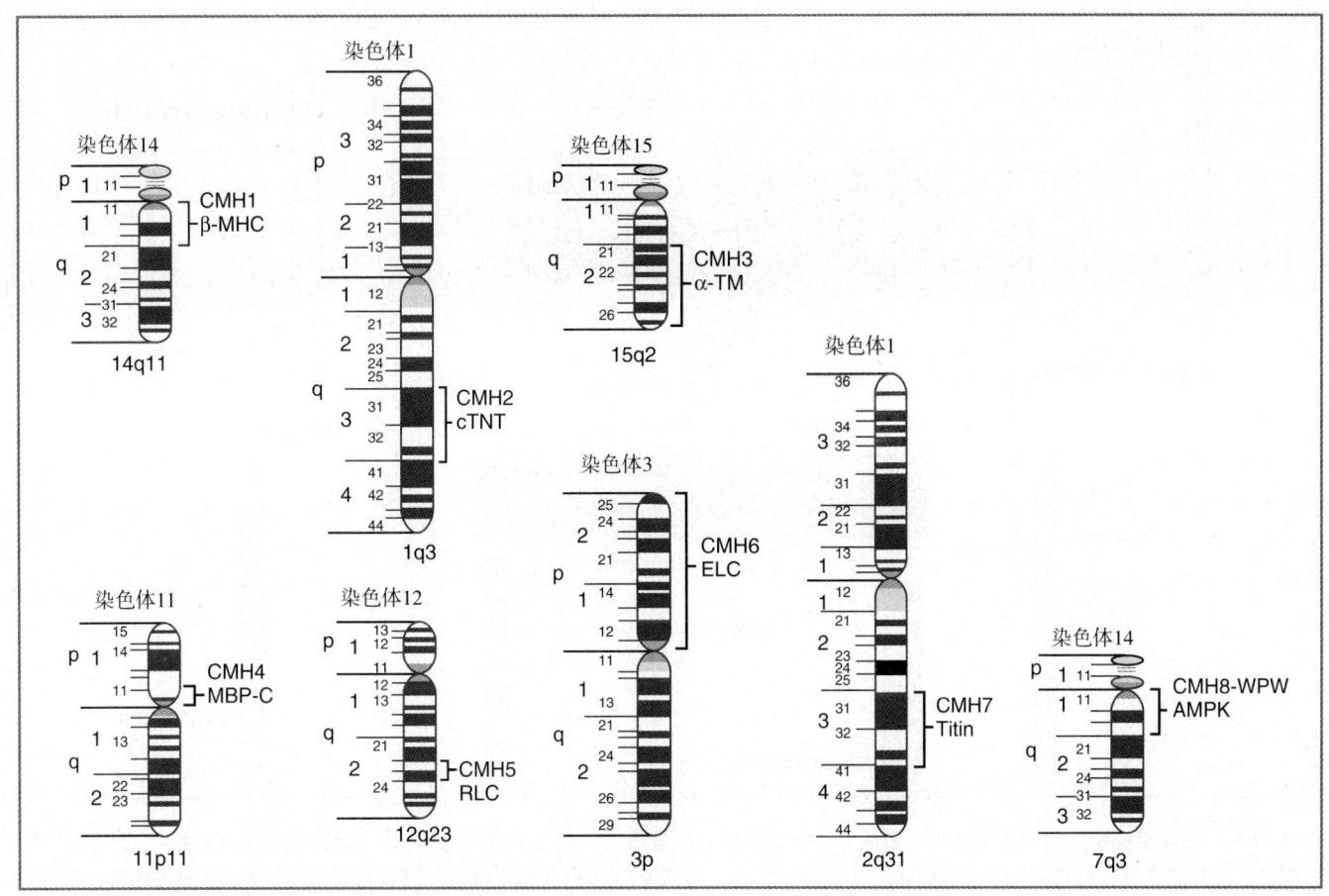

图 49-4 肥厚型心肌病的基因图谱 图示目前已知的遗传基因位点及相关基因共有 8 个。β-MHC：β 肌浆球蛋白重链；cTNT：肌钙蛋白 T；TαTM：α 原肌球蛋白；MBP-C：肌球蛋白结合蛋白 C；RLC：调节轻链；ELC：必需轻链；AMPK：AMP 活化的蛋白激酶

态下的粗肌丝肌球蛋白横桥，表明 cMyBP-C 可改变已活化心肌的能量生成。

多数基因突变对突变蛋白质产生的主要是负性作用[42]，另一种可能是部分糖基化蛋白的生成缺陷或降解加速。这种蛋白质的快速降解可能是阻断肌原纤维生成和扰乱肌丝形成（而不是聚集）的关键环节。

4. 细肌丝蛋白

细肌丝蛋白包括肌动蛋白、肌钙蛋白复合体和原肌球蛋白（见图 49-5）[42]。肌钙蛋白复合体和原肌球蛋白组成钙敏感的通道调解心肌纤维的收缩。在 α-TM 和肌钙蛋白复合物的两个亚单位上均已发现了突变：cTnI-抑制性亚单位，cTnT-原肌球蛋白结合亚单位。另外，肌动蛋白突变也有报道[42]。

α-TM 由 *TPM1* 编码，其心脏亚型在心室肌和骨骼肌中均表达。cTnT 由 *TNNT2* 基因编码，在人类心肌中有多种 cTnT 亚型，可表达于胎儿、成人和患病心脏，源于 *TNNT2* 单基因的选择性剪切。CTnI 由 *TNNI3* 基因编码，cTnI 亚型仅在心肌表达。cTnI-肌钙蛋白-原肌球蛋白的共同结合是心脏独一无二的特性。已证实 α-心脏肌动蛋白也可作为致病原因[42]。

5. 家族性肥厚型心肌病基因型-表型之间的联系

家族性肥厚型心肌病患者左室肥厚的类型和程度差异很大，即使是在一级亲属中也是如此。在患病的家族中猝死发生率很高。因此明确家族性肥厚型心肌病的基因型异质性是否与疾病表型分布有关很重要。关于 *MYH7*、*TNNT2* 和 *MYBPC3* 基因突变曾有报道。已证实，*MYH7* 基因不同类型突变的患者其预后也大不相同[42]。例如 R403Q 突变与低生存率明显有关，其他突变如 V606M 预后就好一些。*TNNT2* 突变所致疾病约有 20% 不外显，心肌肥厚相对较轻，有时是亚临床的，但是猝死发生率高，无明显临床心肌肥厚也可发生猝死。有报道一个 *TNNT2* 突变的家族

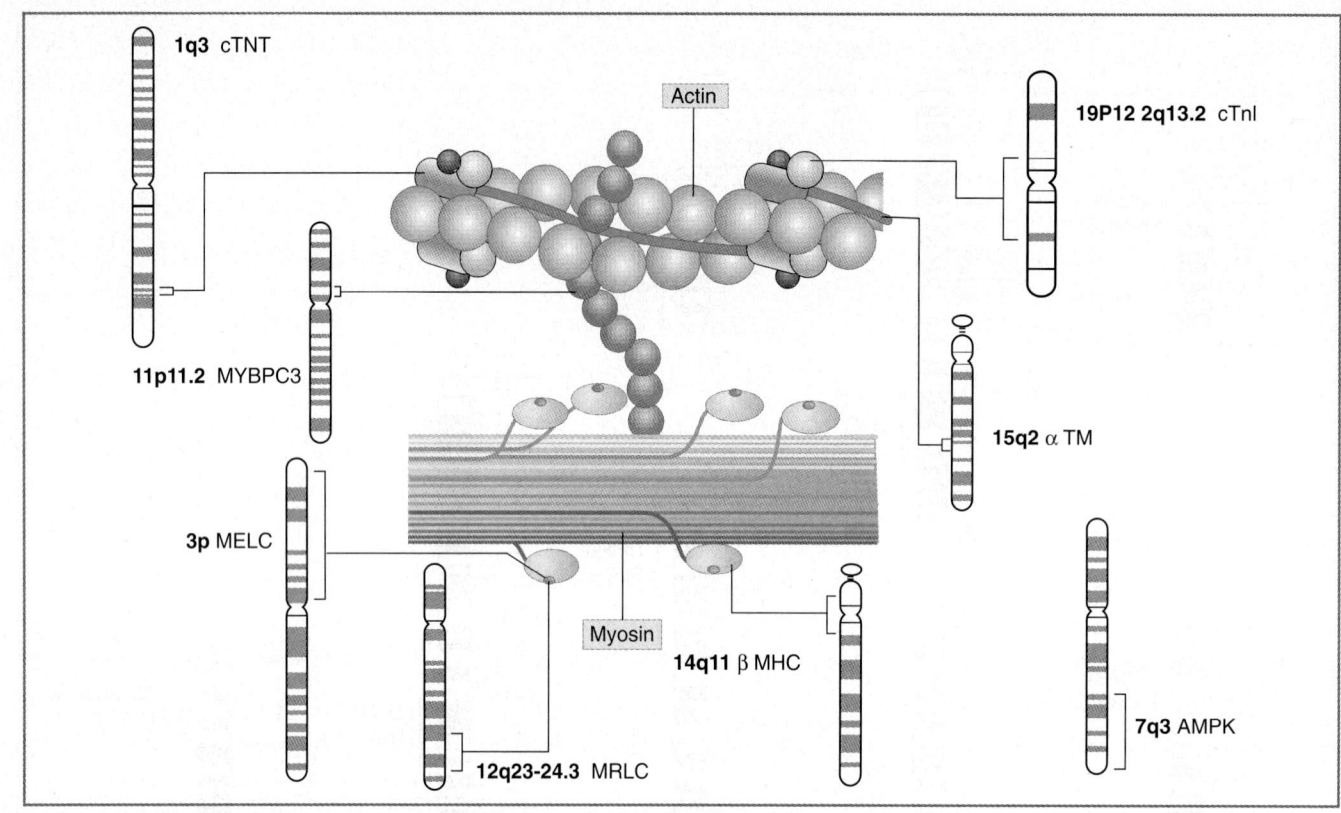

图 49-5　肥厚型心肌病的分子遗传学　显示了致病基因编码的蛋白质。除 AMPK 以外，其余蛋白质可相互影响，这些蛋白质都属肌小节的成员，包括细肌丝（肌钙蛋白 T、肌钙蛋白 I、α 原肌球蛋白和肌动蛋白）以及粗肌丝复合物（β 肌浆球蛋白重链，肌球蛋白调节蛋白以及肌球蛋白结合蛋白）。cTnT：肌钙蛋白 T；cTnI：肌钙蛋白 I；αTM：α 原肌球蛋白；MYBPC3：肌球蛋白结合蛋白 C；MELC：肌球蛋白必需轻链；MLRC：肌球蛋白调节轻链；β-MHC：β 肌浆球蛋白重链；AMPK：AMP 活化的蛋白激酶

有完全外显率，超声心动图所示的心肌肥厚变化范围很大，而且无猝死发生。MYBPC3 基因突变具有特殊的临床特点，年轻患者表型较轻，出现症状时间晚，40 岁之前预后良好[43]。

遗传研究还揭示，存在有携带突变等位基因的临床健康个体，不论是哪个基因受累，在其一级亲属中均有典型疾病表型的患者。突变的表型表达有如此大的差异，其机制可能有：不同环境、后天的习性（如不同的生活方式、危险因素、锻炼）、修饰基因或多态性均可调整疾病表型的表达。到目前为止所知的最显著的就是，血管紧张素 I 转换酶插入/缺失（I/D）多态性对肥厚型心肌病的影响[45]。相关研究表明，与对照组人群相比，D 等位基因在肥厚型心肌病患者中常见，在猝死高发的患者中较常见。

6. 利用遗传模型阐明发病机理

基于在肥厚型心肌病遗传动物模型的在体和离体研究，已明确该病的基本病变是心肌收缩力受损[46]。目前被大家所接受的肥厚型心肌病病因假说是：突变的蛋白混入肌小节并作为有害蛋白使细胞的收缩力受损，然后该细胞又提供促有丝分裂的刺激（可能是几种生长因子）引起代偿性肥厚。在后天疾病过程中，生长刺激多由自分泌或旁分泌因子介导，导致许多患者表现出心肌肥厚，其主要发生于心室间隔。生长因子还刺激成纤维细胞增生增加基质形成。心肌肥厚和组织纤维化与猝死和心律失常的关系还有待明确。有人提出，纤维化组织可导致电传导延迟，使患者易发生心律失常和猝死。是否直接或间接影响到离子通道尚不清楚。

7. 肥厚型心肌病和 Wolff-Parkinson-White 综合征

在正常心脏，心房和心室仅通过房室结一条通路进行电传导。在预激综合征，存在一条副房室旁路，成为快速型心律失常的基础[47]。预激综合征旁路的电传导特性更接近于心室肌而不是房室结的特性，可以在短不应期内快速传导。在窦性心律，心室在房室结兴奋到达之前已经通过旁路激动了部分

心肌,这称为预激。预激的特征性心电图表现为:短 PR 间期、"delta 波"即 QRS 波群升支粗钝。预激综合征患者最常见的心律失常是顺向型房室折返性心动过速(atriventricular reciprocating tachycardia, AVRT),它是通过房室结前传,而旁路进行逆传。这种快速性异位心律常会引起心悸、胸痛、头晕、气短,有些患者可发生晕厥。如果持续发作,AVRT 会转为房颤,因其可通过旁路快速传导而导致室颤,发生这种情况时可有生命危险。因而这些患者是有猝死风险的。

8. 临床遗传学和治疗

多数预激综合征为散发,但属于常染色体显性遗传的也不少见[48]。据报道一级亲属内发生预激的不到 1%,普通人群的患病率大约为 0.15%[48]。值得注意的是,在一级亲属中有多个旁路的患者其预激的发病率增加到大约 1.7%。预激综合征也可发生于先天性心脏病,特别是艾伯斯坦畸形(Ebstein's anomaly)或心肌病(即 HCM)。原发性预激综合征合并伴有常染色体显性遗传家族性肥厚型心肌病家族的突变位点(如图 49-4 所示)定位于 7 号染色体 7q3,最近已经明确这个难以捉摸的基因是磷酸腺苷活化蛋白激酶基因(adenosine monophosphate kinase-activated protein kinase,AMPK 基因),可见表 49-1[49-51]。

目前预激综合征的首选治疗措施是射频消融,在大多数患者可以永久打断旁路。对于少数未行射频消融的患者可考虑采用药物治疗。

9. 分子遗传学

1995 年,肥厚型心肌病和预激综合征的连锁就已确定在 7 号染色体 7q3,但是对这个基因的具体功能还不完全清楚。Gollob 等第一次将 PRKAG2 基因与这个疾病联系起来(见图 49-5),它编码 AMPK 的 γ2 调节亚单位[50]。AMPK 活化可促进 AMP 向 ATP 转化。这个活化过程需要 AMP 直接结合和通过 AMP 活化蛋白激酶激酶(AMPK kinase)的磷酸化以及环 AMP 浓度的升高,AMP/ATP 比率升高是由 β-肾上腺素受体激动所致。这个蛋白质具有不同功能:非经典 ATP 利用通路的失活,调节肌酸激酶,通过脂肪酸氧化储存 ATP,可满足细胞生命所需如适当的离子通道活性、肌小节收缩功能,它入核以后还可调节基因转录。

Gollob 小组观察的患者均有预激综合征的证据[50],于是研究者们认为 PRKAG2 就是预激综合征的基因。但有一些患病个体有左室肥厚的证据,这与最初的报道是一致的。Blair 等几乎在同一时间也发现了这些突变,他们观察的患者有显著的左室肥厚,其中一些合并预激综合征,推断其临床特性归因于能量失常[49]。近来,Arad 等提出该疾病为糖原储存疾病,与婴儿的 Pompe 病相似[51]。究竟是什么引起预激及其所致快速异位心律失常目前仍不明确。

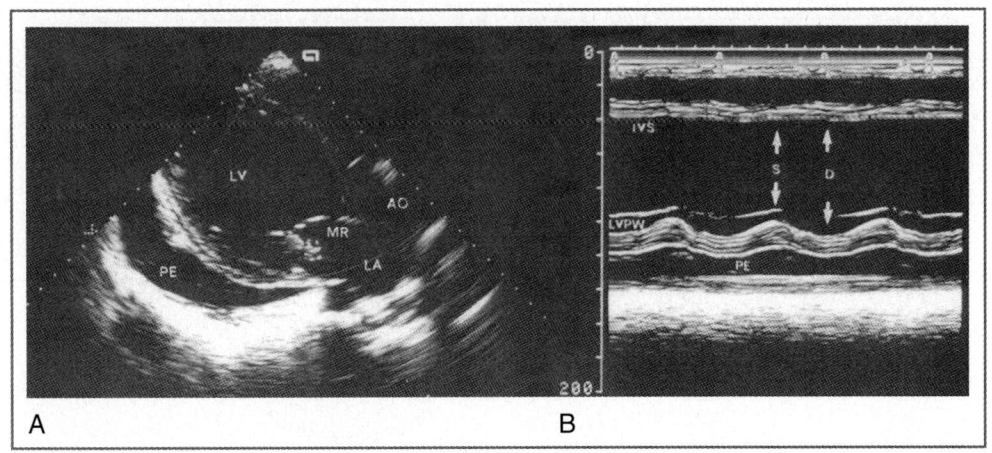

图 49-6 扩张型心肌病超声心动图表现 左室长轴面显示左室(LV)扩大和二尖瓣反流(MR),而左房(LA)及主动脉根部(AO)大小正常,伴中等量心包积液(PE)。M 型超声显示左室扩张伴收缩功能下降,以及心包积液。IVS:室间隔;LVPW:左室后壁;S:收缩期;D:舒张期(见彩图 25)

(二) 扩张型心肌病

1. 临床特点

扩张型心肌病（dilated cardiomyopathy，DCM）以心室腔增大、室壁重量减少、收缩功能受损为特点，也可有继发性舒张功能不全[43]。因左心室扩张，可导致二尖瓣瓣环扩大而出现二尖瓣反流（见图49-6）。当二尖瓣出现明显反流时，左房开始增大，随后出现肺动脉高压。最常见的临床表现是充血性心力衰竭：静息时心动过速（很可能是因交感神经张力的增高所致）、肺水肿所致呼吸困难、肝肿大、因心输出量减低所致的低灌注。可见晕厥和猝死，且多数患者由室速/室颤所致。许多患者也可出现心包或胸腔积液。除了室性心动过速，还可见室上性心动过速，有些患者以传导障碍为主[43]。

2. 遗传学

特发性扩张型心肌病的发病率约40/10万[52]。家族性扩张型心肌病占特发性扩张型心肌病的30%～40%。家族性扩张型心肌病多为常染色体显性遗传，X-连锁、线粒体遗传、常染色体隐性遗传也可见[7,43]。我们确定的第一个常染色体显性遗传基因在1号染色体1q32。许多其他的染色体等位基因也已明确，"单纯性"扩张型心肌病包括10q21-23，5q33，9q13，15q14，2q31等位基因（见图49-1）；复杂扩张型心肌病包括另外3个等位基因：1p1-1q1，1q11-1q21，3p22-25，在合并有传导异常（传导系统疾病合并扩张型心肌病[CDDC]）的家族中还有6q23，有一个6q23连锁的家族合并肢体肌肉营养不良，两个家族合并感觉神经性耳聋。

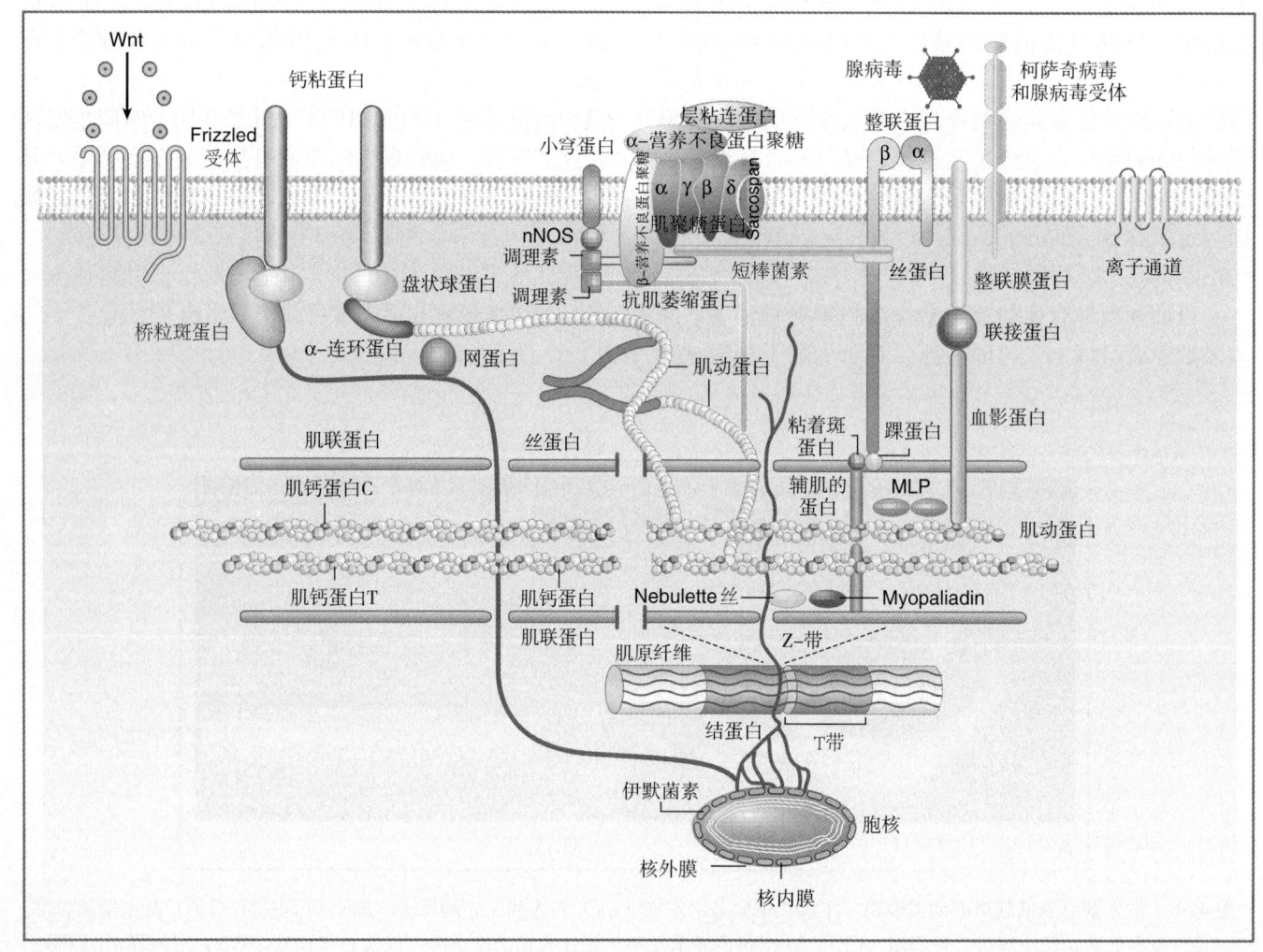

图49-7　心肌的细胞结构　在细胞外基质、肌膜、肌小节和核膜之间可相互联系。值得注意的是，有许多重要的蛋白质来维持正常心脏内的这种联系。在扩张型心肌病时，一些结构蛋白发生了病变，细胞间联系以及肌小结结构也都可能出现异常。nNOS：神经性一氧化氮合酶；MLP：肌LIM蛋白

(三) X-连锁扩张型心肌病

1. 临床特点

Berko 和 Swift 报道了一个扩张型心肌病的五代家系,呈 X-连锁遗传(X-linked inheritance,XL-CM),但无骨骼肌病的临床证据[14]。男性在十几岁或二十几岁发病,超声心动图可见有 DCM 表现及二尖瓣反流。数名患者有发作性室速。其中男性患者病情进展迅速,在1～2年内死亡或做心脏移植。有症状的女性携带者在四五十岁时发生轻度心肌病,疾病进展缓慢。右室心内膜活检有轻度间质纤维化,尸检证实有显著扩张、广泛分布的斑点状纤维化,以后壁最严重,电镜下线粒体正常。除了有明显 X-连锁遗传特点,以及男性患者和女性携带者血清肌酸激酶的肌肉亚型升高外,该心肌病和其他扩张型心肌病之间未发现有特异性病征。

2. 遗传学

Towbin 等在上文提及的家族以及在另一个家族中证明了 Xp21 *dystrophin* 等位基因(即 Duchenne-Becker 肌无力的基因)和 X 连锁遗传性扩张型心肌病之间的联系[15]。X 连锁遗传性扩张型心肌病的蛋白缺陷为抗肌萎缩蛋白 N 端和杆状部的缺失或低表达(见图 49-7)。然而骨骼肌总蛋白正常。这种与肌营养不良蛋白相关的 156kD 糖蛋白,被称作 α-肌营养不良蛋白聚糖,它是一个抗肌营养不良蛋白相关糖蛋白复合物(Dystrophin-associated glycoprotein,DAG)的膜结合结构,它和整个 DAG 在肌组织中表达水平均减低。这一点后来被其他研究者进一步证实。在所有病例中,扩张型心肌病的发生都是由于肌细胞膜失去力学稳定性。

3. 治疗

充血性心力衰竭和室性心律失常的治疗很重要,心脏移植也很常见。药物治疗包括口服药,如地高辛、利尿剂和血管紧张素转化酶抑制剂如卡托普利、依那普利等。近来加用 β 受体阻滞剂,如美托洛尔、卡维地洛成为了标准治疗。因为收缩功能极差,患者有潜在的形成血栓和栓塞的可能,故可考虑加用阿司匹林或其他药物。一些患者需要静脉用药以增强心肌收缩功能,常用治疗药物有小剂量的多巴胺、米力农以及其他药,如多巴酚丁胺、肾上腺素、去甲肾上腺素。心室辅助装置或主动脉内球囊反搏可用于严重心

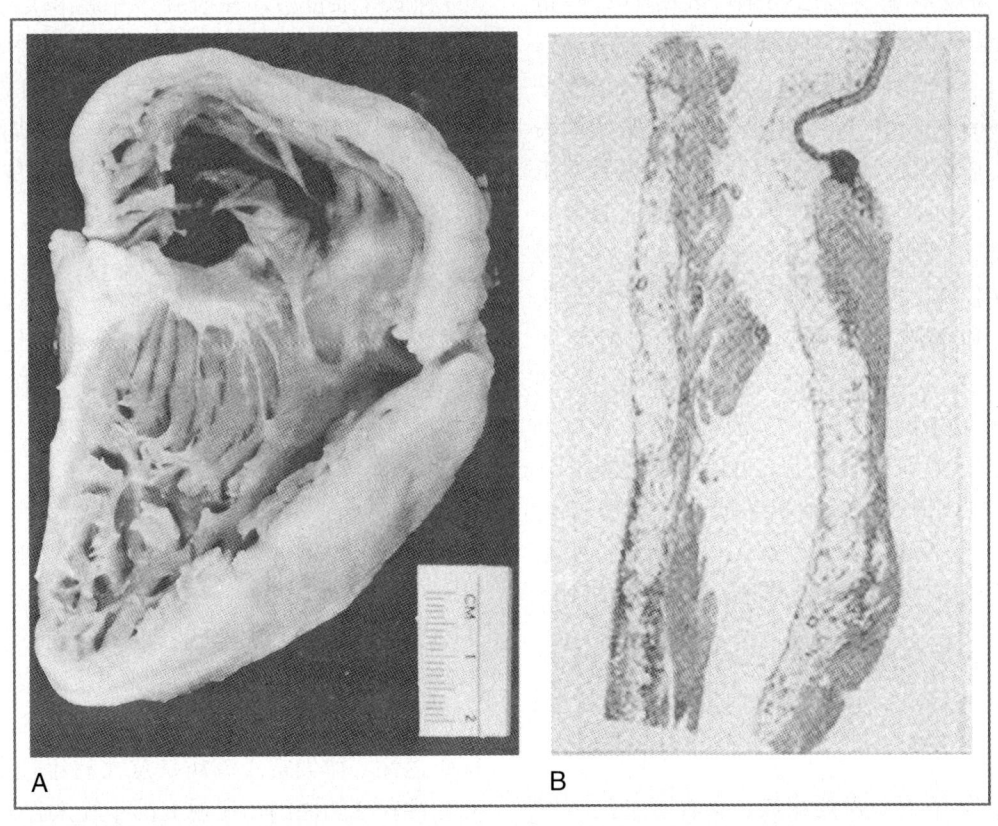

图 49-8 致心律失常性右室发育不良/心肌病 A:大体标本,左侧是正常室腔,右室壁变薄,呈纤维脂肪化。B:组织学证实心肌组织内有纤维脂肪浸润

衰患者等待心脏移植的过渡阶段。心室辅助装置可改善病情。另外一些患者需要抗心律失常治疗,对于有致命性心律失常的患者可植入植入型心脏复律除颤器(Implanted cardioverter defibrillator,ICD)。

(四) 常染色体显性遗传扩张型心肌病和最终共同途径

常染色体遗传扩张型心肌病致病基因的确定显著晚于肥厚型心肌病和心律失常综合征致病基因的确定。肥厚型心肌病是肌小节蛋白突变所致,心律失常是离子通道异常所致,以此为基础我们提出假说:扩张型心肌病通过另一条连接肌膜和肌小节的共同途径最终发病[43]。因为已经发现了这些结构的重要联系蛋白,抗肌营养不良蛋白可引起X连锁遗传性扩张型心肌病,我们沿着这些交叉蛋白进行研究,明确了δ-肌聚糖的突变,它是一个常见于年轻危重患者,与膜结合5q33连锁的抗肌营养不良蛋白相关蛋白复合物(dystrophin-associated protein complex,DAPC)(见图49-1)[43]。对基因敲除小鼠和具有相同病理改变的心肌病田鼠的研究结果也支持这一观点。和肌营养不良基因一样,这个基因的突变可导致一种肌营养不良-肢带肌肉营养不良(limp-girdle muscular dystrophy,LGMD)。β-肌聚糖的突变也已明确,表明DAPC蛋白对肌肉的功能很重要。另外,细胞骨架蛋白结蛋白相连的丝蛋白(desmin intermediated filament protein)和Metavinculin都可导致扩张型心肌病(见表49-1)。结蛋白也可引起骨骼肌病,有些患者也会发生传导异常和限制型心肌病。在肥厚型心肌病中的重要基因——编码肌小节蛋白的基因突变也可引起扩张型心肌病。据推测,扩张型心肌病的肌力障碍是由于肌小节蛋白突变和细胞骨架突变所致的肌力传导障碍[43]。

心律失常的发生机制未明。但是如图49-7所指出的,离子通道位于心肌细胞膜上,可以想象胞膜的分解会引起通道的结构改变,导致功能异常和心律失常。许多通道,包括SCN5A和minK,与诸如抗肌萎缩蛋白的蛋白质都有直接的相互作用。

(五) 伴有传导障碍的扩张型心肌病

1. 临床特点

在患心脏传导障碍疾病的家族,患者于二三十岁出现短暂的心律失常,到三四十岁变成持续发作的心律失常。心律失常包括二度或三度房室阻滞、房颤或显著心动过缓,常需要植入起搏器。扩张型心肌病多发生于四五十岁,一般没有严重心律紊乱。猝死常发生于疾病终末期。尸检可见显著的左、右室扩张,间质纤维化,胞浆空泡样变心肌变性,房室结细胞被纤维组织代替。

2. 遗传学

在过去十年里,对几个家族进行的基因连锁分析,发现了一个突变基因。证实了多个突变位点,包括1q21,2q14-q22,3p22-p25,6q23(见表49-1)。1q21连锁的伴传导障碍的扩张型心肌病基因是 lamin A/C[43](见表49-1)。这个基因编码细胞骨架蛋白中中间丝蛋白质组(intermediate filament class)的两个蛋白质。这些家族的患者也有不同程度的骨骼肌病。该基因还引起具有相同表型的常染色体显性遗传Emery-Dreifuss肌营养不良,骨骼肌病是该病诊断的要点。伴传导障碍的扩张型心肌病的一些患者,包括年轻患者,可以发生快速心律失常、非持续性室速、室上性心动过速、房颤等。

尽管3p22-p25和6q23连锁的基因还未明确,对另一群患者的研究表明,在2q连锁的基因结蛋白(一种肌纤维蛋白,在肌纤维中蓄积)上有突变。在骨骼肌和心肌,正常的结蛋白紧紧环绕Z带与肌动蛋白肌丝,沿心肌纤维协助传导张力,在肌纤维的反复收缩中保护其结构的完整性。突变的结蛋白使肌纤维变脆、收缩障碍。结蛋白缺失的小鼠具有同样表型,但发病较晚。

3. 治疗

传导系统疾病的治疗原则是有症状的心动过缓,需植入起搏器,有充血性心力衰竭的患者,其治疗应遵循充血性心力衰竭的标准治疗方案。

(六) 致心律失常性右室发育不良/心肌病

致心律失常性右室发育不良/心肌病(arrhythmogenic right ventricular dysplasia/cardiomyopathy,ARVD/ARVC)的特点是:右室脂肪浸润、纤维化,最终导致右室室壁变薄,心腔扩大(图49-8)[43]。残余的心肌细胞被纤维组织包绕,这种基质容易发生右室折返性心律失常。该病是意大利年轻人中最常见的心源性猝死的原因,据说美国年轻人猝死大约有17%是由该病所致[53]。

1. 临床特点

ARVD/ARVC 的临床表现有很大差异，包括心悸、晕厥、右心（或全心）衰竭和猝死[53]。有些患者无症状。在青春期前几乎无临床发病，典型发病年龄是 12～45 岁之间，猝死常是首发症状。估计 3%～4% 的患者可发生运动性猝死（占年轻人猝死的 17%）。众所周知这种疾病的节律异常多发生于运动中。

因为缺乏心脏结构、功能和心电表现的诊断标准，ARVD/ARVC 的临床诊断很难。结构改变可包括：右室腔内径增大、流出道深裂隙和小梁形成，局部运动消失或减弱、膨出（特别是在漏斗部顶部和三尖瓣后叶下部区域），局部右室壁变薄。

形态学上，最显著的特点是右室游离壁心外膜和中层心肌组织被脂肪组织替代，而心内膜和室间隔多无此改变[53]。随着疾病进展，左室也可被累及，特别是心外膜。右室局部变薄，特别是在漏斗部，膈面下壁或顶部最典型。组织学检查可见严重营养不良的心肌细胞散在分布于纤维和脂肪组织之间。约 70% 患者可见心脏有细胞坏死和局灶淋巴细胞浸润的急性斑片状炎症。

该病在临床上最重要的特征就是易发心律失常。由于右室壁浦肯野系统传导速度减慢（即壁阻滞，parietal block），在窦性心律时可见异常 QRS 波形。另外，由于右室游离壁解剖异常和室腔增大，心室复极也可出现异常。这些异常包括：（1）右侧胸前导联（$V_1 \sim V_3$）QRS 波时限延长，反映了右室游离壁的传导延迟，它是心脏除极的最后部分；（2）ε（epsilon）波，是于 QRS 波群结束处出现的小电位，反映了右室除极延迟；（3）信号平均心电图可表现为晚电位阳性，也反映了右室除极延迟，并与右室射血分数的降低有关。（4）12 岁以上患者出现的除 V_1 导联以外的 T 波倒置，倒置程度与右室受累程度相关。（5）室性心律失常。因这些病变以右室游离壁为主，故多表现为左束支阻滞图形。有研究提示，心律失常的多发主要是由于心交感神经支配异常和心肌 β-肾上腺素受体密度显著减少。

2. 遗传学

ARVD/ARVC 多是遗传性的，30%～50% 患者有家族史[43]。除了在纳克索斯岛（Naxos）、希腊和委内瑞拉为隐性遗传外，该疾病多为显性遗传，其临床表现程度可不同。其显性遗传具有遗传异质性，目前确定 ARVD/ARVC 有 6 个致病基因，染色体定位于 14q24.3（ARVD1），1q42-q43（ARVD2），14q12-q22（ARVD3），2q32，1-q32.3（ARVD4），3p23（ARVD5），10p12-p14（ARVD6），见表 49-1。还发现了一个与肌原纤维肌病有关的 ARVD/ARVC 等位基因，该病是一种骨骼肌病，表现为躯干及四肢肌无力，肌电图异常，组织活检也有异常表现：边缘空泡（rimmed vacuoles）形成；结蛋白、肌萎缩蛋白和肌聚糖的堆积；肌原纤维结构破坏等。这个基因定位于 10q22.3。

ARVD/ARVC 隐性遗传型，即 Naxos 病，基因定位在染色体 17q21。这种复杂疾病包括与 ARVD/ARVC 相关的弥漫性非表皮掌跖皮肤角质层松解、羊毛状头发，发现于希腊的纳克萨斯（Naxos）岛。该病的致病基因为盘状球蛋白（表 49-1），这是一种桥粒蛋白。有趣的是，常染色体显性的肌原纤维肌病有结蛋白样成分，提示将来可能会发现与该致病基因和纯合型 ARVD/ARVC 基因有相似的基因产物。另外对于委内瑞拉型，即 Carvajal 综合征，它可累及左室，其致病基因 Desmoplakin 在染色体上定位于 6q24。Desmoplakin 同桥粒蛋白一样，为连接蛋白（见图 49-7）。

常染色体显性型 ARVD/ARVC 研究最近有所突破，已明确 AVRD2 基因为 1q42 连锁的兰尼定受体（R_yR_2）[54]。另外也证实了 Desmoplakin 也可导致常染色体显性遗传的 ARVD/C，但可没有 Carvajal 综合征表现[55]。

3. 治疗

药物治疗包括，采用抗心律失常药物控制室性心律失常，如最常用索他洛尔，其他如胺碘酮、氟尼卡、普罗帕酮。虽然索他洛尔对预防室速再发有效，但它是否对预防猝死有效尚属未知。有些患者可行导管消融，但复发并不少见，可能因为是疾病的自然进程。近来对曾有过心脏骤停或具有晕厥/猝死高风险或有多形性室速的患者可行 ICD 植入。但因为心肌组织的病理改变是脂肪浸润，ICD 的植入效果可能还是个问题。

（七）线粒体疾病

线粒体是细胞内细胞器，参与多种代谢途径，包括氧化磷酸化合成 ATP[7,18]。线粒体是独特的细胞器，因为它包含有基因组，编码氧化磷酸化途径中的一些蛋白质和tRNA、rRNA，还有其他的线粒体蛋白质。卵母细胞的线粒体可自身复制，因此线粒体基因突变是母系遗传[19,20]。

1. 临床特点

线粒体肌病的心脏异常比较常见，包括传导缺陷、肥厚型心肌病、扩张型心肌病和混合性心肌病，后者可能是部分肥厚型心肌病发展到晚期的结果[7]。Leber遗传性视神经病（Leber hereditary optic neuropathy，LHON），是由视网膜神经节细胞和视神经轴突退化导致的中枢性视力丧失，常与预激综合征相关[18,20]。其他线粒体疾病也与预激综合征相关，包括MELAS综合征（肌病、脑病、乳酸酸中毒和卒中样发作）和MERRF综合征，即伴有肌阵挛脑病和蓬毛样红纤维（ragged red fibers）[7]。另一个有心脏病变的线粒体肌病是Kearns-Sayre综合征，常并发扩张型心肌病和传导性疾病[21]。

2. 遗传学

人类线粒体基因组是母系遗传的环状DNA分子[7,18-20]。线粒体DNA（mitochondrial DNA，mtRNA）编码氧化代谢所需63种蛋白质中的13种，编码翻译这些蛋白质所需的22种tRNA和2种rRNA。mtDNA远不如核基因组（其中含来自双亲的基因）那么多，tRNA和rRNA以多拷贝形式存在，故线粒体基因是突变引起人类疾病的优选靶点[18-20]。线粒体的许多结构成分依赖细胞核和细胞质，但它确实提供了对细胞呼吸至关重要的蛋白质。产生细胞ATP的电子传递链，将复合体I合成复合体IV和ATP合酶（复合体V）。13 mtDNA编码呼吸链中的酶，包括七种复合体I亚型（ND1、ND2、ND3、ND4L、ND4、ND5和ND6），一种复合体III亚型（细胞色素b），三种复合体V亚型（ATPase 6和8）。每个细胞包含大量线粒体，每个线粒体又包含多拷贝的mtRNA。在大多数线粒体疾病中，患者既有突变线粒体又有正常线粒体，表现出一定的异质性，不同组织之间、同一家族不同个体之间这种正常与异常比例的不同，决定了表型的严重程度。

线粒体肌病常于婴儿时期或童年早期就出现脑和肌肉的功能紊乱。在呼吸链缺陷中心脏病最常见。mtRNA缺陷时，肌肉活检常常可见蓬毛样红纤维（见表49-1），表明已存在ATP生成障碍。与呼吸链复合体有关的各种临床综合征中，部分是由于组织特异的呼吸链复合体受累，也有是非组织特异性呼吸链复合体受累，还有部分与受累组织中某些酶的活性有关。与线粒体缺陷有关的心脏疾病有肥厚型心肌病和DCM[7]。

线粒体基因的定位，不需要基因连锁。在一个患病家族中，每个患者都是由母亲遗传，而不是由父亲遗传的。因为在基因突变中存在许多有害的多态性，因此必要时要对线粒体基因测序以明确其突变。

3. 治疗

这些疾病的治疗通常是对症治疗。传导性疾病多需安装起搏器，心衰按常规治疗。β受体拮抗剂可能对一些患者有效。肥厚性心脏病的治疗常与肥厚型心肌病相似。针对线粒体的治疗包括辅酶Q10、卡尼丁、维生素，但这些治疗不能改变疾病的临床进程。

（八）Kearns-Sayre综合征

典型的线粒体疾病包括上睑下垂、慢性进行性眼外肌麻痹、视网膜色素沉着、心脏传导性疾病和扩张型心肌病[21]。听力丧失和肢体无力常伴有内分泌疾病，如糖尿病、甲状旁腺机功能减退、生长激素缺乏。大约20%的Kearns-Sayre综合征患者有心脏受累，这些患者中大多数有传导障碍，可呈进行性心脏传导阻滞。患者常有大量不同的线粒体基因缺失，其中tRNA$^{leu(UUR)}$-3243最常见。

临床上的传导异常，包括双束支阻滞和进行性高度阻滞，常需要安装起搏器。也有用辅酶Q10作为针对线粒体的治疗。辅酶Q10在线粒体的主要功能是在呼吸链复合体形成时，由复合体I和II向复合体III传递电子。维生素如维生素K_1、维生素K_3、维生素C用于直接向细胞色素C提供电子。内分泌疾病和心力衰竭可按常规治疗。

六、总　结

在过去的十多年里，我们对人类疾病遗传基础的复杂性已有了更深刻的认识，心血管疾病遗传学取得了非常显著的进步，包括对致心律失常疾病病因的认识，例如长QT综合征、Brugada综合征、多形性室速以及近来对房颤的认识。另外，心肌病的致病原因也逐渐被揭示。发现和分析基因突变的方法已经成熟，在以后的章节中将论述心律失常的分子基础。

（张幼怡　张敏丽　龚开政　译）

参考文献

1. Hoffman JIE: Incidence of congenital heart disease: II. Prenatal incidence. Pediatr Cardiol 16:155–165, 1995.
2. Collins FS, Patrinos A, Jordan E, et al: New goals for the U.S. Human Genome Project: 1998–2003. Science 282:682–689, 1998.
3. Brower V: News in science. Nat Biotech 16:895, 1998.
4. Brower V: Genome II: The next frontier, Nat Biotech 16:104, 1998.
5. Collins FS: Shattuck lecture—Medical and societal consequences of the human genome project. N Engl J Med 341:28–37, 1999.
6. Roberts R, Towbin J: Principles and techniques of molecular biology. In Robert R (ed): Molecular Basis of Cardiology. Cambridge, UK, Blackwell Scientific Publications, 1993, pp 15–112.
7. Towbin JA: Molecular genetic aspects of cardiomyopathy. Biochem Med Metab Biol 49:285–320, 1993.
8. Towbin JA, Li H, Taggart RT, et al: Evidence of genetic heterogeneity in Romano-Ward long QT syndrome. Analysis of 23 families. Circulation 90:2635–2644, 1994.
9. Vatta M, Li H, Towbin JA: Molecular biology of arrhythmic syndromes. Curr Opin Cardiol 15:12–22, 2000.
10. Timchenko LT: Myontonic dystrophy: The role of RNA CUG triplet repeats. Am J Hum Genet 64:360–364, 1999.
11. Maron BJ: Hypertrophic cardiomyopathy. Lancet 350:127–133, 1997.
12. Towbin JA: Molecular genetics of hypertrophic cardiomyopathy. Curr Cardiol Rep 2:134–140, 2000.
13. Schwartz PJ, Priori SG, Napolitano C: Long QT syndrome. In Zipes DP, Jalife J (eds): Cardiac Electrophysiology: From Cell to Bedside, 3rd ed. Philadelphia, WB Saunders, 2000, pp 597–615.
14. Berko BA, Swift M: X-linked dilated cardiomyopathy. N Engl J Med 316:1186–1191, 1987.
15. Towbin JA, Hejtmancik F, Brink P, et al: X-linked cardiomyopathy (XLCM): Molecular genetic evidence of linkage to the Duchenne muscular dystrophy (dystrophin) gene at the Xp21 locus. Circulation 87:1854–1865, 1993.
16. Barth PG, Scholte HR, Berden JA, et al: An X-linked mitochondrial disease affecting cardiac muscle and neutrophil leukocytes. J Neurol Sci 62:327–355, 1983.
17. Cox GF, Kunkel LM: Dystrophies and heart disease. Curr Opin Cardiol 9:329–343, 1997.
18. Kelly DP, Strauss AW: Inherited cardiomyopathies. N Engl J Med 330:913–919, 1994.
19. Smeitink J, van den Heuvel L: Human mitochondrial complex I in health and disease. Am J Med Gent 77:395–400, 1998.
20. Wallace DC: Mitochondrial diseases in man and mouse. Science 283:1482–1488, 1999.
21. Tveskov C, Angelo-Nielsen K: Kearns-Sayre syndrome and dilated cardiomyopathy. Neurology 40:553–554, 1990.
22. Haines JL, Perricak-Vance MA: Sibpair analysis. In Haines JL, Perricak-Vance MA (eds): Approaches to Gene Mapping in Complex Human Diseases. New York, Wiley-Liss, 1998, pp 273–303.
23. Serrato M, Marian AJ: A variant of human paraoxonase/arylesterase (HUMPONA) gene is a risk factor for coronary artery disease. J Clin Invest 96:3005–3008, 1995.
24. Yu QT, Safavi F, Roberts R, et al: A variant of β-fibrinogen is a genetic risk factor for coronary artery disease and myocardial infarction. J Invest Med 44:154–159, 1996.
25. Haines JL, Perricak-Vance MA: Lod score analysis. Haines JL, Perricak-Vance MA (eds): Approaches to Gene Mapping in Complex Human Diseases. New York, Wiley-Liss, 1998, pp 253–272, 1998.
26. Zhau LP, Aragaki C, Hsu L, Quiaoit F: Mapping of complex traits by single-nucleotide polymorphisms. Am J Hum Genet 63:225–240, 1998.
27. Hagmann M: A good SNP may be hard to find. Science 285:21–22, 1999.
28. Weissenbach J, Gyapay G, Dib C, et al: A second generation linkage map of the human genome based on highly informative microsatellite loci. Gene 135:275–278, 1994.
29. Cooperative Human Linkage Center (CHLC): A comprehensive human linkage map with centimorgan density. Science 265:2049–2054, 1994.
30. Cooper NG (ed): The Human Genome Project: Deciphering the Blueprint of Heredity. Mill Valley, CA, University Science Books, 1994.
31. Wang Q, Keating MT: Isolation of P1 insert ends by direct sequencing. Biotechniques 17(2):282, 284, 1994.
32. Orita M, Iwahana H, Kanazawa H, Sekiya T: Detection of polymorphisms of human DNA by gel electrophoresis as single strand conformation polymorphisms. Proc Natl Acad Sci U S A 86:2766–2770, 1989.
33. O'Donovan MC, Oefner PJ, Roberts SC, et al: Blind analysis of denaturing high-performance liquid chromatography as a tool for mutation detection. Genomics 52:44–49, 1998.
34. Oefner PJ, Underhill PA: Comparative DNA sequencing by denaturing high-performance liquid chromatography (DHPLC). Am J Hum Genet 57:A266, 1995.
35. Keating MT, Sangunetti MC: Molecular and cellular mechanisms of cardiac arrhythmias. Cell 104(4):569–580, 2001.
36. Tristan-Firouzi M, Jensen JL, Donaldson MR, et al: Functional and clinical characterization of KCNJ2 mutations associated with LQT7 (Andersen syndrome). J Clin Invest 110(3):381–388, 2002.
37. Chauhan VS, Tuvia S, Buhusi M, et al: Abnormal cardiac Na$^+$ channel properties and QT heart rate adaptation in neonatal ankyrin(B) knockout mice. Circ Res 86(4):367–368, 2000.
38. Chen Q, Kirsch GE, Zhang D, et al: Genetic basis and molecular mechanism for idiopathic ventricular fibrillation. Nature 392:293–296, 1998.
39. Priori SC, Napolitano C, Tiso N, et al: Mutations in the cardiac ryanodine receptor gene (hR$_y$R$_2$) underlie catecholaminergic polymorphic ventricular tachycardia. Circulation 103:196–200, 2001.
40. Postma AV, Dnjoy I, Hoorntje TM, et al: Absence of calsequestrin 2 causes severe forms of catecholaminergic polymorphic ventricular tachycardia. Circ Res 91:e21–e26, 2002.
41. Schott J-J, Alshinawi C, Kyndt F, et al: Cardiac conduction defects associated with mutations in SCN5A. Nat Genet 23:20–21, 1999.
42. Arad M, Seidman JG, Seidman CE: Phenotype diversity in hypertrophic cardiomyopathy. Hum Mol Genet 11(20):2499–2506, 2002.
43. Towbin JA, Bowles NE: The failing heart. Nature 415:227–233, 2002.
44. Schiaffino S, Reggiani C: Molecular diversity of myofibrillar proteins: Gene regulation and functional significance. Physiol Rev 76:371–423, 1996.
45. Marian AJ, Yu QT, Workman R, et al: Angiotensin-converting enzyme polymorphism in hypertrophic cardiomyopathy and sudden cardiac death. Lancet 342:1085–1086, 1993.
46. Dalloz f, Osinska H, Robbins J: Manipulating the contractile apparatus genetically defined animal models of cardiovascular disease. J Mol Cell Cardiol 33:9–15, 2001.
47. Mehdirad AA, Fatkin D, DiMarco JP, et al: Electrophysiologic characteristics of accessory atrioventricular connections in an inherited form of Wolff-Parkinson-White syndrome. J Cardiovasc Electrophysiol 20:629–635, 1999.
48. Vidaillet HJJ, Pressley JC, Henke E, et al: Familial occurrence of accessory atrioventricular pathways (preexcitation syndrome). N Engl J Med 317:65–69, 1987.
49. Blair E, Redwood C, Ashrafian H, et al: Mutations on the γ2 subunit of AMP-activated protein kinase cause familial hypertrophic cardiomyopathy: Evidence for the central note of energy compromise in disease pathogenesis. Hum Mol Genet 10:1215–1220, 2001.
50. Gollob MH, Green MJ, Tang AS-L, et al: Identification of a gene responsible for familial Wolff-Parkinson-White syndrome. N Engl J Med 344:1823–1831, 2001.
51. Arad M, Benson DW, Perez-Atayde AR, et al: Constitutively active AMP kinase mutations cause glycogen storage disease mimicking hypertrophic cardiomyopathy. J Clin Invest 109(3):357–362, 2002.
52. Manolio TA, Baughman KL, Rodenheffer R, et al: Prevalence and etiology of idiopathic dilated cardiomyopathy (Summary of a National Heart Lung and Blood Institute Workshop). Am J Cardiol 69:1458–1466, 1992.

53. Thiene G, Basso C, Calabrese F, et al: Pathology and pathogenesis of arrhythmogenic right ventricular cardiomyopathy. Herz 25:210–215, 2000.
54. Tiso N, Stephan DA, Nava A, et al: Identification of mutations in the cardiac ryanodine receptor gene in families affected with arrhythmogenic right ventricular cardiomyopathy type 2 (ARVD2). Hum Mol Genet 10:189–94, 2001.
55. Rampazzo A, Nava A, Malacrida S, et al: Mutation in human desmoplakin domain binding to plakoglobin causes a dominant form of arrhythmogenic right ventricular cardiomyopathy. Am J Hum Genet 71:1200–1206, 2002.

第 50 章

长 QT 综合征、Brugada 综合征和其他离子通道疾病的遗传学

Silvia G. Priori, Ilaria Rivolta, Carlo Napolitano

本章目录

- 电压依赖性心脏离子通道疾病 459
- 锚定蛋白疾病 464
- 细胞内钙调节蛋白疾病 465
- 基因检测和临床实践：展望和提示 465

20世纪90年代早期，Keating 等的研究引出了这样的一个概念：编码心脏离子通道基因的异常是心律失常致心源性猝死的病理基础[1-3]。虽然 Keating 等主要是指长 QT 综合征（LQTS），但很快就发现其他几种心脏结构正常、被称作"特发性室颤"的遗传学基础也是编码离子通道的基因变异。

感谢几个遍布全球的研究队伍在过去十年中的一致努力，使得在遗传性致心律失常综合征领域的主要观念得以革新。目前发现，至少有十个基因与心脏遗传性电不稳定的形成有关，证实了致心律失常性疾病的高度遗传异质性。现在已经认识到，对于每一个临床疾病（LQTS、儿茶酚胺敏感性室性心动过速等）均可能同时有多个基因变异。特别需要指出的是，基因型-表型关系的研究表明，遗传性心律失常疾病的遗传变异可以不同，因此每个疾病都应被看作是独立的疾病。例如：尽管所有 LQTS 均有 QT 间期延长的心电图特点，但不同表型具有不同基因型，这种表型上的差异要比它们的相似性更为重要。相应的，产生了基因特异的危险分层方法和治疗方法，这表明只要基因检测成为常规程序，遗传病的诊断和治疗就会实现个体化。这也需要建立结合表型、结合分子基础和基因功能的遗传性心律失常综合征新的分类和命名规则。这里，我们提出一个基于遗传缺陷而不是临床表现的新遗传性心律失常疾病的分类方法。在这个分类中，基于相似的亚细胞途径（跨膜动作电位控制、细胞内钙调节蛋白、靶蛋白或锚定蛋白）将疾病分为三大类：（1）电压依赖性离子通道疾病；（2）细胞内钙调节蛋白疾病；（3）锚定蛋白疾病。根据异常蛋白的功能特征，每一类中包括一个或多个疾病。于是我们将编码 HERG（human ether-a-go-go）和 MiRP（MinK 相关蛋白）的基因存在缺陷的患者称为"I_{Kr}病"患者。为区别每一个特定的基因突变，确立了疾病亚型：例如在 I_{Kr} 疾病中，LQT2 和 LQT6 分别表示 KCNH2 和 KCNE2 的突变，见表 50-1。这种分类反映了心律失常疾病的复杂性，也提供了一个含义广泛的诊断方案，它纳入了更大范围的信息，从基因缺陷到受累蛋白质的功能，乃至临床表型。

除了分类方法，我们还将详细论述不同疾病的分子基础、功能序列、不同亚型间表型特征的鉴别。与临床治疗相关的临床问题将在本书的其他章节讨论（第 67、68、70、71 章）。

一、电压依赖性心脏离子通道疾病

（一）常染色体显性遗传 I_{Ks} 疾病/常染色体隐性遗传 I_{Ks} 疾病

心脏延迟整流钾电流（I_K）是心脏动作电位3相复极的主要决定部分。离体猪心肌实验表明它包含两个独立成分：快速的部分称 I_{Kr}，缓慢的对儿茶酚胺敏

表 50-1　遗传性心律失常肌病的分类

疾病群	分型	亚型	基因位点	基因	蛋白质	蛋白质功能	参考文献
电压门控离子通道疾病	I_{Ks}疾病	LQT1	11p11.5	KCNQ1	KVLQT1	I_{Ks}通道（α亚单位）	1
		LQT5	21q22.1-p22.2	KCNE1	MinK	I_{Ks}通道（β亚单位）	7
		LQT-JLN1	11p15.5	KCNQ1	KVLQT1	I_{Ks}通道（α亚单位）	4
		LQT-JLN2	21q22.1-q22.2	KCNE1	MinK	I_{Ks}通道（β亚单位）	5
	I_{Kr}疾病	LQT2	7q35-q36	KCNH2	HERG	I_{Kr}通道（α亚单位）	2
		LQT6	21q22.1-p22.2	KCNH2	MiRP1	I_{Kr}通道（β亚单位）	16
	I_{Na}疾病	LQT3	3p21-p23	SCN5A	Nav1.5	I_{Na}通道	3
		Br-S1	3p21-p23	SCN5A	Nav1.5	I_{Na}通道	35
		Lenegre	3p21-p23	SCN5A	Nav1.5	I_{Na}通道	45
		混合型	3p21-p23	SCN5A	Nav1.5	I_{Na}通道	49
	I_{k1}疾病	And-S1	17q23	KCNJ2	Kir2.1	I_{k1}通道	53
锚定蛋白疾病	锚蛋白疾病	LQT4	4q25-q27	ANK2	锚蛋白B	锚蛋白	59
细胞内钙处理蛋白疾病	兰尼定受体疾病	CPVT1	1q42-43	RyR2	RyR2	兰尼定受体	61
	肌集钙蛋白疾病	CPVT2	1p11-13.3	CASQ2	CASQ2	肌集钙蛋白	67

感的部分称作 I_{Ks}。KCNQ1 编码心脏延迟整流电流缓慢部分 I_{Ks} 通道的 α 亚单位，KCNQ2 编码其 β 亚单位。KCNQ1 和 KCNQ2 突变的异质性与 LQTS 的亚型相关（LQT1 和 LQT5）。KCNQ1 基因突变是 Romano-Ward LQTS 最普遍的基因缺陷，约一半患者是该基因的突变。KCNQ1 突变有 100 多种（多为单个氨基酸置换）。相反，KCNE1 突变少见，LQT5 是一种不常见的 LQTS 类型，所占比例不到 5%。同时包括了 KCNQ1 和 KCNE1 的纯合或复合杂合突变导致的 Jervell-Lange-Nielse 常染色体隐性遗传型（分别为 JLN1 和 JLN2），其特征包括心脏表型（长 QT 间期和室性心律失常）和神经感觉性耳聋[4-5]。因为缺乏 50% 的心脏野生型蛋白的等位基因，JLN 患者临床心脏表型与他们的 Romano-Ward 型父母相比，通常更为严重。JLN 综合征的致死率比 LQT1 和 LQT5 要高。

1. 遗传缺陷及其功能影响

I_{Ks} 病患者基因缺陷包括错义突变、框内缺失、阅读框移位、无义突变和拼接错误，见表 50-2，而以错义突变最为重要，更多信息可访问 http://pc4.fsm.it:81/cardmoc。

关于 KCNQ1 和 KCNE1 突变蛋白质的研究表明其机制有多种，包括电流密度的减小以及在动力学和门控上的异常，见表 50-2[6-9]。一个突变引起多种电生理异常并不多见。缺陷蛋白可能成为"毒性多肽"，从而以负显性效应改变通道的功能。这些突变累及野生型蛋白，故可导致 50% 以上的电流减少。其他突变不影响野生型蛋白的功能，故它们的作用与单倍体不足（haploinsufficiency）有关（即：功能损失 ≥ 50%）。KCNQ1 和 KCNE1 突变引起 I_{Ks} 病的机制包括有：细胞内蛋白运输障碍[10]，同时缺乏 minK-KvLQT1 共组装[9,11]，minK/KvLQT1 和 Yotiao 蛋白相互作用的改变[12]。总之，KCNQ1 和 KCNE1 相关的基因缺陷，减少复极 I_{Ks} 电流，因此延长了动作电位时限和 QT 间期。

2. I_{Ks} 疾病的表型特征

作为 LQTS 的一种，多数基因型缺陷携带者的特点都是 QT 间期延长，发生多形性室性心律失常和猝死的风险增加。

一些表型特征与 LQTS 亚型 I_{Ks} 病有关。有鉴别意义的心电图特点是宽大低平的 T 波[13]，心脏事件多由与情感和运动有关的肾上腺素能诱发[14]。在对性别和 QTc 进行校正后，对 I_{Ks} 病患者的自然病程分析提示，在 40 岁之前，无论男女，QTc 在 500 ms 以上的患

表 50-2　与遗传性心律失常有关的基因，蛋白及其机制

疾病群	分型	基因	蛋白质	突变的编码作用	细胞表型/功能障碍	参考文献
电压门控离子通道	I_{ks}疾病	KCNQ1	KvLQT1	错义突变	电流密度的减少	6
				拼接错误	激活减慢	9
				缺失	在稳态时的正向转变	8，9
				阅读框移位	激活	
				无义突变	失活率增加	8
					电压依赖失活的正向转变	9
					与β亚单位共组装的相互作用	9，11
					毁坏与Yotiao结合的LZ基序	12
		KCNE1	MinK	错义突变	电流密度的减少	7，8
				无义突变	运输缺陷	10
				缺失	电压依赖激活的转变	7
				阅读框移位	激活	
					快速失活	7
	I_{kr}疾病	CNH2	HERG	错义突变	电流的减少或抑制	18～20
				无义突变	抑制	
				拼接错误	快速激活	22，23
				缺失	快速失活	22，23
				阅读框移位	从失活状态快速恢复	23
					电压依赖失活的正向转变	22
					电压依赖失活的负向转变	20，21
					运输缺陷	23～26
		KCNE2	MiRP1	错义突变	快速失活	16
					电压依赖失活的正向转变	16
					电压依赖失活的负向转变	16
	I_{Na}疾病	SCN5A	Nav1.5	错义突变	迟发的持续性电流	30，52
				无义突变	失活率减慢	31，47
				拼接错误	从失活状态快速恢复	33，46
				缺失	快速失活	31，41，46，51
				阅读框移位	电压依赖激活的负向转变	32
				插入	与β1亚单位关系的变化	34，42
					电流的减少或抑制	38，47，49，50
					从失活状态缓慢恢复	39，47
					电压依赖失活的正向转变	33，41，46，52
					电压依赖失活的负向转变	31，46，49，52
					电压依赖失活的正向转变	33，40，47
					关闭状态失活的减少	47
					显著的关闭状态失活	51
					缓慢失活的增强	40，51
					运输缺陷	39
	I_{k1}疾病	KCNJ2	Kir2.1	错义突变	电流的减少或抑制	54，55
锚定蛋白		ANK2	锚蛋白B	错义突变	未知	无资料可利用
Ca^{2+}处理蛋白	肌浆网Ca^{2+}通道疾病HRyR2		兰尼定受体	错义突变	通道基础活性的增加 增加咖啡因作用下钙瞬变	64
	细胞内Ca^{2+}储积疾病CASQ2		肌集钙蛋白	错义突变 无义突变 无义突变		无资料可利用

注：表内的细胞表型都是文献所报道的。值得注意的是，多数情况下，一种突变会导致一种以上的异常。因此，可以讲对某种电生理现象其突变是独特的。另外，在SCN5A突变病例中，具有不同临床表型的患者其功能异常存在交叉。

者都有发生心脏事件的高风险，40岁之前发生第一次心脏事件的累积可能性为70%。然而有趣的是，QTc在500 ms以上的男性I_{Ks}病患者发生心脏事件要早于女性患者。在I_{Ks}病患者，QTc是否大于500 ms，其在40岁之前出现症状的风险相差20%[15]。

（二）I_{Kr}疾病

位于染色体7q35-q36的KCNH2基因最早在1994年被克隆，并称之为HERG，这个名字仍被保留用作该基因编码的蛋白质名称，该蛋白参与形成I_{Kr}电流通道的α亚单位。Curran等证明了它是LQTS（LQT2）的一个致病基因。该通道的β亚单位称作MiRP，是由一个称为KCNE2的无内含子基因编码，该基因位于染色体21q22.1-22.2，与KCNE1基因相邻[16]。

1. 遗传缺陷和功能影响

关于KCNH2突变在过去5年中的报道相对较多，可登陆http://pc4.fsm.it:81/cardmoc获取更多信息，包括错义突变、无义突变、缺失、阅读框移位和拼接错误，见表50-2。KCNH2突变的患病率数据表明，在LQTS患者中，该突变占所有导致LQTS突变的30%~35%，为第二常见的突变。在曾经报道的一个家族中有两个纯合子携带者[17]，他们的心脏临床表型均很严重，但是和KCNQ1突变纯合子携带者不同的是，他们无心脏以外的异常表现，这个现象的重要性在于，它意外地证实了这样一个事实：纵然是有严重的心律失常，没有I_{Kr}电流的患者也可以活下来。

KCNH2突变可引起轻型LQTS（见表50-2），患者有获得性LQTS的易感性，可登陆http://pc4.fsm.it:81/cardmoc获取更多信息。在我们的研究中，250名LQTS先证者中有1例为KCNH2突变携带者，在所预测的拓扑结构中，蛋白质跨膜片段的重要部分因9个碱基对的缺失而导致了该蛋白质的序列缺失（S. G. Priori和C. Napolitano，未发表的资料）。

KCNH2和KCNE2突变蛋白质的研究已证明了蛋白质功能不全的多种机制[16,18-26]，包括电流密度的减小；门控异常通道蛋白的生成，如电压依赖性的活化和失活的转化；活化和失活的加快；从失活状态恢复的加快；还有一些突变体不发展为成熟型而滞留在内质网（见表50-2）。缺陷蛋白可对野生型蛋白产生负显性效应，从而导致更严重的功能异常。

KCNH2突变具有一个有趣的特性，当暴露于某些化学试剂如丙三醇、E-4013时，可以挽救突变体的功能[27-29]。不同物质其恢复的能力具有突变特异性。

2. I_{Kr}疾病的表型特征

I_{Kr}疾病和其他LQTS一样，具有QT间期延长和快速性室性心律失常的易患性。但是KCNH2具有其自己的临床特点。I_{Kr}疾病具有鉴别意义的体表心电图是平坦的或有切迹的T波[13]。与I_{Ks}疾病不同，肾上腺素触发的心脏事件不常见（50%），心脏事件可发生于运动或休息时[14]。有趣的是，听觉刺激（如噪音、电话铃或闹铃声）常会触发心律失常。对I_{Kr}疾病的自然病程分析表明QTc>500 ms的患者在40岁之前出现症状的风险更大，在40岁之前出现第一次心脏事件的几率为75%；QTc≤500 ms的患者在40岁之前发生心脏事件的可能性与性别有关，女性有40%的可能性，具有同样QTc的男性可能性仅为15%[15]。

（三）I_{Na}疾病

心脏钠通道在1992年被克隆并定位于染色体3p21。多数电压依赖性心脏离子通道既可以形成同源多聚体又可形成异源多聚体，SCN5A蛋白的结构不同于它们。钠通道蛋白是大分子蛋白，它可自身折叠环绕通道的孔径。因此一个基因就可以生成一个有功能的通道。已经明确SCN5A基因有几种不同类型的突变，包括错义、无义、拼接错误、缺失、阅读框移位和插入等突变。

在建立了LQTS家族和染色体带3p21-p23的联系后，不久就明确了SCN5A基因的突变。最近，又有两个基因型与I_{Na}疾病联系起来，Brugada综合征的BrS1变异体，可解释大约15%~20%的Brugada综合征和进展性传导障碍，或Lenègre病。而且，临床表型交叉的家系也有报道。本章讨论I_{Na}疾病的四种独立亚型。

（四）I_{Na}疾病：LQT3亚型

1. 遗传缺陷及其功能影响

Wang等在LQTS患者中发现了第一个SCN5A突变，它位于与钠通道失活功能有关的区域（delKPQ，R1623Q，N1325S）[3]。最近明确了引起这种疾病的突变对心肌电生理活动有不同的影响：如迟发的持续电流、失活减慢、失活后恢复加快、门控方式改变（见表 50-2）[30-33]。另外，与 $β_1$ 亚单位的异常相互作用也有报道[34]。总之，功能研究支持以下观点：通道的突变通过引起蛋白"获得功能"使内向电流增强而延长动作电位时程，从而引起 LQTS 的表型。

相对较少的 SCN5A 突变，可登陆 http://pc4.fsm.it：81/cardmoc 获取更多信息。已有报道，与其相关的 LQT3 发病率约占 LQTS 患者的 10%～15%（S. G. Priori 和 C. Napolitano，未发表的资料）。

2. I_{Na} 表型特征：LQT3 病

在 I_{Na} 疾病患者中，有鉴别意义的 LQT3 其体表心电图特征表现为：ST 段延长和窄而高尖 T 波[13]。与其他类型的 LQTS 不同的是，在休息时更易发生心律失常[14]。从这一点看，与 Brugada 综合征患者类似。LQT3 患者的自然病程已明确[15]。与 I_{Ks} 和 I_{Kr} 疾病患者不同，QT 间期的时限不是 LQT3 患者临床表现严重程度的主要标志。QTc＞500 ms 的男性患者在 40 岁之前发生心脏事件的可能性累计可达 80%，而女性不论 QTc 时限，与 QTc≤500 ms 的男性一样发生心脏事件的可能性相对较低（55%）。

（五）I_{Na} 疾病：Ⅰ型 Brugada 综合征

Brugada 综合征有鉴别意义的特征是：心电图右侧胸前导联 ST 段抬高，与发生室颤的风险增加相关。

1998 年发现 Brugada 综合征的第一个基因变异体（BrS1），是一个新型的 I_{Na} 疾病亚型[35]。我们实验室的数据表明不到 20% 的 Brugada 综合征患者属于Ⅰ型 Brugada 综合征变异体，且这个疾病有遗传异质性。但是，目前还没有报道有其他与 Brugada 综合征相关的基因，尽管已有报道此病是与 3 号染色体连锁的[36]。

1. 遗传缺陷及其功能影响

运用单链构象多态性和 DNA 测序技术得以明确了最先发现的三个 SCN5A 突变是：两个截断突变（truncation）（一个阅读框移位和一个拼接错误突变）导致氨基酸序列的提前终止和一个 SCN5A 跨膜拓扑结构的第四个结构域的错义突变[35]。还有一些突变在文献中陆续报道，可登陆 http://pc4.fsm.it：81/cardmoc 获取更多信息。目前有证据表明，导致Ⅰ型 Brugada 综合征的突变可能涉及整个蛋白质，特别是其羧基末端是突变的多发区[37]。

在Ⅰ型 Brugada 综合征中，SCN5A 突变的体外功能特性显示了常见临床表型的几种机制，包括钠电流抑制、钠通道失活的恢复减慢、电压依赖的失活向更正的电位或更负的电位转化、中间型的失活增强[31,38-42]。SCN5A 突变可以改变与钠通道 β 亚单位的相互作用而导致通道功能不全。最近，发现了Ⅰ型 Brugada 综合征的一种新的发病机制——运输缺陷。

多数基因突变可导致上述的多种异常，有趣的是所有与Ⅰ型 Brugada 综合征有关的突变均导致钠电流的减弱，这会影响动作电位的形态。其对心室壁的影响也存在不均一性，对心外膜细胞的影响大于对心内膜细胞的影响，对右室细胞的影响又大于对左室细胞的影响。这种影响的差异可能与 I_{to} 传导（I_{to}-conduction）通道在心室不同部位的表达差异有关。心外膜细胞，特别是位于右室的心外膜细胞，具有很强 I_{to} 复极电流。因此，动作电位的生理时程很大程度上依靠钠内向电流。如果 I_{Na} 减弱，正如在Ⅰ型 Brugada 综合征中，I_{Na} 电流不足以抵消 I_{to} 复极电流，因此动作电位时程缩短，细胞丧失正常动作电位形态，从而易于发生 2 相折返[43]。

2. I_{Na} 表型特征：Ⅰ型 Brugada 综合征

Ⅰ型 Brugada 综合征患者的自然病程与其他类型 Brugada 综合征患者有所不同，其心电图所表现的 ST 段抬高并无差异。但是Ⅰ型 Brugada 综合征患者的房室功能异常比其他类型 Brugada 综合征患者更为常见[44]。

（六）I_{Na} 疾病：Lenègre 病

1. 遗传缺陷及其功能影响

1999 年，Schott 等在两个传导障碍家族的 SCN5A 基因上均发现了一个突变，从而第一次证明进行性传导障碍是钠通道疾病的一个新亚型[45]。

与进行性心脏传导障碍（Lenègre 病）有关的 SCN5 基因突变包括三个错义突变和一个拼接突变。

Lenègre 病的基因突变引起电生理学改变，包括电流减弱；失活时间的改变、电压依赖门控参数的改变、从失活状态恢复的改变；缓慢失活的增强[46,47]。有趣的是，具有 Brugada 综合征基因型患者的突变也明确了以前所提及的一些功能异常。在具有 Lenègre 基因型的患者中证实的一个基因突变（G514C），表现为从失活状态的恢复加快和关闭状态的失活减少，即在原来有 LQT3 表型的患者中发现的特征，这又增加了 I_{Na} 疾病基因型与表型相关性的复杂性。Clancy 和 Kass 最近的研究表明，I_{Na} 疾病 Lenègre 病的突变以激活曲线右移为特点[48]。他们推测这种缺陷可导致动作电位升支最大速率的减小，因而导致传导的进行性延迟。

2. I_{Na} 的表型特征：Lenègre 病

I_{Na} 疾病 Lenègre 亚型的临床特点还未定论。其心电图特点是心室内传导延迟，主要为右束支阻滞，伴有房室传导延迟甚至传导阻滞。这种患者的长期预后和最佳治疗还不清楚。

(七) I_{Na} 疾病的交叉临床表型

1. 遗传缺陷及其功能影响

具有交叉临床表型的家族，其基因突变包括一个框内插入、一个框内缺失和一个错义突变。研究显示，这些基因突变可导致所编码的通道功能异常，包括电流减小或抑制、失活加快、激活及效应曲线向相反方向移位，出现缓慢失活和显著的关闭状态失活[49-52]。在 1500 位的一个阅读框缺失可导致由通道爆发模式的增强（bursting mode）所致的持续电流的发生。门控参数也受影响，故这种缺失导致效应曲线的负极移位和电压依赖的激活曲线右移，见表 50-2。

2. 具交叉临床表型的 I_{Na} 疾病的基因型特点

LQTS3 和 Brugada 综合征的交叉表型已有报道[49,50,52]。Bezzina 等报道了一个 SCN5A 基因（InsD1795）框内缺失的家族[49]，同时具有 QT 间期延长和 ST 段抬高[52]。这个家族中的几个突变基因携带者表现出窦房阻滞而造成超过数秒的间歇。在 1500 位的突变导致窦房阻滞的机制目前还不明确。

Kyndt 等报道了具有 SCN5A 突变和交叉表型的 Brugada 综合征和传导障碍[50]。有趣的是，不是所有的基因缺陷的携带者都同时表现出两种表型，到目前为止，还没有可以解释影响该家族成员中表现差异的原因。

(八) I_{K1} 疾病：Andersen 综合征

1971 年 Andersen 等报道了一个 8 岁患者，表现为身材矮小、五官距离宽、鼻根宽、软腭和硬腭缺损。1994 年"Andersen 综合征"首次被用于描述具有以下三个特征的临床疾病：钾敏感的周期性麻痹、室性心律失常、营养不良外貌。

1. 遗传缺陷及其功能影响

Plaster 等[53]最近运用基因组（genome-wide）连锁分析方法阐明了 Andersen 综合征的遗传背景，他们成功地在一个大家族中将该病与 17q23.-24.2 等位基因联系起来。在重点区域上进行候选基因的筛选，KCNJ2 基因中的一个错义突变被确定。Tristani-Firouzi 等[54]随后明确了另外的一些突变，为 KCNJ2 基因是某些 Andersen 综合征病例的病因提供了证据，可登陆 http：//pc4.fsm.it：81/cardmoc 获取更多信息。KCNJ2 基因编码一种内向整流钾通道，即 Kir2.1，作为在 4 相复极和静息膜电位的决定因素在心脏中高表达。Plaster 等报道 16 例先证者中有 3 例在该基因无缺陷[53]，提示可能存在遗传异质性，但大多数 Andersen 综合征患者还是存在 KCNJ2 基因突变。该病的平均外显率为 86%，28 个携带者中有 4 例无临床表现。

最近有报道其他突变，包括错义突变和框内缺失。一些突变的功能特性最近也已明确，突变通过引起 I_{K1} 减弱或抑制而影响通道功能（见表 50-2）。与 I_{Ks} 和 I_{Kr} 疾病的突变相似，这些突变可导致单倍体不足，并表现出负显性效应[54,55]。

有趣的是，因为异常的面部表现是 Andersen 综合征的特征性特点，Plaster 等的资料也表明 Kir2.1 可能也参与生长发育信号。

2. I_{K1} 疾病的表型特征

QT 间期不同程度的延长是该病首要的表型特征[56]，除 QT 间期延长外，Andersen 综合征患者还表现复极异常，由一个类似巨型 U 波的晚复极成分组成。

尽管有猝死的报道，但心律失常不是 Andersen 综合征的主要死因，该病的表现常为良性。到目前为止已报道的 Andersen 综合征病例还很少，故也不可能列出 Kir2.1 基因突变患者的表型特征。

二、锚定蛋白疾病

(一) 锚蛋白 B 病

1. 遗传缺陷及其功能缺陷

在明确了一个家族和染色体 4（4q25-27）的联系

后，锚蛋白（ankyrin）基因的一个突变被报道[57]。但近来未再有比较有意义的资料报道来证实这种突变的病理意义。近来在锚蛋白基因敲除的小鼠上得到的数据表明这个蛋白与钠通道的功能有关[58]。如果这个结果被证实，并证实锚蛋白B突变蛋白可导致心脏钠通道的功能障碍，那么锚蛋白病将被归为I_{Na}疾病的第四个亚型。

2. 锚蛋白B病的表型特征

1995年报道了一个QT间期延长的锚蛋白B病法国家族与染色体4（4q25-q27）相关联。这个家族的多数患者表现为QT间期延长、多相T波、明显的窦性心动过缓和阵发性房颤，后者可在该家族50%以上的成员出现[59]。

近来，同一研究者在原家族确定了在锚蛋白基因（ANK2）上的一个突变（E1425G）。但在最近7年未再有资料验证锚蛋白疾病与4号染色体的联系，因此在基因型/表型的关系方面也没有可提供的数据[57]。

三、细胞内钙调节蛋白疾病

（一）兰尼定受体疾病

1. 遗传缺陷及其功能影响

1999年Swan等报道了两个临床表型为儿茶酚胺敏感性多形性室速（catecholaminergic polymorphic ventricular tachycardia，CPVT）的家族和1号染色体长臂（1q42-43）的联系[60]。我们随后又证明了人类兰尼定受体（RyR2）基因是一个CPVT基因[61]。RyR2突变发生于40%的CPVT患者，据此我们推断CPVT是另一种具有遗传异质性的疾病[62]。

RyR2是调节细胞内钙流动和兴奋-收缩耦联的主要成分。该蛋白分布遍及肌浆网膜；在动作电位2相，钙通过L型通道流入，RyR2随即反应性地从肌浆网释放出钙离子。

在CPVT患者中，所有的RyR2突变均已证实为错义突变，可登陆http://pc4.fsm.it:81/cardmoc获取更多信息，它们主要集中在决定蛋白质功能的重要区域：跨膜功能域（位于蛋白质的羧基末端）、钙结合位点、FKBP12.6结合功能域[62,63]。近来只有一个位于4497位的突变明确了功能特性，我们最初在一个有7名患者（包括两个少年发生心脏性猝死）的家族中研究了这个突变。Jiang等研究表明，这种突变使RyR2通道的跨膜功能域在暴露于咖啡因时表现出高反应性[64]。于是作者推测，当突变的通道被磷酸化时，会释放过多的钙，导致钙超载。很明显，这些数据支持如下假说：CPVT患者的心律失常由触发激动导致的钙超载引起。

2. 兰尼定受体疾病的表型特征

已经证明RyR2疾病患者的自然病程与非基因型的CPVT患者不同[62]。然而有趣的是，RyR2病患者的临床表型因性别不同而有所不同。男性患者的疾病表现更严重一些，发病早于女性患者[62]。这与I_{Ks}疾病情况类似，即男性发病比女性早得多，多在青春期前发病。因为两种疾病均有对儿茶酚胺敏感性增高的特点，故有理由推断年轻男孩比女孩对肾上腺素能激活更为敏感。关于兰尼定受体在68章中详述。

（二）肌集钙蛋白（calsequestrin）疾病

1. 遗传缺陷及其功能影响

肌集钙蛋白疾病以常染色体隐性遗传方式遗传，由位于1号染色体（1p11-13.3）的肌集钙蛋白基因（CASQ2）突变引起[65]。肌集钙蛋白在心脏可高度表达（见表50-1）。在心脏，它是主要的钙储池，也是兰尼定受体功能相关的大分子蛋白复合物的一部分，参与兴奋收缩耦联的调节。近来共报道了CASQ2的4个突变，包括两个错义突变、一个拼接错误和一个无义突变[66,67]。还没有比较充分的资料证实这种突变会导致患者的蛋白质功能异常。这可从逻辑角度来推测，基因突变减少钙的蛋白结合特性，从而导致细胞内游离钙增多。

2. 肌集钙蛋白疾病的表型特征

该病患者临床表现与RyR2相似。由于在世界上确诊的患者很少，无论是建立该病的基因型-表型关系，还是确定CASQ2是否为与常染色体隐性遗传的儿茶酚胺性室速相关的唯一基因，都是不可能的。

四、基因检测和临床实践：展望和提示

致心律失常疾病的基因检测还没被列为常规，然而可以提供患者DNA分子鉴定的实验室正在增加。多数情况下，心脏病专家要求基因筛选是因为他们认为这些

信息有助于先证者及其家庭成员的治疗。因此对基因筛选的意义和价值进行研究是很重要的。正如先前所讨论的，对所有疾病作特定遗传缺陷的危险分层目前还不可行。遗传研究对临床的意义还局限于LQTS，包括I_{Ks}病、I_{Kr}病和I_{Na} LQT3病，以及RyR2病。因此，遗传分析目前对患者治疗方面的最大意义在于，可明确先证者的家族成员是否属于患病个体，克服了与遗传性致心律失常性疾病不完全外显有关的局限性。将来可望对这些家族成员在症状发生前进行诊断，提供预防性治疗，这对该类遗传性疾病的处理是非常重要的。相反，对于那些尚不能提供减少猝死风险治疗的疾病，症状前诊断的价值还有争议。

目前，可进行遗传诊断的实验室数目有限、完成检测需要很长时间、检测费用高，都是使患者不能接受遗传检测的原因。随着更多危险分层信息的获得和更多基于遗传缺陷治疗的开展，对遗传学诊断的需求会逐渐增加，在大的医学中心设置基因检测服务也会更合理、更有需求。

（张幼怡　龚开政　张敏丽　译）

参 考 文 献

1. Wang Q, Curran ME, Splawski I, et al: Positional cloning of a novel potassium channel gene: KVLQT1 mutations cause cardiac arrhythmias. Nat Genet 12:17–23, 1996.
2. Curran ME, Splawski I, Timothy KW, et al: A molecular basis for cardiac arrhythmia: HERG mutations cause long QT syndrome. Cell 80:795–803, 1995.
3. Wang Q, Shen J, Splawski I, et al: SCN5A mutations associated with an inherited cardiac arrhythmia, long QT syndrome. Cell 80:805–811, 1995.
4. Neyroud N, Tesson F, Denjoy I, et al: A novel mutation in the potassium channel gene KVLQT1 causes the Jervell and Lange-Nielsen cardioauditory syndrome. Nat Genet 15:186–189, 1997.
5. Schulze-Bahr E, Wang Q, Wedekind H, et al: KCNE1 mutations cause Jervell and Lange-Nielsen syndrome. Nat Genet 17:267–268, 1997.
6. Kubota T, Horie M, Takano M, et al: Evidence for a single nucleotide polymorphism in the KCNQ1 potassium channel that underlies susceptibility to life-threatening arrhythmias. J Cardiovasc Electrophysiol 12:1223–1229, 2001.
7. Splawski I, Tristani-Firouzi M, Lehmann MH, et al: Mutations in the hminK gene cause long QT syndrome and suppress IKs function. Nat Genet 17:338–340, 1997.
8. Huang L, Bitner-Glindzicz M, Tranebjaerg L, et al: A spectrum of functional effects for disease causing mutations in the Jervell and Lange-Nielsen syndrome. Cardiovasc Res 51:670–680, 2001.
9. Franqueza L, Lin M, Shen J, et al: Long QT syndrome-associated mutations in the S4-S5 linker of KvLQT1 potassium channels modify gating and interaction with minK subunits. J Biol Chem 274:21063–21070, 1999.
10. Bianchi L, Shen Z, Dennis AT, et al: Cellular dysfunction of LQT5-minK mutants: Abnormalities of IKs, IKr and trafficking in long QT syndrome. Hum Mol Genet 8:1499–1507, 1999.
11. Chouabe C, Neyroud N, Richard P, et al: Novel mutations in KvLQT1 that affect Iks activation through interactions with Isk. Cardiovasc Res 45:971–980, 2000.
12. Marx SO, Kurokawa J, Reiken S, et al: Requirement of a macromolecular signaling complex for beta adrenergic receptor modulation of the KCNQ1-KCNE1 potassium channel. Science 295:496–499, 2002.
13. Moss AJ, Zareba W, Benhorin J, et al: ECG T-wave patterns in genetically distinct forms of the hereditary long QT syndrome. Circulation 92:2929–2934, 1995.
14. Schwartz PJ, Priori SG, Spazzolini C, et al: Genotype-phenotype correlation in the long-QT syndrome: Gene-specific triggers for life-threatening arrhythmias. Circulation 103:89–95, 2001.
15. Priori SG, Schwartz PJ, Napolitano C, et al: Risk stratification of the long-QT syndrome. N Engl J Med 348:1866–1874, 2003.
16. Abbott GW, Sesti F, Splawski I, et al: MiRP1 forms IKr potassium channels with HERG and is associated with cardiac arrhythmia. Cell 97:175–187, 1999.
17. Hoorntje T, Alders M, van Tintelen P, et al: Homozygous premature truncation of the HERG protein: The human HERG knockout. Circulation 100:1264–1267, 1999.
18. Li X, Xu J, Li M: The human delta1261 mutation of the HERG potassium channel results in a truncated protein that contains a subunit interaction domain and decreases the channel expression. J Biol Chem 272:705–708, 1997.
19. Sanguinetti MC, Curran ME, Spector PS, et al: Spectrum of HERG K+-channel dysfunction in an inherited cardiac arrhythmia. Proc Natl Acad Sci U S A 93:2208–2212, 1996.
20. Nakajima T, Furukawa T, Tanaka T, et al: Novel mechanism of HERG current suppression in LQT2: Shift in voltage dependence of HERG inactivation. Circ Res 83:415–422, 1998.
21. Roden DM, Balser JR: A plethora of mechanisms in the HERG-related long QT syndrome. Genetics meets electrophysiology. Cardiovasc Res 44:242–246, 1999.
22. Nakajima T, Furukawa T, Hirano Y, et al: Voltage-shift of the current activation in HERG S4 mutation (R534C) in LQT2. Cardiovasc Res 44:283–293, 1999.
23. Paulussen A, Raes A, Matthijs G, et al: A novel mutation (T65P) in the PAS domain of the human potassium channel HERG results in the long QT syndrome by trafficking deficiency. J Biol Chem 277:48610–48616, 2002.
24. Petrecca K, Atanasiu R, Akhavan A, et al: N-linked glycosylation sites determine HERG channel surface membrane expression. J Physiol 515:41–48, 1999.
25. Furutani M, Trudeau MC, Hagiwara N, et al: Novel mechanism associated with an inherited cardiac arrhythmia: Defective protein trafficking by the mutant HERG (G601S) potassium channel. Circulation 99:2290–2294, 1999.
26. Zhou Z, Gong Q, Epstein ML, et al: HERG channel dysfunction in human long QT syndrome. Intracellular transport and functional defects. J Biol Chem 273:21061–21066, 1998.
27. Zhou Z, Gong Q, January CT: Correction of defective protein trafficking of a mutant HERG potassium channel in human long QT syndrome. Pharmacological and temperature effects. J Biol Chem 274:31123–31126, 1999.
28. Rajamani S, Anderson CL, Anson BD, et al: Pharmacological rescue of human K(+) channel long-QT2 mutations: Human ether-a-go-go-related gene rescue without block. Circulation 105:2830–2835, 2002.
29. Isbrandt D, Friederich P, Solth A, et al: Identification and functional characterization of a novel KCNE2 (MiRP1) mutation that alters HERG channel kinetics. J Mol Med 80:524–532, 2002.
30. Bennett PB, Yazawa K, Makita N, et al: Molecular mechanism for an inherited cardiac arrhythmia. Nature 376:683–685, 1995.
31. Rivolta I, Abriel H, Tateyama M, et al: Inherited brugada and LQT-3 syndrome mutations of a single residue of the cardiac sodium channel confer distinct channel and clinical phenotypes. J Biol Chem 276:30623–30630, 2001.
32. Wang DW, Yazawa K, George AL Jr, et al: Characterization of human cardiac Na+ channel mutations in the congenital long QT syndrome. Proc Natl Acad Sci U S A 93:13200–13205, 1996.
33. Abriel H, Cabo C, Wehrens XH, et al: Novel arrhythmogenic mechanism revealed by a long-QT syndrome mutation in the cardiac Na(+) channel. Circ Res 88:740–745, 2001.
34. An RH, Wang XL, Kerem B, et al: Novel LQT-3 mutation affects Na+ channel activity through interactions between alpha- and beta1-subunits. Circ Res 83:141–146, 1998.
35. Chen Q, Kirsch GE, Zhang D, et al: Genetic basis and molecular mechanism for idiopathic ventricular fibrillation. Nature 392:293–296, 1998.
36. Weiss R, Barmada MM, Nguyen T, et al: Clinical and molecular heterogeneity in the Brugada syndrome: A novel gene locus on

chromosome 3. Circulation 105:707–713, 2002.
37. Priori SG, Napolitano C, Gasparini M, et al: Natural history of Brugada syndrome. Insights for risk stratification and management. Circulation 105:1342–1347, 2002.
38. Deschenes I, Baroudi G, Berthet M, et al: Electrophysiological characterization of SCN5A mutations causing long QT (E1784K) and Brugada (R1512W and R1432G) syndrome. Cardiovasc Res 46:55–65, 2000.
39. Baroudi G, Acharfi S, Larouche C, et al: Expression and intracellular localization of an SCN5A double mutant R1232W/T1620M implicated in Brugada syndrome. Circ Res 90:E11–E16, 2002.
40. Wang DW, Makita N, Kitabatake A, et al: Enhanced Na(+) channel intermediate inactivation in Brugada syndrome. Circ Res 87:E37 E43, 2000.
41. Wan X, Chen S, Sadeghpour A, et al: Accelerated inactivation in a mutant Na(+) channel associated with idiopathic ventricular fibrillation. Am J Physiol Heart Circ Physiol 280:H354–H360, 2001.
42. Makita N, Shirai N, Wang DW, et al: Cardiac Na(+) channel dysfunction in Brugada syndrome is aggravated by beta(1)-subunit. Circulation 101:54–60, 2000.
43. Antzelevitch C, Yan GX, Shimizu W: Transmural dispersion of repolarization and arrhythmogenicity: The Brugada syndrome versus the long QT syndrome. J Electrocardiol 32:158–165, 1999.
44. Smits JP, Eckardt L, Probst V, et al: Genotype-phenotype relationship in Brugada syndrome: Electrocardiographic features differentiate SCN5A-related patients from non-SCN5A-related patients. J Am Coll Cardiol 40:350–356, 2002.
45. Schott JJ, Alshinawi C, Kyndt F, et al: Cardiac conduction defects associate with mutations in SCN5A. Nat Genet 23:20–21, 1999.
46. Tan HL, Bink-Boelkens MT, Bezzina CR, et al: A sodium-channel mutation causes isolated cardiac conduction disease. Nature 409:1043–1047, 2001.
47. Wang DW, Viswanathan PC, Balser JR, et al: Clinical, genetic, and biophysical characterization of SCN5A mutations associated with atrioventricular conduction block. Circulation 105:341–346, 2002.
48. Clancy CE, Kass RS: Defective cardiac ion channels: From mutations to clinical syndromes. J Clin Invest 110:1075–1077, 2002.
49. Bezzina C, Veldkamp MW, van Den Berg MP, et al: A single Na(+) channel mutation causing both long-QT and Brugada syndromes. Circ Res 85:1206–1213, 1999.
50. Kyndt F, Probst V, Potet F, et al: Novel SCN5A mutation leading either to isolated cardiac conduction defect or Brugada syndrome in a large French family. Circulation 104:3081–3086, 2001.
51. Shirai N, Makita N, Sasaki K, et al: A mutant cardiac sodium channel with multiple biophysical defects associated with overlapping clinical features of Brugada syndrome and cardiac conduction disease. Cardiovasc Res 53:348–354, 2002.
52. Grant AO, Carboni MP, Nepliouева V, et al: Long QT syndrome, Brugada syndrome, and conduction system disease are linked to a single sodium channel mutation. J Clin Invest 110:1201–1209, 2002.
52a. Anderson ED, Krasilnikoff PA, Overvad H: Intermittent muscular weakness, extrasystoles, and multiple developmental anomalies. A new syndrome? Acta Paediatr Scand 60:559–564, 1971.
53. Plaster NM, Tawil R, Tristani-Firouzi M, et al: Mutations in Kir2.1 cause the developmental and episodic electrical phenotypes of Andersen's syndrome. Cell 105:511–519, 2001.
54. Tristani-Firouzi M, Jensen JL, Donaldson MR, et al: Functional and clinical characterization of KCNJ2 mutations associated with LQT7 (Andersen syndrome). J Clin Invest 110:381–388, 2002.
55. Ai T, Fujiwara Y, Tsuji K, et al: Novel KCNJ2 mutation in familial periodic paralysis with ventricular dysrhythmia. Circulation 105:2592–2594, 2002.
56. Tawil R, Ptacek LJ, Pavlakis SG, et al: Andersen's syndrome: potassium-sensitive periodic paralysis, ventricular ectopy, and dysmorphic features. Ann Neurol 35:326–330, 1994.
57. Schott JJ, Mohler P, Gramolini AO, et al: Mutation in the ankyrin-b gene causes long QT syndrome and sinus node dysfunction. Circulation 106(suppl II):308, 2002.
58. Chauhan VS, Tuvia S, Buhusi M, et al: Abnormal cardiac Na(+) channel properties and QT heart rate adaptation in neonatal ankyrin(B) knockout mice. Circ Res 86:441–447, 2000.
59. Schott JJ, Charpentier F, Peltier S, et al: Mapping of a gene for long QT syndrome to chromosome 4q25-27. Am J Hum Genet 57:1114–1122, 1995.
60. Swan H, Piippo K, Viitasalo M, et al: Arrhythmic disorder mapped to chromosome 1q42-q43 causes malignant polymorphic ventricular tachycardia in structurally normal hearts. J Am Coll Cardiol 34:2035–2042, 1999.
61. Priori SG, Napolitano C, Tiso N, et al: Mutations in the cardiac ryanodine receptor gene (hRyR2) underlie catecholaminergic polymorphic ventricular tachycardia. Circulation 103:196–200, 2001.
62. Priori SG, Napolitano C, Memmi M, et al: Clinical and molecular characterization of patients with catecholaminergic polymorphic ventricular tachycardia. Circulation 106:69–74, 2002.
63. Laitinen PJ, Brown KM, Piippo K, et al: Mutations of the cardiac ryanodine receptor (RyR2) gene in familial polymorphic ventricular tachycardia. Circulation 103:485–490, 2001.
64. Jiang D, Xiao B, Zhang L, et al: Enhanced basal activity of a cardiac Ca2+ release channel (ryanodine receptor) mutant associated with ventricular tachycardia and sudden death. Circ Res 91:218–225, 2002.
65. Lahat H, Eldar M, Levy-Nissenbaum E, et al: Autosomal recessive catecholamine- or exercise-induced polymorphic ventricular tachycardia:clinical features and assignment of the disease gene to chromosome 1p13-21. Circulation 103:2822–2827, 2001.
66. Postma AV, Denjoy I, Hoorntje TM, et al: Absence of calsequestrin 2 causes severe forms of catecholaminergic polymorphic ventricular tachycardia. Circ Res 91:e21–e26, 2002.
67. Lahat H, Pras E, Olender T, et al: A missense mutation in a highly conserved region of CASQ2 is associated with autosomal recessive catecholamine-induced polymorphic ventricular tachycardia in Bedouin families from Israel. Am J Hum Genet 69:1378–1384, 2001.

第51章

心律失常的药物基因组学及对药物治疗的影响

Dan M. Roden

本章目录

- 药代动力学 ……………………………… 468
- 药物相互作用的机制 …………………… 470
- 遗传学对药代动力学和药效动力学的
  作用 ……………………………………… 471
- 总结和展望 ……………………………… 473
- 致谢 ……………………………………… 473

不同个体对药物的反应存在着很大的差异。实践中，个体之间对于抗心律失常药物反应的差异很大，对其机制的研究已经大大地促进了对于人群中存在药物治疗反应差异的理解。从药物服用至产生效果的一系列过程中，有两个关键的步骤。第一，药物必须进入体循环并到达其作用的分子部位（受体、离子通道等）。靶效应的强度受药物浓度的影响，也和药物剂量与药物（及其代谢产物）在血浆组织或其他部位如尿液、胆汁等中的浓度相关，即与药代动力学有关。第二个决定药物作用的重要过程称为药效动力学。广义上讲就是两种以上药物联合应用时，一种药物通过影响特殊的分子靶，干扰了另一种药物的药理效应，这种药理效应可以表现在分子、细胞、器官和整个机体水平。由于药物作用发生在一个复杂（且常为异常）的生物学环境中，个体之间药效的明显差异可能与药效动力学机制有关。

药代动力学和药效动力学的理论已经认识了数十年，现在也已经明确了它们就是个体分子的高级调整的表现。因此，药物在肝脏代谢的同时也可以认为是药物与某一特异的肝脏酶的相互作用，这种酶的功能和表达受多种遗传和环境因素的调控。与此相似，药物起作用的生物学环境的差异也可以被认为是多种分子功能的差异，这些分子的整合决定着正常或异常细胞和整个器官的功能。对药代动力学和药效动力学分子基础的认识已经到了能够识别与这些分子表达相关的基因时代。不同个体之间存在着成千上万种DNA变异，其中有一些是罕见的，可以导致特殊的疾病如长QT综合征，此种变异被称为突变。更常见的变异被称为多态性，可以伴有编码蛋白功能的改变；如果这种多态性导致了一级氨基酸结构或者基因转录的mRNA量的改变，蛋白质的功能也将改变。单核苷酸的变化，即单核苷酸多态性，是其中最常见的形式。近来的观点认为多态性可能是一种生理性的"静止"，一直持续到某种环境应激出现，例如高血压、急性心肌缺血或服用某些药物等。在这种情况下，DNA多态性可能决定了不同个体对这些病理生理情况的不同反应[1,2]。

遗传因素决定着某些药物治疗反应存在差异的观点实际上已经存在了一个多世纪。数十年前就曾发现在同一家系里存在着孤立的、通常由特殊突变所致的药物异常反应的个体，并启动了药代动力学研究的新领域。描述DNA变异所导致的不同个体对药物作用的差异的时候，经常提到一个新词汇——药物基因组学[3]。

一、药代动力学

(一) 循环前清除率

药物在体内经历了四个过程：吸收、分布、代谢和排泄。当某种药物经非静脉途径给药时，进入体循环的量可能会少于100%，药物进入体循环的量与静脉注射相等剂量的药物后进入体循环量之比即生物利用度。对于口服药物来说，生物利用度的降低主要有两个原因：(1)药物未能完全溶解从而不能通过肠道粘膜；(2)存在循环前清除，说明见图51-1。肠上皮细胞和肝细胞(药物在进入体循环之前必须经过的途径)内存在药物摄取分子、药物代谢酶和药物排出分子，因此药物在进入体循环之前可能在这两个地方被代谢或者被分泌到肠道或胆汁中。

(二) 药物转运是一个主动过程

既往认为药物出入细胞是一种被动过程，但是过去的十余年来，人们已经逐渐认识到这是一种特异的依赖能量的药物转运过程，是细胞正常功能的体现[4,5]。对于肝细胞和肠上皮细胞，药物的摄取和排出都是与不同位点的特殊药物转运分子密切相关的，这些转运分子可以集中在细胞顶部或外侧基底部的表面。目前只能在分子水平判别调控这些过程的特殊转运分子。现已明确，在药物代谢过程中每一种药物均为数目有限的转运分子的底物。研究最多的药物转运载体是P-糖蛋白，MDR1基因的表达产物。P-糖蛋白是一种在肠上皮细胞腔面膜、脑和睾丸的毛细血管内皮细胞腔面膜高水平表达的排出泵[6]。在这些部位，P-糖蛋白介导的外排作用会使细胞和组织内的药物浓度下降。肠上皮细胞中的P-糖蛋白将药物排泄至肠

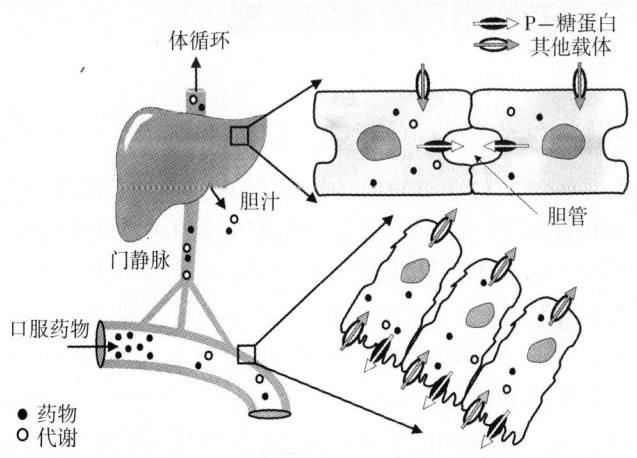

图51-1 循环前清除的现代观点。 口服药物首先必须通过肠上皮。插图下部可见，肠上皮细胞的顶部和基底面均存在着药物转运载体；这些细胞还表达与药物代谢有关的CYPs。药物排泄至肠道(通过P-糖蛋白完成)，从而限制了体循环的利用度。一旦药物越过肠道的障碍，就到达了肝细胞，通过进一步的药物代谢后被排泄至胆汁

腔，使生物利用度下降；而肝细胞中的P-糖蛋白将药物排泄至胆汁，见图51-1。对于脑毛细血管内皮细胞来说，P-糖蛋白能够限制药物进入中枢神经系统，构成了血脑屏障的重要成分。P-糖蛋白是一大类包括12个跨膜片段和2个与细胞内ATP结合位点结构相似的膜相关蛋白家族中的一员[7]。ATP结合盒(ATP-binding cassette，ABC)转运载体蛋白超家族成员还包括：其他药物转运体、囊性纤维化跨膜传导调节器(其突变可以导致囊性纤维化)、磺酰脲受体(一种重要的I_{K-ATP}成分，见第13章)、突变导致Tangier病的胆固醇转运分子。至今尚未在心肌细胞中分离出特异的药物摄取和排出转运载体，关于药物如何到达细胞内作用部位的机制也不明确。

(三) 分子介导的药物代谢

大部分药物在肝脏代谢。在肝脏，大部分通过氧化作用转化成另一种或多种代谢产物[8,9]。代谢产物的极性通常增加，直接或者与配体结合(最常为葡萄糖醛酸)后经肾脏或胆道排泄。药物在转运过程中，每一种药物都是相应的一种或数种特异的药物代谢酶的底物。氧化反应通常由细胞色素P450(CYP)超家族中的成员完成，其中和药物代谢有关的最重要的成员包括CYP3A家族(CYP 3A4和CYP3A5)、CYP2D6、CYP2C9和CYP2C19，肠道中主要的药物代谢酶为CYP3A5。而结合反应则与葡萄糖醛酸转移酶[10]、N-乙酰转移酶或甲基转移酶[11]等有关。

(四) 药物处置状态

药物的吸收、分布、代谢和排泄四个过程的研究可通过数学方式进行，可以采用房室模型。将身体视为一个有若干房室的系统，药物通过一级速率常数进出房室。一级速率指的是体内药物在单位时间内消除的药物量与血浆药物浓度成正比，零级速率是指药物在体内以恒定的速率消除，即不论血浆药物浓度高低，单位时间内消除的药物量不变。由此可以用不同的方程式来分析服药后任一时刻和任一房室模型中药物的浓度。利用房室模型获得的血浆浓度-时间关系的资料可以分析药物处置状态，如分布容积(中央容积、总容积、稳态容积)，还可以通过一级速率常数分析房室间药物的转运。非房室模型的方法与此不同，它利用时间-浓度的数据衍生出一系列不同的参数，例如清除和消除半衰期，来描述药物处置状态。房室模型和非房室模型方法互相补充，可以结合这两

种方法来分析药物的处置状态。

1. 半衰期

描述药物分布的最重要的参数包括生物利用度、分布和消除半衰期、清除率以及分布的中央容积等。当经静脉快速给予单剂药物后,其在血浆中的消除大多符合双指数函数模型。短半衰期的指数项通常与分布有关,而长半衰期的则与消除有关。比如,静脉注射利多卡因后的分布半衰期为8分钟和消除半衰期为120分钟。单次静脉给药后的一个消除半衰期后血浆浓度将下降50%,两个半衰期后为75%,三个半衰期后为87.5%,四个后为93.75%。实际工作中,4~5个半衰期后就认为完全消除了。若为长期给药,当每个单位时间内药物消除量等同于服用量时就认为达到了稳态。每次开始药物治疗、改变药物剂量或者停止药物治疗的时候,达到药物血浆浓度稳态的时间均为4~5个半衰期(图51-2)。

口服药物进入体循环后浓度逐渐升高,其时间-浓度的分布相常常是不够明确的。另一方面,静脉快速给药后经常出现药物浓度的迅速降低,其实是药物在组织的快速分布而非药物清除所致,由此还可以测定分布半衰期。

在某些情况下,药物的代谢清除可以为零级速率。如给予大剂量阿司匹林或普罗帕酮时,其代谢就遵循零级速率消除,而不是一级速率。此时,剂量的轻微增加就有可能导致血药浓度和药效的不适宜增加。

2. 负荷剂量

稳态并不等同于稳定的血浆浓度。在某些情况下,可以通过负荷剂量很快达到接近稳态的血药浓度(图51-2)。不利之处在于药物的副作用可能增加(尤其当负荷剂量过大时)。除非需要快速达到治疗所需的血浆浓度(例如控制心律失常时),给予负荷量治疗仅仅增加了副作用,并没有缩短血药浓度达到真正稳态的时间。

清除率指的是单位时间内药物容积(通常为血浆容积)的清除。除总体清除率以外,器官特异清除率(例如肾清除率或肝清除率)也能被计算出,以判断器官的特异性排泄功能。

传统的药代动力学的数学分析方式不宜来分析药效动力学的差异。体外,很多药物在靶点的相互作用可以用S型关系来描述。然而,人体内药物的浓度

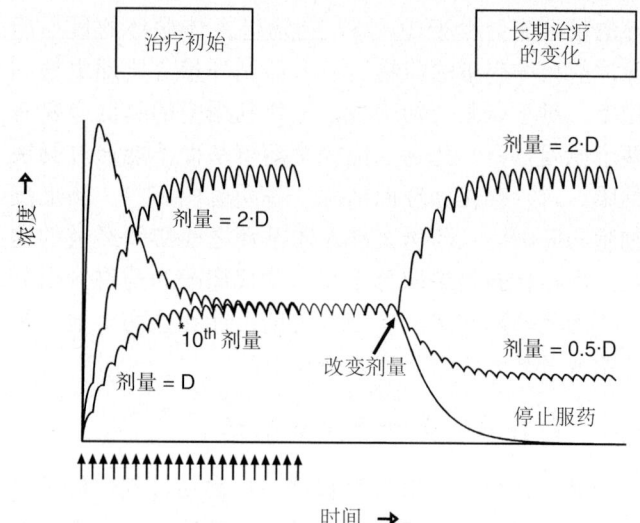

图51-2 模拟的时间-浓度曲线 分别为口服药物治疗起始阶段(左)和血药浓度达到稳定继之改变剂量后(右)的时间-浓度关系曲线。横坐标下箭头所指时间为血药浓度达到稳定之前。图例中的两次服药间隔为50%消除半衰期。大约5个消除半衰期,即第10剂(*记号)后接近稳态。一般在一级速率时,若剂量加倍,所达到的血药浓度也将加倍。服用负荷剂量后可以有更高的初始浓度,但是稳态后血药浓度与无负荷剂量者一样。剂量改变(增加或降低剂量,或者完全停止服药)约5个消除半衰期后产生新的稳态

范围一般明显低于体外试验,从而大部分人的浓度-效应关系表现为线性或对数线性。

二、药物相互作用的机制

(一) 高危药代动力学

揭示药物作用的分子机制有助于进一步理解药物的相互作用,尽管仍然是较机械的和主要依赖经验的理解,但对于预见新的药物相互作用仍很重要。药物的相互作用可以表现为对正常代谢或排泄方式的干扰,这一认识对那些有效剂量和毒性反应剂量之间界限很窄的和仅有一种主要消除途径的药物尤有药物临床意义。过去十年来,最引人注目的例子就是CYP3A4参与的药物相互作用,尤其是抗组胺药物特非那丁[12]和促肠蠕动药物西沙比利[13,14]。它们均为高效能的I_{Kr}阻滞剂,可以通过CYP3A有关的非常广泛的循环前代谢(而且没有其他的主要途径),变成非I_{Kr}阻滞的代谢产物。当同时服用抑制CYP3A的药物时,循环前代谢将受到抑制,进入体循环的特非那丁

和西沙比利量将明显增高,增加了与 I_{Kr} 阻滞有关的尖端扭转型室速的危险。对药物介导的尖端扭转型室速的研究促进了关于基因变异性及其对于药物副作用影响的研究。另外一种主要通过单一分子机制消除的药物是地高辛,其在肾脏和肝脏的排泄主要靠 P-糖蛋白[15]。奎尼丁、胺碘酮、维拉帕米和其他很多药物(例如琥乙红霉素、依曲康唑和环孢霉素)等被明确认为能够提高地高辛的浓度,可能也反映了对这种 P-糖蛋白介导的排泄方式的干扰。氟卡胺为一种 CYP2D6 底物,但由于也通过肾脏排泄,CYP2D6 活性的缺乏(遗传基础或药物干扰导致)通常不会产生问题。但是对于肾功能衰竭的病人,CYP2D6 成了氟卡胺代谢的主要途径,CYP2D6 活性的缺乏就可能导致氟卡胺的毒性作用[16,17]。

与此类似,某些药物也能通过提高基因转录来提高某些药物代谢酶或转运分子的活性。这些相互作用导致了母体药物浓度在血浆中的降低,通常减弱了效果。在某些情况下,药物代谢的结果并非药物失活而是产生更有活性的代谢产物,这些活性代谢产物可能具有与这些母体药物相似的或不同的药理学特性。

(二)药效动力学与药物相互作用

药物的相互作用也可以由药效动力学机制产生。药物能够在同一效应位点产生干扰,使用 β 受体拮抗剂的患者需要大大提高异丙肾上腺素的剂量才能达到增加心率的效果,这就是激动剂和拮抗剂同时作用于同一分子靶点($β_1$ 肾上腺受体)的例子。药物对同一受体的干扰也可能产生协同作用(例如两种具有不同解离特性的钠通道阻滞剂),或者是在增加药效的同时还可以减少服用大剂量的单一药物引起的心脏外副作用。

更多的情况下,药效动力学机制是通过对终末器官的不同分子靶点的调控产生药物的相互作用。I_{Kr} 阻滞剂和拟交感药物并非作用于同一靶点部位,但两者具有增加长 QT 间期相关的心律失常风险的协同作用,因为它们都能影响动作电位,增加了致心律失常的效应。细胞外低钾增加 I_{Kr} 阻滞剂的作用[18],因此,排钾利尿剂和 I_{Kr} 阻滞剂的协同作用是延长 QT 间期。此外,某些利尿剂也能够阻滞 I_{Kr},进一步延长 QT 间期[19]。

三、遗传学对药代动力学和药效动力学的作用

(一)突变

单核苷酸变异可以影响基因的表达产物蛋白质的功能,导致戏剧性的生理学变化,如:长 QT 综合征或遗传性代谢紊乱(如内源性褐黄病)。事实上,一个多世纪以前对内源性底物的生物转化存在缺陷的先天性代谢紊乱的认识已经让人们意识到,在这些患者外源性底物(如药物)可能同样不能被正常代谢和产生异常反应[3]。对特异基因编码的药物代谢酶缺陷的个体和家族的研究也促进了这一认识。当缺乏药物消除的其他途径和母体药物蓄积会导致明显副作用的时候,这些缺陷对于药物相互作用来说就变得非常重要。因此,存在 CYP2D6 活性缺陷的个体使用普罗帕酮治疗时可能会产生母体药物的蓄积,明显增高 β 受体阻断作用(包括支气管痉挛和缓慢性心律失常)[9,20]。与此类似,CYP2C9 活性缺陷的个体可以表现出对华法林的异常敏感[21]。更多的例子见表 51-1。

(二)多态性

对于少见的单基因疾病(长 QT 综合征和先天性代谢紊乱)来说,特异的突变和患者的表型之间、关联的基因分析和体外的生理学实验结果之间的关系,都有很好的一致性。没有外源性应激(药物)的情况下,存在药物生物转化缺陷的个体表型可以正常。这种情况下,遗传缺陷和异常药物反应之间的关系可以通过异常的药物浓度升高和患者及其家族中其他成员也有明确的基因缺陷的证据来证实。这些例子说明了 DNA 变异的共同机制——突变,严重干扰了蛋白质功能,从而在受到外源性应激之后或基础状态下就表现为显型。

相对而言,DNA 的多态性更为常见。尽管多态性和突变之间的区别有时候会不易确定,但一般认为在界定的研究人群中发生率超过 1% 的变异就称为多态性。近年来对人类基因的多态性做了大量的工作,希望能明确导致蛋白质功能改变的途径和多态性与特殊表型的关系[22-25],并开创一个"个体化医学"的新时代,使每个患者的多态性都将用于疾病的诊断和选择最佳的治疗方案。达到这样一个目标是非常有挑战性的,涉及到伦理[26]、试验的规模、遗传学相关的性价比等等问题。DNA 变异、突变或多态性,可以通过 3 条主要机制影响药物的反应:(1)药代动力学改变;(2)药物作用的分子靶点的改变;(3)药物靶分子干扰所发生的生物学大背景的改变。

表 51-1　药物代谢和相互作用

	CYP3A4	CYP2D6	CYP2C9	P-糖蛋白
底物	奎尼丁 多种 HMG CoA 还原酶抑制剂（他汀类药物，除了帕伐他丁） 多种钙通道阻滞剂 环孢霉素 昔多芬	普罗帕同 可待因 噻吗洛尔 美托洛尔 普萘洛尔 卡维洛尔 氟卡胺	华法林	地高辛 多种抗肿瘤药物
抑制剂	胺碘酮 维拉帕米 地尔硫䓬 琥乙红霉素，克拉红霉素（阿齐红霉素不是） 酮康唑 依曲康唑 非常大量的葡萄柚汁	奎尼丁 普罗帕酮 三环类抗抑郁药 百忧解 胺碘酮	胺碘酮	奎尼丁 胺碘酮 维拉帕米 环孢霉素 琥乙红霉素 酮康唑 依曲康唑
诱导剂	利福平 苯妥英 苯巴比妥 匹格列酮			利福平

仅列出主要的心血管药物，更完全列表见 http://medicine.iupui.edu/flockhart/。
HMG CoA，3-甲基-3 羟基戊二酰辅酶 A。

1. 多态性和药代动力学

存在细胞色素 P450 缺陷的患者对药物反应的增强见上述及表 51-1。当存在这些缺陷时，杂合子仍保持蛋白质的功能，但是表达水平降低。影响药物处置状态的最重要的酶 CYP3A4 的活性在不同个体之间存在差异，但是其机制仍未完全明了，多态性并没有改变蛋白质的一级结构。另外，启动子也还有潜在的重要的多态性[27]。此外，在肠上皮细胞和肝细胞表达的 CYP3A5 基因的编码区也还存在着重要的多态性[28]，更令人感兴趣的是，功能缺失的等位基因在美籍非洲人中较白人更为常见。

控制着信使 RNA 量的复杂机制决定于单一基因的转录，按规整的 DNA 顺序结合多个转录因子（由独立的基因所编码的蛋白质）。因此，DNA 变异可能不仅仅改变编码蛋白质的氨基酸顺序，还可以改变由转录控制所产生的正常功能的蛋白质的量。由此看出，产生药物代谢酶（或其他任何蛋白质）量的变异的另一种机制是由于编码转录因子的 DNA 变异，这种情况如今也已基本明确[29]。

虽然已经认识了基因断裂小鼠在基础状态下可以不表现为显型，但还没有关于 P-糖蛋白功能完全缺陷的患者报告。由于 P-糖蛋白具有维持有效血脑屏障的重要功能，当给予某些药物如地高辛时，这些小鼠就可以表现出明显的中枢神经系统药物蓄积和毒性作用。调控 P-糖蛋白体外功能的多态性已被知晓，而且确实与血清地高辛浓度的变异有关系[31-33]。

2. 多态性和药物靶

导致药物靶分子功能产生重要改变的 DNA 多态性是异常的，例如 KCNE2 基因的多态性。有一部分研究提示 KCNE2 能够联合和修饰 HERG 的功能，后者的表达可以产生 I_{kr}[34]。KCNE2 的多态性意味着在 T8A 位置丙氨酸代替了苏氨酸，对 I_{kr} 阻滞剂敏感性提高了近3倍,这与药物介导的尖端扭转型室速的易感性联系在一起了[35]。

3. 多态性和药物作用的生物学环境

基因多态性研究快速发展,观察药物反应变异的指标也逐渐增多,但均来自于药物作用所发生的生物学背景的变异。对尖端扭转型室速发生机制的研究也与此密切相关。事实上所有导致尖端扭转型室速的药物均为I_{kr}阻滞剂[36]。I_{kr}阻滞剂作用的生物学背景包括其他动作电位成分、控制正常自律功能的机制和血清钾。因此,调控这些过程的任何基因的变异理论上都能够影响I_{kr}阻滞剂延长QT间期的程度和导致尖端扭转型室速的作用。我们和别人都曾经报道过这一类家族,长QT综合征有关的突变在基础状态下没有显现,但对延长QT间期的药物的使用存在危险[37,38]。而且,我们已经鉴定出了一种KCNE1基因(编码minK,生成Iks所需的一个辅助的蛋白)的多态性,其对基础状态时的I_{ks}没有大的影响,但早后除极所致心律失常的风险明显增加[39]。近来,Splawski及其同事鉴定出了钠通道基因上的一种多态性,Y1103S,仅存在于美籍非洲人,影响心律失常发生的风险[40]。大部分接受I_{kr}阻滞剂治疗后产生明显QT间期延长和尖端扭转性型室速的病人还存在着其他的一些临床危险因素,例如低血钾或心动过缓。对于这些危险因素,现在可以添加某些DNA的变异体进行干预。我们和其他人都有这个推论:个体对维持短QT间期的调控作用由于受遗传和环境因素的影响而变化,这些因素使复极化储备下降[41],同时对I_{kr}阻滞剂作用的敏感性增加,易导致尖端扭转型室速的发生。

四、总结和展望

遗传基质和环境的相互作用,决定着机体对外源性应激如药物的反应。另一个与单基因疾病、DNA多态性和环境应激的相互作用有关的情况是猝死。大量证据说明,由于遗传机制(Brugada综合征)[42]或药理学的影响(如Cardiac Arrhythmia Suppression Trial 的结果),引起钠通道功能的缺失可以导致心律失常的发生。与此相似,来自于大型临床数据库和离体的研究均支持急性心肌缺血时潜在存在着钠通道功能下降并易发生心律失常[43]。因此,细胞表面钠通道蛋白的量的细微变异也许是一种重要的调整,并非基础状态的电生理特性的调整,但具有预测急性心肌缺血后发生致命性心律失常的作用[44,45]。总之,应该认识到个体具有对药物反应的变异性,并且有临床的、细胞的和分子的机制。对人类基因多样性的理解,为这些问题的研究提供了空前的机会,不仅仅为了提高药物的治疗效果,还应该更全面的理解人类对外界应激反应的变化方式。

五、致 谢

此工作得到了美国公共健康服务机构的部分支持(HL46681,HL49989和HL65962)。

(周益锋 译)

参 考 文 献

1. Collins FS, Jegalian KG: Deciphering the code of life. Sci Am 281:86–91, 1999.
2. Collins FS: Shattuck lecture—Medical and societal consequences of the Human Genome Project. N Engl J Med 341:28–37, 1999.
3. Roden DM, George AL Jr: The genetic basis of variability in drug responses. Nat Rev Drug Discov 1:37–44, 2002.
4. Ambudkar SV, Dey S, Hrycyna CA, et al: Biochemical, cellular, and pharmacological aspects of the multidrug transporter. Annu Rev Pharmacol Toxicol 39:361–398, 1999.
5. Zhang L, Brett CM, Giacomini KM: Role of organic cation transporters in drug absorption and elimination. Annu Rev Pharmacol Toxicol 38:431–460, 1998.
6. Mayer U, Wagenaar E, Dorobek B, et al: Full blockade of intestinal P-glycoprotein and extensive inhibition of blood-brain barrier P-glycoprotein by oral treatment of mice with PSC833. J Clin Invest 100:2430–2436, 1997.
7. Dean M, Rzhetsky A, Allikmets R: The human ATP-binding cassette (ABC) transporter superfamily. Genome Res 11:1156–1166, 2001.
8. Guengerich FP: Cytochrome P-450 3A4: Regulation and role in drug metabolism. Annu Rev Pharmacol Toxicol 39:1–17, 1999.
9. Meyer UA, Zanger UM: Molecular mechanisms of genetic polymorphisms of drug metabolism. Annu Rev Pharmacol Toxicol 37:269–296, 1997.
10. Innocenti F, Iyer L, Ratain MJ: Pharmacogenetics: A tool for individualizing antineoplastic therapy. Clin Pharmacokinet 39:315–325, 2000.
11. Weinshilboum RM, Otterness DM, Szumlanski CL: Methylation pharmacogenetics: Catechol O-methyltransferase, thiopurine methyltransferase, and histamine N-methyltransferase. Annu Rev Pharmacol Toxicol 39:19–52, 1999.
12. Woosley RL, Chen Y, Freiman JP, Gillis RA: Mechanism of the cardiotoxic actions of terfenadine. JAMA 269:1532–1536, 1993.
13. Wysowski DK, Bacsanyi J: Cisapride and fatal arrhythmia. N Engl J Med 335:290–291, 1996.
14. Drolet B, Khalifa M, Daleau P, et al: Block of the rapid component of the delayed rectifier potassium current by the prokinetic agent cisapride underlies drug-related lengthening of the QT interval. Circulation 97:204–210, 1998.
15. Fromm MF, Kim RB, Stein CM, et al: Inhibition of P-glycoprotein-mediated drug transport: A unifying mechanism to explain the interaction between digoxin and quinidine. Circulation 99:552–557, 1999.
16. Funck-Brentano C, Becquemont L, Kroemer HK, et al: Variable disposition kinetics and electrocardiographic effects of flecainide during repeated dosing in humans: Contribution of genetic factors, dose-dependent clearance, and interaction with amiodarone. Clin Pharmacol Ther 55:256–269, 1994.
17. Evers J, Eichelbaum M, Kroemer HK: Unpredictability of flecainide plasma concentrations in patients with renal failure: Relation to side effects and sudden death? Ther Drug Monit 16:349–351, 1994.
18. Yang T, Roden DM: Extracellular potassium modulation of drug block of I_{Kr}: Implications for Torsades de Pointes and reverse use-dependence. Circulation 93:407–411, 1996.

19. Fiset C, Drolet B, Hamelin BA, Turgeon J: Block of I_{Ks} by the diuretic agent indapamide modulates cardiac electrophysiological effects of the class III antiarrhythmic drug DL-sotalol. J Pharmacol Exp Ther 283:148–156, 1997.
20. Lee JT, Kroemer HK, Silberstein DJ, et al: The role of genetically determined polymorphic drug metabolism in the beta-blockade produced by propafenone. N Engl J Med 322:1764–1768, 1990.
21. Aithal GP, Day CP, Kesteven PJ, Daly AK: Association of polymorphisms in the cytochrome P450 CYP2C9 with warfarin dose requirement and risk of bleeding complications. Lancet 353:717–719, 1999.
22. Kalow W: Pharmacogenetics, pharmacogenomics, and pharmacobiology. Clin Pharmacol Ther 70:1–4, 2001.
23. McLeod HL, Evans WE: Pharmacogenomics: Unlocking the human genome for better drug therapy. Annu Rev Pharmacol Toxicol 41:101–121, 2001.
24. Evans WE, Relling MV: Pharmacogenomics: Translating functional genomics into rational therapeutics. Science 286:487–491, 1999.
25. Roses AD: Pharmacogenetics and the practice of medicine. Nature 405:857–865, 2000.
26. Rothstein MA, Epps PG: Ethical and legal implications of pharmacogenomics. Nat Rev Genet 2:228–231, 2001.
27. Wandel C, Witte JS, Hall JM, et al: CYP3A activity in African American and European American men: Population differences and functional effect of the CYP3A4*1B5'-promoter region polymorphism. Clin Pharmacol Ther 68:82–91, 2000.
28. Kuehl P, Zhang J, Lin Y, et al: Sequence diversity in CYP3A promoters and characterization of the genetic basis of polymorphic CYP3A5 expression. Nat Genet 27:383–391, 2001.
29. Schuetz EG, Strom S, Yasuda K, et al: Disrupted bile acid homeostasis reveals an unexpected interaction among nuclear hormone receptors, transporters and cytochrome P450. J Biol Chem 276:39411–39418, 2001.
30. Schinkel AH, Smit JJM, van Tellingen O, et al: Disruption of the mouse *mdr1a* P-glycoprotein gene leads to a deficiency in the blood-brain barrier and to increased sensitivity to drugs. Cell 77:491–502, 1994.
31. Hoffmeyer S, Burk O, von Richter O, et al: Functional polymorphisms of the human multidrug-resistance gene: Multiple sequence variations and correlation of one allele with P-glycoprotein expression and activity in vivo. Proc Natl Acad Sci U S A 97:3473–3478, 2000.
32. Kim RB: Drugs as P-glycoprotein substrates, inhibitors, and inducers. Drug Metab Rev 34:47–54, 2002.
33. Kim RB, Leake BF, Choo EF, et al: Identification of functionally variant MDR1 alleles among European Americans and African Americans. Clin Pharmacol Ther 70:189–199, 2001.
34. Abbott GW, Sesti F, Splawski I, et al: MiRP1 forms I_{Kr} potassium channels with HERG and is associated with cardiac arrhythmia. Cell 97:175–187, 1999.
35. Sesti F, Abbott GW, Wei J, et al: A common polymorphism associated with antibiotic-induced cardiac arrhythmia. Proc Natl Acad Sci U S A 97:10613–10618, 2000.
36. Mitcheson JS, Chen J, Lin M, et al: A structural basis for drug-induced long QT syndrome. Proc Natl Acad Sci U S A 97:12329–12333, 2000.
37. Donger C, Denjoy I, Berthet M, et al: KVLQT1 C-terminal missense mutation causes a forme fruste long-QT syndrome. Circulation 96:2778–2781, 1997.
38. Yang P, Kanki H, Drolet B, et al: Allelic variants in long QT disease genes in patients with drug-associated Torsades de Pointes. Circulation 105:1943–1948, 2002.
39. Wei J, Yang IC, Tapper AR, et al: *KCNE1* polymorphism confers risk of drug-induced long QT syndrome by altering kinetic properties of I_{Ks} potassium channels. Circulation 100:I-495, 1999.
40. Splawski I, Timothy KW, Tateyama M, et al: Variant of SCN5A sodium channel implicated in risk of cardiac arrhythmia. Science 297:1333–1336, 2002.
41. Roden DM: Taking the idio out of idiosyncratic—Predicting Torsades de Pointes. Pacing Clin Electrophysiol 21:1029–1034, 1998.
42. Alings M, Wilde A: "Brugada" syndrome: Clinical data and suggested pathophysiological mechanism. Circulation 99:666–673, 1999.
43. Akiyama T, Pawitan Y, Greenberg H, et al: Increased risk of death and cardiac arrest from encainide and flecainide in patients after non-Q-wave acute myocardial infarction in the Cardiac Arrhythmia Suppression Trial. Am J Cardiol 68:1551–1555, 1991.
44. Spooner PM, Albert C, Benjamin EJ, et al: Sudden cardiac death, genes, and arrhythmogenesis: Consideration of new population and mechanistic approaches from a National Heart Lung and Blood Institute workshop, part I. Circulation 103:2361–2364, 2001.
45. Roden DM: The problem, challenge, and opportunity of genetic heterogeneity in monogenic diseases predisposing to sudden death [editorial]. J Am Coll Cardiol 40:359, 2002.

第十部分
临床心律失常：机制、表现和处理

第 52 章

窦性心律失常

David Lin and David J. Callans

本章目录
- 概述 ·········· 475
- 正常窦性激动 ·········· 475
- 不适宜性窦性心动过速 ·········· 476
- 窦房结功能不良 ·········· 477
- 窦房结折返 ··········

一、概述

窦房结的结构错综复杂，是人类赖以生存的心脏激动的最高频率的起源部位。最早于 1906 年由 Martin Flack 和 Arthur Keith 首先报告，指出窦房结位于右房侧壁的心外膜，走行于界嵴相对应的心内膜的界沟内，被脂肪填充。正常成人中，窦房结厚约 3mm，长约 10mm。在多数人群中，窦房结上端起自右心耳侧壁的顶端，尾端指向下腔静脉[1,2]。窦房结主要由结缔组织构成，显微镜下显示为胶原和纤维组织形成的致密核样结构。窦房结中心的 P 细胞又称"典型的"结细胞，是窦房结的起搏细胞，这些细胞是由随机分布的微量线粒体和肌浆网的肌丝组成[3]。窦房结结构和功能的不均一性在确保窦房结功能方面起到重要作用，主要包括：①避免了周围心房肌超极化对其的影响；②有助于窦房结对周围心房肌的驱动；③对窦房结以外的动作电位侵入的保护；④通过起搏点的移位能够保证在不同的情况下窦房结仍能连续发放冲动。窦房结功能不良（SND）总体上包括窦房结的异常反应和非生理性改变，以及心动过速性心律失常，也包括心动过缓性心律失常。围绕在窦房结周围的传

导的不均质性也为包括窦房结在内的不同心律失常提供了起病的基础。

二、正常窦性激动

窦房结含有丰富的神经支配，包括交感神经和副交感神经，使得窦房结在不同的情况下能够改变心率和利用不同的心率去适应环境的变化。由于副交感神经作用减弱，正常个体的心率在运动开始的时候骤然升高；在运动过程中由于交感神经和体液的联合作用心率逐渐升高；在运动结束后由于交感神经作用减弱，心率很快恢复到基线水平[4]。支配窦性激动起源的细胞群受自主神经影响在界嵴上的波动范围可达 3cm 以上[5]，交感神经激动时起搏点位于界嵴的上端，而迷走神经刺激窦房结的激动沿界嵴向其下部移动[6]。

本章侧重于系统讨论窦性激动的细胞电生理机制，1980 年 Bleeker 及其同事描述了兔窦房结动作电位的多重变化。在窦房结的中心，其除极速度较低（<10V/s），除极幅度也较低（<10mV），动作电位时程长（约 150ms），最大舒张期电位低（-60～-70mV），其起搏电位呈骤起骤降型。从窦房结中心到周边乃至界嵴心房组织，动作电位均有变化，在窦房结中心时动作电位逐渐上升到达最高振幅和最大舒张电位，随着冲动向周边组织的传出，其动作电位时程的逐渐缩短，表现为起搏电位呈骤起骤降型。因此越接近窦房结中心的起搏点，动作电位时程越长，离开中心起搏点的各个方向其动作电位时程逐渐缩短。进一步的详细讨论请读者参阅 Boyett 等的文章[3]。

1970 年 Jose 和 Collision 首先报道了"固有心率"，并通过应用非选择性 β 受体阻滞剂普萘洛尔

（0.2mg/kg）和胆碱能受体阻滞剂阿托品（0.04mg/kg）完全阻断自主神经后来测定，每个人固有心率是固定不变的，固有心率的正常值＝118.1－（0.57×年龄）。若缓慢性心律失常患者固有心率正常，提示自主神经不平衡，如果固有心率降低，提示存在窦房结功能不良。该试验也用于评价不适宜性窦性心动过速患者，这些病人应用阿托品和普萘洛尔阻断自主神经后其固有心率是升高的。

早在1963年，Donald和Shepherd已经提出了在正常人群中，安静状态下心率的维持是副交感神经占优势，并通过对支配狗窦房结的副交感神经切除后和切除前的比较，发现去除副交感神经后心率明显增快。Jose和Collison也通过对人体药物阻断和未阻断副交感神经的比较证实阻断后心率明显增快，这些研究均提示副交感神经在安静状态下占优势。心脏移植后的病人，由于供体心脏含有供体的窦房结，但自主神经被完全去除了，特别是副交感神经的影响被去除，因而心脏移植病人的基础心率是升高的[4]。然而，临床也发现心脏移植后病人常发生心动过缓和缓慢性心律失常，使人们认识到窦房结可能的确主要受迷走神经的影响。

三、不适宜性窦性心动过速

1979年Bauernfeind及其同事首先报告了不适宜性窦性心动过速是由于窦房结的自律性增加所致，是交感神经和迷走神经对静息状态下心率影响的结果，可伴有或不伴有固有心率的增加。最近，Morillo及其同事认为不适宜性窦速是固有心率增加的原发性窦房结自律性异常，以及心脏迷走反应下降和肾上腺素受体敏感性增加的结果。不适宜性窦速是一种排他性诊断，该综合征的临床特点表现为慢性过程、无休止发作，也常伴有严重乏力。病人常主诉心悸，运动耐量下降和晕厥先兆。已有的报道认为接近90%的不适宜性窦速患者为女性，尤其多见于从事医疗保健工作的女性。

不适宜性窦速最常用的诊断标准包括：①P波形态和电轴与窦性P波相似或相同；②静息状态或轻微活动心率超过100次/分；③排除继发性窦速[4]。窦房结自律性异常增加和β肾上腺素受体的高敏感性是导致不适宜性窦速发生的机制。24h动态心电图检测其平均心率大于90次/分，采用标准Bruce方案踏车试验，轻度负荷即可在90s内使心率超过130次/分[6]。不同的不适宜性窦速病人其慢性过程、心悸症状和晕厥先兆的表现各不相同。临床上似乎有两种不同的表现：一种病人表现为静息状态下心率持续性增快，另一类病人主要表现在运动后心率异常反应增快。不适宜性窦速最主要的症状与后者相关，这类病人常对消融疗效反应较好。

异丙基肾上腺素试验是评价β肾上腺素受体的高敏感性的十分有用的无创检查手段。首先，在基础状态下静脉内注射0.25μg异丙肾上腺素，之后每分钟追加0.25μg，直至心率较基础心率提高35次/分，或最高心率达到150次/分。不适宜性窦速心率达到靶目标的异丙肾上腺素的剂量（0.29±0.1μg）比正常对照组（1.27±0.4μg）明显减少。

心脏电生理检查常用来鉴别起源于窦房结周围的窦房结折返性心动过速和房性心动过速，与窦房折返性心动过速比较，不适宜性窦速不能被心房程序刺激诱发。沿界嵴摆放的多极界嵴电极导管有助于鉴别不适宜性窦速和界嵴上部的房速。鉴别不适宜性窦速和房速的其他方法包括心动过速对肾上腺素和迷走刺激的反应，是否有突发突止的特点。的确，局灶起源的房速和不适宜性窦速经常很难鉴别。

β受体阻滞剂、钙通道阻滞剂、IC类药物或上述几种药物的联合应用是治疗不适宜性窦速的主要手段。如果是儿茶酚胺敏感的不适宜性窦速，β受体阻滞剂治疗常常有效。然而，如果心动过速继发于迷走神经张力低下，该心率则很难被控制。由于不同病人对药物治疗的反应不同，对那些不能耐受药物治疗和尽管药物治疗有一定效果，但症状较重的患者必须找到更理想的治疗方法。有趣的是，不适宜性窦速患者射频消融治疗几年后的随访结果显示了射频消融术的重要价值。通过对窦房结上部的导管消融可明显改善药物治疗无效患者的临床情况。另外，激动标测法、其他标测手段如电解剖标测（Biosense Webster）和心腔内超声已直接应用于导管射频消融术中。应用常规导管消融治疗不适宜性窦速的早期经验显示，导管消融几乎可完全摧毁窦房结，大多数病例必须植入永久起搏器治疗。对界嵴高侧处局部消融的窦房结改良术是可行的射频消融治疗手段。

尽管可以将界嵴高侧处作为靶点进行消融，但不适宜窦速的消融也是非常困难的，常需对局部周围进行多点消融。通过激动标测寻找较P波起点最领先的双电位区为消融靶点，其成功率也是有限的[12]。Kalman及其同事和Lee及其同事[13]均报道了采用心脏电生理方法和解剖标测相结合的消融方法。随着标测技术和超声影像质量的提高，已研制出一种以超声为基础的消融方法。

超声心动图指导下消融不适宜性窦速是一项安全和有效的治疗手段，可使消融过程更容易[14]。一种容易操控的 8mm 非温控消融导管也已被应用于解剖指导下的消融。心腔内超声导管可以进入到高位右房上腔静脉和右心耳交界处，指引消融导管定位和观察消融中消融导管的稳定性。判定消融成功的标准是心率突然下降，消融中窦性心率下降大于或等于 20 次/分，且持续存在，Ⅲ导联 P 波仍保持直立。射频消融损伤的程度可通过心腔内超声观察到，对损伤区进行超声检查可见密度减低区扩大并可波及到心外膜，可见线性损伤的低回声区和回声消失的间隙。有心率反应的患者出现回声消失间隙时是一项更为有效的预测指标。这些对心率有效反应的心腔内超声影像特点也提示这种损伤是透壁性损伤，可波及到心外膜（图 52-1，图 52-2）。根据解剖学的改变，应用超声心动图技术判定射频消融损伤的程度，具有很好的指导作用。

尽管射频消融术是十分安全的，但也有一些潜在的并发症。偶见上腔静脉阻塞综合征和膈神经麻痹，也有出现持续性交界区心律而需植入永久起搏器的报道[5,15]。此外，在一些无特征性临床症状的病人，尽管心率降低，但家族性自主神经异常也影响窦房结的功能。Lee 及其同事[5]在一系列报告中也观察到极少数病人在窦房结改良术后出现异位性房性心动过速，该结果也意味着某些不适宜性窦速病人可能除窦房结本身存在异常外还有自律性异常。

四、窦房结功能不良

晕厥、晕厥先兆或心率减慢通常是诊断病态窦房结综合征的最早和最重要的线索。病窦综合征病人还可观察到心脏停搏，以及心房超速刺激后窦房传出阻滞和窦房结的自律性被抑制。尽管病窦综合征可被诊断，但其实际上是仅基于临床的一种诊断，还需要完成更多的试验。窦房结恢复时间（SNRT）和窦房传导时间（SACT）是评价窦房结功能最常用的方法。校正的窦房结恢复时间（CSNRT）是通过 SNRT 减去窦性周期获得的。正常成人中 CSNRT 总体上应

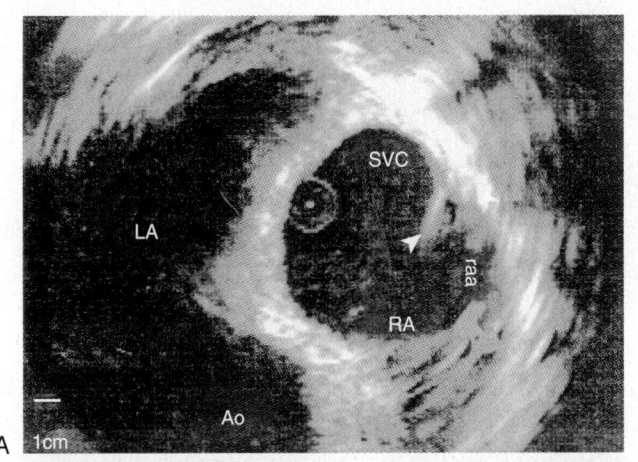

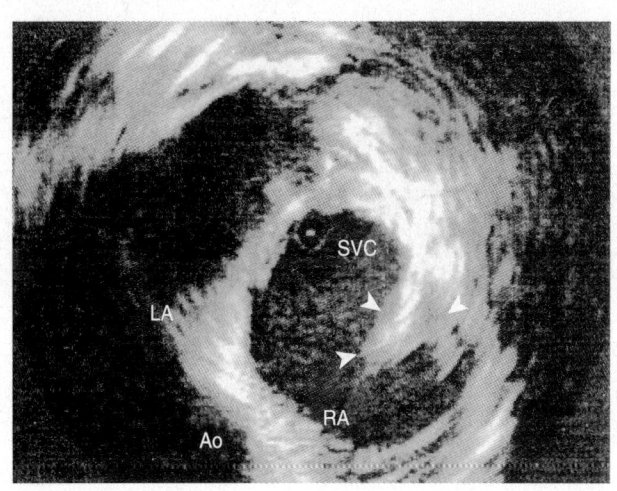

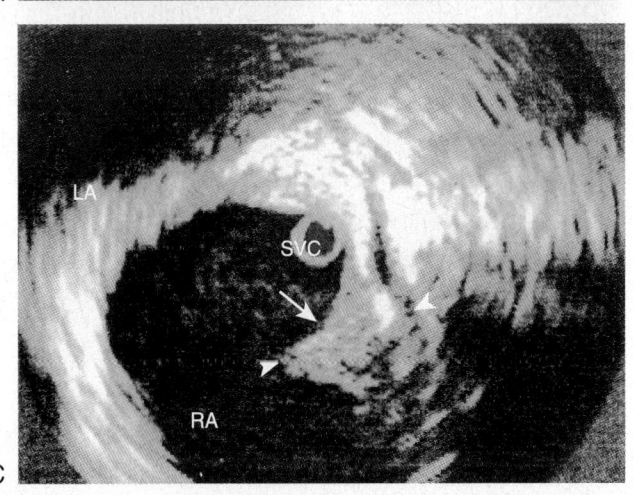

图 52-1 射频消融时心腔内超声显示出现了无回声的线性损伤图像 A：基础状态下的超声影像。B：出现弹坑样无回声的损伤。C：线性消融后损伤波及到心外膜，出现线性无回声区。LA，左心房；RA，右心房；SVC，上腔静脉；AO，主动脉。

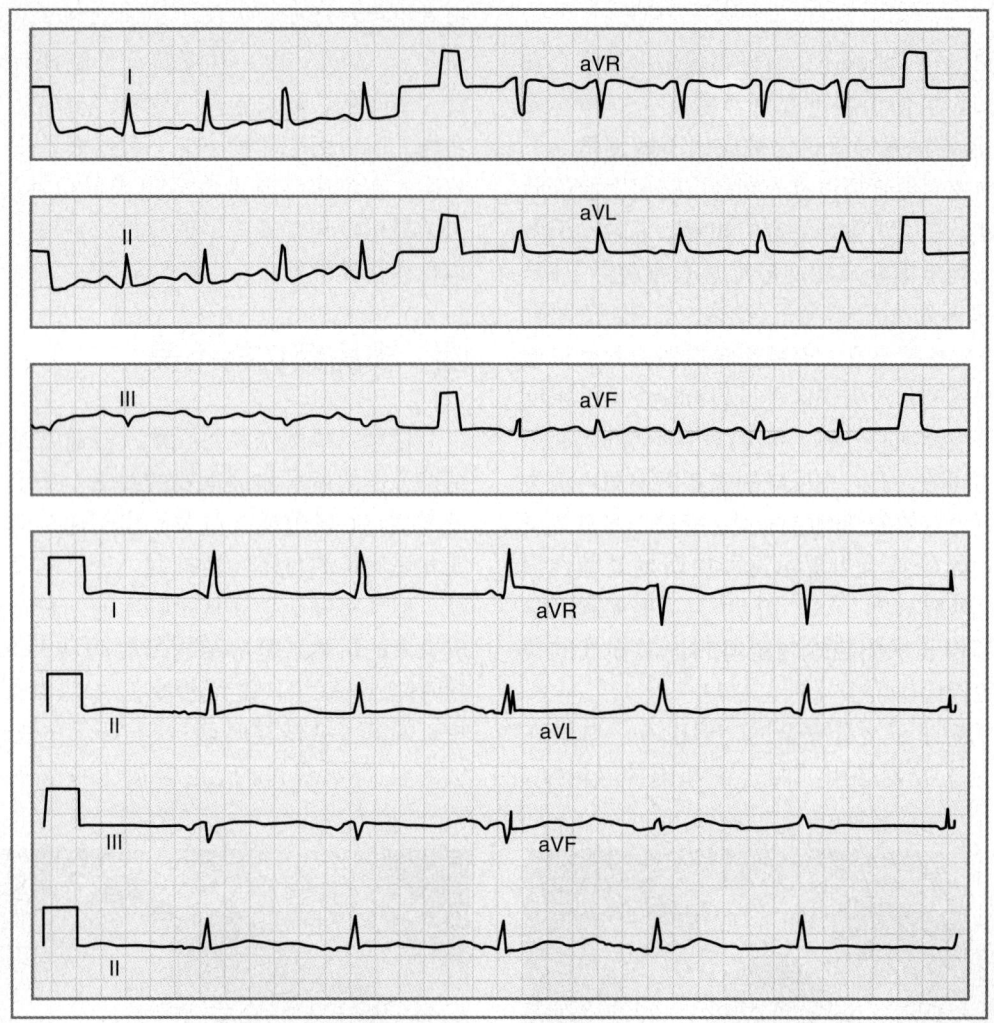

图 52-2 射频消融术后窦性心率下降，体表心电图显示Ⅱ、Ⅲ、aVF 导联的 P 波变为低平，提示窦房结激动的起源部位接近窦房结的尾部区域。

小于 500～550ms。单独应用 SNRT 诊断病窦综合征有很高的特异性，但敏感性偏低。心脏电生理检查大量的研究结果表明，以 CSNRT＞550ms 来诊断病窦综合征的敏感性和特异性分别是 70% 和 90%。当应用腺苷（0.15mg/kg）后，仍采用 CSNRT＞550ms 的诊断标准，其敏感性和特异性分别增加到 80% 和 97%[16]。

SACT 是测定从窦性激动传导至窦房结周围局部心房所需的时间。SACT 包括从心房传导至窦房结，并再从窦房结传回心房的时间，该传导时间是通过应用单个早搏刺激或应用比自主窦性心率高出 20 次/分的频率（通常比窦率快 50～150ms）超速起搏后恢复的第一跳自主心房激动的时间推断出来的。单个房性早搏刺激能穿透至窦房结并使窦房结发生节律重整。反过来，重整的窦房结激动经一定时间又引起局部心房除极。SACT 的总时间为 250～300ms 或更短。关于 SACT 更多的资料请参考前面的章节。

窦房结功能不良分为窦房结本身的异常和窦房结周围的异常，其可以是窦房结本身的病变，也可以是窦房结以外功能异常所致。窦房结功能不良继发的心房颤动也已经被认识多年了（图 52-3），最近的几项研究表明长期的心房颤动可通过缩短心房除极时间和不应期，延长心房的传导时间改变心房的电生理特征[17]。心房不应期的离散和缩短，以及心房内传导时间的延长与房颤的发生直接相关[18,19]。缓慢性心律失常也通过激动恢复后传导速度增加和容易形成折返性心律失常的特点导致房颤的发作和房颤的扩布。另外，窦房结功能不良可能容易发生异位心房激动，产生传导阻滞和折返激动。Manios 及其同事最近的研究证实房颤转复后，每小时异位室上性激动出现的频度对房颤的再发起到了至关重要的作用。该研究与其他研究一致，均提示自律性增强、心房扩大和自主节律的不稳定性有利于频发房性异位激动的出现[17]。

心房起搏较心室起搏有助于降低窦房结功能不良房颤的发生[20-22]。尽管引起房颤的电生理基质还不清楚，但当不应期缩短时折返更容易发生。当不应期未缩短时，发生房颤需要明显的缓慢传导[23]。

窦房结功能不良的临床表现并不清楚，通常称为病窦综合征。病窦综合征的病史较漫长（＞10年），临床表现可从窦性心动过缓到各种程度的窦房阻滞甚至窦性停搏或发生房颤。"低危倾向"的患者是那些：①年龄小于65岁；②左室功能正常或轻微异常；③静息时心率＞40次/分；④动态心电图记录下最慢心率＞35次/分[23]的患者。这些患者有发生晕厥的危险，尤其是那些有晕厥史和CSNRT≥800ms者。在THEOPACE研究结果的基础上，对既往有晕厥史者均应行心脏电生理检查测定CSNRT，若CSNRT≥800ms，且有病史的患者应植入永久性心脏起搏器[25]。

这种房性心动过速的可能机制为窦房折返，但直到1968年才由Han及其同事[26]在离体的兔心肌证实了窦房结折返的存在[27]。在人体上折返环并不是固定的。目前争论的焦点是折返环是仅存在于窦房结，还是有部分界嵴或窦房周围组织参与折返。通过程序刺激易见单次折返或窦房结折返性心动过速。窦房结折返性心动过速的症状可以是典型房速的特点，如心悸、晕厥先兆，很少发生晕厥，原因是其心率通常较慢。为与其他类型的房性心动过速相鉴别，必须进行电生理检查。窦房结折返与其他房速不同的特点是在窦房结附近的心脏程序刺激可反复诱发心动过速。

大多数研究者认为以前高估了窦房折返性心动过速的发生率，其主要原因是缺乏准确的导管标测去证实其为非窦房折返性心动过速。由于程序刺激常诱发窦性回波和持续性窦房折返，但该心律失常既可以被诱发，也可以自主发生，因此这种室上性心动过速可能不是一种常见的发生机制。

（李学斌　译）

五、窦房结折返

尽管早在1943年Barker及其同事通过分析提出

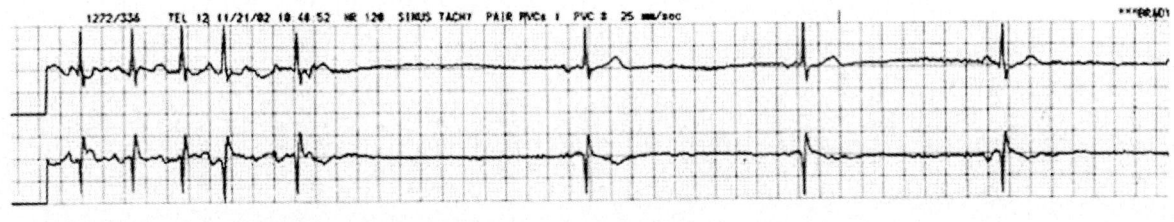

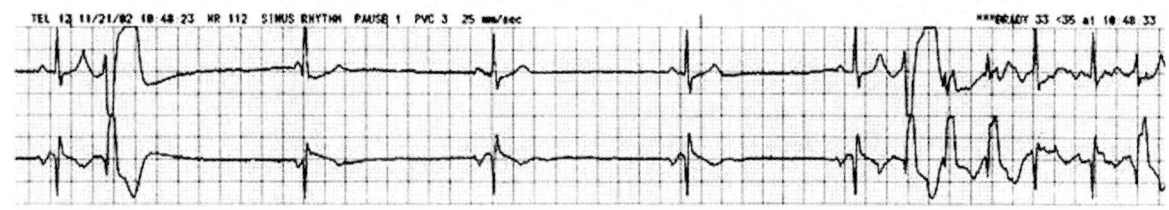

图52-3　心动过缓综合征患者合并房颤时的心电图

参 考 文 献

1. Ho SY, Anderson RH, Sanchez-Quintana D: Atrial structure and fibres: Morphologic bases of atrial conduction. Cardiovasc Res 54:325–336, 2002.
2. Krahn AD, Yee R, Klein GJ, Morillo C: Inappropriate sinus tachycardia: Evaluation and therapy. J Cardiovasc Electrophysiol 6:1124–1128, 1995.
3. Boyett MR, Honjo H, Kodama I: The sinoatrial node, a heterogeneous pacemaker structure. Cardiovasc Res 47:658–657, 2000.
4. Wilson RF, Johnson TH, Haidet GC, et al: Sympathetic reinnervation of the sinus node and exercise hemodynamics after cardiac transplantation. Circulation 101:2727–2733, 2000.
5. Lee RJ, Kalman JM, Fitzpatrick AP, et al: Radiofrequency catheter modification of the sinus node for "inappropriate" sinus tachycardia. Circulation 92:2919–2928, 1995.
6. Lee RJ, Shinbane JS: Advances in supraventricular tachycardia. Cardiol Clin 15:599–605, 1997.
7. Bleeker WK, Mackaay AJC, Masson-Pevet MA, et al: Functional and morphological organization of the rabbit sinus node. Circ Res 46:11–22, 1980.
8. Jose AD, Collison D: The normal range and determinants of the intrinsic heart rate in man. Cardiovasc Res 4:160–167, 1970.
9. Donald DE, Shepherd JT: Response to exercise in dogs with cardiac denervation. Am J Physiol 205:393–400, 1963.
10. Bauernfeind RA, Amat-Y-Leon F, Dhingra RC, et al: Chronic non-paroxysmal sinus tachycardia in otherwise healthy persons. Ann of Int Med 91:702–710, 1979.
11. Morillo CA, Klein GJ, Thakur RK, et al: Mechanism of "inappro-

priate" sinus tachycardia. Role of sympathovagal balance. Circ 90:873–877, 1994.
12. Man KC, Knight B, Tse HF, et al: Radiofrequency catheter ablation of inappropriate sinus tachycardia guided by activation mapping. J Am Coll Cardiol 35:451–457, 2000.
13. Kalman JM, Lee RJ, Fisher WG, et al: Radiofrequency catheter modification of sinus pacemaker function guided by intracardiac echocardiography. Circ 92:3070–3081, 1995.
14. Ren JF, Marchlinski FE, Callans DJ, Zado ES: Echocardiographic lesion characteristics associated with successful ablation of inappropriate sinus tachycardia. J Cardiovasc Electrophysiol 12:814–818, 2001.
15. Leonelli FM, Pisano E, Requarth JA, et al: Frequency of superior vena cava syndrome following radiofrequency modification of the sinus node and its management. Am J Cardiol 85:771–774, 2000.
16. Burnett D, Abi-Samra F, Vacek JL: Use of intravenous adenosine as a noninvasive diagnostic test for sick sinus syndrome. Am Heart J 137:435–438, 1999.
17. Manios EG, Kanoupakis EM, Mavrakis HE, et al: Sinus pacemaker function after cardioversion of chronic atrial fibrillation: Is sinus node remodeling related with recurrence? J Cardiovasc Electrophysiol 12:800–806, 2001.
18. Goette A, Honeycutt C, Langberg JJ: Electrical remodeling in atrial fibrillation: Time course and mechanisms. Circulation 94:2968–2974, 1996.
19. Daoud EG, Bogun F, Goyal R, et al: Effect of AF on atrial refractoriness in humans. Circulation 94:1600–1606, 1996.
20. Lamas GA, Lee KL, Sweeney MO, et al: Mode selection trial in sinus-node dysfunction: Ventricular pacing or dual-chamber pacing for sinus-node dysfunction. N Engl J Med 346:1854–1862, 2002.
21. Anderson HR, Nielsen JC, Thomsen PE, et al: Long-term follow-up of patients from a randomized trial of atrial versus ventricular pacing for sick-sinus syndrome. Lancet 350:1210–1216, 1997.
22. Skanes AC, Krahn AD, Yee R, et al: Progression to chronic atrial fibrillation after pacing: The Canadian Trial of Physiologic Pacing—CTOPP Investigators. J Am Coll Cardiol 38:167–172, 2001.
23. De Sisti A, Leclercq JF, Fiorello P, et al: Electrophysiologic characteristics of the atrium in sinus node dysfunction: Atrial refractoriness and conduction. J Cardiovasc Electrophysiol 11:30–33, 2000.
24. Menozzi C, Brignole M, Alboni P, et al: The natural course of untreated sick sinus syndrome and identification of the variables predictive of unfavorable outcome. Am J Cardiol 82:1205–1209, 1998.
25. Alboni P, Menozzi C, Brignole M, et al: Effects of permanent pacemaker and oral theophylline in sick sinus syndrome the THEOPACE study: A randomized controlled trial. Circulation 96:260–266, 1997.
26. Barker P, Wilson F, Johnston D: The mechanism of auricular paroxysmal tachycardia. Am Heart J 26:435–445, 1943.
27. Han J, Malozzi AM, Moe GK: Sino-atrial reciprocation in the isolated rabbit heart. Circ Res 22:355–362, 1968.

第 53 章

房室阻滞和房室分离

David Schwartzman

本章目录
- 房室阻滞 ······ 481
- 房室分离 ······ 484

房室分离和房室阻滞是有关系的。房室分离意味着心室的激动来源于心房以外，不受心房激动的影响。房室阻滞意味着房室之间存在着病理性传导。房室阻滞由心房、房室结或希浦系统传导延迟所致。在完全性房室阻滞时来源于心房以外的激动使心室除极以维持生命。因此，完全性房室阻滞是房室分离的原因之一。

房室阻滞和房室分离可根据心电图得到诊断，二者均为临床病理学的范畴。对二者正确的评价和治疗有赖于对心脏结构、功能和临床情况的综合考虑。

一、房室阻滞

房室阻滞分为一度、二度和三度阻滞。一度房室阻滞时 PR 间期延长，但每个心房的激动都能下传至心室。二度房室阻滞时一部分来自心房的激动被阻不能下传至心室。三度（完全性）房室阻滞时房室传导关系消失。房室阻滞与心房、房室结、希氏束或双侧束支等部位的组织病理情况有关。特发性纤维化累及到心脏骨架或远端传导系统形成的 Lev 病和 Lenegre 病是房室阻滞的常见病因。心肌缺血或梗死后导致的心肌组织病变也是房室阻滞的病因。其他的病因还包括主动脉瓣或二尖瓣钙化、感染、手术损伤、浸润性疾病（例如淀粉样变性、肉样瘤病和癌症）、炎症（例如血管炎和心肌炎）、神经肌肉性疾病（例如肌强直性肌营养不良、Kearns-Sayre 综合征、腓侧肌萎缩和 Erb 营养障碍）[7] 和先天性疾病。房室阻滞可以是一过性或永久性。一过性房室阻滞的原因包括药物中毒、心肌缺血、迷走神经张力增加和局部损伤（例如消融所致）。

（一）一度房室阻滞

一度房室阻滞心电图表现为正常时间出现的 P 波（非早搏波）后 PR 间期大于 200ms。PR 间期可以发生变化，诸如神经张力的变化可使 PR 间期改变，但每个心房冲动都能经房室传导到达心室。一度房室阻滞可由于心房、房室结和希浦系统传导延迟所致，且每个患者的房室阻滞可能由一个或多个部位的传导延迟所致。在成年人中由房室结传导延迟所造成的房室阻滞占 80% 以上。通过观察 PR 间期和 QRS 波群的时限及变化可以进一步对房室阻滞的部位定位。PR 间期显著延长（大于 300ms）或 PR 间期发生显著变化时表明房室结受累。如果 QRS 波群时限正常，最常见的原因是房室结内传导延迟（>90%）。QRS 波群时限延长时，阻滞部位除仍可能在房室结外，更可能发生在束支和希浦系统，尤其患者有左束支阻滞或右束支阻滞合并电轴左偏或右偏时这种情况更为常见。应该注意到，即使 PR 间期在正常范围内时也不能除外房室传导延迟的可能，特别是当阻滞部位在希浦系统时。确切的阻滞部位的定位可通过心内电图确诊（图 53-1）。

临床上孤立性一度房室阻滞在健康成年人中相对常见，其中大部分的 PR 间期仅轻度延长，很少进展为二度或三度房室阻滞。没有证据表明孤立性一度房室阻滞会增加死亡率。孤立性一度房室阻滞一般没有症状，除非 PR 间期显著延长（大于 300ms）[1]。当 PR 间期明显延长导致心房收缩发生在心室收缩前很短的时间内时，会产生类似起搏器综合征样的症状[2]。

（二）二度房室阻滞

二度房室阻滞分为Ⅰ型和Ⅱ型阻滞、高度房室阻滞和阵发性房室阻滞。

1. 二度Ⅰ型房室阻滞

二度Ⅰ型房室阻滞表现为文氏现象：PR 间期依次逐渐延长，直到一个 P 波被阻滞发生一次心搏脱落；心搏脱落后的第一个 PR 间期缩短，因此包含心搏脱落的长间歇短于两倍的 P-P 间期。这种现象重复出现，房室传导比例一般固定。PR 间期的最大增量一般发生在文氏周期中第二个下传的搏动，随后搏动的 PR 间期增量却是逐渐减少的，这导致心搏脱落前 RR 间期逐渐缩短。临床上，二度Ⅰ型房室阻滞往往不能全部包括文氏现象的典型特征[3]。

二度Ⅰ型房室阻滞可由于房室结、希氏束或希氏束以下水平的传导延迟所致。在有快速的心房激动或没有室内传导延迟表现时，房室结传导延迟是二度房室阻滞最常见的原因（图 53-2）。即使存在室内传导延迟，房室结仍是常见的部位，同时希浦系统阻滞也比较常见[4,5]。阻滞部位可通过心内电图定位。如果阻滞部位在希浦系统，表明传导系统存在弥漫性的器质性疾病。阻滞区位于希氏束或其以下的二度Ⅰ型房室阻滞病例中，大多数文氏周期中的基础 PR 间期和 PR 间期的逐渐增量，都比在房室结内二度Ⅰ型阻滞病例所见的小得多[5]。

临床上，二度Ⅰ型房室阻滞在健康成年人，特别是从事有氧运动的人中相对常见，而且他们的二度Ⅰ型房室阻滞在睡眠时更常见，这与迷走神经张力增加有关。这一点可以用快速阻断迷走神经张力的方法加以证实。在极少数情况下，交感神经张力增高可以导致或加重二度Ⅰ型房室阻滞，这时无论有无室内传导延迟的存在，阻滞区都可能在房室结以下的部位[6]。在心脏结构正常的患者，二度Ⅰ型房室阻滞很少进展为二度Ⅱ型房室阻滞或三度房室阻滞，且这种情况下的二度Ⅰ型房室阻滞病人预后并非不好。而在有器质性心脏病的患者，二度Ⅰ型房室阻滞常常表示心脏病在进展，应警惕患者的预后。

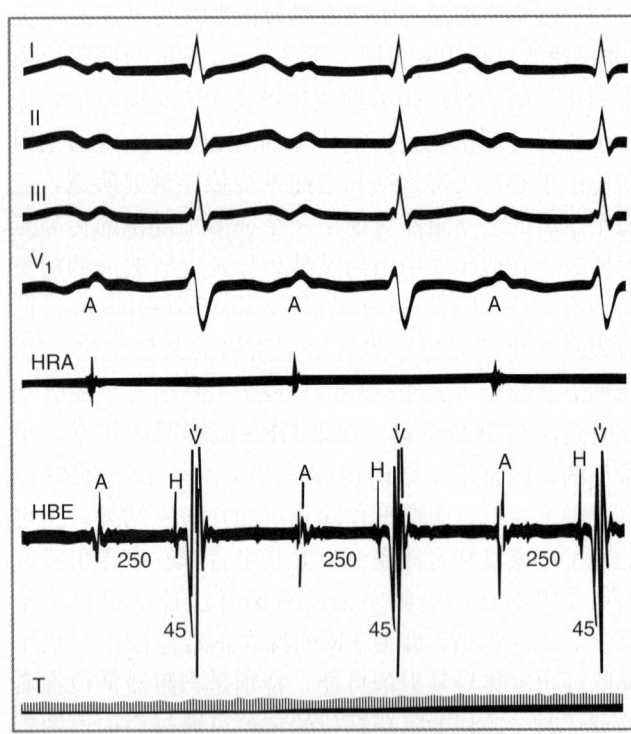

图 53-1 房室结传导延迟导致的一度房室阻滞 AH 间期延长，HV 间期正常。HRA，高位右房；A，心房波；V，心室波；HBE，希氏束电图；HV，希浦系统传导时间；T，时间线。(From Josephson M: Clinical cardiac electrophysiology, 2nd ed. Philadelphia, Lea and Febiger, 1993.)

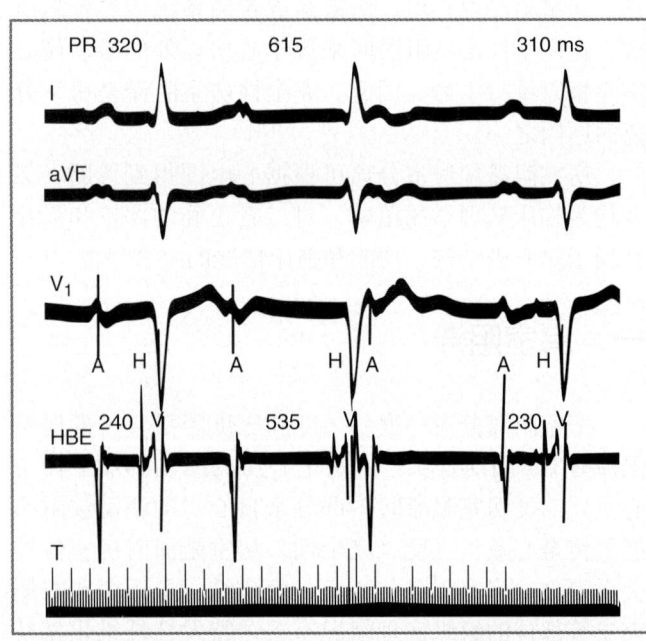

图 53-2 房室结传导延迟导致的二度Ⅰ型房室阻滞 PR 间期和 AH 间期进行性延长，直到第三个 P 波后没有希氏束和心室除极波。A，心房波；V，心室波；HBE，希氏束电图。(From Josephson M: Clinical cardiac electrophysiology, 2nd ed. Philadelphia, Lea and Febiger, 1993.)

2. 二度Ⅱ型房室阻滞

二度Ⅱ型房室阻滞的特征是P波突然受阻不能下传,且无文氏现象存在。发生心搏脱落之前和之后的所有下传搏动的PR间期是恒定的,心搏脱落的长间歇等于两倍的P-P间期。因为二度Ⅱ型房室阻滞的阻滞区几乎均在希浦系统内,预示着希浦系统疾病处在进展期,故Ⅱ型房室阻滞常伴随着室内传导延迟。虽然有报道显示阻滞区在希氏束的二度Ⅱ型房室阻滞伴窄QRS波群,但这种情况更可能的原因是不典型的二度Ⅰ型房室阻滞,而非二度Ⅱ型房室阻滞。

二度Ⅱ型房室阻滞的阻滞区位于希氏束或希氏束以下水平(图53-3)。当已有一侧束支阻滞,再出现二度Ⅱ型房室阻滞时,传导阻滞一般都发生在对侧束支。二度Ⅱ型房室阻滞一般不见于健康人,但应当注意不典型的二度Ⅰ型房室阻滞、隐匿的希浦系统除极和交界区的并行心律可能类似二度Ⅱ型房室阻滞而误诊(图53-4)。

临床上,二度Ⅱ型房室阻滞比二度Ⅰ型房室阻滞少见。不同于二度Ⅰ型房室阻滞,二度Ⅱ型房室阻滞的症状很明显。二度Ⅱ型房室阻滞常进展为三度房室阻滞,这时心室由次级不稳定的逸位起搏点节律所控制。当然,希氏束阻滞如果是功能性(例如房性期前收缩经房室结下传时,房室结的不应期短于希氏束的不应期或某些形式的房室结内折返)或阻滞是暂时性的(例如药物中毒后心脏外科手术)则属于例外。

3. 高度房室阻滞

高度房室阻滞指连续两个或两个以上P波不能下传至心室。

4. 阵发性房室阻滞

阵发性房室阻滞是指本来能正常下传的非心动过速性的P波突然反复性被阻滞不能下传,发作时常有一定时间的心室停搏[6]。虽然阵发性房室阻滞常归类于二度Ⅱ型,即认为阻滞部位在希氏束以下,但应当了解,这与实际情况并非完全符合。虽然阵发性房室阻滞患者的阻滞部位和机制难于确定,但是一般认为其阻滞部位位于希氏束以下,同时次级起搏点不稳定。

5. 发生在急性心肌梗死时的房室阻滞

急性心肌梗死时二度Ⅰ型房室阻滞常见,一般伴发下壁心肌梗死。这种情况下阻滞区在房室结,常为

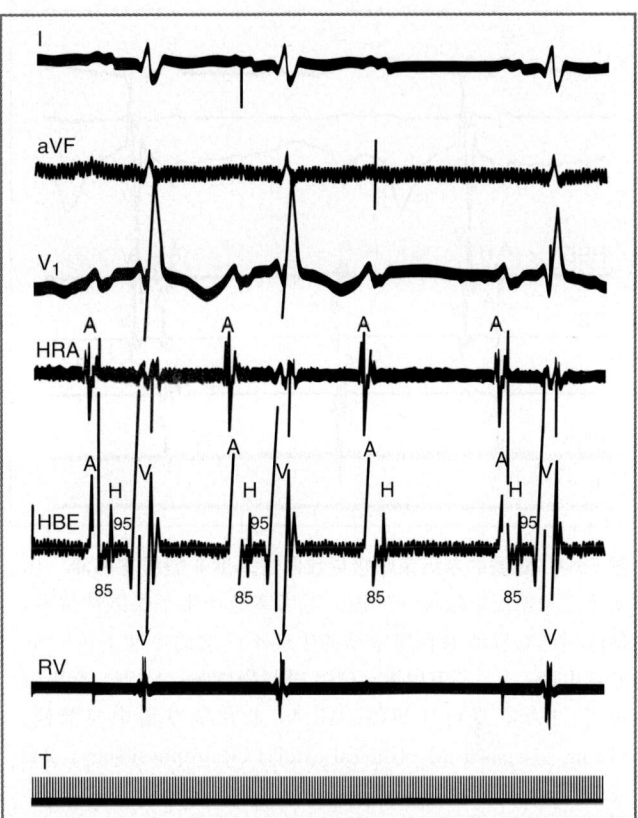

图53-3 希浦系统传导延迟导致的二度Ⅱ型房室阻滞 在下传的激动中,AH间期和HV间期不变。第三个H波后突然出现无心室除极波跟随。而心室波脱落后的所有下传激动间期没有改变。A,心房电图;V,心室电图;HBE,希氏束电图;HRA,高位右房;HV,希浦系统传导时间;RV,右室。(From Josephson M: Clinical cardiac electrophysiology, 2nd ed. Philadelphia, Lea and Febiger, 1993.)

一过性的二度Ⅰ型房室阻滞,很少进展为完全性房室阻滞。

急性心肌梗死时二度Ⅱ型房室阻滞少见,一般和前壁心梗同时出现。这时阻滞区在希浦系统及以远的部位,这可能是其常同时伴束支阻滞的原因。急性心肌梗死合并二度Ⅱ型房室阻滞表示心梗面积较大,且进展为完全性房室阻滞并非罕见。

(三) 三度房室阻滞

三度房室阻滞指所有来自心房的激动都不能传导至心室,即房室分离。阻滞部位下的异位起搏点激动心室,QRS波群的形态和心室率由异位起搏点的位置决定。异位起搏点位于束支及以远部位时,表现为心室率固定,不受自主神经张力的影响。起源于希浦系统和心室组织的逸位起搏点节律很不稳定。

三度房室阻滞时,阻滞区可以位于房室结、希氏

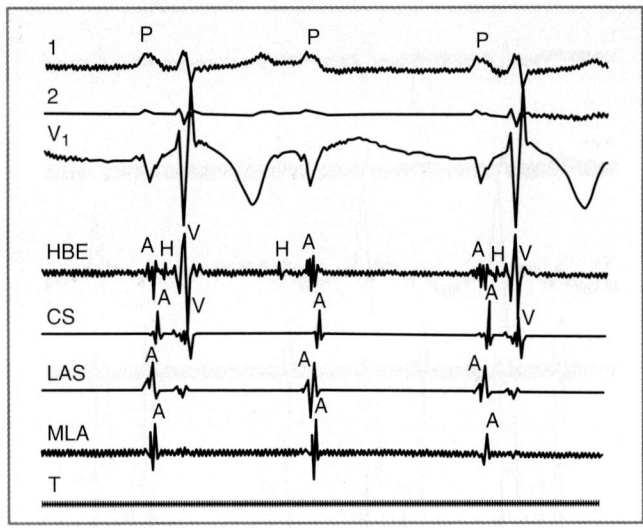

图 53-4　隐匿的希氏束除极导致假性二度 Ⅱ 型房室阻滞　由于第二个希氏束除极（H 波）对房室结产生了隐匿性传导，使随后的心房波遇到房室结的生理不应期而不能下传。A，心房电图；V，心室电图；CS，冠状静脉窦；HBE，希氏束电图；LAS，低位房间隔；MLA，心房前壁偏中左部位。(From Josephson M：Clinical cardiac electrophysiology, 2nd ed. Philadelphia, Lea and Febiger, 1993.)

束或希氏束以下部位。如果 QRS 波群时限正常（过去不存在束支阻滞），阻滞区位于房室结和希氏束的几率大概各占一半。如果 QRS 波群变宽，阻滞区大多数位于希浦系统及其以下的部位。

临床上，三度房室阻滞的症状取决于阻滞的部位和次级起搏点的起搏频率。例如，发生在房室结水平的三度房室阻滞常常没有症状；而有双侧束支阻滞时，几乎所有的患者均有症状。这种阻滞部位的差异往往有助于病因的鉴别，完全性的房室结阻滞一般是先天性的，而希浦系统的阻滞一般是后天获得性的。

（四）先天性房室阻滞

先天性房室阻滞首次表现可以在出生前或出生时，甚至有些直到成年后才被发现。先天性房室阻滞可以独立存在，也可以与器质性心脏病同时存在。当先天性房室阻滞独立存在时，房室阻滞常常是完全性的。因为先天性房室阻滞主要是由于房室结发育异常，少部分由于希浦系统发育异常所致，所以即使开始房室阻滞并非完全，但最终将进展为完全性房室阻滞。先天性房室阻滞中大约 30% 的病例同时发现母亲存在明显的胶原血管病，该病可产生针对细胞内核糖核蛋白的自身抗体，并通过胎盘进入胎儿体内。有趣的是，虽然母体内也存在自身抗体，但母亲的心脏一般不受影响。胎儿同时也合并其他的心外表现，这些心外表现和房室阻滞共存时常诊断为新生儿狼疮综合征。第一次分娩患有新生儿狼疮综合征婴儿的母亲，今后再次分娩时，婴儿患有该综合征的几率明显增加。动物试验表明该病与钙离子通道有关。该病在新生儿时期死亡率最高，在儿童期和青少年期大大减低，成人中病情进展缓慢，后期易出现左室功能不全[8]。但应注意，这种左室功能不全可能是由长期的右室心尖部起搏所致。

（五）急性心肌梗死引起的阻滞

下壁心梗合并完全性房室阻滞时，阻滞区在房室结，是房室结动脉受累和心脏迷走传入神经活性变化共同作用的结果。异位起搏点常在交界区，常伴窄 QRS 波群。下壁心梗合并完全性房室阻滞时短期预后较差，但这种完全性房室阻滞是非持续性的。

前壁心梗合并完全性房室阻滞时，阻滞区在希浦系统。这种情况表示心梗面积较大，其预后较一般前壁心梗差。异位起搏点常来自心室自身，因此非常不稳定。

二、房室分离

房室分离指心房和心室的激动各自独立，根据持续时间分为一过性和持续性的房室分离。房室分离有不同的电生理机制，每种机制与其临床病理基质有关。

1. **心房率过低**：心房率降低至次级起搏点（交界区或交界区下面）频率以下，使得次级起搏点产生逸搏节律，而此逸搏冲动不能逆行激动心房。这种房室分离多出现在心房率和心室率非常接近（心室率仅稍高于心房率）时，并且多为一过性的房室分离。我们称这种房室分离为等率性房室分离。

2. **房室阻滞**：完全性房室阻滞和不完全性房室阻滞都能导致房室分离。心房激动不能下传到心室，导致异位起搏节律出现。一般来说，次级起搏点的频率慢于心房频率，但也有例外情况。

3. **次级起搏点频率加快**：次级起搏点的频率不正常地加快，超过心房率，并且逸位搏动不能逆行激动心房。交界区和室性心动过速形成的房室分离属于这一类。

4. **长间歇引起的房室分离**：任何电活动（房早、

室早和交界区早搏）产生的长间歇的频率低于次级起搏点节律时就可能导致这种房室分离。

5. 上述原因的联合：例如洋地黄中毒导致的房室阻滞（常为二度Ⅰ型房室阻滞）合并交界区心动过速。

（许　原　译）

参 考 文 献

1. Barold SS: Indications for permanent cardiac pacing in first-degree AV block: Class I, II, or III? Pacing Clin Electrophysiol 19:747–751, 1996.
2. Gregoratos G, Abrams J, Epsetin AE, et al: ACC/AHA/NASPE 2002 guideline update for implantation of cardiac pacemakers and antiarrhythmia devices: A report of the American College of Cardiology/American Heart Association task force on practice guidelines. (ACC/AHA/NASPE committee on pacemaker implantation). J Cardiovasc Electrophysiol 13:1183–1199, 2002.
3. Barold SS, Hayes DL: Second-degree atrioventricular block: A reappraisal. Mayo Clin Proc 76:44–57, 2001.
4. Barold SS: Lingering misconceptions about type I second-degree atrioventricular block. Am J Cardiol 88:1018–1020, 2001.
5. Narula OS: Clinical Concepts of Spontaneous and Induced Atrioventricular Block. In Mandel WJ (ed): Cardiac Arrhythmias, 3rd ed. Philadelphia, JB Lippincott, 1995.
6. Barold SS: Atrioventricular block revisited. Compr Ther 28:74–78, 2002.
7. Boutjdir M: Molecular and ionic basis of congenital complete heart block. Trends Cardiovasc Med 10:114–122, 2000.
8. Moak JP, Barron KS, Hougen TJ, et al: Congenital heart block: Development of late-onset cardiomyopathy, a previously underappreciated sequela. J Am Coll Cardiol 37:238–242, 2001.

第 54 章

心房扑动机制、临床表现和治疗

Albert L. Waldo

本章目录
- 房扑的机制 ········· 486
- 房扑的临床特征 ········· 488
- 房扑的治疗 ········· 489
- 总结 ········· 492

1911年Jolly和Ritchie[1]首先描述了心房扑动（房扑），但是房扑的机制比较复杂，直到最近，房扑机制、诊断和治疗才取得了重大进展，新技术的出现，明显改善了房扑急性期和远期的治疗。本章将就这些问题进行阐述。

一、房扑的机制

长期以来，房扑是由单病灶快速驱动引起，还是由折返机制引起一直存在争议。发现触发活动后，人们又认为房扑有可能是由于早期后除极或者晚期后除极引起的。现在大量证据表明房扑主要是由于右房的折返引起来的。

（一）房扑动物模型的启示

多年以来，已建立数种房扑的动物模型。第一项房扑的研究是Lewis和他的同事[1]在正常犬心脏上进行的，他们发现应用法拉第电流能诱发稳定房扑，但是几率不高，他们在几个选定部位记录了心房电图。基于这些研究，结合病人的心电图向量分析，Lewis等提出房扑围绕上腔静脉和下腔静脉折返，在两者之间可能存在传导阻滞（但是并没有特别强调）。但是可以肯定的是，在正常犬心脏很难诱发稳定的房扑。

Rosenbleuth和Garcia-Ramos[1]指出腔静脉之间挤压伤产生的稳定的传导阻滞对于诱发稳定的房扑至关重要，激动顺序标测发现：房扑环绕上下腔静脉和挤压形成的传导阻滞区域。最近，Frame[1]等研究发现腔静脉之间的外科切口和延伸到右心耳的Y字形切口，对于房扑的稳定诱发也很重要，稳定的房扑是围绕三尖瓣环顺钟向或者逆钟向折返。

还有几种犬房扑模型是通过损伤右房游离壁建立的[1]，这些模型中房扑围绕损伤部位形成折返，美中不足的是没有标测房间隔。这些模型很有意义，可以解释临床先心病心脏外科手术术后病人的房扑，比如Mustard、Senning、Fontan[1,2]术后病人的慢性房扑发生率非常高。几个小组的研究还证明[3,6]术后房内折返性心动过速不仅环绕术后的切口或者缝线折返，而且像经典房扑一样，折返环还包括三尖瓣环、下腔、欧氏嵴和冠状窦口之间的峡部。

有趣的是，Tomita[7]等的研究证实，如果正常犬右房游离壁的切口足够长，能形成一个或者两个介于腔静脉之间的固定阻滞线，就会出现典型房扑，房扑围绕间隔和右房游离壁折返。这也许可以解释外科手术切口或者右房缝线形成的腔静脉之间的阻滞线，为经典房扑的形成提供了基质。当然，围绕外科切口或者缝线之间的折返也是可能的。

Cox[8]最新的研究证实肺静脉分离再吻合之后，在这样的犬模型可以诱发房扑，在病人则可以出现自发性房扑[9]，这种情况下，房扑围绕左房的外科切口发生。房扑也是外科Maze手术治疗房颤的常见并发症，由于术中切割线没有连续形成阻滞[10]，激动沿着不完全阻滞的线形成了折返。

也有不依赖原发性心房损伤的房扑模型，Allessie[1]等的犬乙酰胆碱房扑模型显示折返性房扑可以发生在左右房的很多部位，不需要存在解剖的障碍区。值得一提的是这种模型的房扑折返环都很短，小于等于100ms，因此，这种模型可能代表Ⅱ型房扑，这也可以解释为什么临床上Ⅱ型房扑经常演化为房颤[11,12]，这是因为折返周期太短，大部分心房组织不能1∶1激动[12]。其他几个关于犬房扑模型研究显示折返环限于右房，主要是右房游离壁[1,13]。应用无菌型心包炎模型，系统标测房间隔发现无论是单环折返还是8字折返，房间隔都是折返环的关键部位[1]。8字折返过程中，折返环之间有一个共享的枢纽区域，右房游离壁表现为顺钟向转还是逆钟向转取决于共享枢纽区域的激动方向。

（二）人类的房扑研究

很长一段时间，人类房扑的标测位点很有限[1]，但是即使是这样，Puech[1]等的研究还是发现整个房扑环的激动时间可以只用右房的折返时间来计算，包括房间隔和游离壁的激动。以后的研究显示，一过性的拖带和终止房扑说明[1]：人类房扑是心房内的折返，并具有一定的可激动间隙。之后，更加精细的标测发现，正像Puech等认为的一样，人类房扑折返环是右房的反复激动，其方向在间隔部从脚到头，在游离壁从头到脚（图54-1）。Cosio等和Olshansky等的研究显示在折返环的后下部存在缓慢传导区，折返环的中间阻滞区域包括解剖屏障——腔静脉和功能性阻滞部位——界嵴。Cosio[1]等的进一步研究发现折返环可以反转，产生方向相反的典型房扑[14]。

应用拖带标测和心腔内超声技术研究[15-17]进一步确定折返环路。正如我们知道的，三尖瓣环也是房扑折返环的边界，腔静脉和它们之间的阻滞线是折返环的另一个屏障。最近，Firedman等[18]认为这条阻滞线位于冠状窦区域。而且折返环中存在关键的峡部，峡部由三尖瓣环、下腔静脉口、欧氏嵴和冠状静脉窦围成[15,17,19]，峡部是射频消融治疗典型房扑的靶部位。值得注意的是，Kinder等[20]的研究认为房扑峡部并不是缓慢传导的部位，而且，法国Bordeaux等[21]应用三维标测研究进一步定位了折返环，上部环绕上腔静脉，上腔静脉是关键部位。目前在病人身上也记录到8字折返，但是仅限于个别病人[22,23]。我们认为，如果不是标测技术的限制，应该可以在更多病人身上记录到这种8字折返，只是现有的标测技术没有足够的清晰度。

现在发现了各种各样房扑[9,14,22,28]，包括不典型房扑和左房房扑，其中又包括双波折返（两个波同时沿典型房扑折返环折返）、低环折返（折返波通过房扑峡部激动右房后壁，沿着下腔静脉走行，实际上应用了典型房扑折返环的下部）、房间隔折返、上环折返（非峡部依赖的右房上部折返），环绕右房游离壁功能性阻滞线的折返和左房折返。

开胸心脏术后出现的持续性和反复性房扑与手术切口相关[2]，如果右房游离壁的切口足够长，引起了上下腔静脉之间的阻滞，可以形成典型房扑，折返环路呈上行间隔、下行游离壁或者反过来上行右房游离壁、下行房间隔。

令人感兴趣的是，房扑的开始往往是由于一过性的房颤[11]，Shimizu等[1,12]的标测研究显示，房颤过程中，功能性阻滞对于折返环的形成非常重要，特别是在腔静脉之间形成的功能性阻滞线更是至关重要[12]。

（三）房扑的拖带

第一次关于心动过速的一过性拖带的描述见于开胸心脏术后房扑病人的研究[1]，那时，对一过性拖带还不十分理解。现在我们知道，折返性心动过速的一过性拖带中，起搏波进入可激动间隙后双向传导，其中一个反向传导波，即与自发性的心动过速波相反，它与前一次激动的波相撞；而另一个波正向传导，与自发心动过速的波传导方向一致，正向传导使心动过速持续而且重整为起搏频率[29]。这可以泛泛应用于任何有可激动间隙的折返性心动过速的拖带，目前在室速和房扑犬模型的离体标测研究中已经被证实[1]。

只要满足四个标准中的任何一个（表54-1）就说明存在一过性拖带，因此存在有可激动间隙的折返。但是，即使不满足拖带的任一条标准，拖带也可能发生，这叫做隐匿性拖带[1,29]。这是由于起搏点正位于折返环缓慢传导的远端，但是，在另外部位起搏必须能够一过性拖带（图54-2，54-3）[1]，在折返环的峡部起搏能够引起隐匿性拖带，如房扑的峡部。隐匿性拖带时体表心电图的心动过速的图形（QRS波或者P波）以及激动顺序不会变（图54-4）[15,17,29,30]。这项技术不仅有助于证实折返存在，而且有助于定位折返坏的缓慢传导区域，还有助于分析标测部位在环上还是离环很远[15,17,29,30]。这样的定位有助于在房扑射频消融过程中鉴定房扑折返环的关键峡部[15,17,29,30]。

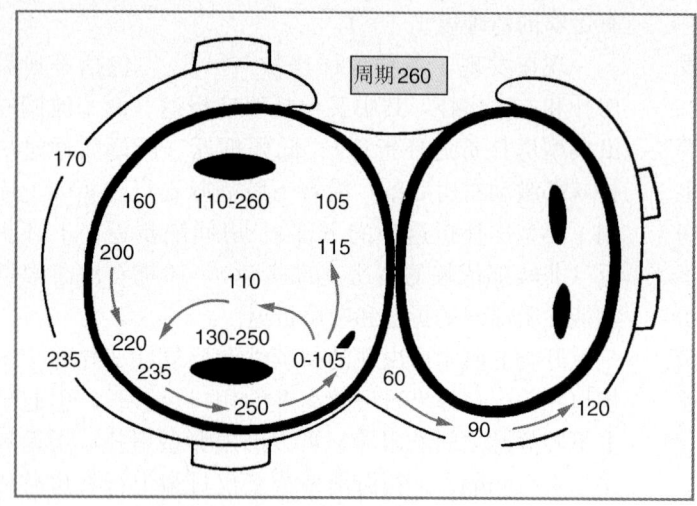

图 54-1 Cosio 所示的典型房扑激动标测图　箭头所示为折返环的方向，图中数字单位为 ms。（引自 Cosio FG, Lopez Gil M, Goicolea A, Et al: Radofrequency ablation of the inferior vena cava-tricuspid valve isthmus in common atrial flutter. Am J Cardiol 71：705-709，1993）

表 54-1　一过性拖带的诊断标准

1. 固定频率快速起搏过程中，心电图表现为稳定的融合波，最后一跳例外，最后一跳拖带了但是没有融合（表现为自发性心动过速的波形）。
2. 表现为进一步的融合，即：任何稳定频率的快速起搏，心电图都表现为稳定的融合波，但是不同的快速频率起搏表现为不同程度的稳定融合。
3. 心动过速终止与一次心跳的一个或多个部位局部传导的阻滞有关，随后阻滞部位产生不同方向的激动，表现为阻滞部位心电图图形的变化，传导时间缩短。
4. 分别用两个高于心动过速的稳定频率起搏时，在另一个部位记录到的传导时间和心电图图形发生了变化，但是没有终止心动过速（心电图进一步融合）。

二、房扑的临床特征

（一）发生率和临床情况

房扑的发病率不详，但男性比女性高发，男女比例为 4.7：1[1]。房扑通常是阵发的，持续时间长短不定，房扑很少是一种持续性心律，持续时间长了，则演变为房颤。外科开胸心脏术后一周，病人好发房扑，这组病人发生室上速的几率 30%，其中三分之一是房扑。而且房扑经常与房颤相关[1,31]，事实上，这两种心律失常经常见于同一个病人，相互转化。房扑也与慢性阻塞性肺病、二尖瓣或者三尖瓣病变、甲状腺疾病、先心病心外科手术涉及右房切开（比如 Mustard、Senning、Fontan 术）相关[1,2]，任何原因引起的心房扩大特别是右房扩大，容易发生房扑[1,8]。

（二）房扑的类型

房扑是由于房内折返引起的快速规则的房性节律，实际上它是最规则的心律失常，逐跳周长几乎完全相同。有两种类型的房扑[1]，Ⅰ型房扑和Ⅱ型房扑。Ⅰ型房扑心房扑动波频率 240～340 或 350 次/分，快速起搏可以拖带或者终止[29]。Ⅱ型房扑不能拖带，

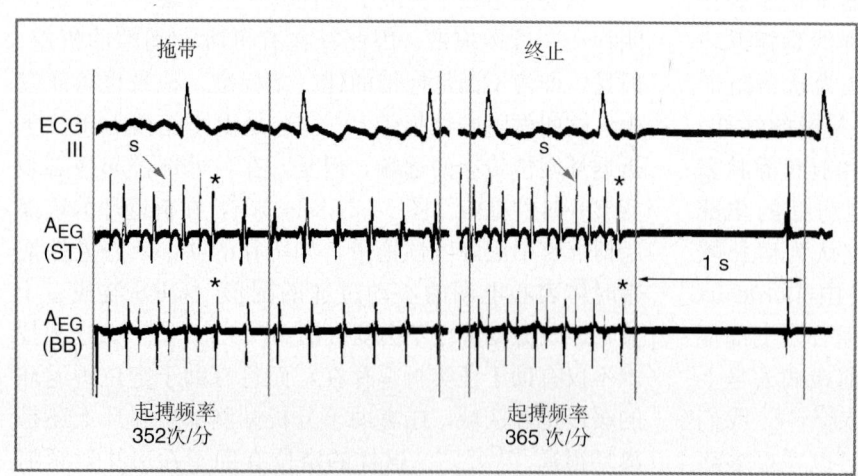

图 54-2　房扑的隐匿性拖带　房扑病人自发性心房扑动频率 320 次/分，在左房后下部快速心房起搏（左，352 次/分，右，365 次/分），起搏 30s 末期同步记录终末嵴（ST）和 Banchmann 束（BB）的双极心内电图（AEG），365 次/分起搏终止房扑，但是每次快速起搏终止都没有拖带，每个记录部位都应用双极电极记录心房电图（AEG），S 代表刺激信号，星号代表最后一个起搏心跳。

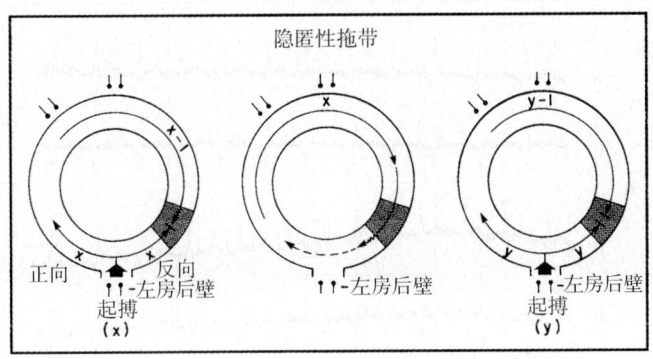

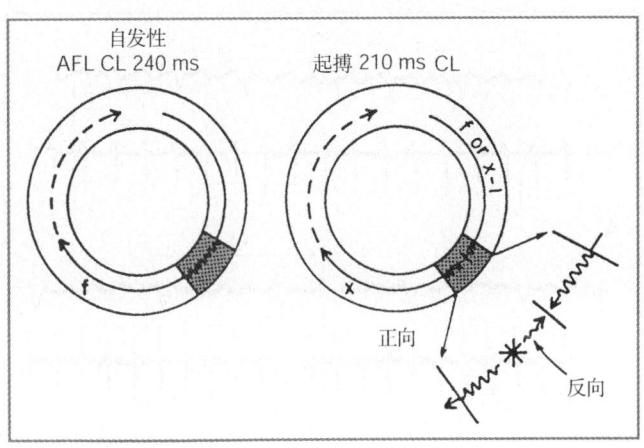

图 54-3　房扑隐匿性拖带的示意图　左图：大箭头所示为起搏脉冲（X）（如图 54-2 所示起搏频率为 352 次/分）从起搏部位（左房后壁）进入折返环，向正反两个方向传导，反向传导波在缓慢传导区发生了阻滞，正传的前一次波（X-1）也在缓慢传导区阻滞，因为落在了起搏心跳 X 的反向传导波的不应期中，正传的波使心动过速持续，并且重整为起搏频率。中图：最后一个起搏波（X）（如图 54-2 所示：352 次/分）完全沿折返环折返，导致房扑重新恢复，这是由于缓慢传导区域没有反向波产生不应期，最后一个波通过了缓慢传导区域，没有拖带的证据。右图：大箭头表示起搏脉冲（Y）（如图 54-2，起搏频率 365 次/分），起搏波进入折返环后，反向传导波在缓慢传导区阻滞，Y-1 的正向传导波也在缓慢传导区阻滞了，这种阻滞与不应期无关。由于正向波和反向波都阻滞了，房扑终止，心电图不容易看出来，因为没有拖带，只有起搏终止才能看出来房扑是否终止了（图 54-2）。

图 54-4　在折返环的峡部和缓慢传导部位起搏，隐匿性拖带房扑　左图：自发性 I 型房扑（AFL）的折返环，心房扑动波周期 240ms（CL），f 代表房扑波。右图：心房扑动波周期＝210ms，在缓慢传导部位起搏（用星号表示），右侧是缓慢传导区的放大，反向传导波在缓慢传导区阻滞，正向传导波就像自发性房扑一样激动心房，前一次心跳不管是房扑（f）或者心房起搏波（X-1），在缓慢传导区域阻滞，另外以前的正传波也可以与反向波相撞，因为反向波只激动心房很小的一部分，因此对心电图没有影响，心房被正向波激动，其传导路径与房扑发作时一样，产生了隐匿性拖带。（引自 Waldo AL：Atrial Flutter：Entrainment characteristics. J cardiovasc Electrophysiol 8：337-352，1997.）

快速起搏可以改变心房电图图形为房颤图形。II 型房扑心房扑动波频率大于 340 或 350 次/分（最快可达 433 次/分），一旦出现，容易演化为房颤，因为心房不能同步 1：1 传导[11,12]，II 型房扑心电图不容易诊断，最好通过心房内电图诊断。欧洲心脏病协会和北美起搏和电生理协会[14]根据房扑机制提出新的分类方法：依赖于峡部的折返；典型房扑或者反向典型房扑，典型房扑激动沿间隔向上传导、沿游离壁向下传导，包括右房峡部；反向典型房扑折返环相同，只是折返的方向相反。在左前斜位分别呈顺钟向传导或者逆钟向传导。90% 房扑符合典型房扑或者反向典型房扑。折返环在左房的房扑称为左房房扑；折返环沿着外科切口的称为切口性房扑，所有其他类型的折返性房速，频率符合房扑的都称为不典型房扑。按这种分类，I 型房扑包括所有心房起搏可以拖带或者终止的折返性房扑。

三、房扑的治疗

（一）房扑的诊断

除了致命的心动过速，所有怀疑房扑的，在治疗之前必须明确诊断，房扑通常可以通过心电图的扑动波诊断，特别是 II 导联、III 导联、aVF 导联和 V₁ 导联。心房扑动波形状恒定并有一定的极性，频率 240～340 次/分[1]，典型房扑时下壁导联扑动波为负向，呈锯齿状（图 54-5），反向典型房扑扑动波在下壁导联为正向[1]。房扑的房室传导比例一般是 2：1 或者 4：1，但是可以不规则，很少情况会有 1：1 传导，1：1 传导多见于预激综合征，旁路前传的不应期很短。另外，1：1 传导可见于所谓 LGL 综合征，这种病人窦律情况下 PR 期间很短；1：1 传导还见于运动或者由于其他临床情况接受儿茶酚胺、拟交感药物、苯妥英钠治疗。房扑的频率和心室反应频率都会受到抗心律失常药物的影响，如果病人应用 I 类抗心律失常药物时，房扑的频率会相应减慢，特别是应用 III 类抗心律失常药物时，房扑的频率会降至 180～200 次/分。

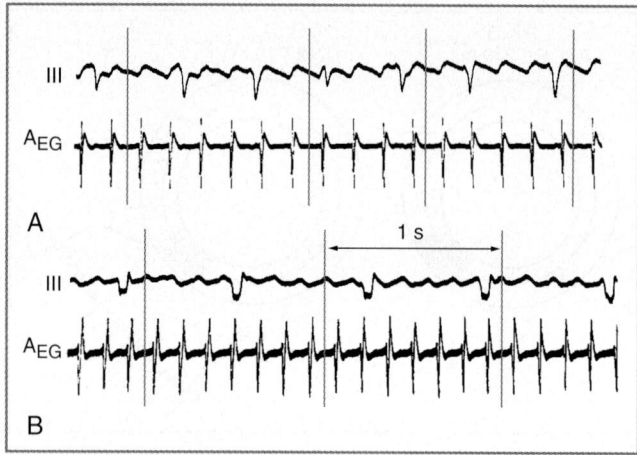

图54-5 A图和B图分别是Ⅰ型房扑心房频率296次/分和Ⅱ型房扑心房率为420次/分时，同步记录Ⅲ导联心电图和双极心房电图（AEG）。每份图均提示房扑的心动周期、极性、形状、心房电图的幅度都是恒定的。（引自Wells JL Jr, Maclean WAH, James TN, Waldo AC: Characteristics of atrial flutter. Studies in man after openheart surgery using fixed atral electrodes. Circulation 60: 665, 1979.）

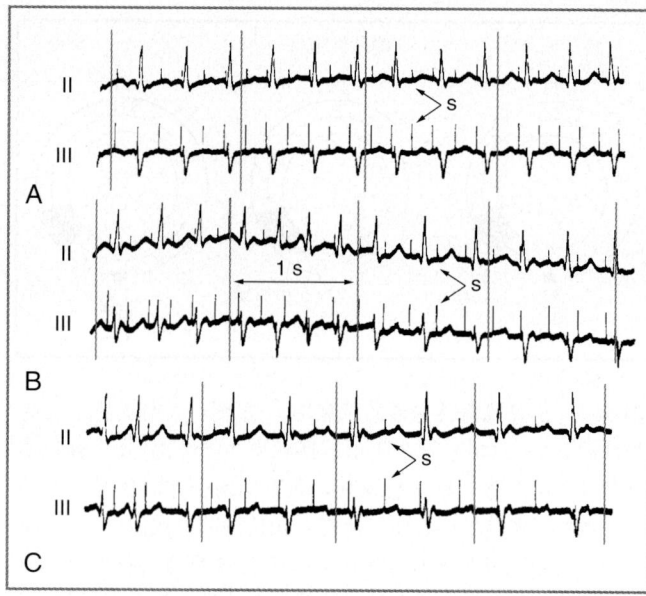

图54-6 A-C图是Ⅰ型房扑，心房率294次/分（心动周期204ms），超速起搏后连续记录的Ⅱ导联和Ⅲ联导心电图。该病人起始超速心房起搏周期为194ms，然后分级递增（起搏频率逐渐递增直至心房波变为正向，然后再降低），起搏周期由171ms降低至157ms（A），在两个导联心房波都是正的。随后起搏周期进一步延长（B、C），即起搏频率减慢，起搏周期长于自发房扑的周期（B图末端），房波仍保持正向波。当起搏周期进一步延长（C），起搏周期长于自发房扑的周期时（B图末端）心房波仍保持正向波。当起搏周期进一步延长（C），房扑没有复发。实际上，心房周期为545ms，起搏频率为110次/分，仍旧能够夺获心房（没有在图中显示）。因此，用分级递增的方法，开始时房扑被一过性拖带，最终被快速起搏终止。时间间隔距为1s。S代表刺激信号。（引自Waldo AL, Maclean WAH, Karp RS, et al: Entrainment and interruption of atrial flutter with atrail pacing, studies in man following open heart surgery. Circulation 56: 737-745, 1977.）

房扑率缓慢，更容易出现1∶1房室传导，导致心室率比用药前更快。

如果标准12导联心电图尚不能明确诊断房扑，情况允许，可应用刺激迷走神经的措施，如按压颈动脉窦、Valsalva动作等方法产生一过性房室阻滞，同时记录心电图。如果是房扑，这些方法可以显露房扑波，如果诊断仍然不清楚，临床情况允许可以采用以下方法：（1）应用食道电极直接记录食道电图，或者在心外科开胸手术过程中在心房放置心外膜电极；（2）或者应用一过性延长房室传导药物，如腺苷、艾司洛尔、维拉帕米、地尔硫䓬、腾喜龙等，可以显露扑动的房波。必须强调的是，宽QRS心动过速（包括室速、室上速伴室内差传及旁路前传的心动过速），用药物鉴别诊断风险较大，通常应该使用同步直流电复律。

（二）急性房扑的治疗

确诊房扑之后，有三种选择来恢复窦律：（1）抗心律失常药物治疗，（静脉应用依布利特，口服氟卡胺300mg，或口服普罗帕酮600mg[1,32]）；（2）直流电复律；（3）快速心房起搏终止房扑[1]。总之，治疗选择取决于病人的临床情况、临床治疗方便与否，以及当时有哪些药物。直流电复律需要应用麻醉剂，对最近刚接受过电复律的病人和严重慢阻肺的病人最好不选择这个方法，可以选择应用抗心律失常药物或快速心房起搏终止房扑，或者用药物控制心室率。对于心外科术后病人的房扑，应用临时心外膜电极快速起搏终止房扑是一个很好的选择[1]。

任何情况下，快速控制房扑心室率都是必要的，可以静脉应用钙通道阻滞剂（地尔硫䓬）或者β受体阻滞剂（艾司洛尔）。如果需要快速恢复窦律，可应用电复律或者快速心房起搏，因为应用抗心律失常药物复律需要时间（依布利特需要1~2h，口服药物需要时间倍增），应用依布利特之前需要注意：（1）血钾必须正常，最好4.0mEq/L以上；（2）QTc小于或等于440ms；（3）心功能不全的患者不建议应用；（4）有可能出现尖端扭转型室速，通常很短暂，不会

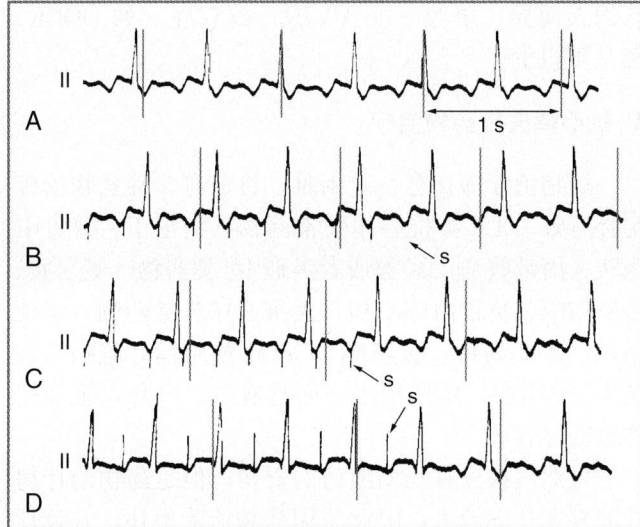

图 54-7 A 图为典型房扑（心房扑动波周期为 264ms）；B 图为高位右房快速起搏，起搏周期分别为 254ms；C 图起搏周期为 242ms；D 图起搏周期为 232ms。所有起搏频率都可以一过性拖带房扑，比较不同周期心房起搏时心房电图的形状，可见心房波逐渐融合。时间线间距为 1s。S 代表刺激信号。（引自 Waldo AL, Maclean WAH, Karp RS, et al: Entrainment and interruption of atrial flutter with atrail pacing, studies in man following open heart surgery. Circulation 56：737-745, 1977.)

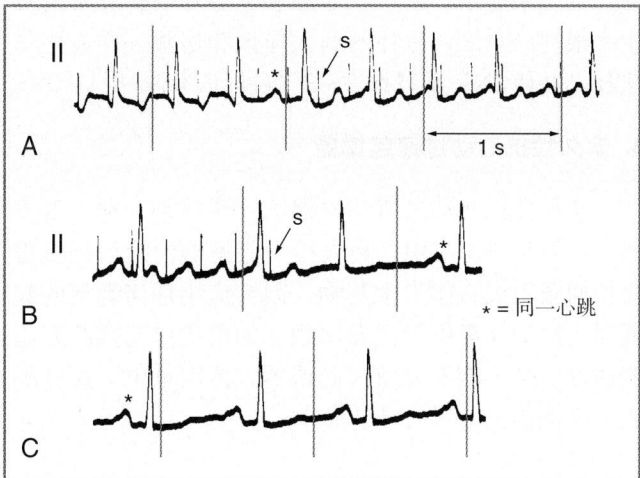

图 54-8 A 图与图 54-7 所示为同一个病人高位右房起搏，心动周期为 224ms 时的 II 导联心电图。注意：第 7 次心房起搏，即：固定频率心房起搏 22s 之后，心房波形突然变正（星号所示）。B 图为同一个病人心房起搏终止时的 II 导联心电图。注意：起搏突然终止之后出现窦律。C 图所示第 1 个心跳（星号所示）与 B 图最后一跳为同一个心跳。时间线间距为 1s。S 代表刺激信号。（引自 WaldoAL, Maclean WAH, Karp RS, et al: Entrainment and interruption of atrial flutter with atrial pacing, studies in man following open heart surgery. Circulation 56：737-745，1977)

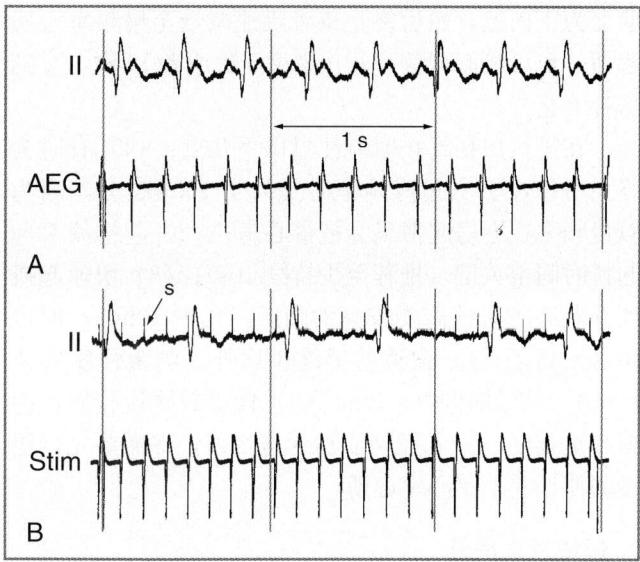

图 54-9 A 图为 I 型房扑，心房率 320 次/分，呈 2∶1 房室传导，心室率 160 次/分时 II 导联心电图及同步记录的心房内电图。该病人行心脏外科手术后，几次偶然的快速心房搏终止了房扑，但是每次房扑都复发了。B 图所示以 450 次/分频率快速起搏心房，可引起房颤，但心室率减慢为 120 次/分，然后应用地高辛，可使心室率进一步减慢。连续快速心房起搏维持房颤以控制心室率，需要 26h，同时应用抗心律失常药物治疗（地高辛和奎尼丁），快速心房起搏终止之后，房颤仍旧存在，但是为一过性的，几分钟之后就转复窦律。时间线间距为 1s。S 代表刺激信号。（引自 Waldo AL, Maclean WAH, Karp RS, et al: Continuous rapid atrial pacing to control recurrent or sustained superventricular tachycardias following open heart surgery. Circulation 54：254，1976.）

引起严重临床后果，但是有时需要电复律、除颤和静脉补充镁剂[32]。电复律和快速心房起搏之前也要应用抗心律失常药物：(1) 增加快速心房起搏转复窦律的成功率（应用奎尼丁、普鲁卡因胺、丙吡胺、依布利特）[1,34]；(2) 抑制电复律后房扑的复发（应用 IA、IC 或 III 类抗心律失常药物）。

1. 快速心房起搏终止 I 型房扑的技术

几种心房起搏技术实用而且有效[1]，任何时候只要可能，尽量选择高位右房起搏，因为 II 导联出现正向波是房扑终止的特征性心电图改变，可以选择分级递增刺激（双极心房起搏，起搏频率比心房频率快 10 次，然后逐渐递增，当 II 导出现正向波，可以突然中止起搏或迅速减慢至慢频率心房起搏）；还可以选择固定起搏频率（图 54-7，54-8）（快速起搏频率是心房频率的 120%～130%，持续 15～30s，或者直到 II 导联变为正向波，然后终止或者迅速减慢至慢频率心房起搏，也可将起搏频率每次递增5次或者10次，直到房扑终止）。

在进行房扑终止时应注意以下几点：（1）有时为终止房扑，心房起搏频率需要大于400次/分，因为较慢频率在心房起搏只会拖带心房；（2）起搏频率和起搏时间很关键（推荐至少持续10s）；（3）快速起搏要夺获心房通常需要较高的强度，至少10mA，但也不必太高；（4）食道起搏终止房扑，刺激强度需要30mA，持续时间9~10s；（5）食道起搏比较痛，起搏越短越好；（6）任何心房起搏之前，都需要先行缓慢起搏证实不是心室起搏。

2. 起搏诱发房颤

在有些病人快速起搏可以诱发房颤，房颤通常持续数秒钟到数分钟，然后自发转为窦律。如果房颤持续发作，心室率也会比房扑时低，而且应用阻滞房室结的药物很容易控制心室率。因而，Ⅰ型房扑反复发作的病人，虽然快速心房起搏可以终止房扑，但也可用持续心房起搏诱发持续性房颤，再用药物控制心室率[1]。

3. 房扑的直流电复律

房扑直流电复律成功率很高，25J可以成功，50J成功率更大，100J是肯定有效的，而且不会有副作用，所以应该首选100J，如果用新的双相波除颤，能量可以再低一些。

（三）慢性房扑的治疗

1. 导管消融术

很多病人房扑反复发作，射频消融可以根治。首先必须标测房扑的折返环，如果房扑折返环包括峡部，峡部消融可以成功治愈房扑[1,19]。然而，有些病人会出现房颤[1,19]。对于那些折返环围绕右房外科手术切口的房扑，消融治疗是可行的，消融线从阻滞中央（外科切口）至传导边界通常是指房室沟[2]。然而，右房切口的心外科术后的瘢痕折返型房扑常常沿经典房扑折返环传导[3,6]。

其他的消融方法还有消融希氏束造成高度房室阻滞（一般为三度房室阻滞），治疗房扑的快速心室率，这种方法适用于消融失败又不耐受药物治疗的病人，需要植入人工心脏起搏器，起搏器的类型应该因人而异，单腔（如VVIR）或双腔（如DDDR）都是可以的。

2. 抗心律失常药物治疗

药物治疗房扑有一定困难，目前有9种药物治疗房扑有效：IA类抗心律失常药物（奎尼丁、普鲁卡因胺、丙吡胺）、IC类或者类似IC类药物（氟卡胺、普罗帕酮、莫雷西嗪）和Ⅲ类抗心律失常药物（索他洛尔、多菲利特、胺碘酮）。没有器质性心脏病，首选IC类药物，副作用小，而且有效，另外，Ⅲ类药物也同样有效。

虽然现在没有长期随访的资料，但是药物治疗房扑的复发几率较大，因此使用药物治疗房扑，有效性应该用复发频率来衡量，如果很少复发，治疗应该是有效的。如果病人需要治疗应该首选消融治疗而不是药物，房扑病人不适宜长期药物治疗。

3. 抗凝治疗

虽然小样本的心外科手术病人的研究证实，房扑很少出现血栓和卒中[1]，其他的研究结果认为房扑发生卒中的几率与房颤相似[1,31,35,37]。而且临床上，房扑和房颤经常并存[31]，另外，房扑病人的食道超声[35-39]结果显示，超声自显影和左心耳明显异常的发生率很高。总之，房扑的病人应该和房颤一样应用华法林，并使INR维持在2~3（目标值2.5）[40]。

4. 永久性抗心动过速起搏器

永久性抗心动过速起搏器治疗房扑是一种有效方法[1]，但是很少应用。病人接受起搏器治疗后仍然需要长期服用抗心律失常药物。因为应用任何类型的起搏器治疗房扑都可能诱发房颤。如果任何起搏的方法能诱发房颤，就不要植入起搏器，再次重申，这样的病人应该首先选择射频消融术。

四、总　结

大量的证据表明房扑是由折返所致，折返环位于右房，房扑很容易诊断，心房起搏、直流电复律或抗心律失常药物单独应用或联合应用都可以终止房扑，长期应用抗心律失常药物抑制房扑复发是没有指征的，导管消融折返环的关键部位可以治愈房扑。

（杨延宗　林治湖　译）

参 考 文 献

1. Waldo AL: Atrial flutter: From mechanism to treatment. In Camm AJ (ed): Clinical Approaches to Tachyarrhythmias. Armonk, NY, Futura Publishing, 2001, pp 1–56.
2. VanHare GF, Lesh MD, Ross BA, et al: Mapping and radiofrequency ablation of intraatrial reentrant tachycardia after the Senning or Mustard procedure for transposition of the great arteries. Am J Cardiol 77:985–991, 1996.
3. Chan DP, Van Hare GF, Mackall JA, et al: Importance of atrial flutter isthmus in post-operative intra-atrial reentrant tachycardia. Circulation 102:1283–1289, 2000.
4. Kanter RJ, Papagiannis J, Carboni MP, et al: Radiofrequency catheter ablation of supraventricular tachycardia substrates after Mustard and Senning operations for d-transposition of the great arteries. J Am Coll Cardiol 35:428–441, 2000.
5. Collins KK, Love BA, Walsh EP, et al: Location of acutely successful radiofrequency catheter ablation of intraatrial reentrant tachycardia in patients with congenital heart disease. Am J Cardiol 86:969–974, 2000.
6. Anne W, van Rensburg H, Adams J, et al: Ablation of post-surgical intra-atrial tachycardia. Predilection target sites and mapping approach. Eur Heart J 23:1609–1616, 2002.
7. Tomita Y, Matsuo K, Sahadevan J, et al: Role of functional block extension in lesion related to atrial flutter. Circulation 102:1025–1030, 2001.
8. Gandhi SK, Bromberg BI, Schuessler RB, et al: Left-sided atrial flutter: Characterization of a novel complication of pediatric lung transplantation in an acute canine model. J Thorac Cardiovasc Surg 112:992–1001, 1996.
9. Gandhi SK, Bromberg BI, Mallory GB, Huddleston CB: Atrial flutter: A newly recognized complication of pediatric lung transplantation. J Thorac Cardiovasc Surg 112:984–991, 1996.
10. Gillinov AM, Blackstone EH, McCarthy PM: Atrial fibrillation: Current surgical options and their assessment. Ann Thorac Surg 74:2210–2217, 2002.
11. Waldo AL, Cooper TB: Spontaneous onset of Type I atrial flutter in patients. J Am Coll Cardiol 28:707–712, 1996.
12. Waldo AL: Mechanisms of atrial flutter and atrial fibrillation: Distinct entities or two sides of the same coin? Cardiovasc Res 54:217–229, 2002.
13. Uno K, Kumagai K, Khrestian C, Waldo AL: New insights regarding the atrial flutter reentrant circuit in the canine sterile pericarditis model [abstract]. J Am Coll Cardiol 229:254A, 1997.
14. Saoudi N, Cosio F, Waldo A, et al: Classification of atrial flutter and regular atrial tachycardia according to electrophysiologic mechanism and anatomical bases. A statement from a joint expert group from the Working Group of Arrhythmias of the European Society of Cardiology and the North American Society of Pacing and Electrophysiology. Eur Heart J 22:1162–1182, 2001; and J Cardiovasc Electrophysiol 12:852–866, 2001.
15. Olgin J, Kalman J, Fitzpatrick A, et al: The role of right atrial endocardial structures as barriers to conduction during human Type I atrial flutter: Activation and entrainment mapping guided by intracardiac echocardiography. Circulation 92:1831–1848, 1995.
16. Olgin JE, Kalman JM, Lesh MD: Conduction barriers in human atrial flutter: Correlation of electrophysiology and anatomy. J Cardiovasc Electrophysiol 7:1112–1126, 1996.
17. Nakagawa H, Lazzara R, Khastgir T, et al: Role of the tricuspid annulus and the Eustachian valve/ridge on atrial flutter. Relevance to catheter ablation of the septal isthmus and a new technique for rapid identification of ablation success. Circulation 94:407–424, 1996.
18. Friedman PA, Luria D, Fenton AM, et al: Global right atrial mapping of human atrial flutter: The presence of posteromedial (sinus venosa region) functional block and double potentials. Circulation 101:1568–1577, 2000.
19. Cosio FG, Lopez-Gil M, Giocolea A, et al: Radiofrequency ablation of the inferior vena cava–tricuspid valve isthmus in common atrial flutter. Am J Cardiol 71:705–709, 1993.
20. Kinder C, Kall J, Kopp D, et al: Conduction properties of the inferior vena cava–tricuspid annular isthmus in patients with typical atrial flutter. J Cardiovasc Electrophysiol 8:727–737, 1997.
21. Shah DC, Jais P, Haissaguerre M, et al: Three-dimensional mapping of the common atrial flutter circuit in the right atrium. Circulation 96:3904–3912, 1997.
22. Shah D, Jais P, Takahashi A, et al: Dual-loop intra-atrial reentry in humans. Circulation 101:631–639, 2000.
23. Kall JG, Rubenstein DS, Kopp DE, et al: Atypical atrial flutter originating in the right atrial free wall. Circulation 101:270–279, 2000.
24. Olgin JE, Jayachandran JV, Engelstein E, et al: Atrial macroreentry involving the myocardium of the coronary sinus: A unique mechanism for atypical atrial flutter. J Cardiovasc Electrophysiol 9:1094–1099, 1998.
25. Cheng J, Scheinman MM: Acceleration of typical atrial flutter due to double wave reentry induced by programmed electrical stimulation. Circulation 97:1589–1596, 1998.
26. Cheng J, Cabeen WR Jr, Scheinman MM: Right atrial flutter due to lower loop reentry: Mechanism and anatomic substrates. Circulation 99:1700–1705, 1999.
27. Scheinman MM, Cheng J, Yang Y: Mechanisms and clinical implications of atypical atrial flutter. J Cardiovasc Electrophysiol 10:1153–1157, 1999.
28. Yang Y, Cheng J, Bochoeyer A, et al: Atypical right atrial flutter patterns. Circulation 103:3092–3098, 2001.
29. Waldo AL: Atrial flutter: Entrainment characteristics. J Cardiovasc Electrophysiol 8:337–352, 1997.
30. Van Hare G, Waldo AL: The atrial flutter reentrant circuit: Additional pieces of the puzzle. Circulation 94:244–246, 1996.
31. Biblo AL, Yuan Z, Quan KJ, et al: Risk of stroke in patients with atrial flutter. Am J Cardiol 87:346–349, 2001.
32. Ellenbogen KA, Stambler BS, Wood MA, et al: Efficacy of intravenous ibutilide for rapid termination of atrial fibrillation and atrial flutter: A dose-response study. J Am Coll Cardiol 28:130–136, 1996.
33. Boriani G, Biffi M, Capucci A, et al: Oral propafenone to convert recent-onset atrial fibrillation in patients with and without underlying heart disease. A randomized, controlled trial. Ann Intern Med 126:621–625, 1997.
34. Stambler BS, Wood MA, Ellenbogen KA: Comparative efficacy of of atrial flutter by atrial overdrive pacing. Am J Cardiol 77:960–966, 1996.
35. Wood KA, Eisenberg SJ, Kalman JM, et al: Risk of thromboembolism in chronic atrial flutter. Am J Cardiol 79:1043–1047, 1997.
36. Weiss R, Marcovitz P, Knight BP, et al: Acute changes in spontaneous echo contrast and atrial function after cardioversion of persistent atrial flutter. Am J Cardiol 82:1052–1055, 1998.
37. Seidl K, Haver B, Schwick NG, et al: Risk of thromboembolic events in patients with atrial flutter. Am J Cardiol 82:580–584, 1998.
38. Grimm RA, Stewart WJ, Arheart KL, et al: Left atrial appendage "stunning" after electrical cardioversion of atrial flutter: An attenuated response compared with atrial fibrillation as the mechanism for lower susceptibility to thromboembolic events. J Am Coll Cardiol 29:582–589, 1997.
39. Irani WN, Grayburn PA, Afridi I: Prevalence of thrombus, spontaneous echo contrast, and atrial stunning in patients undergoing cardioversion of atrial flutter: A prospective study using transesophageal echocardiography. J Am Coll Cardiol 29:582–589, 1997.
40. Fuster V, Ryden LE, Asinger RW, et al: ACC/AHA/ESC Guidelines for the management of patients with atrial fibrillation: Executive summary. Circulation 104:2118–2150, 2001.

第 55 章

房性心动过速

Kenneth A. Ellenbogen, Mark A. Wood

本章目录
- 分类和机制 ········· 494
- 局灶性房性心动过速 ········· 494
- 局灶性房速的心电图定位 ········· 495
- 房速的心脏电生理学鉴别诊断 ········· 499
- 大折返性房速 ········· 502
- 大折返性房速的心电图特点 ········· 503
- 大折返性房速的特殊类型 ········· 503

房性心动过速并不是常见的室上性心动过速。大多数的临床研究发现，在所有因室上性心律失常就诊行心脏电生理检查的成人患者中，房速大约占5%。而在儿童患者中发生率更高，无先天性心脏病的儿童患者中房速大约占10%～15%，而在患先天性心脏病行外科手术后的儿童患者中这个比例还要高。

本章目的是回顾房性心动过速的分类、机制、心电图定位和心脏电生理学特点方面的新进展。

一、分类和机制

欧洲心脏病学会和北美起搏与电生理学会的专家组按照发生机制和解剖定位的不同对房扑和规律性房性心动过速进行了分类[1]。房性心动过速是指起源于心房并有规律心房律的心动过速，进一步分为局灶性或大折返性房速。局灶性房速可能是由于自律性机制、触发机制或微折返机制所引起。局灶性房速是激动由单一兴奋灶呈放射状、圆形或向心性向外传播，而并不存在电活动跨越整个折返环的情况。大折返性房速是由于折返激动通过一个相对较大的并有潜在明确特点的折返环所引起。大折返性房速以电活动环绕整个折返环反复激动模式为特点。已知的激动模式包括单一折返环（如典型房扑）、2个折返环形成的8字折返以及通过临近瘢痕或解剖学屏障处（如三尖瓣）的狭窄通道所形成的折返。典型房扑、低位折返环性折返、双折返环折返、左房大折返性房速、瘢痕性房速、反向典型房扑以及右房游离壁大折返性房速均属于大折返性房速。

按照这种分类方法可能使一部分房速，如不适当性窦速和窦房折返性心动过速不易分类。这种分类方法除了这些局限性以及临床工作中并不使用发生机制来分类等限制外，用局灶性还是大折返性来分类是很有用的。因为大折返性房速需要多点消融并需要使用拖带或标测瘢痕折返环的技术，所以这种分类法对于消融术有重要意义。

二、局灶性房性心动过速

局灶性房速的三个可能机制是微折返机制、自律性异常机制和触发机制。Chen 及其同事使用多种起搏和药物方法研究了 36 例房速患者[2]。其中70%的患者没有器质性心脏病。并根据下述发现将心动过速分为三种类型。

出现下述一个或多个特点者定义为自律性房速：(1) 房速仅能通过输注异丙肾上腺素诱发；(2) 程序刺激不能诱发或终止房速；(3) 房速可被超速起搏一过性抑制但可以逐渐恢复其心房率；(4) 普萘洛尔可终止心动过速；(5) 房速发作和终止有温醒和冷却现象；(6) 腺苷不能终止房速。36 例患者中 7 例患者可能是自律性房速。

36例房速患者中9例可能是触发性房速。触发性房速有下述的一项或几项特点：（1）快速心房起搏或心房期前刺激需要达到临界周长才能诱发房速；（2）房速不能被拖带但可以超速抑制或终止房速；（3）在房速诱发前使用单相电位记录导管可以记录到延迟后除极电位，但在远离心动过速的区域不能记录到；（4）腺苷可以终止房速；（5）诱发房速时很少需要异丙肾上腺素；（6）双嘧达莫、普萘洛尔、维拉帕米、氯化腾喜龙、Valsalva动作和颈动脉窦按压在所有患者中均可终止房速。

20例患者为微折返性房速。微折返性房速有下述特点：（1）使用心房起搏和期前刺激可以重复诱发和终止房速；（2）使用单相动作电位导管不能记录到延迟后除极；（3）心动过速时起搏可显性和隐匿性拖带心动过速；（4）维拉帕米和腺苷可以终止房速；（5）诱发房速的期间刺激联律间期和心动过速第一跳的间期呈反变关系。

这项研究的主要局限性是不同机制的房速其药物反应特点上有重叠。比如，维拉帕米和腺苷均可终止大折返性房速和触发性房速。不同的机制其临床意义并不清楚。Chen及其同事进行文献检索以确定房速的机制是否对成功消融有所帮助[3]。他们将房速分为自律性和非自律性两组。自律性房速在儿童患者中更常见并常为阵发性。右房自律性房速最常见的起源位置在高位右房并沿界嵴分布。多因素分析表明心动过速的起源位置并不能预测其机制。

详细的激动顺序标测可用来确定房速的机制。在一项研究中，对10例曾行心脏外科手术的房速患者的13种房速进行了右房电解剖学标测（CARTO，Biosense Webster）。其中3例患者为局灶性房速，7例患者为大折返性房速。这种标测系统可以快速分辨出局灶性和大折返性房速。在局灶性房速患者中，等时性标测可见激动由最早激动点向各个方向呈放射状传播（图55-1），右房激动时间显著短于心动过速周期，平均大约占心动过速周期的14%。大折返性房速患者的等时性标测中显示激动沿右房呈连续性传播，最早激动点与最末激动点临近（图55-2），右房激动时间与心动过速周期相似，大约占心动过速周期的70%或更多。

Engelstein及其同事仔细研究了腺苷对房速的作用[5]，并在27例患者中检验了腺苷对不同机制房速的作用。其中5例患者为房内折返性房速，7例患者为自律性房速，1例患者为触发性房速（其他14例患者为其他机制——窦房折返性房速或房扑）。腺苷对折返性房速患者没有作用，对自律性房速患者可以一过性抑制或减慢房速的心房率，可终止触发性房速。Kall及其同事[6]在17例房速患者中研究了6～12mg腺苷的作用。结果显示腺苷可以终止3例患者（18%）的房速，一过性抑制4例患者（18%）房速的心房率，在其他10例患者中可以产生完全性房室阻滞但未影响心动过速周期。基于这个发现，作者认为异丙肾上腺素可诱发的自律性房速可以被腺苷一过性抑制。由房性期前刺激诱发和终止的房速患者中不足50%对腺苷敏感，而自发性房速且不能被房性期前刺激诱发的患者中也只有不足50%对腺苷敏感。最后，这些研究者认为房速对腺苷的敏感性并不能说明房速的机制。Lerman及其同事[7]对30例房速患者使用了3～18mg腺苷。其中15例患者终止了心动过速，3例患者的心动过速被一过性抑制。腺苷对其余的患者无效。腺苷的作用是可重复的。腺苷对13例大折返性房速患者中的12例无效。17例局灶性房速患者中14例的心动过速终止，其余3例的房速被一过性抑制。绝大多数的房速起源于界嵴或心房的其他部位并呈无休止性反复发作的形式。Lerman及其同事与Chen及其同事观察结果的不同可能由于两项研究对于判断腺苷终止房性早搏诱发的心动过速以及确定心动过速机制的标准可能有不同。

Chiale及其同事[8]近来报道了8例反复单形性无休止性房速，心动过速发作至终止时可见到心动过速周期逐渐延长。使用比心动过速周期更长的心房周期起搏或静脉推注利多卡因可以终止房速，但静脉应用维拉帕米无效。其中2例患者使用美西律有效。心动过速均位于右房，其确切机制仍有待进一步研究。

自主神经系统可能在一部分房速患者的诱发或触发中起一定的作用，但确切机制仍不清楚，自主神经系统的作用可由心房容量来调节。体位改变、打嗝、吞咽和吸气可触发房速以及由Valsalva动作、氯化腾喜龙或β肾上腺素能阻滞剂可终止房速都表明了自主神经系统的这一作用。

三、局灶性房速的心电图定位

总的来说局灶性房速在所有心电图导联上都可以见到由等电位线所分隔的P波。有大量文献阐述了P

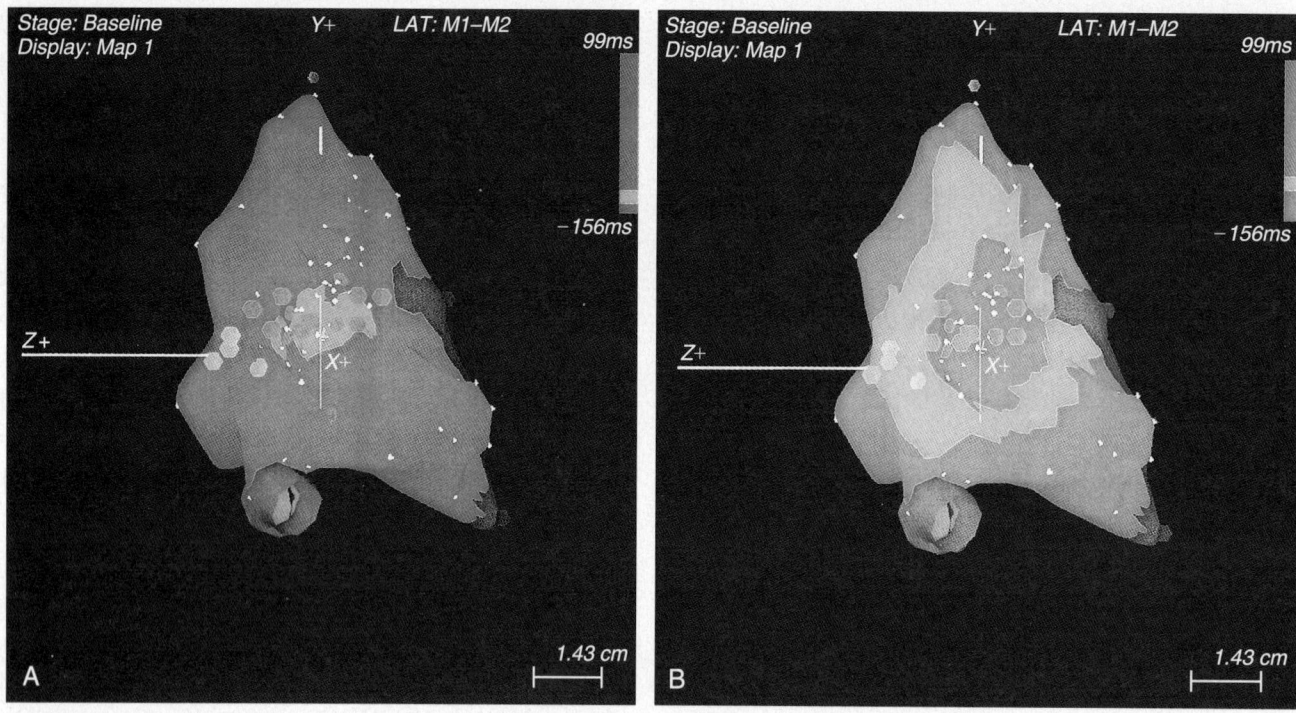

图 55-1　开胸心脏手术后患者的局灶性房速的电解剖标测图序。标测图显示心房激动由局灶起源点呈离心性播散。（见彩图 26）房速起源点位于右房游离壁，图中显示了房速时心房激动的顺

波形态和心房起源位置的关系。本文回顾了在电生理检查时或开胸心脏手术时进行不同部位起搏的早期文献。这种算法虽然在 P 波形态上有重叠，但由于房速的起源位置相对较少所以这种算法仍很有用。P 波形态重叠说明在使用起搏标测研究时空间分辨率有限，只

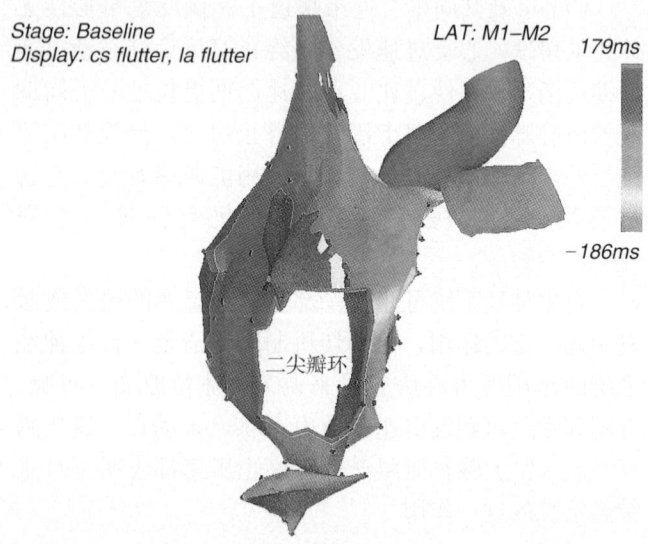

图 55-2　大折返性房速的左房电解剖图　有二尖瓣疾病病史的患者发生了大折返性房速，电解剖图显示房速起源于临近左下肺静脉的折返环。使用由左下肺静脉至二尖瓣环的连续阻滞线成功消融了本例心动过速。（见彩图 27）

有两个不同起搏位置相差 2cm 时方可鉴别 P 波的形态。此外 P 波常常在心动过速时被 T 波和 QRS 波掩盖。最后，鉴别房速的算法主要是从没有器质性心脏病和心房扩张的房速患者中分析得出的（图 55-3 和 55-4）。

房速起源的主要位置包括界嵴区域、肺静脉内或附近（上肺静脉更为常见）、冠状静脉窦内或附近、上腔静脉、房间隔和 Koch 三角。Tang 及其同事[9]建立了进行房速定位的算法。他们研究了 31 例成功标测和消融房速患者的 12 导联心电图，并建立了鉴别右房房速和左房房速的算法，其敏感性为 88%～93%，特异性为 79%～88%。aVL 和 V_1 导联的 P 波形态最有助于鉴别右房房速和左房房速。aVL 导联的 P 波呈正向或双向说明房速起源于右房，而 V_1 导联 P 波正向说明房速起源于左房。但对于起源于右上肺静脉的房速这种算法不能准确预测，起源于右上肺静脉的房速其 aVL 导联的 P 波可呈正向，而按照上述方法其 P 波应是负向，这可能是因为右上肺静脉在解剖位置上更临近高位右心房的缘故。在右上肺静脉起源的房速中，仔细观察窦性心律和房速发作时 V_1 导联的 P 波形态，可以发现其由双向变为正向。Tada 及其同事进一步改进了算法以定位右房房速[10]。按照右房在左前斜位的影像，在消融时进一步将房速分为起源于高侧位、下侧位和下中位。aVR 导联的负向 P 波说明

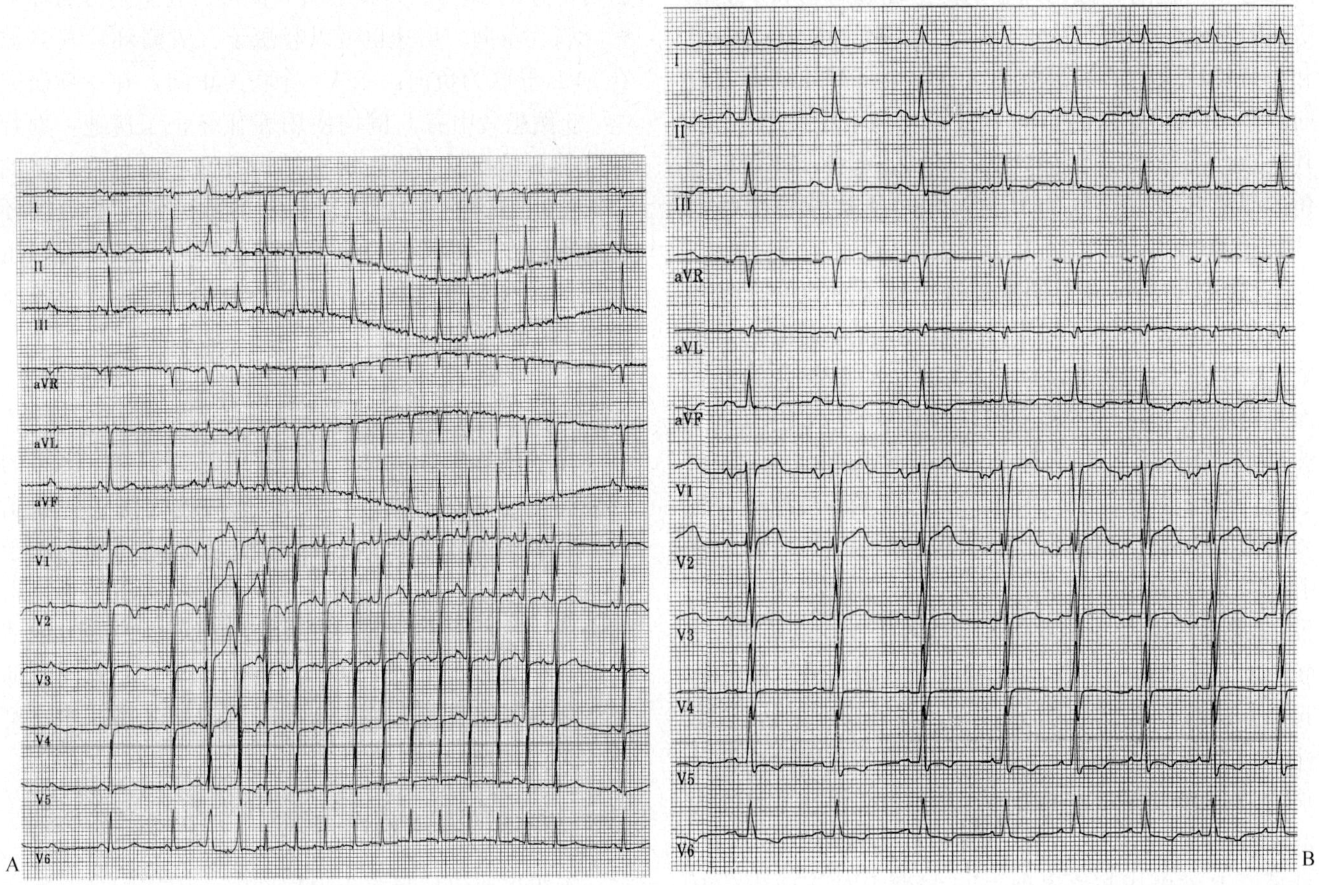

55 房性心动过速

图 55-3 A：起源于二尖瓣的房速。注意其在 V_1 导联的 P 波形态呈正向，而在下壁导联的 P 波形态倒置。B：起源于右房游离壁的房速。注意其在 V_1 导联 P 波倒置。

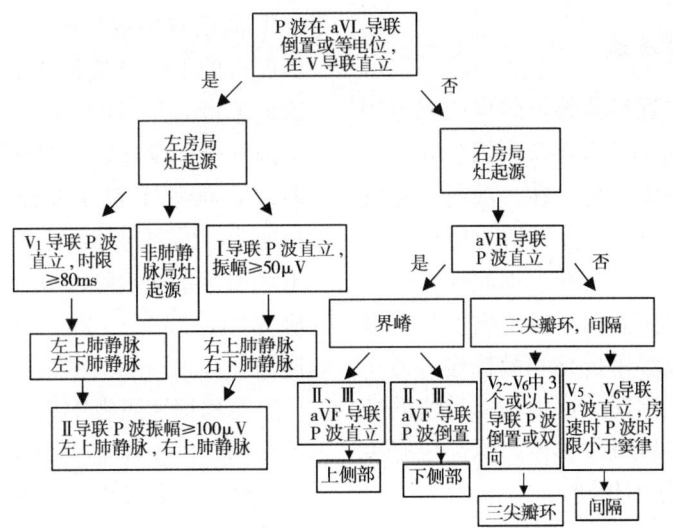

图 55-4 局灶性房速的定位算法（改编自参考文献 9～15）

房速起源于界嵴，其敏感性为100%，特异性为93%。下壁导联的正向P波可以鉴别出上侧位房速和下侧位房速，其敏感性为86%，特异性为100%。在下中位和下侧位房速中P波形态在至少一个下壁导联中为负向。V_5和V_6导联的负向P波说明为下中位的房速，其敏感性为92%，特异性为100%。起源于Koch三角的房速其下壁导联的P波时限短于窦性心律时限（图55-4）。

Haissaguerre及其同事近来报道了对肺静脉起源房速的定位算法[11]。基于30例患者的分析建立了区别左肺静脉和右肺静脉的三条标准。aVL导联的直立而相对较低平的P波和Ⅰ导联的高于$50\mu V$的直立P波表明起源于右上肺静脉，其特异性分别为100%和97%，敏感性分别为38%和72%。这两条标准的阳性预测值为100%和98%。Ⅱ导联有顿挫的P波对于左上肺静脉起源的预测特异性为95%，敏感性为39%。Ⅲ/Ⅱ导联的P波振幅比例大于或等于0.8以及V_1导联的P波时限大于80ms也有助于鉴别左或右肺静脉起源。这两个标准的特异性分别为75%和73%，敏感性分别为96%和85%，对于左肺静脉的阳性预测值分别为79%和76%。左肺静脉起源的特点是在Ⅰ导联为低电压、低平的P波，在aVL导联为负向P波，Ⅱ、Ⅲ导联P波电压与之类似，V_1导联P波正向成分时限延长。上肺静脉起源的房速与下肺静脉起源房速在P波振幅上有显著不同，上肺静脉起源房速Ⅱ导联P波振幅高于或等于$100\mu V$。使用这个标准鉴别上肺或下肺静脉起源特异性为74%，敏感性为81%，其阳性预测值为86%。

（一）起源于界嵴部位的房速

腔内心电图对于鉴别临近界嵴部位的房速很有用处[12]。房速可能产生于界嵴的所有部位，因为其是无器质性心脏病患者房速的好发部位。在一项研究中发现界嵴房速占所有房速的2/3，故称界嵴为房速的点火环。这个区域的房速发作几率高的生理原因是因为界嵴组织内细胞与细胞间的横向耦联较差而使其有显著的各向异性，这可能形成缓慢传导和微折返。另一原因可能是含有自律性的细胞团。这种心动过速的特点上文已经阐述，并与其在界嵴的具体起源部位有关（如界嵴的上部或下部特点各不相同）。

（二）起源于房室瓣环的房速

数个研究报道引起了对这种心动过速的注意[13-15]。起源于三尖瓣环的房速并不常见，一项研究报道其占右房房速的13%。其典型的P波形态在胸前导联和下壁导联为负向。房速也可以起源于二尖瓣环，其P波在aVL导联为负向，于V_1导联为正向。在一项研究中，6例患者中有5例均使用腺苷终止了房速，而且腺苷的剂量均低于终止房室结折返性心动过速剂量的1/2。由于这种心动过速对腺苷的敏感性和临近瓣环的细胞的电生理特性类似于房室结特性并缺少连接蛋白43，所以推测这种心动过速的机制可能是涉及这些结样细胞的微折返。

（三）起源于冠状窦口肌束的房速

在一项右房房速的研究中报道起源于这一区域的局灶性房速大约占12%[16]。多数房速起源于冠状窦口的外缘或紧临口内。在一项报道中发现房速起源于冠状窦内深处，推测可能是起源于冠状窦肌束中，因为心动过速不能由左房心内膜消融而可由冠状窦内消融成功。其致心律失常基质推测是与左房心外膜延伸环绕冠状窦的肌束有关。起源于冠状窦的房速中常可见到V_6导联的负向P波。

（四）起源于房间隔的房速

本组房速包括起源于上房间隔、中房间隔、下房间隔和Koch三角的房速[17-22]。这种房速与起源于三尖瓣环的房速类似，比界嵴处房速对腺苷更敏感。此外，在一项研究中发现45%的间隔房速需要使用异丙肾上腺素诱发，而起源于右房游离壁的房速仅有32%的患者需要。前间隔和中间隔的右房房速在V_1导联上P波呈双向或负向。V_1导联上P波呈双向或负向而所有的下壁导联P波呈正向或双向常支持前间隔房速的诊断；V_1导联上P波呈双向或负向而在至少2个或3个下壁导联上P波为负向支持中间隔房速的诊断。V_1导联P波正向而所有的下壁导联P波均负向说明为后间隔房速。电生理检查对于鉴别这种房速和不典型房室结双路径或间隔部旁道非常重要。在一些研究中，27%~35%的患者为起源于此区域的房速。

右房房速患者中约10%的患者起源于Koch三角的顶部（房室结移行细胞区）。这种心动过速也对腺苷敏感并需要异丙肾上腺素诱发。多数患者可在不损伤房室结的情况下消融成功。心动过速时的P波时限比窦性心律时短20ms。在无器质性心脏病患者仔细标测左房也很重要。在右房单侧心房激动标测不能分辨房速是起源于左或右房，激动经过 Bachmann 束快速跨间隔传播可产生早期的右侧突破点。在左房房速患者，一项研究中发现 P 波在 V_1 导联是正向的，但其他研究中并不是如此[21,22]。在一项 16 例患者的研究中，其最早心房激动位于 Koch 三角，但在 40% 的患者发现房速起源于左房。

（五）窦房折返性心动过速

起源于窦房结区域的房速是由于临近窦房结或结周组织（上位界嵴）的微折返所引起。心动过速时 P 波形态与窦性心律时 P 波形态相同。局灶性房速也可起源于上腔静脉[23,24]。起源于上腔静脉的房速可传导至右房。也有报道在上腔静脉中房颤样传导伴有传出阻滞时表现类似于右房房速。在一例报道中，使用网篮电极证实了上腔静脉至右房连接处的传导延缓在心动过速的诱发中起了一定作用[24]。

（六）不适宜性窦性心动过速

不适宜性窦速并不常见，对其特点了解也较少，可能是一组异质性的疾病。特点是持续性的静息时心率升高，并在较轻的身体活动时心率过度增加。一些患者的固有心率增加，其他患者对异丙肾上腺素的反应增强。心电图特点是 P 波形态与窦性心律时相同。一些患者可能有原发性自主神经系统功能异常、体位性直立性心动过速或原发性窦房结功能异常等疾病。近来一项对 18 例不适宜性窦速患者使用静脉腺苷（0.1 至 0.15mg/kg）的研究发现这类患者对腺苷反应并不敏感，与行电生理检查的年龄匹配的患者相比其窦性周期的延长较少[25]。在行药物自主神经阻滞后也能见到这种现象。说明在这种综合征中窦房结可能存在器质性病变。

四、房速的心脏电生理学鉴别诊断

房速尤其是间隔部房速需要与隐匿性间隔部旁路、房室结折返性心动过速及其变异型以及其他少见心动过速如隐匿性结室旁路、结束旁路折返相鉴别。其中最重要的心脏电生理或心电图特点是房室阻滞。当出现房室阻滞时，即排除了隐匿性旁路的可能。

在室上性心动过速患者中腺苷是十分有用的鉴别诊断方法[26]。在由 Scheinman 及其同事的报道中，229 例室上速患者在电生理检查中静脉弹丸式推注 6~18mg 腺苷。房速患者（53 例）对腺苷的反应与其起源位置无关。56% 的房速患者应用腺苷后心动过速被抑制或终止，但对鉴别自律性或触发以及折返性房速并无帮助作用。使用腺苷前只有房速的患者出现心动过速周期的振荡现象（23%）。在使用腺苷后只有房速患者可以见到房室阻滞现象，但只有 27% 的患者出现。

有许多起搏方法用来鉴别房速和其他类型的室上速（表 55-1 和表 55-2）[27-29]。心室起搏可以鉴别房速与房室折返性心动过速和房室折返性心动过速。于右室发放周期远快于心动过速的 3~6 个猝发刺激（或使用单个或成对心室早搏刺激）可以终止、拖带心动过速或使心室与心动过速分离。如果心室与心动过速分离，可以排除有旁路参与。如果猝发刺激可以反复终止心动过速而并没有传导至心房，可以排除房速。也可以在右室发放较长时间的猝发刺激，并使刺激周期仅略短于心动过速周期。当心房率加速至起搏频率时说明存在 1:1 的室房传导，而且当起搏时心房激动顺序与心动过速时顺序不同时，说明存在房速或有房室旁路作为辅助。如果心房激动顺序一致，并且当停止起搏时，随着最后的心室起搏节律，腔内电图显示 V-A-A-V 顺序（加速至起搏频率的最后一跳房波跟随着另一个房波，并位于下一个室波之前），这说明心动过速为房速[28]。间隔部慢旁路和慢慢型房室结双路径患者有时可以见到假性 V-A-A-V 反应。

心房起搏也有助于鉴别多种不同类型的室上性心动过速。心动过速时以略短于心动过速周期的频率行右房起搏可以终止心动过速或在起搏终止时心动过速继续发作。如果回归周期的 VA 间期与心动过速时 VA 间期差在 10ms 以内，那么心动过速可能是房室结折返或旁路折返。如果 VA 间期多变或不同，那么心动过速可能为房速。第二种方法是在心动过速时以能产生房室阻滞的最小频率超速心房起搏。测量起搏停止时的最后一个心房希氏束间期。如果心动过速终止时，其 AH 间期与心动过速继续发作时的 AH 间期相比较短，心动过速可能是房室结依赖型而不是房速。另一个方法是比较心动过速时以及以心动过速周期或接近周期的频率高位右房起搏时的 AH 间期。如果心房快速起搏时的 AH 间期比心动过速时的 AH 间期长 40ms 以上，不典型房室结折返的可能性更大。对于房速和隐匿性折返性心动过速，AH 间期的差别应在 20ms 以内。

表 55-1 心动过速基本现象和特点的发生率及其在诊断中的价值

基本现象和特点	发生率(%)	敏感性(%) AVNRT	敏感性(%) ORT	敏感性(%) AT	特异性(%) AVNRT	特异性(%) ORT	特异性(%) AT	PPV(%) AVNRT	PPV(%) ORT	PPV(%) AT	NPV(%) AVNRT	NPV(%) ORT	NPV(%) AT
基本现象													
显性预激	15	3	41	4	69	97	83	10	96	3	46	78	86
房室结双径路	55	86	10	36	83	24	42	86	6	8	82	36	82
基础状态下周期大于600ms时出现房室阻滞	11	8	2	50	84	84	84	41	5	55	41	66	93
希氏束起搏时出现结外反应	18	5	47	0	67	96	80	17	83	0	36	80	85
心动过速特点													
诱发需关键的 AH 间期	55	90	16	4	88	26	36	91	8	1	87	42	71
心动过速维持需要异丙肾上腺素	39	47	23	57	68	51	62	65	18	17	56	58	91
心动过速周期≥500ms	3	4	2	0	99	96	97	83	17	0	44	69	87
间隔部 VA 间期大于 70ms	53	16	100	100	0	69	54	17	59	24	0	100	100
向心性心房激动	31	0	74	61	30	89	74	0	76	24	19	88	93
心动过速时有自发房室阻滞	10	11	0	33	91	85	93	60	0	40	44	65	91
有房室阻滞时自发终止	28	33	31	0	78	73	67	66	34	0	48	70	82
出现 RBBB	32	31	36	30	66	69	67	54	35	11	42	71	82
出现 LBBB	12	1	36	4	73	99	87	4	92	4	36	81	87
当有 BBB 时 VA 间期增加大于 20ms	7	0	35	0	69	100	80	0	100	0	51	57	92

AH: 心房希氏束; AT: 房速; AVNRT: 房室结折返性心动过速; BBB: 束支阻滞; LBBB: 左束支阻滞; NPV: 阴性预测值; PPV: 阳性预测值; ORT: 顺向型折返性心动过速; RBBB: 右束支阻滞; VA: 室房。引自 Knight BP, Ebinger M, Oral H 等: Diagnostic value of tachycardia features and pacing maneuvers during paroxysmal supraventricular tachycardia. J Am Coll Cardiol 35; 574-582, 2000。

表 55-2 心动过速时起搏方法的诊断价值

起搏方法/结果	所尝试的心动过速方法%	能掩带的比例	结果出现的频率 AVNRT	ORT	AT	敏感性(%) AVNRT	ORT	AT	特异性(%) AVNRT	ORT	AT	PPV(%) AVNRT	ORT	AT	NPV(%) AVNRT	ORT	AT
以比室上速周期短10～40ms的周期起搏心室固定的VA同期	89	87	87	98	5	97	18	3	27	35	1	64			87	96	17
以出现房室阻滞的房室周期起搏心房在AH水平终止心动过速	69	NA	80	76	8	96	20	11	44	30	1	69			88	65	47
以比室上速周期短10～40ms起搏心室掩带心房	97	78															
心房激动与室搏一致			92	100	0	100	13	0	20	36	0	64			100	100	0
停止起搏出现房室反应			94	100	0	100	89	0	14	37	0	63			100	100	0
VA阻滞周期大于室上速周期			7	0	48	3	89	98	86	0	80	20			41	66	93
心室起搏周期200～250ms	91	NA															
终止室上速			27	37	0	27	78	69	74	43	0	57			44	73	83
不影响心房，心室与室上速分离			16	0	16	11	88	93	95	0	25	75			45	66	89
舒张期心室早搏刺激不影响心房，希氏束处于不应期	80	NA	3	8	0	0	100	97	94	100	0	0			42	71	87
室上速终止，夺获心房，希氏束处于不应期			10	27	0	0	100	92	80	100	0	0			38	75	86
室上速未终止，夺获心房，希氏束处于不应期			12	34	0	0	100	88	76	100	0	0			37	77	86

AH：心房希氏束；AT：房速；AVNRT：房室结折返性心动过速；BBB：束支阻滞；CL：折返环周期；NA：不适用的；NPV：阴性预测值；ORT：顺向型折返性心动过速；PPV：阳性预测值；VA：室房。引自 Knight BP, Ebinger M, Oral H 等：Diagnostic value of tachycardia features and pacing maneuvers during paroxysmal supraventricular tachycardia. J Am Coll Cardiol 35: 574-582, 2000.

新标测方法的影响

标测心律失常的新技术包括网篮标测、电解剖标测和非接触性标测。新的标测技术有肯定的优势，包括标测不稳定、很难重复诱发和非持续性心律失常的能力。使用这些技术，可以标测短阵发作的，只有1跳或几跳的心律失常。许多研究报道了使用这些新技术标测消融房速[30-37]。这些新技术均可减少操作者的射线曝光量。

五、大折返性房速

(一) 分类

大折返性房速可分为峡部依赖型（依赖于三尖瓣环-下腔静脉峡部间的传导）和非峡部依赖型房速[1]。成人中大折返性房速中的绝大多数为峡部依赖性。非峡部依赖型大折返性房速中的绝大多数与瘢痕区域有关，常常是切口性。大折返性房速，包括房扑、低位环形折返、双波折返、起源于右房游离壁的大折返以及与既往手术有关的发生于右或左房的大折返性房速，包括既往心房切开、手术瘢痕、间隔部人工补片、缝合线或其他解剖学障碍。由于近来标测技术的发展对这种心动过速进行了仔细研究。在其他章节将对这种心动过速进行仔细讨论（见54章和60章）。

(二) 机制

早在上世纪90年代早期即有数个研究小组对大折返性房速的电生理学特点、标测和消融进行了阐述，其中包括台湾的Chen及其同事[2,3]以及旧金山的Lesh及其同事[12]。这些学者均强调了使用标准电生理学技术在缓慢传导区记录舒张期心房电位并证实了拖带的重要性。由动物试验资料推断心房局部瘢痕提供了心房内折返的基质。心房内心内膜多点标测技术以及拖带技术用来确定被保护的缓慢传导区。比如，通过某个位点是否可以隐匿性拖带心动过速来确定可能的消融位点。这些研究者还使用这种起搏标测技术来消融室速。研究者通过心房起搏并试图寻找使起搏后的第一个间期与心动过速周期差在10～30ms以内以及起搏信号与体表P波时间等于在此位点的激动时间的绝对值（图55-5）的位点。当存在术后心脏结构异常或房速起源点位于解剖学屏障附近时（如静脉口或瓣环），对此区域的标测应更仔细。这些部位常常有较宽的双电位或其电位常较低。

使用更先进的计算机标测技术可以更精确更快速地确认心律失常的机制。研究大折返性房速的第二种方法主要是研究环绕瘢痕或手术切口后的大折返。这些新技术可以重建心脏各腔室并记录局部激动时间和确定心脏的瘢痕组织，在许多患者中重建等时性标测或全部折返环。Nakagawa及其同事[38]在这一问题上对16例曾行先天性心脏病手术并伴有右房大折返性房速的患者进行了标测和消融研究。在13例患者中使用CARTO电解剖标测系统标测了15种房速。首先，所有的大折返性房速均通过较窄的峡部折返（小于2.7cm），通常是标测系统确定在2个临近的高密度或低密度瘢痕之间的低电压区域。作者的发现符合"无峡部，无折返"的说法。电图的形态、电压和时限并不能鉴别狭窄通道内和通道外的位点。拖带标测不能鉴别位于折返环通道内与通道外的位点。许多患者均未行拖带标测，因为拖带会诱发新的心动过速或终止原有的心动过速。拖带标测其他的局限性在于常常不能准确测量起搏后间期，因为在瘢痕区其心房电压常较低或缺失。拖带标测也可能诱发出房颤。最后，较慢频率心房起搏时可以记录到双电位，表明可能存在有解剖学阻滞的固定部位。总体来说，瘢痕或相关解剖学屏障（如瓣环、上腔静脉、肺静脉或下腔静脉）的位置和大小决定了心动过速折返环的大小和

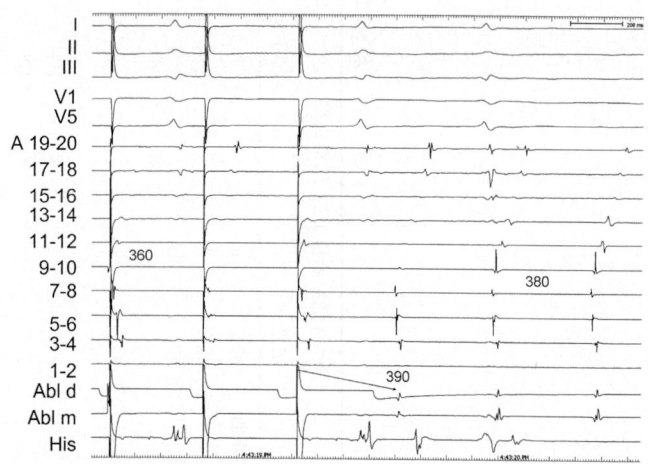

图55-5 起源于冠状静脉窦的大折返性房速的拖带 图示自上而下依次是体表心电图导联，腔内电图分别为沿界嵴放置的Halo电极导管、希氏束导管、冠状窦内的消融导管。由消融导管起搏显示起搏后间期较心动过速周期长10ms，表明大折返环存在并涉及左房。在左房和右房其他部位起搏均存在较长的起搏后间期。

特性。

确定关键峡部的隐匿性拖带的经典标准的敏感性和特异性是建立在对室速研究基础之上的。Morton及其同事研究了这些标准确定心房拖带的敏感性和特异性[39]。他们使用典型房扑模型并使用 4 种不同频率在 7 个不同位点行拖带标测。扑动周期减去 10ms 的隐匿性拖带对峡部位点诊断的敏感性达 100%，但其特异性只有 54%。扑动周期减 40ms 特异性可提高至 98%，但敏感性只有 65%。扑动周期减 30ms，敏感性和特异性分别为 85% 和 90%。10 例患者中 5 例患者可以在非峡部部位见到隐匿性拖带。这项研究说明了 Nakagawa 及其同事[38]研究的重要性，仅仅依靠拖带单一标准来确定消融靶点可能会降低消融的成功率。这些发现也说明了仅仅依靠一种标准来确定复杂大折返性房速的消融位点是很困难的。总的来说，联合解剖学方法和电生理学标测的方法可用来保证这种复杂心律失常的消融成功。

六、大折返性房速的心电图特点

大折返性房速的心电图定位远比局灶性房速的心电图定位复杂。大折返性房速折返环的心电图电位受到心房解剖、手术切口和心房波阵传导的影响。例如，顺钟向和逆钟向房扑以在下壁导联上 P 波的不同极向为特点。这两种房扑的折返环所环绕的路径相同，但 P 波极向受到心房激动方向影响（如脚头位或头脚位）。临近欧氏嵴的大折返环可能会产生与典型房扑类似或相同的 P 波形态[40]。产生于左房后壁或侧壁和涉及左肺静脉的左侧房扑其特点为冠状窦激动顺序为由远端或中段向近端激动并且显示脚头位的激动顺序，在 V_1 导联 P 波低平或正向，在下壁导联常为直立 P 波[41,42]。

七、大折返性房速的特殊类型

近来有 3 个电生理实验室研究了左房大折返性房速或左房房扑的特点。Lerman 及其同事[43]研究了 10 例曾行二尖瓣手术的大折返性房速患者。其中 6 例房速起源于右房，4 例起源于左房，1 例患者双房均有起源点。80% 的患者心动过速折返环由心房切口或管腔位置所决定。其中共标测了涉及左房间隔和右肺静脉的 3 种大折返性房速，在其中 2 例患者为单一折返环，1 例患者为 8 字折返，围绕后壁低电压区的顺钟向环路和围绕二尖瓣环的逆钟向环路以及在 2 个环路中的低电压区作为中央峡部。有意思的是，3 例患者心动过速有局灶起源。另 2 项研究中使用了 CARTO 系统标测了左房房扑并成功消融了 70% 的患者[44,45]。绝大多数患者有器质性心脏病并且 14%～32% 患者有二尖瓣疾病。研究者认为大折返性房速具有连续的心房激动顺序并且心房最早和最后激动点临近，心房激动时间占心动过速折返周长的 90% 或更多。在一部分患者进行拖带标测可确定缓慢传导区的关键峡部。在右心房包括下腔三尖瓣峡部区域和右房游离壁的 3 个或更多位点的研究中发现，如果起搏后间期比心动过速周期的差值大于或等于 40ms，那么即认为可以排除右房的大折返性房速，右房的自发变异大于 100ms，而左房的变异小于 20ms，在超过 8 个点以上的连续导管标测时，右房激动占心律失常环周期不足 50%。典型左房扑动为环绕二尖瓣环、电静止区或临近先天性或获得性解剖学屏障，如手术瘢痕或肺静脉的双电位线的大折返环（图 55-2）。电静止区域是指不能记录到电图或电图振幅小于 0.05mV 的区域。在一项研究中发现 74% 的心动过速为双环折返环路，其他 26% 的患者为单环折返环路。与 Nakagawa 及其同事对右房房速的发现类似，左房房速的峡部相对较窄并且电图电压较低。

对其他大折返性房速的不常见起源点也有研究。例如，Olgin 与其同事在 1 例无器质性心脏病患者的研究中发现其心房大折返环的关键峡部位于冠状静脉窦内。其折返环涉及冠状静脉窦的肌袖，出口在房间隔下部左房侧并重新进入冠状窦。需要在冠状静脉窦内环形消融才能成功消融这个折返环。

（李　鼎　译）

参 考 文 献

1. Saoudi N, Cosio F, Waldo A, et al: Classification of atrial flutter and regular atrial tachycardia according to electrophysiologic mechanism and anatomic bases: A statement from a joint expert group from the Working Group of Arrhythmias of the European Society of Cardiology and the North American Society of Pacing and Electrophysiology. J Cardiovasc Electrophysiol 12:852–866, 2001.
2. Chen S-A, Chiang C-E, Yang C-J, et al: Sustained atrial tachycardia in adult patients: Electrophysiological characteristics, pharmacological response, possible mechanisms and effects of radiofrequency ablation. Circulation 90:1262–1278, 1994.
3. Chen S-A, Tai C-T, Chiang C-E, et al: Focal atrial tachycardia: reanalysis of the clinical and electrophysiologic characteristics and prediction of successful radiofrequency ablation. J Cardiovasc Electrophysiol 9:355–365, 1998.
4. Reithmann C, Hoffmann E, Dorwarth U, et al: Electroanatomical mapping for visualization of atrial activation in patients with incisional atrial tachycardias. Eur Heart J 22:237–246, 2001.
5. Engelstein ED, Lippman N, Stein KM, Lerman BB: Mechanism-

specific effects of adenosine on atrial tachycardia. Circulation 89:2645-2654, 1994.
6. Kall JG, Kopp D, Olshansky B, et al: Adenosine-sensitive atrial tachycardia. Pacing Clin Electrophysiol 18:300-306, 1995.
7. Markowitz SM, Stein KM, Mittal S, et al: Differential effects of adenosine on focal and macroreentrant atrial tachycardia. J Cardiovasc Electrophysiol 10:489-502, 1999.
8. Chiale PA, Franco A, Selva HO, et al: Lidocaine-sensitive atrial tachycardia. J Am Coll Cardiol 36:1637-1645, 2000.
9. Tang CW, Scheinman MM, Van Hare GF, et al: Use of P wave configuration during atrial tachycardia to predict site of origin. J Am Coll Cardiol 26:1315-1324, 1995.
10. Tada H, Nogami A, Naito S, et al: Simple electrocardiographic criteria for identifying the site of origin of focal right atrial tachycardia. Pacing Clin Electrophysiol 21:2431-2439, 1998.
11. Yamane T, Shah DC, Peng J-T, et al: Morphological characteristics of P waves during selective pulmonary vein pacing. J Am Coll Cardiol 38:1505-1510, 2001.
12. Kalman JM, Olgin JE, Karch MR, et al: "Cristal tachycardias": Origin of right atrial tachycardias from the crista terminalis identified by intracardiac echocardiography. J Am Coll Cardiol 31:451-459, 1998.
13. Nogami A, Sugut M, Tomita T, et al: Novel form of atrial tachycardia originating at the atrioventricular annulus. Pacing Clin Electrophysiol 21:2691-2694, 1998.
14. Morton JB, Sanders P, Das A, et al: Focal atrial tachycardia arising from the tricuspid annulus: Electrophysiologic and electrocardiographic characteristics. J Cardiovasc Electrophysiol 12:653-659, 2001.
15. Matsuoka K, Kasai A, Fujii E, et al: Electrophysiological features of atrial tachycardia arising from the atrioventricular annulus. Pacing Clin Electrophysiol 25:440-445, 2002.
16. Tritto M, Zardini M, De Ponti R, Salerno-Uriarte JA: Iterative atrial tachycardia originating from the coronary sinus musculature. J Cardiovasc Electrophysiol 12:1187-1189, 2001.
17. Iesaka Y, Takahashi A, Goya M, et al: Adenosine sensitive atrial reentrant tachycardia originating from the atrioventricular nodal transitional area. J Cardiovasc Electrophysiol 8:854-864, 1997.
18. Lai L-P, Lin J-L, Chen T-F, et al: Clinical, electrophysiological characteristics, and radiofrequency catheter ablation of atrial tachycardia near the apex of Koch's triangle. Pacing Clin Electrophysiol 21:367-374, 1998.
19. Connors SP, Vora A, Green MS, Tang ASL: Radiofrequency ablation of atrial tachycardia originating from the triangle of Koch. Can J Cardiol 16:39-43, 2000.
20. Chen C-C, Tai C-T, Chiang C-E, et al: Atrial tachycardias originating from the atrial septum. J Cardiovasc Electrophysiol 11:744-749, 2000.
21. Frey B, Kreiner G, Gwechenberger M, Gossinger HD: Ablation of atrial tachycardia originating from the vicinity of the atrioventricular node: Significance of mapping both sides of the interatrial septum. J Am Coll Cardiol 38:394-400, 2001.
22. Marrouche NF, Sippens Groenewegen A, Yang Y, et al: Clinical and electrophysiologic characteristics of left septal atrial tachycardia. J Am Coll Cardiol 40:1133-1139, 2002.
23. Ino T, Miyamoto S, Ohno T, Tadera T: Exit block of focal repetitive activity in the superior vena cava masquerading as a high right atrial tachycardia. J Cardiovasc Electrophysiol 11:480-483, 2000.
24. Dong J, Schreieck J, Ndrepepa G, Schmit C: Ectopic tachycardia originating from the superior vena cava. J Cardiovasc Electrophysiol 13:620-624, 2002.
25. Still A-M, Huikuri HV, Juhani KE, et al: Impaired negative chronotropic response to adenosine in patients with inappropriate sinus tachycardia. J Cardiovasc Electrophysiol 13:557-562, 2002.
26. Glatter KA, Cheng J, Dorostkar P, et al: Electrophysiologic effects of adenosine in patients with supraventricular tachycardia. Circulation 99:1034-1040, 1999.
27. Knight BP, Ebinger M, Oral H, et al: Diagnostic value of tachycardia features and pacing maneuvers during paroxysmal supraventricular tachycardia. J Am Coll Cardiol 35:574-582, 2000.
28. Knight BP, Zivin A, Souza J, et al: A technique for the rapid diagnosis of atrial tachycardia in the electrophysiology laboratory. J Am Coll Cardiol 33:775-781, 1999.
29. Man KC. Niebauer M, Daoud E, et al: Comparison of atrial-His intervals during tachycardia and atrial pacing in patients with long RP tachycardia. J Cardiovasc Electrophysiol 6:700-710, 1995.
30. Wetzel U, Hindricks G, Schirdewahn P, et al: A stepwise mapping approach for localization and ablation of ectopic right, left, and septal atrial foci using electroanatomic mapping. Eur Heart J 23:1387-1393, 2002.
31. Zrenner B, Ndrepepa G, Schneider MAE, et al: Mapping and ablation of atrial arrhythmias after surgical correction of congenital heart disease guided by a 64-electrode basket catheter. Am J Cardiol 88:573-578, 2001.
32. Schmitt H, Weber S, Schwab JO, et al: Diagnosis and ablation of focal right atrial tachycardia using a new high-resolution, non-contact mapping system. Am J Cardiol 87:1017-1021, 2001.
33. Natale A, Breeding L, Tomassoni G, et al: Ablation of right and left ectopic atrial tachycardias using a three-dimensional nonfluoroscopic mapping system. Am J Cardiol 82:989-992, 1998.
34. Marchlinski F, Callans D, Gottlieb C, et al: Magnetic electroanatomical mapping for ablation of focal atrial tachycardias. Pacing Clin Electrophysiol 21:1621-1635, 1998.
35. Leonelli FM, Tomassoni G, Richey M, Natale A: Ablation of incisional atrial tachycardias using a three-dimensional nonfluoroscopic mapping system. Pacing Clin Electrophysiol 24:1653-1659, 2001.
36. Schmitt C, Zrenner B, Schneider M, et al: Clinical experience with a novel multielectrode basket catheter in right atrial tachycardias. Circulation 99:2414-2422, 1999.
37. Molenschot M, Ramanna H, Hoorntje T, et al: Catheter ablation of incisional atrial tachycardia using a novel mapping system: LocaLisa. Pacing Clin Electrophysiol 24:1616-1622, 2001.
38. Nakagawa H, Shah N, Matsudaira K, et al: Characterization of reentrant circuit in macroreentrant right atrial tachycardia after surgical repair of congenital heart disease: Isolated channels between scars allow "focal" ablation. Circulation 103:699-709, 2001.
39. Morton JB, Sanders P, Deen V, et al: Sensitivity and specificity of concealed entrainment for the identification of a critical isthmus in the atrium: Relationship to rate, anatomic location and antidromic penetration. J Am Coll Cardiol 39:896-906, 2002.
40. Sehra R, Coppess MA, Altemose GT, et al: Atrial tachycardia masquerading as atrial flutter following ablation of the subeustachian isthmus. J Cardiovasc Electrophysiol 11:582-586, 2000.
41. Ricard P, Imianitoff M, Yaici K, et al: Atypical atrial flutters. Europace 4:229-239, 2002.
42. Della Bella P, Fraticelli A, Tonod C, et al: Atypical atrial flutter: Clinical features, electrophysiological characteristics and response to radiofrequency catheter ablation. Europace 4:241-253, 2002.
43. Markowitz SM, Brodman RF, Stein KM, et al: Lesional tachycardias related to mitral valve surgery. J Am Coll Cardiol 39:1973-1983, 2002.
44. Jais P, Shah DC, Haissaguerre M, et al: Mapping and ablation of left atrial flutters. Circulation 101:2928-2934, 2000.
45. Ouyang F, Ernst S, Vogtmann T, et al: Characterization of reentrant circuits in left atrial macroreentrant tachycardia: Critical isthmus block can prevent atrial tachycardia recurrence. Circulation 1934-1942, 2002.
46. Olgin JE, Jayachandran JV, Engelstein E, et al: Atrial macroreentry involving the myocardium of the coronary sinus: A unique mechanism for atypical flutter. J Cardiovasc Electrophysiol 9:1094-1099, 1998.

第 56 章

心房颤动

Stanley Nattel and Joachim R. Ebrlich

本章目录

- 临床回顾 ... 505
- 房颤的发生机制 ... 505
- 房颤的临床表现、评价和潜在的并发症 ... 511
- 临床处理 ... 511
- 未来的方向 ... 514

一、临床回顾

临床最常见的心律失常是心房颤动（房颤）[1]。房颤对人群致残率、医疗花费甚至致死率均有明显的影响[2,3]。寻找房颤最适合的治疗仍是目前的挑战，这一心律失常有着复杂的发病机制[4]。

临床将房颤分为三种形式（图 56-1）：（1）阵发性，这类房颤的发生和终止均为自发性，可持续数秒至数小时，甚至数天；（2）持续性，这类房颤持续发生直到（电或药物）复律终止；（3）永久性，这类房颤即使经过治疗也无法复律或不适宜复律。房颤最初多为阵发性，逐渐变为持续性或永久性[5]。然而，与"心动过速导致重构"这一理论不同，有一些阵发性房颤患者尽管房颤频繁发作，但始终未发展成持续性。

房颤可以使很多心脏疾病变得复杂（表 56-1）。高血压病、冠心病均是最常见并发房颤的疾病[1]。急性心肌梗死（MI），尤其是累及右冠状动脉的病变，常合并房颤的发生[6]。充血性心力衰竭（CHF）是一个非常常见的并发房颤的疾病，而且房颤的发生率随心力衰竭程度的加重而增高：心功能 II 级的心力衰竭患者的房颤发生率为 10%，而心功能 IV 级的患者房颤发生率在 40%～50%[7]（图 56-2）。心力衰竭患者的血流动力学参数可因房颤的发生而显著恶化，窦性心律的恢复可以改善其血流动力学[8]。大型的心力衰竭治疗试验，如 SOLVD[9] 和 DIAMOND-CHF[10] 结果显示房颤可能影响患者的生存率。目前正在进行的一项临床试验（AF-CHF 研究）前瞻性地评价充血性心力衰竭患者进行房颤治疗对其生存率的影响[11]。房颤也可以发生于没有任何心脏异常的健康人，这种房颤称为"孤立性"房颤（表 56-1）。

二、房颤的发生机制

有关房颤发生机制的概念可以追溯到一百年前的教科书[4,12]（图 56-3）。Garrey 和 Mines 认为多个共存的折返环形成房颤，而另外学者认为单个或多个快速发放冲动的心房局部异位灶维持房颤，Thomas Lewis 则认为单个折返环伴颤动样传导是这一心律失常的基础。多环路折返理论，经过 Gordon Moe 多子波学说的改进，直到最近仍然是房颤机制的主要观点（见第 35～41 章及参考文献 4 有关上述理论的历史回顾）。

（一）多环路折返

1. 生理条件

多环路折返的特征为多个、同时发生的功能性折返环，且其折返部位和时间持续不断变化（图 56-3）。这些多环路折返活动的维持有赖于组织能够同时容纳

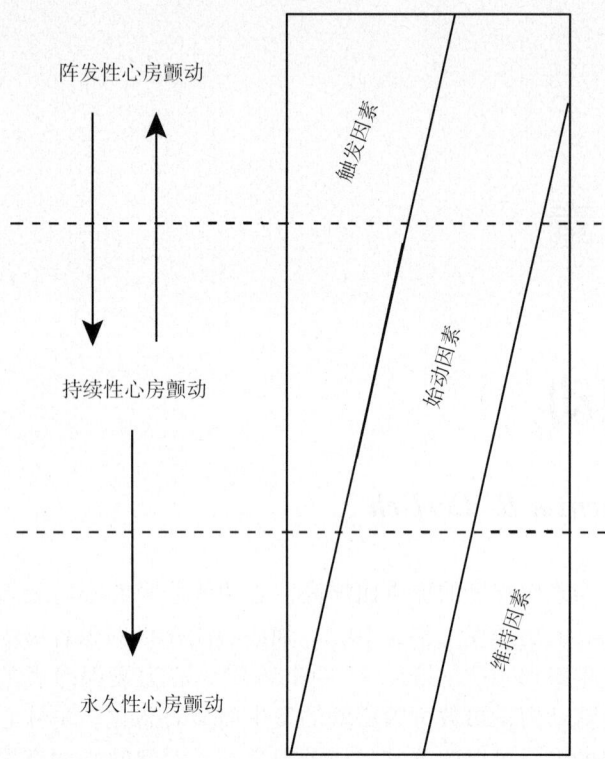

图 56-1 阵发性、持续性和永久性心房颤动的相互关系（左） 在许多患者中，阵发性和持续性房颤可以相互转化，而永久性房颤，顾名思义，是不可转化的。作用在易患基质上的触发因素常表现为一过性因素，如自主神经张力的改变或心肌缺血，而始发房颤。维持因素可以促进房颤的持续。右图显示触发因素、始动因素，以及维持因素在每一种类型房颤中的相对作用。

足够的折返波阵面，不至于使心房中不同部位的活动同时消失。经典的主导环折返理论认为，功能性折返环自发地以最小折返路径——即折返波长，形成折返（图 56-4），而波长等于不应期（RP）与传导速度（CV）的乘积。基于此点，短不应期和传导速度缓慢可以缩短环路大小，利于心房容纳更多的折返环而导致多环路折返和房颤的形成。由此推论，心房扩大也应有利于多环路折返的形成。不应期离散使激动围绕

表 56-1　与心房颤动相关的常见临床病因

心源性病因	非心源性病因
高血压	电解质紊乱
冠状动脉疾病	甲状腺功能异常
充血性心力衰竭	乙醇中毒
心包炎/心肌炎	迷走/交感神经张力失衡
瓣膜性心脏病	肺脏疾病
心脏外科手术	感染性疾病，发热性疾病

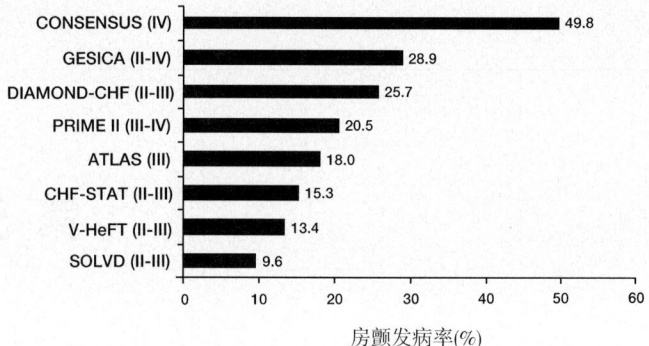

图 56-2　几项大型试验中不同程度充血性心力衰竭患者心房颤动的发病率 心衰的程度越严重，房颤的发病率越高。（改自 Ehrlich JR, Nattel S, Hohnloser SH: Atrial fibrillation and congestive heart failure: Specific considerations at the intersection of two common and important cardiac disease sets. J Cardiovasc Electrophysiol 13: 399-405, 2002.）

不同不应期组织传导，所产生的空间差异有利于多环路折返的形成。一般来说，期前收缩是所有形式折返活动始动的必要条件。

2. 实验和临床证据

多环路折返最初的证据是基于对颤动组织的观察，当组织被切割成小块时颤动会自行终止。Allessie 利用多电极标测胆碱能房颤狗模型，提供了多折返波阵面的证据（参阅参考文献 4）。Maze 术式是利用多环路折返这一理论设计出来的，这是一种外科术式，即将心房分割成多个小区域，仍维持电学的连续性，但心房无法支持折返活动[13]。Maze 术式的高度有效性（慢性房颤＞90%）为多环路折返理论提供了支持的证据（见第 118 章）。

3. 治疗结果和临床相关性

多环路折返房颤的维持有赖于环路的大小（多用波长表示）和心房的大小（见图 56-4）。增加不应期的药物可以增加环路的大小，使房颤不易发生或终止房颤。这一论点与临床观察一致。许多可以增加心房不应期的药物（如 IA 类药物奎尼丁，Ⅲ类制剂多菲利特）在治疗房颤上均有效。药物对快室率房颤的终止有赖于其对房颤波长的作用；而对于窦性心律时房性早搏诱发慢频率房颤的预防有赖于药物对不应期的延长作用。因此，能够延长慢频率时的不应期而较少影响快频率时不应期的药物（如，Ⅲ类药物多菲利特、索他洛尔，具有"负向频率依赖

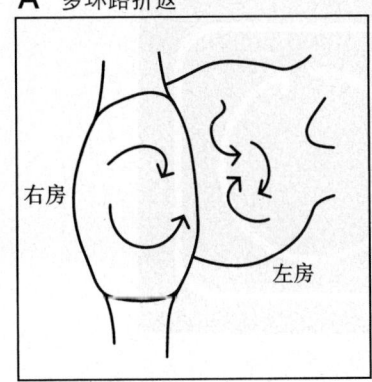 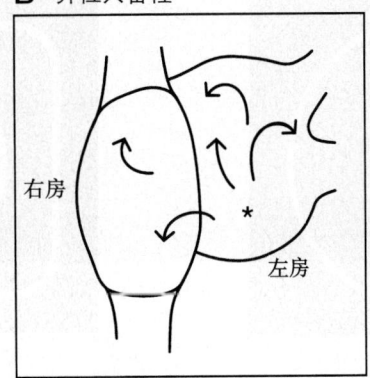 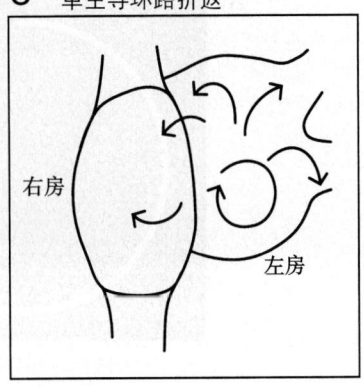

图 56-3　二十世纪初期有关心房颤动发生机制的理论　A：多环路折返（折返波以箭头表示），最初由 G. R. Mines 和 W. E. Garrey 于 1914 年提出。B：由单一的快速发放异位冲动的兴奋灶（星状标记）引起，冲动在心房内呈颤动样传导。C：单主导环路折返伴心房内颤动样传导。单主导环路折返房颤的快速折返过程和不规则的心房传导可以与心房扑动相鉴别，后者为相对缓慢的、规律传导的折返机制。

性"作用），其终止房颤的作用弱于预防房颤的作用[14]。如前所述，Maze 术的有效性与多环路折返理论相一致。多环路折返应该会被强效的钠通道阻滞药物所易化/促进，如 IC 类药物，可以强有力地减缓心房传导。然而临床经验却相反，IC 类药物可以有效预防和终止房颤[15]，这对经典的多环路折返决定因素提出了质疑和挑战。通过靶组织消融治愈房颤是一个高度理想的目标。目前所知，仅有 Maze 术是利用组织破坏方法来改变基质，从而使房颤不能维持。多环路折返的理论提示，任何以导管为基础的治疗方法都需达到外科 Maze 术消除房颤基质的目标。

（二）快速异位活动

1. 生理条件

局灶异位活动可以源于多种机制（见第 12、39 和 40 章）。简而言之，当 4 相去极化加速提前达到阈值，则可以导致快速冲动发放，即正常的自律性增强。延迟后除极（DAD）发生于细胞内钙超载，当舒张期钙从超载的肌浆网中释放出来，激活钙依赖性除极电流（如 Na^+/Ca^{2+} 交换电流），导致 DAD 和触发活动。早期后除极（EAD）是由动作电位过度延长，再激活平台期钙电流，后者继发性地在动作电位 2 相和 3 相产生致心律失常的除极活动。也有证据显示组织牵拉，如发生于充血性心力衰竭时，也可以产生后除极和异位活动。单一的快速发放冲动的心房病灶可能会产生一种规律的心动过速。但是，如果冲动发放频率过快，心房其他组织不能够 1∶1 传导，则可产生心房颤动。另外，由房性心动过速引起的心房重构也可以产生心动过速重构，最终导致多环路折返（在后面讨论）。

2. 实验和临床证据

Gordon Moe 证实可由乌头碱（aconitine）刺激心耳尖部诱发房颤，乌头碱可导致该部位快速发放冲动，维持心律失常。通过钳夹心耳进行隔离，则房颤即刻终止。Haissaguerre 及其同事[16]证实房颤常常是由起源于肺静脉区域的异位活动引发。此后，肺静脉的快速电活动在房颤维持中的作用在临床[17]和实验模型[18]中均得到进一步的证实。

3. 治疗结果和临床相关性

如果房颤起源的局部活动灶能够被识别出来并通过靶目标法进行破坏，则心律失常应该被消除。肺静脉异位灶在房颤中的重要作用得到证实以后，消融的方法被广泛地应用于消除肺静脉异位活动灶，进行房颤治疗。如果局部的活动病灶不能够很好地被识别出来，或呈休眠状态，那么将肺静脉从心房中进行电学隔离，也可有效预防房颤的复发。肺静脉隔离术获得了显著成功，对阵发性房颤较持续性房颤更有效[17]。如果肺静脉仅作为一个触发病灶，而不是房颤基质中的关键因素，则对于潜在同时并存的或从肺静脉以外的心房部位起源的触发活动诱发的房颤，肺静脉消融效果有限。

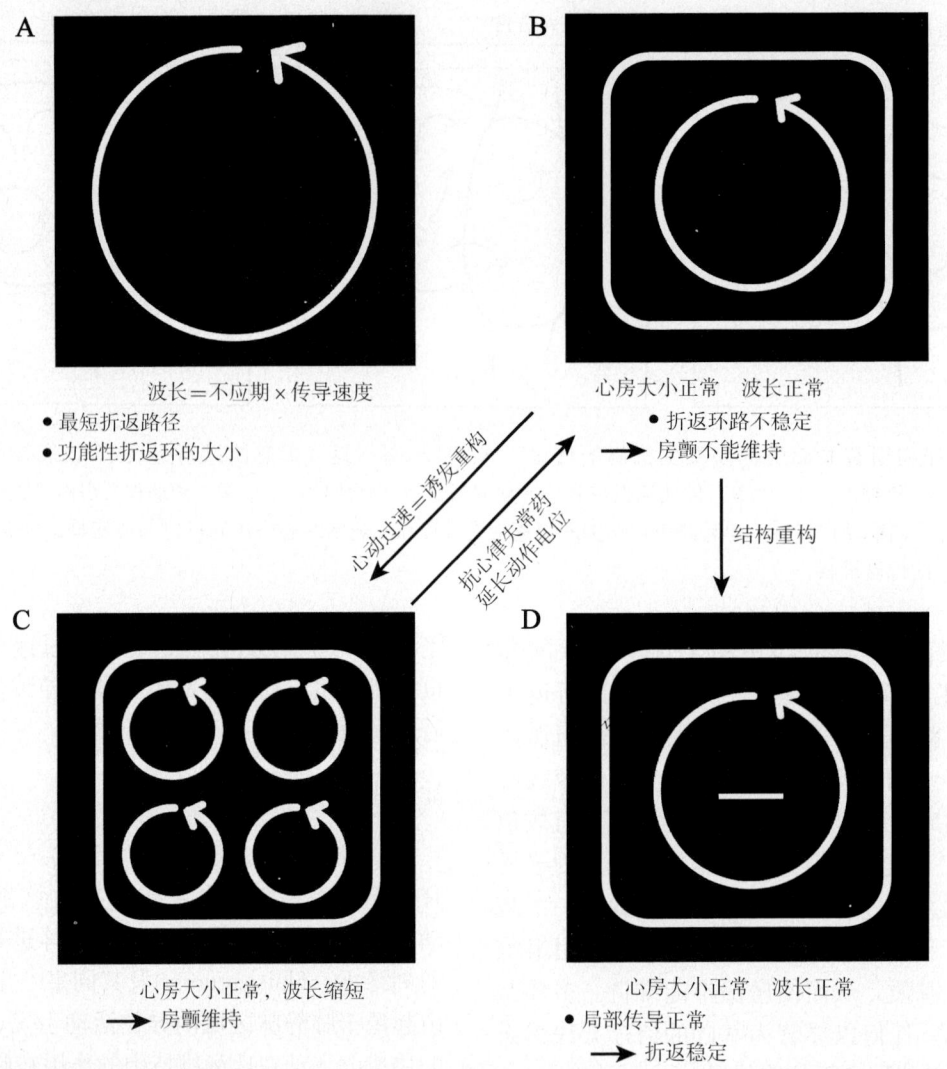

图 56-4 折返（主导环）和多环路心房颤动的条件　A：维持折返和最短环路的条件。波长由箭头表示，等于不应期和传导速度的乘积。B：在一个大小和波长正常的心房，可容纳的环路数目是很少的，而且由于环路的不稳定，房颤易于自发终止。C：在一个大小正常的心房，如果不应期缩短（例如，心动过速导致的重构或者迷走张力加强、甲状腺功能亢进、I_{Ks} 获得性功能突变等，导致外向电流的增加）使波长减小，心房则可以容纳更多的环路同时存在，从而增加了房颤维持的能力。相反，如果抗心律失常药物延长动作电位时程以及相应的不应期，则房颤终止。D：单环路折返由于存在缓慢传导的中心区域或解剖障碍合并缓慢传导区而得以在正常的心房中稳定存在。

（三）单环路折返

1. 生理条件

单环路折返的维持有赖于表 56-4A 中所列的条件。由于单环路折返更不稳定，则需要更特殊的条件来维持心房内单环路折返的稳定性。心房扑动是一种典型的单个稳定的折返环路。如果由单个环路发放的快速冲动在心房内遇到功能性传导障碍，产生多个非 1∶1 传导反应的区域，则可导致心房颤动（所谓的"颤动样传导"）。颤动样传导可以由不应期的空间差异所导致，或者由于心房组织结构特性伴电源-电穴（source-sink）不匹配，形成传导反应空间梯度而产生[19]。

2. 实验和临床证据

标测高浓度乙酰胆碱浸泡的离体狗右心房，显示单个折返环路在房颤中具有重要意义[20]。Mandapati 及其同事研究指出，局限于左心房的病灶，可以形成单个微折返环路，可能是离体动物房颤的基础[21]。数学模型同样提示，单个螺旋波（spiral-wave rotors）常为在模拟狗心房组织乙酰胆碱不均一分布所诱发房颤的基础[22]。与其相类似，在充血性心力衰竭实验模型中，单个大折返环是一部分模型中房颤维持的基础[23]。临床证据提示，在部分同时有房颤和房扑病史的患者中，通过直接消融维持心房扑动的单一折返环可预防房颤的发生[24]。

3. 治疗结果和临床相关性

导管消融术可以有效而安全地治愈不同种类的心律失常，但不包括房颤[14]。然而对于单个折返环形成的房颤，这种折返环关键靶部位的消融治疗（不需要复杂的类 Maze 术）会有效。也有一些这方面的临床研究报道。

（四）房性心动过速诱导的重构及不同房颤机制的相互作用

对房颤病理生理方面的研究发现房颤本身（以及其他形式的房性心动过速）可以改变心房的电生理特性，易于房颤的发生和维持[26]。房颤诱导重构的最特征性电生理表现为不应期的缩短和不应期-频率依赖性的丧失[26]。这种不应期的改变在空间上是不均一的，进而有助于房颤的发生和维持[27]。房性心动过速诱导的重构在人心脏中已经得到充分证实[28,29]，重构可以解释许多临床上的重要现象，如其他形式的室上性心动过速具有发展成房颤的倾向，电复律后房颤早期复发的倾向，长期持续的房颤对抗心律失常药物治疗存在抵抗，以及阵发性房颤演变为持续性房颤的倾向[12,26]。

房颤引起的不应期改变可能主要与 L-型钙电流（I_{CaL}）减少有关。房性心动过速引起心房肌细胞钙离子负荷的变化，后者可以触发 L 型-钙通道短期功能性的（I_{CaL}的失活）[31]和长期基因表达上的（I_{CaL}的 α 亚基 mRNA 的下调）改变[32]。I_{CaL}的降低可预防潜在的致命性的钙超载，也会引起动作电位时程和不应期缩短[33]。缩短的不应期使波长减小，从而促进多环路折返，如图 56-4C 所示。

持续的房性心动过速还可以引起其他一系列的细胞改变。这些改变包括钠电流的减少，传导速度（CV）的降低[34]，心房连接蛋白40（connexin40）表达的非均一性丧失[35]，以及内向整流钾电流（I_{K1}）的增加[36]，以及超微结构的重构导致更加致命的心肌溶解，糖原聚集等[37]。心房钙代谢障碍引起收缩功能不良及潜在的血栓栓塞易患基质，可能均与房颤相关[38,39]。这些改变可以解释房性心动过速时重塑的改变，延迟超过 24～48 小时，而 24～48 小时以内，RP缩短已达最大值，因此房性心动过速的致房颤作用被认为有"继发因素"。

房性心动过速引起重构的理论使我们对房颤机制的认识发生改变，如图 56-5 所示。房颤的机制并不像最初所认为的那样各种机制自成一体，其潜在的基本机制更可能是以一种互动的方式相互联系。房颤可能以快速的异位活动或单个环路折返为始动机制，进而房性心动过速诱导重构，导致有效不应期的空间离散和缩短，使房颤转为多环路折返。有个案报道显示房颤由一个非常明显的局灶演变为多环路折返的整个过程[40]。房性异位活动可以作为触发灶作用于易于发生折返（单个或多环路）的基质，而始动房颤。最后，有证据提示持续性房性心动过速可以促进肺静脉触发房颤局灶源的出现[16,41]。

上述的心律失常机制可以粗略地分为触发因素、始动因素和维持因素，如图 56-1 所示。异位活动是触发因素的主要组成。房颤的维持是由于触发因素的活动发生在一个易形成折返或触发活动的基质上而导致，并共同组成始动因素。一过性因素，如自主神经张力的变化或心肌缺血，也可以成为始动因素。心房重构（包括心动过速相关的和结构上的重构）对心律失常的持续具有重要作用。在阵发性房颤中触发因素和始动因素占主导地位，根据定义阵发性房颤的维持因素一定不足以使其维持，因而呈阵发性，可自行终止。对于永久性房颤，维持因素一般非常强，使房颤难以终止。这一图表显然过于简单，但却是一种实用的概括性显示。

（五）心房结构的重构

各种病理条件下产生的房颤其心房都有一个共同的病理表现，即间质纤维化。在狗充血性心力衰竭模型中，即使不存在波长缩短或自发的异位活动，只要存在广泛的间质纤维化，使心房肌纤维分割伴有明显的局部传导异常，持续性房颤就很容易被诱发出来[42]。在一些病例中，房颤表现为单个环路折返[23]，其稳定性可能主要通过局部传导障碍得以维持，如图 56-4D。房颤患者心房存在着许多生化异常，包括与组织重构相关的血管紧张素转换酶（ACE）和线粒体激活蛋白激酶的活性变化，还有血管紧张素受体的改变，提示肾素-血管紧张素系统的激活[43]。ACE 抑制剂可减弱充血性心力衰竭狗心房组织的纤维化和房颤的持续[44]，提示肾素-血管紧张素系统与临床房颤引起的结构重构密切相关。充血性心力衰竭不仅可以导致结构重构和折返基质的形成，还可以上调 Na^+/Ca^{2+} 交换，促进延迟后除极的产生，导致触发活动和局部异位激动[45]，这些结果表明房颤的病理生理机制十分复杂。

（六）与特殊病理条件相关的房颤发病机制：甲状腺功能亢进，高血压，冠状动脉疾病以及基因综合征

甲状腺功能亢进是一种人们早已认识的房颤的危险因素。人们很早就已知道甲状腺功能亢进可以缩短心房动作电位，进而缩短不应期和波长。动作电位缩短的机制尚不确定，其中缓慢延迟整流钾电流（I_{Ks}）的增加可能起着一定作用[46]。也有实验证据显示在甲状腺素浸泡数小时的肺静脉心肌出现触发性心律失常[47]。尽管高血压是一种常见的与房颤发生相关的临床疾病，但其机制却并不清楚。10%～15%急性心梗患者可发生房颤，冠状动脉疾病是房颤常见的危险因素。心房缺血实验显示缺血对房颤的维持具有非常强的促进作用[48]。其他并发于急性冠状动脉疾病的因素，如充血性心力衰竭、梗死后心包炎、自主神经张力平衡的改变等也可以导致房颤易患基质的形成。

基因性心律失常综合征的识别使我们对各种室性快速性心律失常的分子机制有了进一步的认识。基因突变导致的房颤直到最近才被认识。最近发现，KvLQT1，一种编码 I_{ks} 的 α 亚基的基因，其获得性功能突变与中国人种家族性房颤的发病相关[49]。其可能机制为缩短动作电位时程促进了多环路折返。编码 I_{Ks} β 亚基的 minK 基因多态性也与房颤的好发相关，但其相关的功能基础尚不清楚[50]。一种膜结合（adaptor）蛋白 ankyrin-B 的缺失性功能突变，也被发现与家

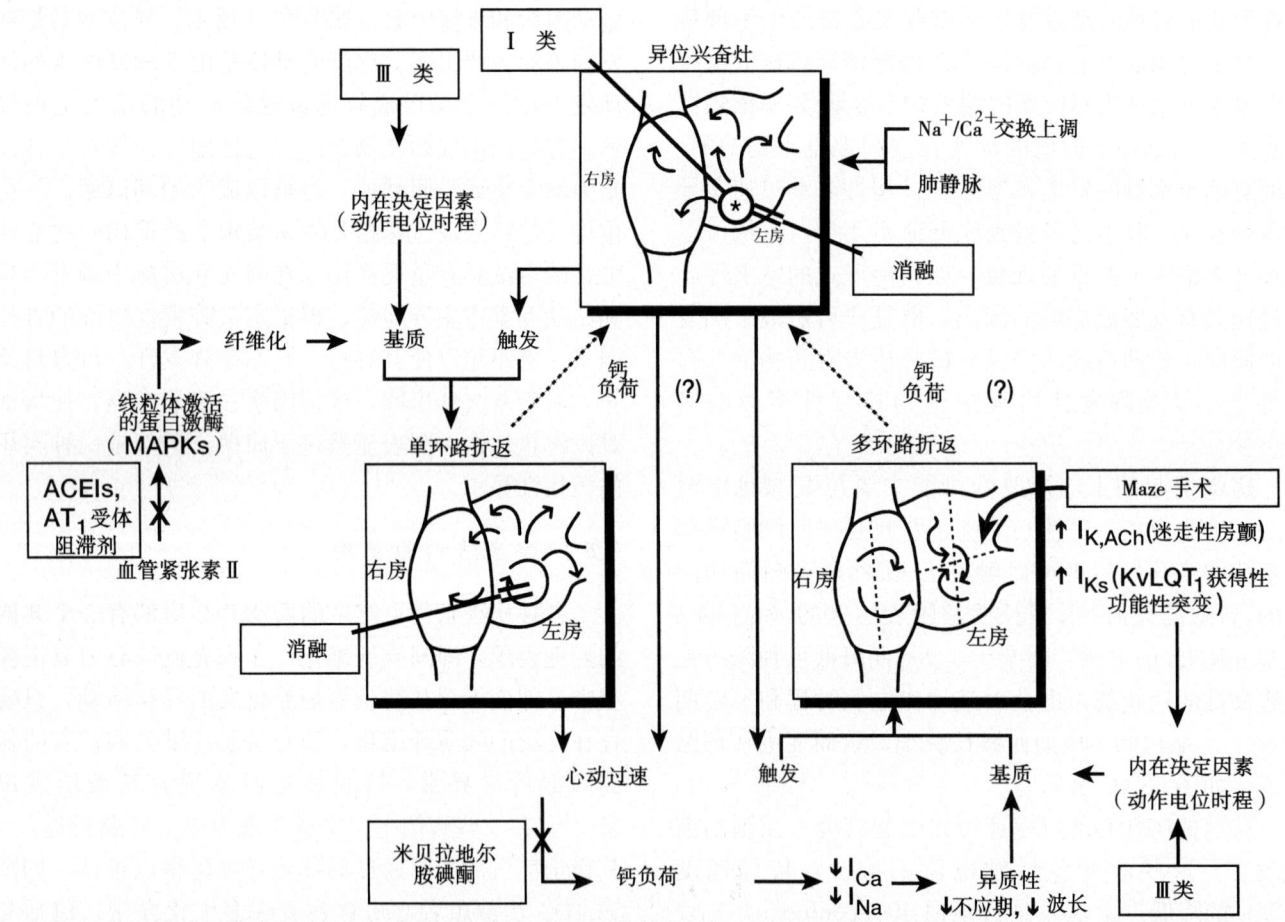

图 56-5 各种心房颤动的机制和基于可能机制的治疗方法之间的相互作用 上图显示一个快速发放冲动的兴奋灶，即起源于肺静脉或由 Na^+/Ca^{2+} 交换上调引起的触发活动。异位灶在适当的心房基质中可以触发单环路或多环路折返（左下或右下图）或引起房性心动过速，进一步引起心动过速-重构，后者与肾素-血管紧张素系统和 MAPK 的激活有关。单环路折返引起的心动过速-重构可以使其向多环路折返转化。迷走性房颤或 KvLQT1 获得性功能突变也可以通过缩短动作电位及有效不应期形成多环路折返。这之间的相互转化用箭头表示，相应的治疗方法显示在方框里。ACEIs：血管紧张素转换酶抑制剂

族性心律失常，包括房颤和先天性长 QT 综合征密切相关[51]。其可能的心律失常机制为异常的钙代谢导致的致心律失常性后除极的发生[51]。

三、房颤的临床表现、评价和潜在的并发症

（一）症状和体征

房颤可以产生相当多的症状，包括心悸、胸痛、呼吸困难、晕厥、头晕以及乏力。在大多数已发表的研究中无症状性房颤患者仅占一小部分，然而症状的发生率有可能被高估，因为有症状才易于引起注意和就诊。即使在有症状的房颤患者中，也有许多房颤发作不伴临床症状。房颤患者的首发临床表现可以是血栓栓塞导致的终末器官的缺血症状，也可以是由于舒张期充盈时间的缩短、氧需求的增加导致的肺水肿，或未控制的心室率相关的心室功能不全引起的呼吸困难。

房颤的典型体征为明显的脉律不齐，常称为"irregularly irregular"。房颤的诊断可以通过典型的心电图表现：快速而不规则的颤动样心房活动来确诊。房颤需与多源性房性心动过速（MFAT）相鉴别，后者表现为一种快速而不规则的房性心律伴房波未下传。两者鉴别的关键在于多源性房性心动过速时可以见到有组织、有规律的心房活动，而房颤时心房活动无规律。

（二）临床评价

详细的病史对发现各种诱发因素、确定可能存在的心脏疾病，评价并发症以及房颤可能持续的时间很重要。对是否为首次发作还是复发，既往发作的次数、频度以及持续时间，既往治疗反应等的确定也很重要。心电图记录房颤和心室反应，以及相关心脏疾病的征象均很重要。动态心电图记录，电话或电信传输事件记录，以及埋置体内的事件记录仪对于有类似房颤症状而就诊时为窦性心律者均有意义。胸片对于评价血管和肺实质疾病、是否存在充血性心力衰竭以及心脏大小均有意义。经胸超声对于评价器质性心脏病和心包疾病是一种非常重要的辅助检查手段，经食管超声对于检测心房内血栓以及血栓栓塞危险尤其有用。所有房颤患者均应行至少一次的血浆甲状腺素（T4）或促甲状腺激素（TSH）检验，因为甲状腺功能亢进在房颤的病因中并不少见，且常为隐匿性。

（三）潜在并发症

如果房颤时心室率未能得到充分控制，经过数周或数月的时间，过快的心室率可引起心室心肌病（有时称为心动过速性心肌病）改变，常可导致充血性心力衰竭[52]。因此，控制心室率不仅可以缓解房颤相关的症状，而且对于预防心室功能的恶化均有重要意义。对于伴有充血性心力衰竭的房颤患者，快速的心室率反应很容易被错误地认为是心脏功能失代偿的表现，而忽略了快速心室率房颤可以是导致心脏功能失代偿的原因。房颤诱发的心动过速性心肌病需要正确诊断和治疗，因为表现为严重充血性心力衰竭的患者可能通过恢复正常心率而得到完全纠正[52]。房颤可以通过引起心动过速性心肌病导致心脏功能不全，还可以由于快速心室率导致舒张期充盈时间的缩短而引起急性心脏失代偿。当存在舒张期充盈不良时，如严重二尖瓣狭窄、肥厚型心肌病以及限制性心脏病等，舒张时间是心脏功能或左房压力的主要决定因素。与逐渐形成的心动过速性心肌病不同，对于有严重舒张期充盈不良的患者，过快的心室率反应可以导致病情在几分钟至数小时内迅速恶化。

血栓栓塞性卒中是房颤最严重的并发症之一。总体上，未服用抗凝药物的非瓣膜性房颤患者发生卒中危险大约增加 6 倍[53]。既往有卒中史、高血压、糖尿病、充血性心力衰竭、冠心病以及高龄是房颤患者发生卒中的危险因素[54]。大于 75 岁的高龄人群中，房颤是卒中唯一的最常见相关因素[55]。房颤患者具有血栓栓塞的易患基质原因尚不清楚。尽管血流淤滞常被认为是其原因之一，新近的一个研究显示房颤患者左房心内膜内皮细胞一氧化氮合成酶下调，使一氧化氮生成减少，而凝血酶原和纤维蛋白溶酶原激活物抑制剂 1（PAI-1）的表达增加[56]。这一改变可以使局部血液凝固性增强，进而导致血栓栓塞性并发症的发生。

四、临床处理

新近发表的 ACC/AHA/ESC 指南对于不同类型房颤的特殊处理都有详尽的论述。本章节主要阐述有关房颤的治疗原则，而不涉及不同类型的房颤患者的特殊治疗建议。治疗的总目的是消除房颤的临床症状和预防相关并发症，而不是通过治疗给患者又增加另

一个同样甚至更加严重的并发症或副作用。

（一）血栓栓塞性并发症的预防

房颤最严重的并发症为血栓栓塞，尤其是脑卒中。口服抗凝药物可降低房颤患者卒中危险约60%[57]。维生素K依赖性抗凝剂，如华法林，预防卒中的有效性直接与抗凝的强度（用国际标准比率INR表示）相关，同样出血的风险也与其直接相关（图56-6）[57]。因此，要达到有效预防血栓栓塞性并发症而不增加出血并发症的风险，必须密切随访。直接凝血酶抑制剂口服制剂的开发，如ximelagatran，也许可以提供一种安全、可控、有效、不需常规监测凝血指标的抗凝治疗[58]。

适宜口服抗凝药物治疗患者的选择是比较复杂的。对于持续性房颤，有血栓栓塞高危因素［年龄大于65岁伴或不伴高血压，糖尿病，冠心病，充血性心力衰竭，或既往有卒中/短暂缺血发作（TIA）］的患者，应予抗凝治疗。小于65岁、不伴危险因素的年轻患者卒中发生率较低，可以不用口服抗凝药物治疗。对于阵发性房颤患者抗凝治疗的指征尚不确切。在心房颤动的卒中预防（SPAF）试验中持续性房颤患者发生缺血性卒中的危险与复发性房颤患者是相近的[59]。但有关阵发性房颤患者房颤发作频率和持续时间与血栓栓塞性风险之间的关系，尚缺乏详细资料。房颤患者在成功复律后应口服抗凝药物治疗多长时间目前仍不确定。在心房颤动节律控制的随访研究（AFFIRM试验）中，血栓栓塞事件主要发生在未能充分抗凝的患者中，且常发生在窦性心律时[60]。

抗凝治疗在接受复律的患者中常需特别关注，以保证患者在复律时达到充分抗凝。血栓脱落和急性血栓栓塞的危险在有效心房收缩恢复时会增加1%～7%[54]。房颤持续时间与血栓形成密切相关，一般认为房颤持续48h以上，血栓形成的可能显著增加。因此，对于房颤持续大于48h的患者应该至少在复律前3周进行有效抗凝，复律后继续抗凝4周，除非术前经过食道超声心动图检查明确排除了心房血栓。

（二）窦性心律的恢复和维持

从理论上讲，窦性心律的恢复和维持是治疗房颤的最佳选择。大多数房颤患者行电复律都能恢复窦性心律，但房颤常常复发。对于复发房颤的处理通常为重复复律或应用抗心律失常药物维持窦性心律。

1. 维持窦性心律的抗心律失常药物

许多治疗剂量的抗心律失常药物，包括ⅠA，ⅠC，和Ⅲ类药物，均有助于房颤患者窦性心律的维持[15]。延长动作电位的药物，如ⅠA和Ⅲ类药物，可以延长不应期和波长，进而使最小环路增长，减少心房可容纳的环路数目，如图56-4所示。钠通道阻滞剂（ⅠC类药物）对房颤治疗有效，但机制尚不十分清楚。ⅠC类药物预防房颤的作用可能与其抑制触发折返的异位激动有关，但这并不能解释临床明确观察到的这类药物并不延长波长却能有效终止房颤的作用[61]。近来有研究显示，钠通道阻滞剂是通过降低兴奋性和主螺旋波产生子波的稳定性来终止房颤的[62]。胺碘酮具有所有四类抗心律失常药物的特点，在窦性心律的维持上优于索他洛尔和普罗帕酮（图56-7）[63,64]。狗房颤模型研究显示，胺碘酮具有阻止由房性心动过速重构所导致的钙通道α亚基蛋白表达和心房不应期的改变以及心房的易颤性，而多菲利特（dofetilide）和氟卡胺（flecainide）则没有这些作用[65]。这些发现提示，胺碘酮预防房颤的作用部分与预防心房重构有关。

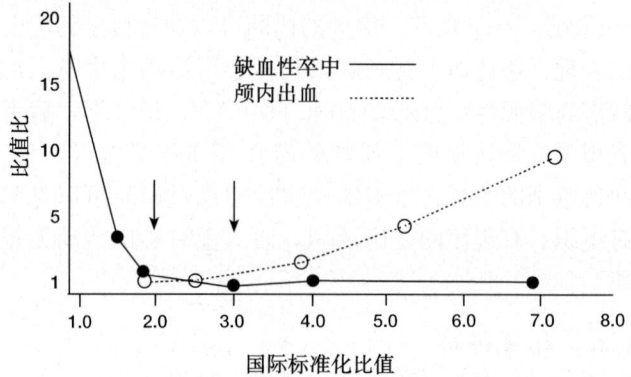

图56-6 房颤患者抗血栓治疗的随机试验中抗凝强度与缺血性卒中和颅内出血的相关性（校正的比值比） 水平轴代表国际标准化比值的治疗范围（2～3之间），可见在2～3之间出血和缺血性卒中的风险最低。（引自 Fuster V, Ryden LE, Asinger RW, et al, ACC/AHA/ESC guidelines for the management of patients with atrial fibrillation: executive summary: A Report of the American College of Cardiology/American Heart Association Task Force on Practice Guidelines and Policy Conferences [Committee to Develop Guidelines for the Management of Patients with Atrial Fibrillation] -Developed in Collaboration with the North American Society of Pacing and Electrophysiology. J Am Coll Cardiol 38: 1231-1266, 2001.) DZ: Last circle for interrupted line should be "open".

虽然抗心律失常药物有助于窦性心律的维持，但这些药物尚有潜在的严重副作用。其中最显著的是致室性心律失常的副作用，治疗药物延长动作电位产生的获得性长QT综合征（LQTS）和促进室性折返活动相一致，尤其是在急性心肌缺血时应用钠通道阻滞剂[66]。维持窦性心律药物的其他电生理副作用包括房颤规律化、快速的心室率反应以及由于缓慢性心律失常而需要埋置起搏器。

2. 维持窦性心律的非药物治疗

如上所述，Maze术对于窦性心律的维持是非常有效的（见第118章）[67]。由于Maze术是一个较大的外科手术，使其在房颤人群中的广泛应用受到限制；但对于需要进行外科瓣膜置换，尤其是二尖瓣病变（常与房颤的发生有关）的患者非常有用。对维持窦性心律最有效的导管治疗是肺静脉隔离术，尤其对阵发性房颤有效（见第113章）[17]。肺静脉狭窄和房颤复发是目前这一治疗的两个主要局限。还有一种更广泛的肺静脉消融，对左房组织进行更广泛的破坏，这种方法对持续性房颤具有较高的成功率[68]。曾有植入式心房除颤器问世，但由于患者对电击的不适反应使其应用受到限制。在需要起搏器治疗的患者中，生理性起搏器（心房起搏或双腔）较心室起搏更能降低房颤的发生率[69]。也有许多种预防房颤的起搏方式研发出来，包括双房起搏以减小心房激动离散的设计以及各种预防异位活动和使不应期离散最小化的起搏功能。这些方法获得一些成功[15]，并还在继续开发。

3. 控制心室率

房颤的许多表现是由于心室率过快引起的，而且在许多患者中单纯控制心率即可有效控制临床症状。一些药物通过延长I_{CaL}依赖性房室结动作电位的不应期增强房室结的滤过功能，可以用于控制心室率。常用的药物有β肾上腺素能受体阻滞剂，钙通道阻滞剂，以及地高辛。地高辛具有正性肌力效应，因而尤其适用于伴有充血性心力衰竭的房颤患者。地高辛的有效性依赖于迷走神经张力的加强，因而对于类似运动时迷走神经张力降低状态下的心室率控制效果有限。对于阵发性房颤患者的心室率控制比较困难。另外，房颤常与心动过缓相伴（慢快综合征），为预防控制心室率引起缓慢性心律失常常需埋藏永久起搏器保护。

对于药物不能充分控制心室率的患者，导管消融可能较有效。房室结消融加起搏治疗可以非常有效地控制临床症状，提高有显著症状的房颤患者的生活质量[15]。还有一种消融方法，通过消融房室结后侧通路（posterior nodal pathway）对房室结传导功能进行改良（仍保留其传导功能）；但起搏器依赖是其一个常见并发症，而且症状的控制程度不如阻断房室结联合起搏治疗[15]。

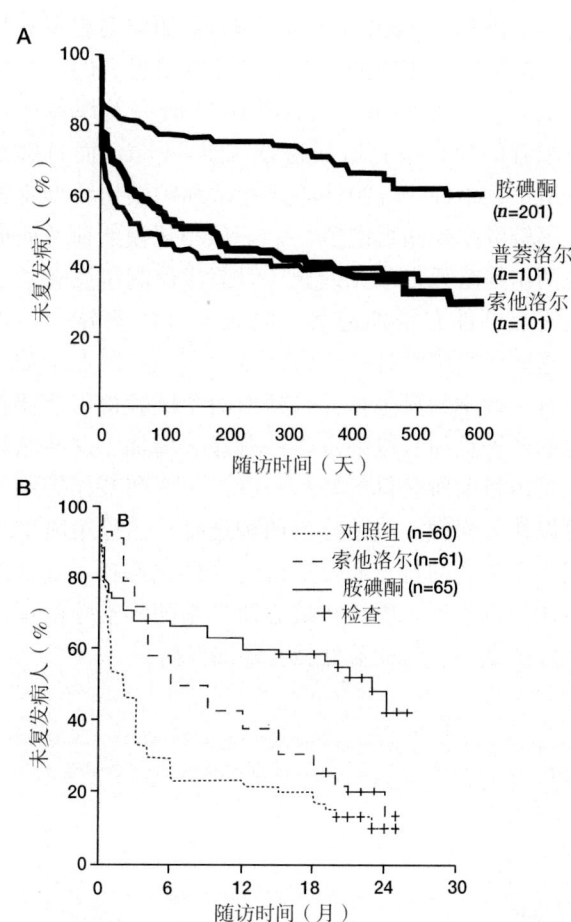

图56-7 A：Kaplan-Meier预测接受胺碘酮或普罗帕酮治疗期间无心房颤动（房颤，AF）复发患者的百分比。随访从随机入组后的第21天开始（记为0）。索他洛尔和普罗帕酮组房颤的复发率几乎相同，且显著高于胺碘酮治疗组。B：Kaplan-Meier曲线。胺碘酮对房颤复发的预防作用高于索他洛尔或安慰剂。（A，改自Roy D, Talajic M, Dorian P, et al: Amiodarone to prevent recurrence of atrial fibrillation: Canadian Trial of Atrial Fibrillation Investigators. N Engl J Med 342：913-920，2000；B，改自Kochiadakis GE, Igoumenidis NE, Marketou ME, et al: Low dose amiodarone and sotalol in the treatment of recurrent, symptomatic atrial fibrillation: A comparative, placebo controlled study. Heart 84：251-257，2000.）

4. 节律与频率控制策略的比较

节律控制使患者真正转为正常窦性心律，从理论上讲应具有优势，但仅有少数房颤患者可以在不用抗心律失常药物的情况下维持窦性心律，而且目前可用的抗心律失常药物存在着较大的副作用，均提示心室率控制可能是房颤的首选治疗。最近几个随机临床试验对房颤节律和频率控制进行了比较。房颤的药物干预试验（PIAF）得出节律和频率控制策略对患者总生活质量的影响是相似的，但节律控制组患者的6分钟行走试验优于对照组[70]。AFFIRM研究发现节律控制组患者的死亡率有增加趋势（图56-8），而且肺及胃肠道不利事件，缓慢性心律失常和尖端扭转型室速发生率较频率控制组增多[60]。一项小规模的荷兰研究发现两组策略死亡率无差异，但节律控制组患者总的负面终点事件有增加趋势，但无显著性差异[71]。总之，这些研究中没有一个研究显示在主要终点参数上两组有统计学的显著差异，其中两个试验得出节律控制组的各种负面二级终点事件有显著增加。这些结果提示，由目前所获得的资料来看，频率和节律控制策略可以作为房颤一线治疗的两种选择，治疗策略应该根据每个患者的特点和反应进行个体化选择。如果选择节律控制治疗，应该将抗心律失常药物治疗的风险与治疗所期望获得的益处相互仔细权衡。

五、未来的方向

定位于基质和预防策略

对房颤发生机制认识的新进展有希望更精确地确定房颤发生的基质，如图56-5所示。由于房性心动过速引起的重构可以增加心房的易颤性以及促进复律后房颤的复发，因而有人尝试应用作用于钙负荷的I_{Ca}拮抗剂来促进房颤复律和复律后窦性心律的维持。研究结果各不相同，显示有益的证据不足[12]。狗试验显示胺碘酮[65]和米贝拉地尔[72]可以有效预防房性心动过速引起的重构，这一结果提示心动过速引起的重构有可能成为治疗的靶目标。ACE抑制剂可以抑制充血性心力衰竭狗模型的心房纤维化和房颤的持续[44]，而且也有研究证实可以预防伴有左室功能不良的心肌梗死患者房颤的发生[73]。随着对房颤机制的深入认识，我们有可能发现更加特异的房颤作用靶点和环节，从而研发出更有效而且安全的治疗方法。

（杨延宗　林治湖　译）

参 考 文 献

1. Wolf PA, Benjamin EJ, Belanger AJ, et al: Secular trends in the prevalence of atrial fibrillation: The Framingham Study. Am Heart J 131:790–795, 1996.
2. Benjamin EJ, Wolf PA, D'Agostino RB, et al: Impact of atrial fibrillation on the risk of death: The Framingham Heart Study. Circulation 98:946–952, 1998.
3. Wolf PA, Mitchell JB, Baker CS, et al: Impact of atrial fibrillation on mortality, stroke, and medical costs. Arch Intern Med 158:229–234, 1998.
4. Nattel S: New ideas about atrial fibrillation 50 years on. Nature 415:219–226, 2002.
5. Sopher SM, Camm AJ: Atrial fibrillation: Maintenance of sinus rhythm versus rate control. Am J Cardiol 77:24A–37A, 1996.
6. Sakata K, Kurihara H, Iwamori K, et al: Clinical and prognostic significance of atrial fibrillation in acute myocardial infarction. Am J Cardiol 80:1522–1527, 1997.
7. Ehrlich JR, Nattel S, Hohnloser SH: Atrial fibrillation and congestive heart failure: Specific considerations at the intersection of two common and important cardiac disease sets. J Cardiovasc Electrophysiol 13:399–405, 2002.
8. Pozzoli M, Cioffi G, Traversi E, et al: Predictors of primary atrial fibrillation and concomittant clinical and hemodynamical changes in patients with chronic heart failure: A prospective study in 344 patients with baseline sinus rhythm. J Am Coll Cardiol 32:197–204, 1998.
9. Dries DL, Aarons D, Exner DV, et al: Atrial fibrillation is associated with an increased risk for mortality and heart failure progression in patients with asymptomatic and symptomatic left ventricular dysfunction: A retrospective analysis of the SOLVD trials. J Am Coll Cardiol 32:695–703, 1998.
10. Pedersen OD, Bagger H, Keller N, et al: Efficacy of dofetilide in the treatment of atrial fibrillation-flutter in patients with reduced left ventricular function: A Danish investigations of arrhythmia and mortality on dofetilide (diamond) substudy. Circulation 104:292–296, 2001.
11. Rationale and design of a study assessing treatment strategies of atrial

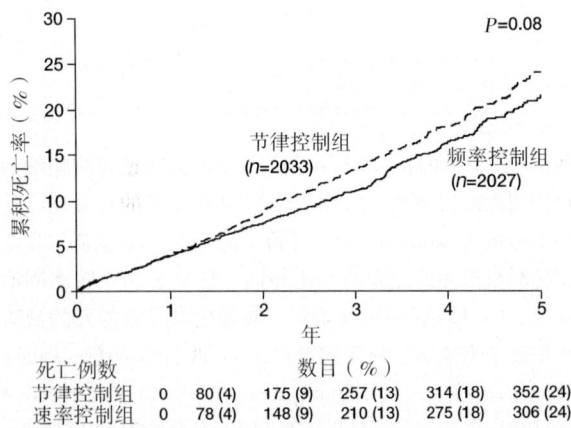

图56-8　节律控制心房颤动随访调查试验（AFFIRM）中节律和频率控制组各种原因导致的累积死亡率　两组死亡率无统计学差异（引自 Wyse DG, Waldo AL, DiMarco JP, et al: A comparison of rate control and rhythm control in patients with atrial fibrillation. N Engl J Med 347：1825-1833，2002）

fibrillation in patients with heart failure: The Atrial Fibrillation and Congestive Heart Failure (AF-CHF) trial. Am Heart J 144:597–607, 2002.
12. Nattel S: Therapeutic implications of atrial fibrillation mechanisms: Can mechanistic insights be used to improve AF management? Cardiovasc Res 54:347–360, 2002.
13. Cox JL, Schuessler RB, Boineau JP: The development of the Maze procedure for the treatment of atrial fibrillation. Semin Thorac Cardiovasc Surg 12:2–14, 2000.
14. Derakhchan K, Villemaire C, Talajic M, Nattel S: The class III antiarrhythmic drugs dofetilide and sotalol prevent AF induction by atrial premature complexes at doses that fail to terminate AF. Cardiovasc Res 50:75–84, 2001.
15. Nattel S, Khairy P, Roy D, et al: New approaches to atrial fibrillation management: A critical review of a rapidly evolving field. Drugs 62:2377–2397, 2002.
16. Haissaguerre M, Jais P, Shah DC, et al: Spontaneous initiation of atrial fibrillation by ectopic beats originating from the pulmonary veins. N Engl J Med 339:659–666, 1998.
17. Oral H, Knight BP, Tada H, et al: Pulmonary vein isolation for paroxysmal and persistent atrial fibrillation. Circulation 105:1077–1081, 2002.
18. Wu TJ, Ong JJ, Chang CM, et al: Pulmonary veins and ligament of marshall as sources of rapid activations in a canine model of sustained atrial fibrillation. Circulation 103:1157–1163, 2001.
19. Berenfeld O, Zaitsev AV, Mironov SF, et al: Frequency-dependent breakdown of wave propagation into fibrillatory conduction across the pectinate muscle network in the isolated sheep right atrium. Circ Res 90:1173–1180, 2002.
20. Schuessler RB, Grayson TM, Bromberg BI, et al: Cholinergically mediated tachyarrhythmias induced by a single extrastimulus in the isolated canine right atrium. Circ Res 71:1254–1267, 1992.
21. Mandapati R, Skanes A, Chen J, et al: Stable microreentrant sources as a mechanism of atrial fibrillation in the isolated sheep heart. Circulation 101:194–199, 2000.
22. Kneller J, Zou R, Vigmond EJ, et al: Cholinergic atrial fibrillation in a computer model of a two-dimensional sheet of canine atrial cells with realistic ionic properties. Circ Res 90:E73–E87, 2002.
23. Derakhchan K, Li D, Courtemanche M, et al: Method for simultaneous epicardial and endocardial mapping of in vivo canine heart: Application to atrial conduction properties and arrhythmia mechanisms. J Cardiovasc Electrophysiol 12:548–555, 2001.
24. Katritsis D, Iliodromitis E, Fragakis N, et al: Ablation therapy of type I atrial flutter may eradicate paroxysmal atrial fibrillation. Am J Cardiol 78:345–347, 1996.
25. Liu TY, Tai CT, Chen SA: Treatment of atrial fibrillation by catheter ablation of conduction gaps in the crista terminalis and cavotricuspid isthmus of the right atrium. J Cardiovasc Electrophysiol 13:1044–1046, 2002.
26. Wijffels MC, Kirchhof CJ, Dorland R, Allessie MA: Atrial fibrillation begets atrial fibrillation: A study in awake chronically instrumented goats. Circulation 92:1954–1968, 1995.
27. Fareh S, Villemaire C, Nattel S: Importance of refractoriness heterogeneity in the enhanced vulnerability to atrial fibrillation induction caused by tachycardia-induced electrical remodeling. Circulation 98:2202–2209, 1998.
28. Franz MR, Karasik PL, Li C, et al: Electrical remodeling of the human atrium: Similar effects in patients with chronic atrial fibrillation and atrial flutter. J Am Coll Cardiol 30:1785–1792, 1997.
29. Manios EG, Kanoupakis EM, Chlouverakis GI, et al: Changes in atrial electrical properties following cardioversion of chronic atrial fibrillation: Relation with recurrence. Cardiovasc Res 47:244–253, 2000.
30. Sun H, Chartier D, Leblanc N, Nattel S: Intracellular calcium changes and tachycardia-induced contractile dysfunction in canine atrial myocytes. Cardiovasc Res 49:751–761, 2001.
31. Courtemanche M, Ramirez RJ, Nattel S: Ionic mechanisms underlying human atrial action potential properties: Insights from a mathematical model. Am J Physiol 275:H301–H321, 1998.
32. Yue L, Melnyk P, Gaspo R, et al: Molecular mechanisms underlying ionic remodeling in a dog model of atrial fibrillation. Circ Res 84:776–784, 1999.
33. Yue L, Feng J, Gaspo R, et al: Ionic remodeling underlying action potential changes in a canine model of atrial fibrillation. Circ Res 81:512–525, 1997.
34. Gaspo R, Bosch RF, Bou-Abboud E, Nattel S: Tachycardia-induced changes in Na^+ current in a chronic dog model of atrial fibrillation. Circ Res 81:1045–1052, 1997.
35. van der Velden HM, Ausma J, Rook MB, et al: Gap junctional remodeling in relation to stabilization of atrial fibrillation in the goat. Cardiovasc Res 46:476–486, 2000.
36. Dobrev D, Graf E, Wettwer E, et al: Molecular basis of downregulation of G-protein-coupled inward rectifying K(+) current (I(K,ACh)) in chronic human atrial fibrillation: Decrease in GIRK4 mRNA correlates with reduced I(K,ACh) and muscarinic receptor-mediated shortening of action potentials. Circulation 104:2551–2557, 2001.
37. Ausma J, Wijffels M, Thone F, et al: Structural changes of atrial myocardium due to sustained atrial fibrillation in the goat. Circulation 96:3157–3163, 1997.
38. Sun H, Gaspo R, Leblanc N, Nattel S: Cellular mechanisms of atrial contractile dysfunction caused by sustained atrial tachycardia. Circulation 98:719–727, 1998.
39. Schotten U, Ausma J, Stellbrink C, et al: Cellular mechanisms of depressed atrial contractility in patients with chronic atrial fibrillation. Circulation 103:691–698, 2001.
40. Hobbs WJ, Van Gelder IC, Fitzpatrick AP, et al: The role of atrial electrical remodeling in the progression of focal atrial ectopy to persistent atrial fibrillation. J Cardiovasc Electrophysiol 10:866–870, 1999.
41. Chen YJ, Chen SA, Chen YC, et al: Effects of rapid atrial pacing on the arrhythmogenic activity of single cardiomyocytes from pulmonary veins: Implication in initiation of atrial fibrillation. Circulation 104:2849–2854, 2001.
42. Li D, Fareh S, Leung TK, Nattel S: Promotion of atrial fibrillation by heart failure in dogs: Atrial remodeling of a different kind. Circulation 100:87–95, 1999.
43. Goette A, Lendeckel U, Klein HU: Signal transduction systems and atrial fibrillation. Cardiovasc Res 54:247–258, 2002.
44. Li D, Shinagawa K, Pang L, et al: Effects of angiotensin-converting enzyme inhibition on the development of the atrial fibrillation substrate in dogs with ventricular tachypacing-induced congestive heart failure. Circulation 104:2608–2614, 2001.
45. Li D, Melnyk P, Feng J, et al: Effects of experimental heart failure on atrial cellular and ionic electrophysiology. Circulation 101:2631–2638, 2000.
46. Bosch RF, Nattel S: Cellular electrophysiology of atrial fibrillation. Cardiovasc Res 54:259–269, 2002.
47. Chen YC, Chen SA, Chen YJ, et al: Effects of thyroid hormone on the arrhythmogenic activity of pulmonary vein cardiomyocytes. J Am Coll Cardiol 39:366–372, 2002.
48. Sinno H, Derakhchan K, Libersan D, et al: Atrial ischemia promotes atrial fibrillation in dogs. Circulation 107:1930–1936, 2003.
49. Chen YH, Xu SJ, Bendahhou S, et al: KCNQ1 gain-of-function mutation in familial atrial fibrillation. Science 299:251–254, 2003.
50. Lai LP, Su MJ, Yeh HM, et al: Association of the human minK gene 38G allele with atrial fibrillation: Evidence of possible genetic control on the pathogenesis of atrial fibrillation. Am Heart J 144:485–490, 2002.
51. Mohler PJ, Schott JJ, Gramolini AO, et al: Ankyrin-B mutation causes type 4 long-QT cardiac arrhythmia and sudden cardiac death. Nature 421:634–639, 2003.
52. Shinbane JS, Wood MA, Jensen DN, et al: Tachycardia-induced cardiomyopathy: A review of animal models and clinical studies. J Am Coll Cardiol 29:709–715, 1997.
53. Echocardiographic predictors of stroke in patients with atrial fibrillation: A prospective study of 1066 patients from 3 clinical trials. Arch Intern Med 158:1316–1320, 1998.
54. Fuster V, Ryden LE, Asinger RW, et al: ACC/AHA/ESC guidelines for the management of patients with atrial fibrillation: executive summary: A Report of the American College of Cardiology/American Heart Association Task Force on Practice Guidelines and the European Society of Cardiology Committee for Practice Guidelines and Policy Conferences (Committee to Develop Guidelines for the Management of Patients With Atrial Fibrillation)—Developed in Collaboration With the North American Society of Pacing and Electrophysiology. J Am Coll Cardiol 38:1231–1266, 2001.
55. Hart RG, Halperin JL: Atrial fibrillation and stroke: Concepts and controversies. Stroke 32:803–808, 2001.
56. Cai H, Li Z, Goette A, et al: Downregulation of endocardial nitric oxide synthase expression and nitric oxide production in atrial fibrillation: Potential mechanisms for atrial thrombosis and stroke. Circulation 106:2854–2858, 2002.

57. Hart RG, Benavente O, McBride R, Pearce LA: Antithrombotic therapy to prevent stroke in patients with atrial fibrillation: A meta-analysis. Ann Intern Med 131:492–501, 1999.
58. Wahlander K, Lapidus L, Olsson CG, et al: Pharmacokinetics, pharmacodynamics and clinical effects of the oral direct thrombin inhibitor ximelagatran in acute treatment of patients with pulmonary embolism and deep vein thrombosis. Thromb Res 107:93–99, 2002.
59. Hart RG, Pearce LA, Rothbart RM, et al: Stroke with intermittent atrial fibrillation: Incidence and predictors during aspirin therapy—Stroke Prevention in Atrial Fibrillation Investigators. J Am Coll Cardiol 35:183–187, 2000.
60. Wyse DG, Waldo AL, DiMarco JP, et al: A comparison of rate control and rhythm control in patients with atrial fibrillation. N Engl J Med 347:1825–1833, 2002.
61. Wijffels MC, Dorland R, Mast F, Allessie MA: Widening of the excitable gap during pharmacological cardioversion of atrial fibrillation in the goat: Effects of cibenzoline, hydroquinidine, flecainide, and d-sotalol. Circulation 102:260–267, 2000.
62. Kneller J, Leon J, Nattel S: How do class 1 antiarrhythmic drugs terminate atrial fibrillation? A quantitative analysis based on a realistic ionic model. Circulation 104:5, 2001.
63. Kochiadakis GE, Igoumenidis NE, Marketou ME, et al: Low dose amiodarone and sotalol in the treatment of recurrent, symptomatic atrial fibrillation: A comparative, placebo controlled study. Heart 84:251–257, 2000.
64. Roy D, Talajic M, Dorian P, et al: Amiodarone to prevent recurrence of atrial fibrillation: Canadian Trial of Atrial Fibrillation Investigators. N Engl J Med 342:913–920, 2000.
65. Shinagawa K, Shiroshita-Takeshita A, Schram G, Nattel S. Effects of antiarrhythmic drugs on fibrillation in the remodeled atrium: Insights into the mechanism of the superior efficacy of amiodarone. Circulation 107:1440–1446, 2003.
66. Nattel S: Experimental evidence for proarrhythmic mechanisms of antiarrhythmic drugs. Cardiovasc Res 37:567–577, 1998.
67. Cox JL, Ad N, Palazzo T, et al: Current status of the Maze procedure for the treatment of atrial fibrillation. Semin Thorac Cardiovasc Surg 12:15–19, 2000.
68. Pappone C, Rosanio S, Oreto G, et al: Circumferential radiofrequency ablation of pulmonary vein ostia: A new anatomic approach for curing atrial fibrillation. Circulation 102:2619–2628, 2000.
69. Skanes AC, Krahn AD, Yee R, et al: Progression to chronic atrial fibrillation after pacing: The Canadian Trial of Physiologic Pacing—CTOPP Investigators. J Am Coll Cardiol 38:167–172, 2001.
70. Hohnloser SH, Kuck KH, Lilienthal J: Rhythm or rate control in atrial fibrillation: Pharmacological Intervention in Atrial Fibrillation (PIAF)—A randomised trial. Lancet 356:1789–1794, 2000.
71. Van Gelder IC, Hagens VE, Bosker HA, et al: A comparison of rate control and rhythm control in patients with recurrent persistent atrial fibrillation. N Engl J Med 347:1834–1840, 2002.
72. Fareh S, Benardeau A, Thibault B, Nattel S: The T-type Ca(2+) channel blocker mibefradil prevents the development of a substrate for atrial fibrillation by tachycardia-induced atrial remodeling in dogs. Circulation 100:2191–2197, 1999.
73. Pedersen OD, Bagger H, Kober L, Torp-Pedersen C: Trandopril reduces the incidence of atrial fibrillation after acute myocardial infarction in patients with left ventricular dysfunction: TRACE Study group—TRAndolapril Cardiac Evalution. Circulation 100:376–380, 1999.

第 57 章

交界区心律和交界区心动过速

Hakan Oral and S. Adam Strickberger

本章目录

- 交界区异位心动过速 …………………… 517
- 手术后交界区心动过速 ………………… 519
- 继发性交界区心律 ……………………… 520
- 总结 ……………………………………… 520

交界区心律是起源于房室交界区的电活动，尽管相对少见，交界区心律却包含了较宽的心律失常范围，其临床表现、意义及治疗策略是不同的。交界区心律可分为四类：(1) 一类是原发于交界区的异常，可引起无休止性或阵发性交界区异位心动过速；(2) 一类是发生在心外科手术后，多见于婴幼儿和儿童；(3) 一类是自主性、代谢性或药物影响出现的交界区心律；(4) 最后一类是在严重心动过缓时出现的逸搏心律。本章将重点讨论前两种交界区心律。

一、交界区异位心动过速

交界区异位心动过速由 Coumel 和他的同事在 1976 年首次提出。交界区异位心动过速是一种窄 QRS 波心动过速，特点是心动过速周期不规则，可见窦性夺获，房室或室房关系可变以及室房分离（图 57-1，图 57-2）。这种心律失常的发生有两种特定的临床形式，一种是无休止性，通常发生在小于 6 个月的婴儿，另一种是阵发性，大多发生在儿童，也可发生在成人。

无休止性交界区异位心动过速是罕见的，发生率不超过儿童心律失常的 1%，常常引起心脏肥大，60% 的患儿出现充血性心力衰竭，死亡率达 35%。交界区异位心动过速有家族性，产前可以作出诊断。

(一) 心电图和心脏电生理特征

在体表心电图上交界区异位心动过速常表现为不规则的窄 QRS 波心动过速（110~230 次/分），窦性夺获及室房阻滞（图 57-1）。P 波通常不易分辨。如果 P 波不能辨别时，体表心电图酷似心房颤动。伴束支传导阻滞时交界区异位心动过速呈现宽 QRS 波，难以同室性心动过速相鉴别。交界区异位心动过速伴室房阻滞是一种特殊情况。

交界区异位心动过速时心脏电生理标志是在每一个 QRS 波群之前有希氏束电位，HV 间期是正常的，除非存在传导系统疾病（图 57-2）。常规地能观察到房室传导和室房传导的变化，几乎总是出现室房传导阻滞和房室分离，但大多数病人能见到室房传导。心动过速的起始和终止是自发的，心室起搏容易诱发心动过速，或在静点异丙肾上腺素时起搏可诱发。有些病人心室起搏或注射腺苷可终止心动过速。沿房间隔的任何地方都能够记录到最早的逆传心房电位。

几乎一半的交界区异位心动过速的病人同时存在其他类型的室上性心动过速，包括房室结折返性心动过速和房性心动过速。交界区异位心动过速同房室结折返性心动过速鉴别是很困难的，两者都可伴有房室或室房分离，但在后者是不常见的。交界区异位心动过速的诱发和终止通常不依赖丁程序刺激，而房室结折返性心动过速则不是，它的诱发依靠临界的 AH 间期（图 57-3）。

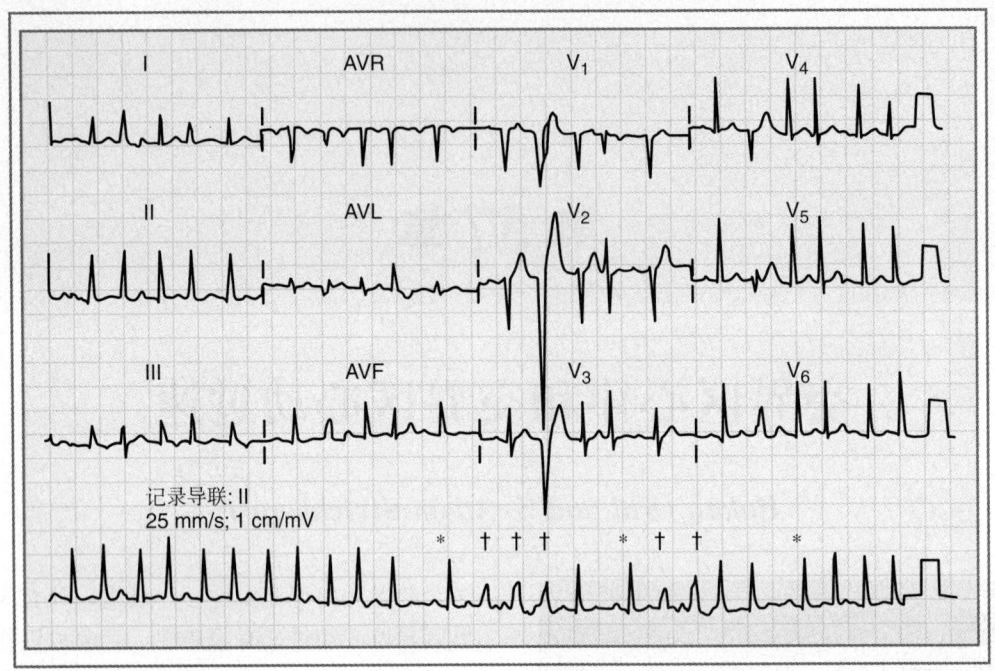

图 57-1 交界区异位心动过速的体表心电图 心动过速是不规则的,有窦性夺获(*)和异常形态的 QRS 波群(+)。(引自 Ruder MA, Davis JC, Elder M, et al: Clinical and electrophysiologic Circulation 73: 930~937, 1986.)

(二) 机制

交界区异位心动过速的机制不清楚,然而,最常见的解释是异常自律性和触发活动。由于大多数发作的起始和终止是自发性的,心动过速相当不规则,用异丙肾上腺素后容易诱发,所以异常自律性似乎是最合适的解释。心室起搏可以诱发心动过速,注射腺苷可终止心动过速,所以说触发活动也是一种可能的机制。

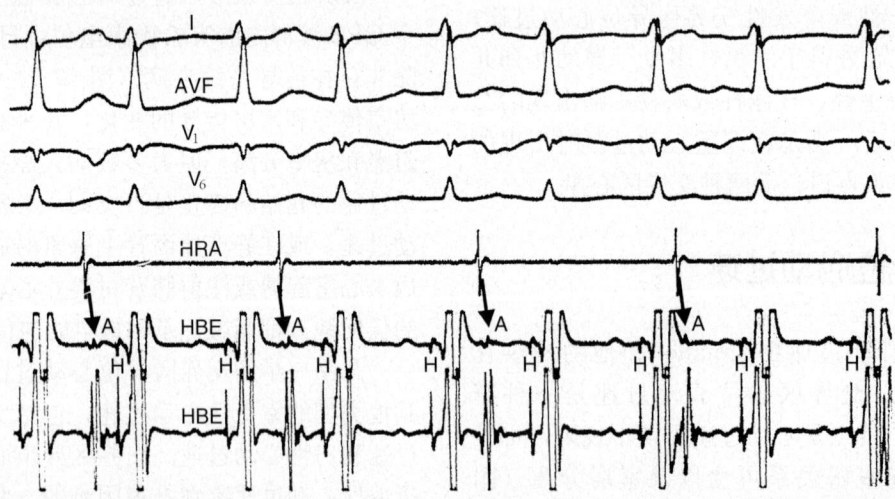

图 57-2 交界区异位心动过速的心腔内心电图 每个 QRS 波前均有希氏束电位,室房分离。心房电位是正常的(箭头所示),发生的顺序是从高位右房(HRA)至低位右房(HBE)。本图记录顺序从上至下分别是 Ⅰ、aVF、V₁、V₆导联和高右房(HRA)以及两条希氏束通道。(引自 Gillette PC, Garson A Jr, Porter CJ et al: Junctional automatic ectopic tachycardia: New proposed treatment by transcatheter His bundle ablation. Am Heart J 106: 619~623, 1983.)

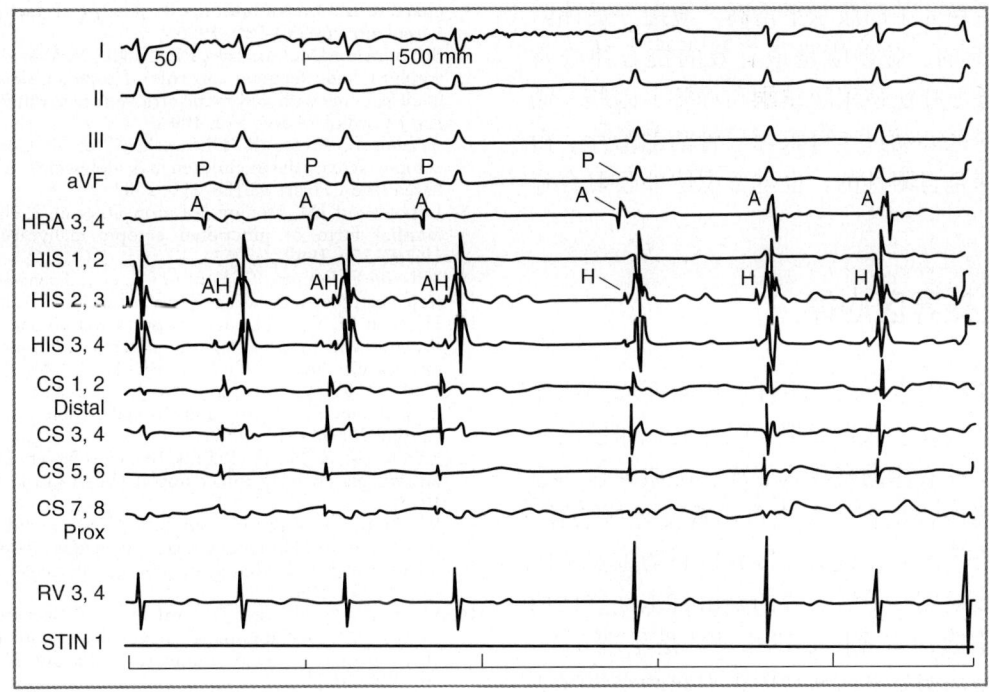

图 57-3 交界区异位心动过速的发生 该图显示，在心动过速诱发时临界的 AH 间期与心动过速的起始没有关系。A：心房除极波；H：希氏束除极波；P：体表心房波。（引自 Hamdan M，Van Hare GF，Fisher W et al：Selective catheter ablation of the tachycardial focus in patients with nonreentrant junctional tachycardial. Am J Cardiol 78：1292-1297，1996.）

（三）治疗

交界区异位心动过速的治疗选择包括异位点的导管射频消融术和房室结消融后植入永久性起搏器。对这些方法的选择在成人比婴幼儿的反应更好一些。地高辛、β受体阻滞剂、普罗帕酮、氟卡胺和胺碘酮等均有小系列的报道用于治疗交界区异位心动过速。对这种心律失常胺碘酮是最好的抗心律失常药，当和普罗帕酮或氟卡胺联合应用时应选择小剂量。交界区异位心动过速病人常伴希浦氏系统疾病，可发生三度房室阻滞。应用抗心律失常药可进一步影响希浦氏系统功能，甚至发生猝死。

导管射频消融术已被用于治疗交界区异位心动过速。Hamdan 和他的同事报道了最多的一组病例，共 11 例，其中 9 例经射频消融治疗得到了长期根治，1 例病人发生了三度房室阻滞。在室房传导存在时，以最早的心房激动点作为靶点。无室房传导时，经验性消融后间隔区域，相当于房室结折返性心动过速时慢径消融区，消融点逐渐地向上直至消融成功。成功的消融点中 3 例位于后间隔，3 例位于中间隔，4 例位于前间隔。如果室房传导不存在，以及消融过程中出现了交界区异位激动，在放电时要完整地监测房室传导，此时心房起搏的频率稍快于交界区异位心律。在射频消融治疗无效时，有症状的交界区异位心动过速可以考虑房室结消融同时植入永久性起搏器。

二、手术后交界区心动过速

手术后交界区异位心动过速常发生在婴幼儿及儿童先天性心脏缺损矫正术后 4 天内，很少见于成人心脏外科手术后。连续观察 343 例先天性心脏缺损修补术后的一系列病人，术后交界区异位心动过速发生率是 10.8%。交界区异位心动过速在法洛四联症术后发生率 22%，房室间隔缺损修补术后 10%，室间隔缺损修补术后 4%。在伴交界区异位心动过速的病人死亡率是 8%，余下的病人死亡率是 3%。从这个大系列的多变量分析中证实法洛四联症的病人右室流出道大部分肌肉切除后其梗阻的缓解和牵拉是交界区异位心动过速的独立预测因素。手术后交界区异位心动过速与房室交界区周围的损伤、渗出性出血和炎症反应等有一定关系。

大多数手术后交界区异位心动过速发作是自限性，并且能引起显著性血流动力学障碍，在手术后早期应积极地治疗。早期治疗是很重要的，主要是维持窦性心律及控制心室率。成功地使全身温度低至 32～35℃ 及避免发热性反应。纠正电解质失衡特别是镁离子。通过镇静避免儿茶酚胺水平增高，应用β-受体阻滞剂也是有帮助的。胺碘酮是最有效的抗心律失常药，结合全身低温疗法使用胺碘酮和普鲁卡因胺。顽固性手术后交界区心动过速可采用导管消融治疗。由于这种心动过速是自限性的，也可考虑体外膜氧合疗法。

三、继发性交界区心律

交界区心律的发生可由自主性、代谢性或药物作用引起。在能增加肾上腺素能神经张力的代谢性疾病可观察到快于窦性心律的交界区心律。心肌缺血、急性风湿性心脏炎及洋地黄中毒也可出现交界区心律。在这些情况下交界区心律比交界区异位心动过速实际上要慢一些且较规则。最后要说的是由自主性、代谢性或药物影响引起的交界区心律几乎总是呈现1∶1室房传导。典型的例外是洋地黄中毒引起的交界区心律伴室房分离。这种情况容易发生在心房颤动的病人，过量的洋地黄减慢了心室率。继发性交界区心律可能的机制是延迟后除极引发的触发活动。交界区逸搏心律发生在严重的病态窦房结综合征或三度房室阻滞患者，是一种正常的心脏自主性节律。

四、总　结

初发的交界区心动过速一般用药物治疗。射频消融治疗由于并发三度房室阻滞的危险一般用于药物治疗无效的病人。手术后交界区心动过速一般发生在婴儿和儿童，最好是预防儿茶酚胺水平增高，应用低温疗法或同时应用抗心律失常药。继发性心律失常是由代谢性或药物作用引起。交界区逸搏心律是严重心动过缓的结果，是心脏自主性节律。

（刘书旺　译）

参 考 文 献

1. Coumel P, Fidelle JE, Attuel P, et al: Congenital bundle-of-His focal tachycardias. Cooperative study of 7 cases. Arch Mal Coeur Vaiss 69:899–909, 1976.
2. Garson A Jr, Gillette PC: Junctional ectopic tachycardia in children: Electrocardiography, electrophysiology and pharmacologic response. Am J Cardiol 44:298–302, 1979.
3. Gillette PC, Garson A Jr, Porter CJ, et al: Junctional automatic ectopic tachycardia: New proposed treatment by transcatheter His bundle ablation. Am Heart J 106:619–623, 1983.
4. Villain E, Vetter VL, Garcia JM, et al: Evolving concepts in the management of congenital junctional ectopic tachycardia. A multicenter study. Circulation 81:1544–1549, 1990.
5. Ruder MA, Davis JC, Eldar M, et al: Clinical and electrophysiologic characterization of automatic junctional tachycardia in adults. Circulation 73:930–937, 1986.
6. Scheinman MM, Gonzalez RP, Cooper MW, et al: Clinical and electrophysiologic features and role of catheter ablation techniques in adult patients with automatic atrioventricular junctional tachycardia. Am J Cardiol 74:565–572, 1994.
7. Sarubbi B, Musto B, Ducceschi V, et al: Congenital junctional ectopic tachycardia in children and adolescents: A 20 year experience based study. Heart 88:188–190, 2002.
8. Lupoglazoff JM, Denjoy I, Luton D, et al: Prenatal diagnosis of a familial form of junctional ectopic tachycardia. Prenat Diagn 19:767–770, 1999.
9. Villazon E, Fouron JC, Fournier A, et al: Prenatal diagnosis of junctional ectopic tachycardia. Pediatr Cardiol 22:160–162, 2001.
10. Hamdan M, Van Hare GF, Fisher W, et al: Selective catheter ablation of the tachycardia focus in patients with nonreentrant junctional tachycardia. Am J Cardiol 78:1292–1297, 1996.
11. Paul T, Reimer A, Janousek J, et al: Efficacy and safety of propafenone in congenital junctional ectopic tachycardia. J Am Coll Cardiol 20:911–914, 1992.
12. Henneveld H, Hutter P, Bink-Boelkens M, et al: Junctional ectopic tachycardia evolving into complete heart block. Heart 80:627–628, 1998.
13. Van Hare GF, Velvis H, Langberg JJ: Successful transcatheter ablation of congenital junctional ectopic tachycardia in a ten-month-old infant using radiofrequency energy. Pacing Clin Electrophysiol 13:730–735, 1990.
14. Ehlert FA, Goldberger JJ, Deal BJ, et al: Successful radiofrequency energy ablation of automatic junctional tachycardia preserving normal atrioventricular nodal conduction. Pacing Clin Electrophysiol 16:54–61, 1993.
15. Young ML, Mehta MB, Martinez RM, et al: Combined alpha-adrenergic blockade and radiofrequency ablation to treat junctional ectopic tachycardia successfully without atrioventricular block. Am J Cardiol 71:883–885, 1993.
16. Wu MH, Lin JL, Chang YC: Catheter ablation of junctional ectopic tachycardia by guarded low dose radiofrequency energy application. Pacing Clin Electrophysiol 19:1655–1658, 1996.
17. Fishberger SB, Rossi AF, Messina JJ, et al: Successful radiofrequency catheter ablation of congenital junctional ectopic tachycardia with preservation of atrioventricular conduction in a 9-month-old infant. Pacing Clin Electrophysiol 21:2132–2135, 1998.
18. Rychik J, Marchlinski FE, Sweeten TL, et al: Transcatheter radiofrequency ablation for congenital junctional ectopic tachycardia in infancy. Pediatr Cardiol 18:447–450, 1997.
19. Braunstein PW Jr, Sade RM, Gillette PC: Life-threatening postoperative junctional ectopic tachycardia. Ann Thorac Surg 53:726–728, 1992.
20. Raja P, Hawker RE, Chaikitpinyo A, et al: Amiodarone management of junctional ectopic tachycardia after cardiac surgery in children. Br Heart J 72:261–265, 1994.
21. Saul JP, Walsh EP, Triedman JK: Mechanisms and therapy of complex arrhythmias in pediatric patients. J Cardiovasc Electrophysiol 6:1129–1148, 1995.
22. Dodge-Khatami A, Miller OI, Anderson RH, et al: Impact of junctional ectopic tachycardia on postoperative morbidity following repair of congenital heart defects. Eur J Cardiothorac Surg 21:255–259, 2002.
23. Dodge-Khatami A, Miller OI, Anderson RH, et al: Surgical substrates of postoperative junctional ectopic tachycardia in congenital heart defects. J Thorac Cardiovasc Surg 123:624–630, 2002.
24. Pfammatter JP, Paul T, Ziemer G, et al: Successful management of junctional tachycardia by hypothermia after cardiac operations in infants. Ann Thorac Surg 60:556–560, 1995.
25. Walsh EP, Saul JP, Sholler GF, et al: Evaluation of a staged treatment protocol for rapid automatic junctional tachycardia after operation for congenital heart disease. J Am Coll Cardiol 29:1046–1053, 1997.
26. Azzam FJ, Fiore AC: Postoperative junctional ectopic tachycardia. Can J Anaesth 45:898–902, 1998.

第58章

房室折返及变异形式

Bradley P. Knight，Fred Morady

本章目录
- 房室折返的特点 521
- 诊断 521
- 治疗 527
- 总结 528

一、房室折返的特点

旁路（或旁道，accessory pathway，AP）是位于房室瓣环的异常心脏肌束，连接心房与心室，常常具有快速的激动传导功能。旁路可能是房室环在胚胎期发育不全的结果，有时也可能是遗传性的[1]。房室折返性心动过速（atrioventricular reentrant tachycardia，AVRT）由大折返引起，其折返环包括心房、房室结、希浦系统、心室和旁路。AVRT发生时，如果激动在房室结的传导方向是前传而在旁路是逆传，这种AVRT称为顺向型房室折返性心动过速，心动过速的心电图表现为窄QRS波群，除非有束支阻滞。顺向型房室折返性心动过速占整个阵发性室上性心动过速（室上速）病例的35%，需与房室结折返性心动过速、房性心动过速（房速）、交界区异位心动过速（junctional ectopic tachycardia）鉴别。参与顺向型房室折返性心动过速机制的近50%的旁路只有逆传功能，因此在窦性心律下的体表心电图上没有预激的表现，这种旁路又称为隐匿性旁路。

AVRT发作时，如果经过旁路的传导为前向，而经过房室结的传导为逆向，这种心动过速称为逆向型房室折返性心动过速，心动过速的心电图表现为宽大畸形的QRS波群。逆向型房室折返性心动过速应与起源于二、三尖瓣环附近的室性心动过速进行鉴别。如果旁路具有前传功能，在窦性心律下心室的预激是显而易见的，这种旁路又称显性旁路。如果房室结的传导速度快，或者旁路的前传速度慢，或旁路位于二尖瓣环的侧壁而远离窦房结时，心电图上的心室预激表现就会不明显。当病人有心室预激并伴随心动过速发作的临床表现时，称为预激综合征（Wolff-Parkinson-White综合征，或WPW综合征）。

AVRT的变异形式包括：具有递减特性的旁路折返、连接心房或房室结与心室或束支之间旁路的折返以及多旁路间的折返。具有递减传导特性的隐匿性旁路常位于后间隔区。因为有两个慢传导肢的心动过速具有较宽的可激动间隙，缓慢传导的旁路会引起无休止性长RP间期心动过速，是交界区房室折返性心动过速（junctional reciprocating tachycardia）的一种持续形式。这种持续性的交界区房室折返性心动过速在儿童更常见，而且常引起心动过速介导性心肌病。另一种旁路的变异形式是心房与右束支之间的连接。这种连接常常位于三尖瓣环的侧壁，而且只有前向的传导功能。虽然房束（支）间的旁路常常称为Mahaim束（Mahaim fiber），但Mahaim最初描述的却是结-束旁路，实际上后者比前者要少得多。通过隐匿性房结（心房-房室结）旁路产生的窄QRS波群心动过速已有报道[2]。

二、诊 断

一个有规律的窄QRS波群心动过速的鉴别诊断包括：顺向型房室折返性心动过速、房室结折返性心动过速、房速和交界区异位心动过速。临床和心电图资料对诊断很有用，但是，大多数病例需要做电生理检查才能确定顺向型房室折返性心动过速诊断。

(一) 临床诊断

AVRT 病人的临床症状表现为阵发性室上性心动过速的特点，包括快速和有规律的心悸、胸痛、气短、先兆晕厥，极少数情况下可出现晕厥。AVRT 的发作和终止常呈突然性。然而，在某些病例，AVRT 终止后继发的窦性心动过速使病人感到心动过速是逐渐终止的。极少数情况下，有无休止性心动过速的病人并没有感觉到心跳过速，而表现为心力衰竭的症状。临床症状对于鉴别 AVRT 与其他类型的阵发性室上性心动过速通常没有帮助。

AVRT 病人通常没有器质性心脏病。然而，对每一个病人仍要进行体格检查和 12 导联心电图记录。因为先天性异常，如肥厚型心肌病、埃布斯坦畸形 (Ebstein anomaly) 常合并旁路，如果体检或心电图的结果异常，应进行超声心动图检查。顺向型房室折返性心动过速（也包括其他类型阵发性室上速）发作时常出现 ST 段压低，但对冠心病诊断没有特异性价值，也不需要进行心导管检查。

旁路介导性心动过速病人的平均年龄为 25 岁[3]，但年龄范围很宽。病人也可能到了 90 岁才出现 AVRT 的首次发作。AVRT 在男性比女性多见。在一个包括 910 例旁路介导的心动过速的病例报道中[3]，左侧旁路的男女比率为 1.7，间隔旁路为 1.2，右侧旁路为 1.1。

(二) 心电图诊断

心电图可以对窄 QRS 波心动过速提供重要的诊断线索。窦性心律下心室预激现象的存在强烈提示心动过速机制为顺向型房室折返性心动过速。前传不应期长的旁路通常在窦性心率比较缓慢时才表现出来。所以，在寻找心室预激的证据时，检查心动过速终止后经过一个间歇而恢复的第一个 QRS 波群可能更有帮助。在房束旁路病人心室预激常常不能表现出来，因为旁路的前向传导速度很慢。

顺向型房室折返性心动过速发作时，心房激动发生在希浦系、心室和旁路激动之后。因此，P 波常常出现在 QRS 波群之后。相反，在典型（慢-快型）房室结折返性心动过速，心房和心室几乎同时除极，因此 P 波落在 QRS 波群中或紧接其后。当逆传的 P 波使 QRS 波群变形，在 V_1 导联出现假性 r' 波，在下壁导联出现假性 s 波，则顺向型房室折返性心动过速可以除外[4]。在顺向型房室折返性心动过速发作时，如果 P 波能够识别，则 P 波形态可用于隐匿性旁路的定位，但是 P 波常常被 T 波掩盖。如果心动过速随着房室阻滞而自发终止，则可除外房速。

心动过速发作时，QRS 波群电压的交替性变化称为 QRS 波群电交替（QRS alternans），在顺向型房室折返性心动过速病人比房室结折返性心动过速病人更常见。然而，QRS 波群电交替是频率依赖性的，并不能提示心动过速的机制。顺向型房室折返性心动过速的频率倾向于比房室结折返性心动过速快，心动过速频率超过 220 次/分时更倾向于顺向型房室折返性心动过速。在一例房室结双路径病人顺向型房室折返性心动过速发作时出现心动周期长短交替时，提示激动通过房室结的慢径和快径交替前向传导。

(三) 心脏电生理检查

虽然现在已有几种新型先进的心脏标测系统应用于临床，但是 AVRT 通过经典的三根电极导管几乎都可以作出诊断。导管放置在高位右房、右心室和三尖瓣环附近的希氏束部位。如果需要记录冠状静脉窦电图，可将希氏束部位的导管向足、向后方向旋转送入冠状窦。心动过速通常由频率递增的心房或心室刺激或心房期前刺激诱发。有时需要静脉点滴异丙肾上腺素来诱发持续性心动过速。

1. 窦性心律时的基础特点

对于可诱发的心动过速，支持 AVRT 诊断的窦性心律下的基础特点为旁路存在的证据（表 58-1），如心室预激（HV 间期＜35ms），或在希氏束旁起搏时出现结外反应，或心房起搏可使心室的预激程度最大化。当预激最大化的 QRS 波群形态与宽 QRS 波心动过速发作时的 QRS 波群形态相同时，提示心动过速的最可能机制是逆向型房室折返性心动过速。

希氏束旁起搏指在记录到高振幅的希氏束电位的部位以不同的刺激强度进行起搏，以达到夺获右心室或同时夺获右心室和希氏束的目的。当希氏束被夺获时，其 QRS 波群比单纯右心室夺获时的 QRS 波群窄。如果存在间隔旁路则可见到旁路反应，其特点为不管有无希氏束夺获，室房间期相同（图 58-1A）。因为不论有无希氏束夺获，在基础右心室起搏期间激动都会通过间隔旁路传导至心房。而房室结的反应则为

表 58-1　阵发性室上速心脏电生理检查时基础和心动过速特点的发生率和阳性预测率

基线或心动过速时特点	发生率（%）	阳性预测率（%）		
		AVNRT	ORT	AT
窦性心律下的预激现象	15	10	86	3
希氏束旁刺激的结外反应	18	17	83	0
基础情况下＞600ms 间期起搏出现 VA 阻滞	11	41	5	55
间隔的 VA 间期＞70ms	53	17	59	24
离心性心房激动	31	0	76	24
心动过速时自发性房室阻滞	10	60	0	40
房室阻滞时心动过速自行终止	28	66	34	0
LBBB 出现	12	4	92	4
束支阻滞时 VA 间期增幅＞20ms	7	0	100	0

VA＝室房，LBBB＝左束支阻滞，ORT＝顺向型房室折返性心动过速

在希氏束夺获时的室房间期短于希氏束未夺获时的室房间期（图 58-1B）。房室结反应产生的机制为：希氏束夺获时，激动通过房室结逆传至心房，而单纯心室夺获时，激动通过右心室基底部至心尖部、浦肯野纤维、希氏束、房室结才逆传至心房。以 600ms 间期起搏心室时，室房阻滞的出现提示病人不大可能诱发顺向型房室折返性心动过速，而合并阵发性室上速的病人仅占 11%[6]。

在决定旁路是否存在的检查中，起搏比药物激发更有价值。例如，在心室起搏时，腺苷诱发的室房阻滞说明存在旁路的可能性不大。然而，极少数旁路对腺苷是敏感的。此外，在注射腺苷时持续存在的室房传导并不能确定旁路的存在，因为注射腺苷时，经过房室结快路径的逆传常常不被阻滞[7]。

支持存在（心）房束（支）旁路、（房室）结束（支）的基础依据包括：在心房频率递增起搏过程中心室预激逐渐明显并伴随房室间期逐渐延长以及沿三尖瓣环出现的旁路电位，这种电位类似希氏束电位（图 58-2）。在多旁路病人，心房起搏以及房颤的诱发可视作预激的变异形式。然而，在多旁路病人的 AVRT 机制上，心动过速发作的前传肢和逆传肢都经旁路的可能性很少，除非旁路相距足够远使一条旁路有足够的时间恢复其可激动性。

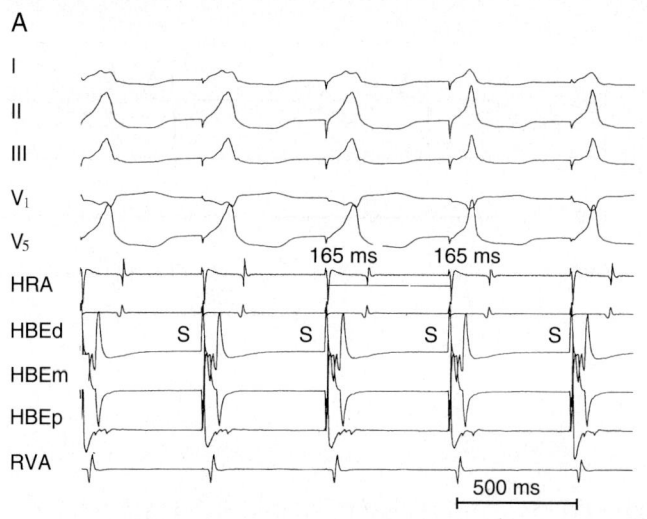 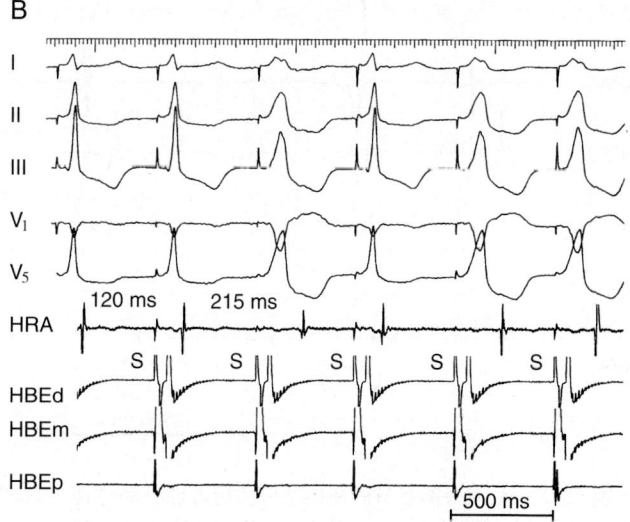

图 58-1　希氏束旁起搏的反应　图示为Ⅰ、Ⅱ、Ⅲ、V₁、V₅ 导联的体表心电图和高位右房（HRA）、远端希氏束（HBEd）、中位希氏束（HBEm）、近端希氏束（HBEp）和右心室心尖部（RVA）记录通道。A：显示有后间隔旁路病人对希氏束旁起搏的反应。在窄 QRS 波群后的室房间期（165ms）与宽 QRS 波群后的室房间期（165ms）相同。B：在后间隔隐匿性旁路消融后的结区反应。当希氏束起搏夺获和窄 QRS 波群（120ms）出现时的室房间期短于希氏束起搏失夺获和 QRS 波群变宽时的室房间期（215ms）。S，起搏刺激。

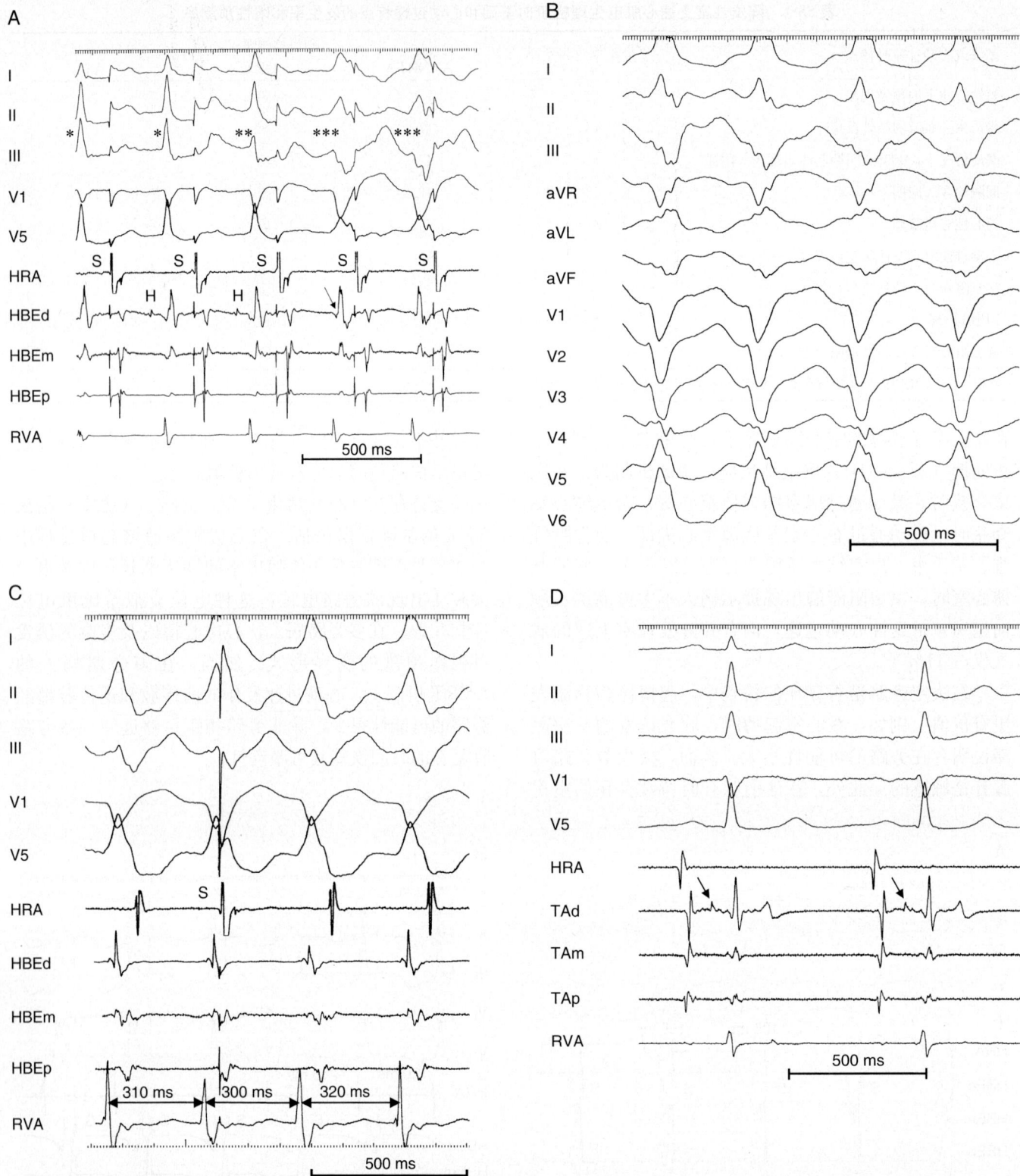

图 58-2 房-束旁路参与的逆向型房室折返性心动过速 格式和标注同图 58-1。A. 心房起搏使 PR 间期和 AH 间期逐渐延长。前两个 QRS 波群（标 *）是窄的，因为心室激动只通过房室结传导。第 3 个 QRS 波群（标 **）为经房室结激动与心室部分提前激动（预激）的融合波。第 4、5 个 QRS 波群（标 ***）呈完全预激图形。第 3 个 QRS 波群的希氏束电图（H）不能分辨，可能隐藏在右室电位的起始部分（箭头所示）。B. 逆向型房室折返性心动过速的体表心电图示 QRS 波群类左束支阻滞图形，胸前导联 QRS 波群过渡区左移至 V_5 导联。C. 在间隔部心房电图出现时同步发放心房期前刺激，引发了心室的提前激动，而此时房室结处于不应期，因此可以确定存在房室结外异常房室传导通路。D. 通过放置于三尖瓣环侧壁的标测导管记录显示有房-束旁路电位（箭头），该电位可作为射频消融的靶点。

2. 心动过速特点

有几个特点提示顺向型房室折返性心动过速为心动过速的机制（表58-1）[6]。在典型的房室结折返（慢-快型）时，间隔部位靠近房室结的心房最先激动，所以心房激动呈"向心性"。在不典型房室结折返（快-慢型或慢-慢型）时，最早的心房激动出现在冠状窦口附近。"离心性"心房激动是指最早的心房激动位于冠状窦的远端或三尖瓣环的侧壁。虽然偏心性心房激动不可能是房室结折返，但是在非典型房室结折返时最早的心房激动点（EAA）可以位于冠状窦内[8]。对于显性预激的病人，重要的是要识别顺向型房室折返性心动过速发作时的最早心房激动点，不应认为显性旁路就是顺向型房室折返性心动过速的逆传肢。同样重要的是，在逆向型房室折返性心动过速时要仔细检查逆传，因为在AVRT发作时，同一个旁路既可作前传肢，又可作逆传肢。

在顺向型房室折返性心动过速发作时，如果旁路侧出现束支阻滞，室房传导时间延长是由于激动通过对侧心室和室间隔传导至旁路出现传导延迟所致（图58-3）。顺向型房室折返性心动过速发作时，如同侧束支阻滞使VA间期延长≥25ms，提示游离壁旁路；右束支阻滞时VA间期延长＜25ms提示前间隔旁路；左束支阻滞使VA间期延长＜25ms时，提示后间隔旁路。VA间期延长也会引起心动过速周期延长，除非存在代偿性AV间期缩短。束支阻滞时VA间期延长支持顺向型房室折返性心动过速诊断，但仅见于7%的室上速病人。

有趣的是，心动过速伴左束支阻滞强烈提示顺向型房室折返性心动过速（阳性预测率92%），而且预测价值独立于心动过速频率。为什么左束支阻滞更常见于顺向型房室折返性心动过速而非房室结折返有两种解释。第一，房室结折返的诱发常常需要房室结传导的明显延缓，从而使H_1-H_2间期延长，使差传变得不太可能。第二，当左侧有旁路时（大多数旁路位于左侧），左束支阻滞有利于顺向型房室折返性心动过速的诱发。

当间隔VA间期＜70ms时，可以除外顺向型房室折返性心动过速，同样心动过速发作时V_1导联上的假R波也有助于除外顺向型房室折返性心动过速。心动过速发作时自发性房室和室房阻滞可以除外顺向型房室折返性心动过速，因为心房和心室都是折返环的必需成分。心动过速通常突然发作和终止。如果心动过速发作依赖于旁路的前向阻滞，则高度提示顺向型房室折返性心动过速（图58-3）。心动过速自发终止并伴房室阻滞则可除外房性心动过速。

如果QRS波群前缺少希氏束电图，则逆向型房室折返性心动过速容易与室上性心动过速伴束支阻滞相鉴别。由房-束或结-束参与的逆向型心动过速表现为类左束支阻滞的宽QRS波心动过速，胸前导联过渡区左移至V_{4-5}导联，右室远端激动领先于近端，希氏束电位处于QRS波群的起始部分内（图58-2）。如心动过速时存在室房阻滞，则支持结-束参与的逆向型心动过速，从而能够与房-束参与的逆向型心动过速鉴别开来。

（四）心动过速的诊断方法

有几种诊断性起搏方法有助于AVRT的诊断[6]。总之，在窄QRS波心动过速时心室起搏更有用，而在宽QRS波心动过速时心房起搏更有价值。

在窄QRS心动过速时一个有用的方法是用比心动过速周期稍短的间期进行心室超速起搏[9]。如果起搏过程中心室激动与心动过速分离，则顺向型房室折返性心动过速可除外。如果心室起搏时心房没有被除极，但心动过速终止，则常常可除外房性心动过速（房速）。然而，在极少数情况下，尽管心房没有被除极，心室起搏通过电机械反馈也可终止房速。

如果在心室超速起搏时心动过速频率被加速到起

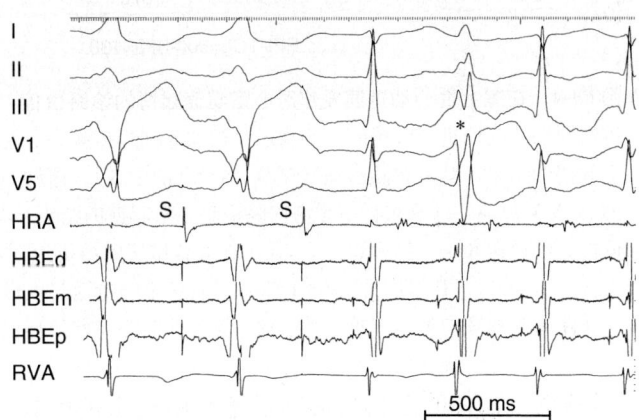

图58-3 心房起搏诱发窄QRS波群心动过速 图的格式和标注与图58-1相同。前两个QRS波群为预激图形，符合后间隔旁路。第3个QRS波群变窄，为旁路前传阻滞引起，同时触发了心动过速。心动过速触发伴旁路前传阻滞高度提示房室折返性心动过速（AVRT）。应注意第4个QRS波群（标*）呈左束支阻滞图形，由于长短周期现象引起。呈左束支阻滞图形的心动过速的VA间期与窄QRS波群的VA间期相同，可以除外左侧游离壁旁路。

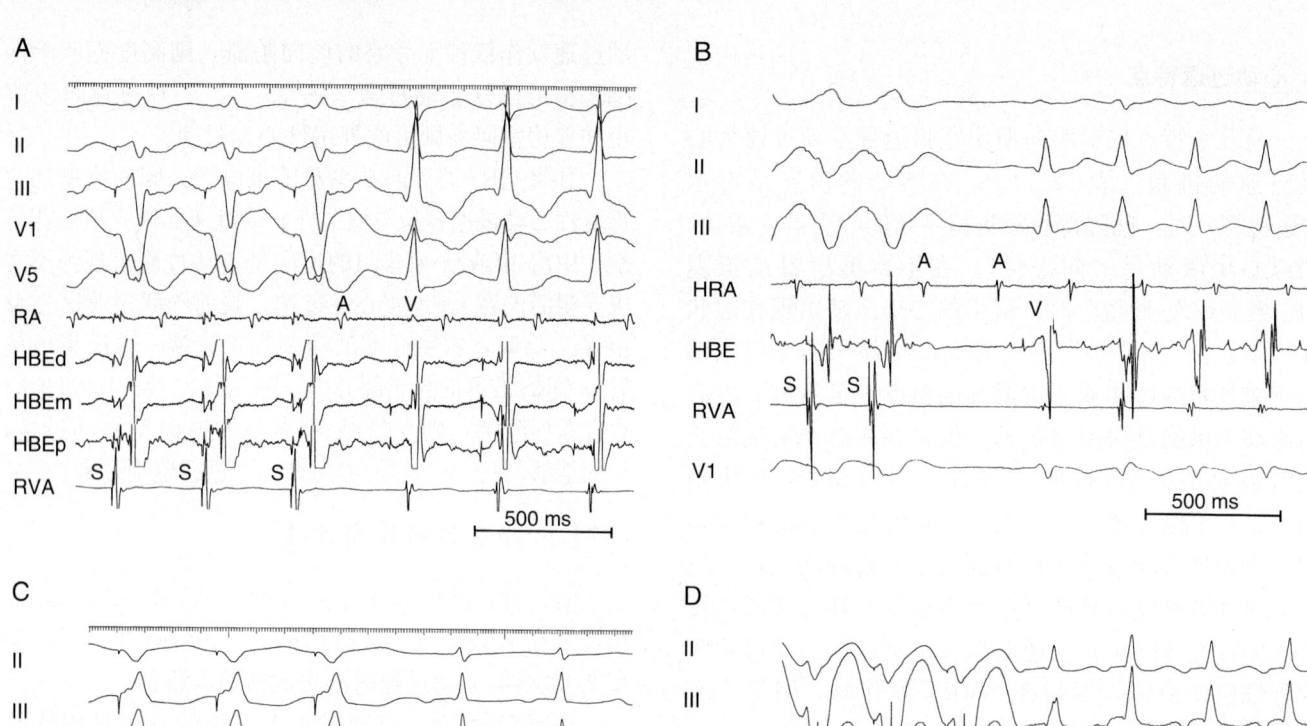

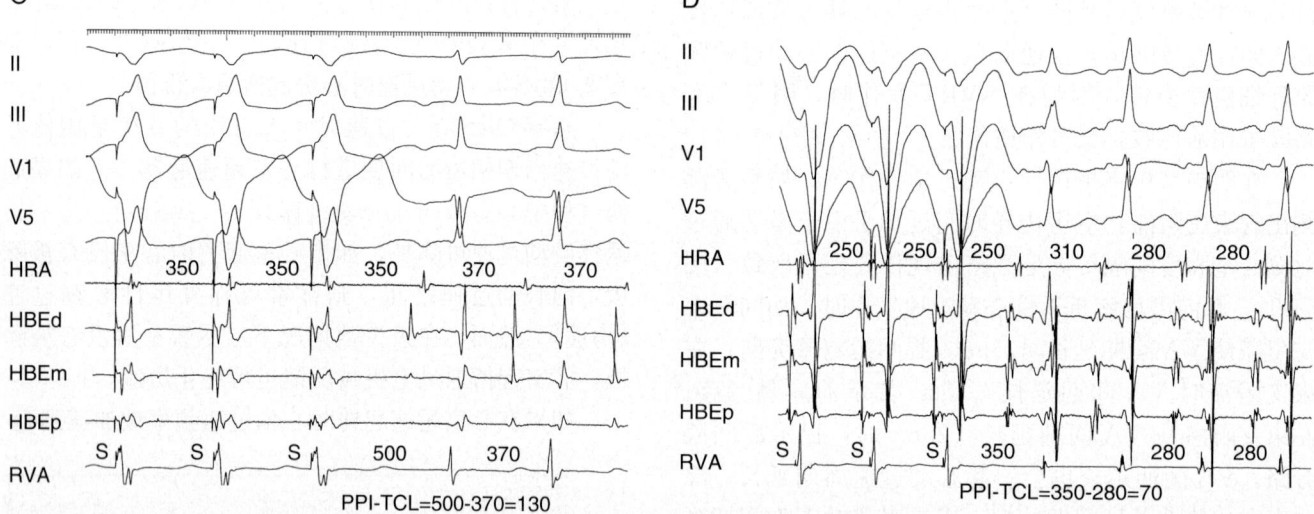

图 58-4 在室上性心动过速发作时心室超速起搏的诊断价值 图的格式和标注与图 58-1 相同。A：在右室心尖部以稍短于心动过速周期的间期进行起搏时，心动过速被加速到起搏频率。在心室起搏停止后的即刻，最后一个心房激动（图中 A）仍然是心室起搏的结果，其后跟随房室（AV）传导（图中 V）。这种 A-V 反应可除外房速。B：显示在房速发作时进行心室超速起搏后的 A-A-V 反应。注意最后一个心房除极是心室起搏的结果，其后伴随房室（AV）阻滞。这种反应形式可以除外顺向型房室折返性心动过速和房室结折返。C：显示在非典型房室结折返时心室起搏后的反应。起搏后间期（PPI）与心动过速周期（TCL）之差为 130ms。PPI-TCL 之差>115ms 可将房室结折返与由慢传导旁路参与的顺向型房室折返性心动过速鉴别开来。D. 由慢传导旁路参与的顺向型房室折返性心动过速发作时心室起搏后的反应，PPI-TCL 之差为 70ms。

搏频率时，而停止起搏后心动过速又恢复原来状态，那么这种心动过速的反应具有诊断价值。根据最后一个心室起搏后的即刻反应可分为 A-V 型和 A-A-V 型。在房室结折返或顺向型房室折返性心动过速发作时，心室起搏后 VA 以 1∶1 比例逆传，由最后一个心室刺激产生的心房除极后面常常跟随 AV 传导，因为心动过速的前传肢没有处于不应期。这种反应又常常称为房室（A-V）反应（图 58-4A）。相反，在房速发作时，心室起搏后伴 1∶1 室房逆传，由最后一个心室除极后产生的心房除极会紧跟出现房室阻滞，因为房室结由于前次逆传的关系而处于不应期中，而房速的第一个心房激动常常跟随房室传导，这种反应形式又称为 A-A-V 反应（图 58-4B）。

在窄 QRS 心动过速发作时另一个有用的起搏方法是用单个心室期前刺激扫描舒张期。如果心房激动由于位于希氏束不应期的心室刺激提前或者延迟，则可确定旁路的存在（图 58-5A、B）。然而，如果这种现象不出现则不能除外游离壁旁路，因为起搏是位于右室心尖部。如果心室刺激正好在希氏束不应期发放，在没有心房除极的情况下终止心动过速，则可以确定心动过速的机制为顺向型房室折返性心动过速（图58-5C）。

由慢传导旁路参与的顺向型房室折返性心动过速与不典型的房室结折返（快-慢型）鉴别困难。在长RP心动过速发作时，心房或心室刺激有助于鉴别诊断。在窦性心律下以心动过速的周期进行心房起搏，如果病人是由慢传导旁路参与的顺向型房室折返性心动过速，则AH间期等于心动过速时的AH间期。反之，如果病人是快-慢型房室结折返，窦性心律下以心动过速周期起搏产生的AH间期长于心动过速时的AH间期，因为心房起搏时激动是通过房室结前向传导的[10]。在长RP心动过速发作时，第二个有用的方法是比较心动过速的周期与通过右室对心动过速进行加速起搏后的间期（PPI）。由于心室是顺向型房室折返性心动过速折返环的一部分，顺向型房室折返性心动过速的PPI-TCL短于房室结折返时的PPI-TCL（见图58-4C、4D）。人们发现，PPI-TCL之差＞115ms时支持非典型房室结折返，可与由间隔旁路参与的顺向型房室折返性心动过速鉴别开来[11]。

通过心脏电生理检查对窄QRS心动过速作出顺向型房室折返性心动过速诊断主要依照几个线索，但常常是排除性诊断。联合两种心动过速发作时的特点（间隔部VA间期和逆向心房激动顺序）和一种起搏方法（心室拖带后的即刻反应）可以对65%的室上速作出诊断，同时还可对27%的室上速发生机制做出排除性诊断[6]。

在宽QRS波心动过速发作时，心房起搏有较大价值。在宽QRS波心动过速发作时，在房室结不应期发放的心房期前刺激引起的心室预激可以确定宽QRS波心动过速的前传肢是旁路（见图58-2C）。在宽QRS波心动过速发作时，如果心房刺激能够夺获心室但未产生室性融合波，则支持逆向型房室折返性心动过速，并除外室性心动过速。

三、治 疗

旁路介导的心动过速病人是否需要治疗取决于预激的存在与否、病人症状的严重性和出现频率以及病人的意愿。大多数无症状的心室预激病人发生心脏停搏的可能性很小，不需要治疗。无心室预激、AVRT也很少发作的病人也不需要预防性治疗。当症状明显或病人要求预防性治疗时，主要的治疗选择是药物治疗或导管消融。导管消融具有根治的优势，对那些不愿意接受药物治疗、担心复发和尽管接受了药物治疗仍有明显症状的病人，消融应成为一线治疗措施。对于有症状的预激综合征病人，如果症状发作频繁、严重，心动过速呈无休止性发作，或有心脏停搏的危险，也应接受导管消融治疗。

（一）药物治疗

静脉注射腺苷和维拉帕米（异搏定）仍然是持续性阵发性室上速的急诊一线治疗。腺苷具有高效、代谢快和不引起低血压等优点，但对哮喘病人可引起支气管痉挛。当腺苷治疗阵发性室上速时，高达12%的病人可诱发心房颤动（房颤）[12]。所以，将腺苷用于机制不明阵发性室上速或已知的预激综合征的病人时，应准备好除颤器。静脉注射普鲁卡因胺或依布利特具有阻滞旁路传导的作用[13]，可用于逆向型房室折返性心动过速或已知的顺向型房室折返性心动过速。持续性ARVT发作的病人极少需要电转复。

门诊病人可使用单次剂量的维拉帕米、普萘洛尔或普罗帕酮[14]有效终止AVRT。对那些有心动过速持续发作但发作频率较少而又不足以日常服药预防的病人，这些所谓"随身携带的药片"或"鸡尾酒疗法"理应成为有效的治疗手段。

有几种药物可用于AVRT病人的慢性预防性治疗。对于没有预激的病人，应首选能阻滞房室结的药物，如维拉帕米、β阻滞剂或地高辛。对那些不接受导管消融或外科手术的显性预激病人，应该选择阻滞旁路传导的药物，如钠通道或钾通道阻滞剂。最近研究显示，多菲利特在预防AVRT复发或减少发作频率方面与普罗帕酮同样有效，但开始用药时需要住院观察[15]。

（二）导管消融

导管消融治疗AVRT具有高效和根治优势[16]。在几个研究中，射频消融治疗旁路的成功率超过90%。在美国密歇根大学医学中心过去12年中，1245例病人（有1315条旁路）接受导管消融治疗，成功率超过95%。用于插管、诊断、消融和X线透视的平均时间分别为21±9min、22±18min、68±62min和47±32min。此外，消融术的并发症发生率很低。在密歇根大学医学中心接受导管消融的1245例病人中，并发症发生率为：心脏压塞0.48%，心包积液0.32%，外周血管损伤0.24%，完全性心脏阻滞0.16%，冠状动脉损伤0.16%，瓣膜损伤0.16%，死

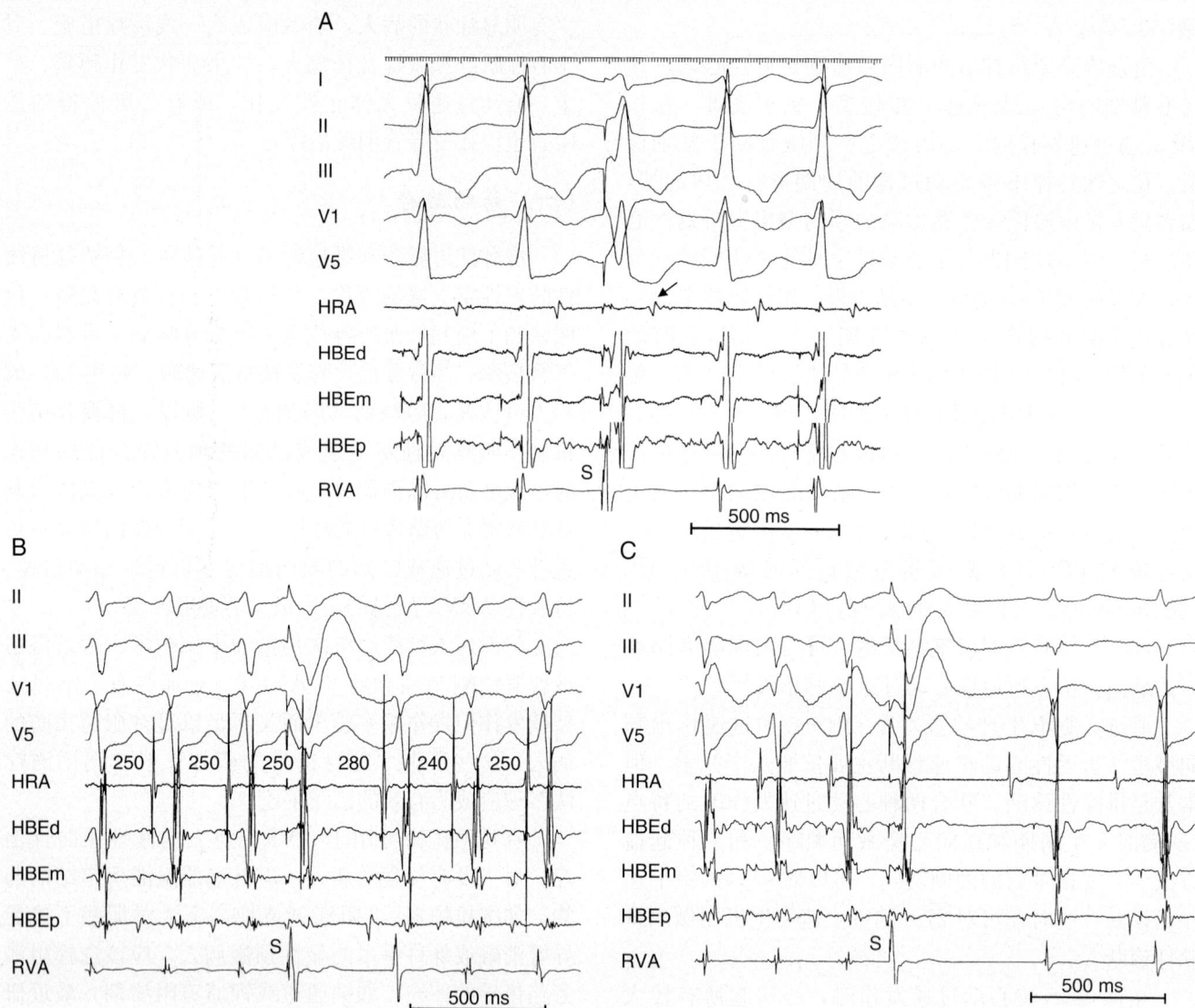

图 58-5 在顺向型房室折返性心动过速发作时在希氏束不应期中发放心室期前刺激的不同反应 图的格式和标注同图 58-1。A: 心室期前刺激引起心房激动提前 (图箭头所示)。这种现象支持旁路逆传存在的证据，但是不能除外在房速和房室结折返中旁路作为"无辜的"旁观者的可能。B: 心室刺激引起心房激动延迟。这反映了具有递减传导特性的旁路的存在。C: 心动过速周期终止而心房没有除极，这种结果支持顺向型房室折返性心动过速诊断。

亡 0.16% (1 例死于心脏穿孔，另 1 例死于大出血)，腹膜后出血 0.08%。一个包括 1050 例病人的多中心消融研究结果与此相似，主要并发症的发生率 3%，死亡率 0.3%[17]。限制透视使用、采用脉冲透视和先进的非透视的导管定位标测系统能够最大限度地降低放射线的曝光量[18]。

和其他心动过速进行鉴别。导管消融是 AVRT 安全和高效的治疗手段，对于有预激综合征、药物治疗效果不好的心动过速、症状严重病人以及要求根治的病人应考虑首选。

(王 斌 译)

四、总 结

旁路是 AVRT 折返环路的关键部分，在心脏电生理检查中联合采用检测和起搏方法可以对 AVRT

参 考 文 献

1. Lu CW, Wu MH, Chu SH: Paroxysmal supraventricular tachycardia in identical twins with the same left lateral accessory pathways and innocent dual atrioventricular pathways. PACE 23:1564–1566, 2000.
2. Zivin A, Morady F: Incessant tachycardia using a concealed atrionodal bypass tract. J Cardiovasc Electrophysiol 9:191–195, 1998.
3. Tada H, Oral H, Greenstein R, et al: Analysis of age of onset of accessory pathway-mediated tachycardia in men and women. Am J Cardiol 89:470–471, 2002.
4. Tai CT, Chen SA, Chiang CE, et al: A new electrocardiographic algorithm using retrograde P waves for differentiating atrioventricular node reentrant tachycardia from atrioventricular reciprocating tachycardia mediated by concealed accessory pathway. J Am Coll Cardiol 29:394–402, 1997.
5. Lam HD, Stroobandt R, Knight BP: Supraventricular tachycardia with alternating cycle length. What is the mechanism? Arrhythmia of the month. J Cardiovasc Electrophysiol 12:1329–1330, 2001.
6. Knight BP, Ebinger M, Oral H, et al: Diagnostic value of tachycardia features and pacing maneuvers during paroxysmal supraventricular tachycardia. J Am Coll Cardiol 36:574–582, 2000.
7. Souza JJ, Zivin A, Flemming M, et al: Differential effect of adenosine on anterograde and retrograde fast pathway conduction in patients with AV nodal reentrant tachycardia. J Cardiovasc Electrophysiol 9:820–824, 1998.
8. Hwang C, Martin DJ, Goodman JS, et al: Atypical atrioventricular node reciprocating tachycardia masquerading as tachycardia using a left-sided accessory pathway. J Am Coll Cardiol 30:218–225, 1997.
9. Knight BP, Zivin A, Souza J, et al: A technique for the rapid diagnosis of atrial tachycardia in the electrophysiology laboratory. J Am Coll Cardiol 33:775–781, 1999.
10. Man KC, Niebauer M, Daoud E, et al: Comparison of atrial-His intervals during tachycardia and atrial pacing in patients with long RP tachycardia. J Cardiovasc Electrophysiol 6:700–710, 1995.
11. Michaud GF, Tada H, Chough S, et al: Differentiation of atypical AV nodal reentry from orthodromic tachycardia using a septal accessory pathway by the response to ventricular pacing. J Am Coll Cardiol 38:1163–1167, 2001.
12. Strickberger SA, Man KC, Daoud EG, et al: Adenosine-induced atrial arrhythmia: A prospective analysis. Ann Intern Med 127:417–422, 1997.
13. Glatter KA, Dorostkar PC, Yang Y, et al: Electrophysiological effects of ibutilide in patients with accessory pathways. Circulation 104:1933–1939, 2001.
14. Reimold SC, Maisel WH, Antman EM: Propafenone for the treatment of supraventricular tachycardia and atrial fibrillation: A meta-analysis. Am J Cardiol 82:66N–71N, 1998.
15. Tendera M, Wnuk-Wojnar AM, Kulakowski P, et al: Efficacy and safety of dofetilide in the prevention of symptomatic episodes of paroxysmal supraventricular tachycardia: A 6-month double-blind comparison with propafenone and placebo. Am Heart J 142:93–98, 2001.
16. Knight BP, Morady F: Catheter ablation of accessory pathways. In Scheinman M (ed): Advances in Supraventricular Tachycardia. Cardiology Clinics of North America. Philadelphia, WB Saunders, 1997, pp 647–660.
17. Calkins H, Yong P, Miller JM, et al: Catheter ablation of accessory pathways, atrioventricular nodal reentrant tachycardia, and the atrioventricular junction: Final results of a prospective, multicenter clinical trial. The Atakr Multicenter Investigators Group. Circulation 99:262–270, 1999.
18. Drago F, Silvetti MS, DiPino A, et al: Exclusion of fluoroscopy during ablation treatment of right accessory pathway in children. J Cardiovasc Electrophysiol 13:778–782, 2002.

第 59 章

房室结折返性心动过速的电生理学特征：折返环路的意义

Deborah Lockwood, Kenichiro Otomo, Zulu Wang, Sara Forresti, Hiroshi Nakagawa, Karen Beckman, Benjamin J Scherlag, Eugene Patterson, Ralph Lazzara, Warren M. Jackman

本章目录

- 房室结双径路的电生理学特征 ········ 530
- 房室结快径路 ················ 531
- 房室结慢径路 ················ 532
- 房室结折返性心动过速的分型 ······ 536
- 房室结折返性心动过速的鉴别诊断和治疗 ················ 543

房室结折返性心动过速（atrioventricular nodal reentrant tachycardia，ANVRT）在阵发性室上性心动过速中最常见[1]，同时它也是心律失常中非常有趣的一种类型。AVNRT 最初被认为由致密房室结内的折返所致[2,3]，然而目前认为典型 AVNRT（慢-快型）的折返环包括房室结、部分心房肌和至少 2 个心房-房室结之间的连接[4-16]。目前对 AVNRT 折返环组成成分的了解主要来自消融方法的不断改进，因为只要一个远离致密房室结的心房-房室结连接被消融成功，AVNRT 就会被根治且不产生房室阻滞[4-12,16-18]。

ANVRT 在女性中更常见[4-9,17]，在 557 例经导管消融 AVNRT 的患者中，436 例（78%）为女性。尽管以往认为 AVNRT 在儿童中不常见，但是本中心 74 例（13%）患者≤16 岁，其中包括 2~5 岁 10 例（1.8%），6~10 岁 8 例（1.4%），11~13 岁 16 例（2.9%），14~16 岁 38 例（6.8%）。

一、房室结双径路的电生理学特征

早期研究者提出 AVNRT 是由于真房室结内功能上的纵向分离而在房室结内形成快、慢径之间的折返的结果[2,3]。这种假设源于以下发现：在心房激动和希氏束激动之间记录不到任何电位，在 AVNRT 的患者中房室结双径路现象很常见（可高达 85%），而在无 AVNRT 的患者中很少见[19]。过去也有人认为心房激动能够从心动过速中分离出来。尽管心动过速与心房分离的病例极其罕见，但是这些病例提示至少在部分病例中，心动过速折返环被局限在一个被保护的区域内[2,3,20]。然而，上述病例并不能排除部分心房组织参与折返环。

房室结双径路的电生理学特征是根据对心房期前刺激试验的反应来定义的，随着局部心房起搏配对间期（A_1-A_2）每缩短 10ms 时，从局部心房电位到希氏束电位的传导时间（A_2-H_2）延长≥50ms，则明确地定义为房室结双径路[21,22]。同样，当以每次周长递减 10ms 刺激心房时，A-H 间期延长≥50ms 也定义为房室结双径路现象[23,24]。这种房室结传导时间的突然延长被解释为房室结快径传导阻滞后，经由慢径传导。当在慢径上传导时间足够长，快径从不应期中恢复，传导就可能通过快径逆传回心房，从而产生心房回波或诱发 AVNRT。

近期较多研究表明在 AVNRT 的折返环内，快、慢径代表不同的心房-房室结连接间的传导，而不是在真房室结内的纵向分离所致[4-17,25-34]。这些研究发现包括：(1) 和Sung等早期描述的结果一样[25]，通过快径路和慢径路逆传时心房最早激动部位不同[4,5,12-14,25]；(2) 在房室结旁到右房后间隔或冠状窦给予晚发的心房期前刺激均可重整心动过速[11-15,27]；(3) 对狗和家兔的房室结折返回波的微电极和细胞外记录以及光学标测的结果[30,35,36]；(4) 在远离真房室结的心房部位消融，可以选择性地阻断快径或慢径传导[4-12,17,18,33,34,37,38]。

二、房室结快径路

快径路和慢径路的心房连接处可以通过在选择性的快径路或慢径路逆传中，标测最早的心房激动部位来确定[4,5,25,39,40]。当快径逆传时，应用传统上的宽间距双极电极（间距5~10mm）所记录到的最早心房激动部位与记录到希氏束电位的部相位同。然而，此宽间距双极电极所记录到的激动分布范围较大，涉及Todaro腱以上（在Koch三角外）到右束支近端的区域。对48位患者的右心房应用短间距电极（1mm间距）标测中发现，最早的心房激动部位位于记录到近端希氏束电位部位的后方5±3mm和上方（三尖瓣环以上）8±3mm（图59-1至图59-3）[39]。在48例患者中有47例，标测导管所记录到的最早逆传心房激动在左前斜位下位于希氏束导管的左侧（图59-2和59-3），表明心房最早激动部位位于Todaro腱的上方和Koch三角外，如图59-3所示[39]。如果标测导管越过Todaro腱，接近三尖瓣环（在Koch三角内），那么在左前斜位置下标测导管将会平行于希氏束电极导管，而不会位于希氏束导管的左侧。

快径逆传时，心房激动在Todaro腱以上，Koch三角以外的区域，由从前向后的方向传导（见图59-2）。在Koch三角内（邻近三尖瓣环），心房激动发生得相对较晚，传导方向为由后向前，其传导开始于冠状窦口外，向Koch三角的顶角方向传导（见图59-2）。在部分患者应用高分辨的电解剖标测系统标测结果证实，Koch三角以内的心房激动较晚，最晚的心房激动位于Koch三角的顶部，比发生在Todaro腱以上区域的最早心房激动约晚50ms[40]。这两种在相反方向上的电传导提示在Todaro腱存在传导阻滞。

在慢-快型AVNRT时，在滤波为30~250Hz的双极标测下，最早心房激动处的心房电位通常包括两种成分：起始的低频、负向电位成分，随后的尖锐、主要为正向、约晚10ms的电位成分（见图59-2）[39]。

因为此处（Todaro腱上方）为真正的房间隔处，起始的低频心房电位有可能为起始于左侧房间隔的远场电位[39]。在部分存在卵圆孔未闭的患者，在左侧房间隔可标测到一个尖锐的电位（近场电位），其激动时间与在右侧房间隔所标测到的起始低频电位成分的时间相同，此部位同时为左侧房间隔所能标测到的最早心房激动的部位[39]。左侧房间隔激动时间最早可能有助于解释在近端冠状窦有相对较早的激动时间。快径逆传时可能的心房激动模式见示意图59-4A。

在右侧房间隔具有最早逆传心房激动的部位消融（恰好在Todaro腱的上方）可以选择性地阻断快径传导，同时治愈90%左右的典型AVNRT患者[5,7-9,17]。在犬的在体及离体灌注心脏（Langendorff心脏制备模型）研究中，在Todaro腱的上方进行射频消融可以选择性地消融房室结快径前传。组织学检查也证实消融所产生的组织损伤局限在Todaro腱上方的区域，而没有累及Koch三角以内的组织[37,38]。这个区域包括移行区细胞，微电极记录证实此类细胞动作电位的特征介于心房细胞和房室结细胞之间。这些移行细胞越过Todaro腱，移向房室结[38,41,42]。家兔心脏的微电极记录结果提示这些前区的移行细胞插入房室束的部相位对邻近中心纤维体（即希氏束）[43]。以上研究结果提示房室结快径的右房部分作为心房肌细胞起始于卵圆窝的前肢，在接近Todaro腱时变成移行区细胞，之后插入到房室束（希氏束），位于大部分真房室结的远端[43]。这种快径插入房室结远端可以解释为

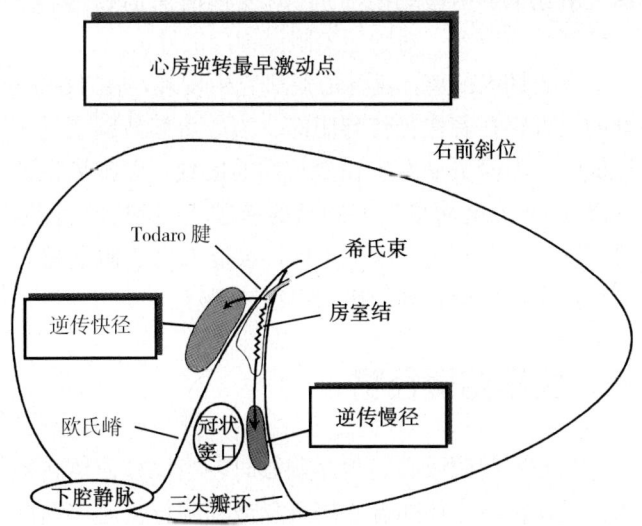

图59-1 房室结快径逆传（逆传快径）和慢径逆传（逆传慢径）时最早逆传心房激动部位示意图

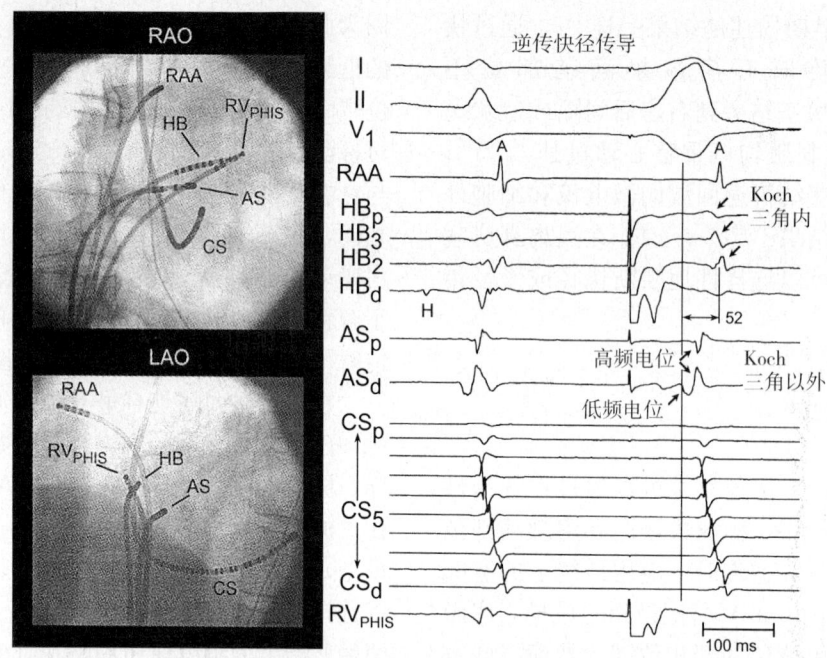

图 59-2　慢-快型房室结折返性心动过速的心房激动特点　左图：为右前斜位（RAO）及左前斜位（LAO）下的导管位置。RAA：右心耳；RV$_{PHIS}$：希氏束旁右室起搏部位；CS：冠状静脉窦。放置 8 极希氏束电极导管（HB）使其最远端双极电极记录到最近端的希氏束电位。调整希氏束导管方向使之大致平行于 Todaro 腱和三尖瓣环，能够沿着 Koch 三角记录局部电信号。标测导管（AS：位于房间隔）放置在有最早心房激动的部位，大约在记录到希氏束电位的部位的上、后方各约 1cm 的地方。在左前斜位下，标测导管（AS）位于希氏束导管的左侧，表明其位于 Todaro 腱的上方。右图：为左图所示电极导管所记录的慢-快型房室结折返性心动过速时的双极心内电图（滤波 30～500Hz）。在 Todaro 腱的上方（位于 Koch 三角以外）所记录到的最早心房激动（AS$_d$）包括两部分：一个起始的低频成分，可能代表房间隔左侧的远场激动，和一个迟发的高频成分，可能代表房间隔右侧的局部激动。希氏束电图上记录了 Koch 三角内由后至前方向上的较晚的心房激动（希氏束电图上箭头所示）。最晚的激动位于 Koch 三角内（见 HB$_2$），比 Koch 三角外所测的最早激动延迟 52ms。

什么相对于慢径来说，快径具有很少的递减传导特征、对典型的房室结阻滞剂（β 受体阻滞剂和钙通道拮抗剂）反应差、对钠通道阻滞剂反应好。

在近期犬的离体灌注心脏研究中发现，在 Todaro 腱的上方存在着快径传导阻滞。当心房起搏频率逐渐增加时，阻滞更易发生在更近端的区域，即阻滞逐渐远离 Todaro 腱而接近卵圆窝的前肢[38]。快径前传阻滞的部位发生在 Koch 三角外，可能有助于阻断慢径逆传，从而可能有利于启动房室结折返。

三、房室结慢径路

在心室起搏或心室程序刺激时，当快径逆传转换为慢径逆传时，伴随着心房最早激动部位从心房前间隔（Koch 三角外）转换到 Koch 三角内或冠状窦近端内。在大多数患者中，最早的逆传高频电位（A$_{SP}$ 电位）可在三尖瓣环和冠状窦口之间记录到（图 59-4B-1 和图 59-5）[4,25]。此与逆传通过房室结右侧后延伸相一致（图 59-6）[42,44]。下一个最早激动点通常在冠状窦口的底部记录到。冲动沿冠状窦肌袖向左侧传导，并激动距离冠状窦口 2～3cm 处邻近二尖瓣环的左房心肌（见图 59-4B-1）。左房激动继续向左、右侧传导至房间隔，从而激动 Todaro 腱上方的右心房（见图 59-4B-2）。右房激动向后传导到欧氏嵴和冠状窦口的后部（图 59-5A 第 2 跳心内电图 PS$_p$），向前传导至 Todaro 腱上方，产生可以在希氏束电图上记录到的心房电位。慢径逆传时激动顺序的假设见图 59-4B 的示意图。

近期两个实验的结果为上述慢径逆传的激动方式提供了证据。首先，我们近期的研究表明冠状窦口心肌袖为在冠状窦口附近的右心房和左心房之间提供了电学连接[45,46]。其次，欧氏瓣形成完全的阻滞线，从而使慢径只能局限在 Koch 三角内逆向传导。此传导阻滞线可能解释为什么逆传 A$_{SP}$ 电位能够从右房激动中分离出来（图 59-7C），同时也可以解释为什么窦性心律时前传 A$_{SP}$ 电位出现较晚。窦性心律时，A$_{SP}$ 电位

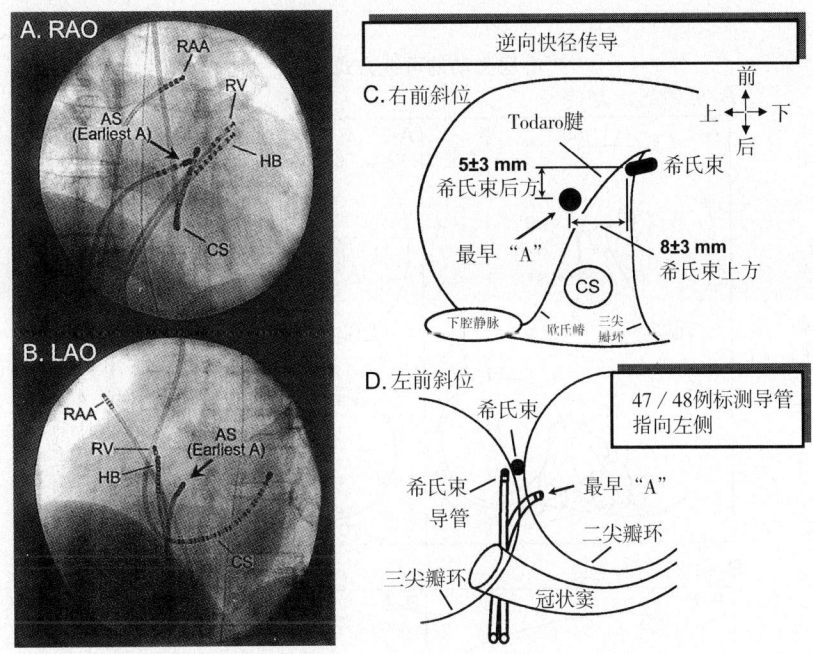

图 59-3 连续 48 例慢-快型房室结折返性心动过速患者最早逆传心房部位的 X-线影像及示意图 左图：在 X-线影像右前斜位及左前斜位下显示希氏束导管（HB）和在房间隔右侧记录到最早逆传心房激动部位（Earliest "A"）的导管（AS）的关系。左前斜位影像示 AS 导管位于 HB 电极的左侧，表明此处位于 Todaro 腱的上方，Koch 三角以外。右图：右前斜位下的示意图示 48 例患者其最早心房激动部位（箭头和大黑点所示）位于记录到近端希氏束电位的上方 8±3mm 和后方 5±3mm。左前斜位下的示意图表明 48 例患者中，47 例其最早心房逆传激动部位位于希氏束导管的左侧。

代表在后间隔三尖瓣环和冠状窦口之间的激动时间，尽管记录到希氏束电位和记录到 A_{SP} 电位的电极导管之间的距离很小，但 A_{SP} 电位在冠状窦近端激动之后出现，更迟发于希氏束电图上的心房激动（见图 59-5B）。A_{SP} 电位明显迟发于希氏束电图上心房激动的原因可能为，希氏束电极的心房电位由 Todaro 腱上方的心房激动产生，尽管右房激动跨过 Todaro 腱，传导至移行区细胞形成快径，但是这些细胞也许并不能够激动位于 Koch 三角内的心房肌（见图 59-4C）[47]。窦性心律时，前传 A_{SP} 电位可能代表了由后向前方向的激动（基于如下面所描述的对消融的反应）。A_{SP} 电位可能来源于 Koch 三角的后部，邻近终末嵴的激动所产生。在产生 A_{SP} 电位的组织激动之前，冠状窦的肌组织可能已被激动（见图 59-4C，图 59-5B）。在一些个体中，窦性心律时 A_{SP} 电位出现很晚，此时，来自左心房的激动可能传导至冠状窦的肌组织，然后激动 Koch 三角内的组织而产生 A_{SP} 电位（见图 59-4D）。

在欧氏瓣/嵴的传导阻滞可能解释在快径逆向传导时 A_{SP} 电位的延迟出现（见图 59-5A，第 1 跳）。快径逆传后，Todaro 腱上方的心房激动也许并不能够直接传导至 Koch 三角内（见图 59-4A-1）。冠状窦的心肌袖被左房心肌激动后，再激动产生 A_{SP} 电位的组织（见图 59-4A-2）。

对消融的反应为"A_{SP} 电位代表慢径（房室结的右侧后延伸）的心房连接端的激动，和在窦性心律时记录到的前传 A_{SP} 电位代表由后向前方向的激动"的假设提供了很强的证据。在三尖瓣环和冠状窦之间的右心房后间隔区域（在冠状窦口中间或更低水平），在记录到高大而尖锐的 A_{SP} 电位（单极电图上）的部位释放射频电流时，可立即产生加速的交界区性心律伴快径逆传[48]。在部分患者中，在出现交界区性心律前可出现 1~3 跳与慢径逆传激动顺序相一致的房性期前收缩。在放电过程中出现的加速性交界区性心律通常伴有慢径前传或逆传功能的改良或消除而不抑制快径传导[4-8]。交界区性自律性的出现表明连接慢径区域组织的受热。在狗的慢径消融实验[49] 和 1 例已行慢径消融的 AVNRT 患者[50] 所做的组织学检查表明射频消融所产生的改良或消除慢径传导的病变仅累及房室结右侧后延伸，而未累及真房室结。当在右心房后间隔三尖瓣环和冠状窦口之间行线性消融时，消融线前方的 A_{SP} 电位消失，而消融线后方的 A_{SP} 电位仍然存在。如果在消融线的前方（上方）释放射频电流，就会产生交界区心律（慢径自律性）；然而，如果放

心房激动的可能方式

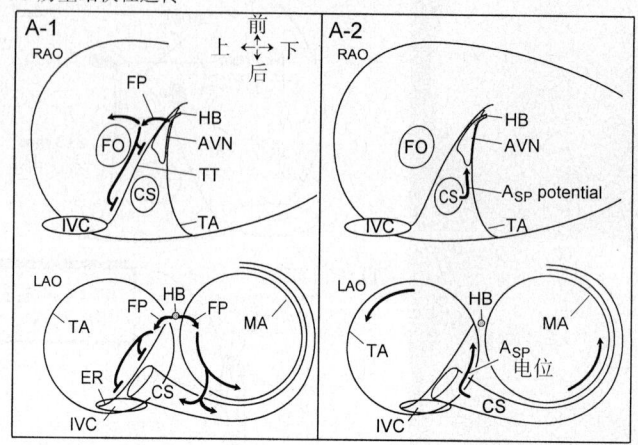

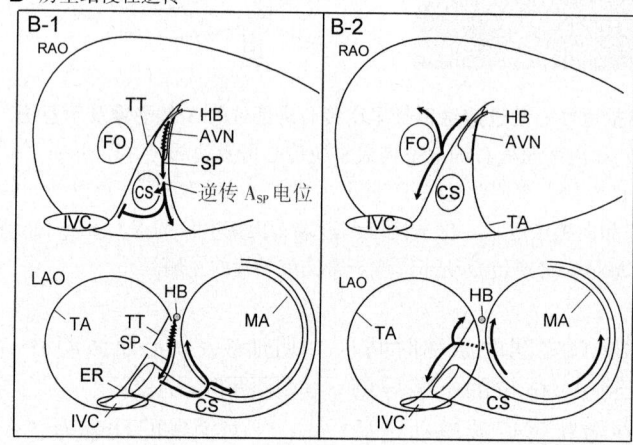

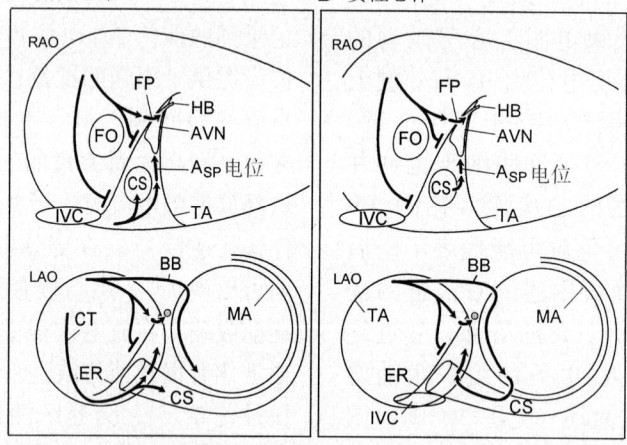

图 59-4　经由房室结快径逆传（A）、房室结慢径逆传（B）和窦性心律下（C 和 D）心房激动的可能方式　A-1：慢-快型 AVN-RT 时，快径逆传激动房间隔左、右两侧（LAO）。间隔右侧的激动发生于 Todaro 腱的上方，可能并不能传导至 Koch 三角内（RAO）。间隔左侧的激动传导到二尖瓣环附近的左房肌，然后激动冠状窦肌袖（LAO）。激动沿着冠状窦心肌组织向右侧传导至冠状窦口。A-2：激动经冠状窦口激动 Koch 三角内的右心房和过渡区细胞纤维。此部分组织由后向前上方激动产生高频（A_{SP}）电位。B-1：逆传慢径（SP）激动向后沿着房室结后延伸传导至产生 A_{SP} 电位的组织。沿着欧氏瓣/嵴的传导阻滞可能使激动只能限制在 Koch 三角内传导（RAO）。然后，激动经由冠状窦心肌组织向左侧传导，激动距离冠状窦口 1.5～3cm 的左房心肌（LAO）。B-2：左房激动向左、向右激动房间隔，并通过房间隔激动 Todaro 腱上方的右心房。C：窦性心律时，房间隔右侧的冲动传导通过 Todaro 腱前部的过渡区细胞而形成快径。来自这些细胞的低电流也许并不能够激动位于 Koch 三角前部的心房肌。激动沿着界嵴（CT）激动冠状窦肌组织和位于三尖瓣环与冠状窦口之间的心肌组织，产生了由后向前方向的 A_{SP} 电位。这一点可解释窦性心律时 A_{SP} 电位出现较晚的现象。D：在窦性心律下出现 A_{SP} 电位明显延迟的患者，可能由左房激动传导至冠状窦肌组织，然后激动产生 A_{SP} 电位的组织。FO，卵圆窝；BB，Bachman 束；TA，三尖瓣环；IVC，下腔静脉；MA，二尖瓣环；ER，欧氏嵴。

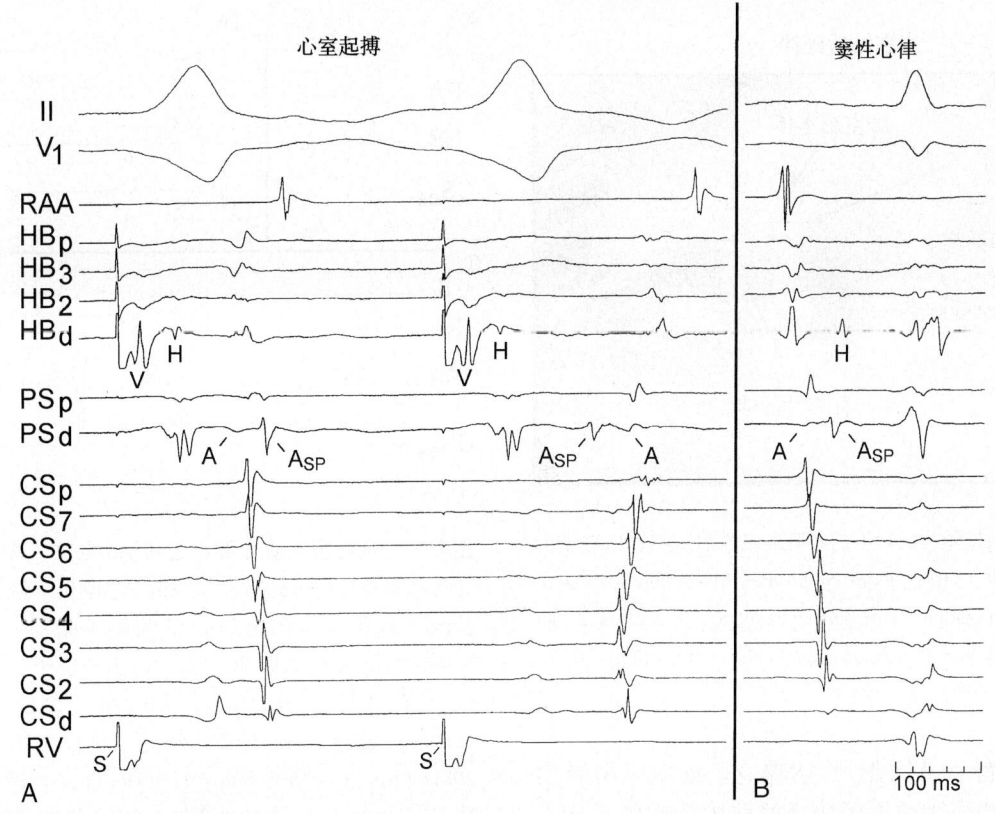

图 59-5　房室结快、慢径逆传时不同的心房激动顺序　A：起搏右心室间隔前基底部（旁希氏束部位）。经由快径逆传时（左侧波群），前间隔（HB2）所记录到的心房激动早于位于三尖瓣环与冠状窦口之间的右房后间隔（PSd）和冠状窦近端（CS5 至 CSp）的心房激动。当快径逆传阻滞，而选择性经由慢径逆传时（右侧波群），在右房后间隔（PSd）可记录到最早的高频电位（ASP电位），随后为冠状窦激动。注意希氏束旁起搏提早局部心室激动和延迟希氏束逆传，从而把希氏束电图上的希氏束电位（H）和局部心室电位（V）分离出来。B：窦性心律时，前传的 ASP 电位晚于冠状窦近端的心房激动时间，更晚于希氏束电图上的心房激动时间。注意当快径逆传时，ASP 电位也同样在希氏束和近端冠状窦的心房激动时间之后（A：左侧波群）。

电位置是在消融线的后方（下方），通常不会出现交界区心律。以上观察与 ASP 电位来自于在 Koch 三角内由上至下方向，垂直于长轴方向纤维的各向异性传导所产生的假设相反[47]。而以上观察恰恰支持以下假设，ASP 电位代表由后向前方向上的传导，基本平行于连接房室结后延伸区域的纤维，而形成房室结慢径。

有很强的证据表明房室结慢径并不是单一的整体。心房期前刺激所产生的多个 A_2-H_2 间期突然延长≥50ms（"跳跃"）很早就被发现[51]。在程序心室刺激时，H-A 间期变化伴随冠状窦上最早心房激动部位的变化并非少见。在慢径消融技术发展的早期，通常在慢径逆传的最早激动部位释放射频电流，当对冠状窦内的一个部位消融后，经常可以见到慢径逆传仍然存在，但伴有不同的 H-A 间期和不同的最早激动部位[4]。目前我们采用在后间隔三尖瓣环和冠状窦口之间行线性消融的方法，通常在此消融线有 2～3 处可产生加速性交界区性心律，包括冠状窦口前缘，提示在消融线上有与慢径的多处连接。尽管沿着这条线消融通常会消除导致心动过速的慢径传导，但是在 75% 左右的患者中，心房期前刺激仍可出现 A_2-H_2 间期的跳跃并出现一次心房回波，提示存在另一条不走行于三尖瓣环和冠状窦口之间区域的、"非致心律失常性"的慢径。这种附加慢径可能代表房室结左侧后延伸的传导（见图 59-6）[42,44]。在犬及家兔的心脏所做的标测研究支持此附加"慢径"进入冠状窦口前方的 Koch 三角区域[28,52]。

心房连接房室结的前、后入口，分别形成快、慢径，在正常的心脏中也同样存在[30,42,44,53]。这表明快径和慢径传导（房室结双径生理学）在大部分人群中也应存在。在连续 200 例消融 1 条房室旁路的患者中（无 AVNRT 病史或在消融术中未诱发 AVNRT），存在前传或逆传两者之一的房室结双径路传导的患者为 168 例（84%）[23,24]。在这组患者中双径路的高发生率

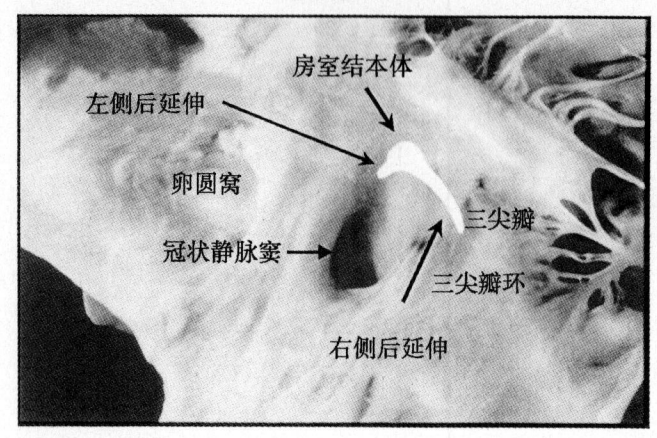

图 59-6 房室结后延伸 图片上的心脏显示真房室结、房室结的左侧和右侧后延伸。(引自 Inoue S, Becker AE: Posterior extensions of the human compact atrioventricular node: A neglected anatomic feature of potential clinical significance. Circulation, 1998, 97: 188-193.)

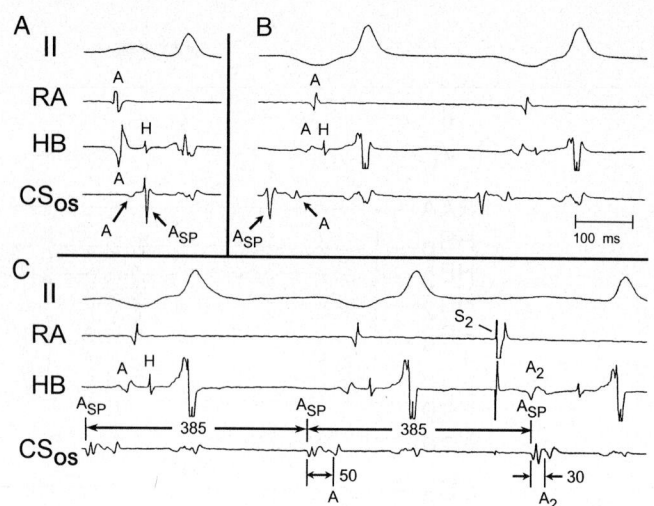

图 59-7 从右房激动分离出逆传 A_{SP} 电位 A:窦性心律时,在冠状窦口外记录到高大尖锐的 A_{SP} 电位(冠状窦口),此电位晚于希氏束电图上所记录的心房激动 40ms。B:周长 360ms 的快-慢型 AVNRT 时, A_{SP} 电位位于右心房激动之前。C:在右心耳处发放的房性期前收缩(RA)提前 Koch 三角外的心房激动 46ms(HB)和冠状窦口电图上的心房激动 20ms(A_{SP}-A 间期从 50ms 缩短到 30ms),然而没有改变在 Koch 三角内的 A_{SP} 电位的激动时间和形态,提示右房激动进入 Koch 三角内受阻。

可能与深度镇静(芬太尼/咪达唑仑,近期应用异丙酚)有关,这些药物减弱了快径的前传及逆传,从而有利于显示慢径传导。低剂量异丙肾上腺素(0.25~0.5μg/min)增加快径传导的作用明显强于增加慢径传导,通常完全地掩盖了慢径的前传和逆传功能(图 59-8)。这种在深度镇静或麻醉患者中应用低剂量的异丙肾上腺素可能模仿了正常静息状态下患者的交感神经活性,这解释了在以前的研究中为什么在不镇静的、无 AVNRT 的患者中双径路的发生率低[19]。关于前传房室结双径路(A_2-H_2 间期跳跃)发生率低的其他可能原因还有在快径阻滞前,快径和慢径之间有相近的传导时间,或在快、慢径之间有一个中间径传导。然而,在多数患者中,A-H 间期或 A_2-H_2 间期长于 200ms 时多为房室结慢径前传。

从快径逆传到慢径逆传平滑的转换也可被观察到。在不同患者中,快径和慢径的 H-A 间期存在较大的重叠。因此,H-A 间期的长短对于鉴别是否有慢径逆传无特殊价值。然而,由于存在逆传心房激动顺序的改变,故从快径逆传到慢径逆传的转换很容易识别(图 59-5A)[24]。

四、房室结折返性心动过速的分型

AVNRT 至少可被分为四型。在我们行导管消融的 658 例 AVNRT 患者中,慢-快型 499 例(76%),左侧变异慢-快型 7 例(1%),慢-慢型("后位型"[12])71 例(11%)[55,56],快-慢型("非常见型")81 例(12%)[9,26,56]。

(一) 慢-快型房室结折返性心动过速

慢-快型 AVNRT 也被称为普通型或典型 AVNRT,它经房室结慢径(可能为房室结左侧后延伸)前传,房室结快径逆传。此型 AVNRT 的典型诱发方式为心房程序刺激时突然出现 A-H 间期延长(大于 50ms),提示前向传导经由房室结慢径[21,22]。然而,有些患者由于快、慢双径在转换时有相近的传导时间,故心动过速诱发时仅出现 A-H 间期的逐渐延长(无"跳跃")[1,21,54,57]。慢-快型 AVNRT 发作时,A-H 间期相对较长(通常大于 200ms),且按我们的经验,A-H 间期可长达 550ms(中位数 290ms)。在希氏束电图上测量的 H-A 间期相对较短,通常在 25~90ms(中位数 50ms)。标测右心房和冠状窦可以鉴别

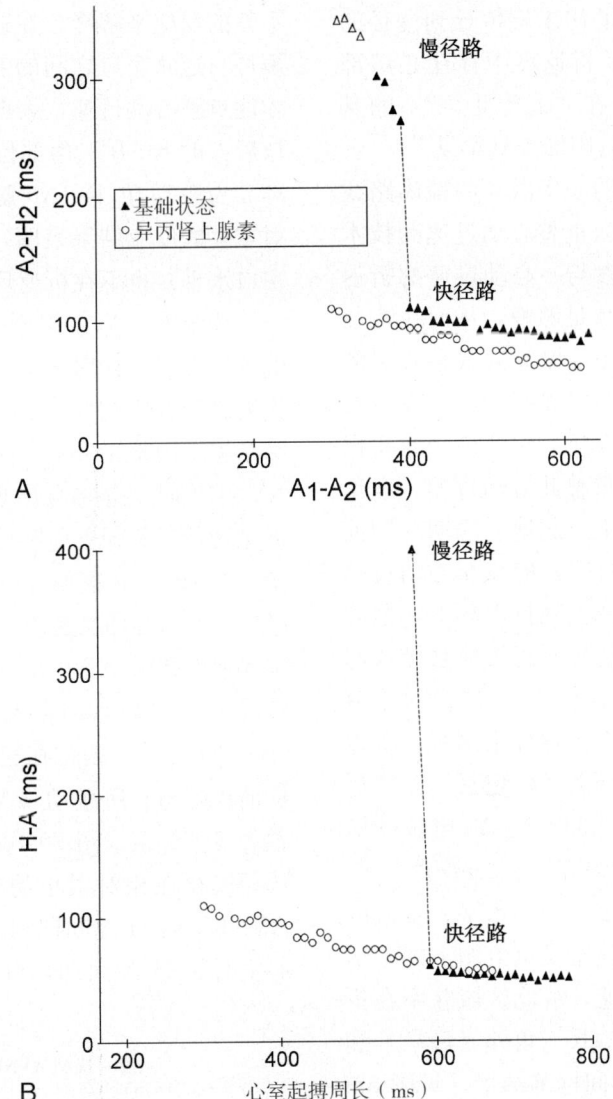

图 59-8　小剂量异丙肾上腺素（0.5μg/min）对房室结双径路的作用　A：心房期前刺激确定房室结不应期曲线。在基础状态下（深度镇静），A_1-A_2 间期从 400ms 缩短至 390ms 时，A_1-H_2 间期增加 155ms（从 110ms 增至 265ms），表明快径前传阻滞，而选择性地从房室结慢径传导（用黑三角形代表）。A_1-A_2 间期的进一步缩短导致 A_2-H_2 间期的逐渐延长至 335ms 或以上时（用空白三角形代表）出现单个心房回波（慢径前传/快径逆传）。给予低剂量异丙肾上腺素后缩短了快径的有效不应期 100ms（从 390ms 至 290ms，用圆圈表示），但没有相应缩短慢径的有效不应期，故完全掩盖了慢径传导的出现。B：心室递增起搏确定房室结逆传曲线。在基础状态下（用黑三角形代表），仅在以 590ms 或以上周长心室起搏时出现房室结快径逆传。在以 580ms 周长起搏时，H-A 间期增加 335ms（从 65ms 增至 400ms），表明快径逆传阻滞，而选择性地从房室结慢径逆传（用黑三角形代表）。房室结逆传阻滞发生在以 570ms 周长起搏时。低剂量异丙肾上腺素明显增强房室结逆向传导功能，1：1 快径逆传周长缩短至 300ms（用圆圈表示）。慢径逆传功能没有相应增强，故被逆传快径传导所掩盖。注意应用异丙肾上腺素下并没有使 HA 间期明显缩短。此患者临床上无 AVNRT 发作，在基础状态下和应用异丙肾上腺素（剂量最高达 4μg/min）时心房和心室程序刺激均不能诱发 AVNRT。

慢-快型与慢-慢型 AVNRT，慢-快型时最早的心房逆传激动部位在 Todaro 腱的上方（逆传快径激动，见图 59-1 和图 59-3）。短的 H-A 间期通常会导致 P 波与体表心电图 QRS 波群相重叠，从而掩盖了 P 波的大部分。然而，在 QRS 波的末端多可区别出 P 波的末端，在 V_1 导联 QRS 波末端产生一个特征性的向上的波（伪 r′波），或在下壁导联产生一个向下的波（伪 S 波）。

快径和慢径的心房连接之间的距离提示慢-快型 AVNRT 的折返环可能含有相对较大的心房部分，在此心房部分折返激动从快径的心房末端传导到慢径的心房末端。在慢-快型 AVNRT 折返环中存在心房部分（即在快径与心房之间不存在"上传共径"）的其他证据是在心动过速时发生心房阻滞极其罕见。

在房室结快径与慢径之间的心房激动的精确路线还没有确定。通过房性期前刺激重整心动过速的技术可用来鉴别心房是否邻近（或参与）心动过速的折返环。此房性期前刺激的发放必须足够晚，从而在快径逆传至最早心房激动部位前，不能激动此最早心房激动部位[13,15,27]。如果某个心房部位邻近折返环或恰好位于折返环上，在此部位的晚发的心房期前刺激将提前下一次的希氏束电位时间并重整此心动过速。理论上，如果一个部位位于折返环上，起搏后间期（期前刺激到下一个局部心房电位的时间）应该与心动过速周长很接近。然而，尽管起搏部位在折返环上，但起搏时所导致的房室结内的额外传导延迟可能会导致起搏后间期的延长（长于心动过速周长），这样对于鉴别此部位是否在折返环内和邻近折返环很困难。重整心动过速时有最短的起搏后间期的部位包括：右房后间隔（在三尖瓣环和冠状窦口之间产生 A_{SP} 电位的区域）和冠状窦近端（距离冠状窦口 1～2cm）[13,15,27]。相反，在欧氏嵴后部（在冠状窦口中心水平）发放的房性期前刺激，如果没有先提前希氏束电图上的心房激动时间，则不能重整心动过速，故此区域并不在折返环上[27]。上述观察，结合 Koch 三角外（最早）和 Koch 三角内（最晚）的激动时间标测结果（见图 59-2），提示慢-快型 AVNRT 的新的折返环假说（图 59-9，折返机制 1）。在这个假说中，快径逆传后激动房间隔的左侧和右侧，但只有左侧房间隔的激动参与折返环。来自左侧房间隔的激动传导至距离冠状窦口约 1～3cm 的冠状窦心肌袖。折返冲动沿着冠状窦上部肌袖传导至冠状窦口，激动连接房室结右侧后延伸的纤维，然后激动房室结慢径（见图 59-9）。在近期的研究中[58]，47% 的慢-快型 AVNRT 患者发生心动过速时，其最早冠状窦激动点在远离冠状窦口的部位记录到，证实在这些患者中，冠状窦的肌袖是被左心房所激动。

慢-快型 AVNRT 的其他 4 种可能折返环见图 59-9 所示。折返环 2（传统假设）的心房部分局限在 Koch 三角内。折返环 3 不能解释在冠状窦发放的晚发房性期前刺激可以重整心动过速或在三尖瓣环与冠状窦口之间释放射频电流可成功消融慢径的心房连接。折返环 4 的心房部分环绕冠状窦口，也不能用对重整的反应来解释。在冠状窦口的后方需要比在三尖瓣环与冠状窦口之间的部位发放更早的心房期前刺激才能重整心动过速，表明在折返环的心房部分冠状窦后方的 Koch 三角部位并不在折返环内[15,27]。折返环 5 为激动在 Todaro 腱以上环绕下腔静脉口传导，对重整的反应结果表明，欧氏嵴的后方心房肌（冠状窦口水平）也不在折返环内[27]。

传统上认为在慢-快型 AVNRT 中，快、慢径远端的连接点是在房室结内，在快、慢双径的远端与希氏束之间存在房室结组织区域（即下部共径）。由房室结组织组成的下部共径的存在能够预测在慢-快型 AVNRT 时，有时可出现在希氏束以上的传导阻滞，但是这种现象却极为罕见。近期较多证据提示在慢-快型 AVNRT 中仅存在很短或者几乎没有下部共径[55,59-61]。心动过速时，晚发的心室期前刺激如果能够提前逆传激动希氏束（与无室性期前刺激时的前传希氏束电位激动时间相比），则能够提前激动心房（图 59-10）[61]。通常在逆传希氏束电位（H_1-H_2 间期）提前程度与心房激动（A_1-A_2 间期）的提前程度上存在着线性关系（图 59-10C），提示在下部共径和逆传快径仅存在相对很小的递减传导。通过比较慢-快型 AVNRT 时 H-A 间期和以与心动过速相同的周长起搏心室时的 H-A 间期，可得到相同的证据。心动过速

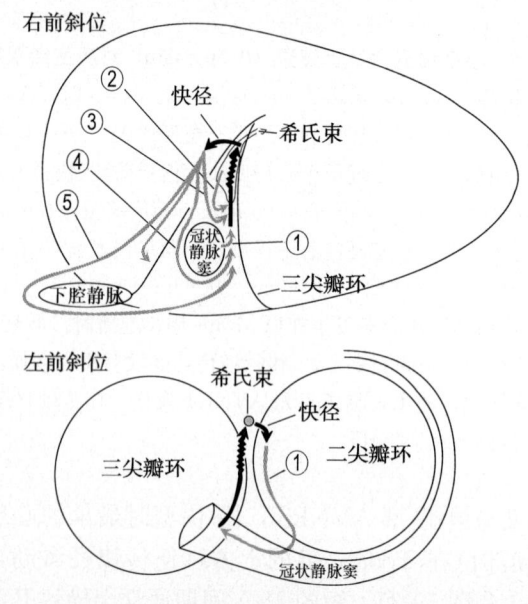

图 59-9 慢-快型 AVNRT 的 5 种可能折返环的示意图　详见正文。

时的 H-A 间期应该等于快径逆传时间减去经由下部共径的前传时间（从快、慢双径的远端连接点到希氏束）。心室起搏时的 H-A 间期，从逆传希氏束电位的末端测量到心房激动的起始，从时间上应等于经由下部共径逆传的时间（从希氏束到快径）加上经由快径逆传的时间。假设心室起搏与心动过速时应用同一条快径逆传，且快径逆传时间相同，则心室起搏时的 H-A 间期减去心动过速时的 H-A 间期就等于经由下部共径的前传和逆传时间之和。重要的是，必须记录到最近端的希氏束电位，因为记录到的希氏束电位越靠近远端，就会错误地增加心室起搏时的 H-A 间期和缩短心动过速时的 H-A 间期，从而错误地提示存在着较长的下部共径。为了记录到最近端逆传希氏束电位的末端，心室起搏必须放置到能把希氏束的激动和局部心室肌的激动区分开的部位。起搏右室间隔前基底部可满足此条件，此部位非常接近右束支近端，但当不夺获右束支近端（希氏束旁起搏）时[62]，就会导致希氏束逆传激动远远晚于局部心室电位（图 59-5，图 59-11）。最精确的比较方法如下，诱发慢-快型 AVNRT 并持续 3min 以上，发放 3~4 跳的心房快速起搏终止心动过速后，立即以心动过速的同样周长来起搏心室。上述方法可使心室起搏和心动过速时的自主神经张力的变化降低到最小程度。使用这种方法，心室起搏时的 H-A 间期（从逆传希氏束电位的末端测量）要比慢-快型 AVNRT 时的 H-A 间期平均短 9ms（图 59-11A）[63,64]。这看上去自相矛盾的发现（心动过速时的 H-A 间期长于心室起搏时的 H-A 间期）有以下可能的解释。一是逆传快径起源于希氏束（即不存在下部共径）。但是这种解释可能性不大，因为对部分已证实具有双路径的人类移植心脏的组织学研究显示没有心房-希氏束旁路，而且这些心脏与"正常"心脏并无解剖学上的差异。此外，一项有 687 例尸解心脏的组织学研究发现，仅有 2 个心脏存在真正的心房-希氏束连接（0.3%）[66]。我们目前认为房室结双径路的心房到房室结有多个入路，并且可能存在于所有心脏[24]，而心房-希氏束旁路仅存在于极少数人群中，不能用来解释发生在大部分人群中的房室结双径路现象。其他对心动过速时的 H-A 间期长于心室起搏时的 H-A 间期的解释包括：所标测到的最近端的希氏束电位实际上为在快、慢双径连接前的最远端的慢径电位（可导致心动过速时 H-A 间期的伪性延长）；或者在心动过速时，由于快、慢双径在连接点上的激动波方向上的改变而导致传导延迟[47]，从而

延长经由快径的传导时间；或者在 AVNRT 和心室起搏时存在不同的传导路线。

几乎不存在下部共径也许可通过在家兔心脏所得到的研究结果来解释。在家兔心脏中，移行区细胞纤维形成跨越 Todaro 腱的快径，插入邻近中心纤维体的房室结（即邻近希氏束）[41,43]。

（二）左侧变异慢-快型房室结折返性心动过速

有一型罕见的慢-快型 AVNRT，其最早的逆传心房激动与慢-快型 AVNRT 一样在 Todaro 腱以上的区域，但是参与折返环的慢径却不能在右房后间隔或是冠状窦口处消融成功[31-34]。在部分患者，参与折返环的慢径可以在冠状窦的顶部（最远可距离冠状窦口 5~6cm）消融成功。本中心有 8 例患者的心动过速可以被在二尖瓣环后壁或后侧壁所发放的左房房性期前刺激所重整；其中 7 例的慢径在二尖瓣环后侧壁能重整心动过速的部位消融成功[33]。在这些部位释放射频电流后，可发生与典型的慢-快型 AVNRT 在右房后间隔放电所产生的同样的加速性交界区性心律（伴快径 1：1 逆传），表明慢径的心房连接部位的受热反应相同。另外 1 例消融靶点位于二尖瓣环后间隔处，在重整心动过速部位的偏间隔处选择性消融逆传快径成功（但是并没有损伤快径前传功能）。这些观察提示房室结的左侧后延伸可能形成了参与折返的前传慢径（见图 59-6）。与普通慢-快型 AVNRT 不同，变异型慢-快型 AVNRT 的整个折返环可能均在心脏左侧。部分此型患者可以出现 2 种不常见的电生理现象：（1）心动过速时很短的 H-A 间期（15ms 或更短），可能代表较长的下传共径；（2）心房程序刺激时，出现"2-for-1 现象"，即一个心房期前刺激可分别通过快径和慢径前传产生两次希氏束电位。后一种特点提示快径前传时缺少慢径的逆传渗透，从而使慢径也能够前传，可能是提示此型 AVNRT 折返环的一个有用的指标。

（三）慢-慢型房室结折返性心动过速

慢-慢型与慢-快型 AVNRT 一样，都是用慢径作为前传支，均有长的 A-H 间期（以我们的经验 A-H 间期可长达 485ms，中位数 240ms）。当进行程序性心房刺激时，心动过速的诱发会伴随 A-H 间期的突然延长。在心房期前刺激时，具有慢-慢型 AVNRT 的患者多表现出多次的 A_2-H_2 间期跳跃，符合多条慢径的存在。通过在心动过速时标测右房和冠状窦，可以区分慢-慢型和慢-快型 AVNRT（图 59-12 至图 59-

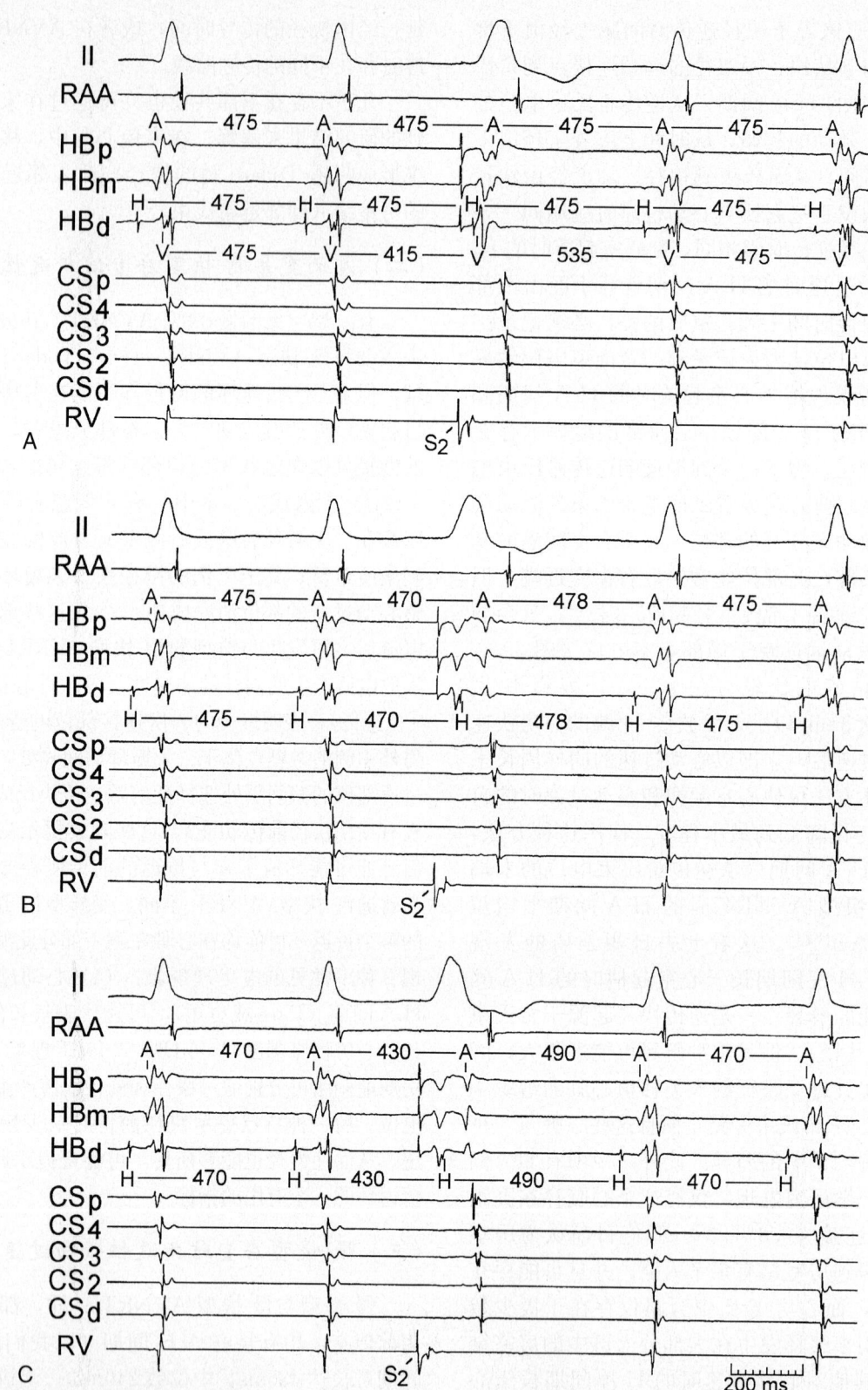

图 59-10　心室期前刺激验证慢-快型房室结折返性心动过速诊断　A：心动过速时，在邻近最早心房激动部位的右室间隔前基底部（希氏束旁部位）发放单个期前刺激（S_2）。S_2 使记录到最早心房激动（希氏束电图）处的心室激动时间提前 60ms（V-V 间期由 475ms 提前至 415ms），但并没有提前希氏束激动（H）时间或逆传心房激动（A）的时间，表明心房激动在心动过速时不依赖于局部心室激动时间，可以除外经由房室旁路传导逆传心房激动和顺向型房室折返性心动过速。B：更提前的室性期前刺激产生希氏束逆向激动，逆传希氏束电位的末端比预期发生的前传希氏束激动提前 5ms（H-H 间期由 475ms 提前至 470ms），致使逆传心房激动时间也相应提前 5ms（A-A 间期由 475ms 提前至 470ms），但不改变心房的激动顺序，表明心房激动依赖于逆传希氏束激动，故可除外房性心动过速而明确 AVNRT 的诊断。C：进一步缩短室性期前刺激联律间期产生更早的希氏束逆传激动，致使逆传心房激动时间有同等程度的提前（H-H 间期＝A-A 间期＝430ms）。

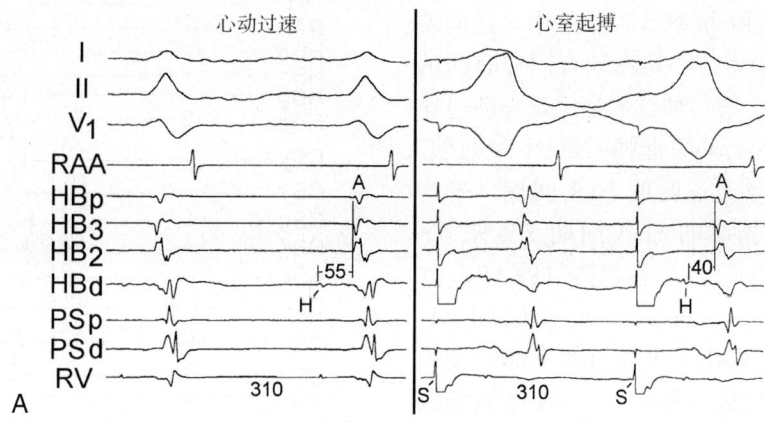

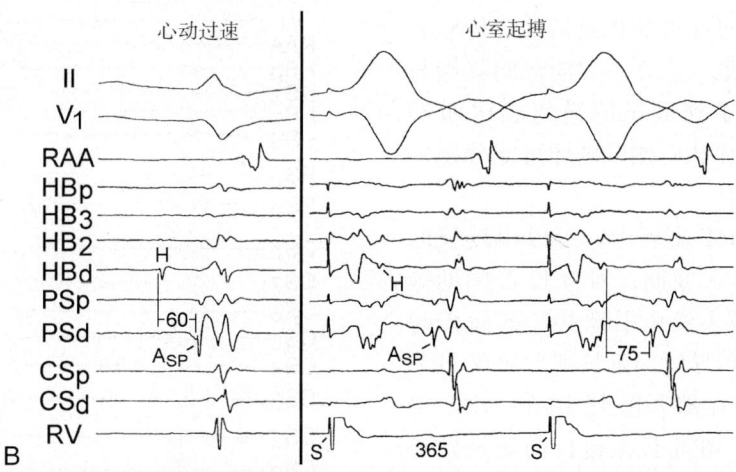

图 59-11 比较慢-快型（A）和慢-慢型（B）房室结折返性心动过速患者心动过速时与心室起搏时的 H-A 间期　A：在周长为 310ms 的慢-快型 AVNRT 时，H-A 间期为 55ms（左图，从前传希氏束电位的起始测量）。右图：终止左图中的心动过速后，即刻以 310ms 周期在希氏束旁起搏心室。从逆传希氏束电位的终点测量 H-A 间期为 40ms，比心动过速时的 H-A 间期缩短 15ms。注意希氏束旁发放心室起搏使希氏束电图上产生很早的心室激动和延迟的逆传希氏束激动，从而使希氏束电图上的希氏束电位（H）和局部心室电位分离，易于鉴别逆传希氏束电位的终点。B：在慢-慢型 AVNRT 时（左图），在右房后间隔记录到最早的心房激动（A_{SP} 电位），H-A_{SP} 间期为 60ms。右图：终止心动过速后，即刻以周期 365ms 起搏心室。H-A_{SP} 间期为 75ms，尽管心室起搏周期比心动过速时的周期延长 15ms，心室起搏时的 H-A_{SP} 间期仍比心动过速时延长 15ms。

14）。从标测中可以显示典型慢径逆传时的心房激动顺序，即可在冠状窦近端的顶部记录到最早逆传心房激动（可能代表逆传激动经由房室结左侧后延伸），或者在少数患者中，可在三尖瓣环与冠状窦口之间的右房后间隔记录到（可能代表逆传激动经由房室结右侧后延伸）。

与慢-快型 AVNRT 相比较，慢-慢型的 H-A 间期有更大的变动范围，我们的经验为－30～260ms（中位数 120ms）[67]。与慢-快型 AVNRT 相似，慢-慢型的 H-A 间期通常较短，导致房室同时激动，故此型 AVNRT 与慢-快型常不易区分，甚至曾被认为是慢-快型 AVNRT 的逆传快径为后部出口的一种变异型（后位型 AVNRT[12,16]）。然而约 50% 的慢-慢型 AVNRT 患者除逆传慢径外还同时存在逆传快径。在程序性心室刺激时，逆传心房激动顺序的转换证实逆传激动并不经由快径（见图 59-13）。在心动过速时房室同时激动的患者，在希氏束旁发放晚发的心室期前刺激可使房室电位分离，从而有助于鉴别逆传心房激动顺序（见图 59-12）。

慢-慢型与慢-快型 AVNRT 之间的另一个不同是在慢-慢型 AVNRT 中有一条明显延长的下部共径。此特点可通过前面已描述的两种技术方法加以证实。一种是在心动过速时发放心室期前刺激，慢-慢型 AVNRT 必须更多地提前逆传希氏束电位（30～60ms

或更多），才能提前逆传心房激动和重整心动过速（见图 59-14B、C）。而在慢-快型 AVNRT 中，逆向希氏束电位的提前通常可使逆传心房激动有同样时间的提前（见图 59-10B、C）。第二种技术是比较心动过速时和以心动过速相同周长行心室起搏时的 H-A 间期。在慢-慢型 AVNRT，心动过速时的 H-A 间期（平均 30ms）明显短于心室起搏时的 H-A 间期（见图 59-11B）；而在慢-快型 AVNRT，心室起搏时的 H-A 间期比心动过速时的 H-A 间期稍短（如图 59-11A）[63,64]。在慢-慢型 AVNRT 中较长的下部共径提示其折返环距离希氏束较远（偏后）。一种可能机制是在房室结右侧后延伸和左侧后延伸之间发生折返（图 59-15）。当在冠状窦的顶部区域记录到最早逆传心房激动时，右侧后延伸可能形成折返环的前传肢而左侧后延伸可能形成逆传肢。当在三尖瓣环间隔侧与冠状窦口之间的区域记录到最早的逆传心房激动（A_{SP} 电位）时，左侧后延伸和右侧后延伸可能分别形成折返环的前传肢和逆传肢。

在许多慢-慢型 AVNRT 患者中，可以用较长的下部共径来解释较短的 H-A 间期，因为 H-A 间期等于经由逆传慢径的时间减去经由下部共径的前传时间，如果经由下部共径的传导时间延长则会导致 H-A 间期缩短。这可用来解释在部分慢-慢型 AVNRT 患者中 H-A 间期可为负值（在希氏束电位前记录到心房激动，见图 59-13）。

至少有两个原因表明鉴别慢-慢型与慢-快型 AVNRT 是必要的。第一，快径消融技术可能仍然被一些医师所应用，如果不鉴别慢-慢型与慢-快型 AVNRT，快径消融对慢-慢型 AVNRT 无效。实际上，有短 H-A 间期的慢-慢型 AVNRT 与慢-快型 AVNRT 非常相似，有报告在典型（慢-快型，早期以短的 H-A 间期为标准）AVNRT 行快径消融后，可出现 5%～10% 的不典型 AVNRT，此不典型 AVNRT 可能为慢-慢型[56]。第二，以我们的经验，慢径消融后慢-慢型 AVNRT 的复发率明显高于慢-快型 AVNRT（分别为 8.3% 和 0.5%），因此在慢-慢型 AVNRT 患者中，在右房后间隔和冠状窦近端进行更广泛的消融可能有助于降低复发率。

（四）快-慢型房室结折返性心动过速

快-慢型 AVNRT（非常见型 AVNRT[9,26,56]）有短的 A-H 间期（我们的经验为 30～185ms，中位数 80ms）和长的 H-A 间期（135～435ms，中位数为

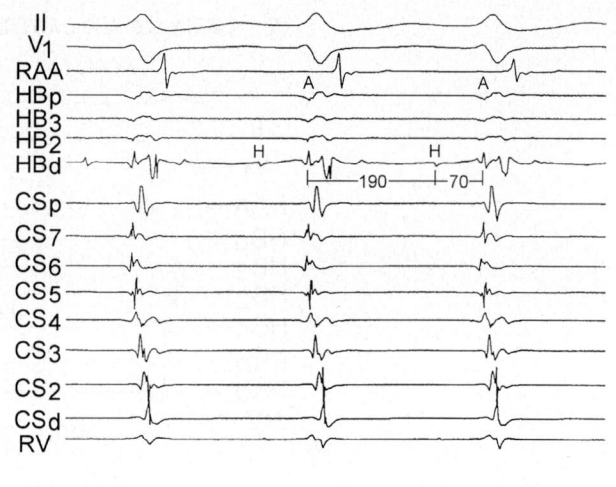

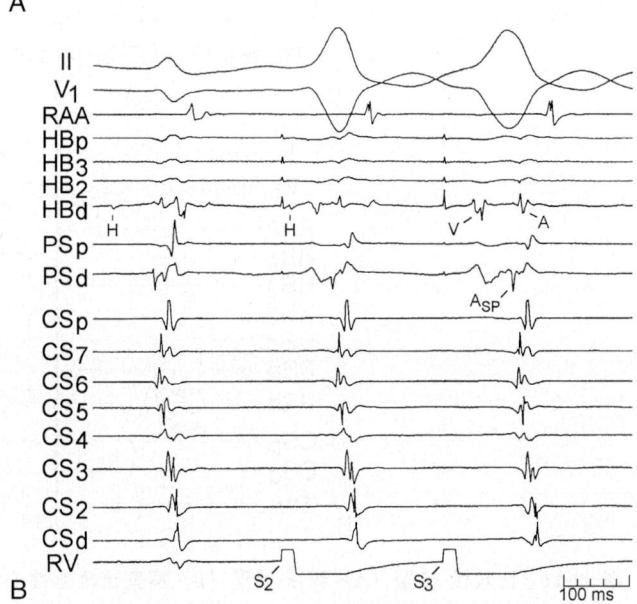

图 59-12 具有短 H-A 间期的慢-慢型房室结折返性心动过速类似慢-快型房室结折返心动过速　A：在慢-慢型 AVNRT 时，短的 H-A 间期（在 HB_d 电图上为 70ms）使房室同时激动，从而使逆传的心房激动顺序难以识别，而与慢-快型 AVNRT 相似。B：在右室间隔前基底部（希氏束旁区域）发放 2 次心室期前刺激。第 2 个心室期前刺激（S_3）提前局部激动心室时间（V），清楚显示出逆传心房激动顺序，最早的逆传心房激动部位在近端冠状窦顶部（A_{SP} 电位），最早激动向两个方向传导（CS_6-CS_p 和 CS_6-CS_d）。

260ms）。心动过速时，最早逆传心房激动与典型的通过房室结慢径逆传激动顺序相同，大多数逆传 A_{SP} 电位在右房后间隔记录到，而少部分患者可在冠状窦内记录到。此型 AVNRT 的 R-P' 间期长于 P'-R 间期，在体表心电图的下壁导联上出现倒置 P 波（图 59-7 和图 59-16）。顾名思义，快-慢型 AVNRT 被认为经由快径前传，慢径逆传，即与慢-快型 AVNRT 有同样的折返环，但却有相反的方向[26,30,68]。由此可推测

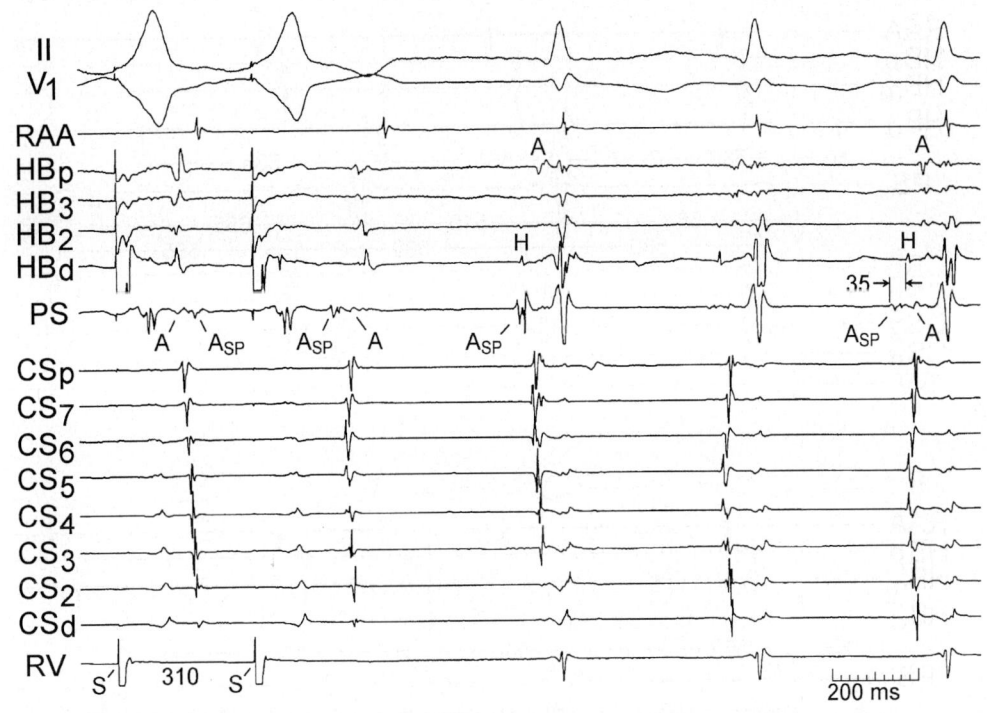

图 59-13 心室起搏诱发慢-慢型房室结折返性心动过速 图中第 1 跳，心室起搏后逆传心房激动顺序符合房室结快径逆传。注意前传的 A_{SP} 电位在冠状窦近端的心房激动时间之后。在第 2 跳中，心室起搏导致快径逆传阻滞而选择性经由慢径逆传（A_{SP} 电位早于其他部位的心房激动）并诱发持续性慢-慢型 AVNRT。心动过速时，希氏束电图上心房激动位于希氏束激动之后，与慢-快型 AVNRT 相类似。然而，在右房后间隔（PS）电图上逆传的 A_{SP} 电位较希氏束激动提前 35ms（负的 H-A 间期）。

快-慢型 AVNRT 将和慢-快型 AVNRT 一样几乎没有下部共径（两条路径的远端连接处到希氏束之间的距离）。然而，发放的心室期前刺激必须使希氏束激动时间提前 30～60ms 或更多才能使随后的心房激动时间提前并重整心动过速（见图 59-16）。此为存在相对较长的下部共径的有力证据，提示快-慢型 AVNRT 的折返环路更接近于慢-慢型而不是慢-快型。一个非常诱人的假说为折返环存在于房室结的左侧和右侧后延伸之间，左侧后延伸为前传肢而右侧后延伸为逆传肢（见图 59-15）。房室结右侧后延伸激动冠状窦的心肌袖，后者激动左心房后传导至房间隔，从而前传激动快径，产生一个短的 A-H 间期和 P-R 间期。在这个机制中，快径仅起旁观者的作用。

支持快-慢型 AVNRT 为慢径间的折返，而快径并不参与的另外一个观察结果为，在程序性心房刺激时快-慢型 AVNRT 的诱发常伴有 A-H 间期的突然增加，提示前传经由一条慢径，随后逆传经由另外一条慢径。

五、房室结折返性心动过速的鉴别诊断和治疗

（一）房室结折返性心动过速与房室折返性心动过速和房速的鉴别诊断

根据不同类型 AVNRT 的心房激动顺序难以同顺向型房室折返性心动过速（前间隔、后间隔或左后游离壁旁路），或起源于间隔或冠状窦周围区域的房速相鉴别。通过心动过速时观察心房的激动时间或在特定时间发放心室期前刺激，可将 AVNRT 与顺向型房室折返性心动过速和房速相鉴别。

在顺向型房室折返性心动过速时，折返冲动通过希氏束-浦肯野系统使冲动在到达旁路前先激动心室，导致室房（V-A）传导时间（从 V 波的起始到逆传 A 波的起始）至少为 50ms，通常大于 60ms[69]。心动过速时逆传 P 波在 QRS 波末端附近或在 ST 段上。在 AVNRT 中，心室部分并不在折返环内。在大多数慢-

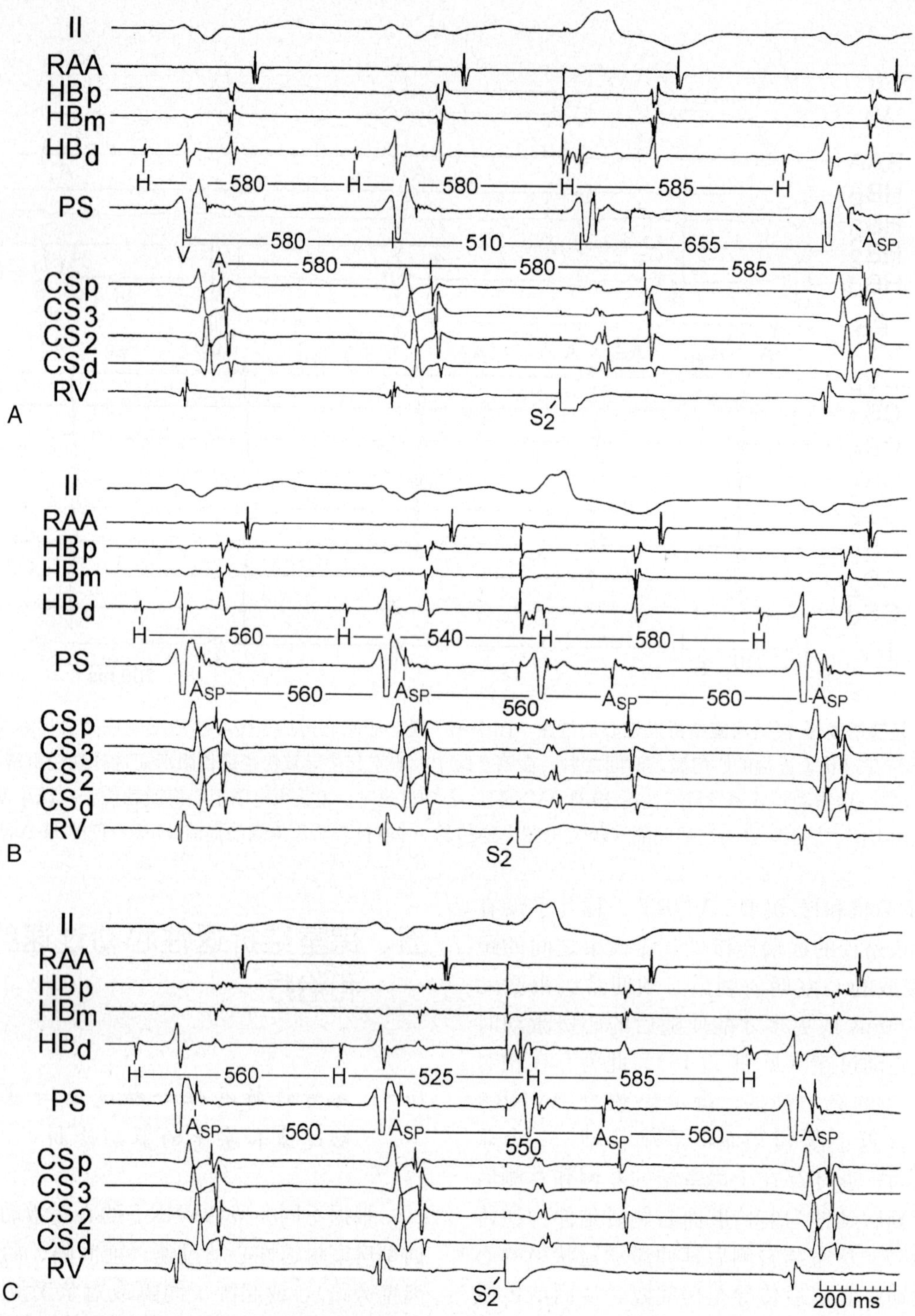

图 59-14 应用心室期前刺激确定慢-慢型房室结折返性心动过速的诊断 A：心动过速时，在右室间隔前基底部发放单个心室期前刺激（S_2），使右后间隔（PS）电图上（此处记录到最早心房激动）的局部心室激动时间提前 70ms（V-V 间期从 580ms 提前到 510ms）。然而，S_2 却没有提前希氏束或心房激动时间，故可排除逆传经由后间隔旁路传导和顺向型房室折返性心动过速。注意心室期前刺激使心室与心房电位进一步分离，使逆传心房激动顺序更容易辨认，包括提前的逆传 A_{SP} 电位。B：更提前的室性期前刺激产生希氏束逆向激动，逆传希氏束电位的末端比预期发生的前传希氏束激动提前 20ms（H-H 间期由 560ms 提前至 540ms）。然而，逆传心房激动时间（A_{SP}-A_{SP}=560ms）并没有提前，支持此心动过速的诊断为有较长的下部共径的 AVNRT 或者为房性心动过速。C：进一步缩短室性期前刺激联律间期产生更早的希氏束逆向激动，逆传希氏束电位的末端比预期发生的前传希氏束激动提前 35ms（H-H 间期由 560ms 提前至 525ms），使逆传心房激动时间提前 10ms（A_{SP}-A_{SP} 由 560ms 提前至 550ms）且不改变心房激动顺序，表明心房激动时间依赖于希氏束激动时间，故可排除房速而明确诊断为 AVNRT。

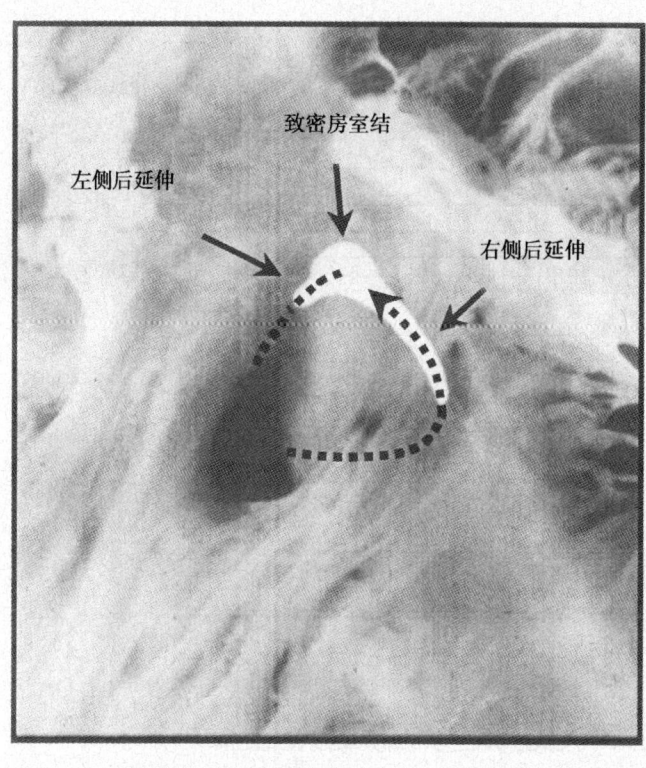 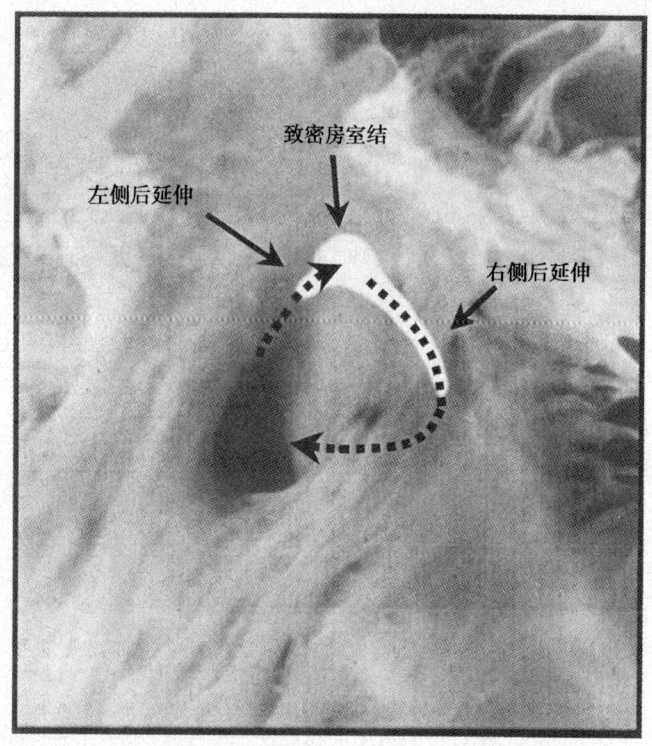

图 59-15　慢-慢型和快-慢型房室结折返性心动过速在房室结左侧和右侧后延伸之间形成折返的假说　逆时针（CCW）折返多伴有长的 A-H 间期，短的 H-A 间期且有典型的慢-慢型 AVNRT 的心房激动顺序（在近端冠状窦的顶部记录到最早激动）。顺时针（CW）折返产生短的 A-H 间期和长的 H-A 间期，最早心房激动在三尖瓣环与冠状窦口之间的部位（A_{SP}电位），为快-慢型 AVNRT 的典型表现。（在 Inoue S，Becker AE：Posterior extensions of the human compact atrioventricular node：A neglected anatomic feature of potential clinical significance. Circulation，1998，97：188-193 发表的图片上修改。）

快型 AVNRT 和一些慢-慢型 AVNRT 患者中，V-A 间期小于 50ms，据此可排除顺向型房室折返性心动过速（见图 59-10 到图 59-13）。

在心动过速时发放单个或 2 个晚发的心室期前刺激可以判定心室肌是否参与折返环，从而鉴别 AVNRT 和顺向型房室折返性心动过速。心动过速时，在希氏束电位起始处以后约 50ms，在逆向激动希氏束前，以每次递减 5～10ms 发放单个（R-S_2）或两个晚发（R-S_2S_3）的心室期前刺激。如果没有首先提前逆向激动希氏束而心房提前激动，表明房室旁路的存在。如果提前激动的心房激动顺序与心动过速时的激动顺序相同，同时心房激动时间的略微提前致使下一次希氏束激动时间也发生变化（重整此心动过速），则表明此时房室旁路参与此心动过速并构成折返环的一部分，同时证实此心动过速的机制为顺向型房室折返。相反，如果在邻近最早的逆传心房激动部位（邻近可能的房室旁路部位）发放心室期前刺激，使心室激动提前 30ms 或更多，而逆传心房激动的时间和激动顺序无变化，则可能不存在房室旁路（见图 59-10A、59-14A、59-16A）。当心动过速时最早的心房激动部位在前间隔时，最好选择在邻近（但不夺获）近端右束支的部位行心室起搏（希氏束旁起搏部位[62]）。当心动过速时最早的心房激动部位在后间隔的三尖瓣环处或冠状窦近端时，最好选择在右室间隔的后基底部靠近三尖瓣环处起搏。这些起搏部位可以最大程度提前邻近最早心房激动部位的心室激动时间而不产生逆传希氏束激动，因为在这些部位起搏时，激动应首先向心尖部传导，然后才能激动希氏束-浦肯野系统。应用短间距的双极电极（电极间距 1mm）记录希氏束电图可减少局部心室电位的时间，从而减少局部心室电位与希氏束电位的重叠，有利于明确前传或逆传希氏束激动（如图 59-10、59-14 和 59-16）。

通过发放早发心室期前刺激可以区分 AVNRT 和房速。在 AVNRT 时，如果室性期前刺激明显提前希氏束逆传的激动时间（30～60ms 或更多），将会改变心房的激动时间（但不改变心房的激动顺序），或者产生 V-A 阻滞并且终止 AVNRT，但在房速时对最早心房激动时间没有影响。通过提前希氏束逆向激动并提前逆传心房激动时间所需的最短时间与下部共径的长度相关（即下部共径越长，希氏束激动时间需要提

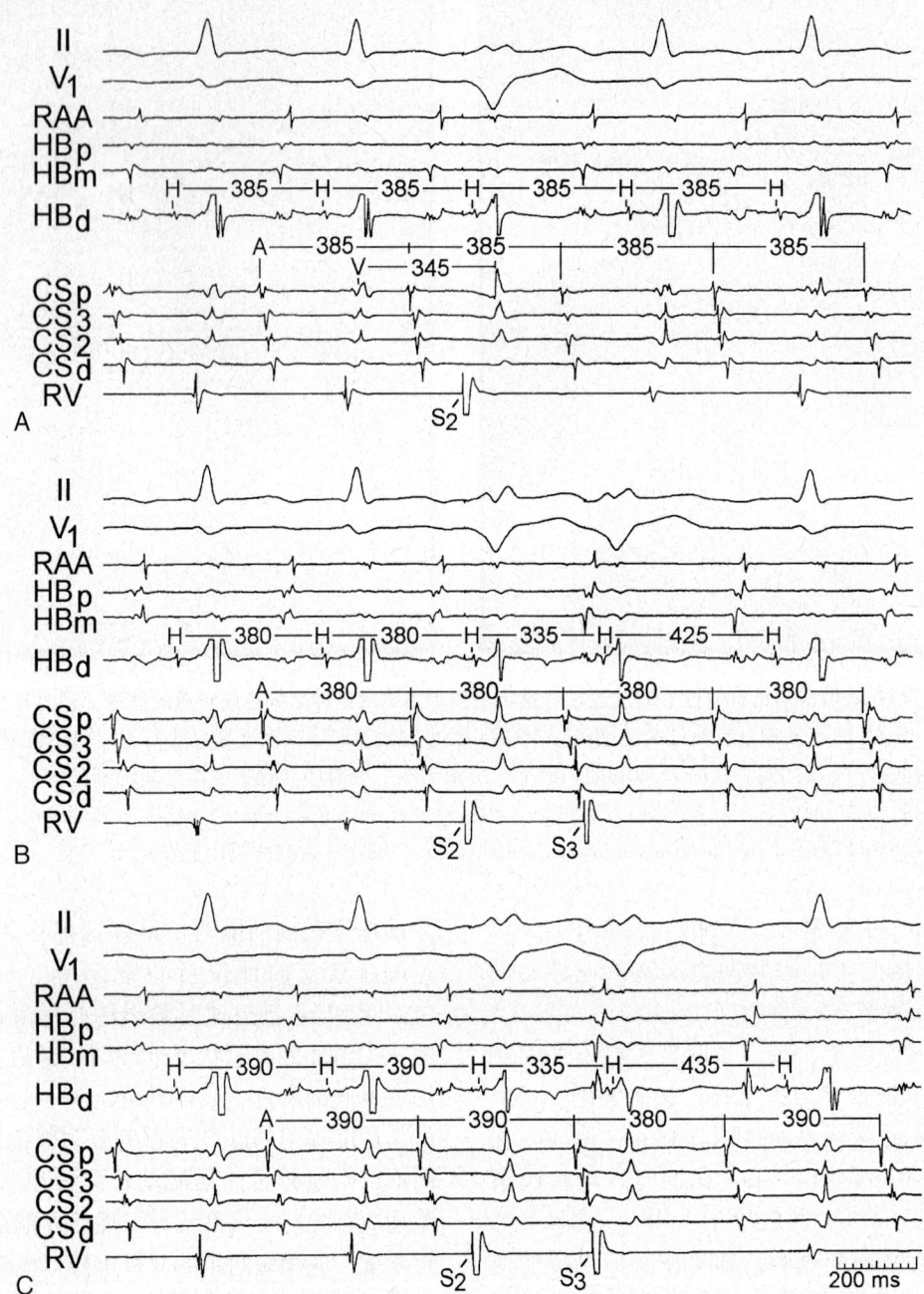

图 59-16 应用心室期前刺激明确快-慢型房室结折返性心动过速的诊断 A：心动过速时，单个心室期前刺激（S₂）提前了邻近最早心房激动部位的近端冠状窦电图（CS_p）上的心室激动时间 40ms（V-V 间期由 385ms 提前至 345ms），但却没有提前希氏束或逆传心房的激动时间，表明在心动过速时心房激动不依赖于局部心室激动，故可除外经由后间隔旁路的逆传和顺向型室折返性心动过速。B：发放 2 个心室期前刺激。第 2 个心室期前刺激（S₃）使希氏束产生逆传激动，逆传希氏束电位的末端比预期发生的前传希氏束激动提前 45ms（H-H 间期由 380ms 提前至 335ms）。然而，S₃ 却没有提前逆传心房激动（A-A＝380ms），支持此心动过速为具有很长下部共径的 AVNRT 或者为房性心动过速。C：进一步缩短室性期前刺激联律间期产生更早的希氏束逆传激动，逆传希氏束电位的末端比预期发生的前传希氏束激动提前 55ms（H-H 间期由 390ms 提前至 335ms），使逆传心房激动时间提前 10ms（A-A 由 390 ms 提前至 380ms）且不改变心房激动顺序，表明心房激动时间依赖于希氏束激动时间，故可排除房速而明确诊断为 AVNRT。

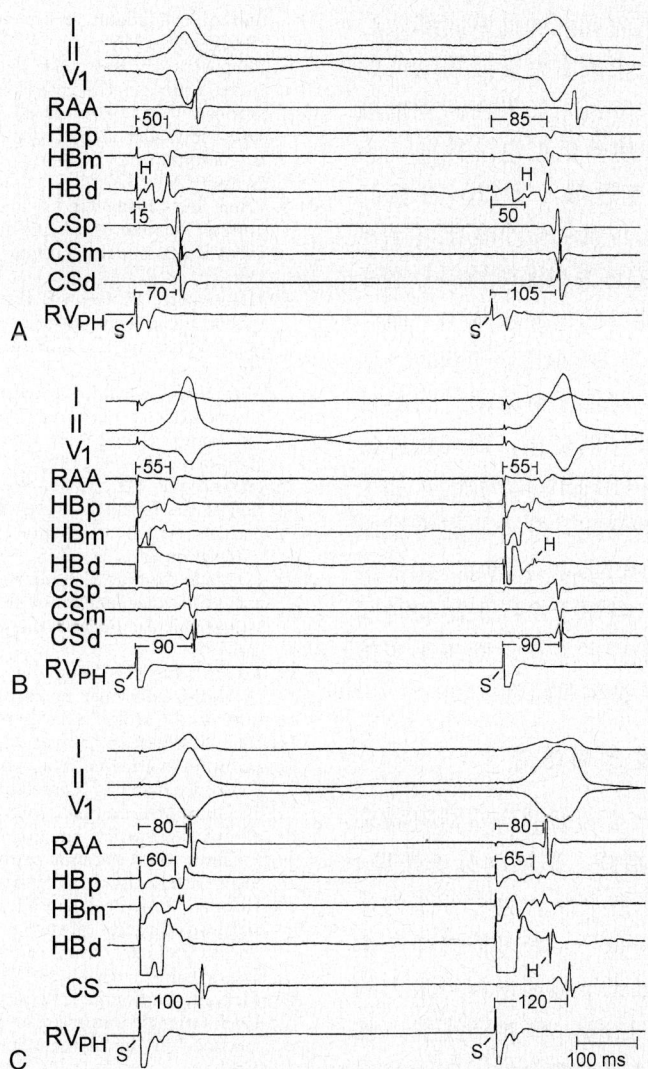

图 59-17 希氏束旁起搏的 3 种基本反应类型 A：逆传完全通过房室结。左侧的起搏刺激（S）同时夺获心室和希氏束或右束支近端（HB-RB 夺获），产生一个相对较窄的 QRS 波和较早希氏束激动（H）。右侧的起搏刺激未夺获 HB-RB，故产生一个较宽的 QRS 波，并使刺激-希氏束间期（S-H）延长 35ms（由 15ms 延长至 50ms），同时使刺激-心房（S-A）间期增加 35ms 而不伴逆传心房激动顺序的改变。恒定的 H-A 间期和心房激动顺序表明逆传只依赖于希氏束的激动，故逆传完全经由房室结。B：逆传完全经由前间隔旁路。左侧波形为 HB-RB 夺获（相对较窄的 QRS 波）而右侧为 HB-RB 失夺获（QRS 波增宽和 S-H 间期延长）。不管 HB-RB 夺获或失夺获，S-A 间期和心房激动顺序均保持恒定，表明逆传依赖于心室激动的时间而不依赖于逆传希氏束激动的时间。C：逆传同时经由前间隔旁路和房室结。当 HB-RB 失夺获时（右侧波形），心房激动顺序的变化表明逆传激动同时经由旁路和房室结（当 HB-RB 夺获与失夺获时，通过旁路和房室结激动心房的数量有所不同）。当 HB-RB 失夺获时（右侧波形），在右心耳（RAA）处所记录到的 S-A 间期保持恒定（80ms），表明此处心房在 HB-RB 夺获与失夺获时均由旁路激动。当 HB-RB 失夺获时，S-A 间期在 HB 电图上延长了 5ms，在冠状窦电图上延长了 20ms，但明显小于 S-H 间期的延长，表明心房的这些部位在 HB-RB 夺获时经由房室结激动，而在 HB-RB 失夺获时经由旁路激动。

前的越多）。需要提前希氏束逆向激动时间的值在慢-快型、慢-慢型和快-慢型 AVNRT 并不相同。在慢-快型 AVNRT，当逆传希氏束电位的末端比预定的前传希氏束电位略为提前，逆传心房激动时间就随之提前（见图 59-10B）[61]。在慢-慢型和快-慢型 AVNRT，心室期前刺激通常必须提前希氏束激动时间 30～60ms，才能改变逆传心房激动时间（见图 59-14B、C，59-16B、C）；通常需要发放多次心室期前刺激或采用比心动过速略短的周长行持续性心室起搏才能达到希氏

束激动明显提前。如果在心动过速时心室期前刺激或心室起搏已使逆传希氏束激动提前 60～80ms 而不改变心房的激动时间和激动顺序，则可以明确房速的诊断。根据心动过速对腺苷的反应也可排除 AVNRT，当出现一段时间的完全性 A-V 阻滞时（超过 2～3 个心动周期）而不改变心房的激动时间和形态，强烈支持房速的诊断。

希氏束旁起搏间断夺获希氏束可以用来鉴别逆传分别是通过房室结的快径、慢径，还是通过前、后间

隔旁路[62]。窦性心律时，在右室间隔的前基底部做心室起搏，此部位距记录到希氏束或右束支近端电位的部位向前和向心尖部方向 3～5mm，如果在高能量输出起搏时出现 QRS 波变窄并使希氏束电位提前，表明已直接夺获希氏束或右束支近端（HB-RB 夺获）。随着呼吸运动出现的起搏电极位置的微小变化可导致 HB-RB 的间断夺获。另一个方法为在保持局部心室夺获的条件下，通过起搏输出能量的增加或减少，而产生 HB-RB 的夺获和非夺获。当 HB-RB 非夺获时，如果出现心房激动时间的延迟（与希氏束激动时间的延迟相同）而不出现心房激动顺序的变化，则表明逆传经由房室结（图 59-17A）。当 HB-RB 非夺获时，如果不出现心房激动时间和顺序的变化，则表明逆传经由房室旁路（图 59-17B）。当 HB-RB 非夺获时，如果出现心房激动时间的部分延迟（略短于希氏束激动时间的延迟）而且出现心房激动顺序的变化，则表明逆传同时经由房室旁路和房室结（如图 59-17C）。

（二）房室结折返性心动过速的治疗

终止 AVNRT 可以通过产生短暂的房室结阻滞来完成。增强迷走神经张力的措施，如颈动脉窦按摩、吸气后屏气（Valsalva 法）或潜水反射通常可作为最先选用的方法用来终止心动过速，一般可使慢径产生传导阻滞而终止心动过速。如果增强迷走神经张力的措施无效，使用腺苷（成人 12mg，弹丸样注射）常可终止 AVNRT。如果心动过速很快复发，应用钙通道阻滞剂（维拉帕米或地尔硫䓬）或先应用 β 受体阻滞剂（艾司洛尔、普萘洛尔、美托洛尔）后再追加一剂腺苷多可终止心动过速。

房室结慢径消融已经成为所有类型 AVNRT 的一线治疗方法，治愈率高（成功率 95%～99%）[4-8]、房室阻滞发生率低（小于 1%），在本书 116 章有详细描述。对那些不接受或不能消融的患者长期药物治疗也可能有效。β 受体阻滞剂和钙通道阻滞剂由于其安全性和易获得性而通常为首选，其主要作用于慢径前传。然而，I 类抗心律失常药物如氟卡胺、普罗帕酮通常更为有效，其主要抑制快径逆传。Ⅲ 类抗心律失常药物索他洛尔和胺碘酮同样有效，但较少用于 AVNRT。

（王祖禄 译）

参 考 文 献

1. Wu D, Denes P, Amat-y-Leon F, et al: Clinical, electrocardiographic and electrophysiologic observations in patients with paroxysmal supraventricular tachycardia. Am J Cardiol 41:1045–1051, 1978.
2. Mignone RJ, Wallace AG: Ventricular echoes: Evidence for dissociation of conduction and reentry within the AV node. Circ Res 19:638–649, 1966.
3. Josephson ME, Kastor JA: Paroxysmal supraventricular tachycardia: Is the atrium a necessary link? Circulation 54:430–435, 1976.
4. Jackman WM, Beckman KJ, McClelland JH, et al: Treatment of supraventricular tachycardia due to atrioventricular nodal reentry, by radiofrequency catheter ablation of slow-pathway conduction. N Engl J Med 327:313–318, 1992.
5. Chen SA, Chiang CE, Tsang WP, et al: Selective radiofrequency catheter ablation of fast and slow pathway in 100 patients with atrioventricular nodal reentrant tachycardia. Am Heart J 125:1–10, 1993.
6. Haissaguerre M, Gaita F, Fischer B, et al: Elimination of atrioventricular nodal reentrant tachycardia using discrete slow potentials to guide application of radiofrequency energy. Circulation 85:2162–2175, 1992.
7. Mitrani RD, Klein LS, Hackett K, et al: Radiofrequency ablation for atrioventricular node reentrant tachycardia: Comparison between fast (anterior) and slow (posterior) pathway ablation. J Am Coll Cardiol 21:432–441, 1993.
8. Jazayeri MR, Hempe SL, Sra JS, et al: Selective transcatheter ablation of the fast and slow pathways using radiofrequency energy in patients with atrioventricular nodal reentrant tachycardia. Circulation 85:1318–1328, 1992.
9. Lee MA, Morady F, Kadish A, et al: Catheter modification of the atrioventricular junction with radiofrequency energy for control of atrioventricular nodal reentry tachycardia. Circulation 83:827–835, aaaa1991.
10. Lo HM, Lin FY, Tseng CD, et al: Selective surgical ablation of the slow atrioventricular nodal pathway by posterior perinodal dissection. Am J Cardiol 71:1457–1459, 1993.
11. Keim S, Werner P, Jazayeri M, et al: Localization of the fast and slow pathways in atrioventricular nodal reentrant tachycardia by intraoperative ice mapping. Circulation 86:919–925, 1992.
12. McGuire MA, Lau KC, Johnson DC, et al: Patients with two types of atrioventricular junctional (AV nodal) reentrant tachycardia: Evidence that a common pathway of nodal tissue is not present above the reentrant circuit. Circulation 83:1232–1246, 1991.
13. Jackman WM, Beckman KJ, McClelland JH, et al: Participation of atrial myocardium (posterior septum) in AV nodal reentrant tachycardia: Evidence from resetting by atrial extrastimuli [abstract]. Pacing Clin Electrophysiol 14:646, 1991.
14. McGuire M, Bourke J, Robotin M, et al: High resolution mapping of Koch's triangle using sixty electrodes in humans with atrioventricular junctional (AV nodal) reentrant tachycardia. Circulation 88:2315–2328, 1993.
15. Yamabe H, Misumi I, Fukushima H, et al: Electrophysiological delineation of the tachycardia circuit in atrioventricular nodal reentrant tachycardia. Circulation 100:621–627, 1999.
16. Ross DL, Johnson DC, Denniss AR, et al: Curative surgery for atrioventricular junctional ("AV nodal") reentrant tachycardia. J Am Coll Cardiol 6:1383–1392, 1985.
17. Kottkamp H, Hindricks G, Willems S, et al: An anatomically and electrogram-guided stepwise approach for effective and safe catheter ablation of the fast pathway for elimination of atrioventricular node reentrant tachycardia. J Am Coll Cardiol 25:974–981, 1995.
18. Oglin JE, Ursell P, Kao AK, Lesh MD: Pathological findings following slow pathway ablation for AV nodal reentrant tachycardia. J Cardiovasc Electrophysiol 7:625–631, 1996.
19. Denes P, Wu D, Dhingra R, et al: Dual atrioventricular nodal pathways: A common electrophysiological response. Br Heart J 37:1069–1076, 1975.
20. Chen J, Josephson ME: Atrioventricular nodal tachycardia occurring during atrial fibrillation. J Cardiovasc Electrophysiol 11:812–815, 2000.
21. Denes P, Wu D, Dhingra RC, et al: Demonstration of dual A-V nodal pathways in patients with paroxysmal supraventricular tachycardia. Circulation 48:549–555, 1973.
22. Goldreyer BN, Damato AN: The essential role of atrioventricular conduction delay in the initiation of paroxysmal supraventricular tachycardia. Circulation 43:679–687, 1971.
23. Moulton KP, Wang X, Xu Y, et al: High incidence of dual AV nodal pathway physiology in patients undergoing radiofrequency ablation of accessory pathways [abstract]. Circulation 82:iii-319, 1990.
24. Hazlitt HA, Beckman KJ, McClelland JH, et al: Prevalence of slow AV nodal pathway potentials in patients without AV nodal reentrant tachycardia [abstract]. J Am Coll Cardiol 21:281A, 1993.
25. Sung RJ, Waxman HL, Saksena S, Juma Z: Sequence of retrograde

atrial activation in patients with dual atrioventricular nodal pathways. Circulation 64:1059–1067, 1981.
26. Sung RJ, Styperek JL, Myerburg RJ, Castellanos A: Initiation of two distinct forms of atrioventricular nodal reentrant tachycardia during programmed ventricular stimulation in man. Am J Cardiol 42:404–415, 1978.
27. Otomo K, Beckman KJ, McClelland JH, et al: Resetting response suggests the absence of an upper common pathway in slow/fast and presence in slow/slow atrioventricular nodal reentrant tachycardia [abstract]. Pacing Clin Electrophysiol 19:730, 1996.
28. Tchou P, Cheng Y, Mowrey K, et al: Relation of the atrial input sites to the dual atrioventricular nodal pathways: Crossing of conduction curves generated with posterior and anterior pacing. J Cardiovasc Electrophysiol 8:1133–1144, 1997.
29. Medkour D, Becker AE, Khalife K, Billette J: Anatomic and functional characteristics of a slow posterior AV nodal pathway: Role in dual-pathway physiology and reentry. Circulation 98:164–174, 1998.
30. Wu J, Wu J, Olgin J, et al: Mechanisms underlying the reentrant circuit of atrioventricular nodal reentrant tachycardia in isolated canine atrioventricular nodal preparation using optical mapping. Circ Res 88:1189–1195, 2001.
31. Altemose GT, Scott LR, Miller JM: Atrioventricular nodal reentrant tachycardia requiring ablation on the mitral annulus. J Cardiovasc Electrophysiol 11:1281–1284, 2000
32. Sorbera C, Cohen M, Woolfe P, Kalapatapu SR: Atrioventricular nodal reentry tachycardia: Slow pathway ablation using the transeptal approach. Pacing Clin Electrophysiol 23:1343–1349, 2000.
33. Tondo C, Otomo K, McClelland J, et al: Atrioventricular nodal reentrant tachycardia: Is the reentrant circuit always confined in the right atrium [abstract]? J Am Coll Cardiol 27:159A, 1996.
34. Tondo C, Beckman KJ, McClelland JH, et al: Response to radiofrequency catheter ablation suggests that the coronary sinus forms part of the reentrant circuit in some patients with atrioventricular nodal reentrant tachycardia [abstract]. Circulation 94:i-380, 1996.
35. Scherlag BJ, Patterson E, Jackman WM, Lazzara R: The elusive extracellular AV nodal potential: Studies from the canine heart, ex vivo. J Interv Cardiac Electrophysiol 7:39–52, 2002.
36. Lin LJ, Billette J, Khalife K, et al: Characteristics, circuit, mechanism, and ablation of reentry in the rabbit atrioventricular node. J Cardiovasc Electrophysiol 10:954–964, 1999.
37. Hirao K, Scherlag BJ, Poty H, et al: Electrophysiology of the atrio-AV nodal inputs and exits in the normal dog heart: Radiofrequency ablation using an epicardial approach. J Cardiovasc Electrophysiol 8:904–915, 1997.
38. Antz M, Scherlag BJ, Patterson E, et al: Electrophysiology of the right anterior approach to the atrioventricular node: Studies in vivo and in the isolated perfused dog heart. J Cardiovasc Electrophysiol 8:47–61, 1997.
39. Otomo K, Antz M, Beckman KJ, et al: Left atrial activation precedes right atrial activation in slow/fast atrioventricular nodal reentrant tachycardia [abstract]. Circulation 94:i-683, 1996.
40. Ashar MS, Otomo K, Wang Z, et al: Late activation in the triangle of Koch suggests block at the tendon of Todaro in slow/fast AVNRT [abstract]. Pacing Clin Electrophysiol 25:II-542, 2002.
41. Janse MJ, Van Capelle FJL, Anderson RH, et al: Electrophysiology and structure of the atrioventricular node of the isolated rabbit heart. In Wellens HJJ, Lie KI, Janse MJ (eds): The Conduction System of the Heart. Philadelphia, Lea & Febiger, 1976, pp 296–315.
42. Becker AE, Anderson RH: Morphology of the human atrioventricular junction area. In Wellens HJJ, Lie KI, Janse MJ (eds): The Conduction System of the Heart: Structure, Function and Clinical Implications. Philadelphia, Lea & Febiger, 1976, pp 263–286.
43. Patterson E, Scherlag BJ: Fast pathway connections to the distal AV node: Evidence for partial AV nodal bypass tract [abstract]. Pacing Clin Electrophysiol 21:919, 1998.
44. Inoue S, Becker AE: Posterior extensions of the human compact atrioventricular node: A neglected anatomic feature of potential clinical significance. Circulation 97:188–193, 1998.
45. Antz M, Otomo K, Arruda M, et al: Electrical conduction between the right atrium and the left atrium via the musculature of the coronary sinus. Circulation 98:1790–1795, 1998.
46. Sun y, Arruda MS, Otomo K, et al: Coronary sinus-ventricular accessory connections producing posteroseptal and left posterior accessory pathways: Incidence and electrophysiological identification. Circulation 106:1362–1367, 2002.
47. Spach MS, Josephson ME: Initiating reentry: The role of nonuniform anisotropy in small circuits. J Cardiovasc Electrophysiol 5:182–209, 1994.
48. Jentzer JH, Goyal R, Williamson BD, et al: Analysis of junctional ectopy during radiofrequency ablation of the slow pathway in patients with atrioventricular nodal reentrant tachycardia. Circulation 90:2820–2826, 1994.
49. Racker DK: Atrioventricular node and input pathways: A correlated gross anatomical and histological study of the canine atrioventricular junctional region. Anat Rec 224:336–354, 1989.
50. Inoue S, Becker AE, Gaita F: Interruption of the posterior extension of the compact atrioventricular node underlies successful radiofrequency ablation of atrioventricular nodal reentrant tachycardia [abstract]. Pacing Clin Electrophysiol 21:796, 1998.
51. Kuck KH, Kuch B, Bleifeld W: Multiple anterograde and retrograde AV nodal pathways: Demonstration by multiple discontinuities in the AV nodal conduction curves and echo time intervals. Pacing Clin Electrophysiol 7:656–662, 1984.
52. Antz M, Scherlag BJ, Otomo K, et al: Evidence for multiple atrio-AV nodal inputs in the normal dog heart. J Cardiovasc Electrophysiol 9:395–408, 1998.
53. Janse MJ, Anderson RH, McGuire MA: AV nodal reentry: Part I. AV nodal reentry revisited. J Cardiovasc Electrophysiol 4:561–572, 1993.
54. Sheahan RG, Klein GJ, Yee R, et al: Atrioventricular node reentry with "smooth" AV node function curves: A different arrhythmia substrate? Circulation 93:969–972, 1996.
55. Baerman J, Wang X, Jackman WM: Atrioventricular nodal reentry with an anterograde slow pathway and retrograde slow pathway: Clinical and electrophysiologic properties [abstract]. J Am Coll Cardiol 17:338A, 1991.
56. Goldberger J, Brooks R, Kadish A: Physiology of "atypical" atrioventricular junctional reentrant tachycardia occurring following radiofrequency catheter modification of the atrioventricular node. Pacing Clin Electrophysiol 15:2270–2282, 1992.
57. Tai CT, Chen SA, Chiang CE, et al: Complex electrophysiological characteristics in atrioventricular nodal reentrant tachycardia with continuous atrioventricular node function curves. Circulation 95:2541–2547, 1997.
58. Anselme F, Papageorgiou P, Monahan K, et al: Presence and significance of the left atrionodal connection during atrioventricular nodal reentrant tachycardia. Am J Cardiol 83:1530–1536, 1999.
59. Li YG, Bender B, Bogun F, et al: Location of the lower turnaround point in typical AV nodal reentrant tachycardia: A quantitative model. J Cardiovasc Electrophysiol 11:34–40, 2000.
60. Anselme F, Poty H, Cribier A, et al: Entrainment of typical AV nodal reentrant tachycardia using para-Hisian pacing: Evidence for a lower common pathway within the AV node. J Cardiovasc Electrophysiol 10:655–661, 1999.
61. Thibault B, Beckman K, McClelland J, et al: Use of ventricular stimuli to examine lower common pathway in S/F AVNRT [abstract]. Circulation 90:i-214, 1994.
62. Hirao K, Otomo K, Wang X, et al: Para-Hisian pacing: A new method for differentiating retrograde conduction over an accessory AV pathway from conduction over the AV node. Circulation 94:1027–1035, 1996.
63. Heidbüchel H, Beckman K, McClelland J, et al: Presence or absence of a lower common pathway differentiates slow/slow from slow/fast AV nodal reentrant tachycardia [abstract]. Pacing Clin Electrophysiol 17:759, 1994.
64. Heidbüchel H, Ector H, De Were FV: Prospective evaluation of the length of the lower common pathway in the different diagnosis of various forms of AV nodal reentrant tachycardia. Pacing Clin Electrophysiol 21:209–216, 1998.
65. Ho SW, McComb JM, Scott CD, Anderson RH: Morphology of the cardiac conduction system in patients with electrophysiologically proven dual atrioventricular nodal pathways. J Cardiovasc Electrophysiol 4:504–512, 1993.
66. Brechenmacher C: Atrio-His bundle tracts. Br Heart J 37:853–855, 1975.
67. Thibault B, Beckman K, McClelland J, et al: Variation in H-A interval suggests a lower common pathway in slow/slow AVNRT [abstract]. Pacing Clin Electrophysiol 17:840, 1994.
68. Yamabe H, Shimasaki Y, Honda O, et al: Demonstration of the exact anatomic tachycardia circuit in the fast-slow form of atrioventricular nodal reentrant tachycardia. Circulation 104:1268–1273, 2001.
69. Benditt DG, Pritchett EL, Smith WM, Gallagher JJ: Ventriculoatrial intervals: Diagnostic use in paroxysmal supraventricular tachycardia. Ann Intern Med 91:161–166, 1979.

第 60 章

先天性心脏病的房性心律失常

John K. Triedman

本章目录
- 临床背景 550
- 房内折返性心动过速 550
- 先心病房颤 557
- 心动过缓 558
- 总结 558

随着先天性心脏病（congenital heart disease, CHD）外科技术的不断发展，因典型的心脏疾病而存活的儿童和青少年人口逐渐增多。在美国约有1百万人患有某种类型的先心病，其中15%~20%需要手术干预。在先心病患者中房性心律失常是普遍存在的，尤其是在经历过大范围心脏手术后并且长期生存的患者中更为常见。不典型的房性折返性心动过速和继发于窦房结功能障碍的缓慢型心律失常十分常见。而这些心律失常在心脏解剖结构正常的青少年中却很少见，这些心律失常与发绀和长期血流动力学负担加重造成的心肌肥厚和纤维化有关。这些心律失常的自然病程和处理已成为临床医师在处理这些病人时的重要问题。

先心病患者合并心律失常可显著影响患者的症状，医师必须对这种心律失常的潜在危险和不同疗法的安全性、可行性进行评估。因此，除了分析患者的心律失常，临床医师必须对患者心血管系统解剖以及该种解剖结构的改变以及手术矫正对心功能的影响有完整和准确的认识。

本章回顾了先心病合并房性心律失常的病理生理、自然病程、评估和处理。

一、临床背景

对于成年获得性心脏病患者，通过大规模、前瞻性的临床研究已经获得了有效的、准确的评估心源性猝死危险性的办法。这些病人可以分为大的、相对同质的、有着相似危险性增高的亚组（例如：心梗后1年射血分数降低的病人）。与之相反的是，很难为先心病定义准确的危险因素，或以相对明确的终点来评价干预措施的效果，如存活率。先心病病人人群小、解剖异常变化多，猝死率相对较低，即使在"高危组"其死亡率也低于每年2%[1]。虽然先天性心脏缺陷的解剖分型是复杂的，但是由于在人群中的高发病率以及与心律失常的高相关性，三种主要类型的心脏缺陷占伴有心律失常的先心病患者的多数（表60-1）。在年长的先心病病人中，心律失常和死亡的自然病程仍不十分清楚，部分原因是手术治疗方法的不断发展。但是，对这些类型病人的研究清楚地表明：同获得性心脏病一样，心律失常在先天性心脏病中是常见的，而且心源性猝死是其总死亡率的一个主要因素[3]。这些临床发现也与多种解剖缺陷的不同结局有关，包括残留的血流动力学缺陷、手术修补时机较晚以及较长的随访时间。

二、房内折返性心动过速

关于先心病患者常见的房性折返性心动过速的命名，曾经提出过多种命名，包括房扑、不典型房扑、大折返性房速和切口性房速。这反映了调查者们尝试通过仔细的描述性命名法去阐明这些问题的临床和

表 60-1　与心律失常相关的先天性心脏缺陷

Mustard 和 Senning 手术	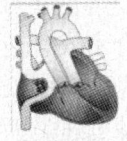	从 20 世纪 70 年代到 90 年代早期，通过使用合成材料（Mustard 手术）或折叠和强化心房壁（Senning 手术）来建立房内隔板治疗患有大动脉转位的患者。重建的腔静脉血和肺静脉血都可纠正发绀，将右心室作为体循环的心室。
Fontan 手术	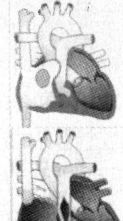	许多先心病有类似的解剖特点即先期手术清除了室间隔，造成单心室的生理状态。分期手术通常的终点是 Fontan 手术，将单心室作为系统的心室并将系统的静脉血导回肺动脉。已有多种改进型，目前，已创新出上腔静脉和肺动脉的连接，并使用心外隧道或心房内隔板连接腔静脉。
法洛四联术		法洛四联症的非手术者儿童时期较高的生存率和发现年龄较早使得修补手术变得可行，出现了大量的、有相同的临床经历的病人。修补包括室间隔缺损（VSD）的闭合和减轻右心室负荷，经常需要双心室切开和心房切开。

（修改自：Triedman JK：Arrhythmias in adults with congenital heart disease. Heart 87：383-389，2002.）

电生理表现。在这一章里将采用房内折返性心动过速（intra-atrial reentrant tachycardia，IART）这一术语。

虽然在正常心脏中少见，房内折返性心动过速是许多先心病患者的晚期并发症。与房扑类似，房内折返性心动过速有稳定的周长和 P 波形态，说明它由固定的心肌参与形成。图 60-1 给出了一个典型的、连续的房内折返性心动过速心电图的示例，表现为常见的窦房结功能障碍合并多变的房室传导阻滞。房内折返性心动过速通常被认为是右心房的心律失常，反之，心房颤动（atrial fibrillation，AF）则通常是左房疾患的表现。通过比较先心病患者术后右心房异常和成人获得性心脏病患者左房大小、功能异常，可以认为这是一个可信的概念。然而，已有关于来自左房的有序折返的描述[4]，右房也已被认为与某些类型房颤的发生和维持有关。这种先心病相关的快-慢综合征的发生导致了一系列临床表现：从良性、无症状的心律失常到猝死。持续性或反复发作的心律失常可逐步导致血流动力学恶化，反之亦然，在临床上形成失代偿的恶性循环。血栓形成和栓塞事件也与房内折返性心动过速有关。这些症状常需要住院治疗和使用仪器、抗心律失常药物等进行处理，对生活质量造成了显著影响。

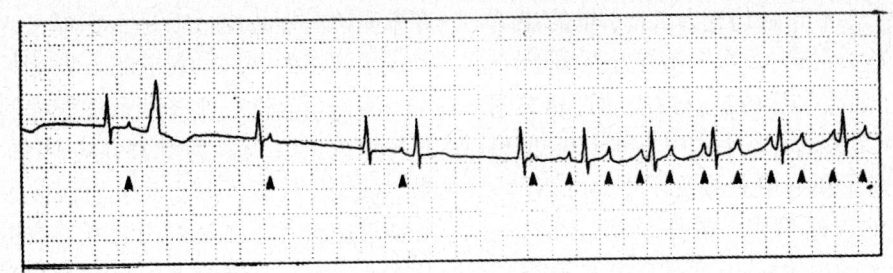

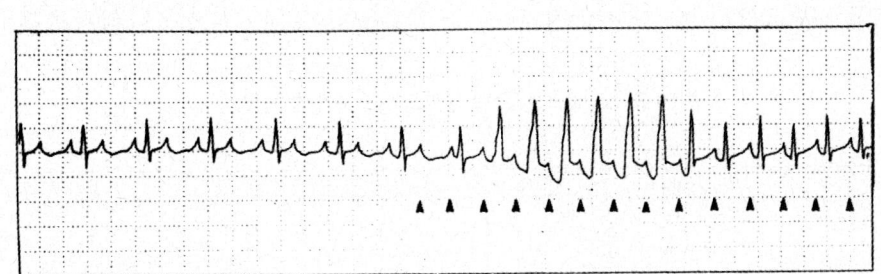

图 60-1　1 例伴有窦房结功能障碍和结性逸搏心律的患者房内折返性心动过速发作的典型的、连续的心电图记录　房室传导是多变的，而且在本例中 QRS 波畸形伴传导速度的突然加快，类似于室性心动过速。

观察性和实验性的研究已经描述了数个导致房内折返性心动过速发生的致病过程。房内折返性心动过速普遍发生于接受过包括大范围的心房切割和修补的外科手术病人中，提示这种房速与手术损伤高度相关。动物模型清楚地模拟了手术后的房内折返性心动过速，形成了与临床观察相似的心动过速。

(一) 流行病学和自然病程

房性心动过速在先心病患者中很常见，房内折返性心动过速在小儿心脏病治疗中经常遇到。一个早期、回顾性、多中心的研究表明，80%以上的年轻的"房扑"患者曾有修补或未修补的先天性心脏病病史，而只有8%来自解剖和功能正常的心脏[5]。虽然房内折返性心动过速被认为是几乎所有类型心脏手术的术后长期并发症，但先心病外科手术似乎导致其发生率大幅度的增加。相关的这些手术包括心房切开或其他的明显对心房进行的手术，例如房间隔缺损修补术、大动脉错位矫正的Mustard手术和Senning手术、单心室重建的Fontan吻合手术、法洛四联症手术、肺静脉畸形引流矫正术等。

四分之一到三分之一的接受Mustard手术和Fontan手术的病人可以诱发出持续性房性心动过速[6]，这与手术多年后自发产生房性心动过速病人的比例相似。一项近500例Mustard手术早期生存者的研究表明：在20年的随访期内，房内折返性心动过速发生率为27%；60%患者有窦房结功能低下，通常伴有房内折返性心动过速。在平均随访超过11.6年的患者中，猝死的发生率为6.5%[1]。在一些较小的研究中也观察到了Mustard手术和房内折返性心动过速之间的联系。对来自于4个大的心脏手术中心共1200例患者的回顾性研究描述了单心室并接受了Fontan手术患者房性心律失常的自然病程。数据显示，25%～50%接受Fontan手术的患者在10年的随访中有房内折返性心动过速的记录（表60-2）[7-10]。房内折返性心动过速的危险因素包括手术时年龄较大和较长的随访时间。使用心外隧道腔肺吻合的改良Fontan手术患者比使用吻合术或管道的全心房与肺动脉连接的经典Fontan手术患者较少出现房性心律失常[7,11]。有观点认为这些心动过速是手术瘢痕的副产物，于是对Fontan术进行了合理改良，采用了腔静脉间管状补片和最小范围的心房操作。这也许是过分简化了房内折返性心动过速的原因，因为这些病人有的在随访的早期即有房性心动过速的报道[12]。最近，Roos-Hesselink和合作者进行了53例法洛四联症患者术后房扑的回顾性研究[13]。他们发现，平均随访18年后，患有窦房结功能障碍和房内折返性心律失常的患者各占1/3，比室性心动过速更多发，而且更可能与症状相关。

对Fontan手术后的房内折返性心律失常的一项早期研究表明，房内折返性心律失常既是慢性心律失常复发的预测因素，也是围术期死亡率最主要的危险因素[14]。一项先心病术后回顾性的随访研究显示，在6.5年后猝死占到总死亡率的10%[5]。虽然房内折返性心律失常的发生与充血性心衰和血栓形成有显著的相关性，但在最近的一项多因素分析研究中未能确认房内折返性心律失常为死亡率增加的危险因素[3]。

关于先心病患者房内折返性心律失常电复律后卒中的报道很少，但Fontan手术常与血管内和心脏内的血栓形成有关[15]。若同时发生房内折返性心动过速可能更容易形成血栓，有报道电复律前作超声心动图的患者心内血栓的发生率可达42%（图60-2）[16]。但并未明确房性心动过速是否能促进此类事件发生，或仅仅是病态的、过早衰老的心脏发生的伴随问题。

房内折返性心律失常自然病程的特点是心动过速日益频繁的复发。为观察抗心律失常药物治疗的效果，回顾性检查了波士顿儿童医院的一组房内折返性心动过速患者。在这组未公开的数据中，无论何种治疗方式，2年随访记录的复发率仍高达60%～80%。Triedman及同事观察了行射频消融术以控制心律失常

表60-2　Fontan术后房内折返性心律失常的发生

研究，时间（引文）	病例数	Cond	APC	TCPC		随访时间
Gelatt, 1994 (9)	269	11%	30%	17%	S	3.8年
Cecchin, 1995 (10)	132	——	42%	26%	S	3.2年
Durongpisitkul, 1996 (8)	499	——	17%	22%	NS	5.0年
Fishberger, 1997 (7)	278	38%	28%	5%	NS	5:1年

APC，房肺连接；Cond，右房-右室或右房-肺动脉管道；TCPC，全腔肺连接。NS，手术方式间无显著的统计学差异；S，显著的统计学差异。

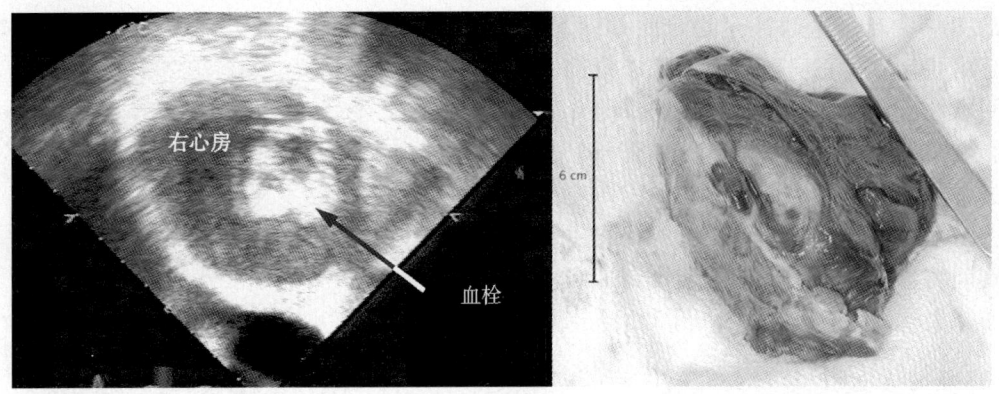

图 60-2　Fontan 术后伴慢性反复性房内折返性心动过速患者晚期随访时观察到巨大的右房血栓　左图：超声发现的漂浮血栓。右图：Fontan 修改手术时去除的附着于右房壁的大血栓。

患者的术后房内折返性心动过速复发的时间模式[17]。在这些病人中，在射频消融前 12～24 个月心律失常复发率逐渐增加，尤其在前 6 个月增加明显。

（二）房内折返性心动过速的心电图表现

先心病患者发生的房内折返性心动过速有时与 I 型房扑有相同的心电图特点——基线呈锯齿波状，周长为 200ms～250ms，伴 2∶1 或更高度的房室阻滞。不典型的心电图形态是普遍的，大约占房内折返性心动过速心电图记录的 70%[18]。P 波经常是可辨别的，P 波之间有较长的等电位线。周长通常比典型房扑中遇到的显著延长，尤其是 Fontan 术后的病人，经常可以长到能允许 1∶1 房室传导（表 60-3）。Hamilton 检查了多种先心病患者心动过速时的 P 波电轴，观察到在 Fontan 手术后的病人中 P 波电轴相对左偏，而 Mustard 手术和 Senning 手术后病人则表现为额面 P 波电轴左偏或不偏[19]。在窦性心律时，P 波时限可能增加，与在这类病人的心内检查中得到的右房激动时间显著延长的数据相一致[17]。

虽然某一次发作时房内折返性心动过速的心电图通常是稳定的，但是在同一病人记录到多样的、不同的房内折返性心动过速，有着截然不同的周长、P 波电轴和形态，也是常见的[20]。这表明不同的心房激动方式可以是同一折返环路的相反激动或沿着其他的环路以及心律失常折返环以外的心房组织被动激动所致。这个特性连同折返周长和 P 波形态对临床上评估同一病人某一特定心动过速的激动环路是否与以前发作时记录的相同是有价值的。

Schoels 和合作者对无菌性心包炎动物模型诱导的多种不典型房扑进行了高密度的心外膜标测[21]。在对这些心律失常进行了心动过速的分类后，他们发现等电位线与心房组织慢传导区的激动相关，而"扑动波"心动过速的标测很少有这样的性质。因此，辨别心电图上扑动波和 P 波形态对于房内折返性心动过速的消融是有用的。

（三）房内折返性心动过速的机制

我们对先心病手术方式以及他们与正常和不正常心房解剖之间关系的详细理解，使得我们能够以一种独特的方式推测房内折返性心动过速电生理和解剖结构的联系。先心病患者的心房肌从出生起即受到不同的压力和不正常的条件影响。除了基础的与先心病有关的心房和瓣膜的解剖异常，心房切开和隔板造成的手术瘢痕可产生完全的传导阻滞或不正常的传导。许多先心病手术形成了心房表面新的不连续（如：房间隔缺损、右房与肺动脉吻合、肺静脉重建），而且转流术的套管插入点可能在房腔交界处附近。结果导致非传导区的几何形状相当复杂，能够形成多种形式的折返环路。

手术形成的传导障碍对维持房内折返性心动过速的重要性和充分性已经很明确（见后），但其他因素如：炎症或心肌肥大或二者联合导致的纤维化以及心动过缓介导的不应期离散度改变的重要性仍不清楚。虽然房内折返性心动过速通常见于术后，但也可见于

表 60-3　房内折返性心动过速的心电图表现

- 畸形但单一形态的 P 波或扑动波
- 周长恒定，但经常比普通房扑长
- 同一患者可有多种心电图表现
- 多变的房室阻滞，可能 1∶1 传导
- 突发突止
- 可被起搏、拖带诱发和终止

尚未行手术的患者中。自出生起甚至是自胎儿期起，先心病可造成心房肌乏氧、心房壁压力增加以及与手术操作有关的间歇性心包炎症。由此导致的纤维化和心肌肥大可能影响了心房内细胞与细胞间的传导，并且形成致心律失常的基质。此外，继发的窦房结功能障碍是常见的。手术合并心动过缓和心脏的去自主神经化效应毫无疑问将影响心房不应期离散度，而且可能进一步导致心律失常发生。

（四）房内折返性心动过速的动物模型

为模仿与先心病相关的外科手术解剖，设计了两种犬心房折返的手术模型，特别有助于我们对手术后心房折返性心动过速的认识（图60-3）。第一个是大动脉错位Mustard假手术模型[22]。这个模型显示：扩展的心房缝合线本身即具有很高的致心律失常性，为心律失常折返环的形成提供了多个可能的传导障碍。多数心动过速中观察到的共同通路是右房游离壁，而且在心房切口和三尖瓣环之间作切割线可毫无例外地终止心动过速。经典的和改良型的Fontan手术的急性和慢性模型也得到了研究[23,24]。在那些有高致心律失常性和经历了仔细标测的标本中发现，环绕补片的长环形缝合线是心律失常环路的首要决定因素。将界嵴包含在缝合线内大大增加了心律失常的易发性。在Mustard手术模型中，致心律失常的基质可通过创造"阻断性"的损伤，将缝合线锚定到三尖瓣环的非传导区，从而"治愈"。当界嵴、假手术缝合线和心房切口都合并在一起并作为潜在的传导障碍除去时，这些损伤的抗心律失常效应可达到最大[25,26]。

（五）临床机制的研究

房内折返性心动过速的血流动力学耐受性通常较好，所以可以运用最新的临床标测技术进行详细的心动过速机制研究。这可以评估从动物模型和早期电生理观察中得到的关于机制的假说。随后，经验性的基于解剖学的房内折返性心动过速治疗和预防方法也得到了发展和检验。这些方法包括在不同程度的直接电生理指导下利用射频和冷冻制造线性损伤。

心脏消融术的研究大大增加了我们对心房解剖特点和电生理机制之间联系的认识。射频消融可即时中断心动过速环路，为消融位点是心动过速环路的关键组成部分提供了强有力的证据。对先心病房速病人成

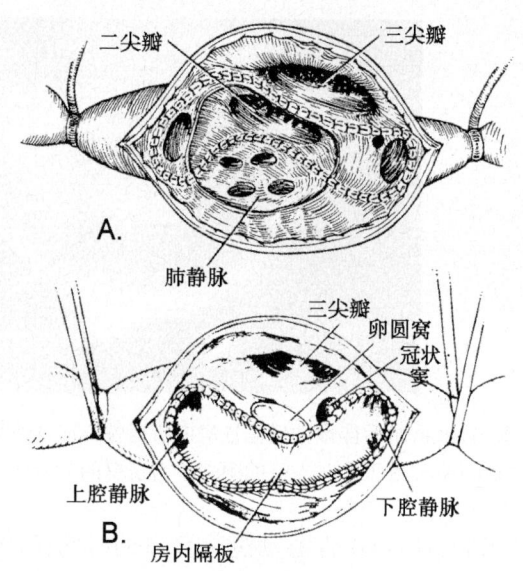

图60-3 从术者的视角看术后房内折返性心律失常犬模型

A图：用假手术线和心房切开模拟Mustard手术的效应，使用房内隔板来引导腔静脉血穿过房间隔（已去除）到二尖瓣和肺静脉，再回到三尖瓣。B图：用假手术线和心房切开模拟常见的"心外隧道"改良型Fontan术的效应，使用心房隔板来引导下腔静脉血流向上腔静脉，然后通过腔肺吻合（图中未显示）流向肺动脉。（引自Rodefeld MD, Bromberg BI, Schuessler RB, et al: Atrial flutter after lateral tunnel construction in the modified Fontan operation: A canine model. J Thorac Cadiovasc Surg 111: 514-526, 1996; 和Gandhi SK, Bromberg BI, Schuessler RB, et al: Characterization and surgical ablation of atrial flutter after the classic Fontan repair. Ann Thorac Surg 61: 1666-1678, 1996.）

功消融位点的初期评估对这些位点进行了初步的归类[27]。随着经验的增加和更精确的临床标测技术的运用，可以发现，能否打断折返环路的关键性位点在某种程度上取决于原始的先天性心脏损伤。对存在右侧房室瓣的病人（如：双心室修补、Mustard手术、Senning手术后的病人），其消融成功的靶点可能位于三尖瓣和下腔静脉间的峡部，与普通型房扑病人相似[28,29]。相反的，Fontan手术后的病人，其消融位点广泛分布于整个心房，但某种程度上集中于右房后壁。图60-4提供了电解剖标测房内折返性心动过速的两个例子。

对右房后壁成功消融位点的详细分析，增加了我们对右房切口导致的传导阻滞在"切口性"房速发生中的重要性的认识[30]。直观地看到这些非解剖性的传导阻滞位点的确切位置是困难的，但根据前面回顾过的信息，这样的概念是合理的，即：先前的手术瘢痕

内的心房肌传导特性是固定的。确定这些瘢痕位置的一个方法是明确"碎裂电位"或"双电位"线,即是在同一位点同时记录到多发的离散的电活动信号。Baker 和合作者[31]成功地运用双电位作为房内折返性心动过速消融术的"靶点"。此方法的成功基于这样的推论:双电位的集中标志着连续的心房瘢痕,而瘢痕作为"中心障碍"或传导屏障,限定房内折返性心动过速的折返环路,可以用射频消融的方法将其延伸到非传导的边界,从而功能性地除去。Love 和合作者[32]分析了多种使房内折返性心动过速折返环固定下来的解剖学和电生理学的中心障碍的特点,包括右侧房室瓣(当存在时)、房间隔缺损和位于右房游离壁上的手术瘢痕。在基于拖带刺激的解剖标测中,许多这类房内折返性心动过速病例的折返环以其完整性为特点[33]。最近,有研究描述了局部的折返活动和围绕下腔静脉口的折返环(腔静脉周围折返)[34]。

已经明确,界嵴和欧氏嵴在普通房扑的机制中起关键作用[35,36]。仔细的心内标测技术可以发现跨越界嵴的缓慢横向传导,但是在房扑发作时,跨界嵴的传导被有效地阻滞了,将右房游离壁的前半部分和后半部分隔开,促使形成一个长的、稳定的大折返环。许多先心病房速病人的激动模式与普通房扑并无区别,那么界嵴可能在这些房速中起了类似的作用。但是,它在其他类型的房内折返性心动过速中的作用尚未被阐明。

在大多数右房的房内折返性心动过速折返环中,少数几个峡部起主要作用。其中包括下腔静脉和右侧房室瓣间的峡部、卵圆窝上部与上腔静脉之间的边缘带、存在于右房游离壁上的瘢痕与右侧房室瓣环或位置较为靠后的界嵴之间的空隙。先心病病人右房标测到的总的心内电信号振幅显著降低[37],特别是环绕界嵴的区域和手术损伤附近的位点。用简单的电压标准可确定穿行于复杂的岛状心房"瘢痕"中心肌激动的关键通道,并已成功地作为射频消融的靶点[38]。多位研究者记录到,折返环在解剖上与房间隔或左房的修补有关,如异常肺动脉连接或 Maze 术后房内折返性心动过速复发的病人。

(六) 房内折返性心动过速的治疗

比较房内折返性心动过速不同的治疗方式的结果是困难的,特别是数据来源于一组样本量相对较少的、病变程度不同的病人的回顾性分析。这是因为先心病病人的房速经常是短暂发作,症状多变,而且治

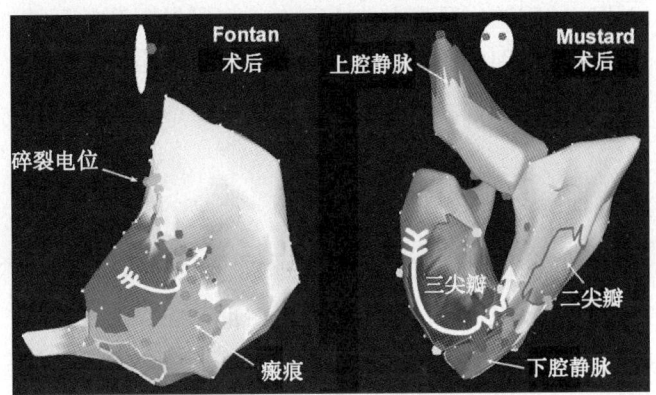

图 60-4 先心病患者房内折返性心动过速(IART)电解剖标测 彩色标记代表心内膜表面双极电极测量的不应期;成功消融位点用暗红色点表示(译者著:原书缺彩图)。左图:一个 Fontan 手术病人心房游离壁的右后面观,房内折返性心动过速依赖于右心房下部表面的狭窄走廊的传导,下部与电静止区域(推测代表瘢痕)相邻,上面有一条双电位线(蓝色点),须与界嵴传导阻滞线或手术瘢痕的效应相鉴别。右图:一个 Mustard 手术病人左、右心房左前斜位观,显示了手术隔板的上腔静脉和下腔静脉"肢"的少见的解剖和更靠后的肺静脉、心房和环绕隔板脚分叉处侧缘的三尖瓣之间的联系。房内折返性心动过速依赖于腔静脉三尖瓣峡部,类似于普通房扑环绕三尖瓣的逆钟向折返,消融邻近三尖瓣环的肺静脉侧隔板可成功阻断折返环。

疗性干预措施的抉择取决于临床判断。要对抗心律失常治疗作出更有效的评估,需要结合心律失常的发作频率、相关症状的严重性和与死亡相关的危险进行综合考虑和确认。

1. 药物治疗

一般把抗心律失常药物作为房内折返性心动过速的第一线治疗。各类抗心律失常药物都曾被用作慢性、预防性治疗,但是没有前瞻性的研究显示其有效性和安全性。小样本、无对照的、回顾性证据提示某些药物如索他洛尔和胺碘酮可以降低心动过速的复发率[39,40]。但是,其他数据表明没有抗心律失常药物可以延长先心病患者房内折返性心动过速复发的间隔时间(见图 60-5)。根据心房折返的实验模型显示的电生理机制,IC 类和Ⅲ类药物可能有有益的作用,而且有时在个别病人中使用这些药物可抑制有症状的心律失常发生。但致心律失常作用和对心室、房室结功能的不利作用限制了其应用。

成年先心病房速患者经常有血栓形成,说明华法林和其他有力的抗凝剂应该用于大部分的这类病人中。这类治疗对 Fontan 手术术后病人来说是正在积

极研究的问题，但尚未被证实[41]。房室结阻断的药物也可能被用到，但很难准确地掌握，因为房内折返性心动过速时经常见到相对较慢的周长和固定的传导比例。

2. 起搏治疗

心房超速起搏对房内折返性心动过速的急性终止经常是有效的。心房起搏器是房内折返性心动过速治疗的重要辅助手段，而且在有些病例中是首要的治疗手段。在窦房结功能低下的患者中，仅仅单用心房抗心动过缓起搏有时就可以改善症状，降低心动过速发生频率[42]。心率、良好的心房激动模式和适时的心房激动带来的血流动力学改善在其中所起的作用尚不清楚。因为快速的心房起搏可暂时阻断心动过速折返环从而终止房内折返性心动过速，现已开发了具有自动心动过速识别和短阵快速刺激功能的起搏器，并已证明在部分病人中有效。但是，无论抗心动过缓或抗心动过速起搏对房内折返性心动过速只是相对有效，而且 AAIT 模式起搏在此类病人中有产生致命性心律失常的记录[42]。这些研究使用的是现在已过时的心房抗心动过速装置，更先进装置包含 DDD 起搏和增强的检测算法，其安全性和有效性，还没有在此人群中得到研究。在此类患者中电极的放置也是显著的技术难题（见后文）。

目前，在房颤治疗中已发展了其他创新性的装置，如双部位起搏和植入性心房除颤器，但其在先心病患者中应用的潜力还未得到探索。植入性除颤器（AICD）对有基础先心病的患者会增加发作频率并有致室性心律失常的危险。因为这类病人中室速和房速常同时发生，如有可能应考虑放置双腔起搏系统，并进行合理的程控以尽可能的监测各种形式的心律失常。

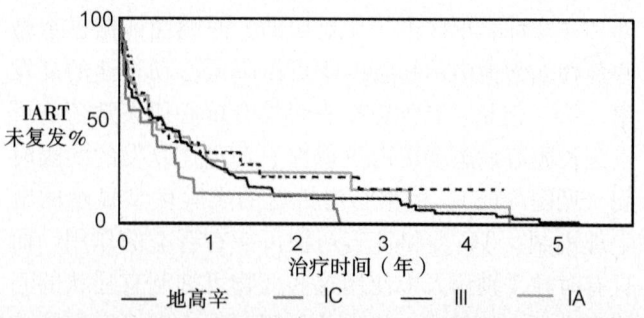

图 60-5 接受地高辛和其他类抗心律失常药物治疗的房内折返性心动过速（房内折返性心动过速）患者的时间-复发率曲线（译者著：原图有误。）

3. 导管消融

心房的解剖特点和手术方式给我们重要的启示：以心房肌作为治疗的靶点，以导管或手术的方法消融易诱发心律失常的关键区域。房内折返性心动过速的消融治疗包括形成非传导性的损伤或大折返环路和心脏解剖之间的损伤。在临床上有导管射频消融室速和 Maze 术治疗房颤的先例。手术损伤被用来标定特定的心律失常环路，从而实施更为经验性的、解剖性的术式以使心房不易发生房内折返性心动过速。

经导管射频消融术通常以个体的大折返环路为靶点，寻找易于实施射频损伤的位点。回顾房内折返性心动过速射频消融的经验发现，在有右侧房室瓣的病人中，瓣膜与下腔静脉之间的峡部通常对房内折返性心动过速起支持作用，与普通房扑类似[27,29]。当这个峡部存在时，如 Mustard 手术和 Senning 手术[28,43]、法洛四联症手术[29]和其他的双心室修补术后，临床上在房扑消融术中用到的判断消融终点的技术如峡部传导阻滞的判定，可以类似地运用于房内折返性心动过速消融中以评估消融的有效性。但是，房内折返性心动过速时可经常观察到多个折返环路同时存在，加上其他的与消融相关的解剖或手术特征，环路可能很难被定位。在某些病例中为了打断折返环，需要获得大的、连续的透壁损伤，这可能也是很困难的。临床对房内折返性心动过速的标测显示大多数（虽然不是全部）折返环位于解剖学的右房。然而，由于外科手术的影响，解剖学右房可能位于房间隔靠肺静脉的一侧，认识到这一点很重要，这可能使标测和消融变得复杂。

虽然有这么多困难，房内折返性心动过速射频消融治疗的成功率仍不断增加。运用常规的透视和消融技术，最初的即时消融成功率为 55%～90%[27,31,43,44]。由于近期在标测和消融技术上的革新，即时手术成功率显著提高了。这些革新包括精确的三维标测和导航系统的出现，它能够确定折返环的解剖位置、分析电位特点和心房组织对拖带的反应以及指引消融损伤的位置（图 60-4）[45,46]。此外，通过在导管尖端内部提供散热装置，冷灌注导管消融系统加强了消融产生更大的损伤程度。由于在消融时心内血流对导管尖端不足以产生的足够的对流散热，冷灌注导管消融系统增强了能量的输送和损伤的形成，改善了房速和室速消融的即时结果[48,49]。在伴有长期的、复杂的先心病患者中实施这些复杂的手术，围手术期的发病率和死亡率是低的，而且，虽然 2～4 年随访后约50%的患者房内折返性心动过速会复发,大多数房内折返性心动过速射频消融病人的发病频率、心律失常症状的严重性、电复律和抗心律失常药物的需要大大降低了。这些重要的临床结果的改善使我们对心律失常基质的认识深入和诊治技术得到提高。

4. 外科手术治疗

由于血流动力学原因而尝试将早期Fontan手术术式的路径修正为腔肺动脉型连接,其围术期和早期随访中死亡率为10%左右[50,51]。在伴有房内折返性心动过速的病人中,如无特殊的预防心律失常手术的介入,这种修正本身并不能可靠地预防房内折返性心动过速复发[52]。因此,虽然一期的心外隧道或以外的修补可能与较低的晚期心律失常发病率有关,后来转为心外隧道术式本身对已表现出心律失常的病人并无治疗作用。最近,几个中心已尝试将行成人心房Maze术的经验用于房肺连接型Fontan手术病人的房内折返性心动过速中。这些中心单独或同时运用外科手术或冷冻消融技术,以达到对右房和某些病例中左房的损伤,来预防术后房内折返性心动过速发生,并且已取得了有希望的早期结果。某中心已报道了接受此类Fontan改良手术以预防心律失常复发的前40个病例术后短期随访结果[53]。图60-6显示了一个在右房制造损伤的例子,如病人术前已发生过房颤,损伤还包括肺静脉的隔离、左心耳切除术和如同房颤病人的Maze术一样的左房损伤。在这一组病人中,大部分可不用服药,似乎已无相关的临床房内折返性心动过速,复发率小于13%。对本组病人中术前无房颤病史、手术损伤仅限于右房的亚组进行分析表明房内折返性心动过速的复发率更低,该研究显示了腔静脉间及其边缘损伤的重要性,如同阻断下腔静脉和三尖瓣间峡部的重要性一样。这表明Fontan手术的Maze改良型能够被采用,其手术风险可以接受,可显著降低术后房内折返性心动过速的复发。但是,在这些研究中分流术的效果和再次手术对血流动力学和Fontan手术病人寿命的影响还未得到评估,而且还需要进行更多的随访以确定此类手术是否有长期的益处。

标准的手术术式的改进被作为预防性的手段来阻止晚期的、自发的房内折返性心动过速发生,特别是在Fontan术后的病人中。这与从动物模型中观察的结果相符,位于界嵴上的心房切口可增加心律失常的发生,而连接心房切口和右侧房室瓣环的"特定损伤"可使房内折返性心动过速不易诱导。将切口从界嵴移开可导致较低的房内折返性心动过速发病率[8]。但是,"特定损伤"的手术实验的早期结果已显示:此类方法在房内折返性心动过速动物模型中的成功可能并不能在临床手术中得到重复。对此类方法的评价是困难的,因为术后房内折返性心动过速的发病率在更先进的改良型Fontan手术中似乎降低了。

三、先心病房颤

25%~30%的先心病房速患者会发生心房颤动,在残留有左侧闭塞性损伤或未修补的心脏疾患的患者中更为常见[55]。这种相对的倾向提示我们,右房承受的慢性血流动力学超负荷加上手术瘢痕促进了先心病人右房心律失常的发生,然而,左房和左室扩大能促进伴有获得性心室功能障碍患者房颤的发生。处理的原则可参考普通成年人群的治疗措施,包括抗凝和控制心室率,因为这些病人血栓栓塞的危险可能会增加。先心病的患者经常对房室失同步的耐受能力下降,如果可能的话需要尽可能使用电复律、预防性给予抗心律失常药物和心房起搏来预防转为永久性房颤。房颤伴有房内折返性心动过速的先心病患者,分别针对各个心律失常的治疗并不获益,需要使用抗心律失常药物或外科Maze手术。

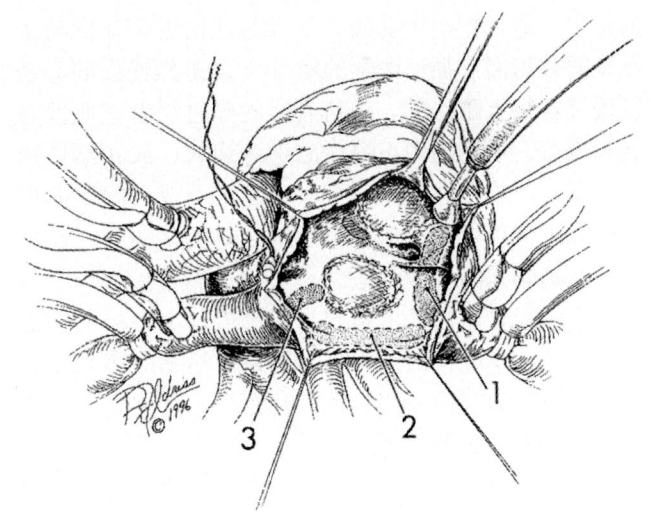

图60-6 Mavroudis和合作者[66]在Fontan改良手术中使用的经验性的右房冷冻Maze术,术后可预防房内折返性心律失常发生 手术线路包括腔静脉间消融和连接上腔静脉到房间隔缺损间(3区)、腔静脉间区域(2区)下腔静脉到冠状窦和右侧房室瓣环(如果存在的话)(1区)间的线性消融。(引自Mavoudis C,Deal BJ,Backer CL,Johnscrude CL:Fontan conversion to cavopulmonary connection and arrhythmia circuit cyroablation. J Thorac Cardiovasc Surg 115:547-556,1998.)

四、心动过缓

在先心病手术中,围术期早期窦房结功能障碍和晚期临床随访中逐步的、进行性的窦性节律的丧失均是常见的[56]。这个问题在手术范围较大、对右房进行改造的患者中尤为常见,如 Fontan、Mustard 和 Senning 手术。为了使这种并发症降到最低,这些术式均进行了改进[57-59]。患有窦静脉缺损或内脏异位综合征特别是左房异构的患者,可能已有先天性的窦房结功能异常,这与手术无关[60]。阵发性房速通常伴有窦房结功能障碍,而且失去窦性节律似乎增加了猝死的危险。对早期的 Fontan 手术术后病人的电生理研究已经发现心房电生理的异常包括窦房结恢复时间、房内传导时间和心房不应期的延长。对窦房结的直接手术损伤已是 Mustard 手术病人窦房结功能异常的一个原因。然而,在更长的随访中观察到进行性的窦性节律丧失提示还有额外的病理生理过程,可能与慢性的血流动力学异常有关。

三度或高度以及二度传导阻滞是先心病患者永久性心脏起搏的明确适应证。但是,由于缺少明确的有症状的心动过缓记录,关于对孤立性窦缓或结性逸搏心律者进行心房起搏的合理适应证,现有的指导性数据很少,而且指南中 II 级、III 级的证据更多地反映了专家的共识而非循证医学的结果[61]。虽然慢性的心动过缓经常是可耐受的,起搏有时的确可缓解充血性心衰和疲劳、运动耐力下降、眩晕等症状,或在结性逸搏心律、严重窦性停搏、变时功能不全或长间歇的患者中减少晕厥发作。为了应用抗心律失常药物,起搏也可能是必需的。

临床经验显示了房室同步的价值,主张植入能提供生理性频率应答的起搏器。但是,频率应答和双腔起搏与简单的起搏模式相比,其在先心病患者中并未体现出良好的特殊价值[62]。Fontan 手术后进行房室同步化起搏的患者,与单心室起搏相比,长期的临床结果似乎有所改善[63]。如前所述,在既有心动过速又有心动过缓的病人中,心房抗心动过缓起搏有时会使心动过速事件的发作频率下降。

面对电极安置和维护问题,实践中经常需要根据特定患者选择合适的起搏系统,心房起搏可能因电极植入困难而未受益[64,65]。先天性和获得性的心血管异常和心内的吻合可能限制了心内膜电极放置,迫使我们选择心外膜电极甚至混合途径。例如装有老式的经静脉电极系统的病人患获得性血管异常,以及 Fontan 手术病人,其心室腔和大部分或全部心房肌因手术而被排除在系统的静脉途径之外。在经过多次手术和遗留有心房壁纤维化、与周围的心包粘连的病人中,心房肌的分隔状态使得寻找既有合适的起搏阈值又有稳定的心房感知位点具有极大的挑战性,有时是不可能的。偶尔,可以通过左侧开胸术将起搏系统植入到左侧心外膜表面。假定在完全 Fontan 手术中没有从右至左的分流,病人也是经静脉途径进行起搏,但应该考虑到心外膜起搏也是可行的选择。但是,无对照的经验显示,在心内膜表面找到一个合适的起搏位点是相当困难的,而且作为异物,起搏器电极的存在使得 Fontan 病人产生右房血栓的倾向可能会大大增加。

五、总　　结

房性心律失常已经成为先心病患者一个主要的长期后遗症。这些病人的预后差,但是病例规模小、解剖异常多变,很难判定控制心律失常是否能带来在寿命上和健康上的获益。由于对病人在初始手术多年后长期自然病程的认识的加深,加上已在无先心病的患者中检测过的诊断治疗技术的革新,使我们对于此类心律失常的认识加深了。动物模型、手术术式的改进和先进介入技术的运用,给我们提供了对先心病患者心律失常的解剖基质有价值的洞察。对导致此类心律失常发生的心肌潜在病理生理有了更广泛的理解,将有助于制定预防和治疗该类心律失常的策略和方法。

(郑强荪　译)

参 考 文 献

1. Gelatt M, Hamilton RM, McCrindle BW, et al: Arrhythmia and mortality after the Mustard procedure: A 30-year single-center experience. J Am Coll Cardiol 29:194-201, 1997.
2. Triedman JK: Arrhythmias in adults with congenital heart disease. Heart 87:383-389, 2002.
3. Ghai A, Harris L, Harrison DA, et al: Outcomes of late atrial tachyarrhythmias in adults after the Fontan operation. J Am Coll Cardiol 37:585-592, 2001.
4. Jais P, Shah DC, Haissaguerre M, et al: Mapping and ablation of left atrial flutters. Circulation 101:2928-2934, 2000.
5. Garson A Jr, Bink-Boelkens MTE, Hesslein PS, et al: Atrial flutter in the young: A collaborative study in 380 cases. J Am Coll Cardiol 6:871-878, 1985.
6. Law IH, Fischbach PS, Goldberg C, et al: Inducibility of intra-atrial reentrant tachycardia after the first two stages of the Fontan sequence. J Am Coll Cardiol 37:231-237, 2001.
7. Fishberger SB, Wernovsky G, Gentles TL, et al: Factors that influence the development of atrial flutter after the Fontan operation. J Thorac Cardiovasc Surg 113:80-86, 1997.
8. Durongpisitkul K, Porter CJ, Cetta F, et al: Predictors of early- and

late-onset supraventricular tachyarrhythmias after Fontan operation. Circulation 98:1099–1107, 1998.
9. Gelatt M, Hamilton RM, McCrindle BW, et al: Risk factors for atrial tachyarrhythmias after the Fontan operation. J Am Coll Cardiol 24:1735–1741, 1994.
10. Cecchin F, Johnsrude CL, Perry JC, Friedman RA: Effect of age and surgical technique on symptomatic arrhythmias after the Fontan procedure. Am J Cardiol 76:386–389, 1995.
11. Stamm C, Triedman JK, Mayer JE, et al: Long-term results of the lateral tunnel Fontan operation. J Thorac Cardiovasc Surg 121:28–41, 2001.
12. Amodeo A, Galletti L, Marianeschi S, et al: Extracardiac Fontan operation for complex cardiac anomalies: Seven years' experience. J Thorac Cardiovasc Surg 114:1020–1030, 1997.
13. Roos-Hesselink J, Perlroth MG, McGhie J, Spitaels S: Atrial arrhythmias in adults after repair of tetralogy of Fallot. Correlations with clinical, exercise, and echocardiographic findings. Circulation 91:2214–2219, 1995.
14. Peters NS, Somerville J: Arrhythmias after the Fontan procedure. Br Heart J 68:199–204, 1992.
15. Coon PD, Rychik J, Novello RT, et al: Thrombus formation after the Fontan operation. Ann Thorac Surg 71:1990–1994, 2001.
16. Feltes TF, Friedman RA: Transesophageal echocardiographic detection of atrial thrombi in patients with nonfibrillation atrial tachyarrhythmias and congenital heart disease. J Am Coll Cardiol 24:1365–1370, 1994.
17. Triedman JK, Bergau DM, Saul JP, et al: Efficacy of radiofrequency ablation for control of intraatrial reentrant tachycardia in patients with congenital heart disease. J Am Coll Cardiol 30:1032–1038, 1997.
18. Muller GI, Deal BJ, Strasburger JF, Benson DW Jr: Electrocardiographic features of atrial tachycardias after operation for congenital heart disease. Am J Cardiol 71:122–124, 1993.
19. Hamilton R: Electrocardiographic features of atrial flutter: Differences between congenital lesions. In Liebman J (ed): Electrocardiology '96: From the Cell to the Body Surface. Singapore, World Scientific, 1997, pp 333–336.
20. Triedman JK, Alexander ME, Love BA, et al: Influence of patient factors and ablative technologies on outcomes of radiofrequency ablation of intra-atrial re-entrant tachycardia in patients with congenital heart disease. J Am Coll Cardiol 39:1827–1835, 2002.
21. Schoels W, Offner B, Brachmann J, et al: Circus movement atrial flutter in the canine sterile pericarditis model: Relation of characteristics of the surface electrocardiogram and conduction properties of the reentrant pathway. J Am Coll Cardiol 23:799–808, 1994.
22. Cronin CS, Nitta T, Mitsuno M, et al: Characterization and surgical ablation of acute atrial flutter following the Mustard procedure. A canine model. Circulation 88:II461–II471, 1993.
23. Rodefeld MD, Bromberg BI, Schuessler RB, et al: Atrial flutter after lateral tunnel construction in the modified Fontan operation: A canine model. J Thorac Cardiovasc Surg 111:514–526, 1996.
24. Gandhi SK, Bromberg BI, Schuessler RB, et al: Characterization and surgical ablation of atrial flutter after the classic Fontan repair. Ann Thorac Surg 61:1666–1678, 1996.
25. Rodefeld MD, Gandhi SK, Huddleston CB, et al: Anatomically based ablation of atrial flutter in an acute canine model of the modified Fontan operation. J Thorac Cardiovasc Surg 112:898–907, 1996.
26. Gandhi SK, Bromberg BI, Rodefeld MD, et al: Lateral tunnel suture line variation reduces atrial flutter after the modified Fontan operation. Ann Thorac Surg 61:1299–1309, 1996.
27. Collins KK, Love BA, Walsh EP, et al: Location of acutely successful radiofrequency catheter ablation of intraatrial reentrant tachycardia in patients with congenital heart disease. Am J Cardiol 86:969–974, 2000.
28. Kanter RJ, Papagiannis J, Carboni MP, et al: Radiofrequency catheter ablation of supraventricular tachycardia substrates after Mustard and Senning operations for d-transposition of the great arteries. J Am Coll Cardiol 35:428–441, 2000.
29. Chan DP, Van Hare GF, Mackall JA, et al: Importance of atrial flutter isthmus in postoperative intra-atrial reentrant tachycardia. Circulation 102:1283–1289, 2000.
30. Kalman JK, Van Hare GF, Olgin JE, et al: Ablation of 'incisional' reentrant atrial tachycardia complication surgery for congenital heart disease. Circulation 93:502–512, 1996.
31. Baker BM, Lindsay BD, Bromberg B, et al: Catheter ablation of intraatrial reentrant tachycardias resulting from previous atrial surgery: Locating and transecting the critical isthmus. J Am Coll Cardiol 28:411–417, 1996.
32. Love BA, Collins KK, Walsh EP, Triedman JK: Electroanatomic characterization of conduction barriers in sinus/atrially paced rhythm and association with intra-atrial reentrant tachycardia circuits following congenital heart disease surgery. J Cardiovasc Electrophysiol 12:17–25, 2001.
33. Triedman JK, Alexander ME, Berul CI, et al: Electroanatomical mapping of entrained and exit zones in patients with repaired congenital heart disease and intraatrial reentrant tachycardia. Circulation 103:2060–2065, 2001.
34. Mandapati R, Walsh EP, Triedman JK: Pericaval and periannular intra-atrial reentrant tachycardias in patients with congenital heart disease. J Cardiovasc Electrophysiol 14:119–125, 2003.
35. Nakagawa H, Lazzara R, Khastgir T, et al: Role of the tricuspid annulus and the eustachian valve/ridge on atrial flutter. Relevance to catheter ablation of the septal isthmus and a new technique for rapid identification of ablation success. Circulation 94:407–424, 1996.
36. Kalman JM, Olgin JE, Saxon LA, et al: Activation and entrainment mapping defines the tricuspid annulus as the anterior barrier in typical atrial flutter. Circulation 94:398–406, 1996.
37. De Groot NM, Kuijper AF, Blom NA, et al: Three-dimensional distribution of bipolar atrial electrogram voltages in patients with congenital heart disease. Pacing Clin Electrophysiol 24:1334–1342, 2001.
38. Nakagawa H, Shah N, Matsudaira K, et al: Characterization of reentrant circuit in macroreentrant right atrial tachycardia after surgical repair of congenital heart disease: Isolated channels between scars allow "focal" ablation. Circulation 103:699–709, 2001.
39. Beaufort-Krol GC, Bink-Boelkens MT: Sotalol for atrial tachycardias after surgery for congenital heart disease. Pacing Clin Electrophysiol 20:2125–2129, 1997.
40. Maragnes P, Villain E, Iselin M, et al: Late supraventricular arrhythmia complicating Fontan or cavopulmonary type procedures. Apropos of 7 cases. Arch Malad Coeur Vaisseaux 89:605–609, 1996.
41. Seipelt RG, Franke A, Vazquez-Jimenez JF, et al: Thromboembolic complications after Fontan procedures: Comparison of different therapeutic approaches. Ann Thorac Surg 74:556–562, 2002.
42. Rhodes LA, Walsh EP, Gamble WJ, et al: Benefits and potential risks of atrial antitachycardia pacing after repair of congenital heart disease. Pacing Clin Electrophysiol 18(pt I):1005–1016, 1995.
43. Van Hare GF, Lesh MD, Ross BA, et al: Mapping and radiofrequency ablation of intraatrial reentrant tachycardia after the Senning or Mustard procedure for transposition of the great arteries. Am J Cardiol 77:985–991, 1996.
44. Triedman JK, Saul JP, Weindling SN, Walsh EP: Radiofrequency ablation of intra-atrial reentrant tachycardia after surgical palliation of congenital heart disease. Circulation 91:707–714, 1995.
45. Dorostkar PC, Cheng J, Scheinman MM: Electroanatomical mapping and ablation of the substrate supporting intraatrial reentrant tachycardia after palliation for complex congenital heart disease. Pacing Clin Electrophysiol 21:1810–1819, 1998.
46. Paul T, Windhagen-Mahnert B, Kriebel T, et al: Atrial reentrant tachycardia after surgery for congenital heart disease: Endocardial mapping and radiofrequency catheter ablation using a novel, noncontact mapping system. Circulation 103:2266–2271, 2001.
47. Otomo K, Yamanashi WS, Tondo C, et al: Why a large tip electrode makes a deeper radiofrequency lesion: Effects of increase in electrode cooling and electrode-tissue interface area. J Cardiovasc Electrophysiol 9:47–54, 1998.
48. Jais P, Hocini M, Gillet T, et al: Effectiveness of irrigated tip catheter ablation of common atrial flutter. Am J Cardiol 88:433–435, 2001.
49. Soejima K, Delacretaz E, Suzuki M, et al: Saline-cooled versus standard radiofrequency catheter ablation for infarct-related ventricular tachycardias. Circulation 103:1858–1862, 2001.
50. van Son JA, Mohr FW, Hambsch J, et al: Conversion of atriopulmonary or lateral atrial tunnel cavopulmonary anastomosis to extracardiac conduit Fontan modification. Eur J Cardiothorac Surg 15:150–157, 1999.
51. Marcelletti CF, Hanley FL, Mavroudis C, et al: Revision of previous Fontan connections to total extracardiac cavopulmonary anastomosis: A multicenter experience. J Thorac Cardiovasc Surg 119:340–346, 2000.

52. Deal BJ, Mavroudis C, Backer CL, et al: Impact of arrhythmia circuit cryoablation during Fontan conversion for refractory atrial tachycardia. Am J Cardiol 83:563–568, 1999.
53. Mavroudis C, Backer CL, Deal BJ, et al: Total cavopulmonary conversion and maze procedure for patients with failure of the Fontan operation. J Thorac Cardiovasc Surg 122:863–871, 2001.
54. Deal BJ, Mavroudis C, Backer CL, et al: Comparison of anatomic isthmus block with the modified right atrial maze procedure for late atrial tachycardia in Fontan patients. Circulation 106:575–579, 2002.
55. Kirsh JA, Walsh, Triedman JK: Prevalence of and risk factors for atrial fibrillation and intraatrial reentrant tachycardia among patients with congenital heart disease. Am J Cardiol 90:40–43, 2002.
56. Valsangiacomo E, Schmid ER, Schupbach RW, et al: Early postoperative arrhythmias after cardiac operation in children. Ann Thorac Surg 74:792–796, 2002.
57. Cohen MI, Bridges ND, Gaynor JW, et al: Modifications to the cavopulmonary anastomosis do not eliminate early sinus node dysfunction. J Thorac Cardiovasc Surg 120:891–900, 2000.
58. Manning PB, Mayer JE, Wernovsky G, et al: Staged operation to Fontan increases the incidence of sinoatrial node dysfunction. J Thorac Cardiovasc Surg 111:833–839, 1996.
59. Kirjavainen M, Happonen JM, Louhimo I: Late results of Senning operation. J Thorac Cardiovasc Surg 117:488–495, 1999.
60. Wu MH, Wang JK, Lin JL, et al: Cardiac rhythm disturbances in patients with left atrial isomerism. Pacing Clin Electrophysiol 24:1631–1638, 2001.
61. Gregoratos G, Abrams J, Epstein AE, et al: ACC/AHA/NASPE 2002 Guideline update for implantation of cardiac pacemakers and antiarrhythmia devices: Summary article. J Am Coll Cardiol 40:1703–1719, 2002.
62. Paridon SM, Karpawich PP, Pinsky WW: The effects of rate responsive pacing on exercise performance in the postoperative univentricular heart. Pacing Clin Electrophysiol 16:1256–1262, 1993.
63. Fishberger SB, Wernovsky G, Gentles TL, et al: Long-term outcome in patients with pacemakers following the Fontan operation. Am J Cardiol 77:887–889, 1996.
64. Cohen MI, Vetter VL, Wernovsky G, et al: Epicardial pacemaker implantation and follow-up in patients with a single ventricle after the Fontan operation. J Thorac Cardiovasc Surg 121:804–811, 2001.
65. Warfield DA, Hayes DL, Hyberger LK, et al: Permanent pacing in patients with univentricular heart. Pacing Clin Electrophysiol 22:1193–1201, 1999.
66. Mavroudis C, Deal BJ, Backer CL, Johnsrude CL: Fontan conversion to cavopulmonary connection and arrhythmia circuit cryoablation. J Thorac Cardiovasc Surg 115:547–556, 1998.

第 61 章

冠心病相关性室性心动过速

David J. Callans and Mark E. Josephson

本章目录

- 病理生理基质 ……………………… 561
- 持续性室性心动过速的发生机制 …… 562
- 对程序刺激的反应 ………………… 562
- 临床表现和治疗 …………………… 564
- 长期治疗对策 ……………………… 564
- 未来发展方向 ……………………… 565

持续性室性心动过速常发生在陈旧性心肌梗死患者，其临床表现多样，严重程度不一，可以是偶然发现室速、也可表现为晕厥和心源性猝死（SCD）。随着心脏电生理技术的发展，对动物模型和患者进行的研究以及多中心随机试验的结果极大地增加了我们对持续性室性心动过速病理生理机制的认识以及治疗方法的选择。

一、病理生理基质

持续性单形性室速常发生在有广泛解剖基质异常的陈旧性心肌梗死患者。心肌坏死的范围、室间隔受累的程度以及左室功能障碍的程度是心肌梗死后是否发生心律失常最重要的决定性因素。可耐受性室性心动过速患者与非持续性室速或心源性猝死（SCD）患者相比，其心肌梗死范围更大，形成左室室壁瘤的几率更多，左室功能障碍程度更重。例如，持续性室速患者与猝死和非持续性室速患者相比，射血分数最低（分别为 27%、35%、37%）[1]。一般情况下，心肌梗死后患者出现持续性单形性室速的发生率约为 3%。

现代治疗手段使梗死面积越来越小，室壁瘤形成的机会减少，在心肌梗死相关血管成功再通的患者中室速的发生率也明显下降，不到 1%[2]。虽然此比例降低，但由于更多高危存活患者的老龄化，总体人群的室性心律失常和猝死的发生率无明显变化，仍保持相对稳定的水平[3]。

室性心动过速常起源于大面积心肌梗死的存活心肌细胞中[2]。虽然在心肌梗死瘢痕区周边的细胞中可记录到正常的钠离子依赖性动作电位，但很可能由于缝隙连接的分布和功能异常，导致动作电位传导缓慢且不连续[4]。窦律时，从室速起源部位可持续记录到低振幅、传导延缓、多个碎裂的电位（图 61-1）。这些碎裂电位中的每个独立成分可能都由孤立的心肌细胞群组成的个体化心肌细胞"岛"所产生。局部电位的持续时间代表电极记录范围内某一特定部位异常缓慢传导的延迟激动。

室性心动过速的电生理基质常在心肌梗死后的最初 2 周逐渐形成，基质一旦形成，仍有可变性。虽然目前还未充分了解能诱发的室速与自发性室速之间的关系，但可诱发的室速预示着患者存在一个室速发生的解剖学基质，它可增加心律失常事件的易感性，这一点已被证实[5]。多种心律失常的触发因素，如急性心肌缺血、自律性异常、心力衰竭，都与可诱发的室速和自发性室速有关[6]。虽然室速事件可由这些能够逆转的临床情况所促发，但是认识室速发生的解剖基质是非常重要的[7]。发生持续性室速时，即使是急性心肌缺血和心力衰竭症状已被很好地控制，心律失常的危险性仍不能确定。

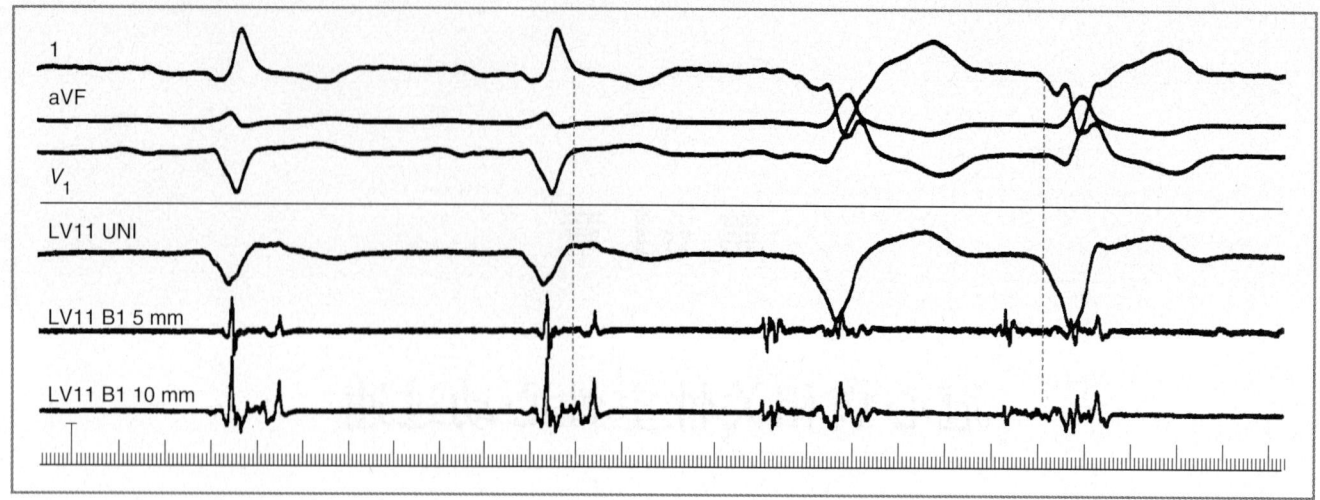

图 61-1 窦性心律和室性心动过速时出现的异常电位　图中显示 3 个体表导联心电图和从左室前壁记录的 3 个心内通道电图。窦性心律时，记录到一个碎裂的多成分信号（电位）；该电位的最后一部分出现在体表心电图 QRS 波群结束之后。而在室性心动过速发作时（记录的最后 2 次心搏），该部位记录到一个提前于 QRS 波群 90ms 的电位。(自 Josephson ME: Clinical Cardiac Electrophysiology: Techniques and Interpretations, 3rd ed. Philadelphia, Lippincott Williams & Wilkins, 2002.)

二、持续性室性心动过速的发生机制

有证据强力支持折返是陈旧性心肌梗死患者持续性室性心动过速的发生机制[1,8]。心室程序刺激可反复诱发和终止室速被认为是折返的必要条件。程序刺激不能诱发正常或异常自律性机制促发的心律失常，延迟后除极引起的触发性活动常能通过超速起搏和静滴儿茶酚胺而诱发[9]。据我们的经验，95%的陈旧性心肌梗死患者和自发性持续性室速患者都可通过程序刺激诱发室速。

冠心病室速的其他特征也支持折返机制。诱发冠心病患者室速需刺激某些特殊部位（即诱发部位特异性）；22%的室速在右室心尖部程序刺激诱发失败后在右室流出道诱发成功。在触发性心律失常中，则不存在诱发部位的特异性。许多室性心律失常可以观察到期前刺激的联律间期与期前刺激到心动过速开始的第一个波群间的回归间期成反比关系，该现象说明折返形成的一个主要前提条件即缓慢传导是诱发室速的必需条件（联律间期较短时更为明显）。在室速起源部位标测到舒张中期电位或明显的收缩期前电位与局灶性起源的心律失常发生机制不符。心动过速的诱发和维持有赖于缓慢传导延缓的严重程度，这一事实表明整个舒张期持续的电活动符合折返机制（图 61-2）。

三、对程序刺激的反应

证实折返机制最令人信服的事实是室速对程序刺激的反应-重整和拖带。程序刺激技术除用于阐明室速的发生机制外，还被用于研究患者对抗心律失常药物和起搏干预的反应、室速标测以及室速折返环路电生理特性的研究。这些技术一个很大的局限性是它仅适用于血流动力学稳定的、可耐受的持续性室速患者。

重整是单个期前刺激作用于心动过速折返环，产生一个不完全性代偿间期[1,8]。从远离室速起源部位的地方发放期前刺激，85%以上可耐受的持续性室速（心动过速周长＞270ms）可被重整[1]。要重整一个心动过速，刺激脉冲必须到达折返环，遇到可兴奋组织。这意味着刺激波锋侵入心动过速折返环的可兴奋组织，一方面激动的传导方向与原来的心动过速折返方向相反，二者发生碰撞，另一方面激动与原心动过速折返方向相同，顺向传导，维持心动过速（图 61-3）。如果心肌组织完全处于可兴奋期，早搏刺激到达心动过速折返环入口的提前程度决定了心动过速波锋向前扩布的状况。回归周期，定义为从期前刺激到此后心动过速的第一个波群之间的间期，与刺激脉冲到达折返环、激动在折返环内传导以及回到刺激部位所需的时间相一致。回归周期与期前刺激联律间期之间存在 3 种节律重整反应方式，即：平台型、递增型、混合型。平台型反应方式是指在室速折返环的所有部位发

位发

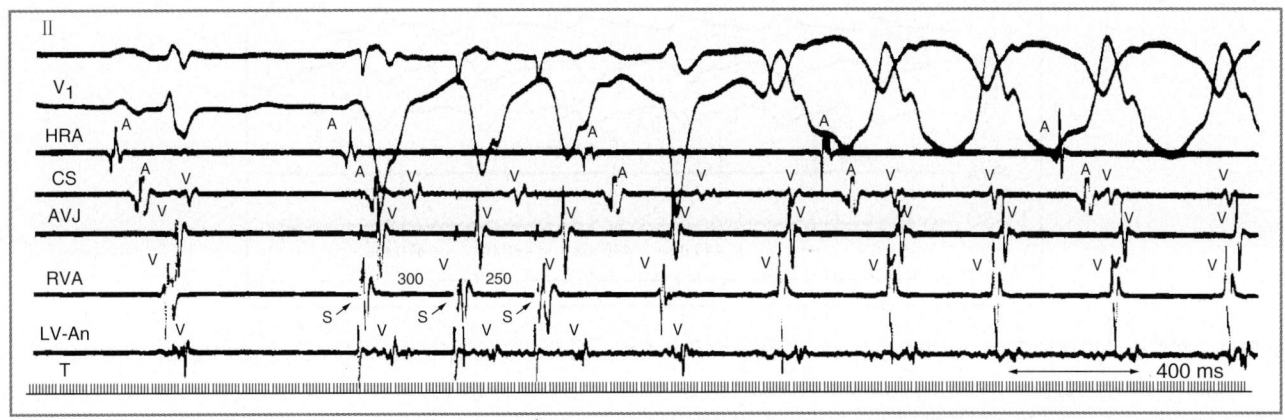

图 61-2　室速期间持续的电活动　图中显示体表 II 导联、V_1 导联和从冠状静脉窦、希氏束、右室心尖部以及左室室壁瘤记录的心内电图。窦性心律时，左室电极导管的远端记录到一个随着刺激频率增加而时限和复合成分增加的一个碎裂电位。室速发生时，该部位可记录到持续的电活动。A：心房电图；V：心室电图。（自 Josephson ME, Horowitz LN, Farshidi A：Continuous local electrical activity：A mechanism of recurrent tachycardia. Circulation 57：659-665，1978.）

放刺激脉冲都可侵入可激动组织（完全性可激动间隙），在大多数冠心病室速患者中（>67%）证实完全性可激动间隙至少要持续一定的时间（>30ms）。递增型反应方式是指回归周期随着期前刺激联律间期的递减而增加。这说明脉冲在全部或部分折返环中遇到部分处于不应期的组织，从而表现为联律间期依赖性传导延缓。混合型反应方式是指在联律间期较长时符合平台型反应与联律间期较短时符合递增型反应的组合。

　　能否发生节律重整本身并不能证明存在折返机制。自律性或触发性心律失常都能被适时的期前刺激

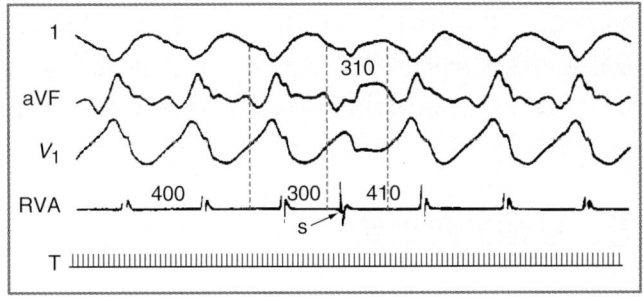

图 61-3　室性心动过速的节律重整　图中显示室性心动过速时从 I、aVF 和 V_1 导联以及右室心尖部记录的体表及心内电图。在体表心电图 QRS 波群的起始部发放一个期前刺激出现一个不完全性代偿间期。请注意，该刺激在体表心电图上引起一个由右室心尖部起搏和室速共同形成的 QRS 融合波。（自 Almendral JM, Rosenthal ME, Stamato NJ：Analysis of the resetting phenomenon in sustained uniform ventricular tachycardia：Incidence and relation to termination. J Am Coll Cardiol 8：294-300，1986.）

所重整。自律性异常机制诱发的心律失常表现为平台型反应方式，其回归周期等于异位自律点的频率间期加上从刺激部位到异位自律点的往返时间。触发性节律表现为一个恒定的回归周期，为室速折返周期长度的 100%~110% 或表现为一种递减型反应。体表心电图或局部左室电图上记录到节律重整和融合是诊断折返存在的重要依据。它表明刺激波锋能够兴奋心动过速已经激动并产生体表 QRS 波群的折返环组织（图 61-3）。节律重整和融合，混合或递增型重整反应方式，或回归周期短于室速周期，都从理论上证明折返是心律失常的发生机制。

　　拖带是心动过速对超速起搏的一种特殊反应，存在拖带现象时，强力支持心动过速为折返机制（图 61-4）。诊断拖带的经典标准有：选择一个既定的起搏周期时，出现固定的 QRS 融合波，随着起搏周期的缩短，融合波越来越明显（起搏夺获的形态成分逐渐增加），当起搏停止时，室速以一个夺获但不融合的回归间期波形恢复原心动过速[1]。拖带伴融合的含意与重整中讨论的内容相似。局灶起源机制的室速在超速起搏时，不会出现固定或渐进性融合波形。此外，起搏可超速抑制或加速心律失常，而不是以一个不变的周期（频率）恢复原来的心动过速。

　　拖带和重整都说明同一个生理现象：起搏脉冲侵入室性心动过速折返环，一方面从逆向阻断心动过速的波锋，同时沿心动过速折返环顺向传导，产生回归周期激动。二者一个重要的区别是，节律重整时，仅 1 个刺激作用于心动过速折返环路（即使是给予 2 个期外刺激），重整心动过速。而拖带时，只要起搏的

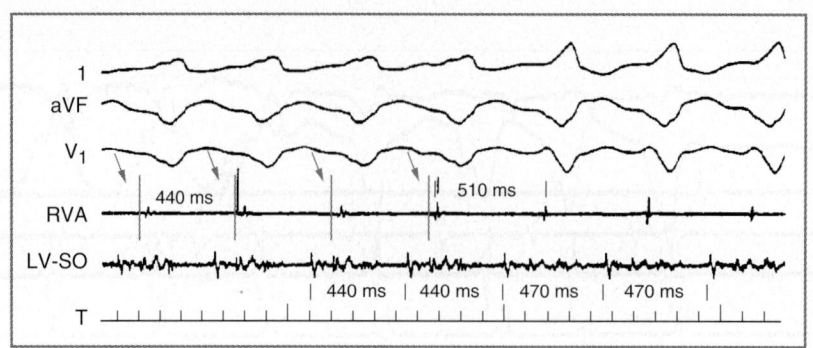

图 61-4 室性心动过速的拖带 图中显示体表心电图导联和从右室心尖部及左室室速起源部位记录的心内电图。从右室心尖部以 440ms 的周期超速起搏时，心动过速的频率暂时加速到起搏频率，QRS 波群表现为介于室速和右室心尖部起搏之间的融合波图形。起搏停止时，室速继续以拖带但不融合的形态恢复到原心率。（自 Almendral JM, Gottlieb CD, Rosenthal ME: Entrainment of ventricular tachycardia: explanation for surface electrocardiographic phenomena by analysis of electrograms recorded within the tachycardia circuit. Circulation 77: 569-580, 1988.）

第一个刺激到达得足够早，就可侵入折返环前面较窄的可激动间隙，随后的起搏刺激作用于前面重整的心动过速折返环路，在一定的配对间期内出现逐渐顺向传导延缓，从而表现为平台型重整曲线[10]。

射频消融术中，拖带技术被广泛用于室速标测。心动过速折返环路保护性峡部内的位点起搏证实存在隐匿性拖带（没有体表和心内融合证据的拖带），其回归周期约等于室速的折返周期[11]。这些技术将在第 118 章作更为详细的论述。

最近对动物和人类进行的研究，其焦点都集中于应用程序刺激技术来观察室速折返环的特性。在犬亚急性心肌梗死的动物模型中，从折返环内或临近折返环的部位发放刺激，可暂时改变折返环路，其本质为功能性的（不应期依赖性）[12,13]。人类室速折返环的屏障似乎可变性较小，推测其原因：至少部分由于解剖上存在较为广泛的心肌梗死瘢痕组织导致折返环屏障固定。窦律下证实在存在孤立晚电位的部位进行起搏常产生一种与室速形态一致的 QRS 波群[14]，这意味着在这些室速患者中，折返环路可能几乎都存在解剖学异常，有明确的折返边界，即使在慢频率起搏时亦如此。然而，我们最近发现人类室速患者的折返屏障可随着与刺激的相互作用而发生变化，表现为一种方向依赖性[15]。这些研究说明决定室速折返屏障特性的解剖因素和功能因素具有很大的变异性。

四、临床表现和治疗

慢性冠状动脉疾病患者的室速可以有多种临床表现，可偶然发现，也可表现为心脏骤停。事件发生时影响血流动力学的关键因素是室速的频率，其他影响因素包括左心功能的基础状态、心肌缺血的进展程度、是否伴有二尖瓣反流。最初的治疗策略取决于血流动力学紊乱的耐受程度[16]。虽然利多卡因一直被认为是慢性心肌梗死患者室速的选择用药，但已证实静脉应用普鲁卡因胺、索他洛尔和胺碘酮的疗效更佳[17]。室速引起严重的心绞痛或血流动力学紊乱时，须用同步心脏电复律治疗。

大多数持续性室速患者其室速发生并不频繁。虽然利多卡因常被用来抑制复发事件，但几乎没有资料推荐这种使用方法。偶尔，患者在伴有危重疾病或急性心肌缺血或心肌梗死时表现出频发或无休止性室速。最近多中心试验结果建议对难治性室速患者可选择静脉注射胺碘酮作为治疗用药[18]。值得注意的是，静脉应用胺碘酮的多中心试验中，30 天的死亡率为 32%～47%，这说明严重的疾病常常诱发难治性室速。

五、长期治疗对策

随机试验的结果对室速患者治疗的影响与日俱增。然而，仍存在一定的问题，这些后面将会讨论。通常，这些试验结果对选择抗心律失常药物还是应用程序刺激来预测其疗效具有直接的影响[19]。同时，随着植入式心脏复律除颤器（ICD）的应用，病人的死亡率和发病率稳步降低，依赖 ICD 治疗的不稳定型室速患者持续增加[20]。抗心律失常药物与 ICD 对比试验（AVID）的研究结果首次证明，对有致命性室性心律失常患者，植入 ICD 与使用最好的抗心律失常药物相比，ICD 治疗可降低病人的死亡率。在 1016 例患者中，ICD 治疗每年可降低总死亡率 39±20%；这个总死亡率的降低得益于 3 年的长期全程随访以及适用于所有患者的亚组分型（根据年龄、射血分数、心脏病的类型和心律失常表现将病人分为不同的亚组）[21]。虽然相对危险性的降低有着重要的临床意义，但 ICD 治疗 3 年（2.7 个月）得出的平均附加生存率并未给人们留下深刻印象。许多人为因素可能降低了这项统计结果的价值（如早期试验观察终点或存在交叉）。AVID 试验中，ICD 治疗存活患者每年的成本费用为 66 677 美元[22]。这项统计结果的解释为社会所承认，这的确不仅仅是一个医学问题。

鉴于上述诸多因素，分析的焦点集中于那些 ICD 治疗可能不会特别受益或根本不能获益的亚组病人。一项 AVID 试验分析结果认为左室储备功能尚可（射血分数＞40%）的患者不会从 ICD 治疗中获益[23]。我们认为 ICD 不适用于这类室速患者有两个原因：第一，AVID 试验中左室具有一定储备功能的患者发生室颤几乎是特有的，尤其在血管重建后的随访过程中事件发生率较低[24]。第二，室速和左室储备功能受损增加患者死亡的几率，可能更得益于 ICD 的治疗[20]。相关的人为试验设计因素，较短的观察时间以及早期试验终点都使得该试验的益处难以在统计学上得到证实。

关于血流动力学稳定、可耐受室速患者的治疗问题仍存有争议。虽然经典的研究表明在这些病人中通过程序刺激指导抗心律失常药物治疗具有较低的危险性，但最近更多的资料表明可耐受室速的患者在心律失常复发时有一定的猝死危险性[25,26]。在这组病例中建议使用射频消融替代 ICD 治疗。然而，基本的导管消融治疗耐受性室速的临床效果还存在争议。可耐受性室速成功射频消融后快速室速、室颤的发病率或猝死的死亡率尚未明确地肯定，其范围约为 1%～10%[20,27]，但是成功消融后停用抗心律失常药物，尤其是胺碘酮，可能是其中的一个影响因素。对程序刺激的反应并不能可靠地预测自发性快速心律失常的危险性。一项近期的研究结果表明，尽管没有其他诱发性（频率快或慢）室速的附加治疗措施，成功消融可耐受、有临床症状的室速后没有发生猝死的病例；在该研究中，所有患者在出现临床症状时都给予抗心律失常药物并维持治疗[11]。针对这类特殊人群确定最佳治疗方案的多中心研究目前正在设计中。

六、未来发展方向

众多前沿学者为探索更好的治疗方法而不断在努力。当室速的电或物理环境能被确定时，预防室速事件的发生可能将成为现实。随着未来技术的进步，ICD 治疗日臻改进，其作为高危亚组人群的一级预防治疗措施，患者的获益将逐渐增加。随着动物室速模型的完善，人们对激动标测的进一步深入了解和提高，导管消融方法将不断改进，它将逐步成为更多患者的基本治疗措施。更重要的是，随着我们识别某些亚组人群对某一既定治疗方案反应能力的逐渐提高，患者可以得到更为个体化和更为特异性的治疗。

（侯爱军 译）

参 考 文 献

1. Josephson ME: Clinical Cardiac Electrophysiology: Techniques and Interpretations, 3rd ed. Philadelphia, Lippincott Williams & Wilkins, 2002.
2. de Bakker JM, Janse MJ: Pathophysiological correlates of ventricular tachycardia in hearts with a healed infarct. In Zipes DP, Jalife J (eds): Cardiac Electrophysiology: From Cell to Bedside, 3rd ed. Philadelphia, WB Saunders, 2000, pp 415-421.
3. Zheng Z-J, Croft JB, Giles WH, Mensah GA: Sudden cardiac death in the United States, 1989 to 1998. Circulation 104:2158-2163, 1998.
4. Peters NS, Coromilas J, Severs NJ, Wit AL: Disturbed connexin43 gap junction distribution correlates with the location of reentrant circuits in the epicardial border zone of healing canine infarcts that cause ventricular tachycardia. Circulation 95:988-996, 1997.
5. Buxton AE, Lee KL, DiCarlo L, et al: Electrophysiologic testing to identify patients with coronary artery disease who are at risk for sudden death. Multicenter Unsustained Tachycardia Trial Investigators. N Engl J Med 342:1937-1945, 2000.
6. Gomes JA, Mehta D, Ip J, et al: Predictors of long-term survival in patients with malignant ventricular arrhythmias. Am J Cardiol 79:1054-1060, 1997.
7. Wyse DG, Friedman PL, Brodsky MA, et al: Life-threatening ventricular arrhythmias due to transient or correctable causes: High risk for death in follow-up. J Am Coll Cardiol 38:1718-1724, 2001.
8. Callans DJ, Josephson ME: Ventricular tachycardia in patients with coronary artery disease. In Zipes DP, Jalife J (eds): Cardiac Electrophysiology: From Cell to Bedside, 3rd ed. Philadelphia, WB Saunders, 2000, pp 530-536.
9. Peters NS, Cabo C, Wit AL: Arrhythmogenic mechanisms: Automaticity, triggered activity, and reentry. In Zipes DP, Jalife J (eds): Cardiac Electrophysiology: From Cell to Bedside, 3rd ed. Philadelphia, WB Saunders, 2000, pp 345-356.
10. Callans DJ, Hook BG, Mitra RL, Josephson ME: Characterization of return cycle responses predictive of successful pacing-mediated termination of ventricular tachycardia. J Am Coll Cardiol 25:47-53, 1995.
11. El-Shalakany A, Hadjis T, Papageorgiou P, et al: Entrainment mapping criteria for the prediction of termination of ventricular tachycardia by single radiofrequency lesion in patients with coronary artery disease. Circulation 99:2283-2289, 1999.
12. Hanna MS, Coromilas J, Josephson ME, et al: Mechanisms of resetting reentrant circuits in canine ventricular tachycardia. Circulation 103:1148-1156, 2001.
13. Peters NS, Coromilas J, Hanna MS, et al: Characteristics of the tem-

poral and spatial excitable gap in anisotropic reentrant circuits causing sustained ventricular tachycardia. Circ Res 82:279-293, 1998.
14. Bogun F, Bahu M, Knight BP, et al: Response to pacing at sites of isolated diastolic potentials during ventricular tachycardia in patients with previous myocardial infarction. J Am Coll Cardiol 30:505-513, 1997.
15. Callans DJ, Zardini M, Gottlieb CD, Josephson ME: The variable contribution of functional and anatomic barriers in human ventricular tachycardia: An analysis with resetting from two sites. J Am Coll Cardiol 27:1106-1111, 1996.
16. Ho RT, Callans DJ: Malignant ventricular arrhythmias. In Antman EM (ed): Cardiovascular Therapeutics, 2nd ed. Philadelphia, WB Saunders, 2002, pp 477-502.
17. Guidelines 2000 for Cardiopulmonary Resuscitation and Emergency Cardiovascular Care: An international consensus on science. Part 6: Advanced Cardiovascular Life Support; Section 5: Pharmacology I: Agents for arrhythmias. Circulation 102:I112-I128, 2000.
18. Levine JH, Massumi A, Scheinman MM, et al: Intravenous amiodarone for recurrent sustained hypotensive ventricular tachyarrhythmias. The Intravenous Amiodarone Multicenter Study Group. J Am Coll Cardiol 27:67-75, 1996.
19. Naccarelli GV, Wolbrette DL, Dell'Orfano JT, et al: A decade of clinical trial developments in postmyocardial infarction, congestive heart failure, and sustained ventricular tachyarrhythmia patients: From CAST to AVID and beyond. Cardiac Arrhythmic Suppression Trial. Antiarrhythmic Versus Implantable Defibrillators. J Cardiovasc Electrophysiol 9:864-891, 1998.
20. Josephson ME, Callans DJ, Buxton AE: The role of the implantable cardioverter-defibrillator for prevention of sudden cardiac death. Ann Intern Med 133:901-910, 2000.
21. A comparison of antiarrhythmic-drug therapy with implantable defibrillators in patients resuscitated from near-fatal ventricular arrhythmias. The Antiarrhythmics Versus Implantable Defibrillators (AVID) Investigators. N Engl J Med 337:1576-1583, 1997.
22. Larsen G, Hallstrom A, McAnulty J, et al: Cost-effectiveness of the implantable cardioverter-defibrillator versus antiarrhythmic drugs in survivors of serious ventricular tachyarrhythmias: Results of the Antiarrhythmics Versus Implantable Defibrillators (AVID) economic analysis substudy. Circulation 105:2049-2057, 2002.
23. Domanski MJ, Sakseena S, Epstein AE, et al: Relative effectiveness of the implantable cardioverter-defibrillator and antiarrhythmic drugs in patients with varying degrees of left ventricular dysfunction who have survived malignant ventricular arrhythmias. AVID Investigators. Antiarrhythmics Versus Implantable Defibrillators. J Am Coll Cardiol 34:1090-1095, 1999.
24. Hallstrom AP, McAnulty JH, Wilkoff BL, et al: Patients at lower risk of arrhythmia recurrence: A subgroup in whom implantable defibrillators may not offer benefit. Antiarrhythmics Versus Implantable Defibrillator (AVID) Trial Investigators. J Am Coll Cardiol 37:1093-1099, 2001.
25. Caruso AC, Marcus FI, Hahn EA, et al: Predictors of arrhythmic death and cardiac arrest in the ESVEM trial. Electrophysiologic Study Versus Electromagnetic Monitoring. Circulation 96:1888-1892, 1997.
26. Pinski SL, Yao Q, Epstein AE, et al: Determinants of outcome in patients with sustained ventricular tachyarrhythmias: The Antiarrhythmics Versus Implantable Defibrillators (AVID) Study Registry. Am Heart J 139:804-813, 2000.
27. Rothman SA, Hsia HH, Cossu SF, et al: Radiofrequency catheter ablation of postinfarction ventricular tachycardia: Long-term success and the significance of inducible nonclinical arrhythmias. Circulation 96:3499-3508, 1997.

第 62 章

扩张型心肌病的室性心律失常

Joseph M. Galvin and Jeremy N. Ruskin

本章目录
- 流行病学 ······················ 567
- 分子遗传学 ···················· 567
- 扩张型心肌病室性心律失常的病理生理 ························ 570
- 总死亡率和室性心律失常的预测因素 ··· 571
- 治疗 ·························· 573
- 总结 ·························· 578

扩张型心肌病是以左室或双心室扩大和收缩功能障碍为特征的综合征（图 62-1）。冠状动脉疾病、瓣膜病、饮酒、高血压、怀孕和感染是最常见的潜在致病因素。特发性扩张型心肌病，根据其定义，虽然有遗传、自身免疫、病毒、代谢原因牵涉其中，但其病因是不明确的。不管其潜在的病因如何，扩张型心肌病的一个共同特征是室性心律失常和猝死的多发。本章重点讨论心律失常的发生机制、猝死的预测因子以及扩张型心肌病特别是特发性扩张型心肌病室性心律失常的处理。

一、流行病学

美国大约有 400 万充血性心力衰竭患者，并且导致了每年 20 万人的死亡。每年超过 1 万人的死因是特发性扩张型心肌病。由于诊断的标准、病例的确认和所处的地理位置的不同，特发性扩张型心肌病的发病率在 4/10 万～8/10 万变化。在明尼苏达 Olmsted 地区，从 1975 年到 1984 年，经性别和年龄校正后其总的年发病率为 6.0/10 万，而 1985 年的发病率增至 36.5/10 万，几乎两倍于肥厚型心肌病。特发性扩张型心肌病发病率将可能一直增长，这或许是由于发病率的增加，或是由于提高了患病病例的确认数量。

特发性扩张型心肌病病人的发病年龄大多介于 18 岁和 50 岁之间，但是儿童和老人也可发病。相对于女性，男性更好发（2.5:1）；非裔美国人比白人好发（2.5:1），但是导致不同性别、不同人群发病率差异的机制并不清楚。特发性扩张型心肌病的存活率是相当低的，而且主要与病人检查确定后的治疗和疾病被确诊的时间有关。其 1 年存活率从轻度临床症状且左室射血分数小于 25% 并拒绝心脏移植亚组的 46% 到总体人群的 95% 之间变化（图 62-2）。当缺血性心肌病和非缺血性心肌病被共同考虑时，1 年存活率从 48% 到 95% 不等，2 年存活率从 19% 到 66% 不等。随着药物治疗的进步，例如：血管紧张素转换酶抑制和 β 受体阻滞剂和介入治疗的进步，如 ICD 和心室辅助装置，存活率已被提高。

二、分子遗传学

大约 35% 的特发性扩张型心肌病病人有家族发病的历史，虽然存在 X 连锁性状遗传、常染色体隐性遗传、线粒体遗传，但大多数病人表现为常染色体显性遗传。过去 10 年，在鉴定扩张型心肌病发病的候选基因方面，已取得了巨大的进展（图 62-3[1]）。线粒体遗传经常见于家族性扩张型心肌病的儿童型，然而 X 连锁性状遗传、常染色体隐性遗传在儿童型和成人型中的比例几乎相等。10 年前对 X 连锁性状遗传形式

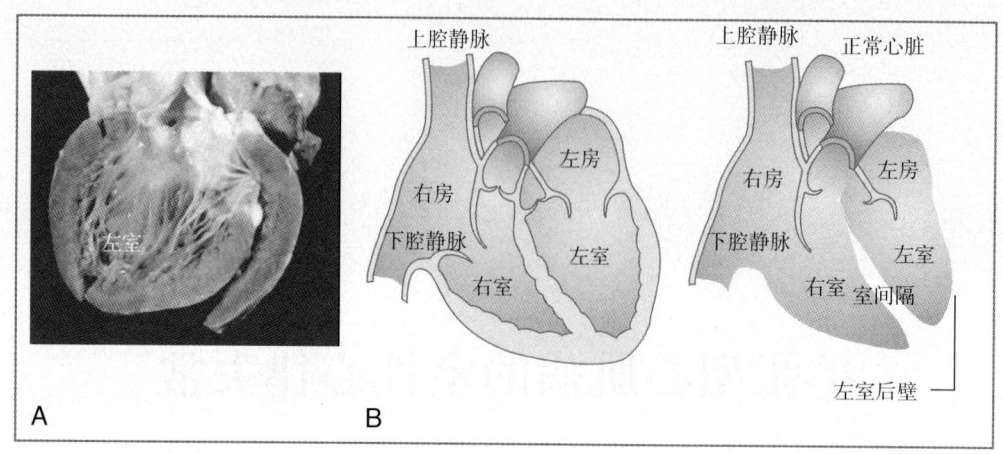

图 62-1 扩张型心肌病

的家族进行研究取得了一些初期进展。最近几年,对常染色体隐性遗传已经有了充分认识。在 X 连锁性状遗传病例,有两种特征性的功能障碍:X 连锁的心肌病,经常出现在青春期和年轻人;Barth 综合征,其特征是经常在婴儿期出现。家族性扩张型心肌病最常见的常染色体隐性遗传有两种类型:"单纯性"扩张型心肌病和扩张型心肌病伴心脏传导系统疾病。

(一) 常染色体显性遗传单纯性扩张型心肌病

在单纯性扩张型心肌病的病例中,已经被确定的突变基因位点包括:1q32,2q31,2q35,4q12,5q33,9q13-22,10q21-23,14q11,15q2 和 15 q14[2-7]。现在已发现七个突变基因:(1) 肌动蛋白 (染色体 15q14)[2],一种肌节蛋白,是细肌丝的成分之一,它由原肌球蛋白和肌钙蛋白相互作用而成;(2) 结蛋白 (染色体 2q35)[3],一种细胞骨架蛋白,形成中间丝,特别在肌肉中;(3) β-肌聚糖 (染色体 4q12)[4];(4) δ-聚糖 (染色体 5q33)[5],是肌萎缩蛋白-配糖蛋白复合物 (DGC,见图 62-1) 亚单位 sarcoglycan 的组成成分;(5) 心脏肌钙蛋白 T (染色体 1q32)[6] 和 (6) α-原肌球蛋白 (染色体 15 q2)[7],是肌节收缩蛋白复合物的关键部分;(7) β-肌球蛋白重链 (染色体 14 q11)[6],包括肌球蛋白的结合部,而且是收缩能量产生的核心部分。

(二) 扩张型心肌病伴随心脏传导系统疾病

对于心脏传导系统疾病也存在遗传异质性。目前为止,心脏传导系统疾病基因已经被定位于染色体 1p1-1q1[8],2q14-21[9],3p22-25[10] 和 6q23[11]。唯一

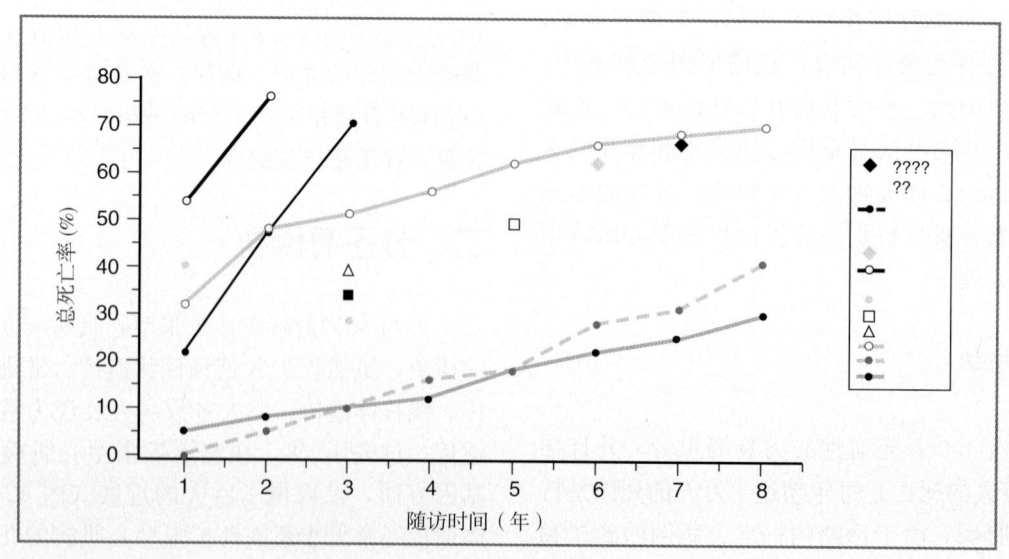

图 62-2 从 1978 到 1996 年报道的一系列扩张型心肌病病人累积的总死亡率 (引自 Tamburro P,Wilber D:Sudden death in idiopathic dilated cardiomyopathy,Am Heart J 124:1035-1045,1992.)

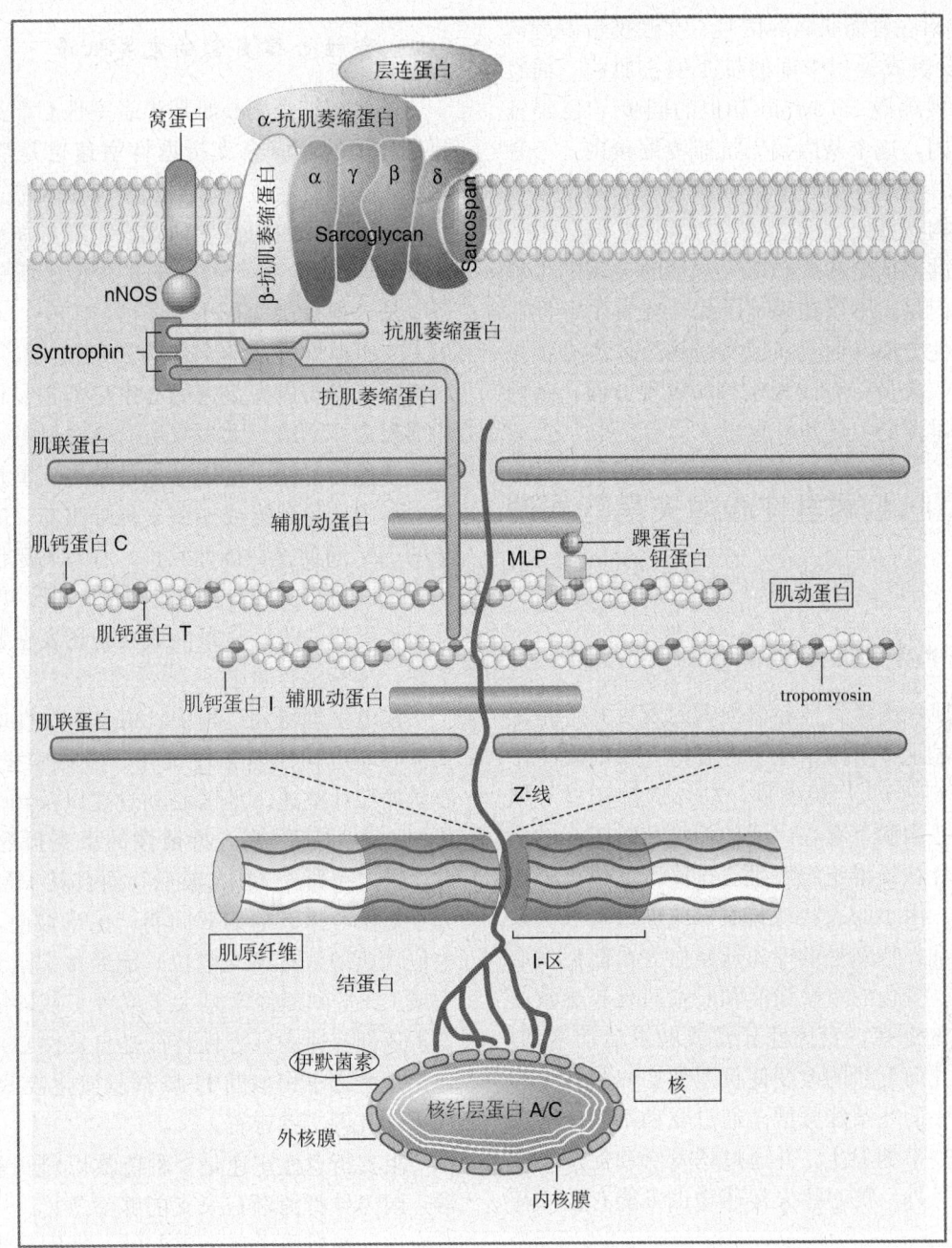

图 62-3 扩张型心肌病发病牵涉的蛋白的概略图[1] 已鉴别的导致扩张型心肌病的基因包括细胞骨架蛋白编码基因：肌膜的 β-sarcoglycan、δ-sarcoglycan，抗肌萎缩蛋白；中间丝蛋白编码基因：结蛋白和核纤层蛋白 A/C；肌纤维蛋白编码基因：肌动蛋白、β-肌球蛋白重链、α-tropomyosin、心脏肌钙蛋白 T 导致了扩张型心肌病或肥厚型心肌病，然而肌钙蛋白 I 和肌球蛋白轻链导致了肥厚型心肌病。Dystrobrevin（一种细胞骨架蛋白）的突变导致了中间物的表现型-左室心肌致密化不合。MLP，肌界核蛋白；nNOS，神经元型一氧化氮合酶。

被确定的基因是位于染色体 1q211[12] 的核纤层蛋白 A/C，它编码中间丝蛋白的核包膜部分。但它导致扩张型心肌病和传导系统不正常的机制当前仍不清楚。

（三）X 连锁扩张型心肌病

这种类型的扩张型心肌病在 1987 年被首次报道，发生在 10 多岁的儿童和 20 岁出头的年轻人，快速从充血性心力衰竭发展到死亡或需要心脏移植。X 连锁扩张型心肌病的显著特征是血清肌酸激酶肌肉亚型增高[13]——一种潜在骨骼肌病的信号。女性携带者趋向于在50多岁发展成轻到中度的扩张型心肌病，而且这种疾病的进展缓慢。Towbin和他的同事[14]已经证实它的发病基因，这个基因编码抗肌萎缩蛋白：一种细胞骨架蛋白，通过在肌膜上形成网格状的网络来提供肌细胞的结构支持。

对于个体的遗传型和致心律失常性的关系的了解仍是很少的。但是，不仅在确定受累个体发生室性心律失常的危险性方面，而且在证实受累个体患有扩张型心肌病的家族成员将有或无疾病的表现方面，基因型将作为一种重要的工具是可能的。

三、扩张型心肌病室性心律失常的病理生理

(一) 致心律失常发生的相关因素

扩张型心肌病患者室性心律失常的发生并不是单一机制，研究显示多个因素在室性心律失常的发生中起着作用（表62-1）。尸检发现，33%的扩张型心肌病病人在左室心内膜下存在广泛的瘢痕化，57%的病人存在区域斑片状纤维组织增生。这些区域也许将成为折返的位点。由小的冠状动脉血栓或栓子造成的缺血和电解质紊乱，特别是低钾和低镁血症可能促发心律失常的发生。变化的室壁强度和心室肌延长导致心室有效不应期的缩短、自律性异常或触发活动增加，心室机械学和几何形状的改变使折返性心律失常更容易发生。循环中的儿茶酚胺增高通过驱动细胞内的钙间接促进心律失常的发生，并通过诱发活动促进心律失常的发生。另外，抗心律失常药物也可能有致心律失常的作用。

表62-1 扩张型心肌病室性心律失常发生的易患因素

1. 低钾血症，低镁血症（经常与利尿剂的使用有关）
2. 持续性心室肌的伸展使有效不应期和动作电位时程缩短形成折返
3. 短的搏动性伸展诱发后除极
4. 肌浆网上钙泵减少导致舒张期钙超载
5. 增强的Na^+-Ca^{2+}交换活动诱发后除极
6. 循环中的儿茶酚胺增加
7. 交感活性增强
8. 心肌纤维化/瘢痕
9. 浦肯野系统传导延迟
10. 心房扩张或心室内膜表面积增加
11. 药物（抗心律失常药物，地高辛，交感系统活性药物，磷酸二酯酶抑制剂）

(二) 室性心律失常的束支阻滞

虽然在扩张型心肌病患者室性心律失常的其他机制是常见的，但束支折返性室速也是最具有特征性的。束支折返通过一个累及希浦系统的大折返环产生室速，通常其前向传导通过右束支，而逆向传导通过左束支。大约6%～41%的扩张型心肌病病人室速的产生是这种机制。在一个系列研究中，对于曾经诱发出束支折返性室速的全部病人来说，45%有扩张型心肌病。束支折返性室速的心室率通常是快速的，其平均周长为279ms。大多数病人伴发晕厥，有进一步发展成室颤的可能。基础电生理检查典型发现为非特异性心室内传导延迟或左束支传导阻滞。窦性心律下记录的HV间期是特征性延长。右室刺激诱发的心动过速表现出左束支传导阻滞图形的特征。期前刺激前一个短长周期的改变是最能成功地诱发室性心动过速的条件，尽管仍有争论。

在电生理研究过程中，束支折返性室速必须和室上性心动过速伴差异性传导、多源性室性心动过速、心肌梗死灶室速、结区心动过速以及经Mahaim束前传的心动过速区别。特征性的束支折返性室速的H波，继之于每个QRS波后，而且其HV间期等于或大于窦性心律下的HV间期。在V波前，右或左束支电位（典型是右束支电位）能经常记录到，而且RB-V或LB-V间期经常是大于或等于基础情况下的。束支折返性室速的标志性特征是自发性心律失常的周长变化是继之于相似的H-H周长变化或RB-RB周长的变化，或者二者皆有。

束支折返性室速是一种能被识别的重要的心律失常，因为导管消融右束支能够治愈它。一些病人将在右束支消融后要求双心室起搏，特别是先前有广泛左束支阻滞患者。根据左室功能障碍的严重程度，植入双腔ICD可能是正当的。

(三) 猝死的机制

随着远距离心脏监测的出现和动态心电图监测的运用，先前被认为是很少发生的室性心律失常已经在50%至60%扩张型心肌病患者中被注意到，而且室性心律失常估计在全部的死亡原因中占到了8%至50%。在发展成充血性心力衰竭的全部病人中，大约50%被报告发生了猝死。死于进展性室性功能障碍的病人数量大致与此相当。虽然心力衰竭症状的严重程度加重导致了死于进行性泵功能衰竭可能

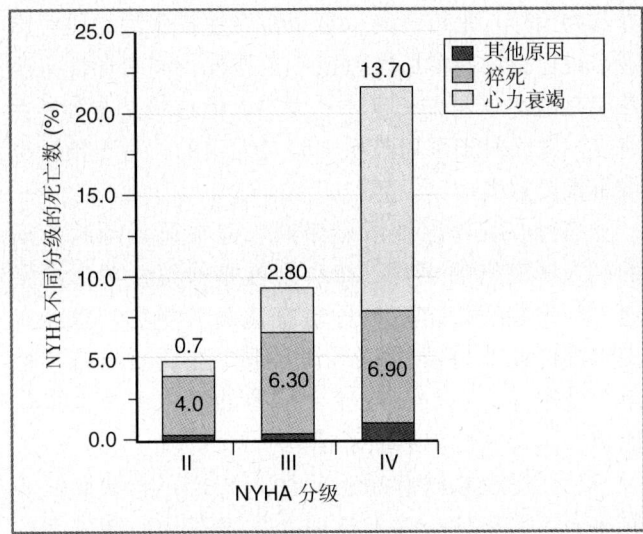

图 62-4 在 MERIT 试验中严重左室功能障碍的病人 NHYA 分级不同的死亡方式 平均随访 12 个月，在随访期内于死于突发心律失常、进展性泵衰竭或其他原因的百分比与不同分级心功能的关系。

性的增加，而不是心律失常所致猝死的可能性增加，但是猝死的绝对可能性增加，多数是心律失常性死亡，与 NYHA 心功能分级相关（图 62-4）。把猝死从泵功能衰竭导致的死亡中区分出来是相当困难的。一组研究表明，根据评价标准不同，猝死的比例从 31% 到 55% 不等。

尽管室性心动过速常见，它并不是猝死的唯一原因。Luu 和他的助手[14a]回顾了 20 个住院接受监护病人的 21 次心脏停搏事件，其终末期心衰均由缺血或非缺血心肌病导致。他们发现，仅 38% 心脏停搏事件是原发性室性心律失常造成的，心动过缓或电-机械分离是 62% 患者的初始事件。相应的，一度和二度房室阻滞已经被作为扩张型心肌病患者不良预后的特征性指标。其他人也指出缺血、继发于急性冠状动脉血栓或栓子也许导致一小部分病人的猝死。肺动脉血栓和高钾血症是心衰病人猝死的其他重要原因。

四、总死亡率和室性心律失常的预测因素

临床上治疗扩张型心肌病伴有室性心律失常病人时最大的挑战，是与其他死亡相比评估其猝死的相对危险度，以及仅从当前相对不完善的预测指标中推定病人的预期寿命。

（一）死亡率的临床预测因素

对于特发性扩张型心肌病合并充血性心力衰竭的病人，左室功能障碍的严重程度是最重要的死亡率预测因素。研究已经表明左室射血分数与存活率强烈相关，射血分数越低，存活率越小。一项研究表明：射血分数小于 35% 的特发性扩张型心肌病病人，39 个月的死亡率平均为 84%，而射血分数大于 35% 的病人死亡率仅为 46%。虽然射血分数是最常用的指标，但其他显示左室、右室功能的指标包括肺毛细血管楔压、心脏指数、每搏指数、每搏量也被用作预测指标，而且右房压也可预测心肌病病人的死亡率。

与左室功能的指标相比，临床表现和心功能分级不是强的死亡率预测指标。然而，NYHA 分级和第三心音与特发性扩张型心肌病合并充血性心力衰竭病人的生存率相关。特发性扩张型心肌病病人的猝死发生率显著高于晕厥病人。预测死亡率的实验室指标包括：低钠、血浆中高去甲肾上腺素、肾素、心房和脑钠素水平。准确的组织形态学分析未发现组织学是生存率的预测指标。左室的大小、心室功能自主性不能预测生存率。大多数包括对缺血性心肌病和非缺血性心肌病病人的研究证明冠心病病人的预后较坏。但也有相反的报道。

（二）心电图、心律失常、心脏电生理的预测指标

1. 心电图

对于特发性扩张型心肌病来说，左束支阻滞和一度、二度房室阻滞与不良预后显著相关。VEST 研究已经证实 QRS 波增宽的程度与死亡率之间有着重要的相关性（图 62-5）。房颤也是一个预后更差的指标。到目前为止与此相关的最大病例组的研究，入选 390 例病人，包括 191 例特发性扩张型心肌病病人。严重心功能衰竭的病人中 19% 发展成阵发性房颤或慢性房颤。房颤病人与窦性心律病人的一年存活率分别是 52% 和 71%（$P=0.001$）；但是，当用升高的肺楔压进行校正后，结果就不显著了。房颤因增加血栓事件或室性心律失常减少生存率，且由于房颤通过短长周期增加了心室不应期的离散性。因此，房颤也可作为严重左室功能障碍的指标。

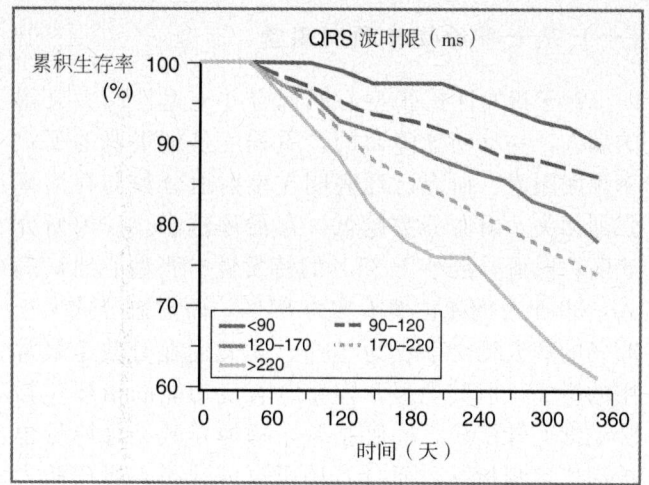

图62-5 VEST研究受试者的累积生存率与12导联心电图QRS波时限的关系（引自Gottipaty et al：JACC 33 [2]：145A [abstract 847-4]，1999.）

2. 自发性室性心律失常

80%～95%的扩张型心肌病病人可出现多种室性早搏、室性早搏二联律和非持续性室性心动过速。在一项24h动态心电图监测研究中发现，53%的病人有超过500个室性早搏，54%有室早二联律，31%有过非持续性室性心动过速事件。在充血性心力衰竭的病人，随着左室功能的恶化，室性心律失常更常见和更复杂。研究表明，在心功能Ⅰ～Ⅱ级的充血性心力衰竭病人非持续性室性心动过速的发生率从15%～20%不等，而心功能Ⅳ级的则为50%～70%。尽管室性异位活动高度频发，但这些心律失常通常是无症状的。由于它们普遍存在，使它们的重要性很难被评估，但一些研究报告（而不是所有研究报告）指出室性心律失常已经被作为整个心源性死亡率或心源性猝死独立的预测因子。DeMaria和他的助手[14b]通过对218例病人研究发现，虽然不如左室射血分数和心脏每搏做功指数有力地预测存活率，但心律失常的复杂性仍是生存率的一个主要预测因子。相反，Romeo和他的同事[14c]发现在104例特发性扩张型心肌病病人中，Lown分级为4级的室性早搏和更高程度的心律失常是猝死的独立预测因子。

3. 心室程序刺激

一直缺乏证据证明程序电刺激是非缺血性扩张型心肌病患者猝死的准确预测指标。对于大多数非缺血性心肌病患者而言，诱发持续性单性形室速的电生理研究是不可信的，由此作出的系列药物试验（据此选择药物治疗）是可疑的。对于特发性扩张型心肌病患者来说，持续性单形性室速不易诱发，而多形性室速却能在高达86%的患者中诱发出，但这些是非特异性终点，进而对于系列药物试验是无用的，对于预后也没有重要意义。

当行心脏程序性电刺激时，存在冠状动脉疾病的病人诱发出的主要心律失常就是持续性单形性室速。与那些有持续性单形性室速病人相比，曾经有心脏骤停或非持续性室速病人很少能诱发出持续性单形性室速。在没有或较少早搏的病人中，也很少能诱发出持续性单形性室速。

与存在冠状动脉疾病的病人相比，非缺血性心肌病病人的室性心律失常的诱发率对于心律失常的复发和猝死的预测价值很小（表62-2）。这些资料表明，在那些诱发出室性心律失常并能被药物控制的病人中，28%的室速病人后来复发，43%的心脏骤停病人后来发生猝死。虽然程序性电刺激中不能诱发出持续性单形性室速的病人与诱发出室性心动过速的病人相比，心律失常的复发率和猝死率较低，但其复发率和猝死率仍然很高。因此，具有严重的左室功能障碍、晕厥或室性心动过速史的特发性扩张性心肌病患者具有高的猝死危险，对这些病人不应仅仅基于阴性的电生理研究结果，而不进行预防性ICD植入。

4. 信号平均心电图

对于存在晕厥或冠状动脉疾病的病人而言，信号平均心电图能鉴别出发展为室性心动过速和猝死的高危病人。尽管扩张型心肌病患者晚电位的发生率很低，有报道信号平均心电图在预测非缺血性心肌病患者的室性心动过速和猝死的敏感性高达100%。然而，也有报道敏感性低到22%～38%。特异性变化在45%～96%之间。Poll和他的同事[14d]发现信号平均心电图的敏感性为83%，特异性为86%。41例非缺血性心肌病患者包括35例特发性扩张型心肌病，12例曾经有持续性室性心律失常或心脏骤停，在这12个病人中，83%有不正常的信号平均心电图。在29例没有持续性心律失常的病人中，仅仅14%有不正常的信号平均心电图。不正常心内膜电图，代表电活动的传导延迟和缓慢传导，发生在近77%的特发性扩张型心肌病病人中，但不能预测猝死的发生。

表 62-2　扩张型心肌病无持续性室性心律失常病史患者的程序性电刺激结果

作者	年	病例数	诱发心律失常				随访		随访期发生心律失常事件	
			NSVT	VES	SMVT	PMVT/VF	月	Ind	MMVT Ind PMVT/VF	Noniucible
Meinertz (99)	1985	42	35%	1~2	0 (0%)	1 (2%)	16+7	0 (0%)	0 (0%)	2 (5%)
Stamato (100)	1986	15	93%	1~2	0 (0%)	0 (0%)	19+4	0 (0%)	0 (0%)	2 (13%)
Poll (37)	1986	20	100%	1~3	2 (10%)	4 (20%)	17+14	0 (0%)	1 (50%)	5 (36%)
Das (101)	1986	24	NA	1~3	1 (4%)	4 (17%)	12+6		1 (100%)	1 (25%)
Gossinger (102)	1990	32	100%	1~3	4 (13%)	0 (0%)	21	1 (25%)		2 (7%)
Brembilla-Perrot (30)	1991	92	46%	1~3	3 (3%)	5 (5%)	24+8	2 (67%)	2 (40%)	3 (4%)
Kadish (103)	1993	43	100%	1~3	6 (14%)	NA	20+14	1 (17%)	NA	6 (16%)
Turrito (104)	1994	80	100%	1-	10 (13%)	7 (9%)	22+26	3 (30%)		6 (10%)
Grimm (105)	1997	34	100%	1~3	3 (9%)	10 (29%)	24+13	1 (33%)	3 (30%)	5 (24%)

Ind，诱发；MMVT，单形性室速；SMVT，持续性单形性室速；NA，没有获得数据；Noninducible，非持续性室性心律失常诱发；NSVT，非持续性室速；PMVT/VF，多形性室速或室颤；VES，心室程序期前刺激的个数。

摘自：Grimm W, Hoffmann J, Menz V, et al: Programmed Ventricular stimulation for arrhymia risk prediction in patients with idiopathic dilated cardiomyopathy and nonsustained ventricular tachycardia. J Am Coll Cardiol 32：739-745，1998.

5. 心率变异性

心率变化的时域或频域分析在评估自主神经系统对心血管系统的影响方面已有一定价值。对于心肌梗死后病人而言，心率变异性的减少与心性猝死和持续性室性心律失常的发生的增加密切相关。关于扩张型心肌病患者的心率变异性仅仅进行了很少的研究。Hoffmann 和他的助手[14e]对 71 例扩张型心肌病患者 24h 心率变化进行了检查，10 例病人在 15 个月的随访过程中发生了室速、室颤或猝死。通过时域和频域分析，发现在两组之间，时域的参数有减低的趋势，但在频域方面无差异。Fei 和他的助手[14f]在 10 例无冠心病的心脏骤停生存者中发现了心率变异性降低，其中只有 3 例被归类于特发性扩张型心肌病。

6. QT 离散度

对于有长 QT 综合征和从心肌梗死恢复后的病人，体表 12 导联心电图反映出的 QT 间期变化与猝死的增加有关。在扩张型心肌病的预测方面，只有很少的数据。到目前为止最大的关于扩张型心肌病的研究中，Grimm 和他的同事[15]发现与年龄和性别匹配的健康对照组相比，107 例扩张型心肌病病人的 QT 间期、QTc 显著延长，而且其校正的 QTc 间期的离散度增加。在 13 个月随访期间发生过持续性室速、室颤或猝死的 12 例病人，其 QT 离散度显著延长（76± 17 vs. 60±26ms，$P<0.03$）。虽然发生过持续性室速、室颤或猝死病人的 QT 离散度延长了，但两组之间在 QTc、校正 QT 离散度的差异未达到统计学意义[15]。

7. T 波电交替

最近发表的两项研究描述了微伏 T 波电交替在预测非缺血性心肌病病人危险性方面的能力。Adachi 和他的同事[16]发现在 58 例非缺血性心肌病病人中，微伏 T 波电交替与自发性室速或室颤高度相关。Kitamura 和他的合作者[17]发现在 104 例非缺血性心肌病病人中，微伏 T 波电交替对于猝死、持续性室速/室颤的阳性预测值为 23.9%，阴性预测值为 97.3%（相对危险度为 8.8）。

五、治　疗

(一) 血管扩张剂治疗

血管扩张剂通过减缓左室功能障碍的进展来提高充血性心力衰竭病人的存活率。与其他血管扩张剂相比，血管紧张素转换酶抑制剂在降低这类疾病猝死的发生率方面也许是独一无二的。在 VHeFT-Ⅱ研究中，应用依那普利可使死亡率下降（18% vs. 28%），依那普利组猝死的发生率减少（37% vs. 46%）。在依那普利组，3 个月内室速发作的频率下降，在 1 年到 2

年内，新的室性心律失常的发生减少。在一个卡托普利与肼屈嗪和异山梨醇比较的更早期的包括106例病人的随机研究中有相似的发现：与肼屈嗪和异山梨醇相比，卡托普利显著降低猝死的发生。相反，CONSENSUS 和 SOLVD 的研究者对253例NHYAⅣ级心衰病人和2569例射血分数低于35%的病人各自随机给予依那普利和安慰剂后，并没有发现心脏性猝死减少。在这些研究中，仅仅SOLVD试验包括了无冠状动脉疾病的病人。

在ELITE试验中，对于一组老年伴症状性心力衰竭和左室收缩功能障碍的病人，与卡托普利相比较，血管紧张素受体拮抗剂洛沙坦降低总死亡率达46%，降低猝死率达64%[18]。这些结果没有被随后的ELITE Ⅱ试验证实。ELITE Ⅱ试验表明在血管紧张素转换酶抑制剂和血管紧张素受体Ⅱ拮抗剂之间，其总死亡率或猝死的发生率没有差异[19]。

（二）肾上腺素能受体阻滞剂

1975年，Waagstein和他的助手[19a]报道了7例特发性扩张型心肌病病人应用β受体阻滞剂后其心室功能和运动耐量得到了改善。自此以后，几个研究表明非缺血性扩张型心肌病病人使用β受体阻滞剂治疗后症状得到了改善。综合9个研究，包括144例病人，观察时间为2~19个月，66%的病人症状得到了改善，19%没有变化，15%病情恶化或死亡。射血分数的提高明显与基础射血分数无关。β受体阻滞剂治疗扩张型心肌病的原理是减少了交感活性增强和循环中的儿茶酚胺的有害作用，如钙超载或收缩蛋白合成的减少。近来发现兰尼丁受体的变异牵涉到舒张期从肌浆网到胞质的钙泄漏，容易触发儿茶酚胺敏感性多形性室速[20]（图62-6）。

卡维地洛，一种非选择性β受体阻滞剂，也具有抗α受体和抗氧化剂的功能。1094例心功能Ⅲ到Ⅳ级、射血分数少于35%的心衰患者被随机分成卡维地洛组或安慰剂加传统治疗组，研究发现卡维地洛显著降低死亡率65%。这个试验的局限性在于预先随机抽样筛选阶段排除了不能耐受这种药物的病人以及收集的数据来自4个不同的试验设计。近来的一个比较卡维地洛和美托洛尔的小型试验未能发现两者在短期改善心功能和血流动力学终点方面存在着差异[21]。MERIT-HF研究将3991例射血分数等于或小于40%且NHYAⅡ~Ⅳ级的心衰病人随机分成美托洛尔组或安慰剂加传统治疗组。在美托洛尔治疗的病人中，全因死亡率在21个月显著地减少了34%，在有无冠心病病人中全因死亡率分别减少40%和30%。心衰相关的死亡减少了49%，心源性猝死减少了41%。在CIBIS Ⅱ研究中，2647例射血分数少于35%且NHYAⅢ、Ⅳ级的病人随机分成比索洛尔组或安慰剂加血管紧张素转换酶抑制剂和利尿剂组。在随访的1.3年内，其全因死亡率显著地减少了34%，主要是1.3年后猝死的死亡率减少了44%，这一结果最终使试验提前终止。

这三个试验结果惊人地相似，显示了卡维地洛显著地减少死亡率可能是多重作用而不是孤立地作用于单一受体，而且进一步增加所有充血性心力衰竭病人应该联合应用血管紧张素转换酶抑制剂和β受体阻滞剂的证据（表62-3）。

（三）抗心律失常药物

CAST试验导致了重新评估经典抗心律失常药物在室性早搏病人中所扮演的角色。特别是恩卡胺、氟卡胺、安慰剂对心梗后伴有室性异位激动和左室功能障碍的病人抑制室性早搏后所带来存活率的益处。这个实验很早提前终止，因为恩卡胺和氟卡胺治疗组心律失常和全因死亡率明显地增加。

表62-3 β受体阻滞剂在充血性心力衰竭作用的三个前瞻性随机化试验的结果

总病人和扩张型心肌病病人的例数	入选标准	药物	相对危险度的减少量（%）		
			总死亡（TD）	猝死（SD）	充血性心力衰竭死亡（CHFD）
Carvediol HFSG, 1094 (570)	NYHA Ⅱ~Ⅳ, (52%) EF≤35%	卡维地洛 3.125~50mg 2次/日	65%	55%	79%
CIBIS Ⅱ, 2647 (317)	NYHA Ⅲ~Ⅳ, (12%) EF≤35%	比索洛尔 1.25~10mg/d	34%	44%	26%
MERIT-HF, 3991 (1385)	NYHA Ⅱ~Ⅳ, (35%) EF≤40%	美托洛尔 12.5~25mg/d	34%	41%	49%

Carvediol HFSG, 卡维地洛心衰群组研究；CHFD, 充血性心力衰竭死亡；CIBIS Ⅱ, 心脏功能不全比索洛尔研究；EF, 射血分数；MERIT-HF, 充血性心力衰竭美托洛尔CR/XL随机化干预试验；NYHA, 纽约心脏协会心功能分级；SD, 猝死；TD, 总死亡。

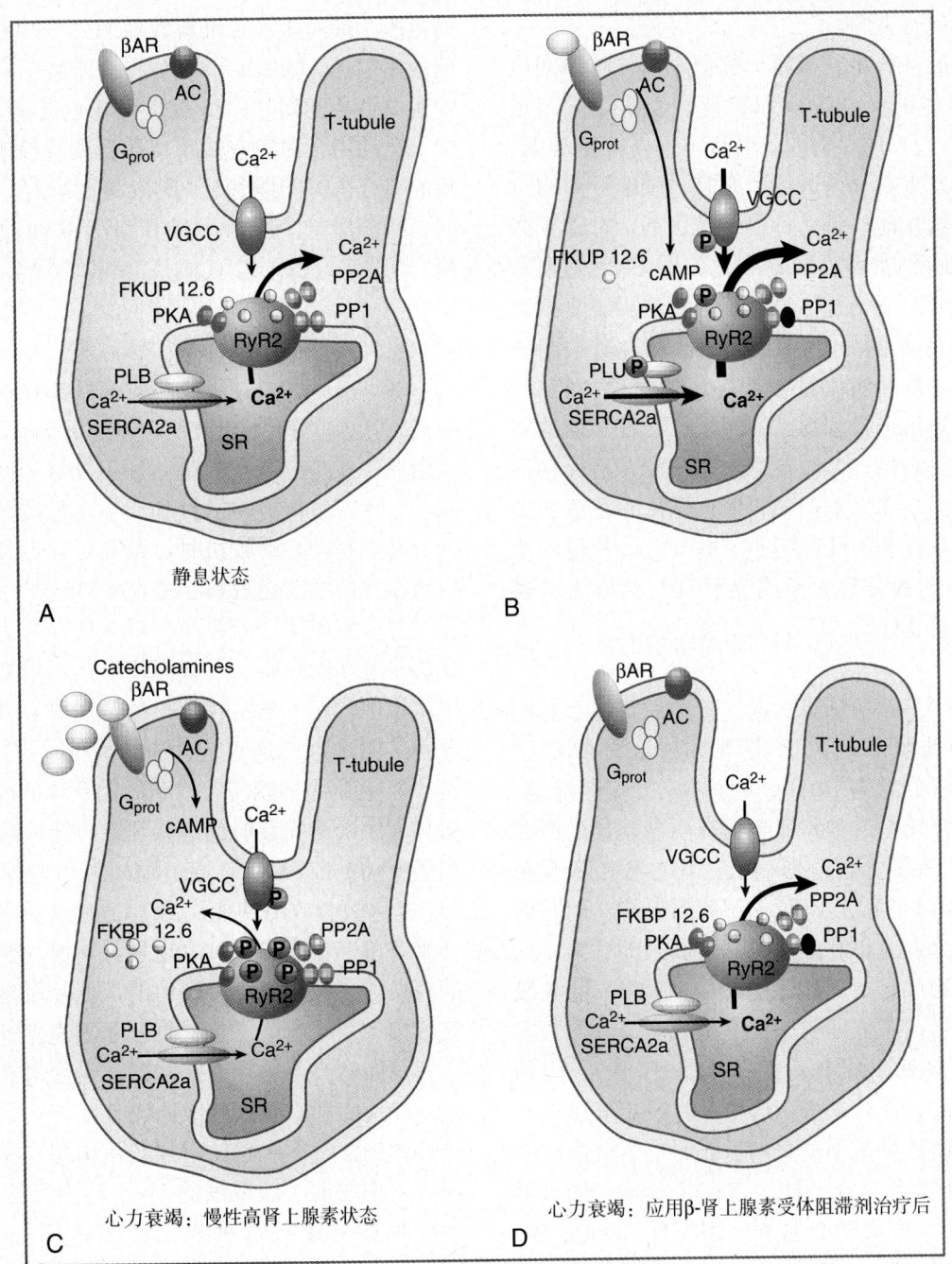

图 62-6 儿茶酚胺诱发的多形性室速 持续的肾上腺素刺激通过 β 肾上腺素受体（β-AR）导致了兰尼丁受体 2（RyR2）动力学的正向改变和舒张期钙泄漏返回至胞质导致了早期后除极和室性期前收缩。这些钙泄漏能被 β 受体阻滞剂减少，通过抑制腺苷酸环化酶（AC）介导的 cAMP 的产生和减少兰尼丁受体 2 的激活。已确定的突变包括肌集钙蛋白 2 基因上的 P2328S，Q4201R，V4653F。Gprot，G 蛋白；PLB，肌浆网磷酸受纳蛋白；SR，肌浆网；VGCC，电压依赖钙通道；T-tubule，T 管；PKA，蛋白激酶 A。

虽然 CAST 试验没有特别地关注扩张型心肌病病人，但它的结果迫使人们重新评估心室功能损害病人的抗心律失常治疗。它很好地建立了一个概念：抗心律失常药物有潜在的致心律失常作用。在 CAST 试验中，与射血分数大于 30% 的病人相比，主要的致心律失常作用在射血分数小于 30% 的病人更易发生。大多数传统的抗心律失常药物能加剧左室功能障碍，特别是丙吡胺和氟卡胺。威胁生命的并发症，包括充血性心力衰竭和导致的心律失常，经常发生在心室功能很弱的病人。最后，对于使用抗心律失常药物治疗的扩张型心肌病病人，没有研究表明猝死的发生率减少。对于这类人群，经验性传统抗心律失常治疗没能证明是有益，甚至是有害的。

一个可能的例外是胺碘酮。数据表明，胺碘酮可以减少病人群体的室性早搏和猝死的发生。低剂量（典型是200mg/d）明显有效，而且不损害心室功能，同时副作用的发生率显著减少。并且，胺碘酮具有抗肾上腺素效应的功能，是一种血管扩张剂，对于扩张型心肌病病人特别有益。Neri和他的同事[21a]发现在64例扩张型心肌病病人中，胺碘酮显著减少了复杂室性心律失常和猝死的发生。一半的病人出现了副作用，但仅仅9.8%的病人是必须终止治疗的。相反，虽然病人不是随机选择，在232例需行心脏移植的特发性扩张型心肌病病人，胺碘酮治疗并没有延长存活率。与传统的抗心律失常药物相似，恶化的左室功能使胺碘酮的有效性和耐受性减少。De Paola和他的伙伴[22]证明左室射血分数大于或等于30%的病人胺碘酮的有效性和耐受性为80%，而射血分数小于30%的则为60%。

CHF：STAT试验随机入选674例症状性心衰病人，将室性期前收缩超过9次/h和射血分数小于40%的病人随机分配至300mg/d胺碘酮或安慰剂组。在两组之间，总死亡率和猝死率没有明显差异。但在193例（29%）非缺血性心肌病人，其总死亡率有减少的趋势（$P=0.07$）。GESICA试验入选516例有症状性充血性心力衰竭和射血分数小于35%的病人，并且在三联药物治疗前提下将病人随机分成300mg/d胺碘酮或安慰剂组，研究证明，胺碘酮治疗组总死亡率下降了28%，猝死率减少了27%（$P=0.16$）。因为冠状动脉造影没有常规进行，这个试验中非缺血性心肌病病人的准确数量是不清楚的。然而，非缺血性心肌病病人的比例也许大于CHF：STAT试验，因为至少20%是特发性扩张型心肌病，10%有Chagas病，支持了对于非缺血性心肌病病人，胺碘酮能有效地减少死亡率的结论。

（四）永久性起搏

短AV间期的双心室起搏已经用于终末期扩张型心肌病病人的治疗。在一个小样本人群，它已经被证明提高了NHYA分级和射血分数，缩小了左室内径、提高了运动耐量和最大氧耗量。导致这些改变的机制是多因素的，而且可能和下列因素相关：（1）消除了二尖瓣、三尖瓣反流的期前收缩成分，改善了心室的充盈量，因而增加了每搏量，改善心输出量；（2）保持心房、心室收缩的同步；（3）增加了舒张期和收缩期血压，提高血管紧张素转换酶抑制剂和β受体阻滞剂使用剂量。Brecker和助手[23]证实了当使用一个非常短的AV间期时，12例扩张型心肌病病人血流动力学、运动耐量和房室瓣膜反流得到急性改善（反流导致心室充盈时间缩短）。反流程度减轻，而且充盈时间、心输出量、运动耐量和最大氧耗量有显著的提高。

（五）双心室起搏

30%～50%的扩张型心肌病病人存在心室内传导障碍，导致QRS间期延长，超过120ms，通常是左束支阻滞。左室游离壁的激动延迟导致与间隔收缩的不同步，使左室每搏输出量和心输出量的减少。除此之外，特别是在心率较快时，激动延迟导致舒张期延迟以致左室的主动充盈和心房收缩同时进行。

双心室起搏已经在几个对充血性心力衰竭伴有严重的左室功能障碍、心室内传导延迟的病人前瞻性随机试验中得到了证实[24,25]。最初左室心外膜起搏需要开胸，但是近来通过应用冠状窦来行左室心外膜起搏[24]。特别是冠状窦导线和传送系统的改进对于大多数病人来讲使安装时间缩短到1～2h。起搏使左室游离壁激动提前：（1）通过缩短机械收缩时间和提高dP/dt来改善收缩功能；（2）通过延长舒张期充盈时间来改善舒张功能；（3）通过提前激动侧壁乳头肌来减轻期前二尖瓣反流。最初的证据显示这些并没有对交感神经系统有负性作用[26]。虽然左室dP/dt和全部心室功能的改善是令人鼓舞的，是否潜在地增加了左室室壁应力和心肌氧耗量同时伴随有害的作用，如室性心律失常发作次数的增加仍不清楚。实际上，猝死的发生率在植入后观察的16个月内高达33%，促使一些观察者建议这种病人应植入双心室起搏除颤器。

到目前公布的9个前瞻性随机试验一致证明了双心室起搏对急性血流动力学[28]、左室dP/dt[29]、左室射血分数[30]、NHYA分级[31]和6分钟步行时间[31,32]的改善，同时使心衰患者住院次数减少。而且在一个研究中，双心室起搏植入1年后医疗费用显著减少。当这些实验结果被统一分析时，在那些随机化分配到双心室起搏的病人中，其死亡率并没有显著减少的趋势，这有可能是入选标准和研究设计的差异所致，这些结论需要小心地对待。除此之外，对于那些被随机分配到双心室起搏加ICD治疗的病人，其ICD电击的次数、要求治疗的次数、非持续性室性室速发作的次数减少了。虽然这些结果是令人鼓舞的,但这种技术的广泛应用将由一项正在进行的观察总死亡率和症状性和功能性终点的前瞻性随机试验的结果决定。

因为在1年内发生泵衰竭的可能性极大,NYHA Ⅳ级心衰病人曾经被认为是ICD植入的禁忌证(除了作为心脏移植的过渡)。因此,双心室起搏将似乎可能是年龄较高不能考虑心脏移植的心衰患者最合适的治疗,然而双心室起搏也许对年轻患者更合适。对于双心室起搏能否持久地改善心衰症状使NHYA分级小于Ⅲ级,特别是能否阻止泵衰竭导致的死亡,需要重新评估。后者在近来完成的COMPANION试验中被部分地强调,该研究显示心功能Ⅲ～Ⅳ级、QRS波时限大于120ms,PR间期大于150ms,射血分数小于35%的病人,双心室起搏加ICD治疗与单用双心室起搏治疗和优化的药物治疗相比,能够显著减少死亡率。与优化的药物治疗相比,单用双心室起搏治疗,可减少死亡率以及住院时间。进一步了解这些问题等待COMPANION研究结果的公布和正在进行的CARE-HF研究的完成。

(六) 植入式心脏复律除颤器

最近10年,ICD的应用经历了一个指数级的增长。已经证明它是一个重要的终止威胁生命的室速或室颤以及预防猝死的装置。技术的发展已从最初需要开胸放置的电击盒,不能或提供很少的诊断信息发展到高度精致的计算机芯片,通过传感器来记录详细的事件并可提供多种特别加强的功能,包括双心室起搏、电图宽度和形态分析、心率稳定性等参数。这些进步,伴随着经静脉系统电极的植入、双线圈导线和小型脉冲发生器的问世,ICD已成为一种越来越令人感兴趣的治疗选择。

在8项针对ICD治疗的前瞻性随机试验中,AVID[33]、CIDS和CASH是二级预防试验,试验对象包括非缺血性心肌病病人。在这些试验中,关于非缺血性亚组的数据只能从AVID中获得。在AVID试验中,162例无冠心病病人(并不是所有都是扩张型心肌病)中,77例被随机分配至传统药物治疗组,75例被分配至ICD植入组来治疗心脏骤停或持续性室性心动过速,心脏骤停或持续性室性心动过速是威胁生命的。在ICD治疗组,总死亡率下降了(1年为9% *vs.* 12%,2年为11% *vs.* 18%,3年为14% *vs.* 38%)。生存曲线在早期就发生了偏离,而且一直持续到为期约3.5年随访期的终末阶段(图62-7)。近来公布的MADIT Ⅱ试验已经澄清了缺血性心肌病病人预防性使用ICD的观念。在MADIT Ⅱ试验中,与最佳药物治疗组包括β受体阻滞剂和血管紧张素转换酶抑制剂相比,随机分配到ICD组(加上最佳药物治疗)射血分数小于30%且先前有心肌梗死的病人,3年后其总死亡率减少了31%。对于非缺血性扩张型心肌病病人来说,这些将同样是正确的,但明确的结论需等待正在进行的SCD-HeFT、AMIVIRT、DEFINITE、DEBUT、PRIDE和CAT研究结果的公布。

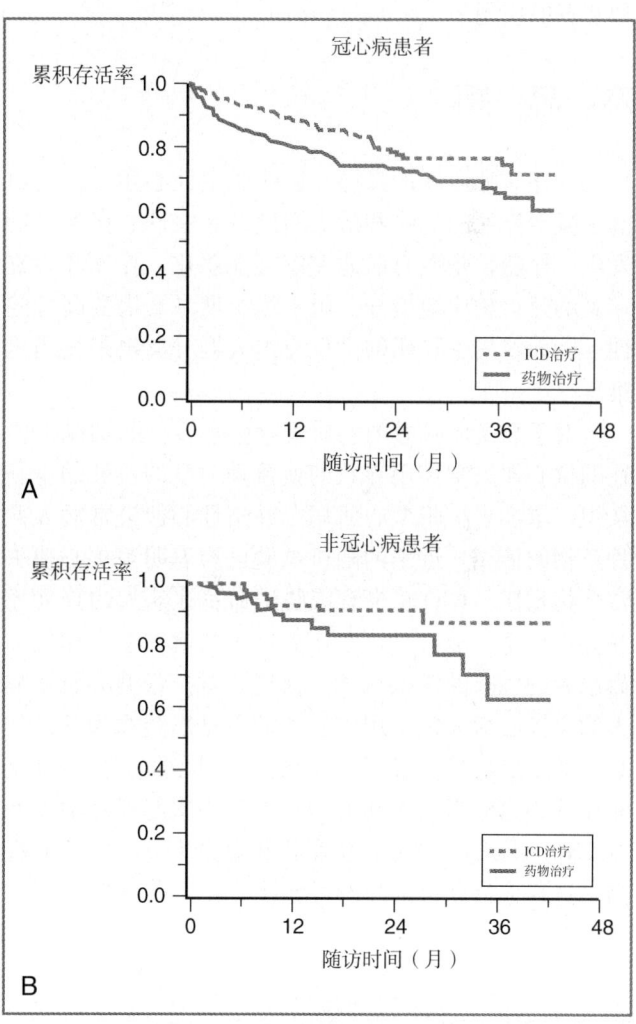

图62-7 在AVID试验中随机分配至ICD或传统治疗组的扩张型心肌病病人死亡K-M分析的自由度 ICD:植入式心律复律除颤器(引自Steinberg JS, Ehlert FA, Cannon DS, et al: Dilated cardiomyopathy vs. coronary artery diease in patients with VT/VF: Differences in presentation and outcome in the antiarrhythmics versus implantable defibrillators [AVID] registry.)[abstract] Circulation 96:1-715,1997.)

(七) 左室辅助装置

左室辅助装置在治疗终末期心衰方面是一项最新的进展。先前主要仅仅被用于心脏移植病人的院内过渡治疗,现在许多病人一直在院外应用,作为即将进行的 HeartMate 和 AbioCor 心室电植入性装置的临床试验一部分[34]。一些安有心室辅助装置的病人对室性心律失常的耐受性大大增加了,因为心输出量是由装置而不是心室决定的。但那些心室功能低下的病人和室颤的病人使用左室辅助装置后可能导致了重要的血流动力学损害。由于它的花费、经皮的动力和驱动的电线感染的危险以及系统性血栓栓塞的危险限制了这种装置的应用。

六、总 结

治疗非缺血性扩张型心肌病和室性心律失常的目的是减少猝死的危险和最大限度减轻室性心律失常的发生。伴随扩张型心肌病左室功能恶化,猝死和心衰相关的死亡相应地增加。由于终末期泵衰竭的高危险性,因而将发生猝死的高危亚组人群分离出来相当困难。

对于β受体阻滞剂和血管紧张素转换酶抑制剂潜在的抗心律失常作用导致的血流动力学的益处的重新认识,增加了扩张型心肌病合并室性心律失常病人两种药物的使用。近来的随机试验已经表明与抗心律失常药物相比,ICD 减少有威胁生命室速病人的猝死率和总死亡率。随着对抗心律失常药物增加左室功能障碍患者的危险的深入认识,促进了对扩张型心肌病病人的室性心律失常采用以装置而不是以药物为基础的治疗的发展趋势。最后,对于扩张型心肌病合并重度充血性心力衰竭病人新的治疗如双心室起搏除颤器和左室辅助装置可改善心衰症状和提高生存率,从而提高对选择人群联合治疗的可能性。

(郑强苏 译)

参 考 文 献

1. Towbin JA, Bowles NE: The failing heart. Nature 415:227–233, 2002.
2. Olson TM, Michels VV, Thibodeau SN, et al: Actin mutations in dilated cardiomyopathy, a heritable form of heart failure. Science 280:750–752, 1998.
3. Li D, Tapscoft T, Gonzalez O, et al: Desmin mutations responsible for idiopathic dilated cardiomyopathy. Circulation 100:461–464, 1999.
4. Barresi R, Di Blasi C, Negri T, et al: Disruption of heart sarcoglycan complex and severe cardiomyopathy caused by β-sarcoglycan mutations. J Med Genet 37:102–107, 2000.
5. Tsubata S, Bowles KR, Vatta M, et al: Mutations in the human δ-sarcoglycan gene in familial and sporadic dilated cardiomyopathy. J Clin Invest 106:655–662, 2000.
6. Kamisago M, Sharma SD, DePalma SR, et al: Mutations in sarcomeric protein genes as a cause of dilated cardiomyopathy. N Engl J Med 343:1688–1696, 2000.
7. Olson TM, Kishimoto NY, Whitby FG, Michels VV: Mutations that alter the surface change of α-tropomyosin are associated with dilated cardiomyopathy. J Mol Cell Cardiol 33:723–732, 2001.
8. Kass S, MacRae C, Graber HL, et al: A gene defect that causes conduction system disease and dilated cardiomyopathy maps to chromosome 1p1-1q1. Nat Genet 7:546–551, 1994.
9. Jung M, Poepping I, Perrot A, et al: Investigation of a family with autosomal dominant dilated cardiomyopathy defines a novel locus on chromosome 2q14-q22. Am J Hum Genet 65:1068–1077, 1999.
10. Olson TM, Keating MT: Mapping a cardiomyopathy locus to chromosome 3p22-p25. J Clin Invest 97:528–532, 1996.
11. Messina DN, Speer MC, Pericak-Vance MA, McNally EM: Linkage of familial dilated cardiomyopathy with conduction defect and muscular dystrophy to chromosome 6q23. Am J Hum Genet 61:909–917, 1997.
12. Brodsky GL, Muntoni F, Miocic S, et al: Lamin A/C gene mutation associated with dilated cardiomyopathy with variable skeletal muscle involvement. Circulation 101:473-476, 2000.
13. Berko BA, Swift M: X-linked dilated cardiomyopathy. N Engl J Med 316:1186–1191, 1987.
14. Towbin JA, Hejtmancik JF, Brink P, et al: X-linked cardiomyopathy (XLCM): Molecular genetic evidence of linkage to the Duchenne muscular dystrophy gene at the Xp21 locus. Circulation 87:1854–1865, 1993.
14a. Luu M, Stevenson WG, et al: Diverse mechanisms of unexpected cardiac arrest in advanced heart failure. Circulation 80:1675–1680, 1989.
14b. DeMaria R, Gavazzi A, Caroli A, et al: Ventricular arrhythmias in dilated cardiomyopathy as an independent prognostic hallmark. Am J Cardiol 69:1451–1457, 1992.
14c. Romeo F, Pelliccia F, Cianfrocca C, et al: Predictors of sudden death in idiopathic dilated cardiomyopathy. Am J Cardiol 63:138–140, 1989.
14d. Poll DS, Marchilinski FE, Falcone RA, et al: Abnormal signal-averaged electrocardiograms in patients with nonischemic congestive cardiomyopathy: Relationship to sustained ventricular arrhythmias. Circulation 72:1308–1313, 1985.
14e. Hoffmann J, Grimm W, Menz V, et al: Heart rate variability and major arrhythmic events in patients with idiopathic dilated cardiomyopathy. Pacing Clin Electrophysiol 19(II):1841–1844, 1996.
14f. Fei L, Anderson MH, Katritsis D, et al: Decreased heart rate variability in survivors of sudden cardiac death not associated with coronary artery disease. Br Heart J 71:16–21, 1994.
15. Grimm W, Steder U, Menz V, et al: Clinical significance of increased QT dispersion in the standard 12-lead ECG for arrhythmia prediction in dilated cardiomyopathy. Pacing Clin Electrophysiol 19(11 pt 2):1886–1889, 1996.
16. Adachi K, Ohnishi Y, Shima T, et al: Determinant of microvolt T wave alternans in patients with dilated cardiomyopathy. J Am Coll Cardiol 34:374–380, 1999.
17. Kitamura H, Ohnishi Y, Okajima K, et al: Onset heart rate of microvolt T wave alternans provides clinical and prognostic value in nonischemic dilated cardiomyopathy. J Am Coll Cardiol 39:295–300, 2002.
18. Pitt B, Segal R, Martinez FA, et al: Randomised trial of losartan versus captopril in patients over 65 with heart failure (Evaluation of Losartan in the Elderly Study, ELITE). Lancet 349(9054):747–752, 1997.
19. Pitt B, Poole-Wilson PA, Segal R, on behalf of the ELITE II Investigators: Effect of losartan compared with captopril on mortality in patients with symptomatic heart failure: Randomised trial-the Losartan Heart Failure Survival Study ELITE II. Lancet 355(9215):1582–1587, 2000.
19a. Waagstein F, Hjalmarson A, Varnauskas E, Wallentin F: Effect of chronic beta adrenergic receptor blockade in congestive cardiomy-

opathy. Br Heart J 37:1022–1036, 1975
20. Marks AR, Reiken S, Marx SO: Progression of heart failure: Is protein kinase a hyperphosphorylation of the ryanodine receptor a contributing factor? Circulation 105:272–275, 2002.
21. Kukin ML, Kalman J, Buccholz-Varley C, et al: A direct comparison of carvedilol and metoprolol in CHF. Circulation 8(I):577, 1997.
21a. Neri R, Mestroni L, Salvi A, et al: Ventricular arrhythmias in dilated cardiomyopathy: Efficacy of amiodarone. Am Heart J 113:707–715, 1987.
22. DePaola AAV, Horowitz LN, Spielman SR, et al: Development of congestive heart failure and alterations in left ventricular function in patients with sustained ventricular arrhythmias treated with amiodarone. Am J Cardiol 60:276–280, 1987.
23. Brecker SJD, Xiao HB, Sparrow J, et al: Effects of dual chamber pacing with short atrioventricular delay in dilated cardiomyopathy. Lancet 340:1308–1312, 1992.
24. Gras D, Mabo P, Tang T, et al: Multisite pacing as a supplemental treatment of congestive heart failure: Preliminary results of the Medtronic Inc. InSync study. Pacing Clin Electrophysiol 21(pt 2):2249–2255, 1998.
25. Krahnfeld O, Vogt J, Tenderich G, et al, on behalf of the Path-CHF study group: Changes in QRS duration in patients with biventricular pacing system for congestive heart failure treatment and clinical outcome. Pacing Clin Electrophysiol 22(pt 2):733, 1999.
26. Saxon L, DeMarco T, Chaterjee K, et al, for the Vigor and Ventak-CHF investigators: Chronic biventricular pacing decreases serum norepinephrine in dilated heart failure patients with the greatest sympathetic activation at baseline. Pacing Clin Electrophysiol 22(pt 2):830, 1999.
27. Leclerq C, Cazeau S, Alonso C, et al: Multisite pacing in advanced heart failure. Current status of the French pilot study. Pacing Clin Electrophysiol 22(pt 2):733, 1999.
28. Daubert JC, Ritter P, Le Breton H, et al: Permanent left ventricular pacing with transvenous leads inserted into the coronary veins. Pacing Clin Electrophysiol 21(1 pt 2):239–245, 1998.
29. Aurrichio A, Salo R: Acute hemodynamic improvement by pacing in patients with severe congestive heart failure. Pacing Clin Electrophysiol 20(pt 1):313–324, 1997.
30. Aurrichio A, Ding J, Kramer A, et al: Acute response of heart failure is best at specific left ventricular pacing sites. Circulation 17:I–302, 1998.
31. Alonso C, Lavergne T, Ritter P, et al: Evolution of electrical and mechanical interventricular synchronization during long-term biventricular pacing. Pacing Clin Electrophysiol 22(pt 2):732, 1999.
32. Klug D, Jarwe M, Lacroix D, et al: Outcome in intention to treat with a biventricular pacing system for severe heart failure. Comparison of monoventricular and biventricular pacing. J Am Coll Cardiol 33:125A, 1998.
33. Zipes DP, Wyse DG, Friedman PL, et al, on behalf of the AVID Investigators: A comparison of antiarrhythmic drug therapy with implantable defibrillators in patients resuscitated from near-fatal ventricular arrhythmias. N Engl J Med 337:1576–1583, 1997.
34. Poirier VL: The HeartMate left ventricular assist system: Worldwide clinical results. Eur J Cardiothorac Surg 11:S39–S44, 1997.

第 63 章

致心律失常性右室心肌病的室性心动过速

Guy Fontaine，Paul Fornes，Jean-Louis Hebert，Catherine Prost-Squarcioni，Xavier Jouven，Jean-Sébastien Hulot，Robert Frank，and Daniel Thomas

本章目录

- 右室心肌病的临床分型 ········· 581
- 非冠状动脉性右室心前区 ST 段抬高（Brugada 综合征） ········· 587
- 鉴别诊断 ········· 588
- 致心律失常性右室心肌病室性心动过速的治疗 ········· 589
- 总结 ········· 590
- 致谢 ········· 590

外科手术治疗室性心动过速引起了对致心律失常性右室发育不良（arrhythmogenic right ventricular dysplasia，ARVD）这一疾病的认识[1]。

时光荏苒，越来越多的顽固性室性心动过速的年轻患者被检出。这些患者有着特殊的解剖结构，其右室表面覆盖着脂肪，并在游离壁上记录到延迟电位。此外，这些年轻患者的心脏其他方面检查均正常，无冠状动脉疾病[2]。因为缺乏特殊的病理标志以迅速作出阳性诊断，故提出了一套主要和次要诊断标准，以对家系中的先证者和家族成员进行诊断。

该疾病被归于心肌病的一个新类型。1996 年，致心律失常性右室心肌病（arrhythmogenic right ventricular cardiomyopathy，ARVC）被国际心脏联盟协会（International Society and Federation of Cardiology，ISFC，现已更名为世界心脏联盟）和世界卫生组织（World Health Organization，WHO）加入到修订版心肌病范畴中[3]。致心律失常性右室心肌病包含了一组不同名称和原发表现不同的疾病。基于我们近 300 例患者的经验，参考大多数国际心脏联盟协会专家的共识，我们提出了致心律失常性右室心肌病的分类[4]。此外，我们历时 27 年从法、美、加、日、澳等 7 个国家收集了 89 例患者的组织样本。绝大部分患者的基本组织结构相同，但由于基因异质性而表现为不同的临床表现和结局。在临床患者中，我们选择了 163 例患者，代表单纯、严重而复杂的致心律失常性右室心肌病类型，对他们进行长期临床跟踪和随访，获得了大量具有统计价值的数据。

然而，在未对心脏进行全面的病理检查或得到特异的遗传标记之前，很难对此病作出明确的诊断。我们的经验是，除非是那些在复查时问题明显加重的病人，否则预测病人的结局亦很困难。环境因素及可能的遗传学影响很可能在这些不同的临床模式中起一定作用。

在本书的前几版中，我们描述了典型致心律失常性右室心肌病患者室性心动过速的特点[5]。在本章，我们将集中探讨涉及不同室性心律失常的右室心肌病的不同形式，尤其是这些不同形式的右室心肌病患者伴发的室性心动过速。

一、右室心肌病的临床分型

（一）单纯孤立性致心律失常性右室发育不良

1. 遗传学

典型的致心律失常性右室发育不良是在生命的早期阶段（可能是胚胎时期）由基因所决定的发育不良，为常染色体显性遗传。根据分子失效技术（molecular invalidation techniques）推测，致心律失常性右室心肌病可能是转录因子 dHAND[6]或人类 ALP 蛋白等位基因突变的结果[7]。这些蛋白主要控制心脏右室的发育。

2. 自然病史

对一例 27 周的胎儿在宫腔内观察到右室动脉瘤和心律失常，尸检示心肌被脂肪浸润，但无纤维化或炎性征象，引起了我们的关注[4]。然而，极少有致心律失常性右室发育不良的儿童病例报告。在潜伏期内常仅表现为心电图异常，早期的临床表现通常是在成年期出现源于右心室的室性心律失常（平均年龄 32 岁，范围 10 岁～76 岁）。在绝大部分病人，各种类型室性心律失常均可出现，包括单发室早、二联律和三联律室早、非持续性和持续性室速。室速多呈左束支阻滞形，偶可呈右束支阻滞形。如心动过速起源于漏斗部，心电轴可不偏或右偏。当心动过速起源于右心室心尖部或膈面，电轴常呈极度左偏。

在我们的病例中，43%的患者出现快速而不能耐受的室速或心脏骤停。意外死亡或猝死也可能是本病的首发表现[2]。在有些患者，室速的临床症状可不表现为"心悸"，而表现为头晕、不适、乏力、出汗、恶心或胃肠道症状。

一例发生猝死的患者，心电图记录到其猝死是由多形性室速引起的心室颤动所致[8]。患者心电图呈右束支阻滞图形，右胸导联 ST 段抬高，QRS 波时限离散明显[5]。致心律失常性右室心肌发育不良被越来越多的病理学家和法医学专家所诊断。但在普通人群中，致心律失常性右室心肌发育不良的流行病学尚不清楚[9]。

接受常规药物治疗后，在接下来的 8.1±7.4 年（平均 6.6 年）中，心源性死亡的发生率为每年 2.3%。这些死亡中的 2/3，即每年 1.5%是发生在 52±19 岁的年龄段，而 60±16 岁年龄段的患者多死于心力衰竭。

3. 致心律失常性右室发育不良的大体组织形态

致心律失常性右室发育不良的心脏大体形态包括右心室扩大和前壁漏斗部、心尖部及后下壁（发育不良三角）的膨突。大部分右室心肌被脂肪组织取代[1]。造影结果表明，约 2/3 的患者存在右心室扩大。

4. 致心律失常性右室发育不良的典型组织形态

致心律失常性右室发育不良的典型组织形态是右室心肌的中层或外层，以及小范围的左室心肌（尤其是心尖部分）被脂肪组织和纤维组织所取代，其内夹杂着条索状或片状心肌细胞，是致心律失常性右室发育不良中的最严重类型[10,11]。

冠状动脉远端中膜增厚也许可解释我们的病例中约 1/3 患者出现非典型胸痛。这种组织学形态与在肥厚型心肌病中检出的小血管病变相似。以前从未见到有关胸痛发作的描述，因为致心律失常性右室发育不良患者绝大多数为年轻人，且在常规冠状动脉造影检查时很少发现冠状动脉受累。在我们报告的系列中，仅 5 例患者有明显的冠状动脉疾病，1 例患者发生左室下壁心肌梗死。因此，现在已将与体力无关的不典型胸痛和夜间胸痛认为是致心律失常性右室发育不良的其他标志性特征。致心律失常性右室发育不良与 X 综合征的关系尚不很清楚，小的冠状血管异常在室性心动过速的发生或维持中是否起一定作用还不清楚。

由于左室很少累及，故左室心力衰竭很少见。然而，在疾病发展的过程中，左室受累是一个转折点，对这些病人必须加强随访，以防止发生双心室心力衰竭。

（二）主要累及右心室的致心律失常性右室发育不良

1. 右室心力衰竭

在我们的病例中，6%的患者以右心衰竭作为本病的最初症状，而不伴任何类型室性心律失常。然而在随访期的后半程，由于疾病的进展及其他因素的影响，24%的致心律失常性右室发育不良患者存在右心衰竭，不论其是否与包括室速在内的室性心律失常有关。严重的右心室扩大可导致植入式心脏复律除颤器

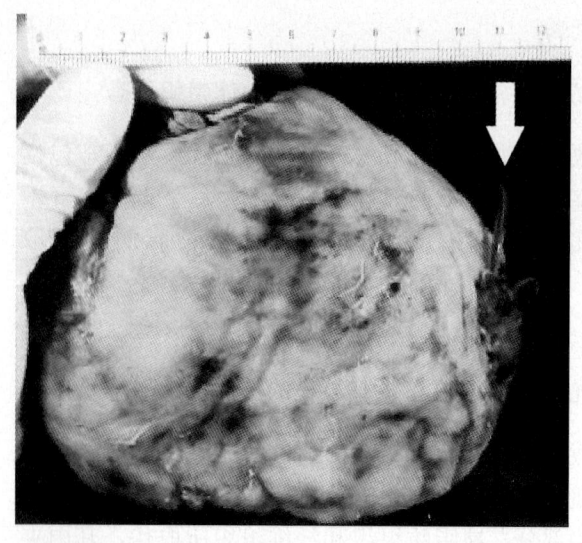 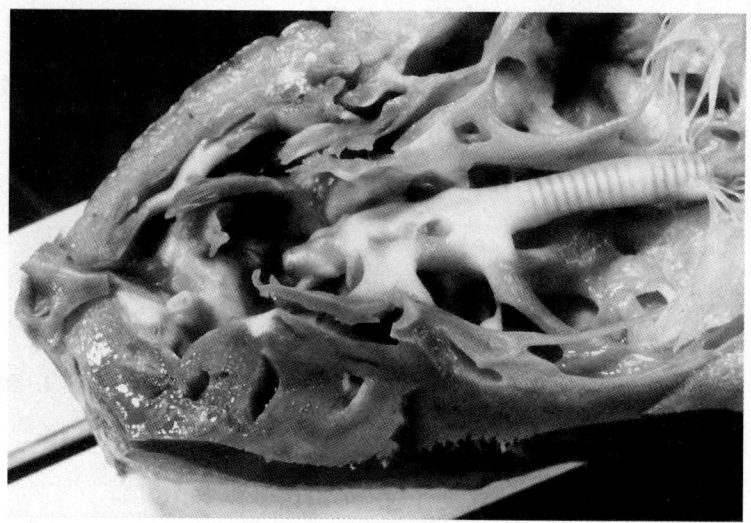

图63-1 右心室严重扩张 左图：一例典型致心律失常性右室发育不良患者进行心脏移植后切下的严重扩张的右心室。可见心肌被脂肪覆盖。箭头所示为因ICD心内膜电极感知不良而置入的心外膜电极。右图：感知不良系由于主动固定电极顶端已不再与心内膜接触，很可能是右心室扩张导致电极导管移位。ICD的"自动增益控制"功能导致不适当放电。（见彩图28）

(implantable cardioverter defibrillator，ICD) 感知不良（图63-1）。

2. Uhl畸形

这种极其罕见的畸形出现在两个年龄组，有着明显不同的临床和病理特征。Uhl畸形常在早年发生充血性心力衰竭并在数周或数月后死亡。在成人组，死亡常由充血性心衰或持续性室性心律失常引发心室颤动所致。Uhl畸形常表现为巨大而近乎透明的右室游离壁（图63-2），脂肪组织在心内膜至心外膜沉积，其内无心肌组织嵌入。在有些病人，畸形仅局限于右室游离壁上的一小部分区域，偶尔可在尸检中发现。因此，Uhl畸形并不代表致心律失常性右室发育不良的晚期形式。

然而近年研究提示，Uhl畸形和致心律失常性右室发育不良可能有着相似的发病机理。Uhl畸形似乎是由于右室心肌广泛和完全凋亡的破坏所致，相反，致心律失常性右室发育不良可能是由于在一段长时间内局灶病变的不断进展所致[12]。

3. 类似Uhl畸形的右室发育不良

这种情况出现于儿童患者，临床表现与典型的Uhl畸形相似，右室极度扩张伴充血性心衰。在心脏移植后进行的组织病理学检查发现右室扩大，右室游离壁非常薄，包含在脂肪的纤维化组织中有存活心肌束，以及炎症细胞浸润等。

（三）累及左室的致心律失常性右室心肌病

1. 单纯双心室发育不良

在单纯双心室发育不良患者，典型的致心律失常性右室发育不良的组织学结构可出现于左右两个心室。因此，左室游离壁也被脂肪组织替代，并有心肌细胞束被纤维组织包裹（图63-3）。然而，致心律失常性右室发育不良病变多始于中膜层，逐渐向心外膜发展。目前的资料表明，在双心室发育不良患者，心肌被纤维脂肪组织替代常始于心外膜层，且不规律地向心内膜发展。由于大量的心肌组织丢失，双心室发育不良可导致心脏功能衰退，并可能被误诊为原发性扩张型心肌病。然而，如发现左室脂肪浸润应不难得出正确的诊断。现今，通过核磁共振显像可能有助于作出此诊断[13]。在有些病人，室性心动过速呈右束支阻滞形态，尤其患者左室功能受损时，提示其发生可能与左室受累有关。

在一例因长期心律失常和心力衰竭进行心脏移植的患者，发现一种独特形式的发育不良变异型。病理检查表明右室心肌完全被脂肪替代，仅在非常细的纤维化边缘有极少量存活的心肌细胞束。左心室肌呈海绵状，大部分被脂肪组织取代，极度分裂了心室纤维。这例病人仅有极少的纤维化包绕的存活心肌，无炎性细胞浸润（图63-4）。据我们所知，文献中尚未见类似报道。

较差[14]。因为仅有极少数致心律失常性右室发育不良患者无炎症浸润，故可推论心肌炎可能加重了基因决定的致心律失常性右室发育不良结构背景。同卵双胞胎的疾病进程截然不同，进一步证实了这一推论，即遗传因素与环境因素共同作用影响疾病的进展过程。

这种炎症过程可由多种原因引起，如病毒、细菌、真菌、中毒、自身免疫等。它较局限，更多呈多灶性或弥散分布，尤其在急性型更是如此。最近的一项报告强调了可引起早期后除极电位的中性粒细胞的活化作用[15]。这些电位可能成为触发致心律失常的基质。心肌炎症可在不同的发展阶段出现，与各种各样的临床症状有关，也可从毫无症状到在数天内由于暴发性心力衰竭而死亡[16]。

事实上，慢性心肌炎症最常见到。其特征是淋巴细胞弥散分布在纤维组织中，两个心室均可出现。纤维化似乎更为严重，平均分布于两个心室。然而，致心律失常性右室发育不良的显著特征仍明显存在，即右心室被大量脂肪组织取代。据推测，心律失常可能是心肌结构异质性的结果。与左心室相比，这种异质性在右心室更为明显。

一般认为器质性心脏病患者比健康个体对心肌炎更加敏感。最近的两项有关运动员猝死的研究把各型心肌病与心肌炎单独进行分析，结果亦支持这一假设[17,18]。除分叶核中性粒细胞外，在典型致心律失常性右室心肌发育不良基因表型病人的心肌中，经常也可见淋巴细胞浸润。这可以归类为致心律失常性右室心肌发育不良的"慢性活动型"。不过，尚不清楚是否这些病人的疾病进展会更快，以及是否与更严重的室性心律失常有关。

如心肌炎累及双心室，充血性心力衰竭可使病人的年死亡率增高1%。在这种疾病的晚期，临床上很难鉴别是原发性扩张型心肌病还是致心律失常性右室发育不良[19]。

如果在非心律失常型发育不良的患者检出心肌炎，则致心律失常性右室发育不良的诊断将更加困难。因此，右室发育不良患者可出现临床显性或隐性心肌炎，以及与原发性扩张型心肌病类似的临床进展。右室游离壁镜下组织学检查可检出发育不良。然而，心肌炎的特征表现可使致心律失常性右室发育不良的诊断变得扑朔迷离，如果不是特意查找，往往易于漏诊[20]。

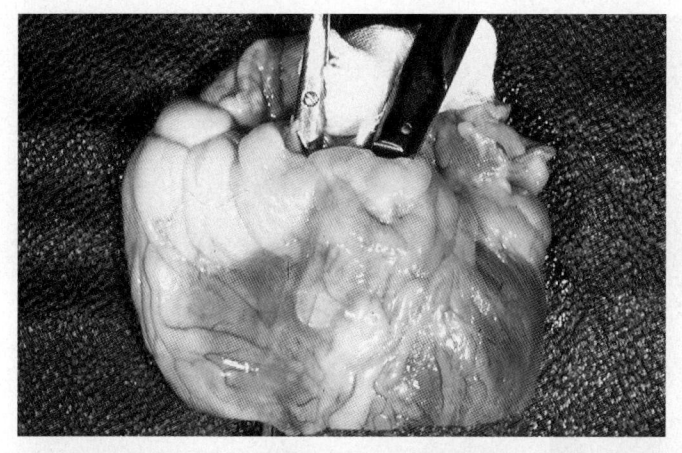
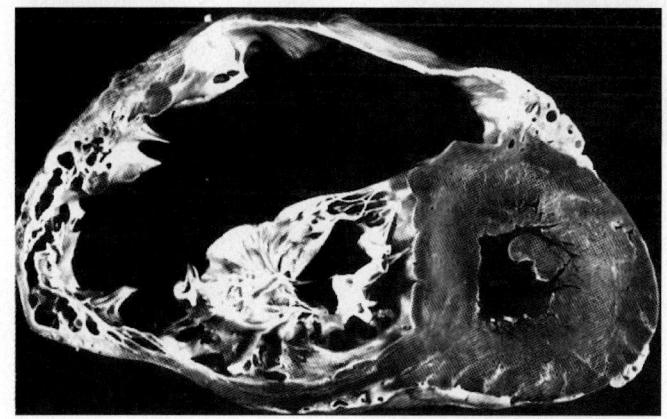
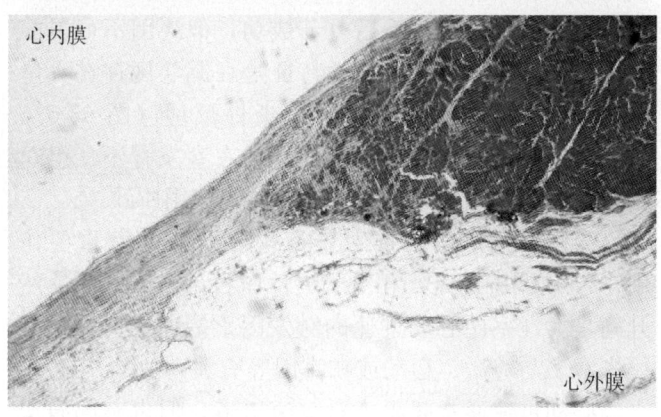

图 63-2　成人典型的 Uhl 畸形　上图：肺动脉内插入剪刀，可见右心室呈透明状。中图：在另一例患者，沿三尖瓣水平切片。可见左心室大小及室壁厚度正常。右心室明显扩张，室壁极度变薄，间隔前部尤为明显。下图："心肌突然断续"，代之以纤维化和脂肪组织。（见彩图 29）

2. 被心肌炎复杂化的发育不良

回顾性的病理分析证实，60%以上的发育不良患者存在炎症反应，因此更为复杂化[10]。心肌炎通常指急性炎症。在一小部分致心律失常性右室发育不良病人，大部分纤维组织被淋巴细胞浸润，提示曾发生过炎症反应。严重的心肌炎症可累及两个心室，且预后

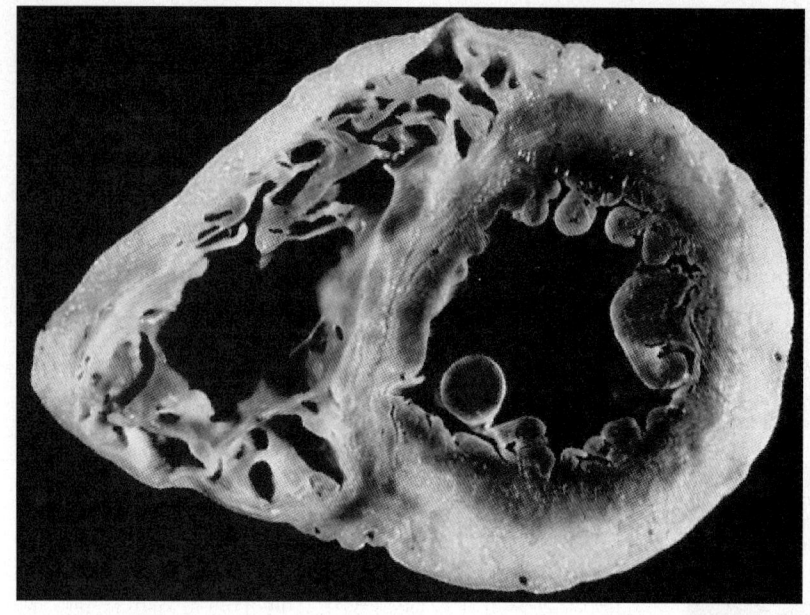
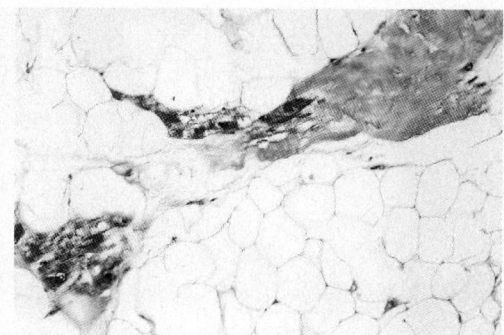
右室纤维组织
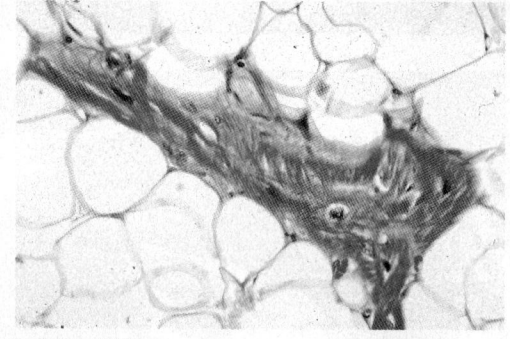
左室心肌细胞

图 63-3 双心室发育不良 患者左心室外壁与右心室一样，表现为同样的疾病过程，心肌被脂肪和纤维化所取代。在这些脂肪组织内可见存活的心肌细胞及纤维条索。（见彩图 30）

（四）右室流出道室性心动过速和良性室性期前收缩

这两种心律失常可能代表同一种疾病的两个不同阶段。右室流出道室性心动过速和良性室性期前收缩均起源于右室漏斗部，是无器质性心脏病患者较常见的心律失常，多在例行体检中发现，临床表现为左束支阻滞图形的单发室早或反复发作的非持续性室性心动过速，Ⅱ、Ⅲ、aVF 导联 QRS 波主波向上，常伴心悸等症状。在疾病的早期阶段，常仅表现为室性早搏。随着时间推移，单发室早逐渐频发，持续时间更长，且越来越明显。有些病人可表现为室早二联律。因血流动力学障碍日益加重而使症状变得明显，尤其是女性患者。女性的发病率是男性的两倍，与致心律失常性右室发育不良的性别分布恰相反。随着疾病的进展，室早变得更为频繁，出现二联律和三联律，并可出现典型的右室流出道室性心动过速。在最严重时，甚至可达到持续性室性心动过速的诊断标准。我们曾见过成为无休止性室性心动过速的患者。

这种反复发作的心律失常多为良性。然而，也有蜕变为心室颤动的报道。

一例十几岁的女性患者，室性期前收缩起源于漏斗部，尽管在心跳骤停后复苏成功，但终因不可逆的脑损伤而死亡。组织形态学特征是在漏斗区存在大量脂肪和间质纤维化组织，伴以炎性反应（图 63-5）。我们认为其死因很可能为炎症伴与右室发育不良组织形态学类似的漏斗区发育不良的共同作用所致。

交感神经兴奋可能对室速反复发作起着重要作用[21]。更明确的是，相对于男性而言，激素水平突然升高是女性室性心动过速的触发因素，而在男性，心律失常多与应激、运动或咖啡因等有关[22]。

心动过速通常起源于右室流出道，但也有起源于高位室间隔及左侧间隔的报道[23,24]。室速的起源点可通过对室速心电图进行完整的分析来推测[25]。对于不典型部位成年或儿童病例的室速，消融治疗常很困难[26]。然而，可通过网篮导管或非接触性标测等先进的导管技术来帮助确定合适的消融部位[27,28]。

在磁共振检查时，有些病人可发现器质性心脏疾病的迹象，部分可通过造影检查得以确认，强烈提示沿右心室前壁漏斗区有局灶性结构异常。其他致心律失常的基质也应考虑。这些患者中致心律失常性右室发育不良的发生率较高，但需进一步研究证实[29]。

我们的初步经验表明，部分因右室流出道室性心

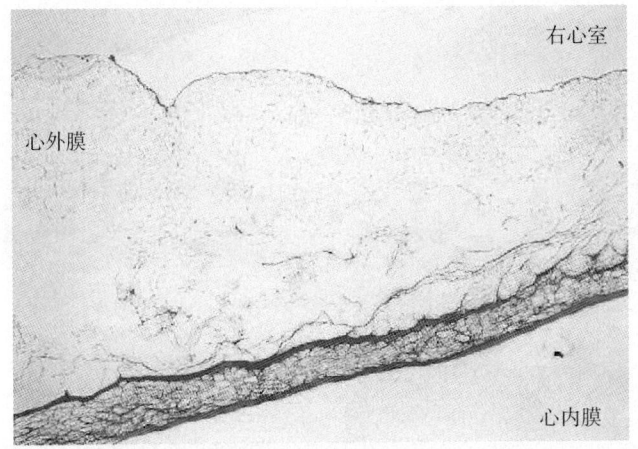
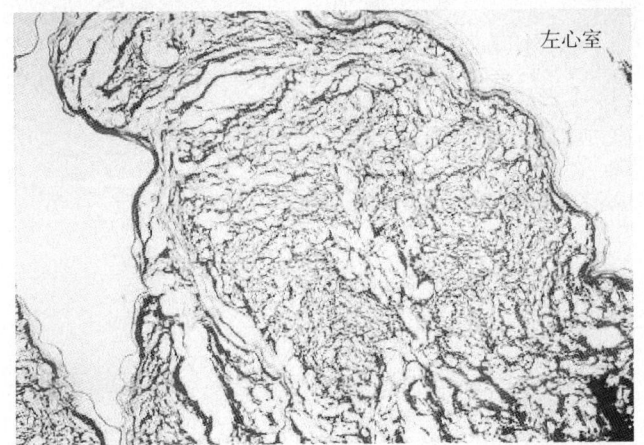
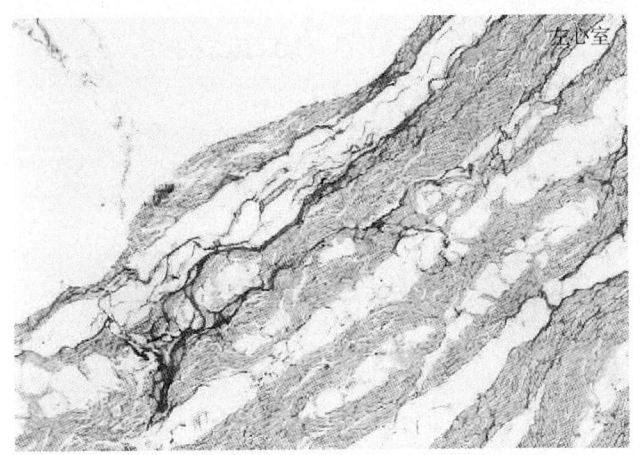

图63-4 双心室海绵样发育不良 上图：右心室壁完全被脂肪取代。两条纤维化线代表残存的心外膜和心内膜。中图：左室大部分心肌纤维被脂肪和小灶纤维化所分隔。下图：左心室游离壁高倍放大图。（见彩图31）

动过速变为无休止持续发作而进行抗心律失常外科治疗的病人，通过带有跨壁针式的多极记录电极，可以记录到高位室间隔的碎裂电位。

（五）威尼斯心肌病

1. 典型的威尼斯心肌病

典型的威尼斯心肌病（曾称为右室心肌病）具有大部分致心律失常性右室心肌发育不良的特征，但在威尼斯地区家族发病率高达50%，而在其他地区发病率不超过15%～25%。尽管为显性遗传，但威尼斯心肌病的家族外显率明显低于纳克索斯病（Naxos disease）。患者及三代家庭成员中以及多数累及左室的患者，猝死的发生率明显增高[30]。最近，遗传学和分子生物学研究又确定了一些新的亚组。

2. 桥粒斑蛋白右室心肌病

桥粒斑蛋白右室心肌病（desmoplakin right ventricular cardiomyopathy）为桥粒斑蛋白突变的显性遗传，最早发现于一个意大利家系[31]。像盘状球蛋白（plakoglobin）一样，主要累及桥粒连接中的细胞浸润粘合蛋白。曾报告一例厄瓜多尔病人存在同种基因的隐性遗传，不过患者为原发性扩张型心肌病，无脂肪浸润[32]。

3. 兰尼丁右室心肌病

兰尼丁（ryanodine）右室心肌病以一个特异基因编码的连接钙通道的蛋白为特征[33]。临床和组织学特征均与致心律失常性右室发育不良相似，包括炎性浸润[34]。

临床表现包括：用力/情绪激动可导致室性心律失常、晕厥和儿童猝死。运动诱发的典型室性心动过速是双向性和多形性室速。尽管病人有晚电位，电生理学检查程序刺激并不能诱发心律失常。在对无症状家族成员的早期诊断中，基因筛查是识别高危患者的唯一可行的方法[35]。

但是，北欧的另一组报道在有些携带相同基因型和临床特征的患者中并未发现器质性心脏病的证据[36]。法国儿科医生持相同观点，将这些病人归类于儿茶酚胺敏感性室性心动过速（见第68章）。无论病理机制如何，检出这些患者是至关重要的，因为给他们终身服用合适剂量的β受体阻滞剂可防止猝死[37]。

4. 纳克索斯病

纳克索斯病（Naxos disease）是另一种具有较强地域性的致心律失常性右室发育不良的亚型。在希腊

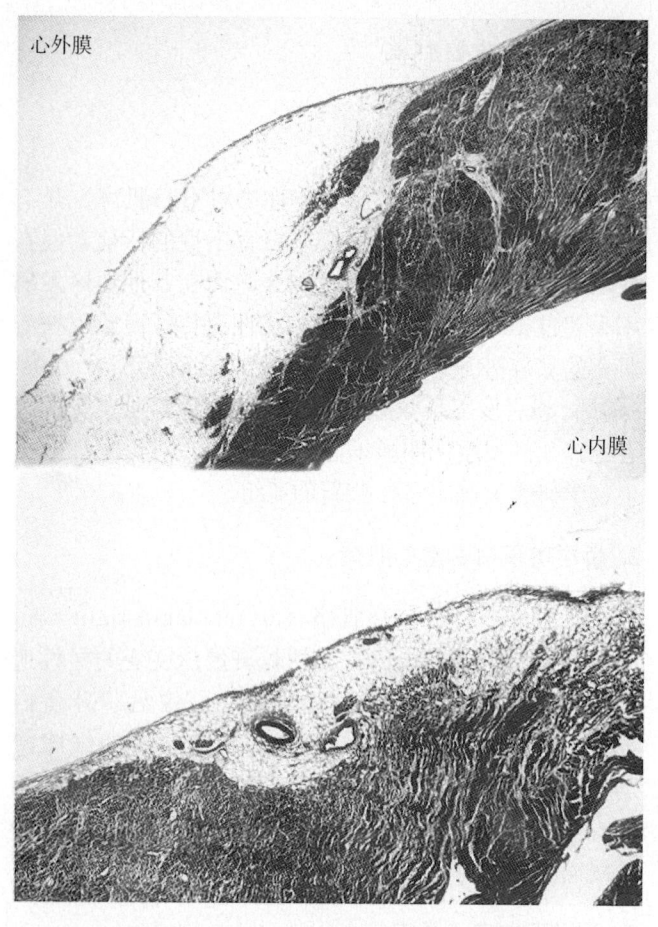
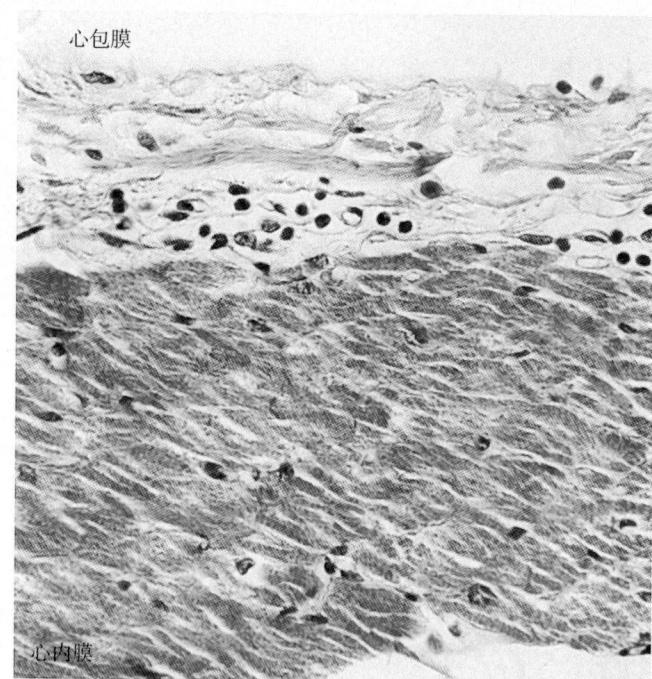
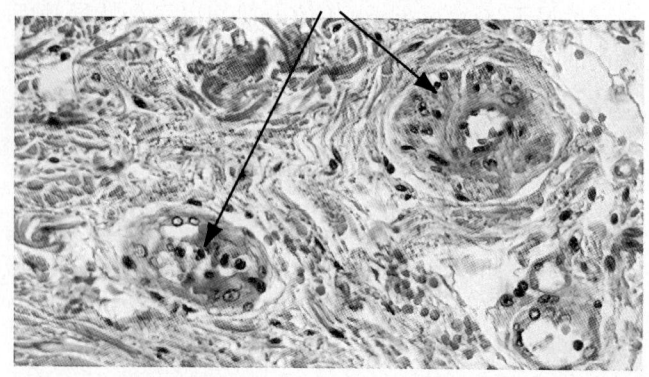

图 63-5　一例既往无症状的 16 岁女孩发生猝死　上三幅图：漏斗部及其邻近的有肌小梁的区域可见心肌被大量脂肪细胞取代，夹以存活的心肌细胞带，提示为致心律失常性右室发育不良的局灶型。下图：小冠状血管壁增厚的典型类型。（见彩图 32）

纳克索斯岛，来自 12 个家系的 26 名患者确诊此病。它是一种隐性遗传疾病，家族外显率 100%。它与另一种类型的发育不良、掌跖硬皮病和羊毛状发有关。临床表现、心电图特点和活检结果与致心律失常性右室发育不良一致。室性心动过速和猝死的发生也与典型的致心律失常性右室发育不良相似。调控此病的基因使盘状球蛋白断裂，而盘状球蛋白是心脏细胞间粘附蛋白的一部分，这种蛋白存在于细胞桥粒和缝隙连接处。心脏细胞间粘附蛋白的变形或可解释纳克索斯病及致心律失常性右室发育不良患者的传导障碍。此推理进一步被缝隙连接蛋白 connexin43 的表达减少所证明，可以解释患者的肌间传导异常[38]。纳克索斯病的典型患者为纯合子，这与右室流出道心动过速的病人（杂合子）恰相反[39]。在这个岛上纳克索斯病的聚集可能来源于近亲繁殖。

（六）临界性右室心肌病

1. 二尖瓣脱垂

对来自意大利威尼斯地区疑诊或尸检发现的二尖瓣脱垂猝死患者进行的一系统病理研究显示，这些病人中约 2/3 存在致心律失常性右室发育不良的右室组织学基质。此发现或许可解释为防止心律失常和猝死对二尖瓣脱垂患者进行二尖瓣换瓣手术结果的不一致性[40]。然而，如同威尼斯心肌病一样，有必要考虑此疾病在世界报道的起源地聚集的可能性。

2. 脂肪分裂综合征

两项研究应用右室心肌形态学和形态测定分析来区分右室游离壁脂肪浸润和作为致心律失常性右室心肌病组织学标志的纤维脂肪浸润[2,10]。除小面积纤维化之外，这两组人群有着相同的心肌组织结构，即心肌间夹杂脂肪组织或被脂肪替代。在猝死病人中，我们发现，即使没有纤维化，脂肪里的心肌纤维束也可能导致猝死。这一结果可能有重要的临床意义，因为大部分看似正常的心脏存在右室心肌脂肪浸润[41]。这些病人的脂肪浸润可能代表在纤维组织出现之前致心律失常性右室发育不良的早期阶段。因此，很大比例的正常人实际上可能存在与猝死高危相关的右室心肌病的潜在背景。大量致心律失常性右室发育不良病人有炎症的组织学证据。一种解释是在脂肪散在浸润的心肌发生心肌炎。被心肌炎侵袭的条状心肌细胞被纤维化替代，形成纤维脂肪浸润。被心肌炎性活化的嗜中性粒细胞可能是心律失常危险性增高的触发因子。这一问题可通过识别基因异常得以解决。

3. 非致心律失常型右室发育不良

世界卫生组织新的心肌病分类"致心律失常性右室心肌病"中包括心律失常这个单词。然而，心律失常只是一种表象，部分通过右室心肌有创性或无创性检查发现的各种右室心肌病患者并未检出室性心律失常。在这些病人中，虽存在致心律失常的基质，却未表现出来。患者的心电图有特征性表现，信号平均心电图也可检出心室晚电位，心室晚电位阳性可解释在"貌似"健康人中出现的心电图假阳性结果，这些患者是发生室性心律失常的潜在人群。

二、非冠状动脉性右室心前区 ST 段抬高（Brugada 综合征）

非冠状动脉性右室心前区 ST 段抬高，又称为 Brugada 综合征（见第 67 章），是一种由于跨膜离子转运异常导致的家族遗传性疾病，有特异的心电图形态。Brugada 综合征可见于休息或睡眠时有猝死风险的年轻人。报告的病例多见于东南亚，包括泰国、老挝、日本等国[42,43]。心电图特征为完全性（或不完全性）右束支阻滞并伴有右心前区导联 V_1 至 V_3 导联 ST 段明显抬高。有两种主要类型：穹隆形和马鞍形，其中以穹隆形相关性最好。在大多数患者，这些心电图特征可间歇出现。但是这种心电图异常可被钠通道阻滞剂诱发出，例如 IA 或 IC 类抗心律失常药物。这些病人易于发展成心室颤动或快速多形性室速，导致头晕、晕厥或猝死。Brugada 综合征是常染色体显性遗传，外显率相对很低。男性患病率是女性的 8～10 倍。

（一）遗传学和电生理背景

业已明确，Brugada 综合征的遗传学背景是一种大分子跨膜蛋白（SCN5A），受钠通道不同基因突变影响[44]。通过对一例患者心内、外膜同步记录的研究，经心大静脉记录心外膜电位，经置于右室流出道的网篮导管同步记录心内膜电位，发现右室游离壁存在电不均一性[45]。这种电不均一性可引起 2 相折返，促发心外膜环形运动，继而引致尖端扭转型室速。由于右室的瞬间外向电流比左室强，故对右室影响较显著[46]。

在一例儿童[47]和一例 69 岁的患者[48]，发现发热可引起 Brugada 综合征的心电图变化[49]。尽管此离子机制可在实验室中复制，然而，此儿童患者体温恢复正常后，应用氟卡胺并未能再激发出 ST 段抬高的心电图图形[47]。

（二）药物

Brugada 综合征的基因背景可以解释为何钠通道阻滞剂可使正常范围心电图揭示出典型的 Brugada 综合征心电图波形。多篇文献报道了心电图的药物激发作用。通常，钠通道阻滞药物能够揭示或加剧 ST 段的抬高[50]。不过，这些药物也可能产生意想不到的结果[51]，且对 Brugada 综合征的诊断并不特异。

(三) 心脏电生理学检查

在心室程序刺激时，Brugada 综合征患者常可诱发出快速持续性或多形性室速，进而导致心室颤动[52]。

心脏电生理学检查的结果主要取决于程序刺激方案，尤其是刺激部位[53,54]。应用异丙肾上腺素并不增加诱发室性心律失常的成功率，反而会抑制心律失常的诱发[55]。这与致心律失常性右室发育不良患者恰相反，致心律失常性右室发育不良电生理检查时如难以通过常规的程序刺激诱发室速，可应用异丙肾上腺素提高诱发成功率。

一项大样本研究随访近 3 年的结果表明，在有症状的患者，应用电生理程序刺激的方法更易于诱发出室性心律失常，提示电生理检查对于有症状的患者可有助于检出发生危险性心律失常的高危人群[52]。

(四) 近期进展

应用信号平均心电图可预测哪些患者易于发生心室颤动，且结果可重复性好。重复记录有助于决定哪些无症状的 Brugada 综合征患者易于发展为危险性心律失常，应当进行电生理学检查[56]。

交感神经分布 ^{123}I-间碘苄胍成像也被用来阐明心脏自主神经功能不良新的电生理学机制[57]。

心电图出现 Brugada 波的病人，体表标测呈 ST 段抬高和信号平均心电图晚电位阳性者均易在程序心室刺激中诱发室速。因此，这两种方法可作为对这些病人进行危险分层的无创性手段[58]。

近期的研究强调了复极和除极异常在评估 Brugada 综合征患者的心室颤动易感性中的作用[59]。为了预测心脏事件的再发，对有症状的 Brugada 综合征患者诱发室颤。随访 3 年的结果表明，对有症状的 Brugada 综合征患者，诱发室颤与否并无预测价值[60]。

通过在心脏外科术中应用接触电极标测心外膜，一组研究人员发现在所有 Brugada 综合征病人的漏斗区均存在"钉样"和"穹隆"样波形，而对照组中无一例出现此种波形[61]。另一组研究人员通过在右冠状动脉圆锥支插入导管，记录单相动作电位，证实了这一结果。这或可解释 Brugada 综合征病人延迟电位的起源。

然而，Brugada 综合征的 SCN5A 突变阳性率已从最初报告的 50% 降至晚近报告的 30% 甚至更低[44]。而 Brugade 综合征的新临床表现，如阵发性心房颤动，有报告可高达 30%[62]。心房不应期和房内传导时间亦延长，或可解释心房易损性增高的原因[63]。

最近，在一些具有典型 Brugada 综合征心电图表现的患者中发现致心律失常性右室发育不良基因型表达的病理改变[64,65]。然而，现有的报告中有关右室解剖结构的影像技术，包括超声、核素、磁共振成像、右室造影术、心内膜活组织切片检查和病理检查等资料尚不够充分[64]。

常用的方法可能不足以检测出某些细微的解剖异常（图 63-6）。因此，对来源于猝死病人或接受心脏移植患者的任何病理标本的研究均极为重要，以进行正确的分类，从而决定哪些病人符合 ICD 的植入标准。

(五) 危险分层

当符合下列条件时，具有永久性 Brugada 心电图表现的患者发生心脏事件的风险增高：

- 心电图异常波形可被抗心律失常药物激发；
- 有晕厥病史[66]；
- 家庭成员早年发生猝死；
- 心脏电生理检查诱发出心室颤动或快速性室性心动过速[52]。

现有的资料推荐这些病人应植入 ICD[67]。然而，如果发生"交感风暴"，心脏移植可能是唯一的替代方法[68]。

三、鉴别诊断

(一) 原发性扩张型心肌病

在原发性扩张型心肌病的早期阶段，如左室功能尚未严重受损，且伴有起源于右室的室性心动过速，可能被误诊为右室心肌病。然而，心脏影像学检查显示全心扩大和双心室壁运动低下，而不是致心律失常性右室心肌病典型的节段性运动障碍。

(二) 孤立性心肌炎

在大部分病人，组织学诊断不会有误，但是当心肌炎伴大量的脂肪细胞时，有可能误诊为致心律失常性右室发育不良。然而，脂肪细胞的区域性分布与致心律失常性右室发育不良明显不同。

不论在急性期还是完全治愈之后，单纯心肌炎本身也可致心律失常。最近已被运动中发生的猝死所证实[18]。

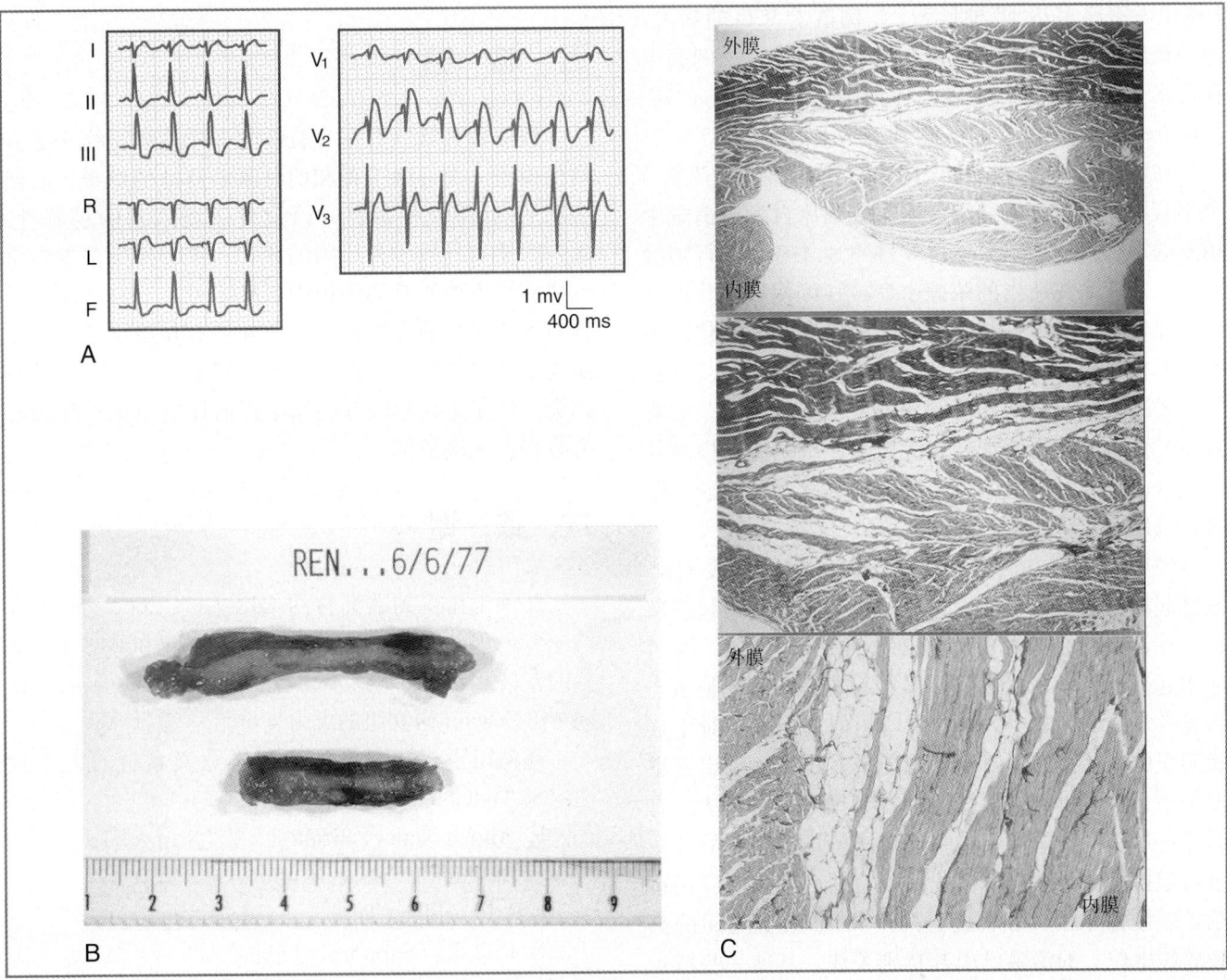

图63-6 具典型心电图特征的 Brugada 综合征 右室游离壁可见心外膜与心内膜之间夹以脂肪组织,此类表现有可能不被常规的影像学检查检出。脂肪带与1977年手术治疗的典型致心律失常性右室发育不良患者相似。此患者在室速起源部位的右室呈"三明治"样结构,心外膜与心内膜两层间夹着厚厚的脂肪层。(见彩图33)

四、致心律失常性右室心肌病室性心动过速的治疗

在所有的致心律失常性右室心肌病患者(不包括 Brugada 综合征),最常见的住院原因为源于右室的持续性室性心动过速。抗心律失常药通常有效,但是,不能确保能预防猝死的发生,迄今为止,ICD 仍是防止猝死的唯一有效方法[69]。不过,当出现下列情况时可以考虑导管消融持续性室速:ICD 频繁放电、无休止性室速、频发的慢频率室性心动过速、抗心律失常药物治疗依从性差或不能耐受抗心律失常药物的不良反应。

以我们通过射频消融或直流电消融治疗室速的经验[70],所有致心律失常性右室心肌病患者中,有一例为酷似 Uhl 畸形的患者,另一例致心律失常性右室发育不良局限于右室心尖部。一例患者曾被诊为右室流出道室性心动过速,另一例为纳克索斯病。随着时间推移,所有这些病人均发展成为严重的致心律失常性右室心肌病,并经右心室造影证实。

研究的全部人群包括38例男性和12例女性患者,初次消融时平均年龄为48±15岁(17～76岁)。44例患者的左室射血分数平均为59±12%,两例患者低于40%。在42例病人中,30例患者两次独立的室速之间的最长间隔≥1年。在47例患者中,17例发作室速1～5次,3例发作5～10次,27例发作大于20次,7例呈无休止性室速。

在45例资料可得的病人中,23例为单形性室速,15例有2种形态室速,6例有3～6种形态室速,更有

1例患者室速多达12种形态。2例植入ICD的病人，因频繁放电不能耐受而寻求导管消融治疗。4例病人在首次射频消融前的第4、5、6、19年曾在La Salpetriere医院进行抗心律失常外科手术治疗。

在消融之前，应至少停用Ⅰ类抗心律失常药物5个半衰期。胺碘酮可继续应用。仅临床自发或消融中诱发的一种或多种单形性持续性室速才考虑进行消融治疗。治疗需在适当的镇静中完成，以使病人获得良好的放松，更好地控制心肌功能和经食管心脏超声来监测血栓的形成。室速通常由程序刺激诱发，有些患者需要短阵超速起搏和静滴异丙肾上腺素诱发。如病人耐受性差，或需经食管超声监测左室功能和检测并发症（心包填塞）时，可应用全身麻醉。多巴酚丁胺可首选用于耐受性差的患者。

经典的标测方法是，在室速时寻找比体表QRS波群起始部提前最早的电位，从而确定室速的起源部位。在器质性心脏病患者，常提前30ms以上。也可应用起搏标测，在室速起源部位起搏可准确复制出与自发性室速心电图12个导联均相似的形态。对于症状明显的良性室性早搏、而未能诱发出右室流出道室速的患者，有时起搏标测是唯一可用的标测方法。有时还可通过用消融导管在室速时进行拖带起搏的方法进行起搏标测，在起搏停止后，室性心动过速应仍持续，缓慢传导区（常表现为两个QRS波群之间的高频碎裂电位）的消融已引起特别关注。其他一些特点也有助于确定缓慢传导区，缓慢传导区是心律失常持续存在的必要环节。

尽管射频消融可作为致心律失常性右室发育不良患者室速的适当的一线治疗方法，然而，初次治疗的有效率尚不足40%；直流电消融对于致心律失常性右室发育不良的室速亦有效，常在初次射频消融失败后实施。但是，直流电消融需要全身麻醉，且在半数患者需多次放电。这两种技术的结合，加上其他药物和非药物治疗的正确应用，包括起搏器和ICD治疗，在连续28例患者中的成功率接近90%。直流电消融疗法的不良声誉是由于对物理和生物物理方法技术问题的误解，包括对射频消融研发的较软且弯度可调导管出现之前所应用导管的误解。而如今，在射频消融不成功后，仍可在同一部位应用射频消融导管进行直流电消融。

在大部分病人，长期随访中新发生的室性心动过速是疾病进展的结果，这时可应用同样的方法进行治疗，成功率与前述相同。我们的经验是，多发的单形性室速对成功消融并无明显影响。

五、总　结

致心律失常性右室心肌病的多样性和宽临床疾病谱是由于人类心肌一种和两种基本特征的结果：心肌被脂肪/纤维化所取代，以及对环境因素的易感性。这些因素可导致多种原因的死亡。致心律失常性右室心肌病远不像原有的认识中那样罕见。对致心律失常性右室心肌病的更好理解，尤其是对其遗传学和分子生物学背景的认识，将有助于更好地将这些患者进行归类，这是进行危险分层和恰当治疗以防止猝死和心力衰竭的先决条件。

六、致　谢

此项工作得到欧洲合约QLG1-CT-2000、法国合约99b 0691、Le Teleton（AFM）5774和Gustave基金的支持和资助，以及Simone Prevot、Geneve、Suisse和Servier研究组的大力支持。

谨向以下提供具有重要科学意义素材的人士致谢：S. Abdelali（Rabat，Morocco），

E. Aliot（Nancy，France），

P. Brugada（Aalst，Belgium），

J. P. Fauchier（Tours，France），

X. Fujioka（Sapporo，Japan），

H. Klein（Magdeburg，Germany），

F. Lobo（Hamilton，Ontario，Canada），

R. Myerburg（Miami，FL），

N. Protonotarios（Naxos，Greece），

Z. Stamenkovic（Belgrade，Serbia），

P. Adragao（Carnaxide，Portugal），

L. Boccon-Gibod（Paris，France），

F. Camerini（Trieste，Italy），

J. Fisher（New York，NY），

L. Kappenberger（Lausanne，Switzerland），

B. Letac（Rouen，France），

F. I. Marcus（Tucson，AZ），

A. Medina（Jerusalem，Israel），

R. Slama（Paris，France），

J. Vohra（Melbourne，Australia）。

（张海澄　译）

参 考 文 献

1. Fontaine G, Fontaliran F, Hebert JL, et al: Arrhythmogenic right ventricular dysplasia. Ann Rev Med 50:17–35, 1999.
2. Burke AP, Farb A, Tashko G, Virmani R: Right ventricular cardiomyopathy and fatty infiltration of the right ventricular myocardium: Are they different diseases? Circulation 97:1571–1580, 1998.
3. Richardson PJ, McKenna WJ, Bristow M, et al: Report of the 1995 World Health Organization/International Society and Federation of Cardiology. Task Force on the Definition and Classification of Cardiomyopathies. Circulation 93:841–842, 1996.
4. Fontaine G, Fontaliran F, Frank R: Arrhythmogenic right ventricular cardiomyopathies. Clinical forms and main differential diagnoses [editorial]. Circulation 97:1532–1535, 1998.
5. Fontaine G, Tonet J, Frank R: Ventricular tachycardia in arrhythmogenic right ventricular dysplasia. In Zipes DP, Jalife J (eds): Cardiac Electrophysiology: From Cell to Bedside, 3rd ed. Philadelphia, WB Saunders, 2000, pp 546–555.
6. Srivastra D, Thomas T, Lin Q, et al: Regulation of cardiac mesodermal and neural crest development by the bHLH transcription factor, dHAND. Nat Genet 16:154–160, 1997.
7. Pashmforoush M, Pomies P, Peterson KL, et al: Adult mice deficient in actinin-associated LIM-domain protein reveal a developmental pathway for right ventricular cardiomyopathy. Nat Med 7:591–597, 2001.
8. Fontaine G, Aouate P, Fontaliran F: Repolarization and the genesis of cardiac arrhythmias. Role of body surface mapping [editorial]. Circulation 12:2600–2602, 1997.
9. Fornes P, Ratel S, Lecomte D: Pathology of arrhythmogenic right ventricular cardiomyopathy/dysplasia. An autopsy study of 20 forensic cases. J Forens Sci 43:777–783, 1998.
10. Basso C, Thiene G, Corrado D, et al: Arrhythmogenic right ventricular cardiomyopathy. Dysplasia, dystrophy or myocarditis? Circulation 94:983–991, 1996.
11. Corrado D, Basso C, Thiene G, et al: Spectrum of clinico-pathologic manifestations of arrhythmogenic right ventricular cardiomyopathy/dysplasia. A multicenter study. J Am Coll Cardiol 30:1512–1520, 1997.
12. James TN, Nichols MM, Sapire DW, et al: Complete heart block and fatal right ventricular failure in an infant. Circulation 93:1588–1600, 1996.
13. McCrohon JA, John AS, Lorenz CH, et al: Left ventricular involvement in arrhythmogenic right ventricular cardiomyopathy. Circulation 105:1394, 2002.
14. Fontaine G, Fontaliran F, Rosas Andrade F, et al: The arrhythmogenic right ventricle. dysplasia versus cardiomyopathy. Heart Vessels 10:227–235, 1995.
15. Hoffman BF, Feinmark SJ, Guo SD: Electrophysiologic effects of interactions between activated canine neutrophils and cardiac myocytes. J Cardiovasc Electrophysiol 8:679–687, 1997.
16. Fontaliran F, Fontaine G, Brestescher C, et al: Signification des infiltrats lymphoplasmocytaires dans la dysplasie ventriculaire droite arythmogene. Arch Mal Coeur 88:1021–1028, 1995.
17. Wesslen L, Pahlson C, Lindquist O, et al: An increase in sudden unexpected cardiac deaths among young Swedish orienteers during 1979–1992. Eur Heart J 17:902–910, 1996.
18. Maron BJ, Shirani J, Poliac LC, et al: Sudden death in young competitive athletes. Clinical, demographic, and pathological profiles. JAMA 276:199–204, 1996.
19. Nemec J, Edwards BS, Osborn MJ, Edwards WD: Arrhythmogenic right ventricular dysplasia masquerading as dilated cardiomyopathy. Am J Cardiol 84:237–239, 1999.
20. Girard F, Fontaine G, Fontaliran F, et al: Catastrophic global heart failure in a case of non arrhythmogenic right ventricular dysplasia. Heart Vessels 12:152–154, 1997.
21. Hayashi H, Fujiki A, Tani M, et al: Role of sympathovagal balance in the initiation of idiopathic ventricular tachycardia originating from right ventricular outflow tract. Pacing Clin Electrophysiol 20:2371–2377, 1997.
22. Marchlinski FE, Deely MP, Zado ES: Sex-specific triggers for right ventricular outflow tract tachycardia. Am Heart J 139:1009–1013, 2000.
23. Jadonath RL, Schwartzman DS, Preminger MW, et al: Utility of the 12-lead electrocardiogram in localizing the origin of right ventricular outflow tract tachycardia. Am Heart J 130:1107–1113, 1995.
24. Yoshida Y, Hirai M, Murakami Y, et al: Localization of precise origin of idiopathic ventricular tachycardia from the right ventricular outflow tract by a 12-lead ECG: A study of pace mapping using a multielectrode "basket" catheter. Pacing Clin Electrophysiol 22:1760–1768, 1999.
25. Krebs ME, Krause PC, Engelstein ED, et al: Ventricular tachycardias mimicking those arising from the right ventricular outflow tract. J Cardiovasc Electrophysiol 11:45–51, 2000.
26. O'Connor BK, Case CL, Sokoloski MC, et al: Radiofrequency catheter ablation of right ventricular outflow tachycardia in children and adolescents. J Am Coll Cardiol 27:869–874, 1996.
27. Aiba T, Shimizu W, Taguchi A, et al: Clinical usefulness of a multielectrode basket catheter for idiopathic ventricular tachycardia originating from right ventricular outflow tract. J Cardiovasc Electrophysiology 12:511–517, 2001.
28. Friedman PA, Asirvatham SJ, Grice S, et al: Noncontact mapping to guide ablation of right ventricular outflow tract tachycardia. J Am Coll Cardiol 39:1808–1812, 2002.
29. Chinushi M, Aizawa Y, Takahashi K, et al: Morphological variation of nonreentrant idiopathic ventricular tachycardia originating from the right ventricular outflow tract and effect of radiofrequency lesion. Pacing Clin Electrophysiol 20:325–336, 1997.
30. Pinamonti B, Miani D, Sinagra G, et al: Familial right ventricular dysplasia with biventricular involvement and inflammatory infiltration. Heart 76:66–69, 1996.
31. Rampazzo A, Nava A, Malacrida S, et al: Mutation in human desmoplakin domain binding to plakoglobin causes a dominant form of arrhythmogenic right ventricular cardiomyopathy. Am J Hum Genet 71:1200–1206, 2002.
32. Carvajal-Huerta L: Epidermolytic palmoplantar keratoderma with woolly hair and dilated cardiomyopathy. J Am Acad Dermatol 39:418–421, 1998.
33. Tiso N, Stephan DA, Nava A, et al: Identification of mutations in the cardiac ryanodine receptor gene in families affected with arrhythmogenic right ventricular cardiomyopathy type 2 (ARVD2). Hum Mol Genet 10:189–194, 2001.
34. Bauce B, Nava A, Rampazzo A, et al: Familial effort polymorphic ventricular arrhythmias in arrhythmogenic right ventricular cardiomyopathy map to chromosome 1q42-43. Am J Cardiol 85:573–579, 2000.
35. Bauce B, Rampazzo A, Basso C, et al: Screening of ryanodine receptor type 2 mutations in families with effort-induced polymorphic ventricular arrhythmias and sudden death: Early diagnosis of asymptomatic carriers. J Am Coll Cardiol 40:341–349, 2002.
36. Swan H, Piippo K, Viitasalo MT, et al: Arrhythmic disorder mapped to chromosome 1q42-q43 causes malignant polymorphic ventricular tachycardia in structurally normal hearts. J Am Coll Cardiol 34:2035–2042, 1999.
37. Leenhardt A, Lucet V, Denjoy I, et al: Catecholaminergic polymorphic ventricular tachycardia in children. A 7-year follow-up of 21 patients. Circulation 91:1512–1519, 1995.
38. Kaplan SR, Protonotarios N, Tsatsopoulou A, et al: Diminished myocardial connexin43 expression and gap junction remodeling in naxos disease [abstract]. Pacing Clin Electrophysiol 24(pt II):525, 2002.
39. Protonotarios N, Tsatsopoulou A, Anastasakis A, et al: Genotype-phenotype assessment in autosomal recessive arrhythmogenic right ventricular cardiomyopathy (Naxos disease) caused by a deletion in plakoglobin. J Am Coll Cardiol 38:1477–1484, 2001.
40. Corrado D, Basso C, Angelini A, Thiene G: Sudden death in young people with apparently isolated mitral valve prolapse [abstract]. Pacing Clin Electrophysiol 20(pt II):1120, 1997.
41. Fontaine G, Fornes P, Mallat Z, et al: Why patients with arrhythmogenic right ventricular dysplasia die suddenly? In Aliot E, Clementy J, Prystowsky EN (eds): Fighting Sudden Cardiac Death: A Worldwide Challenge. Armonk, NY, Futura, 2000, pp 251–263
42. Matsuo K, Akahoshi M, Nakashima E, et al: The prevalence, incidence and prognostic value of the Brugada-type electrocardiogram: A population-based study of four decades. J Am Coll Cardiol 38:765–770, 2001.
43. Furuhashi M, Uno K, Tsuchihashi K, et al: Prevalence of asymptomatic ST segment elevation in right precordial leads with right bundle branch block (Brugada-type ST shift) among the general Japanese population. Heart 86:161–166, 2001.
44. Vatta M, Dumaine R, Varghese G, et al: Genetic and biophysical basis of sudden unexplained nocturnal death syndrome (SUNDS), a disease allelic to Brugada syndrome. Hum Mol Genet 11:337–345, 2002.
45. Shimizu W, Aiba T, Kurita T, Kamakura S: Paradoxic abbreviation of

repolarization in epicardium of the right ventricular outflow tract during augmentation of Brugada-type ST segment elevation. J Cardiovasc Electrophysiol 12:1418–1421, 2001.
46. Brugada J, Brugada P, Brugada R: The syndrome of right bundle branch block ST segment elevation in V1 to V3 and sudden death. The Brugada syndrome. Europace 1:156–166, 1999.
47. Saura D, Garcia-Alberola A, Carrillo P, et al: Brugada-like electrocardiographic pattern induced by fever. Pacing Clin Electrophysiol 25:856–859, 2002.
48. Morita H, Nagase S, Kusano KF, Ohe T: Spontaneous T wave alternans and premature ventricular contractions during febrile illness in a patient with Brugada syndrome. J Cardiovasc Electrophysiol 13:816–818, 2002.
49. Dumaine R, Towbin JA, Brugada P, et al: Ionic mechanisms responsible for the electrocardiographic phenotype of the Brugada syndrome are temperature dependent. Circ Res 85:803–809, 1999.
50. Brugada R: Use of intravenous antiarrhythmics to identify concealed Brugada syndrome. Curr Control Trials Cardiovasc Med 1:45–47, 2000.
51. Miyazaki T, Mitamura H, Miyoshi S, et al: Autonomic and antiarrhythmic drug modulation of ST segment in patients with Brugada syndrome. J Am Coll Cardiol 27:1061–1070, 1996.
52. Brugada P, Geelen P, Brugada R, et al: Prognostic value of electrophysiologic investigations in Brugada syndrome. J Cardiovasc Electrophysiology 12:1004–1007, 2001.
53. Eckardt L, Kirchhof P, Schulze-Bahr E, et al: Electrophysiologic investigation in Brugada syndrome. Yield of programmed ventricular stimulation at two ventricular sites with up to three premature beats. Eur Heart J 23:1394–1401, 2002.
54. Gasparini G, Priori SG, Mantica M, et al: Programmed electrical stimulation in Brugada syndrome: How reproducible are the results? J Cardiovasc Electrophysiology 13:880–887, 2002.
55. Tanaka H, Kinoshita O, Uchikawa S, et al: Successful prevention of recurrent ventricular fibrillation by intravenous isoproterenol in a patient with Brugada syndrome. Pacing Clin Electrophysiol 24:1293–1294, 2001.
56. Masaki R, Watanabe I, Nakai T, et al: Role of signal-averaged electrocardiograms for predicting the inducibility of ventricular fibrillation in the syndrome consisting of right bundle branch block and ST segment elevation in leads V1–V3. Jpn Heart J 23:367–378, 2002.
57. Wichter T, Matheja P, Eckardt L, et al: Cardiac autonomic dysfunction in Brugada syndrome. Circulation 106:e59–60, 2002.
58. Eckardt L, Bruns HJ, Paul MH, et al: Body surface area of ST elevation and the presence of late potentials correlate to the inducibility of ventricular tachyarrhythmias in Brugada syndrome. J Cardiovasc Electrophysiol 13:742–749, 2002.
59. Nanke T, Nakazawa K, Arai M, et al: Clinical significance of the dispersion of the activation-recovery interval and recovery time as markers for ventricular fibrillation susceptibility in patients with Brugada syndrome. Circ J 66:549–552, 2002.
60. Kanda M, Shimizu W, Matsuo K, et al: Electrophysiologic characteristics and implications of induced ventricular fibrillation in symptomatic patients with Brugada syndrome. J Am Coll Cardiol 39:1799–1805, 2002.
61. Kurita T, Shimizu W, Inagaki M, et al: The electrophysiologic mechanism of ST-segment elevation in Brugada syndrome. J Am Coll Cardiol 40:330–334, 2002.
62. Itoh H, Shimizu M, Ino H, et al: Arrhythmias in patients with Brugada-type electrocardiographic findings. Jpn Circ J 65:483–486, 2001.
63. Morita H, Kusano-Fukushima K, Nagase S, et al: Atrial fibrillation and atrial vulnerability in patients with Brugada syndrome. J Am Coll Cardiol 40:1427–1444, 2002.
64. Corrado D, Nava A, Buja G, et al: Familial cardiomyopathy underlies syndrome of right bundle branch block, ST segment elevation and sudden death. J Am Coll Cardiol 27:443–448, 1996.
65. Corrado D, Basso C, Buja G, et al: Right bundle branch block, right precordial ST-segment elevation, and sudden death in young people. Circulation 103:710–717, 2001.
66. Priori SG, Napolitano C, Gasparini G, et al: Natural history of Brugada syndrome: Insights for risk stratification and management. Circulation 105:1342–1347, 2002.
67. Brugada J, Brugada R, Antzelevitch C, et al: Long-term follow-up of individuals with the electrocardiographic pattern of right bundle-branch block and ST-segment elevation in precordials leads V1 to V3. Circulation 105:73–78, 2002.
68. Ayerza MR, de Zutter M, Goethals M, et al: Heart transplantation as last resort against Brugada syndrome. J Cardiovasc Electrophysiol 13:943–944, 2002.
69. Link MS, Wang PJ, Haugh CJ, et al: Arrhythmogenic right ventricular dysplasia: Clinical results with implantable cardioverter defibrillators. J Interv Card Electrophysiol 1:41–48, 1997.
70. Fontaine G, Tonet J, Gallais Y, et al: Ventricular tachycardia catheter ablation in arrhythmogenic right ventricular dysplasia. A 16 year experience. Curr Cardiol Rep 2:498–506, 2000.

第 64 章

肥厚型心肌病的室性心律失常

Barry J. Maron

本章目录	
■ 前言	593
■ 病程发展	593
■ 非持续性室性心动过速	594
■ 猝死的发生机制	594
■ 猝死的预防	595
■ 肥厚型心肌病的危险期	597
■ 总结	598

一、前言

肥厚型心肌病（HCM）是临床表现与自然病史差异较大的一类遗传性心脏疾患[1-4]。自40年前首次报道以来，突然和意外死亡一直被认为是肥厚型心肌病的一个主要而严重的并发症[5]。肥厚型心肌病中室性心律失常（VT）的发生一直是研究的热点，这主要是因为此类心律失常与猝死之间可能存在某种因果关系[6-14]。这一当今流行的观点也解释了为何将室速与猝死相联系以及预防干预的重点所在。

二、病程发展

自 Teare 首次报道该病的病理特征以来[5]，现已认识到在肥厚型心肌病中，仅有部分亚组病人具有较高的心脏性猝死的危险性，该组病人也是多年来引起人们广泛关注于心律失常的作用和危险分层的人数较少的但是非常重要的群体[1,3,4,6-14]。对于能有效预防这些难以预料的灾难性后果的适宜治疗措施，目前仍存有较大争议[15]。近年来，一些学者提出在年轻的无症状肥厚型心肌病患者中，猝死并不少见[2,5,6,11,12,15,16]，据文献报道，在第三诊治中心的研究中，在主要由高危患者组成的人群中，其年死亡率可高达 4%～6%[1,4]。而在多数非选择性病例中，肥厚型心肌病引发的猝死年死亡率仅为 1%[4]。

由于与发生心脏性猝死的危险有关，因而在肥厚型心肌病患者中准确判明室速是十分重要的。在常规 24h 的动态心电监测中，约 90% 的肥厚型心肌病患者可出现室性心律失常。通常表现为频发、多源性室性期前收缩（尤其是室早总数较多，在 24h 记录中，约 20% 以上患者其室早总数大于 200 次），成对室早（见于 40% 以上患者）或非持续性室性心动过速（见于 20%～30% 患者）[9,13,14,17,18]（图 64-1）。在单次 24h 心电记录中，仅有 10% 的患者表现为较多的室早，包括 200 次或以上室性异位搏动，5 个或以上的成对室早，以及非持续性室速。然而，在病人总人群中，肥厚型心肌病患者的室早总数似乎与心脏性猝死的发生率并不成比例[4]。

早在 20 世纪 80 年代初，来自肥厚型心肌病第三诊治中心的两项研究业已证实，偶发或短阵的非持续性室速（通常为 3 至 6 个搏动）是猝死的标志。虽然作为一种自发性心律失常，持续性单形性室性心动过速并不常见，但在肥厚型心肌病患者中，它通常被认为是一个高危因素，且与那些进展至左室心尖部室壁瘤伴流出道梗阻的极少部分亚组病人有关[18-20]。总之，上述临床观察是基于肥厚型心肌病患者室速的研究以及用动态心电图监测作为猝死危险分层方法的研究之上[9,13,21-24]，因而也开创了药物预防性抗心律失常治疗的新纪元。

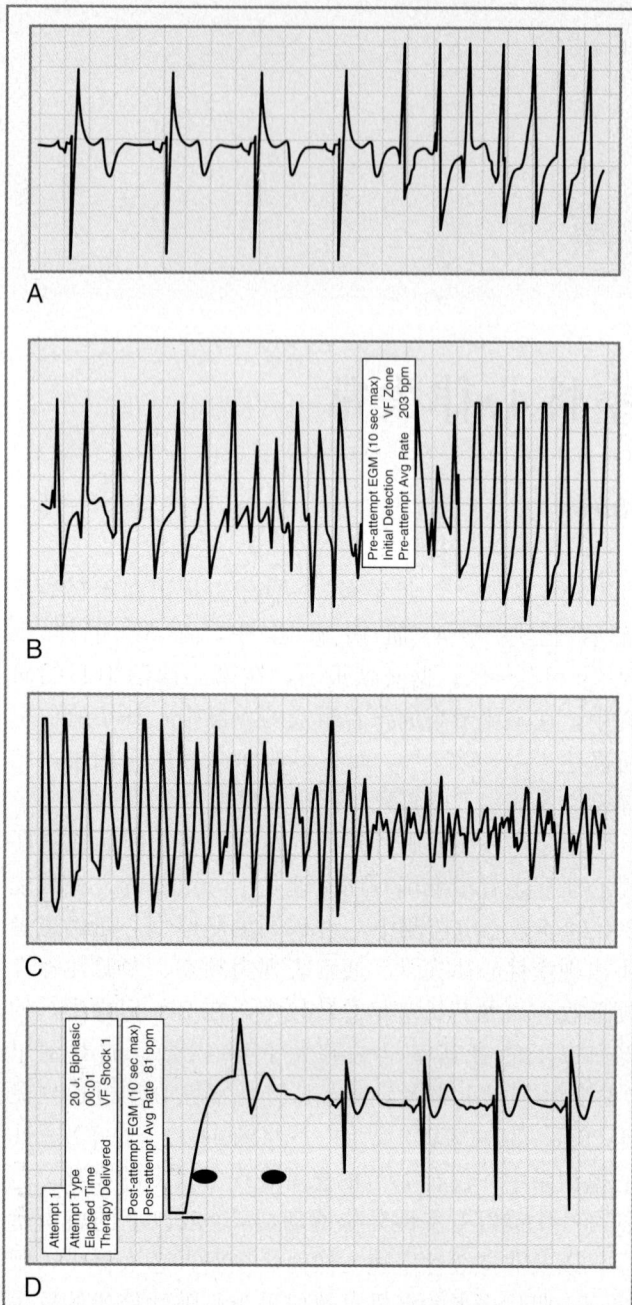

图64-1 肥厚型心肌病（HCM）心脏性猝死的一级预防 这份心电图来自一例35岁的男性患者，因有肥厚型心肌病相关性猝死的家族史和室间隔显著肥厚（室壁厚度为31mm），故预防性植入了植入式心脏复律除颤器（ICD）。在植入4年8个月后（清晨1:20AM，睡眠中）记录到的心内电图。以25mm/s走速连续记录，在4份电图中，每帧均为从左至右记录。A：开始4个心搏均为窦性心律，然后突然发生室速（200次/分）。B：ICD感知室速并开始充电。C：室速蜕变为室颤（VF）。D：室颤时，ICD适时放电（20J电击），立即转复为窦律。（引自 Maron BJ, Shen WK, Link MS, et al. Efficacy of implantable cardioverter-defibrillators for the prevention of sudden death in patients with hypertrophic cardiomyopathy. N Engl J Med. 342：365-373，2000.）

三、非持续性室性心动过速

临床上，在24或48h的心电监测中，肥厚型心肌病患者室性心律失常的发生率变化较大。病人可伴有心悸或轻微头痛。实际上，在动态心电图监测过程中，短阵的非持续性室速可能增加猝死的危险性近8倍，年死亡率约为8%，而在无室速的患者中，仅为1%。其阴性预测值较高，阳性预测值较低（分别为95%和25%）[9,13]。阳性预测值较低可能提示，在肥厚型心肌病患者人群中，猝死的危险因素的遗传机制不同，且心血管事件的发生率相对较低。

尽管动态心电图检测室性心动过速的价值有限，目前人们通常仍将其视为可用于肥厚型心肌病成年患者猝死危险分层的一个有效且实用的无创性检测方法。若在一个成年肥厚型心肌病患者的动态心电图监测中并无室速的发生，临床上可确定患者属于低危人群。在动态心电图监测中证实有非持续性室速，则有助于对此类高危患者做进一步的危险性评估，包括连续的动态心电监测，以便在一段较长的时间内能更好地评价此类心律失常。少数患者在连续心电监测中可记录到多源性反复非持续性室速，该类型的心律失常可能是肥厚型心肌病患者的一个危险因素和表现方式，也是心脏性猝死的一个触发机制。尽管缺乏特异性证据，若在动态心电图中记录到持续较长的非持续性室速（如大于10次心搏），也应将其视为一个高危标志。

四、猝死的发生机制

肥厚型心肌病患者发生心脏性猝死的原因仍不十分清楚。尽管猝死的发生机制可能是一个多因素的复杂过程，但包括室速在内的严重恶性事件可能是主要的因素[7,9,11,13,23,24]。此外，以往要证实这些心律失常与肥厚型心肌病患者突然意外死亡直接相关是极为困难的，这是因为事件发生时往往缺乏心电图记录资料[23]。

然而近年来，在植入并经历ICD适宜放电治疗的肥厚型心肌病患者中，通过ICD存储的心电图资料业已记录到了一些心律失常[11,24]。这些观察结果为了解肥厚型心肌病患者猝死机制提供了一个窗口。一项有关肥厚型心肌病高危患者的多中心ICD试验结果显示，每次临床事件中，室速或室颤均触发ICD的放电治疗[11]。这支持长期以来的假设即原发性室速是此类患者发生意外恶性事件的主要原因[1-3]。然而，由于ICD本身具有基础起搏功能，因而也不能除外在肥厚型心肌病相关性心脏猝死事件中，心动过缓介导性事件发生的可能性。此外，在这些心血管事件中，也可能存在其他类型的心律失常机制[24]。

由于肥厚型心肌病患者中部分ICD放电是由室速所触发，因而一些学者提出，植入前原本可自行终止的短阵非持续性室速（10s内）可能引发了ICD的自动放电。需要强调的是，持续较长的室速（200~250个心搏）已远远超过了在肥厚型心肌病患者中动态心电图所记录到的室速，实际上，在后者，持续仅10~15个心搏的室速即被视为较长的、异乎寻常的高危状态。所以，不能由此断定那些引发ICD放电的非持续性室速是良性的。

肥厚型心肌病室速发生的机制可能主要是因左室心肌结构紊乱所造成的电不稳定和异常电传导的基质[5,25,26]，或可引起心肌坏死和以纤维替代修复为表现的心肌缺血发作（可能是因结构异常或壁内动脉狭窄）所引发[27]（图64-2）。这种心肌基质对无论是内在的（与肥厚型心肌病疾病过程有关的，如流出道梗阻的突然加重）还是外在的（如剧烈的体力活动）各种诱发因素均敏感。个体易感性在决定肥厚型心肌病患者在其疾病过程的某一特定时刻的临床事件中也起着一定的作用。完全性心脏阻滞和其他传导异常如旁路引起的房室传导加快是肥厚型心肌病患者发生晕厥或猝死的已知但特别罕见的原因之一[4]。

五、猝死的预防

（一）药物治疗

目前，肥厚型心肌病高危患者的治疗仍局限于传统的β受体阻滞剂、维拉帕米和抗心律失常制剂如普鲁卡因胺、奎尼丁及近来更多应用的胺碘酮等预防性药物[4,21,22]。然而，仅有极少数回顾性资料支持药物治疗可有效预防肥厚型心肌病猝死[11,21,22]。目前尚无有关β受体阻滞剂或维拉帕米对猝死影响方面的对照研究。此外，由于致心律失常作用，目前临床上已不再应用IA类抗心律失常药物（如普鲁卡因胺、奎尼丁）预防治疗动态心电图监测中存在非持续性室速的肥厚型心肌病患者[1,3,4,7]。

目前认为胺碘酮可能会减低肥厚型心肌病患者猝

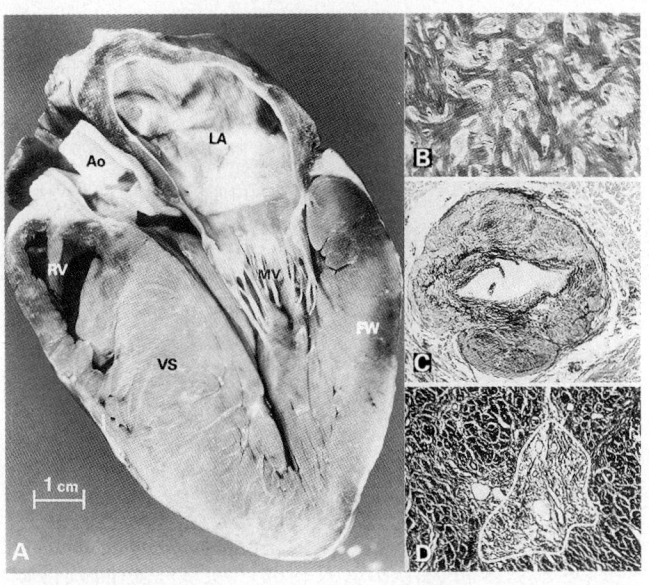

图64-2 肥厚型心肌病电不稳定及猝死的形态学基质 A：与超声心动图胸骨旁长轴切面相似，心脏横切面的大体解剖标本。左室壁不对称性肥厚，主要局限于室间隔，室间隔凸向左室流出道，左室腔变小。左室游离壁如图B，C，D所示。肥厚型心肌病心肌组织形态学特点和致心律失常性基质。B：相邻肥大的心肌细胞以直角和斜角排列，呈明显的结构紊乱。C：肌壁内冠状动脉管壁增厚，主要因中膜肥厚致管腔明显狭窄。D：邻近异常的壁内冠脉的心室肌区域被纤维组织所替代（心肌凋亡后）。AO：主动脉；FW：左室游离壁；LA：左房；RV：右室。（引自 Maron BJ. Hypertrophic cardiomyopathy. Lancet 350：127-133，1997.）

死的危险性[21]。然而，得出胺碘酮对猝死有保护性治疗作用的仅有的一篇文献是发表在15年前，研究对象为伴有非持续性室速且无症状或症状轻微的肥厚型心肌病患者，并且采用的是非随机、回顾对照的试验设计[21]。同样，声称胺碘酮对肥厚型心肌病猝死[21]具有绝对保护作用的研究结果也受到了质疑。一项来自植入了ICD的肥厚型心肌病高危患者的研究结果显示，大约50%因室速或室颤引发ICD放电的肥厚型心肌病患者同时服用胺碘酮[11]。此外，与长期服用胺碘酮相关的严重副作用（主要累及心脏外其他脏器）也大大限制了其在危险期较长的肥厚型心肌病年轻患者中的应用。因此，目前已不再推荐长期使用小剂量胺碘酮（200mg/d）或其他抗心律失常药物预防性治疗动态心电图监测中出现的短阵非持续性室速[7,9,13,21,22]。

（二）植入式心脏复律除颤器

预防肥厚型心肌病猝死仍是近40年来临床医师一直未能解决的主要挑战。自20年前Michel

Mirowski[28]首次在临床中应用 ICD 治疗以来，鉴于其能自动终止致死性室速及延长患者尤其是严重冠心病高危患者的寿命等无可争议的功效，作为预防猝死的措施，ICD 这一植入性装置已获得了广泛的认可[29-31]。近来一些前瞻性、随机的临床试验研究结果显示，在上述病人群体中，ICD 的益处明显优于抗心律失常药物[29-31]。然而，即便是在冠心病亚组病人中，ICD 的应用虽然较为广泛并日趋增加，但在某些少见却具有猝死危险的遗传性疾病中（如长 QT 综合征、Brugada 综合征、致心律失常性右室发育不良和肥厚型心肌病）中[32-36]，则应用得相对较少。

（三）ICD 应用的临床试验

近来，来自美国和意大利的一项多中心回顾性研究，对具有猝死高度危险的肥厚型心肌病患者进行了分析，以评估 ICD 感知并自动终止有潜在致死性的快速性心律失常的功能（图 64-3）[11]。受试者为 128 例肥厚型心肌病患者，所有病人均植入了 ICD，平均随访 3 年。结果显示，由室速触发的 ICD 治疗（电击或抗心动过速起搏）见于 25％ 左右的病人，年放电率约为 7％（图 64-3 和图 64-4）。此外，在整个随访期内，约 60％ 的患者经历了 ICD 多次有效的放电治疗。值得一提的是，尽管肥厚型心肌病患者左心室的重量明显增加，但 ICD 的功效依然显著[37]。来自欧洲心脏骤停存活者的大样本 ICD 登记资料[35]和高危儿童患者的初步报告显示了 ICD 治疗的临床益处[33]。

（四）二级预防

ICD 放电治疗多见于那些用于二级预防的植入患者，即心脏骤停幸存者（记录到室颤）或经历短阵自发的持续性室速患者。在相对较短的 3 年随访期内，约 40％ 以上既往有室颤或持续性室速的患者接受了 ICD 的适当治疗（图 64-3 和图 64-4）。潜在致死性室性心律失常在心脏骤停存活者中的发生频率与以往报道的在 ICD 前时代肥厚型心肌病患者中的发生频率相近[38]。

（五）一级预防

在那些将 ICD 仅用于一级预防的患者中，ICD 治疗的频率约为 5％/年（图 64-3 和图 64-4）。因高危状态而进行的包括预防性植入 ICD 在内的一级预防措施是由于患者存在一个或多个明确的猝死危险因素。这些危险因素有早产儿肥厚型心肌病相关性死亡的家族史，尤其是近亲属猝死或猝死高发史；高选择病例中存在高危突变基因；难以解释的晕厥，尤其是年轻患者在运动时发生的或反复发作的能够证实与心律失常相关的晕厥；连续动态心电图监测中有频发、多源或持续时间较长的非持续性室速；直立运动时异常的血压反应，血流动力学状态不稳定、低血压或 50 岁以下患者存在更高的预测价值；室壁厚度达到 30mm 或以上的极度左室肥厚，尤其是儿童和年轻患者[1,3,4,8,13,15,16]。然而，临床上，仅仅或主要根据低血压或运动时肥厚型心肌病患者血压反应减弱而判定病人属于高危状态

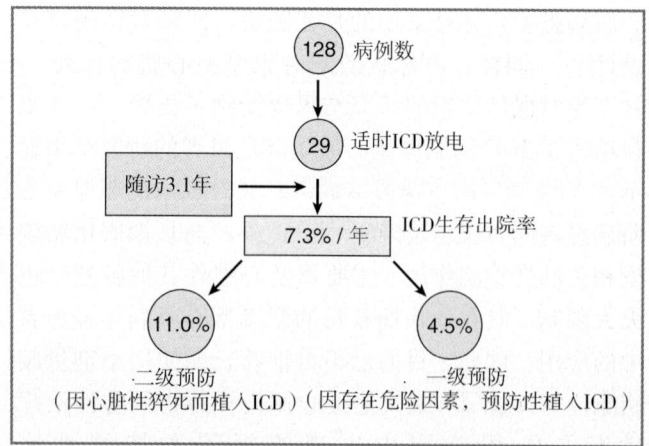

图 64-3　128 例因一级预防（≥1 个危险因素）和二级预防（心脏骤停或持续性室速幸存后）而植入 ICD 的肥厚型心肌病高危患者随访流程图　2 例肥厚型心肌病患者（未列出）死于终末期难治性心衰（尽管已植入了 ICD）。

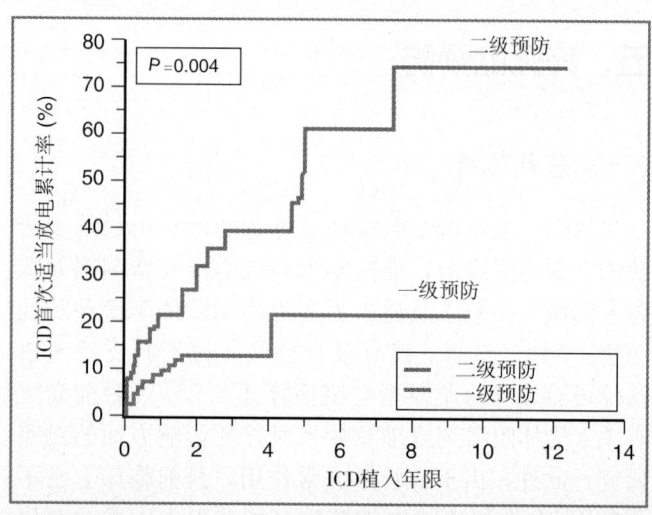

图 64-4　植入 ICD 后首次适当放电累计率，将因存在危险因素而预防性植入 ICD 的一级预防患者与因心脏骤停或持续性室速幸存后而植入 ICD 的二级预防患者分别计算

的情况极为罕见。

对肥厚型心肌病患者危险分层和ICD治疗的个人经验提示，在连续动态心电图监测中记录到多次反复发作的非持续性室速，应推荐ICD干预治疗。目前尚未证实流出道梗阻及梗阻程度是肥厚型心肌病患者发生猝死的强有力独立危险因素[39,40]。

需要强调的是，为防止猝死而给肥厚型心肌病患者预防性植入ICD标志着一种新的纯粹的一级预防形式。它仅仅评估了有自发的或经电生理检查证实的心律失常，且无症状（或症状轻微），无主要心血管事件的患者。

六、肥厚型心肌病的危险期

理解ICD在肥厚型心肌病中作用的关键在于重视ICD治疗在冠心病患者中的人口统计学特征。后者植入ICD时的年龄相对偏大（平均65岁），通常处于陈旧心梗引发的疾病进展期。相对而言，有猝死危险的肥厚型心肌病患者通常较为年轻，症状较轻或无症状，植入ICD或ICD适当放电时的年龄仅为40岁左右，并且近25%的患者不足30岁[11]。然而，重要的是包括中年甚至老年患者，其猝死的危险期较长[6,11,40]。实际上，肥厚型心肌病患者似乎并没有一个猝死危险减少的特殊年龄段。

肥厚型心肌病患者ICD的年放电率低于冠心病患者[29-31]。而且ICD植入时患者年龄更轻，通常并没有合并具有长期潜在危险的明显的充血性心力衰竭。若在ICD的保护下，这些病人可能存活数十年，甚至可以接近或达到正常人的寿命。

通过分析已报道的肥厚型心肌病患者ICD适当放电率[11]，我们估计，10年内对于大约50%预防性植入ICD的年轻患者，ICD可能会干预并成功治疗一次猝死事件。实际上，在已植入ICD的高危亚组患者中，其5%的年放电率极其接近第三诊治中心的高选择性肥厚型心肌病危险患者的猝死率[3]。

特别值得一提的是，从植入ICD到首次适当放电的时间间隔变化较大，延迟至9年后才发生拯救生命的干预治疗并不少见[11]（图64-5）。这些观察结果提示肥厚型心肌病患者猝死时间的不可预测性以及在最终适当干预治疗之前，ICD在很长的时间内均处于静止期。同样，根据危险分层和高危状态的识别时间而决定给肥厚型心肌病患者预防性植入ICD通常也是带有一定的偶然性。例如，一例患者20岁时就已证实存在高危因素（并在同时预防性植入了ICD），由于他很年轻，并且到35岁时危险性更大，即便ICD在这15年内并未进行适当放电，也应当植入ICD。因此，对于一个肥厚型心肌病高危患者，一旦决定给其植入ICD，就应将它作为一个终生预防治疗措施来考虑。

（一）诱发的室性心律失常

应用心室程序刺激进行心脏电生理检查和诱发室速来明确猝死[41]发生基质和机制意义的策略，现已基本被抛弃不用[1,3,4,42,43]。人们认识到该项技术的局限性，包括在肥厚型心肌病患者诱发出的单形性室速较为少见（仅见于10%的患者）。实际上，肥厚型心肌病心脏对心室刺激的电反应似乎更依赖于所用的刺激方案。例如，在相当一部分用3个心室期前刺激的心脏电生理检查方法就可能会诱发出持续性多形性室速或室颤。因此，当患者合并存在多种常见的心脏疾病如冠心病时，这些诱发性心律失常很可能是一种非特异性反应[3,4,42,43]。而对于肥厚型心肌病患者应用2个期前刺激诱发室速的实际临床意义也并不十分明确，而且与该方案本身的危险和操作过程的复杂性有关。因此，有关这些诱发性心律失常的意义可能并不太大。此外，临床中应用除心室程序刺激以外的无创性检测方法也可明确多数高危患者[4]。所以，目前常规

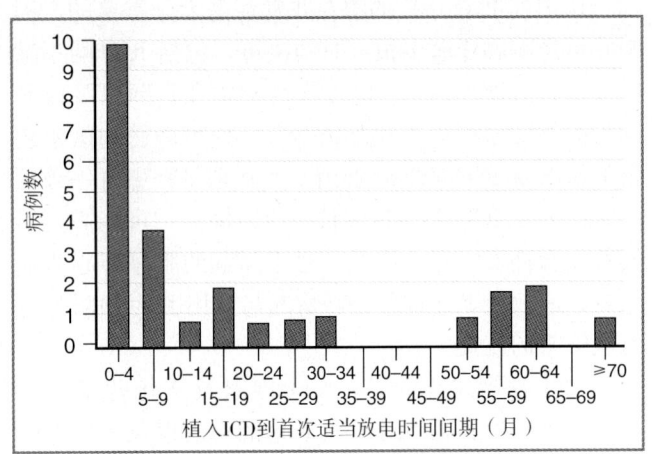

图64-5 29例肥厚型心肌病患者从植入ICD到首次适当放电的时间间期 注意有相当一部分患者在植入ICD 4～9年后才发生ICD的首次适时放电。（引自 Maron BJ, Shen WK, Lin MS, et al. Efficacy of implantable cardioverter-defibrillators for the prevention of sudden death in patients with hypertrophic cardiomyopathy. N Engl J Med. 342：365-373.2000.）

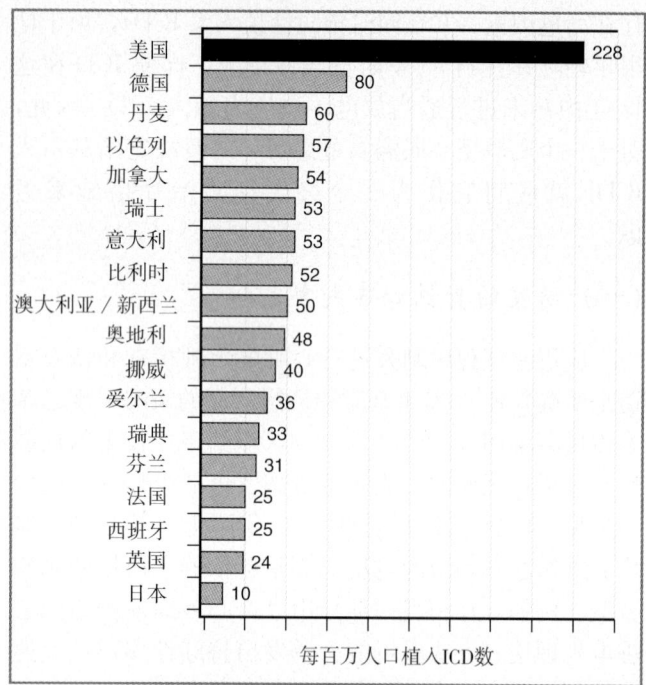

图 64-6 2001 年全球植入 ICD 示意图,以国别表示(每百万人口计) 所有患者均符合 ICD 植入指征,但其中大部分为冠心病。

应用电生理检查复制临床心律失常来预测肥厚型心肌病患者预后的方法的临床实用价值似乎不大。

(二)并发症和其他

认识到 ICD 治疗的潜在并发症是十分重要的,因为它可影响临床医生植入时的决策,包括 ICD 的不适当甚至误放电[11,29-30]、电极导线破损和折断以及极其罕见的静脉血栓形成和感染等。其他可能影响医生决策的情况有 ICD 的实际费用,尤其是年轻患者一级预防时植入了 ICD 并经过较长一段时间后,可能需要更换数个脉冲发生器。因此,对于高危的肥厚型心肌病患者,应权衡上述这些不利情况与应用 ICD 预防猝死可能带来的益处。

同样需要注意的是,由于国家及文化背景的不同,临床医生和患者对植入 ICD 的态度以及医疗保险系统对 ICD 的评估也有很大的差别(图 64-6)[44]。因此,这些均可能影响临床决策,特别是对肥厚型心肌病患者预防性植入 ICD 标准的界定。例如,相对于人口规模的 ICD 植入量,美国最多,约占全世界总量的 75%,为欧洲的 5 倍,为英国的 10 倍[44](图 64-6)。植入量的差别提示即便是同等危险程度的肥厚型心肌病患者能否接受 ICD 的一级预防,主要取决于患者所在的国家。

七、总 结

在肥厚型心肌病患者中,起源于电学特性不稳定心肌基质的原发性室速并不少见,可能也是经目前危险分层方法证实的高危患者发生突然及意外死亡的基础。应用 ICD 治疗此类遗传性心脏疾病,为部分高危患者预防猝死带来了希望。很显然,ICD 可有效治疗肥厚型心肌病患者,挽救病人的生命,并在猝死的一级和二级预防中发挥着十分重要的作用。

(黄卫斌 译)

参 考 文 献

1. Maron BJ: Hypertrophic cardiomyopathy. Lancet 350:127–133, 1997.
2. Wigle ED, Rakowski H, Kimball BP, Williams WG: Hypertrophic cardiomyopathy: Clinical spectrum and treatment. Circulation 92:1680–1692, 1995.
3. Spirito P, Seidman CE, McKenna WJ, Maron BJ: The management of hypertrophic cardiomyopathy. N Engl J Med 336:775–785, 1997.
4. Maron BJ: Hypertrophic cardiomyopathy: A systematic review. JAMA 287:1308–1320, 2002.
5. Teare D: Asymmetrical hypertrophy of the heart in young patients. Br Heart J 20:1–8, 1958.
6. Maron BJ, Olivotto I, Spirito P, et al: Epidemiology of hypertrophic cardiomyopathy-related death: Revisited in a large non-referral based patient population. Circulation 102:858–864, 2000.
7. Spirito P, Rapezzi C, Autore C, et al: Prognosis of asymptomatic patients with hypertrophic cardiomyopathy and nonsustained ventricular tachycardia. Circulation 90:2743–2747, 1994.
8. Olivotto I, Maron BJ, Montereggi A, et al: Prognostic value of systemic blood pressure response during exercise in a community-based patient population with hypertrophic cardiomyopathy. J Am Coll Cardiol 33:2044–2051, 1999.
9. Maron BJ, Savage DD, Wolfson JK, Epstein SE: Prognostic significance of 24-hour ambulatory electrocardiographic monitoring in patients with hypertrophic cardiomyopathy: A prospective study. Am J Cardiol 48:252–257, 1981.
10. Saumarez RC, Grace AA: Paced ventricular electrogram fractionation and sudden death in hypertrophic cardiomyopathy and other non-coronary heart diseases. Cardiovasc Res 47:11–22, 2000.
11. Maron BJ, Shen WK, Link MS, et al: Efficacy of implantable cardioverter-defibrillators for the prevention of sudden death in patients with hypertrophic cardiomyopathy. N Engl J Med 342:365–373, 2000.
12. Spirito P, Bellone P, Harris KM, et al: Magnitude of left ventricular hypertrophy predicts the risk of sudden death in hypertrophic cardiomyopathy. N Engl J Med 324:1778–1785, 2000.
13. McKenna WJ, England D, Doi YL, et al: Arrhythmia in hypertrophic cardiomyopathy: I—Influence on prognosis. Br Heart J 46:168–172, 1981.
14. Savage DD, Seides SF, Maron BJ, et al: Prevalence of arrhythmias during 24-hour electrocardiographic monitoring and exercise testing in patients with obstructive and nonobstructive hypertrophic cardiomyopathy. Circulation 59:866–875, 1979.
15. Elliott PM, Gimeno JR, Mahon NG, et al: Relation between severity of left-ventricular hypertrophy and prognosis in patients with hypertrophic cardiomyopathy. Lancet 357:420–424, 2001.
16. Elliott PM, Poloniecki J, Dickie S, et al: Sudden death in hypertrophic cardiomyopathy: Identification of high risk patients. J Am Coll Cardiol 36:2212–2218, 2000.
17. Adabag AS, Casey SA, Maron BJ: Sudden death in hypertrophic cardiomyopathy: Patterns and prognostic significance of tachyarrhythmias on ambulatory Holter ECG. Circulation 106(Suppl. II):II-710, 2002.

18. Alfonso F, Frenneaux M, McKenna WJ: Clinical sustained monomorphic ventricular tachycardia in hypertrophic cardiomyopathy: Association with left ventricular aneurysm. Br Heart J 61:178–181, 1989.
19. Maron BJ, Hauser RG, Roberts WC: Hypertrophic cardiomyopathy with left ventricular apical diverticulum. Am J Cardiol 77:117–119, 1996.
20. Ando H, Imaizumi T, Urabe Y, et al: Apical segmental dysfunction in hypertrophic cardiomyopathy: Subgroup with unique clinical features. J Am Coll Cardiol 16:1579–1588, 1990.
21. McKenna WJ, Oakley CM, Krikler DM, Goodwin JF: Improved survival with amiodarone in patients with hypertrophic cardiomyopathy and ventricular tachycardia. Br Heart J 53:412–416, 1985.
22. Cecchi F, Olivotto I, Montereggi A, et al: Prognostic value of non-sustained ventricular tachycardia and the potential role of amiodarone treatment in hypertrophic cardiomyopathy: Assessment in an unselected non-referral based patient population. Heart 79:331–336, 1998.
23. Nicod P, Polikar R, Peterson KL: Hypertrophic cardiomyopathy and sudden death. N Engl J Med 318:1255–1256, 1988.
24. Elliott PM, Sharma S, Varnava A, et al: Survival after cardiac arrest in patients with hypertrophic cardiomyopathy. J Am Coll Cardiol 33:1596–1601, 1999.
25. Maron BJ, Roberts WC: Quantitative analysis of cardiac muscle cell disorganization in the ventricular septum of patients with hypertrophic cardiomyopathy. Circulation 59:689–706, 1979.
26. Maron BJ, Anan TJ, Roberts WC: Quantitative analysis of the distribution of cardiac muscle cell disorganization in the left ventricular wall of patients with hypertrophic cardiomyopathy. Circulation 63:882–894, 1981.
27. Maron BJ, Wolfson JK, Epstein SE, Roberts WC: Intramural ("small vessel") coronary artery disease in hypertrophic cardiomyopathy. J Am Coll Cardiol 8:545–557, 1986.
28. Mirowski M, Reid PR, Mower MM, et al: Termination of malignant ventricular arrhythmias with an implanted automatic defibrillator in human beings. N Engl J Med 303:322–324, 1980.
29. A comparison of anitarrhythmic-drug therapy with implantable defibrillators in patients resuscitated from near-fatal ventricular arrhythmias: The Antiarrhythmics versus Implantable Defibrillators (AVID) Investigators. N Engl J Med 337:1576–1583, 1997.
30. Moss AJ, Hall WJ, Cannom DS, et al: Improved survival with an implanted defibrillator in patients with coronary disease at high risk for ventricular arrhythmia. N Engl J Med 335:1933–1940, 1996.
31. Moss AJ, Zareba W, Hall WJ, et al: Prophylactic implantation of a defibrillator in patients with myocardial infarction and reduced ejection fraction. N Engl J Med 346:877–883, 2002.
32. Moss AJ, Daubert JP: Images in clinical medicine: Internal ventricular defibrillation. N Engl J Med 342:398, 2000.
33. Silka MJ, Kron J, Dunnigan A, et al: Sudden cardiac death and the use of implantable cardioverter-defibrillators in pediatric patients. Circulation 87:800–807, 1993.
34. Link MS, Wang PJ, Haugh CJ, et al: Arrhythmogenic right ventricular dysplasia: Clinical results with implantable cardioverter defibrillators. J Interv Card Electrophysiol 1:41–48, 1997.
35. Borggrefe MM, McKenna WJ: Primary and secondary prevention of sudden death with the implantable cardioverter-defibrillator in hypertrophic cardiomyopathy: Results of the European Registry on Implantable Cardioverter-Defibrillators in Hypertrophic Cardiomyopathy [abstract]. Circulation 106:II–710, 2002.
36. Primo J, Geelen P, Brugada J, et al: Hypertrophic cardiomyopathy: Role of the implantable cardioverter-defibrillator. J Am Coll Cardiol 31:1081–1085, 1998.
37. Klues HG, Schiffers A, Maron BJ: Phenotypic spectrum and patterns of left ventricular hypertrophy in hypertrophic cardiomyopathy: Morphologic observations and significance as assessed by two-dimensional echocardiography in 600 patients. J Am Coll Cardiol 26:1699–1708, 1995.
38. Cecchi F, Maron BJ, Epstein SE: Long-term outcome of patients with hypertrophic cardiomyopathy successfully resuscitated after cardiac arrest. J Am Coll Cardiol 13:1283–1288, 1989.
39. Maron MS, Olivotto I, Betocchi S, et al: Effect of left ventricular outflow tract obstruction on clinical outcome in hypertrophic cardiomyopathy. N Engl J Med 348:295–303, 2003.
40. Maron BJ, Casey SA, Poliac LC, et al: Clinical consequences of hypertrophic cardiomyopathy in an unselected regional United States cohort. JAMA 281:650–655, 1999.
41. Fananapazir L, Chang AC, Epstein SE, McAreavey D: Prognostic determinants in hypertrophic cardiomyopathy: Prospective evaluation of a therapeutic strategy based on clinical, Holter, hemodynamic and electrophysiologic findings. Circulation 86:730–740, 1992.
42. Geibel A, Brugada P, Zehender M, et al: Value of programmed electrical stimulation using standardized ventricular stimulation protocol in hypertrophic cardiomyopathy. Am J Cardiol 60:738–739, 1987.
43. Kuck KH, Kunze KP, Schluter M, et al: Programmed electrical stimulation in hypertrophic cardiomyopathy: Results in patients with and without cardiac arrest or syncope. Eur Heart J 9:177–185, 1988.
44. Camm AJ, Nisam S: The utilization of the implantable defibrillator: A European enigma. Eur Heart J 21:1998–2004, 2000.

第 65 章

心脏肥大和心力衰竭的室性心动过速

Marc A. Vos and Harry J. Crijns

本章目录
- 前言 600
- 心脏肥大和心力衰竭的病理生理 600
- 心力衰竭患者心脏性猝死的预防 605
- 总结 608

一、前　言

在西方国家，心力衰竭致死的患者已越来越多。据估计在美国约有 500 万充血性心力衰竭患者，其中每年的住院患者超过 200 万，平均每年新增 40 万病例。实际上，随着人口的老龄化，这个数字仍在上升，例如在 50 岁以下人群中，仅有 1％的人群发生心力衰竭，而在 80 岁以上的人群中，心力衰竭的发生率达到 10％。近几十年来，由于药物治疗的进展，心衰患者的生存率明显提高，但总的死亡率仍然很高。尽管使用了血管紧张素转换酶抑制剂（图 65-1），每年的死亡率仍达 5％～38％。因此，心衰患者的 5 年预后仍然不容乐观，约有 50％以上的患者将在 5 年内死亡，其中心脏性猝死率平均在 40％～50％。对于无症状性心力衰竭的患者，总死亡率是低的，通常多是猝死，表明心脏性猝死可能在临床诊断心力衰竭之前就已经发生。为了更好地理解此类心脏性猝死的发生机制，我们将要讨论心脏肥大患者心律失常方面的内容，但这些患者还无心功能不全的表现。

心力衰竭可由多种疾病引起，常常是多种疾病的协同作用，最主要的病因是高血压和冠心病[1]。需要注意的是，舒张功能不全的发生率在不断上升，其特点是不仅有临床表现，而且多数心力衰竭患者是老年人（>70 岁），此前已有收缩功能不全的表现。在前几章（参见第 61～64 章），我们已经叙述过心律失常性心脏病特别是心肌病的特点。在本章，我们讨论的重点放在心力衰竭时的不同心室重塑过程导致的室性心律失常和心脏性猝死。

二、心脏肥大和心力衰竭的病理生理

（一）心室重塑

心脏在其环境发生改变时就已开始出现适应性反应（获得性病理改变）。这种改变可能是压力负荷增加（高血压）、容量负荷增加（瓣膜性心脏病）、缺血事件（只有很少心肌参与泵血）、神经内分泌信号、缓慢性或快速性心律失常、病毒感染或上述诸因素的结合。上述所有情况都可发生心室重塑。目前广泛研究的内容是针对能引起心力衰竭和心律失常表型的更广泛遗传因素。

心脏的适应性改变包括电激动、收缩功能、代谢和结构特征的改变，并已在完整心脏、多细胞标本和从人移植心脏分离的心肌细胞及心力衰竭动物模型上得到证实。这种心室重塑引起室性心律失常和心脏性猝死的危险性增加[2-11]。为了能给予适当治疗，需要了解疾病的进展和信号转导通路。如仅为了达到这个目标，只用动物模型就可以了。但为了弄清心脏从代偿发展到失代偿的信号转导通路，要求动物模型最好应具备这种转变的过程[12,16]，并可能涉及新的发生机制。必须对逆转不同重塑过程治疗的有效性进行评价。这些研究可以选择患者进行研究，也可以进行动

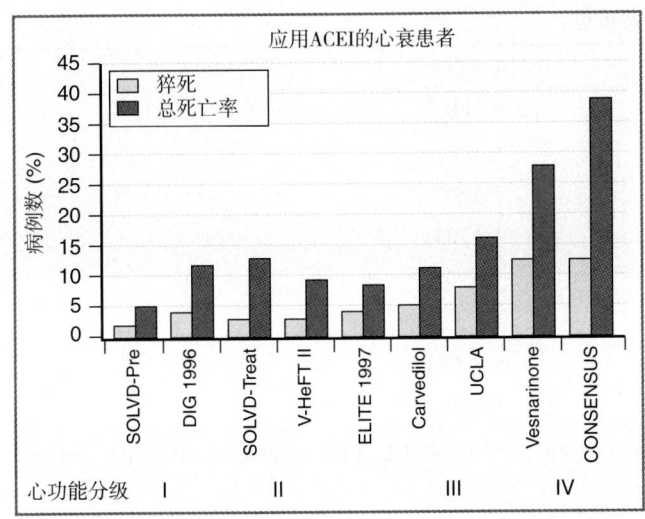

图 65-1 近期心力衰竭试验中的年死亡率和心脏性猝死率

图中这些试验按照心力衰竭的严重程度从左至右依次为：左侧为轻度（NYHA Ⅰ级），右侧为重度（NYHA Ⅳ级）。请注意心脏性猝死和总死亡率之间的比率，当心功能在Ⅰ～Ⅲ级之间时，其比率高达50%，而当心功能在Ⅳ级时，心脏性猝死比率较低。（引自 Stevenson WG, Stevenson LW. Prevention of sudden death in heart failure. J Cardiova sc Electrophysiol, 2001; 12: 112-114.）

物模型实验。

但决定心室动作电位时限的钾电流存在着种属间的明显差异。例如在小型哺乳动物，瞬间外向钾电流（I_{to}）是主要复极电流，而在大型哺乳动物，延迟整流钾电流（I_k）是主要复极电流。本章主要讨论大型动物模型。我们要提出的心室重塑模型的动物是兔，因为兔与人相同，延迟整流钾电流是主要复极电流。

左室肥大是曾被描述过的最早的重塑过程。心室肥大可能是多种心脏病恢复正常室壁张力的代偿机制。心室肥大的特征、时间长短及严重程度，表明心室体积的增大可能是通过其他结构的改变来代偿的，如纤维化（替代性）、细胞间的耦联改变（缝隙间接功能的障碍）、毛细血管/心肌细胞比例下降（心肌缺血）以及胚胎性基因程序再启动而伴随的心肌细胞去分化和退化改变。此外，心室肥大信号通路的慢性激活被认为与心力衰竭的发生有关。

钙离子（Ca^{2+}）是心肌电机械耦联的基本离子。当钙离子从细胞外进入细胞后，即L型钙电流，能诱发肌浆网的钙大量释放进入细胞质，再连接肌丝产生收缩。肌浆网上的兰尼丁受体能完成钙浓度依赖性钙释放。钙也可以通过肌浆网上的 Ca^{2+}-ATP 酶（SERCA2）再泵回肌浆网，而经钙通道进入细胞内的部分钙离子又通过钠-钙交换体泵出细胞外[12]。

当在病理情况下机体需求增加时，机体/心脏要激活许多神经内分泌通路来维持心输出量，并迅速出现钙调基因的改变，来持续增加钙电流，其最终结果是发生充血性心力衰竭、基本收缩功能减弱、对β肾上腺素刺激的收缩反应降低[5]和变时性减低或负性肌力作用[6]。肌浆网可通过向细胞质缓慢排出钙离子而减少钙存储。上述这些因素均能降低和延长细胞内钙电流[4]。降低 Ca^{2+}-ATP 酶（SERCA）作用和增强钠-钙交换泵功能均能引起这种钙处理功能的异常。而通过改变兰尼丁受体功能（过度磷酸化）从肌浆网增加舒张期钙释放也能减少肌浆网钙超载[7]。

不论是人类还是动物模型，与结构或收缩状态无关的重塑心脏的最明显特征是心室动作电位的延长（电重塑，表65-1）。因此，动作电位时限延长所表现的QT间期延长似乎是心脏发生适应性改变的关键。

充血性心力衰竭患者的持续交感神经兴奋能引起肾上腺素能受体下调，特别是 $β_1$ 肾上腺素受体。这可能导致交感神经分布的失衡，引起心律失常。

此外，充血性心力衰竭患者，室上性心律失常，特别是心房颤动，可能引起严重的并发症。心房颤动能导致心房辅助泵功能的急性丧失，不能在快速心室率的情况下维持心输出量，并能诱发心动过速介导性心肌病。换句话说，充血性心力衰竭能够使心房颤动更易发生，因为纤维化能引起缓慢传导[17]。当充血性心力衰竭和心房颤动同时发生时，其因果关系很难确定。

（二）心脏电重塑的离子基础

许多离子通道或离子泵相互密切合作参与心室动作电位的形成[18]。除极电流和复极电流间精密平衡才能引起电-机械耦联。每种通道选择性允许特定离子通过，具有特定的生物物理特性。许多离子通道是由大分子形成，不同的亚单位形成功能单位[19]。这些亚单位是不同基因的产物。如图65-2所示，不同离子通道的构成均有α亚单位（孔形成蛋白）和β亚单位（修饰蛋白）。已证实健康者基因表达水平和电流强度有明显的差异，可用动作电位的形态和时限来描述（图65-2）。心室不同区域间动作电位时限的差异称为复极空间离散，在犬的心脏，左心室存在跨壁复极离散，而且在双室之间及心尖部与心底部之间也存在复极离散。离子通道的表达和功能之间也有差异（参见图65-2下图）。请注意这仅仅是对心室动作电位而言的。

表 65-1 心室重塑

	结构重塑	收缩功能重塑	电重塑	心律失常
CHF 移植心脏	≈/↑	↓	↑APD	(+)
CHF 犬心脏	≈	↓	↑APD	+SCD
CHF 兔心脏	↑	↓	↑APD	?
CAVB 犬心脏	↑		↑↑APD	+SCD
CAVB 兔心脏	↑	=	↑↑APD	++SCD
R+N 兔心脏	↑	?	≈/↑APD	—
AI+AS 兔心脏	↑	↓	≈/↑APD	++SCD
MI 犬心脏	↑	=	↑APD	PES

注：AI，主动脉瓣关闭不全；APD，动作电位时限；AS，主动脉瓣狭窄；CAVB，完全性房室阻滞；CHF，充血性心力衰竭；MI，心肌梗死；R+N，肾结扎和肾切除兔；SCD，心脏性猝死。

对于心脏其他部位来说，请参考最新综述[20]。在充血性心力衰竭和心肌梗死后，也存在浦肯野纤维的电重塑，其可能与早期后除极依赖的触发活动和心律失常有关。

电重塑涉及在表达水平、生物物理或特异离子通道调节和交换水平的缓慢细胞和分子变化，包括脉冲的形成（窦房结功能改变和异位搏动的产生）、脉冲的传导（缝隙连接的表达改变和更严重的纤维化）[21]、或心室的复极（QT 间期延长）。心室动作电位时限的延长常常发生在静息膜电位、动作电位最大上升速度（Vmax）和幅度没有变化的情况下。电重塑的特征并不就是 QT 间期延长，而是存在心室复极不同区域间内在差异，这在代偿性肥大和心力衰竭时更为明显[16,22-25]。不过，在最近几篇研究报告中，在起搏诱发的心力衰竭动物模型上其左室跨壁离散度极小[10,11]。由于动作电位时限的延长，心肌细胞有极小的复极储备，即意味着调节动作电位时限长短的能力明显降低，特别是在动态情况下当心率快速变化时。这种适应能力的丧失可以引起：（1）早后除极和相关的异位触发活动；（2）在连续心搏时，QT 间期的长度明显不同时表现为时间离散。局部早后除极的产生能引起空间离散，而异位触发活动能引起时间和空间离散。

在离子通道水平（离子通道病），时空离散可以用 mRNA 表达或蛋白表达的改变和对特异刺激反应的功能改变来解释。表 65-2 显示，不同动物模型因离子通道改变引起的动作电位时限变化，虽然目前还无详细结论，但很明显取决于模型或疾病。以前，研究报告主要集中在代偿性肥大心脏和心力衰竭时瞬间外向钾电流和 L 型钙电流及钠钙交换泵的改变，最近动物实验主要集中在延迟整流钾电流（I_K）[8-11,13-15,22]。延迟整流钾电流由两种成分组成，即缓慢（I_{Ks}）和快速（I_{Kr}）电流。延迟整流钾电流的功能丧失可能与离子通道亚单位的密度降低或生物物理特性改变有关，能够引起整个细胞电流的降低。这项动物实验研究已经取得进展，也期望从这些技术中了解到更多的知识。

（三）心律失常的发生机制

绝大多数进展期心力衰竭的患者发生猝死的机制可能是室性心动过速或心室颤动（表 65-3）。尽管在心力衰竭终末期，心动过缓、栓塞和电机械分离可能起主要作用[1,11]，但是由于疾病的复杂性，可能有多种致心律失常机制参与，包括异常脉冲的形成和折返。异常脉冲的形成可分为异常自律性和触发活动。

充血性心力衰竭的长期病理改变结果是心室重塑。受累的心肌可能局限在一个心室或两个心室的特定区域。此外，不同类型的适应性反应也可能在同一心室出现，如在心肌梗死时，坏死心肌发生不同的重塑。重塑肥大的心脏更可能面对多种因素的挑战，如药物、缺血、再灌注和电解质失衡。

心肌广泛纤维化可能降低有效传导速度，缓慢传导可能引起单向传导阻滞，进而发生折返性心律失常。除此之外，心肌梗死区的存活心肌可能成为异常传导和晚电位的发生基质，这是由于隐匿性连续脉冲传导所致。

钙调节功能的适应很容易触发异常脉冲。早后除极和迟后除极都被认为是钙调节异常所致[24]。当收缩反应（收缩后）提前于电反应（后除极），可引起细胞内钙清除异常，因而通过钠钙交换泵产生瞬间内向

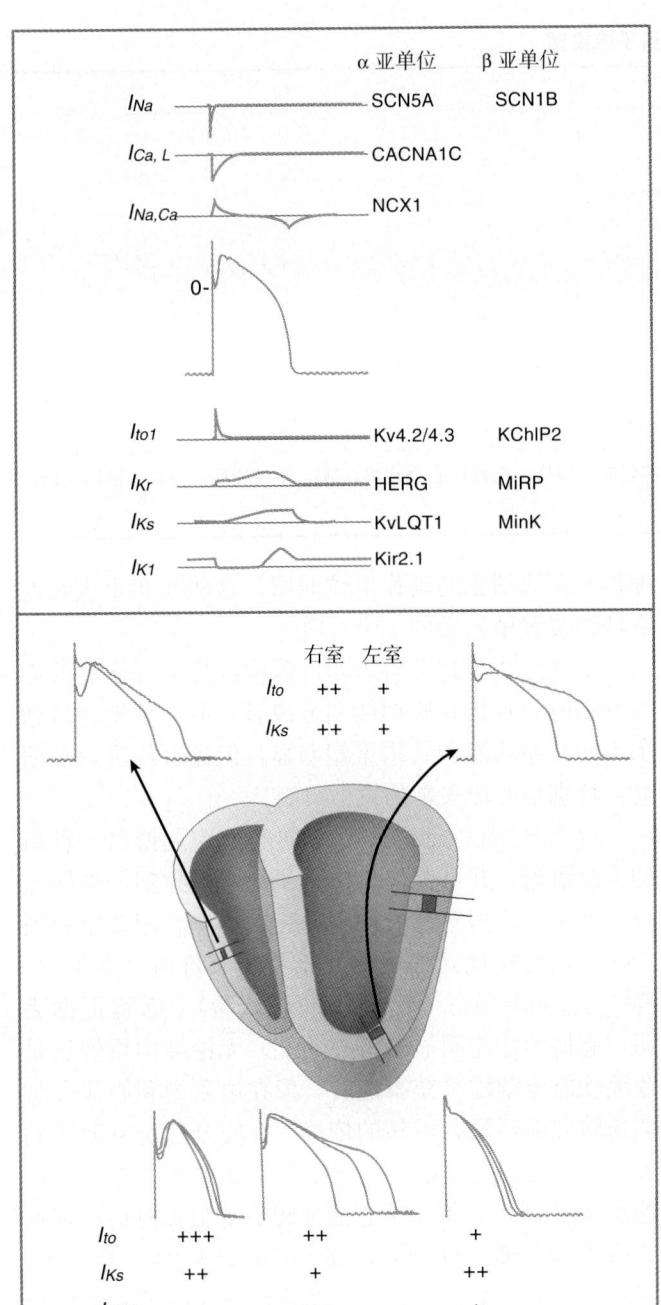

图 65-2 用离子流的分布来解释心室动作电位时限和形态的各向异性 上图显示，编码不同离子流亚单位的基因来解释它们的分布对心室动作电位的影响。下图显示，双室之间（顶图）和左室壁之间（底图，从心外膜至心内膜）动作电位的时限和形态差异，以及表达的离子流相应分布差异。

钾电流。

在充血性心力衰竭的心脏，肌浆网有很少的钙离子可以利用，但触发活动为何能引起充血性心力衰竭患者发生心律失常和心脏性猝死？首先，心脏性猝死可以发生在并不很严重的收缩功能不全的患者。在绝大多数严重心力衰竭的患者，迟后除极依赖性心律失常仍然起主要作用，此时β受体应答反应仍然存在、钠钙交换功能增加以及复极电流降低[9]。此外，并非所有细胞都衰竭，而是有许多细胞过度代偿，其肌浆网有较大的钙池。许多用于临床的正性变时药物有致心律失常作用，如β受体激动剂、钠通道激活剂、磷酸双类固醇抑制剂，所有这些环节都参与钙与心律失常间的连接过程。地高辛也有类似作用，它常常被用于充血性心力衰竭患者的治疗，但是可能引起室性心律失常。

充血性心力衰竭的患者经常出现短暂心肌缺血。而起源于静息膜电位降低的细胞的异常自律性可能引起异位搏动或甚至心动过速。除此之外，还可能发生传导阻滞，易引起单向阻滞和促进心动过速的发生。

复极时间延长的各向异性能产生空间离散，并可通过2相折返引起室性心动过速，因为2相折返能引起触发活动及维持心律失常的折返环。复极时限缩短易于发生药物诱发性尖端扭转型室速[25]。对人心脏的三维标测研究显示，在非缺血性充血性心力衰竭的患者，室速100%是由局灶或非折返机制引起，而在缺血性充血性心力衰竭患者的室速中仅有50%为非折返机制[26]。

（四）心肌重塑过程的演化

心肌重塑的进展和不可逆转的时间是重点研究项目。回答下列问题非常重要：是否不同重塑过程遵循同一演化时间途径；是否在这些适应过程之间有相互联系。已有研究表明，心室重塑过程有不同的信号转导通路。

众多较小型动物模型的实验研究显示，电重塑发生在结构重塑之前。Huang等[27]发现鼠模型的钾通道和钾电流（I_{to}和I_{K1}）下调出现在心肌梗死后3d，此时并无心室肥大。当对鼠心脏进行起搏（程序电刺激诱发的室速）时，钾通道和钾电流的改变引起心律失常。Zobel等[28]已证明，在培养的心肌细胞中，离子通道下调正是心脏结构改变的起始点；同时还证实心室肥大并不是心肌收缩重塑的前提条件[29]。这些有关不同时间途径的研究结果在完全性房室阻滞犬模型上得到验证[30]。收缩功能重塑和电重塑是否享有同一命名还不清楚。研究已证实，在人类，代偿肥大心脏与充血性心力衰竭有不同的信号转导通路：在充血性心力衰竭时，所有的丝裂原激活蛋白激酶（MAPKs）（p38，JNK，ERK）都增加，而在肥大心脏，则不发

表 65-2　左室离子流重塑

	I_{Na}	I_{CaL}	I_{to}	I_{K1}	I_{Kr}	I_{Ks}	NCX
CHF 移植心脏	↑	↓/=	↓	↓		(=)	
CHF 犬心脏		↓/=	↓	↓	=	↓	(↑)
CHF 兔心脏		↓/=	↓	=		↓	↓
CAVB 犬心脏	=	=	=	=	↓/=	↓↓	↑
CAVB 兔心脏	=	=	↑	↓		↓	
R+N 兔心脏	=	↑	↓	↓		=	↓
AI+AS 兔心脏	=		↓	↓		↓	↑
MI 犬心脏	↑	↓	↓	↓	↓	↓	=

注：AI，主动脉瓣关闭不全；AS，主动脉瓣狭窄；CAVB，完全性房室阻滞；CHF，充血性心力衰竭；MI，心肌梗死；NCD，钠钙交换；R+N，肾结扎和肾切除兔。

生这种改变[31]。当从心功能代偿期向左室功能不全转化时，电重塑可能发生。

（五）逆转心肌重塑的干预治疗

关于左室辅助装置疗效的研究资料是十分有价值的，其治疗方法已成为心脏移植的过渡阶段。由于左室辅助装置需要经左室入路植入，所以在植入时获取的心肌组织与心脏移植时所取的心肌组织进行对比，就可得到有价值的研究资料用于研究心室电活动、收缩功能和结构方面的表现，包括压力负荷和容量负荷，其研究结果令人鼓舞[5,32,33]：

1. 逆转结构重塑：通过降低基质金属蛋白酶来逆转心室和心肌细胞肥大、逆转心腔扩张、逆转压力-容量关系曲线、改善左室壁顺应性。

2. 逆转收缩功能重塑：增强心肌细胞的基础收缩功能、提高多数下调钙处理蛋白基因的表达水平、增强对肾上腺素能刺激的收缩反应和增加心率。

3. 逆转神经内分泌信号：增加β受体数量、改善心肌对肾上腺素能刺激的收缩反应、降低血浆中神经内分泌激素和细胞因子以及减少心室利钠肽的表达。

4. 逆转电重塑[33]：控制室率和恢复 QT 间期、缩短心室肌细胞的动作电位时限，这些改变出现在左室辅助装置植入后的 1 个月内。

上述这些研究资料表明，曾被认为不可恢复的心力衰竭的心脏其心肌功能明显改善，但电重塑逆转效果不如收缩功能和结构重塑明显，但还有待进一步研究，特别是心律失常的发生机制。

对充血性心力衰竭的患者进行双室起搏是一种新的治疗措施，并可提供机会来研究心室重塑的逆转过程。近来，许多对充血性心力衰竭的患者用双室起搏治疗并进行长期随访的研究结果很有价值（参见 Yu 等[34]、Linde 等[35]、Companion 试验）。已有证据表明，起搏治疗能明显改善心功能。无论结构重塑还是收缩功能重塑均可获得逆转，但在电重塑和心律失常的逆转方面还没有可靠的依据。在完全性房室阻滞的犬心脏，由起搏重新启动的窦性心律并不能缩短延长的复极时间[30]，提示尽管能逆转心室肥大但仍存在致心律失常基质。同样，Companion 试验的结果表明，双室起搏加用植入式心脏复律除颤器在降低心脏性猝死方面比单纯起搏治疗的效果要好。这表明在收缩功能和致心律失常水平上存在不同的可逆性重塑过程，但收缩功能的改善与心律失常基质减少并不平行。

表 65-3

表示充血性心力衰竭的早期和晚期发生心脏性猝死的各种病理生理机制的相关假说。电解质紊乱、神经内分泌激活和心肌缺血可能是最主要机制

	急性心肌梗死*	栓塞	VT 和 VF	心动过缓	EMD
CHF 早期	++	+	+	−	−
CHF 晚期	−	++	++	++	++

*广泛心肌梗死未进行植入式心脏复律除颤器治疗。
CHF，充血性心力衰竭；EMD，电机械分离；VF，心室颤动；VT，室性心动过速。

三、心力衰竭患者心脏性猝死的预防

(一) 心脏性猝死的机制：循证医学证据

随着充血性心力衰竭程度的加重，心脏性猝死率不断上升，但是从总死亡率角度来讲，心脏性猝死所占比例在下降（图65-1）。迄今为止还不清楚心脏性猝死的发生机制是否随着疾病严重程度的加重而不同。快速性心律失常可能是充血性心力衰竭极早期发生心脏性猝死的主要机制，即多见于左室肥大伴舒张性心力衰竭的患者，其依据是左室肥大引起电重塑，从而引起心律失常。但是，左室肥大的患者可能因其他机制发生猝死，如心肌梗死、严重脑卒中。心律失常多见于充血性心力衰竭早期，但并不能说明抗心律失常措施有效。相反，常规抗心律失常药物可能具有致心律失常的作用，而不是抗心律失常，所以应该避免使用，特别是Ⅲ类抗心律失常药物[25]。在收缩性心力衰竭患者（严重充血性心力衰竭，参见表65-3），各种情况都有作用，包括非心律失常情况[36,37]。相反，心律失常影响最常发生在极严重的收缩性心力衰竭患者，其左室射血分数下降到30%，无论是缓慢性心律失常还是室性心动过速。有证据表明，植入式心脏复律除颤器对严重疾病的患者十分有效，而对收缩功能代偿的患者则效果差[38]。心脏性猝死更多见于严重充血性心力衰竭的患者（缺血性或非缺血性），常有急性冠脉闭塞。但经数年后，所有患者的其余冠状动脉仍然"存活"，而且很少发生斑块破裂、心肌梗死和猝死。除此之外，严重充血性心力衰竭的患者在其生活中既往可能有心肌缺血发作，而且他们可能缺乏在心肌缺血过程中发生心室颤动的遗传易患因素。但是，这些患者有发生大块栓塞和电机械分离的危险。心室颤动和心动过缓的患者可植入植入式心脏复律除颤器。心脏性猝死的其他原因是"血管性"充血性心力衰竭，即主动脉瘤破裂（参见表65-3）。

既然心脏性猝死的发生机制十分复杂，那么要预测心脏性猝死是很困难的。迄今为止，关于左室射血分数方面的资料最多，不仅与心脏性猝死的绝对危险有关，而且与预测植入植入式心脏复律除颤器的治疗反应有关。室性异位激动在充血性心力衰竭的患者常见，有近80%的患者为非持续性室速。但是，这些室性异位激动在预测非缺血性心力衰竭的患者发生心脏性猝死方面没有特异性。已有作者提出，心率变异性和其他功能指标可作为评价指标，可用来反映心率变化和频率一致性。此外，动态心电图记录的QT间期变化提示复极时间缩短与心脏性猝死相关[39]。信号平均心电图能够反映充血性心力衰竭的缓慢传导基质。脑钠肽（BNP）被用来对患者随访监测，据报告它能预测充血性心力衰竭患者发生猝死。但是，除左室射血分数外，上述指标没有一项能用于危险分层。

总之，充血性心力衰竭时需要对心律失常和心脏性猝死的治疗进行探讨。首先，心力衰竭的常规治疗；其次，应针对下列情况进行治疗，如高血压、冠心病和心脏瓣膜病；最后，对充血性心力衰竭合并心房颤动的患者，抗血栓治疗有明确指征，因为大块栓塞能引起心脏性猝死。除上述治疗外，特异的抗心律失常治疗如果需要应该给予（表65-4）。

(二) β受体阻滞剂

慢性肾上腺素能神经过度兴奋在充血性心力衰竭中起重要作用，能引起心肌功能障碍[5,7]。β受体阻滞剂能直接降低肾上腺素能依赖性室性心律失常。β受体阻滞剂具有抗充血性心力衰竭、抗心肌缺血和抗高血压的作用，并起到间接抗心律失常作用。除此之外，许多研究表明，β受体阻滞剂能降低心力衰竭患者的死亡率（表65-5）。而且β受体阻滞剂对心肌梗死后的心力衰竭患者更为有效。联合应用血管紧张素转换酶抑制剂时，β受体阻滞剂能降低左室功能不全时或无充血性心力衰竭症状患者的死亡率[40-43]。除了降低总死亡率以外，β受体阻滞剂还能减少心脏性猝死的发生率以及因心功能不全的住院率。应避免与血管紧张素Ⅱ受体拮抗剂合用[44]。对于植入式心脏复律除颤器的患者，β受体阻滞剂不应该应用，因为它能使心律失常更为复杂，而使植入式心脏复律除颤器很难处理。但植入了植入式心脏复律除颤器的患者也存在非心律失常性猝死机制，β受体阻滞剂具有预防猝死的作用。

(三) 血管紧张素转换酶抑制剂

随机试验入选数千例患者，其研究结果表明，血管紧张素转换酶抑制剂能提高心力衰竭患者的生存率和改善收缩功能不全，其治疗作用与心力衰竭的病因和症状的严重性无关。表65-6列出数项研究。此外，血管紧张素转换酶抑制剂能够有效保护血管完整性，包括内皮细胞、血管运动功能，因而能预防心肌缺血

表65-4 心力衰竭患者的持续性室性心动过速的治疗原则

全球心力衰竭的治疗原则
明确冠状动脉的解剖，对可逆性心肌缺血和存活心肌的功能评估，如有适应证给予血管再通处理
大剂量血管紧张素转换酶抑制剂治疗
应用利尿剂治疗以减轻容量负荷过重，但应注意电解质紊乱
在血流动力学稳定时，尽早应用β受体阻滞剂
考虑抗血栓治疗
抗心律失常治疗措施
绝大多数患者应给予植入式心脏复律除颤器治疗
对不同的患者亚组给予药物治疗（胺碘酮、多非利特、索他洛尔）；Ⅳ级心功能患者也不作为必需心脏移植的对象
对严重左心功能不全患者有轻微症状的心动过速的治疗
对于频发自发性心动过速的患者，考虑用抗心律失常药物治疗（胺碘酮、多非利特、索他洛尔）；对于持续性和无休止性心动过速的患者，应考虑导管消融治疗

表65-5 β受体阻滞剂在充血性心力衰竭中的作用

论文发表（NYHA）	随访（月）	β受体阻滞剂	安慰剂	死亡率	ARR	NNT
CIBIS Ⅱ（Ⅲ～Ⅳ）	16	11.8%	17.3%	34%	5.5%	18
MERIT-HF	12	7.2%	11%	34%	3.8%	26
US 卡维地洛（Ⅱ～Ⅳ）	7	3.2%	7.8%	65%	4.6%	21
Copernicus（Ⅲ～Ⅳ）	10.4	11.2%	16.8%	35%	5.6%	18

ARR，绝对危险下降率；NNT，依据平均随访时间，需要治疗的病例数；RRR，相对危险下降率。

事件的发生，并可用于充血性心力衰竭的患者[45]。心室体积和心力衰竭的严重性也随着这些药物的应用而降低。

在绝大多数研究中，尽管血管紧张素转换酶抑制剂及血管紧张素受体阻断剂对心肌电生理重塑有抑制作用，血管紧张素转换酶抑制剂对自发性室性早搏和非持续性室速无效。

（四）抗血栓治疗

抗血栓治疗在预防心脏性猝死方面的作用还不清楚。这与研究结果有关。循证医学表明，当在窦性心律时，心力衰竭患者比心房颤动患者具有较少发生脑卒中的危险，而心房颤动患者，应该使用华法林治疗[46]。依据几项大规模的研究报告，每年每1000名患者中脑卒中的发生率在1.6～2.5之间[47]。但实际上发生率远远高于这个数字，因为脑卒中事件可能没有报告，而且心脏性猝死通常并不是大块栓塞引起，还有待进一步研究以解决这个问题。

（五）抗心律失常药物治疗

抗心律失常药物已被用来控制有症状的持续性室速，并被用来降低远期死亡率。不过，有几项对照研究显示，抗心律失常药物治疗并不能提高充血性心力衰竭和持续性室速患者的生存率。索他洛尔和胺碘酮可能降低心律失常发生率，且β受体阻滞剂也有同样的效果[48]。然而，尽管降低了室性心律失常，但死亡率仍然很高。因此，药物不能作为对充血性心力衰竭患者预防心脏性猝死的唯一治疗措施。

对于抗心律失常药物在一级预防中的作用，胺碘酮在研究中应用得最广泛（图65-3）。一般来讲，这些试验的入选患者是心肌梗死后患者，并没有表明胺碘酮能降低死亡率。相比之下，胺碘酮可能改善非缺血性心力衰竭患者的生存率，特别是那些有非持续性室速的患者。在一项包括13项预防性使用胺碘酮的随机临床试验的荟萃分析（8项为心肌梗死后，5项为充血性心力衰竭）中，死亡率降低13%。死亡率降低最明显的是充血性心力衰竭患者的试验，特别是非缺血性心肌病患者。但是本组患者中除1例外，胺碘酮似乎对充血性心力衰竭患者的生存率为中性作用。无论如何，这意味着胺碘酮可安全用于其他适应证，如抑制心房颤动和有症状的室性心动过速[49]。

同样，多非利特（dofetilide）也可以用于充血性

表 65-6　血管扩张剂和血管紧张素转换酶抑制剂在充血性心力衰竭中的作用

论文发表	研究人群	研究中每组死亡率（%）		死亡率差异（%）
VHEFT1	充血性心力衰竭	HYD/ISO 组	36.2	10.7（3 年）
	心脏肥大/EF＜45%	安慰剂组	49.9	
VHEFT2	同上	依那普利组	32.8	5.4（2.5 年）
		HYD/ISO 组	38.2	
Consensus Ⅰ	NYHA 分级Ⅳ级	依那普利组	36.2	16.2（1 年）
		安慰剂组	52.4	
SOLVD-T	充血性心力衰竭	依那普利组	35.2	4.5（3.5 年）
	EF＜35%	安慰剂组	39.7	

HYD，肼屈嗪；ISO，硝酸酯类药物。

心力衰竭的患者。如果应用恰当的话，多非利特对患者的生存率有中性作用，但能降低患者因心力衰竭的住院率。此外，它还能降低心房颤动的发生率，甚至能使充血性心力衰竭患者的心房颤动转复为窦性心律[50]。

（六）植入式心脏复律除颤器在心脏性猝死患者中的二级预防

最近有三项研究结果表明，植入式心脏复律除颤器可以用于充血性心力衰竭患者的持续性室速的治疗。这三项研究项目分别是，抗心律失常药物与植入式心脏复律除颤器对照研究（AVID）、加拿大植入式心脏复律除颤器研究（CIDS）和匈牙利心脏骤停研究（CASH）[51-53]。总之，植入式心脏复律除颤器可以降低约 30% 的死亡率。回顾性分析结果显示植入式心脏复律除颤器在心力衰竭中的治疗作用。在加拿大植入式心脏复律除颤器研究中，659 例极高危患者的死亡率降低最明显：NYHA 心功能分级Ⅲ和Ⅳ级，左室射血分数＜35%，70 岁以上老年人。同样，在 AVID 中，植入式心脏复律除颤器对左室射血分数小于 30% 的患者疗效优于胺碘酮（图 65-4）。必须强调一点，不足 50% 的患者服用 β 受体阻滞剂：在所有联合应用药物的研究中，β 受体阻滞剂用于约 40% 随机植入式心脏复律除颤器的患者及 20% 胺碘酮治疗的患者。很明显，依据目前的标准，很多患者没有得到治疗，或至少说这些患者没有得到 β 受体阻滞剂治疗的最佳效果。

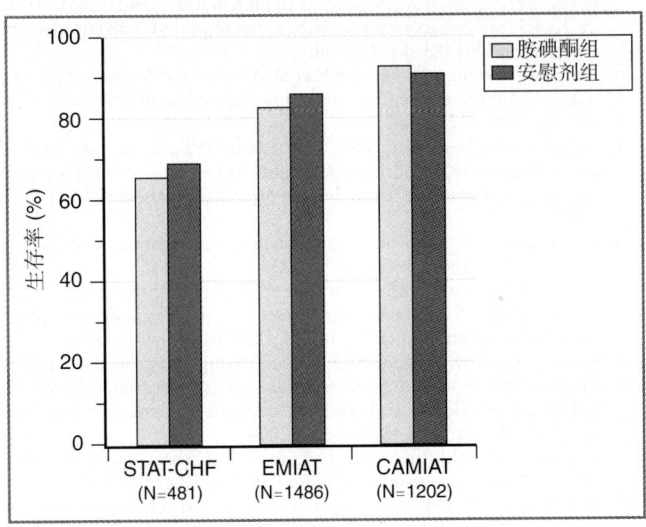

图 65-3　心肌梗死患者胺碘酮预防治疗的三项随机临床试验的两年生存率比较

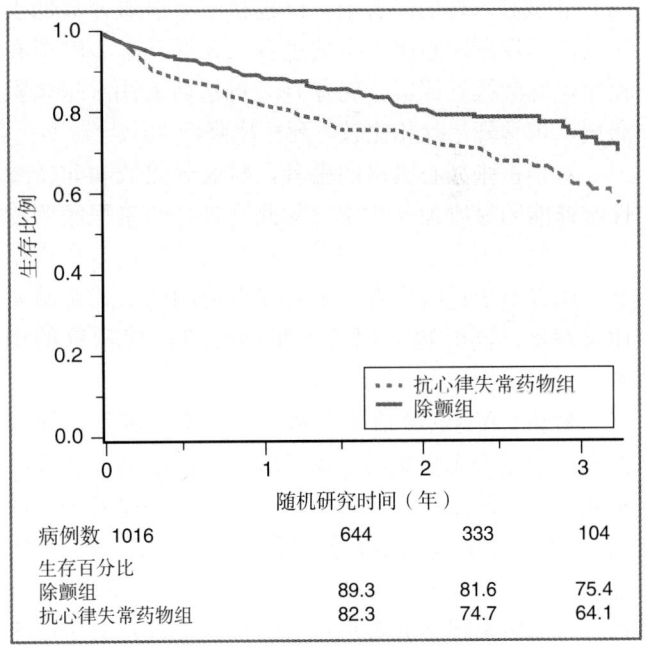

图 65-4　抗心律失常药物与植入式心脏复律除颤器治疗试验中总生存率比较　（引自 The Antiarrhythmics Versus Implantable Defibrillator Investigators: A comparison of antiarrhythmic drug therapy with implantable defibrillators in patients resuscitated from near-fatal ventricular arrhythmias. N Engl J Med, 1997; 337: 1576-1583.）

上述诸项研究中，入选的冠心病患者最多（约80%）。因此，植入式心脏复律除颤器对持续性室速和充血性心力衰竭患者是有效的，因为并不能确定是扩张型心肌病。不过，对于这些患者来说，提倡用植入式心脏复律除颤器作为二级预防。

（七）植入式心脏复律除颤器的一级预防

MADIT-I、MUSTT 和 MADIT-II[38,54,55] 三项研究结果显示，植入式心脏复律除颤器能有效预防缺血性心力衰竭患者的心脏性猝死。前两项研究表明，对于左室射血分数低于 40% 和无症状性非持续性室速的患者，在给予程序性心室刺激时能诱发出致命性心律失常，当采取植入式心脏复律除颤器治疗与抗心律失常药物治疗进行比较时，前者能降低 50% 的死亡率。MADIT-I 试验中的 196 例患者的回顾性分析表明，用植入式心脏复律除颤器治疗的患者其死亡率降低，但主要是左室射血分数低于 26% 的患者。在 MADIT-I、MUSTT 试验中，用 β 受体阻滞剂治疗的患者不足 50%。因此，还不能确定对于用口服 β 受体阻滞剂和大剂量血管紧张素转换酶抑制剂的患者是否用植入式心脏复律除颤器治疗的效果最佳。在 MADIT-II 试验入选的患者中，仅包括左室射血分数低于 30% 而无致命性心律失常的患者，并经动态心电图和程序电刺激检查证实。现有 70% 的患者服用 β 受体阻滞剂，与常规治疗相比较，死亡率降低 30%[38]。

对于扩张型心肌病的患者，射血分数低和非持续性室速能明显增加死亡率。除此之外，心室程序刺激的预测值并不高[56]，而且抗心律失常药物的效果也不好。所以对于这些患者，常常提倡使用植入式心脏复律除颤器，同时也适用于扩张型心肌病伴晕厥的患者。

最新 CAT 试验结果表明，植入式心脏复律除颤器并不适用于无症状的心动过缓、室性心动过速和心室颤动的非缺血性心肌病患者。在 104 例患者中，随访 2~4 年，植入式心脏复律除颤器治疗组与常规治疗组两组之间比较并无差异[57]，而且在这些患者中，植入式心脏复律除颤器也没有保证。此外，对于终末期心力衰竭的患者也不主张用植入式心脏复律除颤器。现在还不清楚是否植入式心脏复律除颤器和双室起搏联合治疗与单纯植入式心脏复律除颤器比较能降低充血性心力衰竭患者的死亡率。

（八）射频消融术

对于频发性反复发作的室性心动过速患者，尽管已用抗心律失常药物治疗，但心动过速病灶的导管消融能够明显降低心律失常的复发率，比药物治疗的效果佳[58]。据报道在随访的 1~2 年中，有近 70% 的缺血性心肌病患者其室速完全被消融[59]。在入选的非缺血性心力衰竭和无休止性室速的患者中，导管消融术不仅治愈了心动过速，而且能明显提高或使左室射血分数正常。束支折返性心动过速的导管消融术是对扩张型心肌病患者的主要治疗方法之一。

四、总 结

心力衰竭患者发生猝死与多种因素有关，其中主要机制是室性心动过速和心室颤动，这也是诸多致心律失常机制的结果。个体化的抗心律失常药物治疗只有在基本原因明确时才能应用。钙调节异常和电重塑导致左室功能障碍、QT 间期改变及致心律失常作用。在这种情况下，预防和逆转不同的重塑过程起重要作用。它们与心律失常有关，而且能够通过导管消融来治疗，并能决定充血性心力衰竭患者将来发生心脏性猝死的预防成功率。药物治疗加植入式心脏复律除颤器是治疗的主要选择。

（张 伟译）

参 考 文 献

1. Stevenson WG, Stevenson LW: Prevention of sudden death in heart failure. J Cardiovasc Electrophysiol 12:112–114, 2001.
2. Beuckelmann DJ, Nabauer M, Erdmann E: Alterations of K currents in isolated human ventricular myocytes from patients with heart failure. Circ Res 73:379–385, 1993.
3. Kaab S, Dixon J, Duc J, et al: Molecular basis of transient outward potassium current downregulation in human heart failure: A decrease in Kv4.3 mRNA correlates with a reduction in current density. Circulation 98:1383–1393, 1998.
4. Jiang MT, Lokuta AJ, Farell EF, et al: Abnormal calcium release, but normal ryanodine receptors, in canine and human heart failure. Circ Res 91:1015–1022, 2002.
5. Ogletree-Hughes ML, Stull LB, Sweet WE, et al: Mechanical unloading restores ß-adrenergic responsiveness and reverses receptor downregulation in the failing human heart. Circulation 104:881–886, 2001.
6. Hasenfuss G, Pieske B: Calcium cycling in congestive heart failure. J Mol Cell Cardiol 34:951–969, 2002.
7. Marx SO, Reiken S, Hisamatsu Y, et al: PKA phosphorylation dissociates FKBP12.6 from the calcium release channel (ryanodine receptor): Defective regulation in failing hearts. Cell 101:365–376, 2000.
8. Tsuji Y, Opthof T, Kamiya K, et al: Pacing induced heart failure causes a reduction of delayed rectifier potassium currents along with a decrease in calcium and transient outward currents in rabbit ventricle. Cardiovasc Res 48:300–309, 2000.
9. Pogwizd SM, Schlotthauer K, Li L, et al: Arrhythmogenesis and contractile dysfunction in heart failure. Circ Res 88:1159–1169, 2001.
10. Li GR, Lau CP, Ducharme A, et al: Transmural action potential and ionic current remodeling in ventricles of failing canine hearts. Am J Physiol 283:H1031–1041, 2002.
11. Lacroix D, Gluais P, Marquie C, et al: Repolarization abnormalities and their arrhythmogenic consequences in porcine tachycardia induced cardiomyopathy. Cardiovasc Res 54:42–50, 2002.

12. Sipido KR, Volders PG, Vos MA, Verdonck F: Altered Na/Ca exchange activity in cardiac hypertrophy and heart failure: A new target for therapy? Cardiovasc Res 53:782–805, 2002.
13. Tsuji Y, Opthof T, Yasui K, et al: Ionic mechanisms of acquired QT prolongation and Torsade de pointes in rabbits with chronic complete atrioventricular block. Circulation 106:2012–2018, 2002.
14. Jiang M, Cabo C, Yao JA, et al: Delayed rectifier K currents have reduced amplitudes and altered kinetics in myocytes from infarcted canine ventricles. Cardiovasc Res 48:34–43, 2000.
15. Rials SJ, Xu X, Wu Y, et al: Regression of LV hypertrophy with captopril normalizes membrane currents in rabbits. Am J Physiol H1216–1224, 1998.
16. de Groot SH, Schoenmakers M, Molenschot MM, et al: Contractile adaptations preserving cardiac output predispose the hypertrophied canine heart for DAD-dependent ventricular arrhythmias. Circulation 102:2145–2151, 2000.
17. Li D, Fareh S, Leung TK, Nattel S: Promotion of atrial fibrillation by heart failure in dogs: Atrial remodeling of a different sort. Circulation 100:87–95, 1999.
18. Antzelevitch C: Drug-induced channelopathies. In Zipes D, Jalife J: Cardiac Electrophysiology: From Cell to Bedside. Philadelphia, PA: WB Saunders, 2004.
19. Marx SO, Kurokawa J, Reiken S, et al: Requirement of a macromolecular signaling complex for beta adrenergic receptor modulation of the KCNQ1-KCNE1 potassium channel. Science 295:496–499, 2002.
20. Schram G, Pourrier M, Melnyk P, Nattel S: Differential distribution of cardiac ion channel expression as a basis for regional specialization in electrical function. Circ Res 90:939–950, 2002.
21. Kanno S, Saffitz JE: The role of myocardial gap junctions in electrical conduction and arrhythmogenesis. Cardiovasc Pathol 10:169–177, 2001.
22. Volders PG, Sipido KR, Vos MA, et al: Downregulation of delayed rectifier K+ current in dogs with chronic complete atrioventricular block and acquired Torsade de Pointes. Circulation 100:2455–2461, 1999.
23. Hsieh MH, Chen YJ, Lee SH, et al: Proarrhythmic effects of ibutilide in a canine model of pacing induced cardiomyopathy. Pacing Clin Electrophysiol 23:149–156, 2000.
24. Volders PG, Vos MA, Szabo B, et al: Progress in the understanding of cardiac early afterdepolarizations and torsades de pointes: Time to revise current concepts. Cardiovasc Res 46:376–392, 2000.
25. Vos MA, van Opstal JM, Leunissen HD, Verduyn SC: Electrophysiological parameters and predisposing factors in the generation of drug induced Torsade de Pointes arrhythmias. Pharmacol Ther 92:109–122, 2001.
26. Pogwizd SM, McKenzie JP, Cain ME: Mechanisms underlying spontaneous and induced ventricular arrhythmias in patients with idiopathic dilated cardiomyopathy. Circulation 98:2404–2414, 1998.
27. Huang B, Qin D, El Sherif N: Early downregulation of K-channel genes and currents in the postinfarction heart. J Cardiovasc Electrophysiol 11:1252–1261, 2000.
28. Zobel C, Kassiri Z, Nguyen TT, et al: Prevention of hypertrophy by overexpression of Kv4.2 in cultured neonatal cardiomyocytes. Circulation 106:2385–2391, 2002.
29. Hill JA, Karimi M, Kutschke W, et al: Cardiac hypertrophy is not a required compensatory response to short-term pressure overload. Circulation 101:2863–2869, 2000.
30. Peschar M, Vernooy K, Vanagt W, et al: Absence of reverse electrical remodeling during regression of volume overload hypertrophy in canine ventricles. Cardiovasc Res 58:510–517, 2003.
31. Haq S, Choukroun G, Lim H, et al: Differential activation of signal transduction pathways in human hearts with hypertrophy versus advanced heart failure. Circulation 103:670–677, 2001.
32. Burkhoff D, Holmes JW, Madigan J, et al: Left ventricular assist device-induced reverse ventricular remodeling. Prog Cardiovasc Dis 43:19–26, 2000.
33. Harding JD, Piacentino V, Gaughan JP, et al: Electrophysiological alterations after mechanical circulatory support in patients with advanced cardiac failure. Circulation 104:1241–1247, 2001.
34. Yu CM, Chau E, Sanderson JE, et al: Tissue Doppler echocardiographic evidence of reverse remodeling and improved synchronicity by simultaneously delaying regional contraction after biventricular pacing therapy in heart failure. Circulation 105:438–445, 2002.
35. Linde C, Leclercq C, Rex S, et al: Long-term benefits of biventricular pacing in congestive heart failure: Results from the MUltisite STimulation in cardiomyopathy (MUSTIC) study. J Am Coll Cardiol 40:111–118, 2002.
36. Pratt CM, Greenway PS, Schoenfeld MH, et al: Exploration of the precision of classifying sudden cardiac death. Circulation 93:519–524, 1996.
37. Epstein AE, Carlson MD, Fogoros RN, et al: Classification of death in antiarrhythmia trials. J Am Coll Cardiol 27:433–442, 1996.
38. Moss AJ, Zareba W, Hall WJ, et al; Multicenter Automatic Defibrillator Implantation Trial II Investigators: Prophylactic implantation of a defibrillator in patients with myocardial infarction and reduced ejection fraction. N Engl J Med 346:877–883, 2002.
39. Berger RD, Kasper EK, Baughman KL, et al: Beat-to-beat QT interval variability: Novel evidence for repolarization lability in ischemic and nonischemic dilated cardiomyopathy. Circulation 96:1557–1565, 1997.
40. Packer M, Bristow MR, Cohn JN, et al: The effect of carvedilol on morbidity and mortality in patients with chronic heart failure: U.S. Carvedilol Heart Failure Study Group. N Engl J Med 334:1349–1355, 1996.
41. The Cardiac Insufficiency Bisoprolol Study II (CIBIS-II): A randomised trial. Lancet 353:9–13, 1999.
42. Effect of metoprolol CR/XL in chronic heart failure: Metoprolol CR/XL Randomised Intervention Trial in Congestive Heart Failure (MERIT-HF). Lancet 353:2001–2007, 1999.
43. Packer M, Coats AJ, Fowler MB, et al: Carvedilol Prospective Randomized Cumulative Survival Study Group: Effect of carvedilol on survival in severe chronic heart failure. N Engl J Med 344:1651–1658, 2001.
44. Cohn JN, Tognoni G; Valsartan Heart Failure Trial Investigators: A randomized trial of the angiotensin-receptor blocker valsartan in chronic heart failure. N Engl J Med 345:1667–1675, 2001.
45. Dagenais GR, Yusuf S, Bourassa MG, et al; HOPE Investigators. Effects of ramipril on coronary events in high-risk persons: Results of the Heart Outcomes Prevention Evaluation Study. Circulation 104:522–526, 2001.
46. Hart RG, Halperin JL: Atrial fibrillation and thromboembolism: A decade of progress in stroke prevention. Ann Intern Med 131:688–695, 1999.
47. Garg RK, Gheorghiade M, Jafri SM: Antiplatelet and anticoagulant therapy in the prevention of thrombo-emboli in chronic heart failure. Prog Cardiovasc Dis 42:225–236, 1998.
48. Steinbeck G, Andresen D, Bach P, et al: A comparison of electrophysiologically guided antiarrhythmic drug therapy with beta blocker therapy in patients with symptomatic, sustained ventricular tachyarrhythmias. N Engl J Med 327:987–992, 1992.
49. Connolly SJ: Evidence based analysis of amiodarone efficacy and safety. Circulation 100:2025–2034, 1999.
50. Pedersen OD, Bagger H, Keller N, et al: Efficacy of dofetilide in the treatment of atrial fibrillation-flutter in patients with reduced left ventricular function: A Danish investigations of arrhythmia and mortality on dofetilide (diamond) substudy. Circulation 104:292–296, 2001.
51. Domanski MJ, Sakseena S, Epstein AE, et al: Relative effectiveness of the implantable cardioverter-defibrillator and antiarrhythmic drugs in patients with varying degrees of left ventricular dysfunction who have survived malignant ventricular arrhythmias: AVID Investigators—Antiarrhythmics Versus Implantable Defibrillators. J Am Coll Cardiol 34:1090–1095, 1999.
52. Sheldon R, Connolly S, Krahn A, et al: Identification of patients most likely to benefit from implantable cardioverter-defibrillator therapy: The Canadian Implantable Defibrillator Study. Circulation 101:1660–1664, 2000.
53. Kuck KH, Cappato R, Siebels J, Ruppel R: Randomized comparison of antiarrhythmic drug therapy with implantable defibrillators in patients resuscitated from cardiac arrest: The Cardiac Arrest Study Hamburg (CASH). Circulation 102:748–754, 2000.
54. Moss A, Hall W, Cannom D, et al: Improved survival with an implanted defibrillator in patients with coronary artery disease at high risk for ventricular arrhythmia: Multicenter Automatic Defibrillator Implantation Trial Investigators. N Engl J Med 335:1933–1940, 1996.
55. Buxton AE, Lee KL, Fisher JD, et al: A randomized study of the prevention of sudden death in patients with coronary artery disease: Multicenter Unsustained Tachycardia Trial Investigators. N Engl J Med 341:1882–1890, 1999.

56. Milner PG, Dimarco JP, Lerman BB: Electrophysiological evaluation of sustained ventricular tachyarrhythmias in idiopathic dilated cardiomyopathy. Pacing Clin Electrophysiol 11:562–568, 1998.
57. Bänsch D, Antz M, Boscor S, et al: Primary prevention of sudden cardiac death in idiopathic dilated cardiomyopathy: The Cardiomyopathy Trial (CAT). Circulation 105:1453–1458, 2002.
58. Strickberger SA, Man KC, Daoud EG, et al: A prospective evaluation of catheter ablation of ventricular tachycardia as adjuvant therapy in patients with coronary artery disease and an implantable cardioverter-defibrillator. Circulation 96:1525–1531, 1997.
59. Rothman S, Hsia H, Cossu S, et al: Radiofrequency catheter ablation of postinfarction ventricular tachycardia: Long-term success and the significance of inducible nonclinical arrhythmias. Circulation 96:3499–3508, 1997.

第 66 章

先天性心脏病术后的室性心动过速

George F. Van Hare

本章目录

- 解剖和手术方法 ……………………… 611
- 自发性室性心律失常 ………………… 612
- 可诱发性室性心动过速和猝死 ……… 613
- 术后室性心动过速的治疗 …………… 614

室性心动过速，以及室速与猝死之间的潜在联系，始终是严重先天性心脏病患者外科修补术后最难处理的问题之一。有人认为在很大程度上，这些患者存在的有生命危险的血流动力学异常，可以通过手术得到成功的控制。但是致死性心律失常通常在数年或数十年后发生，而此类患者发生的猝死更具有毁灭性。最初都认为，这类患者中完全性房室阻滞的发生可能是猝死的原因。但是，尽管一些患者确实存在房室阻滞，但大多数的猝死病例并没有房室阻滞。在主要行心房手术的患者中，如大动脉转位的 Mustard 或 Senning 术，或各种单心室的 Fontan 手术，快速房扑很可能与猝死的发生有关[1,2]。而在法洛四联症以及相似病变，如右室双出口实施完全修补术后，由于室性早搏、阵发性和持续性室速的频发，这种患者中室性心动过速成为猝死的病因之一。有明确报道，在 1～16 岁发生猝死的儿童中[3]，法洛四联症手术术后是最为常见的相关因素，而主动脉狭窄、主动脉缩窄和大动脉转位患者猝死的风险也有增高[4]。

目前为止，与其他先心病相比，绝大多数有关室性心动过速和先心病患者的资料都是关于法洛四联症的。其他病变的患者很少发生室性心律失常[5]。但是为了便于治疗，当其他病变的患者在心室切开术或右室功能不全时出现室性心律失常，可以用法洛四联症作为模型。

在关于室性心律失常和猝死发生中各种危险因素的作用，二者间的确切关系，电生理研究和其他危险分级的方法，以及术后患者室性心动过速最终的合理治疗，都还有很大争论。直到最近，得益于大型多中心的试验，在抗心律失常药物及植入式心脏复律除颤器在冠心病患者中的作用研究上有了大的进展[6]。可以认为，回答这一日趋减少的患者人群的相似问题是一个越来越大的挑战。确实，正如 Bricker 所指出的，不太可能得到足够数目的手术病人来进行充分有力的研究，并对猝死的各种可能因素进行分类[7]。

一、解剖和手术方法

对先心病的解剖和手术方法作详尽回顾不是本章的主要内容。但是，必须认识到这些年来手术方法的改进，才能理解患者年龄、手术年龄以及修补方法在增加心律失常风险中的相互作用。第一例法洛四联症的根治手术是由 Dr. W. C. Lillehei 在 1954 年完成的，并从 20 世纪 60 年代开始逐渐普及。最开始阶段在婴幼儿时期行矫正手术死亡率很高，后来更多的患者都等到晚一些再行修补，多在 20～30 岁时。从 20 世纪 70 年代开始，由于手术方法和术后监护技术的进步，几个中心选择在婴儿期行一期修补取得了好的效果，现在这已成为各地普遍的做法。

法洛四联症的患者存在室间隔缺损，伴有一定程度通常是比较严重的右室流出道梗阻，可导致慢性发绀。姑息性的体肺动脉分流术增加了左室容量超负荷的潜在问题。缺损的矫正包括用补片关闭室间隔缺损及解除右室梗阻。在几乎所有的病人中，这样做需要切除一大块右室心肌，并且在早期的经验中，并不是经右心房手术，而是需要切开心室。最后，肺动脉环通常较小，跨环的补片修补会导致慢性肺动脉瓣关闭不全，这在伴有明显的肺动脉狭窄而造成流出障碍时可能会更严重。推测室性心律失常是多年慢性发绀的结果，也与心室切开，梗阻解除不全造成右室压力的增加，以及严重的肺动脉反流伴有右室功能不全[8-10]有关。这些诸如心壁压力和慢性发绀等因素，随时间的推移可能导致的心肌纤维化，会成为折返性室性心律失常的基础。对突然死亡的法洛四联症病人心脏的组织学研究中，可以见到相当广泛的纤维化[11]，恰好支持这一推测。对在右室进行的分级电扫描和晚电位的电生理研究中，都提示慢传导的存在，亦支持这一假设[12]。尽管在法洛四联症中有5%的冠脉畸形发生率，有可能在根治手术时损伤左前降支或其他大的分支，但这种可能的损害从未被考虑在室性心律失常或猝死的病因中。

对法洛四联症术后发生室速患者精细的电生理研究支持一个观点，心动过速的机制是折返，围绕着右室流出道、右室前壁切开处或室间隔缺损补片处。对折返环的持续消融和在缓慢传导的消融，可得到短暂的复律。对起搏后间期的评价可以强有力地证明右室流出道是一个巨大折返环路的一部分（图66-1和图66-2）。

二、自发性室性心律失常

早期的报道记录了法洛四联症患者术后频发的室性期前收缩。例如，Gillette和他的同事们[13]在18%的患者的常规心电图上见到室性早搏。通过动态心电图监测，报道的结果高达48%[14]。其中一半的患者，其室性异位心律是复杂的，表现为多形波、二联律或室性心动过速。大多数患者的室性异位心律没有症状。

很多研究者曾试着调查与室性异搏发病率相关的各种因素，如发病的年龄、手术修补时的年龄以及各种血流动力学特征。有四个因素看起来是最重要的：初次手术时的年龄，修补术后的时间，残余的右室梗阻症状和明显的肺动脉瓣关闭不全。在Chandar的多中心研究中，年长的手术患者，特别是10岁以后，室性心律失常的发病率接近100%[14]，与其随访的时间长短无关。同一研究中，修补后的时间也可预测室性异搏的发生，4例在婴幼儿时行修补术的患者，在

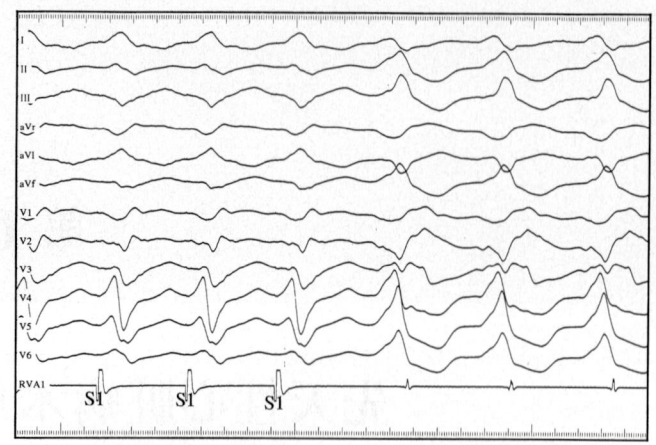

图66-1 曾经在11岁时实施法洛氏四联症修补术的一位35岁男性患者的电生理标测图 用心室期前刺激诱发的室性心动过速，其心动过速周期为435ms。注意到利用起搏周期为280ms的刺激从右室心尖部起搏诱发心动过速时，发生在起搏周期后的第一个非融合波处会产生一个持续的融合波。Dis：远端电极，RVA：右心室心尖部。

16年多以后都发生了室性异搏。但是Walsh及其同事[15]描述的一组18个月以内行手术的患者，其心电图上很少有室性异搏（1%），而在平均随访5年后的动态心电图上则较为常见（31%）。

在一项关于488例法洛四联症修补术后患者的研究中，Garson及其同事[16]指出，右室血流动力学与室性心律失常的发病率密切相关。在右室收缩压大于60mmHg和右室舒张末压大于8mmHg的患者中，室性心律失常的发生率明显增高，提示残余的右室流出道梗阻和肺动脉瓣关闭不全对结果有负面影响。他们同样发现了与手术时年龄的关系，但是不如随访时限重要。在一项对59例11岁前行法洛四联症修补术的患者的前瞻性研究中，Zahka及其同事[8]发现，肺动脉反流的程度是目前自发性室性心律失常频率和严重度最重要的预测因素。而残余右室流出道梗阻的严重度不是预测因素，因为在他们的研究组中几乎没有明显的残余梗阻。在随后的研究中这些观察资料得到了确认，并强调了肺动脉瓣关闭不全的重要性[17,18]。

事实上，作为室性心律失常的一种，自发的持续室性心动过速在法洛四联症修补术后的患者中相当少见。Chandar及其同事[14]在其多中心的研究中发现，359位患者中的9%在动态心电图监测上有室性心动过速，但临床极少有持续性室性心动过速。这方面的最佳数据来自Harrison及其同事的报道，是关于成人先天性心脏病中心的法洛四联症修补术后的患者。通过心电图研究，210例患者中的18例（8.6%）记录

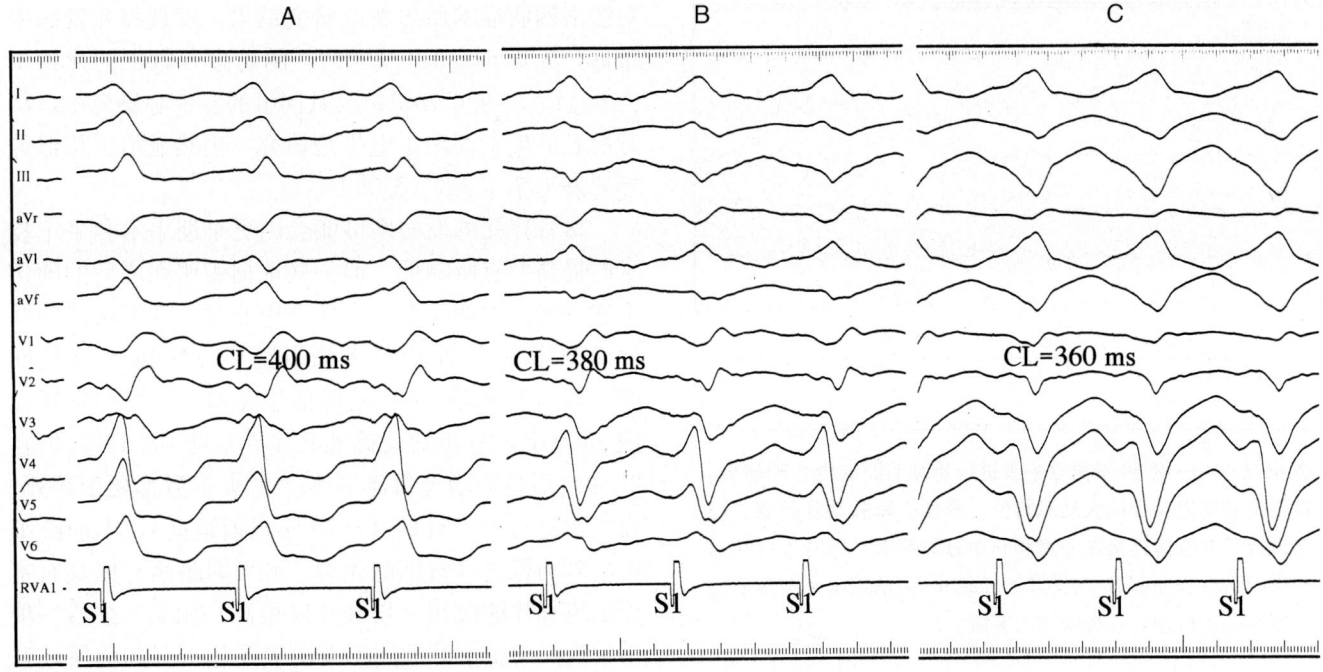

图 66-2 与图 66-1 同一患者的电生理标测图 用（A）400ms，（B）380ms 和（C）360ms 起搏拖带，随着起搏周期的逐渐缩短，可见进展性的融合波。CL：周期长度。

到持续室性心动过速，或者伴有心悸的晕厥/近乎晕厥，并在电生理研究中可诱发持续单一的室性心动过速。术中检测发现室性心动过速起源于右室流出道，并且室性心动过速与右室血流动力学，特别是与右室流出道动脉瘤和肺动脉瓣关闭不全密切相关。Zahka 及其同事[8]的报道与之一致，并强调了肺动脉关闭不全作为室性心律失常高危因素之一的重要性。

三、可诱发性室性心动过速和猝死

先心病修补术后的患者，无论简单的和复杂的自发性室性心律失常的发生率均增高。对这类患者进行持续的观察有时会发现突发的预料之外的死亡，由此得出这一假设：这种患者的猝死是由室性心动过速造成的。当然，在一些患者中，室性心动过速很快就进展到室颤（图 66-3）。从逻辑上可通过抑制室性心律失常防止猝死的发生，抑制自发性或电生理的研究中可诱发的室性心动过速来完成。在 20 世纪 70～80 年代间，为明确可诱发的持续单一室性心动过速，对大部分法洛四联症修补术后或有先天性缺损的患者，进行电生理研究是标准做法。从心律失常的观点来看，几乎所有这样的病人都是没有症状的。但基于上述研究结果，抗心律失常药物治疗还是被应用于这种患者。同时由于缺乏强有力的证据支持通过此方法可以防止猝死发生的观点，这一方法在极大程度上已经被抛弃。而且，抗心律失常药物的致心律失常作用也尚未得到充分评估。

Garson 及其同事[16]推测，早期法洛四联症修补术后患者猝死的发生率高是因为恶性室性心律失常。他们对一组频发室性异搏的患者采取抗心律失常治疗，监测 24h 心电图，试图观察到室性异位搏动被抑制的情况。苯妥英钠、美西律和普萘洛尔可以有效地抑制室性异搏。与早期一组未治疗的室性异搏患者 33% 的猝死率相比，被认为"治疗成功"的患者中无一人猝死。该研究的严重局限性在于采用历史对照组，即在较早期实施的修补术，而未采用前瞻对照组。不过该研究很有影响力，使得一大批无症状患者开始采用苯妥英钠和其他药物进行治疗。

对一大批法洛四联症修补术后患者进行有创电生理检查，其结果是令人不安的，相当大比例的患者，包括几乎所有以前从未有过室性心动过速临床发作的患者，都可诱发室性心动过速。早期的报道和 Garson 等人的数据都提示室性心动过速与猝死之间有直接的联系，使得有创电生理检查在大量无症状患者中得到广泛应用，随后采取抗心律失常治疗，并通过反复电生理检查以指导治疗。但是，随后对于该方法结果的检验并不支持其继续应用。在一个大型多中心的观察

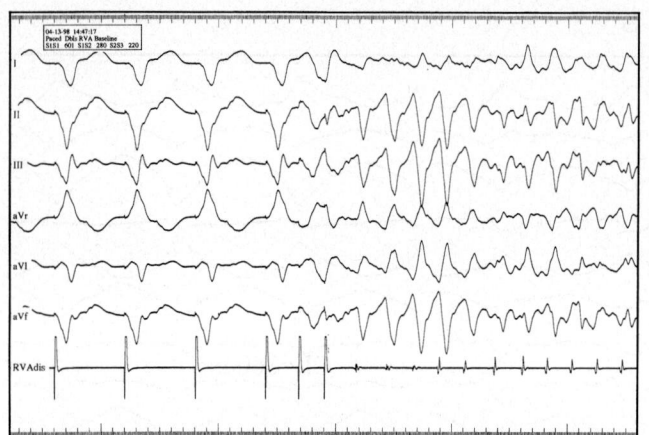

图 66-3 对一例 30 岁男性患者进行持续监测的电生理研究，这位患者有先天性的大动脉转位，异位心和肺动脉闭锁，已经进行了外管道连接左心室和肺动脉的手术 患者进行相对和缓的室性程序刺激（600/290/220ms），诱发出 4 次单形性的室性心动过速，立即蜕变为室颤。

中，Chandar 及其同事[14]报道了他们对于 395 例法洛四联症修补术后患者进行有创电生理检查的经验。17% 的患者可诱发室性心动过速，而在一个无症状并且 24h 心电图正常的患者中却无法诱发。尽管有 5 例患者发生了远期猝死，但没有一例在电生理研究中有可诱发的室性心动过速。Alexander 及其同事[20]报道了 130 例先心病患者程序刺激研究的结果，其中 1/3 做过法洛四联症修补术。尽管阳性结果的患者其后的死亡率较高，但是由于有很高的假阴性率，阴性的结果并不能完全肯定。这些结果质疑对无症状患者进行介入性诊断检查的合理性，也质疑了通过识别和治疗潜在致命的室性心律失常可以预防猝死的观念。

近来的数据表明，室性心动过速的风险率可通过体表心电图的 QRS 波间期得知。Gatzoulis 及其同事[9]仔细研究了 48 例四联症术后患者，发现 QRS 波间期大于 180ms 的患者出现自发室性心动过速、猝死或二者都有的风险显著增高，并且其他研究者[21,22]也已确认了这一观察结果，其原因尚不明确。当然，法洛四联症矫正术后的患者常有右束支阻滞，而使得 QRS 波时限延长。过度延长的 QRS 波可能是肺动脉瓣关闭不全导致右室扩张的标志，或者可能是手术时需要切除右室漏斗部的标志。

事实上，猝死的发生率比以前所担心的要小得多，也可能是有所下降。早期的报道中估计法洛四联症修补术后猝死发生率在 2%～3%[23,24]。随后的报道也显示了同样低的猝死风险率。Wren[25]回顾了 14 个对法洛四联症术后患者的研究结果，发现猝死发病率很低，为 1.6%（49/3006），随访患者每年的死亡率为 0.14%。在 Chandar 及其同事的多中心研究中，尽管所有的患者都做了电生理研究，仍然显示了相似的猝死发生率 1.4%（5/359）。

尽管猝死的发病率可能会因更早期手术和手术技术的提高而有所降低，但一些证据表明在之后的随访中它可能会增加。在一个独立中心对 490 例法洛四联症修补术后存活者的详细研究中，Nollert 及其同事[26]建立了术后 36 年精确的生存曲线。他们发现在前 25 年中，每年的精确死亡率是每年 0.24%，但在 25 年之后显著增至每年 0.94%。大多数都死于猝死。死亡率也与手术日期（1970 年以前最高）、术前红细胞增多的程度（血细胞比容 >48% 时最高）以及右室流出道补片的应用（用补片时最高）相关。最后一项因素当然与肺动脉关闭不全的表现相关（如前所述）。红细胞增多的重要性可能不是一个直接的因素，但它可能与术前发绀的程度和持续时间相关，而这些可导致心肌纤维化。

四、术后室性心动过速的治疗

先心病矫正术后室性异搏的治疗选择可能有两个目标或其中之一：预防猝死以及抑制并终止室性心动过速的发作。治疗方法有抗心律失常药物、射频导管消融、外科冷冻消融，或植入能够提供抗心动过速起搏器和复律除颤器。

很难知道哪一个病人应作电生理研究、治疗或两者都作。事实上，没有任何一个前瞻性研究证明通过某种形式的治疗，可以防止某组术后患者猝死的发生，因而不推荐对大多数有室性异搏的无症状患者行常规电生理研究或治疗。尽管有可能有某一亚组患者通过仔细选择抗心律失常药物治疗，对降低死亡率有良好的效果，但更有可能的是一些群体中，抗心律失常药物治疗的致心律失常作用可能要高于其产生的益处，在 CAST 试验中可看到相似的结果[27]。在同样的前瞻对照性试验完成之前，对大多数无症状患者不推荐用药物治疗，如氟卡胺、奎尼丁和索他洛尔之类。选择特定患者用 β 受体阻滞剂进行预防治疗有一定争论。这样的患者可能包括那些有明显肺动脉反流或残余右室流出道梗阻以及复杂室性异搏的患者。对于这样的患者考虑行心脏手术以纠正血流动力学异常，如残余梗阻，特别是肺动脉分支狭窄，或者考虑行自体瓣膜置换以消除肺动脉关闭不全也同样都有一定争议[28,29]。

如果治疗的目的是为了防止临床证实的室性心动过速的再发，那么就像控制其他形式的室性心动过速一样。通过电生理研究诱发室性心动过速，随后用药物进行治疗的试验是合理的，同时一定要记住应用某些药物治疗可能有致心律失常的风险，尤其是氟卡胺和普罗帕酮。在某些患者中也有用运动试验作为诱发室性心动过速的一种方法。选择长期治疗的药物要基于两点，药物抑制心律失常的能力和药物潜在的致心律失常作用。早先的研究中，有报道一些成功的例子，应用大多数Ⅰ类药物，尤其是奎尼丁、普罗帕酮和氟卡胺，也有用β受体阻滞剂的。近来的研究认为对其致心律失常作用很难评判。Fish及其同事[30]在一项儿科研究中报道，器质性心脏病患者用氟卡胺和恩卡胺有很高的致心律失常发生率。此外，心脏停搏和死亡主要发生在有基础心脏病的患者中。索他洛尔也已知有致心律失常作用，特别是在显著心室功能不全的患者中[31]。这些发现表明，在心室功能不全的法洛四联症修补术后患者中，索他洛尔和ⅠC类药物的使用要极度谨慎。当然就剩下胺碘酮，其优点是很少有致心律失常的报道，即使是在显著心室功能不全的患者中[32]。关于胺碘酮的远期副作用，如肺纤维化、视觉异常、甲状腺功能不全、转氨酶升高以及显著的心动过缓，已经在儿童和年轻成人中观察到[33]，并且在年轻患者中使用该药很可能意味着至少需要服用几十年。这些利害关系自然成为了采取非药物治疗的理由。

如果室性心动过速容易诱发，并且血流动力学可以很好耐受，可以考虑行射频消融。由于大多数证据支持此类易耐受室性心动过速的机制是巨大折返这一观念，则可以实施起搏和标测技术。几位研究者报道了使用射频消融手术[34-36]，特别是Stevenson及其同事[37]，报道了用电压图识别右室瘢痕的位置。

尽管易耐受的室性心动过速可在电生理实验室进行标测定位，但很多患者有心室功能不全或快速的室性心动过速，或二者都有，因此不能耐受。几位研究者报道了在术中标测和消融[38-41]。特别是Downar及其同事，用一个心内球囊电极和一个心外膜的袜状同步电极组，术中在跳动心脏中对右室流出道进行标测，并在常温体外循环心脏跳动时或缺氧停跳时，通过冷冻损伤进行消融，在三位患者中取得了很大成功。

随着近来导线和发生器技术的迅速变化，ICD在先心病修补术后室性心动过速的治疗中成为更加可行的治疗选择[42-46]。Silka及其同事[44]对125例儿科患者的多中心回顾分析显示，先心病修补术后的患者在所有ICD患者中占18％。迄今为止大多数的报道主要研究附于心外膜补片上的装置，但近来的报道包括了经静脉系统的方式[46]。经静脉除颤方式的主要优势是除颤阈值低和避免开胸，在此类患者群中使用经静脉途径更好，因为如果选择心外膜的方式，外科医生在分离心脏和前次手术形成的周围纤维组织时，可能会面对极大困难。然而值得注意的是，心内有分流的患者不能经静脉植入导线，因为有右向左分流导致体循环血栓栓塞的风险。先心病修补术后的患者常有窦房结功能不良、房室阻滞或可诱发的房扑[47]，在法洛四联症修补术后的患者，已有报道他们有很高的房扑发病率[48,49]。最新的ICD发生器，包括一个心房导线和DDD起搏能力，对此类患者群更为适宜。应用心房导线感知房扑并避免不适当的触发，在此类先心病修补术后的患者群中是很有价值的。最终，依据其发生机理，通过ICD完成抗室性心动过速起搏功能也是可行的[50]。

除了关于这些患者ICD植入的技术问题外，患者的选择也是有争议的。很明显，满足通常标准（如室性心律失常导致心脏骤停，反复发生的难以耐受的持续性室性心动过速）的患者都是ICD植入的候选者。其他一些患者是否也适合尚未确定。例如，有一些猝死风险但没有临床证据的心脏骤停或难以耐受的室性心动过速患者是否应该考虑？可以针对特定类型的患者设计一个立项研究。例如，合并有肺动脉瓣关闭不全、右室功能差和频发室性早搏的，有过晕厥而电生理检查阴性的四联症术后患者。与Alexander及其同事[20]的数据相似，Chandar及其同事的资料表明[14]，这类患者虽然电生理检查为阴性，但依旧有猝死的风险。可以针对这些患者预防性植入ICD进行研究。然而基于目前已知的数据，真正无症状的患者，不管其血流动力学状态如何，此时都不应该考虑这种治疗。

（陈 彧 解基严 译）

参 考 文 献

1. Harrison DA, Siu SC, Hussain F, et al: Sustained atrial arrhythmias in adults late after repair of tetralogy of Fallot. Am J Cardiol 87:584–588, 2001.
2. Li W, Somerville J: Atrial flutter in grown-up congenital heart

(GUCH) patients. Clinical characteristics of affected population. Int J Cardiol 75:129–137; discussion 138–139, 2000.
3. Garson A Jr, McNamara DG: Sudden death in a pediatric cardiology population, 1958 to 1983: Relation to prior arrhythmias. J Am Coll Cardiol 5:134B–137B, 1985.
4. Silka MJ, Hardy BG, Menashe VD, Morris CD: A population-based prospective evaluation of risk of sudden cardiac death after operation for common congenital heart defects. J Am Coll Cardiol 32:245–251, 1998.
5. Vetter VL, Horowitz LN: Electrophysiologic residua and sequelae of surgery for congenital heart defects. Am J Cardiol 50:588–604, 1982.
6. A comparison of antiarrhythmic-drug therapy with implantable defibrillators in patients resuscitated from near-fatal ventricular arrhythmias. The Antiarrhythmics versus Implantable Defibrillators (AVID) Investigators. N Engl J Med 337:1576–1583, 1997.
7. Bricker JT: Sudden death and tetralogy of Fallot. Risks, markers, and causes. Circulation 92:158–159, 1995.
8. Zahka KG, Horneffer PJ, Rowe SA, et al: Long-term valvular function after total repair of tetralogy of Fallot. Relation to ventricular arrhythmias. Circulation 78:III14–III19, 1988.
9. Gatzoulis MA, Till JA, Somerville J, Redington AN: Mechanoelectrical interaction in tetralogy of Fallot. QRS prolongation relates to right ventricular size and predicts malignant ventricular arrhythmias and sudden death. Circulation 92:231–237, 1995.
10. Gatzoulis MA, Till JA, Redington AN: Depolarization-repolarization inhomogeneity after repair of tetralogy of Fallot. The substrate for malignant ventricular tachycardia? Circulation 95:401–404, 1997.
11. Deanfield JE, Ho SY, Anderson RH, et al: Late sudden death after repair of tetralogy of Fallot: A clinicopathologic study. Circulation 67:626–631, 1983.
12. Zimmermann M, Friedli B, Adamec R, Oberhansli I: Ventricular late potentials and induced ventricular arrhythmias after surgical repair of tetralogy of Fallot. Am J Cardiol 67:873–878, 1991.
13. Gillette PC, Yeoman MA, Mullins CE, McNamara DG: Sudden death after repair of tetralogy of Fallot. Electrocardiographic and electrophysiologic abnormalities. Circulation 56:566–571, 1977.
14. Chandar JS, Wolff GS, Garson A Jr, et al: Ventricular arrhythmias in postoperative tetralogy of Fallot. Am J Cardiol 65:655–661, 1990.
15. Walsh EP, Rockenmacher S, Keane JF, et al: Late results in patients with tetralogy of Fallot repaired during infancy. Circulation 77:1062–1067, 1988.
16. Garson A Jr, Randall DC, Gillette PC, et al: Prevention of sudden death after repair of tetralogy of Fallot: Treatment of ventricular arrhythmias. J Am Coll Cardiol 6:221–227, 1985.
17. Daliento L, Rizzoli G, Menti L, et al: Accuracy of electrocardiographic and echocardiographic indices in predicting life threatening ventricular arrhythmias in patients operated for tetralogy of Fallot. Heart 81:650–655, 1999.
18. Gatzoulis MA, Balaji S, Webber SA, et al: Risk factors for arrhythmia and sudden cardiac death late after repair of tetralogy of Fallot: A multicentre study. Lancet 356:975–981, 2000.
19. Harrison DA, Harris L, Siu SC, et al: Sustained ventricular tachycardia in adult patients late after repair of tetralogy of Fallot. J Am Coll Cardiol 30:1368–1373, 1997.
20. Alexander ME, Walsh EP, Saul JP, et al: Value of programmed ventricular stimulation in patients with congenital heart disease. J Cardiovasc Electrophysiol 10:1033–1044, 1999.
21. Lucron H, Marcon F, Bosser G, et al: Induction of sustained ventricular tachycardia after surgical repair of tetralogy of Fallot. Am J Cardiol 83:1369–1373, 1999.
22. Neffke JG, Tulevski II, van der Wall EE, et al: ECG determinants in adult patients with chronic right ventricular pressure overload caused by congenital heart disease: Relation with plasma neurohormones and MRI parameters. Heart 88:266–270, 2002.
23. James FW, Kaplan S, Chou TC: Unexpected cardiac arrest in patients after surgical correction of tetralogy of Fallot. Circulation 52:691–695, 1975.
24. Quattlebaum TG, Varghese J, Neill CA, Donahoo JS: Sudden death among postoperative patients with tetralogy of Fallot: A follow-up study of 243 patients for an average of twelve years. Circulation 54:289–293, 1976.
25. Wren C: Late postoperative arrhythmias. In Wren C, Campbell RWF (eds): Paediatric Cardiac Arrhythmias. Oxford, Oxford University Press, 1996, p 251.
26. Nollert G, Fischlein T, Bouterwek S, et al: Long-term survival in patients with repair of tetralogy of Fallot: 36-year follow-up of 490 survivors of the first year after surgical repair. J Am Coll Cardiol 30:1374–1383, 1997.
27. Preliminary report: Effect of encainide and flecainide on mortality in a randomized trial of arrhythmia suppression after myocardial infarction. The Cardiac Arrhythmia Suppression Trial (CAST) Investigators [see comments]. N Engl J Med 321:406–412, 1989.
28. Oechslin EN, Harrison DA, Harris L, et al: Reoperation in adults with repair of tetralogy of fallot: Indications and outcomes. J Thorac Cardiovasc Surg 118:245–251, 1999.
29. Discigil B, Dearani JA, Puga FJ, et al: Late pulmonary valve replacement after repair of tetralogy of Fallot. J Thorac Cardiovasc Surg 121:344–351, 2001.
30. Fish FA, Gillette PC, Benson DW Jr: Proarrhythmia, cardiac arrest and death in young patients receiving encainide and flecainide. The Pediatric Electrophysiology Group. J Am Coll Cardiol 18:356–365, 1991.
31. Waldo AL, Camm AJ, deRuyter H, et al: Effect of d-sotalol on mortality in patients with left ventricular dysfunction after recent and remote myocardial infarction. The SWORD Investigators. Survival With Oral d-Sotalol. Lancet 348:7–12, 1996.
32. Hohnloser SH: Proarrhythmia with class III antiarrhythmic drugs: Types, risks, and management. Am J Cardiol 80:82G–89G, 1997.
33. Daniels CJ, Schutte DA, Hammond S, Franklin WH: Acute pulmonary toxicity in an infant from intravenous amiodarone. Am J Cardiol 80:1113–1116, 1997.
34. Gonska BD, Cao K, Raab J, et al: Radiofrequency catheter ablation of right ventricular tachycardia late after repair of congenital heart defects. Circulation 94:1902–1908, 1996.
35. Horton RP, Canby RC, Kessler DJ, et al: Ablation of ventricular tachycardia associated with tetralogy of Fallot: Demonstration of bidirectional block. J Cardiovasc Electrophysiol 8:432–435, 1997.
36. Papagiannis J, Kanter RJ, Wharton JM: Radiofrequency catheter ablation of multiple haemodynamically unstable ventricular tachycardias in a patient with surgically repaired tetralogy of Fallot. Cardiol Young 8:379–382, 1998.
37. Stevenson WG, Delacretaz E, Friedman PL, Ellison KE: Identification and ablation of macroreentrant ventricular tachycardia with the CARTO electroanatomical mapping system. Pacing Clin Electrophysiol 21:1448–1456, 1998.
38. Ressia L, Graffigna A, Salerno-Uriarte JA, Vigano M: The complex origin of ventricular tachycardia after the total correction of tetralogy of Fallot. Giornale Italiano di Cardiologia 23:905–910, 1993.
39. Frank G, Schmid C, Baumgart D, et al: Surgical therapy of life-threatening tachycardic cardiac arrhythmias in children. Monatsschrift Kinderheilkunde 137:269–274, 1989.
40. Lawrie GM, Pacifico A, Kaushik R: Results of direct surgical ablation of ventricular tachycardia not due to ischemic heart disease. Ann Surg 209:716–727, 1989.
41. Downar E, Harris L, Kimber S, et al: Ventricular tachycardia after surgical repair of tetralogy of Fallot: Results of intraoperative mapping studies. J Am Coll Cardiol 20:648–655, 1992.
42. Kral MA, Spotnitz HM, Hordof A, et al: Automatic implantable cardioverter defibrillator implantation for malignant ventricular arrhythmias associated with congenital heart disease. Am J Cardiol 63:118–119, 1989.
43. Kron J, Oliver RP, Norsted S, Silka MJ: The automatic implantable cardioverter-defibrillator in young patients. J Am Coll Cardiol 16:896–902, 1990.
44. Silka MJ, Kron J, Dunnigan A, Dick M 2nd: Sudden cardiac death and the use of implantable cardioverter-defibrillators in pediatric patients. The Pediatric Electrophysiology Society. Circulation 87:800–807, 1993.
45. Paul T, Luhmer I, Trappe HJ, et al: The automatic implantable cardioverter-defibrillator for prevention of sudden heart death in children and adolescents. Z Kardiol 82:466–473, 1993.
46. Wilson WR, Greer GE, Grubb BP: Implantable cardioverter-defibrillators in children: A single-institutional experience. Ann Thorac Surg 65:775–778, 1998.
47. Garson AJ, Bink BM, Hesslein PS, et al: Atrial flutter in the young: A collaborative study of 380 cases. J Am Coll Cardiol 6:871–878, 1985.
48. Roos-Hesselink J, Perlroth MG, McGhie J, Spitaels S: Atrial arrhythmias in adults after repair of tetralogy of Fallot. Correlations with clinical, exercise, and echocardiographic findings. Circulation 91:2214–2219, 1995.

49. Triedman JK, Jenkins KJ, Colan SD, et al: Intra-atrial reentrant tachycardia after palliation of congenital heart disease: Characterization of multiple macroreentrant circuits using fluoroscopically based three-dimensional endocardial mapping. J Cardiovasc Electrophysiol 8:259–270, 1997.

50. Chinushi M, Tagawa M, Kasai H, et al: Antitachycardia burst pacing for pleomorphic reentrant ventricular tachycardias associated with non-coronary artery diseases: A morphology specific programming for ventricular tachycardias. Jpn Heart J 41:313–324, 2000.

第 67 章

Brugada 综合征

*Pedro Brugada, Ramon Brugada, Charles Antzelevitch, Jeffrey Towbin,
and Josep Brugada*

本章目录	
■ 概要	618
■ 定义	618
■ 历史	619
■ 病因学与遗传学	620
■ 流行病学	620
■ 心脏电生理基质	621
■ 临床表现	621
■ 诊断	621
■ 预后与治疗	621

一、概 要

一个以发作性晕厥或（复苏的）猝死，心电图表现为右束支阻滞（right bundle branch block，RBBB），$V_1 \sim V_3$ 导联 ST 段抬高，而心脏结构正常为特征的综合征于 1992 年首次被提出。该疾病以常染色体显性遗传方式在 50% 的家庭成员中遗传。现已明确一些不同的基因突变影响到钠离子通道的结构、功能和转运。该疾病是普遍存在的，其发病率及流行率很难确定。在南亚每年每 10 000 名居民中可引起 4～10 例猝死，是该地区 50 岁以下男性中最常见的自然死亡原因。婴儿猝死综合征（sudden infant death syndrome，SIDS）和意外猝死综合征（sudden unexpected death syndrome，SUDS）心电图表现及基因突变与 Brugada 综合征相同，故已认为三者之间存在着联系。当心电图表现典型时，很容易诊断，然而对于隐匿性或间歇性心电图改变的患者则很难作出诊断。心电图可因自主神经平衡、体温、血糖水平的变化，以及服用抗心律失常药物、镇静药、抗疟疾药物而发生变化。刺激 β 肾上腺素能受体可使心电图正常化。右室心外膜动作电位穿隆的消失而心内膜动作电位穿隆仍然存在是 ST 段抬高的原因。右室心外膜电不均一性引起成对短间期室早并通过 2 相折返促使发展为室颤（ventricular fibrillation，VF）。抗心律失常药物对有或无症状的患者不能预防猝死的发生。植入自动心脏复律除颤器是目前唯一证实有效的治疗方法。而对常发室颤电风暴的患者，可能需要心脏移植作为最终的治疗手段。

二、定 义

右束支阻滞，$V_1 \sim V_3$ 导联 ST 段抬高及猝死的综合征（Brugada 综合征）是一种建立在心脏结构正常、晕厥或猝死以及特殊心电图特征基础上的临床电生理诊断。心电图表现为[1]：胸前 $V_1 \sim V_3$ 导联 ST 段抬高，心室波（QRS 综合波）形态类似右束支阻滞（图 67-1）。这种心电图特征也可由 J 点抬高引起[2]。当 ST 段抬高为最突出表现时称之为"穹隆型"抬高，若 J 点抬高而不伴 ST 段抬高为特征时则称为"马鞍型"抬高（图 67-1）。在确诊 Brugada 综合征之前，除外其他引起的 ST 段抬高的原因是非常重要的。其他原因如表 67-1 所示。

晕厥及猝死（存活或未存活者）的发生是由快速多形性室速或室颤所引起（图 67-2）。这些心律失常

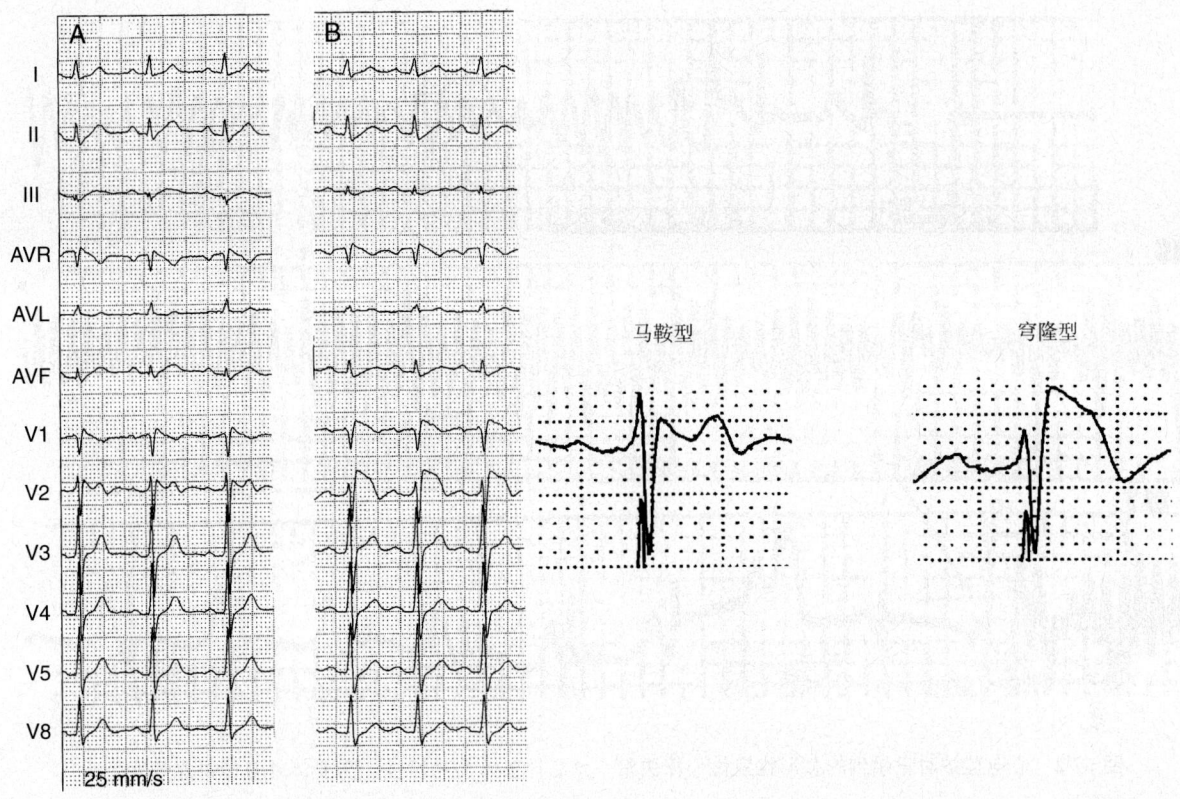

图 67-1 Brugada 综合征典型心电图　B：为"穹隆型"，其在 V_1 导联类似右束支阻滞，$V_1\sim V_3$ 导联 ST 段抬高，PR 间期轻度延长，纸速为 25mm/s。A：为"马鞍型"，该型心电图只有在应用 I 类抗心律失常药物后变为"穹隆型"才认为有诊断意义。

多在无先兆的情况下发生，只有极少数患者在多形性室速发生前心律有长-短交替现象，这种表现是其他心律失常，如长 QT 综合征尖端扭转型室速发生前常见的现象[3]。而不同于儿茶酚胺依赖性多形性室速，它们在发生前常有心率增快现象[4]，是由于兰尼丁（ryanodine）受体突变所致。

三、历　史

Brugada 综合征的首例患者发现于 1986 年。该患者是一名 3 岁的波兰男孩，已经被其父亲成功复苏多次。值得注意的是，多次晕厥或猝死事件发生于患者发热期间。他的姐姐也在多次中止的猝死后于 2 岁时猝死。姐弟两人的心电图相似，都存在异常。1991 年北美起搏与电生理学会（North American Society of Pacing and Electrophysiology，NASPE）会议上报道了另外两名确诊患者初步的资料，而包括 8 名患者的首篇论文于 1992 年发表[1]。此后全球确诊的患者人数呈指数增长。其他作者报道的心电图特征与图 67-1 相似，然而也有人认为这是正常心电图的变异，与猝死之间并无确定联系。

亚洲居民数十年来已认识到该现象的存在。在菲律宾该现象被称为 Bangungut（睡眠猝死的尖叫），在日本被称为 Pokkuri（夜间意外死亡），在泰国这一种死亡

表 67-1　除 Brugada 综合征外其他可导致右胸导联 ST 段抬高的异常情况

右或左束支阻滞，左心室肥大
急性心肌梗死
急性心肌炎
右室心肌梗死
主动脉夹层动脉瘤
急性肺动脉栓塞
各种中枢或自主神经系统异常
大环类抗抑郁药物过量
Duchene 肌营养不良
Frederics 共济失调
维生素 B_1 缺乏症
高钙血症
高钾血症
可卡因中毒
纵隔肿瘤压迫右室流出道（RVOT）
致心律失常性右室发育不良/心肌病

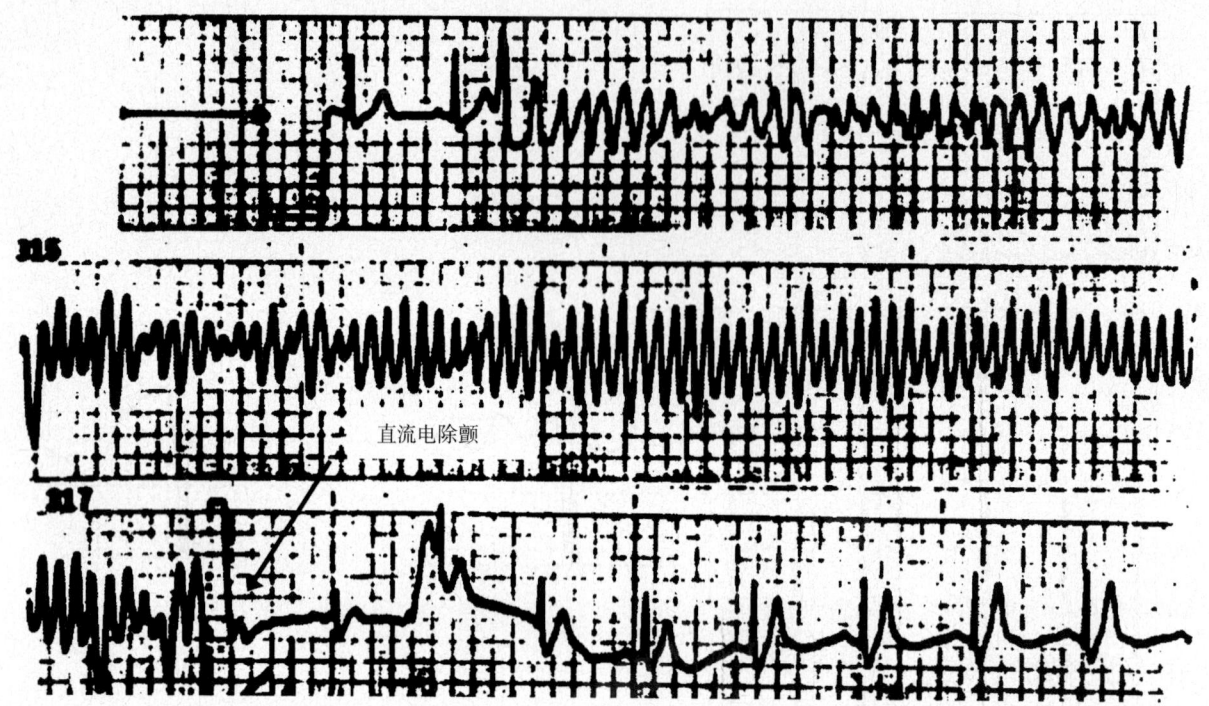

图 67-2 心电监护时记录到的多形性室性心律失常 该心律失常为持续性，需要体外直流电除颤终止。

则被称为 Lai Tai（睡眠之死）或 SUDS（意外猝死综合征）[5]。1997 年发现这些患者患的是同一综合征即 Brugada 综合征。而最近笔者已证实患有 SUDS 的泰国人基因突变与 Brugada 综合征相同[6]。

四、病因学与遗传学

Brugada 综合征通常以散发病例形式发现，但 50% 患者有家族史。Brugada 综合征是否为致心律失常性右室发育不良（arrhythmogenic right ventricular dysplasia，ARVD）的一种类型存在争议。致心律失常性右室发育不良可表现为室性心律失常，典型特征则是右室心肌细胞脂质浸润。基因连锁分析已确定了五个基因位点，包括 ARVD1（14q23），ARVD2（1q42），ARVD3（14q12）及 ARVD4（2q32）[7-9]。而兰尼丁受体突变可能是一个家族发病的原因。

Brugada 综合征遗传学的异常与编码心肌细胞钠通道的 SCN5A 基因突变有关[10]。该基因的突变导致通道功能的丧失或通道从失活状态快速复活的功能丧失。SCN5A 以前被认为是 LQT3 的致病原因，LQT3 是 Romano-Ward 长 QT 综合征中的一种类型。LQT3 与 Brugada 综合征临床表现不同是由于基因突变位点的不同，从而引起不同的生理学表现。不同于 Brugada 综合征，LQT3 的发生是由于 SCN5A 通道介导的末期 I_{Na} 电流增大所致。

尽管 LQTS 与 Brugada 综合征之间存在差异，但亦应注意到两者之间的重要相同点，即两者均可发生由于编码离子通道的基因突变引起的致命性室性心动过速。这一点在某种程度上与家族肥厚型心肌病（familial hypertrophic cardiomyopathy，FHCM）类似。在 FHCM 患者中发现编码肌小节各个组成部分（β-肌球蛋白重链，α-原肌球蛋白，心肌型肌钙蛋白 T，肌球蛋白-结合蛋白-C，肌球蛋白轻链，肌球蛋白调节蛋白轻链，心肌型肌钙蛋白 I）的 7 个基因发生突变，其临床表型，包括预后，皆因突变的基因及特定突变的不同而不同。

五、流行病学

由于该综合征是最近才被确认的，因此很难明确其在世界上的发病率及分布状况。据已发表的不同研究资料，该疾病占所有意外猝死的 4%～12%，而占发生在心脏正常的猝死患者的 50%。

根据现有资料，该疾病为全球分布，而考虑到人群的高流动性及其遗传学基础，这一点亦不足为奇了。随着对该疾病认识的深入，可以预见未来确诊的病例数目将有相当大的增长。一个有关成年日本人群（22 027例）的前瞻性研究显示，有0.05%的心电图表现与该综合征相符（12例）[16]。另一个在日本Awa地区进行的成人研究显示其发生率为0.6%（10 420例中有66例）[17]。而第三个来自日本儿童的研究则显示心电图与该综合征的相符率仅为0.0006%（163 110例中有1例）[18]。这些结果提示该综合征主要在成人阶段发病，这与猝死者的平均年龄（35～40岁）相一致。在笔者的资料库中，猝死年龄最小者为2岁，而最大者为74岁。我们还知道一个Brugada综合征婴儿首发室颤的年龄仅为2天（资料未发表）。

六、心脏电生理基质

有Brugada综合征心电图特征的患者显然有发生快速多形性室速/室颤的倾向。在事件发生前，患者为规则窦性节律（QT间期无变化）。在极少数病例，多形性室速发生前有更明显的ST段抬高。笔者只观察到两例患者，由短-长-短周期触发心律失常。基于大多数有症状的Brugada综合征患者可诱发出多形性室速/室颤的事实，故认为这些患者存在有发生室速/室颤的电生理基质。该综合征患者常伴有延长的希氏束-心室传导时间（H-V间期）。

七、临床表现

完整的综合征表现为，患者发作快速多形性室速，心电图呈右束支阻滞型，V_1～V_3导联ST段抬高。对心律失常发作能自动终止者，仅表现为晕厥发作；当心律失常发作呈持续时将突发心脏骤停，甚至猝死。因此，该疾病临床表现，从无症状患者到猝死者，范围很广。其他症状还包括癫痫发作、濒死状呼吸，夜间睡眠中发作者有呼吸费力、精神激动、尿失禁以及并不常见的近期失忆（可能是由于脑缺氧）。该疾病的许多患者可表现得非常健康和有活力，精力充沛地从事体力活动或运动，体格检查几乎总是正常。首次接诊这些患者的医师常会有强烈的倾向，即相信这些晕厥发作是良性的，可能为血管迷走性。许多患者进行了直立倾斜试验，表现为阳性的患者虽然给予了相应的治疗，但随后仍发生了猝死。与我们所见的其他临床-心电图综合征相比，该疾病表现不同。

无症状患者多在行常规体检时发现不典型心电图，这些心电图与有症状患者心电图并无区别。有一些病人，则是由于其家庭成员因该综合征猝死后，在筛查时记录到典型的心电图改变。另一方面，一组有症状患者被诊断为不明原因或血管迷走性晕厥，或诊断为特发性室颤。有一些患者在随访期间，因心电图自发从正常变为典型综合征心电图时被确诊。还有一些患者则是因为治疗其他的心律失常，如房颤，给予的抗心律失常药物使得该疾病显露出来。

最近的研究表明，表现有该综合征心电图特征的有症状患者，与只有应用钠离子通道阻滞剂才能表现出心电图特征的患者相比，具有相似的心律失常和猝死发生率（图67-3）。

在2～3年的随访期间，可有40%的患者表现出新发或首次多形性室速或猝死发作。然而在无症状患者则并非如此。

八、诊 断

当患者表现有典型的心电图特征（图67-1B）并有多形性室速引起的存活的猝死或晕厥病史时，根据心电图即可作出诊断。V_1～V_3导联ST段抬高伴有右束支阻滞是典型的心电图特征。其ST段改变不同于急性间隔部心肌缺血、心包炎、室壁瘤及一些正常变异，即早期复极综合征时能观察到的改变。然而对那些心电图不典型的患者，只有当医师考虑到该综合征时才可能识别。还有许多患者心电图正常，只有在应用阿义马林、普鲁卡因胺或氟卡胺后连续观察心电图，才表现出典型心电图特征，此时方能作出归类性的诊断（图67-3）。

自主神经或其他影响因素导致的心电图改变会引起其他的诊断问题。Miyazaki等的研究[19]首次显示了该综合征心电图的变异性：刺激肾上腺素能神经可减轻ST段的抬高，而刺激迷走神经则相反。IA、IC及III类抗心律失常药物的使用可增加ST段的抬高，运动可减轻ST段的抬高。但在有些病人，运动后即刻ST段抬高可加重。由心房起搏引起的心率变化可伴随着ST段抬高程度的变化，当心率减慢时，ST段抬高程度增加，而心率增快时ST段抬高程度则减低。

九、预后与治疗

早期的一系列研究表明，发生晕厥或室颤后复苏成功的Brugada综合征患者，在大约2年的时间内约1/3以上的患者会再发多形性室速[20]。同样，无症状

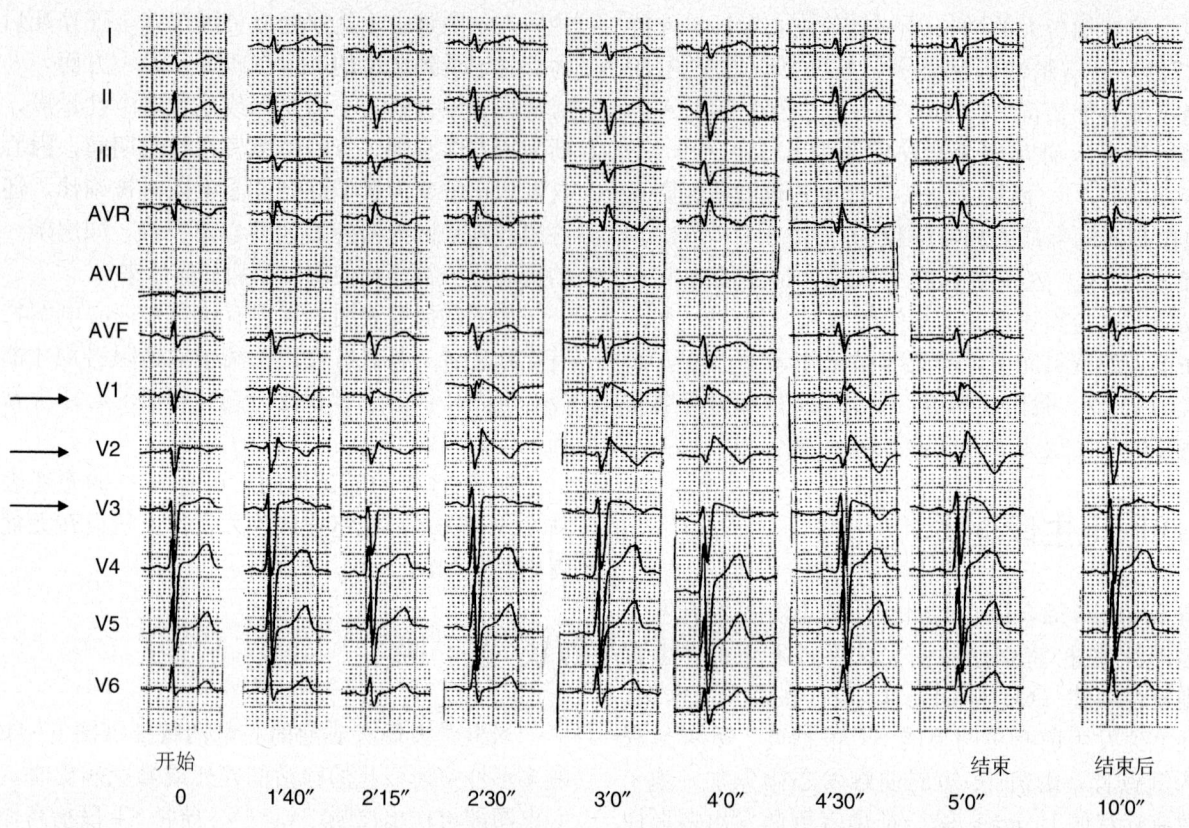

图 67-3 经静脉使用阿义马林对心电图的影响

而心电图特征典型的患者预后亦差。最近对一个667人系列的研究分析（图67-4）进一步证实了这些发现。心电图$V_1 \sim V_3$导联出现终末R'波，J点抬高至少0.2mV，ST段下斜型抬高，T波低平或倒置（穹隆型心电图），被定义为异常心电图（图67-1B）。当静脉应用具有钠通道阻滞剂性质的抗心律失常药，如阿义马林、氟卡胺或普鲁卡因胺后，如上所描述的异常心电图特征变得明显，亦定义为异常心电图。主治医师应通过临床病史，无创性（超声心动图、运动试验、核素磁共振）及有创性方法（冠状动脉造影、左及右室造影剂和组织活检）来谨慎除外器质性心脏病。

667例患者中有120例的异常心电图是在发生猝死幸存后而确定的。124例患者的异常心电图是在一次或多次晕厥发作后而确定的。而另外423例因是该综合征患者的家庭成员，在例行心电图检查或研究时被确定。

心脏电生理检查包括基础的传导间期测定以及心室程序刺激。建议的电生理刺激方案包括1个刺激部位（右室心尖部），3个基础周期（600ms，500ms，430ms）以及外加1个、2个、3个早搏刺激，直到最短的联律间期200ms。如诱发出持续性室性心律失常（室颤，多形性或单形性室速持续超过30s或需紧急干预），则认为该病人是可诱发的。

确诊的平均年龄（第一次确定异常心电图）为41 ± 15岁（2～85岁），男性多于女性（507 vs. 160）。344例患者（51.5%）有可疑阳性家族史。499例（75%）心电图自发异常，168例仅在应用I类抗心律失常药后才显示心电图异常。493例患者进行了电生

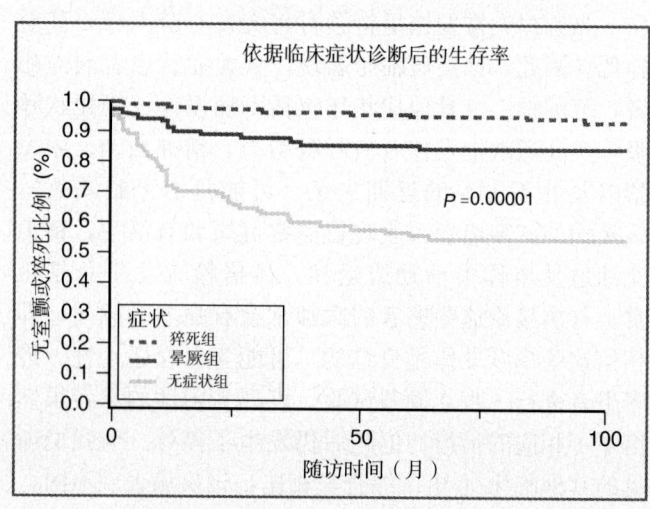

图 67-4 667例基于临床表现诊断的患者的生存曲线

表 67-2　患者的临床特征

临床表现	猝死或室颤	无猝死及室颤	P 值
患者例数	164	503	
男性/女性	141/23	366/137	0.0001
年龄（年）	42±15	43±15	NS
自发异常心电图	150	349	0.0001
心脏性猝死家族史	70	274	0.03
可/不可诱发	95/21	136/241	0.0001

NS，无显著性；P，统计学显著水平。

理检查，其中 231 例（47%）在心室程序刺激过程中诱发出持续性室性心律失常。

共有 164 例患者在一生中至少有一次猝死或室颤发作（120 例症状发作于异常心电图确诊之前，44 例症状发作在确诊之后），人口统计学特征及电生理检查结果如表 67-2 所示。

多因素分析显示，可诱发出持续性室性心律失常，男性及自发心电图异常是心律失常发作的预测因子（表 67-3）。使用这些预测因子不同组合的 logistic 回归模型，研究了事件发生的可能性，见表 67-4。在所有类别中，男性患者预后较女性差。在极端情况下，即一名男性患者，自发心电图异常且可诱发出持续室性心动过速，其发生事件的可能性为 45.1%；在另一种极端情况下，一名女性患者，只有应用抗心律失常药物后才表现出异常心电图，且不能诱发出持续室性心律失常，其发生事件的可能性仅为 3%。

在确诊 Brugada 综合征之后，患者平均随访 38±47 个月。105 例患者新发或再发心脏性猝死，或者有明确的室颤发作。应用多因素分析表明，可诱发出持续性室性心动过速、曾发生过存活性猝死或晕厥是发生事件的最强预测因子（表 67-5）。

以上资料显示：

1. Brugada 综合征的心电图诊断是突发心律失常性死亡的标志：在该系列研究的所有患者中，25% 在一生中发生过猝死或明确的室颤。

2. 男性是猝死的一个危险因素：在所有研究分类中，与女性相比，男性发生（存活性）猝死的风险更高。最近 Di Diego 及其同事的研究[21]证实了这一临床现象的病理生理基础，即男性 Brugada 表现型更为显著——带来临床事件的发生率更高——是由于男性的瞬时外向钾电流（I_{to}）比女性更为显著。

3. 可诱发出持续性室性心律失常是预后最强的标志：与笔者之前的报道[22]相反，在行心室程序刺激研究的病人中，H-V 间期与预后无显著相关。然而随着研究病例的增多，心室程序刺激的预后价值得到了强化。尽管并非所有患者都行心室程序刺激检查，但可诱发持续性室性心律失常的患者发生（存活性）猝死的几率几乎比未诱发者高 4 倍。

4. 家族型病例并不比散发病例预后差：有 Brugada 综合征家族史的患者并不提示预后更差。该系列研究的资料证实了笔者以前报道的观察结果，即猝死家族史或家族型 Brugada 综合征并不比散发病例的预后更差。

5. 自发心电图异常患者比应用抗心律失常药物才显示心电图异常的患者预后更差：自发性心电图异常者在一生中发生心律失常事件的危险是只有应用抗心律失常药物后才显示出具有诊断 Brugada 综合征的心电图患者的两倍。然而这种诊断确定后，这个变量并无预后价值。因此，自发性心电图异常是一生中发生心律失常事件的标志，但作为单一变量，对于无症状患者随访期间并无预测事件的意义，因为其他变量（程序刺激、男性）是更强的预后预测因子。

表 67-3　终生猝死或室颤的可能性

	单因素分析			多因素分析		
	危险比	95%CI	P 值	危害比	95%CI	P 值
可诱发	4.76	3.03~7.69	0.0001	3.85	2.38~6.25	0.0001
不可诱发	1			1		
基础 ECG	3.85	2.17~7.14	0.0001	1.89	1.01~3.70	0.046
AAD ECG	1			1		
男性	2.4	1.56~3.80	0.0001	1.89	1.03~3.45	0.027
女性	1			1		
有家族史	1.05	0.69~1.31	0.787			
无家族史	1					

AAD ECG，应用抗心律失常药物后才显示异常心电图；基础 ECG，自发异常心电图；CI，可信区间；P，统计学显著水平。

表 67-4 终生发生事件的可能性

男性	EPS时不可诱发	EPS时可诱发
AAD后异常心电图	4.4 (2.0~9.3)	23.4 (12.8~38.8)
基础异常心电图	11.0 (7.0~16.8)	45.1 (37.9~52.5)
女性	EPS时不可诱发	EPS时可诱发
AAD后异常心电图	3.0 (1.3~6.9)	17.0 (8.0~32.7)
基础异常心电图	7.6 (3.8~14.8)	35.5 (21.8~52.1)

数据为百分数（95%可信区间）
AAD，抗心律失常药物；EPS，电生理检查

综上所述，这些资料证实了 Priori 及其同事的发现[23]，但是他们并没有发现心室程序刺激可预测事件的发生。

植入式心脏复律除颤器（implantable cardioverter-defibrillator, ICD）仍是唯一有效预防猝死的手段。基于不同的基因背景或病理生理机制，某些患者可能对奎尼丁有较好的治疗反应[24]。不幸的是，笔者对8例有严重的室颤风暴的患者应用奎尼丁治疗，结果却令人失望（未公布）。到目前为止，一例患者已不得不行心脏移植[25]，而另一例也正在等待供体。尚无使用其他 I_{to} 阻断剂的经验，目前只有一例应用西洛他唑（cilostazol）——一种可增加钙电流的磷酸二酯酶抑制剂治疗成功的报道[26]。无论用何种方式，有一种共识就是有症状的患者最好接受除颤器治疗。对于有症状患者来说，主要的问题是，达到何种程度的风险安装除颤器是可接受的。当受影响的患者为儿童时，这一问题就变得尤其突出。然而用笔者提供的资料来评估风险时，不应忘记在作出决定时还要考虑心理及社会因素，即使它们并没有经科学的论证。当面对一个无症状而自发心电图正常且不能诱发出室性心律失常的患者，但因该疾病他已失去6个兄弟姐妹中的4人时，我们该如何处理呢？

（杨新春 译）

表 67-5 临床及电生理因素对确诊后随访期间发生猝死或室颤可能性的影响

	单因素分析			多因素分析		
	危害比	95%CI	P值	危害比	95%CI	P值
可诱发	11.1	4.54~25.0	0.0001	7.14	2.7~20.0	0.0001
不可诱发	1			1		
基础 ECG	3.70	1.75~7.69	0.0001			
AAD ECG	1					
男性	2.94	1.54~5.88	0.0001			
女性	1					
有家族史	1.03	0.68~1.55	0.896			
无家族史	1					
无症状	1		0.0001	1		0.0001
晕厥	2.60	1.43~4.76		2.41	1.16~4.99	
猝死	6.53	4.08~10.4		3.99	2.09~7.60	
HV<55ms	1		0.494			
HV>55ms	1.26	0.66~2.40				

AAD ECG，应用抗心律失常药物后才显示异常心电图；基础 ECG，自发异常心电图；CI，可信区间；HV，窦律时希氏束-心室间期；P，统计学显著水平。

参 考 文 献

1. Brugada P, Brugada J: Right bundle branch block, persistent ST segment elevation and sudden cardiac death: A distinct clinical and electrocardiographic syndrome. J Am Coll Cardiol 20:1391–1396, 1992.
2. Yan GX, Antzelevitch C: Cellular basis for the electrocardiographic J wave. Circulation 93:372–379, 1996.
3. Priori SG, Diehl L, Schwartz PJ: Torsade de pointes. In Podrid PJ, Kowey PR (eds): Cardiac Arrhythmia. Baltimore, Williams & Wilkins, 1995, pp 951–963.
4. El-Sherif N: Polymorphic ventricular tachycardia and torsades de pointes: Beyond etymology. J Cardiovasc Electrophysiol 12:695–696, 2001.
5. Nademanee K, Veerakul G, Nimmannit S, et al: Arrhythmogenic marker for the sudden unexplained death syndrome in Thai men. Circulation 96:2595–2600, 1997.

6. Vatta M, Dumaine R, Varghese G, et al: Genetic and biophysical basis of sudden unexplained nocturnal death syndrome (SUNDS), a disease allelic to Brugada syndrome. Hum Mol Genet 11:337–345, 2002.
7. Rampazzo A, Nava A, Erne P, et al: A new locus for arrhythmogenic right ventricular cardiomyopathy (ARVD2) maps to chromosome 1q42-Q43. Hum Mol Genet 4:2151–2154, 1995.
8. Severini GM, Krajinovic M, Pinamonti B, et al: A new locus for arrhythmogenic right ventricular dysplasia on the long arm of chromosome 14. Genomics 31:193–200, 1996.
9. Rampazzo A, Nava A, Miorin M, et al: ARVD4, a new locus for arrhythmogenic right ventricular cardiomyopathy, maps to chromosome 2 long arm. Genomics 45:259–263, 1997.
10. Chen Q, Kirsch GE, Zhang D, et al: Genetic basis and molecular mechanisms for idiopathic ventricular fibrillation. Nature 392:293–296, 1998.
11. Bonne G, Carrier L, Bercovici J, et al: Cardiac myosin binding protein-C gene splice acceptor site mutation is associated with familial hypertrophic cardiomyopathy. Nat Genet 11:438–440, 1995.
12. Poetter K, Jiang H, Hassanzadeh S, et al: Mutations in either the essential or regulatory light chains of myosin are associated with a rare myopathy in human heart and skeletal muscle. Nat Genet 13:63–69, 1996.
13. Kimura A, Harada H, Park JE, et al: Mutations in the cardiac troponin I gene associated with hypertrophic cardiomyopathy. Nat Genet 16:379–382, 1996.
14. Watkins H, McKenna WJ, Theirfelder L, et al: Mutations in the genes for cardiac troponin T and alpha-tropomyosin in hypertrophic cardiomyopathy. N Engl J Med 332:1058–1064, 1995.
15. Towbin JA: The role of cytoskeletal proteins in cardiomyopathies. Curr Opin Cell Biol 10:131–139, 1998.
16. Tohyou Y, Nakazawa K, Ozawa A, et al: A survey in the incidence of right bundle branch block with ST segment elevation among normal population. Jpn J Electrocardiol 15:223–226, 1995.
17. Namiki T, Ogura T, Kuwabara Y, et al: Five-year mortality and clinical characteristics of adult subjects with right bundle branch block and ST elevation. Circulation 93:334, 1995.
18. Hata Y, Chiba N, Hotta K, et al: Incidence and clinical significance of right bundle branch block and ST segment elevation in V1-V3 in 6-to 18-year-old school children in Japan. Circulation 20:2310, 1997.
19. Miyazaki T, Mitamura H, Miyoshi S, et al: Autonomic and antiarrhythmic modulation of ST segment elevation in patients with Brugada syndrome. J Am Coll Cardiol 27:1061–1070, 1996.
20. Brugada J, Brugada R, Antzelevitch C, et al: Long-term follow-up of individuals with the electrocardiographic pattern of right bundle branch block and ST segment elevation in precordial leads V1 to V3. Circulation 105:73–78, 2002.
21. Di Diego JM, Cordeiro JM, Goodrow RJ, et al: Ionic and cellular basis for the predominance of the Brugada syndrome phenotype in males. Circulation 106:2004–2011, 2002.
22. Brugada P, Geelen P, Brugada R, et al: Prognostic value of electrophysiologic investigations in Brugada syndrome. J Cardiovasc Electrophysiol 12:1004–1007, 2001.
23. Priori S, Napolitano C, Gasparini M, et al: Natural history of Brugada syndrome: Insights for risk stratification and management. Circulation 105:1342–1347, 2002.
24. Belhassen B, Viskin S, Antzelevitch C: The Brugada syndrome: Is an implantable cardioverter defibrillator the only therapeutic option? Pacing Clin Electrophysiol 25:1634–1640, 2002.
25. Rivero-Ayerza M, De Zutter M, Goethals M, et al: Heart transplantation as last resort against Brugada syndrome. J Cardiovasc Electrophysiol 13:943–944, 2002.
26. Tsuchiya T, Ashikaga K, Honda T, Arita M: Prevention of ventricular fibrillation by cilostazol, an oral phosphodiesterase inhibitor, in a patient with Brugada syndrome. J Cardiovasc Electrophysiol 13:698–701, 2002.

第 68 章

儿茶酚胺敏感性多形性室速和短联律间期性尖端扭转型室速

Carlo Napolitano and Silvia G. Priori

本章目录
- 儿茶酚胺敏感性多形性室速 ·············· 626
- 短联律间期性尖端扭转型室速 ·············· 631
- 总结 ·············· 631

一、儿茶酚胺敏感性多形性室速

(一) 背景和定义

对儿茶酚胺在致心律失常方面作用的研究已经有很长的历史了。通过基础实验和临床研究，已有越来越多的关于肾上腺素诱发心律失常的电生理机制被阐明，但直到最近相关的分子机制才被人们所认识。

交感神经系统的突然激活能使有心脏疾病患者产生一系列的致命性心律失常，这些心脏疾病既包括后天获得性疾病，例如心肌缺血和心力衰竭，又包括遗传性致心律失常性疾病，例如长 QT 综合征[1-4]。一些病例中，在患者无任何心脏结构及心电图异常的情况下，儿茶酚胺仍能诱发室性心律失常，这就是儿茶酚胺敏感性室速。该病最初在 1978 年由 Coumel 等首次发现[5]。他们报道的这种心律失常表现为室速、晕厥和猝死，一些有家族聚集现象，但也有散发的病例。他们把具有这种临床特征的疾病称为儿茶酚胺敏感性多形性室速（catecholaminergic polymorphic ventricular tachycardia, CPVT）。Coumel 等发现儿茶酚胺敏感性多形性室速有三个典型的特征：①心律失常的发生与肾上腺素分泌增多（运动或情绪激动）有关；②心律失常发生时表现为典型的双向性室速，而在休息时心电图无明显异常；③心脏结构正常。

最近，儿茶酚胺敏感性多形性室速被认为是一种遗传相关性心律失常，它的病理生理学机制已经越来越多地被阐明。

(二) 临床特征

1. 心电图表现

除一部分表现为轻度的窦性心动过缓外，儿茶酚胺敏感性多形性室速患者休息时心电图无明显异常；患者房室传导正常，信号平均心电图也无明显的异常[6]。

运动或情绪激动是诱发儿茶酚胺敏感性多形性室速患者发生心律失常的重要因素。有趣的是，在运动负荷试验时心律失常的出现是高度可重复的，心律失常的心率阈值一般在 120～130 次/分。随着运动负荷的增加，室性心律失常也变得越来越复杂，从单个室早到室早二联律，最后发展为非持续性室速。如果患者继续运动，室速持续时间也将增加，最终变成持续性室速。双向性室速（相邻的 QRS 波电轴呈 180 度的转换）是儿茶酚胺敏感性多形性室速的典型特征（图 68-1）。但近来研究表明，儿茶酚胺敏感性多形性室速患者也可没有 QRS 波向量规律的变化，而表现为不规则的多形性室速[7,8]。与长 QT 综合征和 Brugada 综合征不同[9]，在儿茶酚胺敏感性多形性室速患者，由运动诱发的非持续性室上性心动过速比较常见[6,10]（图 68-1）。但由于患者血清中儿茶酚胺浓度并未增加，说明心房和心室对生理性交感神经的激动敏感性增加[10]。

因为儿茶酚胺敏感性多形性室速患者心脏结构正常，所以折返机制可能不是肾上腺素诱发的多形性室速的原因。而自律性异常和触发机制更可能是这种心律失常的原因。在运动过程中，随着心率的增加室早联律间期越来越短，这也支持心律失常发生是由延迟后除极和触发机制所致这一假设。

2. 心脏事件和临床表现

由运动或情绪激动诱发的晕厥往往是儿茶酚胺敏感性多形性室速患者的首发表现，但在一些原先无症状的患者中，心源性猝死也可为首发表现[7]。家系调查发现，大概30%的患者家系中有一个或多个成员早期猝死史，猝死多数发生在儿童期，但也有较晚期的猝死（20岁以后）[6,7]。心脏结构无异常患者猝死后，尸检后往往诊断为特发性室颤[7]。

在大多数情况下，即使患者到成年期才发病，但实际上症状在儿童早期就已存在[11]。Leenhardt 等[6]研究表明，儿茶酚胺敏感性多形性室速患者首发症状出现在 7.8±4 岁，这与最近 Priori 等[7]报道的携带有 RyR2 基因突变的儿茶酚胺敏感性多形性室速患者的发病年龄（8±2 岁）相似。

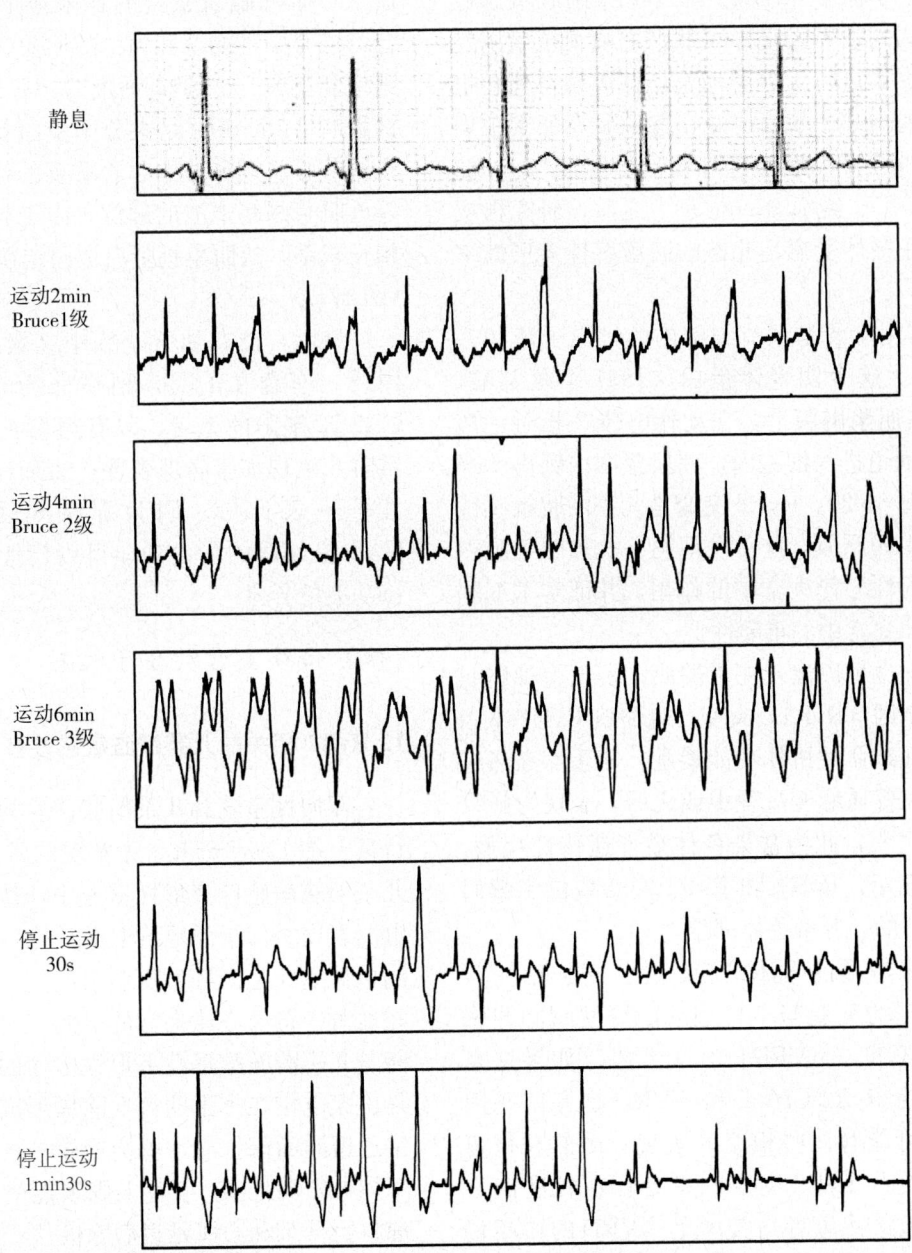

图 68-1 儿茶酚胺敏感性多形性室速的患者进行运动试验　基础心电图无明显异常，采用标准的 Bruce 方案，随着运动负荷的增加，心律失常也变得越来越复杂，双向性室速出现在运动开始后 6min。室上性心律失常在运动早期和停止运动时表现明显。

(三) 基因研究

1. 常染色体显性遗传性儿茶酚胺敏感性多形性室速

有证据表明儿茶酚胺敏感性多形性室速有家族聚集现象[5,6,10,12]。第1例报道的家族性儿茶酚胺敏感性多形性室速的表型分布符合常染色体显性遗传模式[6,10]。最近，Scan等[8]对两个大家系进行基因连锁分析，发现该病的基因位于染色体1q42-43，LOD值（对数）为4.74。

基于这些发现及有研究表明编码人心脏兰尼丁（ryanodine）受体基因（RyR2）位于儿茶酚胺敏感性多形性室速基因的临界区域[13]，我们对负荷试验诱发的双向性室速家族进行了分子筛查，并成功发现和报道了4例患者的RyR2基因突变，这一研究证实常染色体显性遗传性儿茶酚胺敏感性多形性室速与RyR2基因突变有关[14]。继Laitinen等[15]之后，研究再次证实心脏兰尼丁受体受累是儿茶酚胺敏感性多形性室速的原因。

RyR2的作用主要是调节细胞内的钙离子流和兴奋收缩耦联[16]。这个四聚体蛋白（4967个氨基酸，564kD）横跨在肌浆网膜上，在动作电位2相时钙离子经过L型钙通道进入细胞内，使肌浆网内钙离子释放入细胞内（图68-2）。RyR2突变是儿茶酚胺敏感性多形性室速发生的原因，这一发现第一次表明细胞内离子通道在先天性心律失常中的作用，并证实了细胞内钙离子在心律失常中的重要性[16]。

相似的情况也可以出现在骨骼肌，表现为骨骼肌的兰尼丁受体基因（RyR1）突变。骨骼肌RyR1基因突变可引起急性致命性机体功能紊乱，即恶性高热综合征，它出现在普通麻醉过程中或之后，表现为横纹肌溶解和高热[17-19]，此为常染色体显性遗传性疾病。突变位点分析显示，RyR1和RyR2突变点位于编码这两种受体蛋白的同源染色体部位[16]。

近来，越来越多的RyR2突变位点被报道[7,20]，并且提示该基因的突变与不典型或隐匿性致心律失常性右室发育不良（AVRD）有关[20,21]。如果这点被证实，可认为RyR2-CPVT和AVRD是等位基因性疾病，它们可能有一些相似的表现。虽然有报道发现[20-22]，在有些RyR2突变的患者存在轻度的心脏结构异常，但这些患者是否满足AVRD的诊断仍存在争议。另外，二者之间的病理生理性联系（细胞内离子通道的突变与右室心肌纤维脂肪浸润的发展）还远未阐明。

2. 常染色体隐性遗传儿茶酚胺敏感性多形性室速

2001年，Lahat等[22]首次报道了与常染色体显性遗传特征不同的儿茶酚胺敏感性多形性室速。通过对7个有血缘关系的贝多因人家族的研究，他们发现该病的基因在染色体1p23-21上一个长16cM的片段上，其LOD值为8.24。然后他们确定CASQ2是这种儿茶酚胺敏感性多形性室速的突变基因[23]。CASQ2编码肌集钙蛋白（calsequestrin），它是心脏的一种高表达蛋白。肌集钙蛋白是一种钙连接蛋白，位于心肌细胞肌浆网的终末池上，能和大量的钙结合，具有中等的亲和力。故肌集钙蛋白是肌浆网内的钙结合蛋白[24]。肌集钙蛋白、三连体（triadin）和连接蛋白（junctin）是大分子蛋白复合体的核心，可能在调节心肌钙释放中起着重要的作用。这些蛋白位于邻近肌浆网终末池的部位，由于与三连体和连接蛋白相互联系，故肌集钙蛋白被固定在兰尼丁受体附近[25]（图68-2）。

最近，在高加索家族中又报道了少量的突变基因[26]。有意义的是，到目前为止大部分被诊断为CASQ2缺陷的患者，只有当患者一对等位基因都异常时才出现临床病理表现；而杂合子患者的突变基因几乎不表达[26]。因为那条未受损的染色体，使CASQ2编码的蛋白功能得以代偿，而不表现出钙连接功能的异常。

(四) 心律失常的分子机制

1. RyR2相关的儿茶酚胺敏感性多形性室速

双向性室速和儿茶酚胺诱发的心律失常是该病的特征。在Leenhardt[6]等发现的常染色体显性遗传性儿茶酚胺敏感性多形性室速中，他们看到其室速的心电图表现类似于洋地黄中毒时的心电图特征[27]，故猜测该种室速是由触发机制引起的。由于延迟后除极是洋地黄中毒性心律失常的机制，所以延迟后除极也可能是儿茶酚胺敏感性多形性室速的机制。延迟后除极是由膜电位在舒张期自发除极形成的，当电位增大到钠通道激活阈值时，就会产生一次新的动作电位。几个体外实验证实，β肾上腺素能受体激活时，能导致浦肯野纤维和心肌延迟后除极[28]。

与RyR2突变相关的心律失常，可能是由于突变蛋白丧失正常的功能，导致细胞内钙超载[16]。通过改

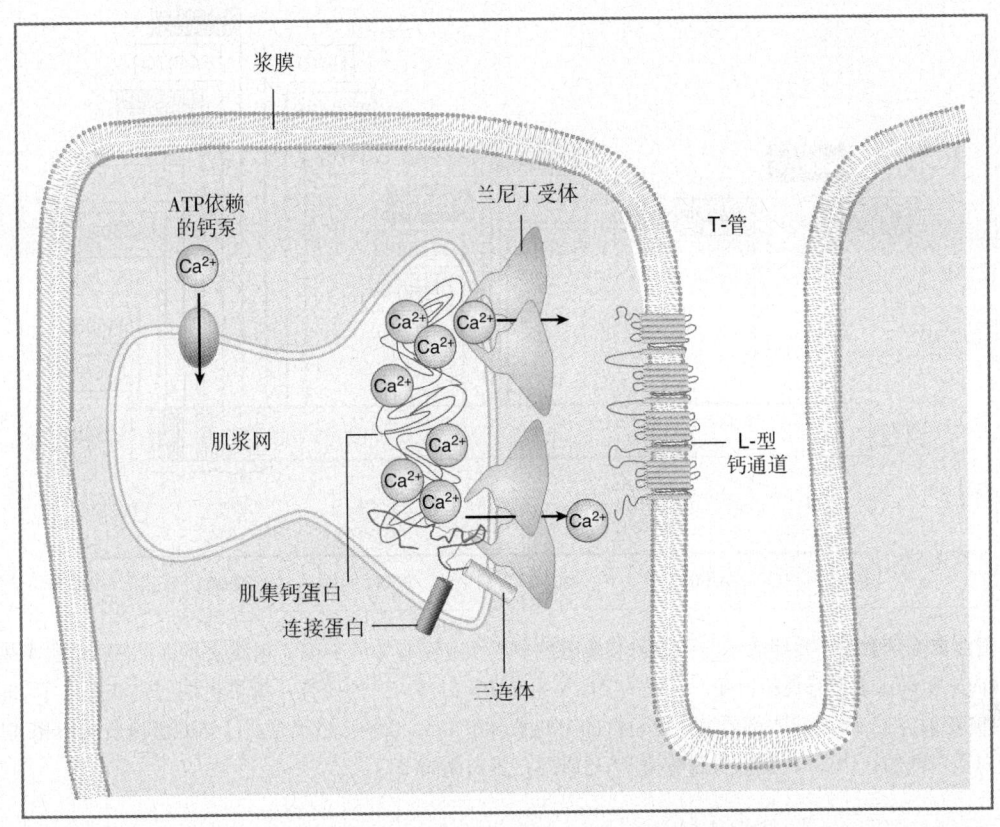

图 68-2　大分子复合物示意图，该复合物参与调控钙离子从心肌细胞肌浆网中释放　ATP：三磷腺苷。

变蛋白质的正常折叠和同源四聚体的正常组合，或通过干扰其与稳定调节分子（例如 FKBP12.6）的结合，突变基因发挥作用，导致舒张期钙释放[14]。另外，通道可能对级联反应变得超敏感。近来报道的儿茶酚胺敏感性多形性室速患者的 RyR2 突变明显集中在蛋白质的重要功能区：跨膜区、钙结合位点、FKBP12.6 结合域（图 68-3）[7,14,29]。

近来，Wehrens 等[30]把已经明确的儿茶酚胺敏感性多形性室速的三个 RyR2 突变基因[14]整合到有 RyR2 通道表达的脂质双分子层中。在基础状态下，其与野生型通道相比无显著性差异。但是，当用蛋白激酶 A（PKA）激活时，在突变体中，单通道开放机率和开放频率明显增加。这表明突变体对 PKA 的激活有高敏感性，在 PKA 激活时单通道活性明显增加。所以当交感激活时（运动或情绪激动），突变的 RyR2 通道触发致命性心律失常。

2. CASQ2 相关的儿茶酚胺敏感性多形性室速

在体外试验中，CASQ2 突变所致的功能变化还不清楚。Lahat 等[23]提出突变可能通过引起蛋白质酸性钙结合中心结构紊乱而干扰 CASQ2 所具有的正常钙螯合作用。这使得肌浆网内游离钙离子浓度增加，导致外向驱动力增加，并可能使钙释放增加。但是，是否 CASQ2 通过这一机制导致儿茶酚胺敏感性心律失常还需要经过功能性研究加以证实。

（五）临床治疗

1. RyR2 相关的儿茶酚胺敏感性多形性室速的基因型和表型的关系

在临床诊断的儿茶酚胺敏感性多形性室速中，大约 50% 的患者有 RyR2 突变[7]。该病是一种基因异质性疾病，而近来没有发现其他基因与这种常染色体显性遗传性儿茶酚胺敏感性多形性室速相关。相关知识的缺乏阻碍了对基因疗法的界定和对其进行危险分层。没有发现 RyR2 基因缺陷的患者发病年龄比存在 RyR2 基因突变的携带者年龄大（20±12 vs 8±2 岁），并且后组中男性患者年轻时发生心脏事件的危险性很高（RR=4.2）[7]。其实，RyR2 突变并非都表现为双向性室速，先证者中大概有 40% 的患者表现为多形性室速[7]。在过去诊断为特发性室颤的患者，RyR2 突变可能是其根本原因[7]。上述两组患者心脏事件的发

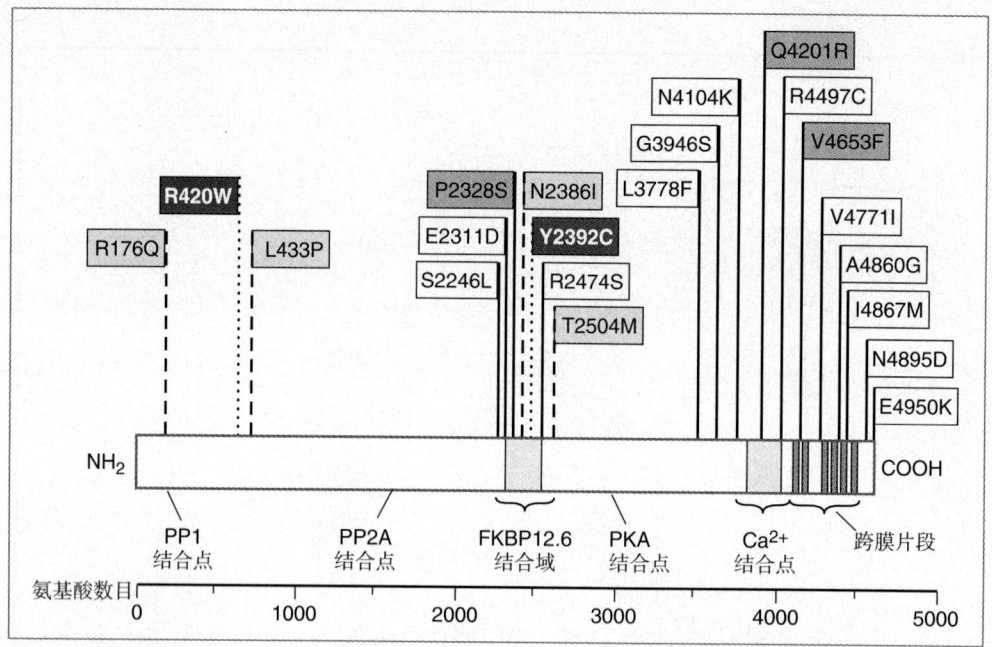

图 68-3　RyR2 蛋白突变示意图　实线表示与儿茶酚胺敏感性多形性室速有关的突变，虚线表示在 ARVD2 患者中发现的突变，点线表示与其他尚未明确的表型有关的突变。白框的突变来自于 Priori 等[7,14]的研究，淡黑色框的突变来自于 Laitinen 等[15]的研究，灰色框的突变来自于 Tiso 等[20]的研究，黑色框的突变来自于 Lahat 等[21]的研究。已知的蛋白质功能相关区域也在图上标明。PP1：蛋白质磷酸酶；PP2A：蛋白质磷酸酶 2A；PKA：蛋白激酶 A。

生率并无差异。两组患者的心脏事件大多数发生在儿童期，60% 以上的患者 20 岁以前有过至少一次心脏事件（晕厥或心脏骤停）[7]。

2. CASQ2 相关的儿茶酚胺敏感性多形性室速的基因型和表现型的关系

由于存在 CASQ2 突变的患者数量有限，无法比较 RyR2 相关的儿茶酚胺敏感性多形性室速和 CASQ2 相关的儿茶酚胺敏感性多形性室速。资料表明，除缺乏双向性室速外，CASQ2 相关的儿茶酚胺敏感性多形性室速与 RyR2 相关的儿茶酚胺敏感性多形性室速的临床特征相同。CASQ2 相关的儿茶酚胺敏感性多形性室速常表现为高度不规则和多形性室速。Lahat 等[23]最初报道的病例中发现 QT 间期轻度延长，但这一特征在随后的病例中没有被证实[26]。有 CASQ2 突变的患者没有任何临床证据表明存在右室结构异常[23]。

3. 儿茶酚胺敏感性多形性室速的危险分层和治疗

β受体阻滞剂是治疗儿茶酚胺敏感性多形性室速的基石[6,7]。有限的经验表明，胺碘酮和Ⅰ类抗心律失常药物治疗无效[6]。程序刺激一般不能诱发儿茶酚胺敏感性多形性室速，故对于该病的诊断和危险分层没有帮助[6,7]。相反，在儿茶酚胺敏感性多形性室速患者，运动能高度重复诱发心律失常，故可用于诊断、调整药物剂量和监测病情。β受体阻滞剂的应用仅限于 RyR2 相关的儿茶酚胺敏感性多形性室速和没有已知突变基因的儿茶酚胺敏感性多形性室速患者[7]，而在 CASQ2 相关的儿茶酚胺敏感性多形性室速患者中的应用经验有限。

长期足量的β受体阻滞剂治疗能防止一些患者再次出现晕厥[6,7]。但是，大概有 40% 的患者即使通过反复的运动试验进行药物优化治疗，仍不能满意地控制心律失常的发生。这时，ICD 治疗可能是有用的，因为有证据表明，在接受药物治疗的患者应用 ICD 后，平均随访 2 年，有一半患者在此期间同时接受过 ICD 的治疗[7]。

分子遗传学发现该遗传性疾病与细胞内钙调控的异常有关。而且，基因检测对该病患者的诊治至关重要。症状发生前获得该病的遗传学诊断可以及时对这种高致命性的疾病进行预防，并采取生活方式的改变[6,7]。因为有效的治疗方法已确定，故对疑似患者的早期诊断和治疗是非常重要的。如果诊断 RyR2 突变，可以进行性别危险分层。证据表明，男性患者预后更差，所以对这组人群应进行更有效的监测和更积极的治疗。

二、短联律间期性尖端扭转型室速

(一) 临床表现和治疗

短联律间期性尖端扭转型室速表现为典型的尖端扭转型室速,且触发心搏为短联律间期。不同于原来由 Dessertenne 描述的尖端扭转型室速,该病表现为 QT 间期正常,首次异位搏动的联律间期都小于 300ms[31]。对这种特殊类型的尖端扭转型室速偶见报道,但只有一项研究对该病进行了系统的描述。目前最大的研究来自 Leenhardt 等[31]人,他们对 14 例患有该病患者的临床特征和心电图进行了描述,并把这种室速命名为短联律间期性尖端扭转型室速。有限的资料表明,人群中该病的发病率较低,且有明显的漏诊。

短联律间期性尖端扭转型室速的患者常发生晕厥,大概 30% 的病例有家族猝死史[31]。短联律间期性尖端扭转型室速的静息心电图无明显异常。心脏的无创和有创检查都没有发现任何有临床意义的器质性心脏病,即使在随访时也没有发生变化。

典型的短联律间期性尖端扭转型室速表现为 QRS 主波在等电位线上下扭转,持续时间从几秒到 10~15s,频率常大于 200 次/分,可蜕化为室颤,甚至猝死。

短联律间期性尖端扭转型室速的治疗有待于进一步研究,大部分患者服用维拉帕米或 β 受体阻滞剂[31,32]。虽然钙离子拮抗剂能明显控制心律失常的发生,但随访 7 个月中,12 例患者中有 6 例心脏事件复发(3 例猝死,3 例受到 ICD 电击)。总之,短联律间期性尖端扭转型室速预后很差,目前没有有效的治疗药物。最近,Haissaguerre 等[33,34]提出射频消融术是治疗该病的新方法。因为该心律失常是由形态一致的异位搏动引起,故对引起室速的室性异位搏动进行消融是可行的。这项研究也包括对常规抗心律失常药物(β 受体阻滞剂、Ⅰ 类抗心律失常药和维拉帕米)治疗无效的特发性室颤和反复发作的多形性室速(酷似短联律间期性尖端扭转型室速)。在 32 个月的随访中,对触发心搏的电生理标测和消融能抑制致命性心律失常的复发。应在得到有关长期预后方面的资料后,再谨慎使用该方法,但这些研究表明射频消融可能成为治疗多形性室速的一种新方法。

(二) 分子机制

短联律间期性尖端扭转型室速的病理生理学机制仍不清楚。因为患者的心脏结构无明显异常,故自律性异常和触发机制更可能是这种心律失常的原因。绝大部分患者不能诱发室性心律失常,更证明了这一假设[31]。儿茶酚胺是儿茶酚胺敏感性多形性室速的特异性触发因素,而短联律间期性尖端扭转型室速中仅有一个亚型,其心律失常是由肾上腺素能介导的[31,35]。在一个案报道中,发现患者的心室不应期不均一及右室流出道不应期较短[32]。

一些短联律间期性尖端扭转型室速患者有家族猝死史,提示该病可能是遗传性疾病,但是,在大多数病例中[35-37]没有家族分布规律。该病的高致死性可解释为何缺少在一个家族中同时有几个患者,而这种家族正是通过基因连锁分析阐明疾病机制所必需的。

总之,短联律间期性尖端扭转型室速的病理生理学机制仍不清楚,发病率低使该病无法得到有关资料,从而无法找到其临床有效的治疗方法。

三、总 结

对儿茶酚胺敏感性多形性室速的病理生理学机制的认识受分子遗传学的影响,而短联律间期性尖端扭转型室速的病理生理学机制远未阐明。二者都发生在心脏结构正常的患者,并且都可发生高致命性的心律失常。因此,早期诊断和治疗是预防致命性事件发生的关键。β 受体阻滞剂是治疗儿茶酚胺敏感性多形性室速的唯一有效的药物。目前,对于短联律间期性尖端扭转型室速和对肾上腺素能阻滞剂无反应的儿茶酚胺敏感性多形性室速,ICD 是唯一可供选择的治疗。

(郭继鸿 张 涛 译)

参 考 文 献

1. Muller JE, Kaufmann PG, Luepker RV, et al: Mechanisms precipitating acute cardiac events: Review and recommendations of an NHLBI workshop. Circulation 96:3233–3239, 1997.
2. Zipes DP, Wellens HJJ: Sudden cardiac death. Circulation 98:2334–2351, 1998.
3. Floras JS: The "unsympathetic" nervous system of heart failure. Circulation 105:1753–1755, 2002.
4. Schwartz PJ, Priori SG, Napolitano C: The long QT syndrome. In Zipes DP, Jalife J (eds): Cardiac Electrophysiology: From Cell to

Bedside. Philadelphia, WB Saunders, 2000, pp 597–615.
5. Coumel P, Fidelle J, Lucet V, et al: Catecholaminergic-induced severe ventricular arrhythmias with Adams-Stokes syndrome in children: Report of four cases. Br Heart J 40:28–37, 1978.
6. Leenhardt A, Lucet V, Denjoy I, et al: Catecholaminergic polymorphic ventricular tachycardia in children. A 7-year follow-up of 21 patients. Circulation 91:1512–1519, 1995.
7. Priori SG, Napolitano C, Memmi M, et al: Clinical and molecular characterization of patients with catecholaminergic polymorphic ventricular tachycardia. Circulation 106:69–74, 2002.
8. Swan H, Piippo K, Viitasalo M, et al: Arrhythmic disorder mapped to chromosome 1q42-q43 causes malignant polymorphic ventricular tachycardia in structurally normal hearts. J Am Coll Cardiol 34:2035–2042, 1999.
9. Priori SG, Napolitano C: Genetic of arrhythmogenic disorders. In Prodrid PJ, Kowey PR (eds): Cardiac Arrhythmia: Mechanisms, Diagnosis and Management, 2nd ed. Philadelphia, Lippincott Williams & Wilkins, 2001, pp 81–107.
10. Fisher JD, Krikler D, Hallidie-Smith KA: Familial polymorphic ventricular arrhythmias: A quarter century of successful medical treatment based on serial exercise-pharmacologic testing. J Am Coll Cardiol 34:2015–2022, 1999.
11. Martini B, Buja GF, Canciani B, et al: Bidirectional tachycardia. A sustained form, not related to digitalis intoxication, in an adult without apparent cardiac disease. Jpn Heart J 29:381–387, 1988.
12. Green JR Jr, Korovetz MJ, Shanklin DR, et al: Sudden unexpected death in three generations. Arch Intern Med 124:359–363, 1969.
13. Otsu K, Fujii J, Periasamy M, et al: Chromosome mapping of five human cardiac and skeletal muscle sarcoplasmic reticulum protein genes. Genomics 17:507–509, 1993.
14. Priori SG, Napolitano C, Tiso N, et al: Mutations in the cardiac ryanodine receptor gene (hRyR2) underlie catecholaminergic polymorphic ventricular tachycardia. Circulation 103:196–200, 2001.
15. Laitinen PJ, Brown KM, Piippo K, et al: Mutations of the cardiac ryanodine receptor (RyR2) gene in familial polymorphic ventricular tachycardia. Circulation 103:485–490, 2001.
16. Marks AR, Priori S, Memmi M, et al: Involvement of the cardiac ryanodine receptor/calcium release channel in catecholaminergic polymorphic ventricular tachycardia. J Cell Physiol 190:1–6, 2002.
17. MacLennan DH, Duff C, Zorzato F, et al: Ryanodine receptor gene is a candidate for predisposition to malignant hyperthermia. Nature 343:559–561, 1990.
18. Quane KA, Healy JM, Keating KE, et al: Mutations in the ryanodine receptor gene in central core disease and malignant hyperthermia. Nat Genet 5:51–55, 1993.
19. Quane KA, Keating KE, Healy JM, et al: Mutation screening of the RYR1 gene in malignant hyperthermia: Detection of a novel Tyr to Ser mutation in a pedigree with associated central cores. Genomics 23:236–239, 1994.
20. Tiso N, Stephan D, Nava A: Identification on mutations in the cardiac ryanodine receptor gene in families affected with arrhythmogenic right ventricular cardiomyopathy type 2 (ARVD2). Hum Mol Genet 10:189–194, 2001.
21. Bauce B, Rampazzo A, Basso C, et al: Screening for ryanodine receptor type 2 mutations in families with effort-induced polymorphic ventricular arrhythmias and sudden death: Early diagnosis of asymptomatic carriers. J Am Coll Cardiol 40:341–349, 2002.
22. Lahat H, Eldar M, Levy-Nissenbaum E, et al: Autosomal recessive catecholamine- or exercise-induced polymorphic ventricular tachycardia: Clinical features and assignment of the disease gene to chromosome 1p13-21. Circulation 103:2822–2827, 2001.
23. Lahat H, Pras E, Olender T, et al: A missense mutation in a highly conserved region of CASQ2 is associated with autosomal recessive catecholamine-induced polymorphic ventricular tachycardia in Bedouin families from Israel. Am J Hum Genet 69:1378–1384, 2001.
24. Yano K, Zarain-Herzberg A: Sarcoplasmic reticulum calsequestrins: Structural and functional properties. Mol Cell Biochem 135:61–70, 1994.
25. Zhang L, Kelley J, Schmeisser G, et al: Complex formation between junctin, triadin, calsequestrin, and the ryanodine receptor. Proteins of the cardiac junctional sarcoplasmic reticulum membrane. J Biol Chem 272:23389–23397, 1997.
26. Postma AV, Denjoy I, Hoorntje TM, et al: Absence of calsequestrin 2 causes severe forms of catecholaminergic polymorphic ventricular tachycardia. Circ Res 91:e21–e26, 2002.
27. Wellens HJJ: The electrocardiogram in digitalis intoxication. In Yu PN, Godwind JF (eds): Progress in Cardiology. Philadelphia, Lea & Fabinger, 2001, pp 271–290.
28. Priori SG, Corr PB: Mechanisms underlying early and delayed afterdepolarizations induced by catecholamines. Am J Physiol 258:H1796–H1805, 1990.
29. Laitinen PJ, Brown KM, Piippo K, et al: Mutations of the cardiac ryanodine receptor (RyR2) gene in familial polymorphic ventricular tachycardia. Circulation 103:485–490, 2001.
30. Wehrens XH, Lehnart SE, Huang F, et al: FKBP 12.6 deficiency and defective calcium release channel (ryanodine receptor) function linked exercise-induced sudden cardiac death. Cell 113:829–840, 2003.
31. Leenhardt A, Glaser E, Burguera M, et al: Short-coupled variant of torsade de pointes. A new electrocardiographic entity in the spectrum of idiopathic ventricular tachyarrhythmias. Circulation 89:206–215, 1994.
32. Shiga T, Shoda M, Matsuda N, et al: Electrophysiological characteristic of a patient exhibiting the short-coupled variant of torsade de pointes. J Electrocardiol 34:271–275, 2001.
33. Haissaguerre M, Shoda M, Jais P, et al: Mapping and ablation of idiopathic ventricular fibrillation. Circulation 106:962–967, 2002.
34. Haissaguerre M, Shah DC, Jais P, et al: Role of Purkinje conducting system in triggering of idiopathic ventricular fibrillation. Lancet 359:677–678, 2002.
35. Eisenberg SJ, Scheinman MM, Dullet NK, et al: Sudden cardiac death and polymorphous ventricular tachycardia in patients with normal QT intervals and normal systolic cardiac function. Am J Cardiol 75:687–692, 1995.
36. Ruan Y, Wang L: Short-coupled variant of torsade de pointes. J Tongji Med Univ 21:30–31, 2001.
37. Viskin S, Belhassen B: Polymorphic ventricular tachyarrhythmias in the absence of organic heart disease: Classification, differential diagnosis, and implications for therapy. Prog Cardiovasc Dis 41:17–34, 1998.

第 69 章

神经系统疾病与心律失常

William J. Groh

本章目录

- 肌营养不良 ················ 633
- Friedreich 共济失调 ········ 637
- 周期性麻痹 ················ 637
- 线粒体脑肌病 ·············· 638
- 脊髓肌萎缩 ················ 639
- 格林-巴利综合征 ·········· 639
- 重症肌无力 ················ 640
- 急性脑血管病 ·············· 640

神经系统疾病合并心律失常的原因与神经系统疾病直接累及心脏以及神经激素异常作用相关。多种神经系统疾病并发心律失常的发病率高，较之神经系统疾病有更高的死亡率。本章我们将重点讨论常伴发心律失常的神经系统疾病：肌营养不良、Friedreich 共济失调、周期性麻痹、其他少见神经肌肉疾病以及急性脑血管病。

一、肌营养不良

肌营养不良是一大组直接对心肌有不同程度影响的遗传性疾病。它包括 X 连锁的 Duchenne 和 Becker 型肌营养不良、强直性肌营养不良、艾-德（Emery-Dreifuss）肌营养不良、肢带型肌营养不良、Friedreich 共济失调。

（一）Duchenne 和 Becker 型肌营养不良

1. 遗传学及心脏病理生理改变

Duchenne 型和 Becker 型肌营养不良均为抗肌萎缩蛋白（dystrophin）基因异常的 X 连锁遗传病。抗肌萎缩蛋白主要存在于骨骼肌、心肌、平滑肌，少量存在于大脑。抗肌萎缩蛋白及其相关糖蛋白在肌细胞骨架和细胞外基质之间起连接作用[1]，在许多与遗传相关的心肌病中，正是由于这些蛋白的缺乏导致了骨骼肌细胞和心肌细胞的凋亡。除了肌营养不良，抗肌萎缩蛋白的缺乏是心肌病包括终末期冠心病等的心肌细胞功能衰竭的重要机制之一[2]。抗肌萎缩蛋白在 Duchenne 型肌营养不良中几乎缺如，而 Becker 型则主要表现为抗肌萎缩蛋白分子量的改变或蛋白含量的减少[3]，而这就是前者病情进展较快，后者相对进展较慢的原因。

不仅仅是 Duchenne 型和 Becker 型肌营养不良患者缺乏抗肌萎缩蛋白，目前发现有一种家族性 X 连锁的扩张型心肌病，同样由于抗肌萎缩蛋白异常而发病，这组临床综合征被称为"抗肌萎缩蛋白缺乏性肌病"[4-7]，临床表现为不同程度肌无力包括心肌病变进行性恶化。

2. 临床特征

Duchenne 型肌营养不良是临床最常见的遗传性神经肌肉疾病，活产男婴的发病率为 1/4000。症状通常在 5 岁前出现，主要表现为近端肌无力，病情呈进行性发展，存活年龄约为 20～30 岁。Becker 型肌营养不良则相对少见（活产男婴的发病率为 3/100 000），主要累及骨骼肌，心肌受累较少，且预后较好，多数能存活至中年以后。

事实上所有的Duchenne型患者都有心肌病的表现，但往往被肌无力症状掩盖。大约四分之一的患者，6岁左右开始出现心脏病变，10岁左右开始出现明显的心肌病临床症状[8]。据观察左室后基底壁及后外侧壁最易受累。约90%的患者存在心电图异常，主要表现为V_1导联R波增高、R/S比值增大及左胸导联深而窄的Q波等局部心肌受损的表现。

Becker型患者心肌受累情况则表现各异，部分患者无心肌受累，而有些患者可伴有严重的心肌病甚至需要心脏移植[9]。该型患者的心脏严重受累可发生于任何年龄且与骨骼肌受累程度无关[9,10]。超过75%的患者心电图改变与Duchenne型相类似，50%的患者有心脏超声改变，心脏扩大往往右室先于左室。

3. 心律失常

Duchenne型肌营养不良患者心脏的节律性和收缩性均可发生改变，常见的心律失常有：

（1）持续性或不稳定性窦性心动过速：这种心律失常最常见[11]，目前其发生机制尚不清楚，是否存在心肌细胞自律性异常改变一直有争议[12-14]，推测可能与心肌细胞的纤维化及脂肪浸润导致窦房结细胞的自律性增高及局部折返形成有关；

（2）房性心律失常：房扑和房颤常常是心肌病变终末期前的主要心律失常[15]；

（3）传导异常：大约超过40%的病人可见P-R间期小于120ms，这可能与部分房室结细胞营养障碍而其余细胞传导异常加快有关。束支阻滞可见于超过10%的病人[16]。完全性房室阻滞目前还未见报道。

Duchenne型肌营养不良患者心肌存在折返的病理基础，大约有三分之一的患者心室晚电位的检查为阳性，监护发现晚电位检出的阳性率与室性心律失常明显正相关，这些心律失常包括了室性早搏及其他复杂室性心律失常，患有严重的骨骼肌病变的患者更多见[11,15,18]。

Duchenne型肌营养不良患者尤其是患严重的骨骼肌病变的患者可发生猝死，死于心脏事件患者约占四分之一，其中严重心力衰竭和猝死约各占一半[11]。目前猝死是否由恶性心律失常引起还未完全确定，已有多个研究通过监护观察到恶性室性心律失常与猝死密切相关[11,18]。也有人报道在Duchenne型肌营养不良患者中观察到单形性室速[19]。

Becker型患者伴发心律失常与心肌病变程度相关，这种心律失常多缺乏特征[20]。Quinlivan R[21]曾报道Becker型肌营养不良患者并发完全性房室阻滞，而室性心律失常的发生率还没有确切资料证实，Negri SM[22]观察到1例病人合并了束支折返性室性心动过速。

4. 治疗及预后

Duchenne型肌营养不良患者通常可存活至30岁，呼吸衰竭和心力衰竭是其主要死因，治疗心律失常并不能提高患者的生存率。静脉注射维拉帕米可以控制房性心律失常但可导致急性呼吸衰竭，Munoz J[19]报道1例室性心动过速因药物抵抗而植入心脏转复除颤器的患者在围手术期死于呼吸衰竭。

对Becker型肌营养不良并发的心律失常应每年定期行心电图和心脏超声的检查[21]，其治疗目前还缺少公认的方法。

近四分之一的Duchenne型肌营养不良的女性携带者或Becker型患者均伴有扩张型心肌病[23]，其心律失常是否与心脏结构异常有关还不明确。

（二）强直性肌营养不良

1. 遗传学及心脏病理生理改变

强直性肌营养不良是一种常染色体疾病，它的主要临床表现为远端骨骼肌反射性及叩击性肌强直、肌无力、肌萎缩，以及秃发、生殖腺萎缩、白内障、智力衰退、心肌受累等症状。近年来已确定多数患者的异常基因位于19q，其核苷酸CTG的重复序列在正常人为5~37个，而强直性肌营养不良患者的重复序列达50至数千个。这种重复序列过度表达导致了该病的发生，并且CTG重复序列数与发病年龄及疾病的严重程度直接相关。该病心脏受累的主要表现为传导异常、心律失常及心脏结构异常，这些表现与患者年龄以及CTG重复序列数直接相关[27-29]。强直性肌营养不良1型患者CTG重复序列过度表达的机制是多因素的[30,31]，Berul[32-34]等发现部分患者心脏传导异常与CTG的重复序列过度表达导致的毗邻蛋白激酶表达下调有关。

强直性肌营养不良2型（即近端强直性肌病）与1型表现类似，但肌肉症状相对稍轻[35,36]。心脏传导异常在2型患者中亦有报道，但似乎没有1型多见[36-38]。临床症候群中，强直性肌营养不良2型的心脏受累表现不一，可能与遗传异质性有关。在较多家系中分离出的致病基因位点位于 3q21[39,40]。

强直性肌营养不良患者中心脏病变十分常见，但发病机制尚不明确，其病理改变主要包括窦房结、房室结、希-浦纤维等传导系统的细胞变性（纤维化和脂肪浸润）。心房和心室的组织变性亦有报道，但很少进展为有症状的心肌病[41,42]。Fragola PV[43]等经心室晚电位检查发现该病患者存在室内传导延迟。Mtta J[44]证实同骨骼肌肌强直类似，心脏在发生变性的病理改变之前，可存在左室舒张早期功能减退[44]。

2. 临床特征

强直性肌营养不良是一种常见的成人遗传性神经肌肉疾病，不同种族其发病率有差别，如法裔加拿大人的发病率较高，而非洲黑人则发病率较低，该病的整体发病率估计为 1/8000[24,25]。强直性肌营养不良的发病年龄平均为 20～25 岁，多数患者可存活至 50～60 岁[46,47]，肌肉症状较轻的年长患者可存活更长时间。通常患者首先是脸部、颈部以及四肢末端肌肉出现肌无力的症状。无症状的患者进行肌电图以及基因学检测通常不难作出强直性肌营养不良的诊断。该病还具有后代较上代发病年龄更早、症状更严重的遗传早现现象，这种现象与遗传 CTG 的重复序列数增加有关[48,49]。

强直性肌营养不良的心脏受累主要表现为心律失常，大部分的成年患者都有心电图的改变，其中最多见的病理改变是传导功能的异常。在美国，一个大型随机的神经肌肉疾病临床研究结果显示，42％的病人存在一度房室阻滞，3％的病人有右束支阻滞，4％的病人有左束支阻滞，12％的病人出现了非特异性的室内阻滞[29]。

3. 心律失常

强直性肌营养不良患者的心律失常表现有多种多样，心内电生理检查研究发现该类患者常有 H-V 间期延长[50,51]。传导功能障碍的加重可引起明显的临床症状以至必需心脏起搏治疗。在不同的研究中心，强直性肌营养不良植入心脏起搏器类型及指征不尽相同，在前述的美国大型随机临床研究中，约 3％的病人接受了起搏器植入治疗，在法国则主张早期预防性植入心脏起搏器，因此接受起搏器植入治疗的病人明显多于美国[51]。ACC/AHA/NASPE 2002 年更新的起搏应用指南中指出，神经肌肉疾病如强直性肌营养不良病人出现无症状的传导障碍（即使是一度房室阻滞）亦可作为安装心脏起搏器的特殊适应证[52]。

房扑、房颤在普通人群中发生率接近 4％，强直性肌营养不良的患者中房扑、房颤也很常见[53]，尤以神经肌肉症状严重的患者更为多见[54]。Lazarus A 等[51]对已有传导功能障碍的患者行心内电生理检查后发现三分之一的患者可诱发持续性房性心律失常。上述病人多同时伴有传导功能障碍，心室频率较慢，因此通常没有自觉症状[55]。

近三分之一的强直性肌营养不良患者会发生猝死或意外死亡[46,54]，这种死亡被认为与心律失常有关。年轻患者猝死也并不少见，但猝死的原因并不清楚。完全性房室阻滞又无逸搏心律代偿的心室静止被认为是主要的死因。已安装心脏起搏器的患者仍发生猝死，提示这部分病人发生猝死的原因可能是快速室性心律失常。强直性肌营养不良的病人出现室性心动过速已有报道，尤其是束支折返性室速多见，这种室速可通过射频消融得到有效的治疗[56-58]。

4. 治疗及预后

关于强直性肌营养不良伴发心律失常目前还无公认的处理方法。临床症状可能与心律失常相关者，必须进行心脏电生理检查以查清症状的原因。对无症状的患者如何进行恰当的筛查尚不明确，有人建议对他们每年进行心电图及 24h 心电监护检查。显著或进行性的心电图异常改变是否需要起搏治疗或电生理干预仍不明确，对强直性肌营养不良伴发心律失常的诊断和治疗进行评估已有一项多中心的研究方法被推荐。

对强直性肌营养不良患者实施麻醉可能增加传导阻滞和其他的心律失常危险。围术期应对患者进行严密心电监护并进行低阈值临时心脏起搏。

有多种复杂心动过速的患者需进行心脏电生理检查，对束支折返性心动过速应进行特别评估。已有报道对一例强直性肌营养不良患者采用了植入式心脏复律除颤器治疗[55]。

猝死对肌营养不良患者的生存率有显著影响，包括那些神经肌肉症状很少的患者。哪些评估和干预措施适合于这类患者及其减少猝死危险的有效性仍不确定。

（三）艾-德肌营养不良及其相关疾病

1. 遗传学及心脏病理生理改变

艾-德肌营养不良是一种罕见的家族性疾病，典型的肌无力症状较轻，但常出现心肌病变和心律失常并危及生命。该病是一种隐性 X-连锁遗传疾病，其基因异常导致了所谓的伊默菌素核膜蛋白缺失[59,60]。

现已确定核纤层蛋白 A、核纤层蛋白 C 两种核膜蛋白编码的基因变异，导致了基因表型为 X 连锁艾-德肌营养不良相关的一系列疾病。这些疾病包括常染色体显性和隐性遗传的艾-德肌营养不良、伴有传导障碍的常染色体显性遗传扩张型心肌病、肢带型肌营养不良以及伴心脏异常的脂肪营养不良[61-65]。

艾-德肌营养不良患者因伊默菌素、核纤层蛋白 A 和 C 的异常导致特征性心肌病变的发病机制仍不清楚。核膜蛋白对细胞核可提供结构支持，并与细胞骨架相互作用，伊默菌素位于心肌的桥粒和筋膜粘着面，对心脏的传导可能存在明显的影响[66]。

病理研究显示此类患者心肌存在明显的纤维化。

2. 临床特征

艾-德肌营养不良具有特征性症状，早期表现为肘部、跟腱和颈后肌群挛缩，缓慢进行性肌无力和肌萎缩以及心肌病变。临床上，该病存在的多种基因表现型可能与艾-德肌营养不良与异常基因的多种突变有关。

艾-德肌营养不良及相关疾病的心脏受累最常表现为心律失常，其中也有不少表现为扩张型心肌病[64]。在起搏治疗后生存期延长的患者中可更多地观察到心肌病的存在。

3. 心律失常

艾-德肌营养不良及相关疾病中，心脏激动的发生和传导异常极为常见，一般在 20~30 岁后出现心电图异常，多表现为一度房室阻滞，心房受累早于心室，表现为心房颤动或扑动，或持续的心房停搏和交界性心动过缓[67]，35~40 岁的典型病例往往需要心室起搏治疗。猝死常见于艾-德肌营养不良及其相关疾病，包括那些已植入起搏器的患者。发生室速、室颤的患者已有过报道。

X-连锁艾-德肌营养不良疾病的女性携带者亦有发生心脏传导障碍和猝死的危险，且特别容易在晚年发生[68]。

4. 治疗及预后

已有心脏受累的患者应仔细监测心电图传导障碍的进展。动态心电图可显示短期监测不易发现的睡眠中的心律失常。一旦证实患者存在传导障碍即应进行起搏治疗。如心房存在电静止，则不能进行双腔起搏。对心脏起搏后仍有猝死危险的患者植入心脏复律除颤器治疗是否有益仍不清楚。呈进行性扩张的心肌病可以导致终末期心衰和死亡[64]。

（四）肢带型肌营养不良

1. 遗传学及心脏病理生理改变

肢带型肌营养不良为一组表现为四肢-骨盆肌带无力，或有遗传异质性及不同临床特征的遗传性疾病。已发现存在常染色体隐性遗传（2型）、显性遗传（1型）及其他散发病例。与染色体 1q11-21（1B 型）连锁的常染色体显性遗传肢带型肌营养不良患者伴有高发的心肌病变[69]。这种疾病与艾-德肌营养不良类似，为编码核纤层蛋白 A 和 C 的基因变异所引起[63]。

常染色体隐性或散发性肢带型肌营养不良（2C-2F 型）的心肌病变（常表现为扩张型心肌病）的发生率很高，它与抗肌萎缩蛋白相关的称之为 Sarcoglycan 蛋白的基因变异有关[70-73]。

2. 临床特征

肌无力发生在不同的年龄，但多在 30 岁前发生。常表现为行走和跑步困难，心脏受累表现通常发生在那些核纤层蛋白 A 和 C 以及 α-Sarcoglycan 出现了基因突变的患者。

3. 心律失常

肢带型肌营养不良可出现心律失常，但仅限于特殊的基因亚型。与染色体 1q11-21 连锁的肢带型肌营养不良与进展性房室阻滞有关，通常需要起搏治疗[63,69,72]。安装了起搏器的患者亦有猝死的报道。有心肌病的患者亦可发生。

由 Sarcoglycan 突变导致的肢带型肌营养不良患者发生心律失常尚未见报道。

4. 治疗和预后

利用心电图和心脏超声检查进行常规筛查对于肢带肌营养不良伴心肌疾病的患者是必要的。对有心肌病变的患者或家族需进一步随访。与染色体 1q11-21 连锁的肢带型肌营养不良伴无症状性的传导障碍的患者可予以起搏治疗。上述干预能否降低猝死的发生率尚不明确。

（五）面肩胛臂型肌营养不良

1. 遗传学及心脏病理生理改变

面肩胛臂型肌营养不良是一种常染色体显性遗传性神经肌肉疾病，其致病基因位于染色体4q-35[74]，具体的编码基因仍未明确。

2. 临床表现

面肩胛臂型肌营养不良是一种更常见的肌营养不良性疾病，发病率为1/20 000[75]，肌无力的症状通常进展缓慢，严重的心脏病变罕见。

3. 心律失常

面肩胛臂型肌营养不良发生心律失常曾有报道，心律失常的发生率及严重程度远不及其他类型的肌营养不良，临床意义不大。在最大的一组遗传性疾病的心脏病变的评估报告中，5%没有心血管危险因素的患者发生了心律失常[76]，每三个有症状的房室阻滞的病人中，即有一个进行起搏器植入治疗。其他的报道因缺少遗传性疾病的诊断依据，其结论的参考价值有限。

4. 治疗和预后

面肩胛臂型肌营养不良患者出现心律失常虽有报道，但具有临床意义的心律失常十分少见，然而对其可能的心律失常仍有必要进行心电图筛查，并就其相关症状进行讨论。

二、Friedreich共济失调

（一）遗传学及心脏病理生理改变

Friedreich共济失调是一种常染色体隐性遗传的脊髓小脑变性疾病，特征表现为四肢和躯干共济失调、构音障碍、深反射消失、感觉异常、骨骼变形和心脏病变。这一疾病与9号染色体上编码210-氨基酸蛋白名为frataxin的基因连锁[77]，其mRNA在心脏高表达。frataxin是一种线粒体蛋白，对维持铁离子稳定和细胞呼吸功能非常重要[78,79]。大多数病人（>95%）编码frataxin的基因的第一个内含子中的放大且不稳定的三核苷酸（GAA）重复序列同源。其序列扩展的程度与患者的发病年龄、神经系统症状的严重性，以及超声显示左室肥大的程度有关[80,81]。

Friedreich共济失调常与一种向心性肥厚型心肌病有关，更少见的是无症状性室间隔肥大，也可出现扩张型心肌病。

（二）临床表现

据估计，Friedreich共济失调的发病率是1/500000，典型的神经系统症状出现在青春期，几乎总是发生在25岁以前。其典型表现是活动功能进行性丧失，病人在症状初发10~20年后需要轮椅助行。除了少数病例，绝大多数病人神经系统症状先于心脏症状出现。95%有神经系统症状的病人进行心电图和超声检查时发现心脏异常，心电图和超声检查结果表现为普遍的T波倒置及典型的心室肥大。

心律失常

Friedreich共济失调可发生心律失常，但其发生较心肌病变的预期发生率更少。房性心律失常包括房扑和房颤，与扩张型心肌病的进展有关[82,83]。尽管病理检查可见传导系统纤维化外，但与临床症状相关的激动异常及传导障碍并未见报道。扩张型心肌病患者可见室性心动过速。Friedreich共济失调也可能会发生猝死但机制尚未完全明确。

（三）治疗和预后

Friedreich共济失调常见进行性神经功能不全。当出现扩张型心肌病后预后差，可快速进入终末期充血性心力衰竭。其心律失常无特殊治疗方法。

三、周期性麻痹

（一）遗传学及心脏病理生理改变

原发的周期性麻痹少见，这种非营养不良性常染色体显性遗传疾病是由于离子通道基因的异常所致。该病分为低血钾型、高血钾型（钾敏感性）和正常血钾型，每一类型又分几种亚型[84,85]。

低血钾型周期性麻痹表现为与血清钾水平下降有关的发作性肌无力。该病在男性呈完全外显性，女性有50%为外显性。低血钾型周期性麻痹致病基因定位于染色体1q-31-32，它导致了对二氢吡啶敏感的钙通道α_1亚单位的序列识别突变[86]。通过对一个低血钾型周期性麻痹和骨骼肌钠通道（SCN4A）突变的家系的研究，发现这种疾病可能具有遗传异质性[87]。

高血钾型周期性麻痹也表现为发作性肌无力，随着钾的补充，症状会进一步加重。据观察该病为完全外显性。患者于发作期血钾水平通常增高，亦可正常。高血钾型周期性麻痹主要是由于 17 号染色体上的 SCN4A 的 α 亚单位突变所致[88]。据报道这一基因存在多种突变，并可能导致对钾敏感的钠通道无法失活[85]。

Anderson 综合征是一种明显的钾敏感性周期性麻痹，患者多有耳朵位置偏低、小下颌、指（趾）弯曲的畸形特征，心电图表现为 QT 间期延长和室性心律失常[89]。Anderson 综合征与染色体 17q-23 连锁，最近发现它是由于编码钾通道的内向调控（Kir2.1）KCNJ2 基因突变所致[90-92]。在心室肌细胞模型中减少 Kir2.1 可延长其 3 相动作电位，并可诱发低血钾时出现的延迟后除极[92]，Anderson 综合征已被命名为长 QT 综合征：LQT7。

（二）临床表现

周期性麻痹的主要临床表现为发作性肌无力。肌无力发作时低血钾型周期性麻痹较高血钾型周期性麻痹症状更严重，持续时间更长。两种类型的周期性麻痹均可在寒冷和运动后休息时诱发。摄入碳水化合物可诱发低血钾型周期性麻痹，对高血钾型周期性麻痹而言则可改善症状。

心律失常

周期性麻痹可出现室性心律失常，绝大多数心律失常出现在低血钾型周期性麻痹和 Anderson 综合征。双向室性心动过速，既可见于非依赖性洋地黄中毒时，亦可在不依赖肌无力发作的情况下出现，其发生通常与血清钾水平无关，可在运动后转为窦性心律。心室异位搏动多见，通常与双向心动过速交替出现。

有些报道中，还观察到间歇性 QT 间期延长，并与肌无力、低血钾或抗心律失常治疗有关，另有一些病人的 QT 间期延长则是持续的。Anderson 综合征典型的表现有 QT 间期延长和频发的心室异位搏动。Anderson 综合征伴严重室性心律失常的情况虽有报道，但与其他长 QT 间期综合征相比，则更为少见[92,93]。

周期性麻痹发生猝死的病例亦有报道。

（三）治疗和预后

肌无力的发作常可用于衡量血钾是否纠正至正常水平[94]，美西律能够改善高血钾型周期性麻痹的肌无力。乙酰唑胺能够改善低血钾型周期性麻痹发作肌无力[95]。对电解质失衡的治疗无助于心律失常的改善，即便是有效，这种改善也只是短时的。β 受体阻滞剂治疗可改善与 QT 间期延长相关的症状性非持续性室性心动过速[96]。I A 类抗心律失常药物可加重肌无力，并导致 QT 间期延长相关的心律失常恶化[97]。Junker J[93] 等报道胺碘酮可减少 Anderson 综合征出现的持续多形性室性心动过速的发作。

四、线粒体脑肌病

（一）遗传学及心脏病理生理改变

线粒体脑肌病是由线粒体功能异常导致的一组异质性疾病[98,99]。疾病的类型有多种多样。线粒体的 DNA 遗传自母亲，大多数线粒体脑肌病均由母亲遗传给下一代，男、女均受累及。另一些疾病则散发存在，或以常染色体显性方式遗传。基于线粒体的重要代谢功能，这些疾病表现出心脏病变是不足为奇的。

线粒体脑肌病有多种临床类型。包括慢性进行性眼外肌麻痹（包括 Kearns-Sayre 综合征），破碎红纤维性肌阵挛性癫痫（MERRF），线粒体肌病、脑病、乳酸病、卒中样发作（MELAS），还有 Leber 遗传性视神经病变[100]。慢性进行性眼外肌麻痹是典型的散发性疾病，上述的其他疾病均是经母亲遗传的。

骨骼肌和心肌组织病理学改变证明线粒体增多。通过骨骼肌活检标本可见破碎的红色纤维，为线粒体异常增多的具体表现[100]。Kearns-Sayre 综合征还可出现心脏传导系统纤维化和脂肪浸润[101]。

（二）临床表现

线粒体脑肌病中常见心肌病变。在 Kearns-Sayre 综合征的典型表现是传导异常，扩张型心肌病虽有报道，但并不常见[101-103]。

在 MERRF 和 MELAS 中，近半数的病人有左室肥大[102]。病情可发展为扩张型心肌病。

1. 心律失常

进行性眼外肌麻痹、色素性视网膜病变和心脏阻滞等是 Kearns-Sayre 综合征的临床特征。症状通常始于少儿时期。心脏阻滞较常见，且通常出现在眼肌病变之后。H-V 间期可以延长。希氏束远端的传导障碍则可伴有反常的短或正常 PR 间期，这可能是由于房室结的传导加快所致，患者在 20 岁前常常需要进行起搏治疗。这种疾病中还有预激合并室上性心动过速的报道。

Leber 遗传性视神经病变，以无痛性、亚急性双侧视觉缺失为特征，在男性更为常见[100]，大多数病人可发生短 PR 间期和预激综合征，室上性心动过速亦见报道，尽管在 MERRF 和 MELAS 中左室肥大频繁出现，心律失常却少见，MELAS 中可有预激综合征[102]。

2. 治疗和预后

在 Kearns-Sayre 综合征中，一旦确认了希氏束远端传导障碍，则需预防性植入心脏起搏器。起搏治疗或许可改善患者的生存率[102]。何种程度的希氏束远端传导障碍需预防性起搏则尚未明确。在 Leber 遗传性视神经病变患者中，用心电图筛查有无预激综合征仍是必要的。

五、脊髓肌萎缩

(一) 心脏病理生理改变和临床表现

脊髓肌萎缩也是一组多种遗传方式的异质性疾病，它是由于脊髓前角运动神经变性导致麻痹和肌萎缩[105,106]。常染色体隐性遗传性脊髓肌萎缩类型有三种（Ⅰ～Ⅲ型），在初发年龄和严重程度上均不相同。Ⅰ型（Werdnig-Hoffman 病）和Ⅱ型在少儿期较早时候发病，存活期严重受限。Ⅲ型（Kugelberg-Welander）发病年龄较晚，且进展较慢，一般可存活至成年。

常染色体隐性遗传性脊髓肌萎缩与染色体 5q-13 连锁[107]。大多数因存活的运动神经元（SMN）和神经元凋亡抑制蛋白（NAIP）两种基因突变导致发病。

常染色体隐性遗传性脊髓肌萎缩的心脏病变包括先天性心脏病、扩张型心肌病和心律失常[108]。

1. 心律失常

心律失常主要见于 Kugelberg-Welander 病，它可能与其他疾病对患者的生存期限制有关。已有报道的心律失常有心房静止、房颤和房扑及房室阻滞[108]。

2. 治疗

对于心房停搏和房室阻滞可能需要起搏治疗。因为本病发生和报道甚少，所以仍未形成明确的治疗指南。

六、格林-巴利综合征

(一) 心脏病理生理改变

格林-巴利综合征是一种急性炎症性脱髓鞘性神经病变，症状表现为外周、脑和自主神经功能障碍[119]。其中 1/2 的病人为急性病毒或细菌感染，典型表现为呼吸或胃肠功能障碍，这些症状较神经系统症状早 5 天～3 周出现。

格林-巴利综合征的心脏异常表现为心律失常[111]，心律失常的出现与自主神经系统病变有关。有证据表明，异常的交感兴奋可表现为不正常的窦性心动过速、高血压、出汗和心率变异性消失。

(二) 临床表现

在发达国家，格林-巴利综合征是造成急性松弛性瘫痪的首要原因[110]。这种疾病通常表现为对称性四肢无力，并可进展为颅神经和呼吸肌无力。近 1/3 的病人需要辅助呼吸。需辅助呼吸的患者中有 20% 的死亡率[112]，常见的死因是心律失常[111]。

(三) 心律失常

危及生命的心律失常几乎都是发生在严重的需辅助呼吸的格林-巴利综合征患者，在一项有 100 例病人的前瞻性研究中，33 例需辅助呼吸的病人中有 11 例发生了严重的心律失常[113]，其中包括 6 例心跳停搏，1 例心动过缓（低于 30 次/分），2 例快速房颤，2 例室性心动过速或室颤。另有一项报道，13 例死亡病例中，有 4 例死于心律失常。所有严重心律失常的病人都表现有自主神经功能障碍，心脏停搏常由气管抽吸所诱发。

(四) 治疗

除了支持治疗以外，早期血浆置换或静脉输入免疫球蛋白可改善预后。需辅助呼吸的患者也需要对心脏节律进行监测。对于严重的心动过缓或心跳停搏的患者可能需要临时或永久性起搏器，这或许可改善患者的生存[113]。阿托品或异丙肾上腺素在气管抽吸之前使用对病人有益。

七、重症肌无力

(一) 临床表现和心脏病理生理改变

重症肌无力是一种自身免疫性疾病，由于体内产生了针对神经细胞突触的烟碱乙酰胆碱受体的抗体，导致神经肌肉接头传递障碍所致。症状一般为波动性肌无力，通常始于眼肌和面肌，然后逐渐累及四肢的大肌肉。这种疾病可出现在任何年龄，以年轻女性和年老男性最为常见。重症肌无力一般与胸腺的不典型增生、良性或恶性肿瘤有关。

心肌炎与重症肌无力有关，特别易出现在胸腺癌中[114]，可能是产生了心肌抗体所致[115]。

(二) 心律失常

在一大组重症肌无力病人的系列研究中[114]，10%的病人伴发心律失常，且不能用其他病因解释。包括房颤、房室阻滞、心跳停搏及不可解释的猝死。在胸腺癌病人中，心脏异常比非胸腺癌病人更常见。活检所见与心肌炎一致。

(三) 治疗和预后

重症肌无力一般用抗胆碱酯酶和免疫抑制剂治疗。常需切除胸腺。抗胆碱酯酶药物可降低心率并导致低血压。免疫抑制治疗或切除胸腺是否能改善心脏病变尚未可知。重症肌无力患者使用奎尼丁和普萘洛尔可能导致肌无力的急性加重，故有必要关注心肌病变的潜在危险。

八、急性脑血管病

(一) 心脏病理生理

急性脑血管病包括蛛网膜下腔出血、其他卒中综合征及头部外伤，它们常合并心脏症状（包括危及生命的心律失常）[116,117]。心脏病变的发生机制与神经系统功能异常有关。一般是由于交感和副交感异常兴奋所致。下丘脑刺激可出现与急性脑血管病同样的心电图改变。刺激下丘脑或蛛网膜下腔出血的相关心电图改变，可通过脊柱横断、星状神经节阻滞、应用抗胆碱能药物和肾上腺素受体阻滞剂而消失。

急性脑血管病的心肌损伤在活检中表现为心内膜下出血或心肌纤维化以及心肌酶的释放[117]。

(二) 临床表现

蛛网膜下腔出血的病人中25%~80%有心电图异常[116,117]。神经损伤越严重，风险就更高[118]。25%~40%的病人有T波高尖、倒置和QT间期延长。50%的蛛网膜下腔出血病人有低钾，因此增加了QT间期延长的可能性[119]。女性发生低钾和QT间期延长的危险更高[120]。其他的心电图改变包括ST段抬高或降低以及T波异常。

其他卒中综合征亦常有心电图改变，但这些心电图改变是否与卒中综合征或潜在的心脏病变有关尚难以确定[116,117]。QT间期延长在蛛网膜下腔出血中要比在其他卒中综合征中更常见。闭合性头部创伤可能引起类似于蛛网膜下腔出血时的心电图异常，包括QT间期延长。

(三) 心律失常

室性心动过速和室颤在蛛网膜下腔出血或头部创伤病人中已有报道[116,117,119]。还有人观察到了尖端扭转型室速。通常认为这些室性心律失常的危险因素是QT间期延长和低钾。

除蛛网膜下腔出血外，其他卒中综合征与室性心律失常的关系较小。房性心律失常在所有卒中综合征中均有报道，一般为房颤[116,117,119]。心动过缓与窦房阻滞、窦性停搏和房室阻滞有关，在约10%的蛛网膜下腔出血的病人中出现[117,119]。其他卒中综合征中，心动过缓并不常见。

(四) 治疗和预后

危及生命的严重心律失常一般发生在神经系统症状出现的第一天[119]。在此期间有必要进行持续的心电图监测。并且有必要监测血钾水平，特别是蛛网膜下腔出血的病人。β肾上腺素能阻滞剂能有效控制室上性和室性心动过速，并能降低与蛛网膜下腔出血和头部创伤有关的心肌损伤[121]。但是β肾上腺素能阻滞剂有增加心动过缓的可能。据报道星状神经节阻滞剂可有效控制折返性室性心律失常。

（蒲晓群　译）

参 考 文 献

1. Towbin JA: The role of cytoskeletal proteins in cardiomyopathies. Curr Opin Cell Biol 10:131–139, 1998.
2. Kaprielian RR, Stevenson S, Rothery SM, et al: Distinct patterns of dystrophin organization in myocyte sarcolemma and transverse tubules of normal and diseased human myocardium. Circulation 101:2586–2594, 2000.
3. Kunkel LM: Analysis of deletions in DNA from patients with Becker and Duchenne muscular dystrophy. Nature 322:73–77, 1986.
4. Beggs AH: Dystrophinopathy, the expanding phenotype. Dystrophin abnormalities in X-linked dilated cardiomyopathy. Circulation 95:2344–2347, 1997.
5. Ortiz-Lopez R, Li H, Su J, et al: Evidence for a dystrophin missense mutation as a cause of X-linked dilated cardiomyopathy. Circulation 95:2434–2440, 1997.
6. Franz WM, Muller M, Muller OJ, et al: Association of nonsense mutation of dystrophin gene with disruption of sarcoglycan complex in X-linked dilated cardiomyopathy. Lancet 355:1781–1785, 2000.
7. Palmucci L, Mongini T, Chiado-Piat L, et al: Dystrophinopathy expressing as either cardiomyopathy or Becker dystrophy in the same family. Neurology 54:529–530, 2000.
8. Nigro G, Comi LI, Politano L, Bain RJ: The incidence and evolution of cardiomyopathy in Duchenne muscular dystrophy. Int J Cardiol 26:271–277, 1990.
9. Melacini P, Fanin M, Danieli GA, et al: Cardiac involvement in Becker muscular dystrophy. J Am Coll Cardiol 22:1927–1934, 1993.
10. Comi GP, Prelle A, Bresolin N, et al: Clinical variability in Becker muscular dystrophy. Genetic, biochemical and immunohistochemical correlates. Brain 117:1–14, 1994.
11. Yanagisawa A, Miyagawa M, Yotsukura M, et al: The prevalence and prognostic significance of arrhythmias in Duchenne type muscular dystrophy. Am Heart J 124:1244–1250, 1992.
12. Miller G, D'Orsogna L, O'Shea JP: Autonomic function and the sinus tachycardia of Duchenne muscular dystrophy. Brain Dev 11:247–250, 1989.
13. Yotsukura M, Fujii K, Katayama A, et al: Nine-year follow-up study of heart rate variability in patients with Duchenne-type progressive muscular dystrophy. Am Heart J 136:289–296, 1998.
14. Lanza GA, Dello Russo A, Giglio V, et al: Impairment of cardiac autonomic function in patients with Duchenne muscular dystrophy: Relationship to myocardial and respiratory function. Am Heart J 141:808–812, 2001.
15. Perloff JK: Cardiac rhythm and conduction in Duchenne's muscular dystrophy: A prospective study of 20 patients. J Am Coll Cardiol 3:1263–1268, 1984.
16. Sanyal SK, Johnson WW: Cardiac conduction abnormalities in children with Duchenne's progressive muscular dystrophy: Electrocardiographic features and morphologic correlates. Circulation 66:853–863, 1982.
17. Kubo M, Matsuoka S, Taguchi Y, et al: Clinical significance of late potential in patients with Duchenne muscular dystrophy. Pediatr Cardiol 14:214–219, 1993.
18. Chenard AA, Becane HM, Tertrain F, et al: Ventricular arrhythmia in Duchenne muscular dystrophy: Prevalence, significance and prognosis. Neuromuscul Disord 3:201–206, 1993.
19. Munoz J, Sanjuan R, Morell JS, Ibanez M: Ventricular tachycardia in Duchenne's muscular dystrophy. Int J Cardiol 54:259–262, 1996.
20. Nigro G, Comi LI, Politano L, et al: Evaluation of the cardiomyopathy in Becker muscular dystrophy. Muscle Nerve 18:283–291, 1995.
21. Quinlivan R, Ball J, Dunckley M, et al: Becker muscular dystrophy presenting with complete heart block in the sixth decade. J Neurol 242:398–400, 1995.
22. Negri SM, Cowan MD: Becker muscular dystrophy with bundle branch reentry ventricular tachycardia. J Cardiovasc Electrophysiol 9:652–654, 1998.
23. Hoogerwaard EM, Bakker E, Ippel PF, et al: Signs and symptoms of Duchenne muscular dystrophy and Becker muscular dystrophy among carriers in the Netherlands: A cohort study. Lancet 353:2116–2119, 1999.
24. Aslanidis C, Jansen G, Amemiya C, et al: Cloning of the essential myotonic dystrophy region and mapping of the putative defect. Nature 355:548–551, 1992.
25. New nomenclature and DNA testing guidelines for myotonic dystrophy type 1 (DM1). The International Myotonic Dystrophy Consortium (IDMC). Neurology 54:1218–1221, 2000.
26. Redman JB, Fenwick RG Jr, Fu YH, et al: Relationship between parental trinucleotide GCT repeat length and severity of myotonic dystrophy in offspring. JAMA 269:1960–1965, 1993.
27. Melacini P, Villanova C, Menegazzo E, et al: Correlation between cardiac involvement and CTG trinucleotide repeat length in myotonic dystrophy. J Am Coll Cardiol 25:239–245, 1995.
28. Tokgozoglu LS, Ashizawa T, Pacifico A, et al: Cardiac involvement in a large kindred with myotonic dystrophy. Quantitative assessment and relation to size of CTG repeat expansion. JAMA 274:813–819, 1995.
29. Groh WJ, Lowe MR, Zipes DP: Severity of cardiac conduction involvement and arrhythmias in myotonic dystrophy type 1 correlates with age and CTG repeat length. J Cardiovasc Electrophysiol 13:444–448, 2002.
30. Tapscott SJ: Deconstructing myotonic dystrophy. Science 289:1701–1702, 2000.
31. Tapscott SJ, Thornton CA: Biomedicine. Reconstructing myotonic dystrophy. Science 293:816–817, 2001.
32. Berul CI, Maguire CT, Aronovitz MJ, et al: DMPK dosage alterations result in atrioventricular conduction abnormalities in a mouse myotonic dystrophy model. J Clin Invest 103:R1–R7, 1999.
33. Saba S, VanderBrink BA, Luciano B, et al: Localization of the sites of conduction abnormalities in a mouse model of myotonic dystrophy. J Cardiovasc Electrophysiol 10:1214–1220, 1999.
34. Groh WJ: A transgenic model of myotonic dystrophy: Will the mouse roar? J Cardiovasc Electrophysiol 10:1221–1223, 1999.
35. Abbruzzese C, Krahe R, Liguori M, et al: Myotonic dystrophy phenotype without expansion of (CTG)n repeat: An entity distinct from proximal myotonic myopathy (PROMM)? J Neurol 243:715–721, 1996.
36. Meola G, Sansone V, Marinou K, et al: Proximal myotonic myopathy: A syndrome with a favourable prognosis? J Neurol Sci 193:89–96, 2002.
37. Ricker K, Koch MC, Lehmann-Horn F, et al: Proximal myotonic myopathy. Clinical features of a multisystem disorder similar to myotonic dystrophy. Archiv Neurol 52:25–31, 1995.
38. Von zur Muhlen F, Klass C, Kreuzer H, et al: Cardiac involvement in proximal myotonic myopathy. Heart 79:619–621, 1998.
39. Ranum LP, Rasmussen PF, Benzow KA, et al: Genetic mapping of a second myotonic dystrophy locus. Nat Genet 19:196–198, 1998.
40. Liquori CL, Ricker K, Moseley ML, et al: Myotonic dystrophy type 2 caused by a CCTG expansion in intron 1 of ZNF9. Science 293:864–867, 2001.
41. Motta J, Guilleminault C, Billingham M, et al: Cardiac abnormalities in myotonic dystrophy. Electrophysiologic and histopathologic studies. Am J Med 67:467–473, 1979.
42. Nguyen HH, Wolfe JT, Holmes DR Jr, Edwards WD: Pathology of the cardiac conduction system in myotonic dystrophy: A study of 12 cases. J Am Coll Cardiol 11:662–671, 1988.
43. Fragola PV, Calo L, Antonini G, et al: Signal-averaged electrocardiography in myotonic dystrophy. Int J Cardiol 50:61–68, 1995.
44. Child JS, Perloff JK: Myocardial myotonia in myotonic muscular dystrophy. Am Heart J 129:982–990, 1995.
45. Thornton C: The myotonic dystrophies. Semin Neurol 19:25–33, 1999.
46. De Die-Smulders CE, Howeler CJ, Thijs C, et al: Age and causes of death in adult-onset myotonic dystrophy. Brain 121:1557–1563, 1998.
47. Mathieu J, Allard P, Potvin L, et al: A 10-year study of mortality in a cohort of patients with myotonic dystrophy. Neurology 52:1658–1662, 1999.
48. Ashizawa T, Dunne CJ, Dubel JR, et al: Anticipation in myotonic dystrophy. I: Statistical verification based on clinical and haplotype findings. Neurology 42:1871–1877, 1992.
49. Ashizawa T, Dubel JR, Dunne PW, et al: Anticipation in myotonic dystrophy. II. Complex relationships between clinical findings and structure of the GCT repeat. Neurology 42:1877–1883, 1992.
50. Prystowsky EN, Pritchett EL, Roses AD, Gallagher J: The natural history of conduction system disease in myotonic muscular dystrophy as determined by serial electrophysiologic studies. Circulation 60:1360–1364, 1979.
51. Lazarus A, Varin J, Ounnoughene Z, et al: Relationships among

electrophysiological findings and clinical status, heart function, and extent of DNA mutation in myotonic dystrophy. Circulation 99:1041–1046, 1999.
52. Gregoratos G, Abrams J, Epstein AE, et al: ACC/AHA/NASPE 2002 guideline update for implantation of cardiac pacemakers and antiarrhythmia devices: Summary article. Circulation 106:2145–2161, 2002.
53. Groh WJ, Lowe MR, Zipes DP: Severity of cardiac conduction involvement and arrhythmias in myotonic dystrophy type 1 correlates with age and CTG repeat length. J Cardiovasc Electrophysiol 13:444–448, 2002.
54. Phillips MF, Harper PS: Cardiac disease in myotonic dystrophy. Cardiovasc Res 33:13–22, 1997.
55. Hadian D, Lowe MR, Scott LR, Groh WJ: Use of an insertable loop recorder in a myotonic dystrophy patient. J Cardiovasc Electrophysiol 13:72–73, 2002.
56. Berger RD, Orias D, Kasper EK, Calkins H: Catheter ablation of coexistent bundle branch and interfascicular reentrant ventricular tachycardias. J Cardiovasc Electrophysiol 7:341–347, 1996.
57. Merino JL, Carmona JR, Fernandez-Lozano I, et al: Mechanisms of sustained ventricular tachycardia in myotonic dystrophy: Implications for catheter ablation. Circulation 98:541–546, 1998.
58. Merino JL, Peinado R, Sobrino JA: Sudden death in myotonic dystrophy: The potential role of bundle-branch reentry. Circulation 101:E73, 2000.
59. Bione S, Maestrini E, Rivella S, et al: Identification of a novel X-linked gene responsible for Emery-Dreifuss muscular dystrophy. Nat Genet 8:323–327, 1994.
60. Nagano A, Koga R, Ogawa M, et al: Emerin deficiency at the nuclear membrane in patients with Emery-Dreifuss muscular dystrophy. Nat Genet 12:254–259, 1996.
61. Bonne G, Di Barletta MR, Varnous S, et al: Mutations in the gene encoding lamin A/C cause autosomal dominant Emery-Dreifuss muscular dystrophy. Nat Genet 21:285–288, 1999.
62. Di Barletta MR, Ricci E, Galluzzi G, et al: Different mutations in the LMNA gene cause autosomal dominant and autosomal recessive Emery-Dreifuss muscular dystrophy. Am J Hum Genet 66 1407–1412, 2000.
63. Muchir A, Bonne G, van der Kooi AJ, et al: Identification of mutations in the gene encoding lamins A/C in autosomal dominant limb girdle muscular dystrophy with atrioventricular conduction disturbances (LGMD1B). Hum Mol Genet 9:1453–1459, 2000.
64. Fatkin D, MacRae C, Sasaki T, et al: Missense mutations in the rod domain of the lamin A/C gene as causes of dilated cardiomyopathy and conduction-system disease. N Engl J Med 341:1715–1724, 1999.
65. Van der Kooi AJ, Bonne G, Eymard B, et al: Lamin A/C mutations with lipodystrophy, cardiac abnormalities, and muscular dystrophy. Neurology 59:620–623, 2002.
66. Cartegni L, di Barletta MR, Barresi R, et al: Heart-specific localization of emerin: New insights into Emery-Dreifuss muscular dystrophy. Hum Mol Genet 6:2257–2264, 1997.
67. Buckley AE, Dean J, Mahy IR: Cardiac involvement in Emery Dreifuss muscular dystrophy: A case series. Heart 82:105–108, 1999.
68. Fishbein MC, Siegel RJ, Thompson CE, Hopkins LC: Sudden death of a carrier of X-linked Emery-Dreifuss muscular dystrophy. Ann Intern Med 119:900–905, 1993.
69. van der Kooi AJ, van Meegen M, Ledderhof TM, et al: Genetic localization of a newly recognized autosomal dominant limb-girdle muscular dystrophy with cardiac involvement (LGMD1B) to chromosome 1q11-21. Am J Hum Genet 60:891–895, 1997.
70. Mascarenhas DA, Spodick DH, Chad DA, et al: Cardiomyopathy of limb-girdle muscular dystrophy. J Am Coll Cardiol 24:1328–1333, 1994.
71. Fadic R, Sunada Y, Waclawik AJ, et al: Brief report: Deficiency of a dystrophin-associated glycoprotein (adhalin) in a patient with muscular dystrophy and cardiomyopathy. N Engl J Med 334:362–366, 1996.
72. Van der Kooi AJ, Ledderhof TM, de Voogt WG, et al: A newly recognized autosomal dominant limb girdle muscular dystrophy with cardiac involvement. Ann Neurol 39:636–642, 1996.
73. Van der Kooi AJ, de Voogt WG, Barth PG, et al: The heart in limb girdle muscular dystrophy. Heart 79:73–77, 1998.
74. Wijmenga C, Sandkuijl LA, Moerer P, et al: Genetic linkage map of facioscapulohumeral muscular dystrophy and five polymorphic loci on chromosome 4q35-qter. Am J Hum Genet 51:411–415, 1992.
75. A prospective, quantitative study of the natural history of facioscapulohumeral muscular dystrophy (FSHD): Implications for therapeutic trials. The FSH-DY Group. Neurology 48:38–46, 1997.
76. Laforet P, de Toma C, Eymard B, et al: Cardiac involvement in genetically confirmed facioscapulohumeral muscular dystrophy. Neurology 51:1454–1456, 1998.
77. Campuzano V, Montermini L, Molto MD, et al: Friedreich's ataxia: Autosomal recessive disease caused by an intronic GAA triplet repeat expansion. Science 271:1423–1427, 1996.
78. Babcock M, de Silva D, Oaks R, et al: Regulation of mitochondrial iron accumulation by Yfh1p, a putative homolog of frataxin. Science 276:1709–1712, 1997.
79. Wong A, Yang J, Cavadini P, et al: The Friedreich's ataxia mutation confers cellular sensitivity to oxidant stress which is rescued by chelators of iron and calcium and inhibitors of apoptosis. Hum Mol Genet 8:425–430, 1999.
80. Durr A, Cossee M, Agid Y, et al: Clinical and genetic abnormalities in patients with Friedreich's ataxia. N Engl J Med 335:1169–1175, 1996.
81. Isnard R, Kalotka H, Durr A, et al: Correlation between left ventricular hypertrophy and GAA trinucleotide repeat length in Friedreich's ataxia. Circulation 95:2247–2249, 1997.
82. Alboliras ET, Shub C, Gomez MR, et al: Spectrum of cardiac involvement in Friedreich's ataxia: Clinical, electrocardiographic and echocardiographic observations. Am J Cardiol 58:518–524, 1986.
83. James TN, Cobbs BW, Coghlan HC, et al: Coronary disease, cardioneuropathy, and conduction system abnormalities in the cardiomyopathy of Friedreich's ataxia. Br Heart J 57:446–457, 1987.
84. Riggs JE: The periodic paralyses. Neurol Clin 6:485–498, 1988.
85. Bulman DE: Phenotype variation and newcomers in ion channel disorders. Hum Mol Genet 6:1679–1685, 1997.
86. Ptacek LJ, Tawil R, Griggs RC, et al: Dihydropyridine receptor mutations cause hypokalemic periodic paralysis. Cell 77:863–868, 1994.
87. Bulman DE, Scoggan KA, van Oene MD, et al: A novel sodium channel mutation in a family with hypokalemic periodic paralysis. Neurology 53:1932–1936, 1999.
88. Ptacek LJ: Channelopathies: Ion channel disorders of muscle as a paradigm for paroxysmal disorders of the nervous system. Neuromuscul Disord 7:250–255, 1997.
89. Sansone V, Griggs RC, Meola G, et al: Andersen's syndrome: A distinct periodic paralysis. Ann Neurol 42:305–312, 1997.
90. Plaster NM, Tawil R, Tristani-Firouzi M, et al: Mutations in Kir2.1 cause the developmental and episodic electrical phenotypes of Andersen's syndrome. Cell 105:511–519, 2001.
91. Ai T, Fujiwara Y, Tsuji K, et al: Novel KCNJ2 mutation in familial periodic paralysis with ventricular dysrhythmia. Circulation 105:2592–2594, 2002.
92. Tristani-Firouzi M, Jensen JL, Donaldson MR, et al: Functional and clinical characterization of KCNJ2 mutations associated with LQT7 (Andersen syndrome). J Clin Invest 110:381–388, 2002.
93. Junker J, Haverkamp W, Schulze-Bahr E, et al: Amiodarone and acetazolamide for the treatment of genetically confirmed severe Andersen syndrome. Neurology 59:466, 2002.
94. Brown RH Jr: Ion channel mutations in periodic paralysis and related myotonic diseases. Ann New York Acad Sci 707:305–316, 1993.
95. Tricarico D, Barbieri M, Camerino DC: Acetazolamide opens the muscular KCa^{2+} channel: A novel mechanism of action that may explain the therapeutic effect of the drug in hypokalemic periodic paralysis. Ann Neurol 48:304–312, 2000.
96. Williams MJ, Hammond-Tooke GD, Restieaux NJ: Hypokalaemic periodic paralysis with cardiac arrhythmia and prolonged QT interval. Aust N Z J Med 25:549, 1995.
97. Tawil R, Ptacek LJ, Pavlakis SG, et al: Andersen's syndrome: Potassium-sensitive periodic paralysis, ventricular ectopy, and dysmorphic features. Ann Neurol 35:326–330, 1994.
98. Simon DK, Johns DR: Mitochondrial disorders: Clinical and genetic features. Annu Rev Med 50:111–127, 1999.
99. Shanske AL, Shanske S, DiMauro S: The other human genome. Arch Pediatr Adol Med 155:1210–1216, 2001.
100. Johns DR: Seminars in medicine of the Beth Israel Hospital, Boston. Mitochondrial DNA and disease. N Engl J Med 333:638–644, 1995.

101. Gallastegui J, Hariman RJ, Handler B, et al: Cardiac involvement in the Kearns-Sayre syndrome. Am J Cardiol 60:385–388, 1987.
102. Anan R, Nakagawa M, Miyata M, et al: Cardiac involvement in mitochondrial diseases. A study on 17 patients with documented mitochondrial DNA defects. Circulation 91:955–961, 1995.
103. Akaike M, Kawai H, Yokoi K, et al: Cardiac dysfunction in patients with chronic progressive external ophthalmoplegia. Clin Cardiol 20:239–243, 1997.
104. Nikoskelainen E, Vilkki J, Huoponen K, Savontaus ML: Recent advances in Leber's hereditary optic neuroretinopathy. Eye 5:291–293, 1991.
105. Stewart H, Wallace A, McGaughran J, et al: Molecular diagnosis of spinal muscular atrophy. Arch Dis Child 78:531–535, 1998.
106. Iannaccone ST, American Spinal Muscular Atrophy Randomized Trials G: Outcome measures for pediatric spinal muscular atrophy. Arch Neurol 59:1445–1450, 2002.
107. Melki J, Lefebvre S, Burglen L, et al: De novo and inherited deletions of the 5q13 region in spinal muscular atrophies. Science 264:1474–1477, 1994.
108. Elkohen M, Vaksmann G, Elkohen MR, et al: Cardiac involvement in Kugelberg-Welander disease. A prospective study of 8 cases. Arch Mal Coeur Vaiss 89:611–617, 1996.
109. Liu YB, Chen WJ, Lee YT: Atrial standstill in a case of Kugelberg-Welander syndrome with cardiac involvement: An electrophysiologic study. Int J Cardiol 70:207–210, 1999.
110. Hahn AF: Guillain-Barré syndrome. Lancet 352:635–641, 1998.
111. Zochodne DW: Autonomic involvement in Guillain-Barré syndrome: A review. Muscle Nerve 17:1145–1155, 1994.
112. Fletcher DD, Lawn ND, Wolter TD, Wijdicks EF: Long-term outcome in patients with Guillain-Barré syndrome requiring mechanical ventilation. Neurology 54:2311–2315, 2000.
113. Winer JB, Hughes RA: Identification of patients at risk of arrhythmia in the Guillain-Barre syndrome. Q J Med 68:735–739, 1988.
114. Hofstad H, Ohm OJ, Mork SJ, Aarli JA: Heart disease in myasthenia gravis. Acta Neurol Scand 70:176–184, 1984.
115. Mygland A, Aarli JA, Hofstad H, Gilhus NE: Heart muscle antibodies in myasthenia gravis. Autoimmunity 10:263–267, 1991.
116. Davis TP, Alexander J, Lesch M: Electrocardiographic changes associated with acute cerebrovascular disease: A clinical review. Prog Cardiovasc Dis 36:245–260, 1993.
117. Sakr YL, Ghosn I, Vincent JL: Cardiac manifestations after subarachnoid hemorrhage: A systematic review of the literature. Prog Cardiovasc Dis 45:67–80, 2002.
118. Zaroff JG, Rordorf GA, Newell JB, et al: Cardiac outcome in patients with subarachnoid hemorrhage and electrocardiographic abnormalities. Neurosurgery 44:34–39, 1999.
119. Andreoli A, di Pasquale G, Pinelli G, et al: Subarachnoid hemorrhage: Frequency and severity of cardiac arrhythmias. A survey of 70 cases studied in the acute phase. Stroke 18:558–564, 1987.
120. Fukui S, Otani N, Katoh H, et al: Female gender as a risk factor for hypokalemia and QT prolongation after subarachnoid hemorrhage. Neurology 59:134–136, 2002.
121. Cruickshank JM, Neil-Dwyer G, Degaute JP, et al: Reduction of stress/catecholamine-induced cardiac necrosis by beta 1-selective blockade. Lancet 2:585–589, 1987.

第 70 章

长 QT 综合征：基因型与表现型的相关性

Peter J. Schwartz and Silvia G. Priori

本章目录

- 长 QT 综合征的相关基因 …………… 644
- 历史回顾 ……………………………… 645
- 体表心电图特点 ……………………… 646
- QT/RR 间期的关系 …………………… 647
- 对儿茶酚胺的反应 …………………… 648
- 心脏事件的触发因素 ………………… 648
- 自然病程和危险分层 ………………… 649
- 对 β 受体阻滞剂的反应/治疗措施 … 651

1995 年 3 月末[1,2]，首先得到确认的两个长 QT 综合征相关基因公开发表。随后，人们在长 QT 综合征基因型-表现型的相关性研究领域中相继取得了许多重要成果。这一发现不仅是心脏电生理学，而且也是整个心脏病学领域的一个重要突破。为人们进一步理解分子心脏病学和临床心脏病学之间的紧密联系奠定了基础。长 QT 综合征患者发生了基因的特异性突变，其心室复极离子调控出现了重要改变，基因的特异性突变和心室复极离子调控异常之间具有密切的相关性，这一事实令人关注。因而，在研究基因型与表现型相关性的特异性和重要价值时，常常把长 QT 综合征作为独特的范例和最好的例证。公正地说，直到 20 世纪 90 年代中期，许多心脏病学家对临床医学与分子生物学的联系并未给予充分的重视。然而，这一领域飞速发展所取得的成果有助于揭示长 QT 综合征这一致命性心律失常的发生机制，更有助于由此解读猝死的机制，这些事实改变了上述学者的观念[3]。同样，许多甚至没有听说过长 QT 综合征的基础科学家也投入到其相关的研究中。因为他们认识到，这方面的研究对于阐明一些更普遍或更复杂的临床疾病的发生机制有很大的帮助。

一些长 QT 综合征相关基因得到了证实（见后）。然而，只有 3 个基因（*KvLQT1*、*HERG*、*SCN5A*）的突变作为致病因素在足够样本量的长 QT 综合征患者中得到证实，可以对其基因型和表现型之间的相关性进行有统计学意义的分析。因而，本章重点介绍相对常见的三个基因亚群：LQT1（*KvLQT1* 基因突变），LQT2（*HERG* 基因突变），LQT3（*SCN5A* 基因突变）。

一、长 QT 综合征的相关基因

长 QT 综合征相关的 6 种基因突变得到了证实（见后）。一些研究者用 LQT7 来表示 Andersen 综合征[4]患者亚群。我们认为这可能误将一部分其他遗传疾病伴有 QT 间期延长的情况归类为长 QT 综合征。因而，本书中未列出不同于长 QT 综合征，而主要与其他疾病相关的基因。

编码慢速激活钾电流 I_{Ks} 通道蛋白 α 亚单位的 *KvLQT1*（又称 *KCNQ1*）基因突变引起 LQT1[5]。编码快速激活钾电流 I_{Kr} 通道蛋白 α 亚单位的 *HERG* 基因突变引起 LQT2[2]。编码心脏钠通道的 *SCN5A* 基因突变引起 LQT3[1]。近年来，据报道，一种具有多态性的细胞膜结合体 ankyrin-B（细胞骨架锚蛋白）突变引起 LQT4[6]。ankyrin-B 突变导致如钠泵、钠/钙交换体、1,4,5 三磷酸肌醇受体（均为 ankyrin-B 锚蛋白）等细胞结构破裂，这减少了受体与横管的连接，减少了总的蛋白水平。编码 I_{Ks} 通道蛋白 β 亚单位的

KCNE1 基因，又称 minK 基因突变引起 LQT5[7]。调节 HERG 基因的 β 亚单位-MiRP1 基因突变引起 LQT6[8]。

值得注意的是，目前，即使在最好的分子学实验室，对于具有典型的临床表现并根据现行的诊断标准[9]诊断为长 QT 综合征患者中的 40%～50%仍无法作出分子水平的诊断。

在两个数据量最大的已明确基因型的长 QT 综合征患者的研究中[10,11]，三种主要基因型与其各自表现型的相关比例分别为 LQT1（44%～54%），LQT2（53%～35%），和 LQT3（6%～11%）。用上述比例作为标准，能够计算出 LQT1、LQT2、LQT3 这三种基因突变患者的总数，加上已确认的、数量相对较少的 LQT5 和 LQT6 患者数，再加上无基因突变患者数，大约占全部长 QT 综合征先证者的 40%。

二、历史回顾

在介绍目前已获得的数据资料之前，我们简单回顾一下为其他研究奠定基础的最初两个基因型-表现型相关性的研究。第一个研究是在确定长 QT 综合征相关基因之前进行的基因连锁的研究。第二个研究结果发表于确定了 HERG、SCN5A 基因分别为 LQT2 和 LQT3 的致病基因后数月之内，发现 KvLQT1 之前。

Moss 等[12]分析了与染色体 3、7、11 连锁的 6 个家系成员的异常心室复极心电图。他们认为：SCN5A 基因突变患者的 QT 间期明显延长，T 波延迟出现，振幅与时限正常；HERG 基因突变患者 QT 间期中度延长，T 波振幅降低，时限延长，这些改变均不同于 11 号染色体异常基因携带患者，后者表现为宽基底 T 波，时限延长（图 70-1）。但他们强调，同一家系中，受累和未受累的（包括致病基因各变异型）的长 QT 综合征的同一家族成员之间，T 波形态有重叠；不同致病基因的各不同基因型之间 T 波形态也有重叠。

Schwartz 等[13]分析了 15 例患者，其中 HERG 基因突变者 7 例，SCN5A 基因突变者 8 例。通过试验，他们验证了一项新的假设：钠通道阻滞剂美西律和运动诱发的心率加快使 LQT3 患者较 LQT2 患者 QT 间期缩短更明显。首先，他们应用模拟 HERG、SCN5A 基因突变所致电生理改变的细胞模型进行观察，而提出这一假设[14]。试验中所实施的两种干预是针对长 QT 综合征患者特殊的基因缺陷设计的，其研究结果表明，长 QT 综合征患者对上述干预的反应具有差异性。钠通道阻滞剂美西律和运动诱发的心率加快使 LQT3 患者出现显著的 QT 间期缩短。对比之下，大多数 LQT2 患者表现为应用美西律后 QT 间期不缩短，QT 间期没有明显的对心率加快的适应性缩短。与对照组比较，结果出人预料：LQT2 患者对心率加快的适应性表现为正常范围内 QT 间期略微缩短，而 LQT3 患者 QT 间期缩短更明显（图 70-2）。

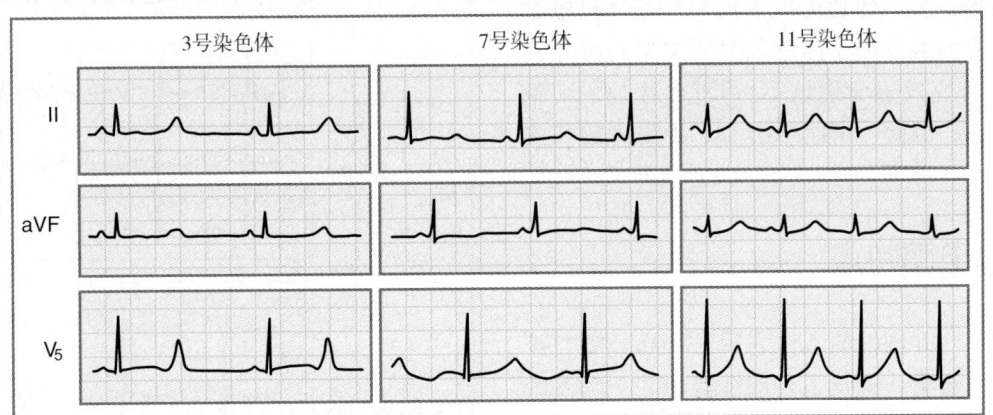

图 70-1 在三个有长 QT 综合征家族史且与染色体 3，7 和 11 基因标记物有关的病人中，记录了 II，aVF 和 V_5 导联心电图 记录心电图的时候均未接受 β 受体阻滞剂治疗。3 号染色体，是一个 15 岁的男孩（家族 1），在他的心脏钠离子通道基因 SCN5A 有突变；他的心率是 42 次/分，QTc 在 II 导联是 570ms，T 波出现较晚，间期和幅度正常。7 号染色体，是一个 21 岁的女性（家族 3）；心率是 57 次/分，QTc 在 II 导联是 583ms，T 波振幅较低。11 号染色体，是一个 31 岁的女性（家族 6）；心率是 79 次/分，QTc 在 II 导联是 573ms，T 波出现较早，T 波基底部宽。（引自 Moss AJ, Zareba W, Benhorin J, et al: ECG T-wave pattern in genetically distinct forms of the hereditary long QT syndrome. Circulation 92. 2929-2934, 1995.）

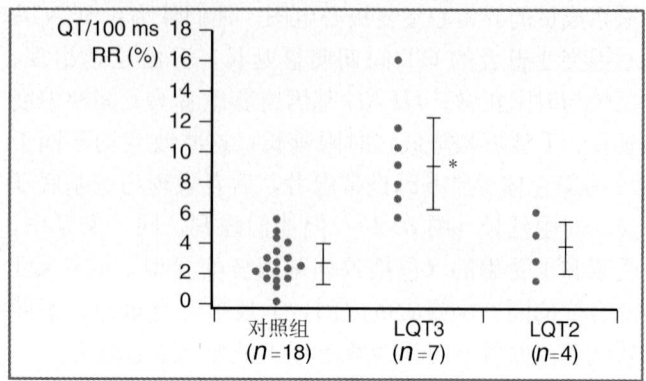

图 70-2 心率加快，QT 间期缩短百分比个体值和均值的散点图 本图表示对照组患者（$n=18$）、LQT3 患者（3 号染色体连锁 $n=7$）、LQT2 患者（7 号染色体连锁 $n=4$）心率加快，QT 间期缩短百分比的个体值和均值。用每100ms RR 间期减少值表示 QT 间期缩短的百分比。* $P<0.05$ 表示对照组和 LQT3 患者相比较差异具有显著性。（引自 Schwartz PJ, Priori SG, Locati EH, et al: Long QT syndrome patients with mutations on the *SCN5A* and *HERG*genes have differential reponses to Na⁺ channel blockade and to inccreases in heart rate. Implications for gene-specific therapy. Circulation 92: 3381-3386, 1995.）

这一研究[13]还得到了另一个出乎预料的结果，扩充了最初的观察结果[15]，并严重影响了治疗的策略。所有 5 例有症状的 LQT2 患者在情绪应激时均出现晕厥发作。与之相比，所有 7 例有症状的 LQT3 患者的心脏事件均发生在静息状态下或睡眠中。还有几位 LQT3 患者在竞技性体育运动中无心律失常事件发生。在上述结果的基础上，作者提出了长 QT 综合征患者致命性心律失常的触发因子因基因突变类型的特异性而不同。这一研究发表于确认 *KvLQT1* 为 LQT1 患者致病基因之前，因而，未能给出 LQT1 患者的相关资料。

三、体表心电图特点

继 Moss 等[12]开创性的工作之后，Zhang 等[16]扩大了研究患者的数量，提供了目前获得的 284 例基因携带者的大量数据。他们在大部分 LQT1、LQT2、LQT3 基因突变患者中确认了一系列典型的心电图表现。

他们认为，LQT1 患者具有以下 4 种典型表现：①所谓"婴儿型"T 波：T 波通常表现为非对称性高耸、基底增宽；②T 波基底增宽，起始点不明显；③T 波形态正常；④T 波延迟出现，形态正常（形态实例见参考文献[12]）。

如前所述[17]，LQT2 患者的心电图特点为 T 波切迹。通常用"双峰"一词来描述 T 波的这一形态，其特点为发生在 T 波波峰之前有一个次波形（"切迹"）。Malfatto 等[18]观察到这一现象常发生于长 QT 综合征患者中。Zhang 等还认为，LQT2 患者具有以下 4 种 T 波形态：①明显 T 波双峰；②微小的 T 波双峰，第二峰出现于 T 波顶部；或③出现于 T 波降支；④振幅低平的双峰 T 波。与这种观点不同，近来，Takenaka 等[19]报告，31 例 LQT2 患者中的 1/3 出现了 LQT1 患者典型的改变——T 波基底增宽。

他们还观察到，LQT3 患者有 2 种 T 波形态改变：①T 波延迟出现，高耸或呈双相；②T 波非对称性高耸。

这些"典型的"T 波表现在 LQT2 患者中的出现率为 88%，在 LQT3 患者中仅有 65%，Zhang 等[16]认为：通过心电图能大致识别基因型，这有助于遗传学研究中确定首先筛选哪个基因。

Moss 等[12]和 Zhang 等[16]的研究为基因型和 T 波形态之间的密切相关性提供了确实的证据。人们对上述结果很感兴趣，但其基本机制，至少部分机制尚未

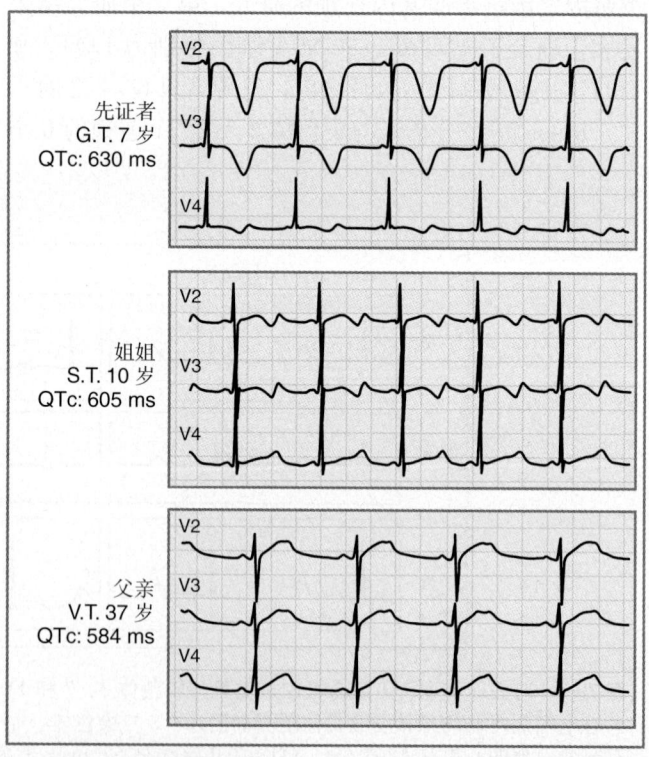

图 70-3 携带了致病基因的、同一家系不同成员的 T 波形态
先证者以心脏骤停作为首发症状。其姐姐无症状，而其父亲有过 2 次晕厥发作。

明确。Shimizu 和 Antzelevition 等[20,21]的研究对其发生机制作出了很好的阐述，常常被人引证，但仍未能解释，甚至在同一家系中，每种基因型患者"典型的"心电图图形具有多样性的原因。图 70-3 描述了一个 LQT2 家系病例，先证者的心电图表现与典型 LQT2 患者截然不同，姐姐 V_4 导联的 T 波包括一个迟发的第二成分，只有父亲的 T 波切迹清楚，符合典型的 LQT2 患者的 T 波形态。如果仅有先证者的心电图，很难就此怀疑这一家系是 LQT2 家系。

心电图对于发现易患心脏事件的条件，增加"罪犯基因"筛选几率均有重要作用。但不能用心电图来给患者进行"基因分型"。

四、QT/RR 间期的关系

心率加快，RR 间期缩短，QT 间期也缩短（QT 适应性）。相对早期的一项临床观察表明：一些长 QT 综合征患者 QT 间期不能适当缩短。基因型和表现型相关性研究不断取得的成果为弄清这一令人困惑的问题提供了机会。

Schwantz 等[13] 1995 年的研究为揭示不同基因型和不同 QT 变化的相关性提供了线索。他们出人意料地提出，LQT3 患者较 LQT2 患者 QT 间期缩短程度更明显。随后，1996 年，人们发现 KvLQT1 基因突变所致的 I_{Ks} 电流减少是 LQT1 的病因，这为解释上述现象提供了新的可能。交感神经激活情况下，I_{Ks} 电流是主要复极电流，心率加快，I_{Ks} 电流加大[22]。从逻辑上讲，I_{Ks} 受损的患者 QT 间期适应心率加快而缩短的能力较正常人差，如运动时的情况。

有三项研究资料提供了与这方面相关的信息。第一项（Schwartz 等，未发表数据），选取对照组 50 例，明确基因型的长 QT 综合征患者 64 例，比较两组在心率增快时 QT 间期缩短的程度。这项研究扩充了 1995 年报道的一些初步观察结果[13]。其主要结果为：尽管有一定程度的重叠，LQT1 患者明显丧失了随心率加快 QT 间期缩短的能力。LQT2 患者与对照组无明显差异，这有些出人意料，但与早期观察结果[13]相一致，LQT3 患者随心率加快，QT 间期较对照组显著缩短。第二项研究中，Swan 等[23]报告 LQT1 患者，而不是 LQT2 患者，在运动后期 QT 间期出现了过度延长。第三项研究中，选取对照组和明确基因型的长 QT 综合征患者各 26 例，比较两组在白天和夜间 QT 间期变化情况[24]（另外一种观察心率增快和心率减慢时 QT 间期变化的方法）。LQT1 患者与对照组无显著性差异，LQT2 患者夜间 QTc 中度延长，LQT3 患者夜间 QTc 显著延长（图 70-4）。LQT3 与对照组，LQT3 与 LQT1 组组间比较统计学差异具有显著性。

图 70-5 列举了这些观察的重要实用价值。一位青年女性例行意大利法律规定的对即将从事竞技性体育运动的人必须进行的常规心脏检查。在运动负荷试验中，医生发现，继发于心率加快的 QT 间期适应性丧失，患者 QTc 显著延长。尽管患者的基础心电图正常，但分子筛选确定存在 KvLQT1 基因突变而确诊为长 QT 综合征。

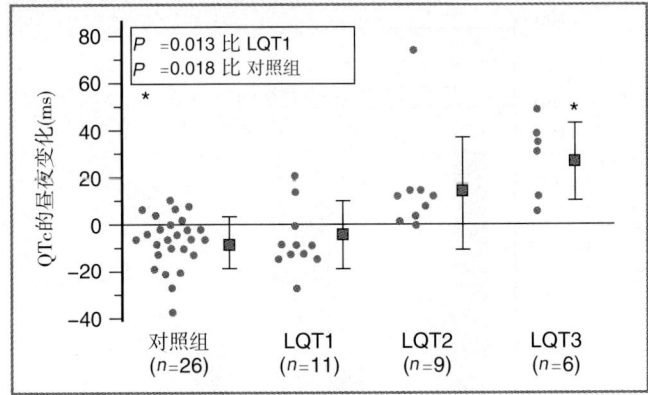

图 70-4　患者睡眠和清醒状态下 QTc 的差异　对照组、LQT1、LQT 2、LQT 3 患者睡眠和清醒状态下 QTc 的差异。显示 QTc 的个体值（开放环）和各组 QTc 的变化，用均值±标准误表示，长 QT 综合征患者夜间 QTc 显著延长。（引自 Stramba-Badiale M，Priori SG，Napolitano C，et al：Gene-specific differences in the circadian variation of ventricular repolarization in the long QT syndrome：A key to sudden death during sleep？Ital Heart J 1：323-328，2000.）

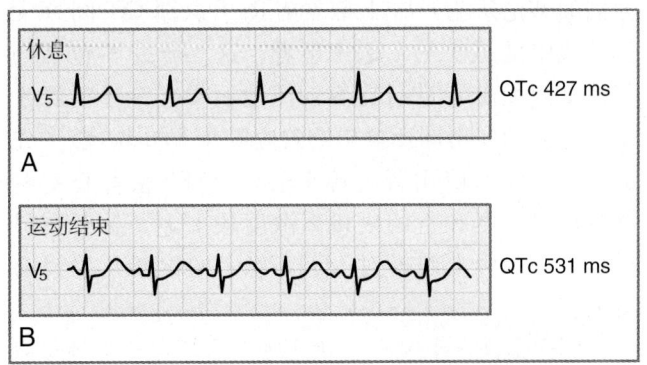

图 70-5　一位 27 岁女性在例行法律规定的从事竞技性体育运动者必须进行的一项常规心脏检查时记录的 V_5 导联心电图　运动试验过程中发现 QT 间期不随心率加快而缩短，使 QTc 延长。立即进行会诊，并行分子筛选，确诊为 KvLQT1 基因突变型长 QT 综合征患者。

近来，据另外一些试验报道：通过分析运动负荷试验中心室跨壁复极离散度（T波顶峰至T波结束的时限）的不同改变，有助于临床区分LQT1和LQT2患者。Takenaka等[19]发现在运动期间，LQT1患者跨壁复极离散度增大，而LQT2患者不增大。

随心率加快，QT间期具有适应性改变，在不同基因型患者，其适应性存在差异，即具有基因相关性的差异，这一发现不仅对基础电生理研究有益，也具有重要的临床意义。当医生发现患者心电图正常或QT间期处于正常临界值时，应注意心率加快时QT间期适应性变化是否正常，这一点对诊断十分重要。当QT间期适应性丧失时，对患者进行详细随访并搜集家族史的同时，应从 $KvLQT1$ 基因开始进行分子筛查。这些数据也有助于我们理解LQT1患者在运动时，LQT3患者在夜间（见后）处于发生心脏事件的高危状态。在这两项研究中，LQT3患者数量有限，应注意从这些观察中得出的推断性结论。

五、对儿茶酚胺的反应

20多年前，Lazzara等[25]首先观察到注射肾上腺素有助于诊断长QT综合征。由于肾上腺素具有促心律失常作用，这一结果并未引起临床重视，但近来，Shimizu等借鉴这一观点研究发现，肾上腺素有助于发现LQT1亚群沉默突变基因携带者。他们观察到[26]：QTc>460ms，也包括一些QTc<460ms的LQT1患者应用肾上腺素后QTc延长，而无突变基因携带的家族成员和正常对照组成员QTc不延长。他们的结论认为：肾上腺素有助于识别QT间期无延长或中度延长的LQT1患者。这一研究不包括与其他基因型患者进行比较，但他们根据β肾上腺素受体阻滞剂在不同亚群中的效应以及Tanabe等[27]先前的报道显示应用肾上腺素后，LQT1患者心室跨壁复极离散度和空间复极离散度较LQT2患者明显增加，提示肾上腺素对LQT2患者的诊断几乎没有帮助。

同样是这一小组[28]，确实观察到，在正常神经张力状态下，应用β肾上腺素受体阻滞剂后，LQT1患者心室跨壁复极离散度（测量从T波顶峰至T波结束的时限）较LQT2患者明显减小。应用肾上腺素后，心室跨壁复极离散度增加。此时，再应用β肾上腺素受体阻滞剂，其抑制离散度增加的作用在LQT1和LQT2患者之间没有差别。

应用肾上腺素和在应用肾上腺素前后分别应用β受体阻滞剂对心室跨壁复极离散度产生了不同的影响，人们已经观察到，LQT1患者对交感神经激活非常敏感，容易发生致命性心律失常，并对β受体阻滞剂治疗反应好。上述试验结果为阐明这一现象的机制提供了附加的证据。然而，是否能将肾上腺素作为常用的诊断工具尚不能确定。

六、心脏事件的触发因素

虽然，在1995年Schwantz等[13]的研究中入选的确定基因型的长QT综合征患者数量较少，但他们得出了新颖的、出人意料的结论：LQT3患者的心脏事件多发生于睡眠或休息时，而LQT2患者心律失常发作在情绪应激时，这一结论暗含着丰富的内涵，有着重要的意义。于是，作者总结并表达了他们的想法：希望在更大的人群中对上述结果重新进行观察，再作定论。

因而，在世界范围内合作的基础上，进行了一个更大规模的研究，确实对长QT综合征患者特异的基因型与触发心脏事件的条件之间作出了最终的结论[15]。该研究入选670例已知基因型的长QT综合征患者（LQT1 371人占55%，LQT2 234人占35%，LQT3 65人占10%）。重要的是，参与数据分析的患

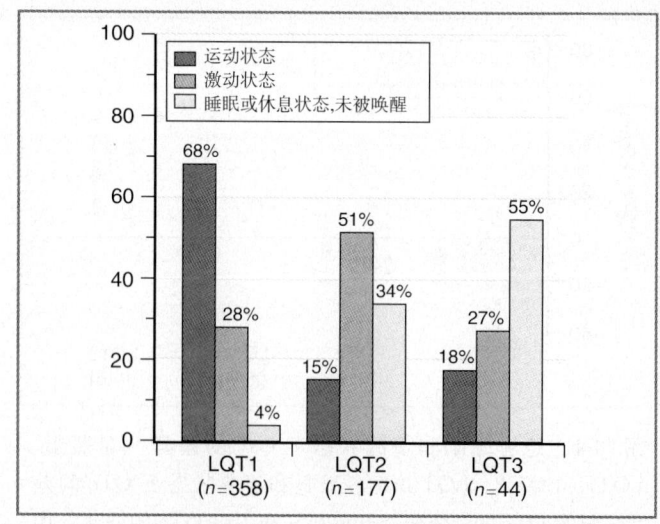

图70-6　三种基因型中所有致死性和非致死性心脏事件的触发因素　（引自Schwartz PJ, Priori SG, Spazzolini C, et al: Gentype-phenotype correlation in the long QT syndrome, Gene-specific triggers for life-threatening arrhythmias. Circulation 103：89-95，2001.）

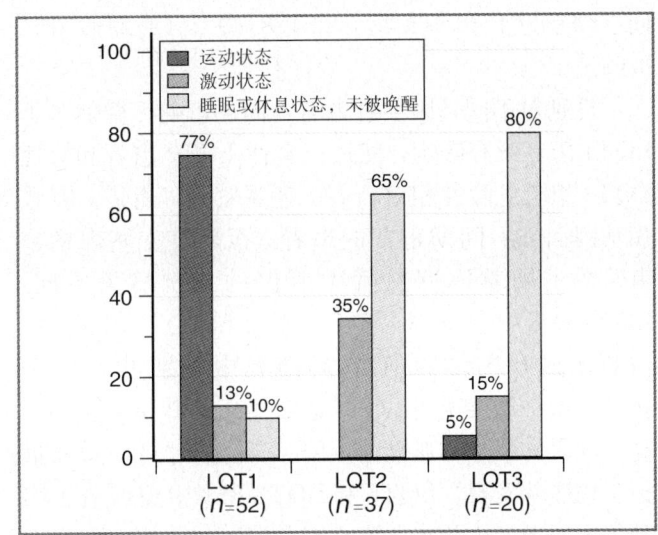

图 70-7 致死性心脏事件（心脏骤停、心源性猝死）的触发因素 资料来自于 579 例明确基因型的患者。（引自 Schwartz PJ, Priori SG, Spazzolini C, et al: Genotype-phenotype correlation in the long QT syndrome. Gene-specific triggers for life-threatening arrhymias. Circulation103：89-95，2001.）

者都有心脏症状（晕厥、心脏骤停或猝死），不包括无症状患者，也不包括 Jervell-Lange-Nielsen 综合征这种长 QT 综合征变异型的患者。确认了三种与心脏事件发生相关的情况或触发因素：运动、情绪应激、休息或持续睡眠（无觉醒）。

观察基因型和三种主要的心脏症状（晕厥、心脏骤停或猝死）之间的相关性，并进行分析。而后，将后两种致命性心脏事件限定为主要症状，对基因型和他们的关系进行分析。第一项分析（图 70-6）显示了基因型与主要心脏症状之间的关系，选择研究症状的范围较大。第二项分析（图 70-7）选择性地将研究症状范围缩小，着重显示了基因型与致死性心脏事件之间的关系。这些数据证实了先前的一些观察结果[13]，并表明在特殊条件下，发生致命性心脏事件的可能性由特定的基因型决定。

最突出的发现如下所述，LQT1 患者在交感神经激活的情况下容易发生心律失常，其中以体育运动为主要触发因素，而在静息状态下心脏事件发生率极小。而 LQT2 和 LQT3 患者在运动中出现心脏事件，仅有中度可能性。LQT2 患者心律失常大多发生在情绪应激时，也发生在休息时。LQT3 患者在休息或睡眠中发生心律失常危险性最大。将研究症状的范围限制在致命性心脏事件范围时（图 70-7），上述趋势更加明显：无一例 LQT2 患者死于运动中，超过 80% 的 LQT3 患者致死性心脏事件发生于休息或睡眠中。

最后，该研究还明确提出：游泳和声音刺激分别是 LQT1 和 LQT2 患者发生致命性心脏事件的特异性触发因素。在游泳时发生的心脏事件中，99% 为 LQT1 患者，高噪音刺激相关的心脏事件中，80% 为 LQT2 患者。前分子时代[29]，游泳和高噪声被认为是长 QT 综合征患者发生心脏事件的重要触发因素。对游泳和 LQT1 患者心脏事件之间的关系大致能够作出解释，因为运动是 LQT1 患者发生心脏事件一个独特的重要触发因素。而声音刺激作为触发因素出乎人们的预料，Wilde 等[30]对这一情况首先做了报道。

在特殊条件下，发生致命性心律失常具有基因特异性，用我们目前对其分子机制的理解，可以解释或部分解释这一现象。在交感神经激活，尤其当心率显著而持续升高时，LQT1 患者危险性更高，运动（心率加快）而不是惊吓更容易触发 LQT1 患者致死性心律失常事件。

由于编码 I_{Ks} 通道蛋白的基因突变致使该通道增加 I_{Ks} 电流的能力受损，无法对 β 肾上腺素受体作出适当的反应[31]。相反，LQT2 和 LQT3 患者运动中发生致命性心脏事件的相对危险性较低，这是由于 I_{Ks} 通道结构完整，而且 LQT3 患者随心率加快能使 QT 间期以超出正常应缩短的程度显著缩短[13]。LQT3 患者睡眠或休息时处于发生致死性心脏事件的高危状态，这与此时患者的 QT 间期较正常延长密切相关[24]。

从这项用于长 QT 综合征患者基因型-表现型相关性研究的最大规模的数据[15]中，我们得到了两方面的启示：一方面，证实了在某些特殊条件下，易患致命性心律失常的长 QT 综合征患者具有基因特异性，即不同基因型的长 QT 综合征患者各自在不同的条件下易患致命性心律失常，并且，应用这些数据对其根本机制进行了深入探讨；另一方面，在同一研究人群中又得出了不同基因型患者心脏事件发生时间的特异性和对 β 受体阻滞剂的不同反应两方面的数据，对原有数据进行了补充，并阐明了一种用来阻止长 QT 综合征患者猝死方法的基本原理，这种方法较以前的方法更新颖、全面、合理。这种新方法是两方面治疗措施的结合，即包括建议患者避免某些能诱发致命性心律失常的行为和针对基因特异性选择的某些治疗。

七、自然病程和危险分层

不同基因型的长 QT 综合征患者自然病程具有基

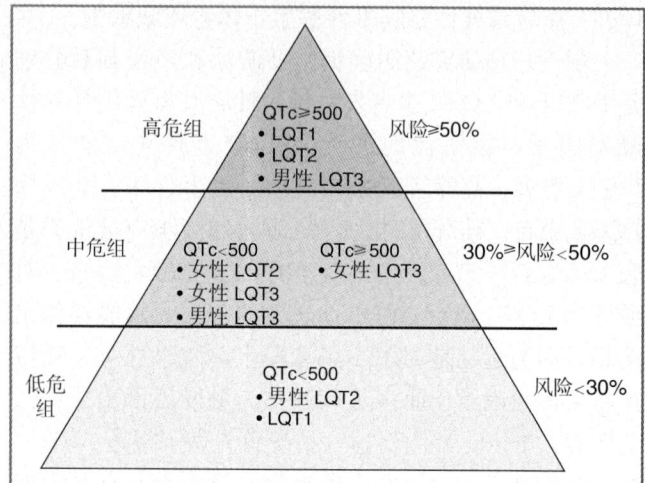

图70-8 根据基因型和性别对长QT综合征患者进行危险分层的方案 根据在40岁之前出现第一次心脏事件（晕厥、心脏骤停或猝死）来划分危险组。其可能性≥50%定义为高危组,可能性在30%～50%之间定义为中危组,可能性<30%定义为低危组。(引自Priori SG, Schwartz PJ, Napolitano C, et al: Risk statification in the long-QT syndrome. N Engl J Med 348: 1866-1874, 2003. Copyright Massachusetts Medical Society, 2003.)

因特异性,主要有三项研究得出的数据为我们提供了有意义的信息[11,15,32]。一个是Schwartz等[15]关于有症状患者的研究。另一个是Zareba等[32]对38个家系（10个LQT1, 22个LQT2, 6个LQT3家系）进行的研究,得到的数据具有特异性,但其特异性十分有限,不足以进行相关性分析。因而,分析时排除了一些小规模家系和一些基因再次突变所致长QT综合征的单个病例,这造成了潜在性的选择偏倚。第三个是Priori等[11]对193个家系（104个LQT1, 68个LQT2, 21个LQT3家系）进行的研究,共647例长QT综合征患者先后确定了基因型。因而,本章对这项最大的、最近期的结果进行详述。

该研究主要观察发生第一次心脏事件的累积可能性。对所有心脏事件（晕厥、心脏骤停、猝死）和致命性心律失常（心脏骤停、发生在40岁之前的猝死、治疗开始前的猝死）进行分析。结果发现,LQT2患者累积生存率低于LQT1患者（P<0.001）。LQT1和LQT3患者累积生存率相似（P=0.07）,也就是说,LQT1患者死亡率低。LQT1患者40岁之前和治疗之前发生第一次心脏事件的危险性确实低,其中,无症状患者占相当大一部分比例。与LQT1患者相比,LQT2和LQT3患者发生心脏事件的相对危险性要高,其相对危险性（RR）分别为1.6 [95%可信区间（CI）为1.16～2.25] 和1.8（95%CI为1.07～3.04）。

性别对不同基因型患者有不同的影响。性别对于LQT1患者没有影响,然而,女性LQT2患者和男性LQT3患者危险性相对较高。还观察到,遗传上有致病基因而QT间期正常的患者（沉默突变基因携带者）在不同基因型患者中所占的比例显著不同。LQT1患者中占36%,多于LQT2和LQT3患者中所占的比例（P<0.001）,后两者中分别占19%和10%。这一结果说明LQT1患者中无症状患者比例较高。在每一个基因亚群中,用四分位数对QTc分布进行了描述并发现,LQT1和LQT2患者中QTc在上四分位中的患者比分布在第一四分位区域内（沉默突变基因携带者）患者的危险性分别高5.3倍（95%CI 2.82～10.13）和8.4倍（95%CI 2.53～27.21）。但LQT3患者中QTc分布没有这种危险性差别。

为了对每个基因型危险性进行综合性的量化,首次用性别和QTc高于和低于500ms（根据最高四分位区域确定的测量指标）进行分析,产生12种不同的量化指标。图70-8显示这12种情况下危险性的区别。

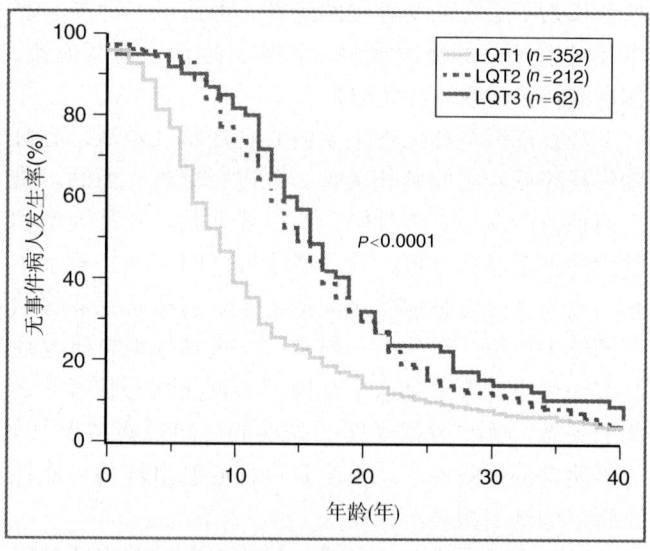

图70-9 Kaplan-Meier累积生存曲线 描述从出生到出现第一次心脏事件（晕厥、心脏骤停复苏、猝死）之间的时间间期。括号中的数字代表患者数量,值得注意的是,这一研究和该图不包括无症状患者。LQT1与LQT2患者相比较P<0.0001; LQT1与LQT3患者相比较P=0.0001; LQT3与LQT2患者相比较,P值无统计学差异。(引自Schwartz PJ, Priori SG, Spazzolini C, et al: Genotype-phenotype correlation in the long QT syndrome. Gene-specific triggers for life-threatening arrhythmias. Circulation 103: 89-95, 2001.)

这一研究得出了一些结论。其中 LQT1 患者致命性心脏事件发生率低这一结论与先前研究结论[32]略有差异。这一研究还证实，QTc 超过 500ms 的 LQT1 患者中，有 30% 无症状发生，并且致命性心脏事件的发生与性别无关。这一结果更支持 LQT1 为恶性度最低的亚型。与之相比，LQT2 患者中，女性危险性高，即使 QTc 低于 500ms，女性患者比男性患者危险性高 4 倍。

关于接受治疗前发生第一次心脏事件时间的分析为制订治疗方案提供了有意义的信息。Schwzrtz 等[15]对一组有症状的已知基因型的人群的研究表明，LQT1 患者出现症状的时间早于 LQT2 和 LQT3 患者（图 70-9）；而且，86% LQT1 患者早在 20 岁时就发生了第一次心脏事件。

长 QT 综合征患者的危险分层并未局限在主要基因亚群水平上进行，对于某些亚群已经扩展到依突变基因的具体位置进行危险分层。Donger 等[33]首次提出长 QT 综合征患者临床症状的严重程度可能与基因突变的特殊位点有关。从一个规模相对较小的研究中得出结论认为：通道基因 C 末端突变较门控区域基因突变的恶性度低。分子水平的研究发现，门控区域基因突变使通道功能下降超过 50%，而非门控区域基因突变主要造成共同组装和转运异常，从而使单体型（亲代任何一方父或母提供的等位基因）不足，使通道功能降低 50%[34,35]。Moss 等[36]的研究对这些发现的重要临床意义作出了最终的解释。他们的研究入选 201 例 LQT2 患者，35 例在 HERG 基因门控区域发生基因突变，166 例在非门控区域发生基因突变。主要结果为：门控区域发生基因突变的 LQT2 患者发生心脏事件的危险性比非门控区域发生基因突变者高。而且，前者在年龄相对较小的情况下就发生了第一次心脏事件，发生心脏事件的频率也高（前者 74%，后者 35%，$P<0.001$），但"流产的"心脏骤停和猝死（前者 15%，后者 6%）二者之间无显著性差异。这些资料证明基因突变位点不同的患者临床结果不同。

从这些研究中，我们获得了一些与临床相关的信息。LQT1 患者中，甚至许多 QTc 显著延长者，都表现为无症状。按目前的观点，在这一人群中，一些"修饰因子"或者增加了心肌的电稳定性，或者使不同突变类型的患者电生理表现之间具有很大的差异。交感神经系统[37]可能是这些"修饰因子"中最具代表性的因子之一。利用一些简单参数，如三种不同的基因型、性别、QTc 时限建立危险分层模型，用这一模型可以分辨不同亚群的危险性。一个重要的进展是，突变位点在确定患者实际危险度方面起着重要的作用。

八、对 β 受体阻滞剂的反应/治疗措施

自从关于长 QT 综合征患者治疗的数据[38,39]首次公布以来，β 受体阻滞剂一直作为首选药物的代表。然而，在明确基因型的患者中应用 β 受体阻滞剂的疗效尚缺乏相关的资料。而且，治疗的主要目的不同时，β 受体阻滞剂常作为次级方案。

三项应用 β 受体阻滞剂的相关信息均不足以证实其安全有效，但有一个例外，就是对 LQT1 患者，它可能有效。第一项是 Moss 等[40]在一个样本量较大的人群中进行的研究，但确定基因型者仅有 139 例。而且，其中只有 67 例在治疗之前出现心脏事件：LQT1 患者 39 例，LQT2 患者 24 例，LQT3 患者 4 例。在 6 年的随访中，LQT1 和 LQT2 患者的心脏事件和心脏骤停，包括死亡的数量显著减少。在 LQT3 患者中没有得出从 β 受体阻滞剂中获益的证据，LQT3 患者数量太少，无法做任何结论。值得注意的是，139 例中，4 例（2.8%）死亡；第 5 位死亡者为一位曾经中断治疗的 LQT3 患者。

表 70-1 基因型与 β 受体阻滞剂治疗

基因型	未再发心脏事件 n(%)	再发心脏事件 n(%)	骤停/心源性猝死（总发生率；再发病人的发生率,%)
LQT1(n=162)	131(81%)	31(19%)	7(4%;23%)
LQT2(n=91)	54(91%)	37(41%)	4(4%;11%)
LQT3(n=18)	9(50%)	9(50%)	3(17%;33%)

引自 Schwartz PJ, Priori SG, Spazzolini C, et al: Genotypephenotype correlation in the long QT syndrome. Gene-specific triggers for life-threatening arrhythmias. Circulation 103:89-95, 2001.

第二项资料来自 Schwartz 等[15]的研究，他们主要研究心脏事件的触发因素。从 270 例已知基因型的患者中（LQT1 患者 161 例，LQT2 患者 91 例，LQT3 患者 18 例），得出了充分的关于 β 受体阻滞剂疗效的数据。这项研究的突出特征为所有入选患者均出现心脏症状，并发生心脏事件。两项观察结果证明 β 受体阻滞剂对心脏事件的复发、心脏骤停和

猝死的发生率有明显的影响（表70-1）。应用β受体阻滞剂防止心脏事件复发，LQT1患者疗效较好，81%LQT1、59%LQT2、50%LQT3患者在随访期间无症状。LQT1和LQT2患者心脏骤停和猝死的累积发生率（均为4%）没有显著差异。在LQT3患者中，尽管已接受治疗，其致命性心脏事件发生率仍较高（17%），但研究中LQT3患者数量较小。

最后一项资料来自一个多中心的试验研究，4个心脏中心入选218例LQT1患者，随访12±7年，其心脏骤停和猝死的发生率在有不适主诉的患者中仅为1.2%[41]。再次证实了β受体阻滞剂能为大多数LQT1患者提供有效的保护。

治疗反应和危险分层均具有基因特异性，这代表了基因型-表现型相关性研究领域中最新的进展。但都还需要更多的样本量和足够长时间的随访加以证实。有关LQT3患者的数据仍面临样本量较小的困境，这是处理这一特殊类型时几乎无法避免的限制。因而，在对这一人群做任何定论时都要十分谨慎。

最确实的数据来自关于LQT1患者多个研究资料的汇总，这类患者的分子缺陷决定其对儿茶酚胺的高度敏感，在交感神经兴奋性增加时，LQT$_1$患者处于高危状态，β受体阻滞剂对这类患者能起到很好的保护作用。

应用β受体阻滞剂治疗LQT2和LQT3患者的疗效尚未确定。足够的数据表明，对这两类患者，其他辅助治疗如植入式心脏复律除颤器（ICD）、左侧心脏交感神经节切除术[42]和起搏器可能有效。尽管，与LQT1患者相比β受体阻滞剂对这两类患者的保护作用弱，但仍没有证据证实，这两类患者可以停用β受体阻滞剂。另外，应尽量避免在患者睡眠时突然出现噪音，在患者的卧室内不要放置电话和闹钟。

（郭继鸿　陈琪　译）

参考文献

1. Wang Q, Shen J, Splawski I, et al: SCN5A mutations associated with an inherited cardiac arrhythmia, long QT syndrome. Cell 80:805–811, 1995.
2. Curran ME, Splawski I, Timothy KW, et al: A molecular basis for cardiac arrhythmia: HERG mutations cause long QT syndrome. Cell 80:795–803, 1995.
3. Zipes DP: The long QT interval syndrome. A Rosetta stone for sympathetic related ventricular tachyarrhythmias. Circulation 84:1414–1419, 1991.
4. Tristani-Firouzi M, Jensen JL, Donaldson MR, et al: Functional and clinical characterization of KCNJ2 mutations associated with LQT7 (Andersen syndrome). J Clin Invest 110:381–388, 2002.
5. Wang Q, Curran ME, Splawski I, et al: Positional cloning of a novel potassium channel gene: KvLQT1 mutations cause cardiac arrhythmias. Nat Genet 12:17–23, 1996.
6. Mohler PJ, Schott JJ, Gramolini AO, et al: Ankyrin-B mutation causes type 4 long-QT cardiac arrhythmia and sudden cardiac death. Nature 421:634–639, 2003.
7. Barhanin J, Lesage F, Guillemare E, et al: KvLQT1 and IsK (minK) proteins associate to form the I_{Ks} cardiac potassium current. Nature 384:78–80, 1996.
8. Abbott GW, Sesti F, Splawski I, et al: MiRP1 forms I_{Kr} potassium channels with HERG and is associated with cardiac arrhythmia. Cell 97:175–187, 1999.
9. Schwartz PJ, Moss AJ, Vincent GM, Crampton RS: Diagnostic criteria for the long QT syndrome: An update. Circulation 88:782–784, 1993.
10. Splawski I, Shen J, Timothy KW, et al: Spectrum of mutations in long-QT syndrome genes. Circulation 102:1178–1185, 2000.
11. Priori SG, Schwartz PJ, Napolitano C, et al: Risk stratification in the long-QT syndrome. N Engl J Med 348:1866–1874, 2003.
12. Moss AJ, Zareba W, Benhorin J, et al: ECG T-wave patterns in genetically distinct forms of the hereditary long QT syndrome. Circulation 92:2929–2934, 1995.
13. Schwartz PJ, Priori SG, Locati EH, et al: Long QT syndrome patients with mutations on the SCN5A and HERG genes have differential responses to Na+ channel blockade and to increases in heart rate. Implications for gene-specific therapy. Circulation 92:3381–3386, 1995.
14. Priori SG, Napolitano C, Cantù F, et al: Differential response to Na+ channel blockade, β-adrenergic stimulation, and rapid pacing in a cellular model mimicking the SCN5A and HERG defects present in the long QT syndrome. Circ Res 78:1009–1015, 1996.
15. Schwartz PJ, Priori SG, Spazzolini C, et al: Genotype-phenotype correlation in the long QT syndrome. Gene-specific triggers for life-threatening arrhythmias. Circulation 103:89–95, 2001.
16. Zhang L, Timothy KW, Vincent GM, et al: Spectrum of ST-T-wave patterns and repolarization parameters in congenital long QT syndrome. ECG findings identify genotypes. Circulation 102:2849–2855, 2000.
17. Dausse E, Berthet M, Denjoy I, et al: A mutation in HERG associated with notched T waves in long-QT syndrome. J Mol Cell Cardiol 28:1609–1615, 1996.
18. Malfatto G, Beria G, Sala S, et al: Quantitative analysis of T wave abnormalities and their prognostic implications in the idiopathic long QT syndrome. J Am Coll Cardiol 23:296–301, 1994.
19. Takenaka K, Ai T, Shimizu W, et al: Exercise stress test amplifies genotype-phenotype correlation in the LQT1 and LQT2 forms of the long-QT syndrome. Circulation 107:838–844, 2003.
20. Shimizu W, Antzelevitch C: Cellular basis for the ECG features of the LQT1 form of the long-QT syndrome: Effects of beta-adrenergic agonists and antagonists and sodium channel blockers on transmural dispersion of repolarization and torsade de pointes. Circulation 98:2314–2322, 1998.
21. Shimizu W, Antzelevitch C: Sodium channel block with mexiletine is effective in reducing dispersion of repolarization and preventing torsade de pointes in LQT2 and LQT3 models of the long-QT syndrome. Circulation 96:2038–2047, 1997.
22. Sanguinetti MC, Jurkiewicz NK: Two components of cardiac delayed rectifier K+ current. J Gen Physiol 96:195–215, 1990.
23. Swan H, Viitasalo M, Piippo K, et al: Sinus node function and ventricular repolarization during exercise stress test in long QT syndrome patients with KvLQT1 and HERG potassium channel defects. J Am Coll Cardiol 34:823–829, 1999.
24. Stramba-Badiale M, Priori SG, Napolitano C, et al: Gene-specific differences in the circadian variation of ventricular repolarization in the long QT syndrome: A key to sudden death during sleep? Ital Heart J 1:323–328, 2000.
25. Schechter E, Freeman CC, Lazzara R: Afterdepolarizations as a mechanism for the long QT syndrome: Electrophysiologic studies of a case. J Am Coll Cardiol 1:1556–1561, 1984.
26. Shimizu W, Noda T, Takaki H, et al: Epinephrine unmasks latent mutation carriers with LQT1 form of congenital long-QT syndrome. J Am Coll Cardiol 41:633–642, 2003.
27. Tanabe Y, Inagaki M, Kurita T, et al: Sympathetic stimulation produces a greater increase in both transmural and spatial dispersion of repolarization in LQT1 than LQT2 forms of congenital long QT syndrome. J Am Coll Cardiol 37:911–919, 2001.

28. Shimizu W, Tanabe Y, Aiba T, et al: Differential effects of beta-blockade on dispersion of repolarization in the absence and presence of sympathetic stimulation between the LQT1 and LQT2 forms of congenital long QT syndrome. J Am Coll Cardiol 39:1984–1991, 2002.
29. Schwartz PJ, Zaza A, Locati E, Moss AJ: Stress and sudden death. The case of the long QT syndrome. Circulation 83(suppl II):II71–II80, 1991.
30. Wilde AAM, Jongbloed RJE, Doevendans PA, et al: Auditory stimuli as a trigger for arrhythmic events differentiate *HERG*-related (LQTS2) patients from *KvLQT1*-related patients (LQTS1). J Am Coll Cardiol 33:327–332, 1999.
31. Marx SO, Kurokawa J, Reiken S, et al: Requirement of a macromolecular signaling complex for beta adrenergic receptor modulation of the KCNQ1-KCNE1 potassium channel. Science 295:496–499, 2002.
32. Zareba W, Moss AJ, Schwartz PJ, et al, for the International Long-QT Syndrome Registry Research Group: Influence of the genotype on the clinical course of the Long QT Syndrome. N Engl J Med 339:960–965, 1998.
33. Donger C, Denjoy I, Berthet M, et al: *KVLQT1* C-terminal missense mutation causes a forme fruste long-QT syndrome. Circulation 96:2778–2781, 1997.
34. January CT, Gong Q, Zhou Z: Long QT syndrome: Cellular basis and arrhythmia mechanism in LQT2. J Cardiovasc Electrophysiol 11:1413–1418, 2000.
35. Huang FD, Chen J, Lin M, et al: Long-QT syndrome-associated missense mutations in the pore helix of the HERG potassium channel. Circulation 104:1071–1075, 2001.
36. Moss AJ, Zareba W, Kaufman ES, et al: Increased risk of arrhythmic events in long QT syndrome with mutations in the pore region of the human ether-a-go-go-related gene potassium channel. Circulation 105:794–799, 2002.
37. Schwartz PJ: Another role for the sympathetic nervous system in the long QT syndrome? J Cardiovasc Electrophysiol 12:500–502, 2001.
38. Schwartz PJ, Periti M, Malliani A: The long QT syndrome. Am Heart J 89:378–390, 1975.
39. Schwartz PJ: Idiopathic long QT syndrome: Progress and questions. Am Heart J 109:399–411, 1985.
40. Moss AJ, Zareba W, Hall WJ, et al: Effectiveness and limitations of β-blocker therapy in congenital long QT syndrome. Circulation 101:616–623, 2000.
41. Vincent GM, Bithell C, Schwartz PJ, et al: Efficacy of beta-blockers in the LQT1 genotype of long QT syndrome (abstract). Circulation 2003 (in press).
42. Cerrone M, Spazzolini C, Priori SG, et al: Left cardiac sympathetic denervation in the management of the long QT syndrome. A worldwide survey. Circulation 106:II–701, 2002.

第 71 章

长 QT 综合征的治疗策略

Arthur J. Moss and Wojciech Zareba

本章目录

- 危险评估 ·············· 654
- 治疗策略 ·············· 655
- 治疗概要 ·············· 660
- 总结 ················ 660

遗传性长 QT 综合征（long QT syndrome，LQTS）是 1957 年由 Jervell 和 Lange-Nielsen 发现有几个耳聋儿童伴有反复晕厥及猝死的一个家族而首先报告的。这些儿童心电图存在 QT 间期延长。几年以后，Romano 和 Ward 分别报告了有晕厥及猝死而无耳聋的几个家族。这些情况曾被认为是癫痫发作，最初使用抗惊厥药物（苯巴比妥和苯妥英钠）治疗。20 世纪 60 年代期间，许多 LQTS 患者被报告，有几例患者是在突然被唤醒时发生晕厥事件及猝死的。少数患者晕厥发作时有动态心电图记录，证实晕厥原因是多形性室性心动过速。70 年代早期，采用外科交感神经切除术和 β 肾上腺素受体阻滞剂等抗肾上腺素能治疗，疗效良好。许多 LQTS 患者存在不适当的窦性心动过缓，80 年代采用起搏治疗，原理是通过生理性起搏减少因长间歇依赖机制发生的异常心室复极而促发的室性心动过速。80 年代中期，植入性心脏复律除颤器开始用于接受了抗肾上腺素能治疗后仍反复发生心脏事件的高危 LQTS 患者。90 年代，揭示了 LQTS 的分子遗传学基础，确认了几个离子通道基因的突变。随着引起 LQTS 的这些基因突变和异常离子通道机制的发现，将会出现针对基因突变的特异性治疗。

根据来自国际 LQTS 注册的大量回顾性观察研究的治疗方案已用于治疗 LQTS 患者。从来没有进行过用来评价 LQTS 治疗方案安全性和疗效的随机、双盲、安慰剂对照试验。因为 LQTS 的严重程度变化极大，甚至在有相同基因突变的 LQTS 家族成员中[1]，无症状或有症状 LQTS 患者的治疗也需要个体化考虑风险与获益。本章概述了近几年来根据积累的 LQTS 临床经验和遗传学知识所推荐的治疗方案。

一、危险评估

国际 LQTS 注册已经登记了 1200 多个家族和近 7000 名家族成员进行前瞻性研究。每个家族由一个先证者确定，即家族中第一个不明原因 QTc（心率校正 QT 间期）≥0.45s 的存活个体。先证者通常由于儿童或青春期晕厥发作提交注册，而大多数证实 QTc 延长的家族成员作为家族评估对象是无症状的。显然，由于在提交注册之前确定的先证者通常都有症状，先证者存在较高危险性（图 71-1）导致存在选择性偏倚。

不论是先证者还是认定的 LQTS 家族成员，心脏事件的危险性直接与 QTc 长度相关，危险率以 QTc 的指数增加（危险率 $=1.052^x$），x 代表 QTc 每延长 10ms 的变化。例如，QTc 为 600ms 的患者发生晕厥或 LQTS 相关死亡的危险性比 QTc 为 400ms 的患者高 2.8 倍（$1.052^{20}=2.8$）。危险性与年龄相关，也受性别影响[2]。男性首次发生心脏事件的危险性在儿童和青春期增加，此后下降；女性首次发生心脏事件的危险性在青春期增加，并持续到成年后数年。这些资料表明 LQTS 患者应在生命的早期就开始预防性治疗，尤其对QTc明显延长的患者更有价值。

LQTS伴有耳聋的患者，即Jervell和Lange-Nielsen综合征患者，发生恶性心律失常的危险性最高。这些患者遗传双倍的突变体等位基因，QTc明显延长，在出生时就应该开始针对LQTS的积极治疗。

传统观念认为先证者存在LQTS的生命威胁将有助于明确认定的家族成员中危险性增加，因为所有认定的LQTS家族成员可能携带相同的突变基因。近期的临床发现不支持这一临床推论。LQTS先证者的临床严重程度不能预测一级家族成员心脏事件的可能性[3]。这些发现与这一遗传性疾病家族内外显率的变异性一致[4]。因此，先证者一级亲属的治疗决策不能依据LQTS先证者的严重程度。

T波的形态可能具有预后意义。T波双峰或切迹，特别是出现在侧壁心前导联时，反映复极不均一性增加，部分研究者认为这些形态的T波伴随着致心律失常基质增加。诊断LQTS的患者应进行运动试验和动态心电图监测，但是在这些检测中记录的QTc变化的阳性预测准确度很低。当发现存在T波电交替和/或短阵扭转型室性心动过速时是一个非常重要的危险标志，但是在检测期间很难发现这些心电事件。几个中心正在进行的研究是采用儿茶酚胺注射，根据诱发的T波形态异常、QTc延长或室性心律失常数量来确定危险性高低，但是诱发这些现象的特异性和预测价值目前并不清楚。

LQTS的临床进程受遗传基因型影响[5]。心脏事件（晕厥、心脏骤停幸存者或死亡）的危险性在含有KCNQ1（LQT1）和HERG（LQT2）基因突变的LQTS显著高于含有SCN5A（LQT3）基因突变的LQTS（图71-2）。虽然不管哪一种基因型累积死亡率都是相似的，但是致命性心脏事件的发生比例在含有SCN5A基因突变的LQTS显著高于含有KCNQ1和HERG基因突变的LQTS。含有HERG通道片段基因突变的LQTS患者，与心律失常相关心脏事件的危险性显著高于无通道突变者，并且危险性取决于QTc间期长短（图71-3）[6]。虽然遗传两种LQTS等位基因突变体的患者极为罕见，但是其QTc显著延长，不论是否伴有耳聋（Jervell和Lange-Nielsen综合征），心脏事件的危险性均极高。

二、治疗策略

（一）左侧颈胸交感神经节切除术

1970年首次报告使用左侧颈胸交感神经节切除术（LCTSG）治疗LQTS，这一技术在世界范围内已用于治疗高危LQTS患者150多例。总的说来，LCTSG似乎在一定程度上可降低心脏事件复发的危险性。在LCTSG临床疗效尚未确定的研究中，出现交感神经节切除术适当性与完整性的问题。最近在世界范围内总结了1970～2001年期间进行的151例LCTSG患者的资料，手术后平均随访8.6±6.1年，采用配对间期分析发现手术后与手术前比较，心脏事件发生率下降80%以上[7]。LCTSG后，LQTS相关死亡率是8.6%，随访期间平均每年1%。

LCTSG最佳外科手术操作为非开胸手术，经锁骨上途径进入左侧星状神经节和高位左侧胸神经节。星状神经节的下半部分和整个第二及第三胸神经节都

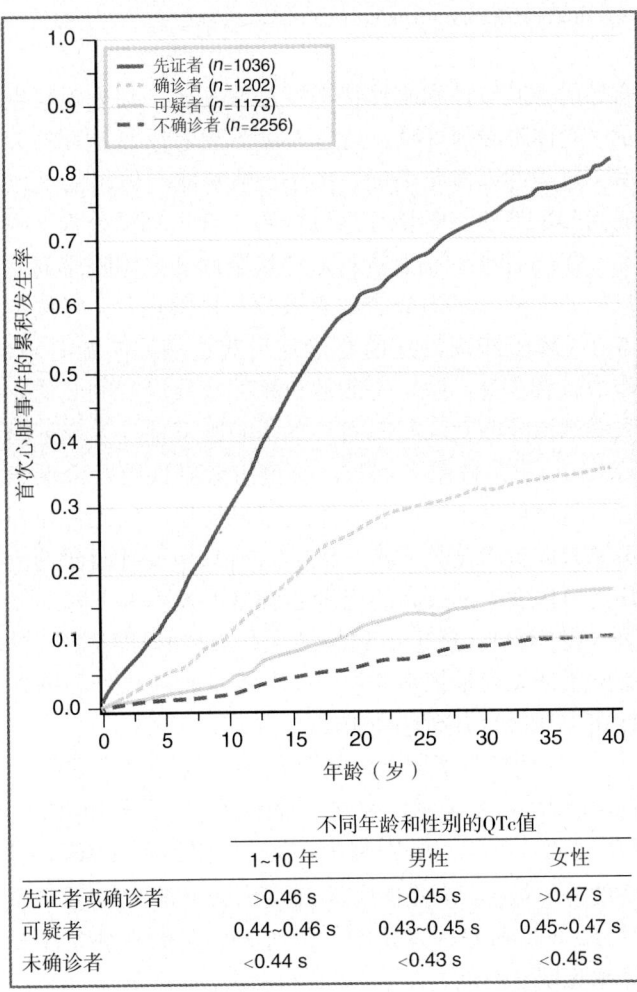

图71-1 国际LQTS注册登记以QTc为标准的先证者和确诊、可疑或不确诊的家族成员从出生开始发生首次心脏事件（晕厥、心脏骤停幸存者或LQTS相关死亡）的累积发生率

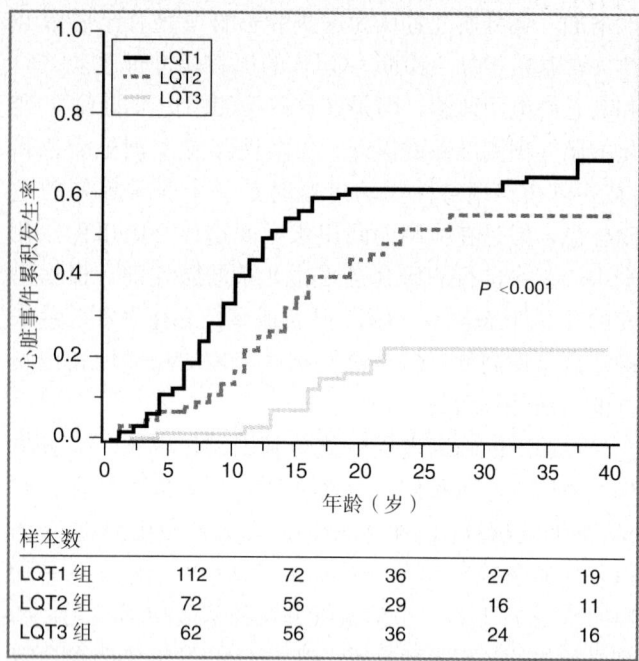

图71-2 LQT1、LQT2和LQT3组从出生开始首次心脏事件（晕厥、心脏骤停幸存者或LQTS相关死亡）的累积发生率

（引自 Zareba W, Moss AJ, Schwartz PJ, et al: Influence of genotype on the clinical course of the long-QT syndrome. International Long-QT Syndrome Registry Research Group. N Engl J Med 339: 960-965, 1998.）

应当被切除。对有经验的外科医生来说，外科手术操作没有困难，切除第二及第三胸神经节是最基本的，外科手术时应通过冰冻切片证实。如果操作适当，外科手术后的患者将有轻度 Horner 综合征，面部左下侧和左上肢出汗减少。

综观现在可以采用的其他各种治疗手段，LCTSG 应当被认为是一种辅助治疗手段，限用于药物及各种装置治疗无效的高危 LQTS 患者。目前，LCTSG 主要用于治疗高危婴幼儿及儿童，因为其身体太小，不适于安置植入性心脏复律除颤器；或用于伴有严重反应性气道疾病的患者，因为其不能够耐受 β 受体阻滞剂治疗。LCTSG 也可用于已经植入心脏复律除颤器和尽管使用 β 受体阻滞剂治疗仍然反复发生危及生命的室性心律失常而接受反复电击的 LQTS 患者。这种情况下，LCTSG 可能减少这些心律失常发作的频率。

（二）β受体阻滞剂

20世纪70年代初期，β受体阻滞剂就已被用于治疗 LQTS 患者。应用 β 受体阻滞剂的机制是由于 LQTS 患者在突然唤醒和体力活动时发生肾上腺素能

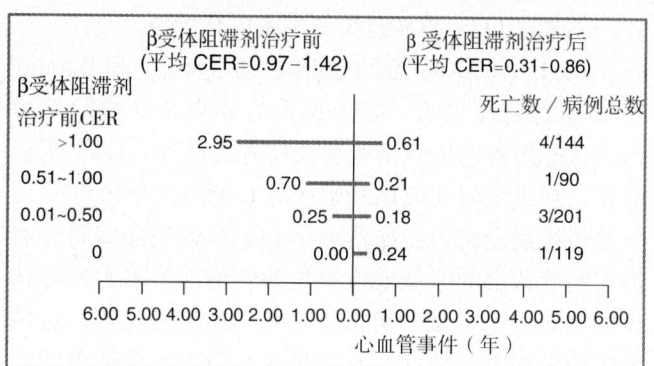

图71-3 581例 LQTS 先证者 β 受体阻滞剂治疗前与治疗后年平均心脏事件发生率（CER）比较 β 受体阻滞剂治疗之前 CER 细分为4个顺序类别。每条水平线的长度代表每一个 CER 类别开始 β 受体阻滞剂治疗之前与之后的平均 CER。β 受体阻滞剂治疗之后平均 CER 明显下降（$P<0.001$）。（引自 Moss AJ, Zareba W, Hall WJ, et al: Effectiveness and limitations of beta-blocker therapy in congenital long-QT syndrome. Circulation 101: 616-623, 2000.）

介导的心脏事件和室性快速性心律失常。临床观察提示 β 受体阻滞剂可减少高危 LQTS 患者反复晕厥的频率。过去的十多年期间，β 肾上腺素能受体阻滞剂已成为 LQTS 患者的治疗选择。2000年，回顾分析了国际 LQTS 注册的临床资料，评价服用 β 受体阻滞剂治疗的869例 LQTS 患者的有效性与局限性[8]。每例患者 β 受体阻滞剂治疗前与治疗后观察相同匹配时间，作为患者自身对照。先证者和相关家族成员的 β 受体阻滞剂治疗前后匹配期间年平均心脏事件发生率见图71-3。心脏事件患者例数、每例患者事件数及每例患者每年事件发生率在 β 受体阻滞剂治疗后先证者和相关家族成员均显著下降（$P<0.001$）。β 受体阻滞剂治疗前事件发生率最高的患者心脏事件发生率下降最显著（图71-4）。意想不到的结果是 β 受体阻滞剂减少心脏事件无剂量依赖关系，β 受体阻滞剂减少心脏事件在小剂量与大剂量是相似的。

139例携带不同基因亚组的患者使用 β 受体阻滞剂后分析结果显示，在主要的3种 LQTS（*LQT1*、*LQT2* 及 *LQT3*）基因型中，β 受体阻滞剂对 QTc 间期的影响最小。β 受体阻滞剂可以明显减少 *LQT1* 和 *LQT2* 的心脏事件发生率，但对 *LQT3* 的心脏事件发生率无明显影响。

评估服用规定剂量 β 受体阻滞剂患者心脏事件发生的影响因素显示，在 β 受体阻滞剂治疗前仅发生过晕厥或心脏骤停存活的患者危险性最高（危险度范围5~6）。服用规定剂量 β 受体阻滞剂患者随着时间推

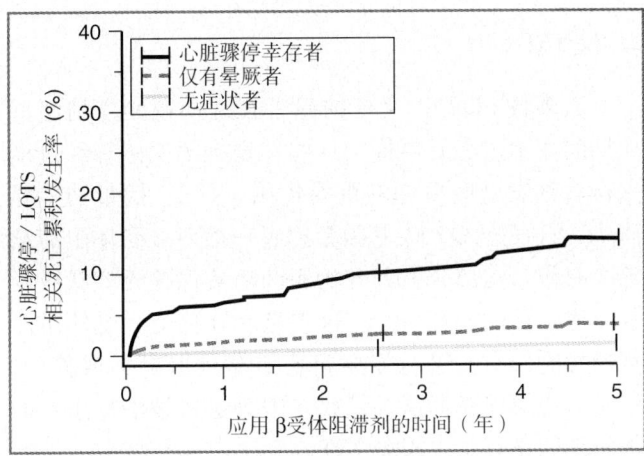

图71-4 无症状或仅有晕厥或心脏骤停幸存的LQTS患者β受体阻滞剂治疗前后心脏骤停幸存或死亡的累积发生率 垂直线代表95%的可信区间。（引自Moss AJ, Zareba W, Hall WJ, et al: Effectiveness and limitations of beta-blocker therapy in congenital long-QT syndrome. Circulation 101：616-623, 2000.）

移，心脏事件和心脏骤停存活或死亡累积发生率见图71-4。服用β受体阻滞剂之前有症状的患者，服用β受体阻滞剂之后，28%患者症状复发或3年内死亡。服用β受体阻滞剂之前经历心脏骤停存活的患者，服用β受体阻滞剂之后，14%患者在5年内经历另一次心脏骤停（存活或死亡）。

我们确定了33例LQTS患者在开始β受体阻滞剂治疗之后死亡，这些患者中76%在死亡时仍在服用规定剂量的β受体阻滞剂。这些死亡病例的平均年龄14±9岁，三分之二是女性，其QTc（QTc=0.53±0.06s）明显长于幸存者（QTc=0.49±0.05s）。总结这些死亡病例提示以下几点：β受体阻滞剂治疗不能绝对预防LQTS死亡；患者存在长期服用β受体阻滞剂的顺应性问题；QTc延长是具有重要意义的危险因素；死亡的危险性在女性较高，特别是在青春期。

所有的β受体阻滞剂治疗LQTS都具有相同的疗效吗？有关这一问题几乎没有科学依据。总之，我们赞成使用非选择性β受体阻滞剂，如普萘洛尔及纳多洛尔等，而不使用相对特异性β$_1$受体阻滞剂，如美托洛尔及阿替洛尔等。后一组药物常常用于LQTS伴有反应性气道疾病的患者或出现非选择性β受体阻滞剂副作用时，如嗜睡、失眠或明显的心动过缓等。虽然我们的β受体阻滞剂研究中没有发现量效关系[8]，但是在儿童必须随着其生长发育按每公斤体重维持适当剂量的β受体阻滞剂。

（三）起搏器

LQTS所伴发的恶性室性快速性心律失常可能是由窦性心动过缓和窦性停搏触发。当然，心动过缓也可能会因使用β受体阻滞剂而更加明显。LQTS的较严重类型由于不应期延长可能引起功能性2：1房室阻滞，特别是伴有窦性心动过缓年龄较小的儿童。不管心动过缓的病因是什么，缓慢的心率和/或长间歇可使心室复极的不均一性更加明显并触发心室后除极，心室后除极引发扭转型室性心动过速。

20世纪80年代后期和90年代初期，几组报告显示伴有不适当心动过缓的症状性LQTS患者生理性起搏后复发性晕厥减少。有些患者起搏频率增加可使QTc缩短。最近，报告了一个β受体阻滞剂治疗和持续起搏的LQTS高危患者的长期随访结果[9]。β受体阻滞剂和起搏（平均起搏频率82bpm）联合治疗的37例患者在平均6年随访期间，76%的患者无症状，但24%的患者在6年随访期间发生猝死或心脏骤停——不利的长期随访结果提示在这一组起搏治疗患者需要植入备用除颤器。

（四）植入式心脏复律除颤器

根据我们采用左侧颈交感神经切除术、β受体阻滞剂和起搏治疗LQTS的经验，单独或联合使用这些治疗手段仍然存在较高的死亡率。现在可以采用经静脉植入式心脏复律除颤器（ICD），其在LQTS患者的使用正在逐渐增加。在个体高危LQTS患者，ICD治疗结果是乐观的，对单个患者ICD可以挽救生命[10]。

我们最近对来自美国国际LQTS注册所登记的125例LQTS患者ICD治疗的临床经验进行回顾性分析[11]。这些ICD治疗患者43%是心脏骤停幸存的高危患者，15%是尽管采用β受体阻滞剂治疗仍有复发性晕厥的患者，42%是由于有症状、QTc间期延长以及近亲家族成员中存在LQTS相关的心脏性猝死而主管医师认定属高危的患者。ICD植入时患者的平均年龄为23岁。平均随访时间3年，125例ICD治疗患者中仅有2例死亡（1.6%）。其中一例6岁男孩是在基础麻醉时死亡，另一例21岁女性死亡病例为ICD植入后1年自杀。采用β受体阻滞剂治疗仍有心脏骤停或反复晕厥发作的植入ICD的LQTS患者（n=73）与未植入ICD的相匹配的另一组LQTS患者比较。这两组患者死亡累积发生率见图71-5。3年随访期间，本研究植入ICD组死亡累积危险度2%，未植入ICD

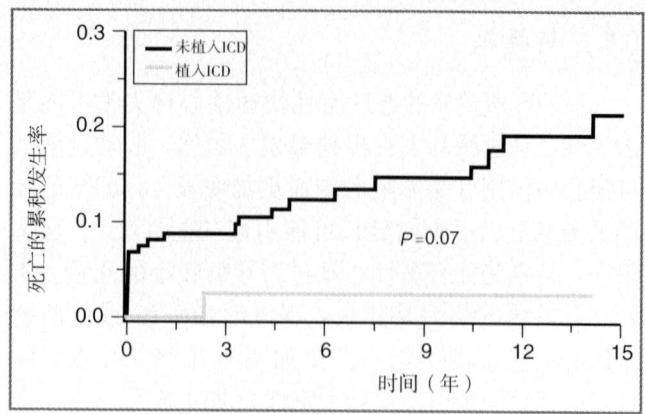

图 71-5 植入式心脏复律除颤器（ICD）治疗的高危 LQTS 患者（$n=73$）与未植入 ICD 相匹配的 LQTS 患者（$n=161$）死亡累积发生率的比较 （引自 Zareba W, Moss AJ, Daubert JP, et al：Implantable cardioverter-defibrillator in high-risk long-QT syndrome patients. J Cardiovasc Electrophysiol 14：337-341，2003.）

组为 11%。

这些来自国际 LQTS 注册的初步研究结果提示 ICD 治疗在高危 LQTS 患者是有效的。从 LQTS 患者相关猝死的不可预测性来看，ICD 治疗将可能在未来几年更广泛地用于治疗这一疾病。LQTS 患者 ICD 治疗潜在的问题包括 T 波超感知、儿童患者 ICD 体积差异、对除颤装置的情绪反应以及 ICD 植入和程控过程发生的外科并发症（如 ICD 植入部位皮肤破溃、伤口感染、静脉血栓形成及导线断裂等）。

偶尔，LQTS 患者可发生心律失常风暴，需反复电击来终止尖端扭转型室性心动过速和/或室颤。静脉追加 β 受体阻滞剂及增加除颤装置的起搏频率通常可使病情稳定，但是需要 24h 或更长时间来强化药物治疗。这种情况增加对心脏病学家治疗技能的要求和患者的情绪反应。尽管存在这些潜在的缺陷，ICD 治疗仍可能成为 LQTS 患者"确保安全"的备用治疗方法，尤其随着针对 LQTS 复极异常而特制的改进型装置的出现和临床经验的增加。

（五）基因特异性治疗

在 5 种 LQTS 基因中已鉴定出近 150 个不同的离子通道突变[12]，几乎每天都能鉴定出新的 LQTS 突变。大部分已鉴定出的 LQTS 突变包括 *LQTS1*、*LQTS2* 及 *LQTS3* 基因，在 3 种离子通道基因的 N 末端、跨膜片段及 C 末端部分广泛分布着突变。目前，仅有少数几个初步研究报告了基因特异性治疗结果。

1. LQTS1

大多数 *LQTS1* 突变的患者在运动或剧烈情绪反应期间发生过心脏事件，这些发现提示交感神经过度兴奋对触发这些事件的重要作用[8,13,14]。携带功能障碍 I_{Ks} 通道的 *LQTS1* 基因型患者一般对 β 受体阻滞剂治疗有效，大部分患者开始服药后或保持无症状或反复晕厥事件明显减少[8]。这些患者在接受 β 受体阻滞剂治疗时仅有少部分发生过心脏骤停而存活或猝死，但是应谨慎地解释这一结果，因为这些被治疗患者的随访期间没有发表相关文献。

2. LQTS2

LQTS2 突变的患者复极 I_{Kr} 电流减少，心脏事件似乎在运动、激动及睡眠/休息时均可发生。对 *LQTS2* 基因型患者，突然的听觉刺激唤醒似乎是特异性心脏事件触发因素[15,16]。增加细胞内 K^+ 浓度的治疗可有助于缩短这些患者的 QTc 间期，减少心脏事件，但是在这种治疗被推荐之前需要进一步研究。总之，β 受体阻滞剂对 *LQTS2* 及 *LQTS1* 突变的患者似乎都有效[8]，而 β 受体阻滞剂在 *LQTS2* 预防高音触发的心律失常可能特别有效。HERG 基因孔区突变的 *LQTS2* 患者心律失常相关的心脏事件风险显著高于无孔区突变的患者（图 71-6）[6]。初步结果提示 β 受体阻滞剂对伴有 *LQTS2* 孔区突变患者心脏事件风险的降低特别有效。

3. LQTS3

携带 *LQTS3* 突变的患者 I_{Na} 电流发生改变。*LQTS3* 基因型患者的心脏事件与其他两种基因型患者比较，似乎更常发生在休息时，心动过缓可能是这种基因型的触发因素。这类患者似乎完全能够耐受运动和活动，伴随心率加快时 QTc 生理性缩短。几项不同的研究提示 β 受体阻滞剂对 *LQTS3* 基因型患者可能不利[8,14]。起搏器可能有利于这类患者，最近对既有 *LQTS3* 基因型又有 Brugada 综合征（氨基酸编码突变位于 SCN5A：1795indD）的一个大家族进行研究发现，起搏器治疗可有效预防猝死的发生[17]。

已经报告了几种不同的 LQT3-SCN5A 突变，携带这种突变的患者的电生理特性和对钠离子通道阻滞剂的反应似乎有突变特异性。SCN5A ΔKPQ 缺失涉及跨膜片段Ⅲ与Ⅳ区域之间的连接点。这种突变损伤降低钠离子通道失活作用，并可使钠离子通道不适当

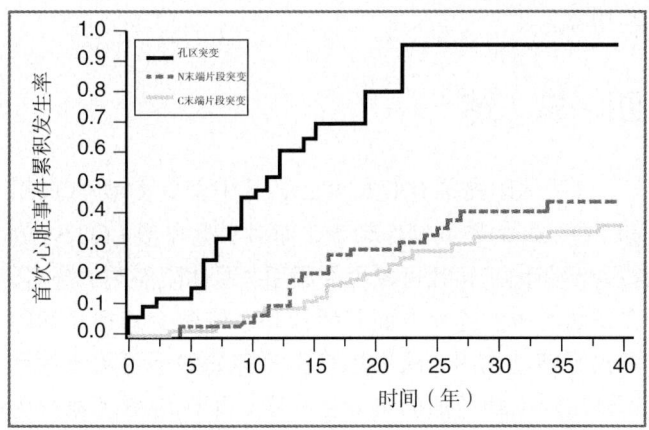

图71-6 *HERG* 基因孔区突变患者（*n*=34）、N 末端片段突变患者（*n*=54）及 C 末端片段突变患者（*n*=91）首次心脏事件累积发生率 曲线之间有显著性差异（*P*<0.001），差异主要是由于孔区突变患者存在较高的首次心脏事件发生率。（引自 Moss AJ, Zareba W, Kaufman ES, et al: Increased risk of arrhythmic events in long-QT syndrome with mutations in the pore region of the human ether-a-go-go-related gene potassium channel. Circulation 105：794-799，2002.）

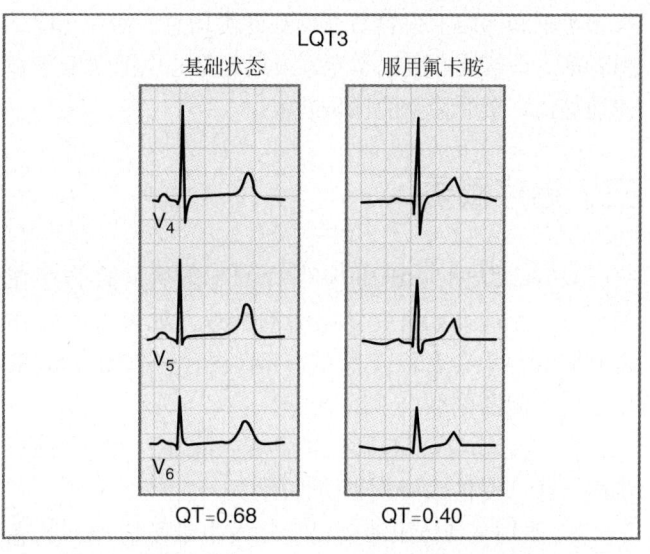

图71-7 *LQT3-SCN5A*（ΔKPQ）突变患者口服 100mg 氟卡胺之前（左图）和之后 8h（右图）心电图 QT 间期和 T 波形态 基础心电图 QT 间期 680ms，T 波明显高尖。服用氟卡胺后，QT 间期缩短至 400ms，T 波振幅正常。

重新开放，导致晚期钠离子内流，延长复极时间。钠离子通道阻滞剂如美西律及氟卡胺等，抑制晚期钠离子内流。5 例 *SCN5A* ΔKPQ 缺失患者短期小剂量服用氟卡胺，使每例患者 QTc 缩短并使 T 波复极形态正常化（图 71-7）[18]。*SCN5A* ΔKPQ 缺失患者的氟卡胺随机、安慰剂对照试验正在进行。

另一个 *LQT3-SCN5A* 突变涉及钠离子通道 α 亚单位 C 末端区域错义突变（D1790G）。这种突变改变钠通道失活动力学，对氟卡胺有特异性反应，与 *SCN5A* ΔKPQ 突变有明显区别[19]。初步研究报告显示，随访从 9 个月延长至 17 个月，氟卡胺使 8 例 *SCN5A* D1790G 突变携带者 QTc 缩短，无心脏不良反应[20]。

同时存在 *LQTS3* 基因型和 Brugada 综合征的 *SCN5A* 1795indD 突变，钳夹研究发现这种突变改变了钠通道的失活门控，使从功能依赖性氟卡胺阻滞恢复的时间延长 4 倍[21]。这一发现可说明氟卡胺在 Brugada 综合征的致心律失常作用是由于存在这一突变。

我们现在处在基因和突变特异性治疗的初期研究阶段。从已揭示的大量单基因突变及根据基因内突变的部位和类型产生的复杂电生理学和药理学作用来看，目前尚无基因和突变特异性药物治疗的特殊建议。

（六）总体建议

明确诊断 LQTS 的患者或根据临床资料、家族史及心电图 QTc 结果高度怀疑 LQTS 的患者，特异性药物和/或装置治疗仅是治疗手段的一部分。不论何种基因类型，LQTS 患者都应建议其避免可能触发致命性心律失常的环境刺激。应该减轻剧烈的门铃和电话铃声，在家里避免使用闹钟。避免暴露在突然出现高音的场合，如摇滚音乐会等。LQTS 患者不应参加竞技运动。应告知患者及其家属晕厥发作是非常严重的事件，应教育发作者在发作后积极寻求医疗关注。如果可能，应在家里配置自动体外除颤仪，家庭成员应接受自动体外除颤仪使用方法的培训。应让学校照顾患儿的主要负责人、保育员及教师了解患儿的情况，学校应配备适当的急救复苏设备。一旦开始 β 受体阻滞剂治疗，必须保持良好的依从性，因为在中断 β 受体阻滞剂时可能由于儿茶酚胺高敏反应性反跳而发生致命性心律失常。

避免使用不必要的药物，特别是兴奋剂、减肥药物、特定的抗生素及非处方药物等。应该指导 LQTS 患者或未成年 LQTS 患者的父母，避免使用可能对心室复极有不良影响的新处方药物。许多网站都有此类信息。因为有些药物的副作用和药物的相互作用可增加 LQTS 患者的危险，应指导患者让他们的医生在开新药处方时随时知道其患 LQTS，应鼓励 LQTS 患者要求其医生仔细地检查任何处方药物对 QT 间期的潜在作用。医师案头参考书和网络上很容易查询到此类信息。所有LQTS患者都应该接受心脏病学专家或最好是心电图学专家规律地随访，接受最新的预防措施。

三、治疗概要

1. 首次发生心脏事件的LQTS患者：除非存在禁忌证，都应开始β受体阻滞剂治疗。如果首次发作是心脏骤停幸存者，或者QTc延长超过520ms，应采用β受体阻滞剂联合ICD治疗。

2. 确诊LQTS的无症状患者：除非存在禁忌证，都应开始β受体阻滞剂预防性治疗。

3. 服用β受体阻滞剂仍反复发生晕厥的LQTS患者：如果患者有大小合适的可植入式除颤器最好给予ICD治疗。ICD治疗的同时应采用生理频率的备用起搏，以预防心动过缓触发的室性心律失常。如果高危婴儿由于身体太小不适合ICD治疗，左侧颈交感神经切除术可作为与β受体阻滞剂联合的辅助治疗。

4. 伴有反应性气道疾病的症状性LQTS患者：应试用保守剂量的心脏选择性β受体阻滞剂，如美托洛尔或阿替洛尔等。如果不能耐受β受体阻滞剂治疗，应改用ICD治疗。

5. 正在或想要妊娠的症状性LQTS患者：在整个妊娠期应持续接受β受体阻滞剂治疗，特别是在高危的产后期[22]。在妊娠期间包括妊娠的前3个月，β受体阻滞剂的益处远远比这类药物可能发生的胎儿畸形的风险更为重要。

6. 伴有Jervell和Lange-Nielsen综合征的高危LQTS婴儿：不论这种患儿是否有症状，致命性心律失常事件的风险都非常高。出生后短期内就应给予β受体阻滞剂和左侧颈交感神经切除术治疗，当患儿的身体生长到能够安全植入较小的ICD时应给予植入。对于很长的心室复极造成功能性心脏阻滞的婴儿，心室起搏可使病情稳定。

7. 植入ICD并经历心律失常风暴（由于反复恶性室性快速性心律失常反复适时电击）的高危LQTS患者：应静脉给予大剂量β受体阻滞剂加上频率80ppm临时心房起搏的辅助治疗，可使绝大多数反复室性快速性心律失常消失，但是需要24h或更长时间。可能需要低水平麻醉和气管插管辅助呼吸。

8. 携带LQT3-SCN5A突变的症状性LQTS患者：应植入ICD治疗，程控适当的生理性起搏频率。无症状的患者，如果窦性心率低于45bpm应植入心房起搏器。

四、总　结

β受体阻滞剂有效减少LQTS中常见类型LQTS1和LQTS2的晕厥发作频率，而对少见类型LQTS3的益处不明确。猝死可发生在服用β受体阻滞剂的患者。在预防心脏性猝死方面起搏器和左侧颈交感神经切除术仅有辅助作用。从LQTS患者猝死的不可预测性和ICD治疗不断增加的有效性来看，ICD应更多地作为这种疾病确保安全的治疗手段。

（吴立荣　译）

参 考 文 献

1. Benhorin J, Moss AJ, Bak M, et al: Variable expression of long QT syndrome among gene carriers from families with five different HERG mutations. Ann Noninvasive Electrocardiol 7:40–46, 2002.
2. Locati EH, Zareba W, Moss AJ, et al: Age- and sex-related differences in clinical manifestations in patients with congenital long-QT syndrome: Findings from the International LQTS Registry. Circulation 97:2237–2244, 1998.
3. Kimbrough J, Moss AJ, Zareba W, et al: Clinical implications for affected parents and siblings of probands with long-QT syndrome. Circulation 104:557–562, 2001.
4. Priori SG, Napolitano C, Schwartz PJ: Low penetrance in the long-QT syndrome: Clinical impact. Circulation 99:529–533, 1999.
5. Zareba W, Moss AJ, Schwartz PJ, et al: Influence of genotype on the clinical course of the long-QT syndrome. International Long-QT Syndrome Registry Research Group. N Engl J Med 339:960–965, 1998.
6. Moss AJ, Zareba W, Kaufman ES, et al: Increased risk of arrhythmic events in long-QT syndrome with mutations in the pore region of the human ether-a-go-go-related gene potassium channel. Circulation 105:794–799, 2002.
7. Cerrone M, Spazzolini C, Priori SG, et al: Left cardiac sympathetic denervation in the management of the long QT syndrome. A worldwide survey. Circulation 106(pt II):701, 2002.
8. Moss AJ, Zareba W, Hall WJ, et al: Effectiveness and limitations of beta-blocker therapy in congenital long-QT syndrome. Circulation 101:616–623, 2000.
9. Dorostkar PC, Eldar M, Belhassen B, Scheinman MM: Long-term follow-up of patients with long-QT syndrome treated with beta-blockers and continuous pacing. Circulation 100:2431–2436, 1999.
10. Moss AJ, Daubert JP: Internal ventricular defibrillation. N Engl J Med 342:398, 2000.
11. Zareba W, Moss AJ, Daubert JP, et al: Implantable cardioverter-defibrillator in high-risk long QT syndrome patients. J Cardiovasc Electrophysiol 14:337–341, 2003.
12. Splawski I, Shen J, Timothy KW, et al: Spectrum of mutations in long-QT syndrome genes. KVLQT1, HERG, SCN5A, KCNE1, and KCNE2. Circulation 102:1178–1185, 2000.
13. Ali RH, Zareba W, Moss AJ, et al: Clinical and genetic variables associated with acute arousal and nonarousal-related cardiac events among subjects with long QT syndrome. Am J Cardiol 85:457–461, 2000.
14. Schwartz PJ, Priori SG, Spazzolini C, et al: Genotype-phenotype correlation in the long-QT syndrome: Gene-specific triggers for life-threatening arrhythmias. Circulation 103:80–95, 2001.
15. Wilde AA, Jongbloed RJ, Doevendans PA, et al: Auditory stimuli as a trigger for arrhythmic events differentiate HERG-related (LQTS2) patients from KVLQT1-related patients (LQTS1). J Am Coll Cardiol 33:327–332, 1999.
16. Moss AJ, Robinson JL, Gessman L, et al: Comparison of clinical and genetic variables of cardiac events associated with loud noise versus

swimming among subjects with the long QT syndrome. Am J Cardiol 84:876–879, 1999.
17. van den Berg MP, Wilde AA, Viersma TJW, et al: Possible bradycardic mode of death and successful pacemaker treatment in a large family with features of long QT syndrome type 3 and Brugada syndrome. J Cardiovasc Electrophysiol 12:630–636, 2001.
18. Windle JR, Geletka RC, Moss AJ, et al: Normalization of ventricular repolarization with flecainide in long QT syndrome patients with SCN5A:ΔKPQ mutation. Ann Noninvasive Electrocardiol 6:153–158, 2001.
19. Abriel H, Cabo C, Wehrens XH, et al: Novel arrhythmogenic mechanism revealed by a long-QT syndrome mutation in the cardiac Na^+ channel. Circ Res 88:740–745, 2001.
20. Benhorin J, Taub R, Goldmit M, et al: Effects of flecainide in patients with new SCN5A mutation: Mutation-specific therapy for long-QT syndrome? Circulation 101:1698–1706, 2000.
21. Viswanathan PC, Bezzina CR, George AL Jr, et al: Gating-dependent mechanisms for flecainide action in SCN5A-linked arrhythmia syndromes. Circulation 104:1200–1205, 2001.
22. Rashba EJ, Zareba W, Moss AJ, et al: Influence of pregnancy on the risk for cardiac events in patients with hereditary long QT syndrome. LQTS Investigators. Circulation 97:451–456, 1998.

第 72 章

非器质性心脏病室性心动过速

本章目录

- 腺苷敏感性室性心动过速 ……………… 662
- 维拉帕米敏感性分支性室性心动过速 … 668

特发性室性心动过速（室速）是泛指起源于结构正常心脏的室性心动过速。此类心动过速在临床上分为几种特殊类型，它们不同的致心律失常机制也被电药理研究资料证实[1,2]。可以根据心动过速的起源部位、对抗心律失常药物的反应、儿茶酚胺的发作依赖性以及 QRS 波的形态对特发性室速进行分类。也可根据其发生机制进行分类（表 72-1）。一般来说，根据心动过速对程序刺激、腺苷、维拉帕米和普萘洛尔的反应，可区分其所属的类型。

一、腺苷敏感性室性心动过速

（一）机 制

起源于右室流出道（RVOT）的室性心动过速是特发性室速的最常见类型。起源于该部位的室速 60%~80% 见于心脏结构正常的患者。特发性右室流出道室速常常表现为两种类型：非持续性、反复发作的单形性室速（RMVT）；阵发性、运动诱发的持续性室性心动过速。上述两种类型的室速都具有腺苷敏感性[3]。

右室流出道室速的共同特征是：QRS 波形态呈左束支阻滞形态（LBBB），电轴右偏。当然，这种形态的心动过速，除 90% 起源于右室流出道外，另有 10% 起源于左室流出道（LVOT）。右室流出道室速的上述两种类型有很大的交叉重叠。例如，运动诱发的阵发性右室流出道室速也可同时出现频繁短阵的相同形态的非持续性室速；反复短阵的右室流出道室速在静脉滴注异丙肾上腺素或心腔内程序电刺激时也可诱发出相同类型的持续性室速。

迄今为止的大多数证据都支持触发活动是腺苷敏感性右室流出道室速的发生机制，而这一触发活动是由儿茶酚胺介导的延迟后除极（delayed afterdepolarizations，DADs）引起的[3-5]。儿茶酚胺刺激 β 肾上腺素受体导致细胞内环磷酸腺苷（cAMP）及 $(Ca^{2+})_i$ 的升高，使 Ca^{2+} 从肌浆网内自然释放至细胞浆内，激活了短暂的内向离子流（I_{Ti}），产生了延迟后除极。I_{Ti} 是由于 Na^+-Ca^{2+}（I_{NaCa}）交换的激活或是非特异性的 Ca^{2+}（$I_{NS[Ca]}$）[6] 激活离子流产生的。由于腺苷酸环化酶的激活和 $I_{Ca(L)}$ 是 cAMP 介导的触发活动的关键，因此触发性心律失常对一些电药理的干预措施是敏感的。如 β 受体阻滞剂、钙通道阻滞剂（维拉帕米）、刺激迷走神经和腺苷可有效终止触发性心律失常（图 72-1）。

除极少数情况外，腺苷均可以终止 cAMP 介导的触发活动所致的室速，这是机制特异性的。在没有 β 肾上腺素能刺激时，腺苷对于心室肌的静息电位、动作电位幅度和时程，或细胞内 cAMP 的水平是没有作用的。然而，cAMP 介导的动作电位变化可被腺苷削弱或完全逆转。由于腺苷可以减弱由异丙肾上腺素以及福斯高林（腺苷酸环化酶激活剂）诱导的 DADs 和 I_{Ti}，但对二丁基 cAMP 诱导的 DADs 和 I_{Ti} 却无减弱作用，说明腺苷的抗肾上腺素能作用发生在 cAMP 之前，即在腺苷酸环化酶的水平[7]。很明显，腺苷的电生理作用是由抑制性 G 蛋白（G_i）介导的，该蛋白质是 A_1 腺苷受体和腺苷酸环化酶的耦联剂，因此可降低细胞内 cAMP 的水平。

表 72-1 特发性单形性室性心动过速的分类

分类	腺苷敏感性室速（触发活动）	维拉帕米敏感性室速（分支性折返）	普萘洛尔敏感性室速（自律性增加）
特征	a. 运动诱发 b. 反复单形性室速	分支性	a. 运动诱发 b. 无休止性
诱发	程序刺激伴或不伴儿茶酚胺诱发	程序刺激伴或不伴儿茶酚胺诱发	儿茶酚胺诱发
形态	LBBB，电轴指向下 RBBB，电轴指向下	RBBB，电轴指向右上 RBBB，电轴指向右下	RBBB，LBBB，多形性
起源	右或左室流出道	左后分支，左前分支	右室/左室
拖带	不能	能	不能
机制	cAMP 介导的触发活动	折返	自律性增加
普萘洛尔	终止	无效	终止或短暂抑制
腺苷	终止	无效	短暂抑制
维拉帕米	终止	终止	无效

注：cAMP：环磷酸腺苷；RBBB：右束支阻滞；LBBB：左束支阻滞。（引自 Lerman BB, Stein KM, Markowitz SM: Idiopathic right ventricular outflow tract tachycardia: A clinical approach. Pacing Clin Electrophysiol 19: 2120-2137, 1996.）

产生延迟后除极有各个不同的因素，但腺苷的作用是特异性的，它对非 cAMP 介导（洋地黄导致 Na^+-K^+-ATP 酶的抑制）的延迟后除极和 I_{Ti} 是没有作用的。而且，腺苷对于奎尼丁和钙通道激活剂 Bay K8644[7] 诱导的 2 相早期后除极（EADs）也没有作用。特别有意义的是，腺苷对儿茶酚胺诱导的器质性心脏病患者的折返性心动过速也无效[8]。与此相似，腺苷对梗死区域浦肯野纤维、部分除极的心室肌或浦肯野细胞的低振幅动作电位也仅有轻微的抗肾上腺素作用。这些组织对腺苷不敏感的机制尚不清楚，可能认为与 A_1 腺苷受体的下调或 G 蛋白与受体的失耦联有关。

除腺苷以外的其他一些药物对鉴别触发活动也具有特异性。例如，维拉帕米可终止触发活动所致的室性心动过速，但该作用不具有特异性，因为它对缺血性心脏病室速、束支折返性室速和异常自律性室速同样有效。氟桂利嗪，可以通过非特异性机制降低细胞内 Ca^{2+} 浓度，被认为具有机制特异性的抗心律失常作用，它对折返性室速和异常自律性室速无效，但可终止延迟后除极触发活动所致的室速[9]。然而，和腺苷不一样，氟桂利嗪还可抑制毒毛花苷 G 介导的早期后除极。

尼可地尔是三磷酸腺苷（ATP）敏感性钾通道开放剂，具有抑制或终止腺苷敏感性室速的作用[10]。钾通道开放剂可以缩短动作电位时程并由此减少缓慢内向钙电流，其抗心律失常作用对于心动过速的机制来讲是非特异性的，因为这类药物同时消除毒毛花苷 G 介导的延迟后除极和早期后除极。这类药物对器质性心脏病折返性室速的作用尚未研究。

cAMP 介导触发活动所致的室速，其生化或分子生物学机制很重要但尚不清楚。几乎所有临床类型的室速均有其解剖学基质。而这一心动过速起源于右室流出道某一局灶组织（直径小于 1cm 的范围内），但并无解剖学异常。曾有假设认为包括 cAMP 在内的各信号转导通路的突变是该室速的电生理基础。在各种类型肾上腺素依赖性的右室流出道室速（非腺苷敏感性室速）患者的体细胞中，已发现抑制性 G 蛋白 $G_{\alpha i2}$ 亚单位的突变[11]。致心律失常病灶活检标本也发现 $G_{\alpha i2}$ 三磷酸鸟苷（GTP）结合区域的点突变（F200L）。这一突变增加了细胞内 cAMP 的水平并减轻了腺苷对于 cAMP 的抑制。由于去除了内源性腺苷的抗心律失

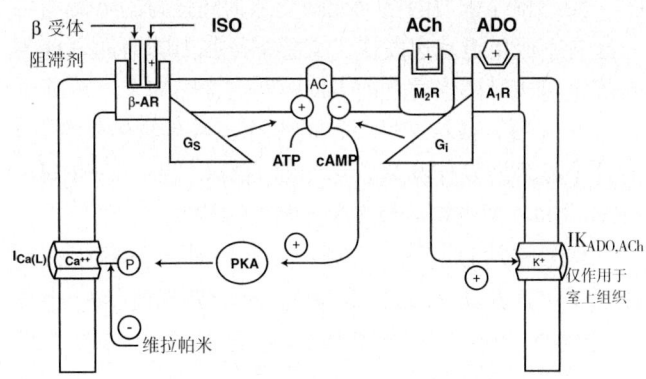

图 72-1 利用药理学方法确定由于细胞内钙超载致使 cAMP 介导心动过速的细胞模型示意图 A_1R：腺苷 A_1 受体；AC：腺苷酸环化酶；ACh：乙酰胆碱；ADO：腺苷；β-AR：β 肾上腺素受体；cAMP：环磷酸腺苷；ISO：异丙肾上腺素；G_i：抑制性 G 蛋白；G_s：兴奋性 G 蛋白；M_2R：毒蕈碱胆碱能受体；PKA：蛋白激酶 A。（引自 Lerman BB, Stein KM, Engelstein ED, et al. Mechanism of repetitive monomorphic ventricular tachycardia. Circulation 92: 421-429, 1995. Copyright 1995, AHA.）

常作用，导致细胞内 cAMP 浓度受肾上腺素刺激而增高，有利于产生室性心动过速（图 72-2）。目前尚未发现心动过速起源部位以外的心肌组织或外周淋巴细胞中 $G_{\alpha i2}$ 的突变。这些结果证明在心肌发育过程中 cAMP 依赖的信号转导通路突变，是一些类型右室流出道室速的病因。

（二）临床特征

右室流出道室速更常见于女性，大部分患者的初始发病年龄在 30~50 岁之间[12]。大多数患者在临床上呈良性病程，提示其潜在的病理过程是非进行性的，心动过速也并非是心肌病的早期表现。右室流出道频繁室性早搏的患者，其临床长期随访的结果也与心动过速患者一致[13]。

窦性节律时的心电图通常无特殊异常。大约有 10% 的右室流出道室速患者有完全性或不完全性的右束支阻滞。90% 的患者超声心动图检查正常。

25%~50% 的患者在运动试验时可以复制出心动过速。阳性结果可有两种类型：一类是在运动试验过程中发作心动过速；另一类是在运动恢复期内发作心动过速[14]。在非持续性反复发作的单形性室速患者，运动试验反而抑制其发作。这两种情况都反映了心动过速的发作依赖于某一关键的窦性心律频率。在运动恢复期内室速发作者，室性心动过速在运动时不被诱发是由于其诱发的频率窗口较窄。

交感神经张力的增加或副交感神经张力的降低均可引起右室流出道室速发作。交感神经张力的增加表现为短阵室速或早搏连发之前 RR 间期逐渐缩短[5]。短阵室速（2~4 跳）或持续性室速的发作也有生物钟性变化，有两个显著的发作高峰，一个是 7AM，另一是 5PM~6PM 之间，两者均可被 β 受体阻滞剂抑制[15]。

信号平均心电图（SAECGs）的时域分析在右室流出道室速患者常无异常发现。在 QRS 波信号滤波后的终末 40ms 或出现异常宽的低频、高幅信号（LAS）时，根据异常的平方根电压（RMS）可发现晚电位。滤波后的 QRS 波时限通常正常[16]。

虽然以往的研究报道特发性右室流出道室速无心脏结构的异常，但是利用核磁共振显像仔细检查右心室的结构和组织学特征时，可见局部室壁变薄、收缩期运动异常和脂肪组织浸润，这些变化在超声心电图检查和右心室造影时是难以发现的[17]。在我们的一组研究中，14 例腺苷敏感性室速患者经核磁共振显像发现 10 例有右室结构的异常，包括室壁变薄、局部室

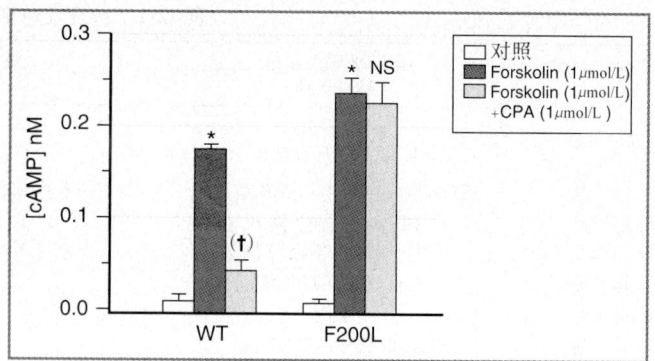

图 72-2　福斯高林（forskolin）和环戊基腺苷（CPA）对于转染人类腺苷 A_1 受体（hA_1R）基因的中华田鼠卵巢细胞 cAMP 水平的影响　被转染的田鼠又分为自然鼠（WT）和 $G_{\alpha i2}$ 变异鼠（F200L）两组。在 WT 转染鼠，福斯高林和对照组的 cAMP 有高度显著差异（$P<0.0001$）（†），而在 F200L 鼠，两组之间无差异（NS）。（引自 Lerman BB, Dong B, Stein KM, et al: Right ventricular outflow tract tachycardia due to a somatic cell mutation in G protein subunit α_{i2}. J Clin Invest 101: 2862-2868, 1998.）

壁运动异常和脂肪组织浸润[18]；而对照组 18 例仅 1 例发现异常。结构异常的最常见部位是右心室游离壁。但总体来说，结构异常部位和室速起源部位并不一定一致，且 30% 的此类室速患者并无结构异常。许多其他的研究也有类似的发现[19,20]。

无创显像技术也用来检测右室流出道室速患者心肌交感神经活性是否异常。大约 50% 的患者 [123]I-次碘苄基胍（[123]I-MIBG）闪烁图显示与铊的摄取不一致，提示有局部区域的交感神经变性[21,22]。但经激动标测和射频消融明确心动过速的起源点后，10 例患者中仅 1 例在邻近心动过速起源点附近区域发现扫描异常[21]。该技术的缺陷在于发现的局部异常局限于左心室，因为右室对 ^{123}I-MIBG 是不显像的。

正电子发射断层扫描（PET）发现，右室流出道室速患者去甲肾上腺素突触前再摄取有异常，这使得心肌神经肌肉接头处突触间隙去甲肾上腺素浓度增加[23]。然而，这些发现仅限于左室并缺乏特异性，因为去甲肾上腺素摄取降低也见于致心律失常性右室心肌病（ARVD）和冠心病室速患者。

右室流出道室速右室活检标本显示各种不同程度的发现，从完全正常到符合非特异性心肌病的各项异常[24]。病理检查发现心肌细胞肥厚、间质和血管周围纤维化、心肌炎症以及小血管内膜和中层硬化、管腔狭窄。但下列几点必须强调：（1）右室流出道室速患者心内膜活检所示的非特异性组织学异常与其无因果关系；

（2）由心肌活检标本来诊断致心律失常性右室心肌病需慎重；（3）正常心肌也可出现一些脂肪成分。

（三）心脏电生理诊断

腺苷、Valsalva 动作、颈动脉窦按压、腾喜龙、维拉帕米和 β 受体阻滞剂（图 72-1、图 72-3 和表 72-1）可终止室速，支持心动过速是由触发活动所致。该室速也可由程序刺激诱发和终止，但不能被拖带。

诱导触发活动依赖于患者当时的自主神经状态。处于深度麻醉状态的患者是很难被诱发。在临床上，该室速可在某次电生理检查时经各种程序刺激不能诱发，而在随后的再次电生理检查时却很容易被诱发，充分反映了此类患者自主神经功能状态的多变性。因此，一次电生理检查不能诱发室速并不能充分证明该心律失常是自律性或非触发活动所致。

为了增加诱发率，并进一步证实细胞内 cAMP 在介导触发活动中的作用，在电生理检查时可使用异丙肾上腺素、阿托品和氨茶碱[5]。如果单静滴异丙肾上腺素不能诱发心动过速，可重复给予快速刺激和程序刺激。若仍不能诱发，可突然终止异丙肾上腺素，有时心动过速可在撤药时发生。这类似于临床上运动时非持续性反复发作的单形性室速不发作，但在停止运动后发生（可能代表心动过速的发作依赖于某一频率窗口）。在再次滴注异丙肾上腺素后，可分别在程序电刺激前后再予以阿托品（0.04mg/kg）和氨茶碱（2.8mg/kg）。这些药物是为了缓解内源性乙酰胆碱和儿茶酚胺的抗心律失常作用，因为它们可能对 cAMP 有抑制作用。阿托品在上述剂量时，主要作为腺苷竞争性的拮抗剂，而不是磷酸二酯酶抑制剂。

（四）治　疗

右室流出道室速是否需要治疗取决于其发作频度和发作时的症状。如果发作少、发作时症状轻微，则并非必须治疗。如果室速发作时出现先兆晕厥或晕厥，或者室速频繁发作影响患者生活，此时可选择导管射频消融术去除致心律失常病灶。临床上大多数患者的症状介于上述两者之间，对于这些患者的治疗，除导管射频消融以外，药物治疗也是方法之一。

抗心律失常治疗有效性的评估依赖于动态心电图监测、运动试验和程序电刺激。然而这些方法都有其局限性，因为右室流出道室速对自主神经的张力有高度敏感性，因此每日发作的变异性非常大。幸运的是，右室流出道室速对各种抗心律失常治疗措施的敏感性远远超过其他器质性心脏病室速。另一值得注意的是此类室速对各类抗心律失常药物都敏感。

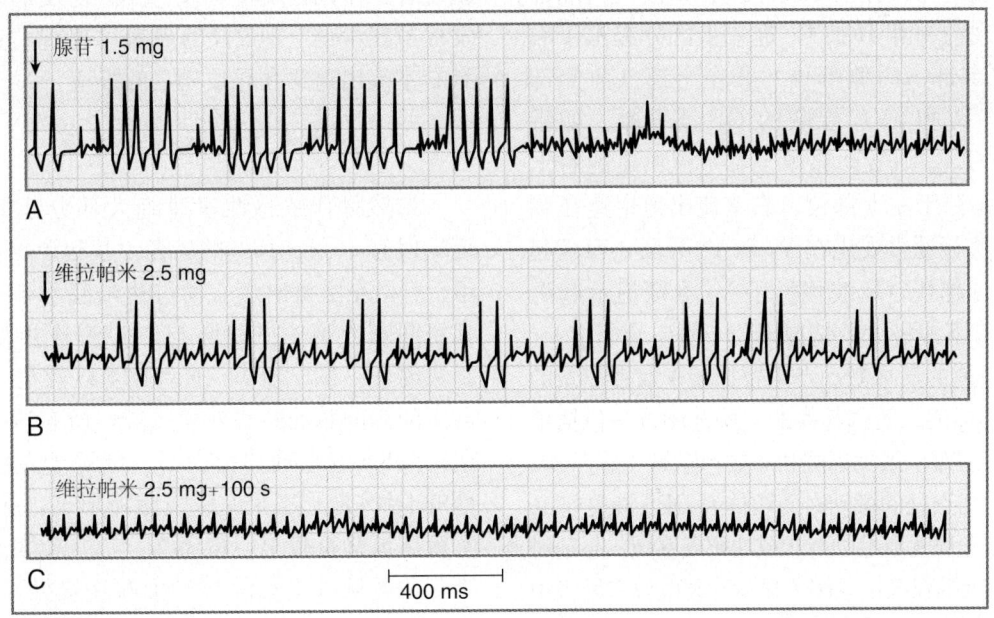

图 72-3　体表心电图连续记录无休止性 RMVT 被药物终止的过程　A：垂直箭头表示推注腺苷并予以生理盐水冲洗完毕。B：无休止性 RMVT 予以维拉帕米静注，箭头处提示注射完毕。C：维拉帕米注射后 100s 心动过速终止。记录导联为体表心电图 Ⅱ 导联。（引自 Lerman BB，Stein K，Engelestein ED，et al：Mechanism of repetitive monomorphic ventricular tachycardia. Circulation 92：421-429. 1995. Copyright 1995，AHA.）

抗心律失常治疗通常首选β受体阻滞剂。约25%～50%的患者该类药物有效且耐受性好。钙通道阻滞剂的有效性在25%～30%，维拉帕米和地尔硫䓬的效果相等。钙通道阻滞剂和β受体阻滞剂联合应用有协同作用。I类抗心律失常药物对右室流出道室速也有效，如IA类药物中的普鲁卡因胺、奎尼丁和IC类药物中的氟卡胺、英卡胺，它们对25%～50%的患者有效。Ⅲ类抗心律失常药物如索他洛尔、胺碘酮的效果更优于上述药物。

右室流出道室速的急性终止可有一系列方法。首先可通过Valsalva动作或颈动脉窦按压增加迷走神经张力来终止心动过速。如此法无效，可静脉推注腺苷（6～24mg）。静脉注射维拉帕米（10mg）也是方法之一，约75%的患者静脉弹丸注射后1～2min有效。另外，利多卡因也是有效药物之一。

右室流出道室速的电生理特征使得该心律失常易于经消融术治愈，因为该心动过速的起源点比较局限，且导管操作容易到位。心动过速的12导联心电图有利于初步判断其起源部位[25]。起源于右室流出道游离壁的室速，其心动过速的QRS波时限常大于140ms，起源于右室流出道间隔部的室速，其QRS波时限小于或等于140ms。因为后者在激动心室时利用了间隔面的浦氏纤维网。相似地，起源于右室流出道游离壁的室速，由于顺序地激动右心室和左心室，其在Ⅱ、Ⅲ导联表现为顿挫的RR′波或Rr波（间隔部起源的室速表现为单相R波）。进一步区分起源于右室流出道的右半部（后侧部位）和左半部（前侧部位）需根据aVR和aVL导联的QS波振幅。如果aVR$_{(QS)}$大于aVL$_{(QS)}$则激动起源于右室流出道的右上部位，反之则起源于左上部位。右室流出道室速在胸前导联的R波移行通常发生在V_2和V_4导联，而且起源部位越高移行越快。R波移行于V_2导联提示起源点紧靠肺动脉瓣下或极少数情况下位于左室流出道。

识别心动过速的最早激动点主要依赖于双极记录的激动标测和起搏标测。还有其他的一些标测方法包括单极心电图记录、三维电解剖标测和非接触标测（图72-4）。一般来说，成功靶点处的激动时间较体表QRS波提前10～45ms，但该领先程度不足以与非成功靶点鉴别。心动过速时，成功靶点处的双极记录图不显示碎裂电位和舒张中期电位。单极记录图对确定各种心律失常的最早激动点也是有效的，最早激动点的单极记录图特征性地显示为起始的负向波（因为激动方向是背离记录电极的）。

虽然起搏标测在识别成功靶点时更为常用，但其精确性尚有不足。心动过速起源点周围8mm范围内都可以获得满意的起搏图形[26]。起搏时既可以用单极也可以用近极距的双极，使用两倍舒张期阈值的起搏强度，这样可排除远场的刺激干扰。起搏标测在窦律下进行，周长与心动过速的周期相一致。通过比较起搏与心动过速时12导联QRS波的R/S比例及微小的切迹变化来计分。满意的起搏标测至少是11个导联图形一致，最好是12导联完全一致。

操纵消融导管时首先将其放置于肺动脉，然后轻轻回撤至右室流出道，紧挨着肺动脉瓣下缘。导管位置的确认可根据局部心内电图或4mA以内的起搏阈值夺获心肌。操作时通过旋转导管可至右室流出道的任何部位。导管放置可在二维影像或三维标测系统指导下进行。

大部分成功消融靶点位于右室流出道的间隔侧，紧靠肺动脉下缘。于成功靶点处放电时可导致快速的心室反应，其QRS波形态与室速时完全一致，随着放电时间的延长该心室节律逐渐减慢并完全消失，此现象类似于慢径消融时的交界性心律。成功靶点处的这一现象具有高度特异性，但敏感性较低[27]。在一些病人，放电后可导致心动过速QRS波形态的轻微变化，同时可伴有标测导管记录时间的轻微变化，这可能是由于同一局灶激动的不同出口或较弥散的局灶激动所致。后者需要在相邻区域作多点消融方能去除致心律失常病灶[28]。90%的患者消融可获成功，而且儿童与青少年同样安全有效[29-31]。复发率可达10%。并发症虽然少见，但2%的患者可出现右束支阻滞，且有右室流出道穿孔导致死亡的报道。

（五）左室流出道室性心动过速

虽然腺苷敏感性室速绝大部分起源于右室流出道，但有10%～15%的患者，其起源点位于左室流出道[2,32]。左室流出道心动过速可起源于多个部位，包括室间隔上部、主动脉与二尖瓣连接处（图72-5）、二尖瓣环（图72-6）、主动脉窦以及位于心大静脉和前室间沟静脉处的心外膜区域，所有这些部位心动过速的QRS波电轴均指向下。起源于左室流出道间隔部的QRS波形态呈左束支阻滞形态，胸导联QRS左室流出道移行较早，位于V_1、V_2导联；起源于左纤维三角区域（主动脉与二尖瓣连接处）的QRS波在V_1呈右束支阻滞形态，全部胸导联为宽而单相的R波。由于主动脉瓣位于右室流出道的右后方，因此起源于主动脉窦的心动过速虽呈左束支阻滞形态，但其V_1、V_2导联的R波较右室流出道心动过速高而宽（R/QRS波时限＞50%，R/S振幅＞30%）[33]。V_2导位。消融结束后必须立即行冠状动脉造影以排除冠状动脉痉挛、夹层或血栓形成。在主动脉瓣下消融其他左室流出道心动过速时，也可引起左冠状动脉主干的闭塞。消融时也可发生主动脉瓣的损伤。

腺苷敏感性左室流出道心动过速很少起源于心外膜。如起源于心外膜，则表现为 V_1 导联高大的 R 波和 V_2 导联的 S 波，胸导联 R 波移行发生于 $V_2 \sim V_4$ 导联，aVL 导联表现为深的 QS 图形和下壁导联高大的 R 波[37]。如在心内膜面不能找到最佳的起搏标测图形，最早激动点处的心室波前有一低幅的远场电位也提示心动过速起源于心外膜。在冠状静脉系统内放置小而柔软并有多个电极的导管可进行心外膜标测（图72-7）。逆行冠状静脉窦造影并双平面显像可观察到冠状静脉的各个分支。在经冠状静脉行心外膜消融时，应同时行冠状动脉和冠状静脉的造影以显示靶静脉和相邻动脉的空间关系。在相邻冠状动脉内行血管内超声检查并监测放电可避免局部热损伤。消融后必须重复冠状动脉造影和心脏超声检查以排除心外膜出血。成功消融靶点常位于后侧静脉（左室侧壁）、心大静脉和前室间沟静脉。经皮穿刺于心包腔内行心外膜标测也是可选择的方法之一[35]。最后，临床上还有一种少见的、变异型的腺苷敏感性室速，它既可呈左束支阻滞形态，也可呈右束支阻滞形态，两者电轴相同。这种心动过速起源于心室间隔内，其激动出口既可以在间隔左侧，也可以在间隔右侧。

（六）鉴别诊断

在排除冠心病以后，左室流出道室性心动过速应考虑以下一些病因。临床医生应首先警惕致心律失常性右室心肌病。致心律失常性右室心肌病患者发病年龄较轻，心动过速易受儿茶酚胺激发，可起源于右室流出道并表现为非持续性反复发作的单形性室速。体表心电图呈右束支阻滞并伴有右胸导联 T 波倒置是致心律失常性右室心肌病的可能线索。因为超声心动图和右室造影不能显示轻微的结构异常，因此需做 MRI 显像。右室活检可以提供纤维组织和脂肪组织沉着的组织学依据。其次需要鉴别的是法洛四联症修补术后的室性心动过速。该心动过速可以被拖带，且对腺苷和维拉帕米不敏感。房束纤维和结室纤维介导的心动过速对腺苷和维拉帕米都敏感，但电轴左偏，且心动过速时希氏束电位在心室激动之后。束支折返性心动过速通常呈左束支阻滞形态，心动过速时的 HV 间期大于或等于窦律时的 HV 间期，该心动过速对腺苷不

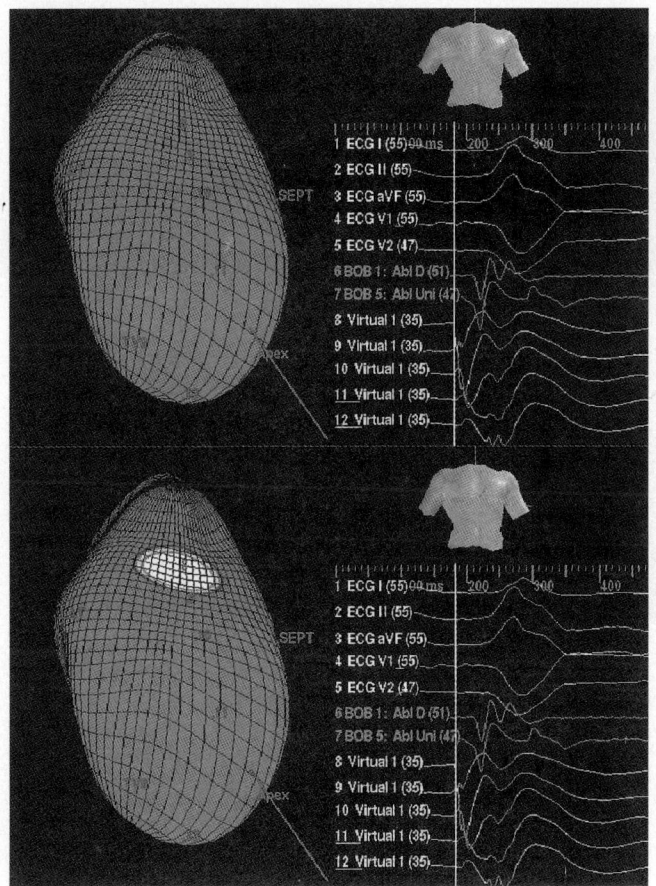

图72-4 起源于右心室流出道室性早搏的非接触标测　上图：示右心室处于电学舒张期，右侧为模型中 8～12 点处的虚拟电图。下图：显示室性早搏的最早激动点处（白色区域），该早搏形态与临床室性心动过速的形态一致。最早激动点处（点 8）的单极虚拟电图呈 QS 图形，而偏离该处的其他点均有起始的 R 波。（见彩图 34）

联 S 波和下壁导联相对高大的 R 波提示心动过速起源点接近于主动脉窦心外膜侧。这种心律失常可能来源于左、右冠状动脉窦基底部的弦月状心肌[34]。相比较而言，无冠状动脉窦的基底部是由结缔组织组成的，它与二尖瓣相连，心动过速极少起源于此处，而多见于左冠状动脉窦，其次为右冠状动脉窦。

左、右冠状动脉窦内消融是可行的，但必须非常谨慎以免伤及冠状动脉。此处起搏标测夺获局部心肌必须用很高的能量输出[35,36]。局部腔内电图可同时记录到心房波和心室波，因为左冠状动脉窦与左心耳非常靠近，右心耳也非常邻近于右冠状动脉窦。消融前应在主动脉根部造影显示右冠状动脉和左冠状动脉主干的开口。在左冠状动脉窦内消融时，左冠状动脉主干必须插管作为影像标志。消融靶点通常必须在离冠状动脉开口 10mm 以上的位置[33]，消融时调整功率在 15～30W 使得局部温度达 55℃。放电时必须连续透视以免导管移

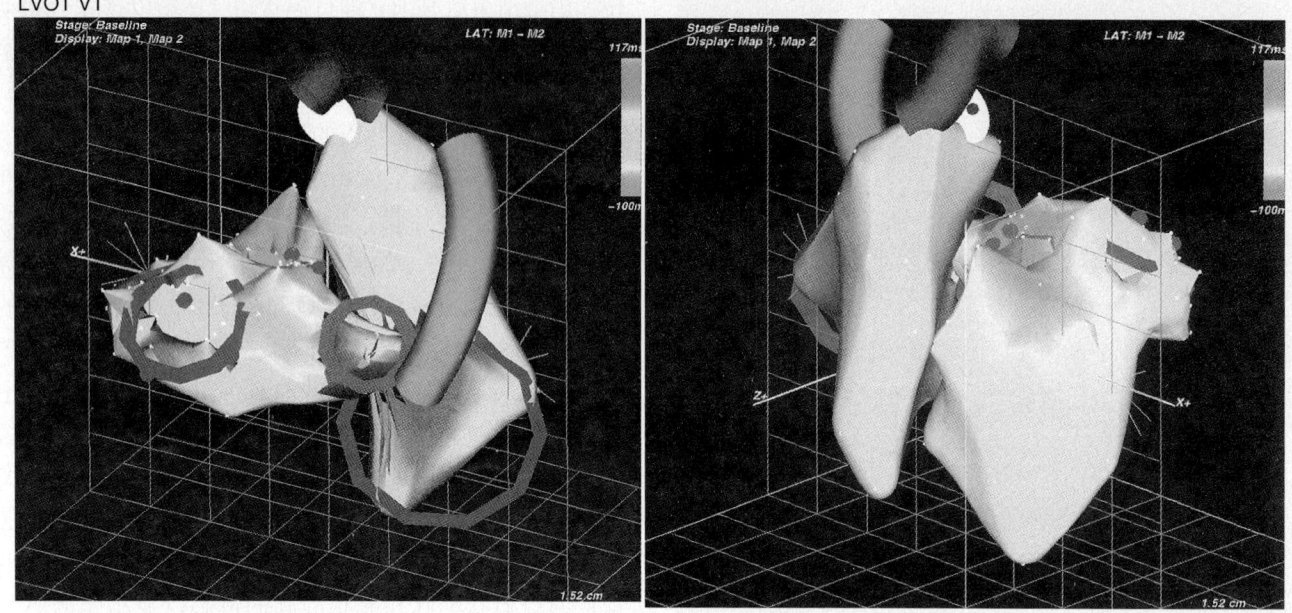

图 72-5 起源于主动脉与二尖瓣连接处的左室流出道心动过速 左图为室性心动过速时电解剖标测图（后前位），三尖瓣环、二尖瓣环及主动脉瓣环均显示在模型中，红色管道为主动脉，灰色区域为肺动脉。心动过速的最早激动点呈红色。右图（前后位）显示消融点位于主动脉与二尖瓣连接处（暗红色点）。（见彩图 35）

敏感。起源于左前分支的心动过速常被误诊为左室流出道室速，其鉴别关键在于前者在多个胸导联具有明显的 S 波、腔内电图有浦氏纤维电位并对腺苷不敏感。

二、维拉帕米敏感性分支性室性心动过速

（一）临床特征

特发性左室室性心动过速的最常见类型是维拉帕米敏感性分支性室速，它起源于左后分支区域，呈

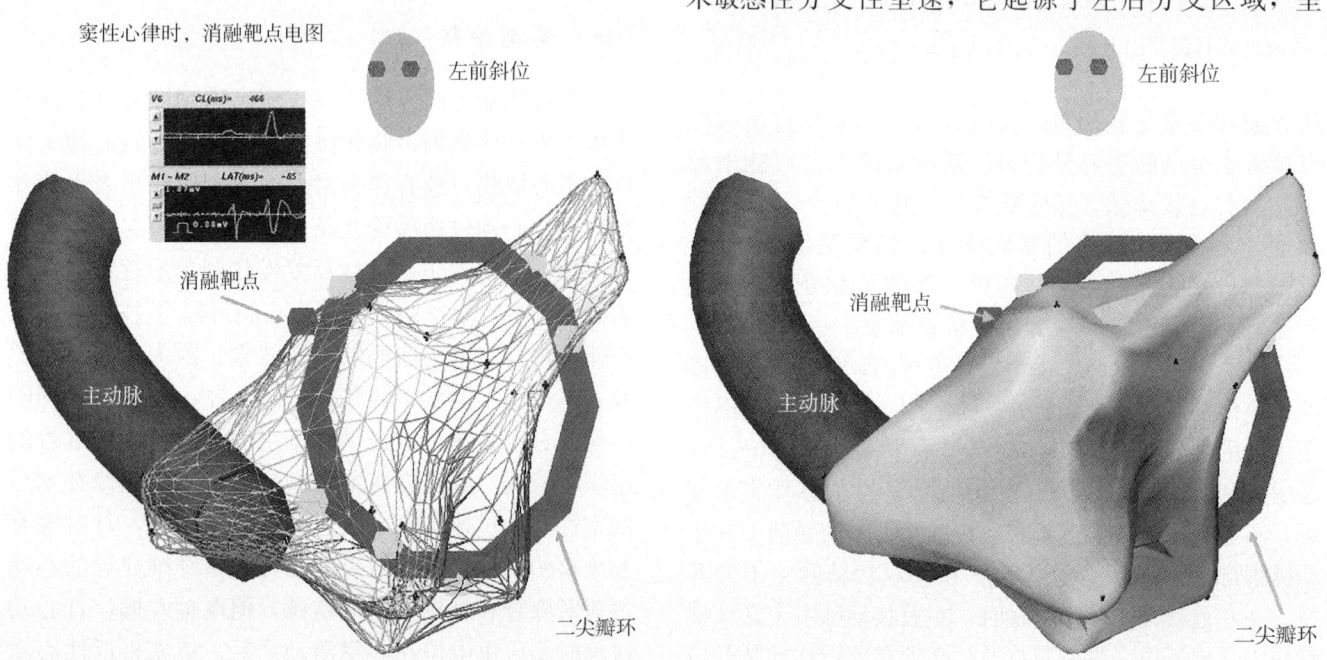

图 72-6 起源于二尖瓣区域的左室室速 左图示窦律下构建的左室栅格状几何图形。成功靶点处的腔内电图显示在左上角有较大的心房和心室波，提示该点邻近二尖瓣环。右图为心动过速时的激动顺序图。（见彩图 36）

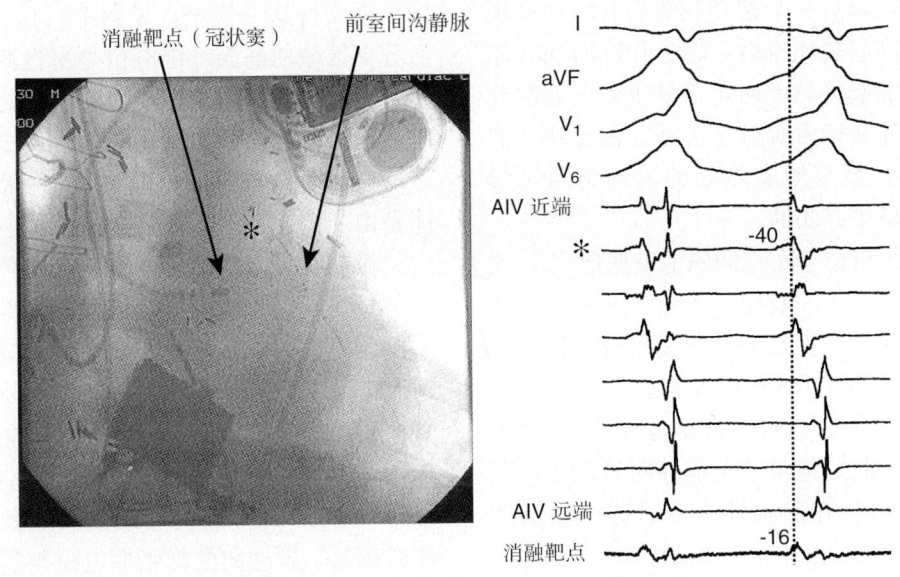

图 72-7　起源于心外膜的左室流出道心动过速　将一多极导管放置于前室间沟静脉（AIV），心动过速时于 AIV 和心大静脉交界处记录到最早的激动，它较左室流出道和右室流出道腔内电图领先 24ms（*处），其次为位于左冠状动脉窦的记录电图。（由于室性心动过速与陈旧性心肌梗死有关，患者已安装 ICD。）

右束支阻滞形态和电轴左偏的特征性形态。分支性室速患者的发病年龄常在 15～40 岁，大约 60%～80% 的患者是男性[12]。窦律时的心电图并无异常，但在心动过速终止后可有下壁和侧壁导联短暂而非特异的 T 波变化。冠状动脉造影和左室功能一般正常。分支性室速可以无休止发作并导致心动过速心肌病。这种类型心动过速一般不引起心源性猝死。

早期都认为分支性室速主要发生于休息时，但该心动过速发作也有儿茶酚胺依赖性（如运动和运动后），并受情绪紧张激发[2,38]。心动过速呈右束支阻滞形态，90%～95% 的患者电轴左偏，提示激动出口位于左后分支区域，紧靠左室间隔的后下部。如心动过速出口位于心尖偏下壁部位时，其电轴显著右偏。剩余部分的分支性室速起源于左前分支区域，激动出口靠近左室间隔面的前上方，其 QRS 波呈右束支阻滞形态，电轴轻度右偏。信号平均电图的时域分析无异常发现。左室活检的组织学检查多无异常发现或显示轻微的纤维化和脂肪组织浸润。

（二）解剖学基质

分支性室速的解剖学基础一度引起广泛的兴趣。心动过速时的心内膜标测发现最早激动点位于左室间隔的后下部。这一发现，结合心动过速时 QRS 波的特征性形态以及短的 VH 间期，提示心动过速起源于左后分支。心动过速时最早心室激动点之前可记录到高频电位，该电位在窦律时也可记录到，这些证据提示心动过速起源于左后分支浦氏纤维网[38]。上述电位被认为是浦氏纤维的激动，并可在左室间隔面三分之一的部位记录到。在浦氏纤维电位领先于心室激动 30～40ms 处放电可成功根治心动过速，提示心动过速起源于浦氏纤维的邻近组织。近来的一些研究认为，分支性室速具有一个大折返环，其一支由左后分支组成，另一支则为具有递减传导功能的异常浦氏纤维。浦氏纤维电位之前的舒张期电位被认为是异常浦氏纤维的电活动[39-42]（图72-8）（见下文"机制"一节）。

心动过速折返环的部分还可来源于左室假腱索或由左室后下部向间隔部延伸的纤维化肌性带。通过激光光凝技术、切除、冷冻腱索的心肌附着端或射频消融腱索的间隔插入端均有根除心动过速的报道。对这些患者手术切除的假腱索行组织学检查发现，浦氏纤维沿腱索的长轴排列并插入心内膜[43]。

假腱索在左后分支性室速有较高的发生率[44]，但这一发现的特异性尚有争议[45]。假腱索作为心动过速折返环的一部分或是左室间隔面浦氏纤维之间的一个连接，均可使心动过速得以发生，这一推测是可能的。

（三）机　制

虽然争论的焦点在于分支性室速的机制是折返还是触发活动（后者的理由是心动过速对内向缓慢钙通道阻滞剂敏感），但绝大多数证据还是支持折返机制。心动过速可被拖带支持折返机制。例如，拖带起搏时产生固定性融合波,最后一个被夺获的心室激动被拖带但没有融合;提高起搏频率时,融合程度增加并趋于固定;进一步增加起搏频率时,最早激动点处的腔内电图提示由正向夺获转为逆向夺获[46]。需要注意的是,在正向夺获时,最早激动点处的激动是通过缓慢、递减传导的区域来夺获的。

缓慢传导区的入口位于左室间隔的基底部[42],这可以解释为什么显性拖带在右室流出道比右室心尖部更容易。在缓慢传导区的近端如右室流出道起搏,容易产生显性拖带并出现 QRS 波的融合。但在距离入口相对远的右室心尖部(与右室流出道相比),由于可激动间隙相对窄,此处拖带的可能性明显减小。这个假定的入口和出口将在隐匿性拖带时进一步阐述(图 72-9)。

根据现有的一些不同研究资料,假设了一个心动过速的折返环路模型。在该模型中,折返激动的前传支是由异常的浦肯野纤维构成,该组织具有缓慢、递减传导的特性,对维拉帕米敏感,其在左室间隔面产生舒张期电位(图 72-10A)。逆传支由左后分支或邻近的其他分支组成,产生浦氏电位。前向传导路径的产生可能与后分支的纵向分离有关,也可能与直接耦联于左后分支区域的邻近组织(如假腱索)有关,该邻近组织与心室肌相连。窦性节律下的折返环路示意图见图 72-10B(心动过速时激动环路恰好相反)。临床证据支持这一模型,见图 72-11。在左图(A),左后分支区域的浦氏纤维电位是窦性激动由近向远前向传导产生的,该电位均在心室激动之前。在心室激动之后,有融合而延迟的正向或负向电位(这很可能是心动过速时的舒张期电位)。这一激动顺序的原因可能是由于左后分支前向传导的速度较快。相比较而言,激动在异常的浦氏纤维内前向传导速度较慢。由于传导速度慢,或传导在近端某一部位受阻,使左后分支的前向激动有机会逆向激动该异常纤维(图 72-10A)。心室程序刺激时,该异常纤维的激动顺序相反并使心动过速发生。心室起搏后,浦氏纤维系统和希氏束均由左后分支来逆向激动(图 72-11B)。基础刺激时(S_1),异常浦氏纤维被双向激动,该顺序与窦律时相反,即逆向的舒张期电位与逆向的浦氏纤维电相位平行;而前向的舒张期电位在逆向浦氏激动完成之后。加入早搏刺激时(S_2),异常浦氏纤维的逆向传导受阻,该纤维由逆向浦氏激动前向兴奋。更提前的早搏刺激使异常浦氏纤维的前向传导足够缓慢,覆盖整个舒张期并逆向激动浦氏纤维使折返激动得以完成,从而发生心动过速(图 72-11C)。因此,心动过速时的舒张期电位代表折返激动前传支的兴奋,而浦氏纤维电位代表逆传支的激动,环路下端两者相接之处的浦氏纤维电位最早(图 72-10A)。

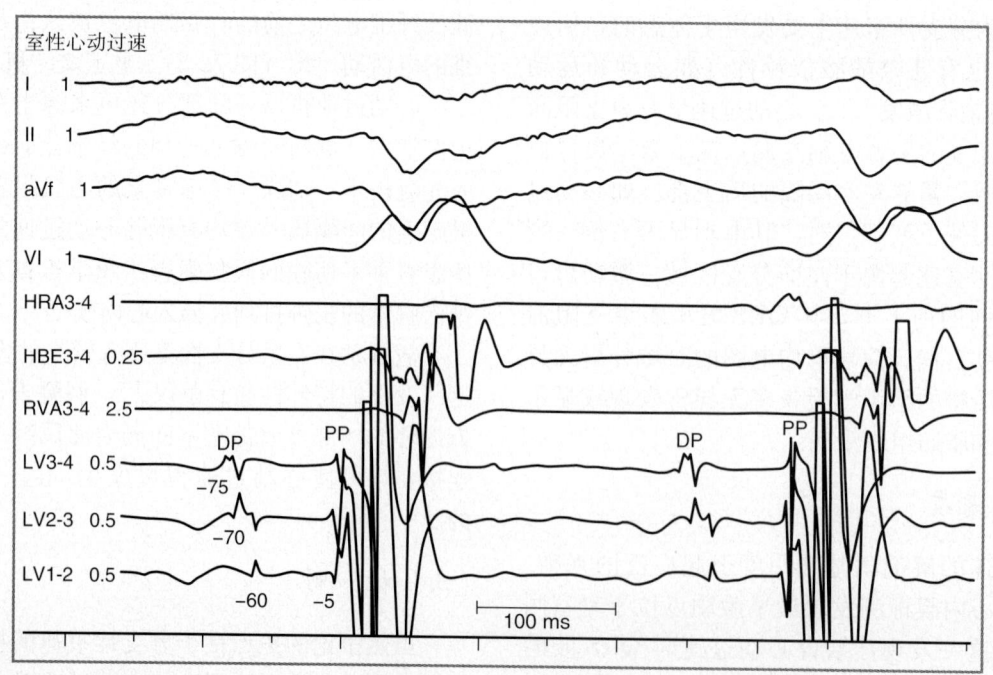

图 72-8 心动过速时于左室间隔中部记录到的浦氏纤维电位　左室记录电极(LV)由近到远,图示舒张期电位(DP)由近向远激动,而浦氏电位(PP)由远向近。HRA:高位右心房;RVA:右室心尖部。(引自 Nogami A,Naito S,Toda H,et al: Demonstration of diastolic and presystolic Purkinje potentials as critical potentials in a macroreentry circuit of verapamil-sensitive idiopathic left ventricular tachycardia. J Am Coll Cardiol 36: 811-823, 2000. Copyright 2000, ACC.)

缓慢传导区的缓慢传导似乎依赖于缓慢的内向钙流，因为心动过速周期延长的程度取决于维拉帕米对缓慢传导区的负性传导作用。利多卡因对心动过速频率的影响程度要小得多[47]。这些结果表明，构成折返环的浦氏纤维在静息时已部分除极，而其除极更多依赖于缓慢内向的钙电流，较少依赖受抑制的快速钠通道。

分支性室速有一特征性的电药理背景。和其他类型特发性室速相似，它对维拉帕米敏感，但又和右室流出道室速不同，腺苷和 Valsalva 动作无效[48]。这些反应有利于在临床上区分不同类型的特发性室速和鉴别其机制。另外这些特点还提示，虽然心动过速的基质是钙依赖性的，但参与心动过速的折返组织是部分除极的浦氏纤维，它们的除极依赖于缓慢内向的离子流。相对而言，右室流出道室速是由触发活动所产生的，其触发活性依赖于细胞内钙离子超载，而这些超载的钙离子是由于 cAMP 刺激和钙离子通透性增加所致。在我们的一组研究与这些理论相一致，26 例左后分支室速无一例被腺苷或三磷酸腺苷终止，而其中 24 例可被维拉帕米终止。这些心动过速在终止前均出现窦律与短阵心动过速相交替的现象，支持心动过速由触发机制引起。只有在一种情况下，该心动过速可被腺苷终止，即心动过速的发作依赖于儿茶酚胺的刺激（静脉滴注异丙肾上腺素）[8]。但绝大多数分支性室速患者在基础状态，其缓慢内向钙流就足以激发和维持心动过速，无需儿茶酚胺刺激，因此对腺苷不敏感。这种对腺苷的双重反应似乎是此类室速所特有的，因为在器质性心脏病室速，即使发作依赖于儿茶酚胺刺激，其心动过速也不能被腺苷终止。

（四）治　疗

虽然分支性室速急性发作时，静脉推注维拉帕米有肯定的疗效，但有关其发作间歇期抗心律失常疗效的临床资料尚较少。维拉帕米 160～320mg/d 对于心动过速中等程度发作的患者可缓解症状，而对于严重发作并伴有心动过速心肌病的患者则效果不佳。

对于分支性室速发作时伴有晕厥或先兆晕厥、心动过速反复发作不能耐受抗心律失常药物治疗或药物治疗无效的患者，应考虑导管射频消融治疗。射频消融的结果与右室流出道室速的消融结果相似，成功率在 90% 左右[38-42]。各种消融并发症尽管罕见，但均有报道，包括消融导管缠绕于二尖瓣瓣叶的某一腱索，

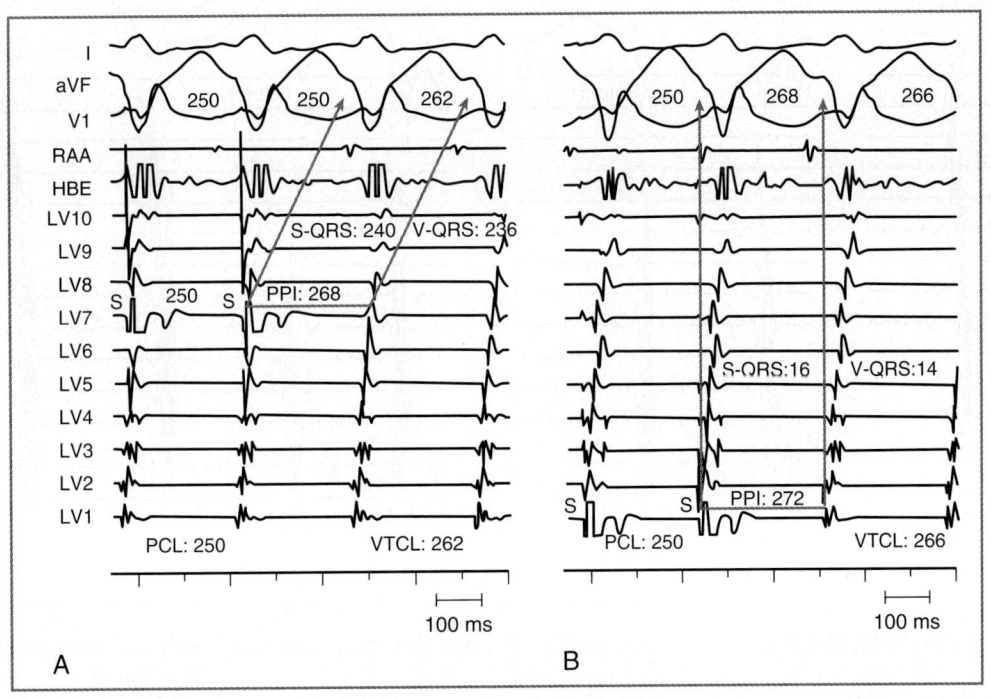

图 72-9　分支性室速缓慢传导区入口附近（A）和出口附近（B）的隐匿性拖带　左室记录电极横跨室间隔的缓慢传导区，入口处起搏点位于间隔中部，出口处起搏点位于间隔近心尖部。图中所有数据均以 ms 表示。PCL：起搏周期；PPI：起搏后间期；S-QRS：刺激信号与 QRS 波起始部的间距；V-QRS：心室局部电位与 QRS 波的间距；VTCL：室速周期。（引自 Maruyama M，Tadera T，Miyamoto S，et al：Demonstration of the reentrant circuit of verapamil-sensitive idiopathic left ventricular tachycardia：Direct evidence for macroreentry as the underlying mechanism. J Cardiolvasc Electrophysiol 12：968-972，2001.Copyright 2001，Futura Publishing CO.）

腱索损伤导致二尖瓣关闭不全；也有由于逆行法操纵导管损伤主动脉瓣导致主动脉瓣关闭不全的报道。

临床上曾应用多种标测策略来寻找最佳消融位点。早期曾用起搏标测寻找起搏图形与心动过速 12 导联心电图形态完全一致的位点，或在心动过速时标测比体表 QRS 波提前 30ms 的靶点。另一标测方法是在左后分支区域最早心室激动前寻找浦氏纤维电位[38]，但这些电位在窦性节律的心室激动前就存在，它代表了左后分支浦氏纤维网的激动，不能完全代表有效靶点。

近年来，临床上越来越重视心动过速时的舒张期电位。这些电位在心动过速时出现在浦氏纤维电位前，可在左室间隔中部 25mm 的范围内记录到。在成功消融靶点处放电时可使舒张期电位和浦氏纤维电位间期逐渐延长，直至传导阻滞使心动过速终止[39,40]。在最早的舒张期电位处消融不一定预示成功。而在最早舒张期电位稍远端消融可致成功，这也降低了损伤左束支主干的风险。另一策略是在窦律下消融尖锐、高频的舒张期电位。窦律下的舒张期电位约在浦氏纤维电位后 150～450ms，仅见于分支性室速患者[49]。

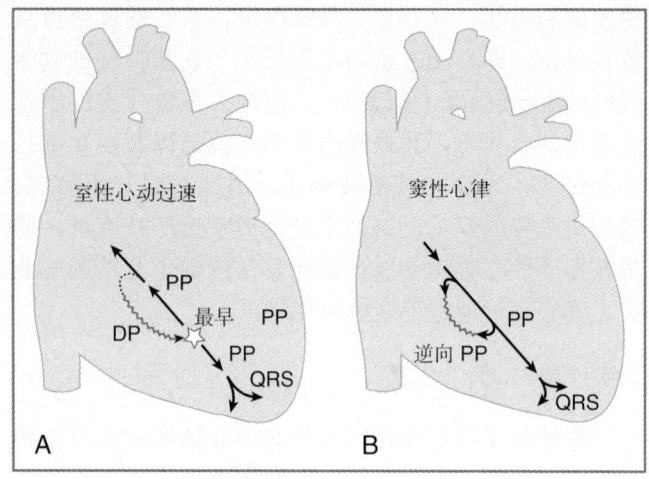

图 72-10　分支性室速折返环的假设模型　A：心动过速时的折返环。激动沿病变的浦氏纤维缓慢前向传导，心电记录图显示舒张期电位（DP）。在其远端激动左后分支出现浦氏电位（PP），该浦氏纤维再逆向激动，构成折返环的逆传支。心室肌不是折返环的必需部分，有时可作为前传支和逆传支之间的桥梁。B：窦律时的激动环路。冲动沿左后分支快速前向激动，邻近部位病变的浦氏纤维可能被部分前向激动，也可能处于不应期而不被激动。冲动至左后分支远端时可逆向激动病变的浦氏纤维，产生逆向浦氏纤维电位。（引自 Aiba T, Suyama K, Aihara N, et al: The role of Purkinje and Pre-Purkinje potentials in the reentrant circuit of verapamil-sensitive idiopathic LV tachycardia. Pacing Clin Electrophysiol 24：333-334，2001. Copyright 2001, Futura Publishing Co.）

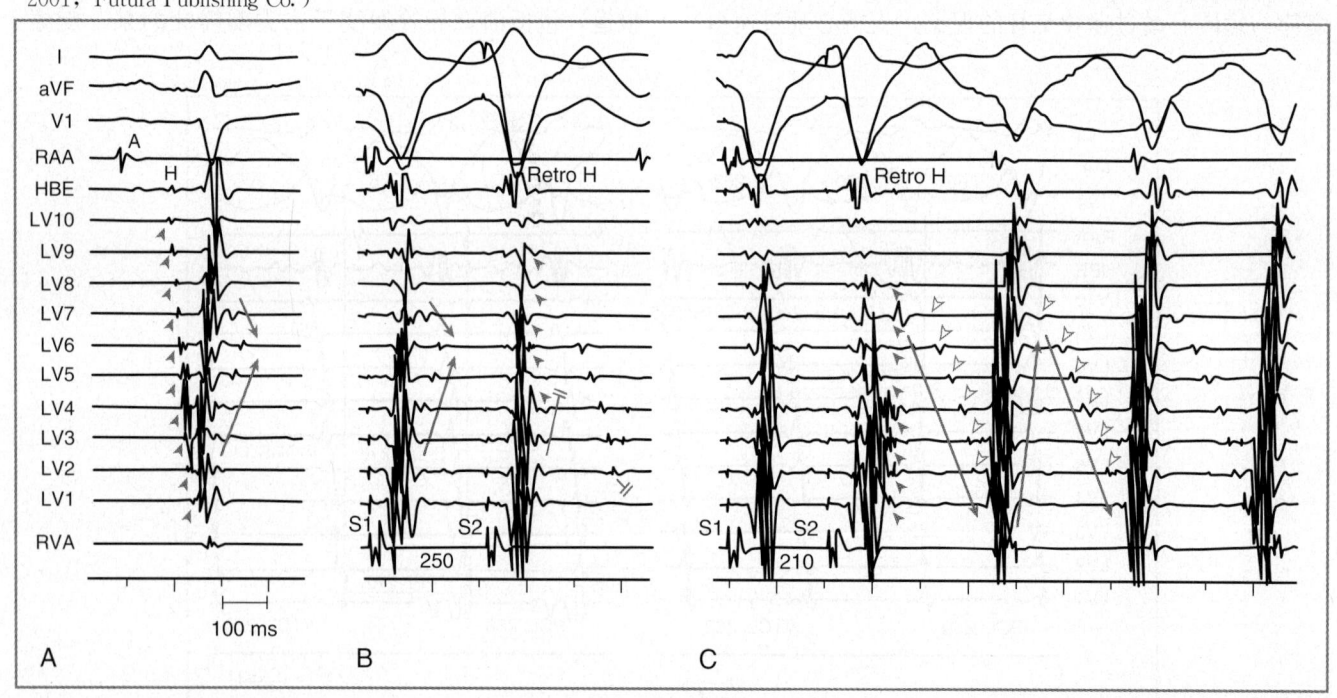

图 72-11　分支性室性心动过速的机制　A：窦性节律时在左室间隔面记录到的由希氏束至左后分支远端前向激动产生的高频电位（短箭头），在心室激动波之后可记录到低频的前向及逆向舒张期电位（长箭头）。B：心室基础刺激（S₁）时，心室激动波之后可记录到低频的舒张期电位，在 250ms 配对的早搏刺激时（S₂），舒张期电位的上行激动受阻，其下行激动一直延续到间隔近心尖处，直至于缓慢传导区远端受阻。C：在配对间期进一步缩短至 210ms 时，缓慢传导区近端的递减传导可使冲动折返进入左后分支，使心动过速得以发生。舒张期电位由近向远的顺序激动可在心动过速的整个舒张期记录到（虚箭头）。图中 Ⅰ、aVL、V₁ 为体表导联，依次向下的双极电图为右心耳（RAA）、希氏束（HBE）、左室记录电极（LV1～LV10）、右室心尖部（RVA）。（引自 Maruyama M, Tadera T, Miyamoto S, et al: Demonstration of the reentrant circuit of verapamil-sensitive idiopathic left ventricular tachycardia: Direct evidence for macroreentry as the underlying mechanism. J Cardiovasc Electrophysiol 12：968-972，2001. Copyright 2001, Futura Publishing Co.）

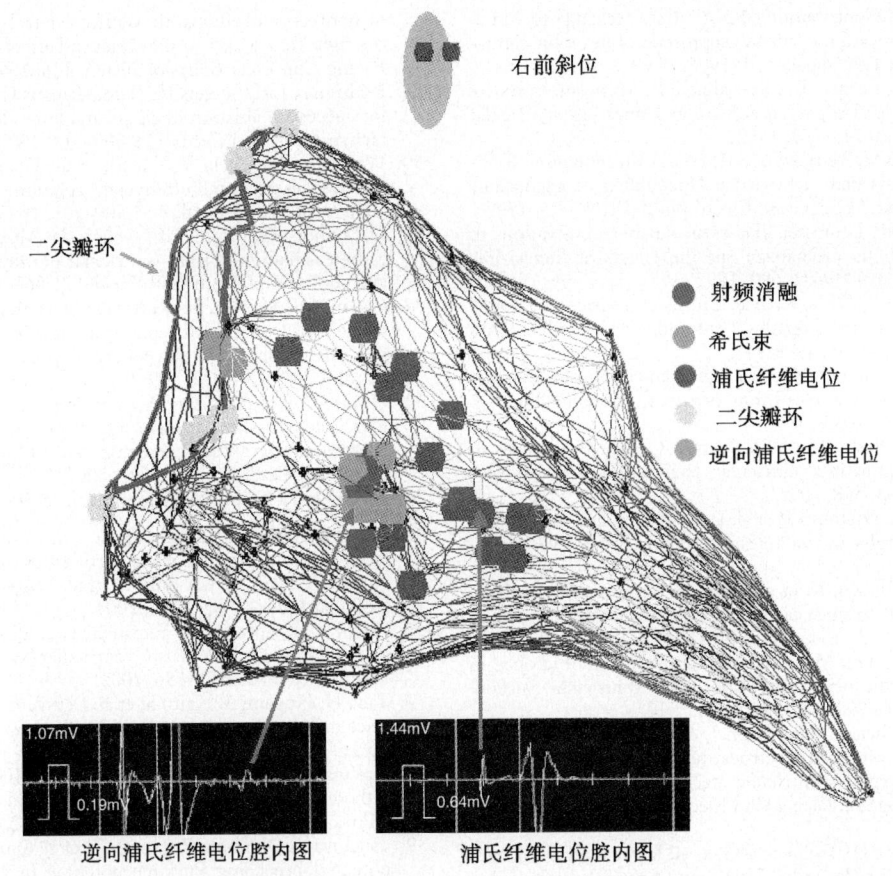

图72-12 分支性室速患者窦性节律下的浦氏纤维电位（PPs）绿色标记表示左后分支区域可记录到浦氏纤维电位的点。右侧插图为该区域记录到的腔内电图，第一个棘波代表浦氏纤维激动，其后为心室激动波。粉红色标记为记录到逆向浦氏纤维电位的点（相当于心动过速时的舒张期电位）。左侧插图为该区域记录到的腔内电图，第一个棘波为浦氏纤维电位（PP），其后为心室激动波，最后为低频的逆向浦氏纤维电位。该点为最早的逆向浦氏纤维电位处，也是成功消融靶点。（见彩图37）

这些电位可在左室间隔的中下部位记录到，位于左后分支或其邻近区域。窦律下的舒张期电位与心动过速时的舒张期电位是相应的，它代表了异常浦氏纤维的激动（图72-10B）。在窦性节律下寻找最早的逆向舒张期电位进行消融可获成功，特别是在心动过速不能诱发时是一个有效的消融方法（图72-12）。

虽然有着独特的电生理特性并在解剖上冠之为分支性室速，但在特发性左室室速的鉴别诊断时仍有必要排除分支间折返性心动过速[50]。分支间折返性心动过速以左束支中一个分支作为前传支，另一个分支作为逆传支，心动过速呈右束支阻滞形态，如伴左后分支阻滞形态则左前分支为前传支；如伴左后分支阻滞形态则左前分支为前传支。尽管窦律下常出现右束支阻滞伴左前或左后分支阻滞，临床上还没有足够的资料来确定分支间折返性心动过速是否一定与心肌病变相关联，是否如束支折返性室速那样，心动过速和扩张型心肌病是伴随疾病。诊断左束支分支间折返性心动过速的标准如下：
(1) 心动过速呈右束支阻滞形，形态与窦律时相似；(2) 心动过速时左束支激动领先于希氏束激动；(3) 心动过速时的HV间期短于窦律时的HV间期；(4) 由于驱使心室激动的束支激动间期变化，可使心动过速的周期自然交替；(5) 心室早搏刺激或射频消融阻断两分支中的任何一支可终止心动过速。

（陈明龙 译）

参 考 文 献

1. Lerman BB, Stein KM, Markowitz SM: Adenosine-sensitive ventricular tachycardia: A conceptual approach. J Cardiovasc Electrophysiol 7:559–569, 1996.
2. Lerman BB, Stein KM, Markowitz SM: Mechanisms of idiopathic left ventricular tachycardia. J Cardiovasc Electrophysiol 8:571–583, 1997.
3. Lerman BB, Belardinelli L, West GA, et al: Adenosine-sensitive ventricular tachycardia: Evidence suggesting cyclic AMP-mediated triggered activity. Circulation 74:270–280, 1986.
4. Lerman BB, Wesley RC, DiMarco JP, et al: Antiadrenergic effects of adenosine on His-Purkinje automaticity: Evidence for accentuated antagonism. J Clin Invest 82:2127–2135, 1988.
5. Lerman BB, Stein K, Engelstein ED, et al: Mechanism of repetitive monomorphic ventricular tachycardia. Circulation 92:421–429, 1995.

6. Han X, Ferrier GR: Contribution of Na(+)-Ca^{2+} exchange to stimulation of transient inward current by isoproterenol in rabbit cardiac Purkinje fibers. Circ Res 76:664–674, 1995.
7. Song Y, Thedford S, Lerman BB, Belardinelli L: Adenosine-sensitive afterdepolarizations and triggered activity in guinea pig ventricular myocytes. Circ Res 70:743–753, 1992.
8. Lerman BB, Stein KM, Markowitz SM, et al: Catecholamine facilitated reentrant ventricular tachycardia: Uncoupling of adenosine's antiadrenergic effects. J Cardiovasc Electrophysiol 10:17–26, 1999.
9. Vos MA, Gorgels AP, Leunissen JD, et al: Further observations to confirm the arrhythmia mechanism specific effects of flunarizine. J Cardiovasc Pharmacol 19:682–690, 1992.
10. Kobayashi Y, Miyata A, Tanno K, et al: Effects of nicorandil, a potassium channel opener, on idiopathic ventricular tachycardia. J Am Coll Cardiol 32:1377–1383, 1998.
11. Lerman BB, Dong B, Stein KM, et al: Right ventricular outflow tract tachycardia due to a somatic cell mutation in G protein subunit$_{\alpha i2}$. J Clin Invest 101:2862–2868, 1998.
12. Nakagawa M, Takahashi N, Nobe S, et al: Gender differences in various types of idiopathic ventricular tachycardia. J Cardiovasc Electrophysiol 13:633–638, 2002.
13. Gaita F, Giustetto C, DiDonna P, et al: Long-term follow-up of right ventricular monomorphic extrasystoles. J Am Coll Cardiol 38:364–370, 2001.
14. Gill JS, Prasad K, Blaszyk K, et al: Initiating sequences in exercise induced idiopathic ventricular tachycardia of left bundle branch-like morphology. Pacing Clin Electrophysiol 21:1873–1880, 1998.
15. Hayashi H, Fujiki A, Tani M, et al: Circadian variation of idiopathic ventricular tachycardia originating from right ventricular outflow tract. Am J Cardiol 84:99–101, 1999.
16. Grimm W, List-Hellwig E, Hoffmann J, et al: Magnetic resonance imaging and signal averaged electrocardiography in patients with repetitive monomorphic ventricular tachycardia and otherwise normal electrocardiogram. Pacing Clin Electrophysiol 20:1826–1833, 1997.
17. Carlson MD, White RD, Trohman RG, et al: Right ventricular outflow tract ventricular tachycardia: Detection of previously unrecognized anatomic abnormalities using cine magnetic resonance imaging. J Am Coll Cardiol 24:720–727, 1994.
18. Markowitz SM, Litvak BL, Ramirez de Arellano EA, et al: Adenosine-sensitive ventricular tachycardia: Right ventricular abnormalities delineated by magnetic resonance imaging. Circulation 96:1192–1200, 1997.
19. Globits S, Kreiner G, Frank H, et al: Significance of morphological abnormalities detected by MRI in patients undergoing successful ablation of right ventricular outflow tract tachycardia. Circulation 96:2633–2640, 1997.
20. White RD, Trohman RG, Flam SD, et al: Right ventricular arrhythmia in the absence of arrhythmogenic dysplasia: MR imaging of myocardial abnormalities. Radiology 207:743–751, 1998.
21. Mitrani RD, Klein LS, Miles WM, et al: Regional cardiac sympathetic denervation in patients with ventricular tachycardia in the absence of coronary artery disease. J Am Coll Cardiol 22:1344–1353, 1993.
22. Wichter T, Hindricks G, Lerch H, et al: Regional myocardial sympathetic dysinnervation in arrhythmogenic right ventricular cardiomyopathy: An analysis using ^{123}I-meta-iodobenzylguanidine scintigraphy. Circulation 89:667–683, 1994.
23. Schafers M, Lerch H, Wichter T, et al: Cardiac sympathetic innervation in patients with idiopathic right ventricular outflow tract tachycardia. J Am Coll Cardiol 32:181–186, 1998.
24. La Vecchia L, Ometto R, Bedogni F, et al: Ventricular late potentials, interstitial fibrosis, and right ventricular function in patients with ventricular tachycardia and normal left ventricular function. Am J Cardiol 81:790–792, 1998.
25. Kamakura S, Shimizu W, Matsuo K, et al: Localization of optimal ablation site of idiopathic ventricular tachycardia from right and left ventricular outflow tract by body surface ECG. Circulation 98:1525–1533, 1998.
26. Green LS, Lux RL, Ershler PR, et al: Resolution of pace mapping stimulus site separation using body surface potentials. Circulation 90:462–468, 1994.
27. Chinushi M, Aizawa Y, Ohhira K, et al: Repetitive ventricular responses induced by radiofrequency ablation for idiopathic ventricular tachycardia originating from the outflow tract of the right ventricle. Pacing Clin Electrophysiol 21:669–678, 1998.
28. Chinushi M, Aizawa Y, Takahashi K, et al: Morphological variation of nonreentrant idiopathic ventricular tachycardia originating from the right ventricular outflow tract and effect of radiofrequency lesion. Pacing Clin Electrophysiol 20:325–336, 1997.
29. Rodriguez LM, Smeets JL, Timmermans C, Wellens HJ: Predictors for successful ablation of right- and left-sided idiopathic ventricular tachycardia. Am J Cardiol 79:309–314, 1997.
30. Wen MS, Taniguchi Y, Yeh SJ, et al: Determinants of tachycardia recurrences after radiofrequency ablation of idiopathic ventricular tachycardia. Am J Cardiol 81:500–502, 1998.
31. O'Connor BK, Case CL, Sokoloski MC, et al: Radiofrequency catheter ablation of right ventricular outflow tachycardia in children and adolescents. J Am Coll Cardiol 27:869–874, 1996.
32. Callans DJ, Menz V, Schwartzman D, et al: Repetitive monomorphic tachycardia from the left ventricular outflow tract: Electrocardiographic patterns consistent with a left ventricular site of origin. J Am Coll Cardiol 29:1023–1027, 1997.
33. Ouyang F, Fotuhi P, Ho SY, et al: Repetitive monomorphic ventricular tachycardia originating from the aortic sinus cusp: Electrocardiographic characterization for guiding catheter ablation. J Am Coll Cardiol 39:500–508, 2002.
34. Anderson RH: Clinical anatomy of the aortic root. Heart 24:670–673, 2000.
35. Kanagaratnam L, Tomassoni G, Schweikert R, et al: Ventricular tachycardias arising from the aortic sinus of valsalva: An under-recognized variant of left outflow tract ventricular tachycardia. J Am Coll Cardiol 34:1408–1414, 2001.
36. Hachiya H, Aonuma K, Yamauchi Y, et al: How to diagnose, locate and ablate coronary cusp ventricular tachycardia. J Cardiovasc Electrophysiol 13:551–556, 2002.
37. Tada H, Nogami A, Naito S, et al: Left ventricular epicardial outflow tract tachycardia: A new distinct subgroup of outflow tract tachycardia. Jpn Circ J 65:723–730, 2001.
38. Nakagawa H, Beckman KJ, McClelland JH, et al: Radiofrequency catheter ablation of idiopathic left ventricular tachycardia guided by a Purkinje potential. Circulation 88:2607–2617, 1993.
39. Tsuchiya T, Okumura K, Honda T, et al: Significance of late diastolic potential preceding Purkinje potential in verapamil-sensitive idiopathic left ventricular tachycardia. Circulation 99:2408–2413, 1999.
40. Nogami A, Naito S, Tada H, et al: Demonstration of diastolic and presystolic Purkinje potentials as critical potentials in a macroreentry circuit of verapamil-sensitive idiopathic left ventricular tachycardia. J Am Coll Cardiol 36:811–823, 2000.
41. Aiba T, Suyama K, Aihara N, et al: The role of Purkinje and pre-Purkinje potentials in the reentrant circuit of verapamil-sensitive idiopathic LV tachycardia. Pacing Clin Electrophysiol 24:333–344, 2001.
42. Maruyama M, Tadera T, Miyamoto S, Ino T: Demonstration of the reentrant circuit of verapamil-sensitive idiopathic left ventricular tachycardia: Direct evidence for macroreentry as the underlying mechanism. J Cardiovasc Electrophysiol 12:968–972, 2001.
43. Suwa M, Yoneda Y, Nagao H, et al: Surgical correction of idiopathic paroxysmal ventricular tachycardia possibly related to left ventricular false tendon. Am J Cardiol 64:1217–1220, 1989.
44. Thakur RK, Klein GJ, Sivaram CA, et al: Anatomic substrate for idiopathic left ventricular tachycardia. Circulation 93:497–501, 1996.
45. Lin FC, Wen MS, Wang CC, et al: Left ventricular fibromuscular band is not a specific substrate for idiopathic left ventricular tachycardia. Circulation 93:525–528, 1996.
46. Okumura K, Yamabe H, Tsuchiya T, et al: Characteristics of slow conduction zone demonstrated during entrainment of idiopathic ventricular tachycardia of left ventricular origin. Am J Cardiol 77:379–383, 1996.
47. Tsuchiya T, Okumura K, Honda T, et al: Effects of verapamil and lidocaine on two components of the re-entry circuit of verapamil-sensitive idiopathic left ventricular tachycardia. Am J Cardiol 37:1415–1421, 2001.
48. Griffith MJ, Garratt CJ, Rowland E, et al: Effects of intravenous adenosine on verapamil-sensitive "idiopathic" ventricular tachycardia. Am J Cardiol 73:759–764, 1994.
49. Ouyang F, Cappato R, Ernst S, et al: Electroanatomic substrate of idiopathic left ventricular tachycardia. Circulation 105:462–469, 2002.
50. Crijns HJ, Smeets JL, Rodriguez LM, et al: Cure of interfascicular reentrant ventricular tachycardia by ablation of the anterior fascicle of the left bundle branch. J Cardiovasc Electrophysiol 6:486–492, 1995.

第 73 章

束支折返性室速

Emile G. Daoud

本章目录
- 机制 ……………………………… 675
- 临床特征 ………………………… 675
- 心脏电生理检查 ………………… 676
- 导管消融 ………………………… 677
- 病人随访 ………………………… 678

希浦系统参与的大折返性反复单形性室速在心脏电生理检查中可被诱发，但伴有希浦系统内传导延迟的病人，大折返性室性心动过速是由右束支和左束支参与的，被称为束支折返性室速（bundle branch reentry，BBR）。认识束支折返性室速是非常重要的，因为这种心动过速对药物治疗的反应差，并有很高的复发率，同时发作时可有晕厥、猝死，经常需要电复律治疗，目前导管消融可以根治这种心动过速。

一、机　制

束支折返性室速是由包括希氏束、右束支、室间隔和浦肯野系统参与的大折返性心动过速。最常见的典型束支折返性室速的图形表现为左束支阻滞的心电图图形。这种心动过速的发生依赖于不应期较长的右束支逆传阻滞和左束支的缓慢逆传（图 73-1），因此，心室最早除极的部位位于右室心尖部。QRS 波群形态呈右束支阻滞形的折返几乎很难见到。

分支间折返性心动过速是希浦系统参与大折返性室速的另一种类型[1-4]。其常见类型为通过左前分支前传和经左后分支逆传，也可发生反方向折返（图 73-1）。QRS 波群形态呈右束支伴左后分支阻滞的图形。这种心动过速不同于分支性或特发性左室室速，因为后者可能的原因是某一分支内微折返所致（如分支性室速）[3]。

二、临床特征

束支折返性室速的患者也引起晕厥和心脏性猝死，引起晕厥的原因是快速心室率，其频率可达 200～300bpm。心电图表现为左束支阻滞形宽 QRS 波心动过速图形（图 73-2）。如果 QRS 波群形态表现为右束支阻滞伴电轴左偏，应考虑分支折返性室速。分支折返性室速和束支折返性室速可以在同一病人共存[1,2]。

持续性束支折返性室速可表现为典型的左束支或右束支阻滞的心电图图形，其 QRS 波形态有一特有的变窄的曲折。这些心电图表现很容易被认做室上速。对于无房室分离，但伴有器质性心脏病的患者应怀疑束支折返性室速的可能。应用阻断房室结的药物不会影响束支折返性室速，并有可能使血流动力学恶化。典型束支折返性室速不受腺苷影响，但亦有 1 例应用腺苷终止束支折返性室速的报告[3]。

对于非缺血性心肌病和希浦系统传导障碍的患者，尤其存在 PR 间期延长和 QRS 波群增宽的患者，一定要考虑束支折返性室速的可能。在一项大系列的研究中，可诱发持续性单形性束支折返性室速的患者 50％以上为非缺血性心肌病病例[5]。另一报告[6]和大多数电生理学家的研究则并未显示出束支折返性室速有如此高的发生率。在缺血性心肌病中，大约仅有 5％病人可诱发室性心动过速。另外，束支折返性室

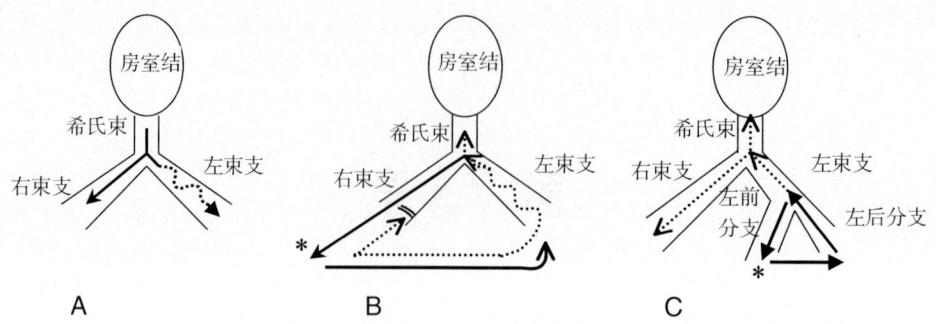

图 73-1　A：窦性心律下为左束支阻滞，而并非完全性阻滞，为左束支下传延缓（虚线表示）。B：束支折返性室速的发生机制显示右束支逆传阻滞而通过左束支缓慢逆传（虚线）。*为右室心尖部的激动的起源点。C：分支折返性室速的机制显示折返激动是前传经左前分支，逆传经左后分支。QRS 波群表现为右束支阻滞合并左后分支阻滞的心电图图形。*为心室除极的起始点。

速的临床特征包括存在器质性心脏病，射血分数较低，左室扩大和充血性心衰。

束支折返性室速的病理生理基础是希浦系统的传导延迟。与非缺血性心肌病相关的弥漫的瘢痕构成了束支折返性室速的基质。影响传导系统的疾病和其他因素还有强直性肌营养不良[7,8]、高血压性心脏病[9]、Ebstein 畸形[10]、瓣膜外科术后[11]，以及钠通道阻滞剂（如氟卡胺）等。然而需要注意的是，有些病人并无心脏病的证据和其他影响希浦系统传导的疾病亦可发生束支折返性室速[3,13,14]。

三、心脏电生理检查

束支折返性室速患者电生理检查中最常见的表现是 HV 间期延长和 QRS 波群增宽。束支折返的诱发依赖于希浦系内的传导延缓和心室的程序刺激。当 R_1 到 R_2 配对间期缩短时遇到了右束支的有效不应期，激动通过左束支缓慢逆传。当通过左束支的逆传传导时间足够长时，右束支的前向传导恢复，束支折返性室速被诱发（图 73-1）。有时，心动过速的诱发需要用短-长刺激诱发，但很少被左室刺激诱发，有报道通过静滴异丙肾上腺素[1,15]、普鲁卡因胺[14]，以及诱发房扑、房颤[1,15]后均可诱发束支折返性室速。心房刺激诱发束支折返性室速也有报道[1]。房性心律失常下诱发束支折返性室速的可能机制是房性心律失常不规则或快速下传心室，进一步导致希浦系统传导延迟所致。

束支折返性室速的诊断要点（表 73-1，图 73-3）：(1) 心动过速时 QRS 波群呈左束支或右束支阻滞图形；(2) 心动过速的诱发依赖于希浦系统的传导延缓；(3) 心动过速终止于希浦系统内的阻滞；(4) 在束支折返性室速发作时，每一个 QRS 波前均有希氏束电位，另外，不论呈左束支阻滞图形还是右束支图形，心动过速时的激动顺序均为希氏束→右束支→左束支→希氏束

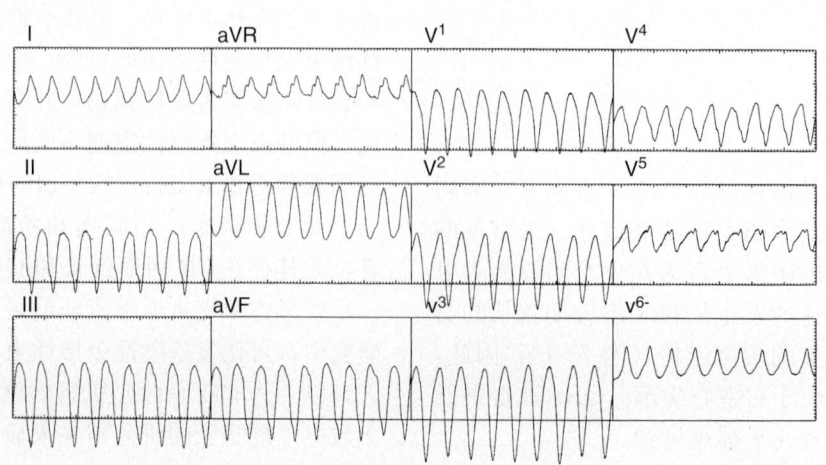

图 73-2　束支折返性室速表现为左束支阻滞的心电图图形（折返周期＝270ms）

表 73-1 束支折返性室速诊断要点

1. 心动过速呈典型的左束支阻滞图形（罕见 RBBB）
2. 心动过速的诱发依赖于希浦系统传导的延迟
3. 希浦系统传导阻滞可终止心动过速
4. 每一个 QRS 波群前均有 H 波
5. 束支折返性室速时的 HV 间期≥窦性心律下的 HV 间期
6. VV 间期的变化随 HH 间期而变化
7. 束支折返性室速时行心房超速起搏的 QRS 波群与室速发作时相同，但并不是真正的心室拖带
8. 右室心尖部起搏拖带起搏后间期-心动过速的折返周期≤30ms

（图 73-3）；（5）心动过速时的 HV 间期通常比窦性心律下的 HV 间期延长或相等[16]。在某些病例中，如果希氏束导管接近希氏束的部位，束支折返性室速时的 HV 间期可能略缩短，缩短间期比窦性心律下的 HV 间期短 10ms 以内。应当注意，分支折返性室速，其心动过速时的 HV 间期通常短于或等于窦律下的 HV 间期，但绝对不会延长；（6）HH 间期变化在 VV 间期变化前；（7）右束支消融后，心动过速不能被诱发。

有时束支折返性室速发作时很难记录希氏束电位，在不要求希氏束电位清楚的情况下，诊断的方法是应用心房和右室心尖部进行起搏拖带，观察 QRS 波群的形态[17]，当心房起搏拖带后右束支前向快速下传，而左束支内发生隐匿性传导阻滞，其 QRS 波群形态与束支折返性室速时的 QRS 波群完全一致。然而，当通过右室心尖部起搏拖带时，其 QRS 波群形态与束支折返性室速时不同。另一种不要求准确记录出希氏束电位的方法是通过起搏右室心尖部拖带后的起搏后间期进行判断[18]。如果起搏后间期与心动过速的折返周期的差值始终在 30ms 以内提示为束支折返性室速。

需要与束支折返性室速相鉴别的心动过速：(1) 心肌内折返引起的室速；(2) 分支间或分支内折返性室速；(3) 伴有室房 1：1 传导的室上性心动过速伴差异性传导；(4) 房束束折返性心动过速（Mahaim 旁路）。心肌内折返性室速的 QRS 波群前没有希氏束电位，HH 间期的变化随 VV 间期而变化，如果通过右室心尖部起搏拖带，起搏后间期与心动过速的折返周期的差值在 30ms 以内，大概可以排除心肌内折返、分支性或分支间折返和室上性心动过速的诊断。房束束心动过速的病人其窦性心律下行心房刺激时，心室预激会更明显。

四、导管消融

由于束支折返性室速和分支折返性室速可以通过导管消融根治，正确的认识该疾病非常重要。这些心动过速可通过抗心律失常药物减慢心率，或常需采用电复律治疗。

导管消融右束支可终止束支折返性室速，右束支

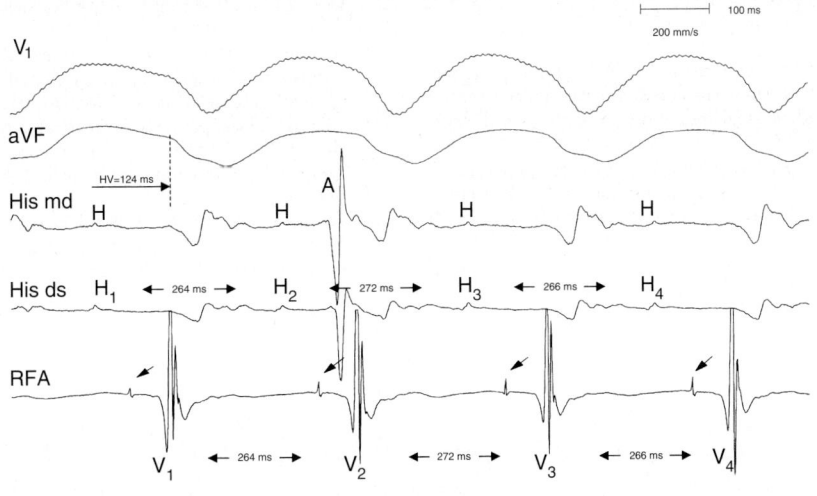

图 73-3　持续性束支折返性室速体表心电图（V_1 和 aVF 导联）和心腔内电图　提示束支折返性室速的特点包括：(1) QRS 波群呈左束支阻滞图形；(2) 有室房（A）分离记录；(3) 每一个 QRS 波群前有一希氏束电位（H），其后有右束电位（箭头所指），这是左束支阻滞图形的束支折返性室速的激动顺序；(4) VV 间期随着 HH 间期的变化而改变；(5) 束支折返性室速的 HV 间期为 124ms，比窦性心律时的 HV 间期 80ms 长。本图为成功消融右束支的靶点图。A：心房电图；ds：远端；H：希氏束；md：希氏束中端；RB：右束支。

的定位需要通过已记录的希氏束电位来确定，在记录到希氏束电位后顺钟向转导管使导管继续向右室间隔送入，典型的右束支电位为一小电位，没有心房电图，右束支电位到V波的间期比HV间期短20ms，并可记录到高大的心室电位（图73-3）。消融右束支有可能在已经存在异常HV间期的病人中使HV间期进一步延长，进一步阻滞结下传导，可能会需要行起搏治疗，尽管也有过1例消融左束支而避免了植入永久起搏器的报告[19]。

对分支折返性室速，消融导管的靶点通常在左后分支区域于窦律下记录到P电位，其位置接近于左室间隔的基底段。

五、病人随访

尽管消融右束支可根治束支折返性室速，但这些病人具有高死亡率。在一项研究中表明，随访16个月的死亡率大约为30%，这些病人多数为充血性心力衰竭的患者[20]。此外，有心源性猝死高危特点的病人，包括：扩张型心肌病或其他类型的器质性心脏病、充血性心力衰竭、射血分数降低、希浦系统传导障碍和宽QRS波群等应考虑植入双腔心脏转复除颤器或行心脏再同步治疗。一些作者建议束支折返性室速复发病例应行心脏电生理检查，以排除其他机制室速的可能。

（李学斌　译）

参 考 文 献

1. Simons GR, Sorrentino RA, Zimerman LI, et al: Bundle branch reentry tachycardia and possible sustained interfascicular reentry tachycardia with a shared unusual induction pattern. J Cardiovasc Electrophysiol 7:44–50, 1996.
2. Berger RD, Orias D, Kasper EK, Calkins H: Catheter ablation of coexistent bundle branch and interfascicular reentrant ventricular tachycardias. J Cardiovasc Electrophysiol 7:341–347, 1996.
3. Rubenstein DS, Burke MC, Kall JG, et al: Adenosine-sensitive bundle branch reentry. J Cardiovasc Electrophysiol 8:80–88, 1997.
4. Crijns HJGM, Smeets JLRM, Rodriquez LM, et al: Cure of interfascicular reentrant ventricular tachycardia by ablation of the anterior fascicle of the left bundle branch. J Cardiovasc Electrophysiol 6:486–492, 1995.
5. Blanck Z, Dhala A, Deshpande S, et al: Bundle branch reentrant ventricular tachycardia: Cumulative experience in 48 patients. J Cardiovasc Electrophysiol 4:253, 1993.
6. Delacretaz E, Stevenson WG, Ellison KE, et al: Mapping and radiofrequency catheter ablation of the three types of sustained monomorphic ventricular tachycardia in nonischemic heart disease. J Cardiovasc Electrophysiol 11:11–17, 2000.
7. Merino JL, Carmona JR, Fernandez-Lozano I, et al: Mechanisms of sustained ventricular tachycardia in myotonic dystrophy. Circulation 98:541–546, 1998.
8. Negri SM, Cowan MD: Becker muscular dystrophy with bundle branch reentry ventricular tachycardia. J Cardiovasc Electrophysiol 9:652–654, 1998.
9. Mittal S, Coyne RF, Herling IM, et al: Sustained bundle branch reentry in a patient with hypertrophic cardiomyopathy and nondilated left ventricle. J Intervent Card Electrophysiol 1:73–77, 1997.
10. Andress JD, Vander Salm TJ, Huang SKS: Bidirectional bundle branch reentry tachycardia associated with Ebstein's anomaly: Cured by extensive cryoablation of the right bundle branch. Pacing Clin Electrophysiol 14:1639–1647, 1991.
11. Narasimhan C, Jazayeri MR, Sra J, et al: Ventricular tachycardia in valvular heart disease. Circulation 96:4307–4313, 1997.
12. Chalvidan T, Cellarier G, Deharo JC, et al: His-Purkinje system reentry as a proarrhythmic effect of flecainide. Pacing Clin Electrophysiol 23:530–533, 2000.
13. Blanck Z, Jazayeri M, Dhala A, et al: Bundle branch reentry: A mechanism of ventricular tachycardia in the absence of myocardial or valvular dysfunction. J Am Coll Cardiol 22:1718–22, 1993.
14. Mehdirad AA, Keim S, Rist K, Tchou P: Long-term clinical outcome of right bundle branch radiofrequency catheter ablation for treatment of bundle branch reentrant ventricular tachycardia. Pacing Clin Electrophysiol 18:2135–2143, 1995.
15. Blanck Z, Jazayeri M, Akhtar M: Facilitation of sustained bundle branch reentry by atrial fibrillation. J Cardiovasc Electrophysiol 7:348–352, 1996.
16. Fisher JD: Bundle branch reentry tachycardia: Why is the HV interval often longer than in sinus rhythm? The critical role of anisotropic conduction. J Intervent Card Electrophysiol 5:173–176, 2001.
17. Merino JL, Peinado R, Fernandez-Lozano I, et al: Transient entrainment of bundle-branch reentry by atrial and ventricular stimulation. Circulation 100:1784–1790, 1999.
18. Merino JL, Peinado R, Fernandez-Lozano I, et al: Bundle-branch reentry and the postpacing interval after entrainment by right ventricular apex stimulation. Circulation 103:1102–1108, 2001.
19. Blanck Z, Deshpande S, Jazayeri MR, Akhtar M: Catheter ablation of the left bundle branch for the treatment of sustained bundle branch reentrant ventricular tachycardia. J Cardiovasc Electrophysiol 6:40–43, 1995.
20. Blanck Z, Akhtar M: Ventricular tachycardia due to sustained bundle branch reentry: Diagnostic and therapeutic considerations. Clin Cardiol 16:619–622, 1993.

第 74 章

尖端扭转型室速

Nabil El-Sherif and Gioia Turitto

本章目录

- 尖端扭转型室速的心电图特征 ········· 679
- 先天性长 QT 综合征和尖端扭转型室速的离子基础 ········· 681
- 药物性长 QT 综合征和尖端扭转型室速 ········· 681
- 尖端扭转型室速：从离子通道到心电图 ········· 682
- 药物性长 QT 综合征和尖端扭转型室速的电生理机制 ········· 684
- 长短周期现象和尖端扭转型室速的发作 ········· 686
- QT/T 波交替和尖端扭转型室速 ······ 687
- 自主神经和长 QT 综合征 ············ 688
- 长 QT 综合征和尖端扭转型室速的临床表现与治疗 ········· 688
- 尖端扭转型室速和多形性室速 ········ 690
- 总结 ········· 690

尖端扭转型室速（torsade de pointes，TdP）是一种引人注目的多形性室速（polymorphic ventricular tarchycardia，PVT）。这个生动形象的术语由 Dessertenne 首先提出[1]，他把这种心电图图形描述为 QRS 波形连续不断地改变，似乎围绕一条假想的基线扭转。这个音乐般的术语和有趣的心电图图形已引起了电生理学家的多年关注，并在一定程度上激起了人们对心律失常遗传学和心脏离子通道病理生理学的兴趣。更重要的是，它有助于我们再次把注意力集中到心室复极离散在恶性快速性室性心律失常形成中的作用。

多形性室速的电生理机制复杂，正确理解这些机制有助于制定适合的个体化治疗方案。多形性室速最恰当的分类方法基于是否合并正常或延长的 QT（或 QTU）间期[2]。这两种类型多形性室速的电生理机制可能不同。TdP 专用于长 QT 综合征（long QT syndrome，LQTS）。然而，并非每一例长 QT 综合征的病人都伴随典型 TdP 形态的多形性室速，而这种典型的心电图形态也可见于无 QT 间期延长的病人。

一、尖端扭转型室速的心电图特征

分析了 26 例有获得性长 QT 综合征病人的 80 次不同的非持续性室速发作的心电图，发现心律失常的发作持续范围从 3 次（非持续性室性心动过速的定义）到 117 次（图 74-1A），平均 15±9 次。心动过速的周期（cycle length）为 193～364ms，平均 286±47ms。室性心动过速之前常有一个多变的二联律间期，这个二联律是由基本心搏的 QT 间期延长合并一个或两个室性早搏引起的（图 74-1A 和 C）。在一次快速性室性心动过速发作终止后，常常能见到比心动过速周期长的单个或多个形态多变的早搏（图 74-1 用星号标记的心搏）。室速发作时 QRS 波形态有多种改变。当快速室性心动过速发作时，整个 QRS-T 波的振幅呈周期性降低并伴有少数的 QRS 电轴明显偏移（图 74-1A）。当室性心动过速心率较慢时，通常可见 QRS 电轴的典型扭转，从正向波占优势的形态变为负

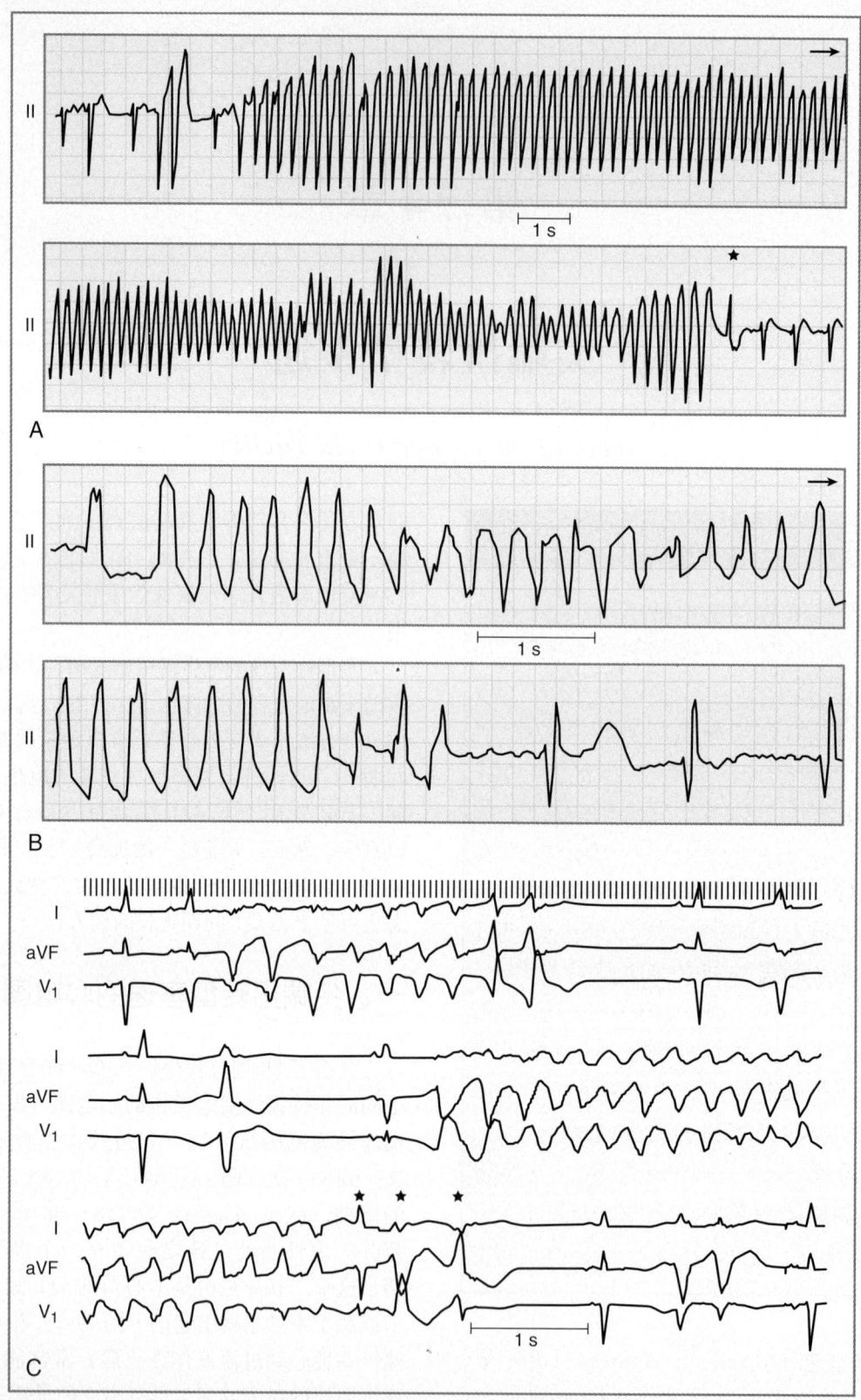

图74-1　3个获得性长QT综合征和尖端扭转型室速的心电图示例　A：一例人类免疫缺陷病毒阳性正在接受喷他脒治疗的23岁女性患者。其入院时有严重的腹泻和低钾血症。B：另一名有高血压和慢性房颤正在接受地高辛和氢氯噻嗪治疗的62岁男性患者，血钾水平3.2mEq/L。在接受总量4片的奎尼丁葡萄糖酸锑钠尝试转复窦性心律12h之后，出现尖端扭转型室速。C：一名正在使用普鲁卡因胺治疗频繁室性期前收缩的64岁男性患者发生了尖端扭转型室速。（引自El-Sherif N，Turitto G：The long QT syndrome and torsade de points. Pacing Clin Electrophysiol 22：91-110，1999.）

向波占优势的形态,并伴有大量过渡性的 QRS 波,反之亦然(图 74-1B)。有时可以见到另一种多形性室速,其缺乏上述的两个特征性的图形(由多个同步导联证实,见图 74-1C,中间的记录)。同一病人在不同次的室速发作时可有不同的形态(图 74-1C)。

二、先天性长 QT 综合征和尖端扭转型室速的离子基础

先天性长 QT 综合征(congenital long QT syndrome, congenital LQTS)(见第 70 章和 71 章)由心脏钾和钠离子通道基因的突变引起,这些特异性基因型如表 74-1 所示[3]。一般认为,LQT1 是由 *KvLQT1* 的 I_{Ks} 钾通道基因突变引起,LQT2 是由 *HERG* 的 I_{Kr} 钾通道基因突变引起。已知基因型的长 QT 综合征的大多数病例(87%)是这两个基因突变所致[4]。LQT3 型占 8%,而 LQT5 和 LQT6 两型极其少见,占长 QT 综合征病例不足 5%。纯合子的 *KvLQT1* 和 *KCNE1* 变异伴有先天性耳聋(Jervell-Lange-Nielsen 综合征),占长 QT 综合征病例的 1% 不到。目前,这些基因大约有 200 个不同的变异[4]。心电图表现的显著改变(T 波形态)、触发心脏事件的因素,及心脏事件的危险性取决于哪个基因发生了哪种突变。因为不是所有已知的长 QT 综合征的事件都是由先前我们讨论的基因突变引起的,因此其他引起这种疾病的基因尚有待被证实。

三、药物性长 QT 综合征和尖端扭转型室速

药物引起复极延长和早期后除极(early afterdepolarization,EAD)的离子机制复杂。一些药物通过影响多个离子电流起协同或拮抗作用。更重要的是,对于关键的复极化延长和 EAD 的发生,常常需要其他因素的协同效应。心率的缓慢和细胞外低钾通常起了重要的协同作用。心率的缓慢很可能通过减少 I_P 起作用。细胞外低钾会降低钾的电导,进而影响许多离子电流,包括 I_K、I_{K1} 和 I_F。

引起长 QT 综合征和尖端扭转型室速的药物不断增加[5](表 74-2)。任何能引起 QT 延长的药物都能导致长 QT 综合征。尖端扭转型室速的发生并不与已知能促发这种心律失常的药物的血浆浓度相关。然而,如果药物剂量过大或代谢减少而造成的高血药浓度,能增加尖端扭转型室速的危险性。代谢减少可能是同时合用了其他干扰细胞色素 P450 酶的药物。干扰药物代谢而诱发尖端扭转型室速的药物包括作用于全身的酮康唑以及结构相似的药物(氟康唑、依曲康唑、甲硝唑),5-羟色胺再摄取抑制剂(氟西汀、氟伏沙明、舍曲林)和其他抗抑郁药物(萘法唑酮),人类免疫缺陷病毒蛋白酶抑制剂(茚地那韦、利托那韦、沙奎那韦),二氢吡啶类钙通道阻滞剂(非洛地平、尼卡地平、硝苯地平),及红霉素和其他大环内酯类抗生素[6]。葡萄和葡萄汁通过干扰细胞色素 P450 酶也会影响一些药物的代谢。尖端扭转型室速也可发生于某些特别条件的病人,诸如肝功不全或先天性长 QT 综合征或电解质紊乱(部分是低钾和低镁),使用了引起 QT 间期延长的药物。电解质紊乱可能是由皮质类固醇、利尿治疗、液体蛋白饮食、严重腹泻或呕吐引起。尽管难以预测哪个病人有发生尖端扭转型室速的风险,但是在使用那些已知能引起 QT 间期延长的药物时应仔细评价风险与效益的比率。

表 74-1 LQTS 遗传形式的基因背景

LQTS 类型	染色体基因座	突变基因	受到影响的离子流
Romano-Ward 综合征			
LQT1	染色体 11p15.5	*KvLQT1*(*KCNQ1*)(杂合子)	钾电流(I_{Ks})
LQT2	染色体 7q35-36	*HERG*	钾电流(I_{Kr})
LQT3	染色体 3p21-24	*SCN5A*	钠电流(I_{Na})
LQT4	染色体 4q25-27	?	?
LQT5	染色体 21q22.1-22.2	*KCNE1*(杂合子)	钾电流(I_{Ks})
LQT6	染色体 21q22.1-22.2	*MiRP1*	钾电流(I_{Kr})
Jervell and Lang-Nielsen 综合征			
JLN1	11Q15.5	*KvLQT1*(*KCNQ1*)(纯合子)	钾电流(I_{Ks})
JLN2	21Q22.1-22.2	*KCNE1*(纯合子)	钾电流(I_{Ks})

表 74-2 能引起 QT 间期延长或尖端扭转型室速的药物

药物种类	药物
抗心律失常药物	
ⅠA 类	双异丙吡胺、普鲁卡因胺、奎尼丁
Ⅲ 类	胺碘酮、溴苄胺、索他洛尔、多非利特、依布利特
抗细菌药物	红霉素、甲氧苄胺嘧啶-磺胺甲基异噁唑、克拉仙霉素
抗真菌药物	氟康唑、酮康唑、依曲康唑
抗组胺药物	阿司咪唑、特非那定、苯海拉明
抗疟疾和抗原虫药物	氯喹、氯氟菲醇、甲氟喹、喷他脒、奎宁
胃肠动力药物	西沙比利
精神活性药物	水合氯醛、氟哌啶醇、锂剂、匹莫齐特、三环抗抑郁药
抗人类免疫缺陷病毒药物	依法韦仑
其他药物	金刚烷胺、吲达帕胺、普罗布芬、他克莫司、血管加压素

最近的数据证实一些由药物引起的 LQTS 和 TdP 的病例中可能有心脏离子通道基因的"沉默型"基因缺陷[7,8]。这可能是患者易患的基质，某种合适的触发因子如 I_{Kr} 阻滞剂，可能会使原来不外显的基因携带者发生长 QT 综合征和尖端扭转型室速。未来随着相关技术的快速发展将能迅速有效地筛选出那些控制心室复极化的编码离子通道的突变基因。

美国食品和药品管理局正在考虑制定对可能引起 QT 延长和尖端扭转型室速的新药研发指南。国际 Holter 和无创性心电学协会（International Society for Holter and Noninvasive Electrocardiology，ISHNE）建议采用心电图评价药物相关的 QT 延长和其他心室复极的改变[9]。

四、尖端扭转型室速：从离子通道到心电图

使用神经毒素海葵素-A（anthopleurin-A，AP-A）能够构建犬长 QT 综合征和尖端扭转型室速的活体模型[10]。这些药物通过在平台期减慢钠通道失活产生一个持续的内向电流而引起动作电位时程（APD）的延长[11]。这个模型构建于最近在 LQT3 病人中发现的钠通道 α 亚单位（SCN5A）遗传变异之前[12]。变异的通道产生了一个除极时持续的内向电流，这与暴露于海葵素-A 或 ATX-Ⅱ 的钠通道相似[13]。尽管模型只代表 LQT3，而 LQT3 是先天性长 QT 综合征中一种相对不常见的形式，但经过改良，这个模型中尖端扭转型室速的基本电生理机制似乎可以应用到所有类型的先天性或获得性长 QT 综合征。在一系列报告中，从离子通道异常到有特征性心电图形态的心律失常，阐述了尖端扭转型扭转型室速的机制[14-17]。

图 74-2 列举了连续记录钠通道的例子。图 74-2A 说明单个暴露于海葵素-A 的钠通道状态。图 74-2B 显示了海葵素-A 对犬心内膜浦肯野纤维（Purkinje fiber，PF）和心肌中层（M）细胞动作电位的影响，中层细胞取自透壁心肌条并置于同室而且使用相同浓度的海葵素-A 灌流。药物引起了浦肯野纤维动作电位时程的延长和一系列早期后除极的出现。相反，药物引起 M 细胞动作电位时程的显著延长以及 2 相末期低振幅的早期后除极。接下来的动作电位显示了 2 相末期电位的出现，这种 2 相末期的电位更能代表电张力的相互影响而不是早期后除极。在图 74-2C 描述了这种现象。该图显示了取自 12 周龄幼犬的左室游离壁并注入海葵素-A 的透壁条，同步记录心外膜下（Epi）细胞、心肌中层（M）细胞和心内膜下（End）细胞的动作电位。记录显示：与心外膜下和心内膜下细胞相比，心肌中层细胞的动作电位时程延长显著[18]；心外膜下细胞和心肌中层细胞出现传导阻滞并在切面出现非同步激动提示为折返激动。

图 74-3 阐述了体内尖端扭转型室速产生的电生理机制的最后一步。此图显示了非持续性尖端扭转型室速 12 次心搏的三维激动走行模式。图 74-3A 显示了尖端扭转型室速起始心搏来自于局灶性心内膜下激动。正如图 74-3 所示，激动的波锋遇到了多个功能传导阻滞区域，这些区域出现在相邻的伴有不同不应期的部位。当再次激动位于等时线♯20 的 3 和 4 部分以引发第一个折返环前，波锋环绕左室腔沿缓慢的逆时针方向路径行进。图 74-3 B1～B4 显示所有接下来的尖端扭转型室速的心搏都是由变化的三维激动模式的折返激动引起的。当前向折返波阻滞时，即终止了折返激动，尖端扭转型室速的心动过速就会终止。当尖端扭转型室速发作时，围绕 QRS 轴的扭转在下壁导

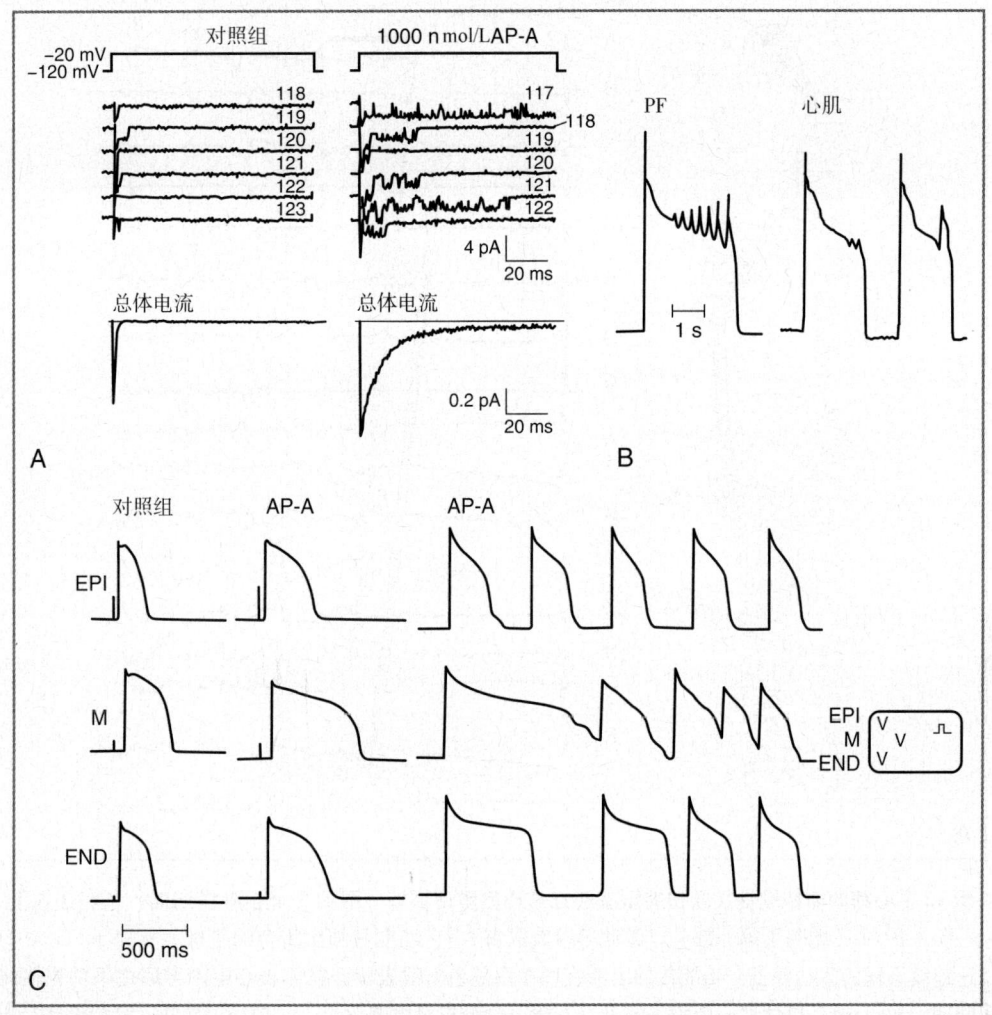

图 74-2　A：单个 Na⁺ 通道对 AP-A 的反应　该图显示了两个兔心肌细胞从－120mV 除极到－20mV 时，单个 Na⁺ 通道电流反应的顺序记录。左图：对照条件下的记录。右图：加入 1000nmol/L 的 AP-A 条件下的记录。在－20mV 时，对照组的 Na⁺ 通道短暂开放，平均仅有一次，在电位平台后非常迅速。相反，加入 AP-A 的 Na⁺ 通道显示长时间的突然发作，包括被短暂关闭所打断的反复的长时间的开放。一些突然的发作可持续整个电位平台期。底下两段显示了总体电流。对照组的总体电流显示快速弛缓。而加入 AP-A 组的 Na⁺ 通道的总体电流显示显著减慢的弛缓，持续 95ms 后，电流仍不能完全松弛。动态分析显示 AP-A 导致 Na⁺ 通道门控状态。**B：心内膜浦肯野纤维（PF）和心肌中层（M）细胞动作电位记录**　标本取自 10 周龄幼犬的左心室，置于相同室内，并用 50mg/L 的 AP-A 灌注。用 3000ms 的周长刺激标本。浦肯野纤维（PF）显示了一系列在最后复极前幅度逐渐增加的早期后除极（EADs）。相反，心肌中层（M）细胞的第一个动作电位显示显著的 APD 的延长和 2 相末期低振幅 EADs。随后的动作电位显示在 2 相末期电位的发生代表电张力的相互作用而不是 EAD。该现象在 C 图中得以描述。**C 图：取自 12 周龄并注射了 50mg/L 的 AP-A 的幼犬的左室心肌条，同步记录心外膜（Epi）细胞、心肌中层（M）细胞和心内膜下（End）细胞的电位**　标本用 4000ms 的周长刺激。与心外膜细胞和心内膜细胞相比，对照记录显示 M 细胞 APD 特征性地延长。AP-A 导致 3 种细胞的 APD 都延长，但在 M 细胞中，这种影响更加显著。在 C 图中，以周长 1200ms 刺激标本可出现自发的规律的激动。在心外膜细胞有 1∶1 的反应，但在心肌中层细胞和心内膜细胞反应不规则。特别是心肌中层细胞 APD 显著延长，显示了 3 相波形，提示电张力的相互作用。也有证据显示标本中存在非同步的激动（很可能是折返激动的基质）。在其他 4 个透壁标本中，心肌中层（M）细胞显示了 APD 和刺激周长之间的特殊关系。然而，与浦肯野纤维（PF）相比，在相似的周长和 AP-A 浓度时，这些细胞中以 EAD 为特征的震荡反应并不常见。（引自 El-Sherif N，Turitto G：The long QT syndrome and torsade de pointes. Pacing Clin Electrophysiol 22：91-110，1999.）

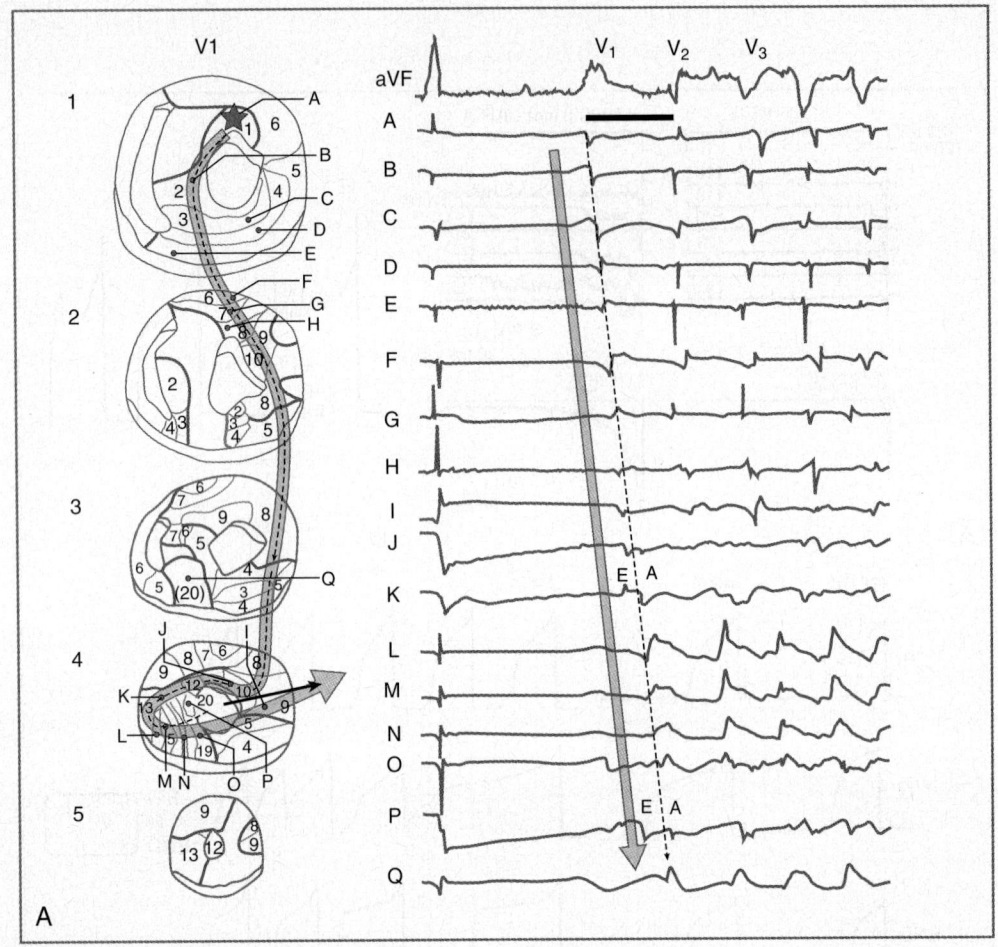

图 74-3 A~B4 示 12 个心搏的非持续性尖端扭转型室速三维心室激动模型 图示 5 个心脏横切面，基底部在上，心尖部在下，并以 1 到 5 标记。B1~B4 中，删除了第一部分。激动等时线以每 20ms 间期被画作闭合的轮廓并标以 1、2、3 等，从而更容易理解室性心动过速连续心搏的激动模型。功能传导阻滞在图中由黑色实线表示。在体表心电图导联之下的粗横线表示由每个三维图覆盖的时间间期。V_1 心搏是局灶性心内膜下激动（在第 1 部分以星号表示）。A，在 V_1 导联，沿折返路径记录的局部心电图，阐述了在第 1 个持续 400ms 的折返周期中完全的舒张期桥联。在第 4 部分的缓慢传导区记录的双极电图有宽的多组分的图形。在功能传导阻滞弧近端记录的电图有双重电位，分别代表电子电位（E）和激动电位（A）。电子电位与功能传导阻滞弧相反侧（心电图 J，K 和 Q）的激动同步。所有接下来的尖端扭转型室速的心搏都是由不同形态的折返环路产生的折返激动引起（B1~B4）。在室性心动过速发作的后半部分，扭转的 QRS 形态在 aVF 导联更明显。QRS 轴的移行（在 V_7 和 V_{10} 之间）与分叉相关，占据主导的单个旋转的波锋成为两个分开并同时围绕左室和右室腔旋转的波锋。QRS 轴最后的移行（在 V_{10} 和 V_{11} 之间）与右室环路的终止和单个左室环状波锋再次建立有关。P，P 波。（改自 El-Sherif N, Chinushi M, Caref EB, Restivo M：Electrophysiological mechanism of the characteristic electrocardiographic morphology of torsade de points tachyarrhythmias in the long QT syndrome. Detailed analysis of ventricular tridimensional activation patterns. Circulation 96：4392-4399，1997.)

联 aVF 更明显。QRS 轴开始的移行（在 V_7 和 V_{10} 之间）与占据主导地位并伴有两个独立但同时围绕左室和右室腔旋转的波锋的分叉相关。QRS 轴最后的移行（在 V_{10} 和 V_{11} 之间）与右室环路的终止和单个左室环状波锋的再次建立有关。

五、药物性长 QT 综合征和尖端扭转型室速的电生理机制

最近，在慢性房室阻滞引起心脏肥大的犬模型[19]中进行了获得性长 QT 综合征电生理机制的研究，这种心室肥厚模型是继发于长期容量负荷过重所致。该

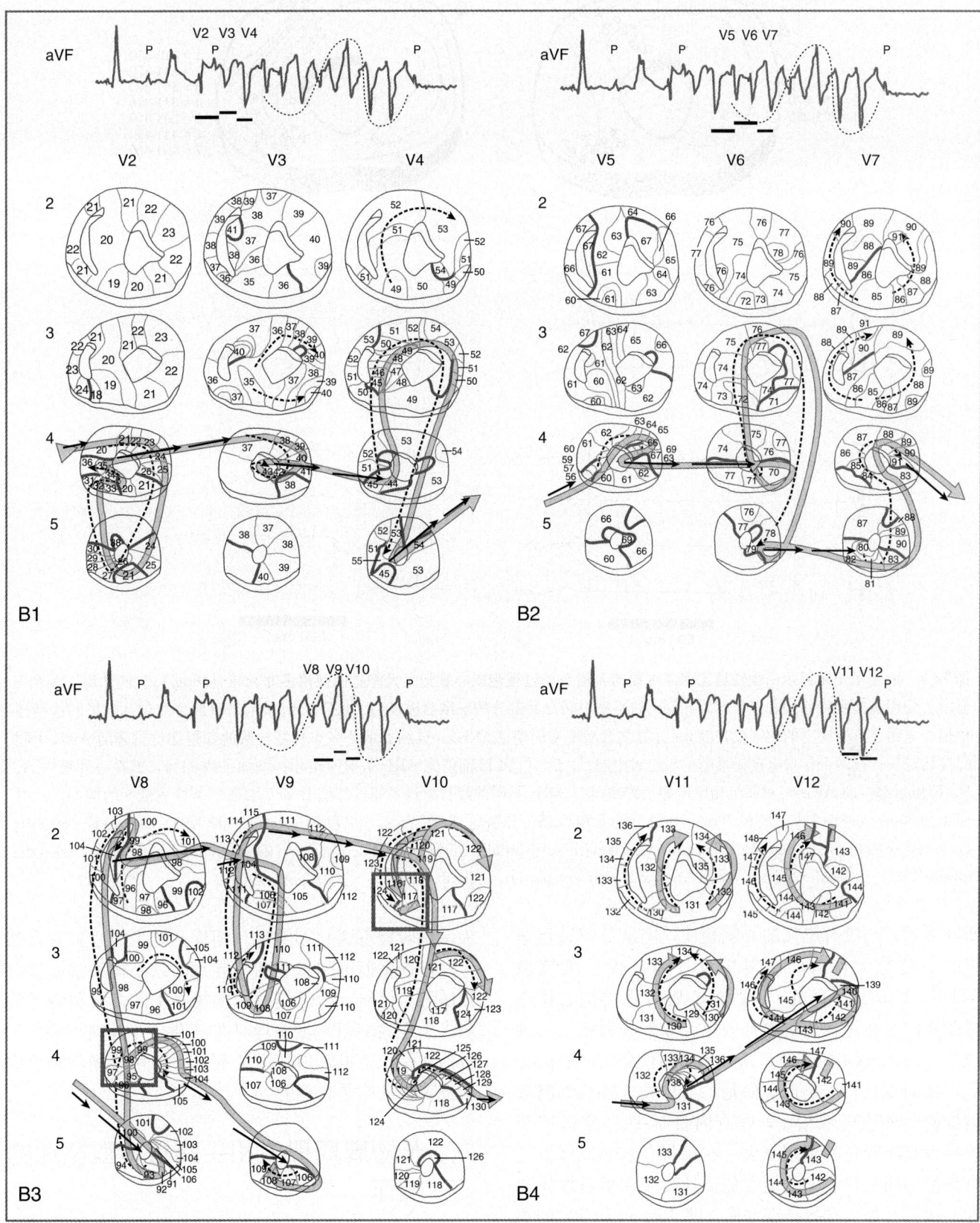

图 74-3 续图

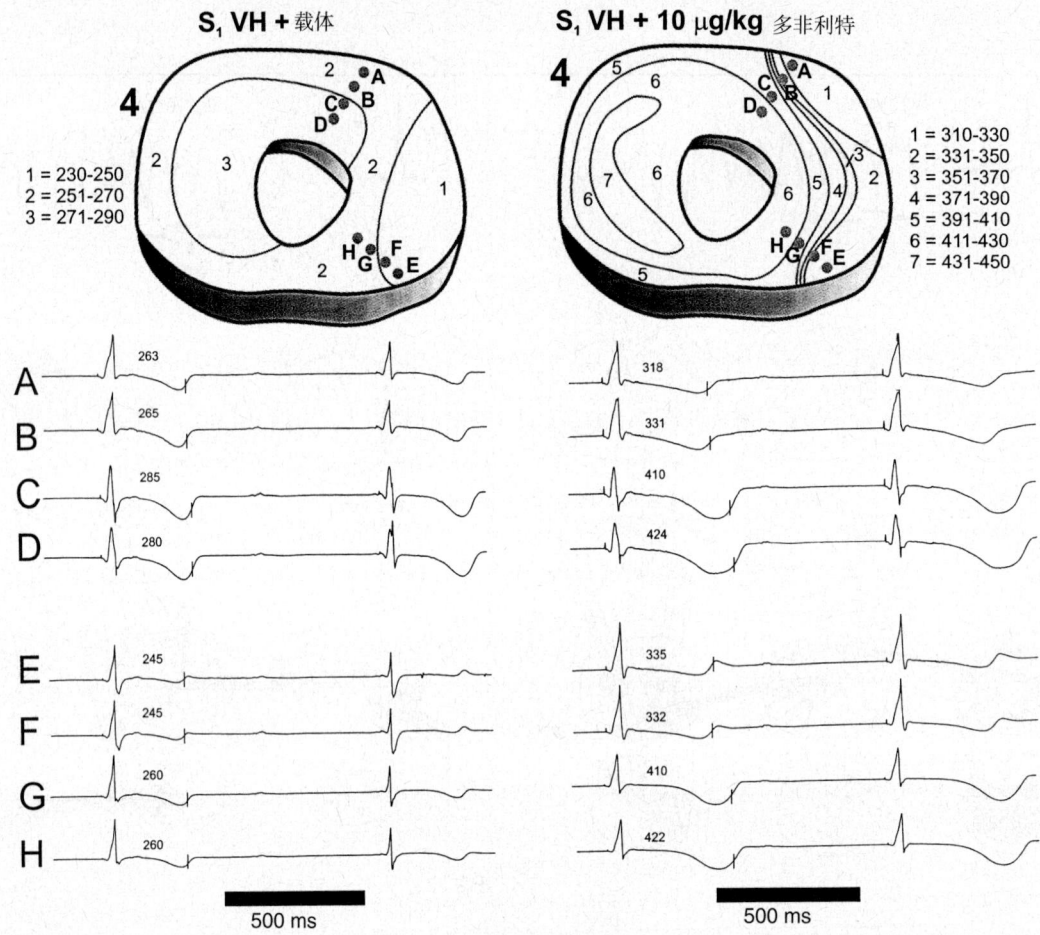

图74-4　心电图记录显示由慢性房室阻滞导致的容量负荷过重造成心脏肥大犬静脉内使用多非利特（10μg/kg）的作用　A 和 B 显示了使用多非利特前后心室起搏波（S_1）的心室中间交叉部分的三维复极模型。底下的记录示来自两个穿刺针电极的选择性单极心电图。心电图上的数字代表以 ms 计算的激动恢复周期（ARIs）。该图显示了多非利特导致的邻近部位显著的 ARIs 不同程度的延长。在两个针状电极记录图中，心肌中层 C、D、G 和 H 部位的 ARIs 与对照组相比增加了约54%，而在心外膜的 A、B、E 和 F 部位的 ARIs 与对照组相比增加了约28%。ARIs 不同的延长导致了邻近部位 B 和 C 显著的复极离散度的增加，从对照组的 20ms 到使用多非利特的 79ms，在邻近的 F 和 G 部位分别是 15 到 78ms。（引自 Kozhevnikov DO, Yamamoto K, Robotis D, et al: Electrophysiological mechanism of enchanced susceptibility of hypertrophied heart to acquired torsade de points arrhythmias: Tridimensional mapping of activation and recovery patterns. Circulation 105: 1128-1134, 2002.）

研究显示，与没有肥大的心脏相比，容量负荷过重造成的心脏肥大伴有心室复极延长和复极三维离散（TDR）的增加。此外，肥大的心脏对Ⅲ类抗心律失常药物的复极延长效应更加敏感，如多非利特是一种选择性的 I_{Kr} 通道阻滞剂。多非利特可使肥大心脏的心室复极明显延长。更重要的是，与造成复极三维离散增加的心外膜区域相比，在心内膜/心肌中层区域药物导致复极延长的差别更大。在相邻心肌部位复极三维离散的增加代表了功能性的传导阻滞和折返性快速性心律失常如尖端扭转型室速（图74-4 和 74-5）的主要电生理基质。该研究显示高剂量的多非利特导致复极的延长，增加复极的三维离散，在正常心脏中引起尖端扭转型室速并不常见。相反，肥大的心脏对在临床允许剂量范围的多非利特导致的致心律失常后果更加敏感。该研究为已报道的剂量相关的多非利特导致病人发生尖端扭转型室速事件提供了电生理基础[20]。目前在临床上推荐逐步增加剂量并密切监测药物效应的建议被证明是合理的。

六、长短周期现象和尖端扭转型室速的发作

一个或更多的长短周期现象，通常是心室早搏二联律的结果，常常出现在恶性室性快速性心律失常发

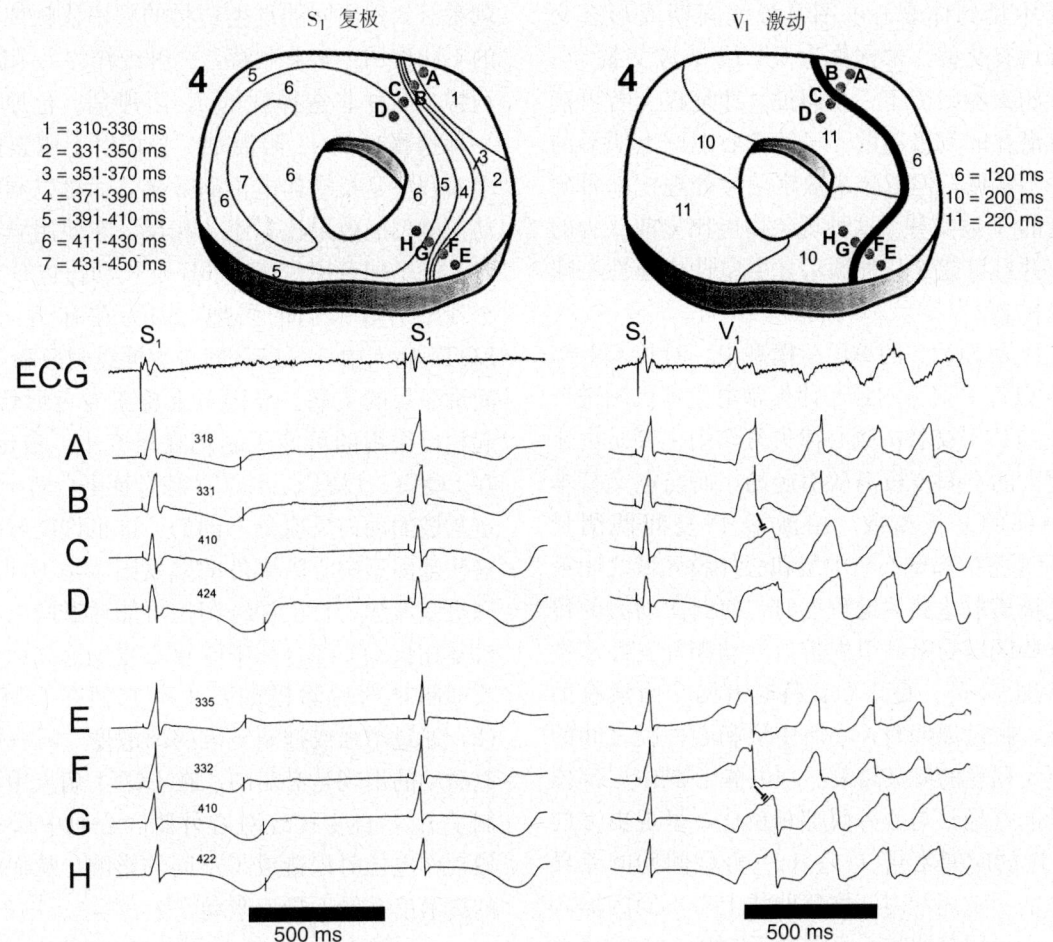

图 74-5 与图 74-1 同一个试验的记录 该图把在引发 TdP 之前的 S_1 刺激引起除极搏动的复极电图与开始 TdP 的 V_1 搏动相并列。基于功能传导阻滞区和折返激动的电生理基质,多非利特增强了关键部位的复极三维的离散度。底下左边,两个在 TdP 之前的 S_1 刺激引起除极心搏。底下右边,同一个心电图,紧跟在 TdP 发作之前的 S_1 刺激引起除极心搏和初始的 4 个 TdP 搏动。该图清楚地显示在邻近的部位 B、C、F、G 出现的由 V_1 心搏导致的功能传导阻滞,并伴有显著的空间复极离散,正如拥挤的复极等时线所描述的那样。所有接下来的 TdP 的搏动都归结于不同的前向波锋。ECG:心电图。 (引自 Kozhevnikov DO, Yamamoto K, Robotis D, et al: Electrophysiological mechanism of enchanced susceptibility of hypertrophied heart to acquired torsade de points arrhythmias: Tridimensional mapping of activation and recovery patterns. Circulation 105: 1128-1134, 2002.)

生之前。在有器质性心脏病而 QT 间期正常[21]的病人和在有先天性[22]或获得性[23]长 QT 综合征的病人中也可以看到这种现象。但电生理机制尚未完全清楚。最近应用犬 AP-A 模型,即代表 LQT3 模型进行了这方面的研究[17]。持续的二联律起源于相同或不同部位的心内膜下局灶激动 (subendocardial focal activity, SFA),而尖端扭转型室速则在复极离散的基质上通过心内膜下局灶激动的侵入导致了折返性心律失常。在多灶性二联律情况下,尖端扭转型室速发生在心内膜下局灶激动之后,心内膜下局灶激动既有起源的关键部位也有与潜在的促使折返的复极离散的模式有关的局部耦联间期。在单灶性二联律情况下,尖端扭转型室速发生的机制如下:(1) 第二个来自不同部位的心内膜下局灶激动侵入了第一个心内膜下局灶激动的复极离散区从而启动了折返;(2) 前面周期的轻微延长导致了关键部位的复极离散度增加,因为与心外膜区域相比心肌中层区域局部复极时间增加不同。这导致了新的功能性传导阻滞弧并且减慢了传导进而引发了折返。因此,从二联律到尖端扭转型室速的移行是促发折返激动的电生理变化的结果。

七、QT/T 波交替和尖端扭转型室速

人们早已熟知,心动过速依赖性的 T 波电交替 (见第 91 章) 出现在先天性和特发性的长 QT 综合征中并可能预示尖端扭转型室速的发作。在不同的实验

和临床工作中见到体表心电图复极波间期或形态交替，或二者均有交替，常常称为 QT 或 T 波交替[24]。对复极交替的兴趣归因于一个假说，即复极交替可能反映了心脏潜在的复极离散。尽管在心电图上明显的 T 波交替并不常见，但近年来数字信号处理技术可确认细微程度的 T 波交替。这种现象可能比先前认为的更加普遍，并且可能是一种预示发生室性快速性心律失常的重要标志。

最近在代表 LQT3 的 AP-A 模型中，对长 QT 综合征病人中 QT/T 交替的致心律失常电生理机制进行了研究[16]。QT/T 交替的致心律失常作用主要是由比心率慢时更大的空间复极离散引起的，而与电交替本身无关。局部的复极离散（由激活/恢复间期测量[ARIs]）在左室游离壁心肌中层和心外膜区域之间最明显。当复极离散达到关键程度时，前向激动波的传播可能在这些区域受阻而引发折返激动和阵发性室性心动过速（图 74-6）。QT/T 交替时有两个因素有助于调节复极，在短周期时，心肌中层和心外膜之间的区域产生更大程度的复极离散：(1) 在心肌中层部位恢复动力学的差异，与心外膜部相位比，呈现更大的 ΔARI 和更慢的时间常量（τ）；(2) 舒张间期的差异导致在相同的固定周期时，恢复曲线上有不同的输入量。在第一个短周期期间心肌中层部位更长的 ARI 导致了更短的舒张间期，并因此造成了更大程度的 ARI 的缩短。这些结论在其后的实验模型中得到了证实[25,26]。

一个重要的发现是，显著的复极交替可以出现在局部电图中而不伴有体表心电图显著的 QT/T 交替。伴心外膜和心肌中层部位复极力度的逆转，在交替周期时心肌内 QT 波极性逆转的短周期中可见体表心电图 QT/T 交替现象[16,25]。这一发现为近年来试图用来确认微伏级 T 波交替的数字信号处理技术提供了理论。

八、自主神经和长 QT 综合征

临床观察显示 Na^+ 通道变异的 LQT3 病人中尖端扭转型室速的发作可能出现在休息或睡眠时，而不是在运动中，这可能与相对的心动过缓有关[27]。相反，K^+ 通道变异的病人，特别是 LQT1 病人，通常在紧张的情况下有晕厥或心脏骤停，可能是儿茶酚胺的致心律失常作用的影响，或者是由于 QT 间期对周期缩短的调节能力包括调节率和调节度的差异，或者二者兼而有之[27]。Schreick 和同事[28]研究了 β 肾上腺素能刺激对 3 种不同的Ⅲ类药物的频率依赖性电生理活动的不同作用：多非利特，一种纯粹的 I_{Kr} 阻滞剂；氨巴利特，一种非选择性的 I_K 阻滞剂；色原烷醇 293B，一种选择性的 I_{Ks} 阻滞剂。异丙肾上腺素能显著降低多非利特延长动作电位的效果，而氨巴利特降低延长动作电位的效果比较小。相反，在使用异丙肾上腺素时，能增加色原烷醇 293B 延长动作电位的效果。这个现象引起人们的兴趣，因为在有 I_{Ks} 通道变异的 LQT1 病人中，可以看到自主神经刺激和 TdP 发作之间最显著的关联。异丙肾上腺素对色原烷醇 293B 引起相反作用的可能机制仍在研究中。最近研究表明，在 LQT1、LQT2、LQT3 综合征中，对于交感兴奋心室复极的动力反应是不同的，这也许能解释为什么在这些基因型中心脏事件的触发因素是不同的。从电生理机制考虑，自主神经调控可能通过两条内在相关的机制在长 QT 综合征中导致心律失常：(1) 通过增强或抑制早期后除极的发生和它们在心脏中的传导；(2) 通过增强或抑制复极的离散度。后一种机制对折返激动的出现是必需的。在 LQT1 病人中可能因为抑制了 I_{Ks}，自主神经对心外膜、心肌中层和心内膜区域动作电位时程造成了不同的影响，从而增加了复极的离散度并触发折返激动[29]。

九、长 QT 综合征和尖端扭转型室速的临床表现与治疗

（一）先天性长 QT 综合征

目前估计长 QT 综合征基因的携带率为 1/10 000[30]。在美国儿童和青年中长 QT 综合征每年引起 3000～4000 人猝死。大约三分之二的基因携带者发生过晕厥，有症状的携带者可能发生过 1 次到数百次不等的事件。在一个拥有相同基因型和变异的家族中，同时存在有症状的和终生无症状的个体。症状出现时间平均在 10 岁前或十几岁，最早可至生命的第 1 天，而迟至 40～50 岁发病的很少见。总的来说，10%～30% 有症状的病人发生猝死，有频繁晕厥或心脏骤停后复苏病史的病人猝死发生风险更高。猝死可能发生在第一次晕厥时，这强调了症状前诊断和治疗的巨大重要性。晕厥和猝死最常出现在运动或情绪激动时，但在 HERG 和 SCN5A 基因型的病人中，晕厥和猝死可能出现在睡眠中。这些事件可在先前无症状的病人中由延长 QT 间期的药物和低钾血症诱发（见

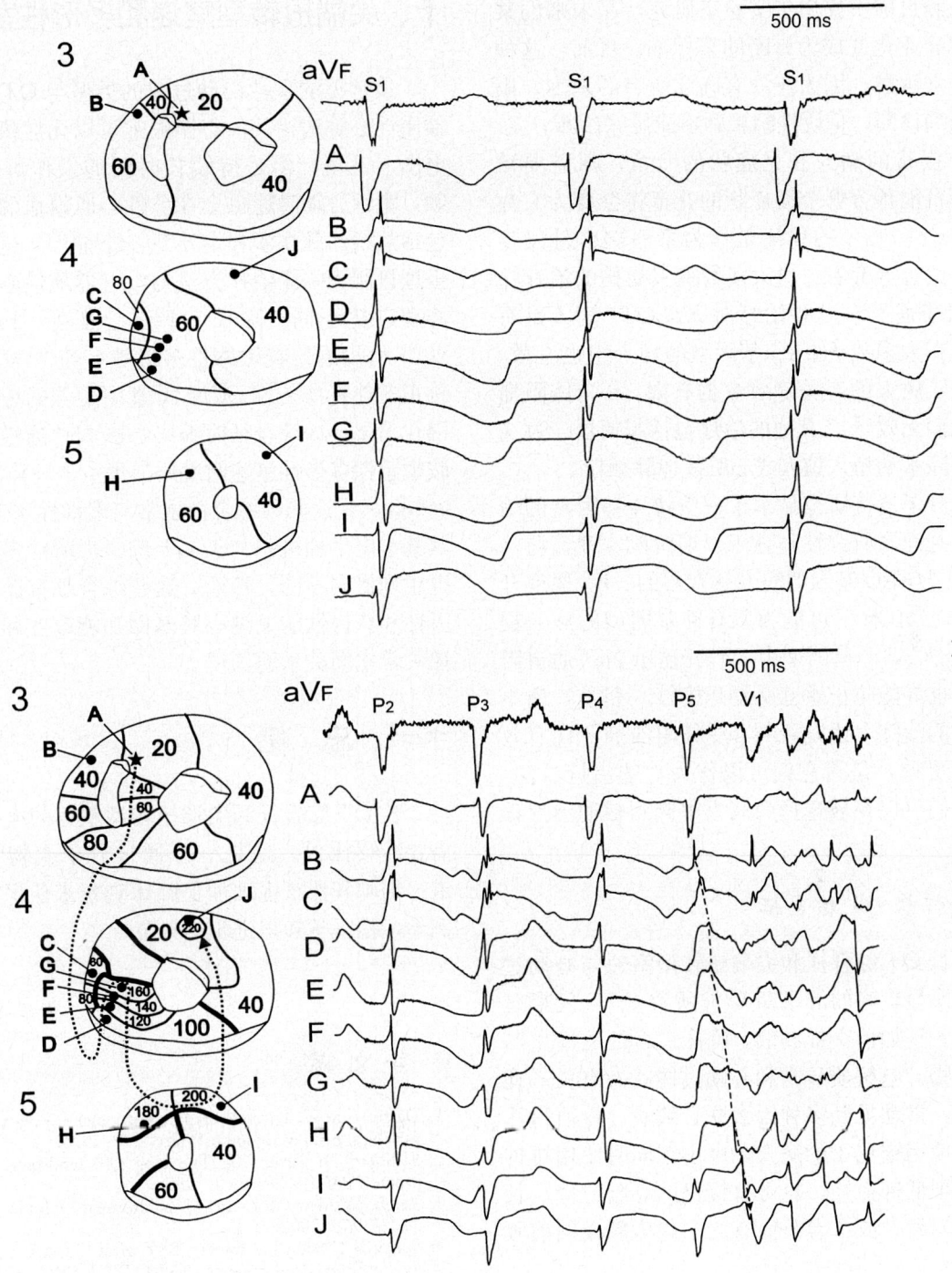

图 74-6　代表 LQT3 模型的 AP-A 犬试验记录　在心电图 aVF 导联的 T 波电交替是由心室起搏的周期长度（CL）从 700ms（上面）到 350ms（底下）突然缩短引起的。随之而来的第 5 个起搏搏动是短周期长度（P_5），多形性室速开始发作，其中第 1 个搏动被标以 V_1。该图显示了起搏节律 700ms 时的三维激动图形（S_1）（上图）。在第 3 部分，激动在起搏部位开始（星号）。总的心室激动时间 80ms，并且没有功能传导阻滞弧。右侧显示的是选择性的单极心电图。在这个周期长度任何部位都没有 QT/T 的交替。底下显示的是来自同一个试验，当周期长度突然缩短到 350ms（P）时的记录。左侧显示的是引起折返激动的 P_5 的激动图形。右侧显示的是沿着折返路径的心电图，显示完全的舒张桥联。与心外膜部位 B、C、I、J 相比，在心肌中层部位 E 到 H 出现 QT/T 交替更为明显。在 220ms 等时线再次激动第 4 部分心外膜下部位前，折返波锋环绕在第 4 和第 5 部分的心外膜和心肌中层之间的功能传导阻滞弧（实线）。（引自 Chinushi M, Restivo M, Caref EB, El-Sherif N: Electrophysiologic basis of arrhymogenicity of QT/T alternans in the long-QT syndrome: Tridimensional analysis of the kinetics of cardiac reporlarization. Circ Res 83：614-628，1998.）

表74-2）。对LQT4病人唯一的发现是阵发性房颤。

遗传检测目前主要用于实验室研究，在未来的某个时候可能商业化并成为诊断的金标准。目前，这种检测并不非常敏感，因为还没有确定所有的基因。阳性结果能明确诊断，但阴性结果并不能排除诊断。

所有有症状的病人和无症状的儿童，都需要治疗。我们不可能预言哪个无症状的儿童将会变为有症状，由于30%~40%的猝死是作为第一次事件发生的，因此不适合等等看。对大多数病人初始的治疗选择β受体阻滞剂[31]。这种治疗对KvLQT1病人是有效的，并且在大多数HERG基因型的病人中也有效。Na⁺通道变异病人的有关疗效数据有限，β受体阻滞剂可能对他们无效[32]。其他的治疗包括起搏器、颈交感神经节切除术和植入植入式心脏复律除颤器。

最近的分子遗传研究显示了一些特异基因型的治疗方法。这些尚属研究性且处于早期阶段。钾负荷治疗[33]可能对HERG基因型病人是有益的。K⁺通道开放剂[34]和维拉帕米[35]可能为所有钾基因型的病人提供帮助。在SCN5A基因型中，研究显示Na⁺通道阻滞剂美西律也许能防止通道反复开放[32]。目前，尚不知道这些新的治疗方法是否与β受体阻滞剂一样有效或是更好或更差，是否它们可以作为首选治疗方法，或者是否它们仅仅在被选择的病人中起到辅助治疗作用。

（二）获得性长QT综合征

获得性长QT综合征和尖端扭转型室速与心动过缓性停搏和明显较晚的舒张期U波所致QTU间期延长密切有关。正如前文提到的，临床综合征的发生与应用某种药物、电解质异常和心动过缓状态有关。在临床实践中，常常见到多种因素联合致病。最值得注意的例子是使用奎尼丁的病人，可由于同时使用排钾利尿剂而出现低钾血症，也可有缓慢的心脏节律、长的心动过缓间歇，或二者兼而有之（如房颤或期前收缩后的间歇）[36]。

对获得性长QT综合征和阵发性室性心动过速病人的治疗需要立即采取措施抑制快速性心律失常。静脉内使用硫酸镁能抑制室性心动过速而并不缩短延长的QTU间期[37]。通过给予阿托品或异丙肾上腺素或采取更加可取的方法如临时心室起搏增加心率，通常能成功抑制心律失常。快速的起搏缩短动作电位时程和QT间期并抑制早期后除极。长期治疗措施包括纠正潜在的电解质异常和停用引起发作的药物。

十、尖端扭转型室速和多形性室速

最常见的室性心动过速的类型与QT间期正常的器质性心脏病相关。心律失常可以无症状而在动态心电图上发现，但是持续长时间的发作可以蜕变为室颤。室性心动过速也会在急性心肌缺血的情况时出现包括冠状动脉痉挛和变异型心绞痛[38]。这些病例的电生理机制和临床治疗方法与没有器质性心脏病的室性心动过速不同。除长QT综合征外，Brugada综合征[39]和儿茶酚胺敏感性多形性室速[40]发生在心脏结构正常伴有遗传性SCN5A基因变异的患者中，该基因在Brugada综合征时编码心脏Na⁺通道，在儿茶酚胺敏感性多形性室速时编码斯里兰卡肉桂碱受体（ryanodine）。这两种综合征也常与多形性室速发生有关，其基本电生理机制与长QT综合征时的多形性室速的电生理机制不同。然而，这些综合征有助于提高对先天性和获得性的关键心脏基因功能改变和恶性室性心律失常之间关系的认识。

十一、总 结

长QT综合征和尖端扭转型室速的电生理机制还需要继续探讨。这是一个通过分子生物学、离子通道、细胞和器官生理加上临床观察来认识疾病的最佳例子，是医学知识进步的典范。

（邹建刚 译）

参 考 文 献

1. Dessertenne F: La tachycardie ventriculaire a deux foyers opposes variables. Arch Mal Coeur 59:263–272, 1996.
2. El-Sherif N, Turitto G: The long QT syndrome and torsade de pointes. PACE 22:91–110, 1999.
3. Zareba W, Moss AJ: Long QT syndrome in children. J Electrocardiol 34:167–171, 2001.
4. Splawski I, Shen J, Timothy KW, et al: Spectrum of mutations in long QT syndrome genes. KVLQT1, HERG, SCN5A, KCNE1, and KCNE2. Circulation 102:1178–1184, 2000.
5. Castillo R, Pedalino RP, El-Sherif N, Turitto G: Efavirenz-associated QT prolongation and Torsade de pointes arrhythmia. Ann Pharmacother 36:1006–1008, 2002.
6. Canadian Adverse Drug Reaction Newsletter: Drugs causing prolongation of QT interval and torsade de pointes. Can Med Assoc J 158:103–104, 1998.
7. Napolitano C, Schwartz PJ, Brown AM, et al: Evidence for a cardiac ion channel mutation underlying drug-induced QT prolongation and life-threatening arrhythmias. J Cardiovasc Electrophysiol 11:691–696, 2000.
8. Sesti F, Abbott GW, Wei J, et al: A common polymorphism associated with antibiotic-induced cardiac arrhythmia. Proc Natl Acad Sci

U S A 97:10613–10618, 2000.
9. Moss AJ, Zareba W, Benhorin J, et al: ISHNE guidelines for electrocardiographic evaluation of drug-related QT prolongation and other alterations in ventricular repolarization: Task Force summary. A report of the Task Force of the International Society for Holter and Noninvasive Electrocardiology (ISHNE), Committee on Ventricular Repolarization. Ann Noninvasive Electrocardiol 6:333–341, 2001.
10. El-Sherif N, Zeiler RH, Craelius W, et al: QTU prolongation and polymorphic ventricular tachyarrhythmias due to bradycardia-dependent early afterdepolarizations. Circ Res 63:286–305, 1988.
11. El-Sherif N, Fozzard HA, Hanck DA: Dose-dependent modulation of the cardiac sodium channel by the sea anemone toxin ATXII. Circ Res 70:285–301, 1992.
12. Wang Q, Shen J, Splawski I, et al: SCN5A mutations associated with an inherited cardiac arrhythmia, long QT syndrome. Cell 80:805–811, 1995.
13. Bennett PB, Yazawa K, Makita N, George AL Jr: Molecular mechanism for an inherited cardiac arrhythmia. Nature 376:683–685, 1995.
14. El-Sherif N, Caref EB, Yin H, Restivo M: The electrophysiological mechanism of ventricular tachyarrhythmias in the long QT syndrome: Tridimensional mapping of activation and recovery patterns. Circ Res 79:474–492, 1996.
15. El-Sherif N, Chinushi M, Caref EB, Restivo M: Electrophysiological mechanism of the characteristic electrocardiographic morphology of torsade de pointes tachyarrhythmias in the long QT syndrome. Detailed analysis of ventricular tridimensional activation patterns. Circulation 96:4392–4399, 1997.
16. Chinushi M, Restivo M, Caref EB, El-Sherif N: Electrophysiological basis of the arrhythmogenicity of QT/T alternans in the long QT syndrome. Tridimensional analysis of the kinetics of cardiac repolarization. Circ Res 83:614–628, 1998.
17. El-Sherif N, Caref EB, Chinushi M, Restivo M: Mechanism of arrhythmogenicity of the short-long cardiac sequence that precedes ventricular tachyarrhythmias in the long QT syndrome. J Am Coll Cardiol 33:1415–1423, 1999.
18. Antzelevich C, Sicouri S: Clinical relevance of cardiac arrhythmias generated by afterdepolarizations: Role of M cells in the generation of U waves, triggered activity and torsade de pointes. J Am Coll Cardiol 23:259–277, 1994.
19. Kozhevnikov DO, Yamamoto K, Robotis D, et al: Electrophysiological mechanisms of enhanced susceptibility of hypertrophied heart to acquired torsade de pointes arrhythmias. Tridimensional mapping of activation and recovery patterns. Circulation 105:1128–1134, 2001.
20. Mazur A, Anderson ME, Bonney S, et al: Pause-dependent polymorphic ventricular tachycardia during long-term treatment with dofetilide: A placebo-controlled, implantable cardioverter-defibrillator-based evaluation. J Am Coll Cardiol 37:1100–1105, 2001.
21. Leclercq JF, Maison-Blanche P, Cauchemez B, Coumel P: Respective role of sympathetic tone and cardiac pauses in the genesis of 62 cases of ventricular fibrillation recorded during Holter monitoring. Eur Heart J 9:1276–1283, 1988.
22. Viskin S, Alla SR, Barron HV, et al: Mode of onset of torsades de pointes in congenital long QT syndrome. J Am Coll Cardiol 28:1262–1268, 1996.
23. Kay GN, Plumb VJ, Arciniegas JG, et al: Torsades de pointes; the long-short initiating sequence and other clinical features; observations in 32 patients. J Am Coll Cardiol 2:806–817, 1990.
24. El-Sherif N, Turitto G, Pedalino RP, Robotis D: T-wave alternans and arrhythmia risk stratification. Ann Noninvas Electrocardiol 6:323–332, 2001.
25. Shimizu W, Antzelevich C: Cellular and ionic basis for T-wave alternans under long QT conditions. Circulation 99:1499–1507, 1999.
26. Pastore JM, Girouard SD, Laurita KR, et al: Mechanism linking T-wave alternans to the genesis of cardiac fibrillation. Circulation 99:1385–1394, 1999.
27. Schwartz PJ, Priori SG, Locati EH, et al: Long QT syndrome patients with mutations of the SCN5A and HERG genes have differential responses to Na+ channel blockade and to increases in heart rate. Implications for gene-specific therapy. Circulation 92:3381–3386, 1995.
28. Schreick J, Wang Y, Gjini V, et al: Differential effect of β-adrenergic stimulation on the frequency-dependent electrophysiologic actions of the new class III antiarrhythmics dofetilide, ambasilide, and chromanol 293B. J Cardiovasc Electrophysiol 8:1420–1430, 1997.
29. Noda T, Takaki H, Kurita T, et al: Gene-specific response of dynamic ventricular repolarization to sympathetic stimulation in LQT1, LQT2, and LQT3 forms of congenital long QT syndrome. Eur Heart J 23:975–983, 2002.
30. Vincent GM, Timothy K, Leppert M, Keating MV: The spectrum of symptoms and QT interval in carriers of the gene for the long-QT syndrome. N Engl J Med 327:846–852, 1992.
31. Vincent GM, Fox J, Zhang L, Timothy KW: Beta-blockers markedly reduce risk and syncope in KVLQT1 long QT patients. Circulation 94(suppl 1):1–204, 1996.
32. Schwartz PJ, Priori SG, Locati EH, et al: Long QT syndrome patients with mutations of the SCN5A and HERG genes have differential responses to Na+ channel blockade and to increases in heart rate. Implications for gene-specific therapy. Circulation 92:3381–3386, 1995.
33. Compton SJ, Lux RL, Ramsey MR, et al: Genetically defined therapy of inherited long-QT syndrome. Correction of abnormal repolarization by potassium. Circulation 94:1018–1022, 1996.
34. Vincent GM, Fox J, Zhang L, et al: Effects of a potassium channel opener in KVLQT1 long QT gene carriers. J Am Coll Cardiol 29:183A, 1997.
35. Shimuzu W, Ohe T, Kurita T, et al: Effects of verapamil and propranolol on early afterdepolarizations and ventricular arrhythmias induced by epinephrine in congenital long QT syndrome. J Am Coll Cardiol 26:1299–1309, 1995.
36. Roden DN, Woosley RL, Prim RK: Incidence and clinical features of the quinidine associates long QT syndrome: Implications for patient care. Am Heart J 111:1088–1093, 1986.
37. Tzivoni D, Keren A, Cohen AM, et al: Magnesium therapy for torsade de pointes. Am J Cardiol 53:528–530, 1984.
38. Wolfe CL, Nibley C, Bandhari A, et al: Polymorphous ventricular tachycardia associated with acute myocardial infarction. Circulation 84:1543–1551, 1991.
39. Brugada P, Brugada J: Right bundle branch block, persistent ST segment elevation and sudden cardiac death: A distinct clinical and electrocardiographic syndrome. J Am Coll Cardiol 20:1391–1396, 1992.
40. Priori S, Napolitano C, Memmi M, et al: Clinical and molecular charaterization of patients with catecholaminergic polymorphic ventricular tachycardia. Circulation 106:8–10, 2002.

第 75 章

加速性室性自主心律和双向性室性心动过速

Wolfram Grimm and Francis E. Marchlinski

本章目录

- 加速性室性自主心律 ············· 692
- 双向性室性心动过速 ············· 693

一、加速性室性自主心律

早在1910年Thomas Lewis就报道了加速性室性自主心律的病例,但直至1950年Harris[1]才第一次详细描述了发生在实验性心肌梗死的异位室性心律。他注意到"心室异位性激动的频率几乎等于窦房结交替地夺获和失夺获的频率"。Harris也认识到这种心律失常是良性的,与心室颤动无关系。后来,这种异位心律曾获几种名称:室性自主性心动过速、缓慢室性心动过速和非阵发性室性心动过速等。最后,Marriott和Menendez[2]通过纯粹地描述性术语称之为加速性室性自主心律,这个名称现在仍被普遍接受。

加速性室性自主心律是3个或3个以上连续的室性早搏、频率快于正常心室固有的逸搏心率30~40bpm,但慢于室性心动过速的异位节律(表75-1)。另外,加速性室性自主心律还有一些与室性心动过速显然不同的典型特征,包括心律失常起始和终止方式,而且其通常为良性过程。异位频率通常和占优势的窦性心率相似,导致等同节律的房室分离(图75-1)。然而,当较长的加速性室性自主心律存在时,也能发生1:1的室房传导(图75-2)。因两个起搏点竞争性控制心室除极,经常在心律失常发作和终止时出现融合波。通常只有一个加速的室性病灶,但在急性心肌梗死[3]和急性心肌炎病人[4]中已有多形性加速性室性自主心律被报告。

对于加速性室性自主心律的上限频率的意见尚不一致。因为具有加速性室性自主心律的典型特征是异位心室律偶然频率高于100bpm,所以我们推荐用120bpm作为加速性室性自主心律的上限频率界限[5,6]。更重要的是,单独频率标准不足以诊断加速性室性自主心律,还有其他特征,包括心律失常开始和终止的方式,都能用来同缓慢的室性心动过速进行鉴别。有时,不可能仅依靠心电图标准做出正确诊断,还需临床提供线索。频率是100~130bpm的缓慢室性心动过速更常发生在应用Ⅰ类或Ⅲ类抗心律失常药物的心肌梗死后的病人。与加速性室性自主心律相反,缓慢的室性心动过速经常持续存在甚至不停止,因为伴有缓慢的室性心动过速的病人通常也有快速性室性心动过速的基础,所以伴随突然心源性猝死的危险性增加。

临床上,加速性室性自主心律更常发生于器质性心脏病,也可见于无明显心脏病的成人和儿童。加速性室性自主心律常见于冠心病、风湿性心脏病、扩张型心肌病、急性心肌梗死、高血压性心脏病、洋地黄中毒和可卡因中毒的病人[7]。9%~46%的急性心肌梗死而没有溶栓治疗的病人能发生加速性室性心律[8],而使用溶栓药物治疗的病人更常发生加速性室性心动过速[9-11]。溶栓药物治疗后加速性室性自主心律可作为再灌注有效的非介入性标志。出现加速性室性自主心律强烈支持再灌注治疗成功(特异性≥80%),但没有加速性室性自主心律也不能排除溶栓成功(敏感性≤50%)。梗死的范围和部位与加速性室性自主心律的起源无明显相关性[12]。

表 75-1　加速性室性自主心律的特征

1. 3 个连续的室性异位节律，频率快于正常心室固有的逸搏频率 30～40bpm，但慢于室性心动过速。
2. 当异位心室病灶加速超过窦性心率，或当室上性节律减慢或窦房阻滞、房室阻滞发生时，允许加速的心室逸搏节律发生时逐渐发作，并通常伴有一个长配对的室性搏动。
3. 通常伴有长串融合波的等同节律的室房分离，但也可发生 1∶1 逆传心房夺获。
4. 通常短暂的和间歇的事件持续 3bpm。
5. 当窦性心律加速和/或异位室性心律减速时逐渐终止。
6. 通常发生在伴急性心肌梗死病人，特别是出现早期再灌注时，但也可能发生在任何其他心脏病，甚至发生在无心脏病的成人和儿童。
7. 通常对血流动力学的耐受性较好，预后良好；除非伴有更多的持续心律失常致房室失去同步而影响血流动力学，一般不需要治疗该心律失常。

在表 75-1 中描述的加速性室性自主心律的心电图特征强烈提示不正常的自律性增强（例如：4 位相心室肌纤维的除极）是很多病例的潜在发生机制[3,13]。有些情况（例如：在急性缺血或洋地黄中毒）触发活动也可以起到加速性室性自主心律的起源作用。与室性心动过速的病人相反，折返在加速性室性自主心律的起源方面并不显示有什么作用，而伴有心肌梗死的室性心动过速病人，在心肌梗死边界的折返是最常见的心律失常的发生机制[3,13]。

一般而言，加速性室性自主心律是良性的，即使呈多形性时也一样[3,4]。因为大多数成串的加速性室性自主心律对血流动力学的耐受性良好而短暂，所以它们无需处理，仅需治疗潜在的心脏病。在极个别情况时加速性室性自主心律伴有洋地黄中毒，该时洋地黄的治疗需要停止。对于心功能处于临界状态的病人，在加速室性自主心律发作时丧失了心房对心室充盈的作用而导致血流动力学的损害。在这种情况下，用阿托品加速窦性心率通常使窦房结重新控制心室律。至于急性心肌梗死病人，加速性室性自主心律不会增加心室颤动的发生率或住院死亡率[12]，在心肌梗死急性期后加速性室性自主心律几乎总是自然消失，因此，这种心律失常不需要治疗。对一组 202 例扩张型心肌病病人进行的前瞻性研究中[6]，我们发现加速性室性自主心律存在于 8% 的病人，随访期间发现对主要心律失常事件或总死亡率没有预后意义[7]。

二、双向性室性心动过速

双向性室性心动过速这个术语是指 QRS 波在室性心动过速时额面电轴逐跳地发生变化。因此，双向性室性心动过速是一组不同类型的心律失常，对有相似的心电图形态及不同电生理机制的单纯的描述性术语。临床上，双向（束支）性室性心动过速最常与洋地黄中毒有关[14,15]，但也见于没有洋地黄中毒的其他临床情况，如：草药的乌头碱中毒[16]、家族性低钾性周期性麻痹[17]和没有明显心脏病的病人[18]。最近，也有报道见于儿茶酚胺敏感性室性心动过速病人（见第 68 章）[19,20]。

在洋地黄中毒时双向（束支）性室性心动过速显示一些典型的心电图特征[14]：（1）心室率通常在 140～180bpm 之间；（2）QRS 波是窄的，通常小于 140ms，

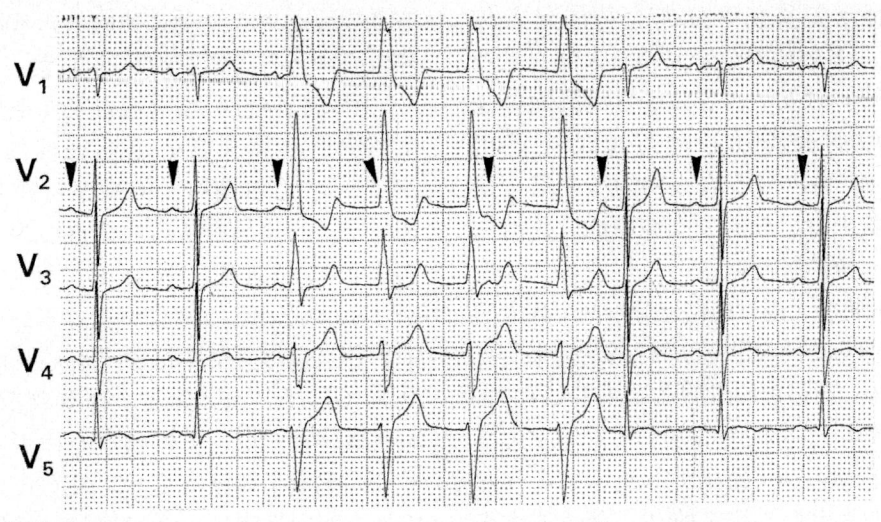

图 75-1　心电图记录（25mm/s）显示一阵 4 跳连串的加速性室性自主心律（88bpm）　箭头指示为窦性 P 波。在加速性室性自主心律期间没有室房传导。

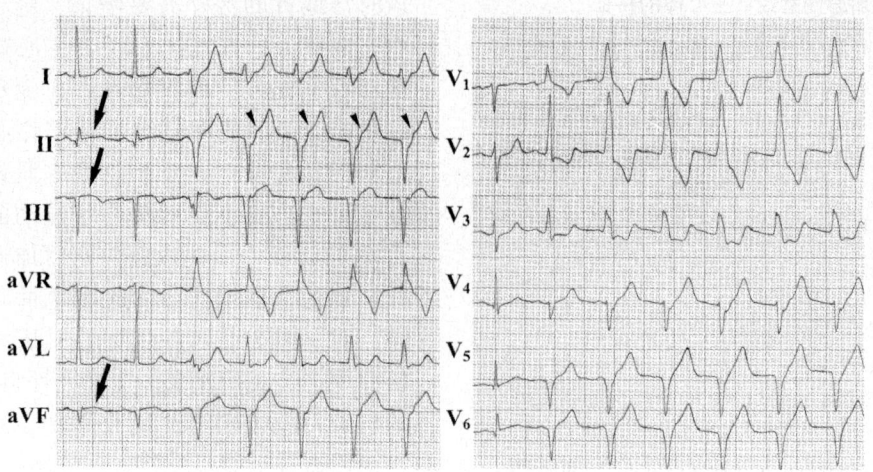

图 75-2 溶栓治疗后再灌注期间的心电图记录（25mm/s），患者发生了急性下壁心梗伴 Ⅱ、Ⅲ、aVF 导联 ST 段的抬高（箭头指示）在加速性室性自主心律期间（小箭头示）有 1∶1 的室房传导。

形态类似右束支阻滞；(3) 在额面导联电轴成左、右交替偏移，在肢体导联表现为"双向"（图 75-3）。因此，洋地黄导致的双向性室性心动过速显示出分支性室性心动过速的所有特征，除了有右束支阻滞形的 QRS 波伴有交替性电轴右偏和左偏外。值得注意的是，诊断双向性室性心动过速通常需要记录至少 3 个平面导联（理想的记录包括全部 12 导联），因为心动过速时在单一导联观察可能都很相似或仅有幅度的变化。

自 1922 年[21]Schwensen 在洋地黄中毒的患者中第一次描述了双向性室性心动过速后，其电生理机制一直是令人感兴趣的课题。在洋地黄中毒导致的双向性心动过速病人进行希氏束检查时证明了心动过速起源于心室，伴两个或多个独立的起源点，或仅有一个起源点却伴有左前分支和左后分支交替的异常传导[22]。到现在为止，多数的实验研究和对人体心电图的观察已有证据表明，触发活动导致的延迟后除极是洋地黄中毒时导致的分支性心动过速的主要机制[14,23-25]。Vanagt 和 Wellens[25] 在犬的模型中通过超速起搏演示了洋地黄中毒引起的分支性心动过速的加速度，加速度值与起搏频率正相关。

我们有一独特的机会，通过透彻地分析两个病人的心电图，观察心动过速对于使用 Fab 片段的治疗来研究地高辛中毒时分支性心动过速的机制[14]。实验研究时，模拟的紊乱情况导致从不同的心室部位自发产生室性早搏和非持续性室性心动过速。使用 Fab 抗原结合片段后，在心动过速转变为窦性心律之前[14]，随着地高辛作用的降低，可以看到心动过速从多形（双向）到单一形态，且心动过速的频率逐渐减慢的变化。我们也观察到在心动过速的不同阶段截然不同的反应；例如对不同的成对自发的心室除极的缓慢反应，对非阵发性室性心动过速短暂的使心动过速加速的反应。对于地高辛中毒的双向性心动过速，这些事实强有力地支持其为触发活动而排除了折返机制[14]。

与良性的加速性室性自主心律相反，即使前文描述的多形性室速，洋地黄中毒引起的室性心动过速包括双向性心动过速，常预后不良。当认识到洋地黄是导致束支性心动过速的原因后应当给予适当治疗，使用地高辛特异的抗原结合片段治疗，预后明显改善，多数病人得以幸存[14,15]。使用地高辛特异抗原结合片段治疗的反应相对迅速，治疗 1 小时内能够终止分支性室性心动过速。因此，对于多数伴有症状的洋地黄中毒导致的束支心动过速病人，地高辛特异抗原结合片段必须被考虑作为治疗的选择。

双向性室性心动过速也是儿茶酚胺敏感性多形性室性快速心律失常心电图表现的一部分（见第 68 章）[19,20]。心电图特有的顺序与肾上腺素的刺激强度相平行。心室早搏从四联律进展为二联律，伴随着短的或长的双向性室性心动过速，进展为多形性室速[19]。而心律失常可随肾上腺素的刺激减少而趋向消失。在这个综合征中已发现有心脏的斯里兰卡肉桂碱受体（RyR2）基因突变。伴有 RyR2 基因突变和儿茶酚胺敏感性多形性室性快速心律失常的病人更多见于男性，生命早期就有症状，且有较高的心脏事件的危险性。双向性室性心动过速的发展似乎并非特别地与 RyR2 基因突变相关。在 Priori 及其同事[20] 的一份报告中评价了临床证实的儿茶酚胺敏感性多形性室性快

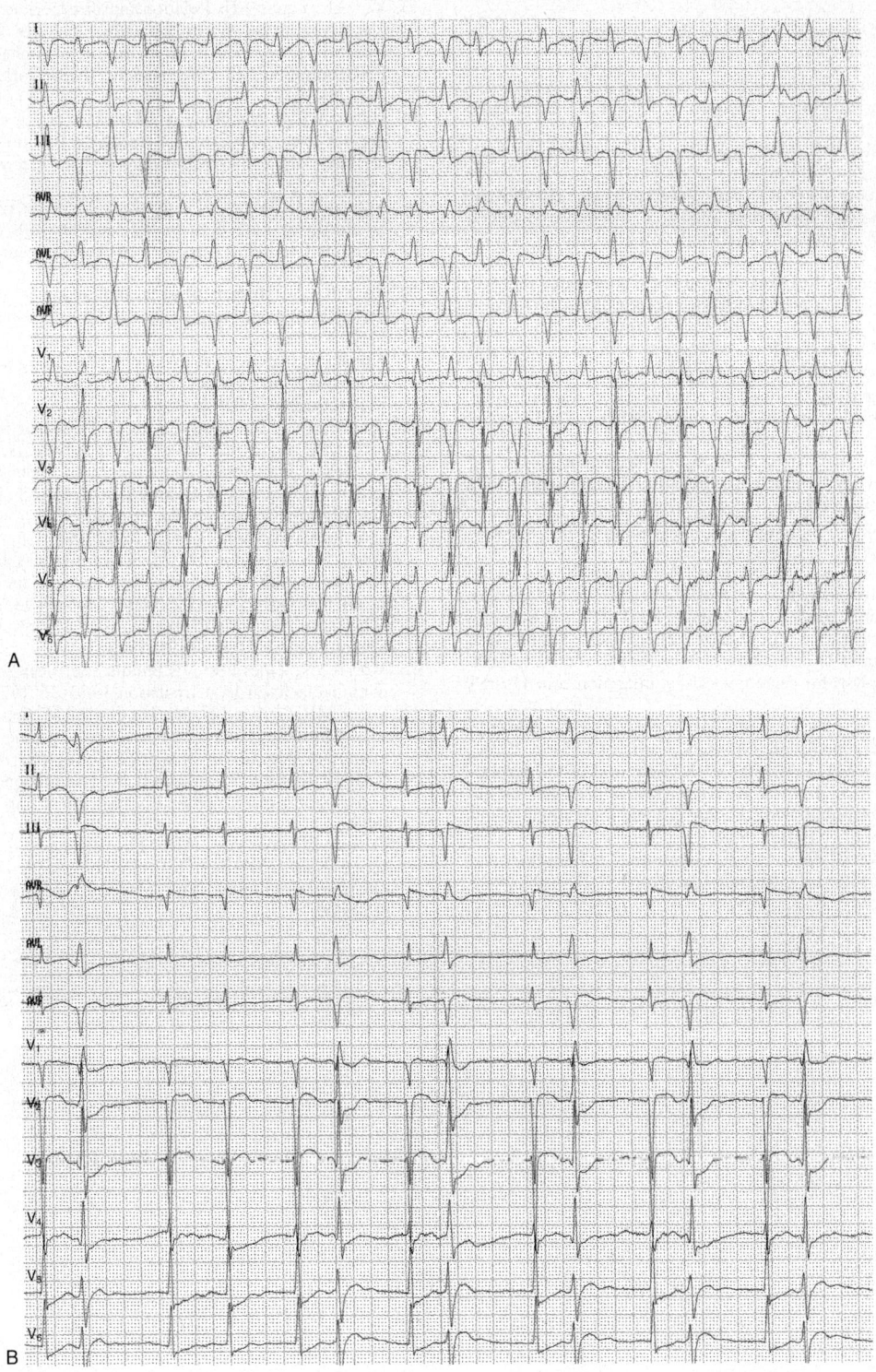

图 75-3　A：12 导联心电图（25mm/s）显示双向室性心动过速，患者 83 岁，其地高辛血浆浓度 86mg/L（正常范围 10～25mg/L）。B：同一病人的心电图（25mm/s），在 A 图开始使用抗原结合片段大约 20min，显示心房颤动伴有偶发的束支搏动。

速心律失常 30 个家系的先证者，这些病人的心律失常分别是双向性室性心动过速（36%）、多形性室性心动过速（58%）、先天的心室颤动（50%），而证明 RyR2 基因突变者有相似的比例。伴有儿茶酚胺敏感性多形性室性快速心律失常的双向性心动过速的理想治疗是 β 肾上腺素受体阻滞剂。因为这一先天的综合征有较高的致死率，有很多病人应植入 ICD 治疗。

（黎　辉　孙志奇　译）

参 考 文 献

1. Harris AS: Delayed development of ventricular ectopic rhythms following experimental coronary occlusion. Circulation 1:1318–1328, 1950.
2. Marriott HJL, Menedez MM: A-V dissociation revisited. Prog Cardiovasc Dis 8:522–538, 1966.
3. Sclarovsky S, Strasberg B, Fuchs J, et al: Multiform accelerated idioventricular rhythm in acute myocardial infarction: Electrocardiographic characteristics and response to verapamil. Am J Cardiol 52:43–47, 1983.
4. Nakagawa M, Hamaoka K, Okano S: Multiform accelerated idioventricular rhythm (AIVR) in a child with acute myocarditis. Clin Cardiol 11:853–855, 1988
5. Denes P, Gillis AM, Pawitan J, et al: Prevalence, characteristics and significance of ventricular premature complexes and ventricular tachycardia detected by 24-hour continuous electrocardiographic recording in the cardiac arrhythmia suppression trial. Am J Cardiol 68:887–896, 1991.
6. Grimm W, Hoffmann J, Menz V, et al: Significance of accelerated idioventricular rhythm in idiopathic dilated cardiomyopathy. Am J Cardiol 85:899–904, 2000.
7. Grimm W: Accelerated idioventricular rhythm. Card Electrophysiol Rev 5:328–331, 2001.
8. De Soyza N, Bissett JK, Kane JJ, et al: Association of accelerated idioventricular rhythm and paroxysmal ventricular tachycardia in acute myocardial infarction. Am J Cardiol 34:667–670, 1974.
9. Goldberg S, Greenspon AJ, Urban PL, et al: Reperfusion arrhythmia: A marker of restoration of antegrade flow during intracoronary thrombolysis for acute myocardial infarction. Am Heart J 105:26–31, 1983.
10. Shah PK, Cercek B, Lew AS, Ganz W: Angiographic validation of bedside markers of reperfusion. J Am Coll Cardiol 21:55–61, 1993.
11. Gorgels APM, Vos MA, Letsch IS, et al: Usefulness of the accelerated idioventricular rhythm as a marker for myocardial necrosis and reperfusion during thrombolytic therapy in acute myocardial infarction. Am J Cardiol 61:231–235, 1988.
12. Rothfeld EL, Zucker IR, Parsonnet V, Alinsonorin CA: Idioventricular rhythm in acute myocardial infarction. Circulation 37:203–209, 1968.
13. Wit AL, Janese MJ: Relationship of experimental delayed ventricular arrhythmias to clinical arrhythmias. In Wit AL, Janese MJ (eds): The Ventricular Arrhythmias of Ischemia and Infarction: Electrophysiological Mechanisms, New York, Futura, 1993, pp 285–291.
14. Wieland JM, Marchlinski FE: Electrocardiographic response of digoxin-toxic fascicular tachycardia to Fab fragments: Implications for tachycardia mechanism. Pacing Clin Electrophysiol 9:727–738, 1986.
15. Antman EM, Wenger TL, Butler VP Jr, et al: Treatment of 150 cases of life-threatening digitalis intoxication with digoxin specific Fab antibody fragments: Final report of a multicenter study. Circulation 81:1744, 1990.
16. Tai VT, Lau CP, But PP, et al: Bidirectional tachycardia induced by herbal aconite poisoning. Pacing Clin Electrophysiol 15:831–839, 1992.
17. Fukuda K, Ogawa S, Yokozuka H, et al: Long-standing bidirectional tachycardia in a patient with hypokalemic periodic paralysis. J Electrocardiol 21:71–75, 1988.
18. Tai VT, Fong PC, Lau CP, et al: Reentrant fascicular tachycardia with cycle length alternans: Insights into the tachycardia mechanism and origin. Pacing Clin Electrophysiol 13:900–907, 1990.
19. Leenhardt A, Lucet V, Denjoy I, et al: Catecholaminergic polymorphic ventricular tachycardia in children: A 7 year follow-up of 21 patients. Circulation 91:1512–1519, 1995.
20. Priori SG, Napolitano C, Memmi M, et al: Clinical and molecular characterization of patients with catecholaminergic polymorphic ventricular tachycardia. Circulation 106:69–74, 2002.
21. Schwensen E: Ventricular tachycardia as a result of the administration of digitalis. Heart 9:199, 1922.
22. Morris SN, Zipes DP: His bundle electrocardiography during bidirectional tachycardia. Circulation 38:32–36, 1973.
23. Rosen MR, Gerband H, Merker C, et al: Mechanisms of digitalis toxicity: Effects of quabain on phase four of canine Purkinje fiber transmembrane potentials. Circulation 47:681–689, 1973.
24. Moak JP, Rosen MR: Induction and termination of triggered activity by pacing in isolated canine Purkinje fibers. Circulation 69:149–162, 1984.
25. Vanagt EJ, Wellens HJJ: The electrocardiogram in digitalis intoxication. In Wellens HJJ, Kulbertus HE (eds): What's New in Electrocardiography? The Hague, Martinus Nijhoff, 1981, pp 315–343.

第 76 章

心室颤动

Andrew E. Epstein

本章目录
- 临床表现 …………………… 697
- 流行病学 …………………… 697
- 心室颤动到死亡的时间 ……… 698
- 特殊的综合征 ……………… 698
- 治疗 ………………………… 700

室颤动（室颤）是心室肌快速、紊乱及不同步收缩。1850 年 Hoffa 和 Ludwig 提到"这些不规律的运动是因为心脏失去了相互关联，收缩不再统一"[1]。1887 年 MacWilliam 将室颤描述为"一种快速连续的不规则的蠕动收缩的状态"，并在 1914 年用心室颤动这个词来描述这种心律失常，并认为其是猝死的原因[2]。

在体表心电图，室颤的特点是无法识别的 QRS 波[3]。室颤最常出现在器质性心脏病患者[4-6]。然而，在某些患者则没有心脏病表现，心律失常的原因不能确定，或仅能被广泛的检查确定（如遗传分析）[6]。室颤是大多数院外心脏停跳患者死亡的主要原因，而且成功复苏的患者在第一年的室颤复发率为 30%[5-8]。由于室颤的特殊病因在其他章节已经讨论，本章仅提供有关室颤临床问题和处理的总观点。

一、临床表现

室颤时心室收缩失去了规则性而使患者产生意识丧失。室颤发作常无预兆，发作时出现脑血流减低、抽搐、呼吸停止，如果不用电除颤终止其发作，则患者很快死亡。在心脏停搏期间，患者无脉搏、无血压，心音消失，全身皮肤苍白。心电图表现为不规则的波浪线。尽管心房不依赖于心室而继续收缩，但 P 波看不到[3]。最终心脏缺氧，心脏所有电及机械功能停止。

表 76-1 概括了室颤的原因。尽管病因学分类大体是按疾病种类划分，但最终室颤的病因是基于细胞和遗传水平。

二、流行病学

通常室颤导致无预兆的突然死亡，病因常是冠心病[4-6]。尽管冠心病引起的死亡在过去几十年有所下降，但猝死的发生率相对没有变。每年在美国有 30 万人发生猝死[6]。

虽然心脏停搏前许多病人有前驱症状[9]，至少在室颤的幸存者中，因急性心梗引起室颤者不到 20%[7]。鉴别十分重要，因为室颤在原有的条件下复发率很高[8]。心脏停搏出现在急性心梗时，1 年的复发率不到 2%。相反，如果心脏停搏出现在慢性心肌缺血而不是急性心肌梗死时，1 年的复发率至少 30%[8]。监测中的心脏停搏很大比例是由心动过缓而不是心动过速引起的[10,11]。

总的来说，室颤及其复发的危险因素主要与冠状动脉疾病相关，还包括高血压、高血脂、吸烟、肥胖、糖耐量损害、左室肥厚、心梗病史、房室阻滞、室内传导阻滞、非特异性 ST-T 异常、非持续性室性心律失常、心肌缺血、使用洋地黄、左室功能损害、年龄增加、种族及摄入酒精[6]。另外，炎性标记物（C 反应蛋白）[12]、特殊长链脂肪酸[13]及家族史[14,15]最近也被认为是危险因素。心理因素包括焦虑、沮丧、压力、社会疏远等也可以是室颤及其复发的危险因素[16,17]。

表 76-1 室颤的病因

器质性心脏病
  冠状动脉疾病
    伴有急性心梗或缺血
    不伴急性心梗
  心肌病
    充血性/扩张型
    肥厚型（梗阻性和非梗阻性）
    致心律失常性右室发育不良
  瓣膜性心脏病
  先天性心脏病，包括冠状动脉异常
  心肌炎
心脏结构正常的离子通道病
  长 QT 综合征
  Brugada 综合征
  家族性/儿茶酚胺敏感性多形性室速
  亚临床的膜缺陷伴有环境因素参与（药物引起 QT 间期延长或引起心动过缓和尖端扭转型室速）
其他
  特发性室颤
  代谢异常（如电解质紊乱）
  室上速，包括 WPW 综合征
  自主神经失衡（如脑卒中后）
  电击伤
  外伤（如心脏震击）
  不适当/非同步心脏转复或除颤放电（心内或体外）

三、心室颤动到死亡的时间

自发性室颤出现前常有室性心动过速，伴或不伴有"先兆性心律失常"如孤立性和非持续性室性异位节律[10,11,18-22]。偶尔，室上性心律失常可以成为室颤的前奏[23-26]。尽管有这些看法，准确确定引起心脏停搏及紧跟着死亡的心律失常常是困难的，事实上心动过缓既可以是死亡时唯一的心律，也可以是室颤的前驱[11,27,28]。Killingsworth 及其同事[28]的心梗诱发猝死的犬模型中提示尽管在所有犬都记录到了室颤，但只有一只犬的室颤自行停止，另两只在室颤前出现窦性心动过缓并最终死亡。在这些动物中，心脏性猝死的促发原因可能已经被错误地认为是快速室性心律失常，正如临床 ICD 只储存心动过速的腔内电图，并不记录心动过速之前的心动过缓（图 76-1）。简而言之，受到记录心律失常开始时间的限制，死亡可能被归于不同的原因，对其发生机制也可做出不同的归类。

四、特殊的综合征

冠状动脉疾病是心脏停搏最常见的基础病，占心

脏性猝死病因的 70%～80%[5,6]。在梗死边缘区，纤维灶散布在心室肌中间，为发生室速进而室颤提供折返环[29,30]。Ursell 及其同事研究了犬心肌梗死愈合时心外膜边缘的结构和电生理变化[29]。在心梗的亚急性期（1～5d），静息电位和动作电位的幅度、上升速度及动作电位时程均显著降低。电活动沿着与左前降支冠状动脉垂直的方向传播，向心底部垂直的方向穿过心外膜下心肌纤维。愈合后，电生理参数恢复正常。2 个月后心肌纤维被结缔组织广泛分开，在这一区域，激动速度减慢，这可能是细胞间的连接消失。可以假定心梗愈合区持续存在的缓慢传导对慢性心律失常的产生有作用。与此相反，Uretsky 及同事[31]指出急性冠状动脉的病变（冠脉内血栓、斑块破裂、出现近期或急性心肌梗死）在冠心病和心衰患者的猝死病例中常常没有诊断，认为急性冠状动脉事件可能是室颤和猝死的促发机制。

心肌病是另一种重要的产生室颤的基础心脏病[5,6,32,33]。不可理解的是随着心衰程度的加重，与非猝死（因心衰）相比猝死的相对发生率下降了[34]。目前，心肌病患者猝死及心律失常性死亡的危险性尚未确定。特别是那些高危的肥厚型心肌病患者，即同时有左室肥厚、非持续性室速、猝死家族史、运动后血压反应异常（年龄小于 40 岁）、可诱发的持续性室性心律失常或特殊的基因型[32]。室颤也可以是致心律失常性右室心肌病及罕见心肌炎的结果[33,35]。

瓣膜病及先心病患者也有猝死的危险。主动脉狭窄的患者死亡的原因不仅是室性心律失常，还有心动过缓、流出道梗阻及缺血[36]。先心病的外科手术瘢痕形成的解剖障碍区为心室形成折返性心动过速提供物质基础[37]。相反没有左、右心功能不全的先心病患者似乎危险较低。其他室颤的原因包括非同步除颤，甚至外伤（如心脏震击）[38]，或胸部重击终止心律失常等（图 76-2）。

药物潜在的毒性作用非常重要，抗心律失常药物本身可以致心律失常[39]。心律失常抑制试验（CAST）[41,42]和 d-索他洛尔存活试验（SWORD）[42]精辟地指出了抗心律失常药物对冠心病患者促心律失常作用的危险。心衰患者使用洋地黄也是引起室性心律失常的重要原因[43]。传导阻滞或药物作用引起的心动过缓可以导致 QT 间期延长、尖端扭转型室速，最后导致室颤。

代谢性酸中毒和电解质紊乱也能导致室颤[44-46]。代谢性酸中毒时室颤的阈值降低，代谢性碱中毒时室

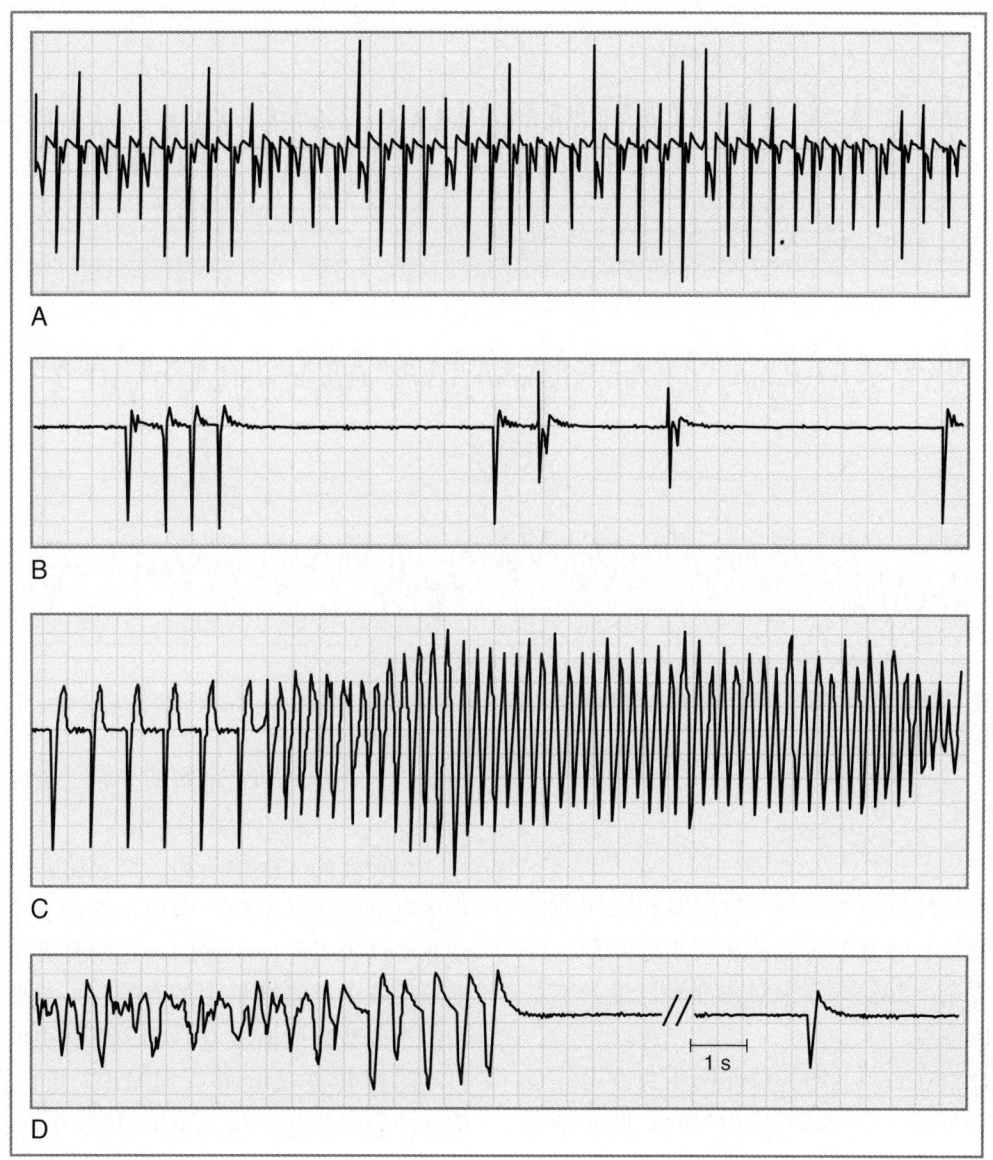

图 76-1 通过心外膜电极记录到狗的心动过缓和心脏性猝死　伴室性异位节律的心率通常 131bpm（A），心动过缓进展前的 5min（B），心动过缓后约 3min，心率到 76bpm 并出现室颤（C），持续 3min 后自行停止。室颤停止后 91s 出现了 1 次心室激动（D），心室收缩停止。（引自 Killingsworth CR, Ritscher DE, Walcott GP, et al: Continuous telemetry from a chronic canine model of sudden cardiac death. J Cardovasc Electrophysiol 11: 1333, 2000.）

颤的阈值升高[45]。酸中毒是如何增加室颤的易发性尚不清楚。有趣的是用碳酸氢钠使血清碱化可以治疗Ⅰ类抗心律失常药物促发的心律失常[47]。相反在心脏停搏时常规使用缓冲剂并未证明有价值[48]。在碱性环境里，抗心律失常药物透过细胞膜及活性通道受阻。低钾作为室颤发生的危险因素已得到共识[44]。

在过去 10 年中，对室颤的遗传基础已经做了很多研究[6,49]。长 QT 综合征、Brugada 综合征、致心律失常性右室发育不良及儿茶酚胺敏感性室速相关的膜缺陷遗传编码都已被确定[6,49,50]。SCN5A 钠通道的变异与非洲裔美国人的心律失常危险增加相关[51]。扩张型心肌病产生的心肌细胞 Na^+-K^+-ATP 酶抗体可能使一些患者出现了电的不稳定性[52]。一些临床上不明显的遗传缺陷仅仅有外部影响如药物或电解质失衡时才有表现[53]。

最后，继发于神经体液和中枢神经系统影响的电生理异常及电不稳定性最近也受到关注[5,54-56]。有证据支持自主神经调节失衡，如心率变异性降低，与心律失常性死亡有关[5,55,56]。院外心脏停搏的出现时间有一定的昼夜变化规律，在 6：00AM 和 12：00PM 之间死亡率增加[57]。

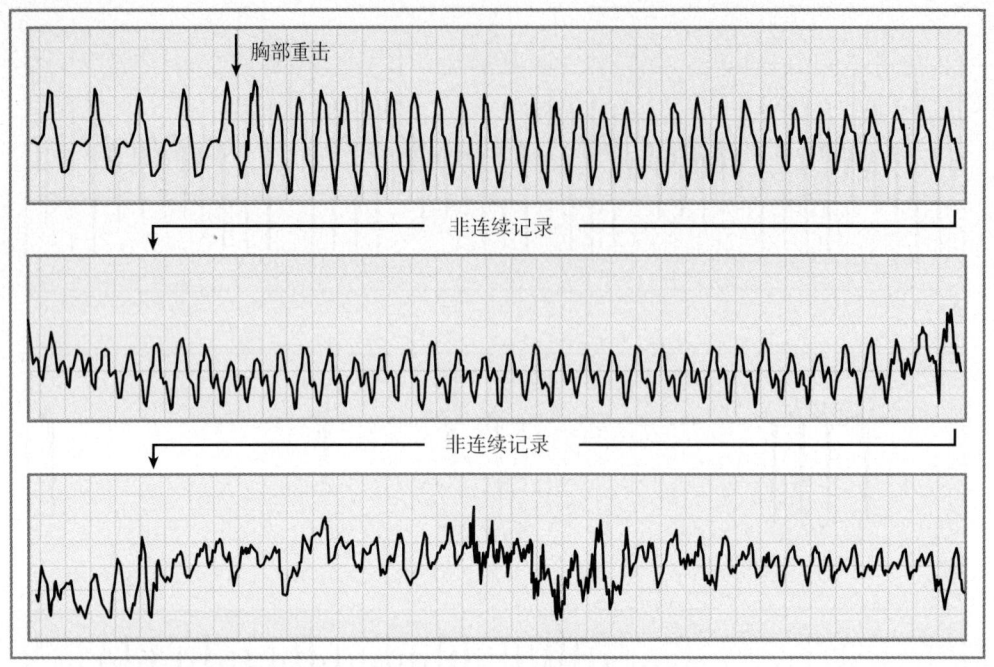

图 76-2　室速时胸部非同步的重击导致室颤　因为体外除颤器已经连接，除颤很容易并成功完成。

五、治　疗

室颤患者的治疗分为两个期：急性期和慢性期治疗。急性期即紧急心肺复苏所需的非同步电除颤。慢性期治疗比较复杂。其他章节中对此都有讨论，本章仅讨论一些总的观点。

室颤的急性治疗必须立即释放非同步直流电。室颤的自行终止很罕见[58,59]。除颤应用早时，低能量即可成功[48]。相反，气管插管、保持酸碱平衡及纠正其他代谢异常（缺氧、高血钾及其他）是成功除颤必需的辅助措施。有时镇静剂或全身麻醉造成的自主神经张力降低有助于室性心律失常的复发。最近，双心室辅助装置已经被用在心脏移植前的过渡治疗[60]。

利多卡因、普鲁卡因胺、奎尼丁及胺碘酮都被用于预防和治疗室颤。但心肌梗死时预防性使用利多卡因可增加死亡率，这种方法已不再应用[61,62]。溶栓、阿司匹林及β受体阻滞剂在急性心梗时的重要性也不必过分强调。

慢性室颤治疗的第一步是确定病因。如果心脏停搏出现在急性心肌梗死时，复发率较低。但停搏出现在慢性心肌缺血时则复发率较高[6-8]。心导管造影、负荷试验及非介入影像检查都是非常重要的诊断手段。如果心脏停搏是由一过性心肌缺血引起的，应当在有指征时给予药物、PCI 术及外科手术等抗缺血治疗[62,63]。当然，纠正电解质异常、撤除促心律失常的药物及可逆性病因治疗是必需的。

对猝死的一级预防和二级预防，可用动态监测和程序电刺激指导治疗，但也不是没有争论。对于冠状动脉疾病患者的一级预防，这两种方法都在最近完成的随机临床试验结果中放弃[64-66]。对那些有心梗病史和射血分数减低而没有心律失常病史的患者，多中心自动除颤转复试验 II（MADIT II）表明与未植入 ICD 的患者相比，植入 ICD 患者的生存时间改善[67]。需要进行进一步的研究以确定哪些患者获益最大。对于非缺血性及扩张型心肌病患者，心肌病试验（cardiomyopathy trial）因 ICD 对该类患者并无益处而终止试验。心衰猝死试验（SCD-HeFt）将为怎样治疗这类患者提供肯定的答案。这个试验随机优化常规心衰治疗方法，单独或联合使用胺碘酮或 ICD[68]。

目前其他的挑战包括筛选有遗传相关的有室颤家族史的家庭成员，及怎样治疗无症状的个体。不清楚的问题还包括突变基因的外显率的重要性、预防性治疗的危险及并发症和相对获益的权重、确定致死危险率的假阳性、无症状患者限制活动与损害公民自由的解释[69]。

心律失常手术仅在不连续的左室室壁瘤及能诱发的可标测室速患者中有可行性[70]。单支血管病变及非室壁瘤区心室功能正常的患者预后较好。室颤本身并不能用室壁瘤切除和心内膜切除治愈，但如果室速促发心室停搏，这种手术则可以考虑。

由于外科手术、药物及植入装置治疗室颤都有缺点，必须对室颤机理及治疗进行深入的研究。研究的起点是基因和导管干预。在识别心律失常的相关基因后，基因工程有望改变和修复细胞膜的缺陷。最近的报告甚至指出在选择的病例中，导管消融可以去除室颤的触发灶[71]。通过不断的基础和临床研究将能确定患者室颤的危险性及治疗室颤幸存者的有效手段。

（王 龙 译）

参 考 文 献

1. Schechter DC: Exploring the Origins of Electrical Cardiac Stimulation. Minneapolis, Minn, Medtronic, Inc, 1983, p 150.
2. Snellen HA: History of Cardiology. Rotterdam, Donker Academic Publications, 1984, p 141.
3. Waldo AL, Akhtar M, Brugada P, et al: NASPE policy statement: The minimally appropriate electrophysiologic study for the initial assessment of patients with documented sustained monomorphic ventricular tachycardia. Pacing Clin Electrophysiol 8:918, 1985.
4. Davies MJ, Thomas A: Thrombosis and acute coronary-artery lesions in sudden cardiac ischemic death. N Engl J Med 310:1137, 1984.
5. Huikuri HV, Castellanos A, Myerburg, RJ: Sudden death due to cardiac arrhythmias. N Engl J Med 345:1473, 2001.
6. Myerburg R: Scientific gaps in the prediction and prevention of sudden cardiac death. J Cardiovasc Electrophysiol 13:709–723, 2002.
7. Cobb LA, Werner JA, Trobaugh GB: Sudden cardiac death: I. A decade's experience with out-of-hospital resuscitation. Mod Concepts Cardiovasc Dis 49:31, 1980.
8. Cobb LA, Werner JA, Trobaugh GB: Sudden cardiac death: II. Outcome of resuscitation, management, and future directions. Mod Concepts Cardiovasc Dis 49:37, 1980.
9. Madsen JK: Ischaemic heart disease and prodromes of sudden cardiac death. Is it possible to identify high risk groups for sudden cardiac death? Br Heart J 54:27, 1985.
10. Wang F-S, Lien W-P, Fong T-E, et al: Terminal cardiac electrical activity in adults who die without apparent cardiac disease. Am J Cardiol 58:491, 1986.
11. Luu M, Stevenson WG, Stevenson LW, et al: Diverse mechanisms of unexpected cardiac arrest in advanced heart failure. Circulation 80:1675, 1989.
12. Albert CM, Ma J, Rifai N, et al: Prospective study of C-reactive protein, homocysteine, and plasma lipid levels as predictors of sudden cardiac death. Circulation 105:2595, 2002.
13. Kris-Etherton PM, Harris WS, Appel LJ, for the Nutrition Committee: Fish consumption, fish oil, omega-3 fatty acids, and cardiovascular disease. Circulation 106:2747, 2002.
14. Friedlander Y, Siscovick DS, Weinmann S, et al: Family history as a risk factor for primary cardiac arrest. Circulation 97:155, 1998.
15. Jouven X, Desnos M, Guerot C, Ducimetière P: Predicting sudden death in the population. The Paris Prospective Study I. Circulation 99:1978, 1999.
16. Engel GL: Sudden and rapid death during psychological stress: Folklore or folk wisdom? Ann Intern Med 74:771, 1971.
17. Brackett CD, Powell LH: Psychosocial and physiological predictors in sudden cardiac death after healing of acute myocardial infarction. Am J Cardiol 61:979 1988.
18. Nikolic G, Bishop RL, Singh JB: Sudden death recorded during Holter monitoring. Circulation 66:218, 1982.
19. Savage DD, Castelli WP, Anderson SJ, et al: Sudden unexpected death during ambulatory electrocardiographic monitoring: The Framingham Study. Am J Med 74:148, 1983.
20. Pratt CM, Francis MJ, Luck JC, et al: Analysis of ambulatory electrocardiograms in 15 patients during spontaneous ventricular fibrillation with special reference to preceding arrhythmic events. J Am Coll Cardiol 2:789, 1983.
21. Bayés de Luna A, Coumel P, Leclercq JF: Ambulatory sudden cardiac death: Mechanisms of production of fatal arrhythmia on the basis of data from 157 cases. Am Heart J 117:151, 1989.
22. Pepine CJ, Morganroth J, McDonald JT, et al: Sudden death during ambulatory electrocardiographic monitoring. Am J Cardiol 68:785, 1991.
23. Bekheit S, Turitto G, Fontaine J, et al: Initiation of ventricular fibrillation by supraventricular beats in patients with acute myocardial infarction. Br Heart J 59:190, 1988.
24. Hays LJ, Lerman BB, DiMarco JP: Nonventricular arrhythmias as precursors of ventricular fibrillation in patients with out-of-hospital cardiac arrest. Am Heart J 118:53, 1989.
25. Wang Y, Scheinman MM, Chien WW, et al: Patients with supraventricular tachycardia presenting with aborted sudden death: Incidence, mechanism and long-term follow-up. J Am Coll Cardiol 18:1711, 1991.
26. Klein GJ, Bashore TM, Sellers TD, et al: Ventricular fibrillation in the Wolff-Parkinson-White syndrome. N Engl J Med 301:1080, 1979.
27. Janse MJ, Vermeulen JT, Opthof T, et al: Arrhythmogenesis in heart failure. J Cardiovasc Electrophysiol 12:496, 2001.
28. Killingsworth CR, Ritscher DE, Walcott GP, et al: Continuous telemetry from a chronic canine model of sudden cardiac death. J Cardiovasc Electrophysiol 11:1333, 2000.
29. Ursell PC, Gardner PI, Albala A, et al: Structural and electrophysiological changes in the epicardial border zone of canine myocardial infarcts during infarct healing. Circ Res 56:436, 1985.
30. Aronson RS, Ming Z: Cellular mechanisms of arrhythmias in hypertrophied and failing myocardium. Circulation 87(suppl VII):VII-76, 1993.
31. Uretsky BF, Thygesen K, Armstrong PW, et al: Acute coronary findings at autopsy in heart failure patients with sudden death. Results from the Assessment of Treatment with Lisinopril and Survival (ATLAS) Trial. Circulation 102:611, 2000.
32. Maron BJ: Hypertrophic cardiomyopathy. A systematic review. JAMA 287:1308, 2002.
33. Corrado D, Fontaine G, Marcus FI, et al: Arrhythmogenic right ventricular dysplasia/cardiomyopathy: need for an international registry. Study Group on Arrhythmogenic Right Ventricular Dysplasia/Cardiomyopathy of the Working Groups on Myocardial and Pericardial Disease and Arrhythmias of the European Society of Cardiology and of the Scientific Council on Cardiomyopathies of the World Heart Federation. Circulation 101:E101, 2000.
34. Uretsky BF, Sheahan RG: Primary prevention of sudden cardiac death in heart failure: Will the solution be shocking? J Am Coll Cardiol 30:1589, 1997.
35. Strain JE, Grose RM, Factor SM, et al: Results of endomyocardial biopsy in patients with spontaneous ventricular tachycardia but without apparent structural heart disease. Circulation 68:1171, 1983.
36. Schwartz L, Goldfischer J, Sprague GJ, et al: Syncope and sudden death in aortic stenosis. Am J Cardiol 23:647, 1969.
37. Downar E, Harris L, Kimber S, et al: Ventricular tachycardia after surgical repair of tetralogy of Fallot: Results of intraoperative mapping studies. J Am Coll Cardiol 20:648, 1992.
38. Maron BJ, Gohman TE, Kyle SB, et al: Clinical profile and spectrum of commotio cordis. JAMA 287:1142, 2002.
39. Ruskin JN, McGovern B, Garan H, et al: Antiarrhythmic drugs: A possible cause of out-of-hospital cardiac arrest. N Engl J Med 309:1302, 1983.
40. Echt DS, Liebson PR, Mitchell LB, et al: Mortality and morbidity in patients receiving encainide, flecainide, or placebo: The Cardiac Arrhythmia Suppression Trial. N Engl J Med 324:781, 1991.
41. The Cardiac Arrhythmia Suppression Trial II Investigators: Effect of the antiarrhythmic agent moricizine on survival after myocardial infarction. N Engl J Med 327:227, 1992.
42. Waldo AL, Camm AJ, deRuyter H, et al: Effect of d-sotalol on mortality in patients with left ventricular dysfunction after recent and remote myocardial infarction. Lancet 348:7, 1996.
43. Vanagt EJ, Wellens HJJ: The electrocardiogram in digitalis intoxication. In Wellens HJJ, Kulbertus HE (eds): What's New in Electrocardiography. Boston, Martinus Nijhoff, 1981, p 315.
44. Surawicz B: Ventricular fibrillation. J Am Coll Cardiol 5:43B, 1985.
45. Gerst PH, Fleming WH, Malm JR: Increased susceptibility of the heart to ventricular fibrillation during metabolic acidosis. Circ Res 19:63, 1966.

46. Gettes LS: Electrolyte abnormalities underlying lethal and ventricular arrhythmias. Circulation 85(suppl I):I-70, 1992.
47. Pentel PR, Goldsmith SR, Salerno DM, et al: Effect of hypertonic sodium bicarbonate on encainide overdose. Am J Cardiol 57:878, 1986.
48. American Heart Association in collaboration with the International Liaison Committee on Resuscitation (ILCOR): Guidelines 2000 for cardiopulmonary resuscitation and emergency cardiovascular care. An international consensus on science. Circulation 102:I-1, 2000.
49. Tobin JA, Vatta M: The genetics of cardiac arrhythmias. Pacing Clin Electrophysiol 23:106, 2000.
50. Priori SG, Napolitano C, Memmi M, et al: Clinical and molecular characterization of patients with catecholaminergic polymorphic ventricular tachycardia. Circulation 106:69, 2002.
51. Splawski I, Timothy KW, Tateyama M, et al: Variant of SCN5A sodium channel implicated in risk of cardiac arrhythmia. Science 297:1333, 2002.
52. Baba A, Yoshikawa T, Ogawa S: Autoantibodies produced against sarcolemmal Na-K-ATPase: Possible upstream targets of arrhythmias and sudden death in patients with dilated cardiomyopathy. J Am Coll Cardiol 40:1153, 2002.
53. Makita N, Horie M, Nakamura T, et al: Drug-induced long-QT syndrome associated with a subclinical SCN5A mutation. Circulation 106:1269, 2002.
54. Schwartz PJ, La Rovere MT, Vanoli E: Autonomic nervous system and sudden cardiac death: Experimental basis and clinical observations for post-myocardial infarction risk stratification. Circulation 85(suppl I):I-77, 1992.
55. Coumel P: Cardiac arrhythmias and the autonomic nervous system. J Cardiovas Electrophysiol 4:338, 1993.
56. van Ravenswaaij-Arts CMA, Kollée LAA, Hopman JCW, et al: Heart rate variability. Ann Intern Med 118:436, 1993.
57. Levine RL, Pepe PE, Fromm RE, et al: Prospective evidence of a circadian rhythm for out-of-hospital cardiac arrests. JAMA 267:2935, 1992.
58. Dubner SJ, Gimeno GM, Elencwajg B, et al: Ventricular fibrillation with spontaneous reversion on ambulatory ECG in the absence of heart disease. Am Heart J 105:691, 1983.
59. Ring ME, Huang SK: Spontaneous termination from prolonged ventricular fibrillation. Am Heart J 113:1226, 1987.
60. Geannopoulos CJ, Wilber DJ, Olshansky B: Control of refractory ventricular tachycardia with biventricular assist devices. Pacing Clin Electrophysiol 14:1432, 1991.
61. Hine LK, Laird N, Hewitt P, et al: Meta-analytic evidence against prophylactic use of lidocaine in acute myocardial infarction. Arch Intern Med 149:2694, 1989.
62. Antman EM, Berlin JA: Declining incidence of ventricular fibrillation in myocardial infarction: Implications for the prophylactic use of lidocaine. Circulation 86:764, 1992.
63. Epstein AE: When is bypass surgery enough? The answer is still uncertain. J Cardiovasc Electrophysiol 5:995, 1994.
64. The AVID Investigators: A comparison of antiarrhythmic drug therapy with implantable defibrillators in patients resuscitated from near-fatal sustained ventricular arrhythmias. N Engl J Med 337:1576, 1997.
65. Connolly SJ, Gent M, Roberts RS, et al: Canadian Implantable Defibrillator Study (CIDS). A randomized trial of the implantable cardioverter defibrillator against amiodarone. Circulation 101:1297, 2000.
66. Kuck K-H, Cappato R, Siebels J, Rüppel R, for the CASH Investigators: Randomized comparison of antiarrhythmic drug therapy with implantable defibrillators in patients resuscitated from cardiac arrest. The Cardiac Arrest Study Hamburg (CASH). Circulation 102:748, 2000.
67. Moss AJ, Zareba W, Hall WJ, et al: Prophylactic implantation of a defibrillator in patients with myocardial infarction and reduced ejection fraction. N Engl J Med 346:877, 2002.
68. Bardy GH, Lee KL, Mark DB, et al: Sudden Cardiac Death in Heart Failure Trial Pilot Study. Pacing Clin Electrophysiol 20:1148, 1997.
69. Estes NAM, Link MS, Cannom D, et al: Report of the NASPE Policy Conference on Arrhythmias in Athletes. J Cardiovascular Electrophysiol 12:1208, 2001.
70. Miller JM, Kienzle MG, Harken AH, et al: Subendocardial resection for ventricular tachycardia: Predictors of surgical success. Circulation 70:624, 1984.
71. Haïssaguerre M, Shoda M, Jaïs P, et al: Mapping and ablation of idiopathic ventricular tachycardia. Circulation 106:962, 2002.

第 77 章

心室复极延长与婴儿猝死综合征

Peter J. Schwartz and Marco Stramba-Badiale

本章目录

- QT 间期假说 703
- 新生儿心电图与婴儿猝死综合征的意大利研究 704
- QT 间期延长与致命性心律失常 705
- 分子机制 706
- 法律学意义 709
- 致谢 710

西方国家，婴儿猝死综合征（sudden infant death syndrome，SIDS）是导致生后第 1 年婴儿死亡的主要原因，同时也给受累者家庭带来了沉重的心理负担。

婴儿猝死综合征的定义是指发生在婴儿或幼儿的突然死亡而没有相关病史，没有能引起突然死亡的病史，全面尸检找不出死亡的原因。死亡当时情况的调查是诊断的必要条件之一。

关于婴儿猝死综合征的研究很多，大多数集中在呼吸或心脏功能异常方面，但婴儿猝死综合征的病因仍然不明确。近年来有观点认为心源性机制占主导，尤其是致命性心律失常可能是婴儿猝死综合征的一个重要病因[1,2]，但对此观点仍有争议。

本章我们将介绍心脏性猝死机制假说的相关理论，根据该假说，一部分婴儿猝死综合征患者可能是由复极延长导致的室颤引起。本文总结了我们长达 20 年的前瞻性研究，收集了 34 000 例婴儿的心电图[3]，并讨论我们正在进行的试验中最新发现[4,5]，即首次从分子水平证实婴儿猝死综合征与长 QT 综合征（long QT syndrome，LQTS）有关。

一、QT 间期假说

有很多理论用来解释婴儿猝死综合征，但没有一个得到证实。共同的观点是婴儿猝死综合征是一个多因素疾病[2,6]，发生在婴儿的突然而不可预料的猝死可能原因各不相同。一种机制并不被另一种机制所否定。因为导致婴儿猝死综合征发生的主要原因是我们不能确定的一种特异性疾病或病因，所以重要的是要找出导致婴儿猝死的容易识别的主要机制。婴儿猝死综合征是一种排除性诊断，当我们用现有的知识，经过全面而专业的尸检之后仍然不能解释一个看起来健康的婴儿为什么突然死亡时，就只能诊断为婴儿猝死综合征。

大多数婴儿猝死综合征的发生是由于呼吸异常，或心脏功能异常[6]，或神经支配异常，这些异常可能是一过性的，但足以触发一次致命事件。

至于所谓的"呼吸暂停假说"，是来自美国国家健康基金协会组织的名为 CHIME 的一项前瞻性试验，入选至少 1000 个婴儿，在生后的最初 6 个月使用家庭心电呼吸监测进行观察，总监测时间接近 720 000h [7]。试验的结论是即使存在"极端事件"（包括呼吸暂停至少 30s 或 10s 内心率下降 50bpm）也不可能是婴儿猝死综合征的前兆。Jobe 对此进行了评论[8]，同时提醒读者注意当前美国仅早产儿监护一项的花费每年达到了 2400 万美元，不包括内科医生的费用及其他费用，也不包括对那些被认为婴儿猝死综合征高危的足月儿的监护费用。Jobe 得出结论：该试验不支持那种认为婴儿猝死综合征高危的婴儿比健康的婴儿有更多心脏及呼吸暂停事件的设想，而认为此类事件不是婴儿猝死综合征前兆。该试验证实了减少使用家庭监护防止婴儿猝死综合征的正确性。

至于心脏假说，Schwartz[1]注意到在西方国家20～65岁成人死亡的主要原因是突发的心源性猝死，相关的机制几乎总是致命性心律失常：室颤。因此设想婴儿的猝死可能也与致命性心律失常密切相关。

1976年，Schwartz[1]提出一些婴儿猝死综合征病例的发病机制可能与长QT综合征患者猝死的机制相似，而长QT综合征是20岁以下年轻人猝死的主要原因[9,10]。一个可能的机制是心交感支配的发育异常使一部分婴儿在生后的第1年内容易发生致命性心律失常[1]。另一个可能的机制是基因突变，而这种基因突变最近仅被证明可以导致长QT综合征[9,10]。临床上可用来检测这些机制的唯一标记是心电图上QT间期的延长。

1976年Schwartz的评论之后[1]，QT间期延长可能是婴儿猝死综合征重要原因的假说得到了充分的重视。但是，除了早期Maron及其合作者支持外[11]，这一理论很快同时也很草率地被一系列表面上似乎阴性的试验结果否定了[12-16]。反对QT间期延长在婴儿猝死综合征中作用的论述指出了这一理论的缺点并进行了详尽的讨论，感兴趣的读者可以参考相关的文章[2,17]。这里我们只做一个简短的评论。

大多数得出所谓阴性结论的试验仅在极小范围的人群中进行，或只针对"婴儿猝死综合征高危患儿"，例如兄弟姐妹死于婴儿猝死综合征的婴儿[13,15]，或发生了所谓"几乎流产"或已流产的婴儿猝死综合征的婴儿[12,14]，在这些婴儿中并未发现QT间期延长。仅凭这些试验得出的结论来评价婴儿猝死综合征的风险与QT间期延长的关系是不合适的，因为婴儿猝死综合征的发病率极低，任何一个危险因素都有很高的假阳性。然而，对于婴儿猝死综合征，即使假定其发生率高达2/1000，任何一个使危险性增高5倍的因素仍会有99%的假阳性。这就意味着尽管试验者研究了100例据称是"高危"的婴儿，也仅有1例（1%）后来死于婴儿猝死综合征，而此例患儿又没有表现出某种预定危险因素，就会得出该因素与婴儿猝死综合征无关的结论。我们提出QT间期延长这一危险因素就是如此被一些小样本的研究否定的。这些"高危婴儿猝死综合征"的研究结论提示QT间期延长在试验中的特殊病人中不重要。然而把这样的结论推广到一般人群甚至真正的死于婴儿猝死综合征的婴儿是毫无根据的。这些基础的统计学概念似乎迷惑了很多婴儿猝死综合征的研究者。

二、新生儿心电图与婴儿猝死综合征的意大利研究

为了验证QT间期延长与婴儿猝死综合征的相关假说，1976年我们设计了一个前瞻性的研究，研究基础是记录出生3～4天婴儿的标准心电图。假定婴儿猝死综合征的发生率较低（每1000例活产中0.5～1.5例），我们必须前瞻性地在一个很大的人群中收集新生儿心电图，然后进行1年的随访，确定患儿发生的是婴儿猝死综合征或其他原因导致的死亡。此研究结果发表于1998年[3]。以下我们总结了本研究的主要发现。

该研究记录了9个产科医院34 442例新生儿的12导联心电图，测量了所有死亡婴儿的QT间期，及来自整个试验人群的9725例随机样本的QT间期。测量者在测量时不知道婴儿是否存活，该研究共进行了19年。

进入研究的34 442例婴儿中，33 034例（96%）完成了1年的随访。失访的主要原因是由于居住地址的变化。平均QTc（根据心率校正的QT间期）400±20ms，男性与女性之间没有差异（401±19ms vs 400±20ms）。QTc在人群中呈正态分布，第97.5百分位数值为440ms。为了达到研究的目的，我们将QTc超过440ms定义为QTc间期延长。

在1年的随访过程中，34例婴儿死亡，其中24例死于婴儿猝死综合征，10例死于其他原因。死于婴儿猝死综合征的婴儿死后尸检结果均为阴性，不能明确死亡的确切原因，而这些死于婴儿猝死综合征的婴儿没有长QT综合征或猝死的家族史。

婴儿猝死综合征组的平均QTc（435±45ms），与非婴儿猝死综合征死亡组相比显著延长（392±26ms，$P<0.05$），同时显著长于健康对照组的QTc（400±20ms，$P<0.01$）（图77-1）。值得注意的是，分析两组婴儿死亡的单个个体的QTc（图77-1），发现死于婴儿猝死综合征组的24人中有12人（50%）的QTc间期超过440ms，而死于其他原因的所有婴儿QTc均小于440ms。

由于新生儿期的心率相当快，用传统的Bazett公式校正短周期长度的QT间期是不合适的。为此，我们把RR间期分成17级，逐级增加20ms，每一级都

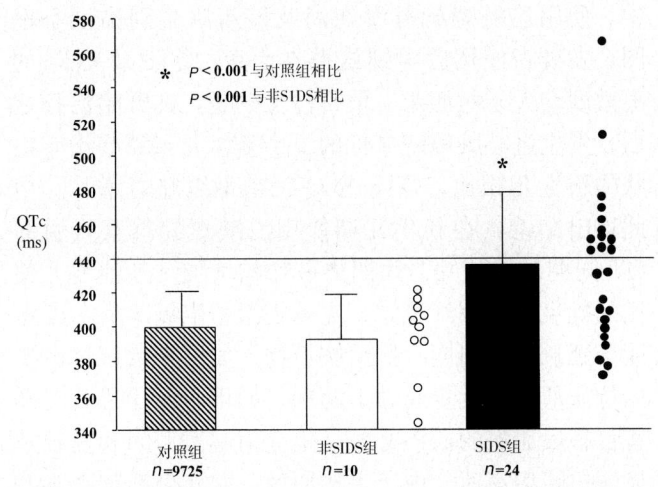

图77-1 在对照组婴儿、死于婴儿猝死综合征（SIDS）的婴儿、因其他原因死亡的婴儿中经心率校正后的平均QT间期 横线代表总人群中97.5％的QTc值并相当于440ms，在平均值的2个标准差之上。实心圆圈和空心圆圈分别代表SIDS组和非SIDS组。（引自Schwartz PJ，Stramba-Badiale M，Segantini A，et al：Prolongation of the QT interval and the sudden infant denth syndrome. N Engl J Med 338：1709-1714，1998.）

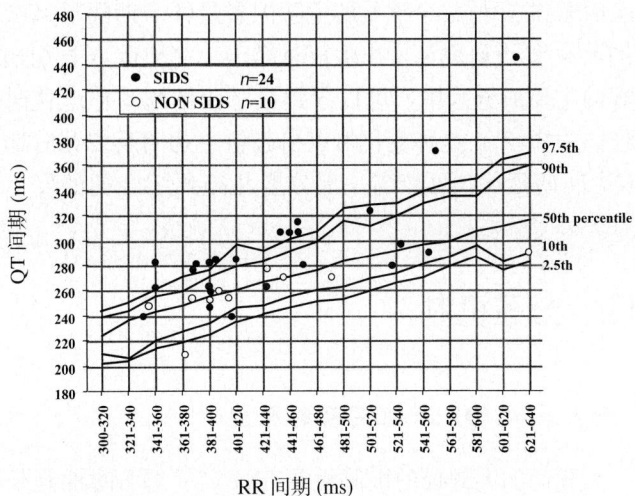

图77-2 QT间期和心脏折返环周长 每一条线代表在相应的RR间期范围其未校正的QT间期。实心圆圈和空心圆圈分别代表因SIDS和非SIDS原因死亡患儿的QT间期数值。（引自Schwartz PJ，Stramba-Badiale M，Segantini A，et al：Prolongation of the QT interval and the sudden infant denth syndrome. N Engl J Med 338：1709-1714，1998.）

根据相应的QT间期值计算百分位数分布，从第2.5百分位数到第97.5百分位数。图77-2显示死于婴儿猝死综合征组24人中的12人每个个体的QT值都处于第97.5百分位数之上，而死于非婴儿猝死综合征组的所有婴儿的该值都在第90百分位数之下。

在我们研究结果的基础上，正常QTc婴儿发生婴儿猝死综合征的绝对危险度是0.37/1000，而在QTc超过440ms的婴儿发生婴儿猝死综合征的绝对危险度达到15/1000。婴儿猝死综合征与QTc延长（>440ms）相关的OR值为41.3（95％可信区间17.3～98.4），显著高于QTc正常的婴儿。

这个包括了至少34 000婴儿的大样本前瞻性研究证实，生后第3天或第4天标准心电图上QT间期延长是预测发生婴儿猝死综合征的重要危险因素。

三、QT间期延长与致命性心律失常

有证据强烈支持婴儿猝死综合征与QT间期延长有关，QT间期延长是心脏电活动不稳定的标志，这表明一部分婴儿可能很容易发生致命性心律失常。

实验和临床研究都表明QT间期延长容易引发致命性心律失常，并且在若干临床情况下与猝死危险性的增加有关[18,19]，但同时也可见于健康个体[20]。在所有临床情况中，与婴儿猝死综合征关系最大的毫无疑问是长QT综合征[9]。

QT间期延长的婴儿可能并不发生婴儿猝死综合征，即出现假阳性率（2.5％），可能至少有两个原因和一个关联。

第一个也是最重要的一个原因是很可能存在"假性QT间期延长"（例如，一个QT间期正常的婴儿在生后3～4天测量到的QT间期恰好在临界点之上，随后测量的QT间期可能恢复到正常）。值得注意的是QT间期的测量是粗略的，存在数毫秒的误差是不可避免的。第二个原因是440ms是人为确定的一个截点值，并不代表测量值超过该界限的婴儿都患有长QT综合征。

一个关联是指婴儿出生后还有引起致命性事件的其他因素。因为QT间期延长只是心律失常事件的"基质"，发生致命性心律失常还需要一个"触发因素"。最为人熟知的在QT间期延长的情况下发生致命性心律失常的触发因素是交感神经激活或其他原因引起的儿茶酚胺释放（包括低钾或药物阻断I_{Kr}离子流，有关的药物包括抗生素、抗组胺药及胃肠动力药如西沙必利），这些情况可进一步延长QT间期[9,21]。值得一提的是，俯卧位睡眠可能是触发婴儿猝死综合征的因素之一。事实上，这种情况[22]与心交感神经活性增加而心迷走神经活性降低有关[23]，而这种自主神经张力的改变已经被证实是触发心律失常性猝死的危险因素[24]。另一个重要的危险因素是怀孕期间母亲吸烟[25]，最近研究证实出生前暴露于一氧化碳（香烟烟雾的主要成分）中，可以导致鼠心肌细胞动作电位时程的缩短[26]，这种变化可以引起新生儿期及婴儿时期QT间期延长，可能与一部分婴儿猝死综合征的发生有关。

四、分子机制

（一）婴儿QT间期延长的原因

我们的大规模的前瞻性研究证实了QT间期延长增加了婴儿猝死综合征的危险性[3]。然而，为什么一个婴儿的QT间期会延长？究竟哪种机制在起作用？很显然如果不能合理解释这些问题会减弱QT间期假说的说服力。心室复极异常的新生儿是一个庞杂的人群，在新生儿期及婴儿期QT间期延长有很多原因，大多数情况下这种异常是一过性的。我们提出了几种不同的可能机制来说明某些新生儿QT间期延长的原因：心脏交感神经支配的发育异常[1]、获得性长QT综合征、某一长QT综合征基因的新生突变、低外显率长QT综合征的发生[27]。

第一个机制的提出是建立在实验的基础上。在心脏正常的3周幼犬，切除右侧星状神经节[28]，造成左优势型的心脏交感神经支配不平衡，引起QT间期延长，这时幼犬在一些状况下容易发生室颤。交感神经支配在出生后继续发育，并在生后接近第6个月时达到功能成熟。偶尔左侧和右侧的交感神经发育速度不同，可能导致暂时的不平衡[29]。交感活性的突然增加，尤其是与左侧致心律失常性的神经有关时[29]，这些电活动不稳定的心脏很容易出现致命性心律失常。我们的关于右侧交感神经节切除、左侧交感神经节注射神经生长因子的资料最近由Chen及其同事发表[30]：具备这种交感不平衡的婴儿，不管是发育性的还是遗传性的，生后的前几个月都是很脆弱的，有较高的发生婴儿猝死综合征的危险性，可以通过观察QT间期延长而被识别。

第二个机制由临床实践得出，在新生儿或婴儿时期常用的几种药物可引起QT间期延长。如：乙酰螺旋霉素，一种在欧洲广泛应用的大环内酯类抗生素，主要用于弓形虫抗体阳性母亲所生的新生儿的预防性治疗，可延长QT间期，并导致心脏停搏[31]。在那些出生后有必要进行弓形虫病预防治疗的新生儿人群中，使用乙酰螺旋霉素期间及停药后分别描记心电图，发现在使用乙酰螺旋霉素期间，QTc及QTc的离散度均大于对照组。值得注意的是，在开始治疗之后，发生过心脏停搏事件的2个新生儿与那些没有症状的新生儿相比，QTc及QTc离散度显著增加。由此得出结论，在新生儿期使用乙酰螺旋霉素将引起QT间期延长及QT间期离散度的增加。其他婴儿使用的抗生素，如红霉素、克林霉素、甲氧苄氨嘧啶可能会延长QT间期。抗组胺药物，如用于治疗过敏症的特非那定，及胃肠动力药，如用于治疗婴儿时期胃食管反流病的西沙必利，也会引起QT间期延长及尖端扭转型室速。由于上述原因，这几个药物在某些国家已经退出了市场。所有这些药物都能够阻断I_{Kr}，都需通过细胞色素P_{450}酶代谢，而这种酶的功能在新生儿并不完善。

最近有人报道了婴儿时期的获得性QT间期延长[32]，并确诊为自身免疫性疾病。抗Ro/SSA抗体阳性的母亲生产的新生儿接近一半以上出现QT间期延长[32]，QTc值有时可超过500ms，而并不出现房室传导异常，这是典型的新生儿狼疮综合征的表现[33]。与先天性心脏传导阻滞不同，这种心室复极异常是一过性的，常在生后6个月时消失，与抗Ro/SSA抗体的消失一致[34]。这种一过性的QT间期延长可能使一些抗Ro抗体阳性的婴儿易于发生致命性心律失常。这个现象的意义有两个方面，当新生儿出现不能用其他原因解释的长QT间期时，需要注意除外母亲患有无症状自身免疫性疾病的可能，而狼疮综合征母亲所产的新生儿需要在生后1年内进行心电图随访。

还有其他两种与长QT综合征有关的可能机制。长QT综合征是一种家族遗传性疾病，但也可表现为散发（没有家族受累的表现），疾病的特征是QT间期延长及猝死的高危险性，通常发生在精神紧张的状况下，但也可发生在睡眠时[9,35]。长QT综合征存在基因异质性，突变最常见于3、7、11及21号染色体[10]。将长QT综合征与婴儿猝死综合征联系在一起的一个困难就是后者不是家族性疾病。这里要提到两个相关的概念。第一，散发长QT综合征患者的新生突变已经在2个基因发现，即HERG及KvLQT1基因，编码I_{Kr}及I_{Ks}钾通道（两个重要的复极离子流）。也发现了心脏钠通道基因SCN5A新生突变，这些新生突变在父母身上没有发现。第二，长QT综合征的外显率低[27]。外显率的定义是基因携带者与表现出疾病所有现象个体的比率。较低的外显率提示临床诊断通常是不充分的,许多受累的个体临床表现可能完全正常。

我们现在已经掌握了这些可能机制中新生突变机制的证据,它很有可能是一部分婴儿猝死综合征的真正原因,能够解释父母QT间期正常而死于婴儿猝死综合征的患儿出现QT间期延长。

(二) 分子水平的证据

我们最近报道的两例独立的病例证实长QT综合征基因新生突变的表现与婴儿猝死综合征的表现难以区别[4,5]。

第一个病例:一个7周大的婴儿出现发绀、窒息、无脉,被其父母发现[4],紧急送到了附近医院,同时他父亲尝试对他进行心肺复苏,急诊室心电图显示患儿发生了室颤(图77-3)。这个婴儿的表现几乎就是典型的婴儿猝死综合征,除颤复苏后,心电图显示QT间期显著延长(QTc为648ms),长QT综合征诊断成立,联合应用β受体阻滞剂及钠通道阻滞剂美西律治疗。该病例的关键点是父母双方的QT间期均正常,血缘关系也是肯定的。分子筛查显示婴儿发生了SCN5A突变,此心脏钠通道基因与3型长QT综合征有关[10]。这个致病的基因突变在父母均未见到,由此可以证实这是一个新生突变(图77-4)。

到达急诊室后记录到的室颤心电图十分重要,常见的情况是"没有人记录到婴儿猝死综合征高危患儿的室性心律失常心电图"[36]。假如这个婴儿死亡,必然也没有复律,没有记录到心电图,而父母的QT间期都正常,长QT综合征的诊断肯定会被除外,而更支持经典的婴儿猝死综合征的诊断。由此可见,一个控制心室复极离子通道的基因出现新生突变的婴儿,在出生后可能表现为QT间期延长。这样的一些婴儿

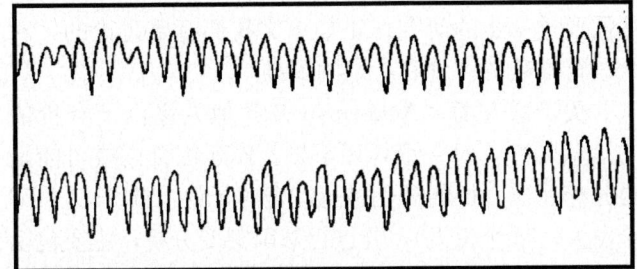

A　44天—未治疗

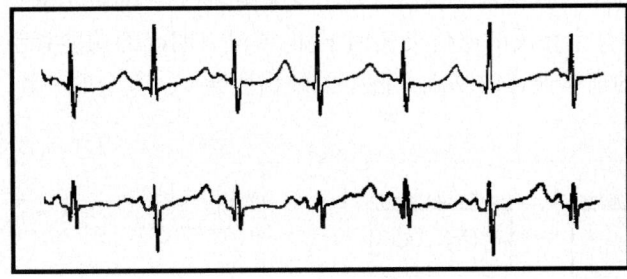

B　44天—QTc648ms—未治疗

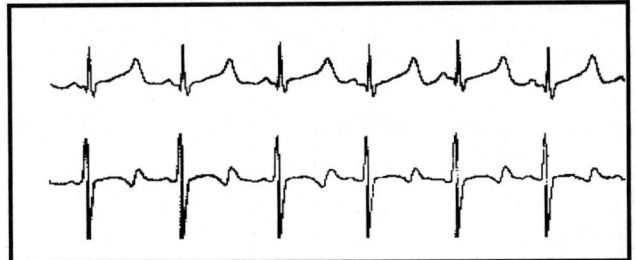

C　3岁—QTc510ms—普萘洛尔+美西律

图77-3　A:为Ⅱ和V₂导联心电图,患者住院期间发生室颤;B:为同天转复为窦性心律后的心电图,显示QT间期延长;C:为最后一次随访时的心电图。(改自Schwartz PJ, Priori SG, Dumaine R, et al: A molecular link between the sudden infant death syndrome and the long QT syndrome. N Engl J Med 343:262-267, 2000.)

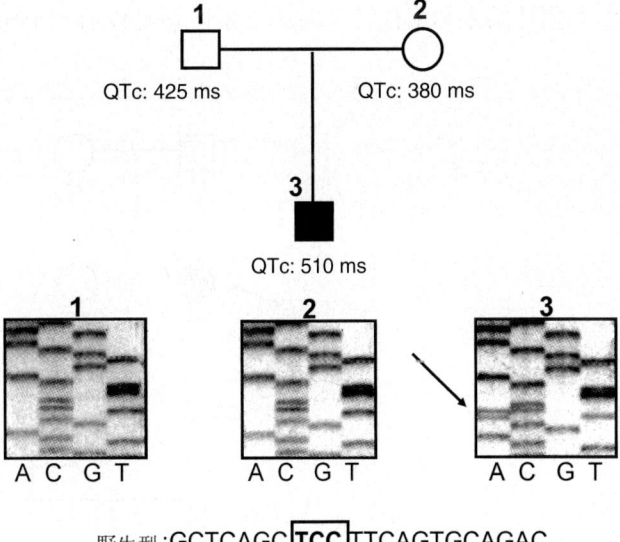

图77-4　家系调查和分子筛查结果　SCN5A基因的第16个外显子DNA序列分析发现如图所示的两个异常条带,表明先证者有杂合突变,而其父母没有此异常条带。(改自Schwartz PJ, Priori SG, Dumaine R, et al: A molecular link between the sudden infant death syndrome and the long QT syndrome. N Engl J Med 343:262-267, 2000.)

可能在宫内时就已经死于室颤,或者在生后的头几个月内死亡,没有获得标志性的心电图而似乎是死于婴儿猝死综合征,其余的可能会在儿童期出现晕厥或非致命性心脏停搏,那时就会被诊断为散发的长 QT 综合征。

第二个病例[5]:一个 4 个月大的婴儿被发现死在她的小床上。她当时仰卧在床上,室温凉爽适宜,父母不吸烟。全面尸检的结果为阴性,因此被诊断为婴儿猝死综合征。然而,在进行分子筛查之后,发现了一个基因突变点导致编码 KvLQT1 蛋白的第 117 位高度保守的脯氨酸被亮氨酸替换。患儿的父母及姐姐的 QT 间期都正常,也没有 P117L 突变,血缘关系能够确定。因此确定患儿出现了新生突变。我们随访的一个长 QT 综合征家族中可以见到相同的突变(图 77-5)。这个病例第一次提供证据表明一个被诊断为婴儿猝死综合征的患者,死后的分子筛查有助于长 QT 综合征的诊断。

迄今为止这些发现的意义超过了通常的单个病例报告,因为它们证明了长 QT 综合征与婴儿猝死综合征相关的观念,第一次明确表明具备几乎所有婴儿猝死综合征特征的婴儿,实际是由于携带一个长 QT 综合征基因的新生突变,发生了室颤而导致猝死。

阴性结果和阳性结果的最主要区别是没有得到充分的正确评价。否定一个假设的机制需要大量的阴性结果。相反,肯定一个假设的机制仅单个阳性结果便足以证实。对于 QT 间期延长与婴儿猝死综合征相关性的评价,我们的大样本前瞻性研究已经获得了足够的信息,证实了 50% 的死于婴儿猝死综合征的患者在生后前几个月 QT 间期是延长的。同时也证实 QTc 超过正常值上限几个毫秒没有必要诊断长 QT 综合征,保守地估计,长 QT 综合征相关的婴儿猝死综合征的发生率为 10%~20%。

我们的研究同样证明,一些死于婴儿猝死综合征的婴儿实际上患有长 QT 综合征。关于长 QT 综合征作为婴儿猝死综合征的一个病因真正的患病率如何仍然需要进一步的研究。正如下文我们将要讨论的,对此进行准确的评价有一定的困难。

关于这方面,Ackerman 及其他人提供了有价值的信息[37,38]。对一系列死于婴儿猝死综合征或可能是婴儿猝死综合征的婴儿进行综合的尸检(共 93 人,59 个白人,34 个黑人),并进行基因突变分析,主要包括 5 个 LQTS 基因:*KvLQT1/KCNQ1*、*HERG/KCNH2*、*SCN5A*、*KCNE1*、*KCNE2*。27 人(29%)5 个基因中的 1 个发生错义突变。4 个受累者发生了在缺乏至少 400 个相关的遗传突变因子和/或没有明确的功能紊乱的离子通道的基础上假定的致病性突变。其余的种族

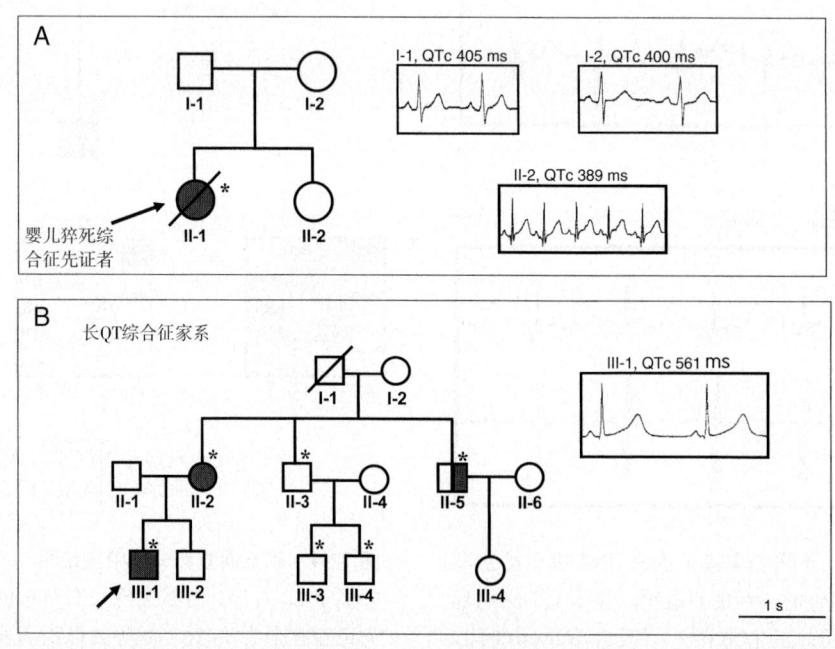

图 77-5 本研究中有 P117L 突变的两个家系及心电图追踪 A:婴儿猝死综合征家系。右图对先证者父母(Ⅰ-1 和 Ⅰ-2)及姊妹(Ⅱ-2)的心电图追踪显示了正常的 QT 间期。B:有 P117L 突变的 LQT1 家系。左边记录了先证者肢导 Ⅱ 导联心电图(Ⅲ-1)。箭头代表先证者。填充标记代表发生过晕厥以及有长 QT 间期的个体。半填充标记代表有 QT 间期延长但没有症状的个体。星号所示为有 P117L 突变的携带者。

相关的遗传突变因子也能够检测到，代表着特异的非同义多态性。这些离子通道的多态性是否减少了复极储备和/或使肾上腺素介导的心律失常更容易发生还需要进一步研究。事实上，单核苷酸多态性（SNPs）未必是无关的"旁观者"。比如：D85N 是 *KCNE1* 中一个相当常见的单核苷酸多态性，编码钾通道的 minK 亚单位，与 *KCNQ1* 或 *KvLQT1* 共同产生 I_{Ks} 离子流。这个遗传突变因子对 I_{Ks} 进行精细的动态调节，因此即使是在部分 I_{Kr} 阻滞的情况下，就像一些常用的药物会引起的那样，会增加 I_{Kr} 阻滞相关的致心律失常性早后除极的危险性，触发致命性心律失常[39]。Ackerman 及其合作者研究了 93 个死于婴儿猝死综合征的婴儿[38]，发现单核苷酸多态性在这些婴儿中有很高的发生率，支持它们中的一部分可能参与了致命性心律失常的发生。

在 Ackerman 及其合作者的研究中，婴儿猝死综合征人群中近 1/3 的人有可识别的离子通道突变，其中引起婴儿猝死综合征的致病性突变接近 5%。即使是在最好的实验室，那些临床上被确诊为长 QT 综合征患者的父母中仅有 50%～60% 能够成功确定基因型；这也提示不论死于婴儿猝死综合征的婴儿中有多少能够确定长 QT 综合征的基因型，可能接近一半的婴儿确实存在长 QT 综合征突变。长 QT 综合征似乎在黑人中发生较少，而黑人占到总研究人群的 37%，没有注意到这一点在寻找可能的长 QT 综合征突变时就已经产生了偏倚。总之，以这些人群为基础的尸检分子学结果为我们之前的发现提供了有力的支持。

结论是有确凿的证据证明心脏离子通道的突变可能诱发婴儿猝死综合征，同时我们假定的一个与婴儿猝死综合征有关的特异机制，也就是新生突变确实是一个致病因子[3-5]。研究结论支持进行广泛的新生儿心电图筛查，并表明至少婴儿猝死综合征高危的婴儿可以在早期被识别，那些迫在眉睫的猝死有可能被阻止，而他们的父母经证实大多数患有长 QT 综合征。

（三）临床意义

在本篇关于 QT 间期延长及婴儿猝死综合征[3]的文章结束前我们将讨论两个问题：诊断中可能存在的困难及临床意义。

第一个问题是 QT 间期延长与婴儿猝死综合征的高度相关性会提高常规新生儿心电图筛查的价值。由于婴儿猝死综合征在一般人群中的发生率低（<0.1%），导致任何与该事件相关的因素的预测价值都很低。因此尽管 QT 间期延长（1.5%）的相对危险度达到 41，显著高于之前报道的任何因素，预测价值也一样不高。除去这点限制，一个简单的心电图筛查就可以识别一部分婴儿猝死综合征高危患儿。

第二个问题是对发现 QTc 延长的婴儿的治疗。我们的研究不包括对新治疗建议的评价，但是 QT 间期延长与婴儿猝死综合征的关系引起人们思索。QT 间期相关的致命性心律失常经常由突然的交感神经激活诱发。在生后的第 1 年，很多条件下可以诱发这种情况[2]，包括突然的噪声、寒冷、快动眼睡眠、呼吸暂停导致的化学感应器反射、唤醒，甚至可能是俯卧。对于长 QT 综合征，抗肾上腺素能药物非常有效[9]。来自将近 1000 个长 QT 综合征家族的数据显示，β 受体阻滞剂治疗可使死亡率下降到小于 3%[9]。这点对在 QT 间期延长的新生儿防止 SIDS 的发生是有意义的。对那些偶然通过新生儿心电图筛查发现确实有 LQTS 的婴儿提供了一种现成的治疗方法，同时提供了一个降低 QT 间期延长婴儿的危险性的有效选择，尽管未被证实，但有一定的理由。

上文提到的发现已经有一定的影响。一些欧洲国家开始考虑将对所有新生儿在生后第 1 个月行心电图检查列入国家健康服务，作为一个心血管筛查项目。一旦新生儿筛查被列为国家健康服务的一部分，那么医院的心脏病专科医师（其中大多数人对新生儿心电图完全陌生），将被要求辨认这些图形。欧洲心脏病协会已经意识到了欧洲心脏病专科医师及卫生保健的需要，相应地开始着手制定解读新生儿心电图的指南[40]。制定指南的主要目的，集中在最有临床意义的异常、随后的治疗及治疗选择。这一文件代表了欧洲心脏病协会关于这个题目的官方意见。

在临床实践中，生后第 3～4 周行心电图筛查，当 QTc 异常时重复进行检查，可以大大减少假阳性病例的数量。当早期发现婴儿的 QT 间期延长而有危险时，就可以考虑预防性的治疗，并持续数月。发育过程中 QT 间期正常后可以停止药物治疗，因为假阳性的婴儿是不可避免的。少数 QT 间期持续延长的婴儿需要继续治疗，对这些婴儿 β 受体阻滞剂可能是挽救生命的措施。

五、法律学意义

上述发现，除了具有相当明显的临床意义外，还有重要的法律学意义。这些法律问题的存在可以解释为什么许多人对 QT 间期延长假说持反对意见。

争论集中在如果医学界接受相当数量（不论 10% 或 20%）的将来可能发生 SIDS 的婴儿在新生儿期心电图上可以识别的概念，加上法律的介入，会有很大的机会防止这部分婴儿猝死。当前普遍的占绝对优势的观念是确定 SIDS 真正高危的婴儿是不可能做到的，除了残酷的命运之外没有人需要为此负责。一旦 QT 假说被接受，这些都会改变。我们提供的证据带来了转折，对一个已经被归类为死于 SIDS 的婴儿而且在没有获得心电图的情况下诊断为 LQTS 是有可能的[5]。死于 SIDS 的婴儿的父母，更确切地说是他们的内科医生，会要求患儿死后接受分子学筛查。那时分子学诊断会显示 LQTS 是猝死的原因。失去孩子的父母及他们的律师就会提出新的问题，为什么他们没有被告知他们的孩子可能患有致命但是可以医治的疾病，而这种疾病通过一个简单的心电图就可以识别，尽管这种疾病非常罕见 [1/（3000~5000）]。

问题到此还没有结束。一旦作出了一份新生儿心电图，就需要有人承担决定 QT 间期是正常、临界，或异常并提出相应建议的责任。在一个诉讼较多的社会，不难想像不得不做大量的新生儿心电图然后评判 QT 间期，还有可能被卷入诉讼程序。这对医生来说是一件令人生厌的事情。因此，我们就可以理解，为什么新生儿心电图对于识别由于心律失常引起早期猝死的高危婴儿是有用的，但儿科学界对这样一个显而易见的现象持反对意见。

六、致　谢

这些关于 SIDS 的研究部分得到 Leducq 基金给予"遗传性心律失常性疾病的分子流行病学"的资助，以及意大利健康研究部门在 1999、2000、2001 年分别给予的资助。

（张　萍译）

参 考 文 献

1. Schwartz PJ: Cardiac sympathetic innervation and the sudden infant death syndrome. A possible pathogenetic link. Am J Med 60:167–172, 1976.
2. Schwartz PJ: The quest for the mechanism of the sudden infant death syndrome. Doubts and progress. Circulation 75:677–683, 1987.
3. Schwartz PJ, Stramba-Badiale M, Segantini A, et al: Prolongation of the QT interval and the sudden infant death syndrome. N Engl J Med 338:1709–1714, 1998.
4. Schwartz PJ, Priori SG, Dumaine R, et al: A molecular link between the sudden infant death syndrome and the long QT syndrome. N Engl J Med 343:262–267, 2000.
5. Schwartz PJ, Priori SG, Bloise R, et al: Molecular diagnosis in a child with sudden infant death syndrome. Lancet 358:1342–1343, 2001.
6. Schwartz PJ, Southall DP, Valdes-Dapena M (eds): The Sudden Infant Death Syndrome. Cardiac and Respiratory Mechanisms and Interventions. Ann NY Acad Sci 533:1–474, 1988.
7. Ramanathan R, Corwin MJ, Hunt CE, et al: Cardiorespiratory events recorded on home monitors: Comparison of healthy infants with those at increased risk for SIDS. JAMA 285:2199–2207, 2001.
8. Jobe AH: What do home monitors contribute to the SIDS problem? JAMA 285:2244–2245, 2001.
9. Schwartz PJ, Priori SG, Napolitano C: Long QT syndrome. In Zipes DP, Jalife J (eds): Cardiac Electrophysiology: From Cell to Bedside, 3rd ed. Philadelphia, WB Saunders, 2000, pp 597–615.
10. Priori SG, Barhanin J, Hauer RNW, et al: Genetic and molecular basis of cardiac arrhythmias: Impact on clinical management. Parts I and II. Circulation 99:518–528, 1999; Part III Circulation 99:674–681, 1999; Eur Heart J 20:174–195, 1999.
11. Maron BJ, Clark CE, Goldstein RE, Epstein SE: Potential role of QT interval prolongation in sudden infant death syndrome. Circulation 54:423–430, 1976.
12. Kelly DH, Shannon DC, Liberthson R: The role of the QT interval in the sudden infant death syndrome. Circulation 55:633–635, 1977.
13. Steinschneider A: Sudden infant death syndrome and prolongation of the QT interval. Am J Dis Child 132:688–691, 1978.
14. Haddad GG, Epstein MAF, Epstein RA, et al: The QT interval in aborted sudden infant death syndrome infants. Pediat Res 13:136–138, 1979.
15. Montague TJ, Finley JP, Mukelabai K, et al: Cardiac rhythm, rate and ventricular repolarization properties in infants at risk for sudden infant death syndrome: Comparison with age- and sex-matched control infants. Am J Cardiol 54:301–307, 1984.
16. Southall DP, Arrowsmith WA, Stebbens V, Alexander JR: QT interval measurements before sudden infant death syndrome. Arch Dis Child 61:327–333, 1986.
17. Schwartz PJ, Segantini A: Cardiac innervation, neonatal electrocardiography and SIDS. A key for a novel preventive strategy? Ann NY Acad Sci 533:210–220, 1988.
18. Schwartz PJ, Wolf S: QT interval prolongation as predictor of sudden death in patients with myocardial infarction. Circulation 57:1074–1077, 1978.
19. Algra A, Tijssen JGP, Roelandt JRTC, et al: QTc prolongation measured by standard 12-lead electrocardiography is an independent risk factor for sudden death due to cardiac arrest. Circulation 83:1888–1894, 1991.
20. Schouten EG, Dekker JM, Meppelink P, et al: QT interval prolongation predicts cardiovascular mortality in an apparently healthy population. Circulation 84:1516–1523, 1991.
21. Napolitano C, Schwartz PJ, Brown AM, et al: Evidence for a cardiac ion channel mutation underlying drug-induced QT prolongation and life-threatening arrhythmias. J Cardiovasc Electrophysiol 11:691–696, 2000.
22. Fleming PJ, Gilbert R, Azaz Y: Interaction between bedding and sleeping position in the sudden infant death syndrome: A population based case-control study. BMJ 301:85–89, 1990.
23. Kahn A, Groswasser J, Sottiaux M, et al: Prone or supine body position and sleep characteristics in infants. Pediatrics 91:1112–1115, 1993.
24. Schwartz PJ, Zipes DP: Autonomic modulation of cardiac arrhythmias. In Zipes DP, Jalife J (eds): Cardiac Electrophysiology: From Cell to Bedside, 3rd ed. Philadelphia, WB Saunders, 2000, pp 300–314.
25. Blair PS, Fleming PJ, Bensley D, et al: Smoking and the sudden infant death syndrome: Results from 1993-5 case-control study for confidential inquiry into stillbirths and deaths in infancy. Confidential Enquiry into Stillbirths and Deaths Regional Coordinators and Researchers. BMJ 313:195–198, 1996.
26. Satriani L, Cerbai E, Lonardo G, et al: Prenatal exposure to carbon monoxide affects postnatal cellular electrophysiological maturation of the rat heart: a potential substrate for arrhythmogenesis in infancy. Circulation (In press).
27. Priori SG, Napolitano C, Schwartz PJ: Low penetrance in the long QT syndrome. Clinical impact. Circulation 99:529–533, 1999.
28. Stramba-Badiale M, Lazzarotti M, Schwartz PJ: Development of cardiac innervation, ventricular fibrillation and sudden infant death syndrome. Am J Physiol Heart Circ Physiol 263:H1514–H1522, 1992.
29. Schwartz PJ: QT prolongation, sudden death, and sympathetic

29. imbalance: The pendulum swings. J Cardiovasc Electrophysiol 12:1074–1077, 2001.
30. Chen PS, Chen LS, Cao JM, et al: Sympathetic nerve sprouting, electrical remodeling and the mechanisms of sudden cardiac death. Cardiovasc Res 50:409–16, 2001.
31. Stramba-Badiale M, Nador F, Porta N, et al: QT interval prolongation and risk of life-threatening arrhythmias during toxoplasmosis prophylaxis with spiramycin in neonates. Am Heart J 133:108–111, 1997.
32. Cimaz R, Stramba-Badiale M, Brucato A, et al: QT interval prolongation in asymptomatic anti-SSA/Ro-positive infants without congenital heart block. Arthritis Rheum 43:1049–1053, 2000.
33. Brucato A, Cimaz R, Stramba-Badiale M: Neonatal lupus. Clin Rev Allergy Immunol 23:279–299, 2002.
34. Cimaz R, Meroni PL, Brucato A, et al: Concomitant disappearance of electrocardiographic abnormalities and of acquired maternal autoantibodies during the first year of life in infants who had QT interval prolongation and anti-SSA/Ro positivity without congenital heart block at birth. Arthritis Rheum 48:266–268, 2003.
35. Schwartz PJ, Priori SG, Spazzolini C, et al: Genotype-phenotype correlation in the long QT syndrome. Gene-specific triggers for life-threatening arrhythmias. Circulation 103:89–95, 2001.
36. Guntheroth WG, Spiers PS: Prolongation of the QT interval and the sudden infant death syndrome. Pediatrics 103:813–814, 1999.
37. Ackerman MJ, Siu BL, Sturner WQ, et al: Postmortem molecular analysis of *SCN5A* defects in sudden infant death syndrome. JAMA 286:2264–2269, 2001.
38. Ackerman MJ, Tester DJ, Bell CM, et al: Cardiac channel mutations in SIDS: A population-based molecular autopsy study. Circulation 106(suppl):II-167, 2002.
39. Wei J, Yang C-H I, Tapper AR, et al: KCNE1 polymorphism confers risk of drug-induced long QT syndrome by altering kinetic properties of I_{Ks} potassium channels. Circulation 100(suppl):I-495, 1999.
40. Schwartz PJ, Garson A Jr, Paul T, et al: Guidelines for the interpretation of the neonatal electrocardiogram. A Task Force of the European Society of Cardiology. Eur Heart J 23:1329–1344, 2002.

第 78 章

心脏性猝死

Robert J. Myerburg，Alberto Interian Jr，Jeffrey Simmons，and Agustin Castellanos

本章目录
- 心脏性猝死的发病率 ········· 712
- SCD 的病因及临床表现 ········ 714
- SCD 的病理解剖 ············ 714
- SCD 危险性的预测策略 ········ 715
- 冠心病 SCD 的一般和特异性危险预测因子 ················ 716
- 扩张型心肌病的危险预测 ······· 718
- 心脏停搏的电生理机制 ········ 718
- 冠心病 SCD 的遗传基础 ······· 718
- SCD 综合系统分析与遗传流行病学 ···················· 719

心脏性猝死（sudden cardiac death，SCD）是指有或无基础心脏病的患者由于心血管原因发生的死亡，其死亡的方式和时间难以预料。目前普遍接受的关于 SCD 的时间定义：从临床症状突然发作到意识丧失不超过 1h[1]。这一时间段的定义，更适合用于人群研究和临床分析，而且与导致最终死亡的病理生理学联系更为紧密。而生物学死亡可发生在中枢神经系统（central nervous system，CNS）损伤后，仍可在生命支持的干预措施下延迟数天到 1 个月，甚至更久的时间。

一、心脏性猝死的发病率

20 多年以来，美国每年估计有 30 万到 35 万例 SCD 发生。然而，这些评估的基础并非来源于直接的流行病学调查，而是来源于观察数据，比如回顾性死亡证明、分析和假定心血管死亡中猝死的比例。在近几年，有关 SCD 发病趋势的不一致观点也被提出。一份基于美国健康统计中心（the National Center for Health Statistics，NCHS）和心肺血液研究所（the National，Heart，Lung，and Blood Institute，NHLBI）的数据，出自美国心脏协会（American Heart Association，AHA）统计手册的评估[2]提出 SCD 的发病率为每年 22 万例。另一份来自西雅图、华盛顿急救系统（Emergency Rescue System，EMS）数据库的分析，推论至全美人群，2000 年时共有 18.4 万例心脏停搏发生[3]，比 1980 年的统计有显著性降低。相反，也正是一份来自 NCHS 的基于死亡证明的研究提示在所有心脏死亡中超过 50% 者为猝死，而且估计 SCD 的年发病率在 46 万例的范围内[4]。两份声明间的显著不一致是基于其采用的 SCD 的定义和人群来源的不同。美国心脏协会的数据仅仅来源于病因为冠心病者，其狭窄的定义建立在所选的 ICD-9 标准（410～414）的基础之上（图 78-1A），而西雅图的数据则仅包含了伴随急救的 SCD（图 78-1B）。在更广泛的 NCHS 研究中，几乎包含了 SCD 的所有病因（图 78-1C），这种包含范围的大大加宽，可能会在一定程度上高估了真实的发病率。而且，众所周知，使用死亡证明数据作为流行病学评估的基础存在着风险[5]，并也受到了限制。虽然如此，全美的 SCD 健康负担更可能是高估，而不是低估了。这种观念在过去 40～50 年间，受到冠心病死亡率的年龄相关危险度显著下降的事实所支持，但当转换为总事件数和未来事件危险度人群大小时，这一观念并不能被解释为疾病的绝对患病率和致死事件的发病率已经降低了[6]。当然，伴

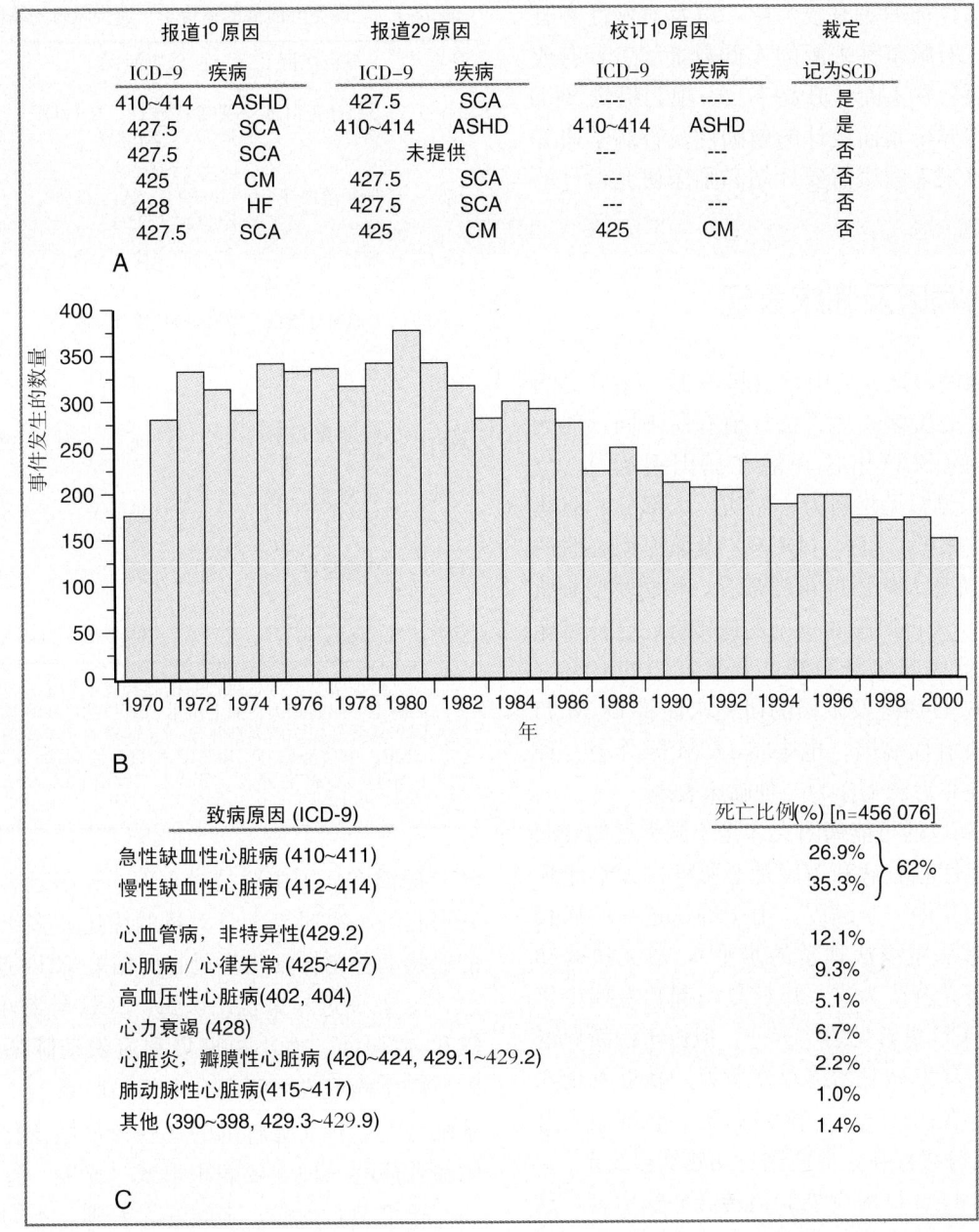

图 78-1 美国心脏性猝死（SCD）发病率评估不一致的基础 最近的评估范围为每年 SCD 从少于 18.5 万到超过 45 万。大多数评估来源于对死亡证明数据的回顾性分析，尚无评估基于全国人群样本的前瞻性分析。每个研究皆采用了不同的纳入标准。A 图：在美国心脏协会（AHA）统计手册所提供的数据中，这些数据只限于诊断为冠心病的院外发生的心脏停搏，采用特殊可植入心脏转复除颤器（ICD）标准（410～414）。这一来源估计年 SCD 的发生为 22 万例。B 图：从 1980 年到 2000 年间，被西雅图急救系统识别的年室颤发病率下降。将这些数据推论到西雅图社区所有的心脏停搏，然后，再依次推论到整个国家，计算出每年有 18.4 万例的 SCD 发病率。C 图：数据发布于美国健康统计中心，其采用了更宽范围的 SCD 病因定义（注释了所采用的 ICD-9 标准），它表明如果采用 AHA 评估所基于的 ICD 标准，在其总 SCD 中只有 62% 可被初步诊断为 SCD。这份数据提示美国每年有超过 45 万例的 SCD 患者。一项采用统一标准的前瞻性研究对于阐明美国 SCD 实际发病率是十分需要的。（A 图，来源于 Myerburg RJ: Scientific gaps in the prediction of sudden cardiac death. J Cardiovasc Electrophysiol 13: 709-723, 2002; B 图，来源于 Cobb LA, Fahrenbruch CE, Olsufka MK: Changing incidence of out-of-hospital ventricular fibrillation, 1980-2000. JAMA 288: 3008-3031, 2002; C 图，来源于 Zheng ZJ, Croft JB, Giles WH, Mensah GA: Sudden cardiac death in the United States 1989 to 1998. Circulation 104: 2158-2163, 2001.）

随对急性冠脉综合征的更有效治疗，以及对慢性心脏病的长期治疗，冠脉事件来源的人群数量（患者有或无已知的心脏病）在不断地升高[7]。一项为提供 SCD 准确计数和其特异机制而设计的前瞻性流行病学研究将是一项有助于未来健康需要计划和临床研究设计的明智投资。

二、SCD 的病因及临床表现

在西方国家的普通人群中，引起 SCD 的最常见病因是冠状动脉性心脏病。尽管估计值有所不同，但大约 75%～80% 的 SCD 由这一潜在病因引起[1]。与 SCD 相关的第二类常见疾病为心肌病。大部分心肌病的定义包含了扩张型心肌病（DCM）及肥厚型心肌病（HCM），但从临床及病因的角度来看，将肥厚型心肌病归入具有发生 SCD 风险的少见的遗传性综合征可能更为恰当。DCM 引起的 SCD 约占全部 SCD 的 10%～15%。许多对 SCD 风险及干预的研究未能将 DCM 归入缺血性或非缺血性病因，也未将 DCM 区分为一种病因或将充血性心力衰竭作为一种临床表现。

其他引起 SCD 的可能病因大多是不同类型的浸润性心脏病、炎症性心脏病和瓣膜性心脏病。无临床症状的心肌炎也是其中一个病因。由于确认这一疾病相当困难（即使是从组织病理学的水平），故无法确知其发病率。有研究者认为这一疾病是引起青春期少年及年轻成年人 SCD 更常见的病因[8]，但由于诊断标准缺乏一致性，对其发病率始终存在争议。新近发现在无炎症标志物存在的情况下，SCD 患者心肌细胞内有病毒 DNA 片段持续存在，更使这一问题变得复杂[9]。

仅有少部分的 SCD 因少见的遗传性疾病引起，这些 SCD 主要发生在青春期少年及年轻成年人中（包括运动员）。这些遗传性疾病有长 QT 综合征（LQTS）、Brugada 综合征、HCM、致心律失常性右室发育不良（ARVD），以及其他非遗传性的先天性疾病，如主动脉瓣狭窄及冠状动脉畸形。总的来说，这些少见疾病占所有 SCD 病例不足 1% 或 2%，但近期逐渐出现的资料显示一些编码离子通道的基因突变，使得某些人在触发条件下易于发生心律失常，尽管这些人在平时的表型是正常的[10]。药物引起的心律失常即为一个例子[11,12]。

三、SCD 的病理解剖

因 SCD 患者获得的大部分病理解剖学资料显示

表 78-1　肥厚型心肌病的遗传学：遗传风险的基因差异模型*

位点	基因产物	SCD 的风险	临床联系
14p11.2-12	β 肌球蛋白重链	突变特异性 [R403Q, R453C, R719W]	显著的 LVH；高危
1q3	肌钙蛋白 T	高 SCD 风险 [Int15G1_A, ΔE160, R92Q, 179N]	中度 LVH
19q13.4	肌钙蛋白 I	高 SCD 风险 [ΔK183]	心尖 LVH
15q22	α 原肌球蛋白	高 SCD 风险 [V95A]	风险不一，多为良性，晚发
11p11.2	肌球蛋白结合蛋白 C	低	
3p21	肌球蛋白轻链-1	低	乳头肌；少见
12q23-24.3	肌球蛋白轻链-2	低	乳头肌；少见
15q14	肌动蛋白	低	一些 DCM 突变
7q3	AMP 活化蛋白激酶 γ2	低	与 WPW 相关

*已经证实 9 个与心肌收缩机制有关编码蛋白的基因位点突变与肥厚型心肌病相关。如上所示，SCD 的发生风险因突变位点而不同。器质性疾病的表型并不一定与 SCD 风险相关。

AMP，单磷酸腺苷；DCM，扩张型心肌病；LVH，左心室肥厚；SCD，心脏性猝死；WPW，Wolff-Parkinson-White 综合征。

SCD 的潜在病因主要是冠心病。关于冠心病的范围及其引起的心室肌异常有大量的描述。多年来公认广泛的冠状动脉粥样硬化是冠心病相关 SCD 的首要解剖标志[13]。然而近年来也认识到，SCD 与粥样斑块存在裂隙和/或侵蚀、血小板聚集和冠状动脉粥样硬化病变内急性血栓形成之间也有密切的联系[14,15]。慢性病变基础之上冠状动脉解剖的这些特征性变化，在急性冠脉综合征的三种主要表现形式（SCD、急性心肌梗死和不稳定型心绞痛）之间并无差别。不同的研究已证实超过 90% 的 SCD 患者中存在一处或多处冠状动脉的活动性病变[16]。

心肌病理学研究显示在心肌梗死后愈合的心肌瘢痕中，普遍存在慢性冠状动脉粥样硬化[17]。急性心肌梗死方面的证据更少。但即使是在溶栓/PCI 前时代对心脏骤停存活者的研究中，衍变为急性透壁心肌梗死的情况也不常见[18]。SCD 患者冠状动脉病变的范围及左心室肥厚的程度间也存在联系[19]。广泛的冠状动脉病变及左心室肥厚间的相关性可能是长期高血压的结果，而长期高血压是冠心病或心肌梗死后心脏重塑的一个危险因子。无论机制如何，心肌瘢痕组织和左心室肥厚是短暂缺血时引起心律失常的危险因子[1,6]。

不太常见的引起 SCD 的其他疾病各有其病理解剖

学特点。在 DCM 中发现非特异性的病理变化，特点是间质纤维化和心肌细胞退行性变。HCM 的解剖学特点与该病的特殊类型有关[20]。对梗阻性、非梗阻性、心尖肥厚型及向心性肥厚型 HCM 均有研究，一些类型与遗传形式的特定基因型有关[20]。在 HCM 观察到的一种普遍现象是心肌细胞的排列紊乱，在大多类型但并非全部 HCM 中均存在。HCM 表型及 SCD 风险间的关系很复杂，因为遗传方式不仅与多个基因位点有关，还存在与突变相关的风险（表 78-1）。

心肌炎引起的猝死可能有不同的组织病理学表现。急性病毒性心肌炎常与心肌的严重炎症反应有关，但有些病毒性心肌炎的心肌细胞浆内存在病毒DNA 残片，其可能表现为广泛的纤维化但无炎症标志物的存在[9]。

四、SCD 危险性的预测策略

SCD 危险性预测的临床实用性和影响很复杂。从个体危险性方面来看，当使用的危险性测量指标不同时，SCD 危险性预测会呈现出一系列不同的预测效能[6,21,22]。传统的流行病学指标为人群危险性提供了很有价值的依据，尤其对冠心病的发展。但是，应用临床预防策略的主要局限发生在对个体危险性的预测上。在不同的流行病学和临床分类中，SCD 发病率和临床事件发生的绝对数量相反（图 78-2），这一点值得注意，特别是当我们的目的是采用治疗性策略时[23]。在群体中，每年 35 岁及以上的人 SCD 的发病率为 0.1% ～ 0.2%，这和美国每年猝死的发病率相同。但是，群体中个体临床事件发病率低以及未进行年龄分层，这限制了治疗策略的使用范围。在冠状动脉粥样硬化高危人群组和未经选择的明确冠心病患者临床事件组中，患病率均有所增加，这对于个体危险性预测的效能仍有一定局限。然而，与之相比的是心力衰竭或射血分数低于 35% 的患者，心源性猝死幸存者以及心肌梗死后高危患者有较高的临床事件发生率。但是，其在人群中绝对发生数量降低，且在总体人群 SCD 疾病负担中占的比例降低[21]。认识到这个原则的重要性与不同的预防性干预措施对人群带来的益处多少有关。比如说，在植入式除颤器临床试验研究中，高危病人组（图 78-3）只占了所有 SCD 患者的小部分，因此其关于安置植入式除颤器的好处的研究报道只能是对于这一小部分亚组人群而言。这就表明了寻找对大部分人群都适用的特异危险性指标十分重要，只有这样才能对更多人群的健康带来益处。

上述观点在冠心病患者心源性猝死前临床表现形式中也可以看出。大量试验表明，30% 或更多的冠心病所引起的 SCD 患者是以 SCD 作为首次临床事件。多于 33% 的人其临床特征显示是发生 SCD 的低危人群（图 78-3）。在此病因类型中，只有小部分发生 SCD 事件的患者有心肌梗死后室性心律失常、低射血分数、心脏功能降低等发生 SCD 的高危因素。作为一个人群问题，能对 SCD 产生重大影响的是获得一个比

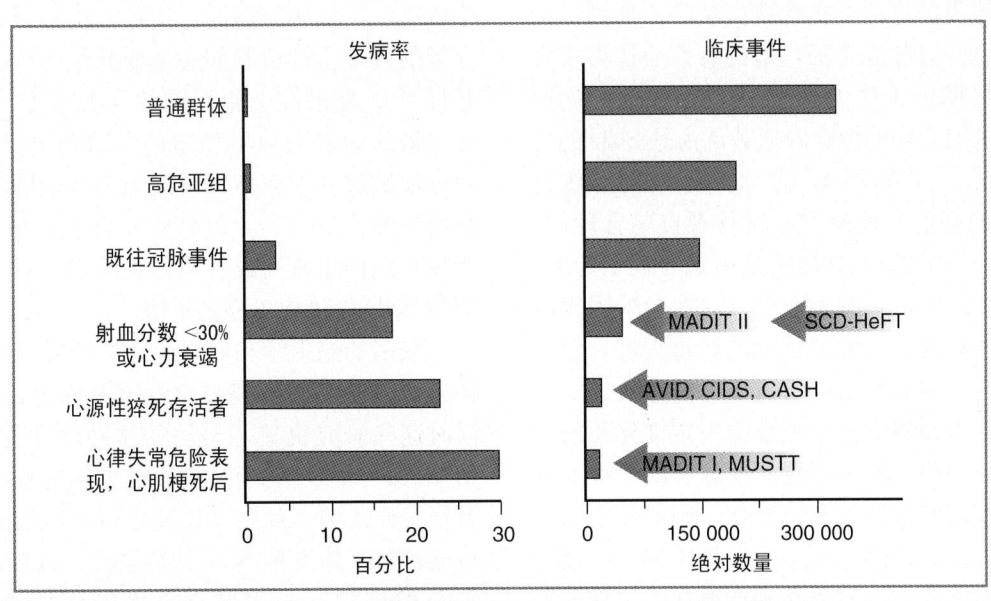

图 78-2 人群亚组心源性猝死发生率和各亚组总体发病人数　根据亚组分析，随着各亚组发病率增加，其相应的心源性猝死发生总体数量减少。这与植入式心律转复除颤器临床试验结果对人群的影响有关。（引自 Myerburg RJ, Interian A Jr, Mitrani RM, et al: Frequency of sudden cardiac death and profiles of risk. Am J Cardiol 80: 10F-19F, 1997.）

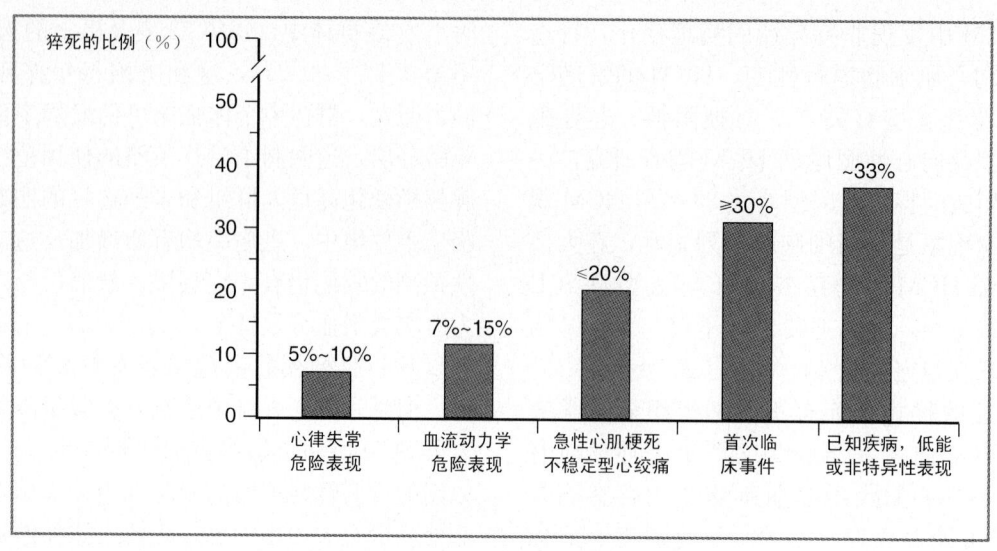

图 78-3　心源性猝死患者的临床情况　有效的预测高危罹患心源性猝死实际很困难，因为几乎近三分之二的心源性猝死患者是以猝死作为首次临床表现，或者是具有临床已知疾病而又没有较强的危险性预测指标的患者。少于25%的罹患者有基于心律失常或血流动力学指标的高危表现。而只有更少部分患者具有发生 SCD 的高危因素。（引自 Myerburg RJ：Sudden cardiac death：Exploring the limits of knowledge. J Cardiovasc Electrophysiol 12：369-381，2001.）

通过现有发病率来预测个体危险性更好的策略。在更广泛的亚组人群中，用这种策略来预测 SCD 有更高的准确性。

五、冠心病 SCD 的一般和特异性危险预测因子

冠心病 SCD 的病变进展包括一系列病理生理的级联变化，经历不同的时间域（表 78-4），包括冠状动脉病变的起始及逐步的进展，血管病变从静止期到活动期转变，发生急性冠脉综合征，最终急性心律失常发作的过程。在早期由于认为 SCD 主要是由冠心病所致，所以传统的冠心病的危险因素被认为是 SCD 的主要危险预测指标[24]（图 78-4，表 78-2）。当然从统计学及公众健康调查的方面来看，这种观点是合理的，因为众多比例和数量的 SCD 确实是由冠心病引起的。但这种观点存在一定的局限性，因为这些危险因素虽然能够预测病变的进展，确定危险的严重程度，但这些对是否进行抗心律失常治疗没有多少参考价值，而且它们也不能作为预测个体发生心律失常性猝死的特异性指标。另外一些用来检查冠状动脉解剖学病变的方法则显示了较高的敏感性和特异性。例如使用电子束 CT 进行解剖病变扫描，已经被推荐作为一种冠心病大规模普查的方法[25]。这项技术能够在一定程度上准确检验出冠状动脉结构的改变，然而结构上的异常并不等同于病变的严重程度及易患病程度，也不是心律失常危险的特异性指标，因此它的价值仍然有限。

如今临床指标已经作为一种预测 SCD 的指标，它主要是验证心肌或者血管的病变程度（表 78-2），虽然准确性较高，但它不能区别心律失常性猝死和其他原因导致的猝死，因此仍是非特异性的。

为了更好地了解心律失常的危险因素，未来以下两种方法可能很有前途。一个是即时危险预测指标，用来鉴别那些短期内存在发生致死性心律失常危险的个体[6,23,26-29]（表 78-2）。这种方法包括自主神经系统介导的病理生理机制如心率变异性[22,30]、压力反射敏感性[31]、复极改变指标例如 T 波交替[32,33]和炎症指标（被认为是斑块不稳定的危险预测指标）。虽然针对斑块破裂的炎症指标可能为急性冠脉综合征提供更高的预测价值[36,37]，但另外一个方法即个体危险预测指标，例如家族性或者遗传性因素，对个体而言，可能为 SCD 提供更可靠的价值。

众多的病理学和病理生理学研究显示冠状动脉粥样斑块侵蚀或者破裂与急性冠脉综合征存在相关性，同时这些研究也显示斑块的这种改变与 SCD 关系密切[14,15]。如果一种有效的途径如果能够在急性冠脉综合征发作之前，预测个体发生斑块破裂的危险性，它也能预测个体发生 SCD 的危险性。最近针对胆固醇水平及炎症指标与冠脉事件可能相关的男性[18]及女性[19]的回顾性研究表明两者都是独立的预测指标，而且两者联合具有最强的预测价值。但在这些调查中，

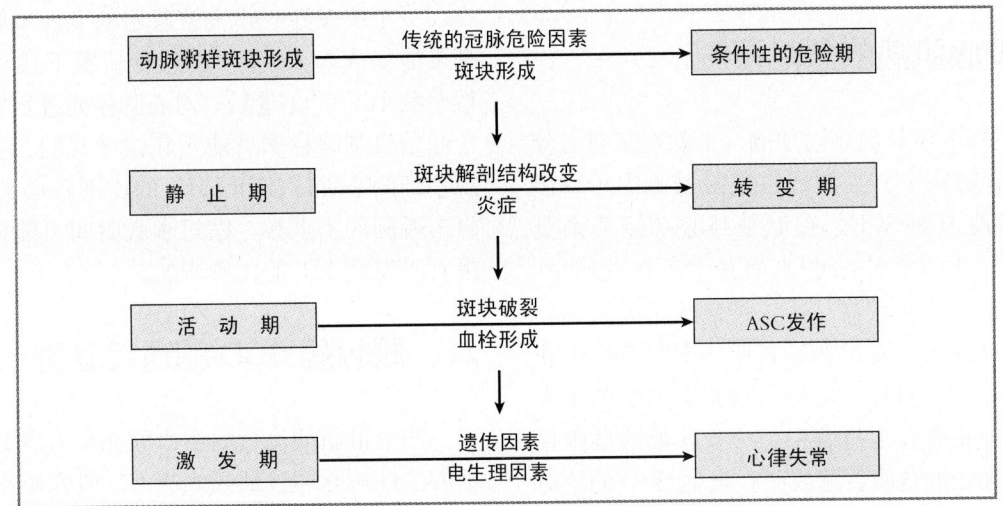

图 78-4 冠心病 SCD 从传统的冠脉危险因素到心律失常产生的过程 这一过程包括 4 步逐步进展的过程：(1) 初期病变及进展，(2) 活动期，(3) 急性冠脉综合征，(4) 致死性心律失常，每一步都有多种危险因素参与其中，包括个人遗传背景。(引自 Myerburg RJ: Scientific gaps in the prediction and prevention of sudden cardiac death. J Cardiovasc Eletrophysiol 13：709-723，2002.)

在其胆固醇及炎症指标浓度水平处于最低百分点而其危险程度却相对增加的个体中，与胆固醇指标相比，炎症指标的绝对预测价值是否更优仍不甚清楚。假如炎症指标优于胆固醇指标，则可能出现一种新的更好的预测指标。最近的研究显示复杂斑块可能是多样的，心梗后病变普遍存在斑块破裂（而不是斑块特异的危险性）及再发率高的特点[40]。这些研究支持炎症易感性的观点。其他直接的和间接的与炎症过程斑块不稳定相关的危险指标也支持这种危险预测理论[41]。

SCD 的家族聚集性是一种不同的存在潜在风险的危险预测指标。在巴黎进行的针对 SCD 危险因素的前瞻性研究[42]数据表明有父母猝死病史的个体发生冠脉事件猝死的可能性比对照组增加两倍，但 SCD 家族史不会增加非猝死性心梗的危险性。一个在华盛顿特区 King 郡进行的对心脏骤停幸存者的回顾性研究得出相似的观点[43]。这种家族群聚现象可能与环境背景或遗传因素有关。King 郡的研究未能区别两者的作用（环境背景或遗传因素）。而来自巴黎的前瞻性研究则认为是遗传因素占主导地位，因为当父母都存在 SCD 家族史时，危险性将增加。

表 78-2 心律失常性猝死的危险因素*

指标	举例	目的	敏感性
ASHD 危险因素	Framingham 危险指数	预测疾病进展	很低
影像学检查	电子束 CT	验证冠心病	很低
临床指标	EF；动态血管造影；EPS；AM/EPS＋EF	检验病变程度 验证心律失常指标 定义高危人群	多变的；病变程度；特异性低 普查特异性低，而特殊人群特异性高 对个体预测价值不甚清楚
即时危险预测指标	T 波电交替；QT 离散度；病理生理机制（如 HRV、BRS）；炎症指标	危险心电图表现 自主神经调节质量 预示斑块不稳定	不清楚，可能很高
个体危险预测指标	家族/遗传背景	在症状发生前预测 SCD 发生	高的预测价值 不太确定；可能有用（？）

*传统的冠脉危险因素及解剖学检查有一定的预测价值，但敏感性很低，且对预测心律失常性猝死无特异性。即时危险预测指标及个体危险预测指标则有希望预测心源性猝死。

AM，动态检测；ASHD，动脉粥样硬化性心脏病；HRV，心率变异性；BRS，压力反射敏感度；EF，射血分数；EPS，电生理检查；SCD，心源性猝死。

(引自 Myerburg RJ：Sudden cardiac death：Exploring the limits of our knowledge. J Cardiovasc Electrophysiol 12：369-381，2001.)

六、扩张型心肌病的危险预测

心肌病患者中 SCD 更难以预测。虽然左室射血分数是 DCM 患者的一个有力的死亡危险预测因子,但是它不能明确地预测 SCD。它似乎与心功能关系更大[44-45]。例如,心功能 I 级的 DCM 患者死亡危险小,但猝死发生的概率相对较高。这一类包括了大量的相对低危患者,这使我们对患者是否能从干预治疗中获益以及干预治疗效果对死亡危险的预测能力受到了限制。而在心功能Ⅲ和Ⅳ级患者中,尽管猝死的危险性相对较低,但死亡的危险普遍较高,发生 SCD 的绝对值也较高[45]。而且,在这一类猝死者中,许多具有继发于血流动力学状态和对电除颤抵触的不能电击的节律和某些可电击的节律,这可能也限制了这类患者从 ICD 获益[46]。

除冠心病以外,对心脏性猝死的这类病因来说,从早期到进展期,以及疾病的全程其危险预测因子是不一致的。这个限制的重要性在于:相对低危亚组中 SCD 的绝对值是高的,但统计学上并未证明积极干预则有好处。未来的研究必须集中在较大的低危人群中进行危险评估[47]。

七、心脏停搏的电生理机制

心脏停搏导致 SCD 最常见的电生理机制是室性快速性心律失常(VT)、室颤(VF)或无脉室速或室颤,但主要的非快速性心律失常事件也很常见,似乎已经超过了以前估计的 20%~30%[1]。后者包括无脉性电活动(PEA)、心脏停搏及可引起脑和其他器官灌注不足的严重心动过缓。快速性心律失常和其他(不能电击的)心律失常之间的机制不同,这一点在临床和流行病学十分重要。快速性心律失常的发生率影响着抗心动过速治疗的评价,例如对植入式心脏复律除颤器(ICD)和自动体外除颤器(AED)的评价。另外,由于 ICD、AED 等的应用使快速性心律失常事件得到有效治疗,患者存活率增加,这一点是鼓舞人心的。

因为 VT/VF 和非快速性心律失常机制之间可发生转变,所以要确定初始节律是困难的,认识到这一点很重要。这可能把基本的电生理机制与结局的关联相混淆。例如,VT 开始和恶化到心脏停搏或无脉性电活动的时间可能很短,限制了干预的可能益处。相反,一个缓慢性心律失常起始的事件不管有没有治疗都可能变成 VT/VF,在这种情况下成功除颤的概率似乎减小了[48]。最后,对心脏停搏进行紧急救护的关于起始机制的数据可能正在误导我们。在初始接触时观察到的心脏停搏和 PEA 的比例较高[49]可能反映了目击者延误了求救,缩短求救时间可能使在初始接触患者时发现 VT 的比例增加。

八、冠心病 SCD 的遗传基础

两个最新的流行病学研究显示,SCD 只发生在个别的急性冠脉综合征病人身上。研究还发现 SCD 存在家族聚集性:如果急性冠脉综合征患者的父母一方有 SCD 家族史,那么,该患者以 SCD 为首发症状的几率就要增加,如果双亲都有 SCD 家族史,首发症状是 SCD 的几率更高。家族聚集性可能是遗传或环境因素造成,或者兼而有之[42]。针对一些心律失常疾病的基因学研究发现,一些基因的变异在生理状况下并不产生什么异常,但发生心肌缺血或其他一过性病理改变时,就可能引起功能改变(表 78-3)。这方面的证据也越来越多[50]。譬如,前不久的一项研究发现,编码心肌钠离子通道的 SCN5A 发生突变(Y1102)后,只有在使用抗心律失常药物时才会增加发生心律失常的危险。美国非洲裔很大部分患者存在这个变异(13.2%;等位基因频率=6.8%),因此发现这部分有发生 SCD 潜在危险的人群有重要的临床意义。然而,目前关于基因突变对 SCD 的影响的研究才刚刚起步,将来或许能促进 SCD 的预测和预防工作的进步。

理论上,如果编码离子通道的 DNA 发生突变的部分并不表达,在病理情况也可能会产生异常表型。这与急性冠脉综合征的病理情况相吻合。导致这些异常表达的机制可能有:病理状态下基因突变或多态性的效应会扩大;只在病理状态下表达的沉默遗传变异如 Y1102(反应性表型表达,表 78-4);发生随机突变[51];离子通道功能在正常范围内发生改变而诱导 DNA 改变,DNA 改变又反馈调节离子通道功能。关于最后一个机制,最近有研究发现心肌细胞核内的某些酶系在缺血损伤时会表达[52],复制 DNA,这样,心肌细胞就可能再生[53]。这促使我们对 DNA 损伤、心肌细胞的再生和疾病之间的关系进行探索。

表 78-3 可能与获得性心律失常相关的基因*

染色体	LQT (R-W)	LQT (J, L-N)	HCM	RVD	Brugada
1			cTnT	RyR2	
2				?	
3	SCN5A		MELC	?	SCN5A
4	?				
7	HERG		?		
10				?	
11	KvLQT1	KvLQT1	MyPBC		
12			MRLC		
14			β-MHC	?	
15			α-TM		
17					Plakoglobin [Recessive]
19	SCN1B {?}	SCN1B {?}	cTnI		
21	minK, MiRP	minK, MiRP1			

*与长 QT 综合征的 Romano-Ward 表型（LQT [R-W]）和 Jervell、Lange-Nielsen 表型（LQT [J, L-N]），肥厚型心肌病（HCM），右室发育不良（RVD）及 Brugada 综合征相关的突变染色体位点和基因。基因位点和疾病的关系如图所示。理论上，这些位点的大多数基因突变和多态性与正常状态时的表型改变无关，却可能与诱导性电活动异常有关。（引自 Myerburg RJ: Scientific gaps in the prediction and prevention of sudden cardiac death. J Cardiovasc Electrophysiol 13: 709-723, 2002.）

表 78-4 基因产物间的相互作用，基因/环境间的相互作用，及心源性猝死的危险因素

几种基因产物间的相互作用	
直接调节物	
α-亚基	β-亚基
KvLQT1 {第 11 对染色体}	minK {第 21 对染色体}
HERG {第 7 对染色体}	MiRP1 {第 21 对染色体}
SCN5A {第 3 对染色体}	SCN1B {第 19 对染色体} [?]
相关调节物	
参与复极的基因产物	钙调节
KvLQT1，minK	RyR2 {第 1 对染色体}
HERG，MiRP1	CASQ2 {第 1 对染色体}
SCN5A，SCN1B	
共同作用	
致心律失常产物	自主神经作用
I_K^+，I_{Na}^+，I_{Ca}^+ 变异	$β_1$-AR 功能多态性
{第 11，7，3，1 对染色体}	{第 10 对染色体}
基因产物/非基因间的相互作用	
分子结构	功能性诱发因素
遗传性离子通道变异	β肾上腺素作用（非基因）
反应性多态性	一过性病理状态
获得性（诱发性）DNA 改变	药物/代谢因素

九、SCD 综合系统分析与遗传流行病学

冠心病流行病学中的一个主要转变开始于对级联瀑布中的多因素表达的新认识，该级联瀑布包括冠状动脉粥样硬化形成、急性冠脉综合征的出现以及 SCD 的触发（图 78-5）。已经证实的冠脉粥样硬化形成[54,55]、斑块活动[56]和血栓形成瀑布[57,58]均受遗传因素控制的理论，加上离子通道的遗传学理论，对个体危险度和导致的病理生理状态有重要影响。对于发生 SCD 的特异危险度，现有的最好的遗传指导理论存在于分子与遗传电生理领域。与遗传学联系最少的是以动脉粥样硬化斑块形成为中心的理论，该理论中动脉粥样硬化斑块形成仍很大程度上取决于传统的危险因素，如糖尿病、高血压、吸烟、高脂血症。这些危险因素的遗传标记的研究正在展开[60,61]，但在病变发生的基础理论方面仍有问题。遗传学对病变进展、活动期的转变、血栓形成瀑布激活等方面的作用正在快速进展。

当用扩展的流行病学方法分析这些资料时，会产生一种概念的转变，就是从连续的病理生理瀑布（图 78-5）到一种复杂系统分析模型的转变[62,63]。这种对

我们可以用基因的一些特征来对从发生冠脉粥样硬化到心源性猝死的临床及流行病学的一系列反应进行预测。基因变异影响电生理功能，从而在急性综合征发生心源性猝死和致命性心律失常的机制中起着复杂作用。某些基因变异会影响离子通道结构和功能的遗传学特点，再加上钙离子调节因素的异常和致心律失常因素的共同作用，以及机体对各种刺激产生的肾上腺素能反应存在个体差异，都会导致 SCD。如果能将离子通道结构和功能的直接调节作用、致心律失常的其他因素和能用遗传学资料预测的其他活动这三者相互作用联合分析，对缺血早期个体发生心律失常的危险性大小的预测会更加准确。某些基因的变异（包括多态性）只在病理状态下表达，及获得性基因改变对缺血早期个体发生心律失常的危险性大小的预测也有一定作用。如是，遗传因素和非遗传因素结合了起来。包括已知的参与调控几条分子过程的基因的染色体如图所示（详见文中细节）。（引自 Myerburg RJ: Scientific gaps in the prediction and prevention of sudden cardiac death. J Cardiovasc Electrophysiol 13: 709-723, 2002.）

新方法的需要源于传统的危险因素从广大普通群体中识别高 SCD 危险个体（或其他冠心病表现）的根本有限性。大部分 SCD 发生在那些没有容易识别的心血管死亡率或总死亡率高的绝对危险的个体（图 78-3），并且这些危险是多因素的（图 78-5），必须找到预测单个病人发生冠心病特别是 SCD 概率的更精确的指标。这就是多风险相互作用的数理分析或综合系统分析。

经过对照干预试验，由单种标记识别的过多的相对危险度和针对特定危险因素的某种干预措施的相对收益在经过挑选的病人组留下深刻印象，但对个体的绝对危险度的减少只提供了有限的预测力。对照组来

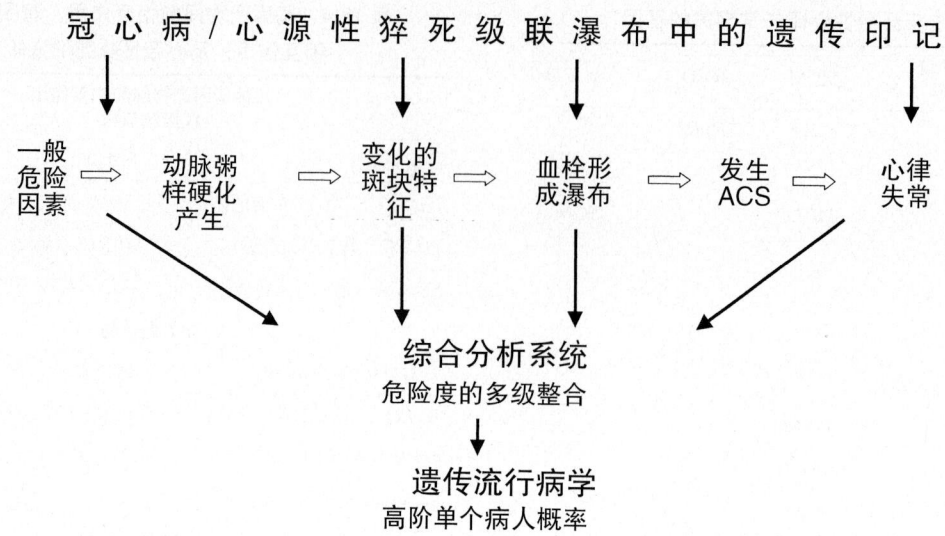

图78-5 冠心病/心源性猝死级联瀑布中的遗传印记 已经证实基因对瀑布从动脉粥样硬化形成的一般危险因素到心律失常导致 SCD 中的多个环节的影响。根据基因分析图，我们已经能识别发生动脉粥样硬化形成，斑块进展，血栓瀑布以及心律失常发生的个体危险度。通过综合分析的方法，多级整合这些个体特征给在遗传流行病学领域中引出高阶单个病人 SCD 概率以希望。通过整合瀑布每步中的危险度，分析图对个体危险度有更高的特异性（详见文中描述）。（引自 Myerburg RJ: Scientific gaps in the prediction and prevention of suddencardiac death. J Cardiovasc Electrophysiol 13：709-723，2002.）

自于大多数的一级预防临床试验，比如 HMG CoA 还原酶降低胆固醇[64]和阿司匹林的预防使用[65]，对这个问题有启发性。在一级预防试验中，治疗组阿司匹林或抑制素（statin）与对照组比较分析证实治疗个体的绝对死亡危险降低率是有限的。这些试验的结果更强调组的效果（相对危险降低率）而不是个体效应（绝对收益）[23,64,66]。在3个抑制素的一级预防试验中[63]，5年死亡率从 3.7% 降到 2.8%，即降低 0.9%。心血管死亡率 5 年降低 0.5%。这些数字来源于一个事实就是安慰剂组绝对死亡危险度相对低（5 年 3.7% 即每年 0.72%），纵然相对来看收益是较高的。然而，由于这些低危险人群分子分母绝对数量较大，用更高阶的预测来得出个体危险，其潜在的收益是巨大的。然而要做到这一点，流行病学的任务就更加艰巨。

想像一下这一综合系统的前景，包括庞大的生物信息，困难与机遇都很明显。遗传、环境以及获得性病理生理状态均在其中发挥作用。以遗传学为基础的危险分析的价值在于能先于临床事件提供危险性的预测。由于实际干预需要足够的进展时间，获得性特征变得更难识别。

这个综合系统组成的轮廓即演变的遗传流行病学模型概括在图78-5中。一般的必要条件包括识别临床表达瀑布多个步骤中存在的突变或多态现象，这些数据综合起来提供的信息可以加强危险度的预测效力。

综合系统列表中的第一条是研究基因之间的相互作用，这可能是直接相关的、功能相关的，或结合有远隔的相关的功能（基因-基因作用）。这种直接关系的例子如控制离子通道结构的基因（如 KvLQT1、HERG、SCN5A）和那些控制它们相关调节多肽的基因（如 minK、MiRP1，SCN1B）[47,67,70]（表 78-4）。一个间接的但与多基因产物间相互作用相关的例子可以想像为离子通道基因变异的表达与调节控制钙调控的基因之间的相互作用。已知后者（如 RyR2 或 CASQ2）的变异与心律失常有关[70-72]。另外，KvLQT1/minK 可能与 RyR2 或 CASQ2 的变异体作用，导致复极化的控制与钙调控耦联，这种关系被认为是心律失常发生的一种机制。最后，一种遗传控制的对 β 肾上腺素受体功能的影响[73,74]与钙离子通道复合体的作用[75]，就是一种远隔的但整合的基因-基因关系的例子。

这个综合系统中的另一个控制离子通道功能的要素是基因影响与非基因因素间的相互作用（基因-非基因相互作用或基因-环境相互作用）。这包括遗传通道病与非基因的 β 肾上腺素能控制，或良性多态现象与短暂的病理生理调节[47]。最具挑战性的是这个病理生理级联瀑布构想自身贯穿了从动脉粥样硬化形成到斑块性质到血栓形成瀑布再到特异的心律失常发作的整个过程。在级联瀑布的每一层里含有进展的遗传影响方面的信息群，它们增加或降低危险度。这些性质使该瀑布进展到一个综合系统。以这样一个系统对多基因影响进行同步的交互式分析，而不是一个由独立变量组成的序列。这时综合系统分析可以将遗传学整合到流行病学中，提供基于个体概率分布对危险预测的多级放大。图78-5勾勒出了连串的遗传印记作用于冠心病/SCD瀑布的概念。从动脉粥样硬化形成危险度转化到活动斑块危险度，随后继之血栓形成瀑布的遗传特征，到最后触发心律失常，瀑布每一元素的遗传影响汇成一个各种特征的总体，这个总体决定了个体的概率。

高阶的单个病人概率（1/10危险度 vs 1/1000危险度）来自于多个病理生理学特征的整合，它将补充SCD瀑布中个体危险度表达的效力（见图78-5底部）。唯一的目标是分析SCD瀑布的多个环节中个体的危险度，所产生概率的特征是有足够大的效力用于远早于临床事件的预防策略中。遗传学作用的分析要达到这个目标所需的水平仍在推测。尽管如此，但要达到这个目标只有通过新的流行病学模型。这要求投入大量专业人员以及生物信息领域的新的科学团队，他们才具有这样的计算处理能力[47,63]。

（姜 建 译）

参 考 文 献

1. Myerburg RJ, Castellanos A: Cardiac arrest and sudden cardiac death. In Braunwald E (ed): Heart Disease: A Textbook of Cardiovascular Medicine, 6th ed. Philadelphia, WB Saunders, 2001, pp 890–931.
2. American Heart Association: 2001 Heart and Stroke Statistical Update. Dallas, American Heart Association, 2000.
3. Cobb LA, Fahrenbruch CE, Olsufka M, Copass MK: Changing incidence of out-of-hospital ventricular fibrillation, 1980-2000. JAMA 288:3008–3013, 2002.
4. Zheng ZJ, Croft JB, Giles WH, Mensah GA: Sudden cardiac death in the United States, 1989 to 1998. Circulation 104:2158–2163, 2001.
5. Every NR, Parsons L, Hlatsky MA, et al: Use and accuracy of state death certificates for clarification of sudden deaths in high-risk populations. Am Heart J 134:1129–1132, 1997.
6. Myerburg RJ: Sudden cardiac death: Exploring the limits of our knowledge. J Cardiovasc Electrophysiol 12:369–381, 2001.
7. Braunwald E: Cardiovascular medicine at the turn of the millennium: Triumphs, concerns, and opportunities. N Engl J Med 337:1360–1369, 1997.
8. Myerburg RJ, Mitrani R, Interian A Jr, Castellanos A: Identification of risk of cardiac arrest and sudden cardiac death in athletes. In Estes NA, Salem DN, Estes NAM III (eds): Sudden Cardiac Death in the Athlete. Armonk, NY, Futura Publishing, 1998, pp 25–50.
9. Pauschinger M, Bowles NE, Fuentes-Garcia FJ, et al: Detection of adenoviral genome in the myocardium of adult patients with idiopathic left ventricular dysfunction. Circulation 99:1348–1354, 1999.
10. Splawski I, Timothy KW, Tateyama M, et al: Variant of SCN5A sodium channel implicated in risk of cardiac arrhythmia. Science 297:1333–1336, 2002.
11. Sesti F, Abbott GW, Wei J, et al: A common polymorphism associated with antibiotic-induced cardiac arrhythmia. Proc Natl Acad Sci U S A 97:10613–10618, 2000.
12. Napolitano C, Schwartz PJ, Brown AM, et al: Evidence for a cardiac ion channel mutation underlying drug-induced QT prolongation and life-threatening arrhythmias. J Cardiovasc Electrophysiol 11:691–696, 2000.
13. Baroldi G, Falzi A, Mariani F, Baroldi LA: Morphology, frequency, and significance of intramural arterial lesions in sudden coronary death. G Ital Cardiol 10:644–656, 1980.
14. Davies MJ: Anatomic features in victims of sudden coronary death: Coronary artery pathology. Circulation 85(Suppl 1):I19–I24, 1992.
15. Taylor AJ, Burke AP, O'Malley PG, et al: A comparison of the Framingham risk index, coronary artery calcification, and culprit plaque morphology in sudden cardiac death. Circulation 101:1243–1248, 2000.
16. Mehta D, Curwin J, Gomes A, Fuster V: Sudden death in coronary artery disease: Acute ischemia versus myocardial substrate. Circulation 96:3215–3223, 1997.
17. Warnes CA, Roberts WC: Sudden coronary death: Relation of amount and distribution of coronary narrowing at necropsy to previous symptoms of myocardial ischemia, left ventricular scarring, and heart weight. Am J Cardiol 54:65–73, 1984.
18. Liberthson RR, Nagel EL, Hirschman JC, et al: Pathophysiologic observations in prehospital ventricular fibrillation and sudden cardiac death. Circulation 49:790–798, 1974.
19. Cooper RS, Simmons BE, Castaner A, et al: Left ventricular hypertrophy is associated with worse survival independent of ventricular function and number of coronary arteries severely narrowed. Am J Cardiol 65:441–445, 1990.
20. Marian AJ, Roberts R: Molecular genetic basis of hypertrophic cardiomyopathy: Genetic markers for sudden cardiac death. J Cardiovasc Electrophysiol 9:88–99, 1998.
21. Myerburg RJ, Kessler KM, Castellanos A: Sudden cardiac death: Structure, function, and time-dependence of risk. Circulation 85(Suppl I):I2–I10, 1992.
22. Huikuri HV, Castellanos A, Myerburg RJ: Sudden death due to cardiac arrhythmias. N Engl J Med 345:1473–1482, 2001.
23. Myerburg RJ, Mitrani R, Interian A Jr, Castellanos A: Interpretation of outcomes of antiarrhythmic clinical trials: Design features and population impact. Circulation 97:1514–1521, 1998.
24. Wilson PW, D'Agostino RB, Levy D, et al: Prediction of coronary heart disease using risk factor categories. Circulation 97:1837–1847, 1998.
25. O'Rourke RA, Brundage BH, Froelicher VF, et al: American College of Cardiology/American Heart Association Expert Consensus Document on electron-beam computed tomography for the diagnosis and prognosis of coronary artery disease. J Am Coll Cardiol 36:326–340, 2000.
26. Moss AJ, Hall WJ, Cannom DS, et al: Improved survival with an implanted defibrillator in patients with coronary disease at high risk for ventricular arrhythmia: Multicenter Automatic Defibrillator Implantation Trial Investigators. N Engl J Med 335:1933–1940, 1996.
27. A comparison of antiarrhythmic-drug therapy with implantable defibrillators in patients resuscitated from near-fatal ventricular arrhythmias: The Antiarrhythmics versus Implantable Defibrillators (AVID) Investigators. N Engl J Med 337:1576–1583, 1997.
28. Connolly SJ, Gent M, Roberts RS, et al: Canadian implantable defibrillator study (CIDS): A randomized trial of the implantable cardioverter defibrillator against amiodarone. Circulation 101:1297–1302, 2000.
29. Buxton AE, Lee KL, Fisher JD, et al: A randomized study of the prevention of sudden death in patients with coronary artery disease: Multicenter Unsustained Tachycardia Trial Investigators. N Engl J Med 341:1882–1890, 1999.
30. Hartikainen JE, Malik M, Staunton A, et al: Distinction between arrhythmic and nonarrhythmic death after acute myocardial infarction based on heart rate variability, signal-averaged electrocardiogram, ventricular arrhythmias and left ventricular ejection fraction. J Am Coll Cardiol 28:296–304, 1996.
31. La Rovere MT, Bigger JT Jr, Marcus FI, et al: Baroreflex sensitivity and heart-rate variability in prediction of total cardiac mortality after myocardial infarction: ATRAMI (Autonomic Tone and Reflexes After Myocardial Infarction) Investigators. Lancet 351:478–484, 1998.
32. Rosenbaum D, Albrecht P, Cohen RJ: Predicting sudden cardiac

death from T wave alternans of the surface electrocardiogram: promise and pitfalls. J Cardiovasc Electrophysiol 7:1095–1111, 1996.
33. Klingenheben T, Zabel M, D'Agostino RB, et al: Predictive value of T-wave alternans for arrhythmic events in patients with congestive heart failure. Lancet 356:651–652, 2000.
34. Ross R: Atherosclerosis: An inflammatory disease? N Engl J Med 340:115–126, 1999.
35. Ridker PM, Glynn RJ, Hennekens CH: C-reactive protein adds to the predictive value of total and HDL cholesterol in determining risk of first myocardial infarction. Circulation 97:2007–2011, 1998.
36. Koenig W, Sund M, Frohlich M, et al: C-Reactive protein, a sensitive marker of inflammation, predicts future risk of coronary heart disease in initially healthy middle-aged men: Results from the MONICA (Monitoring Trends and Determinants in Cardiovascular Disease) Augsburg Cohort Study, 1984 to 1992. Circulation 99:237–242, 1999.
37. Ridker PM, Rifai N, Clearfield M, et al: Air Force/Texas Coronary Atherosclerosis Prevention Study Investigators: Measurement of C-reactive protein for the targeting of statin therapy in the primary prevention of acute coronary events. N Engl J Med 344:1959–1965, 2001.
38. Ridker PM, Cushman M, Stampfer MJ, et al: Inflammation, aspirin, and the risk of cardiovascular disease in apparently healthy men. N Engl J Med 336:973–979, 1997.
39. Ridker PM, Hennekens CH, Buring JE, Rifai N: C-reactive protein and other markers of inflammation in the prediction of cardiovascular disease in women. N Engl J Med 342:836–843, 2000.
40. Goldstein JA, Demetriou D, Grines CL, et al: Multiple complex coronary plaques in patients with acute myocardial infarction. N Engl J Med 343:915–922, 2000.
41. Kuller LH, Tracy RP, Shaten J, Meilahn EN: Reaction of C-reactive protein and coronary heart disease in the MRFIT nested case-control study: Multiple Risk Factor Intervention Trial. Am J Epidemiol 144:537–547, 1996.
42. Friedlander Y, Siscovick DS, Weinmann S, et al: Family history as a risk factor for primary cardiac arrest. Circulation 97:155–160, 1998.
43. Jouven X, Desnos M, Guerot C, Ducimetiere P: Predicting sudden death in the population: The Paris Prospective Study I. Circulation 99:1978–1983, 1999.
44. Kjekshus J: Arrhythmias and mortality in congestive heart failure. Am J Cardiol 65:42I–48I, 1990.
45. Effect of metoprolol CR/XL in chronic heart failure: Metoprolol CR/XL Randomised Intervention Trial in Congestive Heart Failure (MERIT-HF). Lancet 353:2001–2007, 1999.
46. Pires LA, Hull ML, Nino CL, et al: Sudden death in recipients of transvenous implantable cardioverter defibrillator systems: Terminal events, predictors, and potential mechanisms. J Cardiovasc Electrophysiol 10:1049–1056, 1999.
47. Myerburg RJ: Scientific gaps in the prediction and prevention of sudden cardiac death. J Cardiovasc Electrophysiol 13:709–723, 2002.
48. Kudenchuk PJ, Cobb LA, Copass MK, et al: Amiodarone for resuscitation after out-of-hospital cardiac arrest due to ventricular fibrillation. N Engl J Med 341:871–878, 1999.
49. Myerburg RJ, Fenster J, Velez M, et al: Impact of community-wide police car deployment of automated external defibrillators on survival from out-of-hospital cardiac arrest. Circulation 106:1058–1064, 2002.
50. Spooner PM, Albert C, Benjamin EJ, et al: Sudden cardiac death, genes, and arrhythmogenesis: Consideration of new population and mechanistic approaches from a National Heart, Lung, and Blood Institute Workshop, Part I. Circulation 103:2361–2364, 2001.
51. Schwartz PJ, Priori SG, Dumaine R, et al: A molecular link between the sudden infant death syndrome and the long-QT syndrome. N Engl J Med 343:262–267, 2000.
52. Kozlovskis PL, Smets MJ, Strauss WL, Myerburg RJ: DNA synthesis in adult feline ventricular myocytes: Comparison of hypoxic and normoxic states. Circ Res 78:289–301, 1996.
53. Beltrami AP, Urbanek K, Kajstura J, et al: Evidence that human cardiac myocytes divide after myocardial infarction. N Engl J Med 344:1750–1757, 2001.
54. Marenberg MD, Risch N, Berkman LF, et al: Genetic susceptibility to death from coronary heart disease in a study of twins. N Engl J Med 330:1041–1046, 1994.
55. Smithies O, Maeda N: Gene targeting approaches to complex genetic diseases: Atherosclerosis and essential hypertension. Proc Natl Acad Sci U S A 92:5266–5272, 1995.
56. Faber BC, Cleutjens KB, Niessen RL, et al: Identification of genes potentially involved in rupture of human atherosclerotic plaques. Circ Res 89:547–554, 2001.
57. Weiss EJ, Bray PF, Tayback M, et al: A polymorphism of a platelet glycoprotein receptor as an inherited risk factor for coronary thrombosis. N Engl J Med 334:1090–1094, 1996.
58. Anderson JL, King GJ, Bair BS, et al: Associations between a polymorphism in the gene encoding glycoprotein IIIa and myocardial infarction or coronary artery disease. J Am Coll Cardiol 33:727–733, 1999.
59. Topol EJ, McCarthy J, Gabriel S, et al: Single nucleotide polymorphisms in multiple novel thrombospondin genes may be associated with familial premature myocardial infarction. Circulation 104:2641–2644, 2001.
60. Arya R, Duggirala R, Almasy L, et al: Linkage of high-density lipoprotein-cholesterol concentrations to a locus on chromosome 9p in Mexican Americans. Nat Genet 30:102–105, 2002.
61. Jormsjo S, Whatling C, Walter DH, et al: Allele-specific regulation of matrix metalloproteinase-7 promoter activity is associated with coronary artery luminal dimensions among hypercholesterolemic patients. Arterioscler Thromb Vasc Biol 21:1834–1839, 2001.
62. Drew PJ, Ilstrup DM, Kerin MJ, Monson JR: Prognostic factors: Guidelines for investigation design and state of the art analytical methods. Surg Oncol 7:71–76, 1998.
63. Bonow R, Clark EB, Curfman GD, et al: Task Force on Strategic Research Direction: Clinical Science Subgroup key science topics report. Circulation 106:e162–e166, 2002.
64. Hebert PR, Gaziano JM, Chan KS, Hennekens CH: Cholesterol lowering with statin drugs, risk of stroke, and total mortality: An overview of randomized trials. JAMA 278:313–321, 1997.
65. Final report on the aspirin component of the ongoing Physicians' Health Study: Steering Committee of the Physicians' Health Study Research Group. N Engl J Med 321:129–135, 1989.
66. Laupacis A, Sackett DL, Roberts RS: An assessment of clinically useful measures of the consequences of treatment. N Engl J Med 318:1728–1733, 1988.
67. Priori SG, Barhanin J, Hauer RN, et al: Genetic and molecular basis of cardiac arrhythmias: Impact on clinical management parts I and II. Circulation 99:518–528, 1999.
68. Roden DM, Spooner PM: Inherited long QT syndromes: A paradigm for understanding arrhythmogenesis. J Cardiovasc Electrophysiol 10:1664–1683, 1999.
69. Priori SG, Napolitano C, Grillo M: Concealed arrhythmogenic syndromes: The hidden substrate of idiopathic ventricular fibrillation? Cardiovasc Res 50:218–223, 2001.
70. Marks AR, Priori S, Memmi M, et al: Involvement of the cardiac ryanodine receptor/calcium release channel in catecholaminergic polymorphic ventricular tachycardia. J Cell Physiol 190:1–6, 2002.
71. Wu Y, MacMillan LB, McNeill RB, et al: CaM kinase augments cardiac L-type Ca^{2+} current: A cellular mechanism for long Q-T arrhythmias. Am J Physiol 276:H2168–H2178, 1999.
72. Lahat H, Pras E, Olender T, et al: A missense mutation in a highly conserved region of CASQ2 is associated with autosomal recessive catecholamine-induced polymorphic ventricular tachycardia in Bedouin families from Israel. Am J Hum Genet 69:1378–1384, 2001.
73. Sosunov EA, Gainullin RZ, Moise NS, et al: beta(1) and beta(2)-adrenergic receptor subtype effects in German shepherd dogs with inherited lethal ventricular arrhythmias. Cardiovasc Res 48:211–219, 2000.
74. Podlowski S, Wenzel K, Luther HP, et al: β₁-adrenoceptor gene variations: A role in idiopathic dilated cardiomyopathy? J Mol Med 78:87–93, 2000.
75. Pogwizd SM, Schlotthauer K, Li L, et al: Arrhythmogenesis and contractile dysfunction in heart failure: Roles of sodium-calcium exchange, inward rectifier potassium current, and residual beta-adrenergic responsiveness. Circ Res 88:1159–1167, 2001.

第十一部分
心电图的识别

第 79 章

超常传导、隐匿传导和传出阻滞的心电图表现

Michael J. Kilborn and Mark A. McGuire

本章目录
- 超常性 723
- 隐匿传导 725
- 传出阻滞 726

超常传导、隐匿传导和传出阻滞是与心脏传导有关的心电现象。这些术语是在有限的检查技术下提出的，因此前两个术语命名的不恰当是完全可以理解的。隐匿传导可以引起显性超常传导和传出阻滞。

一、超常性

(一) 超常激动

超常激动是一些可兴奋细胞的特性，并最早在神经系统中报道[1,2]。这一名称反映在前一动作电位结束前较小的电流就可引起下一个动作电位，因此第 2 个动作电位是由阈下刺激引起的。超常激动主要出现在动作电位 3 相的后部，持续约 90ms。超常期的长短不受心率或动作电位时限的影响[3]。超常期相当于心电图上 T 波的后半部和 T 波后短暂的等电位间期。超常激动可能的表现见图 79-1。这是一个房室阻滞和植入起搏器患者的心电图，许多起搏器刺激不能夺获，但是落入 T 波后半部的刺激就能夺获心室。同许多超常激动的病例一样，很难证实其机制是超常激动。间歇性夺获的另一种解释是电极植入的位置不稳定。

心房内的 Bachmann 束和浦肯野纤维均存在超常激动[3,4]，而对于希氏束和心室肌是否存在超常性还有争议[3-7]，房室结细胞未发现超常激动[5]。图 79-2 显示在动作电位后部激动浦肯野纤维所需的电流减小[3]，平均减少大约 17%[3]。Spear 和 Moore[3] 证实所需电流的减少是由于阻抗的短暂升高，引起跨膜电压变化的电流变小[3]，但膜阻抗短暂改变的确切机制尚不清楚。

(二) 超常传导

超常传导是一个不恰当的名称，尽管此术语通常表示：（1）传导抑制状态的短暂改善或（2）传导比预期的还好，但超常传导并不意味着传导更好。1924 年，Lewis 首次使用此术语[8]，报道了 1 例完全房室阻滞的病例，当 P 波落在自主心室波 T 波后半部时，就会出现房室传导的短暂改善，他认为其机制可能与超常激动有关，但未证实。

超常激动引起的超常传导称"真超常传导"，其他生理机制引起的超常传导称"伪超常传导"。实验标本证实，浦肯野纤维存在真超常传导，但在人体要得到证实很难。目前，争论的焦点集中在真超常传导是否是人的在体心脏的重要心电现象[5]。有一些心电图现象可能就是由下面描述的真超常传导或伪超常传导所引起的。

1. 高度房室阻滞中的间歇性房室传导

在大多数高度房室阻滞的病例中，只有当 P 波落入前面交界性或室性激动的 T 波后半部时，才会发生房室传导[5,8]，Moe 和同事们[5]认为可以用其他机制解释，如不应期回剥（见后文）[5]。图 79-3 是一名 38 岁男性患者做主动脉瓣置换术后的心电图记录，术后几天出现了高度房室阻滞伴心动周期约 1080ms 的交界性或

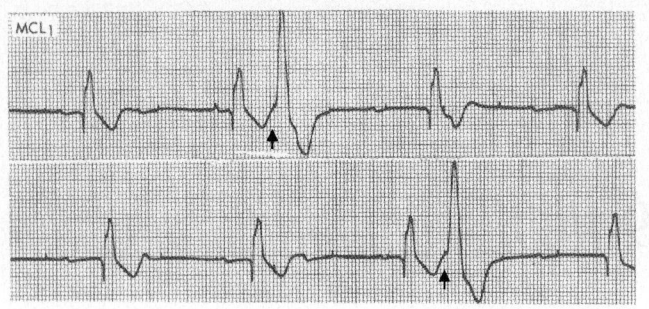

图 79-1　本图是一名房室阻滞植入心脏起搏器患者的心电图　大多数起搏信号失夺获，偶尔有些信号与 T 波后半部重叠（超常期）时能夺获心室（第 3 个和第 8 个 QRS 波，标记了箭头），这种夺获可能因超常激动所致，也可能存在其他机制。（引自 Marriott HJL：Practice Electrocardiography，7th ed. Baltimore，William & Wilkins，1983，358.）

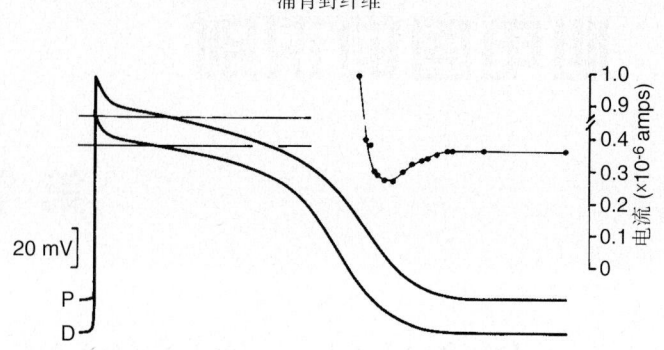

图 79-2　犬浦肯野纤维（上线）动作电位以及形成第 2 个动作电位的微小电流（下线）的微电极记录　在动作电位靠后的部位电流下降，这是一个超常兴奋期（长划线标记）。（引自 Spear JF，Moore EN：Supernormal excitability and conduction in the His-Purkinje system of the dog. Cir Res 35：782-792，1974.）

室性逸搏，第 2、5、10 和 13 个 P 波落在了 T 波的终点或其后部，此时可以经房室结传导到心室，PR 间期 480～560ms，而其他 P 波未引起心室反应，下传的心室波用星号标记，呈 qR 型，这种房室传导就可能是由于房室交界区出现了超常激动所致，但下面的梯形图给出了另一种解释，由于存在 2∶1 房室传导阻滞使第 2、5、10、13 个 P 波下传，第 3、6、8、11、14 个 P 波可能由于房室传导系统中某一部分处在不应期（梯形图中的暗区）而未下传。余下的 P 波未下传可能是由于交界性或室内逸搏节律的竞争抑制所致。

房室传导系统某部分不应期的回剥或后移有助于房室传导（见后文"隐匿传导"部分）[5]。早搏可产生回剥现象，如自发交界性或室性搏动，穿透并提前激动房室传导系统某部，使其不应期提前结束，因此，即使 RP 间期比未传导时仅轻微延长，房早也可下传心室。

2. 房早后 QRS 波群反正常化

窦性心律合并束支阻滞时，短联律间期的房早下传的 QRS 波群形态正常。直观上讲，早搏会遇到束支的不应期，更易出现束支阻滞的图形。QRS 波群正常化的可能机制是当房早进入 T 波终末部的超常期时，束支出现了真超常化。

然而，真超常化不一定是该现象的唯一机制，另外可用裂隙现象解释[5]。例如，房早可引起房室传导系统近侧端即房室结或希氏束（图 79-4）传导延迟。而传导时间延长可使束支不应性恢复，QRS 波群恢复正常。早搏的 PR 间期常比窦律时 PR 间期长，然而，两间期相似也不能除外裂隙现象。体表心电图的 PR 间期包括 PA、AH、HV 间期，因此，PA 间期缩短（例如，从房室结附近发出的早搏）可以减小总 PR 间期的延长。

另一种解释是基础束支阻滞图形是由于束支传导延迟所至，早搏使对侧束支的传导延迟增加，因此心室激动恢复正常形态。这种机制增加 HV 间期和 PR 间期。

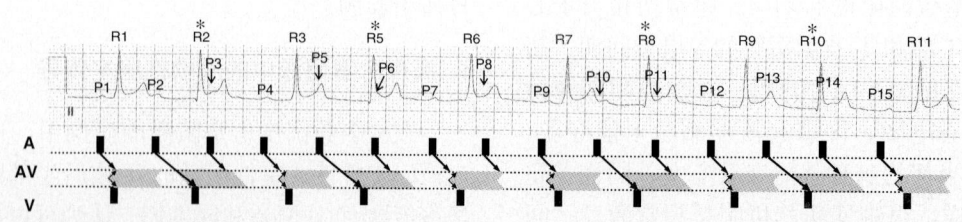

图 79-3　高度房室阻滞伴心动周期 1080ms 的心室逸搏节律　第 2、5、10 和 13 个 P 波落在了 T 波的后半部，并以 480～560ms 的 PR 间期传导至心室，这种心室激动形成的 R 波标记了星号，表现为 qR 型，这种房室传导是超常传导，另一种解释可按下面的梯形图进行。梯形图中的阴影线代表了房室传导的有效不应期。具体解释详见文中。

3. 心房颤动时短 RR 间期后 QRS 波群正常化

早期观察到，心房颤动时可发生束支阻滞，但当 RR 间期缩短后 QRS 波群可恢复正常[9]，虽然很难证实，但这可能是超常性的又一表现。然而应注意到虽然正常的 QRS 波群前有短 RR 间期，但这并不一定意味着两侧束支间激动间期短，可能还有其他的机制如不应期回剥、裂隙现象，或对侧束支的传导延迟增加等。

总之，虽然已证实超常激动是浦肯野系统的特性，并且超常传导已在体外证实，但是否存在真超常传导还不确定。大多数报道超常传导的病例可用其他机制解释。

二、隐匿传导

20 世纪的大多数时期，心电图是了解心律失常的最重要手段，其主要的局限是心脏的许多部分包括窦房结、房室结、希氏束和浦肯野系统的电位不能在体表心电图上表现出来。虽然这些电活动在体表心电图上是隐匿的，但聪明的观察者通过推断这些组织的电活动来解释心脏传导的改变。甚至在心电图使用前，Engelmann[10]就已观察到不能传导到心室的心房波可延缓其后搏动的房室传导。20 世纪中叶，Langendorf、Pick 和 Katz 详细解释并拓展了这一概念，并报道了大量隐匿传导的临床病例[11]。70 年代，临床心脏电生理研究的发展证实了希氏束和浦肯野纤维电活动的存在，并确认了隐匿传导这一概念[12]。若要进一步了解隐匿传导的发展史，参见 Langendorf 的综述[11]。

隐匿传导发生在窦房结和心房中已有描述，但在房室传导系统中最常见。隐匿传导表现为传导阻滞、传导延迟、折返、起搏器重整和传导显著改善。

隐匿传导的临床表现包括：

1. 未传导的早搏可引起 PR 间期延长：早搏可来自心房、心室或希氏束并穿透房室结引起部分组织不应性，可减慢下一次激动的传导。心电图上可以见到心房和心室早搏，但未传导的起源于希氏束的搏动在心电图上看不到[13,14]。

2. 隐匿传导有助于房室传导：这一例证是回剥现象[5]。当早搏穿透房室传导系统时产生回剥，使该系统的一部分提前激动并使不应期也相应提前结束。早搏能缩短长周期依赖的那部分传导系统如希浦系统的

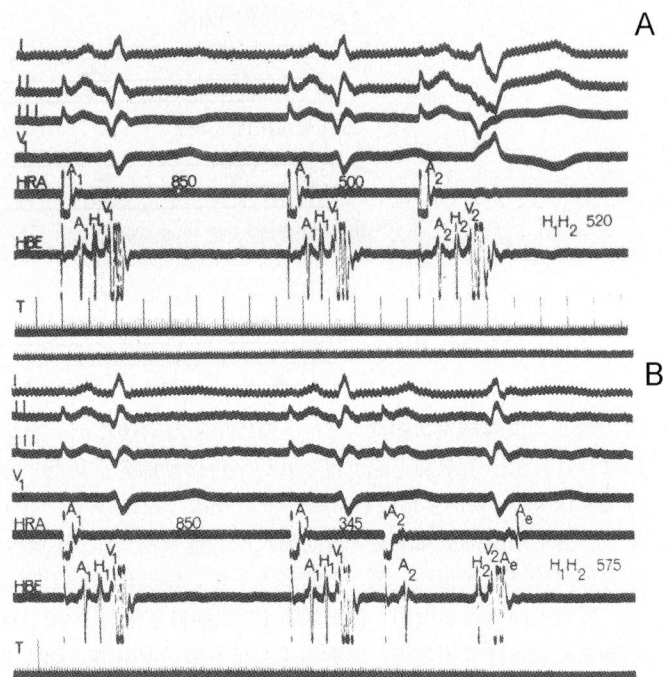

图 79-4 裂隙现象　A图：以基本起搏间期 850ms 连续起搏心房，发放一个联律间期为 500ms 的心房早搏刺激，经房室结传导后形成的 QRS 波群为右束支阻滞图形。B 图：以一个更短的联律间期 345ms 发放心房早搏刺激，尽管刺激联律间期更短，但由于房室传导减慢，HH 间期增加，使右束支从不应期状态下恢复，QRS 波群反而正常化。（引自 Gallagher JJ, Damato AN, Caracta AR, et al: Gap in A-V conduction in man: types Ⅰ and Ⅱ. Am Heart J 85: 78-82, 1973.）

不应期，使房室阻滞或束支阻滞恢复正常。

3. 室上性心动过速或快速心房起搏时，束支隐匿性逆向传导能引起束支阻滞：Moe 和同事们已在实验标本中证实这一机制[5]。室上性心动过速时提前室性激动穿透右束支并阻滞在近端，心电图上表现为右束支阻滞图形。室上性激动由左束支进入心室，激动从左束支扩散穿过间隔，逆行穿透右束支，使右束支对随后由上而来的激动不反应，维持右束支阻滞的图形，直到偶然的室早提前激动右束支，使右束支的不应期在下一次由上而来的激动到达时完全恢复[5]。

4. 心房扑动和颤动时，激动不同程度地穿透房室结，反复发生隐匿传导是缓慢心室率形成的机制。

5. 阵发性房室阻滞时房室传导的恢复（见前文"超常性"）。

6. 折返也是隐匿传导的一个现象。临床中，当房早穿透和阻滞在房室结快径时，激动顺慢径前传然后经房室结快径返回心房形成房室结折返[15]。

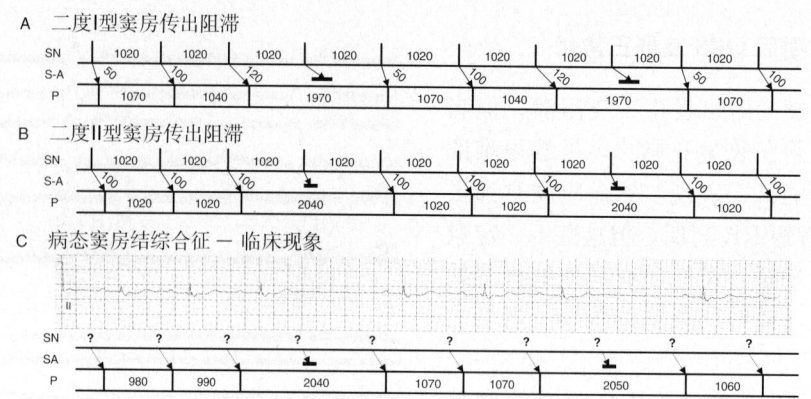

图 79-5 二度窦房传出阻滞 A：Ⅰ型传出阻滞的梯形图。窦房结以固定的周期（本例为 1020ms）发放激动，窦房传导时间逐搏延长，直至一个激动不能下传，其后下传搏动的窦房传导时间恢复至最短值（本例为 50ms），因此，有间歇 PP 间期的长度短于其他 PP 间期的 2 倍，然后循环重新开始。在循环中，由于窦房传导时间的增量逐渐减少，PP 间期逐渐缩短（"文氏现象"）。为了描述得更加清楚，所绘的尺度轻度夸张。B：Ⅱ型传出阻滞的梯形图。窦房结以固定的频率发放激动，每次下传激动的窦房传导时间相同，第 4 个激动未下传，能够传导的 PP 间期相等，有间歇的 PP 间期是其他 PP 间期的 2 倍。C：窦性心动过缓病人的体表心电图。仔细测量 PP 间期显示出与 A 和 B 两种典型模式的细小差别，最合理的解释是Ⅱ型传出阻滞加上与呼吸相关的窦性节律变化，这更像Ⅱ型而不是Ⅰ型阻滞，因为 PP 间期不是逐渐缩短，平均有间歇的 PP 间期是平均 PP 间期的 2 倍，这种节律无可非议被描述为"长达 2.05s 的窦性停搏"。

隐匿传导的心电图表现是多变的，为全面了解这方面的情况，读者可查阅 Langendorf 的综述[16]。

三、传出阻滞

传出阻滞的心电图表现

传出阻滞是从自发或折返电活动点发出的激动不能或延缓传导到心肌的另一位点的现象。

传出阻滞可在各种心脏有电活动的组织，如窦房结、房室结、希浦系统和异位的心房与心室起搏点，以及心房与心室内的折返环中记录到[17,18]。在起搏器电极与心房或心室组织的接触面上也可观察到传出阻滞[19]。通过心内记录已证实窦房传出阻滞至少与窦房结自律性异常同样重要，是病窦综合征中长间歇发生的基本机制，特别是在房性快速性心律失常和快速心房起搏时[20,21]。

无论何时出现"成队搏动"现象，都要怀疑发生了二度传出阻滞，如看到反复出现的 PP 或 RR 图形。成队搏动可表现为Ⅰ型和Ⅱ型周期现象（图 75-5A 和 B）。房室阻滞Ⅰ型（文氏）周期的定义为：在每组搏动中，PR 间期逐渐延长和 RR 间期逐渐缩短；而窦房传出阻滞定义为：SA-P 间期逐渐延长（见第 53 章）。由于 SA-P 间期在体表心电图上看不到，窦房文氏传出阻滞的诊断依靠 P 波典型的成队搏动现象。因此，典型的文氏周期有"文氏现象"的特征——在成队的搏动中，由于 PR 间期或 SA-P 间期增量逐渐减少，表现为 RR 或 PP 间期逐渐缩短，或在两组成队搏动之间出现短于任何两个周期之和的停搏间歇。相反，典型的Ⅱ型传出阻滞的 PP 或 RR 间期是基本周期的 2 倍。

窦房结传出阻滞和房室阻滞不符合典型的Ⅰ型或Ⅱ型周期的图形并不少见[21-25]。引起这种偏差的主要原因是自主神经系统对窦房结和房室结有持续性影响。例如，文氏型房室阻滞时，在整组搏动中 PR 间期的增加可能不逐渐减少或 PR 间期可能不逐渐延长。有时，确定典型房室结Ⅰ型房室阻滞的唯一标准是存在 PR 间期的可变性。对于窦房结传出阻滞，已描述了"非典型"的Ⅰ型周期，但不能与窦性心律失常相区别（图 79-5）。

一度窦房阻滞（1:1 窦房传导，传导时间长于正常范围）用体表心电图不能诊断，必须有心内电图记录[22]才能证实。同样，用心内记录诊断的三度完全窦房阻滞，在体表心电图上也不能与窦性停搏相区别[21]。

由于缺乏缝隙连接，窦房结与心房肌间的电连接有高电阻，防止心房膜静息电相位对超级化，使结区过分电紧张而抑制放电[24]。这使窦房结与心房之间的连接相对薄弱。传出阻滞和窦房结功能障碍与很多疾病相关：包括梗死或其他心肌病（细胞退化、萎缩、纤维化或脂肪浸润)[25-27]，先天性心脏病和随后的手术[28,29]，药物，如地高辛、β受体阻滞剂、钙离子拮抗剂、抗心律失常药或锂剂，运动训练[30]和房性快速性心律失常引起的心肌重塑[25-31]。这些原因或相关疾病的心电图表现可在心电图上看到。

激动从窦房结传出的位点可以变化。窦房结附近的非窦房结组织的逸搏节律点可移动[21,24]。这些变化可由心动过缓时 P 波形态的轻微变化反映出来，但是没有可靠的标准在此水平上判断 P 波的起源。

由于心脏结构的传入阻滞出现异位起搏冲动产生平行收缩，形成两个竞争性心律的特性。这种基质可同时存在短暂的传出阻滞，异位起搏组织的节律显现出长的间期是最短间期的整倍数[17]。

（张　萍　译）

参 考 文 献

1. Adrian ED, Lucas K: On the summation of propagated disturbances in the nerve and muscle. J Physiol 44:69, 1912.
2. Adrian ED: The recovery process of excitable tissue. J Physiol 54:1, 1920.
3. Spear JF, Moore EN: Supernormal excitability and conduction in the His-Purkinje system of the dog. Circ Res 35:782–792, 1974.
4. Childers RW, Merideth J, Moe GK: Supernormality in Bachmann's bundle. Circ Res 22:363–370, 1968.
5. Moe GK, Childers RW, Merideth J: An appraisal of "supernormal" A-V conduction. Circulation 38:5–28, 1968.
6. Moe GK, Mendez C, Han J: Aberrant A-V impulse propagation in the dog heart: A study of functional bundle branch block. Circ Res 16:261, 1965.
7. Moore EN, Spear JF, Fisch C: "Supernormal" conduction and excitability. J Cardiovasc Electrophysiol 4:320–337, 1993.
8. Lewis T, Master AM: Supernormal recovery phase, illustrated by two clinical cases of heart block. Heart 11:371, 1924.
9. Schramroth L: The supernormal phase of intraventricular conduction. Br Heart J 31:337–342, 1969.
10. Engelmann T: Beobachtungen und Versuche am suspendierten Herzen. Plfügers Arch 56:149, 1894.
11. Langendorf R: Concealed conduction, a historical review. In Zipes DP, Jalife J (eds): Cardiac Electrophysiology and Arrhythmias. Orlando, FL, Grune and Stratton, 1985, pp 501–504.
12. Scherlag BJ, Lau SH, Helfant RH: Catheter technique for recording His bundle activity in man. Circulation 39:13–18, 1969.
13. Langendorf R, Mehlman JS: Blocked (non-conducted) A-V nodal premature systoles imitating first and second degree A-V block. Am Heart J 34:500, 1947.
14. Rosen KM, Rahimtoola SH, Gunnar RM: Pseudo A-V block secondary to premature non-propagated His bundle depolarisations. Documentation by His bundle electrocardiography. Circulation 42:367–373, 1970.
15. Goldreyer BN, Bigger JT: The site of reentry in paroxysmal supraventricular tachycardia. Circulation 43:15–26, 1971.
16. Langendorf R: Newer aspects of concealed conduction. In Wellens HJJ, Lie KI, Janse MJ (eds): The Conduction System of the Heart. Structure, Function and Clinical implications. The Hague, Martinus Nijhoff, 1978, pp 410–423.
17. Langendorf R, Lesser ME, Plotkin P, Levin BD: Atrial parasystole with interpolation: Observations on prolonged sinoatrial conduction. Am Heart J 63:649, 1962.
18. Fisch C: Electrocardiography of Arrhythmias. Philadelphia, Lea & Febiger, 1990.
19. King DH, Gillette PC, Shannon C, et al: Steroid-eluting endocardial lead for treatment of exit block. Am Heart J 106:1438–1440, 1983.
20. Asseman P, Berzin B, Desry D, et al: Persistent sinus nodal electrograms during abnormally prolonged postpacing atrial pauses in sick sinus syndrome in humans: Sinoatrial block vs overdrive suppression. Circulation 68:33–41, 1983.
21. Wu D, Yeh SJ, Lin FC, et al: Sinus automaticity and sinoatrial conduction in severe symptomatic sick sinus syndrome. J Am Coll Cardiol 19:355–364, 1992.
22. Reiffel JA, Gang E, Gliklich J, et al: The human sinus node electrogram: A transvenous catheter technique and a comparison of directly measured and indirectly estimated sinoatrial conduction time in adults. Circulation 62:1324–1334, 1980.
23. Denes P, Levy L, Pick A, Rosen KM: The incidence of typical and atypical atrioventricular Wenckebach periodicity. Am Heart J 89:26–31, 1975.
24. Schuessler RB, Boineau JP, Bromberg BI: Origin of the sinus impulse. J Cardiovasc Electrophysiol 7:263–274, 1996.
25. Thery C, Gosselin B, LeKieffre J, Warembourg H: Pathology of sinoatrial node: Correlations with electrocardiographic findings in 111 patients. Am Heart J 93:735–740, 1977.
26. Bharati S, Nordenberg A, Bauerfiend R, et al: The anatomic substrate for the sick sinus syndrome in adolescence. Am J Cardiol 46:163–172, 1980.
27. Shaw DB, Linker NJ, Heaver PA, Evans R: Chronic sinoatrial disorder (sick sinus syndrome): A possible result of cardiac ischaemia. Br Heart J 58:598–607, 1987.
28. Gillette PC, Kugler JD, Garson A Jr, et al: Mechanisms of cardiac arrhythmias after the Mustard operation for transposition of the great arteries. Am J Cardiol 45:1225–1230, 1980.
29. Clark EB, Kugler JD: Preoperative secundum atrial septal defect with coexisting sinus node and atrioventricular node dysfunction. Circulation 65:976–980, 1982.
30. Bjornstad H, Storstein L, Meen HD, Hals O: Ambulatory electrocardiographic findings in top athletes, athletic students and control subjects. Cardiology 84:42–50, 1994.
31. Zipes DP: Electrophysiological remodelling of the heart owing to rate. Circulation 95:1745–1748, 1997.

第 80 章

并行心律

Agustin Castellanos, Nadir Saoudi, Federico Moleiro, and Robert J. Myerburg

本章目录

- 概述 ……………………………………… 728
- 典型的并行心律 ………………………… 728
- 典型的室性并行心律的特征 …………… 729
- 电张性调整的室性并行心律的心电图特征 …………………………………… 730
- 起搏点的湮灭 …………………………… 731
- 并行心律的拖带现象 …………………… 732
- 间歇性并行心律 ………………………… 732
- 并行心律的间歇性：摘要说明 ………… 733
- 并行心律的异化和消退 ………………………………………………………… 734

自从 Kaufman 和 Rothberger 于 1917 年到 1923 年发表了关于并行心律的系列文章后，这种"并行心律"的心律失常备受争议和关注。Scherf 和 Schott[1] 对 1973 年以前的文献做了历史性的回顾和全面的临床综述。本书第二版[2]涵盖了 1973 年至 1995 年这一时期的内容和进展。尽管并行心律可以起源于心脏的任何部位，但本章主要讨论最常见的并行性心律失常：室性并行心律[1-20]。

一、概　述

在常规心电图，典型的和电张性调整的并行心律均有一个"局灶"起搏点，其周围区域可以保护（屏蔽）其不受外界其他节律点激动的侵入[1-3]，即所谓的"传入阻滞"。因而，存在"局灶"起搏点和传入阻滞是室性并行心律的特征。实验研究显示，正常自主节律点、异位节律点、早期后除极和迟后除极引起的触发活动和除极时的自律性，只要在该节律点周围存在传入阻滞[1,2]，均可引起室性并行心律。这些不同的电生理机制可以解释室性并行心律多重的心电图表现。此外，关于传入阻滞的表现和性质，心电学者间争议很大[1-4,21,22]。值得注意的是现已众所周知的 Kaufmann 和 Rothberger 最初的假设：室性并行心律是完全独立而不受外界冲动干扰的一种节律，这一经典概念现已受到冲击[1-4,22]。最有可能的是，任何一个节律点，通过一个兴奋性降低的区域与周围组织相连，产生传入阻滞，同时允许冲动传出，这些都会不同程度受到周围组织除极的电张性调整作用[1-4,22]。

二、典型的并行心律

常见的（非电张性调整的）或典型的并行心律是临床心脏病学和心脏电生理学专著经常讨论的室性并行心律的类型。最近的一次，关于这一问题的全面阐述，可在第五版《Chou's Textbook》中找到，Surawicz[3]几乎重写了该书。3 条经典的标准是：（1）室早的联律间期不等；（2）异位室性搏动之间的间距有数学（公约数）关系；并且（3）有室性融合波。常见的室性并行心律通常被分为：（1）持续性但无传出阻滞；（2）持续性伴传出阻滞；（3）间歇性[1]。传出阻滞已在第 79 章讨论过。虽然常常提到异位搏动之间的间距有稳定的公约数关系，但是，异位冲动的不规则发放，与其说是例外，不如说是惯例，特别是做长时间心电图记录或监测时（比如动态心电图记录）可以发现这点。毫无疑问，诊断室性并行心律（常见的或电张性调整的）最大的障碍是，异位搏动周期存在的内在波动和外界非电张性调整所引起的变化[23]。Castellanos 和同事[2] 在其观察的 90 例并行心律中均发现，并行搏动的频率存在个体变异（变化范围 4.7%~31.3%）。总而言之，随访的时间越长（几个月，甚至几年），变异越明显，但在某些病例，几分钟之内变异就可达 27.6%。异位搏动的周期，除了数分钟（或 1min）内可发生明显不规则变化外，24h 动态心电图的记录显示，还受昼夜节律变化的影响，典型的和电张性调整的室性并行心律可产生频率的上下波动，这很可能是众所周知的自主神经的张力变化造成的[23]。

三、典型的室性并行心律的特征

典型的室性并行心律的数学模型表明，可以对并行节律点的活动规律作出具体的预测[18,19,23,24]，这些活动规律，在心电图上表现为相同的形态和固有节律（如同 VOO 模式起搏节律）[18,19,23,24]。Glass 和同事[24] 报道，在频率没有显著变化的情况下，仅用两个参数就可以对典型室性并行心律的特征做详细的数学描述：异位搏动周期与窦性心动周期的比值，以及心室不应期与窦性心动周期的比值。从这些参数的相互关系得到 3 条规则：（1）在两个并行心律搏动之间，最多可有 3 种数目的窦性搏动（非并行心搏）；（2）仅有一种为奇数；（3）两个较小数的代数和小于另一个较大

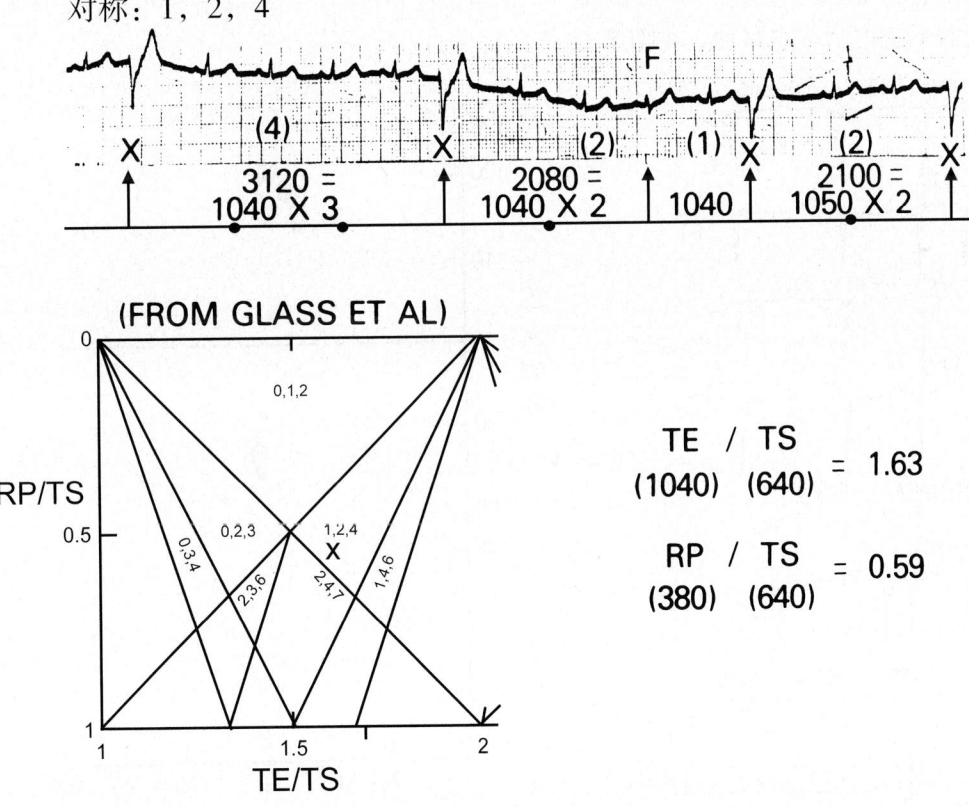

图 80-1 显性的典型的室性并行心律　F，融合波（同样被视为显性搏动）正文下方心电图描绘的是，根据不应期（RP）/窦性周期（TS）、异位搏动周期（TE）/窦性周期（TS）两个比值，数学推算的异位搏动之间窦性搏动的数目。参数之间的 X 位点，对应该格内推算出的窦性搏动的数目。推算出来的窦性搏动的数目（1，2，4）显示在心电图的下方。图 80-1 至图 80-4 中，心动周期值均以毫秒表示。（引自 Castellanos A, Fernandez P, Moleiro F, et al: Symmetry, broken symmetry, and restored symmetry of apparent pure ventricular parasystole. Am J Cardiol 68：256-259, 1991, Copyright 1991, with permission from Excerpta Medica Inc.）

的数[24]。关于自发性和起搏诱发的室性并行心律的几个临床研究已证实了这一点[19,20,23]。

图80-1举例说明多年来所公认的室性并行心律的特征[1-3]。在这份心电图中，上述有关的两个比值分别为0.59和1.63，相应部位"X"标明3个推算出来的结果（1、2和4），它们正好是显性并行心搏之间窦性搏动的数目（括号内，心电图下方）[24]。尽管该研究和其他报道证实可以预测典型室性并行节律点的活动规律，但是，由于窦性周期和异位搏动周期经常出现自发的（有时不规则的）变化[23]，临床心电记录中常见的室性并行节律点的活动规律被打破。事实上，一个完全的、持续存在的对称现象，仅见于持续心房和心室起搏条件下心房率和心室率保持稳定时。

四、电张性调整的室性并行心律的心电图特征

在Jalife和Moe（大约1976年完成）[23,26]及其他研究者经最初的微电极研究之后，观察到，在临床心电图记录中，常发生电张性调整的室性并行心律[2,4,22,26-31]。为了描述这种心律失常的心电图特征，常使用以下几个名称：X＝并行心律的搏动；R＝非并行心律的搏动，X-X＝两个连续的并行心律搏动之间的间期，其间不含任何间位的非并行心律的搏动（即非电张性调整的异位搏动的周期）；X-R＝并行心律搏动和紧随其后的非并行心律搏动之间的间期；以及X-R-X＝两个连续的并行心律搏动之间的间期，其间含有一个间位的非并行心律搏动（电张性调整的异位搏动周期）[2]。

图80-2举例所示，可以看到所有的间期均被标准化为占异位搏动周期（可直接测量）的百分比。异位搏动周期为1200ms（100％），非并行心律搏动发生在X-R间期为42％（图A）和50％（图B）两处，分别使X-R-X间期延长到117％和122％。图C，X-R间期轻度延长为53％，使情况发生逆转，使X-R-X间期缩短为80％。图D中，X-R-X间期进一步缩短，以至于使并行心律的冲动落在非并行心律搏动的不应

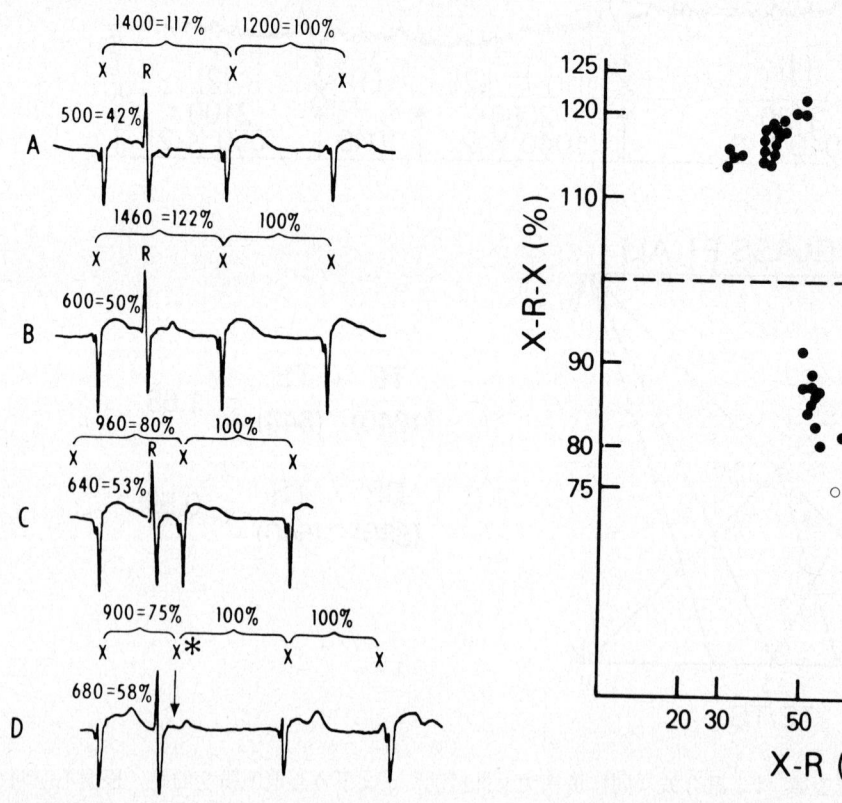

图80-2 电张性调整的室性并行心律 在相应的双相反应曲线（右）中，X-R-X间期（电张性调整的并行心律周期）与X-R间期相关，X-R-X间期标准化为占异位搏动周期的百分比（与水平线的交点处为100％），右图空圈代表隐匿的并行异位激动的发放。（引自 Castellanos A, Luceiro F, et al: Annihilation, entrainment and modulation of ventricular parasystolic rhythms. Am J Cardiol 54: 317-322, 1984, Copyright 1984, with permission from Excerpta Medica Inc.）

期。导致一个隐匿性冲动的发放（X*），发放时间的确定（垂直箭头所示）仅能根据其后非电张性调整的并行心律（要求是显性的）减去100%来推断。

正如实验研究所显示的，非并行搏动的电张性调整作用可以用一条阶段反应曲线来表示，横坐标是X-R间期，纵坐标是X-R-X间期相对于X-X间期的偏离程度（%），最初描述的临床阶段反应曲线与代表X-X间期的水平线呈双相关系[2,4,25-28]。图80-2（右）显示，随着X-R的延长，X-R-X进行性延长（延迟阶段），直到达到最大值。此后，曲线关系反转，直到出现最大幅度X-R-X缩短（往往位于异位搏动周期的中部），此后，曲线转向水平线（加速阶段）。常可见到有重复的（X-R-X）数值，特别是接近或处于拐点时。分析其他已发表的阶段反应曲线，结果显示，非并行搏动的激动靠近下一个并行搏动时可引起：（1）最大延迟；（2）最大加速度；（3）调整作用减小；（4）几乎不起作用；（5）起搏点的消失（见下文）。双相反应曲线依延迟作用或缩短作用孰占优势，可以是对称的或非对称的[2,30]。

三相反应曲线越来越多地见诸报道[2,30,31]，主要见于当非并行搏动发生在异位搏动周期的早期，即在并行搏动的超常期对其进行夺获[2,30,31]。

五、起搏点的湮灭

生物振荡（oscillation）系统在受到来自它周围的外界刺激的干扰时，自律性活动会消失。Jalife和Antzelevitch[32,33]首先报道，应用蔗糖裂解技术，在狗的窦房结和浦肯野纤维的组织片上，当适时的阈下刺激跨越缝隙连接在精确的时间到达作用部位时，可以突然终止其自律性活动（"起搏点的湮灭"）。Rosenthal和Ferrier在具有自律性（在电流作用下产生除极诱发的自律性）的标本上，Gilmour和Zipes在患者的心室肌组织片上，均观察到这一现象[2]。

Jalife和Antzelevitch[32]首先根据Winfree的学说：振荡系统时相重整（phase-resetting）解释他们的发现，在这一学说中微分拓扑学技术得到应用。应

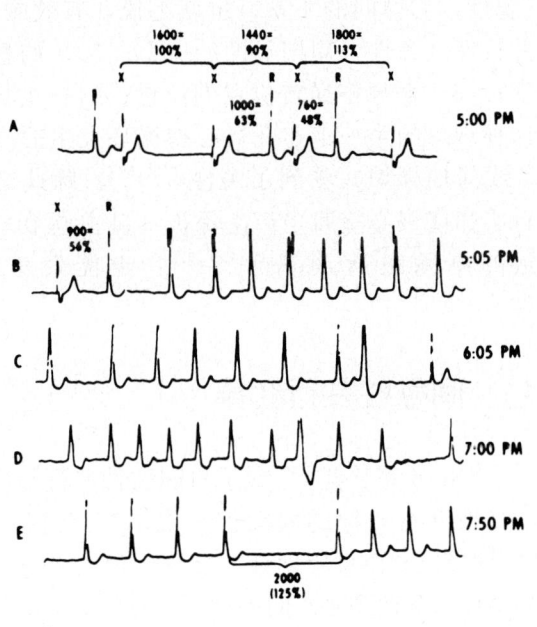
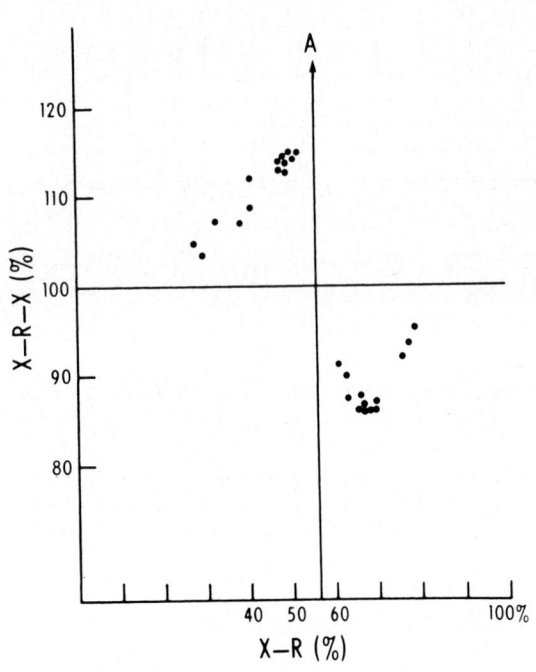

图80-3 一位房颤患者可能出现的起搏点湮灭现象 A图：X-X间期为1600ms（100%），有一个非并行心律搏动发生在X-R间期760ms（48%）处，使X-R-X间期延长至1800ms（113%），而发生于X-R间期1000ms（63%）处，使X-R-X间期缩短为90%。B图：非并行心律搏动发生在一个并行心律搏动之后900ms（56%），明显导致并行心律起搏点湮灭。因为，在此后8h心电监测中未再见到显性的并行心律搏动（B~E图），尽管在这个病人观察到室上性心搏周期存在显著变化，且非并行心律R-R间期比最长的（延长的）异位搏动周期还长（A）。相应的阶段反应曲线揭示，起搏点湮灭现象发生于非并行心律搏动（R）落入异位心搏周期（X-X）的拐点（大约位于异位心搏周期的56%处，即X-R=56%）。（引自Castellanos A, Luceiro F, et al: Annihilation, entrainment and modulation of ventricular parasystolic rhythms. Am J Cardiol 54：317-322, 1984 Copyright 1984, with permission from Excerpta Medica Inc.）

用 Hodgkin-Huxley 模型，在不同膜除极电压时，反复发放刺激，可以验证起搏点的湮灭现象[33]。对某一范围的除极电流强度，相当于含有一个可以终止基本节律的"单一"点（"singular" point）[32,33]。

然而，也有可能，大多数生物节律不会被消灭，理由是这种外界节律根本不会再次出现。在大多数实验研究中，起搏点的兴奋性即使被抑制，也是一过性的。因为，抑制起搏点兴奋性的外界刺激，导致阈下膜电位振荡，振荡持续时间进行性延长，经过一段不确定的时间，再次达到阈电位。在另一些研究中，起搏点兴奋性的抑制似乎是永久的（图80-3）[32,34]，因此，临时抑制可等同于（表现为）较长时间的重整[32-34]。尽管如此，这一现象与其他临床情况（如：病态窦房结或不稳定的室性自主节律）中观察到的持续性重整很可能不一样，在后一种情况时，很可能一个完整的动作电位（非电刺激诱发的除极）会影响未受保护的自律点的节律[2]。时相重整（phase-resetting）、双稳定性（bistabilities）和起搏点湮灭（annihilation）的电模型，对帮助人们理解这些现象，是有启发性的[2]。

六、并行心律的拖带现象

根据振荡学说，与应用于各种实验模型和折返性心律的微电极研究一样，拖带可被定义为：一个自我维系的振荡系统与一个外力振荡的耦联[35-37]。考虑调整后的并行心律，产生的干扰可能是任何一个能调整并行心律的再发非并行心律，这种调整取决于与并行阶段同期的时相[2,26,37,38]。如图80-4描记的病人，非并行搏动与并行搏动间的相互作用导致了阶段性的隐性和显性的1∶1拖带。在此阶段并行心律被改变为和快或慢一些的非并行心律相同。此类拖带与折返性心律失常如房扑、室上速和室速不同。

拖带是一种多因素功能：（1）并行与非并行（窦性）心律间的关系，也就是说，有效的异位/非并行性（窦性）周期长度的比率；（2）调整作用幅度；（3）循环中逆转位点的位置；（4）尤其是导致这种现象的第一个非并行心搏循环发生的时刻（用X线间期标识）受到了关注[2,37,38]。除此之外，并行心律能被心室肌中产生保护（自主调节）部位附近的电除极所调整[2,36,30,37]，也能发生自身拖带[37,39]。

七、间歇性并行心律

Schorf等学者[1,40]最早对间歇性并行心律（不要与显性并行心律的间歇性相混淆）有过以下描述："室性异位节律点周期性的显现与消失……不会被主导节律（窦性节律）的冲动所干扰"（异位节律点自律性间歇性改变所致）。如图80-5所示，在心电记录图80-5B后半部分，突然出现非电张性调整的室性并行心律，而且在心电记录图80-5C中，该异位节律表现为"温醒"现象，随后，在图80-5D中，异位节律逐渐"冷却"，并最后消失（图80-5E）。

近来，间歇性并行心律的概念常用于描述室性并行心律的一种特殊类型，认为在该类型的并行心律中，"完全性"的传入保护只存在于异位节律周期的前半部分，而落入后半部分的主导节律（窦律）冲

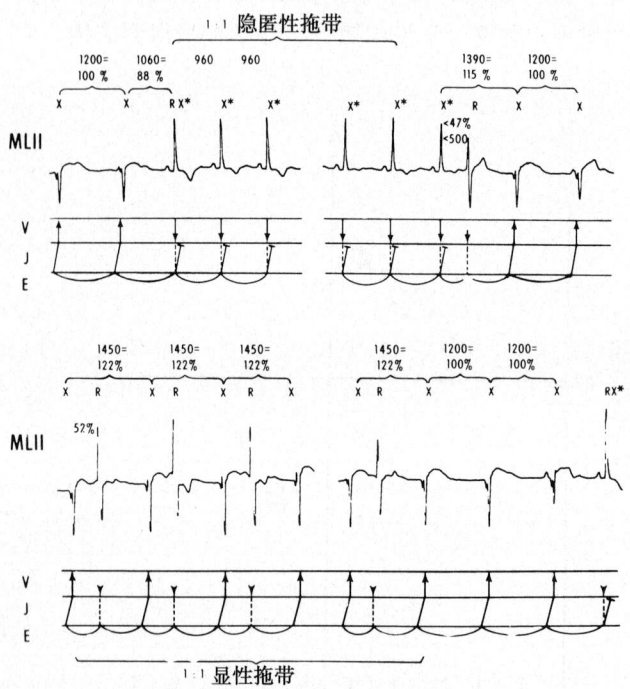

图80-4 调整后室性并行心律的拖带现象　左上，记述了由非并行心律搏动出现在较晚期诱发的一阵隐匿的1∶1拖带，发生在循环的加速阶段。右上，记述的是发生在循环前半阶段一阵非并行心律搏动终止了拖带。在拖带中，并行心律被非并行心律搏动所增加。下面记述的是在循环的早期和延迟阶段分别出现和消失的非并行心律搏动所引起和终止的一阵1∶1拖带。（引自 Castellanos A, Luceri RM, Moleiro F, et al：Annihilation，entrainment and modulation of ventricular parasystolic rhythms. Am J Cardiol 54：317-322，1984，copyright 1984，with permission from Excerpta Medica Inc.）

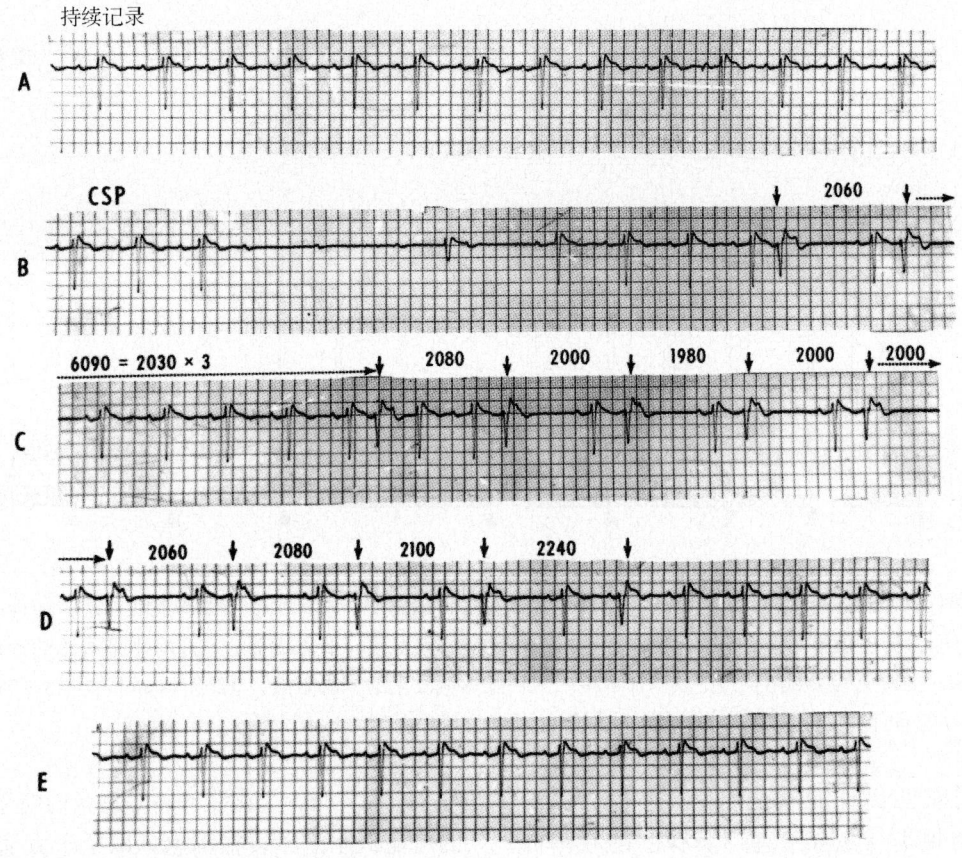

图 80-5 间歇性单纯性室性并行心律 A 图为窦性心律；B 图表示，颈动脉窦按摩（CSP）后出现室性并行心律，周期为 2060ms；C 图表示室性并行心律经过"温醒"阶段，周期缩短为 1980ms；D 图表示室性并行心律逐渐"冷却"；E 图中，室性并行心律消失。尽管可能存在其他的机制，但图中所示为室性并行心律在动态心电图中最常见的表现。

动可以侵入，进而重整或者暂时终止异位节律[2,4,41,42]。

在图 80-6 中，最早出现的 3 个异位搏动中，X-R-X 间期轻微缩短（1180ms 到 1140ms，图上部数字是以百分之一秒作为时间单位）与 X-R 间期的缩短有关。X-R 间期和 X-R-X 间期之间存在着双相关系。因此考虑该异位节律为单纯的、非电张性调整的并行心律，频率为 51~52bpm。第 3 个异位搏动之后，出现 1 个窦性搏动（标记为 X_R），间期为 810ms，该窦性冲动使异位节律点发生节律重整，冲动再次传出后，与前一窦性冲动的配对间期（X_R-X）为 1180ms，与重整前的异位节律周期相似。从图 80-6 底部的时间栏推断异位节律周期的前 750ms 范围存在传入保护。因此，第 4 个异位搏动后出现的窦性搏动，其后在预期时间内并未出现异位搏动（X'）。X_R-X' 间期约为 1140ms，接近异位节律的周期。因为此时心室肌并非处于不应期，异位节律冲动突然不能穿越周围保护区激动心室的原因考虑存在Ⅱ型传出阻滞[8]。但是，窦性冲动也使部分异位节律点周围保护区的心肌处于不应期，从而阻止了后续主导节律的传入（如心电图上第 10 个心搏所示）。在心电图记录的后半部，也能见到相似的现象。因此，通过解释上述现象，推断并行心律并非单纯性，而是间歇性的，其节律周期的前半部存在传入保护和间歇性的Ⅱ型传出阻滞。

上述现象也可以用电张性调整作用的概念解释[30,43]，由于电张性调整作用产生异位节律的夺获加速，使延迟相早期的强度下降到体表心电图不能检测的水平，而此时加速相处于最大水平[30,43]。尽管如此，仍可能存在传出阻滞。而 Kinoshita 等学者[44]提出另外的解释，他们认为二度Ⅰ型和Ⅱ型传入阻滞的并存（而非传出阻滞）可以导致这种现象的发生。

八、并行心律的间歇性：摘要说明

为了正确理解间歇性并行心律的概念，必须了解

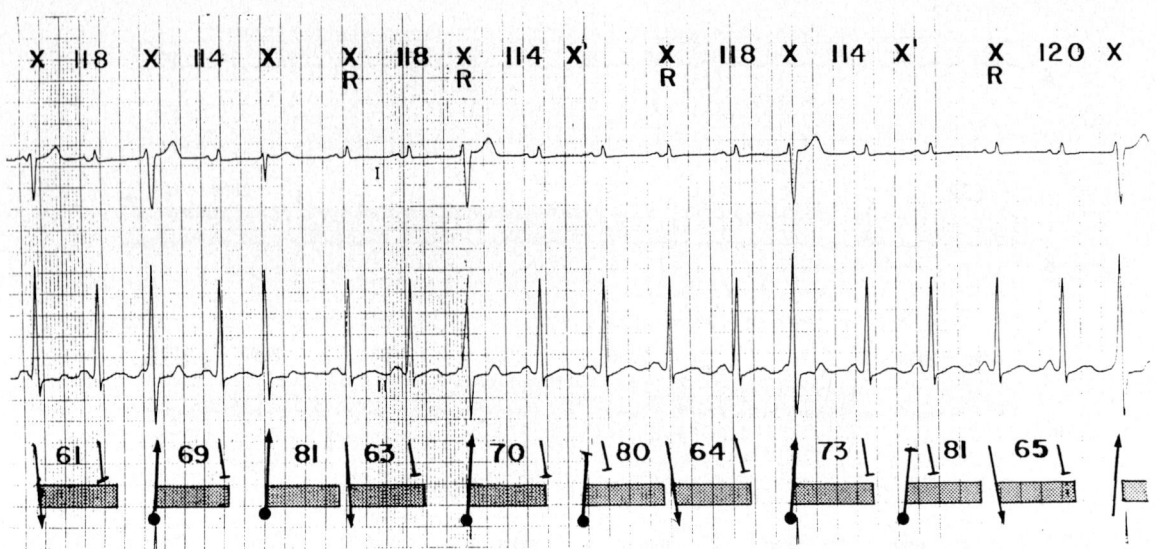

图 80-6　间歇性单纯性室性并行心律，并行心律周期前半部分存在传入保护，即持续电张性调整性并行心律伴延迟相早期强度下降，X 代表并行心律传出阻滞　水平条带代表并行心律存在完全传入保护时的周期部分，此时主导节律的冲动对并行心律的周期无明显的影响。为避免交叉混淆，图中没有标示传入保护区远端发生的传出阻滞。（引自 Castellanos A，Moleiro F，Guerrero J et al：Intermittent parasystole with exit block. J Electrocardial 30：331-335，1997.）

显性并行心律间歇性出现的其他原因，包括：（1）室性并行节律的频率与主导节律（窦律）的频率相等或恰好等于窦性频率的一半时，由于部分异位节律的冲动落入窦性搏动的不应期内，因而表现出显性并行心律的间歇性[2]；（2）由于窦性冲动在周围保护区的隐匿性传导，使异位节律不能传出，称为隐匿的单纯性室性并行心律[2,45]；（3）存在较长时间的传出阻滞；（4）传入阻滞（或传入保护）的消失。此外，动态心电图在诊断"持续性"并行心律中的价值需要重新评估[10,12,22,23]。尽管有些室性并行心律可以发作较长的时间，但是心电图长期监测的结果表明这只是个例，并非常见的情况[2]。何谓"持续性"并行心律呢？举例来说，如果某次发作的并行心律，符合"持续性"的特征，但它具有明显的时间性，只在下午 1 时到 3 时之间发作（其他 22 小时无发作），这应该诊断为"持续性"并行心律，还是并行心律持续两小时呢[22]？在现代医学的大部分领域，专家们的意见是趋向一致的，但对于室性并行心律，情况并非如此。

九、并行心律的异化和消退

2001 年，Surawicz 等[3]强调室性并行心律的发生率目前并不清楚，这是众所周知的，不足为惊奇。在本文，从图 80-1 到图 80-6，学者们对于室性并行心律的可能机制已经备感困惑，以至于大家都避免对并行心律的异化现象进行过多的解释[5]。但并行心律的异化现象不仅具有学术研究价值，也具有临床应用的意义，并可能导致新的技术设备的出现，例如 Takayagani 及同事发明的转速计[11,12]。总之，由于目前认为室性并行心律缺乏重要的临床意义[3]，因此对它的研究主要限于学术研究领域。

（葛堪忆　译）

参 考 文 献

1. Scherf D, Schott A: Extrasystoles and Allied Arrhythmias, 2nd ed. Chicago, Year Book, 1973, pp 269–281.
2. Castellanos A, Saoudi N, Moleiro F, Myerburg RJ: Parasystole. In Zipes D, Jalife J (eds): Cardiac Electrophysiology: From Cell to Bedside, 2nd ed. Philadelphia, WB Saunders, 1995, pp 942–954.
3. Surawicz B, Knilans TK: Chou's Electrocardiography in Clinical Practice. Adult and Pediatric, 5th ed. Philadelphia, WB Saunders, 2001, pp 401–403.
4. Oreto G, Luzza F, Satullo G, Donato A: Parasystole. Revista Latina de Cardiologia 12:268–277, 1991.
5. Castellanos A, Myerburg RJ: Parasystolic alienation: An impression or a reality? J Cardiovasc Electrophysiol 11:178–179, 2000.
6. Grolleau R, Pasquie JL, Macia JC, Leclercq F: Parasystole. Arch Mal Coeur Vasiss 95:5:41–46, 2002.
7. Ren Z, Zhou J, Xu G, et al: The diagnostic criteria for classic parasystole. Chin Med J 112:992–994, 1999.
8. Kinoshita S, Katoh T, Mitsuoka T, et al: Ventricular parasystolic couplets originating in the pathway between the ventricle and the parasystole pacemaker: Mechanism of "irregular" parasystole. J Electrocardiol

纤维化或脂肪浸润)[25-27]，先天性心脏病和随后的手术[28,29]，药物，如地高辛、β受体阻滞剂、钙离子拮抗剂、抗心律失常药或锂剂，运动训练[30]和房性快速性心律失常引起的心肌重塑[25-31]。这些原因或相关疾病的心电图表现可在心电图上看到。

激动从窦房结传出的位点可以变化。窦房结附近的非窦房结组织的逸搏节律点可移动[21,24]。这些变化可由心动过缓时P波形态的轻微变化反映出来，但是没有可靠的标准在此水平上判断P波的起源。

由于心脏结构的传入阻滞出现异位起搏冲动产生平行收缩，形成两个竞争性心律的特性。这种基质可同时存在短暂的传出阻滞，异位起搏组织的节律显现出长的间期是最短间期的整倍数[17]。

(张　萍译)

参 考 文 献

1. Adrian ED, Lucas K: On the summation of propagated disturbances in the nerve and muscle. J Physiol 44:69, 1912.
2. Adrian ED: The recovery process of excitable tissue. J Physiol 54:1, 1920.
3. Spear JF, Moore EN: Supernormal excitability and conduction in the His-Purkinje system of the dog. Circ Res 35:782–792, 1974.
4. Childers RW, Merideth J, Moe GK: Supernormality in Bachmann's bundle. Circ Res 22:363–370, 1968.
5. Moe GK, Childers RW, Merideth J: An appraisal of "supernormal" A-V conduction. Circulation 38:5–28, 1968.
6. Moe GK, Mendez C, Han J: Aberrant A-V impulse propagation in the dog heart: A study of functional bundle branch block. Circ Res 16:261, 1965.
7. Moore EN, Spear JF, Fisch C: "Supernormal" conduction and excitability. J Cardiovasc Electrophysiol 4:320–337, 1993.
8. Lewis T, Master AM: Supernormal recovery phase, illustrated by two clinical cases of heart block. Heart 11:371, 1924.
9. Schramroth L: The supernormal phase of intraventricular conduction. Br Heart J 31:337–342, 1969.
10. Engelmann T: Beobachtungen und Versuche am suspendierten Herzen. Pflügers Arch 56:149, 1894.
11. Langendorf R: Concealed conduction, a historical review. In Zipes DP, Jalife J (eds): Cardiac Electrophysiology and Arrhythmias. Orlando, FL, Grune and Stratton, 1985, pp 501–504.
12. Scherlag BJ, Lau SH, Helfant RH: Catheter technique for recording His bundle activity in man. Circulation 39:13–18, 1969.
13. Langendorf R, Mehlman JS: Blocked (non-conducted) A-V nodal premature systoles imitating first and second degree A-V block. Am Heart J 34:500, 1947.
14. Rosen KM, Rahimtoola SH, Gunnar RM: Pseudo A-V block secondary to premature non-propagated His bundle depolarisations. Documentation by His bundle electrocardiography. Circulation 42:367–373, 1970.
15. Goldreyer BN, Bigger JT: The site of reentry in paroxysmal supraventricular tachycardia. Circulation 43:15–26, 1971.
16. Langendorf R: Newer aspects of concealed conduction. In Wellens HJJ, Lie KI, Janse MJ (eds): The Conduction System of the Heart. Structure, Function and Clinical implications. The Hague, Martinus Nijhoff, 1978, pp 410–423.
17. Langendorf R, Lesser ME, Plotkin P, Levin BD: Atrial parasystole with interpolation: Observations on prolonged sinoatrial conduction. Am Heart J 63:649, 1962.
18. Fisch C: Electrocardiography of Arrhythmias. Philadelphia, Lea & Febiger, 1990.
19. King DH, Gillette PC, Shannon C, et al: Steroid-eluting endocardial lead for treatment of exit block. Am Heart J 106:1438–1440, 1983.
20. Asseman P, Berzin B, Desry D, et al: Persistent sinus nodal electrograms during abnormally prolonged postpacing atrial pauses in sick sinus syndrome in humans: Sinoatrial block vs overdrive suppression. Circulation 68:33–41, 1983.
21. Wu D, Yeh SJ, Lin FC, et al: Sinus automaticity and sinoatrial conduction in severe symptomatic sick sinus syndrome. J Am Coll Cardiol 19:355–364, 1992.
22. Reiffel JA, Gang E, Gliklich J, et al: The human sinus node electrogram: A transvenous catheter technique and a comparison of directly measured and indirectly estimated sinoatrial conduction time in adults. Circulation 62:1324–1334, 1980.
23. Denes P, Levy L, Pick A, Rosen KM: The incidence of typical and atypical atrioventricular Wenckebach periodicity. Am Heart J 89:26–31, 1975.
24. Schuessler RB, Boineau JP, Bromberg BI: Origin of the sinus impulse. J Cardiovasc Electrophysiol 7:263–274, 1996.
25. Thery C, Gosselin B, LeKieffre J, Warembourg H: Pathology of sinoatrial node: Correlations with electrocardiographic findings in 111 patients. Am Heart J 93:735–740, 1997.
26. Bharati S, Nordenberg A, Bauerfiend R, et al: The anatomic substrate for the sick sinus syndrome in adolescence. Am J Cardiol 46:163–172, 1980.
27. Shaw DB, Linker NJ, Heaver PA, Evans R: Chronic sinoatrial disorder (sick sinus syndrome): A possible result of cardiac ischaemia. Br Heart J 58:598–607, 1987.
28. Gillette PC, Kugler JD, Garson A Jr, et al: Mechanisms of cardiac arrhythmias after the Mustard operation for transposition of the great arteries. Am J Cardiol 45:1225–1230, 1980.
29. Clark EB, Kugler JD: Preoperative secundum atrial septal defect with coexisting sinus node and atrioventricular node dysfunction. Circulation 65:976–980, 1982.
30. Bjornstad H, Storstein L, Meen HD, Hals O: Ambulatory electrocardiographic findings in top athletes, athletic students and control subjects. Cardiology 84:42–50, 1994.
31. Zipes DP: Electrophysiological remodelling of the heart owing to rate. Circulation 95:1745–1748, 1997.

第 80 章

并行心律

Agustin Castellanos, *Nadir Saoudi*, *Federico Moleiro*, and *Robert J. Myerburg*

本章目录
- 概述 728
- 典型的并行心律 728
- 典型的室性并行心律的特征 729
- 电张性调整的室性并行心律的心电图特征 730
- 起搏点的湮灭 731
- 并行心律的拖带现象 732
- 间歇性并行心律 732
- 并行心律的间歇性：摘要说明 733
- 并行心律的异化和消退 734

自从 Kaufman 和 Rothberger 于 1917 年到 1923 年发表了关于并行心律的系列文章后，这种"并行心律"的心律失常备受争议和关注。Scherf 和 Schott[1] 对 1973 年以前的文献做了历史性的回顾和全面的临床综述。本书第二版[2]涵盖了 1973 年至 1995 年这一时期的内容和进展。尽管并行心律可以起源于心脏的任何部位，但本章主要讨论最常见的并行性心律失常：室性并行心律[1-20]。

一、概 述

在常规心电图，典型的和电张性调整的并行心律均有一个"局灶"起搏点，其周围区域可以保护（屏蔽）其不受外界其他节律点激动的侵入[1-3]，即所谓的"传入阻滞"。因而，存在"局灶"起搏点和传入阻滞是室性并行心律的特征。实验研究显示，正常自主节律点、异位节律点、早期后除极和迟后除极引起的触发活动和除极时的自律性，只要在该节律点周围存在传入阻滞[1,2]，均可引起室性并行心律。这些不同的电生理机制可以解释室性并行心律多重的心电图表现。此外，关于传入阻滞的表现和性质，心电学者间争议很大[1-4,21,22]。值得注意的是现已众所周知的 Kaufmann 和 Rothberger 最初的假设：室性并行心律是完全独立而不受外界冲动干扰的一种节律，这一经典概念现已受到冲击[1-4,22]。最有可能的是，任何一个节律点，通过一个兴奋性降低的区域与周围组织相连，产生传入阻滞，同时允许冲动传出，这些都会不同程度受到周围组织除极的电张性调整作用[1-4,22]。

二、典型的并行心律

常见的（非电张性调整的）或典型的并行心律是临床心脏病学和心脏电生理学专著经常讨论的室性并行心律的类型。最近的一次，关于这一问题的全面阐述，可在第五版《Chou's Textbook》中找到，Surawicz[3]几乎重写了该书。3 条经典的标准是：(1) 室早的联律间期不等；(2) 异位室性搏动之间的间距有数学（公约数）关系；并且 (3) 有室性融合波。常见的室性并行心律通常被分为：(1) 持续性但无传出阻滞；(2) 持续性伴传出阻滞；(3) 间歇性[1]。传出阻滞已在第 79 章讨论过。虽然常常提到异位搏动之间的间距有稳定的公约数关系，但是，异位冲动的不规则发放，与其说是例外，不如说是惯例，特别是做长时间心电图记录或监测时（比如动态心电图记录）可以发现这点。毫无疑问，诊断室性并行心律（常见的或电张性调整的）最大的障碍是，异位搏动周期存在的内在波动和外界非电张性调整所引起的变化[23]。Castellanos 和同事[2]在其观察的 90 例并行心律中均发现，并行搏动的频率存在个体变异（变化范围 4.7%～31.3%）。总而言之，随访的时间越长（几个月，甚至几年），变异越明显，但在某些病例，几分钟之内变异就可达 27.6%。异位搏动的周期，除了数分钟（或 1min）内可发生明显不规则变化外，24h 动态心电图的记录显示，还受昼夜节律变化的影响，典型的和电张性调整的室性并行心律可产生频率的上下波动，这很可能是众所周知的自主神经的张力变化造成的[23]。

三、典型的室性并行心律的特征

典型的室性并行心律的数学模型表明，可以对并行节律点的活动规律作出具体的预测[18,19,23,24]，这些活动规律，在心电图上表现为相同的形态和固有节律（如同 VOO 模式起搏节律）[18,19,23,24]。Glass 和同事[24]报道，在频率没有显著变化的情况下，仅用两个参数就可以对典型室性并行心律的特征做详细的数学描述：异位搏动周期与窦性心动周期的比值，以及心室不应期与窦性心动周期的比值。从这些参数的相互关系得到 3 条规则：（1）在两个并行心律搏动之间，最多可有 3 种数目的窦性搏动（非并行心搏）；（2）仅有一种为奇数；（3）两个较小数的代数和小于另一个较大

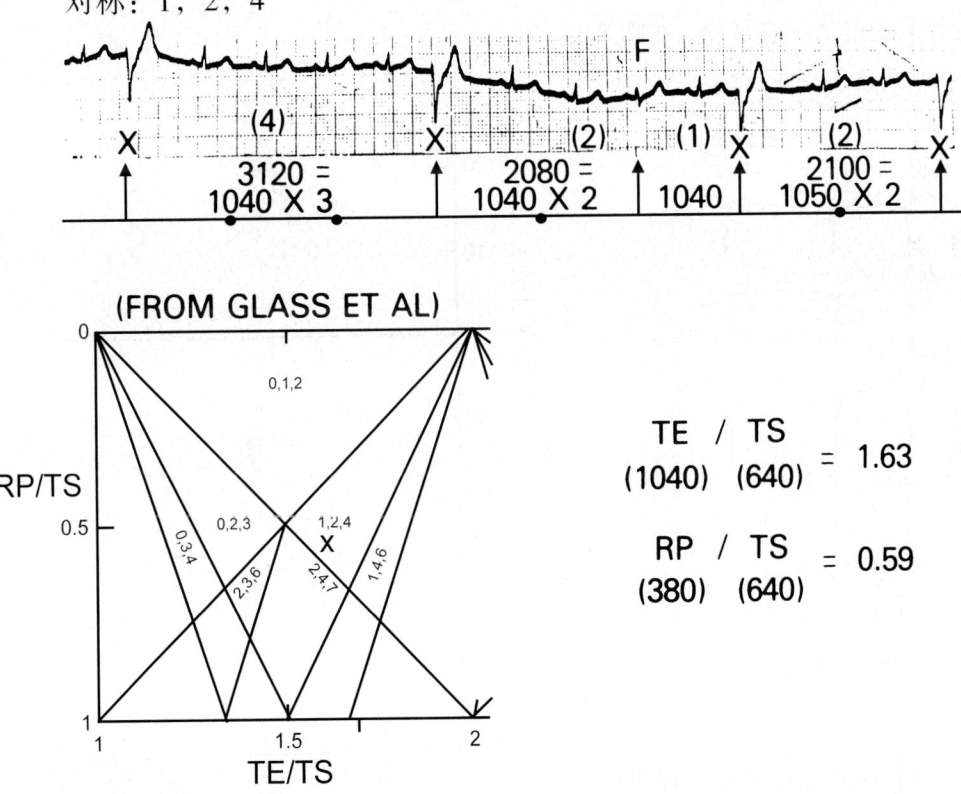

图 80-1 显性的典型的室性并行心律　F，融合波（同样被视为显性搏动）正文下方心电图描绘的是，根据不应期（RP）/窦性周期（TS）、异位搏动周期（TE）/窦性周期（TS）两个比值，数学推算的异位搏动之间窦性搏动的数目。参数之间的 X 位点，对应该格内推算出的窦性搏动的数目。推算出来的窦性搏动的数目（1，2，4）显示在心电图的下方。图 80-1 至图 80-4 中，心动周期值均以毫秒表示。（引自 Castellanos A, Fernandez P, Moleiro F, et al: Symmetry, broken symmetry, and restored symmetry of apparent pure ventricular parasystole. Am J Cardiol 68：256-259，1991，Copyright 1991，with permission from Excerpta Medica Inc.）

的数[24]。关于自发性和起搏诱发的室性并行心律的几个临床研究已证实了这一点[19,20,23]。

图80-1举例说明多年来所公认的室性并行心律的特征[1-3]。在这份心电图中，上述有关的两个比值分别为0.59和1.63，相应部位"X"标明3个推算出来的结果（1、2和4），它们正好是显性并行心搏之间窦性搏动的数目（括号内，心电图下方）[24]。尽管该研究和其他报道证实可以预测典型室性并行节律点的活动规律，但是，由于窦性周期和异位搏动周期经常出现自发的（有时不规则的）变化[23]，临床心电记录中常见的室性并行节律点的活动规律被打破。事实上，一个完全的、持续存在的对称现象，仅见于持续心房和心室起搏条件下心房率和心室率保持稳定时。

四、电张性调整的室性并行心律的心电图特征

在Jalife和Moe（大约1976年完成）[23,26]及其他研究者经最初的微电极研究之后，观察到，在临床心电图记录中，常发生电张性调整的室性并行心律[2,4,22,26-31]。为了描述这种心律失常的心电图特征，常使用以下几个名称：X＝并行心律的搏动；R＝非并行心律的搏动，X-X＝两个连续的并行心律搏动之间的间期，其间不含任何间位的非并行心律的搏动（即非电张性调整的异位搏动的周期）；X-R＝并行心律搏动和紧随其后的非并行心律搏动之间的间期；以及X-R-X＝两个连续的并行心律搏动之间的间期，其间含有一个间位的非并行心律搏动（电张性调整的异位搏动周期）[2]。

图80-2举例所示，可以看到所有的间期均被标准化为占异位搏动周期（可直接测量）的百分比。异位搏动周期为1200ms（100％），非并行心律搏动发生在X-R间期为42％（图A）和50％（图B）两处，分别使X-R-X间期延长到117％和122％。图C，X-R间期轻度延长为53％，使情况发生逆转，使X-R-X间期缩短为80％。图D中，X-R-X间期进一步缩短，以至于使并行心律的冲动落在非并行心律搏动的不应

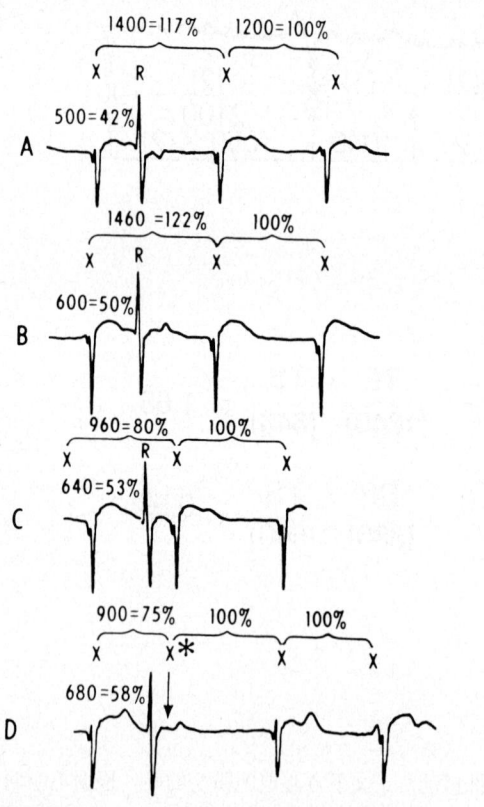
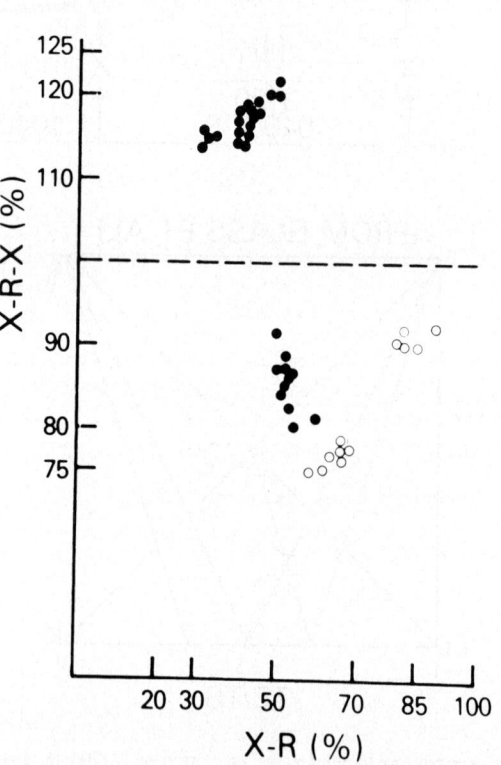

图80-2 电张性调整的室性并行心律　在相应的双相反应曲线（右）中，X-R-X间期（电张性调整的并行心律周期）与X-R间期相关，X-R-X间期标准化为占异位搏动周期的百分比（与水平线的交点处为100％），右图空圈代表隐匿的并行异位激动的发放。（引自Castellanos A, Luceiro F, et al: Annihilation, entrainment and modulation of ventricular parasystolic rhythms. Am J Cardiol 54: 317-322, 1984, Copyright 1984, with permission from Excerpta Medica Inc.）

期。导致一个隐匿性冲动的发放（X*），发放时间的确定（垂直箭头所示）仅能根据其后非电张性调整的并行心律（要求是显性的）减去100%来推断。

正如实验研究所显示的，非并行搏动的电张性调整作用可以用一条阶段反应曲线来表示，横坐标是X-R间期，纵坐标是X-R-X间期相对于X-X间期的偏离程度（%），最初描述的临床阶段反应曲线与代表X-X间期的水平线呈双相关系[2,4,25-28]。图80-2（右）显示，随着X-R的延长，X-R-X进行性延长（延迟阶段），直到达到最大值。此后，曲线关系反转，直到出现最大幅度X-R-X缩短（往往位于异位搏动周期的中部），此后，曲线转向水平线（加速阶段）。常可见到有重复的（X-R-X）数值，特别是接近或处于拐点时。分析其他已发表的阶段反应曲线，结果显示，非并行搏动的激动靠近下一个并行搏动时可引起：（1）最大延迟；（2）最大加速度；（3）调整作用减小；（4）几乎不起作用；（5）起搏点的消失（见下文）。双相反应曲线依延迟作用或缩短作用孰占优势，可以是对称的或非对称的[2,30]。

三相反应曲线越来越多地见诸报道[2,30,31]，主要见于当非并行搏动发生在异位搏动周期的早期，即在并行搏动的超常期对其进行夺获[2,30,31]。

五、起搏点的湮灭

生物振荡（oscillation）系统在受到来自它周围的外界刺激的干扰时，自律性活动会消失。Jalife和Antzelevitch[32,33]首先报道，应用蔗糖裂解技术，在狗的窦房结和浦肯野纤维的组织片上，当适时的阈下刺激跨越缝隙连接在精确的时间到达作用部位时，可以突然终止其自律性活动（"起搏点的湮灭"）。Rosenthal和Ferrier在具有自律性（在电流作用下产生除极诱发的自律性）的标本上，Gilmour和Zipes在患者的心室肌组织片上，均观察到这一现象[2]。

Jalife和Antzelevitch[32]首先根据Winfree的学说：振荡系统时相重整（phase-resetting）解释他们的发现，在这一学说中微分拓扑学技术得到应用。应

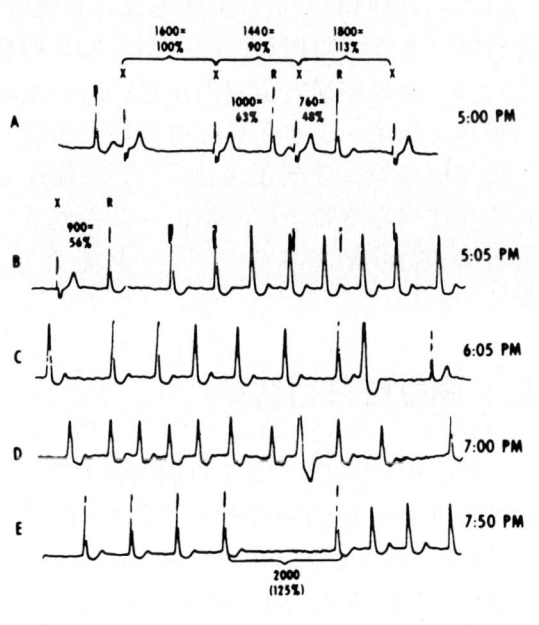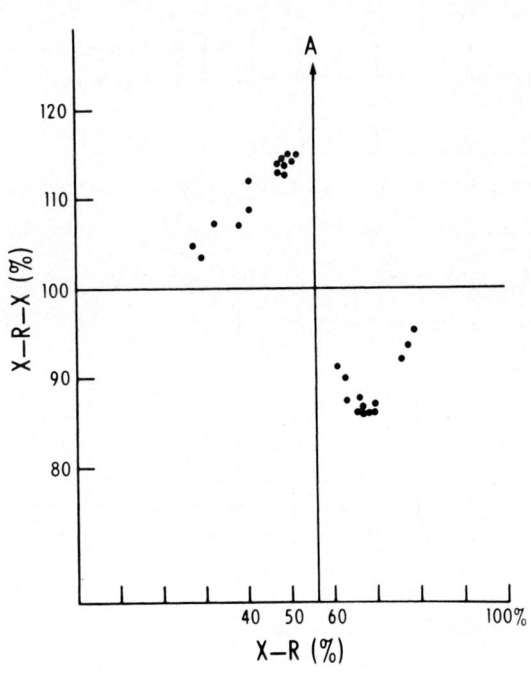

图80-3　一位房颤患者可能出现的起搏点湮灭现象　A图：X-X间期为1600ms（100%），有一个非并行心律搏动发生在X-R间期760ms（48%）处，使X-R-X间期延长至1800ms（113%），而发生于X-R间期1000ms（63%）处，使X-R-X间期缩短为90%。B图：非并行心律搏动发生在一个并行心律搏动之后900ms（56%），明显导致并行心律起搏点湮灭。因为，在此后8h心电监测中未再见到显性的并行心律搏动（B～E图），尽管在这个病人观察到室上性心搏周期存在显著变化，且非并行心律R-R间期比最长的（延长的）异位搏动周期还长（A）。相应的阶段反应曲线揭示，起搏点湮灭现象发生于非并行心律搏动（R）落入异位心搏周期（X-X）的拐点（大约位于异位心搏周期的56%处，即X-R=56%）。（引自Castellanos A, Luceiro F, et al: Annihilation, entrainment and modulation of ventricular parasystolic rhythms. Am J Cardiol 54：317-322，1984 Copyright 1984，with permission from Excerpta Medica Inc.）

用 Hodgkin-Huxley 模型，在不同膜除极电压时，反复发放刺激，可以验证起搏点的湮灭现象[33]。对某一范围的除极电流强度，相当于含有一个可以终止基本节律的"单一"点（"singular" point）[32,33]。

然而，也有可能，大多数生物节律不会被消灭，理由是这种外界节律根本不会再次出现。在大多数实验研究中，起搏点的兴奋性即使被抑制，也是一过性的。因为，抑制起搏点兴奋性的外界刺激，导致阈下膜电位振荡，振荡持续时间进行性延长，经过一段不确定的时间，再次达到阈电位。在另一些研究中，起搏点兴奋性的抑制似乎是永久的（图 80-3）[32,34]，因此，临时抑制可等同于（表现为）较长时间的重整[32-34]。尽管如此，这一现象与其他临床情况（如：病态窦房结或不稳定的室性自主节律）中观察到的持续性重整很可能不一样，在后一种情况时，很可能一个完整的动作电位（非电刺激诱发的除极）会影响未受保护的自律点的节律[2]。时相重整（phase-resetting）、双稳定性（bistabilities）和起搏点湮灭（annihilation）的电模型，对帮助人们理解这些现象，是有启发性的[2]。

六、并行心律的拖带现象

根据振荡学说，与应用于各种实验模型和折返性心律的微电极研究一样，拖带可被定义为：一个自我维系的振荡系统与一个外力振荡的耦联[35-37]。考虑调整后的并行心律，产生的干扰可能是任何一个能调整并行心律的再发非并行心律，这种调整取决于与并行阶段同期的时相[2,26,37,38]。如图 80-4 描记的病人，非并行搏动与并行搏动间的相互作用导致了阶段性的隐性和显性的 1：1 拖带。在此阶段并行心律被改变为和快或慢一些的非并行心律相同。此类拖带与折返性心律失常如房扑、室上速和室速不同。

拖带是一种多因素功能：（1）并行与非并行（窦性）心律间的关系，也就是说，有效的异位/非并行性（窦性）周期长度的比率；（2）调整作用幅度；（3）循环中逆转位点的位置；（4）尤其是导致这种现象的第一个非并行心搏循环发生的时刻（用 X 线间期标识）受到了关注[2,37,38]。除此之外，并行心律能被心室肌中产生保护（自主调节）部位附近的电除极所调整[2,36,30,37]，也能发生自身拖带[37,39]。

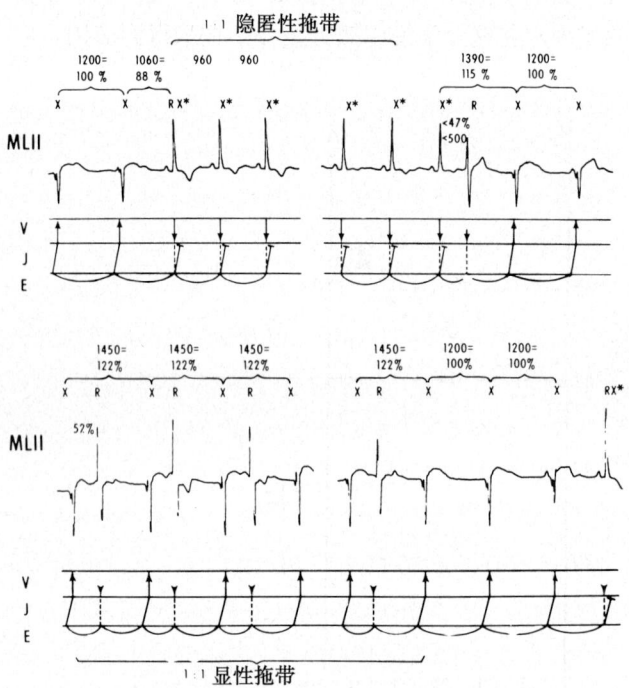

图 80-4 调整后室性并行心律的拖带现象　左上，记述了由非并行心律搏动出现在较晚期诱发的一阵隐匿的 1：1 拖带，发生在循环的加速阶段。右上，记述的是发生在循环前半阶段一阵非并行心律搏动终止了的拖带。在拖带中，并行心律被非并行心律搏动所增加。下面记述的是在循环的早期和延迟阶段分别出现和消失的非并行心律搏动所引起和终止的一阵 1：1 拖带（引自 Castellanos A, Luceri RM, Moleiro F, et al：Annihilation, entrainment and modulation of ventricular parasystolic rhythms. Am J Cardiol 54：317-322，1984，copyright 1984，with permission from Excerpta Medica Inc.）

七、间歇性并行心律

Schorf 等学者[1,40]最早对间歇性并行心律（不要与显性并行心律的间歇性相混淆）有过以下描述："室性异位节律点周期性的显现与消失……不会被主导节律（窦性节律）的冲动所干扰"（异位节律点自律性间歇性改变所致）。如图 80-5 所示，在心电记录图 80-5B 后半部分，突然出现非电张性调整的室性心律，而且在心电记录图 80-5C 中，该异位节律表现为"温醒"现象，随后，在图 80-5D 中，异位节律逐渐"冷却"，并最后消失（图 80-5E）。

近来，间歇性并行心律的概念常用于描述室性并行心律的一种特殊类型，认为在该类型的并行心律中，"完全性"的传入保护只存在于异位节律周期的前半部分，而落入后半部分的主导节律（窦律）冲

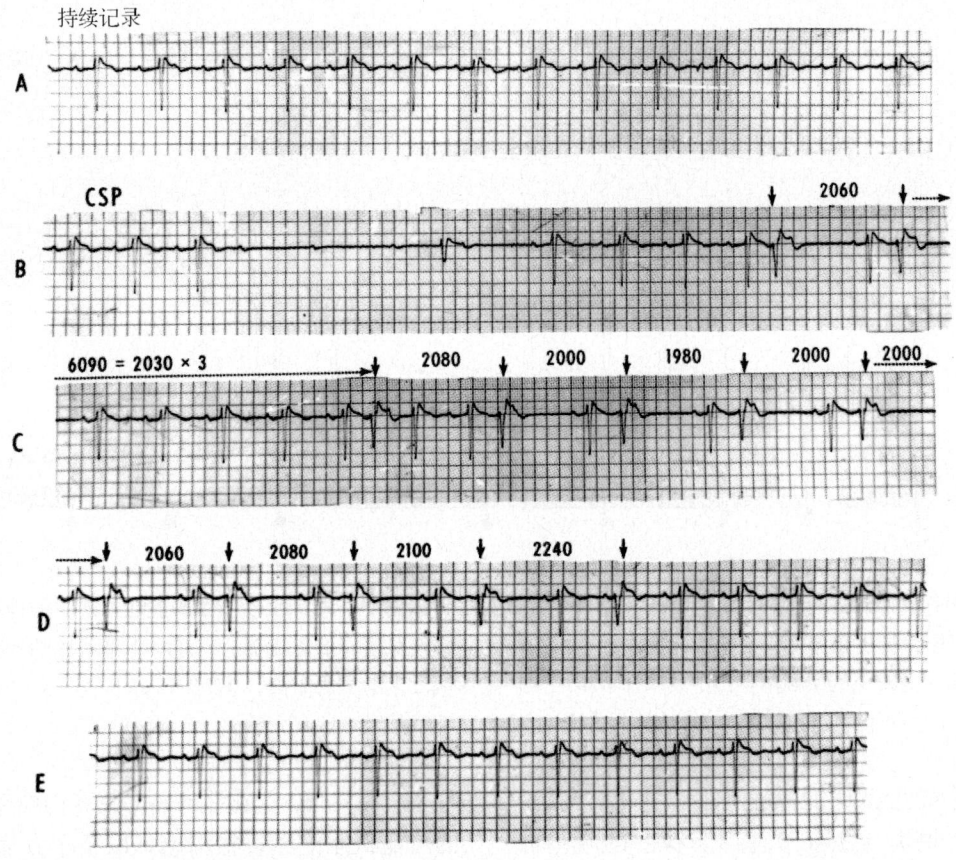

图 80-5　间歇性单纯性室性并行心律　A 图为窦性心律；B 图表示，颈动脉窦按摩（CSP）后出现室性并行心律，周期为 2060ms；C 图表示室性并行心律经过"温醒"阶段，周期缩短为 1980ms；D 图表示室性并行心律逐渐"冷却"；E 图中，室性并行心律消失。尽管可能存在其他的机制，但图中所示为室性并行心律在动态心电图中最常见的表现。

动可以侵入，进而重整或者暂时终止异位节律[2,4,41,42]。

在图 80-6 中，最早出现的 3 个异位搏动中，X-R-X 间期轻微缩短（1180ms 到 1140ms，图上部数字是以百分之一秒作为时间单位）与 X-R 间期的缩短有关。X-R 间期和 X-R-X 间期之间存在着双相关系。因此考虑该异位节律为单纯的、非电张性调整的并行心律，频率为 51～52bpm。第 3 个异位搏动之后，出现 1 个窦性搏动（标记为 X_R），间期为 810ms，该窦性冲动使异位节律点发生节律重整，冲动再次传出后，与前一窦性冲动的配对间期（X_R-X）为 1180ms，与重整前的异位节律周期相似。从图 80-6 底部的时间栏推断异位节律周期的前 750ms 范围存在传入保护。因此，第 4 个异位搏动后出现的窦性搏动，其后在预期时间内并未出现异位搏动（X'）。X_R-X' 间期约为 1140ms，接近异位节律的周期。因为此时心室肌并非处于不应期，异位节律冲动突然不能穿越周围保护区激动心室的原因考虑存在Ⅱ型传出阻滞[8]。但是，窦性冲动也使部分异位节律点周围保护区的心肌处于不应期，从而阻止了后续主导节律的传入（如心电图上第 10 个心搏所示）。在心电图记录的后半部，也能见到相似的现象。因此，通过解释上述现象，推断并行心律并非单纯性，而是间歇性的，其节律周期的前半部存在传入保护和间歇性的Ⅱ型传出阻滞。

上述现象也可以用电张性调整作用的概念解释[30,43]，由于电张性调整作用产生异位节律的夺获加速，使延迟相早期的强度下降到体表心电图不能检测的水平，而此时加速相处于最大水平[30,43]。尽管如此，仍可能存在传出阻滞。而 Kinoshita 等学者[44]提出另外的解释，他们认为二度Ⅰ型和Ⅱ型传入阻滞的并存（而非传出阻滞）可以导致这种现象的发生。

八、并行心律的间歇性：摘要说明

为了正确理解间歇性并行心律的概念，必须了解

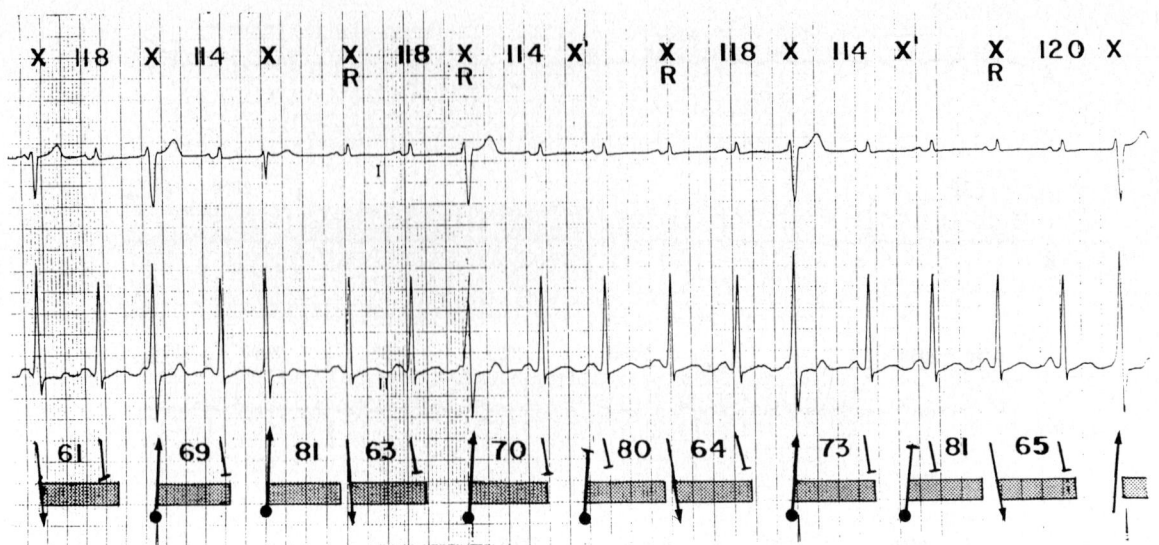

图 80-6 间歇性单纯性室性并行心律,并行心律周期前半部分存在传入保护,即持续电张性调整性并行心律伴延迟相早期强度下降,X 代表并行心律传出阻滞 水平条带代表并行心律存在完全传入保护时的周期部分,此时主导节律的冲动对并行心律的周期无明显的影响。为避免交叉混淆,图中没有标示传入保护区远端发生的传出阻滞。(引自 Castellanos A,Moleiro F,Guerrero J et al:Intermittent parasystole with exit block. J Electrocardial 30:331-335,1997.)

显性并行心律间歇性出现的其他原因,包括:(1)室性并行节律的频率与主导节律(窦律)的频率相等或恰好等于窦性频率的一半时,由于部分异位节律的冲动落入窦性搏动的不应期内,因而表现出显性并行心律的间歇性[2];(2)由于窦性冲动在周围保护区的隐匿性传导,使异位节律不能传出,称为隐匿的单纯性室性并行心律[2,45];(3)存在较长时间的传出阻滞;(4)传入阻滞(或传入保护)的消失。此外,动态心电图在诊断"持续性"并行心律中的价值需要重新评估[10,12,22,23]。尽管有些室性并行心律可以发作较长的时间,但是心电图长期监测的结果表明这只是个例,并非常见的情况[2]。何谓"持续性"并行心律呢?举例来说,如果某次发作的并行心律,符合"持续性"的特征,但它具有明显的时间性,只在下午 1 时到 3 时之间发作(其他 22 小时无发作),这应该诊断为"持续性"并行心律,还是并行心律持续两小时呢[22]?在现代医学的大部分领域,专家们的意见是趋向一致的,但对于室性并行心律,情况并非如此。

九、并行心律的异化和消退

2001 年,Surawicz 等[3]强调室性并行心律的发生率目前并不清楚,这是众所周知的,不足为惊奇。在本文,从图 80-1 到图 80-6,学者们对于室性并行心律的可能机制已经备感困惑,以至于大家都避免对并行心律的异化现象进行过多的解释[5]。但并行心律的异化现象不仅具有学术研究价值,也具有临床应用的意义,并可能导致新的技术设备的出现,例如 Takayagani 及同事发明的转速计[11,12]。总之,由于目前认为室性并行心律缺乏重要的临床意义[3],因此对它的研究主要限于学术研究领域。

(葛堪忆 译)

参 考 文 献

1. Scherf D, Schott A: Extrasystoles and Allied Arrhythmias, 2nd ed. Chicago, Year Book, 1973, pp 269–281.
2. Castellanos A, Saoudi N, Moleiro F, Myerburg RJ: Parasystole. In Zipes D, Jalife J (eds): Cardiac Electrophysiology: From Cell to Bedside, 2nd ed. Philadelphia, WB Saunders, 1995, pp 942–954.
3. Surawicz B, Knilans TK: Chou's Electrocardiography in Clinical Practice. Adult and Pediatric, 5th ed. Philadelphia, WB Saunders, 2001, pp 401–403.
4. Oreto G, Luzza F, Satullo G, Donato A: Parasystole. Revista Latina de Cardiologia 12:268–277, 1991.
5. Castellanos A, Myerburg RJ: Parasystolic alienation: An impression or a reality? J Cardiovasc Electrophysiol 11:178–179, 2000.
6. Grolleau R, Pasquie JL, Macia JC, Leclercq F: Parasystole. Arch Mal Coeur Vasiss 95:5:41–46, 2002.
7. Ren Z, Zhou J, Xu G, et al: The diagnostic criteria for classic parasystole. Chin Med J 112:992–994, 1999.
8. Kinoshita S, Katoh T, Mitsuoka T, et al: Ventricular parasystolic couplets originating in the pathway between the ventricle and the parasystole pacemaker: Mechanism of "irregular" parasystole. J Electrocardiol

34:251–260, 2001.
9. Martinez-Lopez JI: ECG of the month. Contenders. Ventricular parasystole. J La State Med Soc 153:9–11, 2001.
10. Sapoznikov D, Luria MH, Gotsman MS: Enhancing long-term ECG monitoring with graphic analysis of coupling intervals. J Electrocardiol 33:137–145, 2000.
11. Takayanagi K, Tanaka K, Kamishirado H, et al: Direct discrimination and full-day disclosure of ventricular parasystolic heart rate tachograms. J Cardiovasc Electrophysiol 11:168–177, 2000.
12. Takayanagi K, Kamishirado H, Iwasaki Y, et al: Cycle bursts of ventricular premature contractions of more than one minute intervals. Jpn Heart J 40:135–144, 1999.
13. Kuwabara T, Watanabe Y: A case of ventricular parasystole with high-grade exit block. J Cardiovasc Electrophysiol 7:684–687, 1996.
14. Singh VK: Numerology of ventricular parasystole. Chest 109:1663, 1996.
15. Kinoshita S, Ogawa S, Mitsuoka T: Reverse effects of exercise on the sinus and parasystolic cycle length. J Electrocardiol 29:131–137, 1996.
16. Itoh E, Aizawa Y, Washizuka T, et al: Two cases of ventricular parasystole associated with ventricular tachycardia. Pacing Clin Electrophysiol 19:370–373, 1996.
17. Tomcsanyi J, Tenczer J, Horvath L: Effect of adenosine on ventricular parasystole. J Electrocardiol 29:61–63, 1996.
18. Castellanos A, Moleiro F, Interian A Jr, Myerburg RJ: A different approach to the analysis of pure ventricular parasystole. Chest 107:1463–1464, 1995.
19. Saoudi N, Letac B, Castellanos A: An electronic model for evaluating the dynamics of perfect pure parasystole the human heart. Am J Cardiol 75:739–742, 1995.
20. Castellanos A, Moleiro F: Numerology of ventricular parasystole. Chest 119:1663, 1996.
21. Kinoshita S: Concealed bigeminy. Irregular parasystole and allied arrhythmias. In Kinoshita S (ed): A Collection of Papers Published in American and European Journals 1991–2000, 2nd ed. Sapporo, Japan, 2001.
22. Satullo G, Oreto G, Cavallaro L: Le molte facce del ritmo parasistolico. G Ital Cardiol 23:699–712, 1993.
23. Castellanos A, Fernandez P, Moleiro F, et al: Symmetry, broken symmetry, and restored symmetry of apparent pure ventricular parasystole. Am J Cardiol 68:256–259, 1991.
24. Glass L, Goldberger AL, Belair J: Dynamics of pure parasystole. Am J Physiol 251:H841–H847, 1986.
25. Jalife J, Moe GK: Effect of electrotonic potentials on pacemaker activity of canine Purkinje fibers in relation to parasystole. Circ Res 39:801–808, 1976.
26. Jalife J, Moe GK: A biological model of parasystole. Am J Cardiol 43:761–772, 1979.
27. Satullo G, Carbone V, Calabro MP, Oreto G: An irregular escape rhythm: What is the mechanism? J Cardiovasc Electrophysiol 13:1056–1057, 2002

28. Satullo G, Donato A, Busa G, Cavallaro L: Irregular sinus parasystole due to intermittency and modulation of parasystolic activity. J Cardiovasc Electrophysiol 7:259–262, 1996.
29. Kasaoka Y, Ajiki K, Hayami N, Murakawa Y: His-Bundle parasystole masquerading as exercise-induced 2:1 atrioventricular block. J Cardiovasc Electrophysiol 12:965–967, 2001.
30. Antzelevitch C, Jalife J, Moe GK: Electrotonic modulation of pacemaker activity: Further biological and mathematical observations on the behavior of modulated parasystole. Circulation 66:1225–1232, 1982.
31. Oreto G, Satullo G, Luzza F, et al: Supernormal modulation of ventricular parasystole: The triphasic phase-response curve. Am J Cardiol 58:283–290, 1986.
32. Jalife J, Antzelevitch C: Phase resetting and annihilation of pacemaker activity in cardiac tissue. Science 206:695–697, 1979.
33. Jalife J, Antzelevitch C: Pacemaker annihilation: Diagnostic and therapeutic implications. Am Heart J 100:128–130, 1980.
34. Cranefield PF: The causes of arrhythmias. In Cranefield PF (ed): The Conduction of the Cardiac Impulse. Mount Kisco, NY, Futura, 1975, pp 267–268.
35. Winfree AT: Oscillatory glycolysis in yeast: The pattern of phase resetting by oxygen. Arch Biochem Biophys 149:388–401, 1972.
36. Guevara MR, Glass L: Phase locking, period doubling bifurcations and chaos in a mathematical model of a periodically driven oscillator: A theory for the entrainment of biological oscillators and the generation of cardiac dysrrhythmias. J Math Biol 14:1–23, 1982.
37. Moe GK, Jalife J, Mueller WJ, Moe B: A mathematical model of parasystole and its application to clinical arrhythmias. Circulation 56:968–979, 1977.
38. Castellanos A, Luceri RM, Moleiro F, et al: Annihilation, entrainment and modulation of ventricular parasystolic rhythms. Am J Cardiol 54:317–332, 1985.
39. Castellanos A, Mendoza IJ, Saoudi N, Jalife J: Ventricular tachycardia with alternating cycle lengths: Self-entrainment of parasystolic rhythm? Pacing Clin Electrophysiol 11:1291–1295, 1988.
40. Scherf D, Boyd LJ: Three unusual cases of parasystole. Am Heart J 39:650–663, 1950.
41. Satullo G, Donato A, Busa G, Cavallaro L: Irregular sinus parasystole due to intermittency and modulation of parasystolic activity. J Cardiovasc Electrophysiol 7:259–262, 1996.
42. Castellanos A, Moleiro F, Guerrero J, et al: Intermittent parasystole with exit block. J Electrocardiol 30:4:331–335, 1997.
43. Jalife J, Antzelevitch C, Moe GK: The case for modulated parasystole. Pacing Clin Electrophysiol 5:911–926, 1982.
44. Kinoshita S: Mechanisms of intermittent ventricular parasystole due to type II second degree entrance block. J Electrocardiol 16:7–14, 1983.
45. Oreto G, Scimone IG, Satullo G: Failure of parasystolic impulses to appear on schedule: Exit block due to concealed conduction of sinus impulses. J Electrocardiol 25:355–359, 1992.

第 81 章

宽 QRS 波心动过速的鉴别诊断

John M. Miller, Mithilesh K. Das, Rishi Arora, Cesar Alberte-Lista, and Jianyi Wu

本章目录

- 宽 QRS 波心动过速的鉴别诊断 …… 736
- 宽 QRS 波心动过速：诊断策略 …… 743
- 宽 QRS 波心动过速：特殊情况 …… 745
- 总结 …… 745

临床经常会遇到这种情况，一位医生拿着一份宽 QRS 波心动过速的心电图说："我该如何鉴别清楚！"。对临床医生来说，宽 QRS 波心动过速的诊断确实是一个难题，因此建立一套诊断标准和流程有着重要意义。无论对正在发作中的心动过速的终止，还是以后的长期治疗，作出正确的诊断都十分重要。例如：很多医生会将一个血流动力学稳定的宽 QRS 波心动过速确认为室上性心动过速，因为传统的观点认为"室速患者的血流动力学是不稳定的"。病人发生了室速就会出现收缩功能减退，此时，如果按照室上速的治疗给予维拉帕米注射，可能会导致严重的低血压，原本稳定的状态很快就会恶化。初始不正确的诊断会导致随后误入歧途的治疗，因此对宽 QRS 波心动过速的机制作出正确的诊断至关重要。

已有几个指标有助于宽 QRS 波心动过速的鉴别诊断，尽管没有一项完美，但还是能够指导医生对大多数病人作出正确的诊断。本章将阐述宽 QRS 波心动过速的病因，以及用来正确诊断的标准。由于宽 QRS 波心动过速病人的状态不允许医生从容地去分析心电图资料，因此这些诊断标准不仅要精确，还应容易记住。

本章中宽 QRS 波心动过速的定义：心动过速的频率≥100bpm，QRS 波时限≥120ms。室速是指起源于希氏束以下的心动过速；室上速是指起源于希氏束以上的心动过速；左束支阻滞（LBBB）形态的心动过速：是指 QRS 波时限≥120ms，V_1 导联主波为负向；右束支阻滞（RBBB）形态的心动过速：是指 QRS 波时限≥120ms，V_1 导联主波为正向。左束支阻滞和右束支阻滞只是描述 QRS 波的形态，并不代表实际的希浦系统疾病。

一、宽 QRS 波心动过速的鉴别诊断

临床表现为宽 QRS 波心动过速的心律失常有几种，广义区分即室性心动过速、室上性心动过速伴室内传导异常和心室起搏节律（图 81-1）。

1. 室性心动过速：是人群中最常见的宽 QRS 波心动过速，占宽 QRS 波心动过速约 80% 以上[1]，这一发生比率对于宽 QRS 波心动过速的患者已具有诊断意义。

2. 室上性心动过速伴室内传导异常：所占的比例比室速低，约为 15%～30%，其包括多种异常。

a. 室上性心动过速伴室内差异性传导：束支阻滞可以是永久或"固定"的（在正常窦性心律时就已存在），也可以是"功能性"的（只在心动过速时出现）。功能性差异性传导是指心率增快到一定程度时，希浦系统已处于递减传导状态之中，而出现部分或不完全性激动。

b. 存在房室间异常连接的室上性心动过速（WPW 综合征时的预激性心动过速）：由于连接心房和心室的通路位于房室瓣环处，预激性心动过速需要与起源于基底部的室性心动过速鉴别，其心电图的胸前导联 R 波表现为正向同向性和进行性变化，而不是

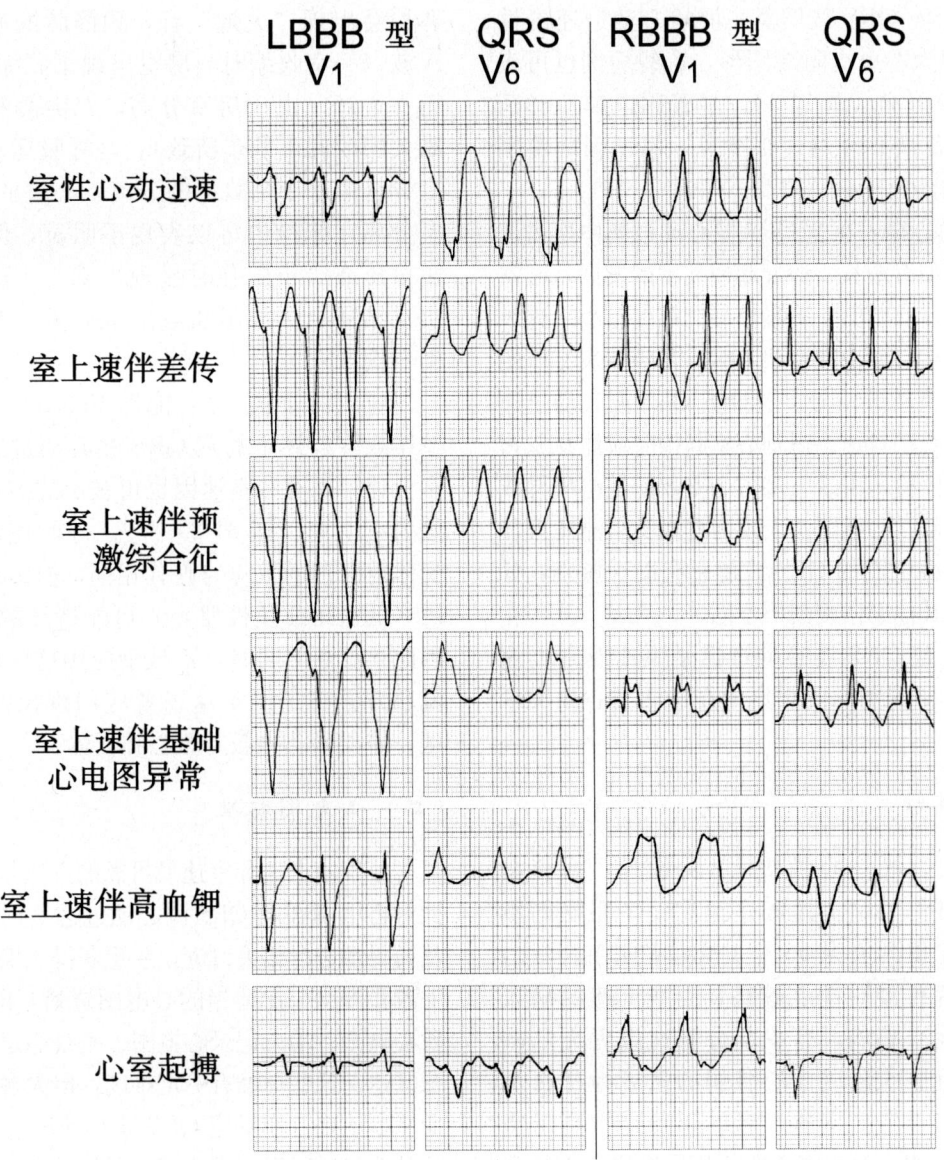

图 81-1 不同类型宽 QRS 波心动过速的右束支阻滞（RBBB）和左束支阻滞（LBBB）时 V_1 和 V_6 导联 QRS 波的形态　不同情况时，QRS 波形态的相似和差别可以识别。

负向同向性（只在少见的房束旁路相关性心动过速时可见）时[2]，预激性心动过速占宽 QRS 波心动过速的比例较小，约为 1%~5%。

c. 由于心室肌内激动传导异常导致的宽 QRS 波室上性心动过速：在这种情况下，希浦系统的传导相对正常，但在窦性心律时就出现右束支阻滞、左束支阻滞或非特异性的室内传导障碍。以右室切开术后病人的右束支阻滞图形为例（如：法洛四联症修补术），右室传导延迟是右室流出道的心室肌间传导延迟所致；而扩张型心肌病病人的左束支阻滞图形是弥漫的左室心肌内的传导延迟所致，而不是希浦系统疾病[3]。在先心病或心肌病中，宽 QRS 波的形态复杂多样。

d. 因药物或电解质紊乱导致的伴宽 QRS 波的室上性心动过速：大剂量的钠通道阻滞剂可引起非特异性的 QRS 波增宽，这可以使原本是窄 QRS 波的室上性心动过速出现宽 QRS 波形态，可误诊为室速。IA 类药物（普鲁卡因胺、奎尼丁和双异丙比胺）、IC 类药物（氟卡尼、英卡尼和普罗帕酮）和胺碘酮均可产生此类效应。另外，在无器质性心脏病和室性心律失常病史的年轻人群中[4]，IC 类药物可以在运动试验中触发持续性单形性室性心动过速。IC 类药物还能通过减慢房扑时的心房率而使房扑呈 1∶1 传导，并伴 QRS 波的增宽。鉴别这种心律失常对治疗十分重要。高血钾也能使 QRS 波增宽，混淆心动过速的性质，典型者表现为左束支阻滞图形，有些病例也可表现为右束支阻滞图形（图 81-1）。尽管因电解质和药物引起的宽 QRS 波心动过速很少见，但正确地鉴别并给病人适宜的治疗十分重要[5]。

3. 心室起搏心律：在宽 QRS 波心动过速中所占比例很小，但近年却有增长。随着起搏技术的发展，心室夺获的能量变小，心电图上刺激信号的幅度较小。这种病人发生室上速或心室快频率跟随时，常规体表心电图不容易识别出起搏脉冲信号。这种宽 QRS 波心动过速容易被误为室性心动过速。识别心室起搏时应注意起搏器相关的病史、体检，由于大多数心室起搏的电极导线植入在右室心尖部，心电图常表现为左束支阻滞图形伴电轴左偏。起搏心电图的 QRS 波形态有助于鉴别，如果起搏电极位于其他部位则图形不同。

由于大多数宽 QRS 波心动过速是室速或室上速伴束支阻滞，所要鉴别的要点集中在这两类心律失常上。

(一) 病史和体检

心脏病病史（既往心肌梗死、心绞痛，或充血性心力衰竭）可作为室上速和室速的一个粗略的鉴别指标，其阳性预测值为 95%（相对室速而言）[6]，大多数室速患者有器质性心脏病，而室上速的病人则有或无器质性心脏病。有少部分室速患者无基础心脏病，而有明显的器质性心脏病的患者为什么不易患室上速原因不清。室速患者的年龄通常高于室上速患者（>35 岁）。室上速的患者既往常有心律失常发作病史，如果病人心动过速的发作史在 3 年以上，室上速的可能性大于室速。而那些既往有心肌梗死病史，初次发作宽 QRS 波心动过速者，则室速的可能性更大[7]。

在宽 QRS 波心动过速发作时，病人的整体状况并不是一个准确的诊断指标，大多数室上速患者的血流动力学稳定，但有相当比例的室速患者血流动力学也是稳定的，他们的主诉可能就是胸闷和轻度头晕[8]。大多数的观点认为宽 QRS 波心动过速时，如果血流动力学稳定则应诊断室上速，这是错误的，甚至会导致有损害性的错误治疗。如前所述，血流动力学稳定的室速患者当作室上速推注维拉帕米进行终止治疗时会出现血流动力学的恶化。

随后我们将会讨论的房室分离是鉴别宽 QRS 波心动过速十分有用的一项指标。当房室存在分离时，体检会出现"大炮"音，颈静脉的波形可以表现出 A 波（心室收缩时心房也出现了收缩）、不同强度的第一心音（由于房室分离，二尖瓣和三尖瓣的开放和关闭时间不同步所致）、与呼吸运动不相关的血压变异（由于心房收缩的分离，心室的灌注不同）。房室分离在体检中可以表现不明显，但在进行颈动脉窦按压或给予腺苷时显现出来[9]。这些方法可产生房室结逆向传导阻滞或房室分离，有助于室速的诊断（图 81-2）。

应用物理学方法：能经 Valsalva 动作、颈动脉窦按压或腺苷终止的宽 QRS 波心动过速则强烈提示为室上速。而有些室速因也可被上述方法终止，常被误诊为室上速（图 81-2）[10-14]。静脉应用维拉帕米或 β 受体阻滞剂的效应与腺苷相同，但是这些药物的副作用（低血压或负性肌力）可能持续数分钟至 1 小时，因此在诊断不明时，不鼓励应用这些药物。有报道血流动力学稳定的室速患者应用维拉帕米后出现低血压，需要紧急抢救乃至心肺复苏[15]。

(二) 心电图标准

鉴别室上速和室速最可靠的方法是心电图。下面将针对心电图在宽 QRS 波心动过速鉴别诊断中的标准以及局限性进行相关讨论。要想获得正确的分析，临床医生需要提供一份适当的心电图资料，即高质量的 12 导联心电图、动态记录心电图、基线稳定。在心脏急症状态下达到这些标准有一定难度，但大多数可以做到，至少基本达到。如果宽 QRS 波心动过速是由于室上速伴差异性传导所致，那么 QRS 波的形态一定与束支阻滞或分支阻滞时 QRS 波的形态相似，如果 QRS 波的形态与束支或分支阻滞的形态不可比，则可能不是差异性传导，应考虑室性心动过速[16,17]。因此要求临床医生尽可能熟悉束支阻滞和分支阻滞的各种心电图图形，就可以在宽 QRS 波心动过速时进行心电图的比较，确定是否存在差异性传导。可以应用下列标准鉴别室速和室上速伴差异性传导：

1. QRS 波的时限：Wellens 和他的同事[18]发现 69% 室速的 QRS 波时限大于 140ms，而室上速的 QRS 波时限很少大于 140ms。由于左束支阻滞差传的 QRS 波时限大于右束支阻滞，当类右束支阻滞图形的 QRS 波时限大于 140ms，类左束支阻滞图形的 QRS 时限大于 160ms 时，室速诊断的可能性大。抗心律失常药物可以非特异性地增宽 QRS 波，在这种情况时，这一鉴别标准的价值就会降低。少数情况下，室速患

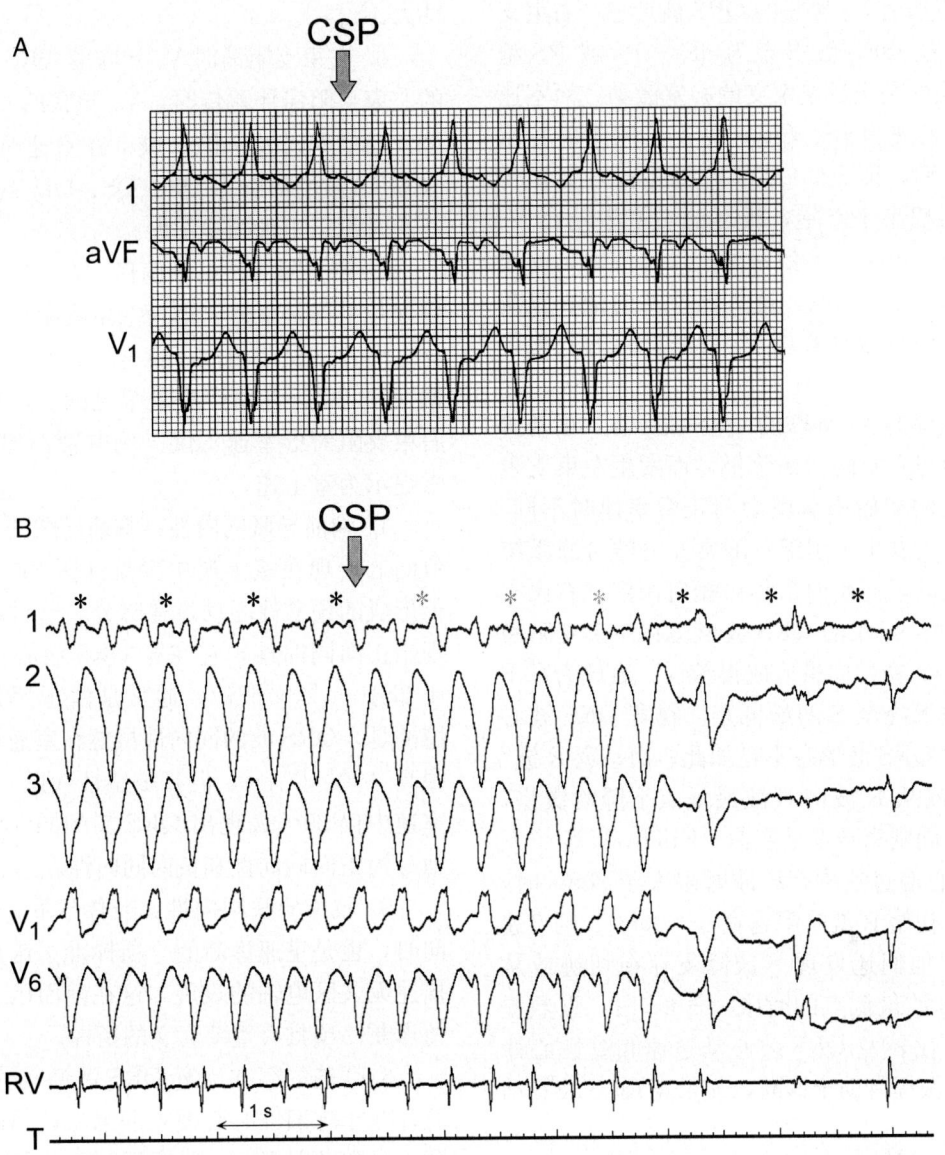

图81-2 室性心动过速经颈动脉窦按压（CSP）的效果 A：左侧为宽QRS波心动过速伴1∶1室房逆传；随后进行颈动脉窦按压，可见室房逆传呈文氏现象，诊断为室速。B：颈动脉窦按压终止了室速，是一种不常见的反应。图自上至下为Ⅰ、Ⅱ、Ⅲ、V_1、V_6导联和心内右室电图的记录。T为时间标记线，星号表示的是P波，淡色星号代表的是未能见到P波的位置。

者的QRS波相对较窄（120～140ms），这常见于不伴器质性心脏病患者。

2. QRS波电轴：一般情况下，电轴越向左偏，室速的可能性比室上速越大。在真正的左前分支阻滞时，QRS波电轴为$-30°\sim-90°$，左后分支阻滞时，QRS波电轴为$+110°\sim+150°$。而在额面电轴有一个象限为$-90°\sim\pm180°$，任何束支阻滞伴左前分支阻滞都不可能达到。因而宽QRS波心动过速伴这种电轴右偏或"西北象限电轴"时，不可能是室上速，而应诊断室速。有人提出窦律下和宽QRS波心动过速时，如果电轴偏差大于40°，提示室速，但不是绝对的[19]。

3. 宽QRS波心动过速时V_1和V_6导联的特殊形态（图81-3）。

a. 右束支阻滞时V_1导联的QRS波形态：心室在正常的初始激动，右室不参与除极，而QRS波初始部分不受右束支差异性传导的影响，V_1导联的QRS波形态在差异性传导时应表现为rSr'、rR'、rsr'或rSR'型。如果QRS波形态呈现单相R波、RS型时R波的时限大于30ms或qR型时，则高度怀疑为室速。后面提到的这些QRS波形态与正常左束支激动的形态不同。

b. 右束支阻滞时 V_6 导联的 QRS 波形态：右束支差传时 V_6 导联的 QRS 波形态为 qRs、Rs 或 RS 型（R/S>1），反映的是经过左束支的心室激动。而室速时 QRS 波形态表现为 rS、Qrs、QS、QR 或单相 R 波，如果为 RS 型，R/S<1。在真正的右束支差传时，因右室的面积小于左室，延迟的右室激动在 V_6 导联形成小 S 波。由于大多数室速起源于左室，室速时 V_6 导联可见较大的 S 波，这不仅反映的是心室激动的右室部分，还有起自背离 V_6 导联部位的其他部分左室激动。

c. 左束支阻滞时 V_1 导联的 QRS 波形态：正常传导时，左束支参与心室的初始除极，而发生左束支阻滞后，心室除极的初始向量就会与正常窦律时不同。然而，尽管左束支发生了阻滞，通常左室的希浦系统被快速传导而激动，初始向量仍可相对保留（右束支参与），这就使 V_1 导联的 QRS 波形态在左束支阻滞时呈 rS 或 QS 型，初始向量形成得较快，表现为窄 R 波、快而平滑地下降至 S 的最低点。在宽 QRS 波心动过速时，如果 QRS 波形态不是如此，而呈宽 R 波/深 S 波、QS 型或从 R 波向 S 波最低点下降时缓慢，与正常激动的不同则意味着是室速。Kindwall 等[20]发现在宽 QRS 波心动过速中，R 波时限大于 30ms 时，可以诊断室速。初始 R 波时限越宽（>30ms）则室速的可能性越大。他们还发现 S 波降支存在切迹或从 QRS 波起始至 S 波最低点的时限≥60ms 时，强烈提示室速。另外，比较宽 QRS 波心动过速和窦性心律时 V_1 导联 R 波振幅有助于诊断，如果宽 QRS 波心动过速时 V_1 导联 R 波振幅高于窦律时，则室速的可能性大。

d. 左束支阻滞时 V_6 导联的 QRS 波形态：在典型的左束支阻滞伴差传时，V_6 导联的 QRS 波初始无 Q 波，而呈 RR' 或单相 R 波。在室速时，常见的 V_6 导联 QRS 波的形态为 QR、QS、QrS 或 Rr' 型，而室上速有时也可出现同样图形。

e. 束支阻滞伴电轴偏移：左束支阻滞图形伴电轴右偏几乎都是室速，因为左束支阻滞性差传永远不会与左后分支阻滞相伴，换言之，右束支阻滞伴电轴不偏（0~90°）在室速中是罕见的（一项研究中 109 例右束支阻滞形室速，仅 3 例电轴不偏[21]），这种情况常提示为室上速。

4. 胸前导联同向性：胸前导联的主波均为正向或负向的表现在室上速中少见（图 81-4），但经旁路前传形成的预激性心动过速除外，这种心动过速可以表现出正向同向性，它在宽 QRS 波心动过速中仅占一小部分（1%~6%），通常是由于 WPW 综合征。遗憾的是，QRS 波的同向性虽然在室速诊断中的特异性很高（90%以上），但其敏感性较低，多数研究显示，室速中仅 20%表现出 QRS 波的同向性[18,21,22]，粗略地分为正向同向性和负向同向性。

5. 肢体导联同向性：肢体导联的 QRS 波均为负向时，也是室速诊断的一项标准。这是从另一个角度描述无人区电轴的表现，这在前面已经强调过，是室速诊断一项具有重要意义的指标。

6. Q 波的存在：宽 QRS 波心动过速时出现的 Q 波存在于陈旧性心肌梗死的患者，因而室速有可能诊断。通常情况下，心肌梗死后发生室速时的 Q 波在心动过速和窦性心律时均存在。这种 Q 波在窦律和心动过速时出现的导联也相似（例如：前壁心肌梗死的患者室速时的 Q 波发生在前壁导联）[24]。有一些扩张型心肌病的患者在室速发作时心电图上也会出现 Q 波，但窦律下却不存在。一些"假性 Q 波"也可以出现在一些室上速中（如：房室结折返性心动过速时，逆传 P 波落在 QRS 波的起始，伪似 Q 波），但较罕见。一些后壁旁路所形成的心室预激可表现为下壁导联的 Q 波。

7. 房室分离：最常用的鉴别室速和室上速的标准仍然是房室的关系。20%~50%的室速中存在完全性房室分离[1,18,25]（敏感性 20%~50%，特异性近 100%），P 波少于 QRS 波的房室分离在室上速伴差传中罕见。房室分离发生率的差异很大，原因是：

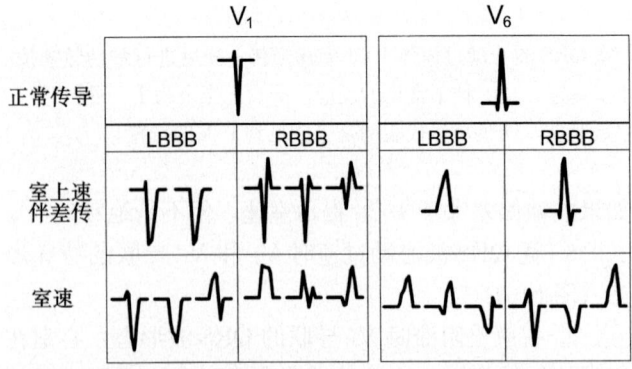

图 81-3 常见的室速和室上速伴差传时 QRS 波的形态　左束支阻滞（LBBB）和右束支阻滞（RBBB）时 V_1 和 V_6 导联 QRS 波形态，注意正常和差异性传导的 QRS 波初始的形态，与室速时 QRS 波形态不同。RS 波形在左、右束支阻滞时均可以见到。

（1）与心动过速的频率有关。心动过速的频率越快，房室分离越不容易分辨，由于舒张期过短，位于 T 波和 QRS 波之间的 P 波不容易识别；（2）受心电图记录时程的影响。在频率较慢的室速中房室分离不易识别的原因，可能与心电图记录的太短有关；（3）与心电图观察者的经验有关。有些病例中，P 波只能被有经验的分析者仔细观察时发现，而容易被无经验者遗漏；（4）与观察者的信心有关。有些心电图的分析过程中，观察者根据个人经验和意愿作出房室分离的诊断。

房室分离是鉴别室速和室上速的最常用指标，室速时房室比例小于 1。除了 20%～50% 的室速患者存在房室分离外，15%～20% 的室速存在二度房室阻滞（呈 2∶1 或文氏传导）。尽管这些表现有助于诊断室速，但在心电图中较难识别。有时，P 波需要将肢体导联放在不同肋间才能记录到（称为 Lewis 导联）。

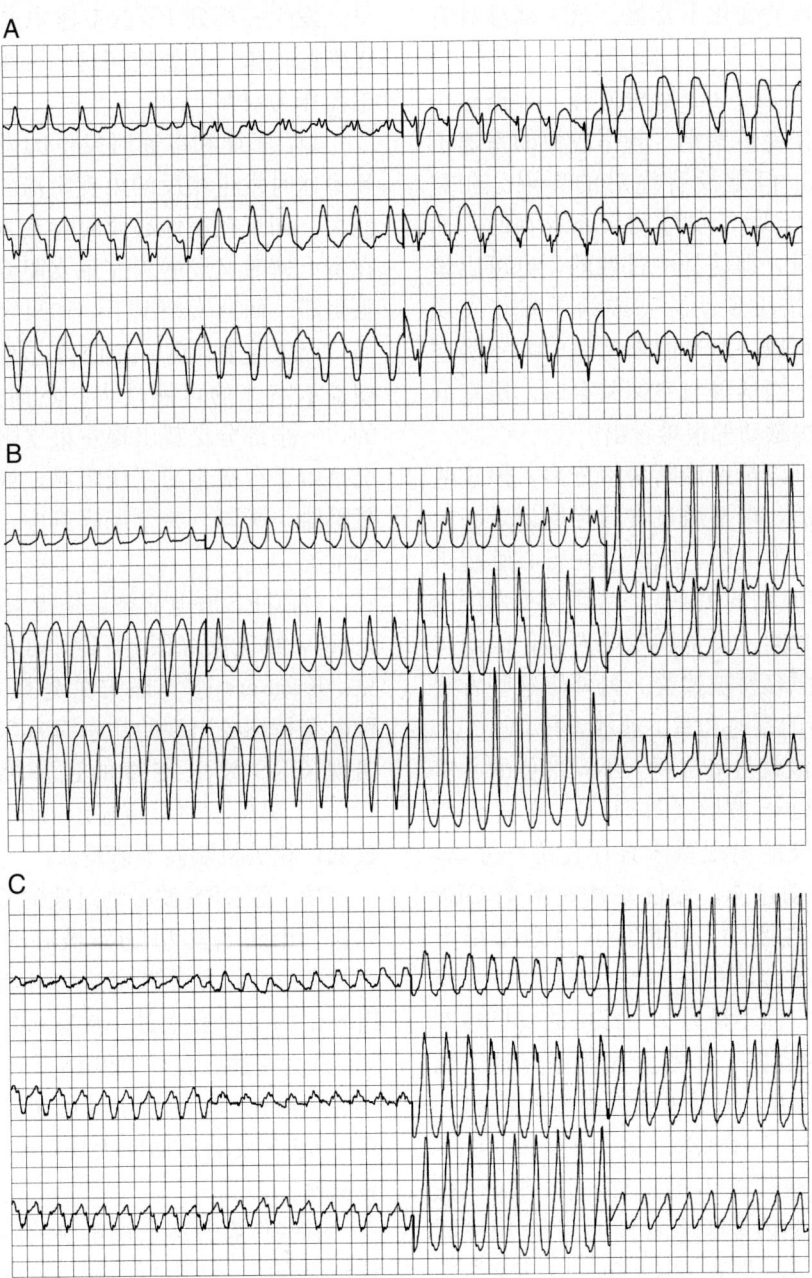

图 81-4　胸前导联 QRS 波的同向性　A：以前有心肌梗死的患者在室速中 QRS 波存在负向同向性，并有房室分离。B：以前有心肌梗死的患者室速时存在胸前导联 QRS 波的正向同向性。在 Ⅱ、Ⅲ、aVF 导联可见 QRS 波振幅交替。C：这是一例预激综合征的患者，发生预激性房扑伴 2∶1 传导。B 图和 C 图的心电图相似。

有些导联的心电图中可见 P 波重叠在 QRS 波的终末部，易被诊断为室上速。在同步记录的心电图各导联中，注意比较 QRS 波的终末时间，可能会减少"假 P 波"的诊断。

房室分离存在的另外一个证据就是在宽 QRS 波心动过速时 QRS 波的振幅发生变异。这是由于 P 波和 QRS 波发生了重叠，或由于房室分离导致心室充盈的变化所致[26]。后者的说法未被验证，有些房室分离模棱两可，R 波振幅的变化不常见，这一标准具有一定的局限性。

将近 30% 的室速具有 1:1 室房逆传，根据这一标准不容易与室上速伴差传鉴别。频率较快的室速不容易存在 1:1 逆传，但是没有绝对的界限。在宽 QRS 波心动过速时，当 1:1 的室房关系存在时，而这种关系又能被改变时，即使是一过性的，也可以诊断室速。这可以通过按压颈动脉窦或给予腺苷实现（图 81-2）。这些方法可以一过性阻断室速时的室房逆传，并且准确率较高。当房颤与室速共存时，房室分离不能诊断，任何心房激动都很难看出。

非心电图方法也可以帮助诊断房室分离，但这些可能会给病人带来不适，包括通过食管导联记录心电图、经静脉电极记录心内电图，或经肋间行心脏超声（评价右房收缩与心室收缩的关系）。尽管这些方法的准确性较高，但需要时间、设备和专业人员，因而这些方法不像心电图那样容易被接受。另外用这些方法也不易鉴别 1:1 逆传的室速和室上速伴差传。

8. 融合波：融合波就是来自两个不同部位的心室激动所形成的混合性 QRS 波形（图 81-5）。在宽 QRS 波心动过速时，融合波的出现意味着存在房室分离，常见于频率较慢的心动过速，允许室速时两个 QRS 波之间出现一次室上性激动，并能经正常房室结下传。具有诊断意义的融合波是室上性 QRS 波与室速 QRS 波形成的融合波，而不是另一个部位的室早与室速的 QRS 波形成的融合波。在室上速伴差传时出现的室早也可以形成融合波，因而可能被误诊为室速。

9. 胸前导联无"RS"型 QRS 波：Brugada 等[27]提出由于大多数室上速伴差传至少有一个导联存在 RS 波，如果任何一个胸前导联均无 RS 波，就应诊断室速。在一项入选 554 例宽 QRS 波心动过速病人的研究中（384 例室速，170 例室上速），83 例无 RS 波形（15%），均为室速。在任何呈 RS 波形的胸前导联中，从 R 波的起点到 S 波最低点大于 100ms 时，则诊断室速。有 175 例存在这种表现，并且均诊断为室速。仅用这两项标准就能够对 554 例中的 258 例室速（47%）作出正确诊断。这种无 RS 波形的诊断标准无法概念化，但临床实践中很有应用价值，可见图 81-6。可以这样讲，对于一份宽 QRS 波心动过速的心电图，如果看起来不像差传，最大的可能就是室速。

10. 室速时 QRS 波形态比窦律时窄：窦性心律存在束支阻滞时，如果发生宽 QRS 波心动过速，但 QRS 波形态比窦律时窄，提示是室速。这种情况较罕见，发生在不到 1% 的室速中[28]，但是室上速时不易见到此现象。若想应用这一标准，必须有一份基础心电图作为对照。

11. 窦律和室速时发生的束支阻滞相反：当窦律和室速时发生相反的束支阻滞，强烈提示室速的可能性大。如果在窦性心律时存在真正的右束支阻滞，而在室上速时又发展为左束支阻滞，将会发生完全性心脏阻滞。而通常情况下，如果窦性心律下是右束支阻滞，而发生宽 QRS 波心动过速时为左束支阻滞，强烈提示室速的可能性大。然而这项标准并不是绝对的，一小部分交替出现左束支阻滞和右束支阻滞的情况是由于存在希浦系统阻滞，或心肌内传导延迟而不是阻滞，所以一些罕见病例中，室上速可能会出现这种情况。

12. QRS 波电交替：是指 QRS 波振幅的变化大于 0.1mV 的现象（图 81-4），在窄 QRS 波室上速中常见。Kremers 等[29]证实在宽 QRS 波心动过速中，这种电交替现象出现的几率约为 25%，室上速伴差传中出现 QRS 波电交替的比率略高于室速（平均为 7:4），另外一些报道显示 QRS 波电交替发生的几率较低，相关机制尚不清楚。

13. 宽 QRS 波心动过速的 QRS 波形态呈多形性：如果一个病人发生 QRS 波心动过速时，QRS 波的形态为多形性，则诊断室速的可能性大。我们分析了一组 861 例至少发生过一次宽 QRS 波心动过速的患者，524 例为室速，其中 266 例（51%）QRS 波形态为多形性，而在 392 例室上速的患者中仅 31 例（8%）出现了 QRS 波的多形性表现，55 例患者既有室上速也有室速。

有些作者分析上述重要的因素，通过多因素相关分析得到了一些简单而较为准确的方法，鉴别室上速伴差传和室速。这些方法中最为简单的应属 Griffith 等[19]提出的。他们发现有 3 个特征可以鉴别宽 QRS 波心动过速，即 aVF 和 V_1 导联 QRS 波的形态、心动过速时电轴比窦律时偏移大于 40°，以及心肌梗死的

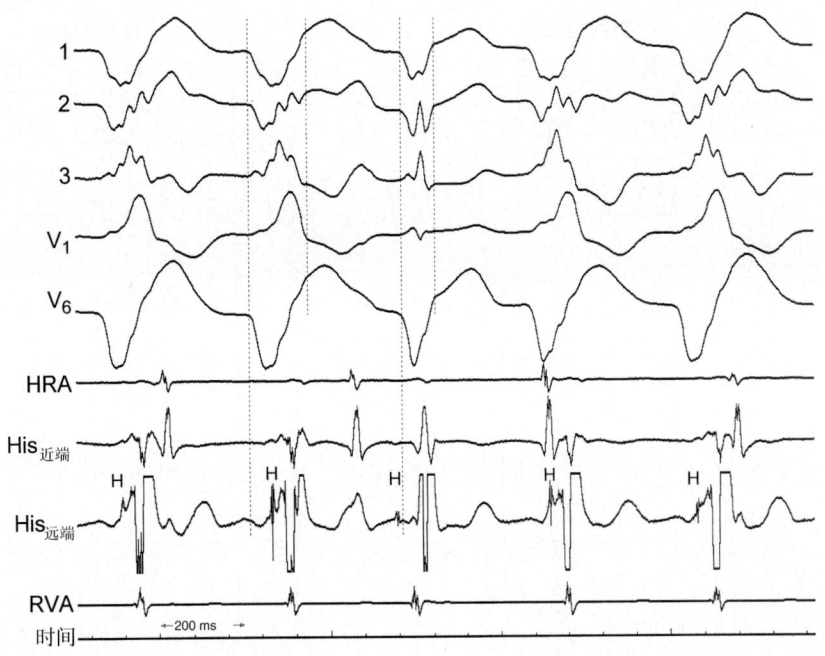

图 81-5 室速时的心室融合波 图中自上而下依次为体表心电图 Ⅰ、Ⅱ、Ⅲ、V_1、V_6 导联和心内高右房（HRA）、希氏束电图近端、希氏束电图远端和右室心尖部（RVA）电图。H：希氏束电位。中间有一跳 QRS 波比其他窄，这是由于分离的心房波经正常的房室结和希氏束传导到心室，与心动过速的心室激动在心室的某一部相位融合形成。

病史，后者鉴别室上速和室速的特异性可达 90% 以上。如果存在两个或两个以上特征，就可以诊断室速，而少于两个特征时，就有可能是室上速。目前已经有计算机程序对宽 QRS 波心动过速的机制作出诊断，但还需更进一步完善[30,31]。

如果窦律心电图中就存在束支阻滞和电轴偏移，上述多数标准的可用性则会明显减小。只有房室分离时这项标准不受影响。有些作者已经意识到：胸前导联 QRS 波的同向性、无人区电轴、V_1 导联呈单相 R 波是室速诊断的可行性标志，即使是窦律下存在束支阻滞[25]。而在这种情况下，胸前导联缺乏 RS 波形这一标准也可能有诊断价值。尽管窦性心律时心电图中有异常，但这些标准仍然有用。如果宽 QRS 波心动过速时 QRS 波形态不符合束支阻滞或分支阻滞的特征，则可能是室速。还可以将以往具有束支阻滞的心电图与宽 QRS 波心动过速的形态相比较，也有助于校正诊断，如果两份心电图的图形一致，则诊断室上速，如果有差异则诊断室速[22]。有一种罕见的情况是窦性心律下束支阻滞的图形与室速发作时一致[32-34]。在这种情况下要想作出正确的室速诊断只能寻找非 1：1 的房室关系。所有已报道的窦律和室速时心电图表现一致的病人中，几乎没有右束支阻滞，窦律时有或没有电轴偏移。

尽管比较基础状态和宽 QRS 波心动过速时的心电图有助于鉴别室上速伴差传和室速，但并不是所有宽 QRS 波心动过速发作时，都能得到基础心电图。

二、宽 QRS 波心动过速：诊断策略

临床急诊情况时，面对一个宽 QRS 波心动过速的患者，通常需要一个快速、直接、准确的方法作出诊断。复杂的流程具有准确的价值，但很难被想起，不适合快速用于宽 QRS 心动过速的鉴别诊断。尽管房室分离是最特异的鉴别标准，但有时模棱两可，不易确定，特别是在快频率心动过速时（>170bpm）。因此我们需要提出一个简单的诊断步骤，像 Brugada 和其同事做的那样[27]。我们前面提到过一个简单的概念性鉴别方法：如果宽 QRS 波心动过速的心电图图形不符合任何已知的差异性传导的图形，那么就可能不是室上速伴差传，而是室速。在应用这一方法时，在心动过速时需要进行心电图比较，识别 V_1 和 V_6 导联差异性传导的图形（图 81-3）。我们应用这一方法时，前两步是按照 Brugada 的流程（胸前导联上无 RS 波形和 RS 间期>100ms），分析了 300 份已作出正确诊断的宽 QRS 波心动过速的心电图。在分析中我们应用了 Brugada 宽 QRS 波心动过速鉴别诊断流程中的前两步，因其内容简单明了，而该流程随后的两个步骤已并入其他更为详细的传统的相关标准。结果，

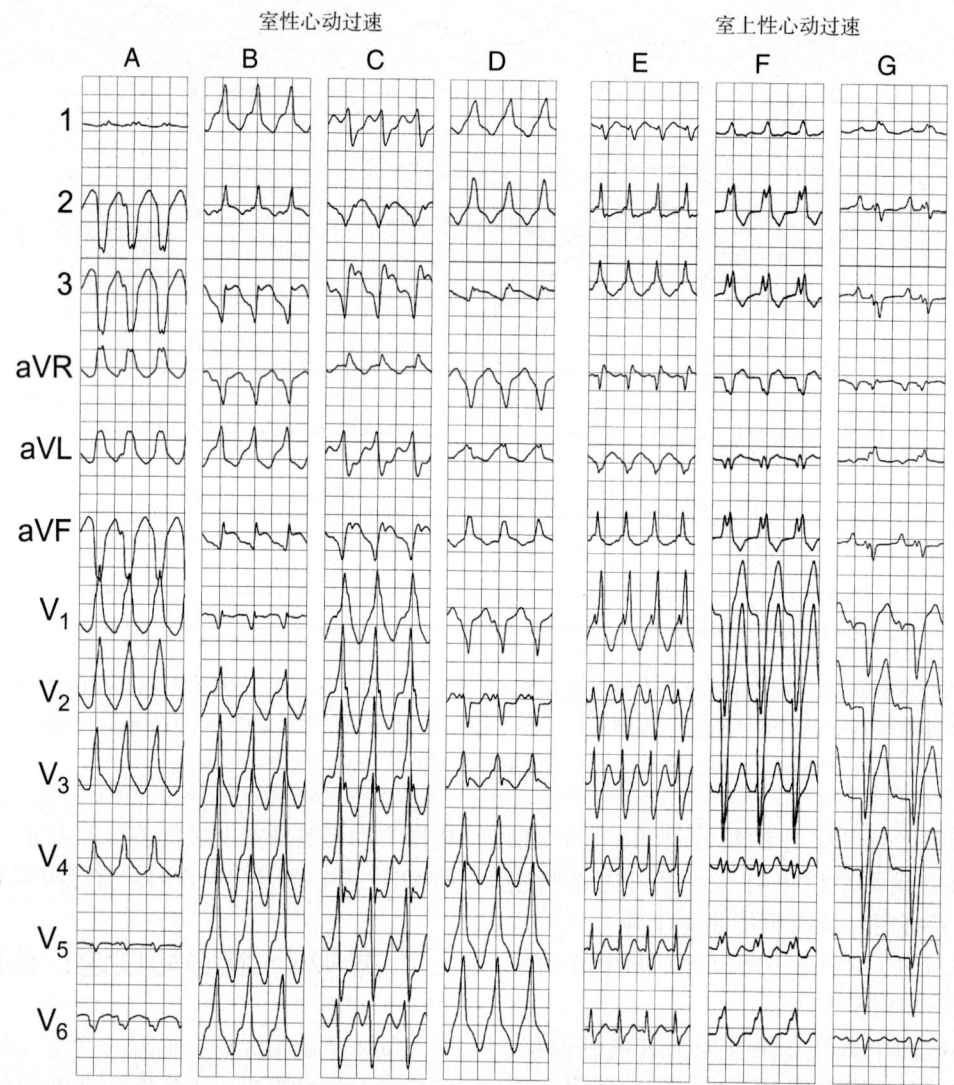

图 81-6 宽 QRS 波心动过速时应用 "RS 标准" 的实例 图中均为 12 导联同步心电图，A~D 图为室速，E~G 图为室上速。在 A 和 B 图中，胸前导联没有一个导联存在 RS 波，C 和 D 图中存在 RS 波形（C 图中的 $V_3 \sim V_6$ 导联，D 图中的 $V_2 \sim V_3$ 导联），RS 间期大于 100ms。E 图（右束支阻滞）和 F 图（左束支阻滞）为室上速伴胸前导联存在 RS 波，但是 RS 间期小于 100ms，G 图为左束支阻滞的宽 QRS 波心动过速，在任何胸前导联均无 RS 波形，提示诊断室速。但实际是室上速。C 图可见假性 P 波（Ⅱ、Ⅲ、aVF 导联 QRS 波终末部可见负向波），病人存在房室分离。

前两步标准应用中其"差异性传导可能性"的敏感性、特异性和阳性预测值分别达到了 96%、65% 和 87%，而应用"RS 标准"时上述参数分别是 83%、56% 和 83%。这两种方法作出正确诊断的能力相似，而 Brugada 的诊断流程简单，但与常规心电图分析方法相比具有概念性区别。我们的诊断方法，需要实施者非常熟悉典型差异性传导的生理特征，以便识别是否存在差异性传导。因而每一种方法都有利有弊，无法说这一方法超过其他方法。那些需要对宽 QRS 波心动过速进行鉴别诊断的医生应该熟悉这些鉴别方法中的一种，以便在急诊情况时能够快速、准确地作出诊断。

尽管很多鉴别室上速伴差传和室速的标准得到了临床的全面验证，但如果医生不能准确反复应用，最佳的标准也不能帮助作出正确的诊断。例如：Isenhour 等[35]要求两位急诊医生和两位心血管医生应用 Brugada 流程诊断 157 例宽 QRS 波心动过速，结果，心血管医生作出正确诊断的敏感性为 85%~91%，特异性为 55%~60%，而急诊医生作出正确诊断的敏感性为 79%~83%，特异性为 43%~70%（原作者分别达到 98.7% 的敏感性和 96.5% 的特异性）。

三、宽 QRS 波心动过速：特殊情况

偶尔情况下，会出现即使正确应用了上述标准依然得不到正确答案的特殊情况。如前所述，预激性室上速的心电图图形有时就可能与室速相同。另一种情况，就是心电图的标准提示是室上速，但实际是室速，对这一情况将进行如下讨论。

（一）束支折返

大多数束支折返性室速，心室激动的最早传出部位起于右束支，心动过速的图形表现为左束支阻滞。尽管实际上是室速，但心电图既有左束支阻滞图形，又与室上速伴差传的心电图标准符合。如果存在房室分离，则有助于作出正确诊断。

（二）不规则性室速

宽 QRS 波心动过速时 QRS 波的规则性对鉴别室上速和室速并无帮助，因为通常情况下这两种心动过速都是规则的。明显的心动周期的变化强烈提示为房颤伴束支阻滞，然而室速也可能不规则，特别是心动过速发生的前 30s[36]。室速伴明显的心动周期不规则常见于那些服用抗心律失常药物的患者。

（三）窄 QRS 波的室速

如前所述，室速的 QRS 波时限可以 <140ms。在一项 702 例室速的分析中[28]，88 例（12%）QRS 波时限 >140ms，28 例（4%）QRS 波时限 <120ms（从定义上讲这已不符合宽 QRS 波心动过速）。这种现象可能的解释有几种：（1）间隔起源的室速，可使左右心室同步激动；（2）激动很早就侵入希浦系统，激动沿着希浦系统快速激动心室。罕见的情况是患者室速发作时 QRS 波比窦性心律时还窄，这一现象在 702 例室速中仅有 2 例（1%）。心动过速时相对短的 QRS 时限也可见于室上性心动过速中。

四、总　　结

尽管有充足的方法可以对大多数病人作出正确的鉴别诊断，但对于很多临床医生来说，鉴别室速和室上速还有一定的困难。要记住简单的法则：当宽 QRS 波心动过速时 QRS 波形态与任何差传的形态都有差异时，可能是室速。然而，这要求医生熟悉所有的差异性传导的心电图图形。在临床应激状态下，记住这些标准和记起其他心电图标准有时一样是很困难的。少见的情况下，如预激性心动过速时，或窦律下心电图不正常的宽 QRS 波心动过速时，心电图的形态学诊断标准就没用了，而此时只有非 1∶1 的室房关系有助于诊断。如果所有的这些方法均不能作出诊断，就将心动过速按室速对待，因为室速是最常见的宽 QRS 波心动过速[1,37]。切记有些治疗方法可能会恶化病人状态，例如对一个由于抗心律失常药物过量所致宽 QRS 波心动过速患者，给予静脉推注普鲁卡因胺或维拉帕米时就会恶化病人状况。

（张　萍　译）

参 考 文 献

1. Akhtar M, Shenasa M, Jazayeri M, et al: Wide QRS complex tachycardia. Reappraisal of a common clinical problem. Ann Intern Med 109:905–912, 1988.
2. Bardy GH, Fedor JM, German LD, et al: Surface electrocardiographic clues suggesting presence of a nodofascicular Mahaim fiber. J Am Coll Cardiol 3:1161–1168, 1984.
3. Vassallo JA, Cassidy DM, Marchlinski FE, et al: Endocardial activation of left bundle branch block. Circulation 69:914–923, 1984.
4. Ranger S, Talajic M, Lemery R, et al: Amplification of flecainide-induced ventricular conduction slowing by exercise. A potentially significant clinical consequence of use-dependent sodium channel blockade. Circulation 79:1000–1006, 1989.
5. Nathan AW, Hellestrand KJ, Bexton RS, et al: Proarrhythmic effects of the new antiarrhythmic agent flecainide acetate. Am Heart J 107:222–228, 1984.
6. Baerman JM, Morady F, DiCarlo LA, de Buitleir M: Differentiation of ventricular tachycardia from supraventricular tachycardia with aberration: Value of the clinical history. Ann Emerg Med 16:40–43, 1987.
7. Tchou P, Young P, Mahmud R, et al: Useful clinical criteria for the diagnosis of ventricular tachycardia. Am J Med 84:53–56, 1988.
8. Morady F, Baerman JM, DiCarlo LA, et al: A prevalent misconception regarding wide-complex tachycardias. JAMA 254:2790–2792, 1985.
9. Rankin AC, Oldroyd KG, Chong E: Value and limitations of adenosine in the diagnosis and treatment of narrow and broad complex tachycardias. Br Heart J 62:195–203, 1989.
10. Waxman MB, Wald RW, Finley JP, et al: Valsalva termination of ventricular tachycardia. Circulation 62:843–851, 1980.
11. Belhassen B, Rotmensch HH, Laniado S: Response of recurrent sustained ventricular tachycardia to verapamil. Br Heart J 46:679–682, 1981.
12. Hess DS, Hanlon T, Scheinman M, et al: Termination of ventricular tachycardia by carotid sinus massage. Circulation 65:627–633, 1982.
13. Lerman BB, Belardinelli L, West A, et al: Adenosine-sensitive ventricular tachycardia: Evidence suggesting cyclic AMP-mediated triggered activity. Circulation 74:270–280, 1986.
14. Grubb BP: Termination of ventricular tachycardia by carotid sinus stimulation. Int J Cardiol 23:397–399, 1989.
15. Buxton AE, Marchlinski FE, Doherty JU, et al: Hazards of intravenous verapamil for sustained ventricular tachycardia. Am J Cardiol 59:1107–1110, 1987.
16. Miller JM: Ventricular tachycardia: ECG manifestations. In Zipes DP, Jalife J (eds): Cardiac Electrophysiology: From Cell to Bedside, 2nd ed. Philadelphia, WB Saunders, 1994, pp 990–1008.
17. Griffith MJ, Garratt CJ, Mounsey P: Ventricular tachycardia as default diagnosis in broad complex tachycardias. Lancet 343:386–388, 1994.
18. Wellens HJJ, Bär FWHM, Lie KI: The value of the electrocardiogram in the differential diagnosis of a tachycardia with a widened QRS complex. Am J Med 64:27–33, 1978.

19. Griffith MJ, De Belder MA, Linker NJ, et al: Multivariate analysis to simplify the differential diagnosis of broad complex tachycardia. Br Heart J 66:166–174, 1991.
20. Kindwall KE, Brown J, Josephson ME: Electrocardiographic criteria for ventricular tachycardia in wide complex left bundle branch block morphology tachycardias. Am J Cardiol 61:1279–1283, 1988.
21. Miller JM, Marchlinski FE, Buxton AE, Josephson ME: Relationship between the 12-lead electrocardiogram during ventricular tachycardia and endocardial site of origin in patients with coronary artery disease. Circulation 77:759–766, 1988.
22. Dongas J, Lehmann MH, Mahmud R, et al: Value of preexisting bundle branch block in the electrocardiographic differentiation of supraventricular from ventricular origin of wide QRS tachycardia. Am J Cardiol 55:717–721, 1985.
23. Reddy GV, Leghari RU: Standard limb lead QRS concordance during wide QRS tachycardia. A new surface ECG sign of ventricular tachycardia. Chest 92:763–765, 1987.
24. Coumel P, Leclercq JF, Attuel P, Maisonblanche P: The QRS morphology in post-myocardial infarction ventricular tachycardia. A study of 100 tracings compared with 70 cases of idiopathic ventricular tachycardia. Eur Heart J 5:792–805, 1984.
25. Kremers MS, Black WH, Wells PJ, Solodyna M: Effect of preexisting bundle branch block on the electrocardiographic diagnosis of ventricular tachycardia. Am J Cardiol 62:1208–1212, 1988.
26. Curione M, Fuoco U, Borgia C, et al: An electrocardiographic criterion to detect AV dissociation in wide QRS tachyarrhythmias. Clin Cardiol 11:250–252, 1988.
27. Brugada P, Brugada J, Mont L, et al: A new approach to the differential diagnosis of a regular tachycardia with a wide QRS complex. Circulation 83:1649–1659, 1991.
28. Miller JM: The many manifestations of ventricular tachycardia. J Cardiovasc Electrophysiol 3:88–107, 1992.
29. Kremers MS, Miller JM, Josephson ME: Electrical alternans in wide complex tachycardias. Am J Cardiol 56:305–308, 1985.
30. Slocum J, Byrom E, McCarthy L, et al: Computer detection of atrioventricular dissociation from surface electrocardiograms during wide QRS complex tachycardias. Circulation 72:1028–1036, 1985.
31. Widman LE, Tong DA: Validation of the EINTHOVEN model-based computerized electrocardiogram rhythm analysis system with three classes of clinical arrhythmias. Am J Cardiol 78:927–31, 1996.
32. Halperin BD, Kron J, Cutler JE, et al: Misdiagnosing ventricular tachycardia in patients with underlying conduction disease and similar sinus and tachycardia morphologies. West J Med 152:677–682, 1990.
33. Olshansky B: Ventricular tachycardia masquerading as supraventricular tachycardia: A wolf in sheep's clothing. J Electrocardiol 21:377–84, 1988.
34. Weiss J, Stevenson WG: Narrow QRS ventricular tachycardia. Am Heart J 112:843–847, 1986.
35. Isenhour JL, Craig S, Gibbs M, et al: Wide-complex tachycardia: Continued evaluation of diagnostic criteria. Acad Emerg Med 7:769–73, 2000.
36. Volosin KJ, Beauregard LA, Fabiszewski R, et al: Spontaneous changes in ventricular tachycardia cycle length. J Am Coll Cardiol 17:409–414, 1991.
37. Steinman RT, Herrera C, Schuger CD, Lehmann MH: Wide QRS tachycardia in the conscious adult. Ventricular tachycardia is the most frequent cause. JAMA 261:1013–1016, 1989.

第十二部分 诊断与评价

第 82 章

心律失常的评估

Douglas P. Zipes and William M. Miles

本章目录
- 病史采集 ·············· 747
- 体格检查 ·············· 748
- 实验室检查 ············ 749
- 总结 ·················· 751
- 致谢 ·················· 751

对怀疑有心律失常的患者作出评估是临床心脏电生理医生的重要基本工作。虽然评价的方法因人而异，并受病人的临床表现及症状的影响，但可以建立一个总的框架，这也是本章的目的。通常评估从仔细的病史询问及体格检查开始。

一、病史采集

不同类型的心律失常临床表现非常相似，由此影响从病史判断临床意义的准确性。即使这样，仍可应用病史对心律失常患者或拟诊心律失常患者的初步评价提供方向和诊断线索，可以说，病史是心律失常最重要的信息源。

(一) 症状

患者对不规则心跳的感觉存在个体差异。许多患者可以清楚地感觉到心跳不规则，而有些人甚至在发生短阵快速室性心动过速时仍无感觉。无症状的患者通常是由于其他原因需要做心律失常评估时被偶然发现。例如：运动员参加体育比赛前，成年人保险前的体格检查或手术前的常规体检。病人最常诉说的症状是心悸。心悸是一种有力的、不规则的、快速的心跳不适感，患者的描述各异。最常形容为胸部有蹦蹦跳或坠落感，喉、颈、胸部发胀或心跳暂停（似乎心脏停跳了）。后一个感觉很有可能是由于室性早搏的代偿间歇或房性早搏后窦性节律的重整所致。推测，早搏特别是过早出现的室早，心室充盈时间不足，在心室收缩时会产生感觉。由于代偿间歇后的心室有力收缩或心脏在胸部的运动增加可引起突发的心悸。患者常因此而感焦虑，并以此为主诉而就诊。

房早或室早是心悸最常见的原因，病人常诉说心脏蹦蹦跳或坠落感。如果早搏频繁特别是出现持续的心动过速时，病人会出现头晕、晕厥或先兆晕厥、胸痛、疲劳，或气短。当病人并存其他的心血管疾病时常能导致不同的症状，例如：室上性心动过速频率超过 180bpm，对冠心病患者可能诱发胸痛，对主动脉瓣狭窄患者可导致晕厥，但对正常的青年人可能仅仅感觉气短。

需要强调的是，室性心动过速的患者发作时可以完全没有症状或仅有轻微不适，特别是年轻人或健康人，没有症状不能排除室速的诊断。缓慢性心律失常通常表现为晕厥、先兆晕厥和疲劳等一些特有的征候群。

(二) 晕厥

对于有晕厥的患者仔细询问病史有助于诊断。心律失常导致的晕厥，发生迅速，持续时间短，没有发作先兆，没有发作后的精神异常。如果病人意识丧失后摔倒可以导致身体外伤。像舌头咬伤、尿失禁这样的癫痫样发作较少见，但如果心律失常导致的晕厥持续时间较长时则可出现。当病人在晕厥发作数秒内就出现癫痫样发作，则中枢神经系统疾病所致的可能性大而非心源性心律失常。

血管迷走性和心脏抑制性晕厥通常起病更慢，发作前常有迷走神经过度激活的表现，如恶心、腹部痉挛、腹泻、出汗和打哈欠。恢复时，病人有心动过缓、面色苍白、出汗和疲劳。这些表现不同于阿斯发作或室速后恢复的患者。后者通常有面色潮红和窦性心动过速（见第61至78章）。常见的引起晕厥的心律失常包括：缓慢性心律失常和快速性心律失常。缓慢性心律失常多为窦房结功能不良或房室阻滞（见第52、53章）。快速性心律失常最常见的是室性心动过速，偶见室上性心动过速（见第54至60章）。患慢快综合征的患者可在心动过缓后出现心动过速，二者都需要治疗。非心源性晕厥如低血糖可通过仔细询问病史后排除。其他非心律失常性晕厥如主动脉瓣狭窄可结合病史和体格检查后排除。

（三）心动过速

了解心动过速发作和终止的情况有助于诊断。例如房室结折返性心动过速常表现为突然发生的阵发性的心动过速（见第59章）；而逐渐加速和减慢的心动过速则更可能为窦性心动过速（见第52章）。心动过速可被Vasalva动作或颈动脉按摩终止时，提示心动过速的折返环路径与窦房结或房室结有关，如窦房结折返、房室结折返或房室折返性心动过速（见第58、59章），但不能完全排除室性心动过速。病人从心悸发作到终止的期间能感觉出心跳的节奏对诊断常很有帮助。通过这种方式，临床医生可以了解心动过速发作和终止的性质、心室律是否规则及心动过速的频率。

未经过治疗的心动过速频率对诊断有一定的帮助，应指导病人如何计算他们的桡动脉或颈动脉率。心室率150bpm常提示为房扑伴2：1房室阻滞（见第54章），而大多数室上速如房室结折返性心动过速或房室折返性心动过速的心室率常超过150bpm，室速的频率与室上速有重叠。

（四）心脏疾病

应了解病人有无器质性心脏病的病史，疾病的诊断和严重程度等对心律失常的诊断很重要。某些临床诊断和特殊的心律失常有特定关系。例如：二尖瓣狭窄的病人，发生房颤的可能性大。有心肌梗死或法洛四联症修补术史的患者发生室速的可能性大，甲状腺功能亢进者房性心律失常和窦性心动过速的可能大。询问家族史中类似病史和获得家庭成员如双亲同胞兄弟或孩子的心电图可能会有助于诊断。例如：近亲心电图上有长QT间期的表现明显时，则比有晕厥发作史更有助于诊断。

（五）诱发因素

采集病史时，医生应寻找心律失常可能的诱发因素。病人通常不能指出特别的诱因，但医生应询问有关心脏潜在刺激性药物的使用情况，如支气管扩张药、H_1受体阻滞剂、抗组胺药、扩血管药或其他非处方药物，以及饮酒或摄入含有过多咖啡因食物的情况。在有些病人，症状可能被某些活动诱发或加重，或在一天或一个月的某段时间发生（例如月经来潮时）。有趣的是，一些房性心律失常患者能通过先出现的胃肠道症状预测其复发。长QT综合征（见第70、71章）的患者，LQT1型常在运动或情绪激动时诱发室性心律失常；LQT2型患者则在运动、情绪紧张和睡眠与休息时室性心律失常的发生率基本相当；LQT3型的患者，其心律失常事件特别容易被声音刺激所诱发并常发生在休息时。

二、体格检查

体格检查可以获得有关并存的器质性心脏病的重要信息，如果体检时心律失常存在，可了解其性质。尽管众所周知，正常心脏可以发生室上速，但较少认识到结构无异常的心脏也可以发生室速，并偶可危及生命。因此体检正常者不能排除室速诊断，特别是年轻人。很有可能这些病人中至少一部分存在器质性心脏病但没有被发现。

病人的性别对判断心动过速的性质也是有用的线索。例如：反复规整的心动过速发作多年，如发生在年轻女性很可能是房室结折返性心动过速，相反发生在年轻男性可能为WPW综合征所致的房室折返性心动过速，有症状的长QT综合征患者常为女性，而Bruguda综合征常见于男性（见第67章）。

（一）房室分离

如果体检时病人正发作心动过速，当时间和病人临床状态允许时，应做12导联心电图检查。如果没有心电图机时，仔细的体格检查也能获得有用的信息。如：发现规则的颈静脉A波，可能是连续的1：1

室房逆传所致。这种情况可见于几种心动过速：房室折返性心动过速、房室结折返性心动过速、一些交界性心动过速或室性心动过速。反之，体检时也可发现病人有房室分离的征象，包括间断的颈静脉A波、第一心音强度不一、收缩压变化和发生在心动周期不同时期的类似奔马律的心房音，这种心音常在心尖部使用钟形听诊器听诊最清楚。常见的房室分离的心律失常包括没有逆传夺获心房的室速和非阵发性交界性心动过速（见第57章）。伴2：1阻滞或文氏阻滞型逆传心房的室性或交界性心动过速可有规则出现的间歇性颈静脉A波。束支阻滞（BBB）时可产生受呼吸影响的第二心音的反常分裂，右束支阻滞使吸气时第二心音的分裂变宽，但呼气时不成为单一心音。

（二）房室阻滞

二度房室阻滞的病人，观察其颈静脉搏动有助于发现阻滞的特性，但这种搏动的变化常太微弱以致难以识别。二度Ⅰ型（文氏型）房室阻滞时静脉搏动A-C间期逐渐延长，直至P波不能下传，室率逐渐加快，第一心音强度逐渐减弱。二度Ⅱ型房室阻滞的病人，阻滞前PR间期固定，所以A-C间期、第一心音强度不变。完全性房室阻滞时可较早见到房室分离。

（三）颈动脉窦按摩

在体格检查时通过颈动脉窦按摩而调节自主神经张力有助于发现颈动脉窦反射高敏的患者。临床医师首先需要仔细听诊双侧颈动脉，确定无血管杂音，轻轻触诊判断颈动脉搏动正常时，然后轻压或按摩颈动脉窦，轻轻按摩5s或更短的时间，通常使易感病人产生明显的窦性停搏或房室阻滞。

观察心动过速对颈动脉窦按摩或其他迷走刺激的反应对于鉴别心动过速的类型很有帮助。最有诊断价值的反应为，颈动脉窦按摩时心动过速终止，见于房室折返、房室结折返、窦房结折返性心动过速。窦性心动过速时心率可逐渐减慢但不被终止。房速、房扑、房颤的心室率可减慢（见第55、56章），但也不能终止发作（这时可暴露心房活动）。持续性房室交界性折返性心动过速可被暂时终止（见第58章），但在颈动脉窦按摩停止后容易再发。对室性或交界性心动过速无影响。但应注意上述心动过速并不都呈现这种"教科书"模式的反应，它们之间的反应有交叉重叠。

三、实验室检查

如前述，对病人最初的评价开始于仔细询问病史和体格检查。一些非侵入性和侵入性检查帮助医生更好地评估心律失常。在检查之前，必须权衡检查所能提供信息的重要性与它的风险和费用比，尽可能选择敏感性、特异性和预测准确性高的检查。每个病人都应做12导联心电图，24h动态心电图或30天的事件记录仪（见第84、85章）。运动试验（见第83章）也有助于检出心律失常。胸部X线和超声心动图对是否存在器质性心脏病可提供有用的信息。对拟诊心律失常的病人，评价和治疗可分步进行，常常从简单、非侵入性、检查费用低的检查到复杂、昂贵、侵入性检查。根据心律失常的性质和对病人的影响来决定需要做哪些检查。某些心律失常，如持续性室速或室颤，本身具有危险性，而其他心律失常如房室折返性心动过速、房室结折返性心动过速必须根据病人的综合情况进行评估。房室折返性心动过速、房室结折返性心动过速时心率180bpm，在青年人可能仅感心悸或轻微不适，但在冠心病患者则可能诱发心绞痛，在主动脉瓣狭窄患者可发生晕厥，在周围血管疾病患者引起跛行。应该强调临床医师采取的决定必须建立在对心律失常心电图的分析并对病人综合评估的基础上。医生评价和治疗的是一个有心律失常的病人，而不是孤立的心律失常。

对有症状无心律失常记录证据的患者，诊断和治疗原则显而易见：仅需要在症状发作时记录一份心电图并判断心律失常和症状的因果关系。但说起来容易做起来难，多种方法可用于达到这样的目的。

（一）动态心律记录仪

频发的心律失常自然比那些偶发的心律失常容易被记录到。对非致命性心律失常的病人进行早期诊断常用的一个方法是在门诊行动态心电图记录（见第84章）。患有致命性心律失常的病人，需要住院并行上述检查。动态心电图记录是评价心律失常最直接的检查方法，过程简单，常是评估心律失常首选和非侵入性的检查方法。在病人日常活动时记录动态心电图可提供心律失常的形态学，心律失常的频度定量和确定其复杂性，分析症状与心律失常的关系，评价抗心律失常药物的效果，而且也可记录QRS波、ST段和T波的改变。

但是，如果心律失常出现的频率不高，仅记录24h，甚至48h的动态心电图也很难捕捉到心律失常时，30d的事件记录仪通常有帮助。病人在症状发生时自行激活记录，储存30s或更长时间的心电图记录（内设滚桶式记录装置，激活之前数秒的心律失常的心电图信息可被记录），并通过电话传送到中心监测站。此外，一些装置可自动记录超过预设范围的节律。事件自动记录仪对于那些无症状的心律失常或由于发生快速加剧的晕厥或其他原因不能自己激活记录系统的病人非常有效。

病人的症状与心律失常必须同时发生，这样的一段记录才有特异性。如果症状出现时没心律失常，则心律失常不是引起症状的原因。记录到心律失常而没有症状，可以排除心律失常和症状之间的因果关系，降低检查的特异性。检查的敏感性随心律失常的患病率有很大的变化。很小的记录仪植入皮下可更长时间监测心律失常（见第85章），在不久的将来或许能同步记录和提供血流动力学信息。这些记录仪可以对心脏猝死危险的病人提供重要信息。

（二）电生理检查

通常，对多数病人进行有创性电生理检查的目的是诱发心律失常（见第93章）。如果诱发出特定的心律失常并且病人产生相应的症状，该检查就能提供重要的诊断依据。然而在某些情况下，临床上存在快速心律失常表现但不能被电生理检查所诱发。这种情况发生时，并不能排除在其他情况时快速心律失常发作的可能性，也不能说明其与病人的症状不相关。由于心律失常性质不同，电生理检查的敏感性可能较低。电生理检查阴性时不等于没有心律失常。

理想的结果是，电生理检查仅能诱发出与自发性心律失常危险性相关的心律失常，这些心律失常有临床和预后意义，而无危险性的病人则不被诱发。但实际情况并非如此，电生理检查需要应用一定数量的期前刺激，有时也能诱发非特异性的快速性心律失常，特别是心房或心室的扑动或颤动。对某些心律失常，电生理检查的特异性很高。例如：对于没有持续性房室折返性心动过速、房室结折返性心动过速临床表现的病人，电生理检查时很少诱发出这些心律失常。同样，临床没有持续性单形性室速病史的病人，电生理检查也常很难诱发。

（三）负荷试验和其他无创性检查

运动负荷试验有助于诊断，特别当病人诉说症状发生在运动时（见第83章）。约1/3的正常人在做运动试验时能记录到室性早搏，通常是偶发单形性室性早搏。这些室早多发生在心率较快时，而且在下次检查中不再发生。正常人在运动中较少发生多形性室早、成对室早和室速。然而这些单形性室早也能见于正常人，所以其出现时并不等于存在心肌缺血或心脏疾病。与正常人相比，冠心病患者的室早常发生在心室率较低时（<130bpm），而且常在恢复早期发生，其室性心律失常在重复检查时容易复制而且常为频发室早（>10bpm）、多形性室早或室速。休息时的室早在运动后被抑制也可见于冠心病患者，所以观察到这种现象并不表示预后良好或无潜在心脏疾病。在正常人，运动试验的结果不易被复制，而冠心病患者则易被复制，但这不能作为诊断依据。运动试验也有利于检出非典型长QT综合征病人的心电图异常。

多种无创性检查用来鉴别病人出现致死性心律失常的危险度。包括信号平均心电图（见第86章）、心率变异性分析（见第89章）、QT离散度、T波电交替（见第91章）、压力感受器敏感性反射（见第89章）。尽管这些试验有助于鉴别病人出现心源性猝死危险性的高低，但都不能明确预测具体病人致命性心律失常的发生。

（四）特殊症状的检查

1. 晕厥

评价怀疑有心脏抑制或血管迷走性晕厥病人的检查常包括直立倾斜试验（见第88章）。对于没有器质性心脏病的晕厥患者使用动态心电图或心脏电生理检查结果常为阴性。尽可能找到晕厥的原因十分重要。因为非心源性晕厥的预后通常良好，而心源性晕厥者心脏猝死率较高。

对于进行包括神经系统检查、动态心电图检查在内的完整评估后仍原因不清的晕厥或先兆晕厥的病人，进行电生理检查十分必要。由于心动过缓或心动过速都可能导致晕厥，因此不能推测患者晕厥的原因。只有记录发作时的心电图，或在电生理检查时复制出有相同或相似症状的心律失常或其他心律失常发生时伴发相同或相似症状时方可鉴别。例如：一度房室阻滞或左束支阻滞的病人可能发生室速，导致晕厥的原因有可能不是发生了更严重的房室阻滞。

2. 缓慢性心律失常

很多病人存在无症状性心动过缓，在决定治疗前确定心动过缓所产生的症状很重要。相反，如果病人出现症状的同时证实有心动过缓，就没有必要做进一步的检查。可能病人在心律失常时症状轻微，但有助于确定治疗措施。例如，病人有二度Ⅱ型房室阻滞及希浦系统阻滞的证据，即使症状轻微或可能无症状，也有足够的证据提示患者应植入起搏器，因为它们有进展为完全性房室阻滞的可能（见第53章）。

患有窦房结功能不良的病人可产生晕厥或先兆晕厥，也可以出现因持续性的心动过缓导致的心排血量减少产生的症状，如疲劳，甚至出现充血性心力衰竭的症状（见第52章）。有些病人可伴有心动过速，称为慢快综合征。对窦房结功能不良者，电生理检查的敏感性低而特异性相对较高。确定心动过缓和病人症状的关系非常重要。只有在反复的无创性检查也不能确定心动过缓与病人症状的因果关系时才需要行有创的电生理检查。应记住心率在35～40bpm的无症状性窦性心动过缓、停搏2～3s的窦性心律失常、二度文氏型房室阻滞（特别发生在睡眠时）、窦性游走节律、交界性逸搏可能是完全正常的，特别是对于青年人。

对有房室阻滞的病人，画出梯形图十分重要（见第53章），因为阻滞的部位通常决定临床进程和是否需要起搏器治疗。分析梯形图常可判断阻滞的部位，很少需要进行有创的电生理检查。自主神经刺激有助于判断阻滞部位。阿托品或异丙肾上腺素可以缩短房室结传导时间和不应期，而迷走刺激反之，对正常希浦系统的传导无大影响。所以，运动、阿托品或异丙肾上腺素可以缩短PR间期，增加文氏型房室阻滞时P波的下传率，而加重二度Ⅱ型房室阻滞P波的阻滞程度。但二者之间可有重叠。

3. 快速性心律失常

如前所述，心动过速发作时，只要病人情况稳定，必须做12导联心电图检查。如果QRS波正常且与窦性节律时相同，则为室上性心动过速，应对其相关的发生机制做鉴别诊断。12导联心电图可提供许多诊断线索。如果无P波或房性激动的心电图表现，而RR间期规整时，最可能是房室结折返性心动过速。如果在ST段上可见逆传P波，可能是房室折返性心动过速。如果心动过速伴长RP和短PR间期，P波在QRS波之前，PR间期短于200～300ms时，可能的诊断是不典型房室结折返性心动过速或持续性交界性折返性心动过速或房速。窦性心律或心动过速时出现旁路传导提示WPW综合征的旁路参与了心动过速。室速时，特殊的QRS波图形和房室分离有助于诊断（见第52～78章）。

四、总 结

对患有或疑有心律失常的病人进行认真检查是临床心脏电生理医生的重要工作。无创性检查可以提供很多有用的信息，并避免不必要的电生理检查。然而当有指征时，特别是与射频消融术结合治疗时，电生理检查可对心律失常的确诊和治疗提供决定性的信息。

五、致 谢

本研究受印第安纳州、印第安纳波利斯市Herman C. Krannert基金会支持。

（林荣 吴兵译）

第 83 章

运动性心律失常

Ruey J. Sung, Chi-Tai Kuo, and Wen-Ter Lai

本章目录
- 运动引发心律失常的机制 ………… 752
- 临床表现 ………………………… 752
- 基因学和分子学依据 …………… 756
- 治疗 ……………………………… 757
- 总结 ……………………………… 757

运动性心律失常是指发生在人体剧烈运动时或之后的心律失常。其临床表现不一，从心悸、头晕、晕厥、心绞痛、急性心肌梗死和充血性心力衰竭，甚至到心脏性猝死[1,2]。运动性心律失常可见于易患心肌缺血患者，比如那些患有动脉粥样硬化性心脏病以及那些患有原发性或继发性心肌病的患者。然而，它们也可能发生在各年龄段表面上似乎健康的个体。在后一组人群中，运动性心律失常可能是良性的，也可能由于获得性（如药物诱发）或先天性（如先天性长 QT 综合征或致心律失常性右室发育不良）心脏电活动或结构的异常而呈恶性[1]。这种潜在病理生理学机制的复杂性，使运动性心律失常的诊断和治疗成为临床医学面临的一个挑战。

一、运动引发心律失常的机制

心血管对运动作出的反应首先是迷走神经张力减低，然后是交感神经活性增强，进而导致心率增快、心脏收缩力增强和收缩压升高[2]。由此引起的心脏负荷增大，导致需氧量增加，进而可造成心肌缺血。心肌缺血则能引发室性心律失常，并伴随着心肌缺血使室颤阈值降低，这种室性心律失常可能会触发或恶化为心室颤动。

在其他因素当中，运动引发交感神经活性增强后，刺激 α、β 肾上腺素受体。β 拟交感神经激动剂与心肌细胞膜上的 β 肾上腺素能受体结合，刺激一种特殊的细胞内 G 蛋白，该 G 蛋白活化酶将激活腺苷酸环化酶/环磷酸腺苷（cAMP）系统，导致各种心脏跨膜离子流的增加或活化，这些跨膜离子流包括：电压依赖性钙离子流（I_{Ca}）、起搏离子流（I_f）、瞬时内向电流（I_{Ti}）和外向电流（I_{To}）及延迟的整流性钾离子流（I_K），尤其是其缓慢成分（I_{Ks}）。α 肾上腺素能受体活化的效应似乎是通过 G 蛋白调节，但不涉及 cAMP 系统的活化。α 拟交感神经的刺激增加了 I_{Ca} 和胞浆内 Ca^{2+}，并由此改变肌醇磷脂和蛋白激酶 C 系统调节的 I_K 的效应。在一定的环境下，由 α、β 拟交感神经刺激而引起跨膜电流和细胞内 Ca^{2+} 的变化，这些可以改变细胞动作电位的持续时间和不应期，有利于引发激动的折返，还可以促进正常或异常的自律性以及早期和延迟的后除极相关的触发活动（表 83-1）[1]。

二、临床表现

运动可引发各种类型的心律失常（表 83-2）[1]。运动性房性或室性早搏通常无预后价值。然而，房性或室性早搏可引发非持续或持续性快速心律失常的发作。一般而言，与室上性快速心律失常相比，室性快速心律失常的预后更为不良[2]。室性快速心律失常多见于有器质性心脏病患者，其对药物和导管消融术的治疗效果均不理想。此外，还有一个不易充分理解的

表 83-1　运动引发的代谢、血流动力学及电生理学效应

↓迷走神经张力，↑交感神经张力和儿茶酚胺分泌
↑心率 ⎤
↑心脏收缩力 ⎬ 心肌需氧量
↑收缩压 ⎦

↑腺苷酸环化酶／cAMP 系统
↑肌醇磷脂和蛋白激酶 C 系统
↑细胞内钙离子　　　　↑折返性
↑跨膜离子流　　　　　↑自律性增高
↑舒张期（4 相）除极　↑触发活动
↓心脏组织的不应期

事实是：运动还可能导致缓慢性心律失常如窦性心动过缓、窦性停搏和房室阻滞[1]。

（一）多形性室性快速心律失常

引发和维持单形性和多形性室性心动过速可能的电生理机制是折返、心室异位自律性和触发活动，也可能是三者兼而有之[3]。此外，在心肌缺血或非心肌缺血情况下都能引发单形性和多形性室性心动过速[3]。多形性室性心动过速是多部位局灶性电活动以及反复地激动传导的综合因素造成的，或是由不稳定性的（变换的）旋涡状的（螺旋的）激动折返造成，而这种折返性活动与心室肌不应期的不一致（离散）造成的快速心室反应有关[3]。由于心室率很快，这种心律失常容易恶化成心室颤动，进而导致心脏性猝死。

表 83-2　运动引发的快速心律失常

室性快速心律失常
　多形性
　单形性
　心室颤动
室上性快速心律失常
　AF，AFL，AT，AVNRT
　AVRT
缓慢性心律失常
　窦性心动过缓，窦性静止
　阵发性 AV 传导阻滞

AF（心房颤动）、AFL（心房扑动）、AT（房性心动过速）、AVNRT（房室结折返性心动过速）、AVRT（房室折返性心动过速）。

除增加心脏负荷外，运动可促使动脉粥样硬化性心脏病患者的血栓形成和不稳定的斑块破裂[4]，也会加剧原发性（肥厚型、扩张型和限制型）和继发性（高血压性、瓣膜性和酒精性等）心肌病患者正常与异常心脏组织间的非同步收缩[1,5]。由此，运动可以引发心肌缺血，从而导致心脏解剖结构异常以及瘢痕、肥厚、扩张、心脏纤维变性引起的心脏重构导致心脏电生理基质异常的这两种人群发生室性快速心律失常（包括心室颤动）（图 83-1），因为在这两种患者的心脏细胞常能见到离子通道活性（I_{Na}，I_{Ca}，I_{To}，$I_{Na/Ca}$ 等）及细胞内 Ca^{2+} 的转运不正常[6]。

虽然运动引发的快速多形性室速潜在的临床病因可能是心肌缺血，但这绝不具有诊断的特异性。可以导致多形性室速的其他临床疾病[1,7-12]包括：(1) 先天性和获得性长 QT 综合征（尖端扭转型室性心动过速，Torsades de Pointes）；(2) Brugada 综合征（右束支阻滞和 V_1～V_3 导联持续性的 ST 段抬高）；(3) 儿茶酚胺敏感性多形性室性心动过速；(4) 特发性心室颤动。有上述 4 种临床疾病的患者主要是存在心电不稳定，而其心脏结构可能正常。除先天性长 QT 综合征 3 型和获得性（如药物所致的）长 QT 综合征以及 Brugada 综合征之外，上述患者可能出现运动引发的多形性室性快速心律失常和／或心脏性猝死[1,7-12]。

（二）单形性室性心动过速

运动性单形性室性心动过速可见于动脉粥样硬化性心脏病患者、原发性或继发性心肌病患者[1]。正如前面所提到的，心律失常的始发因素既可以是缺血性的，也可以是非缺血性的。如同多形性室速一样，运动性单形性室性心动过速也可发生在无器质性心脏病的患者。这就是所谓的"特发性"室速（图 83-2）[1,13-15]。

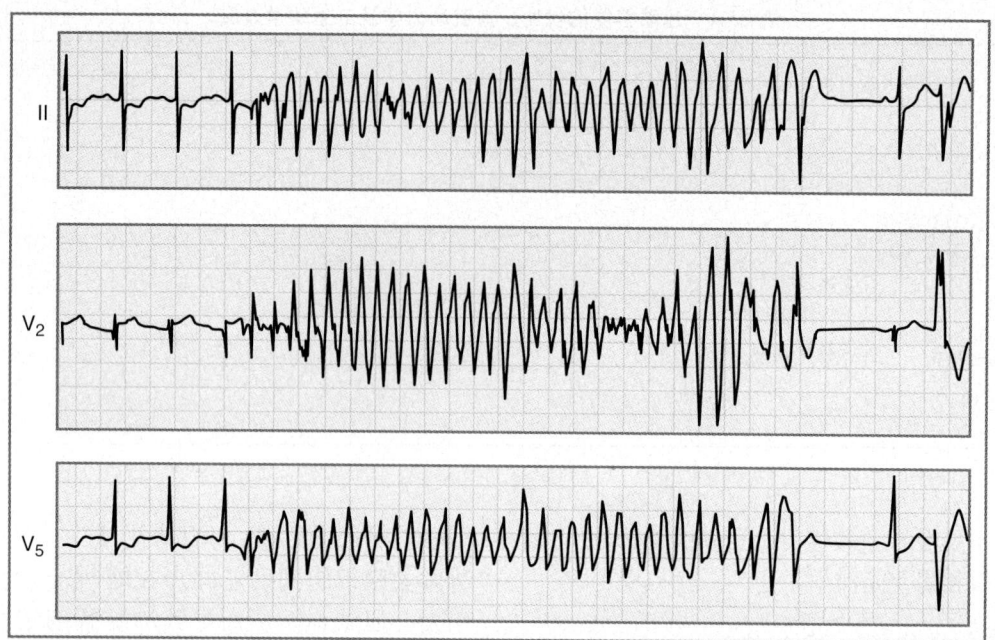

图 83-1 心肌缺血导致的运动性多形性室性快速心律失常 一位 46 岁男性患者在平板运动试验中感到胸闷，随后出现多形性室性心动过速。在室性心动过速发作前记录到心电图 Ⅱ 导联和 V₅ 导联的 ST 段压低。随后在冠状动脉造影术中显示，冠状动脉回旋支近端有一处 90% 的局限性狭窄，随后成功实施了经皮冠状动脉腔内成形术。在成形术后的 5 年随访中，反复地进行平板运动试验未再诱发室性心动过速。

特发性单形性室性心动过速的起源常位于右心室流出道，尤其是漏斗部，QRS 波表现为伴有电轴右偏的完全性左束支阻滞图形，另一种常在左心室基底部到中上部的间隔处起源，QRS 波表现为伴有电轴左偏的完全性右束支阻滞图形。电生理学特征和药理学反应提示特发性单形性室性心动过速的机制是折返性、自律性和触发性的（表 83-3）[1,13-15]。特发性单形性室性心动过速很少情况下发生于右心室间隔上部（电轴左偏）或左心室流出道（电轴右偏）[1]。在临床，具有完全性左束支传导阻滞波形的特发性单形性室性心动过速，应与致心律失常性右室发育不良相关的右心室心动过速、各种类型的心肌病相关的束支折返性心动过速、房室结逆传的房室折返性心动过速以及动脉粥样硬化性心脏病和室间隔缺损或法洛四联症外科手术后引起的心动过速相区别（表 83-4）[3]。

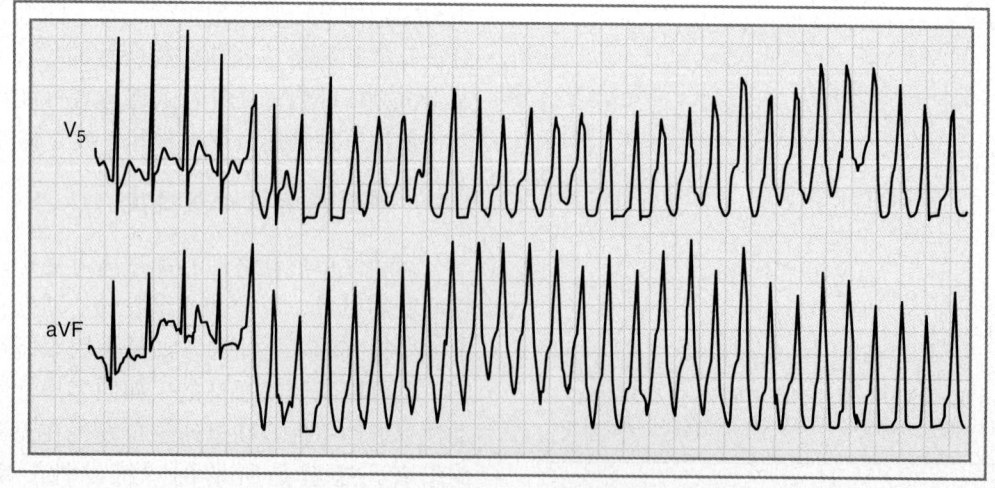

图 83-2 无器质性心脏病的 18 岁男性患者进行平板运动试验时出现持续性室性心动过速 心电图同步记录 V₅ 导联和 aVF 导联。在频率 190 bpm 的室性心动过速发作前，窦性心律的频率增快到 150 bpm。心电图纸速＝25mm/s。（引自 Sung RJ, Shen EN, Morady F, et al: Electrophysiologic mechanism of exercise-induced sustained ventricular tachycardia. Am J Cardiol 51: 525-530, 1983.）

表 83-3　特发性室性心动过速的电生理及药理学特性

	维拉帕米敏感性				非维拉帕米敏感性	
	儿茶酚胺依赖性		非儿茶酚胺依赖性		儿茶酚胺依赖性	非儿茶酚胺依赖性
QRS波形	RBBB	LBBB	RBBB	LBBB	LBBB	LBBB
周长依赖性	+	+	+	+	?	?
超速起搏可终止	+	+	+	+	?	?
维拉帕米	+	+	+	+	?	?
腺苷	+*	+	−	+	?	?
艾司洛尔（或普萘洛尔）	+	+	−△	−△	+	?
普鲁卡因胺	−△	−△	−△	−△	+	+
可能的机制	T, R	T	T, R	T	A	A

* 仅为小部分对维拉帕米具有反应性，且为右束支传导阻滞图形的室性心动过速。
△减慢室性心动过速的频率，但对室性心动过速的诱发没有影响。
+，是或有反应性的；−，否或无反应性的；A，自律性；LBBB，左束支传导阻滞；RBBB，右束支传导阻滞；T，触发活动；R，折返性。

有或没有器质性心脏病患者，应用抗心律失常药物后进行运动可暴露或诱发出原有的心律失常。运动时心率的加快，加强了钠（Na^+）通道的阻滞效应[1,16]。因此，钠（Na^+）通道阻滞引起缓慢传导和不应性的弥散，尤其在病变心肌有利于折返的发生[1,16]。临床上，运动后出现原有的心律失常可见于服用ⅠA类和ⅠC类抗心律失常药物如奎尼丁、普鲁卡因胺、恩卡尼、氟卡尼和普罗帕酮的患者。服用钾（K^+）通道阻滞剂如索他洛尔和胺碘酮的患者，运动通常不能诱发出原有的心律失常，因为当服用这类药物出现心动过缓伴 QT 间期显著延长时可发生尖端扭转型室性心动过速[1]。从理论上讲，选择性阻断儿茶酚胺敏感性 I_{Ks} 通道的 K^+ 通道阻滞剂（如 azimilide）可能导致运动期间出现原有的心律失常，它还能诱发出先天性长 QT 综合征 1 型患者的临床征候群[7]。

（三）室上性快速心律失常

运动可能会引发各种形式的室上性快速心律失常，包括心房颤动、心房扑动、房性心动过速、房室结折返性心动过速以及房室折返性心动过速（表 83-2）[1,14,17]。上述心律失常的出现通常是运动时房性早搏诱发的（图 83-3）。

（四）缓慢性心律失常

如若原来就有或药物性房室结或希浦系统的功能障碍，运动可以引发心动过速依赖性房室阻滞[1]。在阻塞性肺部疾病或冠状动脉粥样硬化性心脏病患者，运动引起窦房结缺氧和／或缺血，可能会引发窦性心动过缓[1]。运动很少引起运动之后（在恢复阶段）因迷走神经张力过度增强的严重窦性心动过缓或窦性静止，从而造成运动后晕厥（图 83-4）[1]。

表 83-4　室性心动过速伴有左束支阻滞 QRS 波形的鉴别诊断

	特发性 ARVD				心肌病；	VSD/TF	逆向性	
	TA	A	R	A	BB 折返性	S／P 外科手术	AVRT	ASHD
QRS 额面轴向	右下		可变		左上	右下；左下	左上／下	可变
PES 诱发和终止	+	−	+	−	+	+	+	+
腺苷	+	−	−	−	−	−	+	−
维拉帕米	+	−	−	−	−	−	+	−

+，是或有反应性的；−，否或无反应性的；A，自律性；ARVD，致心律失常性右室发育不良；ASHD，动脉粥样硬化性心脏病；AVRT，AV 折返心动过速；BB，束支；PES，程序刺激；R，折返性；TA，触发活动；TF，法洛四联症；VSD，室间隔缺损。

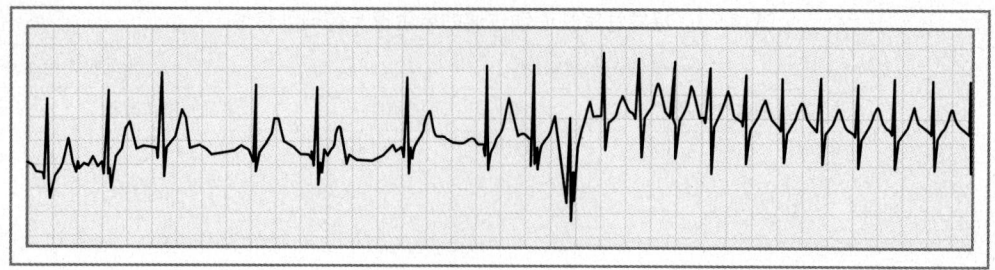

图 83-3 活动时发作心悸、头晕和晕厥症状的 26 岁女性患者在运动中诱发室上性心动过速　平板运动试验时引发了阵发性室上性心动过速,心率 190 bpm(见心电图记录的 Ⅱ 导联)。做 Valsalva 动作后心动过速终止,但在随后又重新出现。室上性心动过速是由房性期前收缩诱发的(第 9 个 QRS 波)。心脏电生理检查证实,在滴注异丙肾上腺素的条件下可诱发房室结折返性心动过速。心电图纸速=25mm/s。

三、基因学和分子学依据

最近,基因学的研究揭示了许多遗传性疾病致心律失常的分子学依据[18-20]。先天性长 QT 综合征潜在的病因是基因的异质性,至少有 7 种基因已被证实,其中有 5 种已表明可编码 K^+ 或 Na^+ 通道蛋白(离子通道病学)[7-9]。在 KCNQ1(长 QT1 综合征)和 KCNE1(长 QT5 综合征)的患者,突变的载体影响 I_{Ks} 的功能,而 I_{Ks} 可被 β 肾上腺素受体调节,因此从事使交感神经张力增强的活动如跳水和游泳时,常出现临床事件(晕厥或心脏性猝死)[3,7]。那些有 HERG 或 KCNH2(长 QT2 综合征)基因突变的患者具有影响 I_{Kr} 的功能性缺陷,在休息和运动时,都可能出现临床事件。值得注意的是,患有长 QT2 综合征的病人中,一部分人会发生由闹钟或电话铃声引发的临床事件。相比之下,那些有 SCN5A(长 QT3 综合征)基因突变并伴有 Na^+ 通道功能增强的患者,由于在休息或睡觉时心率缓慢,QT 间期过度延长而处于高危险状态[7-9]。在患有儿茶酚胺敏感性多形性室性心动过速且不伴有 QT 间期延长的患者,已证实至少 21 种基因突变影响斯里兰卡肉桂碱受体(RyR2)基因(在染色体 1q42-43 上)并与紧张诱发的心脏性猝死相关[21-26]。据推测,这些 RyR2 突变基因可使变异的通道对 β 肾上腺素能信使通路的系列效应超敏(蛋白激酶 A 的超级磷酸化作用),从而导致 Ca^{2+} 从肌浆网中释放出来(细胞内 Ca^{2+} 超负荷)。这与心力衰竭患者心脏性猝死的分子病理生理学机制相似[6]。然而,儿茶酚胺性多形性室性心动过速的范围尚待进一步确定,可能会扩展到包括散在的、无法解释的、由紧张或运动诱发的婴儿、儿童、青少年和成人的猝死病例。

一些遗传性心肌病中已发现有收缩蛋白、结构蛋白以及细胞骨架蛋白存在突变。在家族性肥厚性心肌病,发生突变的有 12 种心脏肌原纤维蛋白(β 重链肌球蛋白,肌球结合蛋白 C,α 肌动蛋白,肌钙蛋白 I、C 和 T,α 原肌球蛋白,心脏必需蛋白和调节蛋白轻链,心脏 elusule LIM 蛋白,titin 蛋白,AMP 活化蛋白激酶)[27,28]。在有传导障碍的遗传性扩张型心肌病

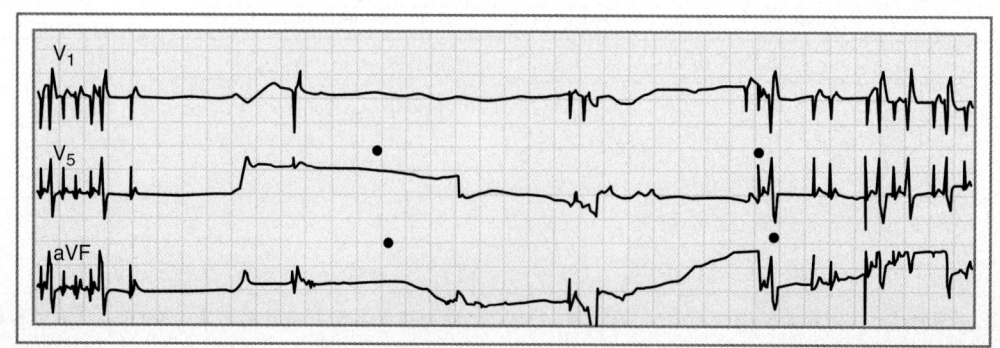

图 83-4 有活动后晕厥史的 22 岁男性患者在运动后即刻的连续性心电图记录(V_1、V_5 和 aVF 导联的同步记录)　运动停止后从窦性心动过速(150 bpm)突然转变成一个长时间窦性静止或传出阻滞(其间仅有几个窦性搏动),然后逐渐恢复了窦性心律伴室性二联律。心电图纸速=25mm/s。(引自 Huycke EC, Card HG, Sobol SM, et al: Postexertional cardiac asystole in a young man without organic heart disease. Ann Intern Med 106: 844-845, 1987.)

患者，则可能与细胞骨架蛋白（肌细胞增强蛋白、结蛋白、α肌动蛋白、核膜蛋白及核纤层蛋白A和C）发生突变有关[29,30]。

在致心律失常性右室发育不良患者，已发现结构蛋白中血小板溶球蛋白[31]和桥粒血小板溶素[32]有隐性突变。这些蛋白在结构和功能上都与细胞间连接或传导有关，因此，它们的缺陷可能造成了心律失常和进行性右心室肌的结构改变。然而，相比之下，在原发性或自律性疾病，主要是致心律失常性右室发育不良，已经发现至少6种基因独特型突变。其中，致心律失常性右心室发育不良2型患者的心脏RyR2基因存在突变（染色体1q42-43），这种病人类似于儿茶酚胺敏感性多形性室性心动过速的患者，常发生心脏性猝死[21-25,33,34]。在将来的研究中，造成此病更多的基因缺陷将被发现和确定。

四、治 疗

应用β肾上腺素受体阻断剂治疗仍然是预防运动性心律失常的基础[1]。但是，临床上有严重症状如眩晕、晕厥、胸痛和充血性心力衰竭的患者以及心脏性猝死高危人群，需要选择介入性的治疗方案。

由动脉粥样硬化性心脏病而造成活动性心肌缺血的患者，有必要行经皮冠状动脉腔内成形术及植入或不植入支架或进行主动脉与冠状动脉间的旁路移植术以获得完全的血管再通。另一方面，因心肌梗死或原发性及继发性心肌病而左心室功能受损的患者，保证最佳的血流动力学和电解质平衡极为重要。通常，这些患者需要利尿剂治疗；若无禁忌证，可用一种血管紧张素转换酶抑制剂或血管紧张素Ⅱ受体阻滞剂和低剂量β肾上腺素受体阻滞剂减轻后负荷；控制高血压；外科手术纠正瓣膜的病变。

患有特发性单形性室性心动过速的患者，除β肾上腺素受体阻断剂（表83-3）外，维拉帕米可能将有效抑制心律失常。导管射频消融对消除特发性单形性室性心动过速（≥80%）、心房扑动、房性心动过速、房室结折返性心动过速及房室折返性心动过速有很好的疗效[1]。

对患有恶性室性心律失常而不适于做导管射频消融术的患者，不管是否伴有器质性心脏病，均应建议植入心律转复除颤器。例如，通常对有RyR2突变的患者建议预防性使用β肾上腺素受体阻断剂。然而，约有30%的儿茶酚胺敏感性多形性室性心动过速的患者，需要植入心律转复除颤器才能有效预防心脏性猝死[26]。

最后，通过对许多遗传性疾病基因特征的了解，将允许更准确地作出症状前筛查和诊断，这非常有利于将来研制和开发针对性强的药物与基因治疗[35,36]。

五、总 结

运动可能诱发各种形式的、不同电生理学机制的心律失常。这些心律失常可能会产生严重的征候群。虽然β肾上腺素受体阻断剂治疗有效，但仍需选择介入性治疗来改善心肌供血和改善血流动力学。对有适应证的患者，还应考虑导管射频消融术和／或植入ICD治疗。随着人类基因组研究的开始，在不久的将来，诊断和治疗方式有望在分子水平获得重大进展。

（柳 茵 译）

参 考 文 献

1. Sung RJ, Lauer R: Exercise-induced cardiac arrhythmias. In Zipes DP, Jalife J (eds): Cardiac Electrophysiology: From Cell to Bedside, 2nd ed. Philadelphia, WB Saunders, 1995, pp 1013–1023.
2. Fletcher GF, Balady GJ, Amsterdam EA, et al: Exercise standards for testing and training. A statement for healthcare professionals for the American Heart Association. Circulation 104:1694–1740, 2001.
3. Sung RJ, Lauer MR: Polymorphic ventricular tachycardia and long QT syndromes. In Sung RJ, Lauer MR (eds): Fundamental Approaches to the Management of Cardiac Arrhythmias. Boston, Kluwer Academic, 2000, pp 732–746.
4. Burke AP, Farb A, Malcom GT, et al: Plaque rupture and sudden death related to exertion in men with coronary artery disease. JAMA 281:921–926, 1999.
5. Rivenes SM, Kearney DL, Smith EO, et al: Sudden death and cardiovascular collapse in children with restrictive cardiomyopathy. Circulation 102:876–881, 2000.
6. Marks AR: Ryanodine receptor/calcium release channels in heart failure and sudden cardiac death. J Mol Cell Cardiol 33:615–624, 2001.
7. Towbin JA, Vatta M: Molecular biology and the prolonged QT syndromes. Am J Med 110:385–398, 2001.
8. Veldkamp MW, Viswanathan PC, Bezzina C, et al: Two distinct congenital arrhythmias evoked by a multidysfunctional Na$^+$ channel. Circ Res 86:e91–e104, 2000.
9. Noh CI, Song JY, Kim HS, et al: Ventricular tachycardia and exercise related syncope in children with structurally normal hearts: Emphasis on repolarization abnormality. Br Heart J 73:544–547, 1995.
10. Leenhardt A, Lucet V, Denjoy I, et al: Catecholaminergic polymorphic ventricular tachycardia in children: A 7-year follow-up in 21 patients. Circulation 91:1512–1519, 1995.
11. Viskin S, Belhassen B: Polymorphic ventricular tachyarrhythmias in the absence of organic heart disease: Classification, differential diagnosis, and implication of therapy. Prog Cardiovasc Dis 41:17–34, 1998.
12. Kasanuki H, Ohnishi S, Ohtuka M, et al: Idiopathic ventricular fibrillation induced with vagal activity in patients without obvious heart disease. Circulation 95:2277–2285, 1997.
13. Kottkamp H, Chen X, Hindricks G, et al: Idiopathic left ventricular tachycardia: New insight into electrophysiological characteristics and radiofrequency catheter ablation. Pacing Clin Electrophysiol 18:1285–1297, 1995.
14. Fauchier JP, Fachier L, Babuty D, et al: Idiopathic monomorphic ventricular tachycardia. Arch Mal Coeur Vaiss 89:897–906, 1996.
15. Gill JS, Prosad K, Blaszyk K, et al: Initiating sequences in exercise-

15. ...induced idiopathic ventricular tachycardia of left bundle branch-like morphology. Pacing Clin Electrophysiol 21:1873–1880, 1998.
16. Levi AJ, Dalton GR, Hancox JC, et al: Role of intracellular sodium overload in the genesis of cardiac arrhythmias. J Cardiovasc Electrophysiol 8:700–721, 1997.
17. Tse HF, Lau CP, Ayers GM: Detection of atrial fibrillation during sinus tachycardia induced by exercise in patients with implantable atrial defibrillators. Pacing Clin Electrophysiol 21:247–252, 1999.
18. Keatnig MT, Sanguinetti MC: Molecular genetic insights into cardiovascular disease. Science 272:681–685, 1996.
19. Priori SG, Bahranin J, Haver RNW, et al: Genetic and molecular basis of cardiac arrhythmias: Impact on clinical management, Part I and Part II. Circulation 99:518–528, 1999.
20. Chen Q, Kirsch GE, Zhang D, et al: Genetic basis and molecular mechanism for idiopathic ventricular fibrillation. Nature 392:293–296, 1998.
21. Lahat H, Pras E, Olender T, et al: A missense mutation in a highly conserved region of CASQ2 is associated with autosomal recessive in Bedouin families from Israel. Am J Hum Genet 69:1378–1384, 2001.
22. Swan H, Piippo K, Viitasalo M, et al: Arrhythmic disorder mapped to chromosome 1q42-q43 causes malignant polymorphic ventricular tachycardia in structurally normal hearts. J Am Coll Cardiol 34:2035–2042, 1999.
23. Priori SG, Napolitano C, Tiso N, et al: Mutations in the cardiac ryanodine receptor gene (hRyR$_2$) underlie catecholaminergic polymorphic ventricular tachycardia. Circulation 103:196–200, 2001.
24. Laitinen PJ, Brown KM, Piippo K, et al: Mutations of the cardiac ryanodine receptor (RyR2) gene in familial polymorphic ventricular tachycardia. Circulation 103:485–490, 2001.
25. Marks AR: Clinical implications of cardiac ryanodine receptor/calcium release channel mutations linked to sudden cardiac death. Circulation 106:8–10, 2002.
26. Priori SG, Napolitano C, Memmi M, et al: Clinical and molecular characterization of patients with catecholaminergic polymorphic ventricular tachycardia. Circulation 106:69–74, 2002.
27. Seidman CE, Seidman JG: Gene mutations that cause familial hypertrophic cardiomyopathy. In Haber E (ed): Scientific American: Molecular Cardiovascular Medicine. New York, Scientific American, 1995, pp 193–210.
28. Bonne G, Carrier L, Richard P, et al: Familial hypertrophic cardiomyopathy: From mutation to functional defects. Circ Res 83:598–593, 1998.
29. Fatkin D, MacLae C, Sasaki T, et al: Missense mutations in the rod domain of the lamin A/C gene as causes of dilated cardiomyopathy and conduction system disease. N Engl J Med 341:1715–1724, 1999.
30. Muchir A, Bonne G, Vander Kooi AJ, et al: Identification of mutations in the gene encoding lamin A/C in autosomal dominant limb girdle muscular dystrophy with atrioventricular conduction disturbances (LGMD1B). Hum Mol Genet 9:1453–1459, 2000.
31. Li D, Ahmad F, Gardner MJ, et al: The locus of a novel gene responsible for arrhythmogenic right ventricular dysplasia characterized by early onset and high penetrance maps to chromosome 10p12-p14. Am J Hum Genet 66:148–156, 2000.
32. Alcalai R, Metzger S, Rosencheck S, et al: A recessive mutation in the desmoplakin gene causes arrhythmogenic right ventricular dysplasia, skin disorder and wooly hair [abstract]. Circulation 106:II–203, 2002.
33. Rampazzo A, Nava A, Erne P, et al: A new locus for arrhythmogenic right ventricular cardiomyopathy (AVRD2) maps to chromosome 1q42-43. Hum Mol Genet 4:2151–2154, 1995.
34. Tiso N, Stephan DA, Nava A, et al: Identification of mutations in the cardiac ryanodine receptor gene in families affected with arrhythmogenic right ventricular cardiomyopathy type 2 (ARVD2). Hum Mol Genet 10:189–97, 2001.
35. Spooner PM, Albert C, Benjamin EJ, et al: Sudden cardiac death, genes, and arrhythmogenesis: Consideration of new population and mechanistic approaches from a National Heart, Lung, and Blood Institute Workshop, Parts I. Circulation 103:2361–2364, 2001.
36. Spooner PM, Albert C, Benjamin EJ, et al: Sudden cardiac death, genes, and arrhythmogenesis: Consideration of new population and mechanistic approaches from a National Heart, Lung, and Blood Institute Workshop, Parts II. Circulation 103:2447–2452, 2001.

第 84 章

动态心电图的应用

Harold L. Kennedy

本章目录

- 心律失常的病理生理及动态心电图的应用原理 ………………… 759
- 动态心电图的临床应用 ……………… 761

动态心电图（Holter）或称为长程心电图是一项应用广泛的无创性心电检查方法，用于评价各种心脏病患者的心电异常。动态心电图的临床应用基础在于其能够在一定时间内连续观察患者的心电图，并且在检查期间允许患者自由活动，有利于记录患者日常各种环境因素（包括生理和心理两方面）对疾病的影响。与普通心电图不同，后者记录患者短时间（<30s）内的 12 导联心电图，而连续记录 24h 的动态心电图一般仅能记录 2～3 个导联的心电图，但其记录时间长，从而能够记录心电现象的动态变化，有些心电现象常常是一过性的，持续时间很短。近来发明的技术已经可以记录 12 导联的动态心电图，但是其确切价值尚未肯定[1]。虽然现在已经有了电话连续监测心电的技术，但动态心电图可记录较长时间的心电信息，并且能对动态变化或一过性的心电事件进行详细分析。与其他心电学检查方法相比，临床研究已经证实动态心电图在诊断自发性心律失常方面有着更高的敏感性[2]。

动态心电图已经成为临床记录快速性和缓慢性心律失常（包括传导异常）的重要诊断方法，历经 30 余年，动态心电图现还可用于评价 ST 段改变（用于诊断心肌缺血）、RR 间期变化（用于评价心率变异性）和 QRS 波测量（用于评价复极异常，如 QT 间期），以及信号平均心电图（用于记录碎裂电位，如晚电位）[3]。这些后期发展的参数提供了更多的心电数据，用于研究一些特殊心律失常发生和持续的机制。

40 余年的临床经验显示，动态心电图已经成为一项最具投效比的无创性临床检查方法，用于诊断和评价心脏症状、预后评估或各种心脏病人群的危险分层，以及对各种治疗手段的疗效进行评价。本章阐述心律失常的病理生理机制、动态心电图记录的电生理参数以及动态心电图的临床应用。

一、心律失常的病理生理及动态心电图的应用原理

心律失常的发生机制包括冲动起源异常和冲动传导异常。快速性或缓慢性心律失常均由这两种机制形成[3]。心律失常的电学基础一般由 3 个重要因素决定：（1）心脏基质，最常见的是心室肌器质性异常；（2）电触发，例如室性早搏，最初曾认为室早是致命性心律失常的主要诱发因素，后来认识到室早仅仅是心律失常机制中的一个因素，而且并非必需；（3）生理的或病理生理的触发因子，其可能导致心肌处于电不稳定状态，从而对致心律失常因素或时间敏感（图 84-1），这些触发因子可能是短暂的异常，如心肌缺血、电解质紊乱、酸中毒、组织缺氧、中毒或致心律失常药物、心肌细胞离子通道的遗传变异或其他系统的疾病。但是，总体来说，最为重要的因素是交感神经和副交感神经张力[3]。近期我们才认识到自主神经张力的重要性以及心肌细胞离子通道遗传变异和遗传性心律失常的关系[4,5]。同样，新近对血管内皮功能异常与缺血时间关系的认识改变了我们过去的心肌缺

血概念[6]。这一进展也支持动态心电图记录的应用,因其在很多情况下能够提供更多的与自主神经张力或导致严重心脏事件的缺血发作等诊断和预后的数据。

20世纪60年代和70年代期间,临床一般认为触发性室性早搏是心律失常发生的主要机制,从而导致动态心电图的广泛应用,接受动态心电图检查期间猝死患者的检查资料提示最常见的心脏性猝死原因是室性快速性心律失常,最终蜕变为室颤并导致死亡[3]。

随后20年间,大量的研究是利用有创性电生理检查阐明心肌基质在心律失常发生中的作用和地位。在此期间,很多研究者利用动态心电图研究发现,有关触发的数据并不能预测患者的治疗效果,有关药物晚期致心律失常的研究进一步证实了这一发现,此即心律失常抑制试验(CAST试验)。该试验发现,药物成功地控制室早并不能减少心脏性猝死[3]。临床患者的抗心律失常治疗难以抉择得到了进一步的重视,开始争议何种评价方法(以及该方法指导的治疗)最为有效,是动态心电图还是有创性电生理检查?

这一争议持续了10年,特别是恶性室性心律失常及心肌梗死后患者的管理方面。为解决这一问题,人们进行了电生理检查和动态心电图的对比试验(ESVEM试验)[3]。这是第一个大规模、前瞻性、随机对照试验,用来对比在预测恶性室性心律失常及既有自发性频发室性心律失常又能诱发室性心动过速的晕厥患者的远期预后方面,电生理检查和动态心电图检查哪一种更为优越[3]。尽管该试验是在高选择人群完成的,但ESVEM试验证实了动态心电图评价药物疗效的应用范围更广,

而且费用更低[3]。另外,动态心电图预测的准确性与电生理检查类似,所以,动态心电图和运动试验等无创性检查方法再次成为有效且投效比高的管理恶性室性心律失常患者的检查方法[3]。

20世纪90年代,几个因素促使人们再次探询猝死的发生机制,对过去发现的现象有了新的理解。左室功能减退与终末期心衰患者心脏停搏或缓慢性心律失常导致死亡率增加之间相关性的重要意义得到证实[3]。而且,随着心脏病患者的存活期越来越长,合并其他致命性疾病的可能性也就越高(例如致命的肺栓塞、主动脉瘤破裂、严重的脑血管意外),而这些情况可能误诊为心律失常引起的心脏性猝死[7]。

无论如何,对心脏性猝死的理解上,一个巨大的改变是对粥样硬化斑块破裂以及与内皮、血管、血液流变学之间关系的认识[8,9]。不稳定的粥样硬化斑块对一些外部因素或自主神经介导的应激十分敏感,这些机制已经证实与心脏性猝死有关。Leor及其同事[10],Spaulding及其同事[11]的研究结果均支持这一观点,即有三分之一到一半的心脏性猝死都是继发于急性斑块破裂(图84-2)。在理解心脏性猝死中第二个巨大改变是随着发现家族性猝死而产生的,它们包括肥厚型心肌病、长QT综合征、Brugada综合征及家族性多形性室速,这些疾病均与异常的基因突变有关,包括肌浆网、肌钙蛋白和肌球蛋白或细胞离子通道[12,13]。

考虑到以上因素,目前心脏性猝死的概念必须综合心电、缺血、机械(泵衰)以及最近提出的心肌细胞遗传变异因素(图84-2)。根据这一观点,常常是首先由一些外部事件激活自主神经系统,交感张力增加,副交感张力减低[3],这些改变导致血压增高、血流剪切力增加、心率增快、血小板聚集增加,血液黏度增加,同时抑制纤溶系统[14]。而且,自主神经张力的改变降低心率变异性和室颤阈值,这些改变引起了斑块破裂、破损的倾向以及随后的血小板聚集,后者导致心肌缺血(心绞痛或心肌梗死)或心电紊乱、心脏性猝死[3,8]。

一些有心脏性猝死危险的患者,如心室肥厚、瘢痕或纤维化,心肌细胞异常(如缺血、坏死或发育异常)以及遗传性疾病,自主神经张力异常可能导致异常的细胞内钙诱发的后除极或异常的跨膜电位,结果导致室性快速性心律失常,或者导致严重的房室阻滞或心脏停搏(图84-2)。所以,心脏性猝死的广义概念必须包含经典的触发、异常的基质、调节因子和基因变异,这些因素由自主神经系统调节,后者受很多内部和外部事件影响,从而通过心电、缺血、机械或

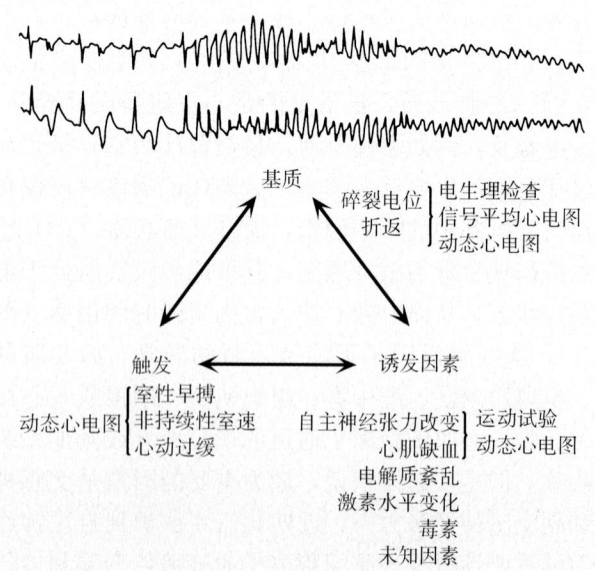

图84-1 心律失常的发生机制

遗传机制等介导严重不良事件的发生（图 84-2）。

动态心电图可以提供很多信息，可以了解导致心脏性猝死事件的心电紊乱或心肌缺血。动态心电图及相关技术能够证实心律失常、缺血性 ST 段改变、晚电位（信号平均心电图）、复极异常（测定 QT 间期和 T 波电交替），以及自主神经张力异常（心率变异性）。这些内容的深入讨论不在本章。在第七部分，"诊断评估"一章中会有进一步的讨论。而在其他专著中可见现代动态心电图技术的深层讨论[2,3,15]。

二、动态心电图的临床应用

近 30 年来，动态心电图的主要临床应用没有明显改变，但现在其应用范围已明显扩展。目前，动态心电图主要用于：（1）心脏症状的诊断与评估；（2）心脏病人群的预后评估和危险分层；（3）疗效评价[3]（表 84-1）。虽然动态心电图的诊断用途没有明显变化，但由于结合了很多新的有预测价值的参数，动态心电图用于心脏病患者危险分层的功能已经从根本上改进。无症状心肌缺血和缺血总负荷[16,17]、自主神经张力异常导致的心率变异性异常[18-20]、平均叠加法记录的晚电位异常[21]，以及心率振荡现象等指标，在各种心脏病患者均有判断预后和危险分层价值。同样，动态心电图这些参数的拓展也增强了其评估疗效的功能（表 84-1）。

然而，目前的临床工作要遵循指南进行[3,22,23]，似乎应该按照以下方式讨论动态心电图的临床应用，即所谓 3 类适应证：Ⅰ类：有证据支持或一致认为动态心电图是有价值或可信赖的检查；Ⅱ类：对动态心电图的价值或效果有不一致的证据或观点，其中ⅡA 类指证据或观点倾向于有价值/有效，ⅡB 类指证据或观点倾向于无价值/无效；Ⅲ类：有证据或一致认为无价值/无效，有时可能有害。近期的指南中还规定了证据等级，A 类：来自多中心随机临床试验；B 类：来自单中心随机临床试验或非随机对照研究；C 类：专家意见。最近的动态心电图指南[22]尚未包含这一内容。

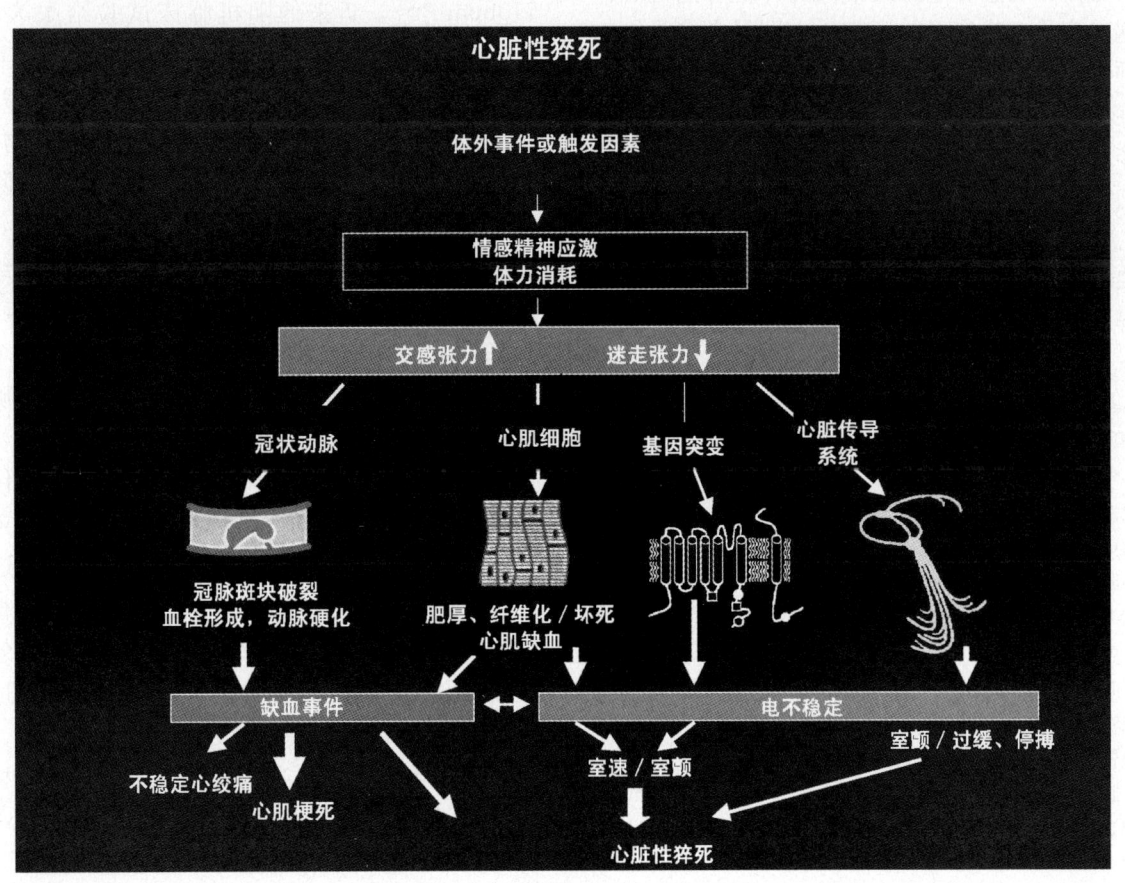

图 84-2 心脏性猝死的病理生理学

动态心电图的应用应该考虑这种证据级别的观点（如心脏症状的诊断与评估、心脏病人群的预后评估和危险分层以及疗效评价，见表84-1）。而且，指南中提出[22]，由于动态心电图的应用存在多样性，不可能列出适用于所有情况的精确条例，也许有时原本属于Ⅰ类适应证，由于情况变化而变为不必要或不适当，或原本属于Ⅲ类适应证，情况改变后临床应用恰当而且有效。心血管专家必须记住这一概念，随着动态心电图检测参数（如心律失常、心率变异性、信号平均心电图和复极异常）的进展，其应用范围也在逐渐变化。而且，虽然常常把美国心脏病学会（ACC）和美国心脏协会（AHA）制订的指南作为权威，但其受某一个国家医生的观点所限，未考虑其他国家的诊断技术和资源，所以，应用动态心电图时眼界应放宽，并要有一定的灵活性[22]。

（一）诊断和评估可能起源于心脏的症状

1. 评价心律

（1）心悸：动态心电图最常用的评价可能是心律失常引起的症状。临床经验证实心电图异常多是短暂的，必须确认心电图异常与症状的关系。根据症状的特点、症状的持续时间和发作频度以及在事件发生前后（发作和终止）心电图资料的重要性而决定是否应该选择心电图记录技术。而在多数情况下，应用24或48h（决定于症状的严重程度）的动态心电图可适于所有患者，以评价心脏节律和可能存在的心律失常或传导异常，可判断日常活动中出现的症状与其主诉

的相关性。这种检查常常可以排除心律失常作为患者主诉的原因。少见的情况是，经电话传输心电监护适用于间歇或偶尔发作症状的患者。相反，如果症状严重而且可能威胁生命，则应该住进冠心病监护病房，在院内安全的环境下进行动态心电监护。如果院内检查未能确诊，根据症状的严重程度（晕厥或抽搐），植入式Holter可以连续监护14个月，可能有助于这类患者的诊断[24,25]。

（2）房颤：随着人们对慢性房颤以及持续性房性心动过速危害认识的加深，动态心电图记录越来越多地用于评价持续性心动过速[3,26]。虽然动态心电图早已用于评价慢性房颤、甲亢以及β受体高敏状态患者的心室率，但近来研究提示控制不佳的慢性房颤及不适当性窦性心动过速也会导致心功能异常，进而导致扩张型心肌病，故对这些异常有了新的认识，现在要求应当严格控制这些患者的心室率（心率<100bpm），这是动态心电图应用的一个新领域。目前已有的数据提示房颤患者的静息心室率应控制在80~90bpm，6min步行试验时的运动心室率不应超过110bpm[28,29]。近来的随机临床试验结果表明[28,29]，对于持续性房颤患者，节律控制治疗（维持其窦性心律）在提高生存率方面并不优于频率控制治疗，而且频率控制治疗还有其他优点，如减少了药物副作用，降低住院率。给所有患者应用抗凝治疗，去除那些停用华法林或华法林治疗力度不够的患者[28,29]，两种治疗方案的卒中发生率相同。根据这一试验的结果，考虑到慢性房颤患者需要数十年而非仅仅数年的治疗，动态心电图检查对其是适宜的，可以观察整个记录过程中（包括白天和黑夜）心动过速的特点，确认心室率控制的效果，指导进一步的治疗（图84-3、84-4）。

（3）头晕或先兆晕厥：对于一些不常发作或难以预测的严重症状（如先兆晕厥或晕厥），直立倾斜试验或心内电生理检查、运动试验并不适合，这些患者可以进行动态心电图检查[30,31]。过去已经有很多研究证实动态心电图检查对诊断上述症状十分有效，尽管早期研究的患者主要症状是心悸或清醒时不适。近来很多研究观察了有血流动力学异常的患者，如头晕、先兆晕厥或晕厥，约25%~50%患者在24h检查过程中出现了不适，约2%~15%患者证实了心律失常，35%~58%患者发作不适时未见心电图异常[3]。对于先兆晕厥或晕厥患者，如果将记录时间延长为3天时，一半患者会有症状发作，而如果记录时间延长到5~21天（平均9天）时，75%患者会有症状发作[3]。

表84-1 动态心电图的临床应用

1. **诊断和评估可能起源于心脏疾病的症状**
    评价心悸的主诉
    评价快速性心律失常和房颤
    评价自觉不适（如短暂的头晕、眩晕或先兆晕厥）
    提示心肌缺血的症状
2. **心脏病人群的预后评估和危险分层**
    心梗后患者
    肥厚型心肌病患者
    心衰患者
    周围血管疾病患者
    新发心脏病患者
3. **评价疗效**
    抗心律失常治疗
    评价起搏器和植入式心脏复律除颤器
    抗缺血治疗
    房颤和不适当窦速的控制

但是，研究结果并非完全一致。Bass 及其同事[3]研究了95名晕厥患者，记录3次24h动态心电图后，只有27%的患者发现了心律失常。对于那些住院期间（经过动态心电图、直立倾斜试验和心内电生理检查）未能确诊的患者，植入式"Holter"提供了进一步的诊断方法，在一个小规模研究中证实了这种长时间监测检查的方法有助于发现心律失常或心跳骤停，这些事件有时难以和神经系统的异常相鉴别[24,25]。

近来人们发现院内和院外患者主诉上的差别[3]。306名住院患者中，6.3%患者原本知道有室性心律失常，24h动态心电图记录对其中95%（20名患者中的19名）证实了相关的心律失常，而278名院外患者的55%有不适主诉者中，只有43.5%（154名患者中的67名）记录到了心律失常。另外，Nwasokwa 及同事[3]发现，住院人群中（研究了1010例患者），年龄、性别、症状与动态心电图检查的异常发现有关，特别是症状有很强的预测意义，所有患者可根据有或无晕厥分为两组，无晕厥组患者在动态心电图检查期间要记日记，报告症状，这一组患者中年龄和性别的意义不大，而在晕厥患者组中则不然，小于60岁女性患者常常报告非晕厥的症状，而60岁以上男性则少4倍[3]。

由于检查人群不同，检查时间不同，心电图异常的定义不同，同时可能未判定症状与心律失常的关系，难以精确分析上述数据。而且，健康无症状人群也可出现窦性心动过缓、窦性停搏、室上性及室性心律失常，所以，这些心律失常未必与一过性的不适有关。所以，如果检查期间出现症状或心律失常，或二者同时出现，而且有临床意义，24h动态心电图检查的准确性最高为76%。相反，如果症状与检测到的心律失常无关，动态心电图检查的准确性只有16%[3]。

（4）晕厥：判断心律失常为相关病因的标准是人为规定的，而且在不断修正。许多作者认为2.0~2.5s的窦性停搏是异常的，而另外的资料表明3.0s甚至更长的窦性停搏不会引起症状或影响预后，这种观点认为，只有窦性停搏的同时伴有症状才需要治疗。Kapoor 及同事[3]研究了心律失常与预后的关系，提示伴有频发和复杂室性心律失常的晕厥患者猝死发生率高，反复发作晕厥并不是判断预后的可靠终点，所以对于有频发和复杂室性心律失常的晕厥患者，不论其心律失常是否与症状有关，都应给予相关的治疗。

Linzer 及其同事[30,31]的研究证实，对于判断哪些不明原因晕厥患者应该接受心内电生理检查，动态心电图检查是有价值的，他们建立了一种模型，用以预测这些患者的电生理检查结果。连续应用于141个不明原因晕厥患者后，结果显示，综合患者的临床表现、心电图和动态心电图结果能够预测电生理检查结果。器质性心脏病和动态心电图发现非持续性室速预示着严重的室性心律失常（敏感性100%），而心电图发现窦性心动过缓、一度房室阻滞或束支阻滞则预示缓慢性心律失常（敏感性79%）[3]。有缓慢性心律失常的"中危"患者可以利用电话传输动态心电图监测的方法进行评价。无上述临床危险因素的患者实际上无严重室性心律失常的危险，缓慢性心律失常的危险也很低[3]。结合这一研究结果及一些支持这一"金标准"的随机临床试验结果，对于晕厥诊断的专家共识认为[30,31]：第一，病史、体格检查、心电图（包括普通心电图和动态心电图）是晕厥诊断的基础（联合诊断率50%）；第二，除非有神经系统的症状或体征，很少应用神经系统检查；第三，器质性心脏病是不良预后的高危因素，相关患者应该进行心脏检查（无创和有创，诊断率5%~35%）；第四，老年人的晕厥常常是多种药物所致或异常的生理反应；第五，对于反复发作的无器质性心脏病的晕厥患者，动态心电图（诊断率25%~30%）和直立倾斜试验（诊断率达60%）是最有用的检查方法；第六，精神病学检查能够在25%的病例中发现伴随晕厥的精神异常；第七，心源性晕厥的高危患者（有器质性心脏病证据）或出现神经系统体征的患者应该住院[30,31]。虽然其他指南可能有所不同[32]，但一般应从常规应用的简单检查着手进行诊断[33,34]。

（5）心律失常分析：动态心电图适合于评价自发性心律失常的各种特点（定性或定量），可以确定各种早搏的形态，了解各种缓慢性或快速性心律失常发作和终止的特点，可以检测多种心律失常指标（如联律间期、频率依赖性、QT间期的变化），推测心律失常起源或折返环的部位，特别是阵发性室上性心动过速，其发作或终止特点对于心律失常机制的确定有重要价值[3]。这些心律失常的P波位置和电轴常能提供有关电生理异常的线索，三导动态心电图记录常可确定诊断[3]。动态心电图评价和诊断心律失常的建议见表84-2。

2. 评价心肌缺血

最近30年来，动态心电图用于检测心肌缺血一直存有争议。开始的争议在于通过动态心电图测量ST段改变是否准确，使用AM或M记录器，以及敏感的双极导联的选择[3]。这些问题解决之后，有关诊

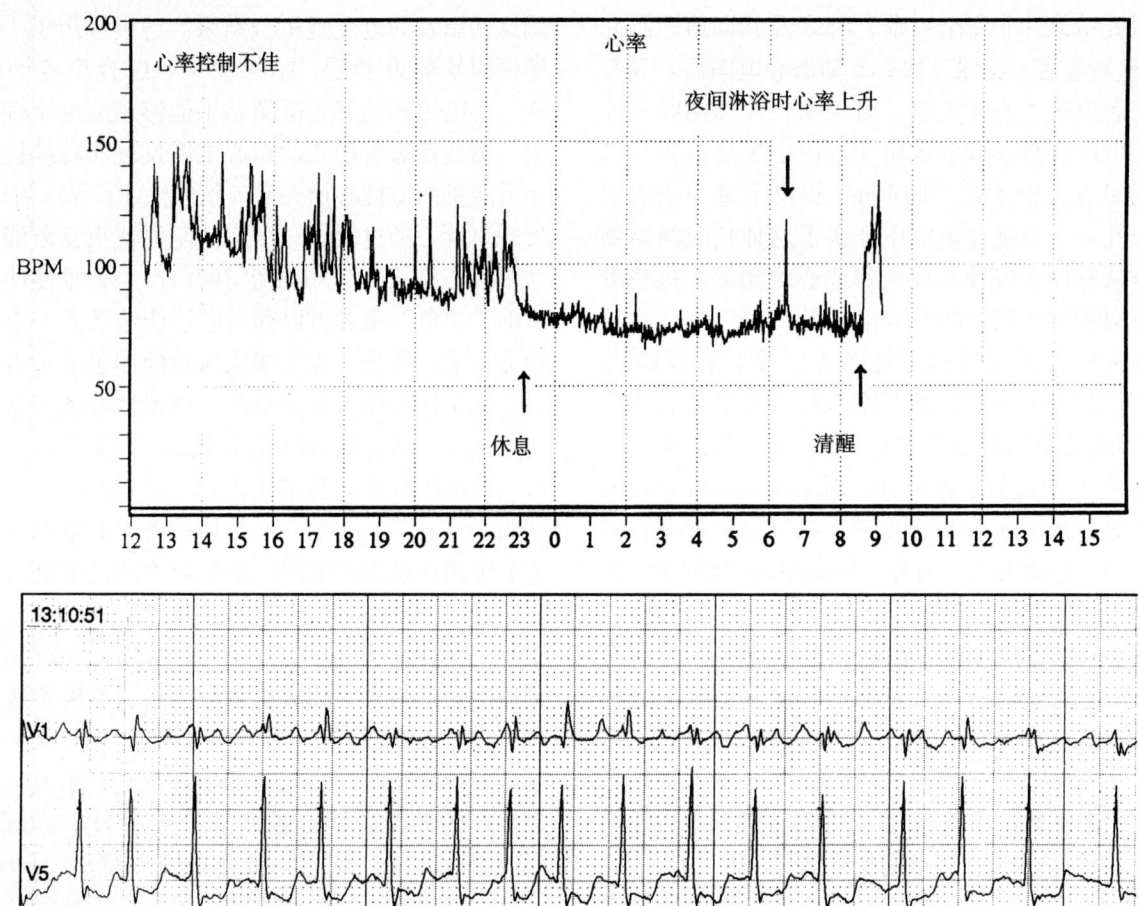

图 84-3 心房颤动 上图:动态心电图的 24h 趋势图显示日常活动及清醒时心室率控制不佳;下图:13:10 的实时打印心电图显示房颤患者心室率约 150bpm。

断标准、伪差识别以及健康人假阳性的鉴别等又出现了争议[3]。在 20 世纪 80 年代和 90 年代间,由于不了解动态心电图所提供信息的意义,专家指南不支持应用动态心电图评价无症状或有症状心肌缺血[3]。进入 21 世纪以后,许多精心设计的临床研究证实动态心电图对诊断心肌缺血的价值和优点,而且证实了其在已确诊的冠状动脉疾病患者的价值[3]。虽然仅是有限的资料支持动态心电图对未确诊冠心病或周围血管疾病患者无症状心肌缺血的诊断价值,但研究已经证实了其在部分有心脏高危因素老年人群的预测价值[3,17]。

相反,对于"稳定"的冠心病患者,其经常发作的无症状心肌缺血事件可能占所有缺血事件的 60%~80%,动态心电图用于评价这种患者非常有价值[3,37]。即使接受了似乎恰当的抗心绞痛药物治疗,仍然可能出现无症状心肌缺血[35]。同样,在急性冠脉综合征患者,动态心电图可以发现残余的心肌缺血,而进行中的缺血发作有很高的预测预后价值[3,36]。在那些没有条件进行再血管化治疗的情况下,这些资料仍然很有意义。对于不明确或不典型胸痛或不适的患者,运动试验无法确诊或无法诱发原有的不适(如变异型心绞痛或 X 综合征),动态心电图也有其价值。由于有了核素和超声心动图(多巴胺试验)等方法,无需运动即可评价心肌灌注状态,所以对于有急性炎症或其他不适于运动的疾病,不必使用动态心电图作为心肌缺血的主要评价方法,但如果无此检查条件时可能不然。

新近,有报告认为,血管疾病患者进行术前评估时,动态心电图是一种投效比较高的检测隐匿性心肌缺血的方法[3,38,39]。9%~39%患者存在异常的无症状

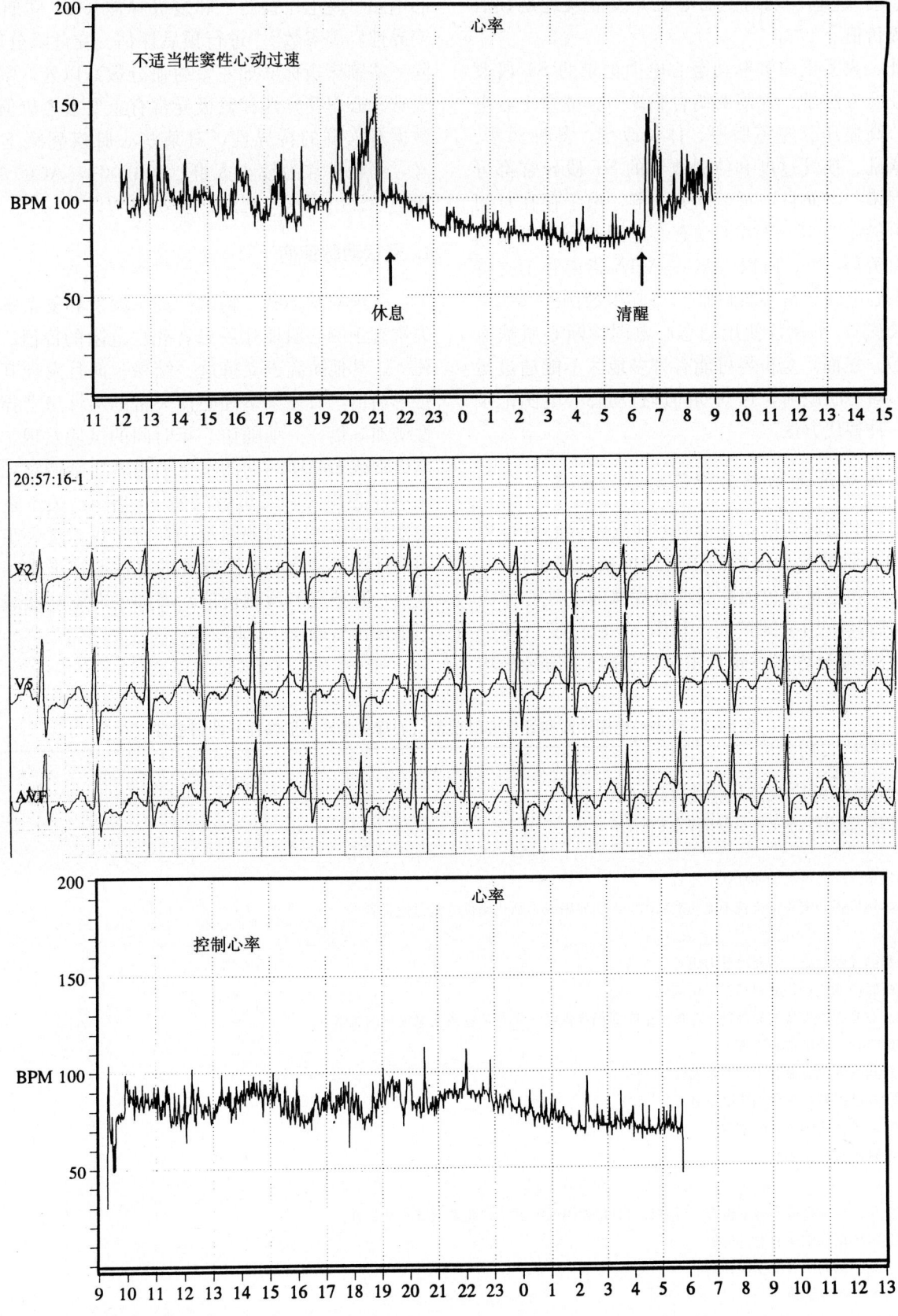

图 84-4 不适当性窦性心动过速 上、下图：动态心电图记录的 24h 趋势图显示 β 受体阻滞剂治疗前（上图）、后（下图）日常活动和清醒状态时均有不适当窦性心动过速；中图：20∶57 患者的实时打印心电图为不适当的窦性心动过速。

ST 段改变，这些发现对术后心脏并发症及远期预后均有预测价值[3,38,39]。

除此，为了正确解释动态心电图记录的 ST 段改变还需注意方法学，并需要结合临床[3]。继发于心电图异常、高血压、左室肥厚、体位改变、各种药物、电解质紊乱、换气过度和体温改变的 ST 段异常都可能引起混淆[3]。而且，对于部分人群，由于存在日间差异，可能需要 48～72h 的动态心电图检查方可正确评价缺血负荷[3,40]。所以，ACC/AHA 指南并不支持使用动态心电图评价心肌缺血[22]。除少数例外（如变异型心绞痛），不建议使用动态心电图诊断心肌缺血（表 84-2）。然而，全世界可能有许多地区不能通过运动试验诊断心肌缺血，运动期间进行动态心电图记录可能是一种替代方法。

（二）心脏病患者的预后评价和危险分层

动态心电图起初用于评价有心律失常或心脏性猝死危险的心肌梗死后患者的预后评价或危险分层[3]，其可以定性和定量评价无症状或有症状的室性心律失常，但随后其应用范围扩大，利用 ST 段改变（评价缺血）、心率变异性（评价自主神经功能）、信号平均心电图（晚电位检测）和复极异常（QT 间期和 T 波变异性）等参数[2,3]进行预后评估。在危险分层方面，除一些临床指标（如左室射血分数）以外，室性心律失常、心率变异性和复极异常有重要参考价值。这些数据有人群的特异性，对某些心脏疾病缺乏完整定义，而且常常为较小人群（＜1000），ACC/AHA 的指南中提出了这一观点（表 84-3）[22]。

1. 冠状动脉疾病

一项冠状动脉药物试验提示频发和复杂室性心律失常有预测心肌梗死后患者死亡危险的价值，包括猝死[3]。其他研究也支持这一结果，而且发现其增加死亡率两倍，有复杂室性心律失常的男性患者猝死危险性增加 3 倍。一项随访 5 年时间的试验发现，室性心律失常或短联律间期的室早男患者年龄调整死亡率是无室性心律失常男患者的 4～5 倍[3]。关于室性心律失常是否为独立预测因子仍存有争议，进一步的研究明确证实了动态心电图发现的室性心律失常（频发或复杂）有独立的预测价值，增加了左室功能减退患者的不良预后的发生风险[3]。

表 84-2　动态心电图诊断和评估心脏疾病（心律失常和心肌缺血）的适应证

Ⅰ类
1. 不明原因晕厥、先兆晕厥或无明显诱因头晕患者
2. 不明原因反复心悸，病史提示为心律失常的患者

ⅡA 类
1. 有冠脉痉挛或变异型心绞痛症状的患者
2. 病史、体格检查和实验室检查不能明确病因的不明原因或不适当窦性心动过速患者*

ⅡB 类
1. 无法解释的呼吸困难、胸痛或乏力患者
2. 怀疑有短暂房颤或房扑的神经系统疾病患者
3. 已经证实有非心律失常的病因且正在接受治疗而仍有晕厥、先兆晕厥或头晕发作的患者
4. 评价不能进行运动的胸痛患者
5. 不能进行运动的患者血管手术的术前评估
6. 已知冠状动脉疾病的不典型胸痛患者
7. 评价持续和慢性房颤患者的心室率*
8. 评价睡眠呼吸暂停患者*

Ⅲ类
1. 根据病史、体格检查或实验室检查已经确诊为其他原因的晕厥、先兆晕厥或头晕患者
2. 无心律失常依据的脑血管意外患者
3. 能进行运动的胸痛患者的初步评估
4. 无症状人群的常规筛查
5. 存在心电图异常（如束支阻滞、室内阻滞），ST 段改变无法评价心肌缺血*

*美国心脏病学会/美国心脏协会（ACC/AHA）指南未分类[22]。

而且，溶栓治疗并不影响这一预测因素，GISSI二期研究了8552名接受溶栓治疗的急性心肌梗死患者，动态心电图发现的频发和复杂室性心律失常仍然使各种原因的总死亡率增加2～3倍，猝死危险增加3～4倍[3]。在此研究期间，CAST试验提示接受抗心律失常药物治疗的左室功能正常的心肌梗死后患者，致心律失常危险增高，而且从抗心律失常获益较小。所以，目前的ACC/AHA指南没有建议左室功能正常的心肌梗死后患者接受动态心电图检查[22]（表84-3）。

由于动态心电图对ST段改变检测的可靠性，临床开始研究其评价冠状动脉疾病患者无症状和有症状心肌缺血的发生率和预后的敏感性[3]。因为动态心电图在检测日常活动及应激状态心肌缺血时有其独特的优点[41,42]，在稳定和不稳定冠状动脉疾病患者，缺血发生率为20%～50%[3]。已经证实动态心电图发现的缺血事件中60%～80%是无症状的，而且动态心电图检查可以识别高危者[3,43]。近期的研究表明，在运动试验的基础上，动态心电图发现缺血性ST段改变提高了预后评估价值。同样，虽然小规模的临床研究发现隐匿性缺血性心脏病患者进行血管手术时，动态心电图检查发现的ST段改变是围手术期事件的预测因子[3]。然而，动态心电图的有关指南还没有广泛接受这些试验结果[22]（表84-2和表84-3）。这可能是由于政府出于经济因素对指南制定专家的影响所致。虽然这在某些国家（如美国）是合适的，但在其他一些国家，动态心电图可能是最具投效比而且是唯一可以进行的检查，因此这种决定可能并不恰当。

动态心电图也可用于心肌梗死后患者，通过检测RR间期评价心率变异性，后者是独立于室性心律失常和左室功能的预后评价因素[3]。研究显示心率变异性差的患者迷走神经张力减低，而交感神经张力增高，心律失常和各种原因所致的死亡率增高[3,45]。

最后，根据动态心电图记录的信号平均心电图也能用于评价心肌梗死后患者的预后[3,46-48]。这种来自于异常心肌的微小电位（晚电位）是形成折返的基础。心肌梗死后患者晚电位阳性时高度提示存在闭塞的梗死相关动脉及心律失常事件，心肌梗死后人群中最有预测价值的信号平均心电图参数是QRS波的宽度超过120ms[46,47]。虽然这些数据来源于实时和长程信号平均心电图的研究，但使用长程信号平均心电图进行危险分层的有效性及投效比还未确定。

近来，心率震荡作为一个新的指标在心梗后危险分层中有一定的价值。从动态心电图得到的心率震荡有两个评价指标：震荡初始（TO）和震荡斜率（TS），TO用于检出单个室早后有无早期加速，TS用于检出单个室早后有无晚期减速。TS和TO作为独立的变量，与左室射血分数、心率变异性和压力反射过敏相比，有更多的预测价值[49,50]。在ATRAMI研究中[50]，对1212名心梗后幸存者进行了检查和平均持续20.3个月的随访。在多变量分析中，异常的TO和TS及左室射血分数仍为独立预测指标。对于所有的异常因素来说，复合的自主指数（TO、TS、压力反射过敏和NN标准差）是最强的多变量危险预测因素（相对危险度8.7；置信区间2.7～7.7；$P=0.0003$）。目前，这个新的变量正在几个疾病人群中进行观察[51]。

总之，动态心电图以及其许多参数已经应用于许多缺血性心脏病患者的研究，多变量联合应用时，其阳性预测准确率一般为15%～50%，敏感性60%～80%，特异性70%～95%[22]。

2. 特发性肥厚型心肌病

动态心电图检查发现三分之二的特发性肥厚型心肌病患者有频发的复杂室性心律失常，约25%的患者存在室性心动过速，与猝死相关[3]，有证据表明胺碘酮治疗可以降低这组患者的猝死发生率，但尚有争议。近期一项随访长达9.6年，观察了368例患者（14～65岁，男性239名）的多中心研究结果提示，发生非持续性室性心动过速的猝死危险率是1.9（可信区间0.7～5.0，$P=0.18$），存在其他危险因素时更为明确。ACC/AHA指南承认动态心电图在肥厚型心肌病患者的判断预后价值，但是由于并没有针对动态心电图发现异常的有效治疗，指南并没有强烈建议进行此项检查[22]。

3. 心衰

80%～90%的缺血性心肌病或原发性扩张型心肌病导致的充血性心力衰竭患者动态心电图检查可发现复杂频发的室性心律失常，虽然有研究者认为这些心律失常与预后无关，但也有研究认为与预后有关。Bigger及其同事[3]研究了766名心肌梗死后患者的室性心律失常、左室功能异常和死亡率的关系，发现室性心律失常是独立的危险因子。其后，Doval及其同事[3,53]报告，根据GESICA试验的资料，非持续性室性心动过速是总死亡率和猝死的独立危险因素，去除其他临床因素影响后仍

表 84-3　动态心电图进行预后评估或危险分层的适应证

I类
无
IIA类
1. 左室功能异常的心肌梗死后患者*
2. 慢性充血性心力衰竭患者*
3. 特发性肥厚型心肌病患者*
IIB类
1. 未进行运动试验的有冠心病危险因素的老年患者△
2. 随访已知窦房结或心脏传导系统疾病的患者△
3. 有症状的二尖瓣脱垂、长QT综合征及预激综合征患者
4. 未进行再血管化治疗且有缺血发作（或有症状）的已知缺血性心脏病患者△
5. 已知血管疾病患者进行外科手术前△
III类
1. 心肌梗死后左室功能正常者
2. 非心脏手术前心律失常评估
3. 评价糖尿病神经病变
4. 血管疾病患者
5. 左室肥厚的原发性高血压患者
6. 睡眠呼吸暂停患者
7. 心脏外伤患者
8. 不能分析心率变异性的心律失常患者（如房颤）

* ACC/AHA 分类为IIB；
△ACC/AHA 指南未分类[22]。

然如此，而且与心肌病（缺血性或非缺血性）的类型无关[53]。以后的两项入选病例更多的研究仍支持动态心电图检查识别高危充血性心衰患者的价值。

目前的资料显示，基于动态心电图的短期或长期心率变异性测定可以评估慢性心衰患者的预后[54-56]，对179例充血性心衰患者的回顾性分析发现，在多因素模型中，SDNN小于65.3ms是生存率的唯一独立预测因子（$P=0.00001$），与猝死显著相关（$P=0.016$）[54]。La Rovere及同事[56]分析了慢性心衰患者的短期心率变异性与猝死的关系，在标准化的记录条件下，清晨平卧休息30min，匀速呼吸，分析5min的心电图记录，进行时域和频域分析，开始202名患者用于确定截断值（cutoff values），然后前瞻性分析242名患者，约一半患者为缺血性心肌病。左室功能减退、心率变异性低频区域（0.04～0.15Hz）以及24h动态心电图中每小时室性早搏83次以上是猝死的预测因素，同时存在这两项危险因素的患者占37%，其3年猝死危险率为23%，而其余63%的患者3年猝死危险率为3%[56]。其他研究也支持心率变异性可以增强其他参数（如射血分数）在充血性心力衰竭患者的预测价值[54,55]。

4. 新发的心脏疾病

许多心脏疾病不会在疾病早期出现症状。有时，患者出现症状前可能应该接受动态心电图检查，特别是早期的病窦综合征患者，在出现明显的窦性心动过缓（35～45bpm）且有症状或慢快综合征（病窦综合征）前，其可能仅仅为无症状性窦性心动过缓（约50bpm），动态心电图可用于随访并评估患者以提供需要起搏治疗的依据，按照这种方案，许多病窦患者在出现症状前可以维持多年而不需植入起搏器。

虽然还没有这方面的临床资料，动态心电图常用于房室阻滞、有症状的二尖瓣脱垂、预激综合征及长QT间期患者的管理。在检查一些猝死患者家族（如长QT综合征、Brugada综合征以及家族多形性室速）时，动态心电图也有其用途，虽然这方面报告较少[57,58]。现在是强调投效比的年代，一些费用高昂的关键性治疗（如ICD）常常需要明确的心电图证据，动态心电图不能完全满足此类需要，ACC/AHA指南也未证实[22]。

（三）疗效评价

动态心电图广泛应用于评价抗心律失常的疗效，其为无创性检查，无风险，可以定性和定量评估心律失常，可以将症状与心电图现象相联系。评价起搏器和ICD植入患者时也有这些优点，虽然起搏器和ICD技术已经可以自行记录心电信息。临床上，动态心电图已经用于评价接受治疗患者的心肌缺血[43]、自主神经张力改变[59]、慢性房颤患者[26]心室率控制情况等（表84-4）。

1. 抗心律失常药物治疗

动态心电图评价抗心律失常药物的疗效基于心脏病

患者心律失常抑制的类型和频率与临床致病率和死亡率的关系。早期的研究为非随机非对照研究，所以，心律失常本身的多变性给动态心电图的评估带来了障碍[3]。如果动态心电图检查证实了抗心律失常有效，必须用统计学方法排除室性心律失常本身频率和形态的变化[3]。而且，25%～27%的良性或潜在致命性室性心律失常患者在12～17个月的随访期内自行缓解，不需治疗[3]，研究发现这种室性心律失常的变异性有时间依赖性，而且在冠心病及频繁室速发作的患者更为明显[3]。影响心律失常变异性的因素很多，与疾病状态、观察时限等有关[3]。另外，对于接受抗心律失常治疗患者的自然病史研究发现：(1)疗效有但短暂丧失；(2)有时需增加药量；(3)对治疗剂量的药物无反应；(4)晚期致心律失常作用出现；(5)治疗期间室性心律失常自行缓解；(6)由于出现延迟的副作用而必须停药；(7)致心律失常作用和延迟出现的副作用可能使医生停止抗心律失常的药物治疗。

近年来，多中心的CAST试验研究了抗心律失常药物治疗的效果。试验发现，尽管I类抗心律失常药（如英卡胺、氟卡胺、莫雷西嗪）可以明显减少频繁发作的室性心律失常，但是与安慰剂组相比，接受抗心律失常药物治疗的患者心脏性和心律失常相关的死亡率增加[3]。然而，其他临床试验仍然在研究Ⅲ类抗心律失常药（如胺碘酮、索他洛尔）对一些心脏病亚组人群心律失常的治疗作用[53,60]。主要研究手段是连续记录24～48h动态心电图，可以在院内或院外进行，一般认为室总早数目减少70%～90%，成对或连续室早消失为抗心律失常治疗有效。根据CAST试验的结果，出现了"健康反应者"和"抗心律失常治疗者"的概念，即对药物有反应的患者与无反应的患者预后不同，这一发现强调了解释无安慰剂组试验资料的重要性。

经电话传输心电监护也用于评价抗心律失常药物治疗，以及监护特殊的高危人群[3]。虽然有研究观察电话传输心电监护评价抗心律失常药物疗效的价值，但目前的试验尚未纳入高危亚组人群。

虽然恶性室性心律失常患者抗心律失常药物治疗的安慰剂对照试验结果仍存争议，两个临床试验对比了动态心电图与电生理检查，研究了存活的有血流动力学紊乱的室速或室颤患者。一项小规模研究提示电生理检查指导的诊断效果更佳[3]，而更大规模的ES-VEM研究证实两种方法指导的治疗预后无差别，而动态心电图更具投效比（住院时间短，诊断费用低）[3]。两项研究中均有部分患者（分别为32%和11%）动态心电图检查未见可疑的室性心律失常。最近，AVID试验研究了1016名有恶性室性心律失常或室颤病史的患者，随机分为ICD治疗或抗心律失常药物治疗（胺碘酮或索他洛尔）组，结果证实ICD治疗有益[61]。所以绝大多数有恶性室性心律失常危险的患者应首选接受ICD治疗，其次才选择动态心电图指导的药物治疗。其后的MADIT试验[62]和MUSTT试验[63]显示冠心病患者、左室收缩功能减退（EF值分别≤0.35和0.40）患者、非持续性室性心动过速患者和可诱发室速患者均可获益于预防性ICD治疗。过去的试验中用动态心电图识别高危患者，MADIT二期试验没有把室性心律失常作为危险因素，而把射血分数低于0.30的心肌梗死后患者作为研究对象，结果显示在现代抗心力衰竭治疗基础上，包括转换酶抑制剂（使用率68%）、β受体阻滞剂（使用率70%）和他汀类降脂治疗（使用率67%），仍可获益于ICD治疗[64]。根据这一发现，对于射血分数低于0.30的患者，动态心电图检查非持续室速和信号平均心电图鉴别高危患者的价值优于电生理检查[65]，所以，动态心电图在识别恶性室性心律失常方面仍有其价值。

2. 起搏器和ICD

虽然90%植入起搏器患者有其私人医生或起搏器随访机构管理，但最近由于技术进步，这一工作应由电生理医师或专门的起搏器随访门诊进行[66,67]。过去，这种门诊主要依靠病史、体格检查、胸片、普通心电图和透视进行，也应用运动试验（检查植入频率是否适应起搏器患者）、电话传输监测设备和动态心电图。由于传统门诊就诊时间有限，动态心电图可以连续检测24h，且在日常活动时检测，其可以发现更多的起搏器功能异常。刚刚植入起搏器的患者，住院期间进行动态心电图检测有助于发现更多的起搏器功能异常，并得以及时治疗。动态心电图检测功能增强不仅仅是由于其延长了检测时间，也得益于能够通过特殊通道检测、识别、放大、记录起搏信号的动态心电图技术[3,68]，其可提供有关失夺获、感知不良、无输出以及起搏信号数量等信息，从而评价起搏器功能。

有证据表明动态心电图检查有助于分析双腔起搏器患者的心电图，目前，只有传统的连续记录心电图记录可以应用于此。NASPE官方建议使用电话传输心电图作为起搏器随访的常规方法[3]，这种方法常仅仅用于评价起搏心率，但现代可程控模式下可以改变监护形式。

尽管有这些优点，动态心电图技术已经落后于起搏器技术的进展。起搏器技术的进展使其拥有了部分"心电图记录"功能,有这种功能的起搏器可以记录所有感知和起搏事件,提供起搏间期的直方图,记录并分析心内电图,所以具有了评价心律失常的功能。虽然大多数起搏器有这种心电图记录功能,但由于其无法参考时间、患者状态及相关症状,其作为无症状起搏器植入者的随访功能仍然有限。

在过去的20年中,ICD已经进展为一种多功能的治疗及监护装置[69-71],目前的ICD具有心房起搏、频率应答、抗房速起搏及除颤功能。新的诊断程序能够可靠地鉴别并治疗室上性和室性心律失常。ICD的诊断和监护功能使其能够评估起搏器功能状态并自动进行功能测试,记录心律失常事件并进行治疗,并存储患者及心律失常的有关资料。与普通起搏器相比,ICD能够记录更详细的激活ICD事件的心电信息。但是,其记录时间有限(通常每一事件5~30s,总记录时间一般为5~10min)。一种新的抗心动过速ICD可以循环式记录抗心动过速起搏或放电前、中、后各50次心内电图。虽然这些记录可以提供更多信息并打印供医生分析,但其记录时间有限且不能提供体表心电图以分析QRS波形态。为了评价ICD抗心动过速起搏或放电是否恰当以及同时进行的药物治疗是否有效,动态心电图仍然是有效的方法,这样可以更佳地调整ICD功能,保证设定的心动过速检测频率与日常生活中可能出现的最大心率间没有重叠。由于近期开发的双腔ICD,双部位右房起搏以及双心室起搏,其功能评价很复杂[72],动态心电图仍然是评价起搏器和ICD功能的有效方法。

3. 缺血性心肌病的治疗

几项研究观察了经过再血管化治疗的冠心病患者,应用动态心电图检测临床稳定患者的心肌缺血,用以评价治疗效果[43,73-75]。在治疗前或开始药物治疗(并非再血管化治疗)时动态心电图检测到的心肌缺血程度(发作次数和持续时间)是以后缺血相关不良预后事件的独立预测因子[35,43,74]。目前,与药物治疗相比,这类患者进行再血管化治疗约可减少不良临床事件45%[43],而且,如仅仅根据症状,临床鉴别生物学稳定的冠脉疾病常常是不可靠的[76]。动态心电图检出的无症状心肌缺血可以识别冠脉病变不稳定的亚组患者,包括斑块溃疡、血栓形成及内皮功能异常[76]。ACIP试验研究了无症状心肌缺血患者的冠脉造影资料,证实这些患者存在复杂或开口部位的冠脉病变[44]。治疗性临床试验的资料提示[73,74,77],动态心电图检测到心肌缺血的患者经药物控制(非再血管化治疗)后其临床预后改善。然而,由于缺乏大规模前瞻性随机对照的临床试验支持,目前的ACC/AHA指南[22]并未确切建议动态心电图的此类应用。但是这一亚组患者似乎应该接受再血管化治疗,尤其在那些资源有限的国家。

4. 其他治疗评估

虽然动态心电图已经用于评估其他能影响自主神经功能(由心率变异性反映)的治疗效果(如睡眠呼

表84-4　动态心电图评价疗效的适应证

Ⅰ类
1. 评估患者对抗心律失常药物的反应,已明确其基础心律失常发作频度且可重复,其发作频繁,可以检测分析
2. 评价频繁发作的心悸、晕厥或先兆晕厥,从而评价植入装置的功能,以排除肌电位抑制和起搏器介导性心动过速,为更好地程控频率适应性及自动模式转换等功能提供帮助
3. 当仅仅程控起搏装置难以诊断时,可用于评价可能存在的装置失灵或功能异常
4. 评价ICD植入者对同时接受的药物治疗的反应
5. 评估未接受再血管化治疗且有进行性缺血发作患者的抗缺血治疗*

ⅡA类
检测高危患者抗心律失常药物治疗时致心律失常作用

ⅡB类
1. 评价房颤患者的心室率控制
2. 证实院外治疗患者反复发作的有症状或无症状的非持续性心律失常
3. 起搏器或ICD植入后即刻进行的术后评估,代替或辅助连续心电监护
4. 评估植入除颤装置患者的室上性心律失常的心率
5. 评估不适当性窦性心动过速、β受体高敏状态及二尖瓣脱垂患者的心率控制情况*

Ⅲ类
1. 当程控资料、心电图及其他可获得的资料(如胸片等)足以确定诊断或明确原因时,评价ICD及起搏器功能异常
2. 有植入装置患者的常规随访

*美国心脏病学会/美国心脏协会(ACC/AHA)指南未分类[22]。
ICD,植入式心脏复律除颤器。

吸暂停)[78-80]，但仅仅进行了初步研究，未证实能改善患者预后。同样，循证医学研究结果也不支持利用动态心电图评价控制慢性房颤患者心室率低于 100 次/分的治疗。但是，以后可能出现支持动态心电图用于评价部分人群心率变异性及房颤患者心室率控制的新依据。

（许多数据的原始文献可见上一版的该章节以及文献 2 和 3）。

（浦 奎 译）

参 考 文 献

1. Kolb C, Nurnerger S, Ndrepepa G, et al: Modes of initiation of paroxysmal atrial fibrillation from analysis of spontaneously occurring episodes using a 12-lead Holter monitoring system. Am J Cardiol 88:853–857, 2001.
2. Kennedy HL: Ambulatory (Holter) electrocardiography recordings. In Zipes DP, Jalife J (eds): Cardiac Electrophysiology: From Cell to Bedside, 2nd ed. Philadelphia, WB Saunders, 1995, pp 1024–1010.
3. Kennedy HL: Use of long-term (Holter) electrocardiographic recordings. In Zipes DP, Jalife J (eds): Cardiac Electrophysiology: From Cell to Bedside, 3rd ed. Philadelphia, WB Saunders, 1999.
4. Roden DM: The problem, challenge, and opportunity of genetic heterogeneity in monogenic diseases predisposing to sudden death. J Am Coll Cardiol 40:357–359, 2002.
5. Kurita T, Shimizu W, Inagaki M, et al: The electrophysiologic mechanism of ST-segment elevation in Brugada Syndrome. J Am Coll Cardiol 40:330–334, 2002.
6. Vita JA, Keaney JF Jr: Endothelial function. A barometer for cardiovascular risk. Circulation 106:640–642, 2002.
7. Pratt CM, Greenway PS, Schoenfeld MH, et al: An exploration of the precision of classifying sudden cardiac death: Implications for the interpretation of clinical trials. Circulation 93:519–524, 1996.
8. Falk E, Shah P, Fuster V: Coronary plaque disruption. Circulation 92:657–671, 1995.
9. Libby P: Current concepts of the pathogenesis of the acute coronary syndromes. Circulation 104:365–372, 2001.
10. Leor J, Poole WK, Kloner RA: Sudden cardiac death triggered by an earthquake. N Engl J Med 334:413–419, 1996.
11. Spaulding CM, Joly LM, Rosenberg A, et al: Immediate coronary angiography in survivors of out-of-hospital cardiac arrest. N Engl J Med 336:1629–1633, 1997.
12. Priori SG, Barhanin J, Hauer RN, et al: Genetic and molecular basis of cardiac arrhythmias: Impact on clinical management. Study group on molecular basis of arrhythmias of the Working Group on Arrhythmias of the European Society of Cardiology. Eur Heart J 20:174–195, 1999.
13. Priori SG, Aliot E, Blomstrom-Lundqvist C, et al: Update of the guidelines on sudden cardiac death of the European Society of Cardiology. Eur Heart J 24:13–15, 2003.
14. Kennedy HL: Role of Holter monitoring for arrhythmia (bradyarrhythmia and tachyarrhythmia) assessment and management. In Podrid PJ, Kowey PR (eds): Cardiac Arrhythmia, Mechanisms, Diagnosis and Management. Baltimore, MD, Williams & Wilkins, 1995, pp 219–232.
15. Heilbron EL: Advances in modern electrocardiographic equipment for long-term ambulatory monitoring. Card Electrophysiol Rev 6:185–189, 2002.
16. Deedwania PC, Stone PH: Ambulatory electrocardiographic monitoring for myocardial ischemia. Curr Prob Cardiol 26:680–727, 2001.
17. Aronow WS, Ahn C, Mercando AD, et al: Prevalence of and association between silent myocardial ischemia and new coronary events in older men and women with and without cardiovascular disease. J Am Geriatr Soc 50:1075–1078, 2002.
18. Molnar J, Weiss JS, Rosenthal JE: Does heart rate identify sudden death survivors? Assessment of heart rate, QT interval, and heart rate variability. Am J Ther 9:99–110, 2002.
19. Bilchick KC, Fetics B, Djoukeng R, et al: Prognostic value of heart rate variability in chronic congestive heart failure (Veterans Affairs' Survival Trial of Antiarrhythmic Therapy in Congestive Heart Failure). Am J Cardiol 90:24–28, 2002.
20. Kruger C, Lahm T, Zugck C, et al: Heart rate variability enhances the prognostic value of established parameters in patients with congestive heart failure. Z Kardiol 91:1003–1012, 2002.
21. Roche F, DaCosta A, Karnib I, et al: Arrhythmic risk stratification after myocardial infarction using ambulatory electrocardiography signal averaging. Pacing Clin Electrophysiol 25:791–798, 2002.
22. Crawford MH, Bernstein SJ, Deedwania PC, et al: ACC/AHA Guidelines for Ambulatory Electrocardiography. A report of the American College of Cardiology/American Heart Association Task Force on Practice Guidelines. J Am Coll Cardiol 34:912–948, 1999.
23. Kadish AH, Buxton AE, Kennedy HL, et al: ACC/AHA Clinical Competence Statement on Electrocardiography and Ambulatory Electrocardiography. A report of the ACC/AHA/ACP-ASIM Task Force on Clinical Competence. J Am Coll Cardiol 38:2091–2100, 2001.
24. Mieszczanska H, Ibrahim B, Cohen TJ: Initial clinical experience with implantable loop recorders. J Invasive Cardiol 13:802–804, 2001.
25. Krahn AD, Klein GJ, Yee R, Skanes AC: Randomized assessment of syncope trial: Conventional diagnostic testing versus a prolonged monitoring strategy. Circulation 104:46–51, 2001.
26. Zipes DP: Atrial fibrillation: A tachycardia-induced atrial cardiomyopathy. Circulation 95:562–564, 1997.
27. Frey B, Heinz G, Binder T, et al: Diurnal variation of ventricular response to atrial fibrillation in patients with advanced heart failure. Am Heart J 129:58–65, 1995.
28. The Atrial Fibrillation Follow-up Investigation of Rhythm Management (AFFIRM) Investigators: A comparison of rate control and rhythm control in patients with atrial fibrillation. N Engl J Med 347:1825–1833, 2002.
29. Van Gelder IC, Hagens VE, Bosker HA, et al: A comparison of rate control and rhythm control in patients with recurrent persistent atrial fibrillation. N Engl J Med 347:1834–1840, 2002.
30. Linzer M, Yang EH, Estes NA, et al: Diagnosing syncope: Part 1. Value of history, physical examination, and electrocardiography. Clinical Efficacy Assessment Project of the American College of Physicians. Ann Intern Med 126:989–996, 1997.
31. Linzer M, Yang EH, Estes NA, et al: Diagnosing syncope: Part 2. Unexplained syncope. Clinical Efficacy Assessment Project of the American College of Physicians. Ann Intern Med 127:76–86, 1997.
32. Brignole M, Alboni P, Benditt D, et al: Task Foce on Syncope, European Society of Cardiology. Part 2. Diagnostic tests and treatment: Summary of recommendations. Europace 3:261–268, 2001.
33. Croci F, Brignole M, Alboni P, et al: The application of a standardized strategy of evaluation in patients with syncope referred to three syncope units. Europace 4:351–355, 2002.
34. Krahn AD, Klein GJ, Yee R, Skanes AC: Randomized assessment of syncope trial: Conventional diagnostic testing versus a prolonged monitoring strategy. Circulation 104:46–51, 2001.
35. Madjlessi-Simon T, Mary-Krause M, Fillette F, et al: Persistent transient myocardial ischemia despite beta-adrenergic blockade predicts a higher risk of adverse cardiac events in patients with coronary disease. J Am Coll Cardiol 27:1586–1591, 1996.
36. Gill JB, Cairns JA, Roberts RS, et al: Prognostic importance of myocardial ischemia detected by ambulatory monitoring early after acute myocardial infarction. N Engl J Med 334:65–70, 1996.
37. Schang SJ, Pepine CJ: Transient asymptomatic S-T segment depression during daily activity. Am J Cardiol 39:396–402, 1997.
38. Fleisher LA, Rosenbaum SH, Nelson AH, et al: Preoperative dipyridamole thallium imaging and ambulatory electrocardiographic monitoring as a predictor of perioperative cardiac events and long-term outcome. Anesthesiology 83:906–917, 1995.
39. Mangano DT, Goldman L: Preoperative assessment of patients with known or suspected coronary disease. N Engl J Med 333:1750–1756, 1995.
40. Patel DJ, Mulcahy D, Norrie J, et al: Natural variability of transient myocardial ischaemia during daily life: An obstacle when assessing efficacy of anti-ischaemic agents? Heart 76:477–482, 1996.
41. Gabbay FH, Krantz DS, Kop WJ, et al: Triggers of myocardial ischemia during daily life in patients with coronary artery disease:

Physical and mental activities, anger and smoking. J Am Coll Cardiol 27:585–592, 1996.
42. Jiang W, Babyak M, Kranz DS, et al: Mental stress-induced myocardial ischemia and cardiac events. JAMA 275:1651–1656, 1996.
43. Pepine CJ, Sharaf B, Andrews TC, et al: Relation between clinical, angiographic, and ischemic findings at baseline and ischemia-related adverse outcomes at 1 year in the Asymptomatic Cardiac Ischemia Pilot Study. J Am Coll Cardiol 29:1483–1489, 1997.
44. Sharaf BL, Williams DO, Miele NJ, et al: A detailed angiographic analysis of patients with ambulatory electrocardiographic ischemia: Results from the Asymptomatic Cardiac Ischemia Pilot (ACIP) study angiographic core laboratory. J Am Coll Cardiol 29:78–84, 1997.
45. La Rovere MT, Bigger JT Jr, Marcus FI, et al: Baroreflex sensitivity and heart rate variability in prediction of total cardiac mortality after myocardial infarction: ATRAMI (Autonomic Tone and Reflexes After Myocardial Infarction) Investigators. Lancet 351:478–484, 1998.
46. El-Sherif N, Denes P, Katz R, et al: Definition of the best prediction criteria of the time domain signal-averaged electrocardiogram for serious arrhythmic events in the post-infarction period: The Cardiac Arrhythmia Suppression Trial/Signal-Averaged Electrocardiogram (CAST/SAECG) Substudy Investigators. J Am Coll Cardiol 25:908–914, 1995.
47. Roche F, DaCosta A, Karnib I, et al: Arrhythmic risk stratification after myocardial infarction using ambulatory electrocardiography signal averaging. Pacing Clin Electrophysiol 25:791–798, 2002.
48. Steinbigler P, Haberl R, Bruggemann T, et al: Postinfarction risk assessment for sudden cardiac death using late potential analysis of the digital Holter electrocardiogram. J Cardiovasc Electrophysiol 13:1227–1232, 2002.
49. Schmidt G, Malik M, Barthel P, et al: Heart-rate turbulence after ventricular premature beats as a predictor of mortality after myocardial infarction. Lancet 353:1390–1396, 1999.
50. Ghuran A, Reid F, La Rovere MT, et al: Heart rate turbulence-based predictors of fatal and nonfatal cardiac arrest (The Autonomic Tone and Reflexes After Myocardial Infarction substudy) Am J Cardiol 89:184–190, 2002.
51. Guzik P, Schmidt G: A phenomenon of heart-rate turbulence, its evaluation, and prognostic value. Card Electrophysiol Rev 6:256–261, 2002.
52. Elliott PM, Poloniecki J, Dickie S, et al: Sudden death in hypertrophic cardiomyopathy: Identification of high risk patients. J Am Coll Cardiol 36:2212–2218, 2000.
53. Doval HC, Nul DR, Grancelli HO, et al, for the GESICA-GEMA Investigators: Non-sustained ventricular tachycardia in severe heart failure. Circulation 94:3198–3203, 1996.
54. Bilchick KC, Fetics B, Djoukeng R, et al: Prognostic value of heart rate variability in chronic congestive heart failure (Veterans Affairs' Survival Trial of Antiarrhythmic Therapy in Congestive Heart Failure). Am J Cardiol 90:24–28, 2002.
55. Kruger C, Lahm T, Zugek C, et al: Heart rate variability enhances the prognostic value of established parameters in patients with congestive heart failure. Z Kardiol 91:1003–1012, 2002.
56. La Rovere MT, Pinna GD, Maestri R, et al: Short-term heart rate variability strongly predicts sudden cardiac death in chronic heart failure patients. Circulation 107:514–516, 2003.
57. Priori SG, Napolitano C, Gasparini M, et al: Natural history of Brugada Syndrome. Insights for risk stratification and management. Circulation 105:1342–1347, 2002.
58. Wilde AAM, Antzelevitch C, Borggrefe M, et al: Proposed diagnostic criteria for the Brugada Syndrome. Eur Heart J 23:1648–1654, 2002.
59. Zuanetti G, Mantini L, Hernandez-Bernal F, et al: Relevance of heart rate as a prognostic factor in patients with acute myocardial infarction: Insights from GISSI-2 study. Eur Heart J 9(Suppl F):F19–F26, 1998.
60. Cairns JA, Connolly SJ, Roberts R, Gent M: Randomized trial of outcome after myocardial infarction in patients with frequent or repetitive ventricular depolarization: CAMIAT. Lancet 349:675–682, 1997.
61. The Antiarrhythmias Versus Implantable Defibrillators (AVID) Investigators: A comparison of antiarrhythmic-drug therapy with implantable defibrillators in patients resuscitated from near-fatal ventricular arrhythmias. N Engl J Med 337:1576–1583, 1997.
62. Moss AJ, Hall WJ, Cannom DS, et al: Improved survival with an implanted defibrillator in patients with coronary disease at high risk for ventricular arrhythmia. N Engl J Med 335:1933–1940, 1996.
63. Buxton AE, Lee KL, Fisher JD, et al: A randomized study of the prevention of sudden death in patients with coronary artery disease. N Engl J Med 341:1882–1890, 1999.
64. Moss AJ, Zareba W, Hall WJ, et al: Prophylactic implantation of a defibrillator in patients with myocardial infarction and reduced ejection fraction. N Engl J Med 346:877–883, 2002.
65. Bigger JT: Expanding indications for implantable cardiac defibrillators. N Engl J Med 346:931–933, 2002.
66. Levine PA, Sanders R, Rankowitz HT: Pacemaker diagnostics: Measured data, event marker, electrogram, and event cunter telemetry. In Ellenbogen KA, Kay GN, Wilkoll BL (eds): Clinical Cardiac Pacing. Philadelphia, WB Saunders, 1995, pp 639–655.
67. Jeffery K, Parsonnet V: Cardiac pacing, 1960–1985: A quarter century of medical and industrial innovation. Circulation 97:1978–1991, 1998.
68. Nowak B, Middledorf T, Housworth CM, et al: Holter recordings with continuous marker annotations: A new tool in pacemaker diagnostics. Pacing Clin Electrophysiol 19:1791–1795, 1996.
69. Saksena S, Prakash A, Madan N, et al: New generations of implantable pacemaker defibrillators for ventricular and atrial tachyarrhythmias. In El-Sherif N, Lekieffre J (eds): Practical Management of Cardiac Arrhythmias. Armonk, NY: Futura Publishing, 1997, pp 321–332.
70. Gregoratos G, Cheitlin C, Connil A, et al: ACC/AHA guidelines for the implantation of cardiac pacemakers and antiarrhythmia devices: A report on the American College of Cardiology/American Heart Association Committee on Pacemaker Implantations. J Am Coll Cardiol 31:1175–1209, 1998.
71. Gregoratos G, Abrams J, Epstein AE, et al: ACC/AHA/NASPE 2002 Guideline Update for Implantation of Cardiac Pacemakers and Antiarrhythmia Devices: Summary Article: A Report of the American College of Cardiology/American Heart Association Task Force on Practice Guidelines. (ACC/AHA/NASPE Committee to Update the 1998 Pacemaker Guidelines). Circulation 106:2145–2161, 2002.
72. Saksena S, Madan N: Management of the patient with an implantable cardioverter-defibrillator in the third millennium. Circulation 106:2642–2646, 2002.
73. Von Arnim T, for the Tibbs Investigators: Prognostic significance of transient ischemic episodes: Response to treatment shows improved prognosis. Results of the Total Ischemic Burden Bisoprolol Study (TIBBS) follow-up. J Am Coll Cardiol 28:20–24, 1996.
74. Rogers WJ, Bourassa MG, Andrews TC, et al, for the ACIP Investigators: The Asymptomatic Cardiac Ischemia Pilot (ACIP) Study: Outcome at 1 year for patients with asymptomatic cardiac ischemia randomized to medical therapy or revascularization. J Am Coll Cardiol 26:594–605, 1995.
75. Dargie HJ, Ford I, Fox KM, on behalf of the TIBET Study Group: Effects of ischaemia and treatment with atenolol, nifedipine SR and their combination on outcome in patients with chronic stable angina. Eur Heart J 17:104–112, 1996.
76. Pepine CJ: Prognostic implications of silent myocardial ischemia [editorial]. N Engl J Med 334:113–114, 1996.
77. Stone PH, Chaitman BR, Forman S: Prognostic significance of myocardial ischemia detected by ambulatory electrocardiography, exercise treadmill testing, and electrocardiogram at rest to predict cardiac events by 1 year (The Asymptomatic Cardiac Ischemia Pilot [ACIP] Study). Am J Cardiol 80:1395–1401, 1997.
78. Otzenberger H, Gronfier C, Simon, et al: Dynamic heart rate variability: A tool for exploring sympathovagal balance continuously during sleep in men. Am J Physiol 275:H946–H950, 1998.
79. Roche F, Gaspoz JM, Court-Fortune I, et al: Screening of obstructive sleep apnea syndrome by heart rate variability analysis. Circulation 100:1411–1415, 1999.
80. Kop WJ, Verdino RJ, Gottdiener JS, et al: Changes in heart rate and heart rate variability before ambulatory ischemic events. J Am Coll Cardiol 38:742–749, 2001.

第 85 章

植入式"Holter"

Andrew D. Krahn，George J. Klein，Allan C. Skanes and Raymond Yee

本章目录

- 装置和植入 …………………… 773
- 临床试验 ……………………… 774
- 植入式"Holter"的其他应用 ……… 776
- 总结 …………………………… 777

对于不明原因的晕厥最理想的检查诊断方法是能得到患者症状发生时综合性的生理资料。检查诊断方法应当容易实施，对病人无伤害的危险，费用低廉，而且不需依靠概率的方式解释各种结果。显然，这种理想的诊断方法是不存在的，尽管植入式"Holter"（植入性环式记录器）代表着对患者自主症状出现时的长程生理检测迈出了最初的一步。由于不明原因晕厥的发作，绝大多数不能预测其发生的时间，而且能够自行缓解，因而成了确定病因的最大障碍。不明原因晕厥的其他诊断手段包括超声心动图和脑电图，但检查结果只能为鉴别诊断和预后的估计提供一般的床边检查的公式化结果，很少能提供特异性的诊断意见。直立倾斜试验、电生理检查方法能够对晕厥相关的病因提供线索或能诱发出异常所见，但是这两项检查的预测价值很低。尽管这样，临床判断仍需要这些激发试验的结果。目前的这些检查的显而易见的局限性，使我们十分重视这种动态检测心律的技术，即向着自主症状发生时提供综合的生理性评估这一金标准迈出重要的一步。

一、装置和植入

植入式"Holter"或称植入性环式记录器（implantable loop recorder）是近年新出现的一种诊断技术，其不需要额外的电极就能长时间地检测患者的心律。其最适合应用于拟诊为心律失常相关晕厥，而发作又不频繁的病人。最新一代的植入式"Holter"具有一对感知电极，间距 3.7cm，位于外壳上。其体积为 6.1cm×1.9cm×0.8cm，形状像一块口香糖，重 17g，内置电池寿命 14 个月（图 85-1）。植入式"Holter"记录的双极单通道心电图记录后保存在一个环状缓冲器中，能够记录 21min 未被压缩的心电信号，或者被压缩后 42min 的心电信号，记录可分成 1 次或 3 次分别记录。其有记忆功能的环式记录器能够记录 21 或 42min 心电图，心脏事件发生后经"激活"记录功能，记录的心电资料可以被永久地保存起来备用。由于被压缩的心电信号与不压缩的信号间差别细微，因此临床中最常应用的是该装置的最大记忆容量，即 42min。当病人发生了一次症状时，该记忆缓冲器用手控触发而被激活和冻结。在植入时已经教会病人触发器的应用方法（图 85-1 右侧）。植入式"Holter"储存的资料可经美敦力公司标准的 9790 起搏器程控仪下载（图 85-2）。最新一代的植入式"Holter"能在心率过缓、过速或停搏时自动检出后自动启动记录（图 85-3）。

植入式"Holter"的植入方法与一般永久起搏器的植入方法相同。只是植入的囊袋更小。手术可经心脏内科或外科医师实施。植入术可在手术室或心电生理检查室或在心导管室进行。在患者的右胸前区域都能得到一个适当的心电信号，而不需要仔细标测[1]。经过术前标测，能够得到最佳的感知信号，注意应当防止发生 T 波的超感知，从而发生 QRS 波和 T 波的双感知和双倍计数。对于有心脏停搏的患者，植入术时，应当将触发器的应用方法教会其家属或朋友。与

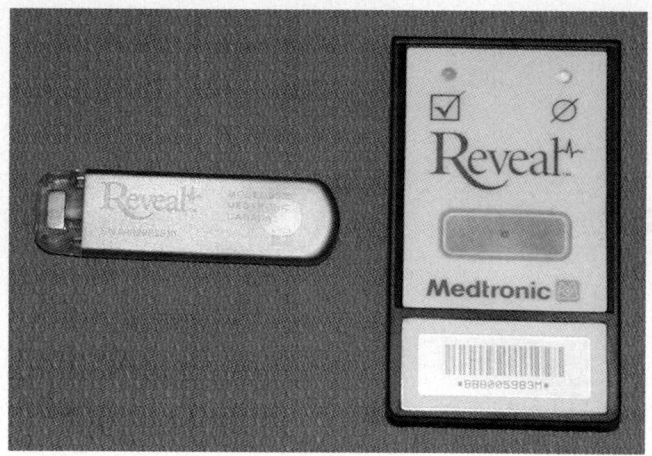

图 85-1 植入式"Holter"的实物照片　图中左为植入式"Holter",其感知的两个电极位于外壳,该装置等病人局麻后,植入在其左胸前区,可供长期心电监测。右为病人应用的记录触发器。

永久起搏器植入术相同,常建议预防性应用抗生素预防囊袋感染。

二、临床试验

目前已有几项研究证实,在长期的心律监测中,植入式"Holter"在确定与症状相关的心律方面十分有用[2-6]。这些研究中最大的一组资料是来自3个中心的206例病人的资料[7]。其中绝大多数的入组病人植入前均进行了无创性检查及选择性的有创性检查,包括直立倾斜试验和心脏电生理检查。全组症状发生时心律失常的检出率为22%,除外心律失常与症状同时发生者42%,有31%的病人在植入后的长期心电监测中症状(晕厥)一直没有发生。检测到的心律失常中,心动过缓多于心动过速(17%比6%),常需植入人工心脏起搏器。重要的是,有4%的病人晕厥发生后,不能适当地激活植入式"Holter"进行记录,因而未能得到与晕厥发生相关的心律记录。多变量的分析不能确定植入前的预测因子与植入后心律失常的发生有明显的预测关系,仅仅与年龄的增长和心动过缓的加重之间有微弱的相关性。不幸的是,没有一个年龄组的患者心动过缓的发生率高于30%,提示对于不明原因的晕厥人群中,给予经验性的起搏治疗作用的局限性。

应用植入式"Holter"的几项近期研究证实了在有选择的人群中长期心电监测的价值。3项研究来自不明病因晕厥的国际性研究(ISSUE),在3组不同的晕厥患者植入了该类"Holter"[10,11]。在该组研究中,

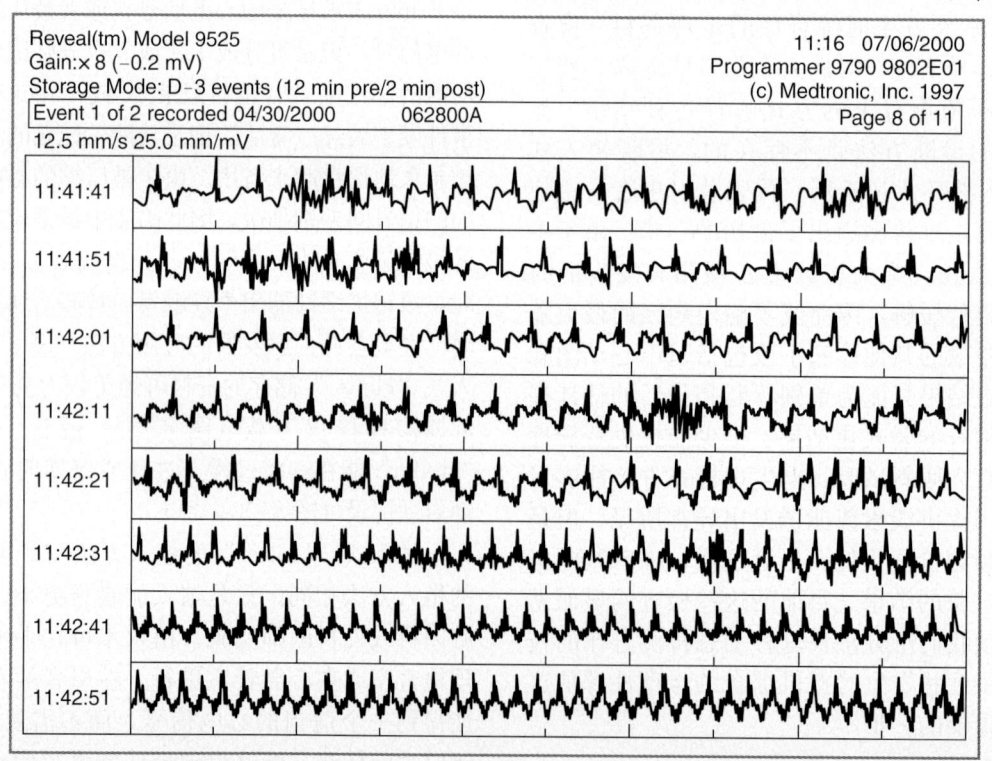

图 85-2 从植入式"Holter"下载的心电图证实这位78岁女性病人明显的先兆晕厥与心率从105bpm突然升到230bpm有关
有趣的是病人否定发作时有心悸的感觉,但在发生先兆晕厥和摔倒后1min记录器被激活,记录到这帧心电图,P波难以辨认,在上半部分心电图中偶有人工伪差。

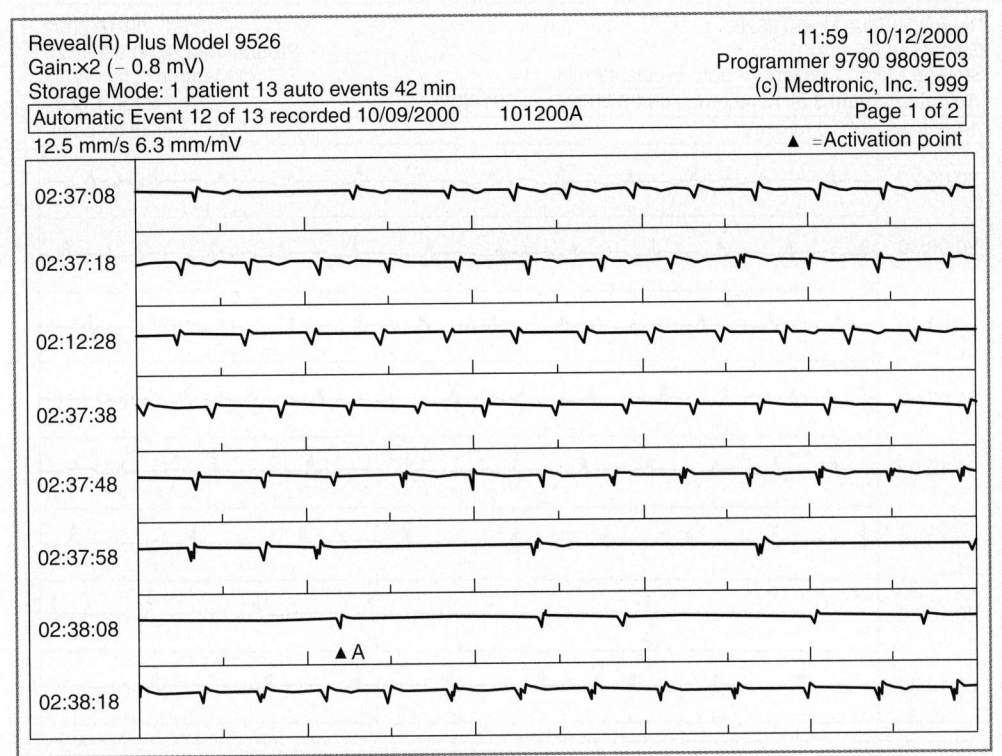

图 85-3 从植入式"Holter"下载的心电图，取自一位 69 岁、有明显先兆晕厥的男性患者，其在植入前 18 个月当中有两次晕厥发作 图中每条为 10s 的单导心电图，在箭头 A 处因明显的心动过缓而触发该装置的自动记录。3min 后当病人找到了手动触发记录器之后，应用手动使记录器开始记录，记录中未能清楚地看到 P 波，病人植入永久起搏器后，晕厥不再发生。

直立倾斜试验阳性和阴性者中 34% 再次发生晕厥，随访期中，明显窦缓或停搏是最多被记录到的心律失常，两者发生率分别为 46% 和 62%。而且证实，直立倾斜试验时的心率反应不能预测晕厥发生时的自主心率反应。自主性晕厥发生时，检测到心脏停搏要比根据统计学及直立倾斜试验结果预期的发生率高。这一研究提示直立倾斜试验预测自发性晕厥中心律结果的能力较低，而且在这一人群组中，心动过缓的发生率比以前认为的更高。图 85-4 是心脏抑制引起神经性心脏晕厥的一个病例。

在另一项 ISSUE 研究中，52 例有晕厥及束支阻滞的患者，其植入小型"Holter"后进行的心脏电生理检查为阴性。52 例有传导系统疾病者中，22 例有晕厥的复发。长期的心电监测证实，其中 17 例患者存在的完全性房室阻滞引起明显的心动过缓，而另 2 例排除了房室阻滞，余 3 例晕厥发生后未能适当地激活小"Holter"的记录，因而无资料获得。这一研究证实了目前的一个重要观点，即心脏电生理检查阴性时，不能除外间歇性完全性房室阻滞的可能。对这组人群，监测时间较长，应当考虑植入永久起搏器。这项研究也表明心脏电生理检查的作用也能部分被长期心电监测可靠地替代。

ISSUE 的第 3 项研究检查了 35 例晕厥患者发作时的自主心率情况[12]，该 35 例患者均有明显的器质性心脏病，电生理检查结果阴性，基础心脏病主要为冠心病、肥厚型心肌病伴中等程度的左心功能不全。虽然目前的研究结果认为，电生理检查结果阴性者的预后较好，但对这组病人仍要考虑室速发生的可能性。结果全组 35 例中，19 例 (54%) 发生了晕厥，4 例为心动过缓，5 例为阵发性室上性心动过速，1 例发生了室速，在 16±11 个月的随访期内无猝死发生。

晕厥的随机评估试验 (randomized assessment of syncope trial, RAST) 是一项单中心回顾性系统研究，其对比分析了动态心电监测的植入式"Holter"的早期应用与常规的不明原因晕厥的各项检查结果[4]。入组的 60 例病人中 33 例男性，27 例女性，年龄 66±14 岁，随机进入常规检查组（包括体外动态小"Holter"检查、直立倾斜试验、电生理检查），或另一组植入式"Holter"组观察 1 年。如果病人左室 EF 值 < 35% 或有心脏神经性晕厥病史不能入组。如果在本组检查中晕厥原因仍然不能诊断时则交叉进入

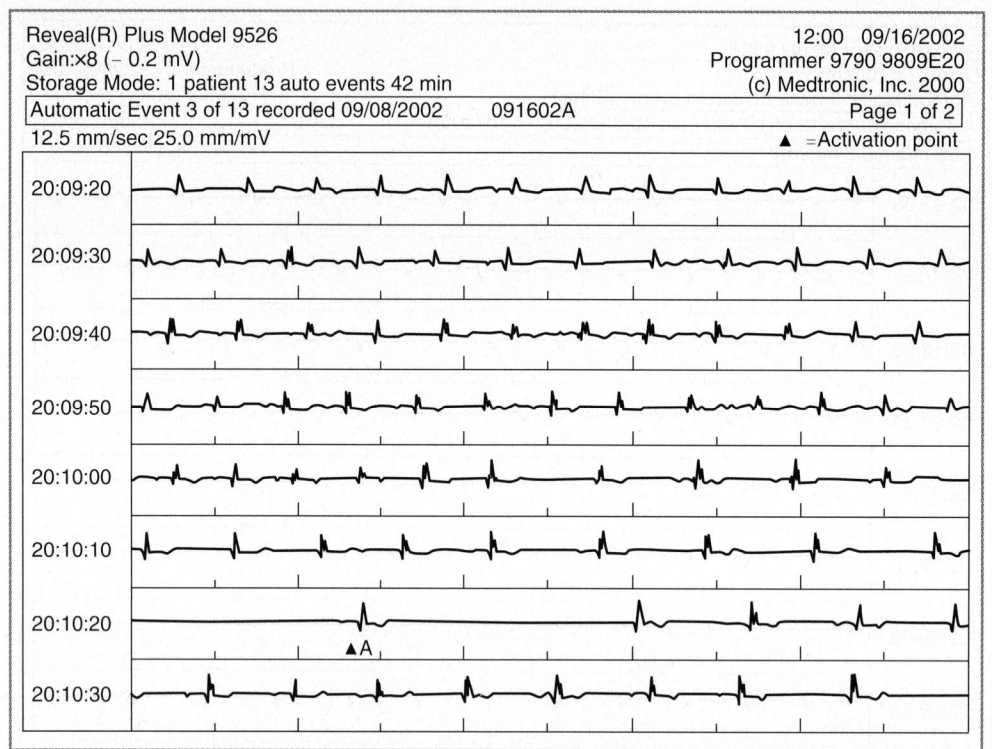

图 85-4 植入式"Holter"下载的心电图证实，这位 48 岁反复发生不明原因的晕厥与神经介导性晕厥发作时心脏显著抑制有关

患者此前的直立倾斜试验阴性，图中可见窦性心动过速，随后发生了 2∶1 的传导阻滞，心率显著性减慢，并自动触发了记录器的记录，在房室阻滞发生前的心电图中可看到 PR 间期的延长，这与自主神经在房室结引起了神经介导性的阻滞一致。此后病人植入了 DDD 起搏器，当患者发生频率骤降时，起搏器能自动给予高频率的起搏，防止晕厥发生。

另一组。结果 27 例进入植入式"Holter"组的患者中 14 例明确了晕厥病因，30 例进入常规检查组的患者仅 6 例获得诊断（$P=0.012$）。交叉后的结果为：进入常规检查的 6 例患者中，1 例获得诊断，13 例进入动态监测（即植入式"Holter"）的患者 8 例获得晕厥原因的诊断。总之，动态心电监测比常规检查组更可能获得晕厥原因的诊断（55% 对 19%，$P=0.0014$）。其中经动态监测而获得诊断者中 14 例存在过缓性心律失常，而经常规检查获得诊断者中 3 例有缓慢性心律失常。这些资料揭示了晕厥的不同病因，也说明了常规各项检查对晕厥原因诊断的局限性。虽然存在着明显的选择偏倚，即不明原因晕厥的病人常经心脏电生理医师处理，但是这一研究说明，直立倾斜试验对于晕厥病人病因的筛选有一定的应用价值，也证实心电生理检查对左室功能尚好的患者应当作为有限制的应用。北美多中心的研究结果与未进行交叉的 RAST 的结果相似。

还有其他两项令人兴奋的结果。第一，在晕厥病人应用植入式"Holter"检查的所有研究中，尽管受检病人在植入"Holter"之前有频繁的晕厥发作，但几乎 1/3 的病人植入后的长期心电监测中无晕厥的发作。这一结果提示，晕厥的原因有时具有自限性，或者是一过性生理性异常引起的。第二，应用植入式"Holter"研究的所有报告目前发现：应用较长时间的心电监测过程中，致命性心律失常的发生和显著发病率较低，这提示：无严重左室功能不全及电生理检查结果阴性的患者，尽管有着不明原因的反复晕厥，其预后是好的，应用长时间的心电检测技术是安全的。这在 ISSUE 研究中，电生理检查结果阴性的人群中尤其显著（见前文讨论）。

三、植入式"Holter"的其他应用

长期的心脏监测最适合用于偶发并怀疑发作的症状与心律失常相关的患者。虽然不明原因的晕厥是这种检测技术的最重要的适应证，但临床还有很多其他的疾病能从这种长期心电监测中获益。一项研究入组了 74 例服用抗癫痫药物治疗后仍有发作或不能解释的反复癫痫发作的病人。Zaidi 及同事[8,9]经过各种检查对病人评估：包括所有病人都做了直立倾斜试验及颈动脉窦按摩试验，其中 10 例植入了小"Holter"。结果 27% 的病人直立倾斜试验阳性，颈动脉窦按摩试

验 10% 阳性。10 例植入 "Holter" 病人中 2 例经长期心电检测证实，癫痫发作前有明显的过缓性心律，1 例为房室阻滞，1 例为窦性停搏。该研究提示，对于不典型的癫痫或对治疗的反应不典型者中，大约有 42% 的人是因心血管病引起的。几项正在进行之中的研究中，囊括大量的不典型或治疗无反应的癫痫患者正在进行心律的评估。

植入式小 "Holter" 的另一个可能的应用与该装置的自动检出心律失常的特征相关。几项研究正在给左心功能不全的患者植入该装置以检出患者的无症状性非持续性室速。这种长期的心电监测也正在用于正处于进行性传导系统疾病和猝死危险之中的肌强直性营养不良的患者。此外，由于对房颤检出的极大兴趣，几项研究开始应用这一技术检测无症状性房颤。目前正在进行的几项研究都是依赖心率的提高而检出房颤的发作，结果则会导致较高的假阳性检出率，因为房颤的心室率与生理性心室率有重叠。将来，功能更加完备的新一代产品将使其具有更多诊断特征，这将使其有更加广泛的应用。

四、总　结

植入式 "Holter" 大大提高了医师对于不明原因晕厥患者自行发作时所获资料的客观性，对于有疑问的晕厥患者，或者存在左心功能不全的晕厥患者，这项检查已成为这些情况时的重要选择的检测手段，体外或植入式长时间心电监测装置能够大大提高临床医生诊断间歇发生的心律失常的能力。毫无疑问，正在进行之中的几项临床试验，将把这项技术应用拓宽到其他疾病中去。

（郭继鸿　译）

参 考 文 献

1. Krahn AD, Klein GJ, Yee R, Norris C: Maturation of the sensed electrogram amplitude over time in a new subcutaneous implantable loop recorder. Pacing Clin Electrophysiol 20:1686–1690, 1997.
2. Krahn AD, Klein GJ, Yee R, et al: Use of an extended monitoring strategy in patients with problematic syncope. Reveal Investigators. Circulation 99:406–410, 1999.
3. Krahn AD, Klein GJ, Yee R, Norris C: Final results from a pilot study with an implantable loop recorder to determine the etiology of syncope in patients with negative noninvasive and invasive testing. Am J Cardiol 82:117–119, 1998.
4. Krahn AD, Klein GJ, Yee R, Skanes AC: Randomized Assessment of Syncope Trial: Conventional diagnostic testing versus a prolonged monitoring strategy. Circulation 104:46–51, 2001.
5. Kenny RA, Krahn AD: Implantable loop recorder: Evaluation of unexplained syncope. Heart 81:431–433, 1999.
6. Alboni P, Brignole M, Menozzi C, et al: Diagnostic value of history in patients with syncope with or without heart disease. J Am Coll Cardiol 37:1921–1928, 2001.
7. Krahn AD, Klein GJ, Fitzpatrick A, et al: Predicting the outcome of patients with unexplained syncope undergoing prolonged monitoring. Pacing Clin Electrophysiol 25:37–41, 2002.
8. Zaidi A, Clough P, Cooper P, et al: Misdiagnosis of epilepsy: Many seizure-like attacks have a cardiovascular cause. J Am Coll Cardiol 36:181–184, 2000.
9. Zaidi A, Clough P, Mawer G, Fitzpatrick A: Accurate diagnosis of convulsive syncope: Role of an implantable subcutaneous ECG monitor. Seizure 8:184–186, 1999.
10. Moya A, Brignole M, Menozzi C, et al: Mechanism of syncope in patients with isolated syncope and in patients with tilt-positive syncope. Circulation 104: 1261–1267, 2001.
11. Brignole M, Menozzi C, Moya A, et al: Mechanism of syncope in patients with bundle branch block and negative electrophysiological test. Circulation 104:2045–2050, 2001.
12. Menozzi C, Brignole M, Garcia-Civera R, et al: Mechanism of syncope in patients with heart disease and negative electrophysiologic test. Circulation 105:2741–2745, 2002.

第 86 章

高分辨心电图

Edward J. Berbari

本章目录

- 方法 778
- 心室晚电位 779
- 急性心肌梗死后信号平均心电图的预测价值 781
- 不明原因晕厥患者的评价 783
- 非缺血性心肌病患者的评价 784
- 非持续性室性心动过速患者的评价 784
- P 波的高分辨分析 784
- 总结 785

随着计算机的发展,出现了以计算机为基础的心电图记录系统,这些新的记录系统增加了许多重要功能,对过去在 12 导联心电图上不能作出标准测量的心电图分析起了非常重要的作用。其中包括减低噪声技术的发展,如信号平均和应用傅立叶分析的频谱测量技术。这些新方法揭示了常规技术看不到和手工测不到的心电图特征。因此高分辨心电图的定义是体表记录的标准心电图上看不到或表现不出来的心电信号。它常暗示该记录系统包含着以计算机为基础的心电信号的处理过程。信号平均心电图(signal-averaged electrocardiogram,SAECG)是最常见的高分辨心电图,但不是唯一的高分辨心电图。

心电图的许多应用,包括无创的希氏束电图记录器(His-Purkinje recordings)[1],晚电位的检测和分析[2-4],P 波的放大[5,6],QRS 波的分析[7,8],都是在这些技术的基础上产生的。本章主要讨论晚电位的分析,对房颤患者 P 波的高分辨分析以及与传导障碍有关的 QRS 波群的异常信号的量化及新的信号处理过程也将予以探讨。

一、方 法

用来减少噪声和确定微弱心电信号的主要方法是信号平均法。关于信号平均法有许多技术和临床报道[9-11]。此外,还有专门的专著[12-14],及两个专业学会报告[15,16],报告概括了应用高分辨心电图的方法和临床意义。下面的章节就信号平均法和分析心脏晚电位的有关技术作一简短概述。这些方法要求使用程序化的计算机,现在应用商业化并已进入心电图系统的微型处理器很容易完成。

应用信号平均心电图有许多前提条件,包括目标信号本身性能的可重复性、干扰噪声的随意性、目标信号和干扰噪声之间的独立性。在高分辨心电图的研究中遇到的噪声有 3 种形式:(1) 电子器械本身的噪声;(2) 干扰能量线(北美 60Hz);(3) 来源于胸壁肌肉的生理性噪声。肌电噪声是最有意义的噪声源,而其他如果存在的话,常提示有需要纠正的技术问题,例如电极片松脱。

大多数的高分辨心电图采用未校正的、正交的 XYZ 导联,用这 3 个导联的原因在于它能减少计算机必须处理的信号量,这个程序虽然必要但消耗时间。有了现代技术,计算机处理信息的速度和获得通道的数量就不存在问题了。

图 86-1 是一个 SAECG 方法学的简略图。随着时间变化,心电图的电压经模拟数字转换器转换成数字的形式,该转换器允许计算机处理心电图信号。一旦这些信号数字化,数据可储存在计算机的硬盘上,硬

盘可连续储存获得的数据，以后这些数据资料可被进一步分析。当然，更常见的方式是在线处理，即记录设施与患者相连时，信号被数字化而且进行逐搏的分析。第一个方法的益处是所有的原始资料都被储存并能为将来的分析所用。第二个方法的益处是可以立即获得结果。储存这些经过平均和分析的心电波形很常见，一般来说可能会阻止新的分析。但这些数据资料被压缩处理，并不出现大量数据处理的问题。

一旦心电图信号数字化，计算机将会自动识别，或者与用户相互作用，形成一个用来识别和排列连续心搏的QRS模板以便为平均法使用。一旦被平均后，信号被高通滤波去掉低频信号，经过这个过程使较高频的信号表现出来。晚电位的基本原理就是激动传导通过梗死区域存活的心肌细胞时由于其方向不一致，导致激动的波锋发生方向的改变所致。

高分辨心电图系统主要的硬件设备如下：（1）一个低噪声前终端放大器；（2）一个以数字信号化的模拟数字转换器；（3）具有滤波和平均功能的信号处理能力；（4）显示、打印经处理后的心电图；（5）有长期的储存、记录设施。商业化的心电图设备都具有这些功能，它通过计算机软件将所有这些功能整合在设备系统内。高分辨心电图除了功能上具备以上要求外，还要有一个容易操作使用的用户界面，因为使用方便是用户易于接受的一个关键因素。

其他分析方法，如提供一个质量控制的噪声分析[17,18]，用来对高分辨信号进行频谱分析的傅立叶分析[19-22]都是重要的。这些方法，都加载在软件和硬件结构中，并通过软件来完成。

二、心室晚电位

到目前为止，高分辨心电图最常见的用途是用于心室晚电位的记录（ventricular late potentials, VLP）。晚电位是心脏内发生病变组织的激动晚于正常组织而产生的。常见的原因是梗死区域内和梗死区周围组织心肌细胞除极延迟而引起。犬梗死模型的标测研究表明，在梗死带内有存活的心肌细胞区域并且在这些复杂的死亡和存活的细胞基质之间有曲折的小路径存在传导速度的缓慢和延长，引起QRS波终末的极化电位延长，并形成晚电位。下壁心肌梗死患者比前壁心肌梗死患者更易记录到晚电位，这是因为下壁心肌梗死时心室的激动顺序正常的缘故。由于心室前壁原来就激动较早，因而该处除极的延迟电位并不像下壁延迟的除极电位那样比整个的QRS波群除极时间明显靠后，故可能融合在QRS波群中而未能显示。同样，有束支阻滞或室内传导阻滞的患者因传导障碍引起除极电位出现较晚，与梗死相关的延迟可能并不比整个QRS波群持续的时间长而在最后出现。

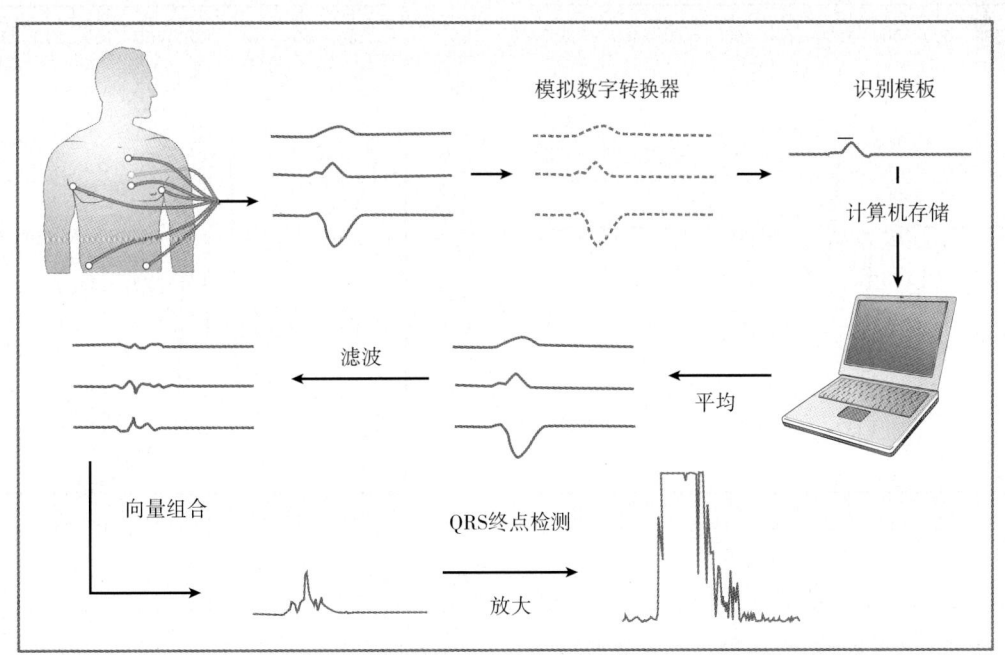

图86-1 记录信号平均心电图的各个步骤 XYZ三个导联的信息经计算机处理后转化成数字形式，计算机对QRS波群进行识别检测、排列、平均和滤波，向量组合，最终作出是否存在晚电位的测量。（引自Vatterott PJ, Hammill SC, Bailey KR, et al: Signal-average electrocardiography: A new noninvasive test to identify patients at risk for ventricular arrhythmias. Mayo Clin Proc 63: 931-942, 1988.）

图 86-2 举例说明最常见的记录和量化心室晚电位的步骤。图 86-2A 表明正常节律时双极 XYZ 导联的条形图。图 86-2B 显示经适当的排列和信号处理后这 3 个导联的 QRS 波群，与图 86-2A 比较，时间刻度减少 10 倍，垂直纵坐标的刻度约减少 5 倍。经过这些处理后，在 QRS 波群后或终末部有可能看到振幅低而持续时间相对较短的波形，与 QRS 波群本身比较是相对高频的成分，用传统的高通电子滤波可以考虑分离这些较高频的信号。然而，由于相对较大的 QRS 波群的低频成分不能完全去掉，这将导致相当大的时相失真造成晚电位的假阳性。Simson[3] 用计算机编码的软件滤波器对 QRS 波群进行向前和相反时相的滤波，这样可能在 QRS 波群中央部分失真的情况下限制了 QRS 波群终末和起始时相的失真，是一种能让人接受的交替换位，因为大多数的晚电位参数要求准确探查 QRS 波的终点。图 86-2C 与图 B 相比又进一步放大 10 倍，显示 XYZ 导联的高通滤波，QRS 波群是多相的并在其末端修剪，在 Z 导联上 QRS 波群起始后 148ms 时观察到晚电位。下一步的分析方法是由 Simson[3] 提出的综合向量（vector magnitude，VM）法。VM 是用 Pythagorean 的理论经 XYZ 导联的转型而形成。

$$VM=\sqrt{X^2+Y^2+Z^2}$$

图 86-2D 是经向量转型得出的波形。注意所有的波形成分有两个极性，有 3 个常用的晚电位参数，总 QRS 时限或 QRSd（QRS duration），其包括晚电位，是心室激动总的时间，在本例中该值是 205ms－67ms ＝138ms。QRS 终末 40ms 电压的平方根，即 RMS40，代表晚电相位应的幅度，是图 86-2D 中的阴影区域，为 20μV。低振幅信号（low amplitude

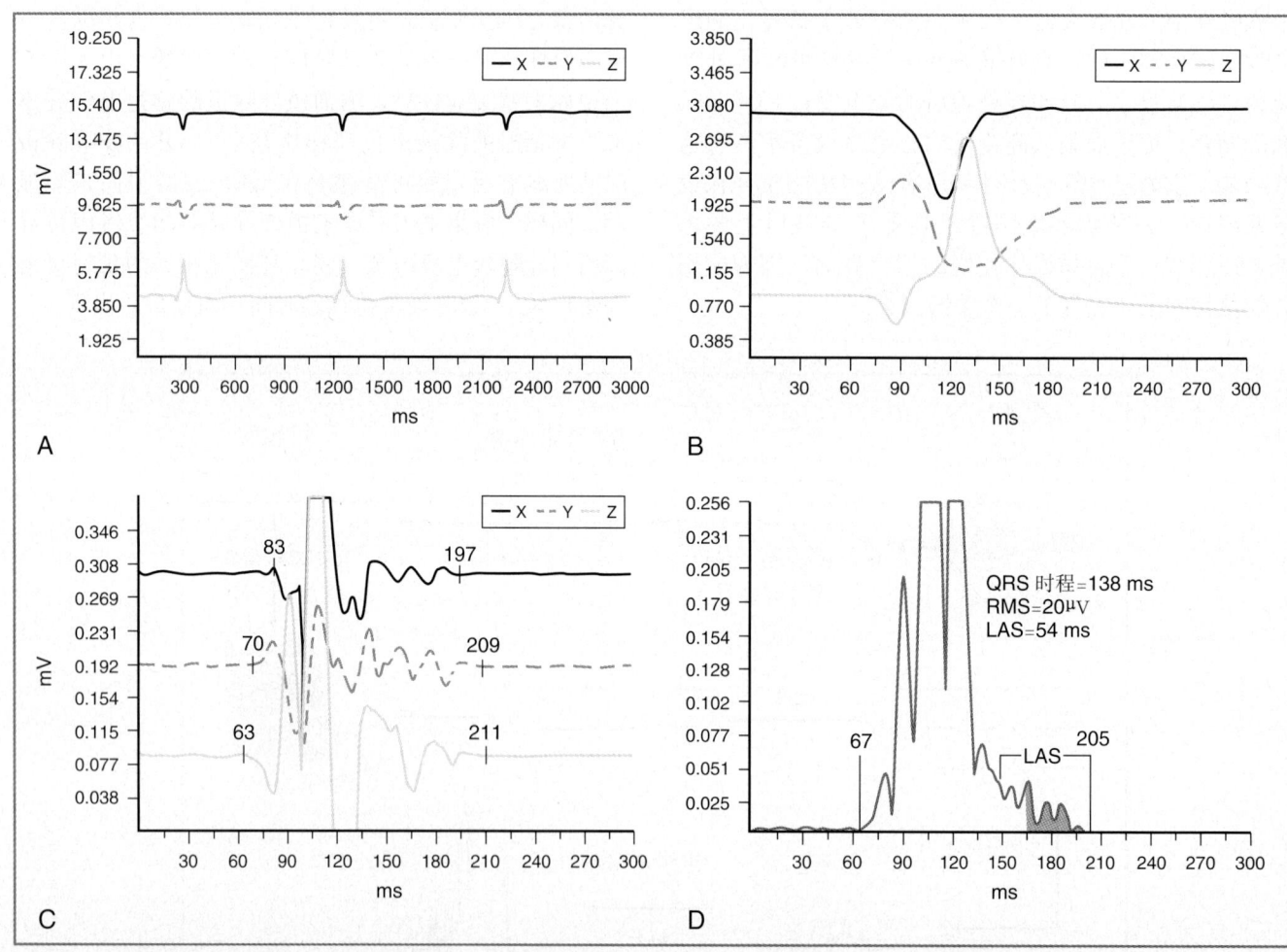

图 86-2 滤波后的综合向量及晚电位参数的信号处理过程 A：XYZ 导联的节律条图。B：信号平均的 QRS 波，时间刻度是 A 图的十分之一，纵轴的刻度是 A 图的五分之一。C：25Hz 时 B 图的信号经高通滤波后获得的图形。D：滤波的向量用三个晚电位参数表示。QRS 时限，终末电压的平方根（RMS；阴影部分）和低振幅信号（LAS）。（选自 Berbari EJ, Lazzara R: An introduction to high-resolution ECG recordings of cardiac late potentials. Arch Intern Med 148：1859-1863, 1988. © 1988 American Medical Association.）

signal，LAS）是信号的持续时间，其起始值小于40μV，图86-2D中括号指的是54ms。许多研究利用这些参数为心肌梗死患者进行分类。有些病例在电生理检查中可诱发室性心动过速，或在随访期间有心律失常事件。这些病例在以后的章节中还要讨论。SAECG检查异常的标准常为QRSd大于114ms，或RMS40小于20μV，或LAS大于38ms[15]。

图86-3说明综合向量导联的弱点。注意自动分析确定的各个导联和综合导联之间QRS波群的起点和分支点不同。通过各导联与综合导联的结合，每个导联产生独立的信号噪声比与单独在综合导联产生的不同，这些因素已被系统地进行了研究，研究从理论[23]和170例以上患者的临床研究[10]两方面实施。实际上，在综合导联QRSd一般小于单个XYZ导联上最大的间期，对于检出室性心动过速的患者有更高的敏感性。然而单独用综合导联与用其他导联相比，有较大的特异性。通过两种测量的结合，表中产生了5个区域，误差区是指在这个区域两种测量方法间至少有20ms的差异，标注1~4的区域对应将来发生室性心动过速的危险形成4个级别。1~4的区域分别代表正常、正常边界、异常边界和异常。应用这个图表时，应该考虑到最初研究中的描述，包括表中原来统计成分的完整描述。

由Lander及同事[10]所做的研究得出的其他有意义的结果是QRSd、RMS和LAS 3个指标的测量缺乏独立性。许多其他的研究也证实了这一点，包括Savard及同事[24]所作的大样本多中心的晚电位研究。此外这些研究也证实了妇女的QRS异常阈值较小，比男性短7~10ms，导致性别差异的最大可能是心电图测量及平均的结果。女性QRS波群比男性短7~10ms，因此人们认识到独立测量晚电位的QRSd最有意义，而对同时合并的性别差异尚无广泛的认识。

临床研究中，常需确定QRSd、RMS和LAS的正常值，这样才能将正常对照组与研究组进行比较。Nakazato及同事[25]确定了滤波的QRSd（FQRS）和LAS的正常分布范围，该研究结果也提出了RMS40的正常分布。图86-4显示了200例健康人获得的这些资料的分布。

三、急性心肌梗死后信号平均心电图的预测价值

临床已有数百篇文章应用信号平均心电图（SAE-

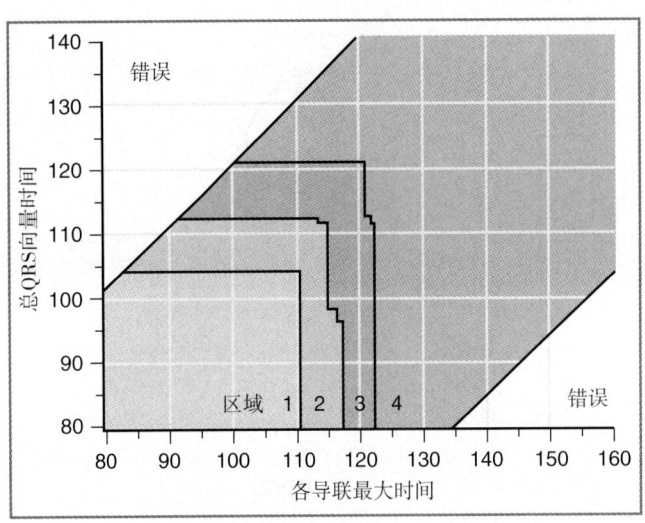

图86-3 QRS向量时间与各导联最大的向量时间　区域1~4分别代表正常、正常分界、异常分界和异常。（选自Lander P，Berbari EJ，Rajagopalan CV，et al：Critical analysis of the signal-averaged electrocardiogram：Improved identification of late potentials. Circulation 87：105-117，1993.）

AG）量化晚电位。这些文章大多数集中在心肌梗死后的病人。早在20世纪80年代就开始了这方面的研究，心肌梗死后的患者成为心脏性猝死的研究对象。由Simson[3]所作的landmark研究不仅系统阐述了研究方法（这个方法目前仍在沿用），而且与Breithardt及同事[4]一起清晰地证明了利用晚电位的出现可确定室性心动过速的患者。以后的研究证明了晚电位对室性心律失常预测的重要价值[26-30]。其他一些指标也可用来进行危险评估，包括动态心电图记录的高级别的异位搏动和室性早搏，显著的射血分数（ejection fraction，EF）下降等。

表86-1概括了自20世纪80年代以来对心肌梗死后患者晚电位评价预后意义的4个研究，Breithard及同事[4]测量了晚电位时程并证实晚电位持续时间长时（>40ms），猝死和室性心动过速的危险性可增加3倍。同期的其他研究也证实与其他危险因素结合能提高对室性心律失常患者的预测价值。表86-2概括了4个这样的研究，它们单独一个因素或结合几个因素比较了晚电位、心室功能和室性早搏的预测价值。这些研究已经证实，与其他许多危险因素一起进行预测，晚电位是一个独立的危险因素。这样晚电位作为一种心律失常基质的标志不依赖于心律失常的触发因素，如室性早搏，或通过EF值或室壁运动异常测量的心室机械功能而独立存在。

然而，自20世纪80年代以来，随着溶栓治疗，

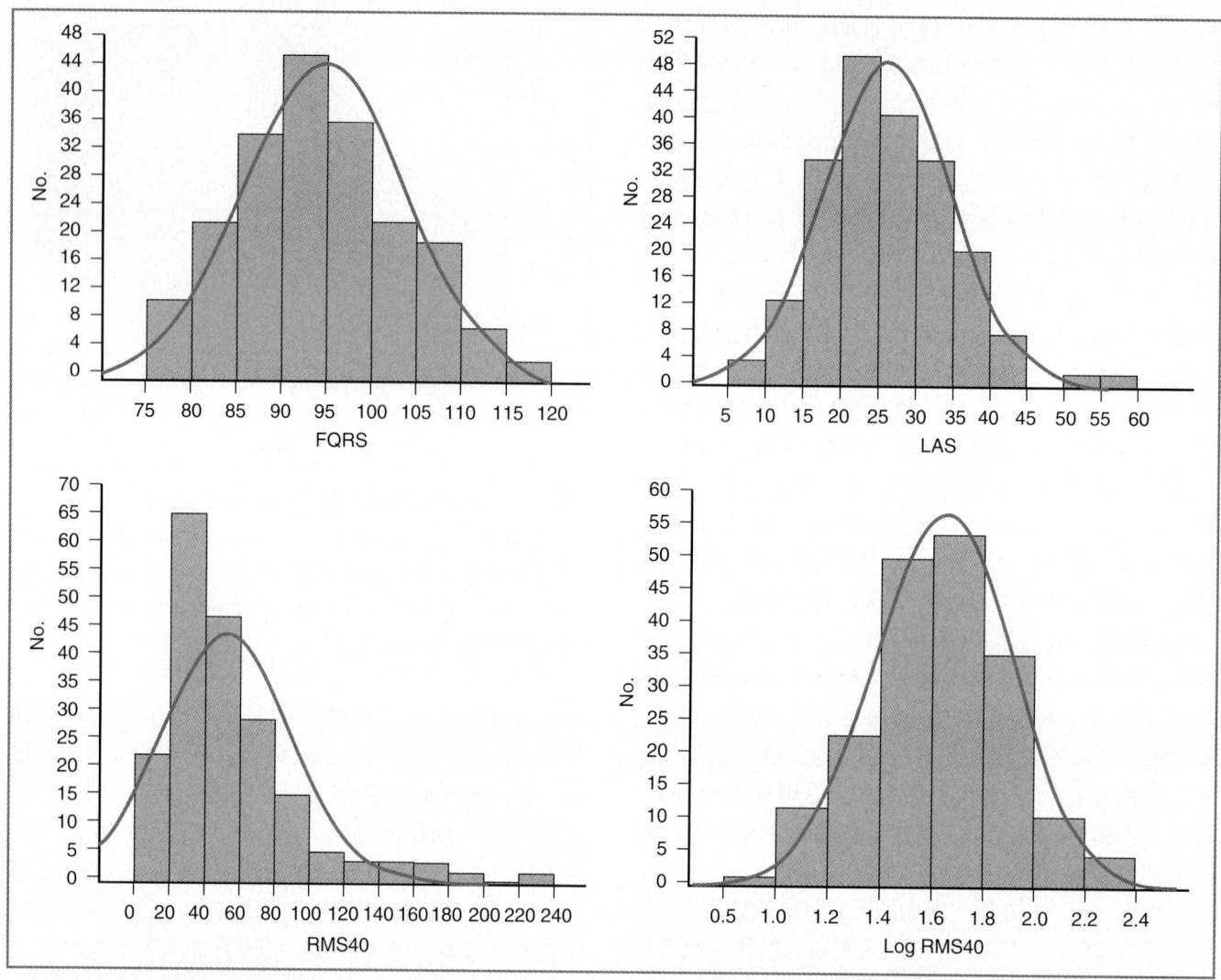

图 86-4 200 例健康人的滤波 QRSd (FQRS)，低幅信号 (LAS)，终末 40ms 电压的平方根 (RMS40)，logRMS40 的分布范围（引自 Nakazato Y, Nakata Y, Nakazato K, et al: Normal values for time-domain, frequency-domain, and spectral turbulence analyses of signal-averaged electrocardiograms in healthy subjects. Ann Noninvasive Electrocardiol 5：139-146，2000.）

冠脉血管成形术、植入式心脏复律除颤器的应用和抗心律失常药物作用的变化，传统的治疗已发生了相当大的改变。几项研究已经做了利用 SAECG 和心室晚电位对接受溶栓治疗的部分患者的定量分析（表 86-3）[31-34]。这些结果表明心律失常事件的发生率大大降低了，很可能与心肌梗死后死亡率降低的趋势一致（发生率降低的原因是多方面的，超出了本章讨论的范围）。当然，在研究中并不是所有的患者都接受了溶栓治疗，但这些因素可能准确地反映了心脏病学治疗的一般规律。心律失常事件率是低的，而患者的数量必须真正达到有统计学意义的水平。Savard 及同事[24]的研究开始于 1983 年，经过 15 项前瞻性信号平均心电图的研究，用图表说明了心律失常的发生率，该研究在文章中作了更详细的表述。前 7 个研究于 1983～1990 年完成，心律失常的发生率 9.6%，而 1990～1995 年完成的 8 个研究中心律失常的平均发生率约 5.8%。尽管有很大的差异，溶栓时代的研究证实 SAECG 和晚电位检测的敏感性和特异性与早先报道的范围相似。同样比较这两个阶段的阳性预测值也无变化（约 20%），而且阴性预测值仍然很高（97%）。晚电位的阳性预测值比较低，因此单独以晚电位的出现为基础提议临床给予猝死预防干预是不适宜的[15,16]。

Savard 及同事[24]作的心肌梗死后 SAECG 测量晚电位的多中心、多变量的研究已经发表。这些报道是心肌梗死加拿大评价（CAMI）研究的一部分，其资料来源于 9 个研究组织的 2461 例无束支阻滞的患者。这些大病例组的研究再一次证实了 QRSd 参数的重要

表 86-1　心肌梗死后晚电位的预后意义

第一作者，年	病人，n	平均随访，月	晚电位	发生率% 猝死	VT-S
Breithardt, 1983[4]	160	7.5	none	3.8	0
			LP<40ms	3.2	4.8
			LP>40ms	11.1	16.6
Denniss, 1986[26]	306	12	正常	2	4
			异常	15	19
Gomes, 1987[27]	102	12	正常	3.5	3.5
			异常	28.9	28.9
Kuchar, 1987[28]	210	14	正常	0.8	0.8
			异常	16.7	16.7

LP，晚电位；VT-S，持续性室性心动过速。

表 86-2　晚电位、心室功能和室性早搏预测室性心动过速的统计

方法	Kanovsky 及同事 1984[29]	Buckingham 及同事 1987[30]	Kuchar 及同事 1987[28]	Gomes 及同事 1987[27]
LP	Sn89%，Sp69%	Sn64%，Sp79%	OR, 23.6	Sn87%，Sp63%
VP	NR	Sn71%，Sp65%	OR, 17.9	Sn80%，Sp54%
VE	NR	NR	OR, 7.6	Sn80%，Sp42%
LP+VP	Sn90%，Sp72%	Sn64%，Sp79%	Sn80%，Sp89%	Sn100%，Sp59%
LP+VE	Sn94%，Sp61%	NR	Sn65%，Sp89%	Sn100%，Sp45%
LP+VP+VE	Sn81%，Sp90%	NR	NR	Sn100%，Sp53%

LP，晚电位；NR，未报道；OR，odds ratio；Sn，敏感性；Sp，特异性；VE，室性早搏；VP，心室功能。

表 86-3　溶栓时代晚电位的预后价值

第一作者，年	病例总数/TRx 例数	+LP	随访，月	心律失常事件 SCD	VT-S	Sn	+LP 预测值% Sp	+PV	−PV
Pedretti, 1992[31]	174/106	41 (24%)	14	4	4	75	82	18	98
Malik, 1992[32]	331/130	48 (15%)	20	12	13	48	88	25	95
McClements, 1993[33]	301/205	61 (20%)	13	11	2	64	81	11	98
Denes, 1994[34]	787/363	97 (12%)	10	31	2	90	61	21	98

+LP，晚电位；+PV，阳性预测值；−PV，阴性预测值；SCD，心脏性猝死；Sn，敏感性；Sp，特异性；TRx，溶栓治疗；VT-S，持续性室速。

价值、总 RMS 和 LAS 参数作为一个独立的心律失常危险标志的价值。性别、年龄和梗死部位也影响着 SAECG 的解释。这项研究结果发现女性 QRSd 值较小，并且将患者分成 4 个年龄组（<50 岁、50～59 岁、60～69 岁和 70～75 岁）和两个梗死部位（非 Q 波和下后壁与前壁）。图 86-5 是 Kaplan-Meier 生存曲线图，它表明了考虑性别、年龄和梗死部位后，24 个月内无心律失常事件的可能性[24]。SAECG 阴性和 SAECG 阳性间曲线的差异具有显著意义（$P<0.0001$）。

四、不明原因晕厥患者的评价

不明原因的晕厥常是一个令人困惑的难题，它可能因心动过缓或心动过速引起。作为一种筛查手段，SAECG 检测晚电位阳性时，提示有可能是室性心动

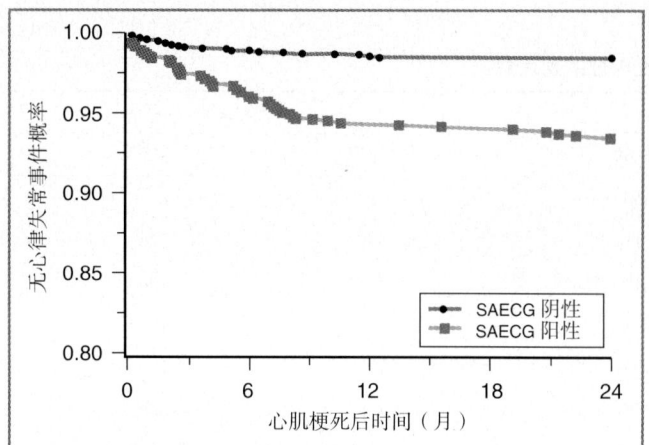

图86-5 校正年龄、性别和梗死部位后信号平均心电图（SAECG）阳性和阴性患者24个月内无心律失常事件的Kaplan-Meier曲线 （引自 Savard P, Rouleau JL, Ferguson J, et al: Risk stratification after myocardial infarction using signal-averaged electrocardiographic criteria adjusted for sex, age, and myocardial infarction location. Circulation 96: 202-213, 1997.）

过速引起。然而晚电位阴性不能排除室性心律失常引起的晕厥。据统计，15%～35%的晕厥患者由持续性室速引起[11]。应用SAECG检查有助于明确晕厥的原因。几项研究已经证实 SAECG 在晕厥患者诊治中的作用[35-38]，并表明对明确的可诱发的室性心动过速的患者有较高的阳性率。缺血性心脏病的晕厥患者，美国心脏病学会（ACC）的资料一致认为 SAECG 检查对这些患者的诊断有明确的价值[15]。对这些患者 SAECG 检查结果阴性时预测值更加有用，阴性预测值的特异性大于90%。

五、非缺血性心肌病患者的评价

缺血性心脏病患者晚电位的基质位于梗死组织内或其周围。然而，在非缺血性心肌病时，疾病的过程通常是弥漫性的，影响着整个心室肌。表现为弥漫的间质纤维化而导致传导异常包括束支阻滞和非特异性室内传导阻滞。经导管活检确定的心肌纤维化程度与 SAECG 测定的心室晚电相位关[39]。该病到最严重的阶段时应考虑心脏移植。Mancini 及同事[40]和 Middlekauff 及同事[41]将 SAECG 结果阳性作为需要立即行心脏移植或死亡预测的指标。Mancini 及同事[40]的研究中，为期12个月的生存曲线表明 SAECG 结果是一个强有力的心律失常事件预测因子。12个月后，SAECG 正常患者（$n=66$）的生存率95%，SAECG 异常患者（$n=20$）的生存率39%（$P<0.0001$）。然而 Middlekauff 及同事[41]的研究并没有发现在相似的条件下有预测死亡的价值。

致心律失常性右室发育不良可能是最早被确立有晚电位的疾病[42]。多数致心律失常性右室发育不良患者存在起源于右室的室性心律失常。这些患者中，常有晚电位阳性的表现，该病越来越多的电生理资料大大激发了研究者日益增加的兴趣。

六、非持续性室性心动过速患者的评价

几项研究已经证明 SAECG 结果对心肌梗死后伴有非持续性室性心动过速[43-46]患者的预测作用。在许多病例中，这些患者可能需行心脏电生理检查以明确他们是否存在可诱发的持续性室性心动过速。对这些患者，SAECG 检查的结果具有较高的阴性预测价值（>90%）。在这些患者中，用 SAECG 结果作为一种筛查工具可免除部分患者经受心导管有创检查，因此有很大的实用性。对于100个患者，心律失常可诱发率25%，Steinberg 和 Berbari[11]预计 SAECG 检查将筛出54%的阴性结果的患者不需做电生理检查，其中可能仅有2～3人存在可诱发的室速。另一方面，电生理检查的22个病人中，21例将诱发不出室速，而仅1例电生理检查结果为阳性。当然这个前提是假设电生理检查是预测心律失常的"金标准"。

多中心非持续性室性心动过速试验（MUSTT）[46]研究了冠状动脉疾病伴非持续性室性心动过速，射血分数小于40%的患者。这些患者常有治疗方面的难题，最近公布了晚电位的研究结果，入选的患者不包括束支阻滞和室内传导阻滞。该研究最初入选2202例患者，完成试验者1268例（66%）。在该组患者中，有QRSd（FQRS）延长的患者在2～5年内心脏性猝死或心律失常性死亡的事件率明显增大（$P<0.01$）。心脏性死亡率和所有原因引起的死亡率具有统计学的差异。最强的预测因子是FQRS>114ms和EF<30%两者的结合。图86-6表明了FQRS和EF值两者结合在确定心脏性猝死或心律失常性死亡的Kaplan-Meier曲线。

七、P波的高分辨分析

信号平均法应用于P波的分析是 SAECG 技术的一个新用途[5,6]。房颤的反复发生，特别是老年人，十分需要确定其复发的危险性。尽管晚电位被认为是一个真

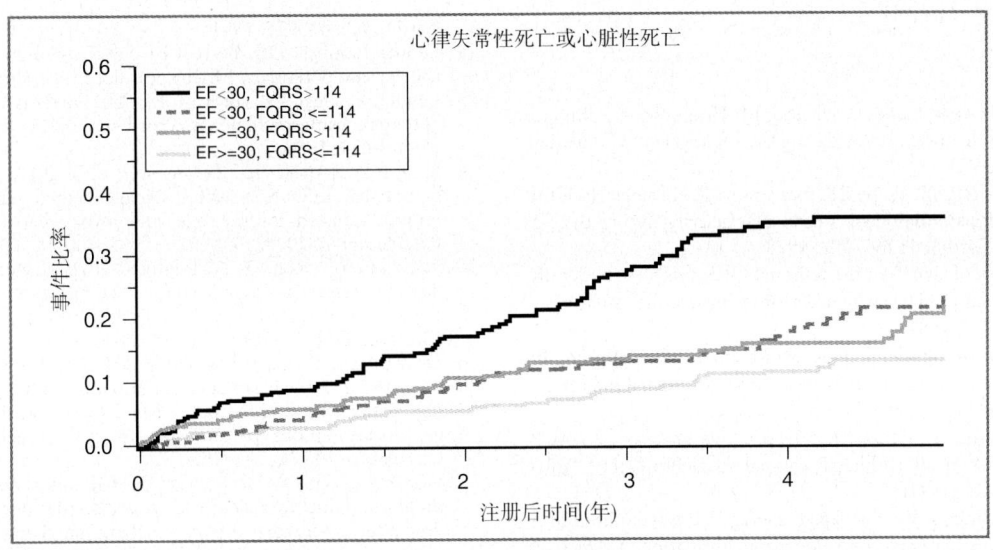

图 86-6 多中心非持续性室性心动过速（MUSTT）实验中，用射血分数和延长的 QRSd（FQRS）绘制的 Kaplan-Meier 生存曲线 （引自 Gome JA，Cain ME，Buxton AE，et al：Prediction of long-term outcomes by signal-averaged electrocardiography in patients with unsustained ventricular tachycardia, coronary artery disease, and left ventricular dysfunction. Circulation 104：436-441，2001.）

正的潜在的心电图成分，但 P 波肯定不是。然而，P 波是一个低振幅的波，通常用节律性来分析。它的出现和消失非常重要。在 12 导联心电图上详细分析 P 波的形态，包括精确确认起点和终点，比较困难。用高分辨精确的 SAECG 技术进行 P 波分析是有可能的。图 86-7 是用信号平均和高通滤波后记录 P 波的两个例子。上图来源于一个健康对照者，P 波时限 116ms，下图是一位房颤患者的记录，P 波时限 162ms，显著延长。对房颤患者，这个记录是在窦性心律时获得的。随着文献的增加，能证明 SAECG 技术可用来预测患者是否容易发生房颤，这是一个很有意义的新用途[47,48]。

八、总 结

信号平均的高分辨心电图的出现，是心电图分析史上一个重要的发展。作为一种临床诊断工具，它是许多无创的危险预测因子之一。晚电位的病理生理基础已被确立，晚电位的阴性预测价值很高。这种方法与其他临床预测指标结合应用时，可用来预测猝死的高危患者。大量的多中心研究（CAMI 和 MUSTT）仍在继续研究和证实其预测猝死高危患者的价值。然而，对假阳性患者没有真正有效和安全的治疗措施也使这项技术和其他筛选指标不能成为单独指导治疗的指标。

（黄织春 译）

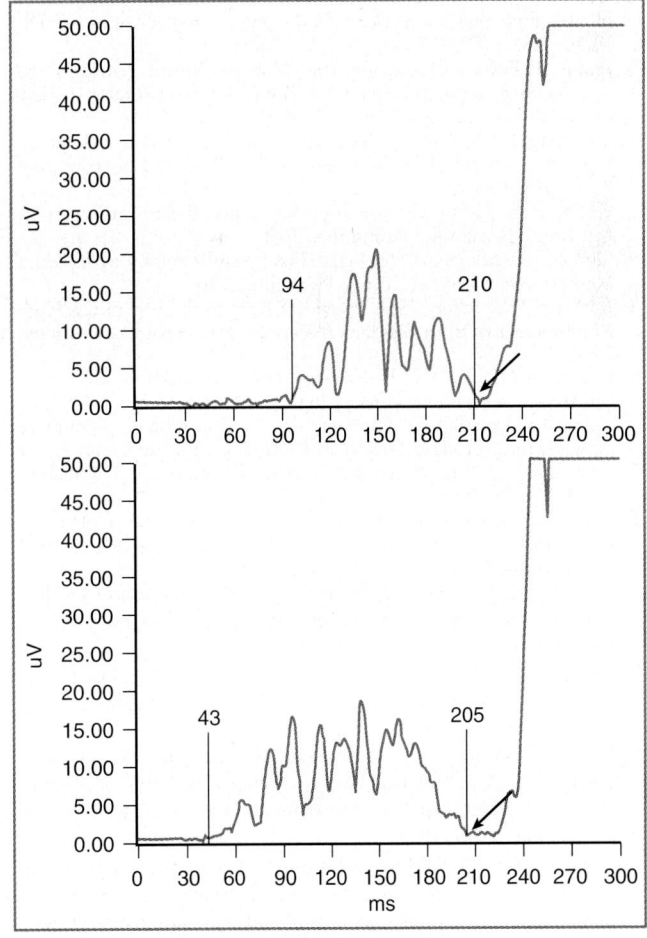

图 86-7 健康人（上图）和房颤患者窦性节律时（下图）获得的信号平均的 P 波 （引自 Guidera SA，Steinberg JS：The signal-averaged P wave duration: A rapid noninvasive marker of risk for atrial fibrillation. J Am Coll Cardiol 21：1645-1651，1993. Reprinted with permission from the American College of Cardiology.）

参 考 文 献

1. Berbari EJ, Lazzara R, Samet P, Scherlag BJ: Noninvasive technique for detection of electrical activity during the PR segment. Circulation 48:1005–1013, 1973.
2. Berbari EJ, Scherlag BJ, Hope RR, Lazzara R: Recordings from the body surface of arrhythmogenic ventricular activity during the ST segment. Am J Cardiol 41:697–702, 1978.
3. Simson MB: Use of signals in the terminal QRS complex to identify patients with ventricular tachycardia after myocardial infarction. Circulation 64:235, 1981.
4. Breithardt G, Schwarzmaier J, Boggrefe M, et al: Prognostic significance of late ventricular potentials after acute myocardial infarction. Eur Heart J 4:487–495, 1983.
5. Stafford PJ, Turner I, Vincent R: Quantitative analysis of signal-averaged P waves in idiopathic paroxysmal atrial fibrillation. Am J Cardiol 68:751–755, 1991.
6. Guidera SA, Steinberg JS: The signal-averaged P wave duration: A rapid noninvasive marker of risk for atrial fibrillation. J Am Coll Cardiol 21:1645–1651, 1993.
7. Lander P, Gomis P, Goyal R, et al: Analysis of intra-QRS late potentials: Improved predictive value for arrhythmic events using the signal-averaged electrocardiogram. Circulation 95:1386–1393, 1997.
8. Gomis P, Jones DL, Caminal P, et al: Analysis of abnormal signals within the QRS complex of the high resolution ECG. IEEE Trans Biomed Eng 44:681–695, 1997.
9. Lander P, Berbari EJ: Principles and signal processing techniques of the high-resolution electrocardiogram. Prog Cardiovasc Dis 35:169–188, 1992.
10. Lander P, Berbari EJ, Rajagopalan CV, et al: Critical analysis of the signal-averaged electrocardiogram: Improved identification of late potentials. Circulation 87:105–117, 1993.
11. Steinberg JS, Berbari EJ: The signal-averaged electrocardiogram: Update on clinical applications. J Cardiovasc Electrophysiol 7:972–988, 1996.
12. El-Sherif N, Turrito G (eds): High Resolution Electrocardiography. Mt. Kisco, NY, Futura Publishing, 1992.
13. Gomes JA (ed): Signal Averaged Electrocardiography. Dordrecht, Netherlands, Kluwer Academic Publishing, 1993.
14. Berbari EJ, Steinberg JS: A Practical Guide to the Use of the High Resolution Electrocardiogram. Armonk, NY, Futura Publishing, 2000.
15. Breithardt G, Cain ME, El-Sherif N, et al: Standards for analysis of ventricular late potentials using high resolution or signal-averaged electrocardiography. A statement by a Task Force Committee between the European Society of Cardiology, the American Heart Association and the American College of Cardiology. Circulation 83:1481–1488, 1991.
16. Cain ME, Anderson JL, Arnsdorf MF, et al: American College of Cardiology Expert Consensus Document: Signal-Averaged Electrocardiography. J Am Coll Cardiol 27:238–249, 1996.
17. Vatterott PJ, Hammill SC, Berbari EJ, et al: The effect of residual noise on the reproducibility of the signal averaged ECG. J Electrocardiol 20(Suppl):102, 1987.
18. Steinberg JS, Bigger JT: Importance of the endpoint of noise reduction in analysis of the signal-averaged electrocardiogram. Am J Cardiol 63:556–560, 1989.
19. Cain, ME, Ambos HD, Witkowski FX, Sobel BE: Fast-Fourier transform analysis of signal-averaged electrocardiograms for identification of patients prone to sustained ventricular tachycardia. Circulation 69:711, 1984.
20. Haberl R, Jilge G, Pulter R, Steinbeck G: Comparison of frequency and time domain analysis of the signal averaged electrocardiogram in patients with ventricular tachycardia and coronary artery disease: Methodologic validation and clinical relevance. J Am Coll Cardiol 12:150–158, 1988.
21. Kelen GJ, Henkin R, Stares AM, et al: Spectral turbulence analysis of the signal averaged electrocardiogram and its predictive accuracy for inducible sustained monomorphic ventricular tachycardia. Am J Cardiol 67:965–975, 1991.
22. Lander P, Albert DE, Berbari EJ: Spectro-temporal analysis of ventricular late potentials. J Electrocardiol 23:95–108, 1990.
23. Lander P, Deal RB, Berbari EJ: The analysis of ventricular late potentials using orthogonal recordings. IEEE Trans Biomed Engr 35:629–639, 1988.
24. Savard P, Rouleau JL, Ferguson J, et al: Risk stratification after myocardial infarction using signal-averaged electrocardiographic criteria adjusted for sex, age, and myocardial infarction location. Circulation 96:202–213, 1997.
25. Nakazato Y, Nakata Y, Nakazato K, et al: Normal values for time-domain, frequency-domain, and spectral turbulence analyses of signal-averaged electrocardiograms in healthy subjects. Ann Noninvasive Electrocardiol 5:139–146, 2000.
26. Denniss AR, Richards DA, Cody DV, et al: Prognostic significance of ventricular tachycardia and fibrillation induced at programmed stimulation and delayed potentials detected on the signal-averaged electrocardiograms of survivors of acute myocardial infarction. Circulation 74:731–745, 1986.
27. Gomes JA, Winters SL, Stewart D, et al: A new noninvasive index to predict sustained ventricular tachycardia and sudden death in the first year after myocardial infarction: Based on signal-averaged electrocardiogram, radionuclide ejection fraction, and Holter monitoring. J Am Coll Cardiol 10:349–357, 1987.
28. Kuchar DL, Thorburn CW, Sammel NL: Prediction of serious arrhythmic events after myocardial infarction: Signal-averaged electrocardiogram, Holter monitoring and radionuclide ventriculography. J Am Coll Cardiol 9:531–538, 1987.
29. Kanovsky MS, Falcone RA, Dresden CA, et al: Identification of patients with ventricular tachycardia after myocardial infarction: Signal-averaged electrocardiogram, Holter monitoring, and cardiac catheterization. Circulation 70:264–270, 1984.
30. Buckingham TA, Ghosh S, Homan SM, et al: Independent value of signal-averaged electrocardiography and left ventricular function in identifying patients with sustained ventricular tachycardia with coronary artery disease. Am J Cardiol 59:568–572, 1987.
31. Pedretti R, Laporta A, Etro MD, et al: Influence of thrombolysis on signal-averaged electrocardiogram and late arrhythmic events after acute myocardial. Am J Cardiol 69:866–872, 1992.
32. Malik M, Kulakowski P, Odemuyiwa O, et al: Effect of thrombolytic therapy on the predictive value of signal-averaged electrocardiography after acute myocardial infarction. Am J Cardiol 70:21–25, 1992.
33. McClements BM, Adgey AA: Value of signal-averaged electrocardiography, radionuclide ventriculography, Holter monitoring and clinical variables for prediction of arrhythmic events in survivors of acute myocardial infarction in the thrombolytic era. J Am Coll Cardiol 21:1419–1427, 1993.
34. Denes P, El-Sherif N, Katz R, et al: Prognostic significance of signal-averaged electrocardiogram after thrombolytic therapy and/or angioplasty during acute myocardial infarction (CAST substudy). Am J Cardiol 74:216–220, 1994.
35. Gang ES, Peter T, Rosenthal ME, et al: Detection of late potentials on the surface electrocardiogram in unexplained syncope. Am J Cardiol 58:1014–1020, 1986.
36. Kuchar DL, Thorburn CW, Sammel NL: Signal-averaged electrocardiogram for evaluation of recurrent syncope. Am J Cardiol 58:949–953, 1986.
37. Winters SL, Stewart D, Gomes JA: Signal-averaging of the surface QRS complex predicts inducibility of ventricular tachycardia in patients with syncope of unknown origin: A prospective study. J Am Coll Cardiol 10:775–781, 1987.
38. Steinberg JS, Prystowsky E, Freedman RA, et al: Use of the signal-average electrocardiogram for predicting inducible ventricular tachycardia in patients with unexplained syncope: Relation to clinical variables in a multivariate analysis. J Am Coll Cardiol 23:99–106, 1994.
39. Yamada T, Fukunami M, Ohmori MD, et al: New approach to the estimation of the extent of myocardial fibrosis in patients with dilated cardiomyopathy: Use of signal-averaged electrocardiography. Am Heart J 126:626–631, 1993.
40. Mancini DM, Wong KL, Simson MB: Prognostic value of an abnormal signal-averaged electrocardiogram in patients with nonischemic congestive cardiomyopathy. Circulation 87:1083–1092, 1993.
41. Middlekauff HR, Stevenson WG, Woo MA, et al: Comparison of frequency of late potentials in idiopathic dilated cardiomyopathy and

ischemic cardiomyopathy with advanced congestive heart failure and their usefulness in predicting sudden death. Am J Cardiol 66:1113–1117, 1990.
42. Fontaine G, Gallais-Hamonno F, Frank R, et al: High amplification electrocardiography in cardiac arrhythmias and conduction defects. In Varenne A, Demartini J (eds): High Amplification Electrocardiography. Nice, JM Vidal, 1980.
43. Buxton AE, Simson MB, Falcone RA, et al: Results of signal-averaged electrocardiography and electrophysiologic study in patients with nonsustained ventricular tachycardia after healing of acute myocardial infarction. Am J Cardiol 60:80–85, 1987.
44. Winters SL, Ip J, Deshmukh P, et al: Determinants of induction of ventricular tachycardia in nonsustained ventricular tachycardia after myocardial infarction and the usefulness of signal-averaged electrocardiogram. Am J Cardiol 72:1281–1285, 1993.
45. Turitto G, Fontaine JM, Ursell SN, et al: Value of the signal-averaged electrocardiogram as a predictor of the results of programmed stimulation in nonsustained ventricular tachycardia. Am J Cardiol 61:1272–1278, 1988.
46. Gomes JA, Cain ME, Buxton AE, et al: Prediction of long-term outcomes by signal-averaged electrocardiography in patients with unsustained ventricular tachycardia, coronary artery disease, and left ventricular dysfunction. Circulation 104:436–441, 2001.
47. Hiraki T, Ikeda H, Ohga M, et al: Frequency and time domain analysis of Pwave in patients with paroxysmal atrial fibrillation. Pacing Clin Electrophysiolgy 21:56–64, 1998.
48. Yamada T, Fukunami M, Shimonagat T, et al: Prediction of paroxysmal atrial fibrillation in patients with congestive heart failure: a prospective study. J Am Coll. Cardiology 35:405–413, 2000.

第 87 章

体表电位标测

Bruno Taccardi and Bonnie B. Punske

本章目录

- 体表电位图表达的诊断信息 ············ 788
- 体表电位图的信号采集和判解中的难题 ············ 789
- 心脏电学事件经体表电位图判解：逆解法 ············ 790
- 从测量或重建的心外膜和心内膜电位图推断室壁的电活动 ············ 791
- 总结 ············ 793
- 致谢 ············ 793

体表电位标测图（body surface potential map，BSPM），简称体表电位图，反映了心脏电位在躯干表面的空间分布。通过躯干表面的多单极心电图可获得体表电位图[1,2]。在PQRSTU间期内的某一瞬间测量每幅心电图的振幅，将这些数值转换为毫伏，并在代表躯干表面的图上相应标记，然后在图上画出等电位线（一般应用线性内插法）。在1个或多个心搏中每一瞬间重复上述相同的过程，每次相隔1ms或2ms，序列400～800帧瞬间图反映了PQRSTU间期中电位的变化。通常情况下，20～50帧适当选择的标测图足以反映体表电位场随时间变化的基本特点。

体表电位图比常规12导联心电图表达更多的电学和诊断性信息：（1）只要有足够的电极数，就能从体表获得完整的电学信息；（2）在常规12导联心电图无法采集信号的区域获得具有诊断价值的电学信息；（3）常能显示在心脏中同时发生的2个或更多事件的不同电学表现，例如兴奋和复极（图87-1A），或2个激动波分别向右心室和左心室传播（图87-1B）；（4）与心电图不同，体表等电位标测图在一定的范围内与测量体表电位的参考点无关；（5）体表电位图可计算从任何电极对或体表电极组合（即从现行的或未来的导联系统）获得的心电图；（6）体表电位图可通过逆解法无创性重建心外膜电位分布、激动时间和心内电图。新近研究表明从体表电位测量也能重建心内膜激动时间[3]。

过去30年间，从体表电位图和心电图派生出许多新型体表标测图（body surface map，BSM）：等积分图（isointegral map）[4]，主成分分析[5]，激动、复极和激动恢复间期（activation-recovery interval，ARI）标测图[6]，偏差标测图（departure map）[7]，拉普拉斯图（Laplacian map）[8]等。

一、体表电位图表达的诊断信息

近40年来众多实验和临床研究表明不同形式的体表标测图比12导联心电图包含更多的心脏电生理的信息，具有很高的诊断价值。在本书1995年和2000年版本（Zipes和Jalife主编[9,10]）中，以及Taccardi等[11]回顾的大量文献都支持这一论点，并描述了正常人和心脏病患者的体表标测图。

这里列举几项关于体表标测图的最近诊断成就（1999～2002）：鉴别顺钟向型和逆钟向型房扑[4]；检测非Q波型心肌梗死[7]；在犬WPW综合征合并顺向型心动过速模型中对最早心房逆传激动点的定位[12]；寻找心肌梗死后患者晚电位与室性早搏起源部位的相关性[13]；鉴别心肌梗死患者有无室性心律失常[14,15]；对室速和房速起源点的定位[16]；诊断先天性心脏病[17]；心脏记忆在体表电位图的表现[6]等。

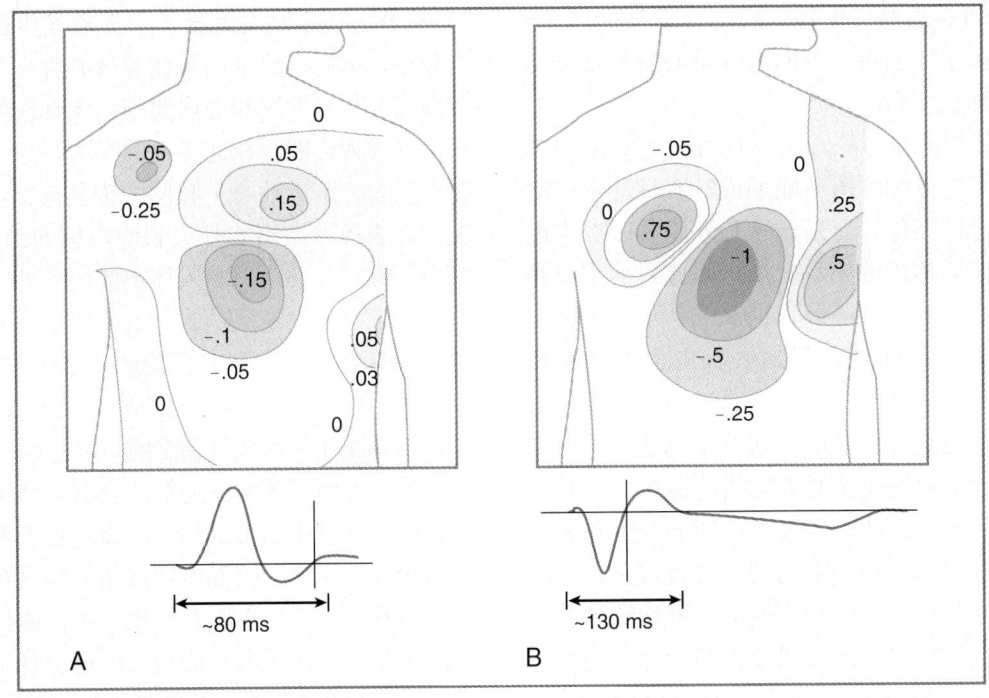

图87-1 A：**正常人的体表电位图** 图中采集的是图下方的心电图（VR导联，仅有QRS波群）中纵线标记的瞬间电位。从QRS波群至ST间期移行时，仍可见激动电位（+0.15mV和−0.15mV），复极电位开始出现（−0.05mV和+0.05mV）。此前的标测图（图中未显示）提示激动电位的极值降低，而随后的标测图（图中未显示）发现激动电位的极值消失，复极电位的极值增加。B：**右束支阻滞患者的体表电位图** 标测图显示的是心电图中（aVR导联）纵线所标记的瞬间电位。右上胸电位极大值（0.75mV）在QRS波群起始后55ms出现，持续到QRS波群的终末部（右心室传导延迟），而左胸电位极大值（0.5mV）代表正常的左心室激动，大约在QRS波群起始后80ms消失。（A图引自Taccardi B：Body surface distribution of equipotential lines during atrial depolarization and ventricular repolarization. Cir Res 19：865-878，1966. B图引自Taccardi B, de Ambroggi L, Riva D：Chest maps of heart potentials in right bundle branch block. J Electrocardiol 2：109-116，1969.）

二、体表电位图的信号采集和判解中的难题

尽管有上述优点，体表电位图至今还没有成为临床常规的标测和检查方法。关于体表标测图、心脏电场、相关数学模型的论文层出不穷，而关于体表标测图临床研究的论文在20世纪80年代中期达到高峰后已经逐年减少，主要原因于下。

1. 技术困难：主要的技术困难是从每个患者放置数十个甚至数百个记录电极（使用的体表电极数为32～219个），各中心采用的导联系统极为复杂[1]。显然，从不同的电极系统获取的信息量不同，因此各系统间电极的数目、位置及可观察电位的幅度（如极大值与极小值）不同。有学者已提出同一患者用不同记录系统相互转换的记录并相互比较的方法[1,18]。

2. 应用问题：检查者很难记住每次心搏中体表电位图的数十个或数百个瞬间电位特点，以及正常人和心脏病人的体表电位图的变异范围。通过体表标测图的积分图或等时图可部分解决这个问题[6,9,10]，这样对每个患者只需要记忆几幅图，但失去了序列电位分布所表达的时间和空间的信息。

3. 失去了电信号从心脏向体表传导的信息：心脏产生的电信号在向体表传导的过程中，必然存在着衰减、失真和滤波[11]。因此，在心脏表面或心室壁观察到的电生理事件并不一定能在体表观察到。所以，多个突破点（breakthrough）、提示激动波锋（也称波阵面）形状和位置的密集排列的等电位线、显示心外膜激动和复极顺序以及心外膜激动传导速度变化的等时图、室速或房速的折返途径、心脏的螺旋形各向异性的影响等在体表电位图几乎不能观察到，而心外膜标测却清晰可辨。

4. 判解体表标测图的困难：影响体表电位标测图临床应用的最大障碍之一是难以将体表标测图随时间变化的多个特点（数目、位置、运动、电位的极大值、极小值、鞍、嵴、盆、谷等）与心腔内事件（即

激动波锋的数目、形状、位置、激动与复极的顺序）相联系。这是由于体表每个点的电位是心脏各部分电位体表分布的加权总和。

与多数心脏影像学方法（超声心动图、X线、CT等）不同，体表电位标测图不能形成具有良好定位的电源和电穴的心脏图像，而是显示心外膜和心腔内电活动在经过衰减后体表的失真投影，因此目前主要是根据正常人与心脏病患者图形识别及统计学处理结果[7]、根据实验和临床研究获得的心脏电生理学知识（包括"起搏标测"获取的数据[16]），以及根据既往和现今的心脏发生器模型的理解（如单个电偶、单个移动电偶、均匀的电偶层和其他更复杂的模型[19,20]）进而分析体表电位图。因此对体表电位图的观察与测量本身不能对心脏单个或多个电活动进行直接定位，因为它们发生在心脏中。在一些病例中，可见到体表标测图中复杂的电位特点及随时间发生的变化，提示心脏中同时存在多个电学事件（图87-1），但确定其位置、形状和时程仍然困难。

三、心脏电学事件经体表电位图判解：逆解法

大量研究表明，心外膜和心内膜的心电标测图是直接从心脏记录心电信号，这要比体表标测图能获得更多的电生理学和诊断性信息。因此，临床心脏电生理学医生常规通过外科途径或用导管的方法从心外膜或心内膜直接记录心腔内电图。过去30年，问世的新方法可以通过无创性方法（始于体表测量）部分获得心外膜或心内膜的心电信息，这些"逆解法"是当前研究的目标，也是今后电生理学的一个重要研究方向[21]。

从体表心电图重建心腔内电活动的演绎方法没有唯一的解，因为从理论上心脏可以有无数个电源产生相同的体表电位分布。但如果对解法加以适当的限定条件，规定所有电流的电源位于心脏表面，则能部分解决这个问题。通过应用这样的限定条件，我们可以计算出具有唯一解的公式，通过体表电位重建心外膜活动，在一些病例还能重建心内膜电活动。

一些研究小组得出了其中一个公式"等时图逆解法"[3,22-27]。这种方法的理论依据是假定在某瞬间心脏产生电位的体表分布与均匀电偶层产生电位分布可以确定，类似于心脏单一电偶层沿心房或心室表面的激动部位排列（心外膜加心内膜）[21]。该电偶层也称

"心脏表面"等效发生器[28]。等效发生器产生体表电位分布，据此可以逆向重建等效心脏发生器。该方法使得确定与心外膜和心内膜表面激动波锋界面的形状和位置成为可能。在此界面的线为一条等时线，通过在心房和心室激动每一瞬间的重复操作，应用"等时线"方法就可绘出心外膜和心内膜的等时图（图87-2）[3]。研究人员在很多人体中应用"等时线"方法并与CARTO方法记录的真正心内膜电图相比较[3]。等时图逆解法是根据等效电源逆解法的一个特例，该方法需要心外膜和心内膜解剖学的知识，对心肌梗死患者，还需要梗死区域解剖学的知识[3,24,29]。

另一方面，等时图逆解法也有一些不足。根据定义，其不能表达心室壁内的波锋，也不能准确重建心内膜和心外膜的电位和电图或给心肌梗死定位。在梗死的心脏，若不从心脏几何模型中去除梗死区而完成逆解法能导致在无激动的梗死区也出现本来不存在的等时线，而在正常区域出现错误的等时线[29]。

另一种方法旨在根据体表心电图重建心外膜电位（电位逆解法）。该方法有唯一解，不需假定心脏电源的性质或位置或动作电位的形状，而且接近心外膜实际电位的分布。该方法寻找在心外膜和躯干电位之间的转换矩阵，这样计算心脏表面每一点的电位可以从躯体表面测量的加权电位值进行线性组合[21]。在数学上该问题很不好解（"等时方法"也是如此[3]），因此，心脏和机体表面几何形状的轻度误差以及机体表面电位测量时小的误差导致解法的严重不稳定性。人们推出了很多调整方法进行稳定地解绎，但失去了一部分信息。关于逆解和调整方法有大量的文献[21,24-26,28-30]（见Dössel的综述[27]）。新近，Ramanathan等[31]提出了调整的新方法，不需要选择调整因素。

逆解的两种方法（等时图和电位法）与12导联心电图和体表标测图相比均有产生三维（3D）影像的优点，这对临床医生很有意义，因为其给出了医生熟悉的解剖特点如心外膜和心内膜表面，并附有激动等时图（图87-2）或激动和复极电位、等时图、心腔内电图（图87-3）。因此，逆解法将心电图转换为电活动的影像，这些方法与显示心脏结构和功能的其他方法如超声心动图、闪烁照相图等相似。

近25年来很多学者研究和应用电位的逆解法[11,30-37]，大多数研究是在实验标本或数学模型中进行，该方法也在一小部分人体中进行了实验。1995年，MacLeod等[32]在7例行PTCA患者观察了短暂

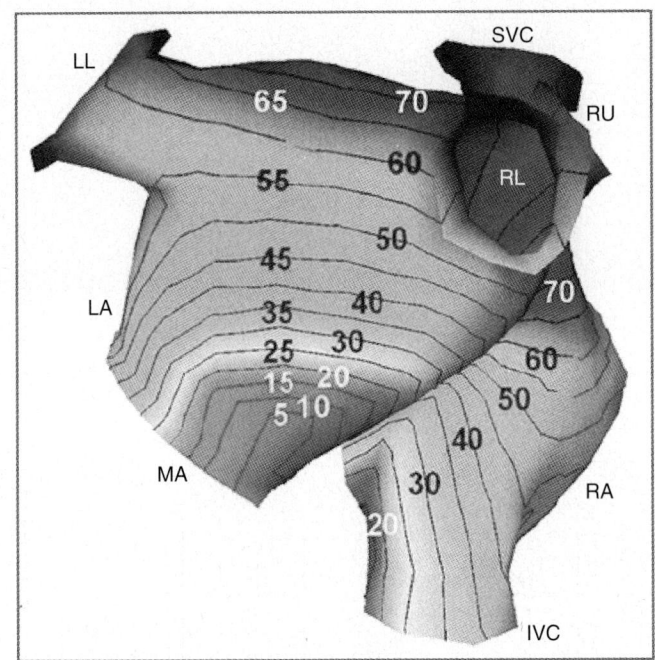

图87-2 一例正常人用导管在冠状窦进行刺激时用逆解法重建心内膜激动的时间图 图为后壁左侧观。IVC：下腔静脉；LA：左心房；LL：左下肺静脉；MA：二尖瓣环；RA：右心房；RL：右下肺静脉；RU：右上肺静脉；SVC：上腔静脉。（引自 Tilg B, Fischer G, Modre R, et al: Model-based imaging of cardiac electrical excitation in humans. IEEE Trans Med Imaging 21：1031-1039, 2003.)（彩图38）

性冠状动脉闭塞引起缺血的心外膜表现及定位。其他研究也对 WPW 患者的预激区进行定位。

意大利 Parma 大学生理研究所（E. Macchi）、意大利 Pavia 市 P. Colli Franzone 领导的研究小组、美国犹他大学心血管研究和培训研究所、在克利夫兰的 Case Western Reserve 第大学的 Y. Rudy 研究小组等长期合作，将离体犬心放在圆柱体或躯干形状的电解箱中，进行逆解法重建心外膜的电活动（图 87-3A～E）[30-37]。通过躯干表面记录的信号重建心外膜电位、等时图和电图，并通过与测量的心外膜电位比较与核实，重建标测图实际显示了 1 个或 2 个起搏点的心外膜部位[36]（图 87-3D、3E）、梗死区域的解剖图[34]（图 87-3F、3G）、单形性或多形性室速心外膜折返环的形状和定位（图 87-4）[33,35]。

目前，根据心外膜电位的逆解法不能反映心内膜电活动（虽然从理论上可以计算出转换系数）。通过从心腔内非接触式电极记录的信号逆解可以解决这个难题[38]。

（一）复极

最近 Van Oosterom[39] 提出并证实了应用"表面等效电源"模型重建复极等时图的可能性。另一方面，Ghanem 等[40] 应用"心外膜电位"法证实可经体表心电图定位心外膜加热和冷却产生的早复极与晚复极区域。在该研究中，通过心电图影像准确反映了与复极有关的电生理特点：（1）加热区 ARI 缩短，QRST 积分增加；（2）冷却区 ARI 延长，QRST 积分减少；（3）在冷热移行区 ARI 和 QRST 积分梯度高。这些作者推断心电图影像可以准确地重建复极的特性，并无创性地定位心脏复极离散的区域。

（二）非均质躯干电阻率

文献中常讨论非均质躯干电阻率对体表和心外膜电位正解和逆解的影响[21]。最近，克利夫兰的研究小组[41] 报告通过含有血液、肺、骨和具有各向异性肌肉的躯干模型进行心外膜电位的重建优于均质性躯干。然而，若忽视躯干的不均质性进行重建后心外膜电位的特点、心内电图、等时图、起搏点的定位准确度等也是相似的。

四、从测量或重建的心外膜和心内膜电位图推断室壁的电活动

上文所述的逆解法可以提供正常心搏、起搏、室速和其他心脏状态下，心外膜和心内膜电活动的信息。反之，从测量或逆运算重建的心外膜或心内膜数据推断室壁激动和复极顺序尚不令人满意。

本研究所及其他实验室以前的研究证明掌握心肌纤维结构及其各向异性特征的知识有助于从测量或逆运算的心外膜或心内膜电位获得室壁电活动的信息[19,42,43]。

众所周知，左心室心肌纤维方向从心外膜至心内膜平均逆时针旋转120°。由于心肌电的各向异性，波锋沿肌纤维纵向的传导比横向传导的速度快。心外膜刺激产生类椭圆形的等时图和四极电位图形，后者也呈类椭圆形，中心区为负，2个极大值位于椭圆长轴的两极外侧（图87-5G）。在激动传播的区域，2个极大值之间的连线平行于心肌纤维的走行方向。在心室壁内刺激产生经心肌纤维传导的波锋，其旋转方向也是逆时针，与起搏深度有关。四极图形的方向也呈逆钟向旋转，随着室壁内肌纤维旋转，而且此图形中心

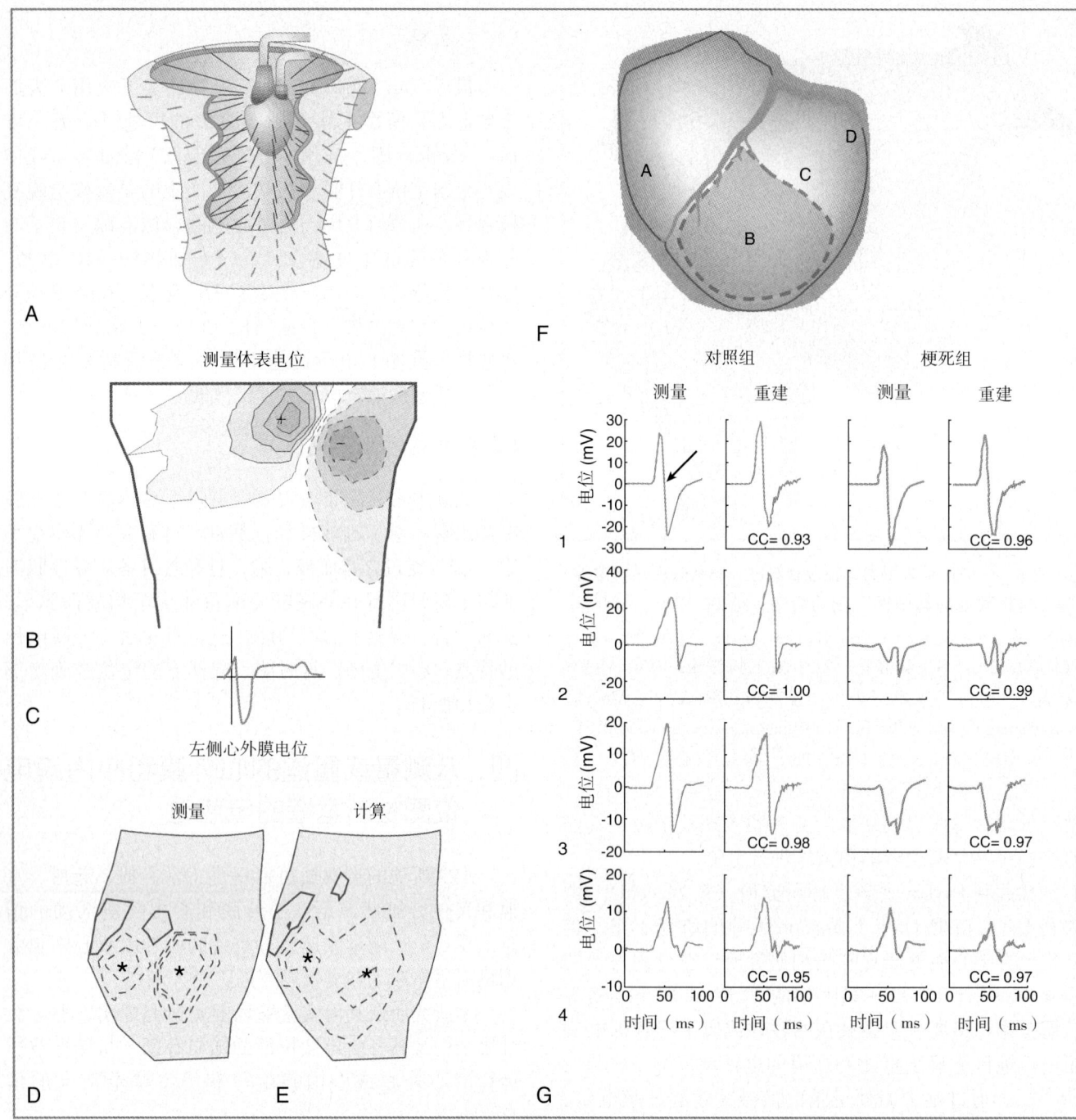

图 87-3 A 图：躯干形状电解箱示意图　离体心脏悬浮在电解箱中，数百个电极杆插入心脏 1cm。所有电极杆的尖端穿过的表面构成了"心外膜封套"。B 图：**从 D 图中星号所示两个部位进行左侧心外膜刺激时在电解箱表面记录的体表电位图（BSPM）**　标测图反映的是 C 图中心电图的纵线所示的瞬间。D 图和 E 图：**在 C 图中所示的瞬间测量的和逆运算的"心外膜"电位分布**　虽然体表电位标测图并不提示存在 2 个激动，逆解重建的心外膜电位图（E 图）清楚显示 2 个电位极小值与 D 图中测量分布的实际起搏部分相近。F 图：**在犬心左前降支的第一对角支注射乙醇引起急性心肌梗死后的犬心前表面**　深灰色区域提示坏死区的大致位置与形状。G 图：**在 1 和 4 部位的电图**　注射乙醇前正常，通过逆解法很好地重建。注射乙醇后，相同部位的电图显示梗死区出现 Q 波，在 B 和 C 部位也出现一些"尖峰"电位，提示坏死的边缘区存在持续的激动。(A～E 图引自 Oster HS, Taccardi B, Lux RL, et al: Electrocardiographic imaging: Noninvasive characterization of intramural myocardial activation from inverse-reconstructed epicardial potentials and electrograms. Circulation 97：1496-1507，1998；F～G 图引自 Burnes JE, Taccardi B, MacLeod RS, et al: Noninvasive ECG imaging of electrophysiologically abnormal subnormal substrates in infracted hearts: A model study. Circulation 101：533-544，2000.)

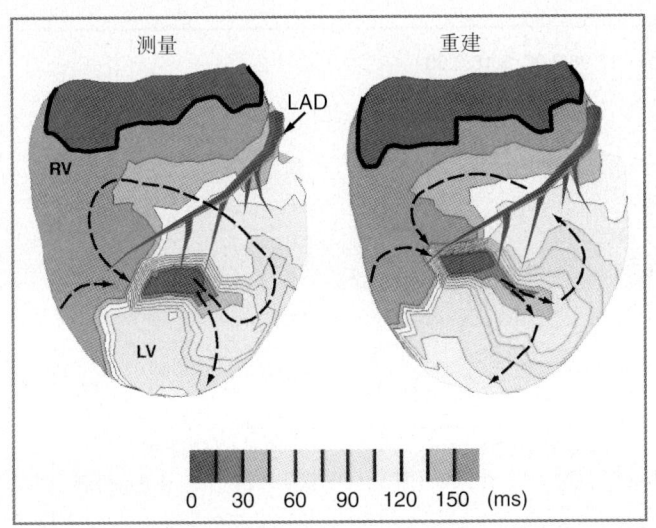

图 87-4 心肌梗死 5 天的心脏 程序刺激诱发了折返性的类单形性室速,在测量的心外膜等时图上(左图)和经计算机逆运算法重建的心外膜电图(右图)上清晰可见。(引自 Burnes JE, Taccardi B, Rudy Y: A noninvasive imaging modality for cardiac arrhythmias. Circulation 102: 2152-2158, 2000.)(彩图 39)

外膜远场反射也旋转,因而提示起搏的部位和深度(图 87-5A~F)。Oster 等[36]也在经逆运算重建的心外膜电位图上观察到这些旋转特点,这显示了起搏点或异位兴奋灶的部位和深度。而且,心外膜刺激产生的长的波锋通过全层室壁传导时呈左手螺旋式旋转。这使壁内阳性区呈螺旋式扩展,而心外膜远场发射引起心外膜阳性区逆钟向旋转式扩展。因此,在测量或逆运算重建的心外膜电位图中,阳性区逆钟向旋转提示波锋自心外膜向心内膜传播(图 87-5I)。反之,顺钟向旋转提示波锋自心内膜向心外膜传播。关于激动波锋产生的电位和电流分布的更完全和更严格的公式,见参考文献[19,20,43,44]。

各向异性的电效应并不限于心脏,通过在躯干容积导体标测电位和电流分布也可检测到(图 87-6)。但通过观察体表电位图却很难区分。然而,这些效应一定存在于体表,因为通过体表电位逆运算得出其在心外膜电位分布中也存在。

新近,一些学者,特别是 Auckland 大学 Hunter 指导的小组深入研究了最早由 Horst 在 20 世纪 60 年代提出的心室壁裂隙与不连续性[45]。他们发现心室壁心肌纤维的结构呈板层状[55],因此室壁内传导性张力的分布呈正交各向异性,而不是通常人们假定的轴向各向异性。正交各向异性是指心脏激动在 3 个正交方向上具有不同的传导速度。最近 Colli Franzone 等[46]通过计算机模拟方法,观察了正交各向异性对激动传播、电位和电图的影响。

掌握心肌的解剖和生物物理特性有助于了解心脏的激动传播及相关的电位场的规律,也有助于解释采用测量或逆运算方法重现室壁电活动的心外膜和心内膜标测图。如果根据心肌的各向异性和肌纤维结构分析这些标测图,可显示起搏点的部位和室壁内深度、异位兴奋灶附近心肌纤维的方向、激动在心室内的螺旋式传播[37]、在心室内是否存在微小的非透壁性坏死灶[42]、"重合角(imbrication angle)"(即心肌纤维的心外膜-心内膜斜率)对激动三维传播和相关电位分布的影响等[11,42]。

数学模拟

显示心室壁激动的三维传播及相关电位的数学模型可提供关于心外膜与室壁内活动相互关系的大量信息[19]。研究显示,虽然通过将心脏当作一个各向异性单域的数学模型可正确地模拟激动的传播,但只有建立在各向异性比例不等的各向异性双域模型才能准确地模拟出心脏及其表面的电位分布、相关的电图、躯干和体表电位和电流的分布(图 87-6)[20,47]。

五、总 结

大量研究表明各种形式的体表心电图标测所包含的信息量及其诊断价值优于标准的 12 导联心电图。然而,体表电位图仍主要用于研究而不是作为常规的诊断方法,可能因为其没有形成心脏的影像来显示心房和心室激动的传播、复极顺序、梗死的定位和面积及其他电学特点。本文总结的近期研究工作提示不同的逆解法形成了心脏科医生易判解的影像,可以成为良好的具有诊断价值的新型影像学方法。

六、致 谢

本研究得到 Nora Eccles Treadwell 基金会的资助和国立卫生研究院的资助(No. RO1-HL 43276-10)。Case Western Reserve 大学的 Charulatha Rhamanathan 博士和 Yoram Rudy 博士帮助分析逆运算法形成的三维数据。

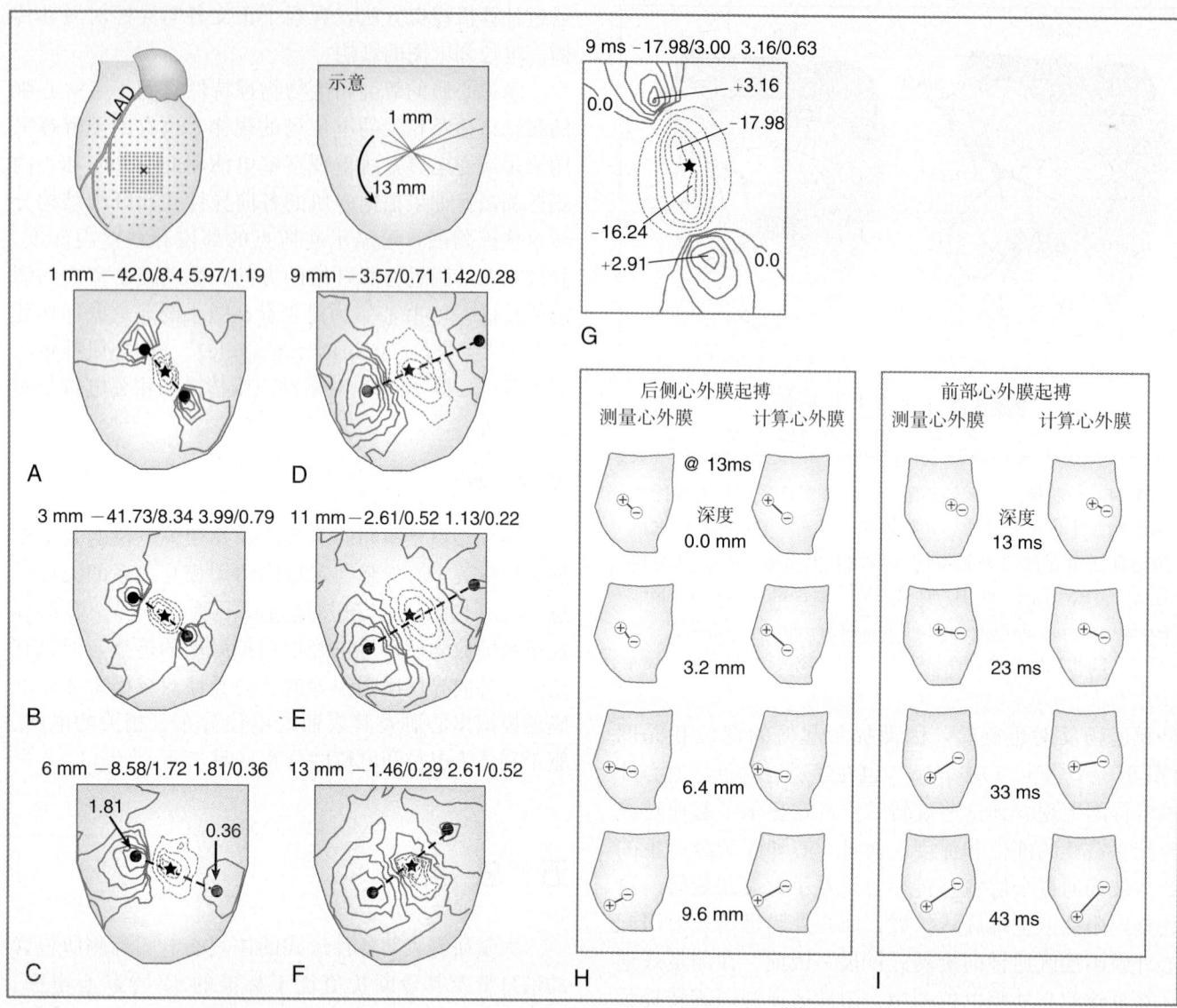

图 87-5　A～G 图：通过壁内针插入左心室壁并逐渐增加深度，进行左心室起搏 13ms 后测量的心外膜电位分布　G 图更详细地描绘了典型的电位特点，中心区为负，并有 2 个极大值。A～F 图中，当起搏点在壁内深度从 1mm 移向 13mm 时，图形逆时针旋转大约 100°。H 图：**逐渐增加起搏深度引起相似旋转的变化示意图**　在 H 图的右侧，逆运算重建的示意图显示相似的旋转。I 图：**心外膜极大值的旋转**　左侧图显示一个心外膜极大值的旋转是心外膜刺激后的时间函数。右侧图显示逆运算能准确模拟这种旋转。（A～G 图引自 Taccardi B, Macchi E, Lux RL, et al: Effect of myocardial fiber direction on epicardial potentials. Circulation 90：3076-3090，1994；H～I 图引自 Oster HS, Taccardi B, Lux RL, et al: Electrocardiographic imaging: Noninvasive characterization of intramural myocardial activation from inverse-reconstructed epicardial potentials and electrograms. Circulation 97：1496-1507，1998.）

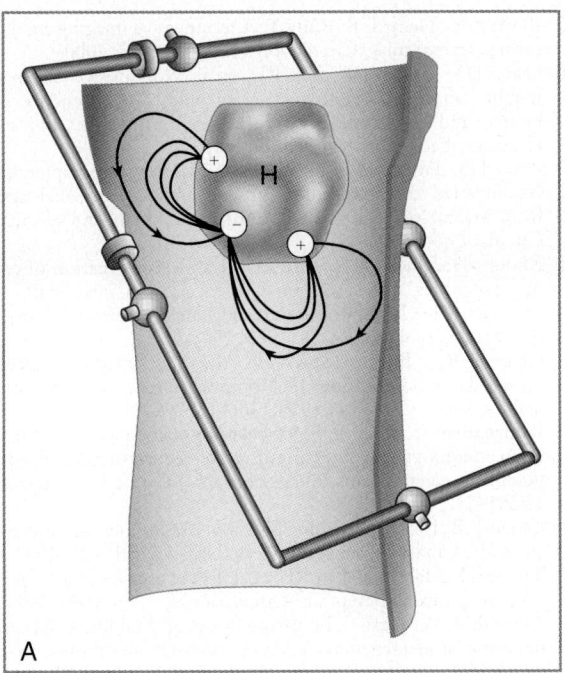 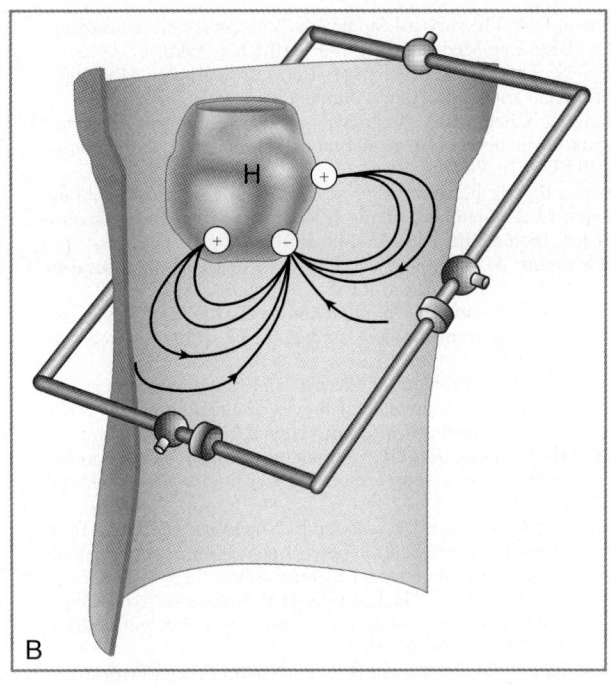

图87-6　A图：**心外膜起搏引起胸腔内电流的三维观**　电流线簇从2个电位极大值（沿着浅表纤维方向排列）向起搏点与中心极小值汇聚。B图：**用心外膜起搏的壁内针进行心内膜刺激**　2个极大值沿着心内膜纤维排列，波锋从心内膜向心外膜传播。然而，电流线仍从2个极大值流向中心极小值，进入了波锋，流向心外膜。（引自Taccardi B，Punske BB，MacLeod RS，et al：Extracardiac effects of myocardial electrical anisotropy. Biomed Tech 46：216-218，2001.）

（洪　江　译）

参 考 文 献

1. Hoekema R, Uijen GJ, Stilli D, et al: Lead system transformation of body surface map data. J Electrocardiol 31:71–82, 1998.
2. Hoekema R, Uijen GJ, van Oosterom A: On selecting a body surface mapping procedure. J Electrocardiol 32:93–101, 1999.
3. Tilg B, Fischer G, Modre R, et al: Model-based imaging of cardiac electrical excitation in humans. IEEE Trans Med Imaging 21:1031–1039, 2003.
4. SippensGroenewegen A, Lesh MD, Roithinger FX, et al: Body surface mapping of counterclockwise and clockwise typical atrial flutter: A comparative analysis with endocardial activation sequence mapping. J Am Coll Cardiol 35:1276–1287, 2000.
5. De Ambroggi L, Aime E, Ceriotti C, et al: Mapping of ventricular repolarization potentials in patients with arrhythmogenic right ventricular dysplasia: Principal component analysis of the ST-T waves. Circulation 96:4314–4318, 1997.
6. Takada Y, Inden Y, Akahoshi M, et al: Changes in repolarization properties with long-term cardiac memory modify dispersion of repolarization in patients with Wolff-Parkinson-White syndrome. J Cardiovasc Electrophysiol 13:324–330, 2002.
7. Medvegy M, Preda I, Savard P, et al: New body surface isopotential map evaluation method to detect minor potential losses in non-Q-wave myocardial infarction. Circulation 101:1115–1121, 2000.
8. Lian J, Li G, Cheng J, et al: Body surface Laplacian mapping of atrial depolarization in healthy human subjects. Med Biol Eng Comput 40:650–659, 2002.
9. Flowers N, Horan L: Body Surface Potential Mapping. In Zipes D, Jalife J (eds): Cardiac Electrophysiology: From Cell to Bedside. Philadelphia, WB Saunders, 1995, pp 1049–1067.
10. Flowers N, Horan L: Body Surface Potential Mapping. In Zipes D, Jalife J (eds): Cardiac Electrophysiology: From Cell to Bedside. Philadelphia, WB Saunders, 2000, pp 737–746.
11. Taccardi B, Punske BB, Lux RL, et al: Useful lessons from body surface mapping. J Cardiovasc Electrophysiol 9:773–786, 1998.
12. Pinter A, Molin F, Savard P, et al: Body surface mapping of retrograde P waves in the intact dog by simulation of accessory pathway re-entry. Can J Cardiol 16:175–182, 2000.
13. Wang X, Kamakura S, Matsuo K, et al: Relation between spatial distribution of late potentials and location of origin of premature ventricular complexes on body surface map in patients with postinfarction ventricular tachycardia. Int J Cardiol 72:111–119, 2000.
14. Stroink G, Meeder RJ, Elliott P, et al: Arrhythmia vulnerability assessment using magnetic field maps and body surface potential maps. Pacing Clin Electrophysiol 22:1718–1728, 1999.
15. Meeder RJ, Stroink G, Ritcey SP, et al: Low frequency component of body surface potential maps identifies patients at risk for ventricular tachycardia. Eur Heart J 20:1126–1134, 1999.
16. van Dessel PF, van Hemel NM, de Bakker JM, et al: Relation between body surface mapping and endocardial spread of ventricular activation in postinfarction heart. J Cardiovasc Electrophysiol 12:1232–1241, 2001.
17. Liebman J: The Body Surface Potential Map in Congenital Heart Disease. In Schalij MJ, Janse MJ, van Oosterom A, et al (eds): Einthoven 2002 100 years of Electrocardiography. Leiden, The Einthoven Foundation, 2002, pp 215–220.
18. Wung SF, Lux RL, Drew BJ: Thoracic location of the lead with maximal ST-segment deviation during posterior and right ventricular ischemia: Comparison of 18-lead ECG with 192 estimated body surface leads. J Electrocardiol (Suppl 33):167–174, 2000.
19. Colli Franzone P, Guerri L, Pennacchio M, et al: Spread of excitation in 3-D models of the anisotropic cardiac tissue. III. Effects of ventricular geometry and fiber structure on the potential distribution. Math Biosci 151:51–98, 1998.
20. Muzikant AL, Hsu EW, Wolf PD, et al: Region specific modeling of cardiac muscle: Comparison of simulated and experimental potentials. Ann Biomed Eng 30:867–883, 2002.

21. Gulrajani RM: The forward and inverse problems of electrocardiography. IEEE Eng Med Biol Mag 17:84–101, 122, 1998.
22. Pullan AJ: The inverse problem of electrocardiography: Modelling, experimental and clinical issues. Biomed Tech 46:197–200, 2001.
23. Pullan AJ, Cheng LK, Nash MP, et al: Noninvasive electrical imaging of the heart: Theory and model development. Ann Biomed Eng 29:817–836, 2001.
24. Messnarz B, Tilg B, Modre R, et al: Comparison of transmembrane and epicardial potential patterns reconstructed by a linear inverse approach. Biomed Tech 46:147–149, 2001.
25. van Oosterom A: Genesis of the T wave as based on an equivalent surface source model. J Electrocardiol 34(Suppl):217–227, 2001.
26. Greensite F, Huiskamp G: An improved method for estimating epicardial potentials from the body surface. IEEE Trans Biomed Eng 45:98–104, 1998.
27. Dössel O: Inverse Problem of Electro- and Magnetocardiography: Review and Recent Progress. Int J Bioelectromagnetism 2(2), 2000. Available at http://ee.tut.fi/rgi/ijbem/volume2/number2/toc.htm.
28. Simms HD Jr, Geselowitz DB: Computation of heart surface potentials using the surface source model. J Cardiovasc Electrophysiol 6:522–531, 1995.
29. Oostendorp T, Nenonen J, Korhonen P: Noninvasive determination of the activation sequence of the heart: Application to patients with previous myocardial infarctions. J Electrocardiol 35:75–80, 2002.
30. Brooks DH, Ahmad GF, MacLeod RS, et al: Inverse electrocardiography by simultaneous imposition of multiple constraints. IEEE Trans Biomed Eng 46:3–18, 1999.
31. Ramanathan C, Jia P, Ghanem R, et al: Noninvasive electrocardiographic imaging (ECGI) application of the generalized minimal residual method (GMRes) method. Ann Biomed Eng 31(8):981–994.
32. MacLeod RS, Gardner M, Miller RM, et al: Application of an electrocardiographic inverse solution to localize ischemia during coronary angioplasty. J Cardiovasc Electrophysiol 6:2–18, 1995.
33. Burnes JE, Taccardi B, Ershler PR, et al: Noninvasive electrocardiogram imaging of substrate and intramural ventricular tachycardia in infarcted hearts. J Am Coll Cardiol 38:2071–2078, 2001.
34. Burnes JE, Taccardi B, MacLeod RS, et al: Noninvasive ECG imaging of electrophysiologically abnormal substrates in infarcted hearts: A model study. Circulation 101:533–540, 2000.
35. Burnes JE, Taccardi B, Rudy Y: A noninvasive imaging modality for cardiac arrhythmias. Circulation 102:2152–2158, 2000.
36. Oster HS, Taccardi B, Lux RL, et al: Noninvasive electrocardiographic imaging: Reconstruction of epicardial potentials, electrograms, and isochrones and localization of single and multiple electrocardiac events. Circulation 96:1012–1024, 1997.
37. Oster HS, Taccardi B, Lux RL, et al: Electrocardiographic imaging: Noninvasive characterization of intramural myocardial activation from inverse-reconstructed epicardial potentials and electrograms. Circulation 97:1496–1507, 1998.
38. Khoury DS, Taccardi B, Lux RL, et al: Reconstruction of endocardial potentials and activation sequences from intracavitary probe measurements: Localization of pacing sites and effects of myocardial structure. Circulation 91:845–863, 1995.
39. Ghanem RN, Burnes JE, Waldo AL, et al: Imaging dispersion of myocardial repolarization, II: Noninvasive reconstruction of epicardial measures. Circulation 104:1306–1312, 2001.
40. Ramanathan C, Rudy Y: Electrocardiographic imaging: II. Effect of torso inhomogeneities on noninvasive reconstruction of epicardial potentials, electrograms, and isochrones. J Cardiovasc Electrophysiol 12:241–252, 2001.
41. Taccardi B, Lux RL, Ershler PR, et al: Anatomical architecture and electrical activity of the heart. Acta Cardiol 52:91–105, 1997.
42. Taccardi B, Macchi E, Lux RL, et al: Effect of myocardial fiber direction on epicardial potentials. Circulation 90:3076–3090, 1994.
43. Taccardi B, Veronese S, Franzone PC, et al: Multiple components in the unipolar electrogram: A simulation study in a three-dimensional model of ventricular myocardium. J Cardiovasc Electrophysiol 9:1062–1084, 1998.
44. Hooks DA, Tomlinson KA, Marsden SG, et al: Cardiac microstructure: Implications for electrical propagation and defibrillation in the heart. Circ Res 91:331–338, 2002.
45. Colli Franzone P, Guerri L, Taccardi B: Modeling ventricular excitation: Axial and orthotropic anisotropy effects on wavefronts and potentials. Presented at BIOCOMP 2002: Topics in Biomathematics and Related Computational Problems, June 3-9, 2002, Hotel Lloyd's Baia, Vietri sul Mare, Italy.
46. Taccardi B, Punske BB, MacLeod RS, et al: Extracardiac effects of myocardial electrical anisotropy. Biomed Tech 46:216–218, 2001.

第 88 章

直立倾斜试验

David G. Benditt, *Cengiz Ermis*, and *Fei Lü*

本章目录

- 直立体位对生理状态的影响 ………… 797
- 血管迷走性晕厥的病理生理学 ……… 798
- 直立倾斜试验评价血管迷走性晕厥
  ………………………………………… 800
- 直立倾斜试验的操作方案 …………… 804
- 利用倾斜试验预测治疗的效果 ……… 805
- 直立倾斜试验应用的建议 …………… 805
- 总结 …………………………………… 806
- 致谢 …………………………………… 806

生理学家和内科医生应用直立倾斜试验已经50余年。该试验一直用于研究体位变换时心率和血压的适应性调整、模拟失血时的机体反应、评价体位性低血压，以及评估在充血性心力衰竭、自主神经功能异常和低血压等状态下的血流动力学和神经内分泌反应。在诸如此类的研究过程中，人们偶然观察到一部分受试者在试验中出现神经反射性介导的低血压和心动过缓，类似于血管迷走性反射。基于上述发现，特别是在1986年Kenny及同事发表相关文章[1]后，被动性直立倾斜试验开始被用于在易感个体中诱发血管迷走性晕厥，进而成为一种诊断方法。最初，采用直立倾斜体位是激发血管迷走事件的唯一手段。后来，药物激发也被引入试验中，以提高检查的诊断检出率。目前，异丙肾上腺素和硝酸甘油是应用最广泛的药物激发剂。

当血管迷走性晕厥发作典型时，单纯通过病史（包括旁观者的观察）就可以确定诊断[2]，而不需要进一步的试验证明。然而，临床中遇到的情况往往是昏晕（faint）以及类似事件而并非"典型"，甚至连经验丰富的病史采集者也不能确定诊断。此外，还有很多病例（特别是老年人或幼儿）不能提供准确的病史。这些病例中的一部分人没有可靠病史可能是因为患者缺乏洞察力，或者由于先兆事件而出现逆行性遗忘（特别是老年人）。对于这些病例来说，如果能提供具有诊断价值的检查方法就会有很大裨益。直立倾斜试验作为一种颇有价值的检查方法逐渐被广泛接受，用来评价患者是否容易发作血管迷走性晕厥。本章就是回顾直立倾斜试验在评价血管迷走性晕厥中的发展，审视该检查的局限性，并推荐和介绍应用于临床实验室中的方法学。

一、直立体位对生理状态的影响

在直立体位下，由于重力作用使体内循环血容量重新分布而产生直立性压力。最初，当体位刚达到直立时，重力作用导致大约500~1000ml的血液转移到身体的较低部分（图88-1）。绝大多数情况下，这种重新分布发生在最初的10s之内。随后，在接下来的10min内，正常个体的体内还将会有额外的700ml不含蛋白质的体液被过滤到组织间隙中[3]。这两种作用的结果导致静脉回流和每搏量明显减少。

人类机体试图通过增加心率和收缩外周的阻力血管和容量血管来代偿在体位变为直立这一动作过程中每搏量的减少。然而，在这种情况下单纯增加心率并不足以维持心排血量和脑血流的供给。体循环血管的收缩对维持动脉血压至关紧要。防止晕厥的发生需要代偿

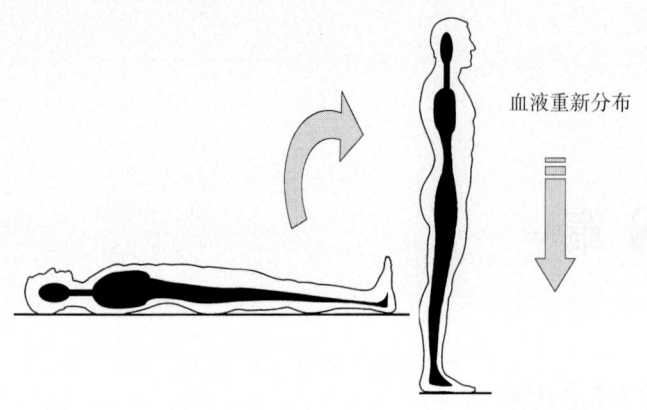

图88-1 当人体由仰卧位变换为直立体位时中心血容量重新分布

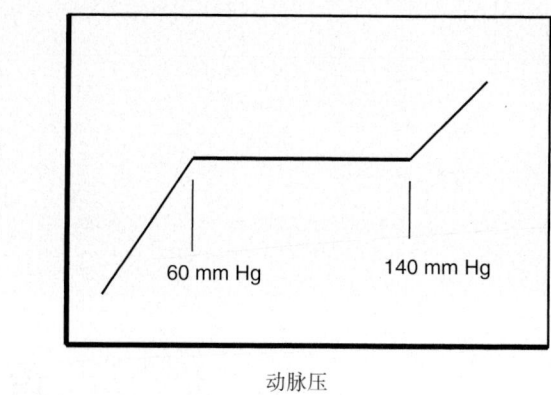

图88-2 脑血流自动调整曲线示意图 横坐标代表动脉压，纵坐标代表脑血流。当血压下降到60mmHg以下时，脑血流明显减少

性的心血管反射使动脉血压（特别是在颈动脉水平的体循环压力）维持一定的数值，使之至少等于足够保证脑部血流所需要的最低数值（大约为60mmHg）。

直立性应激触发的短期心血管调节由自主神经系统专门介导。直立性应激反射调节中的主要感受器是动脉内的机械感受器（即压力感受器对压力、牵张力或两者共同作用发生反应），位于主动脉弓和颈动脉窦。心脏壁内（心房和心室均存在）和肺内（心肺感受器）的机械感受器也起到次要的辅助作用。当直立应激较久时，长期调节中的神经内分泌代偿性机制就开始启动，但在血管迷走性晕厥的病理生理中这些调节作用往往被忽视。

诸如静脉-小动脉反射（venoarteriolar reflex）之类的局部反射以及其他的复合机制，如骨骼肌的泵效应（即使没有明显的运动）和呼吸的泵作用都可以增强交感中枢输出到全身血管的反射活动。上述因素中的任何一种都可以通过促进静脉回流而维持动脉压，从而发挥重要的辅助作用。

如果对直立应激的代偿调节出现异常，就将无法保障中心血容量，导致全身性动脉压下降，并且出现脑血流量不足（图88-2）。最终结果不仅仅是由于全身性低血压引起意识丧失，还有在特定情况下（亦需为敏感个体）所触发的不恰当的神经反射反应（如血管扩张和心动过缓——血管迷走性反射）。后者正是支持应用倾斜试验评估患者是否容易发作血管迷走性晕厥的基础[4,5]。

二、血管迷走性晕厥的病理生理学

神经介导性晕厥的病理生理学尚未完全明晰。然而，我们可以考虑以下4个基本要素：（1）传入支，（2）中枢神经系统，（3）传出支，（4）反馈环路[6,7]。本节内不对这些要素进行详细讨论。概而言之，中枢和外周的机械感受器（见上文）以及偶尔参与作用的化学感受器（如存在心肌缺血时）启动传入感觉神经，传导到位于延髓的心血管调控中枢（孤束核）（图88-3）。目前尚不清楚是通过何种方式对所感受的刺激进行处理而导致不适当的传出反应，但其中部分原因可能是由于几种传入信息不和谐，例如颈动脉窦综合征之类的疾病就可能促进这种情况的发生。无论什么情况，只要交感异常兴奋传出，迷走反射就会发生。引起全身性低血压（如果非常严重最终会导致血管迷走性晕厥）的最主要原因是使腿部骨骼肌内血管收缩的交感神经传出指令明显减少。副交感神经介导的心动过缓（严重时，或相对于血压降低的程度较重时）也参与了此过程，但作用较弱，除非出现长时间的心脏停搏。能够识别并中断这个进程的压力感受器反馈机制出现不明原因的异常似乎在低血压的发生过程中也具有相当重要的促进作用（图88-3）。

在部分患者中，脑血流自动调节反射受损可能也参与了血管迷走性反射的发生。有报道指出在动脉压下降以及脑血管收缩之前即已出现脑血流速度降低，并且有部分病例在未出现全身性低血压的情况下就可能发生脑缺氧。因而，有人提出脑血管痉挛也可能是出现短暂性脑灌注不足的一种发生机制[8,9]，但其发生的几率和重要性还不清楚。

几项观察结果提示，直立倾斜试验阳性所出现的有症状的低血压-心动过缓与自发的神经反射性介导的血管迷走性晕厥具有可比性。首先，无论是自发的还

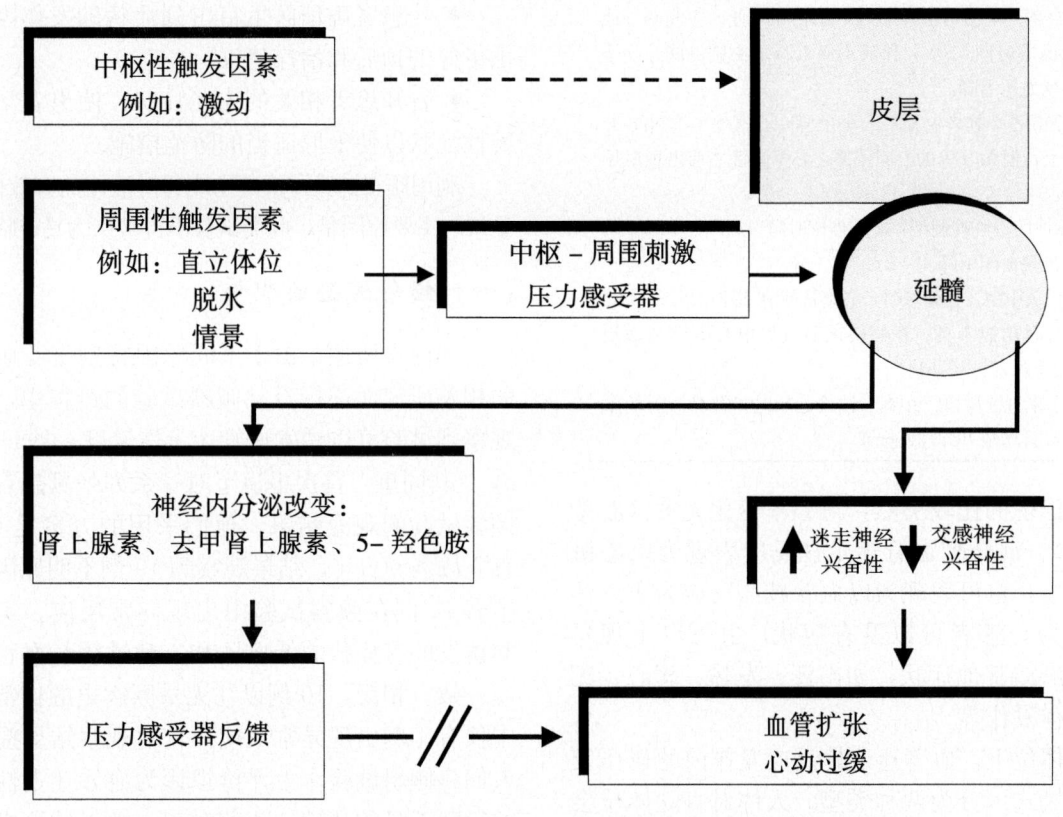

图 88-3 直立体位触发血管迷走性晕厥机制的示意图

是诱发的晕厥发作都有类似的先兆症状（如恶心、出汗）和体征（如明显的面色苍白，保持体位的张力丧失）。其次，在倾斜诱发的晕厥发作过程中血压和心率变化的时间顺序与报道的自主发作类似（图 88-4）。最后，自发晕厥和倾斜诱发晕厥在发作之前及过程中所测定的血浆儿茶酚胺也呈现出显著的相似性。尤其是，无论自发的血管迷走性晕厥还是倾斜试验诱发的低血压-心动过缓，它们的特征都是循环中的儿茶酚胺出现先兆性增加（即在明显的全身性低血压之前）。

根据临床观察，大多数血管迷走性晕厥患者表现为同时具有心脏抑制和血管减压的混合型反应。偶尔可以观察到单纯的血管减压反应。对这些反应进行分类比较困难，目前还存在争议。较为普遍接受的分类方法来自于血管迷走性晕厥国际研究（vasovagal syncope international study，VASIS）工作组（表 88-1）[10,11]。根据定义，单纯的心脏抑制型反应表现为心率骤降超过 20 次/分，伴或不伴心脏停搏、房室传导抑制或血压下降。血管减压反应的定义为显著的血压

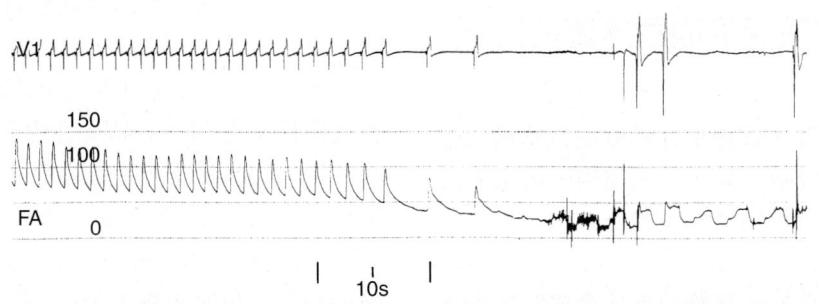

图 88-4 直立倾斜试验诱发血管迷走性晕厥过程中记录的典型心率与血压变化

表88-1　倾斜试验阳性反应的分类

- 1型——混合型：晕厥时心率减慢，但心室率不<40bpm，或心率<40bpm的时间<10s，伴或不伴<3s的心脏停搏。心率减慢之前出现血压下降。
- 2A型：无停搏的心脏抑制型：心率下降，心室率<40bpm并持续10s以上，但无>3s的心脏停搏，心率减慢之前出现血压下降。
- 2B型：伴停搏的心脏抑制型：心脏停搏时间>3s。心率减慢的同时或之前出现血压下降。
- 3型——血管减压型：在晕厥时，心率从峰值下降<10%。
- 特例1——变时功能不良：在倾斜试验过程中心率没有增快（较倾斜前心率增加<10%）。
- 特例2——心率过度增快：在直立体位起始时以及晕厥前的整个过程心率异常增快（>130bpm）。

下降，通常出现的比较突然，与心率变化无关（心率下降<10%）。混合型血管迷走性反应表现为以心脏抑制反应为主，也可表现为以血管减压反应为主。伴随着这些反应，患者可以没有症状，也可以出现晕厥、先兆晕厥或其他症状，如出汗、发热、恶心、无力以及癫痫样发作等。

在直立体位下，血管迷走性反应发作前的血压及心率的变化模式可分为两种类型。人体对直立体位会产生适应性代偿反射，最终维持稳定的血压和心率（这属于正常压力反射功能），如果其初始阶段发生的非常迅速并且完全是典型模式的特征，这种情况将持续到血管迷走性反应突然发作的时候。此类患者中大部分是年轻的健康人。另一类模式的特征是无法适应直立体位并达到稳定状态，所以出现血压和心率的进行性下降直到各种症状发作。这种模式类似于在自主神经功能障碍中较常见的一种反应。就此而言，某些病例中可能存在经典的尽管直立体位触发血管迷走性晕厥的机制尚不清楚，血管迷走性晕厥与更加复杂的自主神经系统功能障碍的相互重叠，但是大多数患者可能不是这种情况[2]。

三、直立倾斜试验评价血管迷走性晕厥

尽管直立体位触发血管迷走性晕厥的机制尚不清楚，直立倾斜试验已经成为揭示不明原因晕厥患者发生血管迷走性晕厥易感性的实验室检查技术。直立倾斜试验可为临床提供：

- 在安全和控制良好的环境中评估个体对血管迷走性晕厥的易感性；
- 确定实验室中诱发的症状是否与自发事件的症状一致；
- 让患者确信医生目击到症状的发作因而能够提供更好的预后和治疗建议；
- 告知患者相关的先兆症状，使患者学会识别预警性症状以便采取适当的防范措施。

利用倾斜试验评价药物或起搏治疗的有效性仍然存有争议。主要原因是，此类试验不再被认为具有临床价值。

（一）倾斜试验的背景

如前文所述，由于不同原因特别是心血管生理学的相关研究而进行直立倾斜试验的过程中，人们偶然观察到试验可以诱发血管迷走性晕厥。1986年，Kenny及其同事[1]首次报道了对一系列晕厥患者进行直立倾斜试验的观察结果。他们采用的方案是60°角度下直立倾斜60min，结果观察到15例不明原因晕厥患者中有10例在倾斜试验中出现异常反应。实质上，试验诱发的有症状的低血压和心动过缓与血管迷走性反应一致。相反，10例以往无晕厥病史的正常对照个体中仅有1例出现异常反应。这组观察结果提供了嗣后人们将倾斜试验作为评价拟诊为血管迷走性晕厥患者的诊断工具的基础。从那时起，倾斜试验成为很多临床研究的课题，并在临床研究中广泛应用。

（二）试验方案

1. 无药物激发的被动倾斜试验

1991年，Fitzpatrick及同事[12]发表文章提出，利用固定在倾斜台上的鞍状物或座位进行试验会导致阳性反应过多（推测是由于腿部的静脉回流减少而引起的静脉受阻所致）。与单独采用脚踏板支持的倾斜台相比，这样的倾斜台配置会降低试验的特异性。他们还提出倾斜角度低于60°会使试验的阳性率下降。他们观察到患者发作晕厥的平均时间为24±10min，从而认为被动倾斜试验的维持时间应当为45min。因此，他们提出了在60°倾斜状态下维持45min的无药物激发方案。据其报道，不明原因晕厥患者采用本方案检查的阳性率为75%，特异性为93%。

Fitzpatrick及其同事的发现[12]有助于确立可供临床应用的倾斜试验方案。随后，主要依据Almquist等[13]和后来的Natale等[14]的报道，绝大多数实验室将倾斜台的角度调整为70°~80°之间。然而，试验时间一直采用45min，直到引入药物激发的方法后才使试验时间得以缩短。

2. 药物激发下的被动倾斜试验

第一个验证利用药物提高倾斜试验诊断率的研究发表于1989年[13,15]。在Almmquist等[13]的报道中提出在被动倾斜试验仅进行10min后就开始输注异丙肾上腺素没有诊断意义。在无药物激发的倾斜试验第一阶段结束后,患者恢复仰卧体位并且给予静脉输注异丙肾上腺素,初始剂量为1μg/min。当患者心率增快达到稳定状态时,再次倾斜。重复这一操作,直至异丙肾上腺素的剂量为5μg/min。采用这种方案,11例不明原因晕厥而电生理检查阴性的患者中9例出现低血压和心动过缓,而18例对照个体中仅2例出现类似反应。

尽管最初应用异丙肾上腺素激发较为流行,但随着时间推移许多弊端逐渐显现。首先,一些学者提出争议,认为这样的激发方案使试验的假阳性率过度增加。其次,异丙肾上腺素可以使很多个体发生不良反应,而且不适于老年人,因为后者可能患有缺血性心脏病。再次,逐级加量输注异丙肾上腺素的方法很费时。最后,2000年在美国由于生产方面的原因,很长时间内无法获得这种药物。因而替代方案(特别是采用硝酸甘油的方案)获得了显现身手的机会。

在异丙肾上腺素假阳性率方面,Kapoor与Brant[16]在1992年报道某些患者加用异丙肾上腺素看起来会使试验的特异性降低到令人无法接受的水平(在45%~65%之间)。他们的方案是在倾斜角度保持80°的情况下,将异丙肾上腺素的剂量从1μg/min逐渐增加到5μg/min,在每次增加剂量之前并不让患者恢复平卧体位。随后,Morillo等[17]提出了低剂量异丙肾上腺素倾斜试验的方案,即15min的基础倾斜之后,不让患者恢复平卧体位而直接逐渐增加异丙肾上腺素输注的剂量(1~3μg/min)。这个方案的阳性反应率为61%,特异性为93%。后一种方案在北美流行了多年,至今仍被广泛应用。

1994年,Raviele等[18]建议以静脉输注硝酸甘油并逐渐增加剂量的方式取代异丙肾上腺素进行激发倾斜试验。采用这种方案,40例不明原因晕厥患者中21例(53%)出现阳性反应,特异性是92%;40例患者中10例(25%)出现不伴心动过缓的进行性低血压。后一种表现被认为不是血管迷走性反应,是药物所致的低血压,而被定义为"过度(exaggerated)"反应。后来,Raviele等[19]采用舌下含服硝酸甘油代替了静脉输注的方法。在基础倾斜45min后,让患者舌下含服硝酸甘油0.3mg。采用这种方案,不明原因晕厥患者的总阳性反应率为51%(基础倾斜试验为25%,给予硝酸甘油后为26%),特异性为94%。硝酸甘油造成的低血压"过度"反应占患者的14%,而占对照个体的15%。

Oraii等[20]比较了异丙肾上腺素激发试验与硝酸甘油激发试验。两种方案的阳性反应率和特异性大致相同,但是硝酸甘油的不良反应发生率较低。硝酸甘油组的敏感性和特异性分别为55%和94.7%,而异丙肾上腺素组分别为58%和89.4%。由于75%的病例反应不一致,如果患者为阴性反应,顺序应用不同的激发试验可以使敏感性增加到84%,而特异性仅有轻度降低(84%)。

给予硝酸甘油舌下含服之前的非药物阶段的最佳时间目前尚未完全确定。Bartoletti等[21]比较非药物阶段分别为45min与5min的效果。他们发现被动倾斜阶段较短的阳性反应率明显降低。根据这个观察结果,似乎被动的无药物激发的基础直立倾斜试验至少需要15~20min。

新近,许多作者采用缩短的直立倾斜试验方案,即在20min的基础倾斜之后给予患者硝酸甘油400μg舌下喷服。其汇集了来自3个采用这种方案的研究数据[22-24],共包含304位患者,阳性率为69%。此阳性反应率与其他3项研究[19,21,25]对169例患者观察的阳性率为62%的结果相似,后者采用的方案是被动倾斜45min之后再给予舌下喷硝酸甘油400μg。因此,我们似乎可以接受在给予硝酸甘油之前维持20min的被动阶段替代45min无药物激发的单纯的被动倾斜试验。

不论采用何种方案,进行倾斜试验时都需要执行一定的措施标准。这些建议发表在1996年的美国心脏病学会专家共识中[26],将在后文中进行总结(见"直立倾斜试验的操作方案")。

(三)直立倾斜试验的特异性:对健康个体的研究

倾斜试验在有症状的血管迷走性晕厥患者与无症状的对照个体之间似乎区别很大。最初研究中的健康个体数目很少($n<30$),结果显示对照组在60°~80°倾斜10~60min的过程中没有出现晕厥患者(阳性率)低于10%。此后的研究显示各个年龄组的基础倾斜和异丙肾上腺素激发倾斜的假阳性率都较低。

一项对202例不明原因晕厥患者的研究发现[22],在基础倾斜阶段(60°倾斜20min)有11%的患者出现倾斜诱发晕厥而对照组为3%，在舌下给予硝酸甘油0.4mg（400μg）之后59%的患者以及3%的对照个体出现晕厥。4%的患者和12%的对照个体出现假阳性反应（也称过度反应，见上文）。总阳性率为70%，特异性为94%。其他研究[27]报道的硝酸甘油激发试验的特异性与此类似。

最大规模的关于健康对照个体进行直立倾斜试验的研究结果由Natale等人[14]报道。150位既往没有晕厥及先兆晕厥病史的健康志愿者进行了直立倾斜试验，倾斜60°、70°及80°维持20min的特异性分别为92%、92%和80%[14]。在给予低剂量异丙肾上腺素使心率平均增快20%后，各组的特异性分别降至88%、88%和60%。低剂量（1.5±0.45μg/min）异丙肾上腺素对特异性的影响（4%）在临床中可以忽略。因此，在进行70°直立倾斜时给予低剂量异丙肾上腺素（1~2μg/min）就有望在保持较高的特异性（大约90%）的情况下提供有效性诊断率。然而，更高剂量的异丙肾上腺素会使试验的假阳性率增高而令人担心。如果以3μg/min和5μg/min的速度输注异丙肾上腺素，试验的假阳性率分别增加到20%和56%。

总体说来，这些特异性数值使倾斜试验在其他被广泛接受的类似的心血管诊断试验（例如用于诊断缺血性心脏病的运动负荷试验）中拥有一席之地。值得注意的是，不论是增加倾斜角度、延长倾斜时间或者使用更大剂量的异丙肾上腺素等激进的激发方法，在本质上都会降低倾斜试验的特异性[14,28]。

概而言之，绝大多数的研究表明在不使用药物激发的情况下角度为60°~70°倾斜试验的特异性大约为90%。由于没有明确的诊断"金标准"，敏感性更加难以评价。将来的研究可能会以"典型"的病史作为"金标准"而进行设计。目前，仅少数几个观察是以这种方式进行的，其结果提示试验的敏感性相当高。试验的特异性可能会因药物激发而降低，而另一方面试验的敏感性可能被提高。如果使用硝酸甘油或较低剂量的异丙肾上腺素，所造成的特异性轻度降低在临床中可以接受。

（四）药物激发试验

药物激发仍然是在基础无药物激发的倾斜试验未能明确诊断之后才采用，是直立倾斜试验中用来诱发低血压-心动过缓的第二个步骤。目前最常使用的药物是异丙肾上腺素和硝酸甘油。

尽管硝酸甘油的应用越来越广泛，但在北美，异丙肾上腺素是最常用的激发药物。异丙肾上腺素激发的根本机制尚不清楚，据推测是通过加强传入神经的活性和β肾上腺素受体介导的外周血管扩张而增强传感器的敏感性。我们已经讨论了几种不同的异丙肾上腺素的激发方法：（1）最初在患者处于仰卧位的情况下，给予剂量为1μg/min的异丙肾上腺素。随后继续输注药物，并使患者倾斜10min。如果需要增加异丙肾上腺素的剂量，则重复相同的步骤，每次增加1μg/min，直至3μg/min；（2）在仰卧位输注异丙肾上腺素10~15min，调整剂量使心率增加20%~30%。重复倾斜试验。这种方法日趋流行；（3）在未能诊断的基础倾斜试验结束时，让患者仍保持直立体位，静脉点滴或弹丸式注射异丙肾上腺素以缩短倾斜时间；（4）不进行无药物激发的被动倾斜试验，而直接进行异丙肾上腺素激发，在得到进一步证实之前不推荐采用这种方法。

人们对在倾斜试验中采用硝酸甘油作为激发药物越来越感兴趣。硝酸盐一般用于扩张静脉。然而，舌下含服硝酸异山梨醇酯可能不会明显增强下肢的静脉潴留作用[29]。硝酸甘油引起肾上腺素水平的升高可能参与了硝酸甘油激发机制。通过静脉以及舌下给予硝酸甘油都可以使倾斜试验阳性率加倍（从25%增加到50%），而保持较高的特异性（>90%）。舌下喷服硝酸甘油400μg的方案诱发晕厥平均需要5min（范围为2~9min）[21]。根据评估硝酸甘油激发倾斜试验的阳性预测值为80%，其敏感性和特异性大约分别为80%和85%。试验时间超过18min后才出现的阳性结果，其特异性降低，在进行分析时需要注意。

与低剂量（1.3±0.5μg/min）异丙肾上腺素相比，硝酸甘油激发试验的敏感性和特异性相似而不良反应发生率更低。舌下给予硝酸甘油的主要优势是不需要建立静脉通道并且节省时间。一些研究显示采用舌下喷服硝酸甘油的激发方案可以将基础倾斜试验的时间由45min减少到20min，而阳性反应率无明显降低（62%对69%）[24]。但是，无药物激发的基础倾斜试验不能完全由硝酸甘油激发试验所取代[21]。舌下给予硝酸异山梨醇酯和硝酸甘油一样，作为激发药物与异丙肾上腺素的敏感性相同。相反，至少有一篇报道提示许多无症状的老年人（60岁以上）出现硝酸甘油诱发的晕厥或先兆晕厥（基础试验的阳性率为9%，而激发后为52%）[30]。这样的调查结果使人们开始质疑在延长的直立倾斜试验之后舌下给予硝酸甘油进行激发试验（基础试验30~40min后再舌下给予硝酸甘油 400μg 并倾斜 15min) 对于诊断老年人的血管迷走性晕厥是否有效。

内源性腺苷的释放可能参与晕厥的触发机制[31]。血管迷走性晕厥时血浆的内源性腺苷水平增高，而且倾斜试验阳性患者的腺苷水平倾向于比试验阴性者高。腺苷与自主神经系统之间既存在直接的相互影响（通过心脏兴奋的传入神经进行），也存在间接的相互影响（通过血管扩张以及交感活动的反射作用进行）。据报道利用腺苷或三磷酸腺苷（ATP，一种腺苷的前体）可以显示患者是否容易罹患神经介导的阵发性房室阻滞，并被推荐作为可以应用的诱发药物[31-38]。然而，使用 ATP 诱发似乎可以鉴别出通常不属于神经介导性晕厥范畴的一个亚组的患者（倾向于老年人更常见），其特征是伴有阵发性房室阻滞或显著的窦性停搏或两者兼有[34,36-39]。因而，ATP 和异丙肾上腺素倾斜试验在诱发阳性反应中可能具有互补作用。

ATP 试验需要在心电图（ECG）监测下迅速地弹丸式注射 20mg ATP。如果停搏超过 6s 或房室阻滞超过 10s 即为异常。目前，多建议在倾斜试验即将结束而没有确定诊断时进行 ATP 试验。ATP 试验阳性的患者需要植入起搏器[36]。然而，当前美国和欧洲正在进行不同的临床研究评估 ATP 在评价晕厥中的确切作用。

其他用于诊断性倾斜试验的药物包括：硝酸异山梨醇酯[40,41]、腾喜龙（抗胆碱酯酶药）[42,43]以及肾上腺素[44]。肾上腺素复制患者症状的敏感性明显低于异丙肾上腺素[44]。其部分原因可能由于异丙肾上腺素对于 α 肾上腺素能受体的激活更强。腾喜龙给药更容易并且明显比异丙肾上腺素节省时间，而诊断作用类似[43]。

（五）直立倾斜试验结果的可重复性

人们通过在同一天内、数日内以及数周内进行多次试验的方法研究了倾斜试验的可重复性。总体看来，无论在同一天内还是在数天内，两次重复进行试验的结果一致性相对较高（约为 80%～85%）。然而，考虑到诱发低血压的病理生理过程（例如心脏抑制与血管减压的各自特征），其可重复性就不那么令人信服了。有趣的是，出现假阳性结果的倾斜试验可重复性也较差[45]。

我们实验室的数据表明，倾斜试验诱发的血管迷走性晕厥在短期内的可重复性对于一种作为诊断试验的方案来说是可以接受的[46]。采用 10min 角度为 80°的直立倾斜试验方案（必要时给予最大剂量 3μg/min 的异丙肾上腺素激发）87% 的病例结果一致。首次倾斜试验结果为阴性的 8 位患者在第二次倾斜时均未出现晕厥（一致性为 100%）。据报道，无论是否使用异丙肾上腺素，年轻患者进行倾斜试验（90°倾斜 15min）的近期可重复性较低（67%）。

倾斜试验在较长时间内的可重复性与近期可重复性相似（70%～80%）。有 21 位患者重复进行倾斜试验，试验的角度为 80°，时间为 30min，必要时再给予异丙肾上腺素激发，结果显示在间隔时间为 3～7d 的倾斜试验的可重复性为 90%[47]。不过其中有 5 例（24%）在两次试验中需要的异丙肾上腺素剂量不同。另一个研究中，46 位患者采用 80°倾斜 10min 以及必要时进行分阶段的异丙肾上腺素激发方案，间隔 1～6 周后重复试验，首次倾斜试验结果为阴性的患者的试验可重复性为 85%，而阳性者的可重复性为 90%[48]。

不明原因晕厥患者进行舌下给予硝酸甘油加强的直立倾斜试验的可重复性（间隔 1～28d）为 80%[25]。在两次试验结果均为阳性的患者中 80% 以上反应的模式相同。同一个体在不同试验中最低心率之间相关性好。然而不同试验中，症状出现的时间却不尽相符。据报道舌下给予硝酸甘油激发的直立倾斜试验（60°倾斜 20min）间隔 1 周的阳性试验的可重复性为 67%，阴性试验的可重复性为 94%[24]。

总体而言，不论在同一天还是一段时间以后重复试验，阳性倾斜试验在短期和中期内出现阳性反应的可重复性大致为 80%。阴性试验的短期和长期可重复性都很高。硝酸甘油或低剂量异丙肾上腺素的剂量对试验的可重复性没有显著影响。

（六）直立倾斜试验的风险和并发症

与直立倾斜试验有关的风险非常小[2]。在晕厥刚发生时就使患者迅速恢复平卧体位，通常足以防止进一步出现与意识丧失相关的不良后果，并能避免低血压时间过长可能伴发的合并症。很少需要进行复苏操作。然而，由于在倾斜过程中可能会突然出现晕厥和意识丧失，在倾斜之前必须进行适当的防护以避免跌倒。

曾有文献报告倾斜诱发的心脏停搏的最长时间为 73s。也有关于在缺血性心脏病或病态窦房结综合征患者中使用异丙肾上腺素激发而引起致命性室性心律失常的相关报道。但是，这些情况非常罕见。我们进行了 1000 例以上的倾斜研究，至今尚未遇到类似情况。目前还没有采用硝酸甘油激发出现并发症的公开报道。一些轻微的不良反应比较常见，例如异丙肾上腺素引起的心悸以及硝酸甘油引起的头痛。在阳性的倾斜试验过程中及结束后可以触发心房颤动。这是一种少见的并发症，与倾斜诱发的过度"迷走风暴"有关。这种心律失常通常是自我限制性并能够自行终止的。

四、直立倾斜试验的操作方案

明尼苏达大学目前所应用的倾斜方案见表88-2。1996年[26]美国心脏病学会（ACC）发表了专家共识报告，并由北美洲起搏电生理协会（NASPE）签署通过，其中详尽介绍了当时被广泛认可的实验室操作方案。随后欧洲心脏病协会（ESC）晕厥特别工作组[2]发表了一篇类似的但更为详细并且补充了更多的近期最新研究的推荐方案（表88-3）。（参见下文中关于实验室问题的完整讨论，其中包括适应证、操作程序以及证据等级。当然，ACC文件中所概述的实验室环境的一些总体特征依然是恰当的。）

表 88-2　明尼苏达大学的倾斜试验方案

患者准备
- 患者应当在空腹、清醒的状态下到电生理实验室检查。
- 对患者进行12导联的心电图（ECG）监测。
- 在局部麻醉下穿刺股动脉插入4F导管以监测血压。
- 动脉穿刺之后，在倾斜试验开始前让患者休息大约30min。
- 在患者休息的过程中，以50ml/h的速度为其输注生理盐水。

倾斜前操作

倾斜试验之前在患者维持仰卧位时需要进行3项操作：
- Valsalva操作
  - 患者经受2次Valsalva操作（40mmHg压力维持15s）。
  - 整个过程中需要监测心率和血压。
- 颈动脉窦按摩（CSM）*
  - 首先记录是否有颈动脉杂音。根据患者的病史和症状确定是否需要进行CSM。
  - 40岁以上的患者需要进行CSM。
  - 先纵向按摩一侧10s，休息3~5min后再按摩另一侧。
  - 重复整个CSM，计算最大反应数据的平均值。
  - 整个过程中需要监测心率和血压。
- 咳嗽试验
  - 指令患者咳嗽（连续迅速咳嗽2次，使收缩压≥200mmHg）。
  - 在咳嗽过程需要使用刻度为300mmHg的血压计来记录血压变化。

倾斜试验
- 基础倾斜（不用药物）：70°倾斜45min或至出现晕厥。
- 必要时，药物激发（腾喜龙、异丙肾上腺素或硝酸甘油）15min。

*颈动脉窦综合征的最常见类型是心脏抑制型反应。颈动脉窦按摩引起心脏停搏或阵发性房室阻滞时能够复制症状，即可以明确诊断。心脏停搏5s或收缩压下降30mmHg，但没有复制症状，则可能有关[49]。

表 88-3　欧洲心脏病协会推荐的倾斜试验方案

Ⅰ类
- 未进行静脉穿刺患者在倾斜前至少平卧5min，进行插管操作的患者至少平卧20min。
- 倾斜角度60°~70°。
- 被动倾斜阶段的最短时间为20min，最长时间为45min。
- 如果被动倾斜试验为阴性时，可以选择静脉给予异丙肾上腺素或舌下给予硝酸甘油进行激发试验。药物激发的时间为15~20min。
- 选用异丙肾上腺素激发时，需要逐渐增加剂量从1μg/min开始到最高3μg/min，使平均心率从基线水平大约增加20%到25%，给药时患者不需要恢复平卧位。
- 选用硝酸甘油激发时，在直立体位下给予固定剂量的400μg硝酸甘油舌下喷服。
- 试验终点的定义是诱发晕厥或者包括药物激发在内的既定倾斜时间结束。如果患者发生晕厥，则判定试验为阳性。

Ⅱ类
- 对于诱发先兆晕厥的判定仍存在分歧。

（一）实验室环境

实验室应当是安静、光线昏暗、温度适宜，并且尽可能消除安全隐患。在试验开始之前，患者应当仰卧位休息至少20min以上，特别是在进行静脉穿刺或有创监测（如静脉内通路、动脉管线）或两者兼有时。如果没有血管通路等操作时更短的休息时间（5~10min）就已足够。

试验前患者需要空腹2~3h。患者可以继续服用平时所服的药物如利尿剂、硝酸盐类及抗高血压药物等。但是，试验前需要停用β肾上腺素阻滞剂以及用来治疗血管迷走性晕厥的其他处方药物至少5个半衰期。

如果有静脉内通路，可根据空腹的小时数给予胃肠外液体补充。如果空腹时间较短（如<4h），则不需要补充液体。

（二）记录

需要持续记录三导联（或以上）同步心电图。最好使用侵入性尽可能小的逐搏式血压记录技术，如手指容积描记技术。如果没有手指容积描记设备，可以采用动脉内记录技术。用血压计来记录压力并不理想，因为可能在测量过程中干扰患者，其本身测量不够精确，并且不能随着每一次心脏搏动观察血压情况。

（三）倾斜台的设计

适宜的电动或手动倾斜台应当可以在10～15s内倾斜60°～90°，并且在试验过程中不会出现摇晃或者位置移动。绝大多数实验室采用的直立倾斜角度为70°。当试验完成或临床情况需要时，倾斜台能够迅速恢复到水平位置（10～15s）。应当对患者进行轻柔地防护以避免跌倒，此外还需要提供具有支撑作用的脚踏板。

（四）倾斜的角度

倾斜60°～80°所产生的生理作用类似，然而角度过低（如30°～45°）时由于引起的体位压力较小因而诊断率有可能会降低。目前被广泛接受的倾斜角度为70°。不应使倾斜角度超过80°。

（五）倾斜试验的时程

不同时期人们主张采用的倾斜试验时程变化范围较宽从（10～60min）。目前认为如果不使用药物激发时，在70°下倾斜试验的最长时间为45min可能最理想。

如果基础试验为阴性，可以使用药物激发以增强试验的敏感性并缩短倾斜的时间（但以降低特异性为代价）。

（六）试验管理

实验室内应当能够提供护理，在同一机构中可以有或没有与心血管运动试验检查室类似的技术支持。医师不必在现场，但要足够接近实验室，如果出现问题能够迅速到场。

（七）影响倾斜试验结果的因素

与临床实验室的环境、由静脉内或动脉插管引起的不适，或者两者兼有，或者先前较长时间的电生理操作有关的忧虑可能会影响倾斜试验的结果。基于同样的原因，在进行倾斜试验评估的同一段时间内不鼓励进行电生理检查。

五、利用倾斜试验预测治疗的效果

许多研究人员以及临床医生已越来越依赖倾斜试验来指导对血管迷走性晕厥患者的治疗决策。但是，用这种方法来确定对患者个体的最佳治疗方案仍然存在争论。很大程度上，这是因为试验的重复性具有可变性，而且关于实验室检查的特定结果与晕厥自主发作之间的联系还有不确定性（例如心脏抑制的程度与血管减压的作用）。

通过患者在随访过程中对治疗的临床反应业已检验了倾斜试验作为评价治疗效果的一种方法的用途。535例患者接受不同药物的治疗[50]，在平均18个月的随访期间91%患者中的倾斜阴性检查与非晕厥发作相关。这个研究的结果倾向于提示直立倾斜试验的结果可能会预测治疗的未来获益。虽然这种结果明显有利，但是由于大多数研究没有进行安慰剂或经验治疗对照，其分析价值有限。为数不多的几个设定安慰剂-对照的研究结果通常不能证实目前的治疗能够获益，倾斜试验的结果一般不具预测性。当前，我们不推荐单纯通过重复倾斜试验来评价治疗的有效性。

六、直立倾斜试验应用的建议

在ACC专家共识报告中已经讨论了倾斜试验的应用[26]。为了实践的目的，对倾斜试验的建议可以分为三类（表88-4）：

Ⅰ类：普遍同意进行倾斜试验。
Ⅱ类：是否进行倾斜试验仍有争议。
Ⅲ类：不建议进行倾斜试验。

从直立倾斜试验的前景来看，除表88-4中列出的应用之外，许多似乎与血管迷走性晕厥并没有关系的其他情况已经引发人们的兴趣。由于还需要更多的研究证实倾斜试验在这些方面的用途[50]，本文中仅进行简要的列举。

1. 不明原因的癫痫发作，神经学检查阴性。
2. 慢性疲劳综合征，直立倾斜试验可能有助于识别出患者中的一个亚组，他们将会受益于直接针对神经介导性疾病的治疗。
3. 反复发作的特发性眩晕，临床表现提示可能由神经介导性低血压-心动过缓引起。
4. 某些老年患者出现的反复短暂性缺血发作，如果临床表现提示由神经介导性因素引起并且经适当检查不能发现其原因。
5. 婴儿猝死综合征，数目有限的观察使我们产生这样一个观念，利用直立倾斜试验可能在婴儿猝死综合征幸存者中复制出严重的心动过缓发作。

此外，可以考虑让表现为不明原因晕厥而心电生理

检查无法得出结论的室内传导障碍或者心律失常患者进行直立倾斜试验检查。认真评价此类患者的临床表现会

表 88-4 倾斜试验的应用

Ⅰ类：普遍同意
A. 评估反复发作的晕厥，或者单次晕厥事件伴有身体损伤、机动车事故，或患者的职业或业余爱好具有"高度风险性"，并且可能由血管迷走性反应引起
  1. 无器质性心血管疾病病史或明显证据的患者，并且病史提示有血管迷走性反应的患者
  2. 有器质性心血管疾病病史，但病史提示其发作为血管迷走性反应的患者，以及通过适当检测未能明确引起晕厥的其他原因的患者
B. 对发作背景与上文 A 条所描述一样的不明原因晕厥患者进行评估
  1. 无器质性心血管疾病病史或明显证据的患者，并且血管迷走性晕厥可能是其潜在病因
  2. 伴有器质性心血管疾病，但通过适当的检测排除了引起晕厥的其他原因的患者
C. 已经证实晕厥与缓慢性心律失常有关的患者，如果起因是神经介导性的则可能影响治疗，需要进行进一步评估

Ⅱ类：意见有分歧
A. 鉴别痉挛性晕厥与癫痫
B. 反复的"近似晕厥"发作，推测为神经介导性起源
C. 评估无器质性心脏病证据的运动诱发性晕厥
D. 评估预防晕厥复发的预防性治疗的效果

Ⅲ类：通常不建议进行倾斜试验
A. 不伴身体损伤以及非高危环境下的单次晕厥发作，临床特点提示血管迷走性晕厥
B. 已经明确由其他特异性原因引起的晕厥，即使可能证实神经介导性因素参与晕厥的发作也不影响治疗计划

提示血管迷走机制可能促使晕厥的发作[51,52]。在这类患者中，心率的慢或快不足以引起晕厥的症状。但是，伴随对神经反射性晕厥的敏感可能削弱血管的代偿反应（特别是患者在直立体位下触发心律失常），而紧接着就会发生低血压。这种设想已经通过阵发性折返性心律失常[53]和心房颤动[54,55]得到说明，诸如严重的窦性心动过缓等某些心动过缓同样也可以说明[56]。

最后，倾斜台诱发的体位压力（独立于诱发血管迷走性晕厥）可以用于研究某些看起来在晕厥发作时存在着的原发性心律失常，但需要有辅助资料证明观察到的心律失常与晕厥症状有关联[57]。在这种情形下，倾斜台的体位压力可能产生这种所需要的诊断性关联，并能提供重要的洞察能力，进而有助于为这些患者提供更有效的治疗。

七、总 结

神经介导的反射性晕厥综合征，特别是血管迷走性晕厥，在全部晕厥患者中占相当大的比例（表 88-5）。被动的无药物激发的直立倾斜试验已经被证实是有效的、容易实施的、成本-效益比良好的识别患者对血管迷走性晕厥敏感性的检查。类似检查已经成为很多研究的课题，最终发展形成被广泛接受的试验方案。与许多普遍认可的其他诊断性的心血管检查（如运动试验及核素心肌显像）相比，这些方案具有较好的可重复性、敏感性、特异性以及阳性预测值。

硝酸甘油和低剂量（$1\sim2\mu g/min$）异丙肾上腺素已成为接受最广泛的在倾斜试验过程中联合应用的药物。使用这些药物可以在缩短试验时间的同时提高直立倾斜试验的诊断率，增进了其在临床中的应用。当然，试验的特异性也有轻微下降，这是不可避免的。

最后，在对神经介导的血管迷走性晕厥的发生机制的理解方面也已取得重要进展。关于这一点，直立倾斜试验作出了重要的贡献。终究是从这类试验中获得的深入理解将会促进我们进一步提高诊断水平，并且改善对已受严重影响患者的治疗。

八、致 谢

作者对 Wendy Markuson 以及 Barry L. S. Detloff 在本文撰写准备工作中给予的协助表示谢意。

表 88-5 神经介导性晕厥综合征

血管迷走性晕厥（普通型或情绪性晕厥）
颈动脉窦性晕厥
情景性晕厥（situational syncope）
• 排尿或排尿后晕厥
• 航空刺激诱发的晕厥
• 咳嗽或喷嚏性晕厥
• 胃肠道刺激诱发的晕厥
  • 吞咽性晕厥
  • 排便性晕厥
• 胸腔内压力增加诱发的晕厥
  • 吹奏喇叭
  • 举重
• 舌咽或三叉神经痛
复合性（miscellaneous）晕厥
• 进餐后晕厥
• 与主动脉狭窄有关的晕厥
• 某些快速性心律失常（如房颤、PSVT 以及部分室性心动过速）发作时伴发的晕厥

（王立群 译）

参 考 文 献

1. Kenny RA, Ingram A, Bayliss J, Sutton R: Head-up tilt: A useful test for investigating unexplained syncope. Lancet 1:1352–1355, 1986.
2. Brignole M, Alboni P, Benditt D, et al: Guidelines on management (diagnosis and treatment) of syncope. Eur Heart J 22:1256–1306, 2001.
3. Smit AA, Halliwill JR, Low PA, Wieling W: Pathophysiological basis of orthostatic hypotension in autonomic failure. J Physiol 519:1–10, 1999.
4. Robertson RM, Medina E, Shah N, et al: Neurally mediated syncope: Pathophysiology and implications for treatment. Am J Med Sci 317:102–109, 1999.
5. Schondorf R, Wieling W: Vasoconstrictor reserve in neurally mediated syncope. Clin Auton Res 10:53–55, 2000.
6. Benditt DG, Lurie KG, Adler SW, et al: Pathophysiology of vasovagal syncope. In Blanc JJ, Benditt DG, Sutton R (eds): Neurally Mediated Syncope: Pathophysiology, Investigataon, and Treatment. Armonk, NY: Futura Publishing Company, 1996, pp 1–24.
7. Benditt DG: Neurally mediated syncopal syndromes: Pathophysiological concepts and clinical evaluation. PACE 20:572–584, 1997.
8. Grubb BP, Gerard G, Roush K, et al: Cerebral vasoconstriction during head-upright tilt-induced vasovagal syncope. A paradoxic and unexpected response. Circulation 84:1157–1164, 1991.
9. Grubb BP, Samoil D, Kosinski D, et al: Cerebral syncope: Loss of consciousness associated with cerebral vasoconstriction in the absence of systemic hypotension. PACE 21:652–658, 1998.
10. Sutton R, Petersen M, Brignole M, et al: Proposed classification for tilt induced vasovagal syncope. Eur J Cardiac Pacing Electrophysiol 3:180–118, 1992.
11. Brignole M, Menozzi C, Del Rosso A, et al: New classification of haemodynamics of vasovagal syncope: Beyond the VASIS classification. Analysis of the pre-syncopal phase of the tilt test without and with nitroglycerin challenge. Vasovagal Syncope International Study. Europace 2:66–76, 2000.
12. Fitzpatrick AP, Theodorakis G, Vardas P, Sutton R: Methodology of head-up tilt testing in patients with unexplained syncope. J Am Coll Cardiol 17:125–130, 1991.
13. Almquist A, Goldenberg IF, Milstein S, et al: Provocation of bradycardia and hypotension by isoproterenol and upright posture in patients with unexplained syncope. N Engl J Med 320:346–351, 1989.
14. Natale A, Akhtar M, Jazayeri M, et al: Provocation of hypotension during head-up tilt testing in subjects with no history of syncope or presyncope. Circulation 92:54–58, 1995.
15. Waxman MB, Yao L, Cameron DA, et al: Isoproterenol induction of vasodepressor-type reaction in vasodepressor-prone persons. Am J Cardiol 63:58–65, 1989.
16. Kapoor WN, Brant N: Evaluation of syncope by upright tilt testing with isoproterenol. A nonspecific test. Ann Intern Med 116:358–363, 1992.
17. Morillo CA, Klein GJ, Zandri S, Yee R: Diagnostic accuracy of a low-dose isoproterenol head-up tilt protocol. Am Heart J 129:901–906, 1995.
18. Raviele A, Gasparini G, Di Pede F, et al: Nitroglycerin infusion during upright tilt: A new test for the diagnosis of vasovagal syncope. Am Heart J 127:103–111, 1994.
19. Raviele A, Menozzi C, Brignole M, et al: Value of head-up tilt testing potentiated with sublingual nitroglycerin to assess the origin of unexplained syncope. Am J Cardiol 76:267–272, 1995.
20. Oraii S, Maleki M, Minooii M, Kafaii P: Comparing two different protocols for tilt table testing: Sublingual glyceryl trinitrate versus isoprenaline infusion. Heart 81:603–605, 1999.
21. Bartoletti A, Gaggioli G, Menozzi C, et al: Head-up tilt testing potentiated with oral nitroglycerin: A randomized trial of the contribution of a drug-free phase and a nitroglycerin phase in the diagnosis of neurally mediated syncope. Europace 1:183–186, 1999.
22. Del Rosso A, Bartoletti A, Bartoletti P, et al: Shortened head-up tilt testing potentiated with sublingual nitroglycerin in patients with unexplained syncope. Am Heart J 135:564–570, 1998.
23. Natale A, Sra J, Akhtar M, et al: Use of sublingual nitroglycerin during head-up tilt-table testing in patients >60 years of age. Am J Cardiol 82:1210–1213, 1998.
24. Del Rosso A, Bartoletti A, Bartoli P, et al: Methodology of head-up tilt testing potentiated with sublingual nitroglycerin in unexplained syncope. Am J Cardiol 85:1007–1011, 2000.
25. Foglia-Manzillo G, Giada F, Beretta S, et al: Reproducibility of head-up tilt testing potentiated with sublingual nitroglycerin in patients with unexplained syncope. Am J Cardiol 84:284–288, 1999.
26. Benditt DG, Ferguson DW, Grubb BP, et al: Tilt table testing for assessing syncope. American College of Cardiology. J Am Coll Cardiol 28:263–275, 1996.
27. Mussi C, Tolve I, Foroni M, et al: Specificity and total positive rate of head-up tilt testing potentiated with sublingual nitroglycerin in older patients with unexplained syncope. Aging (Milano) 13:105–111, 2001.
28. Carlioz R, Graux P, Haye J, et al: Prospective evaluation of high-dose or low-dose isoproterenol upright tilt protocol for unexplained syncope in young adults. Am Heart J 133:346–352, 1997.
29. Koole MA, Aerts A, Praet J, et al: Venous pooling during nitrate-stimulated tilt testing in patients with vasovagal syncope. Europace 2:343–345, 2000.
30. Kumar NP, Youde JH, Ruse C, et al: Responses to the prolonged head-up tilt followed by sublingual nitrate provocation in asymptomatic older adults. Age Ageing 29:419–424, 2000.
31. Sinkovec M, Grad A, Rakovec P: Role of endogenous adenosine in vasovagal syncope. Clin Auton Res 11:155–161, 2001.
32. Shen WK, Hammill SC, Munger TM, et al: Adenosine: Potential modulator for vasovagal syncope. J Am Coll Cardiol 28:146–154, 1996.
33. Mittal S, Stein KM, Markowitz SM, et al: Induction of neurally mediated syncope with adenosine. Circulation 99:1318–1324, 1999.
34. Brignole M, Menozzi C, Alboni P, et al: The effect of exogenous adenosine in patients with neurally-mediated syncope and sick sinus syndrome. PACE 17:2211–2216, 1994.
35. Brignole M, Gaggioli G, Menozzi C, et al: Adenosine-induced atrioventricular block in patients with unexplained syncope: The diagnostic value of ATP testing. Circulation 96:3921–3927, 1997.
36. Flammang D, Church T, Waynberger M, et al: Can adenosine 5'-triphosphate be used to select treatment in severe vasovagal syndrome? Circulation 96:1201–1208, 1997.
37. Flammang D, Chassing A, Donal E, et al: Reproducibility of the adenosine-5'-triphosphate test in vasovagal syndrome. J Cardiovasc Electrophysiol 9:1161–1166, 1998.
38. Flammang D, Erickson M, McCarville S, et al: Contribution of head-up tilt testing and ATP testing in assessing the mechanisms of vasovagal syndrome: Preliminary results and potential therapeutic implications. Circulation 99:2427–2433, 1999.
39. Brignole M, Gaggioli G, Menozzi C, et al: Clinical features of adenosine sensitive syncope and tilt induced vasovagal syncope. Heart 2000; 83:24-8.
40. Ammirati F, Colivicchi F, Biffi A, et al: Head-up tilt testing potentiated with low-dose sublingual isosorbide dinitrate: A simplified time-saving approach for the evaluation of unexplained syncope. Am Heart J 135:671–676, 1998.
41. Zeng C, Zhu Z, Hu W, et al: Value of sublingual isosorbide dinitrate before isoproterenol tilt test for diagnosis of neurally mediated syncope. Am J Cardiol 83:1059–1063, 1999.
42. Lurie KG, Dutton J, Mangat R, et al: Evaluation of edrophonium as a provocative agent for vasovagal syncope during head-up tilt-table testing. Am J Cardiol 72:1286–1290, 1993.
43. Voice RA, Lurie KG, Sakaguchi S, et al: Comparison of tilt angles and provocative agents (edrophonium and isoproterenol) to improve head-upright tilt-table testing. Am J Cardiol 81:346–351, 1998.
44. Calkins H, Kadish A, Sousa J, et al: Comparison of responses to isoproterenol and epinephrine during head-up tilt in suspected vasodepressor syncope. Am J Cardiol 67:207–209, 1991.
45. Sumiyoshi M, Mineda Y, Kojima S, et al: Poor reproducibility of false-positive tilt testing results in healthy volunteers. Jpn Heart J 40:71–78, 1999.
46. Chen MY, Goldenberg IF, Milstein S, et al: Cardiac electrophysiologic and hemodynamic correlates of neurally mediated syncope. Am J Cardiol 63:66–72, 1989.
47. Grubb BP, Wolfe D, Temesy-Armos P, et al: Reproducibility of head upright tilt table test results in patients with syncope. PACE 15:1477–1481, 1992.
48. Sheldon R, Splawinski J, Killam S: Reproducibility of isoproterenol

tilt-table tests in patients with syncope. Am J Cardiol 69:1300–1305, 1992.
49. Benditt DG: Syncope. In Topol EJ (ed): Comprehensive Cardiovascular Medicine. Philadelphia, Lippincott-Raven Publishers, 1998, pp 2027–2051.
50. Benditt DG: Head-up tilt table testing: Rationale, methodology, and application. In Zipes DP, Jalife J (eds): Cardiac Electrophysiology: From Cell to Bedside. Philadelphia, WB Saunders Company, 2000, pp 746–753.
51. Sagrista-Sauleda J, Romero B, Permanyer-Miralda G, et al: Clinical usefulness of head-up tilt test in patients with syncope and intraventricular conduction defect. Europace 1:63–68, 1999.
52. Shinohara M, Kobayashi Y, Obara C, et al: Neurally mediated syncope and arrhythmias: A study of syncopal patients using the head-up tilt test. Jpn Circ J 63:339–342, 1999.
53. Leitch JW, Klein GJ, Yee R, et al: Syncope associated with supraventricular tachycardia. An expression of tachycardia rate or vasomotor response? Circulation 85:1064–1071, 1992.
54. Leitch J, Klein G, Tee R, et al: Neurally mediated syncope and atrial fibrillation. N Engl J Med 324:495–496, 1991.
55. Brignole M, Gianfranchi L, Menozzi C, et al: Role of autonomic reflexes in syncope associated with paroxysmal atrial fibrillation. J Am Coll Cardiol 22:1123–1129, 1993.
56. Brignole M, Menozzi C, Gianfranchi L, et al: Neurally mediated syncope detected by carotid sinus massage and head-up tilt test in sick sinus syndrome. Am J Cardiol 68:1032–1036, 1991.
57. Hammill SC, Holmes DR Jr, Wood DL, et al: Electrophysiologic testing in the upright position: Improved evaluation of patients with rhythm disturbances using a tilt table. J Am Coll Cardiol 4:65–71, 1984.

第 89 章

心率变异性与压力反射敏感性

Marek Malik

本章目录
■ 心率变异性的测定 …………… 809
■ 压力反射敏感性的评估 ………… 812
■ 心率变异性的生理学解释 ……… 813
■ 临床应用 ……………………… 814

最初提出缺乏呼吸性心律失常可能具有临床意义的文献发表于 25 年前[1]。此后，人们对有关自律性规律、调节作用以及心动周期的生理性变异等题目进行了广泛的研究。目前，心率变异性（heart rate variability，HRV）以及压力反射敏感性（baroreflex sensitivity，BRS）被确立为评估心脏自主神经状态的工具[2,3]。

一、心率变异性的测定

尽管心率变异性一词意味着被测定的是心率的变化性，但在大多数情况下研究的是每个心动周期的变化性。由于心率与心动周期之间为非线性的倒数关系，一些从心动周期衍生出的复杂的 HRV 测定值（例如频谱组成部分的比例）与从心率采样衍生出的测定值并不平行。本文中的 HRV 仅指心动周期的变异性。

（一）心电图处理

通过测定每一个 RR 间期，就可以根据任何一份记录时间足够长的心电图（ECG）来评估 HRV。但是：(1) 心电图的信号噪声比应当达到能够确切地识别全部 QRS 波群的要求；(2) 对心电图信号的数字采样必须规则而且足够稳定从而能够确定每个 QRS 波群的基点；(3) 应当对全部 QRS 波群的形态及节律特点进行分类，从而能够区分窦性节律与其他起源的搏动；(4) 只对正常窦性节律下的心搏 RR 间期（也称为正常-正常或 NN 间期）进行分析。可以通过许多不同的方法对 NN 间期序列进行分析。对于评价 HRV 来说，通常以时域（time-domain）、频域（frequency-domain）以及非线性方法最为杰出。

（二）时域方法

时域方法是将 NN 间期序列作为一组无序的间期（或间期对）并采用不同的方法来表示这类数据的方差（variance）。已经有大量方法被推荐用来评价 NN 间期数据的方差及其替代参数。因为这些方法中有许多结果实际上是等同的，被选择的只有那些已经被推荐为"金标准"的时域方法[2]。包括 3 种以标准差（standard deviation）公式为基础的统计学方法，并且用时间单位来表示其结果。

SDNN 测算的是全部 NN 间期的标准差；SDANN 是将原始心电图进行分段（每段之间相互没有交叉重叠），然后计算出所有各段平均 NN 间期的标准差（尽管可以考虑不同的时间分段方法，但目前的标准方法是以 5min 进行分段计算的）；RMSSD 计算的是相邻的 NN 间期差值的均方根（即相邻 NN 间期之间差值的标准差的替代参数）。RMSSD 实际上与通常所应用的 pNN50 等同，后者是指与其前紧邻的 NN 间期差值大于 50ms 的 NN 间期个数所占的比例[2]。SDNN 和 RMSSD 方法可以用于任何实际记录的心电图，而 SDANN 方法通常仅用于长时间（如

24h）的心电图记录。心电图记录的时间长度是 HRV 的重要决定因素。随着心电图记录时间的增加，SDNN 和 RMSSD 值增加（SDANN 也同样）。根据记录时间长度不同的心电图计算出的 HRV 之间不能进行比较。

统计学方法对 NN 间期数据质量的依赖性非常强。心电图记录时间较短时，获取高质量的 NN 间期数据并不难，这种情况下可以通过人工观察来验证对每次搏动的自动分析。但是，对于如何保证从长时间记录的心电图中获取高质量的 NN 间期序列，常常还存在着疑问。当对这样的长时间记录仅是偶尔进行分析时，通过统计学方法提供的 HRV 数值其实质往往并不正确。

为了克服这个困难，人们提出采用几何学的方法来评价 HRV。这些方法利用 NN 间期序列构建一个几何图形并通过一个参数或图形的形状表示 HRV。由于错误的 NN 间期序列通常会落在几何图形的轮廓之外，它们可以被轻易剔除。HRV 三角指数（triangular index）在这方面的经验最丰富。HRV 三角指数构建了全部 NN 间期的样本密度直方图，并根据计算 NN 间期的总数（即直方图的"面积"）与间期的众数时间（modal duration）的数目（即直方图的"高度"）之间的比值来估算基线宽度（为 NN 间期标准差的一个替代参数）。这种方法对于构建直方图的横坐标时间单位的依赖非常强。当采用的时间单位为 1/128s（≈7.8ms）时，与通常的模拟型 Holter 设备所采用的采样率一致，并且用于编辑适当的 NN 间期序列时，此方法获得的结果与 SDNN 的一致性相当好（HRV 三角指数的 1 个单位＝SDNN 的 2.5ms）。

（三）频域方法

功率频谱密度的分析可以提供功率（即方差）作为一个频率的函数是如何分布的基本信息。与采用的方法无关，能够获取的只有一个确定的信号真实频谱密度。

用于计算功率频谱密度的方法总体可以分为非参数法和参数法两类。绝大多数情况下，两种方法的结果类似。非参数法的优点是应用的算法简单（多数采用快速傅立叶转换）并且处理速度快；参数法的优点是频谱成分更加光滑并能够不受预选频率带的约束而被识别，利用对低频和高频功率成分的自动计算使频谱后处理简便，容易识别每一种成分的中心频率，假定信号保持稳定时即使样本数目少也能准确评估功率频谱密度。参数法的基本缺点是需要检验所选择的模型及其命令是否适宜。

根据 2min 以上的短时记录所计算出的频谱可以识别出 3 种主要的频谱成分[4,5]。它们分别为极低频（very-low-frequency，VLF）成分（＜0.04Hz）、低频（low-frequency，LF）成分（0.04～0.15Hz）和高频（high-frequency，HF）成分（0.15～0.4Hz）。功率的分布以及 LF 和 HF 成分的中心频率不是固定的，但是其变化与心脏周期中的自主神经调节改变有关。没有共同的特性并且受到基线算法或趋势消除影响的非和谐成分，通常被认为是 VLF 的主要构成成分。因而利用短时记录所评估得出的 VLF 成分令人置疑。VLF、LF 以及 HF 功率成分通常用功率的绝对值（ms^2）进行计量。LF 和 HF 成分也可以用标化单位（normalized units）进行计量[5]，其代表每种功率与总功率减去 VLF 成分的差值之比的相对值。推荐采用标化单位表示 LF 和 HF 成分是为了强调自主神经系统两个分支的平衡行为。这种标准化也倾向于最大限度地减少总功率值的变化对 LF 和 HF 数值的影响。

谱分析也被用于分析完整的 24h 内的 NN 间期序列。其结果在 VLF、LF 及 HF 成分的基础上还包括超低频（ultra-low-frequency，ULF）成分（＜0.0033Hz）。也可以通过绘制对数-对数比例的坐标图，使频谱数值拟合线性规律以评估 24h 频谱的斜率。对于长程记录而言，必须认真考虑信号的稳定性问题。如果在记录的整个过程中负责心脏周期性调节机制按照某种频率始终不变，可以利用 HRV 中相应的频率成分来测定这些调节功能。如果调节不稳定，对于频率分析结果的解释就不好定义了。特别是，影响 LF 和 HF 功率成分的心脏周期性调节的生理学机制在 24h 内不能被认为是稳定的。因而，根据整个 24h 记录进行的谱分析与根据在 24h 基础上平均计算的较短片段所获得的频谱结果一样，提供的是引起 LF 和 HF 成分变化的平均调节作用。这样的平均值使本来通过更短的时间记录就能得到的关于 RR 间期自动调节的详细信息变得模糊不清。

一般而论，HRV 的频谱成分提供了对自主神经调节程度的测量方法，但不是测量自主神经张力水平。特别是调节的平均值并不代表神经张力的平均水平。

（四）非线性分析

在 HRV 的起源中必然包含着非线性现象。它们是由血流动力学、电生理学以及体液变化之间复杂的相互作用所决定的，同样也受到自主神经和中枢神经系统的调节。傅立叶谱分析的 $1/f$ 计算法、H 等级指数以及粗粒化谱分析已经被用来测量非线性 HRV 特性的参数。庞加莱截面（Poincaré sections）、低维吸引子散点图（low-dimension attractor plots）、奇异值分解（singular value decomposition）以及吸引子轨迹（attractor trajectories）也被推荐用于进行描述。其他被用来定量描述数据的有 D_2 关联维数、Lyapunov 指数、Kolmogorov 熵等[6]。

庞加莱散点图（Poincaré plots，译者注：又称洛伦兹散点图 Lorenz plots），它是反映相邻 NN 间期对的坐标关系的点图，由于推测它可能使对这些散点的分类简化而在一些临床研究人员中引起一定程度的关注。一部分作者提议根据散点呈现的"鱼雷状"、"雪茄状"、"彗星状"及"蝴蝶状"的图形种类进行分类。然而，这种分类方法的主观性比较强，并且从未经过真正的前瞻性盲法研究证实。因此，在实践中庞加莱散点图主要用于评价 NN 间期序列的质量。这些散点图通常可以使坏点和干扰显示得很清楚（图 89-1）。

（五）心率变异性分析的最佳方式

由于被分析的心电图的记录时间长短以及在何种条件下获得的记录等缘故，HRV 的评估特别需要标准化。时域方法可供测量的数值的数目随着记录的时间而增加，而生理学与 LF 及 HF 频谱间的关联依赖于基础自主神经调节的稳定性。因此两种主要方案可以说是泾渭分明。

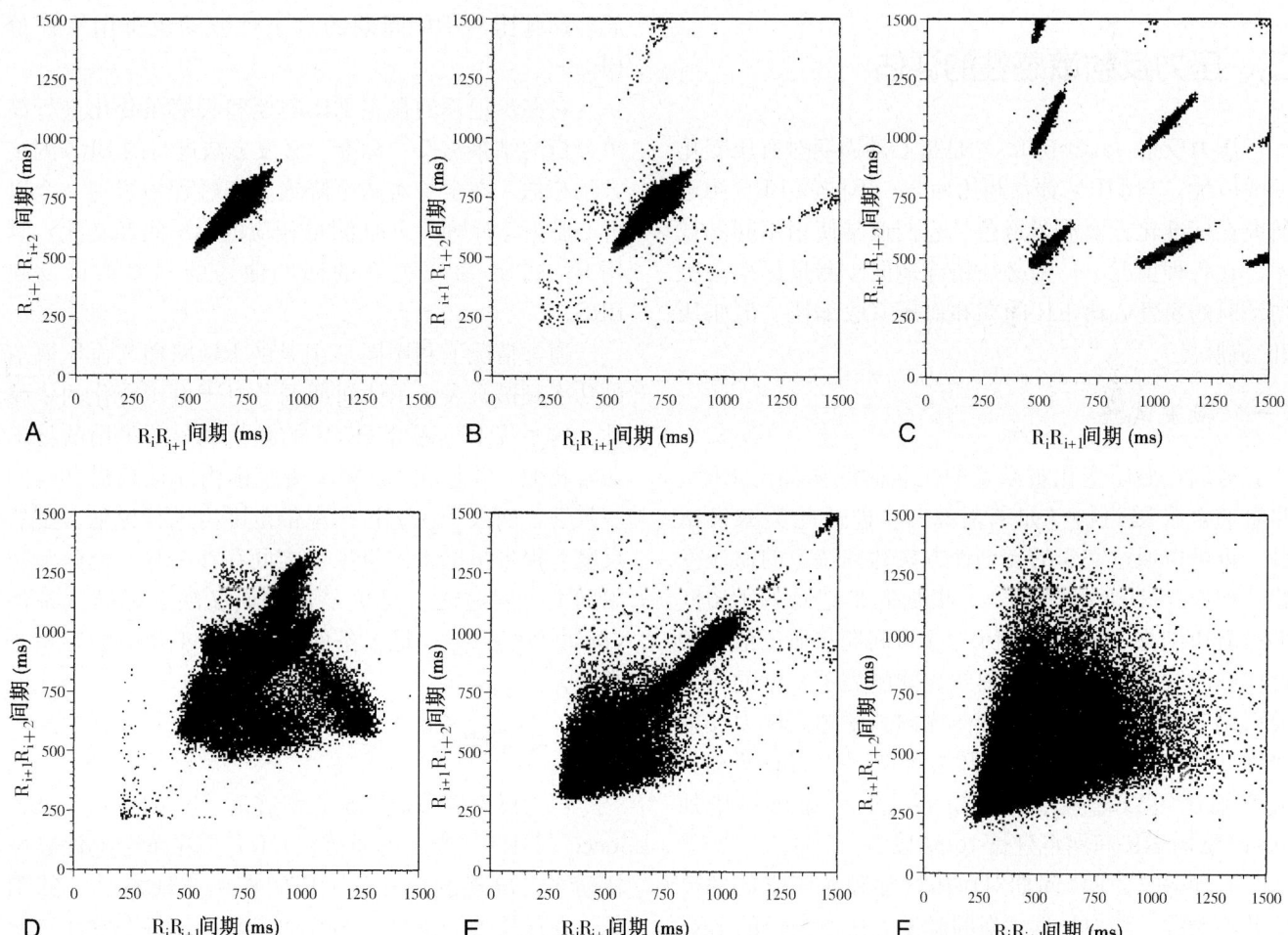

图 89-1　庞加莱散点图（图中显示的散点是分别以 R_iR_{i+1} 与 $R_{i+1}R_{i+2}$ 间期作为横纵坐标而绘制）用来评估 24h 记录中正常-正常 RR 间期序列的质量　A：编辑适当的 RR 间期序列的图形。B：未去除由于干扰和 Holter 识别错误所造成的坏点的同一 RR 间期序列的图形。C：自动系统未能识别出一部分 QRS 波群时所生成的图形，某些 RR 间期测量值实际上是由两个或更多个心动周期所组成。D：根据 Holter 系统对没有锁相时间磁道的磁带记录进行分析所生成的图形；由于磁带绕转的不规则使测量的 RR 间期被扭曲。E：根据伴有阵发性心房颤动发作的 Holter 磁带绘制的图形。F：慢性心房颤动的图形

心脏自主神经状态的生理学研究细节最好通过对较短时间（5min 更为适宜）的谱分析进行，并在稳定状态下记录心电图，即调节心率的生理过程应当保持在一种平稳的状态。相反，对周围环境的自主"应答性"的最佳评估是以 24h 的心电图记录为基础的，通常规定至少包含 18h 可以进行分析的白天和夜晚心电图。这些长时间的记录应当通过时域和/或非线性方法被更好地分析。尽管通过长时间心电图记录所获得的 NN 间期序列也可以利用频域方法进行处理，但其内在的调节机制并不能在长时间段内保持稳定不变。

两种情形下记录的条件都会明显地影响心率调节机制，因此应当对其认真加以控制和/或监测。例如，将卧位和立位混杂的情况下得到的短程记录中 HRV 频谱成分进行比较就不恰当。同样，将住院患者与那些行动完全自由的个体的 24h HRV 测量值进行比较也不恰当。

二、压力反射敏感性的评估

压力反射（baroreflex）是指心动周期对血压变化的适应性。与 HRV 评估相比而言，不同的 BRS 测定研究在标准化方面略显逊色，它们通常使用不同的技术。在各种情况下，都必须精确地同步测量逐次心脏搏动时的窦性心律 RR 间期和血压（收缩压、舒张压和/或脉压）。

（一）激发试验

可以在血压变化被激发的短暂时间内测定 BRS。尽管通常采用药物（如苯福林[7]）进行此类激发试验，也可以通过完全的无创性方法达到特定的血压变化（例如 Valsalva 手法）[8]。根据同步记录的 RR 间期与血压结果，BRS 可表示为 RR 间期与血压值相关性回归曲线的斜率。回归曲线越陡峭提示心率的压力反射调节越强，因而，回归曲线的斜率越大压力反射越强（图 89-2）。正常人静脉给予 25~100μg 苯福林后收缩压可以增强 20mmHg 以上，而血压每增加 1mmHg 时 RR 间期将延长 10ms 以上。

有趣的是，RR 间期对血压增加和血压降低的反应并不对称，相应根据这样的激发方法所测定的 BRS 值本质上就不同。

（二）颈部气室（neck chamber）

颈部气室装置可以通过在颈部局部增加气体压力或抽吸气体而使颈动脉压力感受器激活和/或失活[9]。增加颈部周围压力可使压力感受器感知为动脉压力降低，进而刺激血压增高。由于临床实践中的各种原因，颈部气室抽吸是一种更为理想的刺激方法，因为这样可能使患者更容易接受。

尽管有可能在颈部进行抽吸时对血压和 RR 间期进行同步谱分析，但更常采用在几次重复给予负压过程中延长最大的 RR 间期进行 BRS 量化分析。反应的强度、高度依赖于对不同个体进行抽吸的时间及重复的频率，在每个研究中这些都必须进行标准化。已报道的方案各不相同，抽吸压 5~40mmHg，时间则从单个心搏到 10s 不等。

（三）频谱相关性（spectral coherence）

压力反射不仅对血压的突然变化发生应答，并且主要的是对动脉收缩压的生理性改变进行应答。因此，动脉压与 RR 间期的自主性波动也可用来评价 BRS。

对同步记录的自主 RR 间期和收缩压变化进行简单分析的结果与按"标准"激发方法进行的 BRS 测定大致相似。在全身血压下降或升高过程中识别 3 个以上心脏搏动序列，并且测量相应的 RR 间期变化，利用 RR 间期/血压关系的回归曲线的斜率即可反映 BRS。

通常情况下利用同步记录的 RR 间期与血压调节的功率频谱来表示 RR 间期调节对于血压变化的依赖性。这个技术与评价 HRV 的频谱成分所采用的技术非常相似，并且在 LF 频率带范围内评估频谱之间的一致性，而很少在 HF 频率带范围内进行评估。虽然反复有报告指出不同组患者之间存在差异，但此项技术的主要问题之一是重复性差而又缺乏标准化条件（例如呼吸频率）。记录条件的差异对于结果的影响非常大[10]。

（四）心率震荡

压力反射调节似乎是心率震荡（heart rate turbulence, HRT）产生的原因。HRT 是在单个室性异位搏动之后出现的特殊的 RR 间期调节现象[11]。特别是，在保持着心脏自主调节的患者中，每个室性早搏都跟随着 RR 间期明显缩短（异位搏动之后的最初 2~4 个心动周期）和随后的 RR 间期逐渐延长（异位搏动之后的 5~20 个心动周期）。最初的 RR 间期缩短被描述为"震荡开始"（turbulence onset），它将异位

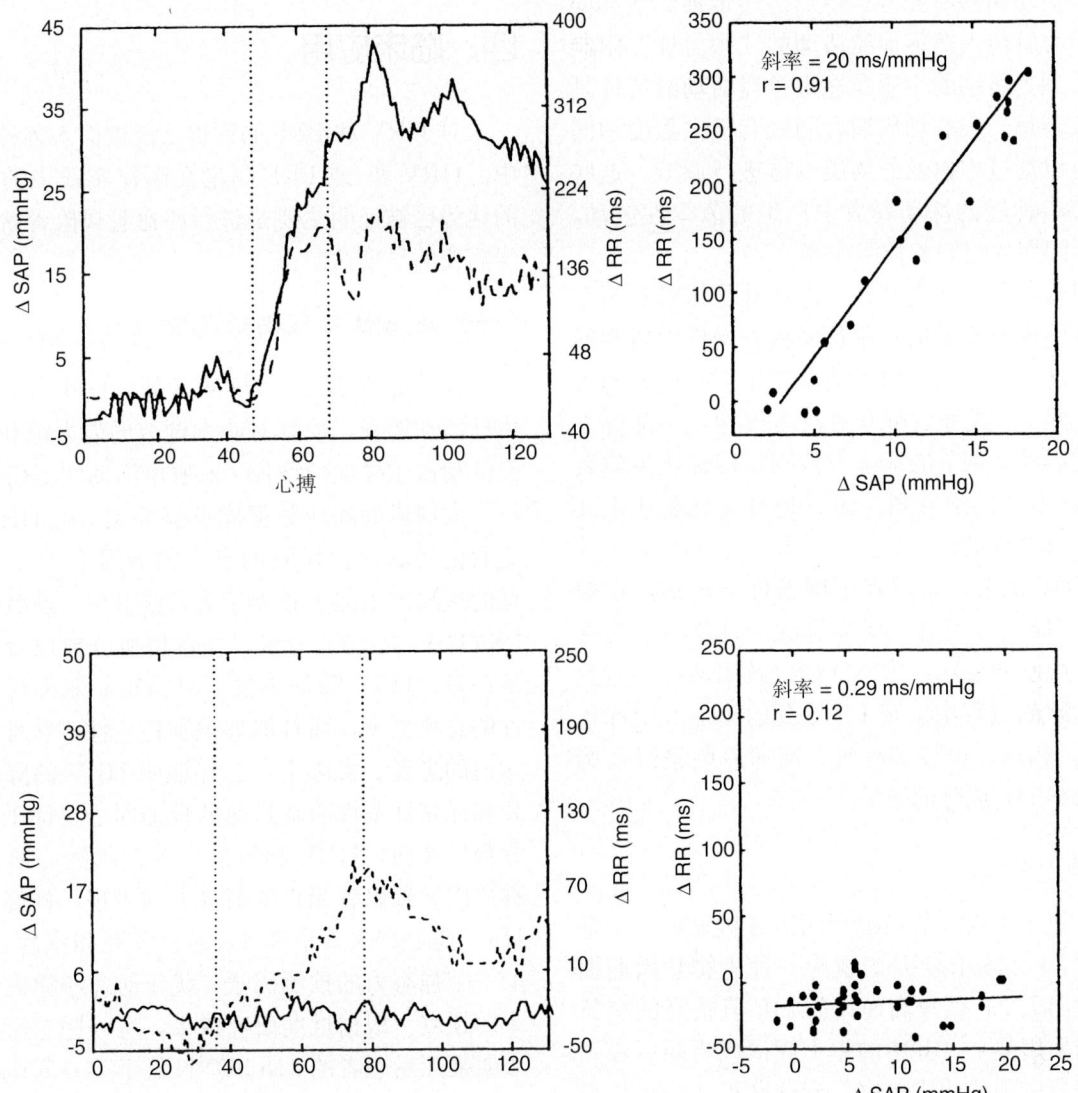

图 89-2 应用苯福林后测定压力反射敏感性的示例 左栏，收缩压（SAP）（虚曲线）以及 RR 间期（实曲线）随每次心脏搏动的变化情况。图中参照基线的数值来显示变化情况。仅对动脉收缩压出现的第一次明显升高（虚线之间的区域）进行分析。从这个区域看，与 ΔSAP 和 ΔRR 值相应的点被用来构建右栏中所显示的回归曲线斜率。上面的一组图形所示为 BRS 正常个体的记录情况；下面的一组图形所示为一位重度充血性心力衰竭患者较差的 BRS。(摘自 La Rovere MT，Pinna GD，M 顺向型房室折返性心动过速 ara A：Assessment of baroreflex sensitivity. In Malik M [ed]. Clinical Guide to Cardiac Autonomic Tests. Kluwer Dordrecht，1998.)

搏动后的最早 2 个 RR 间期与异位搏动前的 RR 间期联系起来。随后的心率逐渐缩短则用"震荡斜率"（turbulence slope）进行测量，后者指 RR 间期与从异位搏动后的最初 20 个心动周期的顺序号之间最陡峭的阳性回归曲线[11]。

这似乎是心室对于异位搏动导致的短暂动脉压下降所作出的代偿性行动，随后跟随着反射性血压升高，而这些改变先于 RR 间期变化[12]。因此，HRT 现象似乎应归因于内源性"激发"的压力反射。有趣的是，一项大型的同时调查 HRT 及压力反射激发的血管活动（采用苯福林方法）的研究显示无论采用任何有意义的方法 BRS 与震荡斜率之间都不具有相关性[13]。

三、心率变异性的生理学解释

(一) 短程记录

迷走神经的传入刺激导致迷走传出活动的反射性激活，并抑制交感神经的传出活动。相反的反射由交感神经传入活动刺激所介导。传出的迷走神经活动同样看似处于心脏传入交感神经活动的"张力性"限制内。直接传到窦房结的交感及迷走神经活动的特征是冲动的释放与每一次心动周期之间具有极大程度的同步性,这可以通过中枢及外周震荡器进行调节。这些震荡器在传出神经的冲动释放中产生的节律性波动,表现为RR间期的短期和长期震荡。

正如对像电刺激迷走神经、毒蕈碱受体阻滞剂及迷走切除等临床及实验的自主神经检查操作中所观察到的那样,迷走神经的传出活动是产生HF成分的主要贡献者。对LF成分的解释更具争议性,一部分人认为它是交感神经调节的标志(特别是用标化单位表示时),而许多其他学者则认为它是对交感和迷走共同作用的综合性测量。

LF和HF成分,可以在不同条件下增加。在健康人进行90°倾斜、站立、精神应激,以及清醒犬在中度运动、中度低血压、体力活动以及闭塞一支冠状动脉或颈动脉的过程中出现LF成分的增加(用标化单位表示)。相反,由控制呼吸、面部冷刺激以及旋转刺激等引起HF成分的增加。

(二) 长程记录

对24h记录中较短节段进行的谱分析显示,正常个体的标化LF和标化HF表现为一种生物学周期模式并且出现白天LF值较高而夜间HF值较高的交替性波动。当采用整个24h中的单个频谱或将随后较短节段的频谱分析平均化则观察不到这些模式。在长程记录中,HF和LF成分大约仅占到总功率的5%左右。尽管ULF和VLF成分约占总功率的其余95%,但似乎这些成分并不代表真正与特殊调节机制有关的谐波成分。确切地说,它们表现的可能是LF和HF成分在较长记录时间内的动态变化,是针对环境变化而需要进行改变的反应。同时,一些刺激和环境条件可能会作用于VLF的节律,包括出血、主动脉缩窄、酸中毒、血管活动药物以及窒息等。但是,操纵VLF的直接调节机制的生理学细节尚不清楚。

尽管缺乏详尽的生理学解释,但这种对24h HRV的整体测量方法的确提供了测量心脏对环境刺激作出自主性反应的敏感途径。因此,这些测量能够反映心脏为适应标准的生理需求而进行自主神经调节的能力。

四、临床应用

对HRV和BRS的评价已经被引入各种临床研究中。HRV和/或BRS测量在医疗实践中的一个明确的优势已被证明主要是进行心血管风险评价以及对神经病变的早期诊断。

(一) 缺血性心脏病的风险

急性心肌梗死后HRV降低,反映出交感神经张力性活动增强,使其对心率调节的能力饱和,交感神经活动占主导地位增加了心脏电活动的不稳定性[14]。

大规模的随访数据库反复证实24h HRV降低是心肌梗死后死亡风险的有力预测因子[15-17]。HRV降低的预测能力似乎独立于人口统计学、纽约心脏协会(NYHA)心功能分级、左室射血分数以及室性异位活动等。HRV降低不仅能够预报心肌梗死后心脏事件的总死亡率,而且能够识别持续性症状性室性心动过速的患者。实际上,已经证明HRV的降低作为猝死和症状性室性心动过速的预测因子要优于左室射血分数。然而,HRV和射血分数在预测心肌梗死后各种原因导致患者死亡的效果方面表现一样好。这提示HRV是心律失常事件(心脏性猝死和室性心动过速)的一个强有力的预测因子,优于对非心律失常性死亡率的预测。根据近期研究成果,有一些专家普遍认为心肌梗死后患者的24h SDNN低于50~70ms或HRV三角指数小于20单位(NN间期以7.8ms为计量单位)为特别高危[2],尤其有其他风险因子并存时(图89-3)。最近,关于风险评估的研究集中在对长程记录的非线性分析。已有报道,采用这些指数进行风险评估的强度增大,并且不依赖于临床变化以及包括左室射血分数在内的其他风险因子[18]。

BRS(苯福林评价法)也具有潜在的风险预测作用,而以HRV和BRS为基础的风险预测已显示出相互独立及附加性[7,19]。此外,潜在风险评估(即导致更高相对风险与标准HRV或BRS指数获得的结果相比[11])可通过HRT获得。

尽管对HRV或BRS降低的预测准确性还有保留意见,但与其他风险预测因子相结合后有可能对心肌梗死后的高危患者进行有效分层[20]。事实上,将不同风险预测因子结合起来似乎能够识别出患者是倾向死于心律失常事件还是非心律失常事件[21]。心律失常性死亡主要与HRV降低和室性心律失常的连续发作有

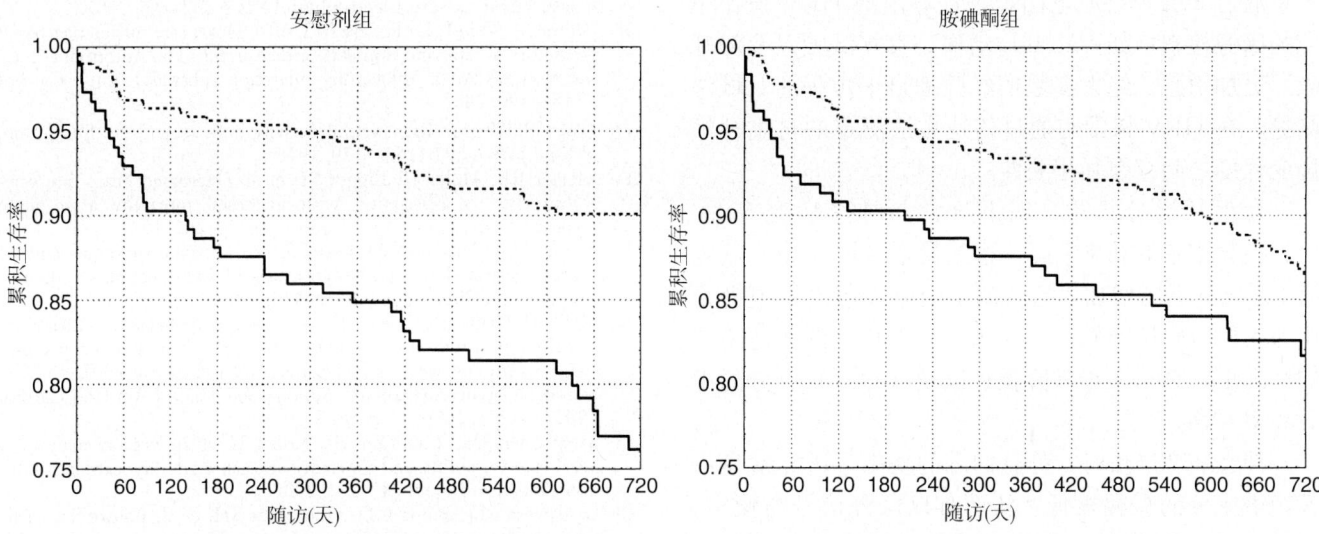

图 89-3　急性心肌梗死患者出院后的累积存活率　图中所示为根据 24h HRV 三角指数值低于（实线）及高于（虚线）20 单位（NN 间期以 7.8ms 为计量单位）进行分组的患者存活曲线。数据来源于欧洲心肌梗死胺碘酮试验（EMIAT）[17]。左图为安慰剂组，右图为胺碘酮组。注意接受安慰剂和胺碘酮治疗的 HRV 正常患者和 HRV 降低患者存活率之间的差异[17]。

关联，而射血分数降低、室性异位搏动以及 HRV 降低则引起非心律失常性死亡。这与目前对于风险预测的病理生理学的理解是一致的。射血分数降低反映出现心力衰竭的倾向性，并且可能区分出发生非猝死性死亡的风险。另一方面，HRV 降低意味着缺乏对室性心律失常的自主神经保护作用，因而也可以更有效地识别具有猝死或心律失常并发症的高危患者。

（二）心力衰竭

先前对慢性心力衰竭患者记录到的自主神经功能障碍的研究与心肌梗死后所见到的副交感神经张力减低同时伴有肾上腺素能系统慢性激活及 BRS 受损相似。

NYHA 心功能分级恶化的心力衰竭患者似乎都有明显的进行性 HRV 降低（无论采用时域法分析还是频域法分析）[22,23]。针对这种 HRV 随着心力衰竭的加重而进展变化的研究也发现采用不同方法测量的 HRV 与左室射血分数的降低具有强相关性[23]。与此类似，人们还观察到氧耗量的峰值（peak oxygen consumption）与 HRV 之间相关联[23]。所有这些都提示心力衰竭时 HRV 降低主要是由于全身性的交感活动过度而不是由于迷走活动撤退所致。

几个研究显示 HRV 在预测慢性心力衰竭患者的总生存率方面具有独立价值[24]。例如，24h SDNN 低于 100ms 以及氧耗量峰值低于 14ml/（kg·min）的患者预后特别差，1 年内死亡率为 37%[25]。因此，对于中度到重度充血性心力衰竭患者来说，HRV 具有重要的预后意义。与其他参数（如左室射血分数及氧耗量峰值）联合起来，可能对于识别需要考虑进行心脏移植的心衰患者具有一定作用。

最近，已有关于 HRT 在充血性心力衰竭患者中的预测能力的报道[26]。

（三）心血管外科手术

对于 HRV 的传统分析和非线性分析都已应用到评估心血管外科手术后患者的自主神经调节功能[27-29]。研究显示 HRV 的降低与高龄及胰岛素依赖性糖尿病都是手术后住院时间延长（>7d）的独立预测因子。HRV 的变化与冠状动脉搭桥后患者出现心肌缺血的发作有关。

（四）糖尿病性神经病变

尽管在包括严重头部外伤及脑死亡、急性脑干卒中、格林-巴利综合征及其他各种不同的神经异常中都进行过 HRV 研究，但经验最多的还是对糖尿病性神经病变的研究。

作为糖尿病的一个并发症，自主神经病变的特征是早期而又广泛的交感及副交感小神经纤维的神经退行性变。糖尿病神经病变的临床表现与 5 年内大约死亡率为 50% 有关。因此，早期检测到亚临床的自主神经病变很重要，而对短程和/或长程 HRV 的分析有助于监测神经病变已经被证实[30]。

通过24h动态心电图记录计算出的HRV值比单纯的床旁检查（如Valsalva动作、直立试验以及深呼吸）更加敏感。绝大多数的经验来自于短程的时域法测量。在HRV异常与通过传统方法测定的自主神经病变程度之间存在强相关性。

短程频谱分析中，以下异常与神经病变有关：（1）各频谱带的功率下降，这是最常见的；（2）站立时LF成分不能增加，这反映了交感反应受损或者是压力反射敏感性降低；（3）在LF/HF比例保持不变的情况下，总功率异常降低；以及（4）LF成分的中心频率左移。

神经病变严重时，静息仰卧的功率频谱经常显示各频谱成分的振幅极低，从而难以区分信号与噪声。这时需要给予诸如站立或倾斜等干预措施。

（王立群 译）

参 考 文 献

1. Wolf MM, Varigos GA, Hunt D, Sloman JG: Sinus arrhythmia in acute myocardial infarction. Med J Aust 2:52–55, 1978.
2. Task Force of the European Society of Cardiology and the North American Society of Pacing and Electrophysiology: Heart rate variability—Standards of measurement, physiological interpretation, and clinical use. Circulation 93:1043–1065, 1996.
3. Berntson GG, Bigger JT Jr, Eckberg DL, et al: Heart rate variability: Origins, methods, and interpretative caveats. Psychophysiology 34:623–648, 1997.
4. Pomeranz M, Macaulay RJB, Caudill MA, et al: Assessment of autonomic function in humans by heart rate spectral analysis. Am J Physiol Heart Circ Physiol 248:H151–H153, 1985.
5. Malliani A, Pagani M, Lombardi F, Cerutti S: Cardiovascular neural regulation explored in the frequency domain. Circulation 84:1482–1492, 1991.
6. Schmidt G, Monfill GE: Nonlinear methods for heart rate variability assessment. In Malik M, Camm AJ (eds): Heart Rate Variability. Armonk, NY, Futura, 1995, pp 87–98.
7. La Rovere MT, Specchia G, Mortara A, Schwartz PJ: Baroreflex sensitivity, clinical correlates, and cardiovascular mortality among patients with a first myocardial infarction. A prospective study. Circulation 78:816–824, 1988.
8. Kautzner J, Hartikainen JE, Camm AJ, Malik M: Arterial baroreflex sensitivity assessed from phase IV of the Valsalva maneuver. Am J Cardiol 78:575–579, 1996.
9. La Rovere MT, Pinna GD, Mortara A: Assessment of baroreflex sensitivity. In Malik M (ed): Clinical Guide to Cardiac Autonomic Tests. Dordrecht, the Netherlands, Kluwer, 1998, pp 257–281.
10. Wichterle D, Melenovsky V, Necasova L, et al: Stability of the noninvasive baroreflex sensitivity assessment using cross-spectral analysis of heart rate and arterial blood pressure variabilities. Clin Cardiol 23:201–204, 2000.
11. Schmidt G, Malik M, Barthel P, et al: Heart-rate turbulence after ventricular premature beats as a predictor of mortality after acute myocardial infarction. Lancet 353:1390–1999, 1396.
12. Wichterle D, Melenovsky V, Malik M: Mechanisms involved in heart rate turbulence. Card Electrophysiol Rev 6:262–266, 2002.
13. Ghuran A, Reid F, La Rovere MT, et al: Heart rate turbulence-based predictors of fatal and nonfatal cardiac arrest (The Autonomic Tone and Reflexes After Myocardial Infarction substudy). Am J Cardiol 89:184–190, 2002.
14. Lown B, Verrier RL: Neural activity and ventricular fibrillation. N Engl J Med 294:1165–1170, 1976.
15. Kleiger RE, Miller JP, Bigger JT, et al: Decreased heart rate variability and its association with increased mortality after acute myocardial infarction. Am J Cardiol 59:256–262, 1987.
16. Zuanetti G, Neilson JMM, Latini R, et al: Prognostic significance of heart rate variability in post-myocardial infarction patients in the fibrinolytic era. Circulation 94:432–436, 1996.
17. Malik M, Camm AJ, Janse MJ, et al: Depressed heart rate variability identifies postinfarction patients who might benefit from prophylactic treatment with amiodarone: A substudy of EMIAT (The European Myocardial Infarct Amiodarone Trial). J Am Coll Cardiol 35:1263–1275, 2000.
18. Tapanainen JM, Thomsen PE, Kober L, et al: Fractal analysis of heart rate variability and mortality after an acute myocardial infarction. Am J Cardiol 90:347–352, 2002.
19. La Rovere MT, Pinna GD, Hohnloser SH, et al: Baroreflex sensitivity and heart rate variability in the identification of patients at risk for life-threatening arrhythmias: Implications for clinical trials. Circulation 103:2072–2077, 2001.
20. Redwood S, Odemuyiwa O, Hnatkova K, et al: Selection of dichotomy limits for multifactorial prediction of arrhythmic events and mortality in survivors of acute myocardial infarction. Eur Heart J 18:1278–1287, 1997.
21. Hartikainen JEK, Malik M, Staunton A, et al: Distinction between arrhythmic and nonarrhythmic death after acute myocardial infarction based on heart rate variability, signal-averaged electrocardiogram, ventricular arrhythmias and left ventricular ejection fraction. J Am Coll Cardiol 28:296–304, 1996.
22. Casolo GC, Stroder P, Sulla A, et al: Heart rate variability and functional severity of congestive heart failure secondary to coronary artery disease. Eur Heart J 16:360–367, 1995.
23. Szabo BM, van Veldhuisen DJ, Brouwer J, et al: Relation between severity of disease and impairment of heart rate variability parameters in patients with chronic congestive heart failure secondary to coronary artery disease. Am J Cardiol 76:713–716, 1995.
24. Boveda S, Galinier M, Pathak A, et al: Prognostic value of heart rate variability in time domain analysis in congestive heart failure. J Interv Card Electrophysiol 5:181–187, 2001.
25. Ponikowski P, Anker SD, Chua TP, et al: Depressed heart rate variability as an independent predictor of death in chronic congestive heart failure secondary to ischaemic or idiopathic dilated cardiomyopathy. Am J Cardiol 79:1645–1650, 1997.
26. Koyama J, Watanabe J, Yamada A, et al: Evaluation of heart-rate turbulence as a new prognostic marker in patients with chronic heart failure. Circ J 66:902–907, 2002.
27. Laitio TT, Makikallio TH, Huikuri HV, et al: Relation of heart rate dynamics to the occurrence of myocardial ischemia after coronary artery bypass grafting. Am J Cardiol 89:1176–1181, 2002.
28. van De Borne P, Neubauer J, Rahnama M, et al: Differential characteristics of neural circulatory control: Early versus late after cardiac transplantation. Circulation 104:1809–1813, 2001.
29. Stein PK, Schmieg RE Jr, El-Fouly A, et al: Association between heart rate variability recorded on postoperative day 1 and length of stay in abdominal aortic surgery patients. Crit Care Med 29:1738–1743, 2001.
30. Bellavere F, Balzani I, De Masi G, et al: Power spectral analysis of heart rate variation improves assessment of diabetic cardiac autonomic neuropathy. Diabetes 41:633–640, 1992.

第 90 章

单相动作电位的记录

Michael R. Franz

本章目录
- 单相动作电位记录的发展史 ………… 817
- 单相动作电位的产生 ………………… 817
- 单相动作电位的记录设备 …………… 818
- 单相动作电位记录的准确性 ………… 819
- 单相动作电位记录的临床应用 ……… 820

通过接触电极导管可以安全方便地记录人体心脏的单相动作电位（MAP）。与心电图及普通腔内电图记录不同，后者是心脏电活动的间接或总体反映，而单相动作电位直接反映的是局部心肌细胞除极和复极的真实信息，能为研究人员提供在体心脏电活动更加直观的信息。不论是正常或病理状态，单相动作电位的记录是临床电生理学和细胞电生理学相互联系的重要桥梁，本章讨论单相动作电位记录的方法学和相关临床应用。

一、单相动作电位记录的发展史

历史上首次记录心脏单相动作电位远远早于跨膜动作电位的发现，当时的记录技术能导致心肌损伤，以前发表的一篇综述详细讨论了有关这一记录技术的发展历程。第一次在人体心内膜记录到单相动作电位是利用吸附电极导管完成的，由于技术和患者的安全问题，这一技术未能广泛应用于临床。吸附电极需要吸引泵、三通阀、气泡过滤器以及其他安全措施，临床应用时很麻烦，更重要的是吸附电极可能损伤记录部位的心肌组织，而且有空气栓塞的危险。由于上述原因，吸附电极不能用于人体左室的电生理研究。Franz 及同事发明的接触电极技术是一种简单且安全的单相动作电位记录技术，不必应用吸附电极，仅仅利用一个特殊设计的电极轻轻接触心内膜即可记录到单相动作电位。这种接触电极记录技术不仅安全而且简单有效。由于其避免了损伤心肌及随后的愈合效应，利用这种技术能长时间稳定地记录单相动作电位，一般可以在人体右心室和左心室同一部位连续稳定地记录数小时。

二、单相动作电位的产生

尽管接触电极记录单相动作电位技术已经广泛应用，但单相动作电位的发生机制尚未完全清楚。一根比单细胞大很多倍的记录电极如何能够进入细胞并且精确地描记细胞动作电位的电压时间曲线呢？

由于单相动作电位首先是直接在损伤的心肌细胞记录到的，所以开始称单相动作电位为"损伤电位"，并认为其发生是损伤细胞膜和邻近的正常细胞膜间的电位差所致。这种假说认为：记录动作电位的细胞外电极之间的电解液分流导致了正常细胞膜动作电位的降低，这种电位差导致了单相动作电位的产生。

"损伤电位"理论无法解释接触电极可以记录到更加稳定的单相动作电位。由于快速愈合效应及损伤组织间电的失耦联效应，损伤电位存在时间短暂，损伤电流很快消失。另外，无论心肌表面是相对干燥状态还是浸润于液体或血液中，接触电极记录的单相动作电位电压相同，与细胞外分流无关。

所以，Franz 提出假说，接触电极记录到的单相动作电位是电流起源的。这种假说认为：接触电极下方一定数量的心肌细胞由于机械压力的作用而除极并保持于不可兴奋状态，而其周围的细胞保持正常的膜电位和兴奋性，并与除极组织间形成电偶。新近，这种假说有了直接实验证据。利用鼠的右室游离壁很薄的标本，能从心外膜连续记录全层心肌细胞的动作电位，直至邻近单相动作电位记录电极处，在接触电极周围的心内膜下层记录到正常的静息膜电位（-78±4mV)，但随着微电极深入到接触电极下方的心肌，除极电位从正常逐渐下降到-23mV。

利用计算机处理上述实验数据，为了解释与单相动作电位记录电极周围电场有关的跨膜电流变化原因，建立了一个简单的三维细胞模型，模型研究支持电流起源假说。所以可以认为单相动作电位起源于记录电极顶端周围除极和正常细胞间形成的强电场。根据上述实验和模拟数据，在接触电极边缘的跨膜电位变化最大，产生了单相的细胞外电位。

三、单相动作电位的记录设备

（一）前置放大器和记录系统

单相动作电位信号包含低频成分，特别是在平台期和舒张期，为了保证信号的真实度，应使用高带宽放大器记录单相动作电位，其频响范围应在 0~5000Hz。为了减少干扰信号，记录带宽应设置为 0.05~500Hz，绝大多数电生理记录系统能做到这一点，传统的心内电图记录通道（30~300Hz）不适用于单相动作电位记录。

（二）单相动作电位的记录电极

单相动作电位记录电极导管的设计参见图 90-1A，导管顶端为半球形探测电极，其材料为非极化银-氯化银合金，另一个银-氯化银电极位于距顶端 5mm 处，作为参照电极。电极远端部分有弹力装置，保证顶端与心内膜在整个心脏收缩舒张期均可稳定接触。端电极与阳极相连，近段电极与记录系统的阴极相连。与传统电极导管不同，起搏电极不在远端，而是位于两个记录电极之间，这种电极分布方式保证了最低的起搏阈值（0.02~0.25mA，平均为 0.09mA），这样能最大限度减少起搏信号对单相动作电位记录的干扰。这些设计是为了方便而精确地测量动作电位时程和不应期。

可利用 Seldinger 穿刺技术经股静脉或股动脉将单相动作电位电极导管送入体内，到达右心室或左心室，将导管与电生理记录系统相连，进一步操纵导管时可监控心电信号。将导管顶端轻轻地接触心内膜，可记录到单相动作电位信号，通常在数个心动周期内其振幅逐渐稳定。单相动作电位信号在舒张期为负向，在收缩早期为正向。一旦达到稳定的接触，即连续记录单相动作电位，同时记录心内和体表心电图（图 90-2）。最佳的记录条件是：顶端电极与心内膜垂直，有弹性的导管可随着心脏收缩舒张而摆动。起初的单相动作电位记录电极导管含有一个控制杆，允许医生在 270°范围内在各个方向旋转导管远端，这有助于使导管通过弯曲的血管。为了使导管通过主动脉瓣，可使导管远端弯曲为半猪尾管形态，使导管顶端以最佳方向接触心内膜，以及在右室或左室的多部位记录单相动作电位。

（三）心脏手术时记录单相动作电位

心脏外科手术时允许直视下记录人体心外膜的单相动作电位，可以利用一个手持的接触电极探针，如图 90-1B 所示。两个非极化电极位于一个扁平带子（flat ribbon）的顶端，其中一个电极可以直接接触心外膜，而另一个电极位于探针顶端圆盘的下方，圆盘利用特殊的合金制成，探针有一定弹性且可控制弯曲度，这样使得外科医生能够迅速调整圆盘的弯曲度从而将探针通过心外膜和心包之间的腔隙到达心室记录点的后方或下方，这样端电极可以垂直地接触心外膜。在人体心外膜许多部位均可记录单相动作电位，例如，可以描记心室的复极顺序，或者研究局部缺血心肌。只有电极直接接触存活心肌才可以记录到单相动作电位，在瘢痕组织处无法记录单相动作电位，所以单相动作电位记录也可以作为诊断方法。但是，人体心脏的心外膜常常被脂肪包被而不能记录单相动作电位。

（四）动物实验中记录单相动作电位

已经有几种单相动作电位记录技术用于实验研究。利用一个装有弹簧的悬臂式探针可以控制电极，可在开胸动物实验中记录狗、猪或其他大动物的心外膜单相动作电位，电极顶端直接接触心外膜，而参考电极由一个盐水浸润的海绵包围在电极顶端。使用一个小的手持式探针，可以在 Langendorff 灌流的小动物例如兔心脏记录单相动作电位。还有装置可以同步记录心外膜和心内膜多点的单相动作电位，同时记录 12 导联心电图。这种技术用于研究心室兴奋和复极过

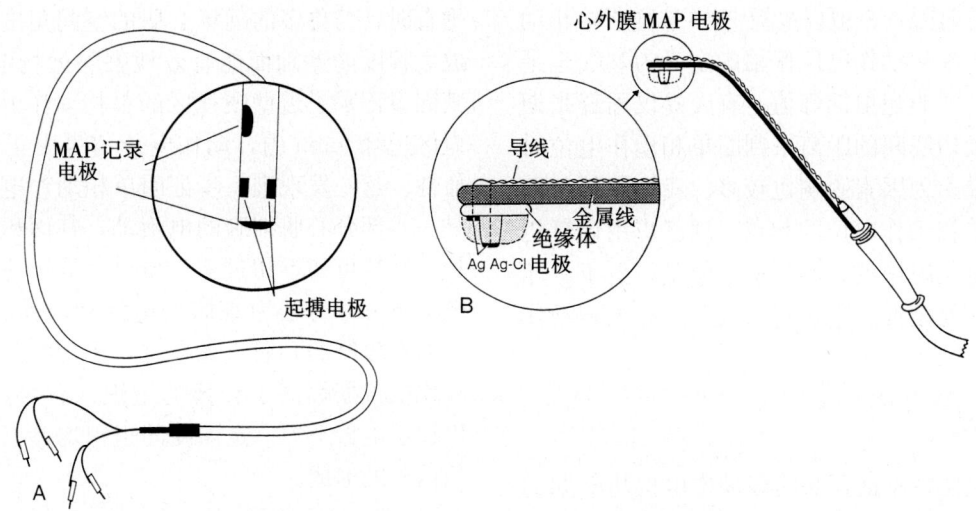

图90-1 A图：用于记录心内膜单相动作电位的接触电极导管　图中所示的模式应用最广泛（单相动作电位记录-起搏联合导管），顶端面积很小的起搏电极距导管顶端2mm，与导管垂直，这种导管可以双向弯曲（未显示）。B图：用于心脏手术时记录单相动作电位的接触电极导管的草图　（引自 Franz MR, Chin MC, Sharkey HR, et al: A new single catheter technique for simultaneous measurement of action potential duration and refractory period in vivo. J Am Coll Cardiol 16: 878-886, 1990; and Franz MR, Bargheer K, Raffenbeul W, et al: Monophasic action potential mapping in human subjects with normal electrocardiogram: Direct evidence for the genesis of T wave. Circulation 75: 379-386, 1987.）

程特别有价值，例如，可以研究直流电除颤的机制，或长QT综合征动物模型早期后除极的发生与动作电位时限及其离散的关系。新近，我们发明了一种更为小型的单相动作电位记录探针，可记录分离的大鼠心脏心外膜或心内膜单相动作电位，其端电极直径仅有0.25mm，能够准确记录鼠心室肌类似跨膜动作电位的单相动作电位。与光学描记技术不同，单相动作电位记录可以在跳动的心脏进行，而无需电机械失耦联，后者会影响动作电位波形。大鼠单相动作电位记录方法对于研究转基因动物模型特别有价值。目前，这种方法已经用于研究携带 *KCNQ1* 和 *SCN5A* 基因的转基因鼠的电生理异常。

四、单相动作电位记录的准确性

在心室肌记录的单相动作电位有其特有的平台期（大鼠、小鼠例外），随后是相对陡峭的3相复极期（图90-2B），相反，心房内膜记录的单相动作电位特点是平台期短或不具平台期，3相复极期较缓慢，从而形成典型的三角形心房肌动作电位（图90-2A）。

（一）动作电位的时限和形态

单相动作电位并不能反映动作电位改变的真实大小。尽管绝对电压不同，单相动作电位可以真实地展现心肌细胞膜的电压时间曲线，经过对比同步记录的邻近心肌的跨膜动作电位和单相动作电位，几个研究

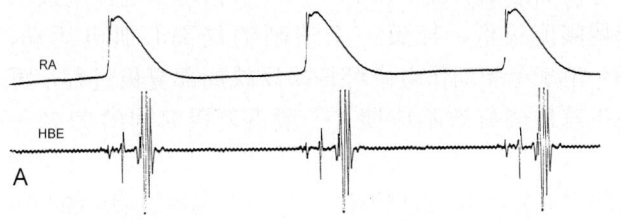

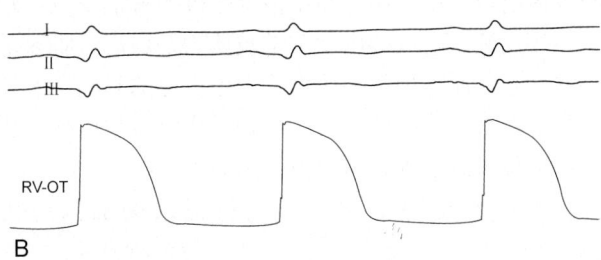

图90-2　接受电生理检查患者心房（A）和心室（B）肌内膜记录的单相动作电位　典型的心房单相动作电位为三角形，而心室肌单相动作电位的特点是有明确的平台期，3相复极陡峭。注意与普通心内电图多相曲折相比，单相动作电位有明确且锐利的超射期。

证实了这一点。由于逐渐完成复极，难以精确测量单相动作电位的总时限，一般以复极 90% 来判断单相动作电位的时限。单相动作电位振幅的定义为基线至平台顶部的距离，并非超射期峰值。有人提议用舒张期基线与 3 相复极切线间的距离来判断单相动作电位时限，这种方法受人为因素影响也较多。我们把超射期开始部位作为单相动作电位的起点。现已应用计算机进行单相动作电位时限的自动分析。但是，由于单相动作电位信号的复杂性，仍然建议人工计算单相动作电位的时限。

（二）超射速度

单相动作电位并不能反映跨膜动作电位超射期的绝对上升速度（V_{max}），单相动作电位的 V_{max} 显著低于跨膜动作电位。犬心室单相动作电位的 V_{max} 平均值为 6.4V/s，远远低于犬心室肌细胞的跨膜动作电位（约 200V/s）。单相动作电位的上升速度低，一方面是因为其绝对电压较低，另一方面是由于其反映的是连续除极的一群细胞的动作电位。另外，与跨膜动作电位不同的是，在单相动作电位的超射期或其前可见小的 Q 波或切迹，反映了邻近细胞的电位，更换参照电极位置或改变放大率可以减小这一干扰。当端电极垂直于心内膜时，参照电极距端电极 5mm 就可以作为无关电极，同时可以最大限度地减少远场电位。远场电位对单相动作电位的影响可能在心室早搏时增强。

（三）静息和动作电位振幅变化

用直流放大器和非极化电极，记录单相动作电位可以反映短暂的静息电位和动作电位的改变。例如，兔室间隔标本急性缺血损伤不仅会导致单相动作电位形态和时限明显改变，而且导致同等程度的静息电位降低，同步记录的细胞跨膜动作电位也证实了这一点。同样，细胞外钾离子浓度从正常值 4.5mmol/L 增加到 9mmol/L 也会导致舒张期跨膜动作电位和单相动作电位同等程度的降低。

（四）单相动作电位的观察范围

决定单相动作电位观察范围的一个重要因素是记录电极顶端面积的大小，其决定了记录电极周围除极细胞与正常细胞的界限，观察空间不会小于电极顶端直径（一般为 1～2mm）；另一个决定因素是端电极与参照电极的距离与夹角，记录人体心脏单相动作电位时，参照电极的距离不应超过 5mm，记录小动物时不应超过 1～2mm。当顶端电极位置适当并与心肌表面垂直时，与更多的远场心肌的空间角度很小，从而因放大程度的差别而能有效地去除远场电位。Franz 及其同事记录了透壁梗死区的单相动作电位，发现在缺血区边缘 5mm 内，动作电位信号由正常突然变为缺血性。这一发现进一步证明单相动作电位信号反映的是一小部分心肌细胞的电活动，其面积不小于电极面积，直径可能不超过 2～3mm。单相动作电位记录了电极下方部分心肌细胞的电活动，其深度尚未确定。因为在较厚的心肌（如左室，大动物）记录到的单相动作电位振幅高于较薄的组织（右房，小动物），所以提示电极下方一定深度的组织均参与了单相动作电位信号的形成。

五、单相动作电位记录的临床应用

（一）一般用途

有起搏功能的接触式单相动作电位记录电极可用于常规电生理检查，包括进行程序刺激，其与传统 4 极电极相比有如下优点：（1）单相动作电位的超射期反映了局部心内膜激动时间，与传统电极记录的常常带有多次曲折的电位不同，使得测量局部激动时间更加方便而准确（图 90-3）；（2）单相动作电位电极的起搏阈值很低，导致一个清晰的局部心肌电活动；（3）由于单相动作电位可直接反映局部复极过程，可以迅速估测有效不应期（一般占复极时间的 75%～85%），不必延长记录时间，有助于了解动作电位的时限对有效不应期的影响；（4）只有电极顶端接触心内膜才能记录单相动作电位，所以应保证持续稳定的电极导管与心内膜接触，这也保证了稳定的起搏阈值，避免与心腔内电位混淆；（5）使用传统电极导管记录时，碎裂、双相及延迟电位的出现常常被认为是瘢痕心肌异常传导的标志，而这种传导异常是发生折返的基础，但是干扰常常带来碎裂电位，对比单相动作电位与传统方法记录的电位可以识别碎裂电位的本质。

以下举例说明单相动作电位记录的临床应用（表 90-1）。

（二）评价抗心律失常药物对复极和不应期的影响

1. 抗心律失常药物对动作电位时程的影响

CAST 试验的结果使得人们更倾向于使用Ⅲ类抗

心律失常药物。单相动作电位记录特别适用于检测和测定Ⅲ类抗心律失常药物延长动作电位时程的效果，不仅比体表心电图更为准确，而且可以在电生理检查时直接测定，而生化测定常常在研究数天之后才能得到结果。

通过以稳定周长起搏时连续记录同一部位的单相动作电位，可以判断延长动作电位时限的药物存在频率依赖性或逆频率依赖性，当心率增加时，如果动作电位时程延长效应增加，则存在频率依赖性，反之则为逆频率依赖性。一般认为，如果一种Ⅲ类抗心律失常药物有效，其延长动作电位时程的作用应随心率增加而增强，从而能够限制或终止心动过速。到目前为止，只有胺碘酮被证实在心率增加时仍能维持其延长动作电位时程作用，胺碘酮延长动作电位时程效应与心动周期呈线性关系，即其无频率依赖效应，是中性的。

2. 复极和不应期的关系

心肌细胞在除极状态对新的刺激没有反应，在动作电位接近结束时恢复其可兴奋性。使用单相动作电位的记录-起搏电极，可以简单和快速地确定同一处心肌动作电位时程和有效不应期的关系（图90-3），利用这种方法，已经确认了在体心肌细胞复极与可兴奋性的相关性。动作电位时程和有效不应期均与起搏周长呈线性关系。所以，药物导致的动作电位时程延长总是导致类似程度的有效不应期延长。心肌疾病，如心肌缺血或抗心律失常药物都会影响复极与不应期的正常关系，与心律失常的发生有关。钠通道阻滞剂可以在不延长甚至缩短动作电位时程的情况下延长有效不应期。抗心律失常药物的作用机制是其延长有效不应期的程度超过了延长动作电位时程的程度，导致复极后的有效不应期延长，防止早搏和快速性室性心动过速。

（三）单相动作电位记录作为研究尖端扭转型室速和后除极机制的方法

很多获得性和先天性长QT综合征患者会发生尖端扭转型室速。早后除极和迟后除极均与触发性心律失常的发生有关，而多形性室速，包括尖端扭转型室速的发生机制为触发活动。单相动作电位记录可用于在体检测后除极。Habbab和el-Sherif报告了普鲁卡因胺诱发的尖端扭转型多形性室速与后除极及U波有关的临床证据（图90-4）。与临床观察一致，心动过缓和长间歇能加强这种后除极，而快速起搏可以抑制这种后除极。尖端扭转型室速的确切电生理机制还在

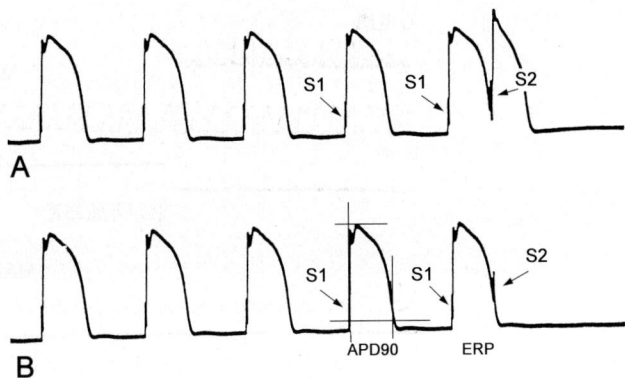

图90-3 用单相动作电位起搏和记录联合电极在体同步测定动作电位时程和有效不应期 S1和S2分别代表基础和期外刺激，上条图显示能引起可扩布兴奋的最短S1-S2联律间期；下条图显示短于最短联律间期5ms的S2刺激未能夺获心肌。S1刺激部分落于单相动作电位的超射期，但不影响单相动作电位起始部位及时程的判断，S2刺激落于复极相，但不影响复极时程。（引自Franz MR, Chin MC, Sharkey HR, et al: A new single catheter technique for simultaneous measurement of action potential duration and refractory period in vivo. J Am Coll Cardiol 16: 878-886, 1990.）

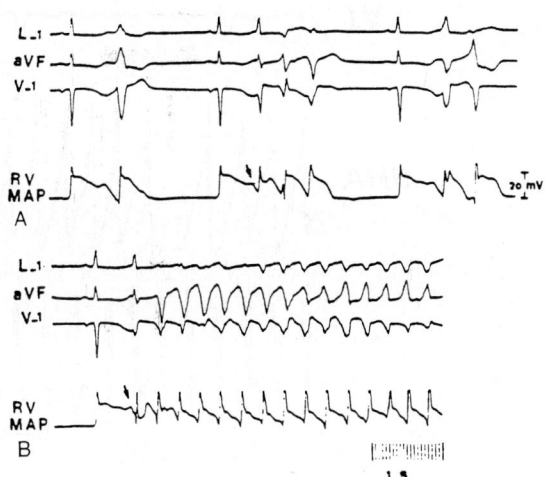

图90-4 用单相动作电位导管在普鲁卡因胺诱发尖端扭转型室速患者右室心内膜记录的早后除极（引自Habbab MA, el-Sherif N: TU alternans, long QTU, and torsade de pointes: Clinical and experimental observations. Pacing Clin Electrophysiol 15: 916-931, 1992.）

研究之中，目前还没有这种心律失常的动物模型。在离体心脏心外膜和心内膜多部位同步记录单相动作电位，同时记录心电图，揭示了获得性或先天性长QT综合征时发生尖端扭转型室速的机制。

（四）在ICD测试过程中鉴别室速和室颤

单相动作电位记录有助于明确鉴别室速和室颤，

822　第十二部分　诊断与评价

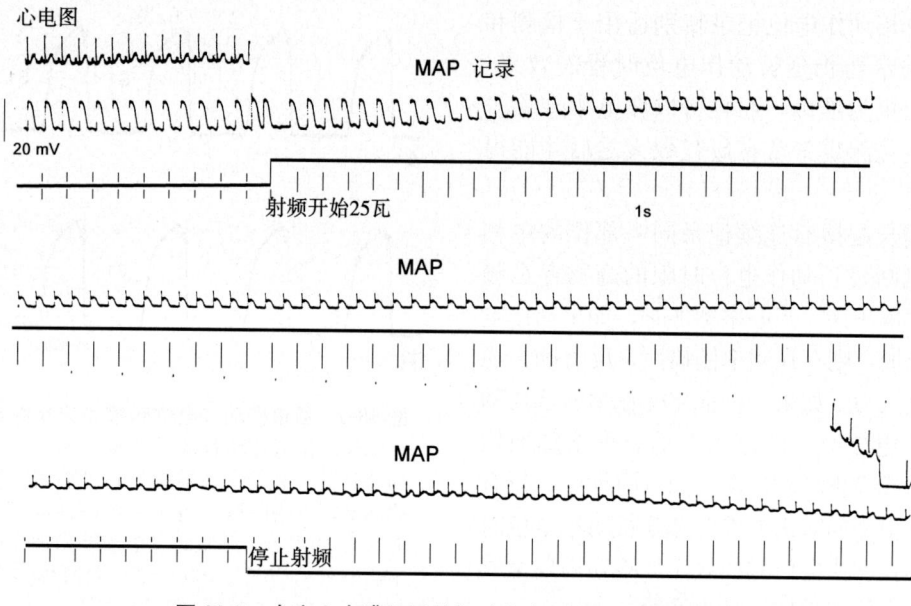

图 90-5　右室心内膜记录单相动作电位时的室速和室颤

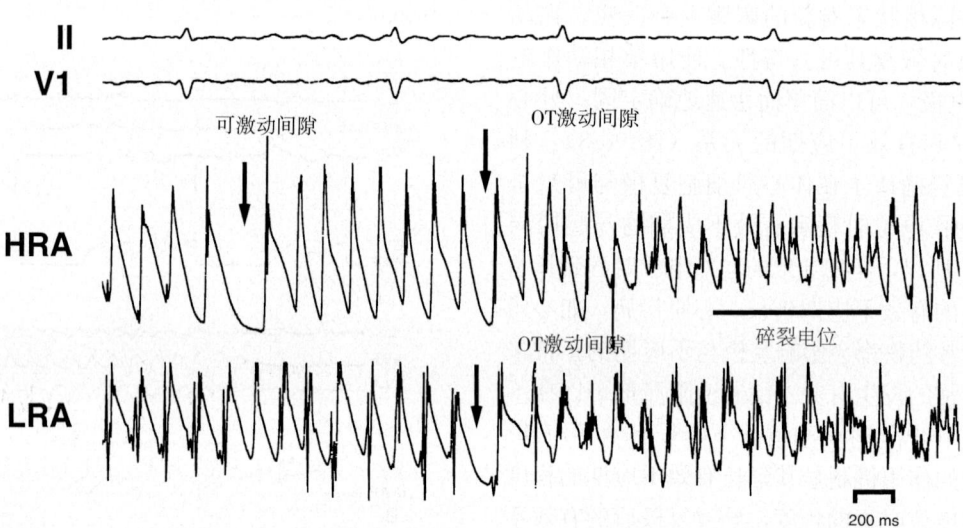

图 90-6　房颤时记录的右房单相动作电位　注意节律高度不规则的激动和复极，偶尔出现舒张期（可激动间隙）。HRA，高位右房；LRA，低位右房。

当体表心电图难以鉴别或由于 ICD 放电而无法记录体表心电图时，这种鉴别方法尤其重要。当除颤器放电后，由于放电引起电极极化和对心电图机放大装置的影响，示波屏幕上心电图曲线常常会消失数秒钟，由于使用的是直流放大器，放电电流和传导电流影响最小的是单相动作电位，其在整个测试过程中均可识别。

（五）射频消融术时利用单相动作电位进行监护

成功的射频消融术由以下几个方面决定，包括心律失常机制的确认、消融电极与靶点心肌的稳定接触以及靶点的成功消融。使用特制的单相动作电位记录

表 90-1　单相动作电位记录的临床应用

研究动作电位时程对频率和节律的影响
后除极和多形室速
先天性或获得性长 QT 综合征
其他形式的触发性心律失常（右室流出道室速？）
抗心律失常药物对动作电位时程的影响
抗心律失常药物对有效不应期/动作电位时程比值的影响
评价 T 波改变
检测心肌缺血和标测梗死区
鉴别存活和非存活心肌
测量复极离散
ICD 测试过程中鉴别室速和室颤
检测房颤的可激动间隙
人体心房的心脏记忆和电重构
ICD，植入式心脏复律除颤器

和射频消融导管，可以实时监控作用于心肌的射频能量产生的效果，利用单相动作电位作为心肌存活的标志，如图90-5所示，在放电数秒钟内单相动作电位的振幅降低。单相动作电位的振幅可以作为反映导管顶端温度的指标，如同温控电极导管一样。单相动作电位振幅降低30%意味着不可逆的心肌破坏。

能够记录单相动作电位的消融电极有助于确认电极与组织稳定而紧密的接触，当单相动作电位微弱或不稳定时，提示电极与组织接触不稳定或不紧密。单相动作电位记录还有助于识别消融靶点，治疗右室流出道室速时，单相动作电位可以发现有早后除极的位点，异位心律常起源于该点，在该点消融可使所有早搏和室速消失。

(六) 房颤和房扑时记录单相动作电位

房颤的特点是高度不规则的激动与复极。与心电图相比，单相动作电位的优点是可以识别除极与复极，并在房颤时显示可激动间隙（图90-6），而可激动间隙是房颤时超速起搏夺获心房的基础。单相动作电位可用于不同类型房颤的鉴别，以及一些房颤与房扑的鉴别。单相动作电位还能发现抗心律失常药终止房扑机制的线索，还可用于确认人体心脏慢性房颤或房扑引起的电重构。近来一项研究显示人体右心房动作电位时程分布不均匀，慢性房颤或房扑患者下腔静脉-三尖瓣峡部区域动作电位时程异常延长，而且频率适应性特征消失。当快速冲动（如房扑、快速超速起搏或来自肺静脉的快速刺激）遇到不应期延长产生的障碍时，电重构的异质性会导致传导途径中出现裂隙，从而出现"房颤样传导"，进而诱发房颤。

（贾忠伟 译）

参 考 文 献

1. Franz MR: Current status of monophasic action potential recording: Theories, measurements and interpretations. Cardiovasc Res 41:25–40, 1999.
2. Franz MR, Chin MC, Sharkey HR, et al: A new single catheter technique for simultaneous measurement of action potential duration and refractory period in vivo. J Am Coll Cardiol 16:878–886, 1990.
3. Franz MR: Long-term recording of monophasic action potentials from human endocardium. Am J Cardiol 51:1629–1634, 1983.
4. Knollmann BC: Microelectrode study of the genesis of monophasic action potentials by contact electrode technique. J Cardiovasc Electrophysiol 13:1246–1252, 2002.
5. Koller BS, Karasik PE, Solomon AJ, Franz MR: The relationship between repolarization and refractoriness during programmed electrical stimulation in the human right ventricle. Implications for ventricular tachycardia induction. Circulation 91:2378–2384, 1995.
6. Koller BS, Karasik PE, Solomon AJ, Franz MR: Prolongation of conduction time during premature stimulation in the human atrium is primarily caused by local stimulus response latency [see comments]. Eur Heart J 16:1920–1924, 1995.
7. Liu XK, Wang W, Ebert SN, et al: Female gender is a risk factor for Torsades de pointes in an in vitro animal model. J Cardiovasc Pharmacol 34:287–294, 1999.
8. Knollmann BC, Katchman AN, Franz MR: Monophasic action potential recordings from intact mouse heart: Validation, regional heterogeneity, and relation to refractoriness. J Cardiovasc Electrophysiol 12:1286–1294, 2001.
9. Casimiro MC, Knollmann BC, Ebert SN, et al: Targeted disruption of the Kcnq1 gene produces a mouse model of Jervell and Lange-Nielsen Syndrome. Proc Natl Acad Sci U S A 98:2526–2531, 2001.
10. Fabritz L, Kirchhof P, Franz MR, et al: Effect of pacing and mexiletine on dispersion of repolarisation and arrhythmias in DeltaKPQ SCN5A (long QT3) mice. Cardiovasc Res 57:1085–93, 2003.
11. Franz MR, Kirchhof PF, Fabritz CL, Zabel M: Computer analysis of monophasic action potentials: Manual validation and clinically pertinent applications. Pacing Clin Electrophysiol 18:1666–1678, 1995.
12. Franz MR, Burkhoff D, Lakatta EG, Weisfeldt ML: Monophasic action potential recording by contact electrode technique: In vitro validation and clinical applications. In Butrous GS, Schwartz PJ (eds): Clinical Aspects of Ventricular Repolarization. London, Farrand Press, 1989, pp 81–92.
13. Franz MR, Flaherty JT, Platia EV, et al: Localization of regional myocardial ischemia by recording of monophasic action potentials. Circulation 69:593–604, 1984.
14. Zabel M, Hohnloser SH, Behrens S, et al: Differential effects of D-sotalol, quinidine, and amiodarone on dispersion of ventricular repolarization in the isolated rabbit heart. J Cardiovasc Electrophysiol 8:1239–1245, 1997.
15. Kirchhof PF, Fabritz CL, Franz MR: Postrepolarization refractoriness versus conduction slowing caused by class I antiarrhythmic drugs: Antiarrhythmic and proarrhythmic effects. Circulation 97:2567–2574, 1998.
16. Bode F, Kilborn M, Karasik P, Franz MR: The repolarization-excitability relationship in the human right atrium is unaffected by cycle length, recording site and prior arrhythmias. J Am Coll Cardiol 37:920–925, 2001.
17. Habbab MA, el-Sherif N: TU alternans, long QTU, and torsade de pointes: Clinical and experimental observations. Pacing Clin Electrophysiol 15:916–931, 1992.
18. Johna R, Mertens H, Haverkamp W, et al: Clofilium in the isolated perfused rabbit heart: A new model to study proarrhythmia induced by class III antiarrhythmic drugs. Basic Res Cardiol 93:127–135, 1998.
19. Liem LB, Swerdlow CD, Franz MR: Distinctive features of ventricular fibrillation and ventricular tachycardia detected by monophasic action potential recording in human subjects. J Electrophysiol 2:484–491, 1988.
20. Franz MR: Bridging the gap between basic and clinical electrophysiology: What can be learned from monophasic action potential recordings? J Cardiovasc Electrophysiol 5:699–710, 1994.
21. Pandozi C, Bianconi L, Villani M, et al: Local capture by atrial pacing in spontaneous chronic atrial fibrillation. Circulation 95:2416–2422, 1997.
22. Stambler BS, Wood MA, Ellenbogen KA: Comparative efficacy of intravenous ibutilide versus procainamide for enhancing termination of atrial flutter by atrial overdrive pacing. Am J Cardiol 77:960–966, 1996.
23. Stambler BS, Wood MA, Ellenbogen KA: Pharmacologic alterations in human type I atrial flutter cycle length and monophasic action potential duration. Evidence of a fully excitable gap in the reentrant circuit. J Am Coll Cardiol 27:453–461, 1996.
24. Franz MR, Karasik PL, Li C, et al: Electrical remodeling of the human atrium: Similar effects in patients with chronic atrial fibrillation and atrial flutter. J Am Coll Cardiol 30:1785–1792, 1997.
25. Narayan SM, Bode F, Karasik PL, Franz MR: Alternans of atrial action potentials during atrial flutter as a precursor to atrial fibrillation. Circulation 106:1968–1973, 2002.

第91章

T波电交替

Stefan H. Hohnloser

本章目录
- 心脏电交替的历史 …………………… 824
- T波电交替的机制 …………………… 824
- T波电交替的检测技术 ……………… 825
- 微伏级T波电交替的分类与结果分析 ……………………………………… 825
- 微伏级T波电交替的临床研究 ……… 827
- 微伏级T波电交替的应用前景 ……… 831

一、心脏电交替的历史

心脏电交替是指心电图各波发生逐波交替。1908年，Hering[1]首先描述了心电图可见的T波电交替（即"肉眼可辨的"T波电交替）。此后不久，Lewis[2]报道T波电交替可以发生在心率显著加快的正常心脏，也可发生在器质性病变或毒性物质损害的心脏。1948年，Kalter和Schwartz[3]分析了6059份心电图，证实了有T波电交替（5例）的患者病死率增加。随后的病例报告描述了在各种临床情况下，如心肌缺血、冠脉痉挛、电解质紊乱、特别是先天性长QT综合征等患者心电图出现T波电交替[4]。事实上，Schwartz和Malliani[5]是首先注意到T波电交替可能与心脏性猝死病理生理学机制相关的学者之一。

1982年[6]，首次报道了应用复杂的计算机分析系统对微伏级T波电交替进行评价。20世纪80年代Cohen等[6,7]在犬模型中，证实了微伏级T波电交替和心室颤动易患性之间紧密相关。Nearing等[8]随后报道了相似的结果。随着这些方法的进一步进展，在微伏级T波电交替的机制、临床应用，以及作为评价患者预后危险性的心电图指标的价值等方面取得了很多新成果。本章旨在对这些新进展进行综述。

二、T波电交替的机制

近来，一些研究应用高分辨率光学图像及电压敏感性染色等方法显示，快速起搏造成的动作电位时程交替在心室肌各层中并不一致[9]。心室肌表现出显著的、连续的动作电位延长和缩短交替波动，但在另一些区域表现出的交替波动则完全相反，这种现象称为心脏的不协调性交替。跨膜电位振幅和方向逐波交替所造成的空间梯度是微伏级T波电交替的基础。Pastore等[9]的研究结果表明，不协调交替能够造成复极空间梯度，这种梯度足以造成单向阻滞和功能性折返，进而产生室颤。用计算机模拟二维心肌组织断层显像[10]的研究结果与这些试验结果[9]一致。同一实验室的工作人员在后来的研究中检测了细胞与细胞之间的失耦联情况，例如在有心脏结构病变的患者中，结构病变使细胞之间绝缘而造成失耦联。存在这些障碍时，各邻近细胞之间更容易表现出其离子基础不同，因为细胞与细胞之间不再有电活动联系。因而，心脏结构障碍导致主导心率显著降低时，不协调性交替容易出现。而且，心脏结构障碍也是稳定性折返的解剖基础，更容易使诱发的单形室性心动过速持续，而不是使室颤持续。Berger[12]指出，这些新发现说明以解剖结构异常为基质的复极不协调性交替是各种折返性心律失常的共同机制。这样，在变时性和代谢性应激状态下，不协调性交替造成的复极梯度足以产生单向阻滞和折返。如果没有心脏结构障碍，表现为功能性折返，产生室颤或多形性室速；如果有心脏结构障碍时，表现为固定解剖结构的折返，容易形成单形性室速。

大量的试验证据表明，微伏级 T 波电交替是产生于单个细胞水平的交替。但至今尚未完全阐明其离子机制。细胞复极交替可能原发于心肌细胞膜离子通道的活动，或继发于细胞内钙循环所致的离子通道交替性变化，或上述 2 种情况均有。近来，Walker 和 Rosenbarm[13]在综述中总结道：已有充分的证据表明，细胞内钙循环在微伏级 T 波电交替机制中发挥着关键性作用。例如，Shimizu 和 Antzelevitch[14]用心室楔形肌块模拟出先天性长 QT 综合征患者的电生理特征。在快速起搏过程中，诱发出 T 波电交替和动作电位时程的交替。应用斯里兰卡肉桂碱（ryanodine）或降低细胞外钙离子浓度能消除这种交替。这表明细胞内钙循环能维持微伏级 T 波电交替。其他证据表明，当用电压钳阻止膜电位交替后，快速起搏过程中的瞬间钙离子流交替仍能发生，因而证实了瞬间钙离子流交替是 T 波电交替的机制，而不是 T 波电交替造成了瞬间钙离子流交替[15,16]。而且，在产生微伏级 T 波电交替过程中，瞬间钙离子流空间不协调性和动作电位时程离散之间的关系也支持上述观点[17]。从临床观点，容易理解钙处理异常在微伏级 T 波电交替产生过程中所起的关键性作用，因为许多不同的心脏疾病都与细胞内钙处理异常有关。

目前，关于细胞交替发生机制的一些重要问题尚未解决。例如，在猝死高危者中，心率较慢时出现显著微伏级 T 波电交替的机制不清，哪些病理性的离子流表达异常、缝隙连接和/或组织重构等原因造成了上述情况尚不清楚。同样，其分子机制也不十分清楚。然而，目前细胞分子生物学进展迅速，相信在不久的将来即可以解答这些问题。

三、T 波电交替的检测技术

检测 TWA 有几种计算方法，如复合波解调分析和自相关统计分析技术等。然而，先前详细讲述的光谱分析技术[18]是应用最广泛的技术。这种方法用 3 个 Frank 正交导联采集至少 128 次窦性心搏心电图，以每两个心搏为一个周期，在 QRS 波群后同一时段内测量 T 波，对心电图信号的向量大小进行分析（图 91-1）。因为这种光谱是逐波进行检测的，其频率用心动周期/搏动来表示。因而，光谱上在 0.5 个心动周期/搏动的位置来检测 T 波电交替的水平（图 91-1）。

交替功率（μV^2）是指交替频率与噪声频率带（计算 0.44~0.49 周/搏之间的频率）的功率之差，这是真正的物理学上检测交替的一个指标。交替值（V_{alt}）是指单数或双数 T 波幅度减去平均 T 波幅度再减去平均噪声幅度，所得结果的平方根。交替率（K 值）是指交替功率除以噪声的标准差，用来衡量电交替是否具有统计学意义。如果 K 值≥3 表示电交替有显著性意义。用这种光谱学方法对微伏级 T 波电交替进行检测的结果很可靠。

正确检测微伏级 T 波电交替依赖于所获得的数据的质量，因为微伏级 T 波电交替是一种低振幅，相对低频率的心电现象，很容易受基线漂移、肌电干扰等伪差影响。因而，微伏级 T 波电交替的检测需要仔细地进行皮肤准备，将电极-皮肤之间的阻抗降低到最小。另外，需要应用特殊电极来记录和处理从各部位记录到的心电信号和阻抗。

确定微伏级 T 波电交替需要提高心率。每一位患者都有一个出现显著微伏级 T 波电交替的阈值心率。在最初的研究中，用心房起搏的方法提高心率，随着检测技术的发展，应用运动平板或踏车等无创方法提高心率[19-22]，用上述起搏或无创检测法获得的微伏级 T 波电交替均具有很高的重复性[20]。近来的研究表明，只有运动试验得出的微伏级 T 波电交替才对冠心病和左心室功能降低的患者具有预后意义[22]。由于这一试验的终点为各种原因所致死亡，而微伏级 T 波电交替仅对于室性心动过速有预测价值，这一结论受到置疑。目前，大多数采用无创方法对微伏级 T 波电交替进行检测。

四、微伏级 T 波电交替的分类与结果分析

随着检测技术的进展，在早期临床研究的基础上，进一步发展了微伏级 T 波电交替的分类方案。近来，发表了解读微伏级 T 波电交替研究目前指南的一个详细报告[23]。简单地说，微伏级 T 波电交替的检出受 T 波振幅大小、交替率和心率变化的影响，并需要排除伪差干扰造成的交替。显著微伏级 T 波电交替是指交替电压≥$1.9\mu V$，K 值≥3（表 91-1）。持续交替是指显著交替至少持续 1 分钟，患者心率在阈值心率-发作心率之上时显著交替一直存在。这些患者从达到发作心率开始到心率降至发作心率之下为止，显著交替一直持续。

微伏级 T 波电交替的结果分为阳性，阴性，不确

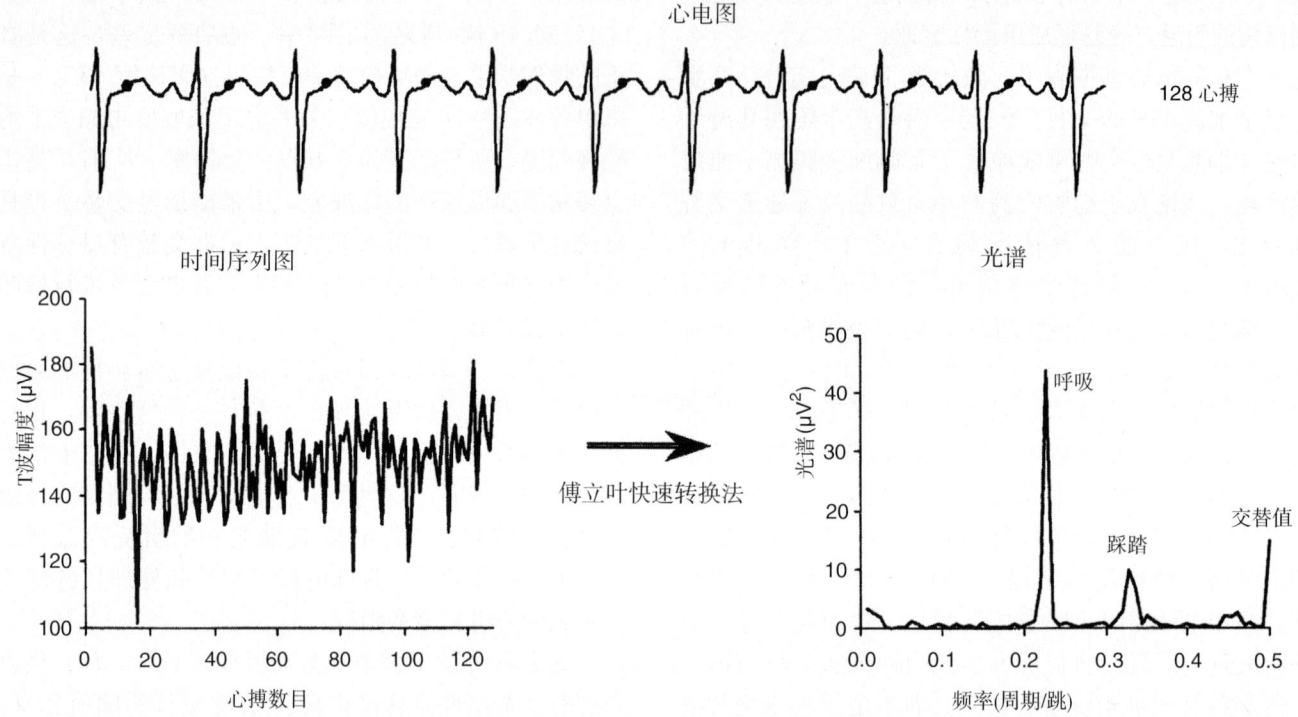

图 91-1 用光谱方法评价微伏级 T 波电交替的原理图　测量 128 个心搏的 T 波相应位置的振幅，建立包括这 128 个振幅的时间序列图，用傅立叶快速转换法计算时间序列的光谱功率。从踏车运动记录得到的光谱功率中，表示出呼吸频率峰值、踩踏频率峰值和交替值。微伏级 T 波电交替表现为 0.5 心动周期时的峰值。将这一峰值和噪音参考值的均数和标准差进行比较。

定性三种（图 91-2）。微伏级 T 波电交替阳性仅需确定 T 波交替是否持续存在，并确定其发作心率。微伏级 T 波电交替阴性和微伏级 T 波电交替不确定性之间的区别在于确定最大阴性心率和最大心率。

（一）微伏级 T 波电交替阳性

当发作心率≤110 次/分时表现为持续性交替，则定义为 T 波电交替阳性。观察正常人心率加快和出现 T 波电交替的关系表明，心率加快时出现微伏级 T 波电交替不具有评价预后的意义，因而将发作心率确定为 110 次/分。当心率≥110 次/分时出现微伏级 T 波电交替，则需要根据患者的最大阴性心率来进一步确定微伏级 T 波电交替为阴性或不确定性。

（二）微伏级 T 波电交替阴性和不确定性

微伏级 T 波电交替阴性和微伏级 T 波电交替不确定性之间的区别在于确定最大阴性心率，最大阴性心率是指没有显著电交替的最大间隔心率。最初确定最大阴性心率≥105 次/分，并将其应用于许多前瞻性的研究中[24,25]。但如果心率大于 95 次/分，有频发早搏或噪声时，不能确定在这一心率下没有微伏级 T 波电交替，不能确定微伏级 T 波电交替阴性，只能确定此时最大阴性心率为 95 次/分，微伏级 T 波电交替为不确定性。也许当早搏或噪声水平降低之后，如心率 100 次/分时，可能出现微伏级 T 波电交替。因而，将最大阴性心率＜105 次/分，没有持续微伏级 T 波电交替定义为微伏级 T 波电交替不确定性。同样，发作心率≤110 次/分时出现微伏级 T 波电交替（无评价预后的价值）而且最大阴性心率＜105 次/分也归类为微伏级 T 波电交替不确定性。

在一些研究人群中，这种分类方法使微伏级 T 波电交替不确定性的比例达到 25%～30%[24-26]。许多情况如患者的最大心率＜105 次/分，不能确定为微伏级 T 波电交替阴性（因为最大心率总是大于最大阴性心率）。为减少微伏级 T 波电交替的不确定性，修正了分类方法（称为 B 法则）来定义微伏级 T 波电交替阴性，即微伏级 T 波电交替未达到阳性标准，或最大心率≥80 次/分，最大阴性心率≥（最大心率－5 次/分）。这一方案已应用于前瞻性试验的研究中，近期有综述对其进行讨论[23]。

表 91-1　微伏级 T 波电交替的分类

定义

持续交替：是指患者心率超过特定心率，持续存在的交替（排除噪音、异位搏动、噪音或心率下降等因素的影响）。
　　至少持续 1 分钟交替电压≥$1.9\mu V$，K 值≥3
　　在任何一个电极正交 X、Y、Z 导联或记录向量的电极，或一个胸前导联和其相邻胸前导联（交替电压≥$0.9\mu V$）
　　在一些时期存在无干扰数据
　　即使当心率大于 120 次/分后微伏级 T 波电交替振幅减低或消失，仍可认为交替是持续性的。

间隔心率：是指间期为 1min 的最低的平稳心率。

最大阴性心率：没有显著交替的最大间隔心率称为最大阴性心率。判断标准：噪音能量在多数导联≤$1.8\mu V$ 或噪音能量的和加上交替能量≤$2.5\mu V$，早搏数≤10%，无导联故障时的最大间隔心率。

发作心率：是指出现持续性交替的最低心率。在确定发作心率时，应该先观察有无能够归因于噪音、早搏或心率下降所致的干扰。

最大心率：间期为 1min 的最高心率。

无干扰数据：如果所得数据符合以下条件则为无干扰数据。
　　异位心搏或早搏数≤10%总心搏数
　　呼吸运动不落在每个心动周期的前 1/4
　　128 次心搏的心率瞬间变化<30 次/分
　　无 RR 间期交替（交替率≥3 的持续时间超过 2s）

分类标准

阳性：发作心率≤110 次/分，或休息时即使心率＞110 次/分存在持续性交替。

阴性：①未达到上述阳性标准；②最大阴性心率≥105 次/分（A 法则）；③最大心率≥80 次/分，且最大阴性心率≥（最大心率－5 次/分）。

不确定性：未达到上述阳性或阴性标准者，试验结果为不确定性。

五、微伏级 T 波电交替的临床研究

（一）微伏级 T 波电交替的临床应用

最初的临床研究应用心房起搏的方法提高心率，以达到诱发微伏级 T 波电交替所需要的目标心率[19-21]。由于这种方法属于相对有创方法，妨碍了微伏级 T 波电交替应用于有严重室性心动过速和猝死危险患者的分层。随后的研究应用踏车运动提高心率直至发生微伏级 T 波电交替的阈值心率。在一项前瞻性的比较运动和起搏诱发的微伏级 T 波电交替的研究中，两种方法的发作心率基本一致，再次强调了不同患者有不同的微伏级 T 波电交替的发作心率[20]。尽管同样心率下，运动峰值时 T 波电交替幅度比起搏时 T 波幅度大，其阳性和阴性结果仍然具有可比性。因而，目前主要应用运动平板或踏车等无创方法提高心率。近来，Bloomfield 等[27]的研究表明，无创性微伏级 T 波电交替试验在短期内具有可重复性。

用这种方法检测出的微伏级 T 波电交替不确定性的比例为 12%～25%[23-26]，限制了其应用。这种情况主要由于患者心率无法超过 105 次/分（心衰或服用 β 受体阻滞剂）。其他原因包括额外的噪声，频发的房性或室性早搏，存在房颤等。然而，用一些方法可以减少不确定性的比例，如认真处理皮肤、应用特殊电极进行记录等。近来还有学者建议[27]，如果最初的试验结果无法确定，可以进行重复试验。

（二）微伏级 T 波电交替和电生理检查预测患者发生室速/室颤的危险

1994 年，Rosenbaum 等[19]完成了具有划时代意义的第一个微伏级 T 波电交替的临床试验。试验入选 83 位接受电生理检查的患者，微伏级 T 波电交替和可诱发的室速/室颤之间密切相关。事实上，有复极交替的患者诱发室速/室颤的相对危险为 5.2。而且，在 20 个月的随访中，微伏级 T 波电交替和室性心动过速的可诱发性是预测无心律失常事件生存率的显著的、等同的指标（$P<0.001$）。近来的一项研究入选 313 位患者进行电生理检查，得到了相似的结论[25]。微伏级 T 波电交替预测主要终点事件（猝死、持续室速、室颤或 ICD 正确的电击治疗）的相对危险为 10.9，电生理诱发室性心律失常的相对危险为 7.1。与 Rosenbaum 等[19]的研究相似，用微伏级 T 波电交替预测电生理检查可诱发室性心动过速的相对危险为

5.7。

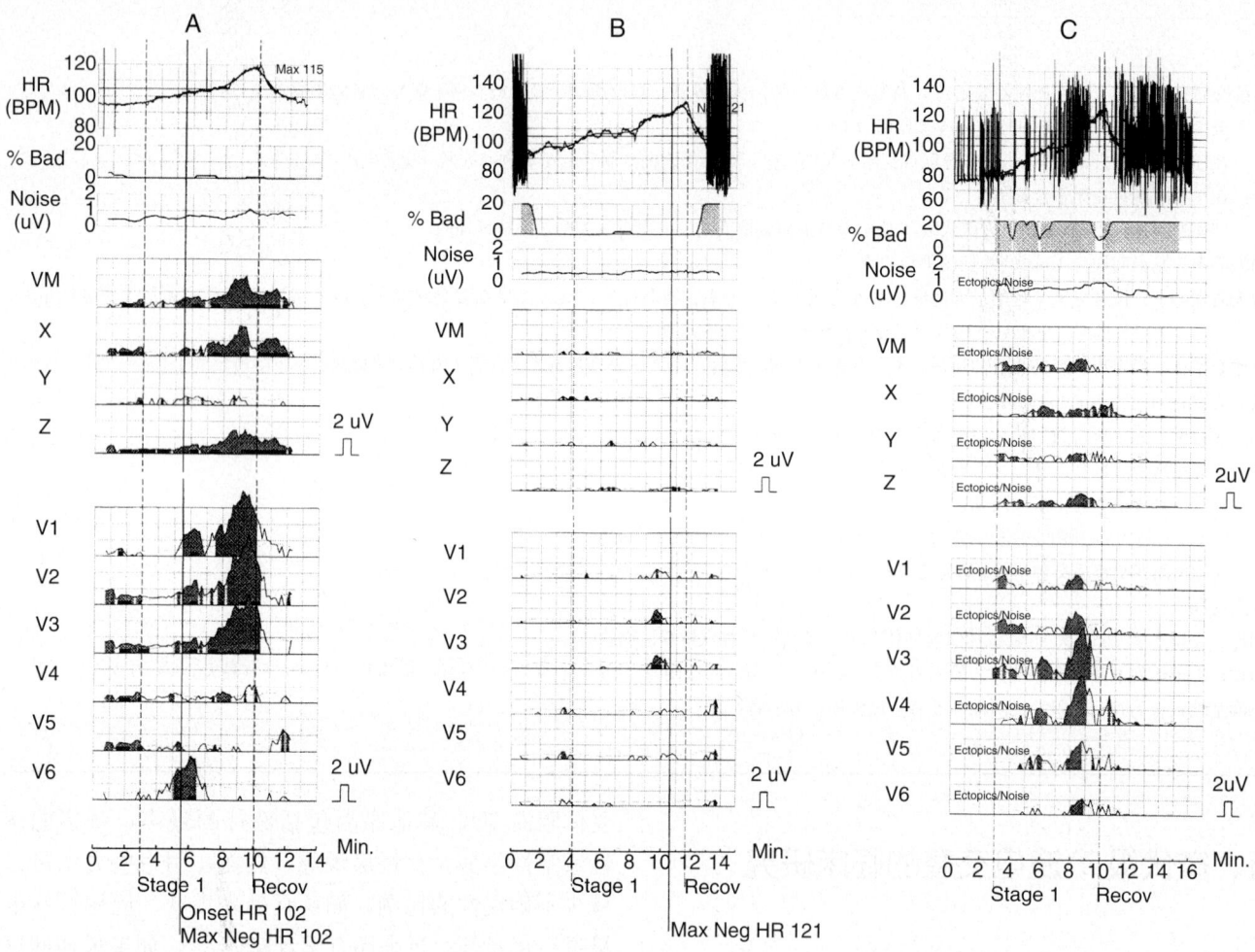

图 91-2 微伏级 T 波电交替阳性、阴性、不确定性结果的图例 从上至下顺序分别为心率趋势图；无价值心率百分比；噪音水平；在心电向量记录导联，正交导联 X、Y、Z，体表心电图 V_1~V_6 导联的微伏级 T 波电交替振幅。图 A 为踏车运动诱发的持续性微伏级 T 波电交替（灰色阴影区域），发作心率为 102 次/分。图 B 为运动试验中最大心率 121 次/分时无微伏级 T 波电交替。图 C 由于有频发的异位搏动，微伏级 T 波电交替为不确定性，在心率趋势图中，用直线来表示这些异位搏动。

Hohnloser 等[24]的一项研究入选 95 例有室性心动过速病史并植入 ICD 的患者，检测微伏级 T 波电交替。另外，同时对其他常用的无创危险分层方法进行了评价，所有患者均接受电生理检查。试验终点是在随访的 442 天内，第一次出现心电图记录证实的、经 ICD 电击终止的室速/室颤。Kapan-Meier 生存分析显示，微伏级 T 波电交替（$P<0.006$）和左室射血分数（LVEF）（$P<0.04$）是仅有的两个有显著性意义的单变量危险分层指标。事实上，多变量 Cox 回归分析表明，微伏级 T 波电交替是心律失常事件的独立预测因子，具有统计学意义[24]。

（三）微伏级 T 波电交替对心梗后患者危险分层的意义

几个研究评价了微伏级 T 波电交替对急性心梗后幸存者心律失常事件，包括猝死的预测价值[28-31]（表 91-2；图 91-3）。一项试验研究入选 448 例患者，心梗后 5~21 天检测微伏级 T 波电交替。18% 微伏级 T 波电交替阳性，55% 阴性，9% 不确定性，17% 患者未完成检测。在随后 4~8 周的随访中，对 184 例患者进行重复检测，结果一致者仅为 67%[28]。这表明，在急性心梗的最初 1 个月中，微伏级 T 波电交替发生了进展。因而，如果将微伏级 T 波电交替作为危险分层指标，需要在心梗急性期之后，微伏级 T 波电交替比较稳定时进行检测。

表 91-2　微伏级 T 波电交替对心梗后患者的危险分层

	ACES，1999[28]	Ikeda 等，2000[29]	Tapanainen 等，2001[30]	Ikeda 等，2002[31]
患者数	448	119	379	834
微伏级 T 波电交替阳性（%）	18	49	15	36
微伏级 T 波电交替阴性（%）	55	46	38	52
微伏级 T 波电交替不确定性/未完成（%）	26	14	47	12
β 受体阻滞剂治疗（%）	未用	31	97	13
评价微伏级 T 波电交替的时间（心梗后的天数）	未用	20±6	8.1±2.4	14～70*
研究的主要终点事件	未用	持续室速，室颤	总死亡率	猝死，室颤
平均随访时间	未用	13	14	25
室性心动过速事件（%）	未用	15	未用	8
敏感性（%）	未用	93	0	92
阳性预测值（%）	未用	28	0	7
阴性预测值（%）	未用	98	未用	99

* 表示 82% 患者；其余 18% 患者在更晚时间评价微伏级 T 波电交替。

近来一些前瞻性的关于微伏级 T 波电交替对心梗预后预测价值的研究出现了有争议的结果。Ikeda 等[29]入选 102 位心梗后幸存者，分析了微伏级 T 波电交替和信号平均电图记录到的晚电位，98% 患者接受了冠脉介入治疗，31% 患者接受 β 受体阻滞剂治疗。微伏级 T 波电交替阳性率高于其他心梗研究中报道的比例（50/102；49%）。在随访的 13±6 个月中，45 位患者出现持续室速/室颤，但其中只有 1 位微伏级 T 波电交替阳性。微伏级 T 波电交替阳性单独预测心律失常事件的危险值为 28%，微伏级 T 波电交替阳性联合晚电位阳性的预测值为 50%。

在另一项前瞻性的随访研究中，入选 379 位心梗后幸存患者，评价微伏级 T 波电交替和其他无创性危险指标预测的价值[30]。其中 133 位患者（35%）未完成试验（56 位不能进行运动试验，77 位目标心率低于 105 次/分）。仅在 14.7%（56 位）患者中检测微伏级 T 波电交替阳性，38%（144 位）阴性，12%（46 位）不确定性。值得注意的是，97% 患者接受 β 受体阻滞剂治疗，2% 接受胺碘酮治疗。微伏级 T 波电交替阳性不是所有致命事件的预测因子，然而，不能完成微伏级 T 波电交替检测是心脏性死亡的一项重要的预测因子[30]。这一研究有两个重要的缺陷。第一，在心梗后 8 天进行微伏级 T 波电交替检测，此时微伏级 T 波电交替尚处于不稳定状态[28]。第二，研究的终点是心脏性死亡，而微伏级 T 波电交替仅对心律失常事件有预测价值（对心衰死亡无预测价值）。

Ikeda 等[31]最近发表了一项大型研究，该项研究入选 850 例患者（平均左室射血分数 51%±13%），在心梗亚急性期对微伏级 T 波电交替和晚电位进行评价。82% 患者在心梗后 2～10 周检测微伏级 T 波电交替，18% 在数月后进行检测。检测时，仅 13% 患者接受 β 受体阻滞剂治疗[31]。36% 患者微伏级 T 波电交替阳性，52% 患者阴性，微伏级 T 波电交替［危险比率

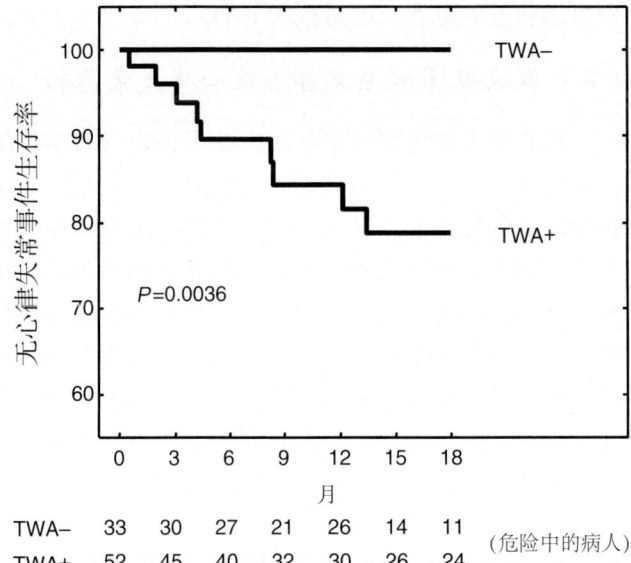

图 91-3　充血性心衰患者微伏级 T 波电交替阳性或阴性对其无心律失常生存（Kaplan-Meier 分析）的影响　（引自 Klingenheben T，Zabel M，D'Agostino RB，et al：Predictive value of T wave alternans for arrhythmic events in patients with congestive heart failure. Lancet 356：651-652，2000.）

11.4%（95%可信区间3.4～37.9）]和左室射血分数［危险比率6.6（95%可信区间3.0～14.6）]是对试验研究终点有显著预测价值的因素，主要试验终点为猝死或室颤并电复律，次级终点为持续室速。微伏级T波电交替和左室射血分数联合应用提高了对主要终点事件预测的准确性。

总之，上述研究结果表明，微伏级T波电交替对心梗后幸存者室性心律失常事件具有预测价值。然而，心梗亚急性期内微伏级T波电交替尚处于进展阶段，用来预测预后的微伏级T波电交替检测应在心梗数周之后进行。因而，在心梗患者的随访过程中检测微伏级T波电交替最为便利。

（四）微伏级T波电交替在充血性心力衰竭患者中的应用

充血性心力衰竭具有很高的猝死率和心律失常性死亡率。但常规的危险分层因素如自发性室性心律失常、自律性检测指标、电生理检查等未能对心律失常事件提供充分可靠的预测信息。另一方面，近期多中心的MADIT Ⅱ（Multicenter Automatic Defibrillator Implantation Trial Ⅱ）试验[32]评价了心梗后左室射血分数≤0.3，无自发性和可诱发性持续室性心动过速病史的患者预防性植入ICD治疗的有效性。在20个月的随访过程中，ICD治疗减少绝对死亡率5.6%（从19.8%降低至14.2%）。在美国，每年确诊的冠心病伴进行性左室功能障碍病例大约为40万。对这些患者常规植入ICD十分昂贵[33]。因而，对这些患者进行有效的危险分层从而筛选出能从ICD治疗中获益的病例有十分重要的意义[33a]。因而，分析微伏级T波电交替有助于筛选出有高危猝死可能的充血性心力衰竭患者，植入ICD治疗。

Adachi等[34]的研究入选58例扩张型心肌病患者，23例微伏级T波电交替阳性，25例阴性，10例不确定性。对有限的室性心律失常记录进行分析，其中包括非持续性室速（14阵），持续性室速（3阵）。结果表明，室性心律失常在微伏级T波电交替阳性患者中更常见。随后，对104例有扩张性心肌病患者进行了21±14个月的随访研究[35]。在发作心率低于100次/分的患者亚群中，微伏级T波电交替是预测患者心律失常事件的最有意义的预测因素（敏感性75%，阳性预测值37.5%）。Klingenheben等[26]进行了一项前瞻性研究，入选107例充血性心力衰竭患者，NYHA分级Ⅱ～Ⅲ级，左室射血分数＜0.46，其中40例为非缺血性心肌病患者，67例为缺血性心肌病患者（图91-3）。在18个月的随访过程中，7位患者突然死亡，5位患者出现持续性室速，1位出现持续室颤并电复律，而3位患者死于难治性心衰。49%患者微伏级T波电交替阳性，31%阴性，21%为不确定性。多变量Cox回归分析显示，所有危险分层因素中，只有微伏级T波电交替是有统计学意义的心律失常事件的独立预测因子。微伏级T波电交替阴性患者发生室速的危险性非常低，这一结果有着同样重要的意义。在另外一个入选34例充血性心力衰竭患者的小型研究中，在随访过程中，比较微伏级T波电交替（测量暂时性复极的指标）和QT离散度（测量空间复极异常的指标）对自发室速（连续5次室早以上）的预测价值[36]。QT离散度没有预测价值，而微伏级T波电交替则是有意义的危险分层指标，微伏级T波电交替阳性预测值为54%，阴性预测值为100%。我们研究所近期的一项研究入选137例扩张性心肌病患者，证实了微伏级T波电交替是心律失常事件的独立预测因子[36a]。

总之，缺血或非缺血因素所致充血性心力衰竭患者中，微伏级T波电交替是重要的危险分层指标，主要用于预测这些患者出现心律失常事件，包括猝死的可能性。微伏级T波电交替试验结果（尤其阴性预测价值高）有助于筛选出能从ICD这种昂贵的治疗方法中可能获益的患者，进而植入ICD。

（五）微伏级T波电交替与抗心律失常药物

抗心律失常药物治疗对微伏级T波电交替能产生一定的调节作用。特别是延长心室复极的抗心律失常药物影响复极交替。Kavesh等[37]前瞻性的研究入选24例可诱发持续室速的患者，评价在未用药物的基础状态下和急性药物负荷状态下，普鲁卡因酰胺对微伏级T波电交替的影响。在窦性心率下，普鲁卡因酰胺使微伏级T波电交替的幅度从0.6±0.8μV降至0.3±0.4μV，在100ppm心房起搏时，从2.0±1.6μV降至0.7±0.7μV；在120ppm心房起搏时，从3.0±2.0μV降至1.7±1.8μV（$P<0.001$）。在心率120次/分时，微伏级T波电交替预测持续性室速的敏感性从87%降至60%。

一项关于植入ICD患者的回顾性研究[38]中，分析了Ⅲ类抗心律失常药物胺碘酮对微伏级T波电交替的影响。在这项研究中，植入ICD并服用胺碘酮的9例患者中，仅有1例（11%）微伏级T波电交替阳性，而植入ICD未服用胺碘酮的22例患者中，14例

（64%）微伏级 T 波电交替阳性。在随访过程中，微伏级 T 波电交替阳性能预测患者将发生室性心律失常，并需要植入 ICD。

在另一个前瞻性随机研究中，入选 54 例患者，评价在未用药的基础状态下和急性静脉应用左旋索他洛尔或美托洛尔情况时，检测微伏级 T 波电交替[39]。用药后，所有入选患者的交替电压比用药前均显著降低，从 $8.4\pm6.4\mu V$ 降至 $4.7\pm3.3\mu V$（$P<0.001$），冠心病亚组患者中，交替电压从 $8.2\pm6.8\mu V$ 降至 $4.5\pm3.5\mu V$（$P<0.001$）。应用美托洛尔的患者中，用药前交替电压为 $7.9\pm6.0\mu V$，用药后降至 $4.9\pm4.2\mu V$（$P<0.001$）。应用左旋索他洛尔的患者中，用药前交替电压为 $8.6\pm6.8\mu V$，用药后降至 $4.4\pm2.3\mu V$（$P=0.001$）。在所有患者中，出现微伏级 T 波电交替的心率在基础状态下和用药后基本一致，应用美托洛尔患者用药前后心率为 94 ± 8 次/分和 95 ± 7 次/分（$P=0.86$），应用左旋索他洛尔患者用药前后心率为 99 ± 10 次/分和 98 ± 12 次/分（$P=0.83$）。48 例基础状态下微伏级 T 波电交替阳性患者中，8 例患者用药后微伏级 T 波电交替转为阴性，其中 5 例应用了美托洛尔，3 例应用左旋索他洛尔。值得注意的是，这 8 例患者基础状态下的交替电压低于应用 β 受体阻滞剂治疗后微伏级 T 波电交替仍为阳性的患者基础状态下的交替电压（分别为 $4.1\pm1.4\mu V$ 和 $9.2\pm6.7\mu V$；$P=0.026$）。应用 β 受体阻滞剂治疗降低患者交替电压的幅度小于 $2\mu V$。

Rashba 等[40]报道了不同的研究结果，对一些可诱发室速或室颤的缺血性心肌病并接受起搏治疗的患者，在基础状态和应用药物后评价微伏级 T 波电交替。20 例患者中，应用艾司洛尔（作用时间极短的 β 受体阻滞剂）前，患者微伏级 T 波电交替阳性率为 70%，用药后降至 35%（$P<0.05$）。这一研究中，应用 β 受体阻滞剂后，最大交替电压幅度降低的结果与 Klingenheben 等的研究结果相同[39]。但 Rashba 等[40]的研究中，应用 β 受体阻滞剂后微伏级 T 波电交替阳性率显著降低，而在 Klingenheben 等[39]的研究中并不显著降低的原因尚不明确。众所周知，β 受体阻滞剂能够减少发生自发性室性心律失常的危险，上述试验证实，β 受体阻滞剂也能减轻微伏级 T 波电交替。由于作用于心脏的药物能改变微伏级 T 波电交替，并能改变自发性室性心律失常的易患性，在用药期间检测微伏级 T 波电交替，并用来对患者进行危险分层具有十分重要的意义。当换用其他药物后，需要重新检测微伏级 T 波电交替，从而确定复极交替是否发生了改变。

六、微伏级 T 波电交替的应用前景

过去几年中，对有室性心动过速危险的患者进行微伏级 T 波电交替检测的方法学方面取得了显著进步。目前，应用运动平板和踏车等无创方法检测微伏级 T 波电交替，而且检测结果十分准确可靠。在多项关于微伏级 T 波电交替的研究中证实，对于一些重要的人群，微伏级 T 波电交替对发生室性心动过速具有重要的预测价值。这些人群包括可能经历室性心动过速的患者，左室功能障碍患者和心梗后患者。研究结果也表明，微伏级 T 波电交替对这些患者具有非常好的阴性预测价值，即微伏级 T 波电交替阴性的患者发生持续室性心动过速的危险性很低，可以进行保守治疗。相反，对微伏级 T 波电交替阳性的患者，需要进一步评价是否需要进行预防性治疗。将来需要进行一些前瞻性的研究来证实，在上述患者中，如果仅以微伏级 T 波电交替阳性作为标准对患者进行预防性治疗，是否能够改善预后还需进一步资料证实。

（陈 琪 译）

参 考 文 献

1. Hering HE: Das Wesen des Herzalternans. Muench Med Wochenschr 4:1417-1421, 1908.
2. Lewis T: Notes upon alternation of the heart. Q J Med 4:141-144, 1910.
3. Kalter HH, Schwartz ML: Electrical alternans. NY State J Med 1:1164-1166, 1948.
4. Amoundas AA, Tomaselli GF, Esperer HD: Pathophysiological basis and clinical application of T-wave alternans. J Am Coll Cardiol 40:207-217, 2002.
5. Schwartz PJ, Malliani A: Electrical alternation of the T wave: Clinical and experimental evidence of its relationship with the sympathetic nervous system and with the long-QT syndrome. Am Heart J 89:45-50, 1975.
6. Adam DR, Powell AO, Gordon H, Cohen RJ: Ventricular fibrillation and fluctuations in the magnitude of the repolarization vector. IEEE Comp Cardiol 241-244, 1982.
7. Smith JM, Clancy EA, Valeri CR, et al: Electrical alternans and cardiac electrical instability. Circulation 77:110-121, 1988.
8. Nearing B, Huang HA, Verrier RL: Dynamic tracking of cardiac vulnerability by complex demodulation of the T wave. Science 252:437-440, 1991.
9. Pastore JM, Girouard SD, Laurita KR, et al: Mechanism linking T-wave alternans to the genesis of cardiac fibrillation. Circulation 99:1385-1394, 1999.
10. Qu Z, Garfinkel A, Chen P-S, Weiss JN: Mechanism of discordant alternans and induction of reentry in simulated cardiac tissue. Circulation 102:1664-1670, 2000.
11. Pastore JM, Rosenbaum DS: Role of structural barriers in the mechanism of alternans-induced reentry. Circ Res 87:1157-1163, 2000.

12. Berger RD: Repolarization alternans. Toward a unifying theory of reentrant arrhythmia induction. Circ Res 87:1083–1084, 2000.
13. Walker ML, Rosenbaum DS: Repolarization alternans: Implications for the mechanism and prevention of sudden cardiac death. Cardiovasc Res 57:599–614, 2003.
14. Shimizu W, Antzelevitch C: Cellular and ionic basis for T-wave alternans under long-QT conditions. Circulation 99:1499–1507, 1999.
15. Chudin E, Goldhaber JI, Weiss J, Kogan B: Intracellular Ca dynamics and the stability of ventricular tachycardia. Biophys J 77:2930–2941, 1999.
16. Hüser J, Wang YG, Sheehan KA, et al: Functional coupling between glycolysis and excitation-contraction coupling underlies alternans in cat heart cells. J Physiol 524:795–806, 2000.
17. Laurita KR, Singal A, Pastore JM, Rosenbaum DS: Spatial heterogeneity of calcium transients may explain action potential dispersion during T-wave alternans [abstract]. Circulation 98(suppl I):I-187, 1998.
18. Zarebra W, Moss AJ, le Cessie S, Hall WJ: T-wave alternans in idiopathic long QT syndrome. J Am Coll Cardiol 23:1541–1546, 1994.
19. Rosenbaum DS, Jackson LE, Smith JM, et al: Electrical alternans and vulnerability to ventricular arrhythmias. N Engl J Med 330:235–241, 1994.
20. Hohnloser SH, Klingenheben T, Zabel M, et al: T wave alternans during exercise and atrial pacing in humans. J Cardiovasc Electrophysiol 8:987–993, 1997.
21. Estes MNA, Michaud G, Zipes DP, et al: Electrical alternans during rest and exercise as predictors of vulnerability to ventricular arrhythmias. Am J Cardiol 80:1314–1318, 1997.
22. Rashba EJ, Osman AF, MacMurdy K, et al: Exercise is superior to pacing for T wave alternans measurement in subjects with chronic coronary artery disease and left ventricular dysfunction. J Cardiovasc Electrophysiol 13:845–850, 2002.
23. Bloomfield DM, Hohnloser SH, Cohen RJ: Interpretation and classification of microvolt T wave alternans tests. J Cardiovasc Electrophysiol 13:502–512, 2002.
24. Hohnloser SH, Klingenheben T, Li YG, et al: T wave alternans as a predictor of recurrent ventricular tachyarrhythmias in ICD recipients: Prospective comparison with conventional risk markers. J Cardiovasc Electrophysiol 9:1258–1268, 1998.
25. Gold MR, Bloomfield DM, Anderson KP, et al: A comparison of T-wave alternans, signal averaged electrocardiography and programmed ventricular stimulation for arrhythmia risk stratification. J Am Coll Cardiol 36:2247–2253, 2000.
26. Klingenheben T, Zabel M, D'Agostino RB, et al: Predictive value of T-wave alternans for arrhythmic events in patients with congestive heart failure. Lancet 356:651–652, 2000.
27. Bloomfield DM, Ritvo BS, Parides MK, Kim MH: The immediate reproducibility of T wave alternans during bicycle exercise. Pacing Clin Electrophysiol 25:1185–1191, 2002.
28. Hohnloser SH, Huikuri H, Schwartz PJ, et al: T-wave alternans in post myocardial infarction patients (ACES Pilot Study) [abstract]. J Am Coll Cardiol 1999; 33:144A.
29. Ikeda T, Sakata T, Takami M, et al: Combined assessment of T-wave alternans and late potentials used to predict arrhythmic events after myocardial infarction. J Am Coll Cardiol 35:722–730, 2000.
30. Tapanainen JM, Still AM, Airaksinen KEJ, Huikuri HV: Prognostic significance of risk stratifiers of mortality, including T-wave alternans, after acute myocardial infarction: Results of a prospective follow-up study. J Cardiovasc Electrophysiol 12:645–652, 2001.
31. Ikeda T, Saito H, Tanno K, et al: T-wave alternans as a predictor for sudden cardiac death after myocardial infarction. Am J Cardiol 89:79–82, 2002.
32. Moss AJ, Zarebra W, Jackson W, et al: Prophylactic implantation of a defibrillator in patients with myocardial infarction and reduced ejection fraction. N Engl J Med 346:877–883, 2002.
33. Bigger JT: Expanding indications for implantable cardiac defibrillators. N Engl J Med 346:931–933, 2002.
33a. Hohnloser SH, Ikeda T, Bloomfield D, et al: T-wave alternans negative coronary patients with low ejection fraction and benefit from defibrillator implantation. Lancet 362:125–126, 2003.
34. Adachi K, Ohnishi Y, Shima T, et al: Determinant of microvolt-level T-wave alternans in patients with dilated cardiomyopathy. J Am Coll Cardiol 34:374–380, 1999.
35. Kitamura H, Ohnishi Y, Okajima K, et al: Onset heart rate of microvolt-level T-wave alternans provides clinical and prognostic value in nonischemic dilated cardiomyopathy. J Am Coll Cardiol 39:295–300, 2002.
36. Sakabe K, Ikeda T, Sakata T, et al: Comparison of T-wave alternans and QT interval dispersion to predict ventricular tachyarrhythmia in patients with dilated cardiomyopathy and without antiarrhythmic drugs: A prospective study. Jpn Heart J 42:451–457, 2001.
36a. Hohnloser SH, Klingenheben T, Bloomfield D, et al: Usefulness of microvolt T-wave alternans for prediction of ventricular tachyarrhythmic events in patients with dilated cardiomyopathy: results from a prospective observational study. J Am Coll Cardiol 41:2220–2224, 2003.
37. Kavesh NG, Shorofsky SR, Sarang SE, Gold MR: The effect of procainamide on T wave alternans. J Cardiovasc Electrophysiol 10:649–654, 1999.
38. Groh WJ, Shinn TS, Engelstein EE, Zipes DP: Amiodarone reduces the prevalence of T wave alternans in a population with ventricular tachyarrhythmias. J Cardiovasc Electrophysiol 10:1335–1339, 1999.
39. Klingenheben T, Grönefeld G, Li YG, Hohnloser SH: Effect of metoprolol and d,l-sotalol on microvolt-level T-wave alternans. J Am Coll Cardiol 38:2013–2019, 2001.
40. Rashba EJ, Cooklin M, MacMurdy K, et al: Effects of selective autonomic blockade on T-wave alternans in humans. Circulation 105:837–842, 2002.

第92章

心脏神经成像

Gary D. Hutchins, Michael A. Miller, and Douglas P. Zipes

本章目录
- 自主神经系统概述 ……………… 833
- 放射性药物 ……………………… 834
- 计算机断层成像原理 …………… 835
- 自主神经系统功能的定量测定 … 836
- 实验和临床观察 ………………… 837
- 参阅文献 ………………………… 841
- 总结 ……………………………… 841
- 致谢 ……………………………… 841

日常正常生理情况下，自主神经系统（ANS）在保证心血管功能的正常运行中起着十分重要的作用。冠心病、心肌肥大、心肌病以及各种电生理异常时，自主神经系统的兴奋与抑制的平衡常遭到破坏。由于缺乏有效的检测工具，很难评价在体心脏的自主神经功能。测定血浆中的儿茶酚胺浓度有助于评价心脏的自主神经功能，但测定时需要长时间心脏放置导管，且不能评价局部自主神经的功能。另一种研究自主神经功能的途径是注射影响心脏生理状态的药物，然后观察心血管系统产生的反应，这种方法也不能将心血管病变引起变化的心肌组织与未受影响的心肌组织区分开来。放射性药物的研究进展不仅有助于传统核医学的发展，同时使正电子发射计算机断层成像技术（PET）评价心脏局部自主神经系统的功能成为可能[1,2]。这些以成像技术为基础，包括心脏病学、放射学、医用化学、医用物理学、药理学、生物化学和生理学等多学科联合的技术，使评价在体心脏生理功能成为可能。应用这些成像技术，可以测定心脏局部自主神经的分布和功能的变化。本章内容在原第三版第89章的基础上进行更新，综述了用于评价心脏自主神经的成像技术以及当前一些实验与临床研究的发现。此外，我们还增加了关于新近研发的示踪剂及其相关的重要文献。

一、自主神经系统概述

自主神经通过交感神经和迷走神经两大系统调节心率、心肌收缩力和心脏传导。交感神经兴奋使心率增加、心肌收缩力增强、心脏传导加速。相反，迷走神经对心脏产生抑制作用，使心率减慢、心肌收缩力减弱、心脏的传导速度减慢。这两大系统都是通过释放心脏神经递质与局部心肌细胞和神经元上的受体相结合而发挥效应的。交感神经、迷走神经释放的神经递质分别是去甲肾上腺素和乙酰胆碱。这些神经递质通过受体介导的过程兴奋（去甲肾上腺素）或抑制（乙酰胆碱）腺苷酸环化酶而发挥其对心脏的作用。神经递质的合成、释放、与蛋白受体位点的结合、神经递质通过代谢降解失活、突触前神经递质的摄取和储存等过程，都为应用放射性药物标记自主神经成像技术提供靶目标。这些过程的原理可用示意图表示（图92-1）。

研究表明和冠状动脉一样，交感神经纤维也是沿着心室外膜表面走行，其分支穿透到心室肌内[3]（图92-2）；相反，迷走神经的分布则是从心室外膜表面直接进入心内膜，主要分布于心内膜（图92-2）。交感神经在左室分布密集，心底部的密度高于心尖部[3]、在左室心内膜的密度高于心外膜[3]。可以通过测定局部去甲肾上腺素的浓度了解心脏交感神经的分布情

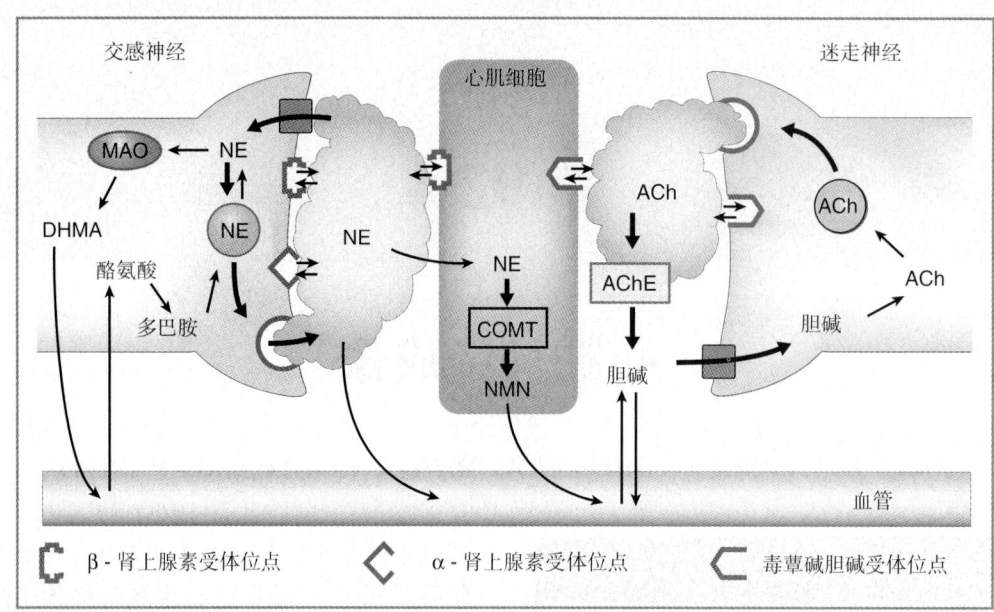

图 92-1 自主神经系统 本原理图显示了自主神经系统的神经递质的合成、释放、再摄取的有关机制。该系统部分控制心率、心肌收缩力和心脏的传导速度。图解上所有的过程都代表了放射性药物探针的靶目标。ACh：乙酰胆碱；AChE：乙酰胆碱酯酶；COMT：邻苯二酚-O-甲基转移酶；DBH：多巴胺-β-羟化酶；DHMA：3，4-二羟扁桃酸；MAO：单胺氧化酶；NE：去甲肾上腺素；NMN：去甲甲基麻黄素。

况。去甲肾上腺素主要的受体（β-肾上腺受体）与突触前神经分布不同，后者在心外膜下层的密度高于心内膜下层，而且从心尖到心底密度逐渐减小。迷走神经主要分布在心房，而在心室内分布稀少。迷走神经的分布可以通过测定乙酰胆碱转移酶的浓度而获得。乙酰胆碱通过作用于毒蕈碱胆碱能受体，抑制心脏的变时性和变力性，心室内的毒蕈碱受体位于肌纤维膜上。

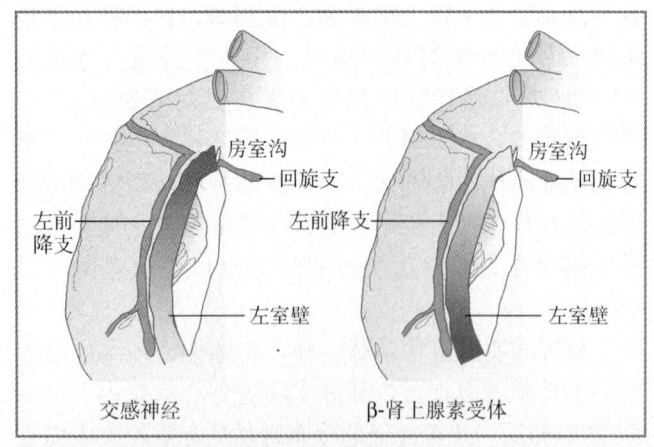

图 92-2 交感神经在左室分布的模式 该图是左室矢状面交感神经元和 β-肾上腺素受体分布的示意图。交感神经在左室心底部分布密集，而在心尖部，其密度有所降低。β-肾上腺素受体的分布则相反，在心尖部密度高而在心底部密度较低。

二、放射性药物

用于自主神经系统成像的放射性药物的特异性靶目标，主要是针对突触前神经递质的摄取和储存、突触后受体位点的相互作用这两个过程。无论哪一种途径，放射性药物需经静脉给药、经血液循环运输到机体组织。一旦这些示踪剂传送至靶器官，它们需经过弥散或特殊的转运机制透过毛细血管膜。在通过毛细血管膜时，示踪剂应该与特异性的、亲和力相对高的靶目标蛋白质位点结合。为能有效地到达特异性蛋白质结合位点、并在组织内具有一定的分布区域和浓聚密度，放射性药物必须具有以下特点[4,5]：

1. 饱和性：无论是用于摄取转运还是用于与受体结合的蛋白质位点的数目都是有限的。因此，当注射高浓度特异性放射性药物时，与这些蛋白质相关的结合必须是饱和的。如果不饱和，示踪剂的聚集程度就不能反映其与特异性蛋白质位点的相互作用情况。

2. 特异性：理想情况下，一种放射性药物只能与一个单一的蛋白质位点结合。如果放射性药物能和多个蛋白位点结合，要分离和量化各种类型的相互作用就会变得相当复杂和困难。

3. 空间选择性：神经递质与蛋白质的摄取转运或

受体位点的相互作用具有特异的空间选择性。相反，非特异性的放射性药物的结合或相互作用不依赖于分子的空间构向。

4. 亲和力：一般情况下，用于成像目的的放射性配体只与高亲和力的目标蛋白质位点结合。蛋白质位点的高亲和力有助于确保该脏器、组织或病变与邻近组织之间形成明显的放射性浓度差。

5. 生物分布：放射性药物的生物分布在组织内部与相邻组织之间必须存在足够显著的差异。例如，对心脏进行成像时，血池清除速率应快于放射性药物在心肌内的代谢速度。邻近器官，如肺和肝脏，应该仅有很少量的示踪剂聚集，以减少背景信号对心脏成像的干扰。

6. 与生物效应的相关性：放射性药物结合率是否与特异性生理反应之间具有良好的相关性，是选择特异性放射药物的一个重要标准。如果二者之间没有良好的相关性，就很难根据生理反应鉴别放射性药物是与特异性还是非特异性蛋白质位点结合。

7. 代谢抵抗：内源性神经递质在内源酶的作用下经过降解而快速失活。如果用于成像的放射性药物降解速率很慢，将有助于简化放射性核素图像的阅读。然而，即使靶器官内放射性标记代谢产物的聚集浓度不够，仍然可以有效地进行成像。

8. 药代动力学：一个理想的用于成像的示踪剂，其摄取和清除速率必须受与特殊蛋白质位点结合频率的限制。许多有希望的放射性药物不能达到预期的效果是由于示踪剂与特殊蛋白质位点的特异性结合速度过快，使得血流或示踪剂的摄取、清除成为主要限速步骤。当然，亲和力过低的放射性核素也不好，这样，示踪剂的特异性聚集不足以使特殊示踪剂与蛋白质位点的相互作用显示出来。因此，示踪剂必须有足够高的亲和力以克服诊断特异性的限制，但却又不能过高，以免示踪剂摄取和清除变成主要的限速步骤。

9. 毒性：在成像研究中注射用的低剂量放射性激动剂或拮抗剂必须无毒。

现已成功将基本或完全符合上述特点的放射性药物用于体内心脏自主神经的成像。目前，用于评估肾上腺系统突触前功能的放射性药物的研发领先于评价突触后功能的药物。目前，已开发的用于评价自主神经功能的放射性药物包括：内源性神经递质或与其密切相关的一类衍生物以及称为假神经递质的一类复合物。其中，作为探针用于评价交感神经突触前功能的化合物包括：^{123}I-间碘苯甲胍、^{11}C-m-对羟麻黄碱（HED）、^{18}F-间羟胺、^{18}F-荧光多巴胺、^{18}F-荧光去甲肾上腺素、^{11}C-去氧肾上腺素[6,7]，[^{11}C]-(-)-α-α-dideutero-去氧肾上腺素、^{18}F-荧光苯甲基胍、^{18}F-para-荧光苯甲基胍、4-[^{18}F]-荧光-3-碘代-苯甲基胍、^{76}Br-bromobenzylguanidine，肾上腺素，^{11}C-去甲肾上腺素、^{11}C-硝基甲烷、^{11}C-多巴胺、^{11}C-metariminol。其中，只有MIBG和HED这两种药物能产生高对比度的心肌成像，目前已广泛应用于人体试验。市场上可供的产品有日本、欧洲生产的[^{123}I]MIBG和美国生产的[^{121}I]MIBG，已有大量的应用这两种产品进行的MIBG心脏成像研究。尽管应用放射性标记的vesamicol和benzovesamicol进行的动物实验，展示其在迷走神经成像这一领域可能具有一定的前景，但尚未能开发出能在人体试验中证实有效地用于标记迷走神经突触前的放射性药物。未能成功研发出迷走神经突触前标记物的部分原因是胆碱代谢为乙酰胆碱并储存在囊泡内的这一过程的高选择性[2]。此外，由于迷走神经在心室内分布很稀疏，也难以从大量的非选择性聚集的示踪剂中区分出来。

作用于突触后受体位点示踪剂的研发最初主要集中在拮抗剂，因为拮抗剂的亲和力一般高于激动剂。已经开发并经过验证的用于PET成像的化合物包括：^{11}C-和^{18}F-标记的醋氨心安、心得安、荧光咔唑心安、^{11}C-CGP 12177，^{11}C-CGP 12388[8]。最近，又致力于合成^{123}I-标记的β-肾上腺素受体拮抗剂[9]。遗憾的是，^{123}I-标记的复合物未能符合一定的前述的放射性药物标准，因此尚未进入临床前试验。目前只有^{11}C-CGP 12177应用于人体PET成像研究。目前，又研发了几种放射性标记的拮抗剂用于研究迷走神经系统的毒蕈碱胆碱受体[2]，其中，仅有亲水配基的^{11}C-N-甲基奎宁环基苯甲酸（MQNB）常规应用于临床。

三、计算机断层成像原理

随着核医学成像技术的发展，目前可应用单光子发射计算机断层成像（SPECT）与正电子发射计算机断层成像（PET）技术，通过测量机体局部放射性药物浓度的动态变化，无创地评价自主神经的分布和功能。这两项技术都是在一系列全身投射成像的基础上形成放射性核素在心脏分布的三维（3D）成像。SPECT成像，把能够放出γ光子的放射性核素或药物注入体内，该物质在体内的分布与局部血流量成正比，即核素浓集于血流丰富的组织中，发出γ射线，由γ照相机接受以确定体内光子的含量（图92-3）。γ照相机围绕躯体作180°或360°的自动旋转，对体内的γ光子进行多角度的探测，计算机采集大量信息，从而能精确重建各种断层影像（图92-3）。现代的SPECT系统具有多个γ照相机，可以同时测量多个投影以减少采集数据所需要的时间。而在PET系统，探测器接收体内正负电子湮没辐射所产生的一对511-keV光子（图92-4）。当正电发射的放射性核素衰减时，细胞核内的光子转变成中子，此时的正电荷释放出来成为正电子（一种和电子有相同的静质量和自旋转的质粒，但带的是正电荷而非负电荷）。正电子发射的放射性核素持续增加，到终点时达最高能量。因此每种放射性核素终点能量不同，据此则可确定放射性核素正电子在组织内运行的平均距离。一般情况下，正电子在组织中最多能运行几个毫米的距离，通过与组织化学成分相关的电子和光子之间静电作用而消耗能量。随着正电子的能量丢失，它们与电子结合的可能性就会增加，从而形成一种氢样实体，称为正电子素（配对的正电子-电子）。正电子素很不稳定，会在数十纳秒内衰变，称为湮没92（完全将质量转化为能量）。在正电子素的湮没中，储存的能量和动能使两个511-keV光子朝180°相反方向运动。PET依靠许多环形排列的探测器，在躯体四周同时进行探测，记录这些光子同时到达放在患者周围的探测系统的情

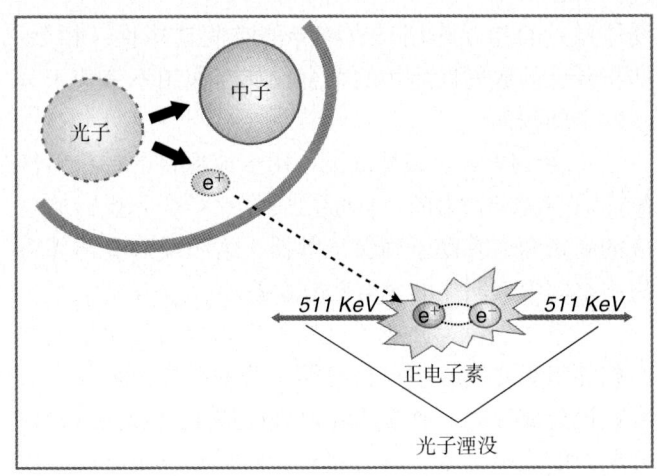

图92-4　正电子发射放射核素衰减过程　正电子发射的放射性核素由于细胞核内有过多的正电荷（即光子/中子混合体不平衡）而很不稳定。这些放射性核素的一种衰减模式是将光子转化为中子释放正电荷后形成正电子，正电子结合一个电子形成正电子素。正电子迅速湮没，质粒的质量转化为能量形成2个朝180°相反方向运动的511-keV光子。

况，能够对产生这种发射的位置进行三维定位，从而得到高质量的图像（图92-5）。PET的独一无二的优势在于可以同时从所有投射角度测量计算机断层影像。通过发展测定光子在组织中分散度技术，SPECT和PET成像技术可以得到放射性核素在组织中分布的定量资料。

四、自主神经系统功能的定量测定

欲隔离特异性的放射性药物与蛋白质相互作用位点，评定蛋白密度和亲和力或者评定神经传递系统的功能，需要运用数学模型[16]。已被用来分离这些相互作用位点的方法包括评定给药后在组织中某个点示踪剂的聚集水平（通常指示踪剂聚集或部分聚集），通过隔离代表实验过程的参数进行参数拟合以描述放射性药物动力学。这两种方法都需要组织放射性核素浓度的定量数据，这些数据通过目前的PET和SPECT成像技术可以获得。通过SPECT成像技术运用参数模型一直有局限，因为在许多SPECT系统中，由于技术的局限阻碍了对组织中快速变化的放射性核素浓度的测定。在PET研究中用来分析动力学的两类参数模型分别是区间模型和弥散模型[10]。弥散模型根据一系列线形或非线形过程描述放射性药物的动力学。对由大量参数组成的弥散模型进行可靠的评估一般比较困难，因为由X线体层摄影系统测量的一系列时间维数据有较高水平的统计干扰。为了克服这些局限

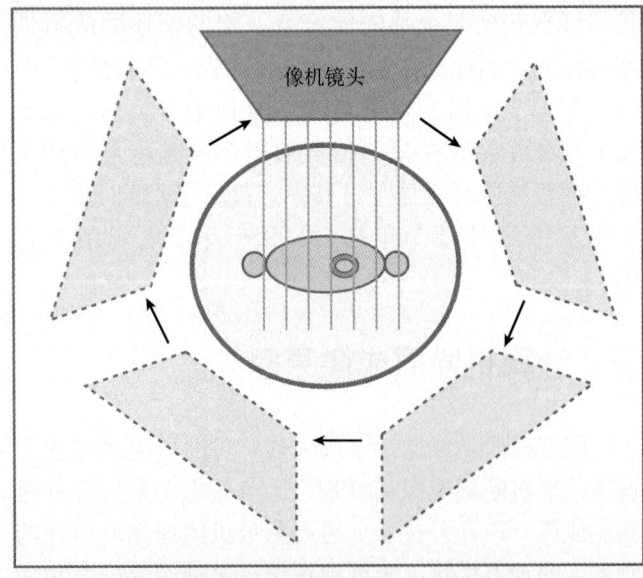

图92-3　单光子发射计算机断层成像（SPECT）的几何示意图　γ照相机成像系统围绕躯体旋转，采集一系列投影影像。这些采集来的投影影像的数据用于产生机体的计算机断层成像。

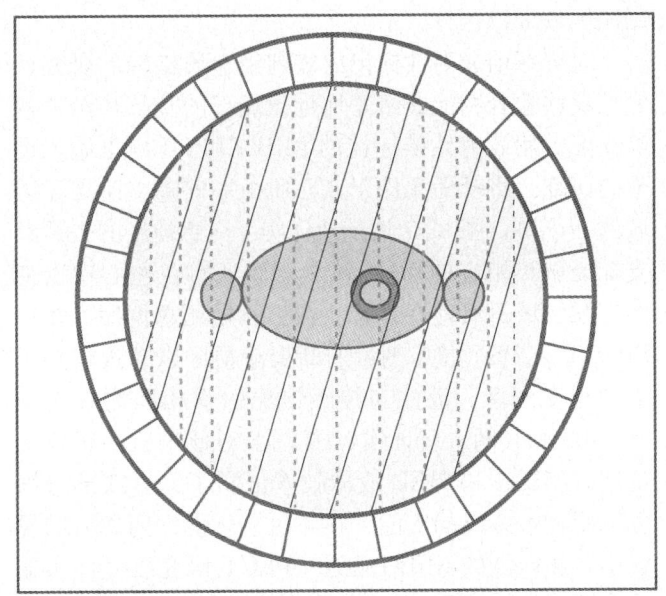

图 92-5 正电子发射计算机断层成像技术（PET）的几何示意图 环形排列的探测器用于探测从正电子-电子湮没时产生的光子同时到达探测系统的情况，能够同时采集和再建计算机断层成像所需的所有投射资料。

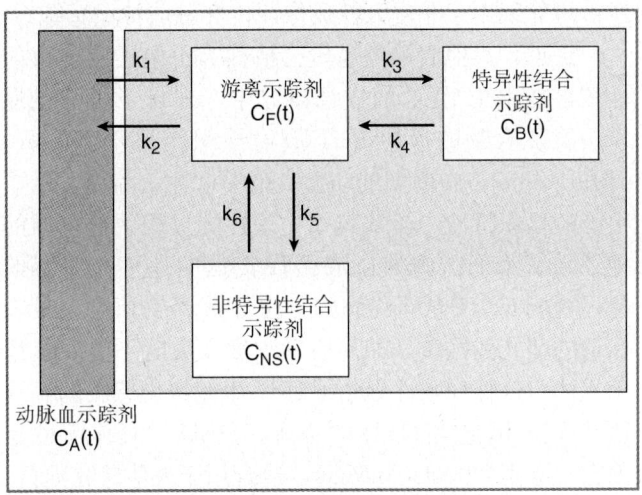

图 92-6 心脏神经成像的区间模型 模型显示了三种典型的组织分区，这些分区分别代表组织内游离的、尚未与组织结合的示踪剂；特异性地与相关的蛋白质位点结合的示踪剂；以及与非特异性蛋白位点结合的示踪剂。$K_1 \sim K_6$ 常数用于描述每一种分区之间的相互转化。常数 K_3 是指用于配基与受体位点结合或可供结合的位点数量的受体研究的结合潜能和结合力常数。在实践中，这一模式常被简化。

性，经常将这些模型简化到代表少量的示踪剂区间，用线性的一相动力学描叙示踪剂在区间的转移。图 92-6 所示为一个典型的常用于心脏神经成像的区间模型。这个模型由四个区间组成：一个区间代表从血液转向到组织的示踪剂浓度（$C_A[t]$），一个区间代表组织中游离的示踪剂浓度（$C_F[t]$），一个区间代表组织中结合的示踪剂浓度（$C_B[t]$），另一个区间代表组织中非特异结合的示踪剂浓度（$C_{NS}[t]$）。说明这些模型的方程式适合于局部组织的放射性核素浓度比时间曲线，可用以发现具体的实验参数。在图 92-6 所示的模型中，参数 K_3 是示踪剂与受体位点的亲和力以及组织中游离结合位点浓度的产物。在受体成像研究中，这个参数常被用来评估结合潜力。在某些情况下，仅知道结合潜力还不够，通过变化受体结合水平以及运用多种示踪剂注射液可以将示踪剂亲和力与受体位点浓度分离，这种模式在概念上类似于散点图的分析。

五、实验和临床观察

（一）突触前放射性示踪剂的研究

用于研究心脏自主神经系统的放射性药物一直主要是以"假神经递质"胍乙啶的放射性标记类似物为基础的。起初，溴苄胺和胍乙啶被证实能选择性地干预肾上腺素能神经的功能。基于这些发现，药物化学家们研制了一些与肾上腺素能系统相互作用有更高效能的化合物，这反过来促进了影像学中替代芳烷基胍的放射性碘的发展。这些化合物和去甲肾上腺素有同样的运输、储存和释放机制。然而，由于受体介导的相互作用，这些化合物激活突触后反应的能力显著下降，因此它们被归类为"假神经递质"。来自于这些化合物在影像学中应用最普遍的放射性药物是苯环结合有放射性碘的 MIBG。这个化合物已经被用于核医学和 SPECT 成像研究中。已经开展了大量的研究以证实 MIBG 对突触前交感神经功能和分布的定位能力。这些研究包括比较 MIBG 和内源性儿茶酚胺的生物学分布，药理性阻断研究量子式和囊泡式摄取机制以证实示踪剂摄取的特异性，进行实验性和药理性的交感神经切除术研究，研究示踪剂周转率评估交感紧张性功能，将局部摄取异常与心脏电生理改变进行联系，以及建立心脏疾病的实验模型进行研究。总的来说，这些研究通过药物阻滞和化学的或者手术的交感神经去神经支配后，证实了 MIBG 的摄取和聚集与散布于左心室的局部去甲肾上腺素水平相平行。然而，MIBG 和去甲肾上腺素的活动也存在一些微妙的差别，这些差别产生的机制有待阐明。尽管如此，MIBG 和去甲肾上腺素之间的相似性多于其差异性，MIBG 已经被可靠地用于非侵入性成像评价突触前神经系统。

最近，其他假神经递质已被称为正电子发射放射性核素并用于PET的成像研究中。来自于假神经递质一类化合物的最初PET放射性配体是6-^{18}fluorometaraminol。在前期的动物实验中这种示踪剂显示了很好的显影特性，能从其他生理性的过程区分特异的神经元示踪剂，例如血液循环转运的速率。遗憾的是，合成6-^{18}荧光间羟胺的方法导致产生相对大量未标记的荧光间羟胺，如果后者浓度太大时不能安全用于人体。这种局限性导致了对N-甲基拟交感胺的调查以及用^{11}C标记的HED的合成。HED的具体活性范围在500到2 000Ci/mM间，适合用于人体研究项目。遗憾的是，HED并没有展示像荧光标记的间羟胺时所观察到的理想特性。在豚鼠中检验HED代谢的研究证实仅仅为代谢的HED在心肌组织中聚集。但是，在血液研究中发现了两种代谢物（α-甲基肾上腺素、α-甲基肾上腺素的3-O-甲基衍生物）。与去甲肾上腺素的储存比较，突触前交感神经元内HED的积聚已被证实对囊泡储存系统的依赖性较小。两个具体的研究对此进行了证实。在第一个研究中，与对照组相比，用利舍平（一种囊泡摄取抑制剂）对心脏进行预处理后仅仅减少HED积聚的50%。在第二个研究中，HED在交感神经元中积聚后加入脱甲丙咪嗪能显著增加HED从组织中的洗脱率。这些研究表明HED在心肌组织中的积聚首先由完整的摄取机制所驱动。因为HED对线粒体单胺氧化酶引起的代谢具有耐受作用，它能不受影响而保存在细胞的胞质中，与去甲肾上腺素不一样。同时这些研究也证实HED从突触前交感神经元释放的终止至少在某种程度上并不依赖于与交感神经紧张密切相关的儿茶酚胺的释放率。HED已被成功运用于与心脏疾病相关的交感神经去神经支配和功能障碍的显影中。

最近对两种与HED相关的化合物进行了研究：[^{11}C]肾上腺素和[^{11}C]脱羟肾上腺素。虽然HED在神经元内出入循环，但[^{11}C]肾上腺素被迅速隔离在神经囊泡后会引起其缓慢代谢成[^{11}C]脱羟肾上腺素[13,14]。[^{11}C]脱羟肾上腺素已成为神经单胺氧化酶的示踪剂。对[^{11}C]脱羟肾上腺素清除的研究表明[^{11}C]脱羟肾上腺素也迅速聚集在囊泡中，但它紧接着又扩布到神经元的胞质中，被单胺氧化酶代谢为[^{11}C]甲胺[13]。这些示踪剂在心脏中清除的限速过程是其从神经囊泡中的逸出而不是单胺氧化酶代谢。因此，这些示踪剂并不能对去神经支配和囊泡功能受抑制的区域加以区分。

对突触前放射性标记的假神经递质摄取的研究证实，这些化合物能够清楚地标识局部的交感神经去神经支配。用放射性碘标记的MIBG和HED也做了类似的研究。将苯酚涂抹于犬心肌由左前降支所支配区域的一小块，图92-7清楚地证实了交感神经的去神经支配区域。相应的NH_3灌聚图像证实在左心室去神经支配区域仍然存在灌聚。在心肌梗死急性期，在用SPECT或PET技术测量的灌聚缺损区以外观察到了去神经支配区。灌注与神经支配的不相匹配首先由Stanton和其同事所证实，图92-8对此进行了很好的证明。MIBG和HED成像技术证实了完全或部分恢复交感神经系统的支配。在心肌梗死慢性期病人的研究中，相匹配的MIBG-灌注SPECT研究已经证实在心梗后2~6个月能部分恢复神经支配以及儿茶酚胺摄取率提高。有意思的是，心梗后交感神经系统复原或者恢复神经支配的时间窗和致死性心律失常高危险密切相关。少量的研究提示在缺血的左心室中，交感神经系统的功能异常存在于梗死区外周。Terada及其同事观察到在运动状态下的研究使静息状态下不相匹配的心肌部分转变为运动状态下相匹配的MIBG灌聚摄取缺损。虽然运动并非在所有病人中都产生这种影响，但该研究还是表明交感神经元和心肌细胞缺血阈并不是相同的。

已经开展了很多研究评估心衰时交感神经系统的功能。在心肌缺血，自发性心肌病，左室和右室肥厚，糖尿病神经损伤以及化疗引起的心脏毒性等病人中已经进行了相关研究。通过这些异常的病人，观察到了MIBG摄取正常或轻微减少的持续模式，接着伴有MIBG从组织中显著增高的洗脱率。用PET研究观察处于心衰期的心肌肥厚病人对HED的摄取和洗脱得到了同样的结果[11]。

与心脏移植相关联的心脏神经横断能引起全面的去神经支配。在对心脏移植受体心的研究中，用MIBG和HED对左心显影发现，与心梗病人恢复儿茶酚胺摄取时间相比，受体在左心需要在更长时间后才能部分恢复神经支配。在心脏移植后及时进行造影研究，发现MIBG和HED在心肌组织中的聚集水平显著降低。在心脏移植后的第13~24个月MIBG和HED的局部摄取增加。在这些研究中，神经支配恢复的模式局限于左室的前部和基底部。DiCarli和他的同事[11]证实接受心脏移植患者的心脏恢复神经支配的区域是功能性的，在冷加压实验引起心肌局部灌聚增

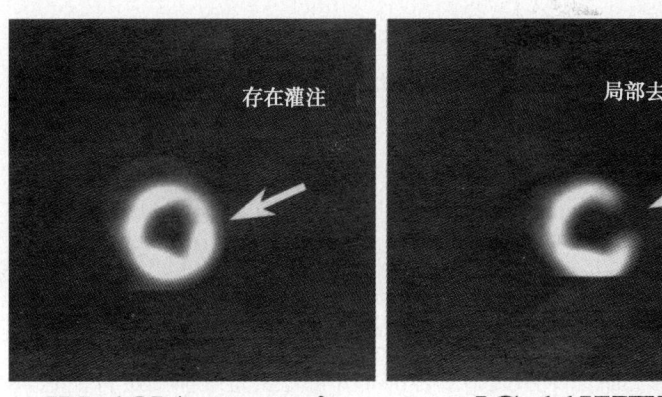

图92-7 犬去交感神经 图像显示在用苯酚局部去交感神经后心室中部短轴面 NH₃（灌注）和对羟麻黄碱（HED）显示交感神经分布的情况。（见彩图40）

加。

有多项旨在阐明患者电生理异常与交感神经恢复神经支配模式间关系的研究。这些研究发现有电生理异常的患者其电生理异质性与 MIBG 聚集的异质性相一致。这些病人包括长 QT 综合征（LQTS）。无器质性心脏病的室性心动过速、心肌病、左心室肥厚、瓣膜疾病、右心室疾病和心梗[1]。评价这些患者时发现：局部去交感神经的患者，核素灌注明显减少，这些患者出现电生理异常的比例增高。同时，局部交感神经分布与灌注比例增加之间不匹配的患者，出现电生理异常的比例也会明显增加。

一项研究[17]通过对缺血性心肌病和特发性心肌病患者进行 SPECT 的 MIBG 成像，以明确 MIBG 成像对预后评估的价值与临床心功能指数（纽约心功能分级、左室收缩和舒张末容积以及左室射血分数）的相关性。在所有心功能指标和定量的成像指标中，无论缺血性还是特发性心肌病组，抑制[123I] MIBG 的活度（心脏到纵隔的比）是预测长期心脏死亡的最强有力的指标。同时评价 MIBG 活度和心功能指标，能提高预测的准确性。动力学变化用于评估初期和后期 MIBG 的活度。死于心源性因素的特发性心肌病患者放射核素的冲刷率明显高于那些存活的患者。而存活的缺血性心肌病患者与死亡患者的核素冲刷率没有差异。

另一项研究[18]调查了非常早期冠心病患者心脏肾上腺素能神经分布的水平。30 例患者分别进行 SPECT 成像（其中 MIBG 用于显示神经分布，[99mTc] sestamibi（MIBI）用于显示冠脉灌注）和定量冠脉造影，假定患者的冠脉狭窄不具有血流动力学意义。结果发现：MIBI 的摄取与冠脉的狭窄程度无关，前降支狭窄程度与后期 MIBI 活度正相关，与 MIBI 冲刷率呈负相关。这表明，即使非常轻的冠脉病变，在任何缺血事件或去神经发生之前，已经使心肌的肾上腺功能受到影响。

先前提到的关于突触前神经分布的研究显示心脏

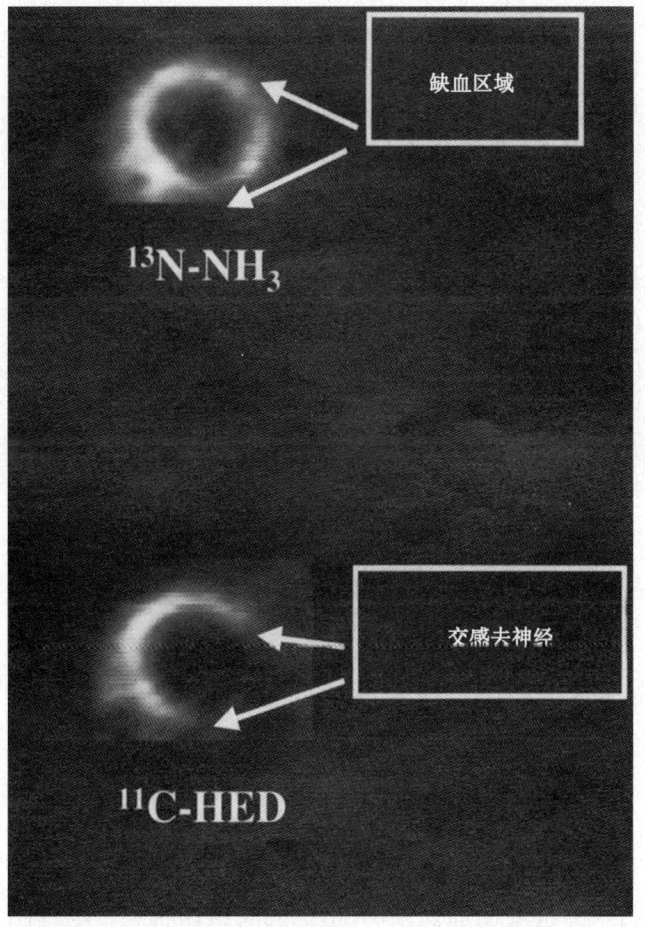

图92-8 冠心病患者去交感神经 图像显示心肌灌注（顶图）和交感神经分布（底图）情况。左室侧部有一相对较大的区域存在中等程度的灌注减少。对羟麻黄碱（HED）成像证实在左室相应的区域存在交感神经系统的受损。（见彩图41）

神经成像能为临床提供很有价值的预后预测。随之而来的问题是：心脏神经成像技术如何评价各种治疗措施的疗效及对疾病神经功能的恢复？有一项研究[19]旨在阐明运动后随着功能的变化，心脏突触前的异常神经分布能否逆转。用[11C] HED，C15O，以及H215O采集基础状态下的PET成像。6个月后在运动试验中重复扫描。通过计算C15O，H215O得出单心腔的平均心肌血流（MBF）。平均HED滞留指数通过[11C] HED成像得出。虽然运动并没有影响平均血流，但确实增加了在基础状态下血流量少的区域血流。运动能明显增加HED的滞留。这些来自影像学的改变与测得的自主神经功能之间具有很好的相关性，提示突触前神经分布的成像可能是慢性心衰患者个体化治疗的一个有效监测工具。

de Jong和他的同事综述[20]了应用PET成像研究心肌β-肾上腺素受体的相关研究。自从半个世纪前首次证实存在β-肾上腺素受体以来，很多研究已表明β-肾上腺素受体对心脏功能的维持和调节具有重要作用。β-肾上腺素受体密度的变化与很多心血管疾病有关，但临床研究受阻于缺乏无创评估体内神经的手段。PET成像技术用β-肾上腺素受体示踪剂获得的图像和动态数据，可以无创地提供心肌β-肾上腺素受体密度在空间上的分布情况。虽然在过去十年间，标记PET同位素的β-受体阻断剂出现，但大多数都不符合前面列举的标准。放射性配体[11C] CGP 12177已成功用于PET研究，但因合成困难而用途有限。仅有2个中心开展了β-肾上腺素受体密度的临床研究。过去几年中，用简单的方法合成了放射性配体[11C] CGP 12388，然而，缺乏β-亚型特异性，限制了[11C]CGP 12177和[11C] CGP 12388的应用。现已研究出具有β1和β2受体亚型选择性的示踪剂，但还需进一步开发。随着多个中心能够开发与合成配体，PET在病理生理研究和临床处理患者等方面将发挥越来越重要的作用。

（二）突触后放射性示踪剂的研究

用于在体心脏受体研究的放射性药物一直以肾上腺素能或毒碱乙酰胆碱受体拮抗剂为主，这些化合物虽然结构相似，但它们与受体位点的亲和力、亲脂性，以及亚型选择等方面都不一样[5]。值得一提的是，符合配体蛋白位点相互作用显影的大多数标准而且在人体研究中沿用至今的唯一化合物是肾上腺素受体[11C]-CGP12177和毒碱乙酰胆碱受体[11C]-MQNB。用SPECT技术对肾上腺素能受体显影一直以来受到放射性药物显影标准的限制。以放射性标记的肾上腺素能拮抗剂吲哚洛尔和碘氰心得舒已被作为造影剂进行了评估，遗憾的是，这些化合物有高水平的非特异性结合吲哚洛尔（pindolol）或显著的肺吸收碘氰心得舒（iodocyanopindolol），限制了作为SPECT造影剂的应用。通过用11C标记的肾上腺素能受体拮抗剂CGP12177，并且运用PET技术进行成像，取得了更有前景的结果。CGP已被证实非特异性结合水平低，达到了早期造影剂标准，并被证实是在体测定肾上腺素能受体密度的示踪剂。11C-CGP12177是一个有力的阻滞剂，对受体位点有高度的亲和力和低水平的非特异性结合。运用替代和阻滞研究已经证实11C-CGP12177对受体位点的高亲和力。另外，研究发现心率的下降和通过受体位点竞争引起的替代水平间有相关性，证实化合物的替代伴随有生物学的变化。在随后的研究中，用in vitro binding分析技术比较活体样本分析时在体的测量值，证实了11C-CGP12177对动物和人体受体密度的定量测定是有用的。用11C-CGP12177进行的PET成像研究证实原发性肥厚性心肌病以及高血儿茶酚胺病人的肾上腺能受体弥散性降低。

业已证实N-甲基符合对在体的受体密度进行定量评估的造影剂所要求标准的绝大部分。它是一个有力的亲水性的拮抗剂，对毒碱胆碱能受体显示了高亲和力。MQNB的动力学特性适合做造影研究，它的肺吸收率低，血池清除率快，使心肌组织和被放射性示踪剂污染的组织产生较好的对照。在置换研究中，AF-DX116置换了心肌组织25%的MQNB，然而加入哌仑西平后未发生置换反应[2]。在狗的研究中，给予丸剂后接着给阿托品大约能置换94%积聚的MQNB，证实在心肌中存在低水平的非选择性MQNB的结合。立体异构特异性也进行了证实。研究证实右苄替米特能将MQNB从结合位点进行置换，但levetimide却不能。生理研究已经证实在研究过程中MQNB与人左心室间隔的结合与心率呈反相关。这些研究支持这样一个假设，那就是毒碱胆碱能神经受体能以两种活性状态存在：一种是激动剂高亲和/拮抗剂低亲和状态，另一种是激动剂低亲和/拮抗剂高亲和状态。随着副交感神经紧张性增强，内源性神经递质结合到激动剂高亲和状态，从而使受体位点转变为激动剂低亲和/拮抗剂高亲和状态，增加了MQNB在组织中的积聚。这些研究中，虽然没有对副交感神经活性进行直接测量，但结果表明MQNB显影能证实毒碱受体的生理活性构像。应用对肾上腺素能受体定量相似的方法，利用 MQNB 的动力学特性能对在体毒碱受体密度进行定量测定。

目前，需要指出的是，除了最近一个受体密度增加的特发性扩张型心肌病病人的研究外，用 MQNB 和 PET 显影对在体毒碱胆碱能神经受体密度和亲和力的评估没有证实有任何变化[12]。对动物模型和人工移植受体进行自主神经去神经支配的认真研究亦未发现毒碱受体密度或亲和力的任何变化。总的来说，目前在体左室毒碱受体密度的影像学价值还不明晰。

六、参阅文献

从本书上一版本发行以来，又有几篇关于心脏神经成像的综述性文章发表[15]。Raffel 和 Wieland 发表了关于应用 PET 技术测定心脏交感神经分布的技术的综述[13]。我们在此重点论述了 PET 技术，Carrio 等[15]就 SPECT 技术的应用进行了较为系统的介绍。此外，DeGrado 及其同事发表了一篇关于核素标记药物动态构型在心脏核医学中的应用[16]。

七、总 结

PET 和 SPECT 是目前唯一可用于自主神经突触前和突触后成像的无创技术。尽管目前尚未研发出理想的特异性标记自主神经的放射性药物，但这些技术可作为研究工具应用于自主神经在心律失常和心脏性猝死中作用的研究工具。全面、系统地评价突触前和突触后自主神经功能，才能获取关于去神经和心脏功能之间关系的准确资料。就目前，临床应用该技术的前景尚不明了。对于存在与电生理异常相关的生理基础的心脏病患者，这些无创的体内成像技术有助于使诊断和治疗变得更为清晰、直观。但是，心脏神经成像技术仅是多种评价和认识自主神经方法学中一个重要的组成部分。

八、致 谢

本研究得到美国 NIH 的资助（NIH HL 52323）。同时感谢 Jeanne Quinn 和 Wendy Winkle 协助。

（易 忠 译）

参 考 文 献

1. Hutchins GD, Zipes D: Imaging the Cardiac Autonomic Nervous System. In Skorton DJ, Schelbert HR, Wolf GL, et al (eds): Marcus Cardiac Imaging: A Companion to Braunwald's Heart Disease. Philadelphia, WB Saunders, 1996, pp 1052–1061.
2. Syrota A: Positron Emission Tomography: Evaluation of Cardiac Receptors and Neuronal Function. In Skorton DJ, Schelbert HR, Wolf GL, et al (eds): Marcus Cardiac Imaging: A Companion to Braunwald's Heart Disease. Philadelphia, WB Saunders, 1996, pp 1186–1203.
3. Zipes D: Autonomic Modulation and Cardiac Arrhythmias. In Zipes D, Jalife J (eds): Cardiac Electrophysiology: From Cell to Bedside, 2nd ed. Philadelphia, WB Saunders, 1995, p 1612.
4. Elsinga PH, van Waarde A, Visser TJ, Vaalberg W: Visualization of β-adrenoceptors using PET. Clin Positron Imaging 1:81–94, 1998.
5. Van Waarde A, Elsinga PH, Anthonio RL, et al: Study of Cardiac Receptor Ligands by Positron Emission Tomography. In van der Wall EE, Niemeyer MG, Paans AMJ (eds): Cardiac Positron Emission Tomography. Dordrecht, Kluwer Academic, 1995, pp 171–182.
6. Raffel DM, Corbett JR, del Rosario RB, et al: Clinical evaluation of carbon-11-phenylephrine: MAO-sensitive marker of cardiac sympathetic neurons. J Nucl Med 37:1923–1931, 1996.
7. Del Rosario RB, Yung YW, Caraher J, et al: Synthesis and preliminary evaluation of [11C]-(-)-phenylephrine as a functional heart neuronal PET agent. Nucl Med Biol 23:611–616, 1996.
8. Elsinga PH, van Waarde A, Jaeggi KA, et al: Synthesis and evaluation of (S)-4-(3-(2′-[11C]isopropylamino)-2-hydroxy-proproxy)-2H-benzimidazol-2-one ((S)-[11C]CGP 12388) and (S)-4-(3-((1′-[18F]-fluoroisopropyl) amino)-2-hydroxypropoxy)-2H-benzimidazol-2-one ((S)-[18F] fluoro-CGP 12388) for visualization of beta-adrenoceptors with positron emission tomography. J Med Chem 40:3829–3835, 1997.
9. Dubois EA, Somsen GA, van den Bos JC, et al: Development of radioligands for the imaging of cardiac beta-adrenoceptors using SPECT: Part II. Pharmacological characterization in vitro and in vivo of new 123I-labeled beta-adrenoceptor antagonists. Nucl Med Biol 24:9–13, 1997.
10. Caldwell JH, Kroll K, Li Z, et al: Quantitation of presynaptic cardiac sympathetic function with carbon-11-meta-hydroxyephedrine. J Nucl Med 39:1327–1334, 1998.
11. DiCarli MF, Tobes MC, Mangner T, et al: Effects of cardiac sympathetic innervation on coronary blood flow. N Engl J Med 336:1208–1215, 1997.
12. Le Guludec D, Cohen-Solal A, Delforge J, et al: Increased myocardial muscarinic receptor density in idiopathic dilated cardiomyopathy: An in vivo PET study. Circulation 96:3416–3422, 1997.
13. Raffel DM, Wieland DM: Assessment of cardiac sympathetic nerve integrity with positron emission tomography. Nucl Med Biol 28:541–549, 2001.
14. Nguyen NT, DeGrado TR, Chakraborty P, et al: Myocardial kinetics of carbon-11-epinephrine in the isolated working rat heart. J Nucl Med 38:780–785, 1997.
15. Carrió I: Cardiac neurotransmission imaging. J Nucl Med 42:1062–1076, 2001.
16. DeGrado TR, Bergmann SR, Ng CK, Raffel DM: Tracer kinetic modeling in nuclear cardiology. J Nucl Cardiol 7:686–700, 2000.
17. Wakabayashi T, Nakata T, Hashimoto A, et al: Assessment of underlying etiology and cardiac sympathetic innervation to identify patients at high risk of cardiac death. J Nucl Med 42:1757–1767, 2001.
18. Simula S, Vanninen E, Viitanen L, et al: Cardiac adrenergic innervation is affected in asymptomatic subjects with very early stave of coronary artery disease. J Nucl Med 43:1–7, 2002.
19. Pietilä M, Malminiemi K, Vesalainen R, et al: Exercise training in chronic heart failure: Beneficial effects on cardiac (11)C-hydroxyephedrine PET, autonomic nervous control and repolarization. J Nucl Med, 43:733–779, 2002.
20. de Jong RM, Blanksma PK, van Waarde A, et al: Measurement of myocardial β-adrenoceptor density in clinical studies: A role for positron emission tomography? Eur J Nucl Med Mol Imaging 29:88–97, 2002.

第 93 章

心脏标测

Vias Markides,*Oliver R. Segal*,*Fernando Tondato*,*and Nicholas S. Peters*

本章目录
- 标测途径 ………………………… 842
- X 线影像 ………………………… 842
- 常规应用的导管 ………………… 842
- 电图的记录和处理系统 ………… 843
- 标测技术 ………………………… 844
- 总结 ……………………………… 850

心脏标测技术就是对心律失常进行识别、判断及定位的过程。虽然偶尔我们也会将诸如解剖学的方法用于某些心律失常（例如典型性心房扑动）的消融术中，但一般情况下，标测技术是指导介入治疗（通常是经皮的消融术）的基础。标测的原则和使用的技术因心律失常的病理基础不同而大相径庭。在操作之前对患者的病史、超声和其他的影像资料以及窦性心律下和临床心律失常发作时的 12 导联心电图进行认真的分析对于选择适当的标测技术大有裨益。

目前应用最普遍的还是常规的心内膜接触式导管标测。可以将导管放置在心脏相应的位置，如高位右房、房室结、三尖瓣环或二尖瓣环（冠状窦）、右心室，有时还会放在左心房或左心室，术者根据这些导管所提供的信息综合判断出在窦性心律、起搏以及心动过速时的心脏激动方式是否正常。此外，还可通过测量心内电图的间期、观察其形态，或用可移动的导管在其他感兴趣的部位起搏来获取额外的信息。这样的标测方法适用于发生在正常心脏的心律失常或者是心律失常病理基础相对简单的情况，而三维标测和其他更先进的标测技术和系统则更适于器质性心脏病或是更复杂的心律失常。

一、标测途径

通过静脉途径可以到达右心房和冠状静脉窦，常用的是股静脉或锁骨下静脉。通过股动脉逆行或经未闭的卵圆孔或房间隔穿刺可以到达左心。此外，比较少见的情况是经皮心包穿刺后进行心外膜标测。

二、X 线影像

X 线影像常用来指导放置诊断性导管以及对可移动导管导航定位（图 93-1）。因为 X 线影像所提供的导管是在二维平面中所处的位置，因而我们可了解对导管的操纵以及如何改变它在相应的三维空间的位置。使用各种不同体位的 X 线影像准确地定位是各个导管位置的基础。

三、常规应用的导管

诊断性心脏电生理检查最常用的是有固定弯度的 4 极导管（电极间距 2～5mm）（图 93-1）。头端可弯曲的电极导管亦可用于标测和消融。目前有很多的电极导管设计，其电极数目、间距、形状、大小以及长度各异。可根据患者需要标测和消融的位置不同加以选择。导管的形状既有简单地可弯曲的能放在任一个心腔里的 4 极导管，也有多达 20 极的一些特殊部位的导管，如三尖瓣环（如 Halo 电极导管），或是肺静脉（如 Lasso 电极导管）（图 93-1）。

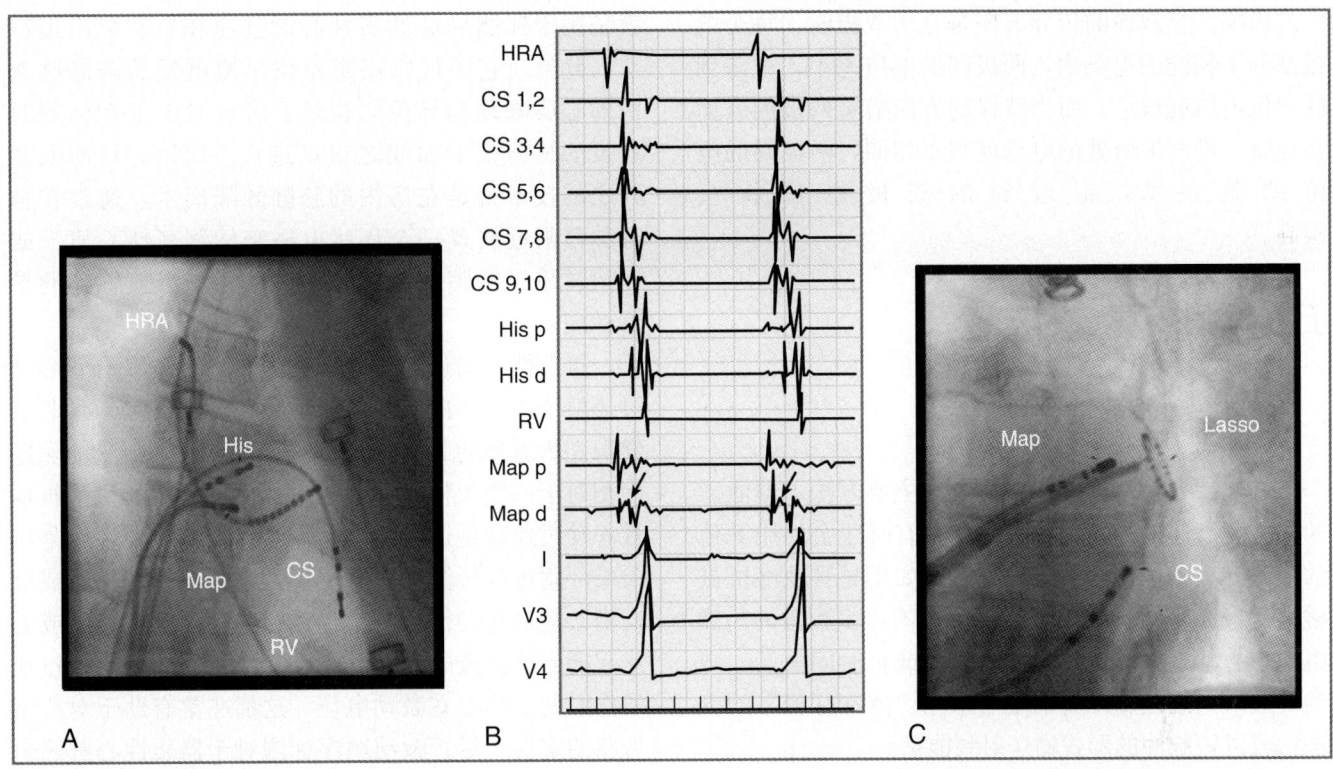

图 93-1　A：预激综合征患者旁路位于中间隔的标测和消融。后前位的 X 线影像上分别可见置于右室心尖部（RV）、希氏束（His）和高右房（HRA）的四极导管，以及放置在冠状静脉窦（CS）的十极导管和放在中间隔房室旁路邻近位置的标测导管（Map）。B：A 图所示导管记录到的相应电位图，以及窦性心律时 I、V_3 和 V_4 导联的心电图。在 V_3 和 V_4 导联上可以很清楚地看到预激 delta 波。标测导管记录到的信号（箭头所指）显示心房和心室电位之间的连续激动，这与导管位置靠近房室旁路是一致的。C：对一个阵发性心房颤动患者的肺静脉的标测和消融。左前斜位的 X 线影像显示置于左上肺静脉的环状标测电极导管（Lasso），以及放在肺静脉口部的标测电极导管（Map）。还有用于从冠状静脉窦（CS）远端起搏的四极导管。

四、电图的记录和处理系统

目前市场上的心脏电生理记录仪都有体表心电图和心内信号的输入通道。这些电信号可以被放大、滤波，还可以被转为数字信号从而可以被显示和记录（图 93-1）。

标测时可能会用到双极或单极记录。记录单极信号时，常以导管上的相关电极作为正极输入端，而以 Wilson 中心接线端或一个血管内的参考电极作为负极输入端。某一波的波锋从别处传向单极记录电极时，就会记录到一个正向的波形；而当波锋的传导背离单极电极而去时，则会记录到一个负向的波形。单极记录大大提高了信号的空间分辨力而不会受到波锋传导方向的影响。单极信号的形态可能会提供额外的有用信息。比如，在一个局灶起源的房性心动过速的起源点，单极电极会描记到一个 QS 波形；而在该起源点一点距离之外，描记到的就是 RS 波形。要想获得如此的记录效果，就要确保标测导管电极和心内膜贴靠良好，而且要将滤波的高通值设置到最小。单极记录电极常能描记到远场电位，这通常是对整个心脏电活动的有效记录，但其大小与到单极记录电极距离的平方成反比。但远场电位可能有的特别问题是，如果想要记录心内某个低振幅的近场电位，毗邻的位置可能有振幅大得多的电位，例如标测缺血性心脏病的梗死心肌灶边缘区域起源的室性心动过速时，远场电位就会形成干扰。而高通滤波有助于减少远场电位的干扰。单极电极比双极电极更易受到噪声的干扰，但如果使用血管内的参考电极能比一个外部的参考电极更有助于减少干扰，尤其当参考电极位于导管的血管内的部位时[1]。

与单极不同的是，双极信号记录是通过多极导管上间距很近的两个电极之间的电位差，而这两个电极都要求与心内膜紧密贴靠（图 93-1），双极记录到的远场电位及噪声是一样的，但双极记录的干扰大大地减少了。但双极记录电极对电信号的空间分辨能力远逊于单极，而且，如果两极相对于某一激动波锋的传导方向所处方位不同的话，对其记录的信号也会有很大的影响。当波锋的传导方向垂直于双极时，每个电极都处于相同的电场内，两极间的电位差小，记录到的双极电位就很小；而当波锋的方向沿着两极的方向传导时，则两极所处的电场就很不相同，两极间的电位差就很大，记录到的双极电位就会很高。

五、标测技术

（一）常规标测技术

常规的导管标测技术基于 3 种主要方法，即激动顺序标测、起搏标测和拖带标测。有时还会加用其他的一些方法，包括使用某种方法（如用导管顶端机械碰撞房室旁路或 Mahaim 旁路），使有心室预激的局部组织在心动过速或窦性心律下暂时或长时间失活，观察其效果；或经皮冷凝消融时采用"冰冻标测"的方法；或以短脉冲的形式输送射频能量。

1. 激动顺序标测

激动顺序标测主要比较可移动导管记录到的每个电位图与参考点（如体表心电图的 P 波、δ 波的起始、QRS 波的起始或是置于心内某固定位置的相关电极记录到的心内电图）之间的时相关系（图 93-1）。这种标测方法多用于心动过速时，但是，对于那些具有心律失常病理基础的病人，在窦性心律下或是心房（或心室）起搏时使用也很可能会获得十分有用的信息。不断移动导管的位置，不断地比较其记录到的电位图与参考点的时相关系，就可能发现最早的心内激动点或是沿着某一固定边界的大折返环的激动传导。这样在术者脑中就可以建立起心腔内或局部区域的激动标测图。激动顺序标测也是电解剖学标测系统（如 CARTO 系统）的基础，这种系统是通过标测导管在每个位点记录到的时相电位图来构建三维的激动标测图。但仅靠时相电位图还是不够的，还应该结合和参考标测时电位图的形态学方面的信息。比如，出现双电位往往代表着该区域是传导阻滞区，且可能就是一个大折返环的缓慢传导区；而一个未被滤波的呈 QS 形的单极电图则提示标测导管正处在一个局灶性心动过速的起源点。

激动顺序标测对于局灶起源或微折返的心动过速最适用，可以在相应的心腔内发现最早激动点，还可结合起搏标测获得更准确的信息。最好的例子就是用于标测局灶性房性心动过速和右室流出道室速。此外，它还可以用来定位早搏诱发的肺静脉起源的心房颤动的异位兴奋灶。但有时由于在标测时自发的早搏很少而使之很难进行。所以，目前取而代之的技术就是左房内的肺静脉隔离术，通常在肺静脉口附近放置一个环状电极来标测窦性心律下或起搏时最早的肺静脉电位，指导下一步消融前的导管标测。

折返性心动过速的一个基本特点是波锋沿着心动过速整个折返环的周长进行循环传导。所以，除非能够识别折返环的关键位点和消融靶点，否则激动顺序标测对于一些大折返的心动过速用处不大。房室折返性心动过速就是这样的一个例子。在二尖瓣环或是三尖瓣环附近进行激动顺序标测，寻找心室起搏时或顺向型心动过速发作时的最早逆行心房激动电位，或心房起搏心室预激成分达到最大时或是逆向型心动过速发作时的最早心室激动电位，这都非常有助于对房室旁路的定位。尽管激动顺序标测对于器质性心脏病也是有用的，如缺血性心脏病的室性心动过速，但不能仅仅靠激动顺序标测来界定折返环。舒张期（在 QRS 波之前）电位可出现于折返环的舒张期通路，也可出现于非折返环组成部分的"盲径"（blind alleys）（无辜的旁观者）通道。这种情况下就应该进一步行拖带标测来明确心动过速的性质。

2. 起搏标测

起搏标测特别适用于标测局灶性或微折返性心动过速的起源点，这些病人的心脏结构大多正常。此外，如前文所述，它还可与激动顺序标测联合使用。起搏标测的基本原理是，如果起搏的位置是在局部心动过速起源点的部位，周长接近自身的心动过速时，就会产生与自身心动过速相同的激动顺序。产生的体表图和心内电图应该和自身心动过速时一致。对于房性心动过速，起搏心电图的 P 波由于受到起搏信号和上一次心跳心室复极 T 波的干扰而无法清楚显示，因此还必须记录相应的心内电信号，才能保证记录到一个足够清楚的起搏标测图。对于右房房速，放置一根 Halo 电极导管就有助于了解起搏是否良好。而对于左房房速，除了放置在右房的导管记录到的信号外，在冠状静脉窦内放置一根多极导管，就可能提供有关起搏标测的足够信息。发生于正常心脏的室性心动过速病通常是局灶起源或微折返性的，这时就适合联合使用激动顺序标测和起搏标测，比较起搏标测时和自身心动过速时的 QRS 波形态能得出最后的结论，而无需分析心内电图。

3. 拖带标测

发生于器质性心脏病的心动过速，如缺血性心脏病的室性心动过速，通常是心室内的大折返所致。这种大折返环理论上有一个可激动间隙，而且心动过速发作时可通过起搏拖带来证实其为折返机制。由于在整个大折返环起到限制作用的传导阻滞区通常在窦性心律时并不存在或并不完全[2]，所以窦性心律下起搏标测时心脏的激动顺序和 QRS 波的形态并不同于自身心动过速发作时，甚至即使在折返环内起搏亦不会相同。在这种情况下，在心动过速发作时进行拖带标测显然要优于在窦性心律下的起搏标测。心动过速发作时行拖带标测，可以在折返环路上的不同部位起搏，就会有相应的各种不同形态的 QRS 波，以便于分析。此外，在一些特定部位行拖带标测还有助于区别折返环路上的某些关键部位，如室速折返环上的舒张期通路，以及无辜的旁观者"盲径"。

折返性心律失常必然存在着一个可激动间隙，刺激脉冲就有可能进入或在折返环路附近夺获可激动的心肌。如果以略低于自身心动过速周长的间期发放一串刺激，这些刺激都会进入折返环的可激动间隙，有可能连续重整或拖带心动过速。在折返环路上起搏产生的刺激进入折返环的可激动间隙后会产生两个方向的波锋，其中一个逆向传导，与自身心动过速的顺向传导激动发生碰撞。与此同时，另外那个顺向传导的波锋就会继续穿越整个折返环并重整心动过速。如果在折返环路以外但是在正向缓慢传导区的近端部位起搏，产生的激动就会穿过其间的心肌组织到达折返环路，并沿两个方向传导，再重整心动过速。

Waldo 和其同事[2a]率先描述了对心房扑动患者的一过性拖带，随后又陆续报道了对许多其他折返性心律失常的起搏拖带，包括折返性房性心动过速、房室折返性心动过速以及折返性室性心动过速。后来也有过对房室结折返性心动过速进行拖带的报道。根据在折返环缓慢传导区近端起搏的观察，提出了有关证实拖带存在的四条标准，具体可见表 93-1。不过，需要强调的是，即使没有符合上述的任一条标准，拖带也有可能存在。起搏拖带的位置与折返环缓慢传导区的关联尤其重要，因为尽管在缓慢传导区的近端或远端起搏都有可能发生拖带，但只有在缓慢传导区的近端进行起搏，才能根据此标准来证实是否符合拖带，而

表 93-1 证实拖带存在的标准

1. 心动过速时以快于自身（且不能终止自身心动过速的）的某一固定频率起搏，除了最后一个被拖带起来而未融合的起搏波外，心电图上可见到固定的融合波。
2. 心动过速时以快于自身的两种不同频率递增起搏时，出现进行性融合但并不终止心动过速。
3. 心动过速时以快于自身的频率起搏会影响到心动过速，这是由于某次起搏时引起了局部的传导阻滞，而其后下次起搏的激动脉冲会沿着另一个方向以更短的传导时间进行传导。
4. 心动过速时在某一固定的位置以两种不同的频率起搏，这两种频率皆快于自身频率且不终止心动过速，则会记录到不同的电位图和传导。

（引自 Henthorn RW, Okumura K, Olshansky B 等：A fourth criterion for transient entrainment: The electrogram equivalent of progressive fusion. Circulation 77: 1003-1012, 1988）

在慢传导区的远端区域起搏则在缓慢传导区产生逆向的波锋阻滞。

由于在折返环路之上或之外起搏都可能产生拖带，所以拖带现象的存在对于定位折返环是毫无价值的。要想确定起搏的位置是否在折返环路上，可以在该部位以比自身心动过速短 10～50ms 的周长起搏，并根据以下三条标准来判断结果：

（1）起搏未能改变心脏的激动顺序，起搏后产生了与自身心动过速相同的波形。如同起搏标测，可以观察大折返性房性心动过速起搏时心电图 P 波形态和心内导联上心房电位的波形以及大折返性室性心动过速所有导联上起搏的 QRS 波形态。所有这些和自身心动过速时的波形都是一致的（隐匿性拖带或是伴有隐匿性融合的拖带）。而唯一可以证实心肌确实被夺获的就是心动过速的周长已缩短到起搏周长。

（2）若拖带的位置在折返环而非"盲径"上，则刺激信号（S）到某个固定的参考点（常取室性心动过速的 QRS 波的起始点）的间期应近似于刺激部位所在位点的自身电活动到同一参考点的间期（差别常不超过 30ms）。起搏时记录到的间期（S-QRS 间期）反映的是起搏产生的顺向冲动到达心动过速折返环路并穿过其而传出到参考点的时间，因此，它应该基本上等同于心动过速时激动经过起搏点所在的位置（由此可记录到一个自身的电活动）后穿过折返环而传出到参考点的时间。

（3）起搏后的回归周期反映的是最后一个起搏波进入并穿过折返环路后，又回到起搏位置的时间。其

测量最好是从最后的那个起搏信号到恢复心动过速的第一个自身电信号起始。若拖带的位置位于折返环上，那么回归周期应基本等于心动过速的周长（差别常不超过30ms）。然而，由于起搏后的除极效应，想要在起搏部位精确测量回归周期还是很困难的。取而代之的方法有：测量双极标测导管上的近端而非一般用于起搏的远端；或是"(N+1)差别"，即在起搏时或起搏刺激刚发放完记录到的电图和QRS波编号为N，那么接下来的自身产生的电位图和QRS波的编号就依次为(N+1)，(N+2)。所谓的"(N+1)差别"就是测量从刺激信号到第(N+1)个QRS波的间期与第(N+1)个电位图到第(N+2)个QRS波的间期的差值。

之所以要以不超过30ms作为拖带位置是否在折返环路上的判断标准，是因为以短于心动过速的周长起搏会在折返环路上导致递减传导，这也是为什么强调要以稍短于心动过速周长的间期进行起搏的原因。

（二）三维立体电学标测

传统的导管标测技术往往都是由术者根据心内固定和可移动导管记录到的电位图，以及X线影像上所见的导管的二维影像在脑中重建出它们的三维空间位置。尽管传统的导管标测技术对于许多常见的心律失常而言已经足够，但是先进的技术使得标测更方便准确，尤其是那些复杂心律失常，而且减少了不必要的射线曝光。

所有这些新型的标测技术都可以提供非X线透视下的导管在三维空间所处位置的信息，这就使得标测更便捷，并能更好地指导消融。其中有些还能够对所标测的心腔进行三维重建，模拟出心腔的轮廓。与传统标测导管相比，这些先进标测技术能提供更多部位的电学信息（无论是同时还是依次的），因而大大提高了标测质量。

CARTO系统和非接触式心内膜标测系统（Ensite 3 000）都是这种先进标测技术，它们都能够把电生理参数、导管定位和导航与解剖信息结合起来，包括对所标测心腔的三维重建。这两种技术之间的一个重要不同点是，CARTO系统需要渐次标测才能获得相关的电生理参数，而非接触式标测系统则要可同步获取。此外，还有一种应用可扩张的篮状电极导管进行标测的系统，可同步标测和重建电极所在心腔的激动电图，但这种系统并不能利用导管进行精确定位，因此存在局限性。这些标测技术的相关软硬件都在不断发展之中，这必将有助于进一步推动它们在临床上的使用。

诸如高频经胸电场定位系统（LocaLisa系统）和实时定位方案（realtime position management，RPM），这些技术主要在三维空间帮助导管进行定位。然而，从局部接触式导管来获得电生理信息的方法可与RPM结合使用，最近也设计出心腔几何重建与激动顺序标测的功能[4]。

1. CARTO系统

CARTO系统（Biosense Webster，Dionand Bar，Calif公司）使用的是7F弯度可控的4极标测和消融导管（NAVI-STAR）。这种导管的顶端轴内有一个磁感器，在手术床下有个外置的磁场发射器不断发射磁场，与处理系统相连的导管就在这个磁场内移动，磁场发射器利用3个线圈来发射超低磁场，通过计算机对患者及其周围作磁场分区编码，使其具有时间和空间特性。在心动周期中人为设置一个参照点，在这个点时大头导管相对于固定在病人背上的外置参考电极的位置会被记录下来，系统通过这样来校正心脏和病人的活动所造成的误差。使用这种磁感应技术，系统能够精确定位并显示导管顶端在三维空间（x，y，z）的位置、方向（前后，左右，上下），还可以记录到局部的心内电图[5]（图93-2）。

放置一些固定位置，如冠状窦、右室心尖部或高位右房的标测导管作为操作者自行定义参考电极，为"感兴趣的窗口"内的标测导管所记录电图的测量提供相对的电学时相参照。无论在图像采集过程中或结束后，都要对在内膜所标测到的每一个点的导管位置、局部激动时间以心动过速周长进行评价。那些不稳定的点就将被拒绝接受或删除。这样渐次采集很多点，每个点都包含着很多的信息，例如其相对于参考点的局部激动时间、导管在心内膜的位置等，系统可以构建这些三维重建的激动顺序图、等电位图以及所标测心腔的激动传导图（图93-2）。

CARTO系统可用于标测任何一个心腔的多种心律失常。该系统对于标测左、右心室起源的室速都很有优势，不仅仅在于它使稳定的心动过速标测起来更方便，而且还可利用电压图来识别瘢痕区，并且指导随后的线性消融[6,7]。对于局灶起源的或是微折返性的，包括那些先天性心脏病外科后瘢痕相关性的心动过速，利用CARTO系统来精确标测的报道也不少。对于典型性心房扑动的病人，使用CARTO系统

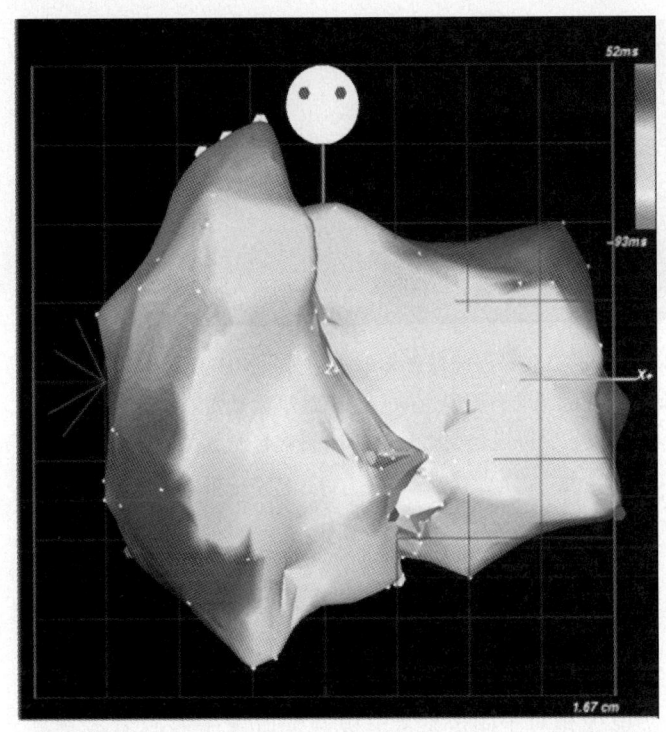

图 93-2 希氏束旁局灶起源的房性心动过速 图示后前位的左右心房激动电图。淡黄色的六边形区域为希氏束，红色区域代表最先激动的区域，其位置邻近希氏束，紫色代表最晚激动的区域。（见彩图 42）

可以有效指导消融并减少 X 线曝光时间[10]。此外最近还有报道利用该系统成功指导小儿右侧房室旁路的消融而完全无需 X 线透视[11]。对于心房颤动的病例，可以利用 CARTO 进行双侧心房的标测[12]以及左房内沿肺静脉口的标测并指导消融[13]。但是，由于该系统要求心动过速稳定发作时才能采集信息，因此，对于那些短阵、多形性或血流动力学不稳定的心律失常除了可进行瘢痕标测以导管定位导航外，其他功能就无法使用。

2. 非接触式标测系统

如前文所述，传统的导管标测技术和一些先进的标测技术如 CARTO 系统和实时定位系统（RPM）的标测都要求在几个心动周期中渐次采集信息点。由于该过程比较费时，尤其是对非持续性心动过速或血流动力学不稳定的患者，可被采集的信息点以及采用这种技术进行标测的方法都会受到限制。例如心梗后的室性心动过速，能够耐受长时间持续性心动过速进行标测的患者不足 20%。这就需要有方法可以同步标测整个心腔的电位图。篮状电极导管和非接触式标测系统可以同时获取整个心腔多部位的电学信息。然而，篮状电极导管使用上存在局限性，主要是在有些心腔比较大的病人，电极导管不能很完全贴靠在心内膜上。

非接触式心内膜标测系统（EnSite 3000，Endocardial Solution 公司）包含有一个可置于预备标测心腔内的网状多电极矩阵，一个专用的记录和放大系统，还有一个 Silicon Graphics 计算机工作站。多电极的矩阵是由一根 9F 导管和一个容量为 8ml 的椭圆形球囊组成。该球囊起到支撑作用，其外包绕 64 根编织成带状的绝缘电线，每根电线上都用激光蚀刻去一小部分的绝缘层，这就使其内部的金属导丝裸露出来起到单极电极的作用。矩阵导管杆的近端常处于下腔静脉或作为外部参考点，其上有一个环状电极，可作为单极的参考电极。系统的放大器有 12 通道的接触式心内电极输入，以及体表心电图的 12 个输入端，也接受来自多电极矩阵的信号。远场电活动也可被放大器接收，取样的频率为 1.2kHz，而且还可以被滤波。

多电极矩阵感知到的远场电活动是低振幅和低频率的，可以通过数学方法予以增强和分辨。Laplace 方程的逆向解析法被用来预测被远方一个点（一个非接触式电极）所探测到的信号将如何被还原于其起源处，并利用界面元素法来逆解这种源于以及位于血液和心内膜交界面的信号矩阵。

一个在传统标测导管和非接触式球囊导管的近、远端的环状电极之间轮流接收 5.68kHz 的低电流定位信号被用来对标测电极进行空间定位。由系统所决定的定位信号角度被用于定位发射源的位置。沿着心内膜面的轮廓拖曳大头导管，系统就会记录下心内膜表面的三维位点，并可用来重建心腔心内膜的三维模型，这适用于任何一个心腔（图 93-3）。这种导管定位系统也可以指引导管到达虚拟心内膜的任何位置，指导进一步的标测和消融而无需 X 线照射（图 93-3）。目前的系统软件有了进一步的发展，可以对一根导管的 4 个电极或是两根不同导管上的一对电极进行定位，进一步增强了几何构建和导航功能。

使用 Laplace 方程的逆向解析法，根据 64 个非接触球囊电极矩阵所探测到的远场电信号，系统可以重建出心腔 3 360 个位点的心内膜虚拟电图。对于球囊所在整个心腔可以同步采集电信号。这样甚至只要有心动过速的一次搏动，即可对心律失常的心内激动模式进行分析。非接触式标测获得的电生理信息可以虚拟电图、连续的等电位图或是等时图的形式伴以体表

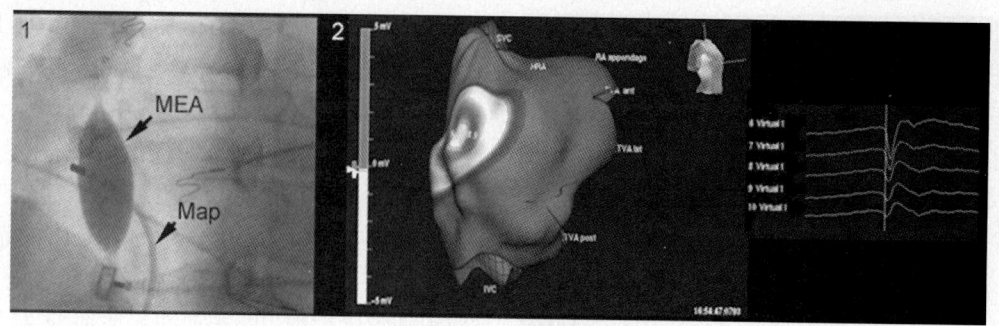

图 93-3 使用非接触式标测对局灶性房性心动过速标测和消融 1. 左前斜位右房内的球囊多电极矩阵（MEA）和单个的标测大头导管（Map）。2. 右心房的等电位图（右侧位）。该等电位图显示局灶起源的右侧房速的心内膜最早激动点（被其他颜色环绕的白色区域），这个区域被尚未除极的心内膜所包绕（用紫色代表）。放置于等电位图上局灶心律失常起源点位置的单极电图（图右侧）呈 QS 型。（见彩图 43）

心电图以及常规接触式导管的电位图同时显示出来（图 93-3）。

该系统的非接触式电位图和导管定位的精确性已经在体外试验[15]、动物试验及人体上反复验证[18,19]。临床上，该系统已被成功地用于四个心腔的标测和消融。对于合并缺血性心脏病大折返环的室性心动过速，非接触式标测能够非常有效地识别舒张期通路，并指导对该部位的消融[20]。此外，该系统对于特发性左室室速[21]和右室流出道室速最早激动部位的标测和导航消融也非常有效[22]。将球囊电极置于左房，就可以识别引发心房颤动的病灶（肺静脉内以及左房内），并能指导对其消融[23]。至于右房，可利用其标测来描述心房扑动和心房颤动的特征[24,25]，并判断房扑线性消融线的完整性[26]。另外，还可利用该系统来指导先心病 Fontan 手术后迟发的瘢痕相关性大折返性房性心动过速的标测和消融[27]。

3. LocaLisa

LocaLisa（Medtronic 公司）是一种非 X 线的导管定位系统。3 个约 30kHz 的高频低强度电场以正确角度作用于体表的 3 对处于三维正交方向（x，y，z）的电极片之间，从每个电极片流过的 30kHz 的电流混合信号被数字化地分离，以分别测定其振幅。根据相应的电场强度来分离电场幅度，这样就能够计算出每个电极相对于固定参考电极（常以置于右心室或是高右房的导管电极中的某一电极作为参考电极）的位置。电极的相对位置每 1～2s 就要平均一次，以减少心动周期的变异，但并不能减少呼吸的变异。一些重要的用于导管定位的和其他的解剖标识，如冠状静脉窦口、希氏束等位置可以在三维网格上用彩色点作标记。在标测过程中，系统会持续显示大头导管的位置变动（图 93-4），可以标记准备消融的靶点，可以是解剖学靶点，如下腔静脉到三尖瓣环之间峡部或是肺静脉口，也可以是电学的靶点，如局灶性房速的最早电信号的产生部位。该系统就可提供非 X 线的导管导航功能，包括线性消融线的标记。

通过在人体的右心房和左、右心室多次验证，该系统的定位精确度在 2mm 以内[28]。在许多的电生理检查和消融过程中，包括对慢路径、旁路、下腔静脉与三尖瓣环之间的峡部以及局灶起源的房颤的消融都

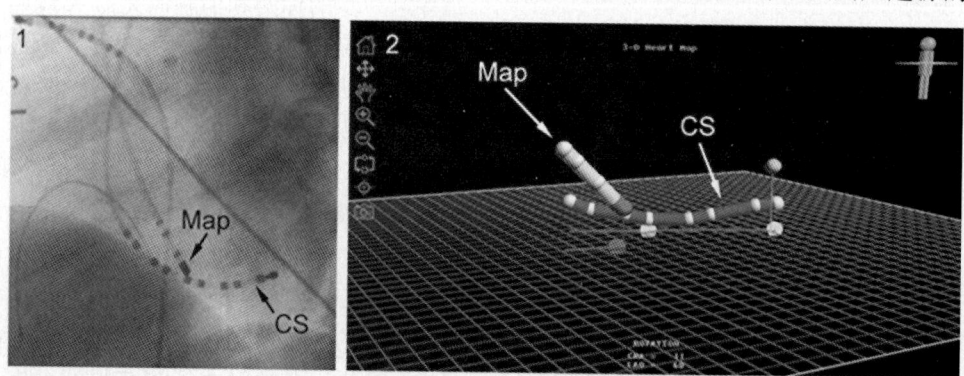

图 93-4 预激综合征患者的左后旁路标测时导管的三维定位 1. 左前斜位时置于冠状静脉窦内的 10 极导管（CS）和沿二尖瓣环的标测导管（Map）。2. 在 LocaLisa 标测显示界面上的冠状窦导管（CS）和标测导管（Map）的三维位置。（感谢 Metronic 公司提供的样图）。（见彩图 44）

显示，使用该系统可明显减少医生和病人的X线照射时间[29,30]。尽管目前LocaLisa系统只是一种导管定位系统，尚不能重建心内膜激动电图或是几何模型，但它可对任何一种导管精确导航并对重要位点进行标记，还能在减少X线照射的情况下指导大头电极消融，而且费用相对较低，这些优势都使得它在电生理实验室具有较大的吸引力。

4. 实时定位系统（realtime position management）

实时定位系统（Cardiac Pathways公司产品）是利用超声扫描来确定大头标测导管相对于两个参考导管位置的技术。这两个参考电极常用的是6F多极固定弯度的导管，一个置于右室心尖部，另一个放在右心房或冠状静脉窦。参考导管上装有4个超声探头。相应的标测和消融大头导管为7F可弯曲导管，上置3个超声探头。由于超声在血流内的传导速度是一个已知的常量，所以标测时发放的超声脉冲信号分别沿着导管输送到参考电极和大头电极，即可根据两探头对脉冲信号接收的时间延迟计算两者之间的距离。计算机根据参考电极上的信息构建出三维框架。据此，利用三角测量法来追踪其他探头（如大头标测导管上探头）的位置。系统可同时处理7个位置的导管、24对双极或48个单极的电图以及12导心电图的信息。电位图经数字化处理并滤波后在计算机显示屏上与其他导管的信号并列出现。在所显示的图像上可以给消融位点和其他需要的部位作相应的标记，这有助于标测和划出相应的消融线。该系统目前已成功地用于房扑、室速和房室旁路的标测和消融[31]。

最近的升级版本已经可以对任何一个心腔进行几何重建和激动顺序标测[32]。所构建的心腔三维模型可随着大头导管的移动而相应地扩展。可根据多个部位对于参考电极的激动时间的先后重建出心内激动顺序电图。目前已经在一小部分房性、交界性及室性心律失常患者中开始使用这种升级版本的系统[33]。

5. 篮状电极导管

如前文所述，可扩张的多极篮状电极导管可进行环心腔的同步标测。标测的效果主要与篮状导管上条索（spline）的数目、电极的数目及与心内膜贴靠的电极数目有关。最常用的导管（Constellation导管，Cardiac Pathways公司产品）由8条弯曲度很高的条索组成，上面分布64个电极，经长鞘送入心腔，通过与一个采集模块及专用的计算机相连后，系统可同时处理56个双极电图的信号（每个条索上顺序排列着7对双极）以及其他导管和体表心电图传来的信号。然后可以在计算机上重建和显示出电位图和彩色激动顺序图。该系统目前已经成功地用于人室性心动过速[34]和各种房性心律失常，包括先心病外科术后的房速[35]以及心房扑动[36]的标测和消融，甚至还可用于肺静脉内[37]和上腔静脉[38]起源的心房颤动的标测和消融。

（三）心外膜标测

尽管多数的室性心动过速起源于心内膜下，但是其折返环的关键部位却可能存在于从心内膜到心外膜的各层心肌中[39]。目前认为5%~15%的折返环位于心外膜下[40]，所以，必须要对其有充分的认识才能指导治疗。

1. 外科标测

外科标测的方法目前已用于难治性室性心律失常的治疗。在多数开胸的情况下，利用手执式探针、指状电极或多部位信号采集系统，如心外膜的鞘状或袜套式电极进行心外膜标测比较简单。但是，有些部位如左心房后侧及房间隔及室间隔，由于解剖结构的原因，用这种方法进行标测比较困难。目前，外科治疗心律失常主要是针对那些药物和射频消融治疗无效的难治性心律失常，或与外科手术有关的如瓣膜置换术或动脉瘤切除术后的心律失常。

2. 非外科方法的标测

目前已经发展出一些技术能够以最小程度的血管或组织介入到达心外膜的表面。经静脉的心外膜标测技术主要是将标测电极导管送入心脏的静脉以记录心外膜的电位。这种技术比外科标测更安全也更易于操作，但在相当程度上受限于心脏静脉系统的解剖结构[41-43]。此外，目前也有经冠状动脉的分支途径对心外膜室性心动过速进行标测的报道[44]。

经皮穿刺到达心外膜的方法也有报道。这种技术先是从剑突下穿刺后送入7F鞘管至心包腔（图93-5）。对病人进行深层麻醉后，即可在心外膜表面使用各种不同的标测和消融导管进行探查，还可以使用那些先进的电解剖标测方法。除去心包反应不说，这种方法的好处是由于心包表面相对光滑，没有什么明显的解剖障碍，可以避免血栓栓塞的合并症而不需要抗凝，并且导管操控相对简单。

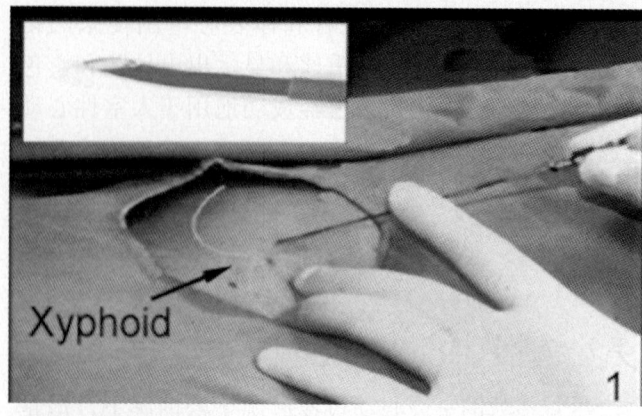
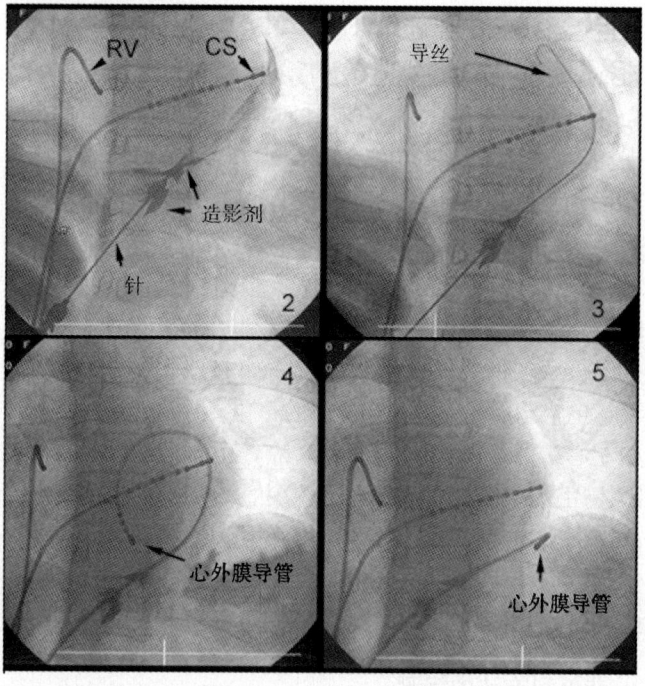

图93-5 将标测/消融导管置入心包腔的技术 根据Kirkorian方法,硬膜外麻醉的穿刺针(图1左上角所示)被用来作为经胸的心包穿刺针,可以引流心包内的渗液(图1、2)。将一根尖端柔软的导引钢丝送入心包腔内(图3)。然后送入8F的鞘管,拔出钢丝。再送入7F的标测导管进行心外膜的标测或消融(图4、5)。(图1左侧的图引自 Sosa E, Scanavacca M, d`Avila et al: Nonsurgical transthoracic epicardial catheter ablation to treat recurrent ventricular tachycardia occurring late after myocardial infarction. J Am Coll Cardiol 35: 1442-1449, 2000. 其余的图引自 Sosa E, Scanavacca M, d`Avila A: Transthoracic epicardial catheter ablation to treat recurrent ventricular tachycardia. Curr Cardiol Rep 3: 451-458, 2001.)

心外膜标测遵循的是和心内膜标测相同的电生理原理,包括识别局灶性心律失常的最早激动部位或是舒张中期电位,以及对折返性心律失常标测时隐匿性拖带的原理。利用这种方法,在确定需要消融区没有冠状动脉主要分支分布的情况下,可成功地进行了射频消融,其风险相对较低。从心外膜标测刺激阈值通常比较高,有时甚至无法夺获。这种现象的机制尚不明了,但可能的解释是导管和局部心肌接触不好,或局部有瘢痕组织的存在[40]。

这种方法尚存在一定的局限性,包括不能从心外膜标测位于间隔部的室速折返环,还可能遇到术后心包愈合困难的问题,虽然这在那些心梗后进行心外膜标测的患者并不常见[40,45]。此外,大多数的室速折返环还是位于心内膜下的,这在一定程度上也限制了该技术在临床上的发展。然而,对于一些有着各种疾病的室速,如缺血性心脏病、Chagas病,以及右室流出道心动过速、儿童的特发性室速,进行心外膜标测和消融的优势是心内膜标测无法取代的[45-47]。尽管目前心外膜标测的确切作用尚需进一步阐明,但它早就被认为是一项安全有效的辅助技术,可用来诊断和治疗心律失常环路,特别是那些位于左室下壁的折返环。

心外膜标测在其他方面(如在实验方面)的应用进一步增加了我们对室性心律失常(包括室颤)的了解。利用多电极系统覆盖心外膜表面同时标测大部分心外膜,使之成为研究复杂心律失常折返环的重要工具。心外膜标测也已广泛用于动物实验[48]及人体外科手术时房颤机制的研究,并能指导消融[49]。

六、总 结

心脏标测技术的发展日新月异。病人的临床病史、有无器质性心脏病史以及术前的12导联体表心电图都有助于对标测方法和设备的选择。自动化的标测系统对于多数普通的心律失常并非必需,但对于复杂的心律失常而言则是标测的利器。而且,非X线导管导航系统不仅极大地方便了导管的标测和消融,而且也大大减少了医生和患者的放射线照射时间。

(姚 焰 译)

参 考 文 献

1. Farre J, Rubio JM, Navarro F, et al: Current role and future perspectives for radiofrequency catheter ablation of postmyocardial infarction ventricular tachycardia. Am J Cardiol 78:76–88, 1996.
2. Stevenson WG, Sager PT, Natterson PD, et al: Relation of pace mapping QRS configuration and conduction delay to ventricular tachycardia reentry circuits in human infarct scars. J Am Coll Cardiol 26:481–488, 1995.

2a. Waldo AL, MacLean WA, Karp RB, et al: Entrainment and interruption of atrial flutter with atrial pacing: studies in man following open heart surgery. Circulation 56(5):737–745, 1977.
3. Soejima K, Stevenson WG, Maisel WH, et al: The N + 1 difference: A new measure for entrainment mapping. J Am Coll Cardiol 37:1386–1394, 2001.
4. Schreieck J, Ndrepepa G, Zrenner B, et al: Radiofrequency ablation of cardiac arrhythmias using a three-dimensional real-time position management and mapping system. Pacing Clin Electrophysiol 25:1699–1707, 2002.
5. Gepstein L, Hayam G, Ben Haim SA: A novel method for nonfluoroscopic catheter-based electroanatomical mapping of the heart. In vitro and in vivo accuracy results. Circulation 95:1611–1622, 1997.
6. Stevenson WG, Delacretaz E, Friedman PL, Ellison KE: Identification and ablation of macroreentrant ventricular tachycardia with the CARTO electroanatomical mapping system. Pacing Clin Electrophysiol 21:1448–1456, 1998.
7. Marchlinski FE, Callans DJ, Gottlieb CD, Zado E: Linear ablation lesions for control of unmappable ventricular tachycardia in patients with ischemic and nonischemic cardiomyopathy. Circulation 101: 1288–1296, 2000.
8. Marchlinski F, Callans D, Gottlieb C, et al: Magnetic electroanatomical mapping for ablation of focal atrial tachycardias. Pacing Clin Electrophysiol 21:1621–1635, 1998.
9. Sokoloski MC, Pennington JC III, Winton GJ, Marchlinski FE: Use of multisite electroanatomic mapping to facilitate ablation of intra-atrial reentry following the Mustard procedure. J Cardiovasc Electrophysiol 11:927–930, 2000.
10. Kottkamp H, Hugl B, Krauss B, et al: Electromagnetic versus fluoroscopic mapping of the inferior isthmus for ablation of typical atrial flutter: A prospective randomized study. Circulation 102: 2082–2086, 2000.
11. Drago F, Silvetti MS, Di Pino A, et al: Exclusion of fluoroscopy during catheter ablation treatment of right accessory pathway in children. J Cardiovasc Electrophysiol 13:778–782, 2002.
12. Pappone C, Oreto G, Lamberti F, et al: Catheter ablation of paroxysmal atrial fibrillation using a 3D mapping system. Circulation 100:1203–1208, 1999.
13. Pappone C, Rosanio S, Oreto G, et al: Circumferential radiofrequency ablation of pulmonary vein ostia: A new anatomic approach for curing atrial fibrillation. Circulation 102:2619–2628, 2000.
14. Khoury DS, Taccardi B, Lux RL, et al: Reconstruction of endocardial potentials and activation sequences from intracavitary probe measurements: Localization of pacing sites and effects of myocardial structure. Circulation 91:845–863, 1995.
15. Gornick CC, Adler SW, Pederson B, et al: Validation of a new non-contact catheter system for electroanatomic mapping of left ventricular endocardium. Circulation 99:829–835, 1999.
16. Gornick CC, Adler SW, Pederson B, et al: Validation of a new non-contact catheter system for electroanatomic mapping of left ventricular endocardium. Circulation 99:829–835, 1999.
17. Kadish A, Hauck J, Pederson B, et al: Mapping of atrial activation with a noncontact, multielectrode catheter in dogs. Circulation 99:1906–1913, 1999.
18. Schilling RJ, Peters NS, Davies DW: Simultaneous endocardial mapping in the human left ventricle using a noncontact catheter: Comparison of contact and reconstructed electrograms during sinus rhythm. Circulation 98:887–898, 1998.
19. Asirvatham S, Packer DL: Validation of non-contact mapping to localize the site of simulated pulmonary vein ectopic foci [abstract]. Circulation 102:II-441, 2000.
20. Schilling RJ, Peters NS, Davies DW: Feasibility of a noncontact catheter for endocardial mapping of human ventricular tachycardia. Circuiation 99:2543–2552, 1999.
21. Betts TR, Roberts PR, Allen SA, Morgan JM: Radiofrequency ablation of idiopathic left ventricular tachycardia at the site of earliest activation as determined by noncontact mapping. J Cardiovasc Electrophysiol 11:1094–1101, 2000.
22. Friedman PA, Asirvatham SJ, Grice S, et al: Noncontact mapping to guide ablation of right ventricular outflow tract tachycardia. J Am Coll Cardiol 39:1808–1812, 2002.
23. Hindricks G, Kottkamp H: Simultaneous noncontact mapping of left atrium in patients with paroxysmal atrial fibrillation. Circulation 104:297–303, 2001.
24. Schilling RJ, Kadish AH, Peters NS, et al: Endocardial mapping of atrial fibrillation in the human right atrium using a non-contact catheter. Eur Heart J 21:550–564, 2000.
25. Schilling RJ, Peters NS, Goldberger J, et al: Characterization of the anatomy and conduction velocities of the human right atrial flutter circuit determined by noncontact mapping. J Am Coll Cardiol 38:385–393, 2001.
26. Schumacher B, Jung W, Lewalter T, et al: Verification of linear lesions using a noncontact multielectrode array catheter versus conventional contact mapping techniques. J Cardiovasc Electrophysiol 10:791–798, 1999.
27. Betts TR, Roberts PR, Allen SA, et al: Electrophysiological mapping and ablation of intra-atrial reentry tachycardia after Fontan surgery with the use of a noncontact mapping system. Circulation 102:419–425, 2000.
28. Wittkampf FH, Wever EF, Derksen R, et al: LocaLisa: New technique for real-time 3-dimensional localization of regular intracardiac electrodes. Circulation 99:1312–1317, 1999.
29. Wittkampf FH, Wever EF, Vos K, et al: Reduction of radiation exposure in the cardiac electrophysiology laboratory. Pacing Clin Electrophysiol 23:1638–1644, 2000.
30. Kirchhof P, Loh P, Eckardt L, et al: A novel nonfluoroscopic catheter visualization system (LocaLisa) to reduce radiation exposure during catheter ablation of supraventricular tachycardias. Am J Cardiol 90:340–343, 2002.
31. de Groot N, Bootsma M, van der Velde ET, Schalij MJ: Three-dimensional catheter positioning during radiofrequency ablation in patients: First application of a real-time position management system [in process citation]. J Cardiovasc Electrophysiol 11:1183–1192, 2000.
32. Schreieck J, Ndrepepa G, Zrenner B, et al: Radiofrequency ablation of cardiac arrhythmias using a three-dimensional real-time position management and mapping system. Pacing Clin Electrophysiol 25:1699–1707, 2002.
33. Schreieck J, Ndrepepa G, Zrenner B, et al: Radiofrequency ablation of cardiac arrhythmias using a three-dimensional real-time position management and mapping system. Pacing Clin Electrophysiol 25:1699–1707, 2002.
34. Schalij MJ, van Rugge FP, Siezenga M, van der Velde ET: Endocardial activation mapping of ventricular tachycardia in patients: First application of a 32-site bipolar mapping electrode catheter. Circulation 98:2168–2179, 1998.
35. Triedman JK, Jenkins KJ, Colan SD, et al: Intra-atrial reentrant tachycardia after palliation of congenital heart disease: Characterization of multiple macroreentrant circuits using fluoroscopically based three-dimensional endocardial mapping. J Cardiovasc Electrophysiol 8:259–270, 1997.
36. Zrenner B, Ndrepepa G, Schneider M, et al: Computer-assisted animation of atrial tachyarrhythmias recorded with a 64-electrode basket catheter. J Am Coll Cardiol 34:2051–2060, 1999.
37. Michael MJ, Haines DE, DiMarco JP, Paul MJ: Elimination of focal atrial fibrillation with a single radiofrequency ablation: Use of a basket catheter in a pulmonary vein for computerized activation sequence mapping. J Cardiovasc Electrophysiol 11:1159–1164, 2000.
38. Shah DC, Haissaguerre M, Jais P, Clementy J: High-resolution mapping of tachycardia originating from the superior vena cava: Evidence of electrical heterogeneity, slow conduction, and possible circus movement reentry. J Cardiovasc Electrophysiol 13:388–392, 2002.
39. Sosa E, Scanavacca M, D'Avila A, Pilleggi F: A new technique to perform epicardial mapping in the electrophysiology laboratory. J Cardiovasc Electrophysiol 7:531–536, 1996.
40. Sosa E, Scanavacca M, D'Avila A, et al: Endocardial and epicardial ablation guided by nonsurgical transthoracic epicardial mapping to treat recurrent ventricular tachycardia. J Cardiovasc Electrophysiol 9:229–239, 1998.
41. de Paola AA, Melo WD, Tavora MZ, Martinez EE: Angiographic and electrophysiological substrates for ventricular tachycardia mapping through the coronary veins. Heart 79:59–63, 1998.
42. Melo WD, Prudencio LA, Kusnir CE, et al: Angiography of the coronary venous system. Use in clinical electrophysiology. Arq Bras Cardiol 70:409–413, 1998.

43. Stellbrink C, Diem B, Schauerte P, et al: Transcoronary venous radiofrequency catheter ablation of ventricular tachycardia. J Cardiovasc Electrophysiol 8:916–921, 1997.
44. Wong T, Chow, AWC, Markides V, et al: Human ventricular tachycardia ablation guided by intracoronary artery guide-wire mapping [abstract]. Pacing Clin Electrophysiol 25(4 Pt II):524, 2002.
45. Sosa E, Scanavacca M, d'Avila A, et al: Nonsurgical transthoracic epicardial catheter ablation to treat recurrent ventricular tachycardia occurring late after myocardial infarction. J Am Coll Cardiol 35:1442–1449, 2000.
46. Arruda M Chandrasekaran, K, Reynolds D: Idiopathic epicardial outflow tract ventricular tachycardia: Implications for RF catheter ablation [abstract]. Pacing Clin Electrophysiol 19:611, 1996.
47. Sosa E, Scanavacca M, D'Avila A, et al: Radiofrequency catheter ablation of ventricular tachycardia guided by nonsurgical epicardial mapping in chronic Chagasic heart disease. Pacing Clin Electrophysiol 22:128–130, 1999.
48. Derakhchan K, Li D, Courtemanche M, et al: Method for simultaneous epicardial and endocardial mapping of in vivo canine heart: Application to atrial conduction properties and arrhythmia mechanisms. J Cardiovasc Electrophysiol 12:548–555, 2001.
49. Yamauchi S, Ogasawara H, Saji Y, et al: Efficacy of intraoperative mapping to optimize the surgical ablation of atrial fibrillation in cardiac surgery. Ann Thorac Surg 74:450–457, 2002.

第十三部分
临床综合征：认识、临床过程和处理

第 94 章

预激综合征

Eric Prystowsky，*Raymond Yee*，*and George J. Klein*

本章目录
- 相关术语 ……………………………… 853
- 解剖和生理学 ………………………… 853
- 临床表现和自然病史 ………………… 855
- 心电图表现 …………………………… 856
- 电生理检查 …………………………… 856
- WPW 综合征的心动过速 …………… 856
- 评价的方法 …………………………… 858
- 治疗 …………………………………… 860

1930 年，Wolff, Parkinson 和 White 报告了 12 例有反复阵发性心动过速的一组病例，患者均为健康的年轻人，其窦性心律时的心电图存在"功能性束支阻滞"和短 PR 间期。目前已明确，这是一种先天性疾病，患者存在附加的房室旁路是其解剖学基础。尽管存在着解剖学变异，但其临床表现相似。对少数病人的研究已证实，心室预激可伴发其他的先天性缺陷，并可伴有心脏肥厚[2-5]。这些患者旁路的电生理特征与孤立性 WPW 综合征的病人相似[5]。这些先天性的旁路为什么会引起心室的预先激动仍需进一步的研究。

电生理检查能够区分和鉴别这些旁路，解释心动过速的发生机制。对该综合征病理生理学基础的更为深入的研究，能使临床医生对其治疗制定合理的分层。除了抗心律失常药物治疗外，现已出现了外科消融术、射频导管消融术等能够根治这一综合征的非药物治疗方法。本章将复习和评述预激综合征的解剖和病理生理学，临床评估及一般治疗原则及方法。

一、相关术语

所谓预激综合征是指患者的心电图有心室预激的表现，同时又有心动过速的发作[1]。如果病人仅有心室预激的心电图表现，但无任何症状，没有心动过速的病史，对于这种情况，常将其简单描述为患者有"心室预激的心电图表现"，而不称其为预激综合征。有症状的病人可能并没有显性心室预激的心电图表现，而经心内电生理检查能够证实其有隐匿性旁路，该旁路仅有逆传功能，通常认为这种病人患有预激综合征。

二、解剖和生理学

(一) 房室旁路

预激综合征的典型心电图是附加的房室旁路存在和传导的结果，这种房室旁路是胚胎时期心管分割成心房和心室腔后残存的组织。组织学上，绝大多数旁路是由类似普通心肌细胞的纤维组成的，其横跨房室环，并在心房肌和心室肌之间产生了电活动的连续。经过旁路的传导与频率无关，这与正常的房室传导系统显著不同。频率无关性传导的特点引起了预激综合征伴房颤时快速的心室率，甚至猝死。不典型的旁路传导形式与正常的房室结组织相似，表现为频率依赖性或称递减性。已被证实，存在一定程度递减传导的旁路约占预激综合征的 7%。多数情况下，旁路的这种递减传导十分轻微，只有通过起搏频率增加时，或期外刺激的联律间期递减时，才能确定旁路的传导时间。旁路的递减性传导常常只表现在前传或逆传一个方向上，而双向传导均有递减传导的旁路实属少见。前传的递减传导几乎不出现在右侧旁路，而多发生在间隔旁路[6]。与其相反，旁路逆传的递减性可见于任何位置的旁路。

根据旁路沿房室环的解剖位置，旁路被分成：右前间隔、右侧游离壁、后间隔、中间隔（希氏束与冠状窦口之间）、左室游离壁等。还有一种倾向是将房室环划为更小、更多的节段，相应出现了左侧或右侧后间隔、后侧壁、间隔旁、前壁、前侧壁、希氏束旁等术语，用来更细微地说明旁路的位置。虽然这有利于讨论，但所有的解剖学分类都是人为的。实际上，房室环很少具有明确标志将某些分类表上列出的部位进行很好的界定。另外，旁路也能发生在静脉的憩室中。旁路最常见的部位是左侧游离壁（50%～60%），其次是后间隔（20%～30%），右侧游离壁（10%～20%）[7]。最少见的是靠近希氏束部位的前间隔和中间隔（<10%）。

旁路电位的记录为了解旁路的生理和解剖提供了重要的信息[8,9]。低振幅的旁路电位通过标准的双极电极能被记录，经仔细的观察能被确认。例如，右前间隔的旁路电位已能和希氏束电极记录的希氏束电位区别（图94-1）。当左侧游离壁和后间隔旁路发生前传或逆传阻滞时，则可发现阻滞的部位十分靠近心室插入端[9]。而对右侧旁路和中间隔旁路，传导阻滞的位置更可能在心房插入端。某些资料提示，左侧旁路的心室插入端的部位比心房插入部位更常靠内侧[10]。旁路电位的记录对确定最佳放电消融的位置提供了重要的标准。

多旁路在预激综合征患者中的发生率5%～20%[11]。但实际发生率比之更高，因为诊断取决于任何两条旁路的空间位置、导管标测技术的空间分析及多条靠近的旁路的诊断标准等。虽然单条旁路最常见的发生部位是左室侧壁，而多条旁路似乎最常见于后间隔和右侧游离壁部位，尤其是Ebstein畸形的患者易发生多旁路。经组织学认定的旁路数量将超过临床检出的旁路的数量，提示并非组织学确定的所有旁路均有功能，或者是电生理检查未能发现某些多旁路。多旁路的存在使电生理检查和研究更为困难，因为心动过速的机制将有更大的变异，激动顺序的融合更复杂[12,13]。已经发现，室颤复苏成功的病例中，多旁路的发生率更高，虽然这可能因为心动过速的机制涉及多个激动的波锋碰撞，并能增加房颤和室颤的

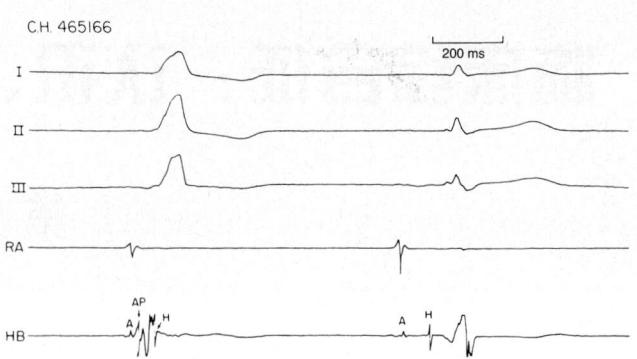

图94-1 电极导管放在希氏束区域记录到旁路电位 图中第一个QRS波为预激性QRS波，心房（A）波后有一个大的AP（旁路）电位和心室电位。此电位后的心室波代表经希氏束前传导发生了阻滞，因其处于不应期内。第二个QRS波自然变为正常化，AH间期与第一个周期相同，但看不到AP电位，因为激动从心房的前向传导未经过旁路

危险，但多旁路患者发生室颤的危险度增大的确切机制仍然不清。

（二）变异性结束和结束旁路

Mahaim和Winston[14]描述了连接房室结和远端束支或邻近心室肌的旁路。这种变异的旁路是WPW综合征变异型的解剖学基础，但在临床相关的问题上仍有争论。当怀疑患者存在结室旁路时，其临床、电生理和心电图可能表现出一种特殊的组合，提示房室结是心动过速折返环的一部分（表94-1）。这些患者的静息心电图正常，预激不明显，预激QRS波的形态类似左束支阻滞和电轴左偏，提示存在右侧旁路。电生理检查提示其结束旁路具有明显的频率依赖性传导，而且旁路只有前传功能。S₂刺激或频率递增性心房起搏，可引起AH间期或A-δ波间期延长，同时预激的成分也增加。绝大多数普通的折返性心动过速的折返环中，经旁路前传，经希氏束或房室结逆传。预激性心动过速发生时进行心室标测能够发现，最早的心室激动点是右室心尖部而不是邻近三尖瓣环的心室肌（右侧房室旁路时也是这样）。而房室结折返，多旁路引起的复杂的心动过速也能伴发这种情况[15]。要想确定是结室或结束旁路引起的反复性心动过速时，需要证实心动过速时存在着房室分离，这一电生理现象不可能出现于其他的解剖变异中（见本章随后的房束和递减性房室旁路中的讨论）。

表 94-1 房束旁路的电生理特点

1. 窦律时预激成分很小或缺如
2. 旁路前向传导时间呈频率依赖性
3. QRS 波呈左束支阻滞形，常伴电轴左偏
4. 应用右房或冠状窦刺激时有利于预激图形的出现
5. 在最大预激图形出现时，右室心尖部电位最早出现
6. 旁路无逆传功能
7. 常共存多旁路及房室结折返

（三）房束旁路

结室旁路的心电图和电生理表现也能由房束旁路引起（表94-1），实际以前认为的结室旁路引发的临床综合征的绝大多数都是房束旁路[16]。该旁路起源于右房心肌，慢频率的右房起搏比左房起搏引发的预激波更明显。其与房室结一样地跨过三尖瓣环，插入右束支远端[16,17]。该旁路与其经过的心室肌呈绝缘状态，典型者具有单向前传和递减传导的特征[16-19]。表现为最大预激 QRS 波的反复性心动过速时，QRS 波呈典型的左束支阻滞的图形，折返环以房束旁路为前传支，右束支、希氏束及房室结为折返环的逆传支。

（四）单向前传、有递减传导的房室旁路

与房束旁路有相似特征的一种解剖学的变异是伴递减前传的房室旁路。当其位于右侧时，预激性 QRS 波呈不典型左束支阻滞形，以及最早心室激动点位于三尖瓣环的心室侧而与房束旁路不同。通过三尖瓣环右室游离壁的射频消融能成功地消除预激和心动过速，可进一步证实诊断的正确性，消融成功的靶点常可记录到旁路电位图。

（五）隐匿性房室旁路（仅有逆传）

这些变异性旁路缺乏或根本没有前传功能。由于没有前传的预激心电图表现，严格地说，这种病人不能充分满足 WPW 综合征最初的诊断标准。这些病人的特征包括：顺向型房室折返性心动过速，其前传经房室结和希氏束，逆传经旁路。就我们的经验，不到一半的阵发性室上速病人无显性心室预激，实际是有一条隐匿性旁路而伴房室折返。当心动过速发生时，心电图上的逆行 P 波落在 ST 段时，则应怀疑患者存在隐匿性旁路，但隐匿性旁路参与了心动过速发生的绝对证据还需心脏电生理检查证实。

（六）束室连接

束室旁路是左束支和心室肌间的连接，这型旁路十分罕见，而且孤立性的束室旁路之间还未能证实能引发折返性心动过速。其特征包括：存在成分很小的心室预激波，伴 HV 间期短而固定，甚至在 AH 间期变化时，HV 间期也是这样。

三、临床表现和自然病史

有预激旁路的患者，其临床表现和自然病史可以迥然不同。旁路属于一种先天性异常，但是，很多有预激旁路的患者可能一直无任何症状，只是偶然的机会被发现。有心室预激但无任何症状者预后常呈良性。罕见情况时，室颤可以是该综合征的首发表现[13,20-22]。这些无心动过速反复发作的患者，心律失常的发生率每年为 1.7%[23]。几项研究结果提示，没有临床或电生理的指标能可靠地预测病人可能发生症状。相反，Pappone 及同事报告[13]，联合应用旁路前传有效不应期≤250ms 及诱发房室折返两个指标，对将来发生心律失常的阳性及阴性预测值分别为 46.9% 和 97.3%。

无症状的患者中，大约 25% 的人旁路无逆传功能，不能发生顺向型房室折返性心动过速。电生理检查时，不能诱发反复性心动过速的患者，诱发房颤时心室率不会太快。而且患者有完整的旁路逆传功能的预测值是低的。无症状的预激患者并有完整的旁路的逆传功能时仅有 11% 的人在随访超过 4 年的时间中发生了折返性心动过速或房颤。旁路传导性质的长期电生理评价结果表明，18%~33% 的无症状人群中，旁路无前传功能[13,24]。这些患者多数年龄偏大，在旁路前传有效不应期的测定中，其值较长。

不到 12 个月的婴儿存在心室预激或发生过折返性心动过速时，心室预激常可自然消失或心动过速者不再发生。但是，在青少年时期发生症状性心动过速者，则在许多年中会长期、反复发生心动过速。有人报告，在青春期和更年期，心动过速发作的情况及频度都会有变化，而在成人期，房颤更为常见。

预激综合征者常主诉有心悸，有时伴胸部不适、呼吸困难、轻度头痛或晕厥。猝死是一个少见的事件，但其可能是以前无症状者的首发症状。猝死在预激综合征患者中的发生率估计每年<0.1%。这种猝死常发生在病人发生了房颤经旁路下传致极快速的心室率，并蜕化为室颤。医学面临的挑战是，在一个数量巨大的无症状和有症状的预激综合征人群中，如何识别处于高危状态中的患者。

目前认为晕厥是一个不祥的先兆,其可能是病人发生了非常快速的心律失常,并引起了血流动力学的不稳定,进而演变为恶性过程引发了晕厥。对某些病人,这可能是事实,在一般的临床和电生理过程中,伴或不伴晕厥病史的人数可能大致相同。Paul 及同事发现[26],在年青患者中,快速房颤有较高的诱发率。Leitch 等[27]建议:折返性心动过速的病人存在晕厥,提示患者对心律失常存在着心血管异常的反应。而且,有心室预激的病人不能除外因其他的原因,如不相关的心律失常引起的晕厥。最后,如果病人伴有器质性心脏病,例如 Ebstein 畸形、二尖瓣脱垂或大血管错位时,这种病人应努力寻求医护人员的关注与保护。

四、心电图表现

存在旁路时的心电图表现变化很大,典型的 WPW 综合征是旁路存在双向传导的结果,前向传导产生了窦性心律时典型的 δ 波,逆向传导将引起顺向型房室折返性心动过速。所谓"心室预激"是指心室激动比预期经房室传导系统下传激动的时间要早,预激的心室 QRS 波实际是室上性激动分别经正常房室传导系统和旁路下传激动心室形成的室性融合波。因此,预激的程度决定于旁路下传和经房室结-希浦系下传激动心室的相对比例,实际这是一个窦房结到旁路之间的距离和经房室结下传时间的一个函数。很小的或微妙的(精细的)预激常发生在心室侧壁旁路,某些旁路不能连续前传,这将使心室预激的图形时隐时现,或在一定心率时预激图形消失(图 94-2)。间歇性预激是指旁路有单薄而不稳定的前传功能,这类病人房颤发生伴快速预激性心室率,进而发生猝死的危险性很低[28]。

体表心电图能给判断旁路大致部位提供重要信息。经心电图为旁路定位主要依据 δ 波的形态,QRS 波的形态,或者两者的形态[29-31]。进行外科消融或射频导管消融术时,则能为旁路精确定位,并能证实旁路部位变化的复杂性,具有实用性和精确度。总之,经 12 导联体表心电图为旁路精确定位仍有一定的局限性。旁路在房室环的位置和心脏在胸腔中的方向最终决定了体表心电图的向量,其他异常心电图的共存、预激的程度、多旁路的存在都能影响旁路定位的精确性。

体表心电图能为旁路的部位提供适度的大致部位的信息。典型的左侧旁路常在 I,aVL 或 V_6 导联有负向 δ 波和假性右束支阻滞图形,并伴 V_1 导联直立的 QRS 波(呈 Rs 型)。对于右前间隔旁路(规定为心室最早激动点靠近希氏束区域),在 II,III,aVF 导联 δ 波直立,V_1 到 V_3 导联 R 与 S 波的比率较低(呈 QS 波或 rS 波),胸前导联的 R 波移行出现较晚。典型的前间隔旁路时,在 II,III,aVF 导联 δ 波为负相或呈等电位线,从 V_1 到 V_2 导联,R:S 比率迅速转换(V_1 导联呈 rS 波,V_2 导联呈 Rs 波)。最后,右侧游离壁旁路时,I 导联的 δ 波直立,类左束支阻滞。作为一般的规律,直立的 δ 波的消失发生在 III 导联,aVF 导联和 II 导联时,提示旁路的位置围绕着房室环从前间隔逆向后间隔。对于右侧旁路,当旁路的位置围绕着三尖瓣环从前移向后时,直立的 δ 波顺序出现在 $V_1 \sim V_4$ 导联。

五、电生理检查

电生理检查对 WPW 综合征及其变异的病理生理学基础的解释是必不可缺少的。对怀疑或已明确 WPW 综合征的所有病例,标准的电生理检查方法是将 4 极电极导管放置在右室心尖部,右室心尖和希氏束部位及冠状窦中(将其近端的一对电极放在窦口)。随后做程序心房和心室刺激,以及递增性心房和心室起搏。这样一个程序刺激,完全能够对房室结和旁路的前传和逆传性质做完整的评估。这些方法包括不同部位的心脏起搏,例如右房及冠状窦起搏,不同部位的心室起搏,特别是鉴别间隔传导是经旁路,还是经正常的房室传导系统,则需要进行希氏束旁起搏;在房室折返性心动过速时,应当使用期前的心室刺激[31-33]。为诱发折返性心动过速,需要时每例都应在电生理检查中给予异丙肾上腺素或阿托品。

六、WPW 综合征的心动过速

WPW 综合征的心动过速能分成两组:(1)旁路

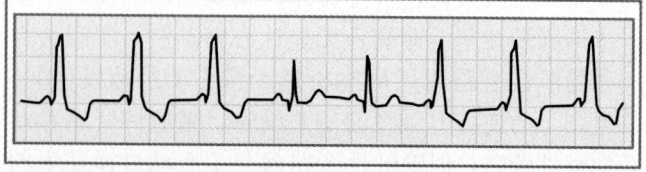

图 94-2 单导联心电图显示间歇性预激 图中前 3 个 QRS 波有心室预激的表现,随后的两个 QRS 波正常化,而后的 3 个 QRS 波又有心室的预激图形。

参与的心动过速，旁路是折返环路的一部分；(2) 心动过速的激动传导经过旁路，但是旁路是旁观者，而不是维持心动过速的必需成分[31]（表94-2）。

（一）顺向型房室折返性心动过速

有症状的预激综合征患者，最常见的过速性心律紊乱为顺向型房室折返性心动过速（图94-3）。发生时的特征是：阵发性、规律的窄 QRS 波（除非伴有功能性束支阻滞），典型者心动过速的频率为每分钟150～250次。功能性束支阻滞发生时，如果影响的束支与旁路同侧时，则心动过速的心动周期将会延长，这能为旁路的定位提供重要线索[31]。当体表心电图可以看到逆传P波时，P波的电轴及形态反映了旁路的部位，因为心房逆向除极是在旁路的心房插入端开始的。例如，左室侧壁的旁路在Ⅰ导联可出现倒置的P波。不幸的是逆向P波的形态常不能被辨认。

顺向型房室折返性心动过速时，前向经房室结和希氏束传导激动心室，而逆传经过旁路激动心房（图94-4）。心动过速的起始需要房室传导系统和旁路的传导和不应期的性质有一定的离散和不同。结果，适时的早搏则能引起折返环的一支出现前传的单向阻滞。

确认旁路是否是折返环的一部分十分重要，心动过速发生的同时，当希氏束处于不应期时，一次室性早搏刺激能引起心房的预激，这能证实患者确实有旁路存在，但不能确定旁路一定参与心动过速的折返。心动过速发生时，4个表现能证实旁路就是心动过速折返环的一部分：(1) 与旁路同侧的束支阻滞时，室房间期增加；(2) HV 间期的增加，将引起 HA 间期的增加；(3) 在希氏束处于不应期时，室早不能逆传到心房，但心动过速能被终止；(4) 希氏束处于不应期时，引入一个室早后，AA 间期延长。

（二）PJRT 综合征

PJRT 综合征是一种无休止性或几乎无休止性的房室折返性心动过速，其可发生于任何年龄组的患者，但多见于儿童及年轻人。Coumel 及同事[34]首先将 PJRT 用于描述这种心律失常。但在当时并不清楚，几乎所有的病例的逆传都是经过旁路而不是房室结。因此，PJRT 实际上是一种误称，最好的术语应当是称为持续性房室折返性心动过速（PAVRT），但 PJRT 已广泛出现在文献之中，典型的 PJRT 旁路均显示有递减性传导的特性。

这种心动过速的心电图特征是非常特殊而明显

表94-2 WPW 综合征时的心动过速

旁路参与的折返性心动过速
　顺向型房室折返性心动过速
　预激折返性心动过速
　逆向型房室折返性心动过速
　多旁路参与的折返性心动过速
旁路呈被动的旁观者，心动过速不需要旁路的参与
　旁室结折返性心动过速
　房室折返性心动过速伴旁观旁路
　心房扑动或心房颤动
　室速

的。P波常增宽，提示是"从低到高"的心房激动顺序。P波在Ⅱ、Ⅲ、aVF 导联倒置，RP 间期长于正常的 PR 间期，这与典型的顺向型房室折返性心动过速恰恰相反（图94-5）。当折返环的逆传支发生传导阻滞时（心电图上无逆P），则可引起心动过速一过性停止。而且逆传支对迷走神经刺激、β受体阻滞剂和钙通道阻滞剂都是敏感的。尽管如此，PJRT 仍对药物治疗的反应差。与房速不同，典型的 PJRT 常能被期外刺激诱发。PJRT 常在一次窦律后发生，而且不需要早搏诱发（图94-5B）。自主神经张力变化或体力活动时，心动过速的频率可反应性增加（100～200次/分）；而频率的变化是 PR 和 RP 间期调整的结果。

（三）逆向型房室折返性心动过速

逆向型房室折返性心动过速时，旁路作为折返环的前传支，而房室结及希氏束作为逆传支（图94-6），

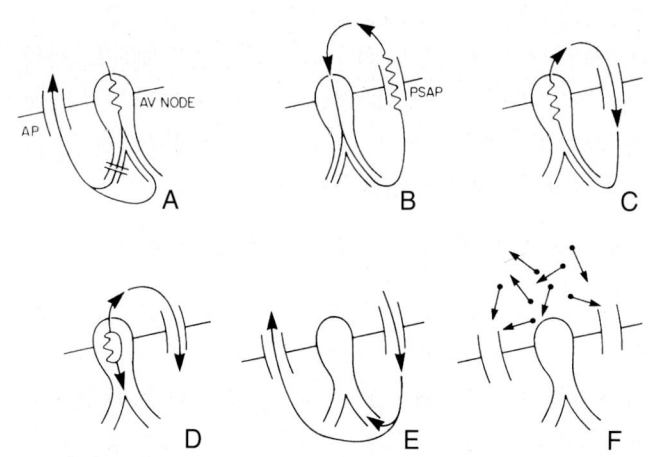

图94-3 预激综合征患者的心动过速谱 A：顺向型房室折返性心动过速不伴或伴功能性束支阻滞；B：PJRT；C：逆向型房室折返性心动过速；D：房室结折返性心动过速伴旁路旁观；E：房室结引起的预激性心动过速；F：房颤伴后间隔旁路。

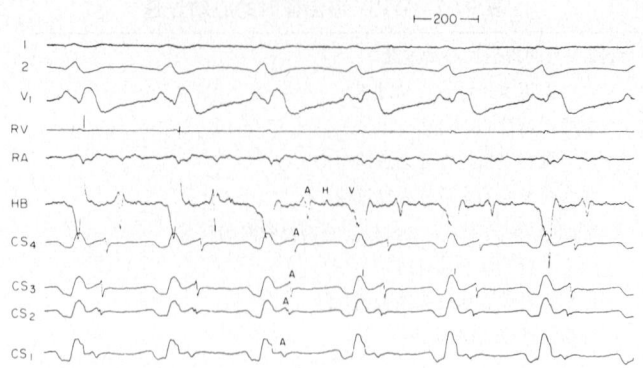

图 94-4 顺向型房室折返性心动过速伴右束支阻滞 房室结及希浦系作为折返的前传支，逆传经左侧游离壁旁路，因为心房最早激动点位于冠状静脉窦的远端。

此型心律紊乱较少见，仅占预激综合征单支旁路患者电生理检查者的 6%[35]。仅有较少的临床特征能将此型心动过速患者与其他类型的心动过速的患者相区分。已注意到，有间隔旁路的患者很少发生逆向型房室折返性心动过速，主要原因就是间隔旁路与房室结距离十分靠近。

当心室激动仅通过旁路下传时，QRS 波群显示最大程度的预激。如果预激综合征的存在并不清楚或仅是怀疑时，则逆向型房室折返性心动过速与室速的鉴别将是困难的，心动过速的机制必须与下述几种情况鉴别：多旁路的其他类型的预激性心动过速，房扑和房速伴有旁观者旁路时。为了鉴别伴有预激 QRS 图形的各种类型的心动过速，常需给患者做电生理检查。在靠近旁路的部位，心动过速发作时，发放一个联律间期较长的心房刺激：(1) 其不会影响间隔的激动；(2) 可引起预激性 QRS 波，但该波与心动过速的 QRS 形态不同；(3) 随后，夺获了间隔部的心房，证实旁路参与了心动过速的折返环。

(四) 多旁路参与的房室折返性心动过速

存在多旁路时，房室折返性心动过速发生时可能有两条旁路参与，而房室结却不参与折返。与顺向型房室折返性心动过速一样，参与折返的两条旁路有不同的前传和逆传的性质，有不同的不应期，这些将有利于折返的形成。当然，这需要一条旁路的前传，另一条旁路可能是隐匿性旁路，充当逆传支。

(五) 心房颤动和心房扑动

预激综合征患者常发生心房颤动，但预激综合征在房颤发生中的作用目前尚不完全清楚[31]。三尖瓣的 Ebstein 畸形，二尖瓣的脱垂常与预激综合征伴发，并认为这些异常可能是患者发生预激综合征的原因。但不能解释无器质性心脏病患者中房颤的发生率增加的原因。能够成为房颤发生的电生理学基础的广泛的心电疾病在预激综合征的病人中又不常见。

预激病人临床房颤的发生常与共存的房室折返性心动过速相关，在电生理检查时能够看到房室折返性心动过速转化为房颤（心动过速诱发心动过速）。这一过程中，房颤常被房早诱发（图 94-7）。典型者，房早的出现时间在高右房电图中最早，其后才是希氏束和冠状窦电图。该种房早可以起源于高右房，实际也可能起源于肺静脉。例如起源于肺静脉的房早，其可能在高右房最早出现，而伪似高右房房早。预激综合征发生房颤的可能机制已经论述很多，但都处于不完全清楚的状态。可能的因素是心房实际存在着异常，心房不应期较短，较快频率的房室折返性心动过速，交替性激动收缩反馈，以及旁路的促发作用[36-38]。所以，预激综合征患者反复发生房颤的原因可能是由多因素引起，这些病人在旁路消融成功后，绝大多数病人房颤不再复发。

预激综合征患者房颤发生的意义是快速的心室率与室颤之间的关系。房颤时，经房室传导系统前传引起的心室率常限于 180～200 次/分。正常时，这一心室率引起室颤的危险性降低。但是，某些旁路的有效不应期更短，其能下传的室上性激动能超过 300～500 次/分并能引起血流动力学的恶化。预激综合征病人猝死的危险与房颤时最短的预激性 RR 间期有关。25 例无器质性心脏病预激患者发生室颤时，该间期无一例外均短于 250ms。快速心室率引起的血流动力学和代谢的变化对室颤的发生起到了很大的作用。

七、评价的方法

为了给予病人最好的评价和治疗，医生应当详细询问病史，包括心动过速时症状的特点、诱发因素、心动过速最早发生时的年龄、伴发的症状，包括是否有晕厥、抗心律失常药物服用史、心律失常或猝死的家族史等。体格检查的结果常为阴性，因为很多预激综合征病人都很年轻，其他方面也十分健康。但部分患者可伴有先天性畸形或异常，例如二尖瓣脱垂、大血管移位、Ebstein 畸形等。我们常规给病人进行二维超声心动图检查，以评价是否患者伴有器质性心脏病。

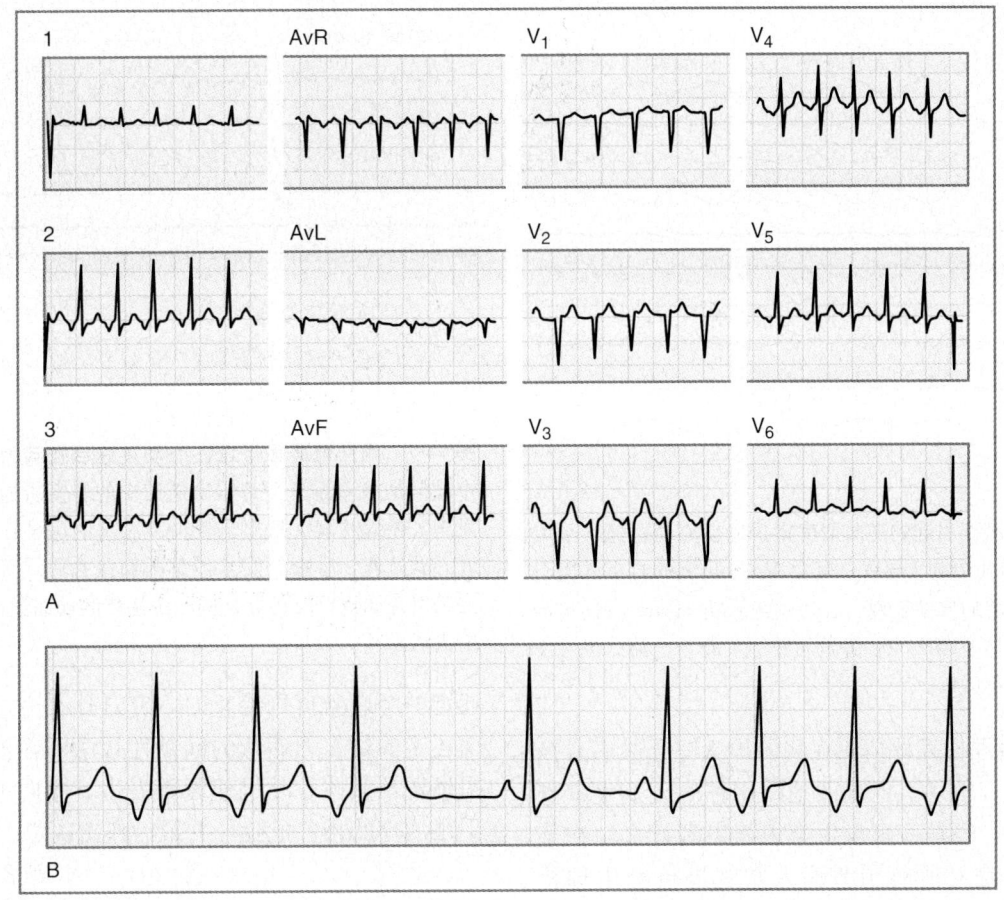

图 94-5　PJRT 患者的体表心电图　A：12 导联体表心电图，心动过速最重要的特征是 Ⅱ，Ⅲ，aVF 导联 P 波倒置，RP 间期长于 PR 间期；B：压迫右侧颈动脉窦可使心动过速暂时终止，终止时无逆向 P 波，说明折返的终止发生在逆传支，而且从图中可以看出，旁路具有类房室结样作用，一旦窦律加速将能自发心动过速。

对有旁路的预激综合征病人的评价中，进行危险分层是一个重要的内容，将危险分层及随后处理的病人常规分成三种情况。

1. 有严重症状：病人有快速房颤或室颤发生史，病人的心动过速发生频繁或严重。
2. 轻到中度症状：病人的房室折返性心动过速常发作不频繁，或能很好耐受。
3. 无症状：病人仅有心电图上的心室预激图形。

房颤伴快速预激性心室率又蜕化为室颤者是发生心脏性猝死的最危险性因素。关于这一观点几乎没有不同的意见，这种情况的病人都应通过导管或外科手术行旁路的根治性消融术。在某些特殊情况时，患者无法接受射频消融术治疗，则应通过系列的电生理检查，以评价Ⅰ类或Ⅲ类抗心律失常药物对抑制旁路传导是否有效；隐匿性旁路和真性间歇性预激综合征患者室颤发生猝死的危险性很低，因为这些旁路的特征提示其有效不应期长[28]。

但是，绝大多数预激综合征病人处于上述两个极端之中的状态。许多人无室颤的发作，但其能有反复的房室折返性心动过速的发生，而且还可能是逆向型的。对这些病人，猝死的相对危险性变异度很大。高危病人的标志包括：存在多旁路，反复发生的房室折返性心动过速或心房颤动，而且房颤发作时预激性 RR 间期小于 250ms。当病人确实属于这种情况时，则属于导管射频根治术的最强适应证，至少要给予药物治疗，而处于较低危险之中的病人可选择其他的治疗。

有创性电生理检查能够全面评估旁路的数量、位置和传导性质，评估心动过速的机制，因此是危险评估的"金指标"。旁路传导性质的特征常与患者猝死的相对危险性相关，这能使医生据此对病人进行危险分层。房颤时短于 250ms 的 RR 间期提示患者处于房颤伴快速心室率及猝死的较高危险状态。因房颤患者常同时有房室折返性心动过速，因此当病人能被诱发房室折返性心动过速和房颤而且预激性室率很快者，则成为有发生室颤的较高危险的亚组[13,31]。

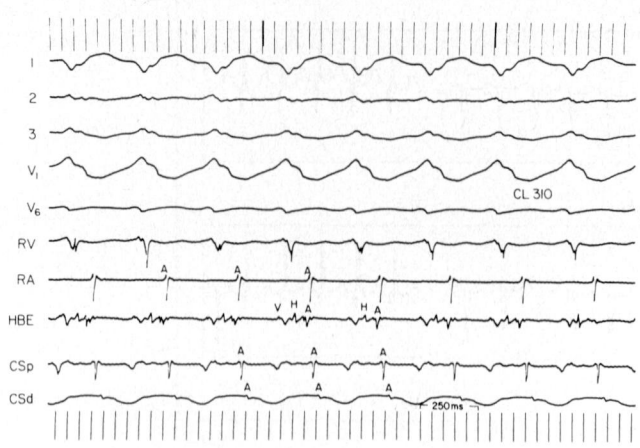

图94-6 左侧壁旁路引起的逆向型房室折返性心动过速 最大的预激性QRS波出现在I导联，以及V_1导联上的右束支阻滞是左侧壁旁路下传的典型表现。心动过速周期310ms时逆传的H波恰好出现在房室结区的心房激动波（A波）之前，说明逆传是经房室结和希氏束。

应用电生理检查评估无症状的预激综合征患者猝死的危险性最有争议。但很清楚，这种病人发生室颤的几率十分低，但是一旦发生常引起患者死亡。在某些中心，并不是对所有预激病人常规进行电生理检查，在电生理检查中大约20%的无症状预激病人能诱发房颤伴快速心室率，其最短的预激性RR间期<250ms[23]。因此，该预后价值的特异性十分低，而且即使其对猝死危险来说是敏感的，但其预测价值是低的。基于上述所见，应用电生理检查的方法对无症状的预激患者进行危险分层十分不妥，应当选择这类病人，其生活模式或职业活动即使发生一个小的危险也不能接受的人，对于这种人应当做心脏电生理检查进行评估。所以决定做电生理检查进行危险分层时，一定是考虑到要降低室颤作为预激患者的第一个症状表现，而且任何一项检查都存在这种危险。更重要的是一定要考虑到这种危险的可能性治疗。因为电生理检查的任何不良所见都不可避免地给予针对性适当治疗。最终，病人都要选择接受电生理检查及射频消融术或心动过速反复发作可能带来的危险。

八、治 疗

此章未对药物和非药物治疗进行详细的讨论，此内容可参考本书其他章节（117章）[31,39,40]。对于WPW综合征中的间歇性预激，如果房室折返性心动过速发作不频繁或短阵发作，患者可耐受，并可通过

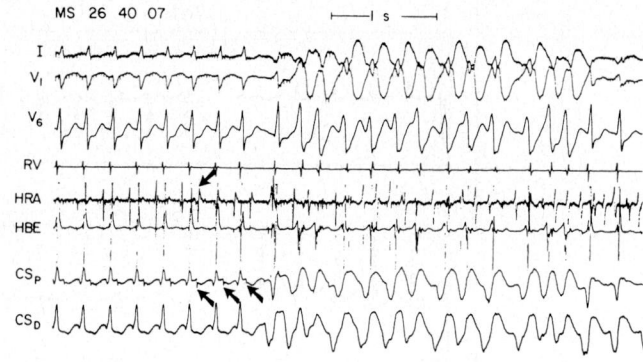

图94-7 顺向型房室折返性心动过速自发转为心房颤动 图中最早是左室侧壁旁路作为逆传支的房室折返性心动过速的发生，顶部的箭头指出自发性高右房的房早终止了房室折返性心动过速，房颤的发生最早限制在右房，而此时较低的左房仍然是原折返环传导来的心房逆传激动而激动。（下行3个箭头指示）

迷走神经刺激自行终止时，究竟什么方法治疗更为合理还不清楚。无症状的间歇性预激不需治疗。但是如果患者预激性心动过速频繁发生，应向患者说明各种干预治疗的相关危险，并最后作出决定。

（郭继鸿 译）

参 考 文 献

1. Wolff L, Parkinson J, White P, et al: Bundle branch block with short P-R interval in healthy young people prone to paroxysmal tachycardia. Am Heart J 5:685, 1930.
2. MacRae CA, Ghaisas N, Kass S, et al: Familial hypertrophic cardiomyopathy with Wolff-Parkinson-White syndrome. J Clin Invest 96:1216, 1995.
3. Gollob MH, Green MS, Tang AS, et al: Identification of a gene responsible for familial Wolff-Parkinson-White syndrome. N Engl J Med 344:1823, 2001.
4. Gollob MH, Seger JJ, Gollob TN, et al: Novel PRKAG2 mutation responsible for the genetic syndrome of ventricular preexcitation and conduction system disease with childhood onset and absence of cardiac hypertrophy. Circulation 104:3030, 2001.
5. Mehdirad AA, Fatkin D, DiMarco JP, et al: Electrophysiologic characteristics of accessory atrioventricular connections in an inherited form of Wolff-Parkinson-White syndrome. J Cardiovasc Electrophysiol 10:629, 1999.
6. Coppess MA, Altermose GT, Jayachandran JV, et al: Unusual features of intermediate septal bypass tracts. J Cardiovasc Electrophysiol 11:730, 2000.
7. Guiraudon GM, Klein GJ, Yee R, et al: Surgery for the Wolff-Parkinson-White syndrome. In Zipes DP, Jalife J (eds): Cardiac Electrophysiology: From Cell to Bedside, 2nd ed. Philadelphia, WB Saunders, 1995, p 1553.
8. Prystowsky EN, Browne KF, Zipes DP: Intracardiac recording by catheter electrode of accessory pathway depolarization. J Am Coll Cardiol 1:463, 1983.
9. Jackman WM, Friday KJ, Scherlag BJ, et al: Direct endocardial recording from an accessory atrioventricular pathway: Localization of the site of block, effect of antiarrhythmic drugs, and attempt at nonsurgical ablation. Circulation 68:906, 1983.
10. Fogel RI, Gest C, Evans JJ, et al: Oblique accessory pathway orientation: New observations and implications for mapping and suc-

diagnosis and localization of multiple accessory pathways. Circulation 81:578, 1990.
12. Teo WS, Klein GJ, Guiraudon GM, et al: Multiple accessory pathways in the Wolff-Parkinson-White syndrome as a risk factor for ventricular fibrillation. Am J Cardiol 15:889, 1991.
13. Pappone C, Santinelli V, Rosanio S, et al: Usefulness of invasive electrophysiologic testing to stratify the risk of arrhythmic events in asymptomatic patients with Wolff-Parkinson-White pattern. J Am Coll Cardiol 41:239, 2003.
14. Mahaim I, Winston MR: Recherches d'anatomic comparée du pathologie experimentale sur les connexions hautes du faisceau de His-Tawara. Cardiologia 5:189, 1941.
15. Ellenbogen KA, Ramirez NM, Packer DL, et al: Accessory nodoventricular (Mahaim) fibers: A clinical review. Pacing Clin Electrophysiol 9:868, 1986.
16. Klein GJ, Guiraudon GM, Kerr CR, et al: "Nodoventricular" accessory pathway: Evidence for a distinct accessory AV pathway with AV node-like properties. J Am Coll Cardiol 11:1035, 1988.
17. Murdock CJ, Leitch JW, Klein GJ, et al: Epicardial mapping in patients with "nodoventricular" accessory pathways. Am J Cardiol 68:208, 1991.
18. Tchou P, Lehmann MH, Jazayeri M, et al: Atriofascicular connection or a nodoventricular Mahaim fiber? Electrophysiologic elucidation of the pathway and associated reentrant circuit. Circulation 77:837, 1988.
19. McClelland JH, Wang X, Beckman KJ, et al: Radiofrequency catheter ablation of right atriofascicular (Mahaim) accessory pathways guided by accessory pathway activation potentials. Circulation 89:2655, 1994.
20. Bromberg BI, Lindsay BD, Cain ME, et al: Impact of clinical history and electrophysiologic characterization of accessory pathways on management strategies to reduce sudden death among children with Wolff-Parkinson-White syndrome. J Am Coll Cardiol 27:690, 1996.
21. Fitzsimmons PJ, McWhirter PD, Peterson DW, et al: The natural history of Wolff-Parkinson-White syndrome in 228 military aviators: A long-term follow-up of 22 years. Am Heart J 142:530, 2001.
22. Goudevenos JA, Katsouras CS, Graekas G, et al: Ventricular pre-excitation in the general population: A study on the mode of presentation and clinical course. Heart 83:29, 2000.
23. Leitch JW, Klein GJ, Yee R: Prognostic value of electrophysiology testing in asymptomatic patients with Wolff-Parkinson-White syndrome. Circulation 82:1718, 1990.
24. Klein GJ, Yee R, Sharma AD: Longitudinal electrophysiologic assessment of asymptomatic patients with the Wolff-Parkinson-White electrocardiographic pattern. N Engl J Med 320:1229, 1989.
25. Auricchio A, Klein H, Trappe H, et al: Lack of prognostic value of syncope in patients with Wolff-Parkinson-White syndrome. J Am Coll Cardiol 17:152, 1991.
26. Paul T, Guccione P, Garson A Jr: Relation of syncope in young patients with Wolff-Parkinson-White syndrome to rapid ventricular response during atrial fibrillation. Am J Cardiol 65:318, 1990.
27. Leitch JW, Klein GJ, Yee R, et al: Syncope associated with supraventricular tachycardia: An expression of tachycardia rate or vasomotor response? Circulation 85:1064, 1992.
28. Klein GJ, Gulamhusein SS: Intermittent preexcitation in the Wolff-Parkinson-White syndrome. Am J Cardiol 52:292, 1983.
29. Haïssaguerre M, Marcus F, Poquet F, et al: Electrocardiographic characteristics and catheter ablation of parahissian accessory pathways. Circulation 90:1124, 1994.
30. Arruda MS, McClelland HJ, Wang X, et al: Development and validation of an ECG algorithm for identifying accessory pathway ablation site in Wolff-Parkinson-White syndrome. J Cardiovasc Electrophysiol 9:2, 1998.
31. Prystowsky EN, Klein GJ: Cardiac Arrhythmias: An Integrated Approach for the Clinician. New York, McGraw-Hill, 1994.
32. Hirao K, Otomo K, Wang X, et al: Para-hisian pacing: A new method for differentiating retrograde conduction over an accessory AV pathway from conduction over the AV node. Circulation 94:1027, 1996.
33. Miles WM, Yee R, Klein GJ, et al: The preexcitation index: An aid in determining the mechanism of supraventricular tachycardia and localizing accessory pathways. Circulation 74:493, 1986.
34. Coumel J, Cabrolo C, Fabiato A, et al: Tachycardie permanent par rhythm reciproque: I. Preuves du diagnostic par stimulation auriculaire et ventriculaire. Arch Mal Coeur 60:1830, 1967.
35. Packer DL, Gallagher JJ, Prystowsky EN: Physiologic substrate for antidromic reciprocating tachycardia: Prerequisite characteristics of the accessory pathway and AV conduction system. Circulation 85:574, 1992.
36. Prystowsky EN: Tachycardia-induced tachycardia: A mechanism of initiation of atrial fibrillation. In DiMarco JP, Prystowsky EN (eds): Atrial Arrhythmias: State of the Art. Armonk, NY, Futura Publishing, 1995, p 81.
37. Chen PS, Pressley JC, Tang AS, et al: New observations on atrial fibrillation before and after surgery in patients with Wolff-Parkinson-White syndrome. J Am Coll Cardiol 19:974, 1992.
38. Iesaka Y, Yamane T, Takahashi A, et al: Retrograde multiple and multifiber accessory pathway conduction in the Wolff-Parkinson-White syndrome. J Cardiovasc Electrophysiol 9(2):141–151, 1998
39. Jackman WM, Wang X, Friday KJ, et al: Catheter ablation of accessory atrioventricular pathways (Wolff-Parkinson-White syndrome) by radiofrequency current. N Engl J Med 324:1605, 1991.
40. Guiraudon GM, Guiraudon CM, Klein GJ, et al: Operation for the Wolff-Parkinson-White syndrome in the catheter ablation era. Ann Thorac Surg 47:1084, 1994.

第 95 章

窦房结功能障碍

Michael O. Sweeney

本章目录
- 对窦房结功能障碍的再认识 ………… 862
- 临床表现和治疗 ……………………… 862

一、对窦房结功能障碍的再认识

窦房结功能障碍于 1968 年首次作为一种临床疾病进行描述[1]，尽管其心电图表现早在 1923 年即被 Wenckebach 报告。窦房结功能障碍是一系列窦房结和心房电活动形成及传导功能异常的总称，包括持续性窦性心动过缓、无明显病因可循的变时性功能不全、阵发性或持续性窦性停搏伴交界性或室性逸搏，以及阵发性或持续性心房颤动。阵发性心房颤动与窦性心动过缓常交替出现，且两者可在短时间内快速转换，并伴有明显的临床症状，称为慢快综合征。

窦房结功能障碍主要见于老年人，推测与窦房结和心房肌的退行性变有关。有关心房起搏治疗窦房结功能障碍的 28 项研究结果表明，这些患者中完全性房室阻滞的年发生率平均为 0.6%（0～4.5%），总发病率平均为 2.1%（0～11.9%）。这一结果提示，尽管退行性变是一缓慢发展的过程，且在疾病发展过程中并不占主导地位，但却可影响整个特殊传导系统[2]。窦房结功能障碍常在六七十岁的老年人中诊断[3]，这也恰恰是因窦房结功能障碍接受起搏治疗的平均年龄[4,5]。窦房结功能障碍也可继发于任何一种导致窦房结细胞受损的器质性疾病，如心肌缺血、感染或心脏外科手术等，其可发生于任何年龄段。

窦房结功能障碍的临床表现可因窦房结受损的程度不同而各异，其中最突出的表现为晕厥。晕厥是由突然发生的长间歇（自发性或继发于房性快速心律失常终止后）引起的脑供血不足所致。这种长间歇导致的血流动力学障碍常因其后的交界性逸搏或室性逸搏不适当出现、延迟出现或未出现而加重。然而，多数窦房结功能障碍患者因其临床表现隐匿而多变，以及对日常活动产生的不适当心率变时性反应，而难以诊断。直到最近几年，心率随日常活动量的改变而发生动态变化的变时性功能的重要性才逐渐得到关注。目前认为，日常活动后正常的心率加快通常为次极量的，但因其频繁发生持续短暂的心率变化从而消耗了大量的心率储备。这种次极量的心率变时性反应不受年龄和性别的影响[6]。

二、临床表现和治疗

未经治疗的窦房结功能障碍患者的自然病程可相差甚远。因窦性停搏和窦性心动过缓发生过晕厥的患者，大多表现为晕厥的反复发作[3]。并不少见的是，窦房结功能障碍患者的自然病程可因某些必需的药物治疗而加剧潜在心动过缓的发生。在起搏方式选择研究（Mode Selection Trial，MOST）[4]中，由≥3 秒的窦性停搏或心动过缓伴变时功能不良而引发症状的患者，使用药物治疗受限的比率分别高达 47% 和 53%。窦房结功能障碍引起猝死的发生率非常低，不论是否接受起搏器治疗，窦房结功能障碍本身不会影响患者的存活率[7,8]。

对于症状性心动过缓唯一有效的治疗是置入永久心脏起搏器。尽管近 20 年来，北美和欧洲对数千名患者进行了研究，窦房结功能障碍的最佳起搏模式和起搏系统的选择仍未确定。尽管凭直觉认为，双腔起搏器的房室同步起搏（DDDR）应优于心室起搏（VVIR），但令人震惊的是，双腔起搏的优势很难被证实。几项大规模临床随机研究的结果均表明，接受DDDR起搏治疗的患者在长期生存率上并未获益[4,9]。然而，即使同一项研究，所得出的起搏模式对不同心血管疾病（如心衰、卒中、房颤）的影响也常相互矛盾。

有关窦房结功能障碍起搏模式选择的临床研究归纳于表95-1。最初的研究为20世纪80年代来自瑞典的两篇连续报道[10,11]，结果表明，与AAI起搏患者相比，接受VVI起搏治疗的窦房结功能障碍患者的心房颤动、卒中和心衰的发生率明显增高。然而，由于大量资料的选择偏倚，使得其结果无法得到合理可信的诠释[12]。Danish研究是对窦房结功能障碍不同起搏模式进行比较的第一项前瞻性随机研究，平均随访3年，结果表明，尽管心房颤动、卒中的发生率及总死亡率在不同治疗组无显著差异，但AAI起搏组卒中和体循环栓塞的联合终点明显低于VVI治疗组（两组分别为5%和20%，$P=0.005$），之后将随访时间延长为5年以上的资料分析进一步证实了此结论[14]。与心室起搏相比，心房起搏可减少心房颤动、卒中、心衰的发生及降低心血管死亡。然而此研究尚缺乏足够的统计学证据明确回答在降低死亡率上房性起搏是否优于心室起搏这一问题[12,15]。

其他有关心脏起搏模式选择的研究结果亦各异。老年患者起搏器选择研究（Pacemaker Selection in the Elderly，PASE）[5]中，因窦房结功能障碍而接受DDDR起搏治疗的患者比VVIR治疗组的生活质量有所改善，临床终点指标（总死亡率、心房颤动、卒中

表95-1 有关起搏模式选择的随机研究

	Danish 研究	PASE	CTOPP	Pac-A-Tach	MOST	UK-PACE
目标人群	窦房结功能障碍房室阻滞	窦房结功能障碍亚组	所有病因导致的心动过缓	窦房结功能障碍	窦房结功能障碍	所有病因导致的心动过缓
治疗模式	比较VVI与AAI/DDD(R)	比较VVIR与DDDR	比较VVI(R)与AAI/DDD(R)	比较VVIR与DDDR	比较VVIR与DDDR	比较VVI(R)与AAI/DDD(R)
患者人数	225	175	2568	198	2010	2000
平均年龄（岁）	76	76	73	72	74	>70
平均随访时间（月）	66	18	36	25	33	50
中途退出率（%）	1.7	28	<5	44	26	<5
状态	完成	完成	完成	完成	完成	完成
心房颤动	AAI/DDD(R) 24% VVI(R) 35% $P=0.07$	DDD(R) 19% VVI(R) 28% $P=0.06$	DDD(R) 5.34%/年 VVI(R) 6.59%/年 $P=0.04$	在一年中 DDDR 43% VVIR 48% $P=0.09$	DDD 22.8% VVI 27.8% $P=0.00$	
卒中	AAI/DDD(R) 12% VVI(R) 23% $P=0.03$	DDD(R) 20% VVI(R) 31% $P=0.07$	DDD(R) 1.09%/年 VVI(R) 1.02%/年	未报告	DDDR 4.2% VVIR 5.6% $P=0.36$	
死亡率	AAI/DDD(R) 35% VVI(R) 50%	DDD(R) 20% VVI(R) 2%	DDD(R) 20% VVI(R) 19%	DDDR 3.2% VVIR 6.8%	DDDR 18.9% VVIR 17.7% $P=0.78$	
年死亡率	AAI/DDD(R) 6.4% VVI(R) 9.0%	DDD(R) 13.3% VVI(R) 8.0%	DDD(R) 6.5% VVI(R) 6.3%	DDDR 3.4% VVIR 1.6%	DDDR 6.3% VVIR 5.9%	
评论	VVI组未充分使用华法林		3年后DDDR组房颤的发生率下降	样本量小交叉率高	DDDR组心衰轻度减少 DDDR组11.0% VVIR组12.4%	

和心衰）的发生亦有减少的趋势。而因间歇性或持续性心脏阻滞而植入起搏器的患者中，这些临床终点指标无显著差异。小规模的 Pac-A-Tach 研究结果表明，植入 VVIR 起搏器的窦房结功能障碍患者死亡率（6.8%）明显高于 DDDR 组（3.2%），而心房颤动的发生率两组无明显差异[16]。加拿大生理性起搏研究（The Canadian Trial of Physiologic Pacing，CTOPP）结果表明，因各种原因（房室阻滞、窦房结功能障碍或两者并存）接受 DDDR 起搏治疗的患者，心房颤动的发生率均低于 VVIR 治疗组，而在卒中和总死亡率联合终点上两者无显著差异[9]。CTOPP 研究还发现，与 VVIR 起搏相比，双腔起搏可以延缓发展至持续性房颤的进程[17]。在 MOST 研究中，与 VVIR 起搏相比，DDDR 起搏组心力衰竭和心房颤动的发生率有一定程度的降低，但死亡率无显著差异[4]。

因此，起搏器治疗虽可消除症状性心动过缓，但并不影响窦房结功能障碍患者的死亡率。由于窦房结功能障碍这一疾病的进程在不断发展，因此，起搏治疗之后，心衰和房颤等决定病情发展程度的因素日益受到愈来愈多的关注。

多项研究表明，在起搏器植入前，窦房结功能障碍患者发生阵发房颤的发生率约 40%~45%[13,18,19]。MOST 研究中，50% 以上的患者在起搏器植入前已有至少一次客观记录的阵发性房颤发作，且 75% 的患者最近一次房颤发生于植入前的 3 周内[4]。窦房结功能障碍患者约 50%~60% 可经起搏器检出房颤，且此发生率随着随访时间的延长而增加[20,21]。在 MOST 研究中，起搏器检出的阵发性房颤是预测卒中、死亡和持续性房颤发生的有力而独立的危险因子，且与动态心电图记录到的房颤吻合良好[21]。由于临床症状并不能可靠地预测哪些窦房结功能障碍患者可经起搏器检出阵发性房颤的发生，因此，起搏器对于检出这些患者的心律失常有重要的作用[22]。

有关起搏器模式选择的临床研究的结果表明，与 VVIR 治疗相比，AAI 或 DDDR 治疗可在一定程度上降低心房颤动的发生率。然而，VVIR 起搏对房颤发生的影响并不如动物实验预期的那么明显，且可延迟发生 3 年以上[9]，这可以从以下两个方面给以解释。

持续性房颤在人和动物均可导致心房电重构，这表现为心房有效不应期缩短及离散、传导速度减慢、房颤易被诱发[23-26]，形成了"房颤诱发房颤的连缀现象"[23]。这种与持续性房颤相关的心房电重构可被心脏电复律所逆转，逆转的程度与复律后窦性心律的维持时间有关[27]。上述心房电重构的作用可能也与心房增大及压力增高有一定关系。

与心房起搏相比，非房室同步的心室起搏患者心房颤动的发生率增高 2~3 倍，主要与类似于慢性房颤的电重构有关。由 VVI 起搏造成的长期房室不同步可使心房有效不应期缩短，窦房结功能恢复时间延长，P 波增宽（传导缓慢）[28]，这种电重构可被房室同步的 DDD 起搏模式逆转[28]。这种电生理异常还常伴有心房内径增大[28,29]。

窦房结功能障碍患者在起搏器植入前房颤的发生率高，提示我们在起搏器植入前，导致房颤反复发作的一定程度的电重构即已存在。在无房颤发作史的窦房结功能障碍患者，心房不应性尚正常，但局部心房传导已有所减慢[30]。在既往有房颤发作且植入双腔起搏器后仍有房颤发作的病人，心房传导障碍更为严重[31]，提示这些患者房颤反复发作的电生理基质不是心动过缓依赖的。部分重构的心房可因持续的 VVIR 起搏而加剧，且间断的 DDDR 起搏也并不会使其得到改善。而在临床中，许多窦房结功能障碍患者并不需要持续性起搏，这使得对起搏模式效果的评价更为困难。例如，静息心律良好且房室传导功能正常的患者，可能仅在窦性停搏时需要启动起搏功能。这些实际情况，尤其是当所设定的心率足够慢而使自主窦性心律占优势时，将减弱持续性 DDDR 起搏的获益，而掩盖 VVIR 起搏的弊端。这与永久性心脏阻滞的患者持续性 VVIR 起搏造成最大化房室失同步的情况迥异。

其次，DDDR 所达到的生理性起搏的效果与 AAI 所达到的效果并不等同。双腔起搏器因其能保持房室同步被认为是生理性起搏，而 VVI 起搏因房室同步丧失而被认为是非生理性起搏。实际上，心房起搏和 DDDR 起搏仅在保持房室同步性方面相似。心房起搏保持了正常生理性的心室激动和收缩方式（室间传导正常的患者），且对心室功能无不良影响。越来越多的证据表明，DDDR 模式的右室起搏尽管保持了房室同步性，但仍属非生理性起搏，可对心室血流动力学、心功能、心肌灌注和心肌细胞结构产生缓慢的不利影响[29,32-38]。

因窦房结功能障碍而接受起搏治疗的患者，包括伴有充血性心力衰竭的病人，大多房室传导功能正常，QRS 波群不宽（室内传导正常），故传统的 DDDR 起搏常可造成强迫性室间失同步。MOST 研究的一项分析表明，尽管 DDDR 起搏保持了房室同步

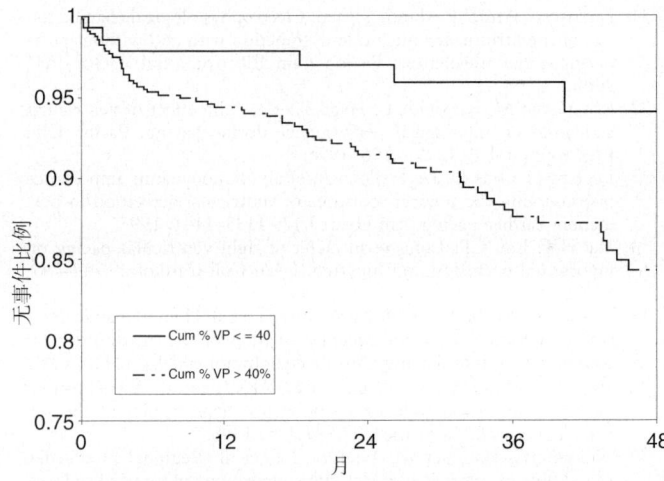

图 95-1　DDDR 工作模式时最初 30 天内心室起搏百分比与随访中不因心衰住院的维持率　Cum%VP，整个随访过程中累积心室起搏的百分比。

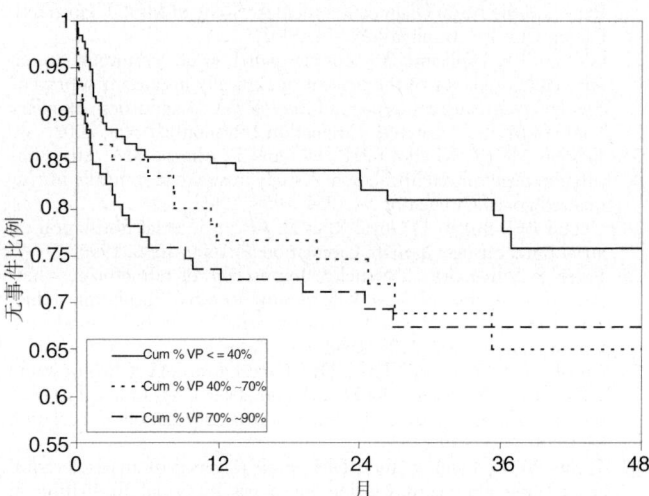

图 95-2　DDDR 工作模式时最初 30 天内心室起搏百分比与随访中不因房颤住院的维持率　Cum%VP，整个随访过程中累积心室起搏的百分比。

性，但与基础状态下 QRS 波群时限正常且心室起搏较少的患者相比，心室起搏比例超过 40% 可使心衰住院的风险增高 2.6 倍[39]。DDDR 模式下心室起搏每增加 1%，房颤发生的危险性亦增高 1%。在对已知的所有关于心衰和房颤的基线预测因子进行校正后，心室起搏是心衰和房颤发生的一个重要的独立危险因素（图 95-1，95-2）。这些研究或可解释此前困扰我们的矛盾性结果：Anderson 等[14]报告 AAI 起搏明显优于 DDDR 起搏，而 Connolly 等[9]、Lamas 等[4]报道 DDDR 起搏更有益。由此得出对于正常室内激动顺序的窦房结功能障碍患者，选择最佳起搏模式的 4 个目标应为：（1）防止症状性心动过缓；（2）必要时能提供生理性变时功能；（3）必要时能保持房室同步；（4）尽可能保持正常的心室激动顺序。

（张海澄　译）

参 考 文 献

1. Ferrer I: The sick sinus syndrome in atrial disease. JAMA 206:645–652, 1968.
2. Rosenqvist M, Obel IW: Atrial pacing and the risk for AV block: Is there a time for change in attitude? Pacing Clin Electrophysiol 12:97–101, 1989.
3. Menozzi C, Brignole M, Alboni P, et al: The natural course of untreated sick sinus syndrome and identification of variables predictive of unfavorable outcome. Am J Cardiol 82:1205–1209, 1998.
4. Lamas GA, Lee KL, Sweeney MO, et al: Ventricular pacing or dual chamber pacing for sinus node dysfunction. N Engl J Med 346:1854–1862, 2002.
5. Lamas GA, Orav EJ, Stambler BS, et al: Quality of life and clinical outcomes in elderly patients treated with ventricular pacing as compared with dual-chamber pacing. N Engl J Med 338:1097–1104, 1998.
6. Mianulli M, Birchfield D, Yakimow K, et al: Do elderly pacemaker patients need rate adaptation? Implications of daily heart rate behavior in normal adults [abstract]. Pacing Clin Electrophysiol 19:681A, 1996.
7. Alt E, Voker R, Wirtzfeld A, Ulm L: Survival and follow up after pacemaker implantation: A comparison of patients with sick sinus syndrome, complete heart block and atrial fibrillation. Pacing Clin Electrophysiol 8:849–855, 1985.
8. Simon AB, Janz N: Symptomatic brady-arrhythmias in the adult: natural history following ventricular pacemaker implantation. Pacing Clin Electrophysiol 5:372–383, 1982.
9. Connolly SJ, Kerr CR, Gent M, et al: Effects of physiologic pacing versus ventricular pacing on the risk of stroke and death due to cardiovascular causes. N Engl J Med 342:1385–1391, 2000.
10. Rosenqvist M, Brandt J, Schuller H: Atrial versus ventricular pacing in sinus node disease: A treatment comparison study. Am Heart J 111:292–297, 1986.
11. Rosenqvist M, Brandt J, Schuller H: Long-term pacing in sinus node disease: Effects of stimulation mode on cardiovascular morbidity and mortality. Am Heart J 116:16–22, 1988.
12. Lamas GA: Pacemaker mode selection and survival: A plea to apply the principles of evidence based medicine to cardiac pacing practice. Heart 78:218–220, 1997.
13. Andersen HR, Thuesen L, Bagger JP, et al: Prospective randomized trial of atrial versus ventricular pacing in sick sinus syndrome. Lancet 344:1523–1528, 1994.
14. Andersen HR, Nielsen JC, Rhomsen PEB, et al: Long-term follow-up of patients from a randomized trial of atrial versus ventricular pacing for sick-sinus syndrome. Lancet 350:1210–1216, 1997.
15. Connolly SJ, Kerr C, Gent M, Yusuf S: Dual-chamber versus ventricular pacing. Critical appraisal of current data. Circulation 94:578–583, 1996.
16. Wharton JM, Sorrentino RA, Campbell P, et al: Effect of pacing modality on atrial tachyarrhythmia recurrence in the tachycardia-bradycardia syndrome: Preliminary results of the Pacemaker Atrial Tachycardia Trial. Circulation XX(suppl I):I-494, 1998.
17. Skanes AC, Krahn AD, Yee R, et al: Progression to chronic atrial fibrillation after pacing: The Canadian Trial of Physiologic Pacing. CTOPP Investigators. J Am Coll Cardiol 38:167–172, 2001.
18. Santini M, Alexidou G, Ansalone G, et al: Relation of prognosis in sick sinus syndrome to age, conduction defects and modes of permanent cardiac pacing. Am J Cardiol 65:729–735, 1990.
19. Simonsen E, Nielsen JS, Nielsen BL: Sinus node dysfunction in 128 patients. A retrospective study with follow-up. Acta Med Scand 208:343–348, 1980.
20. Gillis AM, Morck BA: Atrial fibrillation after DDDR pacemaker implantation. J Cardiovasc Electrophysiol 13:542–547, 2002.
21. Glotzer TV, Zimmerman J, Sweeney MO, et al: Atrial high rate episodes detected by pacemaker diagnostics predict death and stroke:

Report of the Atrial Diagnostics Ancillary Study of MOST [abstract]. Pacing Clin Electrophyiol 25:553, 2002.
22. Glotzer TV, Hellkamp AS, Zimmerman J, et al: Symptoms are an unreliable predictor of the present of clinically important supraventricular tachycardias: Report of the Atrial Diagnostics Ancillary Study of MOST [abstract]. Circulation 106(suppl):II-603, 2002.
23. Wijffels MCEF, Kirchof CJHJ, Dorland R, Allessie MA: Atrial fibrillation begets atrial fibrillation: A study in awake chronically instrumented goats. Circulation 92:1954–1968, 1995.
24. Daoud EG, Bogun F, Goyal R, et al: Effect of atrial fibrillation on atrial refractoriness in man. Circulation 94:1600–1606, 1996.
25. Fareh S, Villemaire C, Nattel S: Importance of refractoriness heterogeneity in the enhanced vulnerability to atrial fibrillation induction caused by tachycardia-induced atrial electrical remodeling. Circulation 98:2202–2209, 1998.
26. Morillo CA, Klein GJ, Jones DL, Guiraudon GM: Chronic rapid atrial pacing: Structural, functional, and electrophysiological characteristics of a new model of sustained atrial fibrillation. Circulation 91:1588–1595, 1995.
27. Hobbs WJC, Fynn S, Todd DM, et al: Reversal of atrial electrical remodeling after cardioversion for persistent atrial fibrillation in humans. Circulation 101:1145–1151, 2000.
28. Sparks PB, Mond HG, Vohra JK, et al: Electrical remodeling of the atria following loss of atrioventricular synchrony: A long-term study in humans. Circulation 100:1894–1900, 1999.
29. Nielsen JC, Andersen HR, Thomsen PEB, et al: Heart failure and echocardiographic changes during long-term follow-up of patients with sick sinus syndrome randomized to single-chamber atrial or ventricular pacing. Circulation 97:987–995, 1998.
30. De Sisti A, Leclerq JF, Fiorello P, et al: Electrophysiologic characteristics of the atrium in sinus node dysfunction: Atrial refractoriness and conduction. J Cardiovasc Electrophysiol 11:30–33, 2000.
31. De Sisti A, Attuel P, Manot S, et al: Electrophysiological characteristics of the atrium in sinus node dysfunction with and without post-pacing atrial fibrillation. Pacing Clin Electrophysiol 23:303–308, 2000.
32. Rosenqvist M, Bergfeldt L, Haga Y, et al: The effect of ventricular activation on myocardial performance during pacing. Pacing Clin Electrophysiol 19:1279–1286, 1996.
33. Leclerc C, Gras D, Le Helloco A, et al: Hemodynamic importance of preserving the normal sequence of ventricular activation in permanent cardiac pacing. Am Heart J 129:1133–1141, 1995.
34. Tse H-F, Lau CP: Long-term effect of right ventricular pacing on myocardial perfusion and function. J Am Coll Cardiol 29:744–749, 1997.
35. Vanderheyden M, Goethals M, Anguera I, et al: Hemodynamic deterioration following radiofrequency ablation of the atrioventricular conduction system. Pacing Clin Electrophysiol 20:2422–2428, 1997.
36. Van Oosterhout MFM, Prinzen FW, Arts T, et al: Asynchronous electrical activation induces asymmetrical hypertrophy of the left ventricular wall. Circulation 98:588–595, 1998.
37. Nielsen JC, Bottcher M, Nielsen TT, et al: Regional myocardial blood flow in patients with sick sinus syndrome randomized to long-term single chamber or dual chamber pacing—Effect of pacing mode and rate. J Am Coll Cardiol 35:1453–1461, 2000.
38. Karpawhich P, Mital S: Comparative left ventricular function following atrial, septal and apical single chamber heart pacing in the young. Pacing Clin Electrophysiol 20:1983–1988, 1997.
39. Sweeney MO, Hellkamp AS, Greenspon AJ, et al: Adverse effect of ventricular pacing on heart failure and atrial fibrillation among patients with normal baseline QRS duration in a clinical trial of pacemaker therapy for sinus node dysfunction. Circulation 107(23):2932–2937, 2003.

第 96 章

晕 厥

Hugh Calkins

本章目录

- 鉴别诊断 ································ 867
- 诊断性检查 ······························ 868
- 病史及体格检查 ························ 868
- 心电图 ·································· 871
- 信号平均电图 ··························· 871
- 动态心电图检查 ························ 871
- 事件监测 ································ 872
- 超声心动图 ······························ 872
- 直立倾斜试验 ··························· 872
- 电生理检查 ······························ 873
- 计算机断层扫描,脑电图,颈动脉扫描和颈动脉造影 ············ 874
- 运动试验和心导管检查 ··············· 874
- 血液学检查 ······························ 874
- 晕厥患者的评估流程 ·················· 875
- 评价晕厥患者时应考虑的其他问题 ···································· 875
- 总结 ······································· 875

晕厥（源于希腊语 synkope，意指停止、暂停）是指突然、暂时的丧失意识和姿势紧张，并可很快自行恢复。意识丧失可能的机制为：流向网状激活系统（脑干中支配意识的烟胺比林网络）的血流可逆性减少。与许多其他器官相比，大脑的代谢更加依赖于灌注。因此，脑血流停止大约 10s 就会出现意识丧失。在晕厥发作停止后，行为和定向力通常立即恢复。逆行性遗忘并不常见。典型的晕厥发作通常短于 20s，但也有报道发现持续数分钟的病例。由于其常见、花费昂贵、常常导致劳动能力丧失、导致受伤并且可能是心源性猝死前的唯一预兆[1]，晕厥被公认为是一种严重的临床病症。晕厥患者中大约有 6%经住院治疗，3%曾赴急诊诊治。统计显示，年龄较小的成人中约有三分之一曾有意识丧失发作史，其中多数为孤立事件，并且未向医务人员报告。Framingham 心脏研究对 7814 人进行了两年的观察，发现首次晕厥的年发生率为 0.62%[2]。每年用于诊断和治疗晕厥患者的费用估计达 8 亿美元[3]。晕厥患者的生活质量明显降低[4]。由于最终诊断各异，晕厥的预后也有很大不同。例如，在 Framingham 心脏研究中，晕厥患者（包括病因不明者）的死亡率高于无晕厥者。其中心脏原因导致的晕厥患者死亡率最高，而由神经调节紊乱导致的晕厥患者（包括直立性低血压和药物相关的晕厥）死亡率并不增加[2]。

本章旨在回顾晕厥的病因，总结其类型，归纳有诊断价值检查的诊断标准，概括晕厥患者的评估流程。由于晕厥的病因诊断没有金标准，因而不可能确定某项检查的敏感性和特异性。由于其他章节已经详细介绍了晕厥的治疗，故本章不再赘述。

一、鉴别诊断

晕厥的病因可归纳为 6 大类：血管性、心源性、神经/脑血管性、心理性、代谢/多种原因以及不明原因导致的晕厥。血管性晕厥可进一步分为反射调节、体位性和解剖异常三种类型。心源性晕厥可进一步分为器质性和心律失常性晕厥。表96-1中显示的是近期

3个前瞻性临床试验中，晕厥的分类及不同类型的相对比例[5-7]。血管性晕厥的发生率最高，其次是心源性晕厥。心理性晕厥的发生率在逐渐升高[5-9]。表96-1中显示的某些晕厥病因并不是"真正晕厥"的一过性脑组织低灌注的原因。这些"非晕厥性"情况包括代谢紊乱、癫痫或醉酒导致的意识丧失（即转换反应）。

尽管医生根据晕厥的常见病因，能够对大多数患者作出诊断，但不能忽视罕见而具有潜在致命性的疾病，如长QT综合征、致心律失常性右室发育不良、Brugada综合征、肥厚型心肌病和肺栓塞[10-12]。此外还应重视晕厥的各种病因在不同年龄段的分布情况。青年患者中，神经调节紊乱是最常见的病因，但在老年患者中相对少见。老年患者的常见病因包括直立性低血压、餐后低血压、药物相关性晕厥、主动脉狭窄、颈动脉窦过敏（CSH）和缓慢性心律失常（如病窦综合征、传导阻滞）。

二、诊断性检查

确定晕厥的引发病因是一项挑战。由于晕厥通常是偶尔发作，很难在发作期间对患者进行体格检查及心电图检查，因此评价晕厥患者的首要目标是针对可能的病因进行检查。可以用来评价晕厥的诊断性检查及其应用将在下文详细阐述。

三、病史及体格检查

病史和体格检查是目前对晕厥患者进行评价的最重要的手段。近期的一些研究显示，25%的晕厥患者可以通过病史和体格检查确定病因[5-7]。通过系统、详细地询问病史，可以最大限度地获得与疾病相关的信息。初步评价应从确定患者是否经历晕厥发作开始。医生应该努力将"真正的晕厥"与"非晕厥性情况"导致的意识丧失如代谢及精神紊乱区别开来。尽管没有意识丧失可区分晕倒与晕厥，但最近的报告显示，二者的症状之间存在重叠[13,14]。这说明，老年人的意识丧失可能包括部分健忘症。评价晕厥患者时，应特别注意以下问题：（1）确定患者有无心脏病史、心脏病家族史、晕厥或猝死发作；（2）确定患者服用的药物是否与晕厥发作有关；（3）确定晕厥和晕厥前状态发生的次数和病程；（4）确定诱发因素，包括体位；（5）确定前驱症状到恢复正常所需的时间及类型。旁观者的细致描述也是非常有用的资料。

多年来，尽管人们认识到临床病史对于评价晕厥患者的重要性，但直到最近，仍无法确定病史中哪些方面的信息对于确定病因最有价值。一项研究对房室传导阻滞、室性心动过速和血管迷走性晕厥患者的病史特征进行了量化和比较[15]。结果表明，房室阻滞与室性心动过速导致晕厥患者的病史相似。这两组患者涉及的32个变量中，只有年龄、前驱症状的持续时间和晕厥前的出汗症状有所不同。与房室阻滞组相比，室速导致晕厥的患者年龄相对较小，前驱症状持续时间较长，晕厥发作前出汗较常见。与之相对比，血管迷走性晕厥患者的病史与上述两组在许多方面都有所不同。房室阻滞和室速导致的晕厥患者的病史中可预测晕厥发作的特征包括男性、年龄大于54岁、晕厥发作少于3次，晕厥发作前的预警时间少于6秒（OR值>5）。非房室阻滞和室速导致的晕厥患者的病史中可预测晕厥发作的特征包括心悸、视觉模糊、恶心、燥热、出汗或晕厥后的疲劳感。在这些变量中，4个最佳预测因子是：年龄、性别、恢复时间和晕厥后的疲劳感。

另一项前瞻性研究对连续341例患者的病史特点进行了标准问卷调查[6]。其中58%为血管性晕厥，23%为心源性晕厥，神经或心理性晕厥为1%，不明原因晕厥为18%。这项研究初步评价了非晕厥特有表现的预测价值，包括：年龄、性别和疑诊心脏病（根据病史和ECG作出的初步评价）。多因素分析显示，疑诊心脏病患者的临床表现是唯一的心源性晕厥的独立预测因子（OR值=16）。对191例疑诊心脏病和146例无心脏病患者病史中的不同特点分别进行了研究（图96-1）。初步评价不考虑心脏病的146例患者中，有142例可排除心源性晕厥（97%）。对不考虑心脏病的患者进行多因素分析显示，心源性晕厥的预测因子包括出现症状的时间≤4年，晕厥前状态和晕厥前有视物模糊。血管性晕厥的预测因子包括出现症状的时间>4年，有晕厥前状态的病史，恶心。在不考虑心脏病的患者中，意识丧失前出现心悸是唯一的心源性晕厥的预测因子，而超过10s的前驱症状是唯一的血管性晕厥的预测因子。作者的结论为，初步评价非可疑的心脏病且晕厥前无心悸的患者，可排除心源性晕厥。尽管疑诊心脏病是心源性晕厥的强预测因子，但其特异性较低。

临床病史对鉴别癫痫和晕厥也非常有价值。临床病史特征包括事件发生后的定向力障碍、口吐白沫、

表 96-1 晕厥的病因

	相对发生率		
	Ammirati 及其同事的研究[5]， n=195 42%	Alboni 及其同事的研究[6]， n=356 58%	Sarasin 及其同事的研究[6]， n=611 62%
血管性			
反射调节			
颈动脉窦过敏	2%	14%	1%
神经调节性晕厥	30%	33%	37%
舌咽反射性晕厥			
环境因素（咳嗽、吞咽、排尿）	4%	7%	
腺苷敏感性		2%	
体位性	6%	2%	24%
自律性减低			
特发性			
低血容量			
药物介导			
解剖异常			
锁骨下窃血			
心源性	21%	23%	11%
心律失常			
缓慢性心律失常	11%	15%	5%
窦房结功能减退/心动过缓			
房室传导阻滞			
快速性心律失常	7%	5%	2%
室上性心律失常			
室性心律失常（包括长 QT 综合征）			
器质性	3%	3%	4%
主动脉狭窄			
主动脉夹层			
心房粘液瘤			
心脏压塞			
肥厚梗阻型心肌病			
二尖瓣狭窄			
心肌缺血/梗死			
肺栓塞			
肺动脉高压			
神经/脑血管因素*	14%	0.7%	5%
Arnold Chiari 畸形			
癫痫（部分发作、颞叶）	3%	0.2%	
脊椎基底动脉功能不全/短暂缺血发作	11%	0.5	
心理因素*	6%	0.2%	1.5%
癔病性			
焦虑/恐慌			
躯体化异常			
转换反应			
代谢/多种原因	1%	0%	2%
代谢*			
毒品/酒精			
过度换气（低碳酸血症）			
低血糖			
低氧血症			
多种原因			
脑源性晕厥			
出血			
不明原因晕厥	18%	18%	14%

*类晕厥样功能障碍

肌肉疼痛、发作后昏昏欲睡和意识丧失超过5分钟等可有效地将癫痫和晕厥区分开。Benbadis及其同事[16]证实了咬舌对诊断癫痫的重要性，他们发现，对于诊断全身强直阵挛性发作的敏感性为24%，特异性为99%。舌侧咬伤对于诊断癫痫大发作的特异性为100%。提示晕厥病因为癫痫的其他表现包括：(1) 有发作先兆；(2) 发作时双眼上翻；(3) 发作时血压升高，脉搏加快；(4) 发作后头痛。大小便失禁既可见于晕厥也可见于癫痫发作，但更常见于癫痫发作时。癫痫大发作时通常伴有强直阵挛。值得注意的是，脑缺血引起的晕厥可导致去皮质僵直伴上肢强直阵挛。通过患者在失去姿势紧张时机体反应性缺失可确认为局限型癫痫或癫痫小发作。颞叶癫痫也容易与晕厥混淆。这些类型癫痫发作的最后几分钟出现意识混乱，清醒程度的变化和自主体征如面红。如果晕厥发作时合并其他脑缺血症状（如复视、耳鸣或感觉减退、眩晕或发音困难），则晕厥的病因可能为椎基底动脉供血不足。偏头痛引发的晕厥通常伴随单侧搏动性头痛，眼冒金星和恶心。最近的一项研究对102例癫痫和569例晕厥患者进行了标准化问卷调查[17]，将癫痫患者与晕厥患者报告的临床症状进行了比较。癫痫患者多在意识丧失前有咬舌、小便失禁、似曾相识的前驱症状、出神、情绪变化、有幻觉或战栗感；发作后意识混乱、肌肉疼痛、头痛；发作时出现抽搐、头部摇摆、对外界刺激无反应；旁观者发现皮肤变蓝。晕厥患者多经历晕厥前状态，在坐或站立较长时间时出现晕厥，或坐位和站立较长时间、在温暖环境中和运动时出现晕厥前状态。晕厥患者多伴有出汗、呼吸困难、胸痛、心悸燥热、恶心和眩晕。据此，有关专家提出了一种区分癫痫与晕厥的简易诊断评分标准，其准确率为85%（表96-2）[17]。

采集详细的病史后，应继续进行体格检查。此外应进行全面的心脏检查，特别注意有无器质性心脏病，检查有无提示自主神经机能异常或脑血管意外的明显的神经系统异常表现。不同体位的生命体征是这项评估的重要组成部分。首先应测量患者卧位时的血压和心率，并在此后3min内，每分钟检测一次。应注意观察3项异常：(1) 早期直立性低血压（站立3min内，出现收缩压降低20mmHg，舒张压降低10mmHg）；(2) 直立性心动过速综合征（站立5min内出现不能耐受的症状，心率加快≥28次/分）。本病的重要性在于其与神经介导性晕厥密切重叠[18]。

(一) 颈动脉窦按摩

通过轻压下颌角处颈动脉搏动可以诊断颈动脉窦过敏综合征（CSH），颈动脉在此处分叉。压迫时间

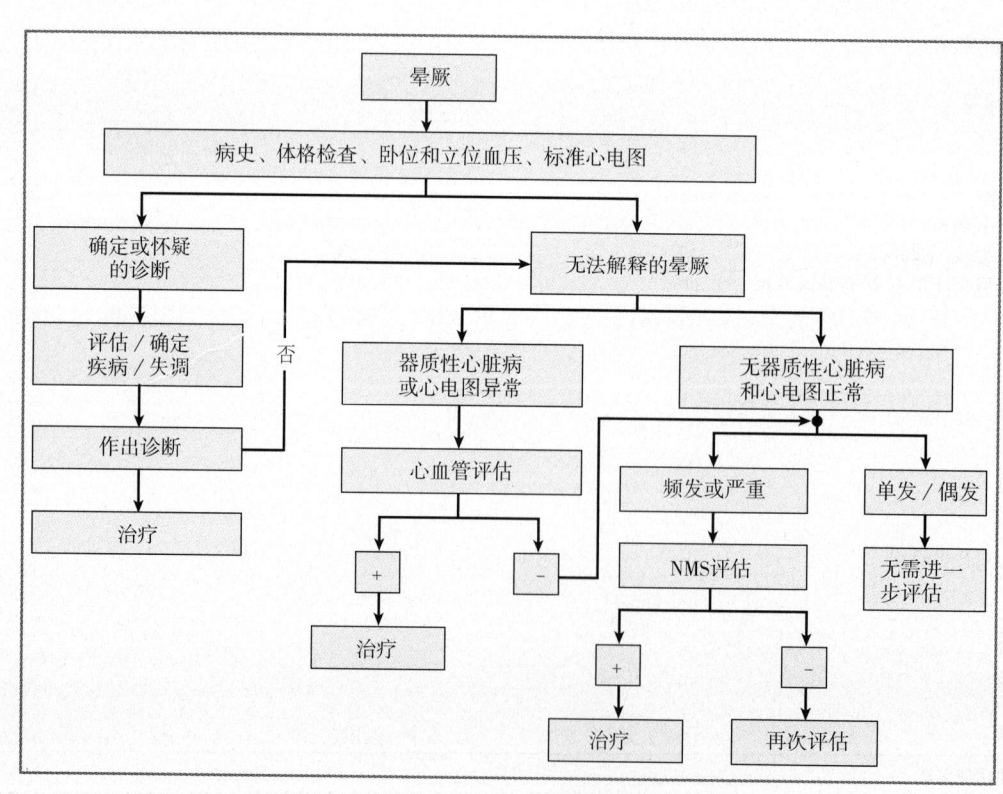

图96-1 欧洲心脏病学会工作组提出的晕厥评估流程

应在5~10s之间。研究表明，在立位和卧位时进行颈动脉窦按摩是很必要的[1,14,19,20]。检查的主要并发症为神经系统表现。一项研究表明，持续的神经系统并发症并不常见，发生比例为1:1 000[21]。因而对于有短暂性脑缺血、近3个月内有脑卒中和有颈动脉杂音的患者应避免颈动脉窦按摩。颈动脉窦按摩的正常反应是，窦性心率短暂降低，或房室传导减慢，或二者同时出现。如果颈动脉窦按摩时出现＞3秒的窦性停搏和收缩压降低≥50mmHg，则可诊断CSH。对颈动脉窦按摩的反应可分为心脏抑制型（停搏），血管抑制型（收缩压降低），或混合型。在中老年晕厥患者中大约三分之一存在CSH。CSH在发生过晕倒的中老年人中也很常见。一项研究显示，279例因晕倒而到急诊室就诊的病人中65例（23%）有CSH[22]。了解这种情况十分重要，但CSH在无症状的老年患者中也很常见，因此CSH的诊断应在谨慎排除晕厥的各种病因后作出。颈动脉窦按摩推荐用于40岁以上的，在病史采集、体格检查和心电图[1]初步评估后仍然无法解释的晕厥患者。一旦作出诊断，对于CSH导致的反复发作的晕厥患者，推荐植入双腔起搏器[23]。

四、心电图

心电图是评估晕厥患者的另一项重要手段。初步的心电图检查结果可对大约5%的患者作出诊断，并建议对另外5%的患者作出诊断[24]。可以确定晕厥病因的特异性表现包括QT间期延长（长QT综合征）、PR间期缩短和delta波（预激综合征）、伴有ST段抬高的类右束支阻滞图形（Brugada综合征）、急性心肌梗死的证据、高度房室阻滞或右胸导联出现T波倒置（致心律失常性右室发育不良）。心电图基础的任何异常都可能是心脏性晕厥或死亡率增加的独立预测因子，应进一步评价可导致晕厥的心脏原因[1]。大多数晕厥患者的心电图检查结果均正常。这是一个很有意义的发现，因为它说明心源性晕厥的发生率很低，晕厥的预后很好，特别是年轻的晕厥患者[6]。尽管通过心电图作出晕厥的病因诊断的可能性较小，但它的价格低廉并且对病人没有风险。因此，心电图成为评价晕厥患者的标准步骤之一[1,24]。

五、信号平均电图

信号平均电图（SAECG）是一种用来检测QRS波终末低振幅信号（晚电位）的非侵入性检查。晚电位可导致室性心律失常。与标准体表心电图相比，在对晕厥患者进行评价的过程中，SAECG的价值还不清楚。有研究显示，在特定的人群中，SAECG预测晕厥患者发生可诱发的室性心动过速的敏感性为73%~89%，特异性为89%~100%[25]。尽管这一结果令人鼓舞，但SAECG对未经选择的病人的应用价值还没有研究报道。此外，还不清楚SAECG是否能替代电生理研究在评价有明显器质性心脏病的晕厥患者中的作用。由于这一现实，以及SAECG无法提供在窦房结功能、房室传导和可诱发的室上性心律失常患者的检查中常规电生理检查（EP）所能提供的附加信息，因此SAECG作为晕厥的诊断工具其作用仍有局限性。此外，这项技术的另一局限是，用于诊断束支阻滞和非特异性室内传导延迟的SAECG标准还未确立。目前并不推荐将SAECG作为评价晕厥患者的标准程序之一[11,26]。

六、动态心电图检查

应用遥测或动态心电图进行持续的心电图监测是检查晕厥患者的常用手段，但不一定能发现晕厥的病因。由于可以确定或排除是否是心律失常导致晕厥，晕厥发作时心电图监测提供的信息极其宝贵。然而，由于晕厥常常是偶尔发作，动态心电图对晕厥和晕厥前状态的诊断率仅为4%[25]。动态心电图的另一用途是检测无心律失常患者的晕厥症状。这一结果是在对超过15%的并且接受持续心电图监测的患者进行研究后发现的[25]。需要强调的是，在持续心电图监测期间无心律失常和晕厥症状发作，并不能排除心律失常导

表96-2 癫痫的诊断评分要点

标准	分值
1. 应激时出现意识丧失	2
2. 头部偏向一侧	2
3. 数数＞30	1
4. 发作时对外界刺激无反应	1
5. 发作前出汗	-1
6. 晕厥前状态	-2
7. 在站立或坐位时间较长时出现意识丧失	-3
诊断癫痫的分值＞0。	

引自 Sheldon R, Rose S, Ritchie D, et al: Historical criteria that distinguish syncope from seizures. J Am Coll Cardiol 40: 142-148, 2002.

致晕厥的可能性。对于那些可能因心律失常导致晕厥的患者，应做进一步的检查，如电生理检查或事件监测。在临床病史、异常心电图或有器质性心脏病表现的基础上，怀疑因心律失常导致晕厥的患者，应进行动态心电图或住院遥测检查[1,25]。对于晕厥或晕厥前状态频繁发作（如每天发作）的患者，动态心电图最有可能作出诊断。

七、事件监测

电话传输心电图监测是一种小型、便携式心电图记录设备，它可由患者长时间携带并由患者启动记录。图形可被记录并随后通过电话线传输。有些事件监测器是闭环事件监测器，其可持续携带并可在事件发生后进行回顾，在事件发生前预先启动心电图记录，而其他类型的监测器只能由患者激活。这些设备通常可进行4分钟回顾性记录或1分钟预测性记录。事件监测器可应用于评价那些发作频率较低的反复发作性晕厥或晕厥前状态的患者，特别是一旦潜在恶性病因被排除以后[1,25,27,28]。当其用于选定的患者时，诊断率可达25%，但在未经严格挑选的患者中，可以预见其诊断率会更低。例如，一项研究报道172例晕厥患者进行监测期间，没有人出现明显的晕厥发作[28]。在出现较轻症状的患者中，有6%发现有心律失常。

有些病人晕厥发作频率很低，仅每年发作1或2次。对这些患者来说，要想成功记录事件发作，就需延长记录时间，所以事件监测器不太可能作出诊断。为了解决这一问题，目前已开发出植入性事件监测器（Medtronic Reveal，Minneapolis，Minn）。该装置重量轻、体积小（61mm×19mm×8mm），设计寿命长达18～24个月，内置检查的双电极，可植入胸部皮下组织。必要时，皮下囊袋可扩大以植入起搏器或ICD。心电图信号存储在循环的闭环记录器之中，其记录时间高达42min。该装置根据程序监测标准，可设定为自动触发，同时具有手动触发器。在使用该装置的最初16例患者中，88%发现心电图相关症状[29]。其中7例为缓慢性心律失常导致的晕厥（窦性停搏4例，传导阻滞2例，病窦综合征1例），2例为快速性心律失常导致的晕厥（房室结折返性心动过速1例，室性心动过速1例）。其余6例患者未发现心律失常。更新的系列报道显示，在10±4个月的随访期内，85例患者中的50例（59%）出现心电图相关症状[30]。其中21例发现心律失常，29例为窦性心律。并发症包括2例感染，1例破溃，1例囊袋疼痛需要重新植入。上述研究的作者，进一步开展了一项随机试验，用来比较Medtronic Reveal装置与传统检查的诊断价值[31]。在经病史、体格检查和超声心动图初步评价后，60例不明原因晕厥患者入选该研究。LVEF<35%的患者被排除。患者被随机分为直接植入Reveal装置组和经外置事件监测器、倾斜试验和电生理检查的标准评价程序组。Reveal装置组27例患者中，14例作出诊断；传统检查组30例患者中，6例作出诊断。尽管植入性监测器为评价晕厥患者提供了新的工具，但这一诊断策略的局限性在于花费昂贵，并且病人需要经历再一次晕厥发作以便作出诊断。目前的指南建议，植入性事件监测器用于高度怀疑心律失常为病因的反复发作性且发作频率较低的晕厥患者[1]。

八、超声心动图

虽然超声心动图常用于评价晕厥患者，但没有证据支持其用于体格检查和心电图正常的患者。对晕厥患者行超声心动检查是为了排除经病史、体格检查和心电图未发现的隐匿性心脏病。只有在怀疑严重的主动脉瓣狭窄和心房粘液瘤时才需行超声心动图检查[1]。一项对128例不明原因的晕厥患者进行的研究显示，88%的病人进行了超声心动检查[32]。52%的病例结果正常，28%存在左室肥厚，13例患者（16%）左室功能减退，其中7例有充血性心力衰竭病史，4例有缺血性心脏病史，2例ECG异常。因此，对不伴器质性心脏病者进行超声心动图的检查影响晕厥患者的评价或治疗的可能性非常低。所以，目前的指南建议，对所有晕厥患者不需要常规进行超声心动图检查，但怀疑心脏病时除外[1]。

九、直立倾斜试验

在过去的10多年中，直立倾斜试验从一种研究性程序演变为现在已被广泛接受的用于评价晕厥患者的标准诊断性检查[1,25,33,34]。由于直立倾斜试验诊断神经介导性晕厥的敏感性很高，故将其作为"金标准"。美国心脏病学会（ACC）的专家意见文件包含施行及解释该试验结果的特别推荐内容[33]。直立倾斜试验的检查时间通常为30～45min，倾斜角度在60°～

80°之间（70°最常用）。当倾斜时间延长、角度更陡、应用激发药物如异丙肾上腺素、硝酸甘油时，可增加敏感性但特异性降低[35-37]。应用异丙肾上腺素时，滴速应每分钟增加 1~3μg，以使心率比基线水平加快 25%。如使用硝酸甘油，应在立位时舌下含服 400μg。应用这两种激发药物的诊断准确率相当[37]。如不采用药物激发，直立倾斜试验的特异性约为 90%[33,34]。目前公认，没有器质性心脏病或已排除其他原因的复发性晕厥或单次晕厥发作的高危患者，以及已经确诊（如心脏停搏）但直立倾斜试验结果表现为神经介导性晕厥的患者，该试验将影响治疗。人们还一致认为，对于仅有单次发作且表现为典型神经介导性晕厥者，晕厥发作时无受伤的患者无须进行直立倾斜试验。

十、电生理检查

对于晕厥患者，电生理检查可提供重要的诊断和预后信息。电生理检查的结果对于作出病窦综合征、CSH、心脏阻滞、室上性心动过速或室性心动过速的诊断很有价值。对晕厥患者进行电生理检查的适应证应依据 ACC/AHA 工作组的报告[38]。人们公认，对于怀疑器质性心脏病和无法解释的晕厥（Ⅰ类适应证）应进行电生理检查；对于已知病因，而电生理检查结果对治疗无指导意义的患者，不应进行该项检查（Ⅲ类适应证）。对于复发的无法解释的无器质性心脏病而且直立倾斜试验阴性的晕厥患者，是否进行电生理检查尚存在争论。

（一）评价窦房结功能

电生理检查评价窦房结功能首先测定窦房结恢复时间（SNRT）。应用 600~350ms 为间期进行右房起搏 30~60s 而测定 SNRT。最后一个起搏脉冲的起点到第一个自发的窦性心房除极的间隔时间为 SNRT。通过减去窦性周期（SCL）可对 SNRT 进行矫正，表达式为 CSNRT=SNRT−SCL。如矫正的 SNRT>525ms，为窦房结功能异常。心房超速起搏停止后，第一个窦性心搏后面的长间歇为继发性停搏，也是诊断阳性的指标。在检查窦房结功能减退的病人时，评价继发性停搏可提高 SNRT 的敏感性。此外，较少应用的评价窦房结功能的指标还包括窦房传导时间和窦房结不应期。虽然窦房传导时间对评价窦房结功能减退很敏感，但因其特异性较低而限制了其判断是否需要植入永久起搏器的诊断价值。窦房结不应期是确定窦房结功能减退的另一项有用的指标，但它对于需要植入起搏器的晕厥患者的价值还有待确定。

通过电生理检查发现的窦房结功能减退导致的晕厥较少见（<5%）。值得注意的是，电生理检查缺乏窦房结功能减退的证据时，却不能排除缓慢性心律失常引起晕厥的可能。例如，Krahn 及其同事[28]报道，通过植入性 Holter 监测发现，在 15 例复发性晕厥患者中，窦性停搏导致晕厥中有 5 例电生理检查和直立倾斜试验结果均正常。

（二）房室阻滞

进行电生理检查时，通过测定心房到希氏束传导时间（AH 间期），希氏束到心室的传导时间（HV 间期）以及心脏对逐级递增的心房起搏频率和心房期前刺激的反应来评价房室传导功能。确定房室阻滞导致晕厥的电生理检查标准包括：HV 间期≥100ms 或出现希氏束下阻滞[34]。通过一项旨在评价 192 例慢性束支阻滞和有或无希氏束下阻滞的晕厥患者临床过程的研究确认了希氏束下阻滞的重要性[39]。在 5 年的随访期中，18 例希氏束下阻滞患者中的 14 例（78%）出现自发性二度或三度房室阻滞，而 174 例无希氏束下阻滞患者中有 15 例（9%）出现类似情况。许多关于应用电生理检查评价晕厥患者的研究发现，房室阻滞导致晕厥的比例约为 10%~15%。Donateo 及其同事[40]报道了对基础心电图有束支阻滞表现的晕厥患者进行系统评价的结果。在总数 347 例患者中，55 例基础心电图有束支阻滞表现。经系统评价（包括电生理检查）发现，25 例（45%）为心源性晕厥：房室阻滞 20 例，病窦综合征 2 例，室性心动过速 1 例，主动脉瓣狭窄 2 例。此外，神经介导性晕厥 22 例（40%），不明原因晕厥 8 例（15%）。

（三）室上性心动过速

室上速导致的晕厥并不常见，除非患者患有心脏病、发作时心室率非常快或有发生神经介导性晕厥的倾向。典型的情况是，在室上性心律失常发作时，由于血压降低而出现晕厥或几乎晕厥状态。不管心律失常是否持续，由于存在代偿机制，患者都将恢复意识。标准的电生理检查可准确诊断导致晕厥的大多数类型的室上性心律失常。在应用异丙肾上腺素以提高检查的敏感性时，特别是在判断是否存在特发性室速或房室结折返性心动过速时，应反复检测。应用电生理检查对不明原因晕厥进行评价发现，室上性心律失常导致的晕厥低于总数的5%。

(四) 室性心动过速

对晕厥患者进行电生理检查时,最常见的心律失常是室速。许多研究报道,经电生理检查发现20%的晕厥患者病因为室速。与持续性室性心律失常患者一样,电生理检查可诱发室速并且安装了ICD的晕厥患者大约50%会发生ICD放电除颤[41]。过去,如果电生理检查可诱发持续性单形性室速,则室速检测定为阳性,而诱发多形性室速或室颤则被认为是电生理检查的非特异性反应。晚近的资料提示,在对晕厥患者进行的电生理检查中,如发现多形性室速和室颤,应考虑为结果异常[42,43]。对最近关于抗心律失常与ICD的比较登记研究(AVID)和AVID晕厥亚组报告的部分数据进行分析表明,可诱发出室速(HR<200次/分)、可诱发出快速室速(HR≥200次/分)与可诱发出多形性室速/室颤的晕厥患者,他们的心律失常发生率无显著差异[42]。与之对比,LVEF值对心律失常事件有很高的预测价值。经1年随访发现,LVEF≥30%的晕厥患者,心律失常发生率为15%;LVEF<30%的晕厥患者,心律失常发生率为38%。

(五) 其他异常的预测价值

大约30%晕厥患者因病因不明而进行了电生理检查,从而明确了诊断。在电生理检查的阳性结果中,具有预测价值的因子包括心室功能受损、男性、既往有心肌梗死病史、束支阻滞、创伤和非持续性室速。

(六) 电生理检查的正常反应

大约70%行电生理检查的晕厥患者结果正常。电生理检查结果阴性的患者通常预示其猝死的风险较低。然而,研究显示,电生理检查对心功能明显受损患者的预测价值较低。一项研究报道,14例伴有晕厥的特发性扩张型心肌病患者中有7例电生理检查结果呈阴性,在24个月的随访期中,为其植入的ICD在室速发作时有效地进行了自动除颤[45]。Fonarow及其同事[46]报道了147例行心脏移植的非缺血性心肌病和晕厥患者的预后。病人的治疗方案(包括是否植入ICD)由心脏病专家决定。医生没有对他们进行电生理检查。对25例植入ICD的患者和122例仅接受传统疗法患者的预后进行比较的结果显示,在平均22个月的随访期中,传统疗法组中31例死亡,18例猝死;ICD组中,尽管2例死亡,但无猝死发生。植入ICD的患者中,40%有恰当的电除颤发生。这一研究的结果表明,对于上述患者,在评价其猝死风险时,可能需要采用敏感性更高的诊断性检查,或更广泛地应用ICD,或二者相结合。

十一、计算机断层扫描,脑电图,颈动脉扫描和颈动脉造影

对于神经系统疾病来说,晕厥很少表现为唯一的症状。由神经系统疾病导致的晕厥低于总病例的5%[5-7]。因此,广泛应用上述检查对神经系统疾病进行筛选,诊断率很低。在许多医疗机构中,对超过50%的晕厥患者过度应用了计算机断层扫描、脑电图、颈动脉扫描和颈动脉造影。如果经详细询问病史及仔细的神经系统检查而未发现异常,经脑电图,颈动脉扫描和颈动脉造影也几乎不会发现神经系统疾病。颈动脉疾病导致的短暂性脑缺血发作不会出现意识丧失。没有研究显示颈动脉多普勒超声检查对晕厥患者有益。目前关于晕厥的指南建议认为:只有在癫痫可能性较高时才需要作脑电图[1]。对于临床表现并不复杂的晕厥患者,不必进行CT和MRI检查。

十二、运动试验和心导管检查

心肌缺血通常不会引起晕厥,而多表现为心绞痛。因此,除非临床高度怀疑心肌缺血,否则对于晕厥患者无须进行运动试验和心导管检查[47]。对于晕厥患者来说,运动试验最适合用于评价那些在劳累时或劳累后立即发生晕厥或晕厥前状态或伴有胸痛的病人。应当注意的是,即使是劳累时出现晕厥的患者,运动试验也很少诱发出另一次事件。怀疑患有严重主动脉瓣狭窄或肥厚梗阻型心肌病的患者不应进行运动试验,因其可以导致心脏停搏。目前的指南建议,运动试验应该用于运动中或运动后短时间内出现晕厥的患者[1],不建议将其用于非运动相关性晕厥;冠状动脉造影推荐用于直接或间接由心肌缺血引起的晕厥。

十三、血液学检查

常规的血液学检查,如血电解质、心肌酶、血糖和红细胞比容等,诊断价值很低[24,48]。因此,不建议对晕厥患者进行常规实验室检查。在少数情况下,患者临床表现的某些方面提示这类检查具有诊断价值。

十四、晕厥患者的评估流程

图 96-1 显示的是欧洲心脏学会工作组提出的评估晕厥的流程[1]。初步评估应从详细的病史采集、体格检查和心电图开始。确定是否有证据表明晕厥患者患有心脏病，应当特别注意搜寻病史中提示特定诊断的线索。在初步评估的基础上，将患者分层为需要急诊处理或门诊处理两类，大约 25% 的患者可以确定病因（如直立性低血压、情景性晕厥和神经介导性晕厥）。在其他病人中，可以通过相关检查推测或确定可能的晕厥病因（如主动脉狭窄、肺栓塞和神经系统疾病）。剩余的未确定病因的患者，下一步的评估依赖于病史或心电图结果或二者是否都提示器质性心脏病或心律失常导致的晕厥。如果怀疑上述两种情况，应该进行进一步的心脏检查，包括超声心动图、运动试验和寻找心律失常线索的检查（如心电监测和电生理检查）。如果心脏检查阴性，下一步应进行神经介导性晕厥的相关检查。如果患者的临床病史和心电图中没有提示器质性心脏病的证据，推荐继续进行神经介导性晕厥的相关检查，特别是对于那些反复发作或严重晕厥患者。如果仍然无法确定诊断，应继续进行其他检查，如事件监测或根据患者病史的严重性和慢性程度进行再次评估和临床治疗。如果怀疑心理原因导致晕厥，应进行心理评估[8,9]。

十五、评价晕厥患者时应考虑的其他问题

（一）晕厥与驾驶

晕厥患者通常向医生询问驾驶风险问题。在驾驶时发生晕厥对患者本人和其他人都很危险。尽管有些人提出，由于理论上存在晕厥复发的可能性，晕厥患者不应该再驾驶汽车，但许多患者不会理睬这种不切实际的观点。对晕厥患者提出建议时要考虑很多因素：（1）晕厥复发的可能性；（2）预警症状的表现和持续时间；（3）晕厥是否仅在坐位或立位时发生；（4）患者是否经常驾车及驾驶能力怎样；（5）各地法律的适用程度。在考虑这些问题时，医生应注意，急性疾病包括晕厥不大可能导致交通事故。AHA 和加拿大心脏病学会发布的指南都考虑到了这一问题[49]。对于非职业性司机，通常建议其限制驾驶几个月，如果患者未再出现症状，可在几个月后恢复驾驶。

（二）运动相关性晕厥

过去几年中，在运动中或运动后立即发生的晕厥被诊断为神经介导性晕厥的病例越来越多。一项研究报道，17 例平均年龄 28 岁，劳累时发作晕厥的患者，经检查后诊断为血管迷走性晕厥[50]。其中 9 例为优秀运动员。所有患者心室功能正常，没有器质性心脏病证据。基于临床病史和直立倾斜试验的结果诊断为神经介导性晕厥。该研究的结果表明，神经介导性晕厥：（1）既可以发生在运动过程中也可发生在运动结束后；（2）既可发生在运动员中，也可发生在普通人中；（3）可以发生在有或没有与运动不相关的典型血管迷走性晕厥患者中；（4）运动试验无法重现症状；（5）伴有与非运动相关的血管迷走性晕厥相似的前驱和恢复症状及相似的治疗反应。该研究中的每一位受试者都继续参加休闲和竞技性体育活动。其他报告也有相似发现。但需要重点强调的是，尽管神经介导性晕厥是运动员晕厥的最常见病因，但晕厥可能是多种致命性心脏疾病的初发表现，包括肥厚型心肌病、先天性心脏病/冠状动脉畸形、早发冠状动脉疾病、致心律失常性右室发育不良、心肌炎、家族性长 QT 综合征、预激综合征和瓣膜病。因此，对患有劳累性晕厥的运动员进行包括运动试验、心电图和超声心动图检查十分必要。

十六、总 结

晕厥是一种常见而重要的临床问题。尽管大多数晕厥患者的预后良好，但晕厥可以是心脏性猝死的唯一预兆。因此，必须进行详细的评估。正确应用诊断工具，可以准确发现晕厥的潜在致命性病因。总之，四分之三的晕厥患者可以明确诊断。一旦确诊，就应开始适当的治疗。

（余 飞 译）

参 考 文 献

1. Brignole M, Alboni P, Benditt D, et al, for the Task Force on Syncope, European Society of Cardiology: Guidelines on management (diagnosis and treatment) of syncope. Eur Heart J 22:1256–1306, 2001.
2. Soteriades ES, Evand JC, Larson MG, et al: Incidence and prognosis of syncope. N Engl J Med 347:878–885, 2002.
3. Nyman JA, Krahn AD, Bland PC, et al: The costs of recurrent syncope of unknown origin in elderly patients. Pacing Clin Electrophysiol 22:1386–1394, 1999.

4. Rose MS, Koshman ML, Spreng S, Sheldon R: The relationship between health-related quality of life and frequency of spells in patients with syncope. J Clin Epidemiol 53:1209–1216, 2000.
5. Ammirati F, Colivicchi F, Santini M, on behalf of the investigators of the OESIL study: Diagnosing syncope in clinical practice. Eur Heart J 21:L935–L940, 2000.
6. Alboni P, Brignole M, Menozzi C, et al: Diagnostic value of history in patients with syncope with or without heart disease. J Am Coll Cardiol 37:1921–1928, 2001.
7. Sarasin FP, Louis-Simonet M, Carballo D, et al: Prospective evaluation of patients with syncope: A population-based study. Am J Med 111:177–184, 2001.
8. Kapoor WN, Fortunato M, Hanusa BH, Schulberg HC: Psychiatric illnesses in patients with syncope. Am J Med 99:505–512, 1995.
9. Ventura R, Maas R, Rüppel R, et al: Psychiatric conditions in patients with recurrent unexplained syncope. Europace 3:311–316, 2001.
10. Wilde A, Antzelevitch C, Borggrefe M, et al: Proposed diagnostic criteria for Brugada syndrome: Consensus Report. Circulation 106:2514–2519, 2002.
11. Nava A, Bauce B, Basso C, et al: Clinical profile and long-term follow-up of 37 families with arrhythmogenic right ventricular cardiomyopathy. J Am Coll Cardiol 36:226–233, 2000.
12. Elliott PM, Poloniecki J, Dickie S, et al: Sudden death in hypertrophic cardiomyopathy: Identification of high risk patients. J Am Coll Cardiol 36:2212–2218, 2000.
13. Close J, Ellis M, Hooper R, et al: Prevention of falls in the elderly (PROFET), a randomized controlled trial. Lancet 353:93–97, 1999.
14. Kenny RAM, Richardson DA, Steen N, et al: Carotid sinus syndrome: A modifiable risk factor for nonaccidental falls in older adults (SAFE PACE). J Am Coll Cardiol 38:1491–1496, 2001.
15. Calkins H, Shyr Y, Frumin H, et al: The value of the clinical history in the differentiation of syncope due to ventricular tachycardia, atrioventricular block, and neurocardiogenic syncope. Am J Med 98:365–373, 1995.
16. Benbadis SR, Wolgamuth BR, Goren H, et al: Value of tongue biting in the diagnosis of seizures. Arch Intern Med 155:2346–2349, 1995.
17. Sheldon R, Rose S, Ritchie D, et al: Historical criteria that distinguish syncope from seizures. J Am Coll Cardiol 40:142–148, 2002.
18. Grubb BP, Kanjwal MY, Kosinski DJ: Review: The postural orthostatic tachycardia syndrome. J Interv Card Electrophysiol 5:9–16, 2001.
19. Morilli CA, Camacho ME, Wood MA, et al: Diagnostic utility of mechanical, pharmacological and orthostatic stimulation of the carotid sinus in patients with unexplained syncope. J Am Coll Cardiol 34:1587–1594, 1999.
20. Tea SH, Mansourati J, L'Heveder G, et al: New insights into the pathophysiology of carotid sinus syndrome. Circulation 93:1411–1416, 1996.
21. Richardson DA, Bexton R, Shaw RE, et al: Complications of carotid sinus massage—a prospective series of older patients. Age Ageing 29:413–417, 2000.
22. Richardson DA, Bexton RS, Shaw FE, Kenny RA: Prevalence of cardioinhibitory carotid sinus hypersensitivity in patients 50 years or over presenting to the accident and emergency department with "unexplained" or "recurrent" falls. Pacing Clin Electrophysiol 20:820–823, 1997.
23. Gregoratos G, Abrams J, Epstein A, et al, Committee Members and Task Force Members: ACC/AHA/NASPE 2002 Guideline update for implantation of cardiac pacemakers and antiarrhythmia devices: Summary article. A report of the American College of Cardiology/American Heart Association Task Force on practice guidelines (ACC/AHA/NASPE Committee to update the 1998 pacemaker guidelines). Circulation 106:2145–2161, 2002.
24. Linzer M, Yang EH, Estes M, et al, for the Clinical Efficacy Assessment Project of the American College of Physicians: Clinical guideline. Diagnosing syncope. Part 1: Value of history, physical examination, and electrocardiography. Ann Intern Med 126:989–996, 1997.
25. Linzer M, Yang EH, Estes III M, et al, for the Clinical Efficacy Assessment Project of the American College of Physicians: Clinical guideline. Diagnosing syncope. Part 2: Unexplained syncope. Ann Intern Med 127:76–86, 1997.
26. Filtered QRS duration on SAECG predicts inducibility of ventricular tachycardia in arrhythmogenic right ventricular dysplasia. Pacing Clin Electrophysiol 10:1955–1960, 2003.
27. Fogel RI, Evans JJ, Prystowsky EN: Utility and cost of event recorders in the diagnosis of palpitations, presyncope, and syncope. Am J Cardiol 79:207–208, 1997.
28. Zimetbaum P, Kim KY, Ho KKL, et al: Utility of patient-activated cardiac event recorders in general clinical practice. Am J Cardiol 79:371–372, 1997.
29. Krahn AD, Klein GJ, Norris C, Yee R: The etiology of syncope in patients with negative tilt table and electrophysiological testing. Circulation 92:1819–1824, 1995.
30. Krahn AD, Klein GJ, Yee R, et al, for the Reveal Investigators: Use of an extended monitoring strategy in patients with problematic syncope. Circulation 99:406–410, 1999.
31. Krahn AD, Klein GJ, Yee R, Skanes AC: Randomized assessment of syncope trial. Conventional diagnostic testing versus a prolonged monitoring strategy. Circulation 104:46–51, 2001.
32. Recchia D, Barzilai B: Echocardiography in the evaluation of patients with syncope. J Gen Intern Med 10:649–655, 1995.
33. Benditt DG, Ferguson DW, Grubb BP, et al: Tilt table testing for assessing syncope. J Am Coll Cardiol 28:263–275, 1996.
34. Natale A, Akhtar M, Jazayeri M, et al: Provocation of hypotension during head-up tilt testing in subjects with no history of syncope or presyncope. Circulation 92:54–58, 1995.
35. Takase B, Uehata A, Nishioka TI, et al: Different mechanisms of isoproterenol-induced and nitroglycerin-induced syncope during head-up tilt in patients with unexplained syncope: Important role of epinephrine in nitroglycerin-induced syncope. J Cardiovasc Electrophysiol 12:791–796, 2001.
36. Calkins H: Isoproterenol-provoked versus nitroglycerin-provoked tilt tests: Do they differ? J Cardiovasc Electrophysiol 12:797–799, 2001.
37. Raviele A, Giada F, Brignole M, et al: Comparison of diagnostic accuracy of sublingual nitroglycerin test and low-dose isoproterenol test in patients with unexplained syncope. Am J Cardiol 85:1194–1198, 2000.
38. Zipes DP, DiMarco JP, Gillette PC, et al: Guidelines for clinical intracardiac electrophysiological and catheter ablation procedures. J Am Coll Cardiol 26:555–573, 1995.
39. Petrac D, Radic B, Birtic K, Gjurovic J: Prospective evaluation of infrahisal second-degree block induced by atrial pacing in the presence of chronic bundle branch block and syncope. Pacing Clin Electrophysiol 19:784–792, 1996.
40. Donateo P, Brignole M, Alboni P, et al: A standardized conventional evaluation of the mechanism of syncope in patients with bundle branch block. Europace 4:357–360, 2002.
41. Andrews NP, Fogel RI, Pelargonio G, et al: Implantable defibrillator event rates in patients with unexplained syncope and inducible sustained ventricular tachyarrhythmias. J Am Coll Cardiol 34:2023–2030, 1999.
42. Steinberg JS, Beckman K, Greene HL, et al: Follow-up of patients with unexplained syncope and inducible ventricular tachyarrhythmias: Analysis of the AVID registry and an AVID substudy. J Cardiovasc Electrophysiol 12:996–1001, 2001.
43. Link MS, Costeas XF, Griffith JL, et al: High incidence of appropriate implantable cardioverter-defibrillator therapy in patients with syncope of unknown etiology and inducible ventricular arrhythmias. J Am Coll Cardiol 29:370–375, 1997.
44. Knigh BP, Goyal R, Pelosi F, et al: Outcome of patients with nonischemic dilated cardiomyopathy and unexplained syncope treated with an implantable defibrillator. J Am Coll Cardiol 33:1964–1970, 1999.
45. Russo AM, Verdino R, Schorr C, et al: Occurrence of implantable defibrillator events in patients with syncope and nonischemic dilated cardiomyopathy. Am J Cardiol 88:1444–1446, 2001.
46. Fonarow GC, Feliciano Z, Boyle NG, et al: Improved survival in patients with nonischemic advanced heart failure and syncope treated with an implantable cardioverter-defibrillator. Am J Cardiol 85:981–985, 2000.
47. Doi A, Tsuchihashi K, Kyuma M, et al: Diagnostic implications of modified treadmill and head-up tilt tests in exercise-related syncope: Comparative studies with situational and/or vasovagal syncope. Can J Cardiol 18:960–966, 2002.
48. Link MS, Lauer EP, Homoud MK, et al: Low yield of rule-out myocardial infarction protocol in patients presenting with syncope. Am J Cardiol 88:706–707, 2001.
49. Epstein AE, Miles WM, Benditt DG: Personal and public safety issues related to arrhythmias that may affect consciousness: Implications for regulation and physician recommendations. An AHA/NASPE Medical Scientific Statement. Circulation 94:1147–1166, 1996.
50. Calkins H, Seifert M, Morady F: Clinical presentation and long-term follow-up of athletes with exercise-induced vasodepressor syncope. Am Heart J 129:1159–1164, 1995.

第 97 章

心房颤动的临床试验

D. George Wyse

本章目录

- 转复窦律 ………………………… 877
- 窦律的维持 ……………………… 878
- 控制心室率 ……………………… 879
- 节律控制与心率控制 …………… 880
- 抗栓治疗 ………………………… 880
- 房颤的主要预防治疗 …………… 880

本章首先对有关定义和内容范围进行说明。临床试验可有不同解释,但有一种特定含义。临床试验是指以人作为研究对象,通过前瞻性研究,比较干预治疗组和对照组的疗效。这个定义的主要条件是:研究是前瞻性的,设有对照组。其他需要考虑的方面包括:对象选择(入选条件)、分配进入治疗组和对照组的方法、接受治疗、是否告知患者、终点的选择、终点评估、伦理学、安全性和副作用的评估、统计方法等等。本书的很多内容都在围绕这个话题,但篇幅所限,有些问题未能详尽叙述。本章讨论的试验都是作者认为符合临床试验定义、符合随机化原则和分配方法适宜的临床试验。本章不是有关房颤临床试验的综述,而是按照教科书的要求编写。因此上述条件中有关房颤的所有试验,不可能面面俱到,而是尽可能广泛地参照相关研究领域发表的著作或述评。

存在的疑问是,临床以房颤患者为研究对象的试验结果是否适用于孤立性房扑患者。临床上,这两种房性心律失常紧密相关,很多试验常常不能清楚将二者鉴别开来。我们将尽可能考虑这两种心律失常的差别。另外,假设试验结果适用于以上两种心律失常,主要是不合并房颤的孤立性房扑临床非常少见。

一、转复窦律

房颤治疗的第一步是决定是否转复窦律或控制心室率。紧急处理时,应考虑到以下多种因素,如房颤持续时间、复律本身出现血栓栓塞并发症的风险、患者的血流动力学情况及其他影响因素。选择长期治疗时,也应考虑到其他因素,如房颤持续时患者的症状。下面将介绍临床试验,探讨上述一些因素对复律或控制心室率决策的影响。篇幅所限,不能对所有这些决策影响因素一一罗列。一旦决定转复窦律,可选择药物复律、电复律或两者合用。临床试验未直接比较药物复律或电复律疗效。

(一)药物复律

临床试验已研究和比较了各种药物转复窦律的疗效[1,2]。这里重点介绍以下几个方面。首先,药物转复对于新近发生的房颤最为有效,新近发生的房颤主要包括阵发性房颤。这类患者自动转复窦律成功率较高(>50%),但既往临床试验是以安慰剂作为对照应该以有治疗作用的安慰剂或有效的药物作为对照。单纯以安慰剂作为对照是一种"不等价"的假设。就是说,这些试验仅考虑到单一方面情况。篇幅所限,这里不进行太多的讨论,但最重要的一点是试验组患者入选标准要与对照组(服用安慰剂)标准一致。

表 97-1 列举了转复窦律疗效较佳的药物,这些药物都经过一个以上的临床试验证实[1]。这里并不排除还存在其他有效转律的药物,但表 97-1 中列举的药物转律的证据最强。其他药物或由于无效,或由于未完

全研究清楚或存在较严重副作用而不在涵盖之列。转复无效（或至少需一周起效）的药物是洋地黄类药物和索他洛尔。胺碘酮、多非利特和依布利特转复持续性房颤（>7 天）有一定疗效[1]。多非利特和依布利特转复房扑比转复房颤更加有效，而心律平和氟卡尼转复房颤更为有效。胺碘酮[3]和多非利特（口服）起效较慢，不适合快速转律。需要强调的是，虽然药物转律已进步到"随身带药"，但所有研究对照组均仅选取住院患者。美国医药食品卫生管理局规定入院患者出现房颤时应用多非利特开始治疗。门诊患者胺碘酮每日最大口服剂量为 600mg，但是这项研究不是临床试验，因为未设立对照组。

（二）电复律

电复律包括电击复律和起搏终止。起搏终止是唯一证实有效转复规则的房性心律（更准确地说，房扑和房速）的方法，不在本章讨论。电复律有许多不同参数。经胸电复律包括不同的转复电击波形，电极的不同尺寸、构型及摆放位置以及不同的电击能量，这些参数都是相互依赖的。它们对电复律的影响已在临床试验证实，一些研究已体现在最近出版的治疗指南中[1]，本章不再介绍。总之，双相波转复所需能量较少，这种波形正在替代其他的电转复波形[5]。电极的摆放位置建议为前后位[1]。其他各种经静脉低能量电转复，不属于经胸电转复范畴。在以往研究中，衰减正弦单相波经胸电转复疗效稍逊于经静脉双相波的转复，但未比较同样波形下经静脉和经胸的转复疗效。

持续性房颤电转律后即刻或亚急性期房颤复发，其疗效欠佳，应用受限。有很多方法可以降低房颤的复发率，目前试验显示预先使用抗心律失常药物，合并使用钙离子通道拮抗剂或血管紧张素受体拮抗剂优于单纯使用抗心律失常药物。早期房颤复发的机制仍不清楚，但已成为研究的热点。

二、窦律的维持

维持窦律[10]的益处还未得到证实，正如下面讨论的，一些既往宣称的益处被证实是不真实的。然而，若干临床试验用来评估维持窦律是否产生较高的优势比。有关维持窦律的优势比还有一些不确定因素；而且，应用常用的方法测定房颤复发还存在很多局限。

（一）药物治疗

临床试验已对大量维持窦律的药物进行评估，这些试验结果已在文献中报道[2,12]。总之，这些药物仅有中等疗效，且有较严重的副反应，特别是对于那些器质性心脏病患者。胺碘酮可能是目前最有效的药物[13]，但仅略好于其他药物，而且有潜在更严重的副作用，特别是对于长期使用胺碘酮的患者[14]。目前并未发现新开发的药物维持窦律优于现有药物[15,16]。药物治疗房颤主要的是安全性，但未经过大量患者的前瞻性研究（可能不同于临床试验研究模式）并不能有效证实其安全性。基于药物安全性考虑，由于一些禁忌和副反应（表 97-2）限制了这些药物在房颤治疗方面的应用。探索更为有效和安全的维持窦律药物需要更深入地了解房颤病理生理机制，更好地进行患者选择及从基因和分子生物学角度发展药物。

（二）非药物治疗

虽然药物治疗一直是维持窦律治疗的主流，但还有新的非药物方法。这些方法在本书的其他篇章已有探讨。目前，这些方法很少经过随机临床试验的检验。很多临床试验评估了起搏治疗[17,18]，但这些结果太繁琐以至于不能对其有效性和应用进行总体评估。同样，起搏器的随机临床试验（防止和终止房颤）仅提供了摘要。

表 97-1 多个试验证明复律有效的药物

药物	Vaughn-Williams 分类	服用方法	常用剂量
胺碘酮	III	静脉，然后口服	5～7mg/kg，然后 1.2～1.8g/d
多非利特	III	口服	0.25～1mg/d
依布利特	III	静脉	10min 内给予 1mg，然后重复 1 次
普罗帕酮	I c	口服	300～600mg，单一次剂量
氟卡尼	I c	口服	100～300mg，单一次剂量

（三）综合治疗

综合治疗是联合采用两个或两个以上的独立治疗方案，通常是将药物和非药物治疗联合，也可以合用两个或两个以上非药物治疗方法。联合治疗控制房颤节律是一种新的方法，但未经过前瞻性临床随机试验评估。然而，一项有关起搏临床试验的亚组分析表明起搏治疗与抗心律失常药物联用最为有效[18]。

三、控制心室率

目前临床试验未能探明控制房颤心室率的良好方法，还需要深入进行这方面的研究。静息心室率和运动时心室率的生理范围有待明确。运动时心室率需要涉及心率加速和心率变时性。最后应认识到，尽可能使心率变得规整是控制心室率治疗的一部分[19]。

（一）药物治疗

多年来，药物治疗一直是控制心室率的主要途径。这方面药物包括β受体阻滞剂、地尔硫䓬、维拉帕米和洋地黄。当其他药物不能奏效时，有时可选用胺碘酮。对控制房颤心室率的药物试验进行荟萃分析[20]。单独使用洋地黄往往不能有效控制心室率，因为后者对运动时心率控制的作用较弱。然而，当一种药物控制心室率不佳时，合用β受体阻滞剂和洋地黄类药物常能有效控制心室率。目前药物趋于有效控制静息时心率，但不能有效控制运动时心率的增加，从而不能避免运动时心率增快带来的不适。

表 97-2　AFFIRM 试验各种抗房颤药物的副作用

	预防	副作用
一般特点	警惕监测药物致心律失常、心动过缓、低钾血症 警惕药物负性肌力作用 应用药物后，QTc≤0.52s 警惕左室肥厚或器质性心脏病 剂量适当，避免房室阻滞 老年患者监测肝肾功能	
特殊		
索他洛尔		哮喘 需要透析 心衰分级≥Ⅱ 慢性心衰史，LVEF≤0.3 LVEF≤0.25
Ⅰ类药	左室收缩功能受损（慢性心衰或低 LVEF） 缺血性心脏病	
普鲁卡因酰胺	12 周内每周验血，然后根据需要验血 每 3~6 个月验血查找狼疮细胞	
丙吡胺		LVEF<0.30 慢性心衰
氟卡尼和 　普罗帕酮		器质性心脏病 心肌病 左室肥厚 心血管疾病 心肌缺血或心梗 左室功能受损 LVEF<0.50 左室壁运动异常

(二) 非药物治疗

目前控制房颤心室率的非药物治疗主要和根本的途径是消融房室交界区，植入永久性起搏器。通过这种心率应答装置，可以为所有患者提供较好的心率控制（尽管不完美）：控制静息和运动时心率，完美的变时性，并使心率规整。通过对房室交界区慢路径消融改良，可作为植入永久性起搏器的替代治疗。然而，随机比较研究显示，慢路径改良和消融稍逊于消融房室交界区，植入永久性起搏器[21]。多项研究，包括随机临床试验评估显示，无论是阵发性房颤[22]，还是持续性房颤[23]，无论是复律，还是控制心室率方面，消融房室结、植入永久性起搏器对症状明显的房颤患者控制心室率疗效均优于药物治疗。但由于接受这种治疗的患者通常中断药物治疗（除了抗凝药物），大部分在第二年可以进展为永久性房颤[24,25]，最适宜起搏方式为VVIR。

(三) 联合治疗

药物控制心率最主要缺陷是当其预防间歇发作的快速心动过速时，常导致静息时心动过缓和变时性不良。而且，药物控制心率不能使心率规整。因此，有必要联合应用起搏器治疗控制心率。虽然在临床中经常联合起搏和药物治疗控制房颤时心率，但还没有经过临床随机试验验证这种联合治疗方法。

四、节律控制与心率控制

近来多个临床试验比较了节律控制和心率控制，并对节律控制进行了深入探讨。对于节律控制，需要恢复并维持窦律；而控制心率，不需要恢复并维持窦律，但需要控制心室率（低或高），理想情况下，心率也应是规整的。上述两种方法均需要抗凝治疗。由于节律控制的众多优点，直到现在，心率控制（仅作为节律控制的替代治疗）仍被认为是稍逊于节律控制[26]。节律控制的好处包括：更好地减轻临床症状，进一步改善心功能，降低死亡率和脑卒中发生率，减少抗凝需要，从而降低出血风险等[27]。但直到现在，节律控制所谓优于心率控制的上述优点还未经临床随机试验证实。这些优点仅是基于临床观察或与不治疗进行比较。这些"证据"忽视了正常的"健康应答"，无论积极治疗还是使用安慰剂，任何窦律下患者都可以带来这些好处[28]。节律控制的不足是现有的药物治疗转复效果欠佳及这些治疗的副作用[27]。目前转复房颤疗效不佳，而抗凝治疗预防脑卒中较有效[29]，这样就造成了困惑：是否节律控制真的优于控制心室率。与节律控制相比，控制心室率公认的优点是相对安全可行，且可通过非药物途径有效治疗（消融房室结，植入永久性起搏器）[27]。

目前有6个大规模临床试验比较节律控制与心率控制的疗效，还有多个试验正在进行中。其中5个试验已公开发表[25,30-33]。这些试验的入选对象主要是具有脑卒中危险因素的老年阵发性或持续性房颤患者（大部分为持续性房颤患者）。4个临床试验（在患者选择上有较大的重叠性）主要结果如图97-1。另外一个正在进行的临床试验正致力于心衰患者研究[34]。数据结果惊人的一致，概括如下：节律控制设想的益处未被证实。就死亡率而言，节律控制不仅没有好处，而且有趋势表明控制心率可带来益处（图97-1）。在患者生活质量方面，两种治疗疗效无明显差异。虽然PIAF (Pharmacological Intervention in Atrial Fibrillation)试验显示节律控制组比心率控制组6分钟步行距离更长，但是仅不足一半的患者进行了6分钟步行试验[30]，且这个结果未在AFFIRM (Atrial Fibrillation Follow-up Investigation of Rhythm Management)试验得到证实[32]。汇总结果是，节律控制组比心率控制组发生缺血性脑卒中更多（但无统计学差异），可能是由于节律控制组患者未连续使用华法林（图97-1）。尽管如此，心率控制组出血发生率仅轻度增高（无统计学显著差异）。节律控制组患者住院和药物副作用更常见。总之，这些试验显示心率控制至少与节律控制同样有效，且在某些方面优于节律控制。同时不能因为心律转复并维持为窦律就中断抗凝治疗。

五、抗栓治疗

虽然本书主要涉及房颤心律控制的电生理内容，但不能疏忽抗栓治疗。抗栓治疗是房颤治疗必不可少的部分，已被一系列临床随机试验所证实。鉴于本章篇幅所限，这里不再赘述。在新近的综述上已概括说明[29]。

六、房颤的主要预防治疗

有关房颤预防的研究较少，目前还不明确。这是一个需要更多关注的领域。如果有更多深入的研究，

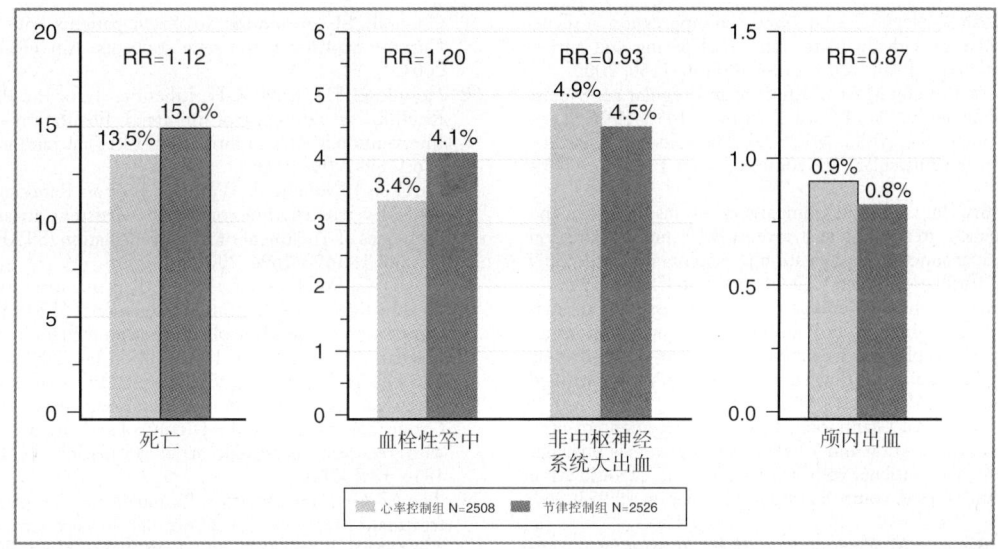

图 97-1 汇总四个临床试验结果，比较节律控制和心率控制临床结果，主要研究对象是具有脑卒中危险因素的老年持续性房颤患者。危险比均无统计学差异。（主要数据来源：PIAF 试验源于 S. Hohnloser，STAF 试验源于 J. Carlsson，RACE 试验源于 I. Van Gelder，AFFIRM 试验源于作者。）

例如 Framingham 心脏研究，将研究靶点定于房颤发生率和房颤发生的危险因素，将有利于房颤的预防。目前这方面数据仅有房颤发病率。例如，房颤多见于高血压和冠心病，但一些房颤患者无明显器质性心脏病。因此，对于既往无房颤患者进行预防房颤治疗，似乎变得谨慎。至少有一个临床试验显示预防房颤富有成效。在这篇报道中，心梗患者随机分为两组，一组给予 ACEI（血管紧张素转换酶抑制剂）药物，另一组给予安慰剂，ACEI 组发生房颤较少[35]。另外两个试验比较心房起搏和心室起搏，均显示心房起搏患者较少发生房颤[36,37]。然而，这些试验不能鉴别是否心房起搏可预防房颤或心室起搏可导致房颤。总之，还需要进一步研究房颤的基因遗传缺陷[38]，并探讨是否这些研究有助于房颤的预防。

（杨延宗　译）

参 考 文 献

1. Fuster V, Ryden LE, Asinger RW, et al: ACC/AHA/ESC guidelines for the management of patients with atrial fibrillation: Executive summary. A report of the American College of Cardiology/American Heart Association Task Force on Practice Guidelines and the European Society of Cardiology Committee for Practice Guidelines and Policy Conferences (Committee to Develop Guidelines for the Management of Patients With Atrial Fibrillation). Circulation 104:2118–2150, 2001.
2. Miller MR, McNamara RL, Segal JB, et al: Efficacy of agents for pharmacologic conversion of atrial fibrillation and subsequent maintenance of sinus rhythm: A meta analysis of clinical trials. J Fam Pract 49:1033–1046, 2000.
3. Chevalier P, Durand-Dubief A, Burri HK, et al: Amiodarone versus placebo and classic drugs for cardioversion of recent-onset atrial fibrillation: A meta-analysis. J Am Coll Cardiol 41:255–262, 2003.
4. Tieleman RG, Gosselink AT, Crijns HJ, et al: Efficacy, safety and determinants of conversion of atrial fibrillation and flutter with oral amiodarone. Am J Cardiol 79:53–57, 1997.
5. Mittal S, Ayati S, Stein KM, et al: Transthoracic cardioversion of atrial fibrillation: Comparison of rectilinear biphasic versus damped sine wave monophasic shocks. Circulation 101:1282–1287, 2000.
6. Levy S, Ricard P, Gueunoun M, et al: Low-energy cardioversion of spontaneous atrial fibrillation. Immediate and long-term results. Circulation 96:253–259, 1997.
7. Crijns HJ, van Noord T, van Gelder IC: Recurrence of atrial fibrillation and the need for new definitions. Eur Heart J 22:1822–1834, 2001.
8. De Simone A, Stabile G, Vitale DF, et al: Pretreatment with verapamil in patients with persistent or chronic atrial fibrillation who underwent electrical cardioversion. J Am Coll Cardiol 34:810–814, 1999.
9. Madrid AH, Bueno MG, Rebollo JMG, et al: Use of irbesartan to maintain sinus rhythm in patients with long-lasting persistent atrial fibrillation. A prospective and randomized study. Circulation 106:331–336, 2002.
10. Waldo AL, for the AFFIRM Investigators: Management of atrial fibrillation: The need for AFFIRMative action. Am J Cardiol 84:698–700, 1999.
11. Wyse DG: Selection of endpoints in atrial fibrillation studies. J Cardiovasc Electrophysiol 13(Suppl):S47–S52, 2002.
12. Nichol G, McAlister F, Pham B, et al: Meta-analysis of randomized controlled trials of the effectiveness of antiarrhythmic agents at promoting sinus rhythm in patients with atrial fibrillation. Heart 87:535–543, 2002.
13. Roy D, Talajic M, Dorian P, et al: Amiodarone to prevent recurrences of atrial fibrillation. N Engl J Med 342:913–920, 2000.
14. Pollak PT: Clinical organ toxicity of antiarrhythmic compounds: ocular and pulmonary manifestations. Am J Cardiol 84:37R–45R, 1999.
15. Pritchett ELC, Page RL, Connolly SJ, et al: Antiarrhythmic effects of azimilide in atrial fibrillation: Efficacy and dose-response. J Am Coll Cardiol 36:794–802, 2000.
16. Singh S, Zoble RG, Yellen L, et al: Efficacy and safety of oral dofetilide in converting to and maintaining sinus rhythm in patients with chronic atrial fibrillation or atrial flutter. The Symptomatic Atrial Fibrillation Investigative Research on Dofetilide (SAFIRE-D) Study. Circulation 102:2385–2390, 2000.
17. Gillis AM, Wyse DG, Connolly SJ, et al: Atrial pacing periablation for prevention of paroxysmal atrial fibrillation. Circulation 99:1843–1850, 1999.

18. Saksena S, Prakash A, Ziegler P, et al: Improved suppression of recurrent atrial fibrillation with dual-site right atrial pacing and antiarrhythmic drug therapy. J Am Coll Cardiol 40:1140–1150, 2002.
19. Daoud EG, Weiss R, Bahu M, et al: Effect of an irregular ventricular rhythm on cardiac output. Am J Cardiol 78:1433–1436, 1996.
20. Segal JB, McNamara RL, Miller MR, et al: The evidence regarding the drugs used for ventricular rate control. J Fam Pract 49:47–59, 2000.
21. Lee SH, Chen SA, Tai CT, et al: Comparisons of quality of life and cardiac performance after complete atrioventricular junction ablation and atrioventricular junction modification in patients with medically refractory atrial fibrillation. J Am Coll Cardiol 31:637–644, 1998.
22. Brignole M, Gianfranchi L, Menozzi C, et al: Assessment of atrioventricular junction ablation and DDDR mode-switching pacemaker versus pharmacological treatment in patients with severely symptomatic paroxysmal atrial fibrillation: A randomized controlled study. Circulation 96:2617–2624, 1997.
23. Brignole M, Menozzi C, Gianfranchi L, et al: Assessment of atrioventricular junction ablation and VVIR pacemaker versus pharmacological treatment in patients with heart failure and chronic atrial fibrillation: A randomized, controlled study. Circulation 98:953–960, 1998.
24. Gianfranchi L, Brignole M, Menozzi C, et al: Progression of permanent atrial fibrillation after atrioventricular junction ablation and dual-chamber pacemaker implantation in patients with paroxysmal atrial tachycrrhythmias. Am J Cardiol 81:351–354, 1998.
25. Brignole M, Menozzi C, Gasparini M, et al: An evaluation of the strategy of maintenance of sinus rhythm by antiarrhythmic drug therapy after ablation and pacing therapy in patients with paroxysmal atrial fibrillation. Eur Heart J 23:892–900, 2002.
26. Falk RH: Atrial fibrillation. N Engl J Med 344:1067–1078, 2001.
27. Wyse DG: The AFFIRM trial: Main trial and substudies—what can we expect. J Interv Card Electrophysiol 4(Suppl 1):171–176, 2000.
28. Pedersen OD, Bagger H, Keller N, et al: Efficacy of dofetilide in the treatment of atrial fibrillation-flutter in patients with reduced left ventricular function. A Danish Investigations of Arrhythmia and Mortality ON Dofetilide (DIAMOND) substudy. Circulation 104:292–296, 2001.
29. Connolly SJ: Preventing stroke in patients with atrial fibrillation: Current treatments and new concepts. Am Heart J 145:418–423, 2003.
30. Hohnloser SH, Kuck K-H, Lilienthal J, for the PIAF Investigators: Rhythm or rate-control in atrial fibrillation—Pharmacological Intervention in Atrial Fibrillation (PIAF): A randomized trial. Lancet 356:1789–1794, 2000.
31. Carlsson J, Miketic S, Windeler J, et al: Randomized trial of rate-control versus rhythm-control in persistent atrial fibrillation: The Strategies of Treatment of Atrial Fibrillation (STAF) study. J Am Coll Cardiol 41:1690–1696, 2003.
32. Wyse DG, Waldo AL, DiMarco JP, et al, Atrial Fibrillation Follow-up Investigation of Rhythm Management (AFFIRM) Investigators: A comparison of rate control and rhythm control in patients with atrial fibrillation. N Engl J Med 347:1825–1833, 2002.
33. Van Gelder IC, Hagens VE, Bosker HA, et al, Rate Control versus Electrical Cardioversion for Persistent Atrial Fibrillation Study Group: A comparison of rate control and rhythm control in patients with recurrent persistent atrial fibrillation. N Engl J Med 347: 1834–1840, 2002.
34. The AF-CHF Investigators: Rationale and design of a study assessing treatment strategies of atrial fibrillation in patients with heart failure: The Atrial Fibrillation and Congestive Heart Failure (AF-CHF) trial. Am Heart J 144:597–607, 2002.
35. Pedersen OD, Bagger H, Koeber L, Torp-Pedersen, for the TRACE Study Group: Trandolapril reduces the incidence of atrial fibrillation after acute myocardial infarction in patients with left ventricular dysfunction. Circulation 100:376–380, 1999.
36. Connolly SJ, Kerr CR, Gent M, et al: Effects of physiologic pacing versus ventricular pacing on the risk of stoke and death due to cardiovascular causes. N Engl J Med 342:1385–1391, 2000.
37. Lamas GA, Lee KL Sweeny MO, et al: Ventricular pacing or dual chamber pacing for sinus node dysfunction. N Engl J Med 346:1854–1862, 2002.
38. Brugada R, Tapscott T, Czernuszewicz GZ, et al: Identification of a genetic locus for familial atrial fibrillation. N Engl J Med 336:905–911, 1997.

第 98 章

有猝死风险患者的自动体外除颤器和植入式心脏复律除颤器临床试验结果

Alfred. E. Buxton

本章目录

- ICD 的二级预防试验 ……………… 883
- ICD 的一级预防试验 ……………… 885
- 自动体外除颤器 …………………… 889
- 总结 ………………………………… 890

植入式自动复律除颤器（implantable cardioverter-defibrillator，ICD）的出现及随后自动体外除颤器（automatic external defibrillator，AED）的问世，使有明确快速室性心律失常和具有这类心律失常风险患者的治疗发生了革命性的变化。

在 20 世纪 80 年早期 ICD 应用于临床及 90 年代早期经静脉植入 ICD 电极导线得以广泛应用之前，快速室性心律失常的治疗仅限于心肌血运重建（主要是冠状动脉旁路移植术）、外科切除致心律失常心肌及抗心律失常药物治疗，前二者只对数量相对小的人群有效，而抗心律失常药物因其疗效低及风险大而使应用受限。相反，ICD 和 AED 具有较高的疗效、较低的并发症。作为一种全新的技术和理念，ICD 在出现之初受到一些人的质疑，但很快受到了公众的认同。目前，似乎可以放心地说，ICD 和 AED 在大多数情况下终止室性心动过速和室颤的效果不容置疑。正因为如此，对发生过不可根治的持续性快速室性心律失常的患者，应用 ICD 治疗已被人们普遍接受。今天，我们面临的挑战是，如何更好地利用这种昂贵的技术预防具有这类事件风险患者的猝死，即Ⅰ级预防。最近几十年进行的许多随机对照试验结果表明，ICD 在降低高危患者群死亡率方面相对获益，前景广阔。AED 方面尚无随机试验，但其效果已在几个观察性分析研究中得到了证实。本章的目的是对该领域最近一些试验结果进行复习。我们将二级预防试验（研究持续性快速室性心律失常和心脏猝死幸存者）结果与一级预防研究分别考虑。

一、ICD 的二级预防试验

从 1997～2000 年，共报告了 3 个对比 ICDs 与抗心律失常药物的随机对照二级预防试验（表 98-1）[1-3]这些研究中，患者的入选条件和治疗上存在细微差别。其中抗心律失常药物与埋藏式除颤器对照（the Antiarrhythmics Versus Implantable Defibrillators，AVID）试验是 3 个之中最大的一个。所入选的患者为心脏骤停幸存者，为持续性室性心动过速伴晕厥、或持续性室性心动过速伴 EF 值<0.40 及提示有严重血流动力学损害症状（几乎晕厥、心力衰竭和心绞痛）的患者。另外，还要求符合条件的心律失常不是因"一过性或可逆的原因"导致的。加拿大埋藏式除颤器研究（the Canadian Implantable Defibrillator Study，CIDS）对除颤或心脏转复后存活的心脏骤停患者、证实有室颤（VF）患者、持续性室速患者、心室频率在 150 次/分以上的持续性或血流动力学不稳定的室性心动过速患者（EF 值≤35%，产生晕厥前症状或心绞痛）、不明原因晕厥但随后发现自发的非持续性室速或可诱发的持续单形性室性心动过速的患者进行随机研究。如果心律失常在急性心

肌梗死72h内发生或有电解质失衡则不能入选。心脏骤停汉堡研究（the Cardiac Arrest Study Hamburg，CASH）对证实因持续室颤引起的心脏骤停患者进行随机研究，如果心律失常发生于急性心肌梗死、心脏外科手术72h内、存在电解质异常或药物致心律失常时，则被排除。

AVID将患者随机分为ICD或抗心律失常药物治疗组。药物治疗选择胺碘酮（经验性给药，不通过试验预测疗效）或索他洛尔（通过电生理检查或动态心电图监测预测疗效）。但是，允许研究者决定患者是否适合用索他洛尔，结果只有2.6%随机接受药物治疗的患者出院时仍服用索他洛尔。CIDS试验将患者随机分配接受ICD或经验性胺碘酮治疗。CASH试验将患者随机分为4个治疗组：ICD、胺碘酮、美托洛尔或普罗帕酮组。药物治疗凭经验给药，尽管也进行动态心电图监测和电生理检查。普罗帕酮组在入选58个患者后，因死亡率过高（是ICD治疗组的2.6倍）而终止。因为研究的样本量小（288个患者），终点分析时将剩下的2个药物治疗组合在一起与ICD组进行比较。

尽管在入选条件和治疗上存在不同，但各个试验的结果非常相似（表98-2）。各个试验中，ICD治疗组具有较高的生存获益。在AVID试验中，平均随访18.2个月后，ICD治疗组15.8%的患者死亡，相比而言，药物治疗组的死亡率为24%。2年随访时ICD治疗组死亡率相对降低27%（$P<0.02$）。CIDS试验中，平均随访3年后ICD治疗组（2年死亡率为14.75%）与胺碘酮治疗组（2年死亡率为20.97%）相比，相对死亡率发生19.7%的非显著性下降（$P=0.142$），2年的相对死亡率下降29.7%。在CASH试验中，平均随访57个月后，美托洛尔与胺碘酮组总死亡率相似（分别为45.5%和43.5%），但ICD组总死亡率（36.4%）下降了23%（无统计学显著差异性，$P=0.081$）。2年随访时，ICD治疗组总死亡率相对下降39.3%。

CIDS和CASH试验中，ICD组与药物治疗组相比，死亡率未达统计学上的显著性降低可能与样本量较小有关，因而没有足够的说服力。然而，这两个试验中，因为随访时间长于AVID试验的时间，因而对试验进行荟萃分析时，二者所提供的死亡病例更多。荟萃分析显示这些研究中入选的患者总体是相似的。很明显，CASH试验中所入选的患者与其他两组相比明显年轻，且具有更高的射血分数（可能因为在CASH试验中，室颤是唯一限定的心律失常）。由于在CASH试验患者中存在这些不同，按理说应该有更好的预后，但有趣的是，CASH试验中所观察到的心律失常死亡风险与其他两组相比没有明显的差异，尽管总死亡率是下降的[4]。虽然许多人表示在这些试验中唯一有效的终点是总死亡率，但在观察ICD疗效时死亡分类还是很重要的。下面我们对ICD降低总死亡率的机制进行一下推理。我们相信ICD对总死亡率的有益影响主要通过有效治疗快速室性心律失常实现。另外可以想象，还有一小部分获益来源于ICD合并的抗心动过缓起搏功能，进一步的获益则是通过减少抗心律失常药物而获得。因此，对死亡率的有益影响应该主要是对猝死或心律失常的作用。事实上，对这些研究的荟萃分析发现，ICD治疗相关的心律失常死亡风险比（hazard ratio，HR）远低于总死亡风险比：0.49（心律失常死亡）比0.73（总死亡）。

表98-1 继发性的预防实验中埋藏式心脏复律除颤器病人的特征

实验（参考）	病人（n）	指数心律失常-VF（%）	CAD（%）	NHD（%）	入选CHF*（%）	EF（%）	BBB（%）
AVID（1）	1016	45	81	3	58	32	24
CIDS（2）	659	47.6	82.6	3	50	34	NA
CASH△（3）	288	100	73.3	10	73	46	20

*纽约心脏协会心功能分级2或3级病人百分数。
△不包括随机服用普罗帕酮的病人。

AVID，抗心律失常与埋藏式除颤器比较；BBB，束支阻滞；CAD，冠状动脉疾病；CASH，心脏停搏汉布格尔研究；CHF，充血性心力衰竭；CIDS，加拿大植入式除颤器研究；EF，左心室射血分数；NA，无入选；NHD，无器质性心脏病；VF，心室颤动。

表 98-2 继发性的预防实验的结果

实验	随机接受 ICD W/植入 (%)	接受胺碘酮 (%)	随访时间 (月)	2年死亡率 药物治疗 (%)	2年死亡率 ICD (%)	危险比率 (ICD)
AVID	98	85 (2年)*	18	24	15.8	0.73
CIDS	95	80 (3年)*	36	20.97	14.75	0.70
CASH	100	90 (研究期间)*	57	22	12	0.61

* 标示处提供了随访信息。

AVID，抗心律失常与埋藏式除颤器比较；CASH，心脏停搏汉布格尔研究；CIDS，加拿大植入式除颤器研究；ICD，埋藏式复律除颤器。

这些试验的研究者试图证明，在某个亚组人群中ICD能使患者获益[4-6]。这些亚组研究证实，具有最大死亡风险的患者最有可能获益。AVID的研究者发现，与胺碘酮治疗相比，EF值≤35%的患者获益最大。事实上，他们并不能证实 EF 大于35%的患者 ICD 与胺碘酮相比有生存获益。同样，CIDS 研究者证实，通过一系列参数包括 EF 值、年龄及心衰程度，可确认胺碘酮治疗患者心律失常复发的最大风险。研究者依据患者所存在的危险因素，将这些患者平分为4部分。以前的研究发现，这些危险因素可预示随机胺碘酮治疗组患者的死亡率。年龄大于70岁，EF 值≤35%，纽约心功能分级（NYHA）Ⅲ～Ⅳ级构成最危险的一组。具有这3种危险因素的患者 ICD 与胺碘酮相比总死亡率下降50%。相反，将3个低危组（没有危险因素，或只有1个或2个危险因素）放在一起，未发现随机 ICD 治疗与胺碘酮治疗组之间生存有何区别。同样，3个试验的荟萃分析证实，只有 EF 值≤35%的患者，ICD 治疗与胺碘酮相比有明显获益，而EF≥35%的患者二者之间的生存率没有区别。

这些观察证实，对于明显左心功能不全和重度心力衰竭患者，快速室性心律失常是最重要的致死原因。他们证实，对这类患者，ICD 可延长生命，应用ICD 治疗并不是仅降低心律失常死亡而将患者置于近似的非心律失常死亡率风险之中。然而，这些分析也提出一个问题，为何在 EF 大于35%的患者中 ICD 与胺碘酮相比无明显获益？是否因为心律失常机制不同，或仅仅是因为左室功能保护得较好时胺碘酮对相同心律失常有更好的抗心律失常作用，才使胺碘酮对EF 较高的患者更为有效呢？有可能是 EF 值较高的患者，因急性缺血导致的室颤在猝死过程中起较大作用，而胺碘酮的β受体阻断作用是疗效得到某种程度改善的原因。对于 EF 值大于35%的患者 ICD 获益相对较小的观察结果还有另一种解释，在这些研究中随访期限相对较短：AVID 试验平均18个月，CIDS 试验平均36个月。EF 值较高的患者心律失常的发作频度似乎较低。因此，如果在研究人群中复发事件的频度足够低、随访期相对较短的话研究不太可能证实一种治疗相对于另一种治疗具有显著获益。

认识到这些试验中的另一个局限性也很重要。每个试验所入选的是符合条件的心律失常患者，无论患者是否有基础心脏病，也不管基础心脏病的类型如何。因此，如果所入选的大多数患者有冠状动脉疾病和陈旧心肌梗死，那么结果主要是应用于有这些特征的患者。没有哪个试验足以证实，如果将这些结果应用于非缺血性心肌病（扩张或肥厚型）是否一样合适。而且，在每个试验中，只有极少数入选患者被分类为有结构性心脏病。因为在这些试验中，入选的时间跨度从20世纪80年代至90年代，而此时，原发性基因性心律失常机制或新近认识的疾病如 Brugada 综合征并未得到人们的广泛认同，因而对是否可将这些试验结果普遍用于心脏骤停幸存者的亚群，人们必定存有疑问。

二、ICD 的一级预防试验

ICD 预防心脏骤停幸存者猝死的价值已被广泛接受，尽管有证据表明这种治疗手段仍然未得到充分使用。相反，对 ICD 在猝死高危患者一级预防中的作用，人们接受起来一直不太积极。这一部分将对新近报告的 ICD 在猝死一级预防中作用的随机试验进行复习（表 98-3）。与二级预防试验不同，每个一级预防试验所关注的是相对同类的患者群。除一个试验外，这些试验都限定于冠状动脉疾病和心功能异常的患者。两个试验对冠状动脉疾病，左心功能不全和无症状的非持续性室性心动过速患者进行了评价。

这些试验中，第一个发表的是多中心自动除颤器植入试验（Multicenter Automatic Defibrillator Implantation，MADIT），该试验对具有以前文献中[11]

所注释特征的患者进行了电生理检查。诱发持续性室速的患者，给予静脉普鲁卡因胺治疗，如果所诱发的持续性室性心动过速持续存在，将随机接受 ICD 或"常规"的抗心律失常药物治疗。而后者是非对照性的，依据研究者的选择而不同。该组中，经验性胺碘酮治疗占 74%，试验不设非治疗对照组，共入选 196 名患者，平均随访 27 个月后，研究者注意到，随机入选 ICD 治疗的患者，总死亡率相对减少 54%。"常规"药物治疗组 2 年实际死亡率为 32%，几个因素限制了对这些结果的解释。这是一个小规模试验，共入选 196 个患者，当发现 ICD 治疗组具有明显生存获益时，试验被提前终止。因而该试验有可能高估治疗的获益，两试验组间 β 受体阻滞剂的应用不平衡：随机"常规"治疗组 8% 的患者出院时服用 β 受体阻滞剂，而随机 ICD 治疗组 26% 的患者接受 β 受体阻滞剂治疗。然而，这种不平衡似乎不太可能对结果产生明显影响，因为 AVID 和多中心非持续性心动过速试验（Multicenter Unsustained Tachycardia Trial，MUSTT）未能显示 β 受体阻滞剂对 ICD 治疗患者的结果会产生明显的影响。该试验在随机分组时不包括未治疗组，因而，如果随机入"常规治疗"组的患者发生了明显的致心律失常作用或其他抗心律失常药物的副作用，ICD 治疗的相对获益可能被高估了。

第二个一级预防试验即 MUST 试验的患者与 MADIT 试验患者具有相似的特征[14]。该随机对照试验的主要目的是评价电生理检查指导下的抗心律失常治疗（包括 ICD 和药物）在降低冠状动脉疾病、左心功能不全和自发性非持续性室性心动过速患者猝死风险方面的作用。该试验将 704 个基础电生理检查（在没有抗心律失常药物治疗情况下进行）诱发出持续性室性心动过速的患者随机平均分为 2 组：一组接受 β 受体阻断剂和血管紧张素转换酶抑制剂（ACEI）的保守治疗，无抗心律失常治疗；另一组应用 β 受体阻滞剂、ACEI 和电生理检查指导下的抗心律失常治疗，先试用抗心律失常药物治疗，对药物无反应（通过电生理检查判断）的患者随后接受 ICD 治疗。共随访 5 年，随机电生理指导治疗的患者心律失常死亡或心脏骤停（试验的一级终点）的风险下降 27%，总死亡率下降 20%，试验未设计 ICD 治疗和抗心律失常药物对降低死亡率效果的对比。然而，试验结束时，评价电生理检查指导的治疗时发现，采用 ICD 治疗的患者与抗心律失常药物治疗者几乎一样多，进一步分析发现，电生理检查指导的治疗对生存的改善作用完全是 ICD 治疗的结果[15]。应用 ICD 治疗的患者特征与药物抗心律失常治疗者非常相似。与 MADIT 试验相反，ICD 治疗与抗心律失常药物治疗者相比具有较低的 β 受体阻滞剂使用率（37% 对 51%）。出院时未植入 ICD 的患者，事件发生率与未治疗对照组相似，而 ICD 降低心律失常死亡或心脏骤停风险近 74%，总死亡率下降 50%。

有趣的是将 MADIT 和 MUSTT 试验的患者特征和研究结果进行比较时，两个试验的入选标准有所不同。MADIT 试验要求患者的左室 EF 值为 26%，而 MUSTT 试验为 30%。此外，因为在 MADIT 试验中，要求患者在电生检查时对普鲁卡因胺没有反应才满足入选条件，因而人们可能预测该研究人群有较大的死亡危险。已知可影响预后的其他因素在两个试验中具有的比例相似。各试验中 2/3 的患者为纽约心功能分级（NYHA）Ⅱ或Ⅲ级，MADIT 试验中 45% 的患者及 MUSTT 试验中 56% 的患者入选前接受过冠状动脉旁路移植术（CABG），各试验中，最近一次心肌梗死的时间距入选时间超过 1 年。MADIT 试验中满足条件的非持续性室性心动过速为 9~10 个心搏，而 MUSTT 试验为 5 个心搏，提示 MADIT 试验中存在某种程度的参考偏差，因为 MUSTT 试验报道的 5 个心搏与心律失常抑制试验（Cardiac Arrhythmias Suppression Trial，CAST）的入选条件是相同的[16]。

MADIT 试验与 MUSTT 试验之间另一个不同之处与既往心肌梗死的病史有关。MADIT 试验要求患者心肌梗死病史至少在入选前 3 个月以上，事实上 75% 的患者最近的心肌梗死至入选的时间超过 6 个月。其中 MUSTT 试验患者有明确的冠心病病史，但不要求有心肌梗死的证据，真正的缺血性心肌病亦可。但 95% 随机入选的患者有明确的心肌梗死，最近一次心肌梗死至入选的平均时间为 39 个月，17% 的患者最近的心肌梗死在 1 个月内。很明显，心肌梗死至入选的时间并不影响室性心动过速的可诱发性，急性心肌梗死后 1 个月入选的患者，42% 存在可随机诱发的室性心动过速；而心肌梗死后 1~6 个月，6~36 个月及超过 36 个月的患者存在上述心动过速的比例分别为 35%、38% 和 43%。因为在 MADIT 或 MUSTT 试验中，心肌梗死后 1 个月内入选的患者很少，还不清楚如果将这些研究中所应用的治疗策略应用于心梗后即刻尚未出院的患者是否能降低死亡率。

表 98-3 冠心病患者的一级预防试验

实验（参考）	病人 (n)	Rx 对照组	CHF (%)*	EF (%)	LBBB (%)	随机接受 ICD 植入 w/植入 (%)	持续时间 f/u（月）	对照组病人 2 年的死亡率 (%)	ICD 组病人 2 年的死亡率 (%)	危险比率 (ICD 治疗)	对照组病人 β 受体阻滞剂的应用 (%)	ICD 组病人 β 受体阻滞剂的应用 (%)
MADIT (10)	196	常规抗心律失常药物治疗	65	26	8	95	27	32	10	0.46	8	26
MUSTT (13)	704	No Rx	63	30	3	—†	39	28	10	0.55	51	37
MADIT-II (20)	1232	No Rx	58‡	23	19	97	20	22	16	0.69	70	70
CABG-Patch (24)	900	No Rx	73	27	11	97	32	17	17	1.07	24	18

* 入选时心功能（NYHA）Ⅱ或Ⅲ级
† MUSTT 试验并非随机分配患者接受 ICD 治疗
‡ MADIT-II 试验中，5%患者为心功能（NYHA）Ⅳ级。
BB，β受体阻滞剂；CABG，冠心病旁路手术；CHF，充血性心衰；EF，左室射血分数；ICD，植入式复律除颤器；MADIT，多中心自动除颤器植入试验；MUSTT，多中心非持续性心动过速试验。

因而，如果想将这些试验结果应用于普通人群，这将是一个重要问题。两个试验中入选的患者都是经过特殊筛选的，目前尚不清楚，这些结果将如何普遍应用于一般临床实践中。应用这些试验结果的关键之处在于，当心肌梗死患者尚在住院治疗时确认其是否是ICD的合适候选者。系统应用这些治疗策略的结果尚不清楚。

尽管在MADIT和MUSTT试验之中，患者特征尚有细微的差别，但与ICD治疗有关的事件发生率和生存获益极为相似。MADIT试验平均随访时间为27个月，而MUSTT试验为39个月，可进行2年事件发生率的合理比较。在MUSTT试验中，随机入选未治疗组的可诱发室性心动过速的患者2年总死亡率为28%，而随机电生理检查指导治疗（未用ICD治疗）组总死亡率为33%，MADIT试验总死亡率为32%，两个试验中，应用ICD治疗组2年死亡率为10%。MUSTT试验中与ICD治疗相关的总死亡率下降55%（与随机非抗心律失常治疗患者相比），而心律失常死亡和心脏骤停风险下降达73%，这些结果为下述概念提供了支持依据，即ICD降低死亡率的原因是其抗心律失常作用。

为了明确MADIT试验中与ICD有关的治疗获益在各亚组之间是否一致，研究者依据是否存在可影响死亡率的各种因素进行分析。作者将试验中所观察的危险因素从中值水平一分为二（左室射血分数<26%对比26%~35%，标准心电图QRS宽度≥120ms对比<120ms，需要治疗的充血性心力衰竭对比无心力衰竭患者）。分析证实低危和高危人群ICD治疗均有较低死亡率，然而，只在具有一个以上高危因素的患者群观察到统计学差异，提示患者受益。因此，EF值在26%~35%之间的患者，"常规"治疗与ICD治疗之间生存率是相等的。QRS宽度<120ms的患者，二种治疗间生存率相同，无充血性心衰病史的患者也是如此。危险因素越多，所观察到的与ICD治疗相关的生存获益越大。如果试验规模较小，人群中近50%的死亡由心律失常引起，且与ICD治疗相关的致死性并发症发生率较低，那么产生这种结果并不令人吃惊。MUSTT试验中也进行过类似的分析，但结果有所不同[19]。在EF值≥30%和<30%的患者中，心律失常死亡和总死亡率都有明显下降，部分原因是因为MUSTT试验的规模较大且随访时间较长。充血性心力衰竭患者应用ICD治疗总死亡率和心律失常死亡风险都是降低的，无心力衰竭的患者，心律失常死亡风险显示出明显降低，但总死亡率没有明显区别。

继这些试验之后，MADIT研究者进行了第2个试验，该试验摒弃了EF测定之外的危险分层[20]。因而该研究入选了冠心病、心肌梗死后至少1个月以上及EF≤30%的患者[21]。患者随机接受抗心律失常药物或植入ICD治疗，试验中β受体阻滞剂的应用比例高于以前的试验，70%的随机患者接受β受体阻滞剂治疗。不进行标准电生理检查，但随机ICD治疗的患者在植入时通过ICD进行刺激，36%的患者诱发持续性室性心动过速，平均随访20个月，研究者发现随机接受ICD治疗的患者总死亡率下降31%（19.8%比14.2%）。因此，尽管研究所入选的患者中近2/3可能诱发不出室性心动过速，但ICD仍明显降低死亡率，虽然降低程度低于MADIT和MUSTT试验。ICD治疗的获益较低可能有几种解释，β受体阻滞剂及I类抗心律失常药应用较少有可能使对照组死亡率下降。无论能否诱发持续性室速都在入选之列，因而使风险下降，尽管该试验中所入选的患者有冠状动脉疾病且EF值较低（平均23%），但未治疗患者的死亡率（20个月时19.8%）明显低于MUSTT试验中可诱发持续性室速的未治疗患者的死亡率（2年28%，平均EF值29%）及MADIT试验中随机"常规治疗"的可诱发持续室速患者的死亡率（2年32%）。事实上，MADIT试验中未治患者的死亡率与MUSTT注册研究试验中入选的未诱发室速患者中所观察到的死亡率相似（2年21%，EF值29%）[22]。后一项研究中只有35%的患者应用β受体阻滞剂，有可能增加其死亡风险。这些观察证明，电生理检查可诱发室性心动过速对危险分层具有很大的作用，同时β受体阻滞剂对因心肌梗死而产生的左室功能异常患者的生存具有有益的影响。

MADIT II试验的结果未被其他研究所证实，目前还不清楚它们将如何应用于临床实践。例如，大多数与ICD治疗有关的生存获益产生于有高危标志的患者：EF值低，标准心电图QRS波最宽的患者[21]。随机入选MADIT II试验的患者，88%最近心肌梗死至入选的时间超过6个月。急性心肌梗死后即刻入选的患者遵循这种试验方案是否能得到相同的结果？诊所经常遇到的10~20年前有过心肌梗死的稳定患者，如果采用这种方案结果是否会一样？心肌梗死确诊的时间对预后有显著的影响。既往二级预防的研究证实，院内心脏骤停存活者的预后明显不如院外心脏骤停者[23]。同样，在MUSTT试验中，在诊所确诊的患者无论治疗与否,其死亡风险明显低于住院时确诊的患者[24]。住院确诊的非持续性室性心动过速患者,冠状动脉病变支数更多,充血性心力衰竭病史更常见,心功能 NYHA 分级更高,最近一次心梗距入选的时间更短,但 2 组间平均左室射血分数是相似的(0.29 : 0.30)。住院确诊非持续性室性心动过速的患者,与院外确诊的患者相比,基础电生理检查时诱发持续单行性室性心动过速的几率更大(35% : 28%,$P=0.06$),未接受抗心律失常药物治疗的 1780 个患者的结果分析(包括可诱发室速但未治疗及未诱发室速的患者)提示:住院确诊的持续性室性心动过速者 2 年及 5 年的总死亡率增加 30%($P=0.018$)。经患者特征变量校正后,心律失常死亡和心脏骤停发生率不明显提高,电生理检查指导的抗心律失常治疗的疗效两组间无差别。此外,即便 ICD 治疗的患者,生存方面也有差别,住院入选的患者 5 年死亡率是院外入选患者的两倍(34% : 17%)。因此,有许多因素可能影响 MADIT II 试验的结果。

2 个一级预防试验已被报道,但它们并未显示 ICD 治疗组与未治对照组相比有生存获益。CABG Patch 试验对如下假设进行了验证,即 EF≤35% 且信号平均电图异常的患者,CABG 术时植入 ICD 将降低死亡率[25]。CABG Patch 试验中 900 个患者在冠状动脉旁路移植术时随机接受 ICD 或非 ICD 治疗。各个治疗组的平均 EF 值为 27%,50% 的患者有心衰病史,似乎是猝死相对高危的研究人群。平均随访 32 个月,对照组和 ICD 组的实际总死亡率分别为 24% 和 27%($P=0.64$)。各治疗组 2 年死亡率近 17%,与 MADIT II 试验中所观察到的结果相似。尽管研究人群具有许多高危特征,但该试验并未显示 ICD 可以改善生存,其原因并不完全清楚,可能是信号平均电图不是心律失常事件强有力的预测因子。如果这是唯一的解释,其结果与 MADIT II 研究的结果相矛盾,因为在后一研究中,当 EF 为 27% 时 ICD 治疗预计有生存获益。然而,MADIT II 试验未入选 3 个月内有心肌梗死的患者。最有可能的情况是,接受 CABG 治疗的患者群有较低的心律失常风险(是外科术后 EF 值提高了吗?)或 CABG 术本身对外科术后 2~3 年的心律失常事件风险有影响。MUSTT 试验中有关 CABG 效果的分析对这一问题作了进一步的阐述[26]。在 MUSTT 试验中,CABG 术后 4~10 天发现非持续性室性心动过速的患者与近期未接受 CABG 的患者相比具有显著降低的总死亡率(2 年为 13%)及心律失常死亡或心脏骤停发生率(2 年为 5%)。非持续性室性心动过速前 10~30 天或超过 30 天之前已接受 CABG 治疗并入选该研究的患者,与从未接受过 CABG 治疗的患者相比,事件发生率具有可比性,后者 2 年的心律失常死亡/心脏骤停发生率及总死亡率分别为 15% 和 24%。因此,在 MUSTT 试验人群中,CABG 治疗对死亡率的任何有益影响似乎不会永久存在。这些结果提示,CABG 术后短期即确认 EF 下降,但未发现有症状的持续性室性心律失常患者,如果没有其他检查如心内电生理检查提示其具有特别高的风险,不太可能从预防性 ICD 治疗中获益。

最近报道的另一个一级预防试验也能证实 ICD 治疗可提高生存率。该试验与前面描述的一级预防试验不同,其研究人群由非缺血性扩张型心肌病患者组成[27]。9 个月内诊断的冠心病(要求作冠脉造影)导致的扩张型心肌病,EF 值≤30%(通过心室造影测量)及 NYHA II-III 级的患者符合入选条件。试验在德国的 15 个心脏中心进行,自 1991~1997 年入选 104 个患者,被随机平均分配接受 ICD 和非 ICD 治疗,2 组间的基础特征匹配良好,所有患者的平均 EF 值为 24%,只有 3.8% 的患者应用 β 受体阻滞剂,96% 接受血管紧张素转换酶抑制剂治疗,平均随访 5.5 年,2 个治疗组间生存率无差别。各组死亡率很低:1 年随访时 ICD 治疗组总死亡率为 8%,对照组 3.7%。2 年随访时 ICD 治疗组死亡率 8%,对照组 7%。该研究中观察到的事件发生率明显低于前面讨论的冠心病患者一级预防试验中所观察到的发生率[28]。以前有关充血性心力衰竭患者的研究显示,因冠心病引起的心衰具有较高的死亡率。虽然该试验规模较小,但随访时间很长。因此,尽管有可能将低死亡率归因于入选试验前发生心力衰竭的时间相对较短,但平均随访 5.5 年对事件产生来说时间已足够。有关 ICD 在非缺血性心肌病患者猝死预防中的潜在作用的进一步信息,待 2003 年 10 月心脏猝死——心衰试验(The Sudden Cardiac Death-Heart Failure Trial,SCD-HFT)完成随访时将会获得。在这些结果出来之前,尚无数据支持 ICD 在非缺血性扩张型心肌病中的应用。

三、自动体外除颤器

自动体外除颤器(automatic external defibrillator,AED)是一种在某些方面比 ICD 更新的技术。

其对猝死的预防作用可能至少与 ICD 一样。因为其花费相对便宜应用前景则更为广泛。目前尚没有 AED 与其他治疗手段对比的随机对照试验。许多证实 AED 能在各种场合有效治疗心脏骤停的观察性研究已有报道。这些场所包括民用飞机场和赌场[29,30]。这些经验证实了旁观者使用 AED 的可行性，立即除颤，室颤者的生存率可高达 59%，远高于依据医务人员急救时所预期的 2%～20% 的生存率。考虑到院外心脏骤停的生存率与心肺复苏开始的时间及除颤的最短延迟时间密切相关，西雅图的研究者证实，给消防人员配备 AEDs，与仅由医务人员使用 AED 的城区相比，可明显缩短除颤的反应时间，因这些地方医务人员反应延迟一直存在[31]。通过将 AEDs 的应用扩展至消防员，除颤的平均延迟时间减少 5 分钟以上，生存率改善 1.8 倍[32]。最近的迈阿密研究证实，给警察配备 AED 时，室颤和室速的生存率与仅由医务人员使用 AED 时提高几乎 2 倍，这种生存率的改善是由于警察的快速反应所致[33]。不幸的是，在迈阿密经验中，61% 的初次记录心律是不可除颤治疗的，明显降低 AED 对生存率总的影响。这些早期的报告扩大了 AED 的使用范围，使其越来越多地应用于繁华的公共场所，如机场、购物中心、运动赛场及健身俱乐部。不幸的是，这些计划总的影响有限，因为 75% 的院外心脏骤停发生在家中[34]。这些观察使个人购买 AED，以便在医生指导下在家中使用成为可能。国家心脏血液研究所（NHLBI）开始了一个前瞻性试验，旨在评价家用 AED 在前壁心肌梗死存活者中的应用情况。

四、总　结

总的来说，我们目前已从众多有关潜在致命室性心律失常存活者和不同程度风险患者的随机对照前瞻性试验中获益，并以此来指导 ICD 的应用。这些结果证实，ICD 能够降低选择性患者群心律失常的死亡风险和总死亡率。我们预期 ICD 在猝死一级预防中将有更为广泛的应用。事实上，将来这方面应用的增长速度将超过二级预防。然而，资料提示，即便对已证实 ICD 可获益的患者，仍有 ICD 使用不足的情况。目前我们面临的主要挑战是：在目前有限的资料环境下，如何精选出有可能从这一治疗获得最大益处的患者。作为 ICD 在最高危患者中应用的补充，有可能对 AED 在中度猝死风险患者中的应用作出评估。

（吴永全　译）

参 考 文 献

1. The Antiarrhythmics versus Implantable Defibrillators (AVID) Investigators: A comparison of antiarrhythmic-drug therapy with implantable defibrillators in patients resuscitated from near-fatal ventricular arrhythmias. N Engl J Med 337:1576–1583, 1997.
2. Connolly S, Gent M, Roberts R, et al: Canadian Implantable Defibrillator Study (CIDS): A randomized trial of the implantable cardioverter defibrillator against amiodarone. Circulation 101:1297–1302, 2000.
3. Kuck K-H, Cappato R, Siebels J, et al: Randomized comparison of antiarrhythmic drug therapy with implantable defibrillators in patients resuscitated from cardiac arrest. The Cardiac Arrest Study Hamburg (CASH). Circulation 102:748–754, 2000.
4. Connolly SJ, Hallstrom AP, Cappato R, et al: Meta-analysis of the implantable cardioverter defibrillator secondary prevention trials. Eur Heart J 21:2071–2078, 2000.
5. Domanski M, Saksena S, Epstein A, et al: Relative effectiveness of the implantable cardioverter-defibrillator and antiarrhythmic drugs in patients with varying degrees of left ventricular dysfunction who have survived malignant ventricular arrhythmias. J Am Coll Cardiol 34:1090–1095, 1999.
6. Sheldon R, Connolly S, Krahn A, et al: Identification of patients most likely to benefit from implantable cardioverter-defibrillator therapy. The Canadian Implantable Defibrillator Study. Circulation 101:1660–1664, 2000.
7. Bansch D, Castrucci M, Bocker D, et al: Ventricular tachycardias above the initially programmed tachycardia detection interval in patients with implantable cardioverter-defibrillators: Incidence, prediction and significance. J Am Coll Cardiol 36:557–565, 2000.
8. Freedberg NA, Hill JN, Fogel RI, et al: Recurrence of symptomatic ventricular arrhythmias in patients with implantable cardioverter defibrillator after the first device therapy: Implications for antiarrhythmic therapy and driving restrictions. CARE Group. J Am Coll Cardiol 37:1910–1915, 2001.
9. Raitt MH, Dolack GL, Kudenchuk PJ, et al: Ventricular arrhythmias detected after transvenous defibrillator implantation in patients with a clinical history of only ventricular fibrillation. Implications for use of implantable defibrillator. Circulation 91:1996–2001, 1995.
10. Ruskin JN, Camm AJ, Zipes DP, et al: Implantable cardioverter defibrillator utilization based on discharge diagnoses from Medicare and managed care patients. J Cardiovasc Electrophysiol 13:38–43, 2002.
11. Moss AJ, Hall WJ, Cannom DS, et al: Improved survival with an implanted defibrillator in patients with coronary disease at high risk for ventricular arrhythmia. Multicenter Automatic Defibrillator Implantation Trial Investigators. N Engl J Med 335:1933–1940, 1996.
12. Ellison KE, Hafley GE, Hickey K, et al: Effect of beta-blocking therapy on outcome in the Multicenter Unsustained Tachycardia Trial (MUSTT). Circulation 106:2694–2699, 2002.
13. Exner DV, Reiffel JA, Epstein AE, et al: Beta-blocker use and survival in patients with ventricular fibrillation or symptomatic ventricular tachycardia: The Antiarrhythmics Versus Implantable Defibrillators (AVID) trial. J Am Coll Cardiol 34:325–333, 1999.
14. Buxton AE, Lee KL, Fisher JD, et al: A randomized study of the prevention of sudden death in patients with coronary artery disease. Multicenter Unsustained Tachycardia Trial Investigators. N Engl J Med 341:1882–1890, 1999.
15. Lee KL, Hafley G, Fisher JD, et al: Effect of Implantable Defibrillators on Arrhythmic Events and Mortality in the Multicenter Unsustained Tachycardia Trial. Circulation 106:233–238, 2002.
16. Denes P, Gillis AM, Pawitan Y, et al: Prevalence, characteristics and significance of ventricular premature complexes and ventricular tachycardia detected by 24-hour continuous electrocardiographic recording in the Cardiac Arrhythmia Suppression Trial. CAST Investigators. Am J Cardiol 68:887–896, 1991.
17. Coromilas J, Buxton AE, Hafley G, et al: How soon after MI should patients with MI and LV dysfunction be screened for NSVT and have electrophysiologic studies done? Circulation 104:II-784, 2001.
18. Moss AJ, Fadl Y, Zareba W, et al: Survival benefit with an implanted defibrillator in relation to mortality risk in chronic coronary heart disease. Am J Cardiol 88:516–520, 2001.
19. Gold M, O'Toole M, Tang A, et al: The effect of ejection fraction and congestive heart failure on the benefit of implantable defibrillators in

MUSTT [abstract]. Pacing Clin Electrophysiol 23:II-493, 2000.
20. Moss AJ, Cannom DS, Daubert JP, et al: Multicenter Automatic Defibrillator Implantation Trial II (MADIT II): Design and clinical protocol. Ann Noninvasive Electrocardiol 4:83–91, 1999.
21. Moss AJ, Zareba W, Hall WJ, et al: Prophylactic implantation of a defibrillator in patients with myocardial infarction and reduced ejection fraction. N Engl J Med 346(12):877–883, 2002. Epub March 19, 2002.
22. Buxton AE, Lee KL, DiCarlo L, et al: Electrophysiologic testing to identify patients with coronary artery disease who are at risk for sudden death. Multicenter Unsustained Tachycardia Trial Investigators. N Engl J Med 342:1937–1945, 2000.
23. Epstein AE, Powell J, Yao Q, et al: In-hospital versus out-of-hospital presentation of life-threatening ventricular arrhythmias predicts survival. Results from the AVID Registry. J Am Coll Cardiol 34:1111–1116, 1999.
24. Pires LA, Lehmann MH, Buxton AE, et al: Differences in inducibility and prognosis of in-hospital versus out-of-hospital identified nonsustained ventricular tachycardia in patients with coronary artery disease: Clinical and trial design implications. J Am Coll Cardiol 38:1156–1162, 2001.
25. Bigger J, The Coronary Artery Bypass Graft (CABG) Patch Trial Investigators: Prophylactic use of implanted cardiac defibrillators in patients at high risk for ventricular arrhythmias after coronary-artery bypass graft surgery. N Engl J Med 337:1569–1575, 1997.
26. Pires L, Hafley G, Lee K, et al: Significance of nonsustained ventricular tachycardia identified postoperatively after coronary bypass surgery in patients with left ventricular dysfunction. J Cardiovasc
27. Bansch D, Antz M, Boczor S, et al: Primary prevention of sudden cardiac death in idiopathic dilated cardiomyopathy: The Cardiomyopathy Trial (CAT). Circulation 105:1453–1458, 2002.
28. Bart BA, Shaw LK, McCants CB Jr, et al: Clinical determinants of mortality in patients with angiographically diagnosed ischemic or nonischemic cardiomyopathy. J Am Coll Cardiol 30:1002–1008, 1997.
29. Page RL, Joglar JA, Kowal RC, et al: Use of automated external defibrillators by a U.S. airline. N Engl J Med 343:1210–1216, 2000.
30. Valenzuela TD, Roe DJ, Nichol G, et al: Outcomes of rapid defibrillation by security officers after cardiac arrest in casinos. N Engl J Med 343:1206–1209, 2000.
31. Holmberg M, Holmberg S, Herlitz J: The problem of out-of-hospital cardiac-arrest prevalence of sudden death in Europe today. Am J Cardiol 83:88D–90D, 1999.
32. Weaver WD, Hill D, Fahrenbruch CE, et al: Use of the automatic external defibrillator in the management of out-of-hospital cardiac arrest. N Engl J Med 319:661–666, 1988.
33. Myerburg RJ, Fenster J, Velez M, et al: Impact of community-wide police car deployment of automated external defibrillators on survival from out-of-hospital cardiac arrest. Circulation 106:1058–1064, 2002.
34. Litwin PE, Eisenberg MS, Hallstrom AP, et al: The location of collapse and its impact on survival from cardiac arrest. Ann Emerg Med 16:787–791, 1987.

第十四部分
心律失常的药物和非药物治疗

第 99 章

Ⅰ类抗心律失常药物：奎尼丁、普鲁卡因胺、丙吡胺、利多卡因、美西律、氟卡胺和普罗帕酮

Anne M. Gillis

本章目录

- ⅠA 类抗心律失常药：奎尼丁、普鲁卡因胺和丙吡胺 ………… 893
- ⅠB 类抗心律失常药：利多卡因和美西律 ………… 896
- ⅠC 类抗心律失常药：氟卡胺和普罗帕酮 ………… 896
- 致谢 ………… 898

Ⅰ类抗心律失常药阻断心脏钠通道。其钠通道阻滞的程度取决于心率、膜电位和每种药物的生化特征，这些生化特征决定了阻断作用的快慢和持续时间长短[1,2]。根据药物对心脏传导的作用程度，Ⅰ类抗心律失常药又可分为几种亚型。ⅠA 类药物包括奎尼丁、普鲁卡因胺和丙吡胺，它们对钠通道有中度阻断作用，通常仅能在心率较快时明显减慢心肌组织的传导性。ⅠB 类药物包括利多卡因和美西律，它们对正常心肌组织的钠通道有轻度阻断作用，但对已去极化的心肌组织则可明显减慢其传导速度。ⅠC 类药物包括氟卡胺和普罗帕酮，它们可明显减慢心脏组织的传导性，在正常心率时这种作用表现为心电图 QRS 波群宽度的增加。此外，许多Ⅰ类药物还可以作用于其他离子通道和/或膜受体，从而介导一些电生理效应（表 99-1）[1,2]。虽然这些药物主要用于治疗室性心律失常，但由于其有致室性心律失常的危险，对有器质性心脏病的患者，这些药物的应用受到了限制[3,4]。

目前，ⅠA 类和ⅠC 类药物主要用于室上性快速性心律失常的治疗[5,8]。

一、ⅠA 类抗心律失常药：奎尼丁、普鲁卡因胺和丙吡胺

（一）药效学

奎尼丁、普鲁卡因胺和丙吡胺可阻断钠离子通道，阻断作用中等。这些药物也可以阻断一种或多种钾离子电流，从而延长动作电位时间（APD）[9-12]。普鲁卡因胺对 APD 的作用是通过它的活性代谢产物氮-乙酰普鲁卡因胺来介导的，它阻断了延迟整流钾电流（I_{Kr}）中的快速激活成分。表 99-1 归纳了在临床相关的药物浓度下，每一种药物对离子通道的特殊作用可能产生的电生理效应[1,2]。这些效应导致心肌兴奋性阈值升高、自律性降低、传导和复极时间延长。奎尼丁也可以阻断 α 肾上腺素能受体，它和丙吡胺都可以抑制胆碱能受体[6]，后者的效应可能加剧它们的迷走介导性致心律失常作用[8]。奎尼丁对心脏的电生理作用与疾病状态相关，对心肌梗死后代偿性肥厚的心肌组织的 APD 的延长作用较小，而且对心力衰竭患者的 QT 间期延长作用也较小[14]。在心室肥厚时，这些效应可能部分是通过下调一种或多种钾离子复极电流来介导的[15]。但在疾病状态下，这些效应的整体不一致性可能导致复极离散度的增加，后者为致心律失常的发生提供了条件[4,16]。对于妇女，奎尼丁可更大程度地延长 APD 并增加复极离散度，因此增加了致室性心律失常的危险[17]。其他Ⅰ类药物可能对病态和正常的心肌组织也会产生不同的效应。

表 99-1　Ⅰ类抗心律失常药物的药效学

	钠通道阻滞后的恢复速度	K$^+$通道	受体
Ⅰ$_A$类			
丙吡胺	中	↓I_{to}，↓I_{kr}，↓$I_{k(ATP)}$	抑制胆碱能受体
奎尼丁	中	↓I_{to}，↓I_{kr}	抑制α肾上腺素能受体和胆碱能受体
普鲁卡因胺	中		
氮-乙酰普鲁卡因胺		↓I_{kr}	
Ⅰ$_B$类			
利多卡因	快		
美西律	快		
Ⅰ$_C$类			
氟卡胺	慢	↓I_{kr}，↓I_{kur}	
普罗帕酮	慢	↓I_{kr}，↓I_{kur}	抑制α肾上腺素能受体

I_{to}：瞬间外向电流；I_{kr}：延迟整流电流的快速激活成分；$I_{k(ATP)}$：ATP敏感的K$^+$通道；I_{ku}：心房组织中超速激活的延迟整流电流。

（二）药代动力学

Ⅰ$_A$类药物主要的药代动力学特征见表99-2[1,2]。奎尼丁和丙吡胺与包括α$_1$-酸糖蛋白在内的血浆蛋白有高度的亲和力。急性应激状态时，包括心肌梗死和充血性心衰，由于体内结合蛋白的增加，可导致有效药物浓度的降低[1,2]。奎尼丁经肝脏氧化代谢，其代谢产物3-羟奎尼丁对钠通道和复极的作用与奎尼丁相同。奎尼丁的代谢取决于细胞色素酶P450 3A4[18]，通过这条途径，促进奎尼丁代谢的药物如苯妥英钠、苯巴比妥可降低其血浆浓度，增加需求剂量，而通过这条途径能减少其代谢的药物有西米替丁和维拉帕米等[1,2,19]。奎尼丁是细胞色素酶P450 2D6强有效的抑制剂，由此可能导致其与许多药物发生相互作用（增加普罗帕酮或β受体阻滞剂的浓度）[1,26]，如奎尼丁可减少地高辛的清除，使地高辛的血浆浓度明显上升[6]。

丙吡胺通过广泛的肝脏代谢转变成无活性的代谢产物。普鲁卡因胺通过与氮-乙酰转换酶结合而转变成氮-乙酰普鲁卡因，它是一种具有电生理活性的Ⅲ类药物，半衰期为6~10个小时[1,2]。在人群中半数以上是快速乙酰化个体，其代谢率各不相同。由于相关的化合物和活性代谢产物可在体内积蓄，并可导致严重的副反应，包括致室性心律失常作用，即尖端扭转型室速。因此，这些药物禁用于肾衰竭的患者。

（三）致心律失常作用

Ⅰ$_A$类药物使QT间期延长，由此可导致尖端扭转型室速的发生[3,4]。据报告，与奎尼丁相关的尖端扭转型室速的发生率为0.5%~8%[6]。这种心律失常通常发生在用药早期血浆药物浓度还很低时。由于与奎尼丁相关的尖端扭转型室速具有不确定性，因此建议开始应用奎尼丁治疗时应在院内持续心电监护下进行[20]。有一项对奎尼丁治疗房颤（AF）随机临床研究的meta分析显示，与服用安慰剂的对照组患者的死亡率0.8%相比，服用奎尼丁的死亡率增加了2.9%[6]。也有报道显示，使用奎尼丁治疗非持续性室速较其他抗心律失常药物具有更高的死亡率（可能是由于其致心律失常作用）[6]。然而，更多的近期研究表明，奎尼丁的致室性心律失常作用很弱。在ES-VEM研究中，在早期药物监测期间，奎尼丁诱发尖端扭转型室速的危险性（0.6%）低于索他洛尔（1.7%），而且在长期的随访过程中，并没有观察到尖端扭转型室速的发生[6,21]。在氟卡胺的多中心房颤研究（FMAFS）中，共观察了239例病人，随机给予奎尼丁或氟卡胺治疗，未发现致心律失常作用[22]。此外，在AFFIRM研究中，使用Ⅰ类药物组（尤其是奎尼丁、普鲁卡因胺或普罗帕酮）导致心律失常而死亡的危险性明显高于胺碘酮组，但并不高于索他洛尔组[23]。虽然许多内科医师认为与其他抗心律失常药物相比，奎尼丁具有更大的危险性，但这种认识的主要依据是回顾性资料，同时在当时对尖端扭转型室速的危险因素并不十分清楚，如电解质异常和药物的相互作用等[6]。而在近期更多的前瞻性研究并不支持这一结论[21-23]。

99 I 类抗心律失常药物：奎尼丁、普鲁卡因胺、丙吡胺、利多卡因、美西律、氟卡胺和普罗帕酮

表 99-2 药代动力学特征

	奎尼丁	普鲁卡因胺	丙吡胺	利多卡因	美西律	氟卡胺	普罗帕酮
血浆浓度达峰时间（小时）	IR 1~3 SR 63±3.2	SK 3.6±3.8	IR 1.9~2.8 SR 4.9		IR 1.7~3.0 SR 4.3~9.2	3	2~3
治疗浓度（μg/ml）	2~5	4~12	2~5	1.5~5.0	0.75~2.0	0.2~1.0	2~10 RM 10~30 PM
生物利用度（%）	70~80	83±16	83±11	只能经非肠道途径给药	87±13	70±11	5~50*
与血浆蛋白结合度	87±5	16±5	28~68%+	70±5	63±3	61±10	85~95
分布容积（L/kg）	2.7±1.2	1.9±0.3	0.78±0.26	1.1±0.4	4.9±0.5	4.9±0.4	3.6±2.1
清除率（ml/min/kg）	4.7±1.8	2.2*	1.2±0.7	9.2±2.4	6.3±2.7	5.6±1.3	17±8
药物原形的肾脏清除率（%）	18±5	67±8	55±6	2±1	4~15	43±3	<1
血浆半衰期（小时）	6.2±1.8	3.0±0.6	6.0±1.0	1.8±0.4	9.2±2.1	11±3	5.5±2.1
活性代谢产物	3-羟奎尼丁	NAPA	消旋的混合物	二甲苯甘氨基乙醇			5-羟普罗帕酮
肝代谢	CYP 3A	NAT2 乙酰化≠			CYP 1A2, CYP 2D6	CYP 2D6	CYP 2D6

* 浓度依赖
+ 浓度依赖性结合
≠ 取决于乙酰化表现型

IR，迅速释放型；SR，轻释型；RM，快速代谢；PM，代谢不良；NAPA，氮-乙酰普鲁卡因胺；NAT，氮-乙酰转化酶；CYP，细胞色素酶 P450
上述资料摘自参考文献 1、2 和 18

(四) 疗效

虽然奎尼丁、普鲁卡因胺和丙吡胺在预防房颤发作方面与其他药物如胺碘酮相比，其效果和耐受性较差[23,24]，但是它们仍是治疗房性快速性心律失常的有效药物。丙吡胺对预防肥厚型心肌病患者房颤的发作是有益的，它通过负性肌力作用减轻流出道梗阻引发的症状。据报道，奎尼丁对房颤的药理学转复作用优于索他洛尔[25]。这些药物也被证实可抑制室性心律失常[1,2,6,19]。联合应用奎尼丁和美西律对室性心律失常有协同抗心律失常作用，然而，药物产生的不可耐受的副反应（表99-3）及其致室性心律失常的危险性抵消了治疗产生的益处[3,4,22]。这些药物禁用于器质性心脏病包括左心室肥大的患者，因为它们可以增加致心律失常死亡的危险性[3,4,8]。这些药物仅被认为对无器质性心脏病或植入式心脏复律除颤器的患者使用是"相对"安全的。因此，这些药物仅作为长期治疗房颤和其他房性快速型心律失常的二线或三线药物。对WPW综合征合并急性房颤的患者，尽管近期研究显示依布利特的有效性，但静脉注射普鲁卡因胺仍然是首选药物[26]。对持续性室速，普鲁卡因胺的疗效优于利多卡因[27]。最近修订的现代心脏病生活支持（ACLS）指南建议，对血流动力学稳定的宽QRS波群心动过速，尤其对那些心功能受损的患者，初始治疗应选择普鲁卡因胺而不是利多卡因[28]。对于Brugada综合征，普鲁卡因胺也可用于显露Brugada波[29]。

(五) 临床应用和副作用

推荐的剂量、副反应以及可能的药物相互作用归纳在表99-3中[1,2,30,31]。

二、I_B类抗心律失常药：利多卡因和美西律

(一) 药效学

利多卡因和美西律阻断钠通道，其阻断作用时间短。当去极化的心肌组织或心率很快时，它们的效果最明显。I_B类药物可通过降低动作电位4相的斜率提高心肌兴奋性的阈值并降低自律性[1,2]。

(二) 药代动力学

利多卡因和美西律主要的药代动力学特征见表99-2[1,2,32]。利多卡因主要通过肝脏进行首过代谢，因此只能通过非肠道途径给药。利多卡因代谢后产生二甲苯甘氨酸和乙醇二甲苯甘氨酸，它们是较弱的钠通道阻滞剂。利多卡因与$α_1$-酸糖蛋白高度结合，后者在心梗或心衰时增加，可导致有效血药浓度的下降。但心衰时利多卡因的分布容积和清除率下降，从而使血药浓度升高。美西律通过细胞色素酶P_{450}系统代谢成无活性的代谢产物。遗传的多样性决定了不同个体对美西律代谢的快慢。

(三) 致心律失常作用

据报道，与利多卡因相关的致心律失常的发生率很低[1,2]。然而，20多个随机试验和5项meta分析对急性心梗预防性使用利多卡因进行了研究，结果显示利多卡因虽可减少室颤的发生率，但可增加急性心梗的死亡率[33]。

(四) 临床疗效

对于急性心梗患者，不推荐常规预防性使用利多卡因。修订的ACLS指南推荐对血流动力学稳定的宽QRS波群心动过速首选胺碘酮或普鲁卡因胺，而不是利多卡因[28]。尽管修订后的指南认为，利多卡因仍可作为治疗顽固性室颤、休克和无脉搏室速的一种抗心律失常药，但支持其有效的证据却很有限，因此不推荐作为首选药物。美西律的应用并不广泛，它对抑制自律性室速可能有效。最近美西律被提倡用于纠正长QT综合征中的钠通道异常所致的QT间期延长。

(五) 临床应用和副反应

推荐的剂量、副反应和可能发生的药物相互作用见表99-3[1,2,30]。

三、I_C类抗心律失常药：氟卡胺和普罗帕酮

(一) 药效学

氟卡胺和普罗帕酮阻断钠通道，其阻断作用时间较长。这两种药物也可阻断钾离子通道（表99-1）。对心房组织，氟卡胺和普罗帕酮在心率较快时可显著地延长APD，这可能是它们治疗房颤有效的原因[10,36]。氟卡胺和普罗帕酮可显著减慢传导，这种作用在去极化的心肌组织中更明显[1,2]。普罗帕酮也有中度β肾上腺素能受体阻断作用。

表 99-3 Ⅰ类抗心律失常药的剂量和副反应

药物	服用剂量	剂量调整	副反应	药物相互作用
ⅠA类 葡萄糖酸奎尼丁[商品名 Biquin Durules（控释型）]	200～250mg PO q8h；若 QTc<460ms 剂量可增加 200～250mg，若 QTc>500ms 则应减少剂量，最大剂量 1g PO q8h	对肾衰竭的患者初始剂量应减少 50%，而且服药间隔应延长至 q12h；在肾衰患者体内，活性代谢产物可积聚，但是监测治疗效应的血浓度不一定有价值；应当通过认真监测 ECG 间期来决定剂量的调整	腹泻、胃痉挛性疼痛、耳鸣、发热、皮疹、血小板减少、溶血性贫血、尖端扭转型室速	地高辛剂量应减少 50%，如果服用华法林，应监测 INR；β 受体阻滞剂剂量应减少；胺碘酮、西咪替丁、地尔硫革、普萘洛尔和维拉帕米可提高奎尼丁浓度
普鲁卡因胺控释片（商品名 Procan 控释片，Pronestyl 控释片）	250mg PO q6h；若 QTc<460ms 可增加 250mg；若 QTc≥500ms，则应减少剂量；最大剂量 1g PO q6h	代谢取决于乙酰化速度，活性代谢产物 NAPA 在快速乙酰化和肾衰患者体内可聚集；必须监测普鲁卡因胺＋NAPA 的水平，使总量＜800μmol/L；监测 ECG 间期改变	粒细胞缺乏症、皮疹、发热、SLE 综合征、尖端扭转型室速	胺碘酮、西咪替丁、普萘洛尔可增加普鲁卡因胺的浓度
普鲁卡因胺（静脉注射）	按 20mg/min 给予负荷量 750～1000mg；维持量为 1～4mg/min			
丙吡胺（商品名 Norpace，Norpace 控释片，Rhythmodan，Rhythmodan-LA）	100mg PO q8h；CR 和 LA：150～250mg q12h；若 QTC<460ms，可增加 100mg，最大剂量 300mg PO q8h	对肾衰患者初始剂量减少 50%，且服药间隔延长至 q12h	尿潴留、视力模糊、便秘、口干、心功能恶化、尖端扭转型室速	
ⅠB类 利多卡因静脉注射	负荷量 1.5mg/kg；维持量 1～4mg/min	对 CHF 患者应减量	肢体麻木、感觉异常、言语含糊、意识改变	普萘洛尔、美托洛尔、西咪替丁可增加利多卡因浓度
美西律（Mexitil）	150～300mg PO q8h		恶心、胃痉挛性疼痛、震颤、视物模糊、共济失调、意识模糊	西咪替丁、奎尼丁可增加美西律浓度
ⅠC类 氟卡胺（Tambocor）	50mg PO q12h，可增加 50mg；最大剂量 200mg PO q12h；若 QRS 波群较基线增宽超过 20%，应减少剂量	对肾衰患者，初始剂量减少 50%，根据 QRS 波群的宽度调整剂量	震颤、视物模糊、头痛、共济失调、CHF、致室性心动过速	胺碘酮、西咪替丁、普萘洛尔、奎尼丁可增加氟卡尼浓度
普罗帕酮（Rythmol）	150mg PO q8h，最大 300mg PO q8h；若 QRS 波群较基线增宽超过 20%，应减少剂量	对肾功能和肝功能衰竭的患者，初始剂量减少 50%，服药间隔时间应延长至 q12h，活性代谢产物可在代谢旺盛的个体中蓄积，服药期间应认真监测 QRS 波群宽度	便秘、眩晕、头痛、金属样味觉、加剧哮喘、致室性心动过速	地高辛服用剂量应减少 25%～50%，西咪替丁和奎尼丁可增加普罗帕酮浓度

PO，口服，max，最大；ECG，心电图；VT，室性心动过速；INR，国际标准化比值；NAPA，N-乙酰普鲁卡因胺；SLE，系统性红斑狼疮；IV，静脉注射；CHF，充血性心力衰竭。

（二）药代动力学

氟卡胺和普罗帕酮在细胞色素酶 P450 2D6 的介导下通过肝脏代谢。氟卡胺的代谢产物无电生理活性。而普罗帕酮的代谢产物 5-羟普罗帕酮是一种和普罗帕酮具有相同效应的钠通道阻滞剂，但对 β 肾上腺能受体的阻断作用较弱[1,2]。普罗帕酮的肝代谢具有可饱和性，从而导致其剂量和稳态平均浓度之间呈非线性关系。在缺乏细胞色素酶 P450 2D6 即代谢不良的个体中，可以发现肝脏的首过代谢较差，血浆中普罗帕酮浓度明显高于代谢旺盛者。代谢率与药物疗效紧密相关，代谢缓慢者较代谢迅速者对房颤的抑制作用较强[17]。

（三）致心律失常作用

心律失常抑制试验（CAST）[3,4]、汉堡心律失常抑制试验（CASH）和多中心非持续性心动过速试验（MUSTT）[39]证实，Ic类药物可增加室性心律失常患者（通常为冠心病患者）发生致命性突发性心血管事件的危险性。在实验模型中，Ic类药物可增加急性缺血或心肌梗死后发生致室性心律失常的危险性[3,4]。因此，这些药物禁用于既往有心肌梗死病史或有持续性室性快速性心律失常的患者。许多临床医师由此推断这些药物也相对禁用于缺血性心脏病或具有缺血性心脏病危险因素以及其他病因致明显左心室功能不全的患者[3,4,8]。但对无器质性心脏病的患者，氟卡胺和普罗帕酮致心律失常的发生率低。氟卡胺和普罗帕酮可以增加房扑患者的心室率，从而可能表现为宽QRS波群心动过速。这种加速现象通常发生在使用了无房室结阻滞作用的药物时。

（四）临床疗效

氟卡胺和普罗帕酮对室上性心动过速有效。这些心动过速包括：房性心动过速、折返性心动过速（含房室折返性心动过速）、房扑、房颤[5,7,8]。氟卡胺和普罗帕酮不推荐用于器质性心脏病人的房性或室性快速性心律失常[2,3,8]。对怀疑为Brugada综合征的病人，氟卡胺可用于暴露右室的传导异常。

（五）临床应用和副反应

推荐的剂量、副反应和可能出现的药物相互作用归纳在表99-3。

四、致　谢

本项工作得到了加拿大健康研究协会和艾伯特心脏和脑卒中基金会的支持。Gillis医生是艾伯特医学研究基金会的一名科学家。

（林　荣　叶志荣　译）

参 考 文 献

1. Stanton MS: Class I antiarrhythmic drugs: Quinidine, procainamide, disopyramide, lidocaine, mexiletine, tocainide, phenytoin, moricizine, flecainide, propafenone. In Zipes DP, Jalife J (eds): Cardiac Electrophysiology: From Cell to Bedside, 3rd ed. Philadelphia, WB Saunders, 2000, pp 890–903.
2. Roden DM: Antiarrhythmic drugs. In Hardman JG, Limberg LE (eds): Goodman and Gilmans's The Pharmacological Basis of Therapeutics, 10th ed. New York, McGraw-Hill, 2001, pp 933–970.
3. Roden DM: Mechanisms and management of proarrhythmia. Am J Cardiol 82:49I–57I, 1998.
4. Gillis AM: Proarrhythmia syndromes. In Electrophysiological Disorders of the Heart. Philadelphia, WB Saunders, in press.
5. Falk RH: Atrial fibrillation. N Engl J Med 344:1067–1078, 2001.
6. Grace AA, Camm AJ: Quinidine. N Engl J Med 338:35–45, 1998.
7. Grant AO: Propafenone: An effective agent for the management of supraventricular arrhythmias. J Cardiovasc Electrophysiol 7:353–364, 1996.
8. Fuster V, Ryden LE, Asinger RW, et al: ACC/AHA/ESC Guidelines for the Management of Patients with Atrial Fibrillation: Executive Summary. A Report of the American College of Cardiology/American Heart Association Task Force on Practice Guidelines and the European Society of Cardiology Committee for Practice Guidelines and Policy Conferences (Committee to Develop Guidelines for the Management of Patients with Atrial Fibrillation) Developed in Collaboration with the North American Society of Pacing and Electrophysiology. Circulation 104:2118–2150, 2001.
9. Paul AA, Witchel HJ, Hancox JC: Inhibition of the current of heterologously expressed HERG potassium channels by flecainide and comparison with quinidine, propafenone and lignocaine. Br J Pharmacol 136:717–729, 2002.
10. Wang Z, Fermini B, Nattel S: Effects of flecainide, quinidine, and 4-aminopyridine on transient outward and ultrarapid delayed rectifier currents in human atrial myocytes. J Pharmacol Exp Ther 272:184–196, 1995.
11. Casis O, Sanchez-Chapula JA: Disopyramide, imipramine, and amitriptyline bind to a common site on the transient outward K^+ channel. J Cardiovasc Pharmacol 32:521–526, 1998.
12. Virag L, Varro A, Papp JG: Effect of disopyramide on potassium currents in rabbit ventricular myocytes. Naunyn Schmiedebergs Arch Pharmacol 357:268–275, 1998.
13. Yuan F, Pinto JM, Li Q, et al: Characteristics of I_K and its response to quinidine in experimental healed myocardial infarction. J Cardiovasc Electrophysiol 10:844–854, 1999.
14. Gillis AM, Mitchell LB, Wyse DG, et al: Quinidine pharmacodynamics in patients with arrhythmia: Effects of left ventricular function. J Am Coll Cardiol 25:989–994, 1995.
15. Gillis AM, Geonzon TA, Mathison HJ, et al: The effects of barium, dofetilide and 4-aminopyridine on ventricular repolarization in normal and hypertrophied rabbit heart. J Pharmacol Exp Ther 285:262–270, 1998.
16. Zabel M, Hohnloser SH, Behrens S, et al: Differential effects of D-sotalol, quinidine, and amiodarone on dispersion of ventricular repolarization in the isolated rabbit heart. J Cardiovasc Electrophysiol 8:1239–1245, 1997.
17. Benton RE, Sale M, Flockhart DA, et al: Greater quinidine-induced QTc interval prolongation in women. Clin Pharmacol Ther 67:413–418, 2000.
18. Thummel KE, Shen DD: Design and optimization of dosage regimens: Pharmacokinetic data. In Hardman JG, Limberg LE (eds): Goodman and Gilmans's The Pharmacological Basis of Therapeutics, 10th ed. New York, McGraw-Hill, 2001, pp 1917–2023.
19. Wilkinson GR: Pharmacokinetics. In Hardman JG, Limberg LE (eds): Goodman and Gilmans's The Pharmacological Basis of Therapeutics, 10th ed. New York, McGraw-Hill, 2001, pp 3–29.
20. Thibault B, Nattel S: Optimal management with class I and class III antiarrhythmic drugs should be done in the outpatient setting: Protagonist. J Cardiovasc Electrophysiol 10:472–481, 1999.
21. Mason JW, Marcus FI, Bigger JT, et al: A summary and assessment of the findings and conclusions of the ESVEM trial. Prog Cardiovasc Dis 38:347–358, 1996.
22. Naccarelli GV, Dorian P, Hohnloser SH, et al: Prospective comparison of flecainide versus quinidine for the treatment of paroxysmal atrial fibrillation/flutter. The Flecainide Multicenter Atrial Fibrillation Study Group. Am J Cardiol 77:53A–59A, 1996.
23. The AFFIRM First Antiarrhythmic Drug Substudy Investigators. Maintenance of sinus rhythm in patients with atrial fibrillation: An AFFIRM substudy of the first antiarrhythmic drug administered. J Am Coll Cardiol 42:20–29, 2003.
24. Roy D, Talajic M, Dorian P, et al: Amiodarone to prevent recurrence of atrial fibrillation. Canadian Trial of Atrial Fibrillation Investigators. N Engl J Med 342:913–920, 2000.
25. Hohnloser SH, van de Loo A, Baedeker F: Efficacy and proarrhythmic hazards of pharmacologic cardioversion of atrial fibrillation: Prospective comparison of sotalol versus quinidine. J Am Coll Cardiol 26:852–858, 1995.
26. Varriale P, Sedighi A, Mirzaietehrane M: Ibutilide for termination of atrial fibrillation in the Wolff-Parkinson-White syndrome. Pacing Clin Electrophysiol 22:1267–1269, 1999.
27. Gorgels AP, van den Dool A, Hofs A, et al: Comparison of pro-

27. cainamide and lidocaine in terminating sustained monomorphic ventricular tachycardia. Am J Cardiol 78:43–46, 1996.
28. Guidelines 2000 for Cardiopulmonary Resuscitation and Emergency Cardiovascular Care. Part 6: Advanced cardiovascular life support: 7B: Understanding the algorithm approach to ACLS. The American Heart Association in collaboration with the International Liaison Committee on Resuscitation. Circulation 102:I140–I141, 2000.
29. Brugada R, Brugada J, Antzelevitch C, et al: Sodium channel blockers identify risk for sudden death in patients with ST-segment elevation and right bundle branch block but structurally normal hearts. Circulation 101:510–515, 2000.
30. Gillis AM, Wyse DG: Supraventricular tachycardia. In Gray JD (ed): Therapeutic choices, 3rd ed. Ottawa, Ontario, Canada, Canadian Pharmacists Association, 2000, pp 241–252.
31. Pinter A, Dorian P: Intravenous antiarrhythmic agents. Curr Opin Cardiol 16:17–22, 2001.
32. Labbe L, Turgeon J: Clinical pharmacokinetics of mexiletine. Clin Pharmacokinet 37:361–384, 1999.
33. Sadowski ZP, Alexander JH, Skrabucha B, et al: Multicenter randomized trial and a systematic overview of lidocaine in acute myocardial infarction. Am Heart J 137:792–798, 1999.
34. Schwartz PJ, Priori SG, Locati EH, et al: Long QT syndrome patients with mutations of the SCN5A and HERG genes have differential responses to Na$^+$ channel blockade and to increases in heart rate. Implications for gene-specific therapy. Circulation 92:3381–3386, 1995.
35. Shimizu W, Antzelevitch C: Cellular basis for the ECG features of the LQT1 form of the long-QT syndrome: Effects of beta-adrenergic agonists and antagonists and sodium channel blockers on transmural dispersion of repolarization and torsade de pointes. Circulation 98:2314–2322, 1998.
36. Seki A, Hagiwara N, Kasanuki H: Effects of propafenone on K currents in human atrial myocytes. Br J Pharmacol 126:1153–1162, 1999.
37. Jazwinska-Tarnawska E, Orzechowska-Juzwenko K, Niewinski P, et al: The influence of CYP2D6 polymorphism on the antiarrhythmic efficacy of propafenone in patients with paroxysmal atrial fibrillation during 3 months propafenone prophylactic treatment. Int J Clin Pharmacol Ther 39:288–292, 2001.
38. Kuck KH, Cappato R, Siebels J, et al: Randomized comparison of antiarrhythmic drug therapy with implantable defibrillators in patients resuscitated from cardiac arrest: The Cardiac Arrest Study Hamburg (CASH). Circulation 102:748–54, 2000.
39. Wyse DG, Talajic M, Hafley GE, et al: Antiarrhythmic drug therapy in the Multicenter UnSustained Tachycardia Trial (MUSTT): Drug testing and as-treated analysis. J Am Coll Cardiol 38:344–351, 2001.
40. Priori SG, Napolitano C, Schwartz PJ, et al: The elusive link between LQT3 and Brugada syndrome: The role of flecainide challenge. Circulation 102:945–947, 2000.

第 100 章

抗心律失常药物：β受体阻滞剂和钙通道阻滞剂

Bramah N. Singh

本章目录

- β受体阻滞剂 ……………………… 900
- β受体阻滞剂治疗室上性心动过速 … 905
- 钙通道阻滞剂 …………………… 906
- 总结 ………………………………… 910

1962年，普萘洛尔和维拉帕米作为抗心绞痛药物经人工合成。随后，它们分别成为β受体阻滞剂和钙通道阻滞剂的原形，广泛用于各种心血管疾病，如高血压、肥厚型心肌病和缺血性心肌病。然而，这两类药物对多种心律失常的治疗作用是逐渐被认识的。人们早已了解，高血压、左心室功能障碍、缺血性或非缺血性心肌病等心脏疾病为室性、室上性心律失常，甚至致命性心律失常提供了发生基质[1,2]。β受体阻滞剂和钙通道阻滞剂重要的治疗价值主要表现在对心律失常相关症状、心律失常相关发病率和死亡率的影响。这两种药物，在很多方面具有相同的特性，但另一些特性则显著不同。本章根据这两种药物的电药理学特性，β受体阻滞剂对其抗心律失常作用进行比较。目前，临床和实验研究中取得的可靠证据表明，β受体阻滞剂对临床多种心律失常具有确实、有效的抗心脏纤维颤动、抗心律失常作用，而钙通道阻滞剂的应用范围相对较局限。

一、β受体阻滞剂

关于β受体阻滞剂的作用，实验观察结果与患者的临床应用情况并非是确定的、一一对应的关系，但人们对β受体阻滞剂全部的抗心律失常作用已经作出了很好的解释。然而，大多数获益于β受体阻滞剂的患者中，β受体阻滞剂发挥作用的电生理机制尚未完全明了[3]。β肾上腺素激动剂能使β受体激活，而产生相应的电生理效应和致心律失常作用，β受体阻滞剂可能从根本上逆转和减轻这些作用而发挥其抗心律失常效应。因而，β受体阻滞剂很可能在受肾上腺能递质影响最显著的细胞和组织中发挥最大的作用。通过治疗心律失常，β受体阻滞剂能降低心肌梗死幸存者、进展性心衰伴左心室功能显著降低者的死亡率，这充分证实了β受体阻滞剂的临床有效性。近年来，由于能降低心衰患者的猝死率和总死亡率，并用于植入式心脏复律除颤器（ICD）的辅助治疗，β受体阻滞剂治疗作用的重要性日益突出。

（一）β受体阻滞剂电药理学作用

关于β受体激动剂、β受体阻滞剂对不同心肌细胞离子流的影响。已经积累了很多资料，但β受体阻滞剂对各种离子流的确切作用与β受体阻滞剂的临床作用并非简单的对应关系。β受体激动剂主要通过L型钙通道加强钙离子流（I_{Ca}），发挥其正变力作用。β受体激动剂对起搏电流（I_f）也有显著的影响，而β受体阻滞剂能减轻这种影响[4]。事实上，预先已经阐明了β受体阻滞剂对起搏电流的影响，这是β受体阻滞剂的药效学特性。

β受体阻滞剂对离体和在体心肌细胞和组织动作电位的作用具有可变性。β受体阻滞剂将动作电位4期自动除极幅度降低致很小程度，并能提高窦房结和房室结细胞的阈电位，这些作用能抑制心肌细胞的自律性。β受体阻滞剂显著影响房室传导（AH间期），延长房室结不应期，增加文氏阻滞出现的几率，这一作用是可以预见的。β受体阻滞剂集中作用于房室结是由于肾上腺素能神经在窦房结和房室结分布密度高。在心房、心室、旁路肾上腺素能神经分布密度相对较低。除非存在心肌缺血，β受体阻滞剂对这些部位的传导和不应期仅有一些影响。从上述观察中可以推断，β受体阻滞剂对转复固定的、持续的房扑或房颤为窦性心律无效。

在离体和整体动物，急性β受体阻滞作用对心脏复极的影响具有可变性。在人体，长期的β受体阻滞作用能增加QTc，但这一作用具有可变性和非持续性，可能无临床意义。唯一例外的是索他洛尔，它兼有β受体阻滞作用和独立的、显著延长动作电位时程的作用[5]。相反，动态心电图记录的数据证实，长期β受体阻滞作用实际上能使患者的QTc缩短超过24h[6]。继发于其他疾病的QTc延长程度越长，β受体阻滞剂使QTc缩短的程度就越大（如心肌梗死时的情况）。β阻滞剂缩短QTc的作用减少了心室肌复极离散，是β受体阻滞产生抗心律失常作用的主要原因之一[6]。

尽管已经十分肯定，β受体阻滞剂的抗心律失常作用主要是通过拮抗儿茶酚胺的致心律失常作用而实现的，但在不同临床情况下，β受体阻滞剂治疗不同心律失常的具体机制也可能不同。β受体阻滞剂这类药物对动态心电图记录的室性和室上性心律失常，尤其是发生在心肌缺血情况下，特别有效，在减少复极离散的同时，增加室颤阈值。但对于已有持续性症状性室速、室颤的患者，β受体阻滞剂不能阻止室速、室颤的诱发。

（二）各种β受体阻滞剂的不同特性

已经合成了很多种β受体阻滞剂，一些作用略有不同的药物已应用于临床。表100-1总结了这些药物的主要药效学、药代动力学作用[7,8]。这些药物的一些作用与临床直接相关。例如，对心肌梗死后患者，降低静息心率对减少死亡率非常有效，而吲哚洛尔具有拟β受体激动剂的作用，对上述心梗患者可能存在不利作用[9]。如吲哚洛尔具有显著的β受体激动剂作用，常增加心率而不是降低心率，这在很大程度上，抵消了其抗心脏纤维颤动、抗心律失常的作用。相反，其内源的拟交感活性对治疗窦房结病变或房室结传导不稳定患者的心动过速有益。一些β受体阻滞剂为相对选择性阻断心脏β₁肾上腺素能受体，如醋丁洛尔、阿替洛尔、比索洛尔、卡维地洛、美托洛尔；其他则为非选择性作用于β₁、β₂受体，如普萘洛尔、纳多洛尔、噻吗洛尔、索他洛尔。

几乎没有证据证实，β受体阻滞剂程度不同的选择性作用显著影响了β受体阻滞剂的抗心律失常和抗心脏纤维颤动作用。然而，如前所述[10,11]，理论上，非选择性β受体阻滞剂对于终止室颤可能更有效，但需要进行大规模前瞻性对照研究对此加以证实。

表100-1 常用β受体阻滞剂的一些特性

药物	β₁效应	β₁选择	脂溶性	辅助作用	半衰期（h）	清除途径
醋丁洛尔	0.3	+	中度	内在拟交感活性、膜稳定作用	3~4（上午8~13点）	肝、肾
阿替洛尔	1.0	++	弱	—	6~9	肾
比索洛尔	10.3	++	弱	—	9~12	肝、肾
布新洛尔	1.0	+	—	直接扩血管作用	—	—
卡维地洛	10.0	+	高度	α受体阻滞作用	7~10	肝
艾司洛尔	0.02	++	弱		9min	血
拉贝洛尔	0.3	0	弱	α受体阻滞作用	3~4	肝
美托洛尔	1.0	++	中度		3~4	肝
纳多洛尔	1.0	0	弱		14~24	肾
吲哚洛尔	6.0	0	中度	内在拟交感活性	3~4	肾
普萘洛尔	1.0	0	高度	膜稳定作用	3~4	肝
索他洛尔	0.3	0	弱	Ⅲ类抗心律失常药物作用	9~10	肾
噻吗洛尔	6.0	0	弱		4~5	肾

引自数据来源 Opie LH: Pharmacologic options for treatment of ischemic heart disease. In Smith TW (ed): Cardiovascular Therapeutics. Philadelphia, WB Saunders, 1996, pp22-57; and Anderson JL: Beta-Blockers. Card Electrophysiol Rev 4: 300-307, 2000.

表 100-2 静脉 β 受体阻滞剂常规应用

药物	$β_1$ 受体选择作用	清除半衰期	静脉注射剂量	适应证*
阿替洛尔	+	6~9h	每 10min 静脉推注 5mg，至 10mg	高血压、心绞痛、心肌梗死
艾司洛尔	+	9min	500μg/kg 负荷剂量，随后以 50~300μg/kg/min 静点	室上性心动过速
美托洛尔	+	3~4h	每 5~10min 给 5mg 至 15mg	高血压、心绞痛、心肌梗死
普萘洛尔	−	3.5~6h	1mg/min 静脉推注，总量 5mg	高血压、心绞痛、心肌梗死、室上性心动过速、室速

*美国药品食品管理局（FDA）许可的适应证

β 受体阻滞剂的抗心律失常作用较预想的要广泛。经过数十年连续的资料积累证实，β 受体阻滞剂是能降低猝死率，延长某些心脏病患者生存率的少数几种药物之一[1-3]。需要强调的是，这种情况下，最有效的两种抗心律失常药物——索他洛尔和胺碘酮是通过竞争和非竞争方式发挥有效的抗肾上腺能作用来治疗室性心动过速的[12,13]。这些发现具有重要的意义，有利于开发新型的具有多方面抗心律失常作用，并能延长患者生存时间的药物。这些药物长期口服有效，静脉注射仅用于治疗心律失常发作等紧急情况（表 100-2）。

（三）β 受体阻滞剂的抗心律失常和抗心脏纤维颤动作用

β 受体阻滞剂具有抗心律失常和抗心脏纤维颤动作用，是减少缺血性心脏病、心力衰竭、左室功能受损患者死亡率的主要药物之一。交感过度激活是心律失常性猝死相关的病理生理机制[12,14,15]。β 受体阻滞剂能通过抑制交感激活以及减少心肌梗死的发生率等途径减少心律失常性猝死。在心肌梗死和心力衰竭患者中，β 受体阻滞剂减少心律失常性猝死的作用是非常显著的。

β 受体阻滞剂的抗心律失常作用与阻断交感激活的程度直接相关，这种阻断作用可以通过心率的降低程度来判断。β 受体阻滞剂作用于窦房结，显著减慢心率，作用于房室结，减慢房室传导，临床可用来终止室上性心动过速，减慢房扑、房颤时的心室率。由于 β 受体阻滞剂影响其他组织传导和不应期的程度不同，因此对这些组织的电生理作用也不同。在离体心肌组织和在体心脏，β 受体阻滞剂对心脏复极的急性影响均具有变异性。长期连续给药，QT 间期可能出现少量延长或缩短的情况也均有报道。与索他洛尔（兼有 β 受体阻滞剂和显著的 Ⅲ 类抗心律失常药物的特性）对心脏的复极作用比较，这些作用较小，无临床意义[12,13]。

（四）β 受体阻滞剂抗心律失常和抗心脏纤维颤动作用及其对死亡率的影响

β 受体阻滞剂能抑制室性和室上性心律失常（室性早搏、房性早搏、非持续性室性心动过速）。而且对缺血心肌，β 受体阻滞剂能增加室颤阈值，降低心室复极离散度。β 受体阻滞剂主要通过抑制交感过度激活发挥其抗心律失常和抗心脏纤维颤动作用[10-14]。交感过度激活包括：（1）缩短心室动作电位时程，缩短心室有效不应期（ERP）；（2）加快心室传导；（3）提高心室的自律性；（4）降低迷走神经活性；（5）降低室性心动过速发生阈值。图 100-1 说明了 β 受体阻滞剂阻止室颤发生的可能机制[11]。β 受体阻滞剂抗心脏纤维颤动试验和临床资料的结果相一致。

规模较小的临床观察结果证实，β 受体阻滞剂能抑制室速发生和减少死亡率。但精确设计和认真执行的大规模临床对照试验的重要研究结果表明，β 受体阻滞剂能有效延长患者生存时间[10,15]。目前，毫无疑问，β 受体阻滞剂能有效减少伴有显著心律失常患者或高危心律失常性死亡患者的死亡率[10,16,17]。例如，β 受体阻滞剂能减少先天性长 QT 综合征患者[16]、心脏骤停幸存者和经选择的室速患者的死亡率[12,17]。这些观察结果得到了临床随机、对照试验的可靠数据的证实，关于 β 受体阻滞剂的这些临床试验主要在两类患者中进行：一类是急性心梗后的幸存者[18-23]，另一类是充血性心力衰竭的患者[24-28]。这些试验显示，只有 β 受体阻滞剂这类抗心律失常药物能持续有效地降低总死亡率，其大部分降低死亡率的作用都或多或少地通过减少可预测的心律失常性死亡而实现。据推断，β 受体阻滞剂阻断 β 受体后所发挥的抗心脏纤维颤动作用是其能够减少死亡率的主要原因。

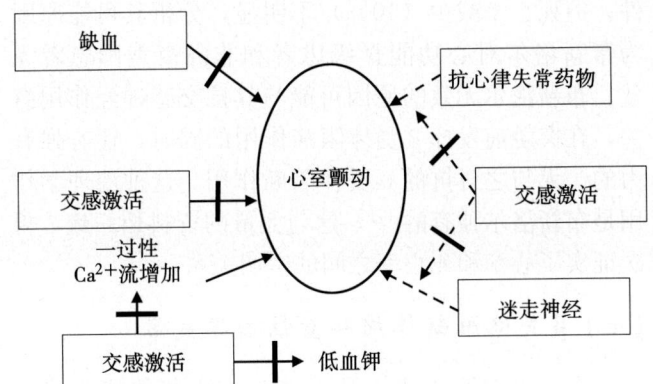

图100-1 β受体阻滞剂抗心脏纤维颤动的可能机制示意图

缺血和肾上腺素能激活可增加（如↑所示）室颤的发生。β₂受体激动剂通过增加一过性钙离子流或加重低钾血症增加室颤的发生。非选择性β受体阻滞剂能阻断上述作用。迷走刺激和抗心律失常药物能阻止（如↑所示）室颤的发生，但交感激活能逆转这一作用。β受体阻滞剂能阻断交感激活的逆转作用，仍然能发挥其抗心脏纤维颤动作用。

（五）β受体阻滞剂降低心肌梗死后猝死和死亡率

已经有资料证实，在心肌梗死院外诊断初期、住院治疗期间[18]和出院后[18,19]，β受体阻滞剂均能减少室颤的发生率和死亡率。也有试验证实，β受体阻滞剂用于对心梗幸存者的二级预防同样能减少室颤的发生率和死亡率，用法为在心梗急性事件后4～28天开始给药，并持续给药90天。第一年降低猝死率和总死亡率分别为18%和39%，据推断，β受体阻滞剂通过抑制室颤而发挥上述作用。在急性心肌梗死早期，给予溶栓药的同时联合应用β受体阻滞剂，先静脉推注，随后口服维持，同样降低了心梗最初10天的死亡率。

用β受体阻滞剂进行心梗后二级预防的药物试验很多[20-22]，尚不包括心律失常抑制试验。许多关于β受体阻滞剂这方面应用的数据使人很感兴趣。β受体阻滞剂降低死亡率的作用独立于年龄、性别、种族、心梗部位和患者的危险因素，猝死越高危者，越能从β阻滞剂中获益[21]。仍需注意的是，β受体阻滞剂试验并非药物抑制试验，但降低心梗和心衰患者死亡率的程度却与心率降低的程度呈线性相关（图100-2）。这在心梗后的试验研究中得到了很好的证实[9]。值得注意的是，有显著内源性拟交感活性的药物降低心率的作用较小，其降低死亡率的作用成比例降低。索他洛尔是唯一例外的药物。与普萘洛尔或美托洛尔同等程度地降低心率，仅降低死亡率18%，可能由于单剂量给予索他洛尔360mg/d。在心梗随访早期可能增加死亡率（由于其促心律失常作用），后期减少死亡率。在这种情况下，需要强调的是动物心率和寿命呈反比关系[4,9]。通过研究新近合成的特殊的窦房结阻断剂伊伐布雷定（ivabradine）可能阐明心率与死亡率之间的确切关系。

还需要强调的是，两个关于心肌梗死后试验研究[21,22]的证据表明，胺碘酮联合β阻滞剂比单用胺碘酮降低总死亡率的作用明显[23]。上述β阻滞剂和胺碘酮的协同作用对β受体阻滞剂用于治疗心血管疾病有着重要的临床指导意义。

（六）β受体阻滞剂在心力衰竭中的作用

尽管应用β受体阻滞剂治疗慢性心衰的历史可以追溯到20世纪70年代，但只是在近10年大型临床试验的结果提供的可靠证据的支持下，β受体阻滞剂才成为临床常规的心衰治疗药物。严格控制β受体阻滞剂用量，并采取逐渐增加剂量的方法能程度不同地显著减少进展性充血性心力衰竭患者的

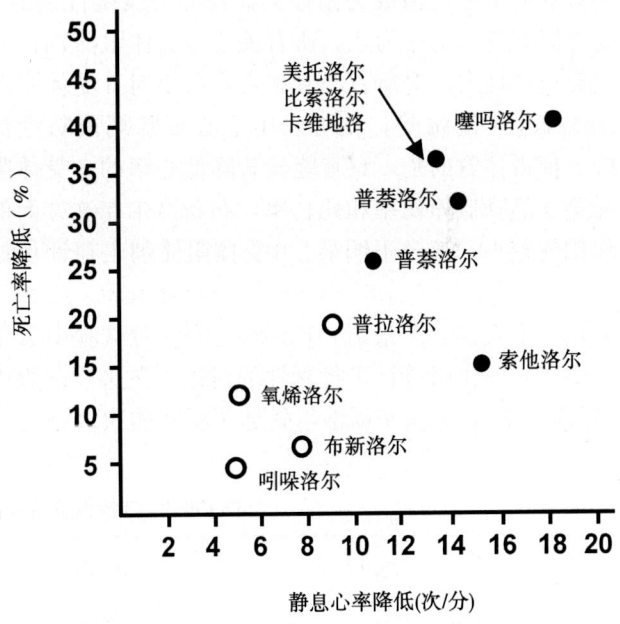

图100-2 静息心率降低和死亡率降低之间的关系，β受体阻滞剂在心肌梗死和充血性心力衰竭患者中的大型前瞻性双盲对照试验 ○代表有内在拟交感活性的β受体阻滞剂；●代表没有内在拟交感活性的β受体阻滞剂。引用的两个研究证实，普萘洛尔使心率降低的程度越大，对患者心衰的影响就越大。值得注意的是美托洛尔、比索洛尔和卡维地洛在减少充血性心力衰竭患者总死亡率方面取得了比较一致的效果，它们产生了几乎一致的使心率减慢的作用。

死亡率[24-29]。β受体阻滞剂不仅能降低死亡率，同时能改善心室功能，能减少伴有房扑或房颤患者的心室率。

表100-3比较了各种β受体阻滞剂近期和先前试验结果，总结了一些重要试验的突出特点[11]。这些研究具有重要的临床意义。关于美托洛尔的研究，入选3 991例NYHA心功能分级Ⅱ～Ⅳ的心衰患者，左心室射血分数<40%，随机分为美托洛尔组（1 990例）和对照组（2 001例），美托洛尔组给予美托洛尔逐渐增加剂量至200mg/d，主要试验终点为个各种原因的死亡率。第一年随访期间，对照组中217例患者死亡（11.0%），而美托洛尔组中147例（7.2%）死亡，具有显著性差异（$P<0.00009$）。美托洛尔组猝死率显著降低44%，与对照组比较具有显著性差异[25]。关于比索洛尔的多中心双盲随机对照研究[27]，入选2 647例患者，比索洛尔组1 327例，对照组1320例，各种原因的死亡率在比索洛尔组为11.8%（156例），在对照组为17.3%，具有显著性差异（$P<0.0001$）。比索洛尔能显著降低猝死率。还有一些相对小型的单样本的关于卡维地洛的研究[28]，但在美国，已经积累的数据使卡维地洛成为治疗充血性心力衰竭首选的β受体阻滞剂。迄今为止，所有关于β受体阻滞剂试验研究资料证实，对所有心衰患者，只要对β受体阻滞剂无禁忌、能耐受，就可以用于心衰常规预防性治疗。值得注意的是，只有能显著降低心率的β受体阻滞剂才能降低猝死率和死亡率，布新洛尔在这方面的作用就较小，甚至不明显。β受体阻滞剂生存评价试验（beta-blocker evaluation of survival trial，BEST）的结果出人预料。最近，Bristow等[15]对试验中关于布新洛尔的作用进行了批判性的讨论。在这一试验中（提前结束），尽管布新洛尔降低了所有的次级终点事件，但死亡率减少（10%）不明显，分析其可能原因为布新洛尔对心功能Ⅳ级患者和非洲裔美国患者无效。布新洛尔无效的原因可能与其抗交感神经作用有关，在突触前发挥β受体阻滞作用的同时，还有强有力的、无与之对抗的α受体阻断作用。这种药理学作用是布新洛尔独有的[15]，这与大量的资料相一致，再次证实了心率和死亡率之间的密切关系。

（七）β受体阻断作用和室性心律失常

有一类室性心律失常可能与或不与临床症状相关，包括室性早搏、频发室性早搏、非持续性室性心动过速等。在有显著器质性心脏病的患者中，这些室性心律失常的存在是猝死的独立危险因素，尤其在急性心梗幸存者和严重充血性心力衰竭伴左室射血分数显著降低的患者中更是如此。很可能，由于心室舒张功能障碍造成的上述室性心律失常（患者射血分数正常），对估计患者的预后有重要临床价值。然而，用β受体阻滞剂或其他抗心律失常药物完全或几乎完全抑制上述室性心律失常后，死亡率无显著降低。患者的预后在很大程度上取决于基础疾病的本质和严重程度。β受体阻滞剂能显著减少心律失常的相关症状，能延长冠心病和心力衰竭患者的生存时间，这些药物抑制室早的作用较弱，而且没有致心律失常作用。β受体阻滞剂长期应用能使心室肌重构、抗心肌缺血、增加心肌电活动的协调一致性、调整肾上腺能受体的反应性。这些药物在降低心率的同时，能增加患者的心率变异性。这类药物所有的有益作用均来自于这种药物的种类特异性[20]。对照试验结果证实，单独应用β受体阻滞剂或联合其他抗心律失常药物对几乎所有室性心律失常有效，能减轻症状和延长生存时间。

表100-3 选择性β受体阻滞剂对心衰患者死亡率的影响

试验（参考资料）	入选病例数	β受体阻滞剂	总死亡率	心脏性死亡率	猝死率	备注
Cardvedilol Multicenter	充血性心衰患者（1 094例）5	卡维地洛	↓65%*	↓65%*	↓55%*	心衰死亡率↓80%*
MERIT HF	心功能Ⅱ～Ⅳ级的充血性心衰患者（3 991例）6	美托洛尔	↓34%*	↓38%*	↓41%*	心衰死亡率↓49%*
CIBIS Ⅱ	心功能Ⅱ～Ⅳ级的充血性心衰患者（2 647例）	比索洛尔	↓34%*	↓29%*	↓44%*	结果与病因无关，因室速/室颤入院率↓70%*
COPERNICUS	心功能Ⅲ～Ⅳ级的充血性心衰患者（2 289例）	卡维地洛	↓34%	无报道	↓41%	平均左室射血分数<↓25%
BEST	心功能Ⅲ～Ⅳ级的充血性心衰患者（2 708例）	布新洛尔	↓8%	↓12%	↓11%	是否具有α受体阻断作用？

注：* 表示差异具有显著性（$P<0.05$）。

尽管室速和室颤可能更容易发生在缺血性心肌病患者中，但直接由阵发性心肌缺血诱发室性心律失常并不常见。心律失常使其他类型的心脏病，如扩张型或梗阻型心肌病的病情更加复杂，在一些可识别的心脏病患者中也可出现。心律失常出现在心脏结构病变时，常常能被心脏程序电刺激诱发。在大多数上述患者中，β受体阻滞剂几乎不能阻止心律失常的诱发，对有症状的、持续单形室速，β受体阻断并非是治疗的重要手段。然而，尽管入选病例相对较少，有一系列的观察研究表明，β受体阻滞剂选择性地对一部分患者的心律失常具有显著治疗作用。据报道，在临床记录到单形室性心动过速的患者中，应用异丙肾上腺素能使程序电刺激更容易诱发室速，而不用异丙肾上腺素时，室速不易诱发。β受体阻滞剂能长期有效控制上述儿茶酚胺敏感性室速。相反的，需要强调的是，目前持续性室速的治疗很少单独应用β受体阻滞剂，在心室功能障碍时，常常联合应用ICD和β受体阻滞剂。

（八）β受体阻滞剂和植入式心脏复律除颤器

抗心律失常药物常用于减少患者不能耐受的ICD放电，常用的药物有β受体阻滞剂、索他洛尔和胺碘酮[31]。目前，没有临床随机试验对上述三种药物的有效性进行评价。然而，已知β受体阻滞剂对室颤阈值无影响，索他洛尔能降低室颤阈值，而胺碘酮对室颤阈值无影响或能使之增加。在非随机的小规模试验中，β受体阻滞剂延长了从ICD植入到ICD首次放电的时间，但并不影响生存率。同样可以估计，在这种情况下，β受体阻滞剂可用于减少不适当的窦性心动过速，并用于控制房颤患者的心室率，能减少ICD放电的次数。近期关于索他洛尔（160～360mg/d）的一项双盲、对照试验表明，索他洛尔能显著减少ICD放电的次数（$P<0.004$），从3.9/年降低到1.4/年；降低ICD放电的危险或死亡危险44%（$P<0.001$）。在其他各种β受体阻滞剂和胺碘酮中，这些数据尚未见报道。因而，关于在植入ICD的患者中，β受体阻滞剂可能用来控制室速或室颤，提出了一些问题：（1）索他洛尔的有效作用在多大程度上归因于β受体阻断作用？（2）β受体阻滞剂在多大程度上通过抑制室速和室颤来减少ICD放电，是否和索他洛尔或胺碘酮同样有效？（3）β受体阻滞剂是否能和抗心律失常药物（Ⅰ类抗心律失常药、胺碘酮和索他洛尔）一样，同等程度地降低室速的频率，使心动过速更容易被抗心动过速起搏终止？（4）β受体阻滞剂和ICD是否对发生室速或室颤（包括心脏骤停幸存者）的患者死亡率的影响是其额外的作用？（5）在植入ICD的患者中，附加小剂量胺碘酮联合β受体阻滞剂治疗室速或室颤，是否优于单独用胺碘酮或β受体阻滞剂治疗室速或室颤？进行认真的详细的临床对照试验才能回答这些问题，而试验的结论可能具有重要的临床意义。

对于β受体阻滞剂在因室速或室颤而植入ICD的患者中的应用，近来一些临床试验资料提出了一些重要的问题。例如，在AVID（Antiarrhythmics versus Implantable Defibrillators）试验中，42.3%的患者在入选后1个月内，开始应用β受体阻滞剂，随访2年后，39.4%的患者仍然服用β受体阻滞剂，应用其他药物（主要为胺碘酮）的比例分别为16%和10.1%[33]。在IDS（Implantable Defibrillator Study）研究中[34]，比较ICD和胺碘酮对室速和室颤的作用，植入ICD组，60%患者服用一种β受体阻滞剂或索他洛尔，而在胺碘酮治疗组只有20%患者服用上述药物。显然，β受体阻滞剂或其等效剂常用于植入ICD的患者，用来控制室速或室颤。这种情况下，近期CASH（Cardiac Arrest Study Hamberg）试验报道的数据更符合临床实际情况[35]。CASH试验是一项前瞻性的随机研究，比较美托洛尔、胺碘酮、普罗帕酮和ICD的疗效，经过11个月随访发现，美托洛尔、胺碘酮和ICD对死亡率无显著影响，由于普罗帕酮可能增加死亡率，而退出试验。在研究结束时，患者数为389例，平均随访3年，仅有6%的患者植入ICD同时应用β受体阻滞剂，而植入ICD同时服用胺碘酮或美托洛尔的患者比例与之相同。试验中[35]三组间单独进行比较时，对总死亡率的影响无显著差异（$P=0.08$），但将服用胺碘酮和β受体阻滞剂的患者作为一组，与植入ICD患者组比较时，二者对总死亡率的影响有显著性差异（$P<0.04$）。值得注意的是，胺碘酮和美托洛尔组之间比较，二者对总死亡率的影响无显著性差异。在某些患者中，选择联合β受体阻滞剂和胺碘酮治疗，与选择单独植入ICD治疗至少具有相同的有效性。显然，对于单用β受体阻滞剂或β受体阻滞剂联合胺碘酮的作用效果，需要更深入的研究。

二、β受体阻滞剂治疗室上性心动过速

众所周知，肾上腺素能神经系统对调整心率具有重要的作用。一般无需采取治疗措施减慢加快的心率，特别是对运动后生理性的心率加快。然而，一些

病理性窦性心率加快需要治疗，如甲状腺毒症和其他一些高动力循环状态时的情况。显然，β受体阻滞剂在这种情况下能发挥作用。目前，需要很好地对特异性窦房结阻滞剂进行定义。过去，静脉应用β受体阻滞剂终止急性阵发性折返性室上速，无论是房室结折返性室上速或旁路参与的反复发作的室上速。现在β受体阻滞剂已经很少再应用于上述情况，基本上被静脉注射腺苷、维拉帕米和地尔硫䓬所替代。β受体阻滞剂能终止50%的折返性阵发性室上速，可能是由于交感激活促使房室结慢径的顺向传导加快，而快径的逆向传导减慢[36]。然而，在预激合并房扑或房颤发作的患者尽量避免用β受体阻滞剂。β受体阻滞剂能增加房室结的不应期，预防阵发性室上性心动过速的复发，也可单独应用β受体阻滞剂，或β受体阻滞剂联合地高辛或具有降低心率作用的钙拮抗剂如地尔硫䓬或维拉帕米。由于多数室上速患者（有或没有旁路）更倾向选择射频消融术治疗[36]，无法对这些药物的确切作用进行研究，可能其作用不如预期的好。

临床上，β受体阻滞剂还可以用来治疗其他类型的心律失常综合征。例如异位房性心动过速，在成人中，这种心律失常并非常见，通常呈阵发性或持续性发作，常受肾上腺素能系统影响。然而，β受体阻滞剂在长期预防性应用过程中终止或抑制房速的有效性并非总是一致[36]。大多数情况下，β受体阻滞剂能通过减慢房室传导而减慢心动过速频率。从有限的对照研究资料中得出的结论来看，β受体阻滞剂对血管迷走综合征的患者也有治疗作用[8]。例如，在一项比较美托洛尔和可乐定的试验中，β受体阻滞剂更有效[37]，吲哚洛尔（具有显著内在拟交感活性）对心脏神经综合征有效[38]。

β受体阻滞剂在房扑和房颤中的应用

β受体阻滞剂对心房无显著的抗心肌纤维颤动的作用，β受体阻滞剂在房扑或房颤中的主要作用是通过减慢房室传导实现的。β受体阻滞剂短期或长期应用，对于转复房扑或房颤无显著疗效，对药物或电转复后窦性心律的维持也无效。

β受体阻滞剂主要通过减慢房室传导减慢房扑或房颤时的心室率。对静息和运动状态下心率的减慢均有作用。在心肌缺血、高血压和肥厚型心肌病患者中，β受体阻滞剂能对这些原发疾病进行治疗，其疗效更加显著[39]。

近几年，很多资料证实了β受体阻滞剂能有效地预防应用于以下两种重要的情况。其中，一种是对于术后容易发生房颤的高危患者，β受体阻滞剂具有显著的预防房颤作用[40]。

从临床实践的角度来看，开胸手术后出现房颤会显著延长患者的住院时间，不可避免地增加医疗费用。目前，还没有系统地发明一种常规方法来阻止胸外科手术后期并发室上性或室性心律失常。有拮抗交感神经激活作用，同时兼具抗心脏纤维颤动的药物可能有效。这些药物有显著的抗肾上腺素能作用，并同时有抗心房和心室纤维颤动的作用（称为Ⅲ类抗心律失常药作用）。已经明确，对于进行手术的患者预防性应用β受体阻滞剂，通常能减少术中心脏并发症[41]。β受体阻滞剂在上述情况下，可作为常规用药。

三、钙通道阻滞剂

钙通道阻滞剂通常作为特异性的冠状动脉扩张剂用来缓解心绞痛，它包括结构各不相同的几类药物，这些药物除了具有阻断心脏慢通道活性的共同特性外，其中一些药物特别作用于房室结，减慢房室传导。钙通道阻滞剂中不同类型的药物具有不同的特性，但其中维拉帕米和地尔硫䓬两种药物表现出的两种特性，从控制心率的作用角度看，具有重要的直接电生理作用。第一种特性为具有显著的抗肾上腺素能活性的作用，能够减慢心率和房室结传导。在一定程度上，特别是其作用于房室结的特性与β受体阻滞剂很相似。这种作用是这类药物阻断室上性心动过速的主要机制[36]，也可以将其用来鉴别窄QRS心动过速。二氢吡啶类钙通道阻滞剂是数量最多的一种钙通道阻滞剂，没有改变房室结传导的作用，对心房和心室不应期也没有特异性的影响，终止房扑/房颤和控制室性心动过速发作的作用很小。近来，引起人们关注的钙通道阻滞剂的第二种特性是其在减慢心率的同时可以缩短心室肌动作电位平台期，并能有效消除浦肯野纤维的早后除极[42,43]。这提出了一个问题：是否钙通道阻滞剂可以阻止药物（如奎尼丁）诱发的尖端扭转型室性心动过速。

目前开发和研制的相对数量很大的钙通道阻滞剂中，只有一小部分（如维拉帕米和地尔硫䓬）具有特异的和直接的抗心律失常作用。因为，这类药物兼具有强有力的抗缺血作用，在改善了冠心病患者的氧供需平衡后，可能间接发挥其抗心律失常作用。一些说法认为，尽管钙拮抗剂在急性心梗幸存者中很好地发挥了抗缺血作用，但在上述情况和其他情况下，其对死亡率的影响尚不清楚。大部分情况下，由于应用患者群不同，个别药物成分和药效学特性不同，钙通道阻滞剂可能无效甚至有害。

（一）电药理学作用

理解了心肌慢通道的特性才能更好地理解钙通道阻滞剂的电生理特点及其抗心律失常作用的机制。L型钙通道阻滞剂和T型钙通道阻滞剂是其中非常重要的两种药物。L型钙通道分布于骨骼肌、心肌和平滑肌细胞，参与正常心肌细胞和血管平滑肌细胞的电机械活动。T型钙通道主要分布于心脏起搏细胞和浦肯野细胞中，在心室肌中少量分布，对β肾上腺素刺激无反应。因而，T型钙通道对心肌收缩力无明显影响，而对起搏和冲动传导有重要作用[44]。选择性地阻断心脏慢通道，并以时间依赖方式增加心脏慢反应纤维的不应期，是心脏慢通道阻滞剂的基本特点。本章主要讨论维拉帕米和地尔硫䓬的抗心律失常特性，以及它们在治疗室性心动过速、室上性心动过速中的作用。

钙通道阻滞剂能有效治疗心律失常的根本原因在于，这类心律失常的发生依赖于心脏慢通道的活性。如心脏直视手术术中活检可见，病变的心房出现慢反应电位；或在室壁瘤术中可见，切除的心室肌出现慢反应电位。尽管已经有充分的试验数据证实慢通道活性异常和各种室上性心律失常相关，但其确切机制尚不清楚。心脏慢通道在临床心律失常，如折返性室上性心动过速，特别是房室折返和窦房折返性心动过速发生过程中所起的作用是研究慢通道和心律失常相关性的最好的依据。腺苷和三磷酸腺苷在折返性室上性心动过速中疗效显著，这一事实支持嘌呤能受体在调整房室传导和房室结不应期方面起着重要作用。正常房室结具有慢通道激活的电生理特点，钙通道阻滞剂通过浓度依赖和剂量依赖的方式抑制房室传导。维拉帕米和地尔硫䓬对心房、心室、浦肯野纤维的不应期或传导速度无显著影响。这两种药物能降低窦房结和房室结4期自动除极，而减慢传导速度，主要影响房室结不应期，使房室结正向、逆向传导的有效不应期、功能不应期显著延长。

表100-4总结了各种钙通道阻滞剂和普萘洛尔（β受体阻滞剂代表药物）的临床电生理作用。一般来说，通道阻滞剂全面的电生理效应可以解释其抗心律失常作用。毫无疑问，钙通道阻滞剂和腺苷通过调整房室结的电生理功能发挥其抗心律失常作用。如表100-4所示，这些药物对房间传导、室间传导或浦肯野纤维传导或不应期没有影响。钙通道阻滞剂对心室肌电生理特性影响较小，对大多数室性心动过速无显著疗效。减慢心率的钙通道阻滞剂在临床上主要用于治疗室上性心律失常，终止室上速发作、预防复发，降低房扑或房颤时的心室率。下面详细讨论和总结维拉帕米和地尔硫䓬的作用特点。

1. 维拉帕米

维拉帕米的电生理特性符合Ⅳ类抗心律失常药物的基本特性。静脉应用维拉帕米（5~20mg 2min内给药），对房室结作用的达峰时间出现于给药后10~15min，疗效持续6h。口服给药时，作用达峰时间出现于给药后3h，半衰期3~7h，疗效持续时间长于给药时间；用于控制心室率的常用剂量为80~120mg，3~4次/d；长期应用时，开始剂量用240~480mg/d。主要的心血管副作用为过度抑制房室结。与地高辛和胺碘酮存在药物的相互作用。

2. 地尔硫䓬

地尔硫䓬的电生理特性与维拉帕米相似，其负性肌力作用相对较小。其抗心律失常作用尚需进一步开发，目前主要用于终止室上性心律失常发作和控制房扑或房颤患者急性、慢性期的心室率。口服吸收率大于90%，但生物利用度仅为45%，起效时间15~30min，作用达峰时间1~2h，半衰期4~7h。仅35%药物经肾脏排泄，其余经胃肠道吸收。为达到迅速控制心室率的目的，在2min内静脉注射给药20mg，15min后可重复给药，继续以5~15mg/h的速度静脉滴注，以延长其作用效果。目前口服常用地尔硫䓬缓释剂（90、120、180、240、300mg/d）。单独应用地尔硫䓬或将其与地高辛、β受体阻滞剂联合用于控制心室率是其主要的抗心律失常作用。地尔硫䓬的副作用与维拉帕米相同，但与地高辛、奎尼丁或胺碘酮没有药物之间的相互作用。

（二）钙通道阻滞剂在室上性心律失常中的应用

静脉注射腺苷转复室上性心动过速的成功率高，副作用很小，射频消融术有效率几乎100%，这些使室上性心动过速的治疗方案发生了变化。目前，静脉应用腺苷是转复室上性心动过速的一线疗法。在一些国家，仍然用药物作为二线治疗，来预防室上性心律失常复发。静脉注射用维拉帕米应用于临床之前，许

表 100-4　钙通道阻滞剂的临床电生理作用

效果	维拉帕米	地尔硫䓬	普萘洛尔
心率	下降+	下降+	下降++++
QRS波群	无影响	无影响	无影响
QT间期	无影响	无影响	增加++
PR间期	增加++	增加++	增加++
A-H间期	增加+++	增加+++	增加+++
H-V间期	无影响	无影响	无影响
心房有效不应期	下降±	下降±	无影响
房室结有效不应期	增加++++	增加++++	增加+++
房室结功能不应期	增加++++	增加++++	增加+++
心室有效不应期	无影响	无影响	无影响
希氏束有效不应期	无影响	无影响	无影响
旁路有效不应期	±	±	±
窦房结恢复时间	无影响	无影响	增加+
心室自律性	无影响	无影响	下降+

注：从+到++++表示药物影响程度从小到大，±表示药物影响有变异性。

多药物曾经用于终止室上性心律失常发作。除高血压和显著左室功能障碍之外，维拉帕米可以用于其他各种情况下室上性心律失常的转复。静脉应用地尔硫䓬和腺苷也是转复室上性心动过速理想有效的药物。如前所述，在迷走神经活性占优势的情况下，可以选择用于转复室上性心律失常为窦性心律的静脉注射药物包括：维拉帕米、地尔硫䓬，尤其目前提倡应用的腺苷。在多数室上速时，心动过速的顺传通路为房室结，其是折返环最薄弱的部位，对静脉注射维拉帕米、地尔硫䓬、腺苷的阻断作用十分敏感。因而，静脉用维拉帕米3～5mg（儿童）、10～15mg（成人），或地尔硫䓬17～25mg，腺苷6～12mg能使快速的、可预测的转复率达到80%～100%[45,46]。有数据表明，地尔硫䓬和维拉帕米终止室上性心动过速发作的疗效相同，然而，地尔硫䓬的负性肌力作用较小。腺苷转复率高，半衰期极短，仅出现一过性副作用的特点使得负性肌力作用不再是药物应用的主要顾虑因素，腺苷已经成为终止阵发性室上性心动过速的首选药物。

多数报道表明，不管应用何种药物转复阵发性室上性心动过速，心动过速终止时的表现基本一致。除Ⅰ类抗心律失常药物具有阻断逆向房室传导终止室上速的作用之外，其他药物均通过逐渐延长AH间期最终达到阻断作用。最常见的终止方式包括：（1）颈动脉窦按压过程中心动过速突然终止；（2）延长房室传导（延长AH间期）增加心动过速周长以终止心动过速，转复为窦性心律前出现短暂心室停搏；（3）转复为窦性心律前出现明显的房室分离和交界区逸搏心律；（4）转复为窦性心律前出现房颤；（5）在转复为窦性心律后出现室性早搏或非持续性室性心动过速；

（6）转复为窦性心律前出现心动过速周长长短交替现象。静脉应用维拉帕米可以用来鉴别体表心电图很难鉴别的房扑2∶1传导和其他类型的室上速。静脉注射维拉帕米后，房室传导减慢，使房扑波显现，从而达到鉴别的目的。地尔硫䓬和腺苷具有与之相同的作用。由于腺苷半衰期极短，经常用于宽QRS心动过速的鉴别诊断。

（三）钙通道阻滞剂在其他类型的室上性心动过速中的应用

钙通道阻滞剂用于房室结折返性室上速和预激综合征合并室上速的情况有足够的经验[36]。钙通道阻滞剂在其他类型的折返性室上速，如房内折返和窦房折返性室上速，以及自律性室上速中的应用十分有限。同样，钙通道阻滞剂在控制异位房性搏动中的作用也不十分清楚。

钙通道阻滞剂在多源房速中的急性治疗作用和预防作用不确定，因为在很大程度上，药物疗效依赖于基础疾病的严重程度。

（四）钙通道阻滞剂减少阵发性室上性心动过速的复发

目前，射频消融术治疗室上速的价值得到充分肯定，药物预防阵发性室上速复发的情况迅速改变。维拉帕米在这方面的应用比较有经验，口服预防复发不如静脉转复的效果好。诱导实验的结果不能预测口服的疗效。长期口服给药（80～120mg，3～4次/天）阻止阵发性室上速复发是否有效，尚无可对比的研究结果。

（五）钙通道阻滞剂在预激综合征中的应用

口服钙通道阻滞剂预防顺向性房室折返性心动过速发作是否有效尚不清楚。随着射频消融治疗的增加，很难进行对照试验。需要强调的是，预激综合征合并房扑、房颤的患者中，缩短旁路不应期的药物（如地高辛）和减慢房室结传导的药物（地高辛和β受体阻滞剂）能加快旁路传导，出现快速心室率，甚至造成室颤。钙通道阻滞剂（如维拉帕米、地尔硫䓬）及其他Ⅰ类抗心律失常药物延长房室结不应期，减慢房室结传导，不能用于预激综合征合并房扑或房颤的患者。

（六）钙通道阻滞剂控制房扑房颤时的心室率

钙通道阻滞剂经常用于控制房扑或房颤时的心室

率。在这种情况下，钙通道阻滞剂的作用和β受体阻滞剂相似。房扑和房颤的治疗一般按照以下原则：首先进行药物或电转复，然后维持窦性心律，并用抗房颤的药物预防房颤复发。可以替代性地仅用药物控制心室率以减轻症状或进行抗凝治疗以防止血栓形成。在近期的一些试验结果的支持下，用后一种方法治疗房颤有增加的趋势[47]。

静脉应用维拉帕米治疗房颤产生三种结果。第一种最常见，减慢房室传导，减慢心室率。药物疗效时间短，静推30min后逐渐失效，心室率开始回升，需要在静脉推注后维持静点。第二种为心室率变规则，可以发生在25%患者中。最后一种，转复房颤为窦性心律，这是一种特殊反应，但在近期发生房颤的患者中比较常见。延长维持缓慢心室率的时间，需要连续静脉滴注或开始口服治疗。

一些研究应用静脉注射地尔硫䓬减慢房扑或房颤时的心室率。Ellenbogen等[48]的试验入选47例房颤或房扑患者，静脉连续滴注地尔硫䓬（15mg/h）观察药物的安全性和有效性。地尔硫䓬20mg或20mg追加25mg静推出现疗效后，再持续静点。47例患者中44例随机分为地尔硫䓬组和安慰剂组。地尔硫䓬24h持续静点对多数患者（83%）有效；药物治疗比安慰剂疗效显著。Heywood等[49]发现，静脉注射地尔硫䓬在充血性心力衰竭的患者中同样起着减慢心室率的作用，平均剂量为25mg（18～50mg）。虽然，上述试验入选的患者数量有限，但试验结果表明，在心室功能受损的患者中应用地尔硫䓬是安全和有效的。应入选不同程度心室功能障碍的患者，进一步扩大研究的范围。

钙通道阻滞剂慢性的控制心室率的作用也主要是通过调整房室结传导和非竞争性肾上腺素能阻断作用而实现的。在静息和运动状态下，在联合应用地高辛或β受体阻滞剂时这种作用更加显著，这种情况在基础疾病不同的患者的众多研究中得到了证实。人们越来越清楚地认识到，钙通道阻滞剂和β受体阻滞剂在已经服用地高辛、无心室功能严重受损的患者中，成为控制心室率的一线治疗药物。近来的一些数据表明，在许多患者中，维拉帕米可以用来控制房扑和房颤患者的心室率。例如，0.25mg或0.5mg地高辛降低运动诱发的心室率加快的比例分别为3%和8%；联合应用地高辛和维拉帕米（240mg）减低心室率加快的比例为29%，单用维拉帕米减少心室率加快的比例为23%。毫无疑问，上述作用是通过钙通道阻滞剂对房室结的直接作用和抗交感激活作用实现的。另外一项研究[49]应用地尔硫䓬（240～360mg/d）联合地高辛有效地控制了房扑和房颤时的心室率，进一步证实了地尔硫䓬控制心室率的有效性。上述药物剂量范围对于静息和运动状态下心率减慢均有效，但剂量越大，副作用的发生率越高。有数据表明，联合应用中等剂量地尔硫䓬和地高辛控制房扑或房颤时的心室率是安全和有效的。

Farshi等[50]选择慢性持续房颤的患者，在静息、运动、日常活动状态下观察5种用药方法控制心室率的疗效。研究者在同一患者群中比较应用钙通道阻滞剂、β受体阻滞剂、地高辛控制心室率的差别。在这项研究之前，在同一患者群静息、运动和日常状态（24h）下，没有对单独应用一种药物或联合应用多种药物控制心室率的作用，进行系统的比较。研究入选12例慢性房颤患者，按每日标准剂量给药，分5组，地高辛0.25mg组（对照组）、地尔硫䓬240mg缓释剂组、阿诺洛尔50mg组、地高辛0.25mg联合地尔硫䓬240mg组、地高辛0.25mg联合阿诺洛尔50mg组，连续服药2周。静息、运动和动态心电图记录的日常状态下的心室率数据用均数±标准差表示。平均24h心室率在单用地高辛时为79.9±17.4次/分。与地高辛组比较，地尔硫䓬组为80.1±16.6次/分，无显著性差异；阿诺洛尔组为73.7±14.2次/分，无显著差异；地高辛联合地尔硫䓬组为68.4±15.6次/分（P<0.0033），有显著性差异；地高辛联合阿诺洛尔组为65.0±11.7次/分（P<0.001），有显著性差异。地高辛联合阿诺洛尔组与单用地尔硫䓬组、阿诺洛尔组比较，也具有显著性差异。5组药物在控制心室节律性方面均具有昼夜节律性（P<0.001）；接受β受体阻滞剂治疗时，心室率变化的昼夜节律性与地高辛组存在显著不同（P<0.001）。运动试验在增加心室率方面呈现出线性趋势（P<0.001）。地高辛组平均心室率为125±27.7次/分。与地高辛组比较，地尔硫䓬组为104.9±14.9次/分（P<0.0152），有显著性差异；阿诺洛尔组为102.1±28.7次/分（P<0.0265），有显著性差异，地高辛联合地尔硫䓬组为93.4±25.5次/分（P<0.0044），有显著性差异；地高辛联合阿诺洛尔组为82.1±9.0次/分（P<0.001），有显著性差异。地高辛组运动峰值心室率为175±36次/分，阿诺洛尔组为130±34次/分，地高辛联合地尔硫䓬组为126±29次/分，后两者与地高辛组比较，心率均显著降低，均具有显著性差异。这

些数据均表明，地高辛单独用于控制房颤患者静息、运动、日常活动时的心室率疗效较差。然而，可以联合地高辛和β受体阻滞剂或钙通道阻滞剂控制24h心室率。而且，地高辛联合阿诺洛尔控制运动时的峰值心室率的作用较单独用地高辛、地尔硫䓬、地高辛联合地尔硫䓬的疗效好。这说明了地高辛的类迷走神经作用和阿诺洛尔的β肾上腺素受体阻断作用对房室结具有协同作用。上述数据为选择最合适的药物用于控制房颤时的心室率提供了依据，在将慢性房颤心室功能障碍降低至最小程度的同时，尽量阻止心室功能恶化。

（七）钙通道阻滞剂在维持窦性心律中的作用

一般认为，钙通道阻滞剂对转复房颤患者为窦性心律和维持窦性心律无效。然而，近来数据表明，维拉帕米联合普罗帕酮或奎尼丁可能对维持窦性心律有显著疗效。上述联合治疗的确实有效性尚需要进行大型的试验研究加以证实。这一看似意外的结果的可能机制尚需要进一步探讨。

（八）钙通道阻滞剂对室性心律失常和减少死亡率的作用

临床试验数据表明，作为抗心律失常药物，钙通道阻滞剂在一些患者中既不增加也不减少死亡率，一些药物如短效硝苯地平几乎不增加死亡率，这与β受体阻滞剂显著不同。尽管，钙通道阻滞剂具有有效的抗心肌缺血作用，但其电生理作用不能减少心肌梗死后猝死高危患者的死亡率。Teo 和 Yusuf 等[51]对24个涉及钙通道阻滞剂的临床试验数据进行了 Meta 分析。从临床实践中，可以得出可靠的结论：仅一小部分心肌梗死后患者能从应用钙通道阻滞剂中获益，而且获益很小。

（九）钙通道阻滞剂和室性心律失常

钙通道阻滞剂在控制室性心律失常中的作用很有限，在所有研究人群中，钙通道阻滞剂对室性早搏的抑制作用均很小。目前，尚无临床研究数据表明，钙通道阻滞剂对肥厚型心肌病、扩张型心肌病和二尖瓣脱垂患者具有抗心律失常作用。

在阐述钙通道阻滞剂减少器质性心脏病患者的室速或室颤发作时，需要注意，钙通道阻滞剂对心室肌或浦肯野纤维的不应期和传导没有影响。钙通道阻滞剂作用的主要机制在于其改善心肌缺血，间接减少了室性心律失常的发生，特别是在复杂的伴有冠脉痉挛的患者中，更是如此。目前获得的数据表明，维拉帕米和地尔硫䓬对致命性心动过速几乎无效，临床上对诱发性室速、室颤、室性早搏或非持续性室性心动过速无效，对后除极造成的室速或室颤无效。

（十）钙通道阻滞剂对无器质性心脏病患者的室性心动过速的作用

发生于无器质性心脏病患者的室速称为特发性室速，其发病机制不清。其中有两类综合征对钙通道阻滞剂有效，目前主要应用射频消融术治疗。

第一种为右室流出道室速，主要发生在年轻患者中（主要为女性），心电图表现为左束支阻滞伴心电轴不偏或右偏[52]，通常呈持续发作，由运动或注射去甲肾上腺素诱发。主要用β受体阻滞剂治疗，但对钙通道阻滞剂和钙通道阻滞剂联合β受体阻滞剂治疗有效。第二种为间隔室速，男性占多数，心电图表现为右束支阻滞图形伴电轴左偏，钙通道阻滞剂治疗有效。电生理检查和心房快速起搏能诱发心动过速，对维拉帕米敏感，对腺苷不敏感。射频消融术为主要的治疗方法，但钙通道阻滞剂在长期治疗中有效。

（十一）钙通道阻滞剂对尖端扭转型室性心动过速的作用

钙通道阻滞剂对阻止尖端扭转型室速可能具有潜在的作用。毫无疑问，慢电流（I_{Ca}）是产生多形室速的基础，临床上胺碘酮所致甲状腺功能减退、严重高钙血症等情况下，可以出现 QT 间期显著延长，但只有电解质紊乱达到十分严重的程度时，才合并尖端扭转型室速。所有上述情况下，慢通道活性显著下降。Hiromasa 等[43]的研究发现，维拉帕米能够消除犬浦肯野纤维动作电位时程显著延长所造成早后除极（尖端扭转型室速最可能的机制）；Gilmour 等[42]也曾经报道过类似现象。尚未进行临床对照试验，钙通道阻滞剂治疗尖端扭转型室速有效性的数据尚缺乏说服力。

四、总　结

β受体阻滞剂和钙通道阻滞剂分别代表了两类主要的抗心律失常药物，二者的电生理特性显著不同，但又有一定程度的相似。二者均降低交感激活，钙通道阻滞剂以非特异性方式，而β受体阻滞剂通过阻断受体而发挥作用。二者均通过产生直接和间接作用抑制某些心律失常，影响或不影响死亡率。β受体阻滞剂的抗心律失常作用主要通过逆转和抵消儿茶酚胺的致心律失常作用而实现，而钙通道阻滞剂的抗心律失常作用机制尚不清楚，这是由于心肌慢通道在临床心律失常发生中的作用尚不清楚。钙通道阻滞剂结构多种多样，具有阻断心肌慢通道的共同特点，对房室结组织作用显著。β受体阻滞剂在结构上比较一致。二者对房室结传导和不应期的影响有些相似。因而，二者均能在房扑和房颤时减慢心室率，均能阻断房室结前传而终止阵发性房室折返性心动过速发作。二者对心房不应期均无显著延长作用，因而，对将房性心动过速转复为窦性心律或转复后窦性心律的维持无效。

尽管β受体阻滞剂和钙通道阻滞剂具有相同的抗心肌缺血特性，二者对室性心律失常作用显著不同。β受体阻滞剂能降低一些不同心脏病患者的死亡率，如心肌梗死幸存者、先天性长QT综合征患者等；可能降低一些疾病患者的死亡率，如持续单形室速患者、心脏骤停幸存者、进行性心力衰竭患者和显著心室功能降低的患者。而钙通道阻滞剂却从本质上缺乏使上述患者受益的作用。理解这两种药物的电药理学特性及这种特性与心律失常产生机制之间的关系，有助于人们更合理地将其用于多种心律失常的治疗。

(郭继鸿　陈琪　译)

参 考 文 献

1. Mangrum JM, DiMarco JP: Acute and chronic pharmacologic management of supraventricular arrhythmias in cardiovascular therapeutics. In Antman E (ed): Cardiovascular Therapeutics: A Companion to Braunwald's Heart Disease, 2nd ed. Philadelphia, WB Saunders, 2000, pp 423–444.
2. Fratt CM, Waldo AL, Camm AJ: Can antiarrhythmic drugs survive survival trials? Am J Cardiol 81:24D–34D, 1998.
3. Singh BN: Antiarrhythmic drugs: A re-orientation in the light of recent developments in the control of disorders of rhythm. Am J Cardiol 81:3D–13D, 1998.
4. Singh BN, Vanhoutte PM (eds): Selective and Specific I_f Inhibition in Cardiovascular Disease. London, Lippincott Williams & Wilkins, 2003, pp 1–134.
5. Singh BN: Overview of trends in the control of cardiac arrhythmias: Past and future. Am J Cardiol 84(9A):3R–10R, 1999.
6. Sarma JSM, Singh N, Schoenbaum MP, et al: Circadian and power spectral changes of RR and QT intervals during treatment of patients with angina pectoris with nadolol providing evidence for differential autonomic modulation of heart rate and ventricular repolarization. Am J Cardiol 74:131–136, 1994.
7. Opie LH: Pharmacologic options for treatment of ischemic heart disease. In Smith TW (ed): Cardiovascular Therapeutics. Philadelphia, WB Saunders, 1996, pp 22–57.
8. Anderson JL: Beta-Blockers. Card Electrophysiol Rev 4:300–307, 2000.
9. Singh BN: Morbidity and mortality in cardiovascular disease: Impact of reduced heart rate. J Cardiovasc Pharmacol Ther 6:313–331, 2001.
10. Reiter MJ, Reiffel JA: Importance of beta-blockade in the therapy of serious ventricular arrhythmias. Am J Cardiol 82(4A):9I–19I, 1998.
11. Reiter MJ: Antiarrhythmic impact of anti-ischemic, antifailure and other cardiovascular strategies. Cardiac Electrophysiol Rev 6:194–205, 2000.
12. Camm AJ, Yap YG: What should we expect from the next generation of antiarrhythmic drugs. J Cardiovasc Electrophysiol 10:307–205, 1998.
13. Singh BN (ed): Approaches to controlling cardiac arrhythmias: focus on amiodarone, the last 15 Years. Am J Cardiol 84(9A):1R–173R, 1999.
14. Meredith IT, Broughton A, Jennings GL, Esler MD: Evidence of a selective increase in cardiac sympathetic activity in patients with sustained ventricular arrhythmias. N Eng J Med 325:618–624, 1991.
15. Bristow M: Antiadrenergic therapy of chronic heart failure. Circulation 107:1100–1102, 2003.
16. Tan HL, Hou CJ, Lauer MR, Sung RJ: Electrophysiologic mechanisms of the long QT interval syndromes and torsade de pointes. Ann Int Med 122:701–704, 1995.
17. Wiesfeld AC, Crijns HJ, Tuininga YS, Lie KI: Beta adrenergic blockade in the treatment of sustained ventricular tachycardia or ventricular fibrillation. Pacing Clin Electrophysiol 19:1026–1035, 1996.
18. Hjalmarson A: Effects of beta blockade on sudden cardiac death during acute myocardial infarction and the postinfarction period. Am J Cardiol 80(9B):35J–39J, 1997.
19. Gottlieb SS, McCarter RJ, Vogel RA: Effect of beta-blockade on mortality among high-risk and low-risk patients after myocardial infarction. N Engl J Med 339:489–495, 1998.
20. Singh BN, Ahmed R: Class III antiarrhythmic drugs. Curr Opin Cardiol 9:12–22, 1994.
21. Julian DG, Camm AJ, Frangin G, et al: Randomized trial of effect of amiodarone on mortality in patients with left ventricular dysfunction after recent myocardial infarction: EMIAT. Lancet 349:667–674, 1997.
22. Cairns JA, Connolly SJ, Roberts RS, et al, and the CAMIAT Investigators: Randomized trial of outcome after myocardial infarction in patients with frequent or repetitive ventricular premature depolarizations: CAMIAT. Lancet 349:675–682, 1997.
23. Boutitie F, Boissel JP, Connolly SJ, et al, and the EMIAT and CAMIAT Investigators: Amiodarone interaction with β-blockers. Analysis of the merged EMIAT and CAMIAT databases. Circulation 99:2268–2275, 1999.
24. Teerlink JR, Bassie BM: Beta-adrenergic blocker mortality trials in congestive heart failure. Am J Cardiol 8:94R–102R, 1999.
25. MERIT-HEFT Study Group: Effect of metoprolol CR/XL in chronic heart failure: Metoprolol CR/XL randomized intervention trial in congestive heart failure (MERIT-HF). Lancet 353:2001–2007, 1999.
26. Packer M, Bristow MR, Cohn JN, et al, for the US Carvedilol Heart Failure Study Group: The effect of Carvedilol on morbidity and mortality in patients with chronic heart failure. N Engl J Med 334:1349–1355, 1996.
27. CIBIS–II Investigators and Committees: The cardiac insufficiency bisoprolol study II CIBIS II). Lancet 353:9–13, 1999.
28. Packer M, Coats AJ, Fowler MB, et al: The carvedilol, prospective randomized cumulative survival study group. N Engl J Med 344:1651–1658, 2001.
29. Design of the Beta-Blocker Evaluation Survival Trial (BEST). The BEST Steering Committee. Am J Cardiol 75:1220–1223, 1995.
30. Kelly RA, Smith TW: The pharmacology of heart failure drugs. In Smith TW (ed): Cardiovascular Therapeutics. Philadelphia, WB Saunders, 1996, pp 176–199.
31. Pinter A, Dorian P: Interactions between implantable devices and antiarrhythmic drugs. Cardiac Electrophysiol Rev 4:222–226, 2000.
32. Pacifico A, Hohnloser SH, Williams JH, et al: Prevention of implantable-defibrillator shocks with sotalol. D,L-Sotalol Implantable Cardioverter-Defibrillator Study group. N Engl J Med 340:1855–1862, 1999.
33. AVID Investigators: A comparison of antiarrhythmic-drug therapy with implantable defibrillators in patients resuscitated from near-fatal ventricular arrhythmias. Antiarrhythmics versus impaltable defibrillators (AVID) trial. New Engl J Med 337:1576–1583, 1997.
34. Connolly SJ, Sheldon R, Robert RS, Gent M: Canadan Implantable Defibrillator Study(CIDS): A randomized trial of the cardioverter defibrillator against amiodarone. Circulation 101:1297–1302, 1999.
35. Kuck KH, Cappato R, Siebels J, et al: Randomized comparison of antiarrhythmic drug therapy with implantable defibrillators in patients resuscitated from cardiac arrest: The Cardiac Arrest Study

Hamburg. Circulation 102:748–754, 2000.
36. Ferguson JD, DiMarco JP: Contemporary management of paroxysmal supraventricular tachycardia. Circulation 107:1096–1099, 2003.
37. Biffi M, Boriani G, Sabbatani P, et al: Malignant vasovagal syncope: A randomized trial of metoprolol and clonidine. Heart 77:268–272, 1997.
38. Iskos D, Dutton, Scheinman MM, Lurie KG: Usefulness of pindolol in neurocardiogenic shock. Am J Cardiol 82:1121–1124, 1998.
39. Falk RH: Control of ventricular rate in atrial fibrillation. In Falk RH, Podrid PJ (eds): Atrial Fibrillation. New York, Raven Press, 1992, pp 255–281.
40. Singh BN, Lopez B, Sarma JSM: Significance of prevention of atrial fibrilltaion occurring after cardiac surgery: A time for fundamental change in strategy? J Cardiovasc Pharmacol Ther 3:259–268, 1998.
41. Mangano DT, Layug EL, Allace A, et al: Effect of atenolol on mortalit and cardiovascualr morbidity after non-cardiac surgery. The Multicenter Study of Perioperative Ischemia Research Group. N Engl J Med 335:1713–1720, 1996.
42. Gilmour RF, Chialvo DR, Jalife J: Calcium-channel blockers. In Singh BN, Dzau VJ, Vanhoutte PM, Woosley RL (eds): Electropharmacological Control of Cardiac Arrhythmias. Mt. Kisco, NY, Futura Publishing, 1994, pp 255–264.
43. Hiromasa S, Coto H, Li ZY, et al: Dextrorotary isomer of sotalol. Electrophysiologic effects and interaction with verapamil. Am Heart J 116:1552–1557, 1988.
44. Frishman WH: Mibefradil: A new selective T-channel calcium antagonist for hypertension and angina pectoris. J Cardiovasc Pharmacol Ther 2:321–330, 1997.
45. Singh BN: Calcium-channel blockers and adenosine as antiarrhythmic drugs. In Singh BN, Dzau VJ, Vanhoutte PM, Woosley RL (eds): Cardiovascular Pharmacology and Therapeutics. New York: Churchill Livingstone, 1994, pp 747–764.
46. Camm AJ, Garratt CJ: Adenosine and supraventricular tachycardia. N Engl J Med 25:1621–1629, 1991.
47. The Atrial Fibrillation Follow-up Investigation of Rhythm Management (AFFIRM) Investigators: A comparison of rate control and rhythm control in patients with atrial fibrillation. N Engl J Med 347:1285–1833, 2000.
48. Ellenbogen KA, Dias VC, Plumb VJ, et al: A placebo-controlled trial of continuous diltiazem infusion for 24-hour heart rate control during atrial fibrillation and atrial flutter: A multi-center study. J Am Coll Cardiol 18:891–897, 1991.
49. Heywood JT, Graham B, Marais GE, Jutzy KR: Effects of intravenous diltiazem on rapid atrial fibrillation accompanied by congestive heart failure. Am J Cardiol 67:1150–1152, 1991.
50. Farshi R, Kistner D, Sarma JSM, et al: Ventricular rate control in chronic atrial fibrillation during daily activity and exercise by five pharmacological regimens. J Am Coll Cardiol 33:304–310, 1999.
51. Teo KK, Yusuf S: Overview of antiarrhythmic drug trials: Implications for antiarrhythmictherapy. In Singh BN, Dzau VJ, Vanhoutte PM, Woosley RL (eds): Cardiovascular Pharmacology and Therapeutics. New York, Churchill Livingstone, 1994, pp 631–643.
52. Wyse DG: Calcum channel blockers. Card Electrophysiol Rev 4:308–311, 2000.
53. Lee SH, Chen SA, Tai CT, et al: Electropharmacologic charcateristics and radiofrequency catheter ablation of sustained ventricular tachycardia in patients in patients without structural heart disease. Cardiology 87:33–41, 1996.

第 101 章

Ⅲ类抗心律失常药物：胺碘酮、依布利特和索他洛尔

Timothy W. Smith，Michael E. Cain

本章目录

- Ⅲ类抗心律失常药的一般特性 913
- 胺碘酮 914
- 依布利特 917
- 索他洛尔 918
- Ⅲ类抗心律失常药的发展趋势 920

折返是临床上房性和室性心律失常最常见的机制。1968年Kaumann和olson[1]报告了能延长心肌动作电位时程的药物可以阻断折返环路。鉴于这类药物作用的重要性及其产生的不应性的增加，促使Singh和Vaughan-Williams[2]于1970年在抗心律失常药分类表中增加了新的一类（Ⅲ类）。

在过去的15年中，Ⅰ类药物在治疗快速性心律失常方面已经失去了它们的重要地位。来自对照试验的数据显示，这类药尽管能控制心律失常，但能增加患有器质性心脏病或心衰患者的死亡率。因此，药物生产者和医生都越来越关注Ⅲ类抗心律失常药。本章将阐明Ⅲ类药的一般特点和典型特性以及胺碘酮、依布利特和索他洛尔的临床应用。

一、Ⅲ类抗心律失常药的一般特性

（一）Ⅲ类药物作用的分子机制

Ⅲ类药物的电生理特性是延长心肌动作电位时程，从而延长不应期。心肌动作电位源于由Na^+、K^+、Ca^{2+}、Cl^-通过特殊的膜通道形成的跨膜电流，这些膜通道可在除极时开放，复极时关闭。通过这些通道的离子运动是由跨膜电化学梯度驱使。心肌细胞的静息膜电位是负的，主要由外向K^+梯度决定。内向离子流I_{K1}主要决定静息膜电位。除极时Na^+和Ca^{2+}通道开放，离子内流从而形成动作电位的除极和平台期。复极是由外向K^+流形成（I_K），它由慢、快、超快三种类型组成（I_{Ks}，I_{Kr}和I_{Kur}）。动作电位时程可通过内向电流增加或外向电流减少而延长。胺碘酮、索他洛尔、多非利特和阿齐利特通过阻滞一个或多个通道而延长动作电位时程。依布利特则引起或增加内向Na^+电流。

延迟整流的快型是选择性Ⅲ类抗心律失常药主要作用靶点，与先天性长QT间期综合性有关的缺陷的I_{Kr}通道是HERG基因突变的产物[3]。胺碘酮和阿齐利特的作用是非特异的，具有慢整流I_{Ks}的慢型的拮抗作用。I_{Ks}是KVLQT1和minK基因的产物，这些基因突变与先天性长QT间期综合征有关（LQT1）[3]。I_{Kr}的拮抗剂是在较慢心率时更有效，这一特征称为逆使用依赖[4]。不幸的是，逆使用依赖在心动过缓时减弱了抗折返作用，此时这一作用是非常有益的。心动过缓时，I_{Kr}拮抗剂延长动作电位时程和QT间期，增加了尖端扭转型室性心动过速发作的风险，它是一种威胁生命的多形性室速。非特异的K^+通道阻滞剂，包括具有重要的I_{Kur}拮抗作用的药物，例如胺碘酮、安巴利特和阿齐利特，有较弱的逆使用依赖效应和较轻的致心律失常作用[5]。

（二）Ⅲ类药物对正常心脏的作用

折返性心律失常需要一个功能性的环路：一个循环着的除极波可绕其运动，环路中非除极的可兴奋的

区域称为可激动间隙。为了维持折返,前行的波锋必须遇到波尾之后的可兴奋组织。通过缩短或去除可激动间隙可终止或阻止折返。波长是同一时间被除极的环路的一部分,是由传导速度和不应期决定的(图 101-1)。在正常心肌,动作电位时程延长可增加折返环路中的波长,缩短可激动间隙,如果可激动间隙被充分缩短,激动的前锋将遇到波尾处于不应期的组织,折返将被终止。只延长不应期和去除可激动间隙的药物可能是理想的抗心律失常药。

延长心房和心室的心肌不应期的药物通过延长动作电位时程而实现之。心室动作电位的延长致使复极延迟和 QT 间期相对延长,药源性 QT 间期延长与尖端扭转型室性心动过速有关。Q-T 间期过度延长,从而引起心律失常是Ⅲ类抗心律失常药的主要副作用,逆使用依赖可能是另外一个副作用。大部分Ⅲ类药有某种程度的逆使用依赖,即心率快时效应降低,心率慢时 QT 间期延长及致心律失常作用增加。作用的非特异性能提高Ⅲ类抗心律失常药安全性,胺碘酮和索他洛尔有重要的 β 肾上腺素能受体阻滞作用,这一作用能降低致心律失常作用。

二、胺碘酮

胺碘酮作为抗心绞痛药物于 1962 年在比利时合成,随后它的抗心律失常作用被发现,1985 年美国 FDA 批准其用于危及生命的室性心律失常的治疗,对其他心律失常包括房颤也是有效的。

(一)基础和临床电生理学

除了对甲状腺代谢有作用外,胺碘酮具有所有 4 类抗心律失常药的电生理特征。在短期和长期给药后引起心肌电生理改变不同[6]。

急性期,胺碘酮抑制内向 Na^+ 和 Ca^{2+} 电流,即 I_{Na} 和 I_{Ca},这分别是 Ⅰ 类和 Ⅳ 类药物的特征[6]。这些作用的强度呈使用依赖性。因此,与慢心率时相比,胺碘酮在快心率时是 Na^+ 和 Ca^{2+} 流的更有效的阻滞剂。对 Na^+ 和 Ca^{2+} 流的阻滞作用呈电压依赖性,通道抑制在除极的舒张期电位作用更强,例如有心肌缺血时,胺碘酮对外向 K^+ 电流有急性的阻滞作用,但对 I_{Na} 和 I_{Ca} 的阻滞作用更显著。当长期用药时,对 K^+ 电流的阻滞作用比对 I_{Na} 和 I_{Ca} 的阻滞作用强[6],除了抑制电压门控 K^+ 电流 I_K、I_{K1} 和 I_{to}(与动作电位 1 期早期复极有关的短暂外向电流)及 I_{Ks} 外,胺碘酮对配

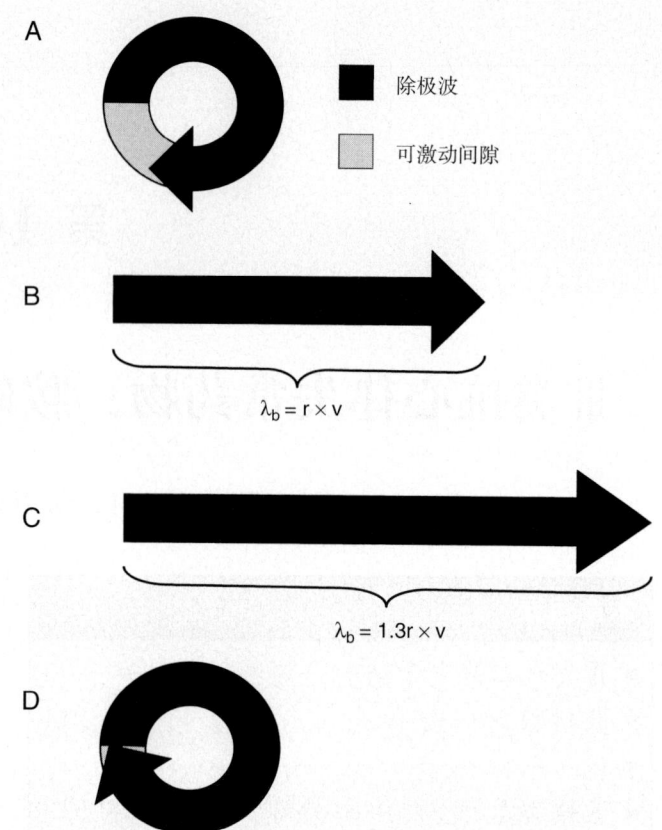

图 101-1 Ⅲ类抗心律失常药的抗折返机制 A 中环形代表折返环,黑色箭头表示除极波,灰色表示可激动间隙。除极波头端总是可激动组织,因而折返可以维持。B:λ 代表除极心肌组织的波长,等于传导速度(v)与不应期(r)的乘积。C:Ⅲ类抗心律失常药的作用。Ⅲ类抗心律失常药使不应期延长 30%,故波长也相应延长。D:由于药物作用,延长的波长在原来折返环中不能存在。可激动间期消失,除极波的头尾相遇,遇到组织不应期,折返消失。

体门控通道也有抑制作用,如 Na^+ 依赖性 K^+ 通道 I_{KNa} 和乙酰胆碱依赖性 K^+ 通道。在活体研究表明,胺碘酮的短期应用对 I_K 有显著作用,对 I_{Ks} 作用较弱,然而长期应用将产生 I_{Ks} 强烈阻滞[7]。通过在正常心脏及临床上胺碘酮短期给药后的观察,其电生理作用源于 Na^+ 和 Ca^{2+} 通道阻滞和 I_{Kr} 的阻滞。在离体心脏,窦房结节律减慢,但是在活体组织窦性节律没有明显降低。房室结传导时间减慢,与 K^+ 通道阻滞有关的作用较少。心室不应期不增加,QT 间期也没有显著延长。

相比之下,在胺碘酮的长期应用时,外向 K^+ 流的抑制对电生理效应有很大的影响[6]。最主要的是对 I_{Kr} 和 I_{Ks} 的影响。K^+ 流的阻滞与动作电位及不应期的延长密切相关,然而不像大多数特异性 I_{Kr} 阻滞剂那

样,长期应用胺碘酮有较少的逆使用依赖性。慢心率作用更显著,正如慢房室结传导一样。QT间期是延长的,至于为什么长期应用胺碘酮的作用与短期应用作用不同,还不清楚。胺碘酮代谢生成脱乙基胺碘酮(DEA),后者能在体内蓄积,胺碘酮和脱乙基胺碘酮的电生理效应相似,表明长期用药的电生理作用不仅仅归因于脱乙基胺碘酮。

两个碘化部分构成了胺碘酮质量的37.3%。200mg胺碘酮包括74.6mg的可吸收碘,在胺碘酮中碘的10%(大约是正常食物摄取的100倍)代谢生成无机碘[8]。通过减少在外周T_4向T_3的转化,抑制T_3进入心肌细胞和抑制T_3与它的核受体结合而影响甲状腺代谢[6]。对甲状腺的抑制表现为对I_{to}以及对持续性K^+流的抑制作用[9]。总之,这些效应部分有助于胺碘酮的临床抗心律失常作用。但是它的电生理效应没有因临床上的甲状腺功能低下而加倍。胺碘酮是有效的非竞争性的α、β肾上腺受体阻滞剂[10]。β肾上腺素能受体阻滞剂显然与腺苷酸环化酶的抑制有关[11]。

(二) 临床效能

胺碘酮已被FDA批准用于危及生命的室性心律失常的治疗,但是它也对有症状的室上性心律失常包括房颤有作用。CASCADE研究确立了胺碘酮对心脏性猝死的二级预防效能[12]。将心室颤动复苏的病人随机分配到胺碘酮组和常规抗心律失常药治疗组中,这些抗心律失常药是通过心室程序刺激或Holter监测筛选的。对于心脏性猝死的幸存者、心室颤动的复苏者以及植入ICD后晕厥者,接受胺碘酮治疗效果显著优于常规药物治疗者。

EMIAT和CAMIAT研究分别评估了对心肌梗死后合并左心室功能不全(EMIAD)或频发室性早搏(CAMIAT)的患者,应用胺碘酮对心脏性猝死和死亡率预防的影响[13,14]。对于参加研究的病人被随机分配到胺碘酮组和安慰剂组,两个研究的数据显示,室颤和心脏性猝死在胺碘酮治疗组比安慰剂治疗组显著降低,但胺碘酮对其他原因引起的死亡率没有有利影响。

其他重要的研究评估了胺碘酮对心衰病人的死亡率的影响。GESICA研究显示,接受小剂量胺碘酮治疗与接受安慰剂治疗相比,非缺血性心肌病病人的死亡率下降28%[15]。相比之下,CHF-STAT研究在胺碘酮和安慰剂治疗组中死亡率没有差别[16]。不过,参加CHF-STAT试验的病人比参加GESICA的病人有更高的缺血性心脏病发生率。对患有冠状动脉疾病的病人进一步分析证实,胺碘酮对生存率无益处。对非缺血性心肌病组胺碘酮的应用对死亡率有降低的趋势。荟萃分析显示具有统计学差异。但是预防应用胺碘酮对死亡率和因心律失常死亡的益处并不显著[17,18]。

基于以上数据,对室性心律失常和猝死的一级预防应用胺碘酮是有争议的。但对有心衰或冠状动脉疾病的患者,为治疗有症状的心律失常如房颤或有症状的非持续室速,死亡率并未增加,故支持应用胺碘酮[19]。

多项研究的数据证明:对有缺血性心脏病和左室功能不全的病人的一级预防和二级预防,ICD治疗优于药物治疗[20-22]。为防止ICD治疗所致的复发性心律失常和休克,许多病人需要抗心律失常药物治疗[19]。胺碘酮和索他洛尔是常用的药物,但是胺碘酮能增加除颤阈值,致使在治疗最初需要反复进行ICD检测。

FDA批准静脉用胺碘酮用于室颤和血流动力学不稳定的室速以及需要胺碘酮治疗但不能口服者[19],对有致命性的室速的患者,胺碘酮的效能可以与溴苄胺相比[23]。除此,在院外心脏骤停的患者,急诊用静脉胺碘酮与安慰剂和利多卡因相比能提高生存率[24]。

虽然没有被FDA批准用于房颤,但胺碘酮对窦性心律的维持也是有效的。患有器质性心脏病或心衰的病人是许多抗心律失常药的禁忌证,但胺碘酮不受此限制,对房颤复发预防的加拿大房颤研究把胺碘酮和普罗帕酮及索他洛尔作了比较,平均随访450天,结果表明接受胺碘酮治疗的病人有65%房颤转复窦律,而接受索他洛尔或普罗帕酮治疗的病人仅有37%的病人房颤转复(图101-2)[25]。

心脏手术后10%~65%病人会出现房颤。这种情况下的房颤很难治疗。它延长了住院时间,增加了发病率和死亡率。心脏手术前给予预防性口服胺碘酮以及手术后立即给予静脉胺碘酮治疗,可以减少手术后房颤的发生率[26]。

(三) 药物代谢动力学和剂量选择

胺碘酮的药理学是复杂的,它是碘化苯基呋喃的衍生物(图101-3),具有很高的脂溶性。它可以在不同的器官组织有不同程度的聚集,特别是在脂肪组织。分布的有效容积大约为5 000L,在负荷剂量后达到稳态浓度需数个星期,渗透到脂肪组织需15g或更大剂量。在停药后,脂肪组织中药物贮存是缓释药物的源泉,清除半衰期为30多天,在停药9个月后,血浆中仍能发现药物存在[27]。

胺碘酮主要在肝脏中代谢生成脱乙基胺碘酮。脱乙基胺碘酮和母链有相似的作用。代谢物的蓄积是胺碘酮长期应用效应改变的根源[6]。肾脏对胺碘酮的代谢或清除作用不明显，因此肾功能不全时不必调整剂量，血液透析和腹膜透析都不能从机体中清除胺碘酮。

为了降低药物不良反应，长期药物治疗需用最低有效剂量，但由于药物蓄积很慢，开始常用负荷剂量。胺碘酮每日可达 1 600mg。对于室性心律失常可用负荷剂量 2～3 周，然后减少到每天 400～600mg，甚至可减少到每天 200mg。对于房颤可用更低的初始剂量[19]。胺碘酮可用于门诊病人等低风险病人，对患有心动过缓和有发展为高度房室阻滞风险的患者应慎用。

静脉给药常以 150mg 一次性静脉注射，然后以 1mg/min 的速度连续静滴几个小时。基于临床反馈，额外的 150mg 一次性注射和连续的点滴通常是必要的。有可能的话，持续滴注应减少到 0.5mg/min。此外，由于药物可能被聚乙烯表面所吸附，所以滴注时应放在玻璃瓶或聚烯烃容器中。为快速输液并预防局部静脉炎，采用中心静脉输液是较好的选择。

（四）不良反应

虽然胺碘酮有较低的致心律失常作用，但对许多脏器都有很多潜在的不良反应。除了肾脏外几乎每个脏器都受影响。通常发生不良反应的风险与每日剂量和蓄积量有关。荟萃分析显示，应用胺碘酮时有 22.9% 的病人因不可耐受的不良反应而停药，而应用安慰剂组停药者占 15.4%[28]。在 CASCADE 研究中，接受胺碘酮治疗组有 29% 的病人停药，而接受常规抗心律失常药物治疗组 17% 的病人停药[12]。在 CHF-STAT、EMIAT 和 CAMIAT 研究中，胺碘酮和安慰剂的停药率分别为 27% 和 23%，38.5% 和 21.4%，36.4% 和 25.5%[13,14,16]。

尽管胺碘酮能延长动作电位时程，但由于其能降低除极的不均一性，因而尖端扭转型室性心动过速并不多见[29]。在 EMIAT 和 CAMIAT 研究中，胺碘酮治疗的病人，此种心律失常发生率分别为 0 和 1%[13,14]。相比之下，在 CAMIT 研究中，安慰剂治疗的病人室性心律失常发生率为 5%[14]。

由于胺碘酮对窦房结或房室结的作用，可引起心动过缓，停药后可恢复正常。如果临床上必须用胺碘

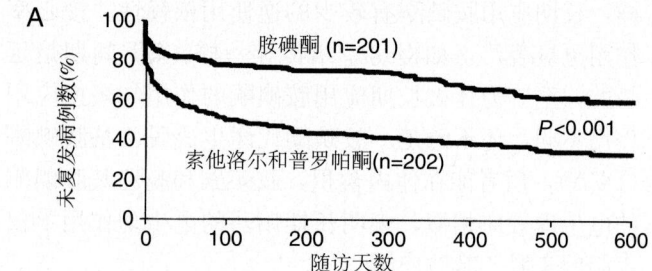

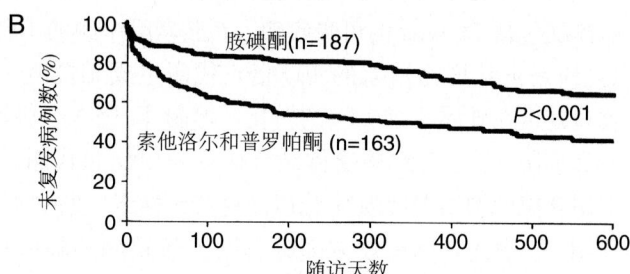

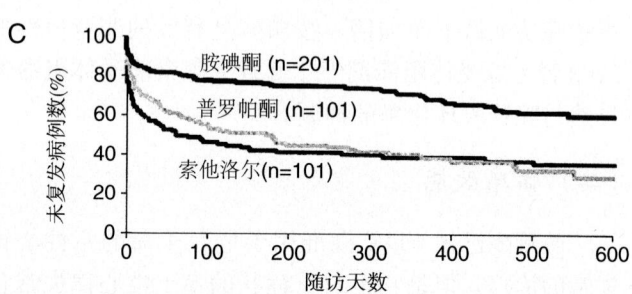

图 101-2 加拿大心房颤动试验中 Kaplan-Meier 评估无房颤复发患者的比率　A：胺碘酮治疗组与索他洛尔和普罗帕酮治疗组对比；B：胺碘酮治疗组与索他洛尔和普罗帕酮治疗组对比，除外当天复发的患者；C：胺碘酮治疗组、索他洛尔治疗组和普罗帕酮治疗组的对比。（引自 Roy D, Talajic M, Dorian P, et al：Amiodarone to prevent recurrence of atrial fibrillation. N Engl J Med 342：913-920，2000．）

酮治疗，可植入埋藏式起搏器。

肺毒性是一个严重的心脏外的副作用，间质性肺炎是常见的表现。细支气管炎和急性呼吸窘迫综合征也可出现。孤立性肺大泡也曾被报道过。肺毒性通常与胺碘酮的蓄积量有关，但它可在治疗的早期出现[30]。肺毒性的体征和体格检查不能说明是胺碘酮所为，诊断困难。胸部 X 线、肺功能检查及支气管镜已被应用，但没有一样是特异性的。用于观察因碘化物沉淀而引起腹膜的高密度损伤的高分辨率 CT 有应用前景[31]。通常停用胺碘酮给予支持治疗，在有些病人，系统应用类固醇激素是必要的[30,32]。

甲状腺功能低下发生率高达 32%[14]。胺碘酮抑制 T_4 在外周的去碘化，增加 T_4 和反 T_3 水平。促甲

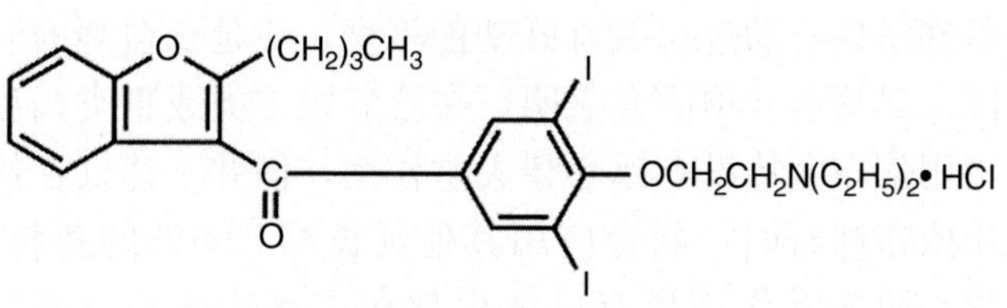

图 101-3 盐酸胺碘酮、富马酸依布利特和盐酸索他洛尔的化学结构

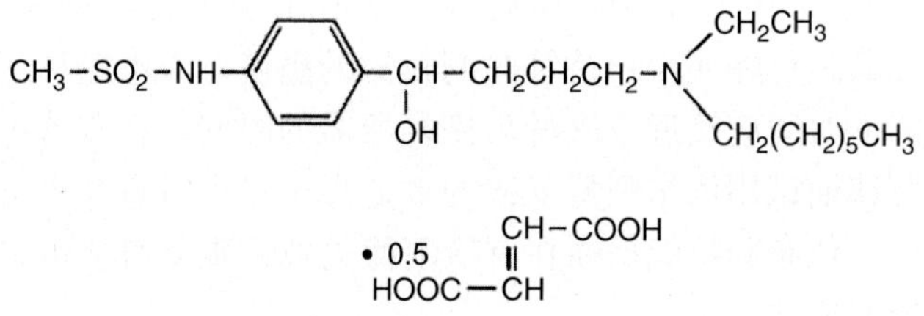

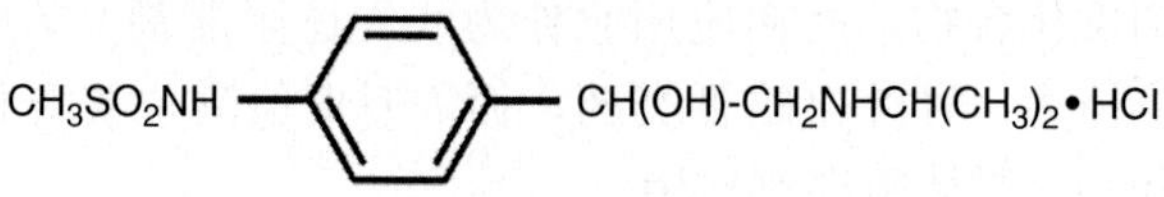

状腺激素水平可轻度升高[8]。停药后，部分病人仍然甲状腺功能低下，可能是甲状腺合成缺陷或自身免疫性甲状腺炎所致[32]。如果必须用胺碘酮治疗，一般需补充甲状腺素。

在美国和世界其他一些碘摄入充分的地区，胺碘酮所致的甲状腺功能亢进比甲低少见[33]。在欧洲，胺碘酮所致的甲状腺功能亢进的发生率为 2%～10%[34]。通常发生在开始治疗后 3～5 年，甲状腺毒症比甲低更难处理，停用胺碘酮并不能使症状缓解。胺碘酮高水平的碘抑制放射性碘的摄取，用 ^{131}I 治疗甲亢将是不可能的。药物治疗包括丙基硫氧嘧啶和甲巯咪唑，但作用迟缓或效果不佳[35]。如果必须继续用胺碘酮治疗可采用甲状腺部分切除[19,32]。

由于泪嵴点液体分泌，胺碘酮沉积在角膜常见。沉积物能通过眼科检查发现，停药后这种作用可逆转。这些沉积物可引起角膜囊肿和脓肿[10]，但很少会直接引起失明[10]。胺碘酮治疗的病人很少有失明报告，原因不明。

胺碘酮能引起皮肤光过敏，患者应避免强光，长期用药也可使皮肤变成灰绿色[36]，停药后可以恢复正常。

肝脏各种酶异常也是常见表现，这些变化是可逆的。中枢神经系统副作用包括头痛、外周神经病变和共济失调。胺碘酮是血管扩张剂，可引起低血压[28,32]，更常见于静脉用药时。该药的 β 肾上腺素受体阻断作用可能起作用，此作用主要在于携带静脉药物制剂的赋形剂——聚山梨醇酯 80。

胺碘酮可以与许多药物相互作用，特别是高蛋白结合率的药物。胺碘酮可增强华法林作用，可使血清地高辛水平增加一倍。目前的指导原则建议，在应用胺碘酮治疗之前，华法林和地高辛应减量。此外，与能延长 QT 间期的药物或其他制剂合用可进一步延长 QT 间期，增加致心律失常的风险。

胺碘酮治疗通常以高剂量的负荷剂量开始，对于那些条件稳定的门诊房颤病人，可用胺碘酮治疗。对于那些由于窦房结或房室结功能障碍而有严重心动过缓风险的住院病人，心电监护是合理的[19]。推荐的治疗方案包括肝功能和甲状腺功能检查、电解质和肌酐检查、胸部 X 线、肺功能检查和心电图。肝功能和甲状腺功能检查应每半年做一次，胸片和心电图应每年做一次。

眼科检查及肺功能检查建议按指征进行[19]。胺碘酮对 ICD 功能的影响不是固定的。长期用药可显著增加能量需求[37]。对植入 ICD 的病人胺碘酮治疗最初应该反复进行除颤测试，尽管这种测试的理想时间还不清楚。

（五）当前治疗学中的作用

胺碘酮是一种有效的抗心律失常药，不良反应在一定程度上限制了它的应用。但医生们逐渐认识到低剂量使用时其不良反应及致心律失常作用少见。因此，如今它已广泛应用于抗心律失常的治疗，包括房颤；在心脏骤停的治疗方面胺碘酮的静脉制剂已成为主要用药。

三、依布利特

1995 年，依布利特获得 FDA 批准，静脉注射用于终止房颤与房扑。

(一) 基础和临床电生理学

依布利特是一类甲醛氨苯磺胺衍生物（图 101-3）。早期研究表明，这类药物可在动作电位平台期诱导一种缓慢钠电流。随后在体外应用不同制剂进行研究表明，依布利特可抑制 I_K 和 I_{Kr} 活性[38,39]。它在人心肌细胞膜的这种作用机制未明。依布利特是通过延长动作电位时程发挥抗心律失常作用的。它可使 QT 间期延长并增加发生尖端扭转型室性心动过速的风险。依布利特不具有逆使用依赖特性[40]。它对窦房结的功能或传导系统无明显影响，不会引起血压的显著变化。

(二) 临床效能

依布利特在终止房颤或房扑和恢复窦性节律方面优于安慰剂[41,42]。其中，转复房扑的效能高于转复房颤（63%比31%）[42]。尽管转复率不及电复律，不过在有麻醉禁忌时，可以应用依布利特。在心律失常持续时间较短时用药，成功率较高[40]。

依布利特也可易化非药理性房颤和房扑的复律。如同普鲁卡因胺，依布利特可增加超速起搏终止房扑的有效性[43]。在初次试用电复律失败的病人中，依布利特可提高重复直流电复律的成功率[44]。

(三) 药物代谢动力学和剂量选择

依布利特只有作为静脉制剂才有效。由于广泛的首过机制，不能口服。药物血浆蛋白结合率低（≈40%）[40]。在肝脏中代谢为 8 种子产物，其中一种有中等抗心律失常活性[40]。代谢物主要经肾清除。消除半衰期从 2～10 小时不等，若肝功能不全会延长[40]。

该药装在一种 10ml 的药水瓶中，其中含有 1mg 依布利特。首次剂量为 10 分钟滴注 1mg。如果在滴注首次剂量 10 分钟后房颤/房扑仍持续，可在 10 分钟内给予第二个 1mg 剂量。如果患者体重低于 60kg，每一次剂量减至 0.01mg/kg。当复律后，同时出现 QT 间期显著延长或出现多形性室性心动过速时，应停止静注。

(四) 不良反应

主要的不良反应是尖端扭转型室性心动过速。在 3.6%～8.3% 的病人中观察到尖端扭转型室性心动过速[41,42]。由于其致心律失常作用，依布利特给药需要在严密监测和有复苏设备的医院里进行。在给予依布利特后，心电图监测至少应持续 4 小时。如果发生多形性室性心动过速或有肝功能不全，应延长监测的时间。尽管有一项研究表明，在已应用 I 类或 Ⅲ 类药后再用依布利特没有致心律失常作用，但并不建议在用依布利特时，联合应用其他延长 QT 间期的药物。致心律失常作用更有可能出现在左室功能不全的患者[44]。

(五) 当前治疗学中的作用

由于直流电复律安全且更有效，依布利特在终止房颤/房扑方面的作用有限。它适用于不希望麻醉，尤其是房颤或房扑持续时间较短的患者。心电监护所需的时间应接近于麻醉后恢复所需的时间。在直流电复律前试用依布利特复律的效益高于只进行直流电复律。依布利特能提高在首次复律失败后重复直流电复律的成功率。

四、索他洛尔

索他洛尔是一种 d 型索他洛尔和 l 型索他洛尔的外消旋化合物。起初应用它作为 β 受体阻滞剂。d 型对应体为一种纯化的 Ⅲ 类药，而 l 型索他洛尔兼有 Ⅲ 类药和 β 受体阻滞剂作用。

(一) 基础和临床电生理学

与胺碘酮相比，l 型索他洛尔为一种竞争性 β 受体阻滞剂。在相对较低的剂量下即可检测到 β 受体阻断作用。这种 β 受体阻断的内在负性变力效应在体内可被与动作电位时程延长相关的正性变力效应所抵消，动作电位时程延长可增加介导收缩力的细胞内钙离子的增加的时间。临床上，索他洛尔可引起中等程度的负性变力效应[4]。

两种对应体都有 Ⅲ 类药物的效应，该效应主要通过阻滞 I_{Kr} 来介导。对其他离子通道在临床浓度下无显著影响。这种抗心律失常效应表现出逆使用依赖，即在较慢的心率下延长动作电位时程，且在心率较快时效应降低。索他洛尔能降低窦房结节律、延长 PR 间期、AH 间期、房室结不应期和 QT 间期。但它不改变 HV 间期或 QRS 波群时间[46]。

(二) 临床效能

在多种室上性和室性快速性心律失常的治疗上，索他洛尔优于安慰剂、β 受体阻滞剂和 Ⅰ 类药物[46]。然而，索他洛尔对心肌梗死恢复期患者发生猝死的一级预防方面的效果令人失望。与安慰剂相比,在开始治疗的早期而非晚期,接受索他洛尔治疗后表现出死亡率增高的趋势(初始剂量每日320mg)。而在口服d型索他洛尔生存试验(SWORD)中,对比d型索他洛尔和安慰剂在患有前壁心肌梗死和左室功能不全的患者的作用。结果显示,在索他洛尔组观察到死亡率上升且具有统计学意义,促使该项试验在早期终止。尽管机制未明,人们猜测l型索他洛尔的β受体阻断作用具有某种程度的保护性。

在预防植入ICDs的患者出现首次除颤和死亡方面,索他洛尔优于安慰剂(图101-4)[48]。由于索他洛尔可防止室上性心动过速,同样可降低因误感知而造成的ICD放电的发生次数。与胺碘酮不同,索他洛尔能持续性降低植有ICDs患者的除颤阈值。索他洛尔的这种降低除颤阈值的作用,以及相对较少的心脏以外不良反应,使它成为植入ICDs患者抗心律失常的一线药(在无禁忌证时)。事实上,人们已提倡用索他洛尔疗法达到降低除颤阈值的主要目的(表101-5)[49]。

索他洛尔在对房颤病人维持窦性节律的效能方面令人失望。在一项研究中,50%病人在4.6个月后复发[50]。另有一项随机安慰剂对照试验中,每日两次给予120或160mg剂量的索他洛尔,在防止房颤复发上比安慰剂更有效;但每日两次给予80mg索他洛尔,效果接近安慰剂[51]。还有一项对索他洛尔、普罗帕酮和胺碘酮治疗房颤的大型随机对照试验,显示胺碘酮在维持窦性节律上优于索他洛尔和普罗帕酮[25]。

(三) 药物代谢动力学和剂量选择

索他洛尔的生物等效性接近100%。口服2~4小时后达到血浆峰浓度,几乎以原形经肾清除。肝功能不全对药物代谢无明显影响。清除半衰期在12~14小时之间。肾功能不全可造成药物在体内蓄积和严重的毒性反应。给药和剂量必须与患者的肌酐清除率相适应。在肌酐清除率低于40ml/min的患者应避免应用索他洛尔[52]。经典的口服剂量为每日两次给予80~320mg。每日两次给予低于120mg的剂量主要表现为β受体阻断作用和轻度Ⅲ类药作用[51]。当更高剂量时必须考虑发生不良反应的风险,特别是QT间期延长和尖端扭转型室性心动过速。索他洛尔通常静脉给药剂量为0.2~1.5mg/kg,该剂量在美国是不采用的[53]。

(四) 不良反应

不良反应与β受体阻断作用和Ⅲ类药的作用有关。β肾上腺素能受体阻滞的不良反应包括心动过缓、疲劳、支气管痉挛和呼吸困难。心衰和肺水肿的发生率为3.3%[54]。尖端扭转型室性心动过速发生率估计为2.4%。上述不良反应大多发生在开始治疗后第一周

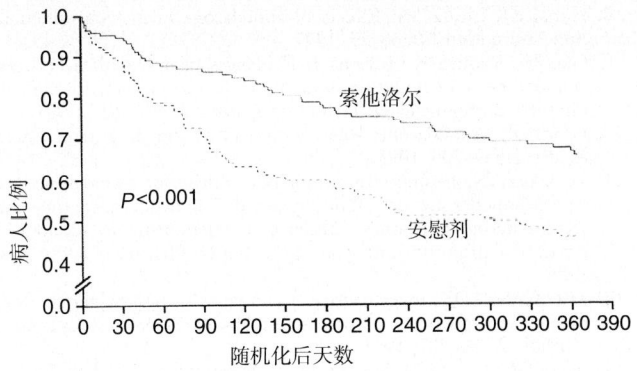

图101-4 索他洛尔对植入ICD的室速和室颤患者可预防电除颤 Kaplan-Meier评估了索他洛尔治疗组与安慰剂组患者的存活率和ICD放电率。两组死亡率都很低(4%),但无显著差异,不过两组发生ICD电除颤的人数有显著差异。(引自Pacifico A, Hohnloser SH, Williams JH, et al: Prevention of implantable-defibrillator shocks by treatment with sotalol. N Engl J Med 340: 1855-1862, 1999.)

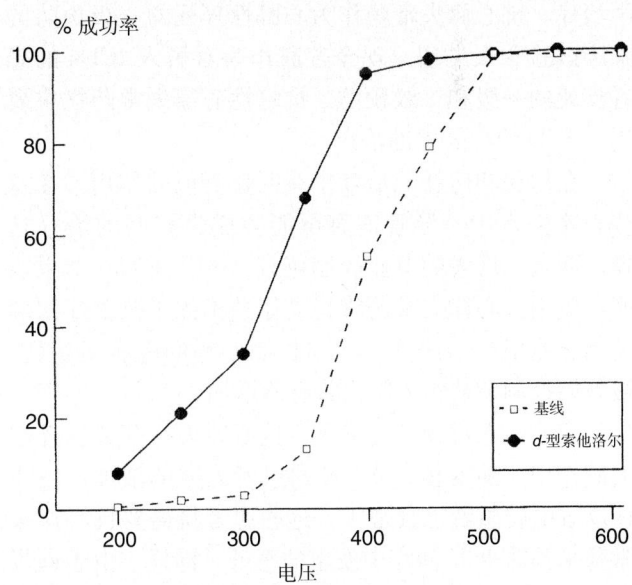

图101-5 右旋索他洛尔对除颤阈值的影响 图为对比右旋索他洛尔前后不同能量的除颤成功率。(引自 Dorian P, Newman D, Sheahan R, et al: d-sotalol decreases defibrillation energy requirements in humans: A novel indication for drug therapy. J Cardiovasc Electrophysiol 7: 952-961, 1996.)

或剂量改变之后。尖端扭转性室性心动过速在女性中更常见。其他易致心律失常的因素包括剂量超过320mg/d、心衰和血清肌酐基线水平升高者[54]。

许多内科医生认为，开展索他洛尔疗法的医院，应该配备有心电监护和具备复苏人员和器械。有资料支持这种建议。该资料表明，在治疗早期发生心动过缓或尖端扭转型室性心动过速的风险最高。对所选择的低风险患者，用索他洛尔治疗可能比较安全[56]。

（五）当前治疗学中的作用

索他洛尔兼有Ⅲ类和Ⅱ类抗心律失常药的效能和不良反应。它可用于房性和室性心律失常，但不如胺碘酮有效。然而，索他洛尔产生的心脏外不良反应更容易控制，并且它的不良反应并非直接与累积量相关，故对可能最终需要数十年疗程的年轻患者来说，作为一线治疗药物与胺碘酮相比更具吸引力。由于它能降低除颤阈值，这使它成为预防植入ICDs病人发生室性心律失常的首选药（在无禁忌证时）。但它有相对较高的致心律失常风险，以及β肾上腺素能阻滞的副作用，要求人们慎用。

五、Ⅲ类抗心律失常药的发展趋势

室性心律失常治疗正在从药物学治疗转向非药物学治疗。抗心律失常药作为心脏性猝死的一级预防的临床试验令人失望。现今普遍作为对植入ICDs的患者猝死的一级和二级预防。抗室性心律失常药物主要用于ICD治疗的辅助治疗。

在房颤和房扑的治疗中有明显类似的作用。在这些心律失常中，导管消融可能会成为较好的治疗选择。而且，房颤的节律控制调查（AFFIRM）结果表明，应用抗心律失常药维持窦律并不优于抗凝疗法和控制心室率[57]。事实上，与控制心率的患者组相比，被施以控制节律组入院人数有所增加。

然而，在可预见的未来，抗心律失常药会发挥更大的作用。随着植入ICDs的患者人数的增加，发生ICD放电的患者也会增加。这些患者将需要抗心律失常药来预防ICD治疗中发生的意外。同样，由于尚没有非药物学治疗房颤的可靠疗法，仍然需要应用抗心律失常药。尽管控制心室率可能在治疗房颤上更有益，但许多内科医生可能更愿选择转复窦律。即使心室率得到适当的控制，一些患者仍表现出症状。某些资料表明，维持窦性心律，患者生活质量会更高[58]。对这些患者来说，仅控制节律的策略并不令人满意，需用抗心律失常药维持窦律。

在对有效的抗心律失常药的需求推动下，Ⅲ类药将继续得到发展。最近多非利特获得FDA批准，用于治疗房颤。阿齐利特、替地沙米、决奈达隆和氨巴利特正在开发研究中。由于这些药物的致尖端扭转型室性心动过速的风险和它们相对较窄的治疗窗，需要慎重选择治疗对象，制订适宜剂量并要进行随访[5]。同时需要研究药物作用的新的分子靶位（如I_{Ks}、I_{to}和I_{Kur}），以期在降低药物致心律失常作用下发挥最大的抗心律失常作用。

（楚英杰　译）

参 考 文 献

1. Kaumann AJ, Olson CB: Temporal relation between long-lasting aftercontractions and action potential in cat papillary muscles. Science 161:293–295, 1968.
2. Singh BN, Vaughan-Williams EM: A third class of anti-arrhythmic action: Effects on atrial and ventricular intracellular potentials, and other pharmacological action on cardiac muscle, of MJ 1999 and AH 3474. Br J Pharmacol 39:675–687 1970.
3. Ackerman MJ: The long QT syndrome: Ion channel diseases of the heart. Mayo Clin Proc 73:250–269, 1998.
4. Kowey PR, Marinchak RA, Rials SJ, Bharucha D: Pharmacologic and pharmacokinetic profile of class III antiarrhythmic drugs. Am J Cardiol 80:16G–23G, 1997.
5. Castro A, Bianconi L, Santini M: New antiarrhythmic drugs for the treatment of atrial fibrillation. Pacing Clin Electrophysiol 25:249–259, 2002.
6. Kodama I, Kamiya K, Toyama J: Cellular electropharmacology of amiodarone. Cardiovasc Res 35:13–29, 1997.
7. Kamiya K, Nishiyama A, Yasui K, et al: Short- and long-term effects of amiodarone on the two components of cardiac delayed rectifier K$^+$ current. Circulation 103:1317–1324, 2001.
8. Harjai KJ, Licata AA: Effects of amiodarone on thyroid function. Ann Intern Med 126:68–73, 1997.
9. Guo W, Kamiya K, Toyama J: Evidences of antagonism between amiodarone and triiodothyronine on the K$^+$ channel activities of cultured rat cardiomyocytes. J Mol Cell Cardiol 29:617–627, 1997.
10. Podrid PJ: Amiodarone: Reevaluation of an old drug. Ann Intern Med 122:689–700, 1995.
11. Venkatesh N, Padbury JF, Singh BN: Effects of amiodarone and desethyamiodarone on rabbit myocardial beta-adrenoceptors and serum thyroid hormones—Absence of relationship to serum and myocardial drug concentrations. J Cardiovasc Pharmacol 8:989–997, 1986.
12. The CASCADE Investigators: Randomized antiarrhythmic drug therapy in survivors of cardiac arrest (the CASCADE study). Am J Cardiol 72:280–287, 1993.
13. Julian DG, Camm AJ, Frangin G, et al: Randomised trial of effect of amiodarone on mortality in patients with left-ventricular dysfunction after recent myocardial infarction: EMIAT. Lancet 349:667–674, 1997.
14. Cairns JA, Connolly Stuart J, Roberts R, et al: Randomised trial of outcome after myocardial infarction in patients with frequent or repetitive ventricular premature depolarisations: CAMIAT. Lancet 349:675–682, 1997.
15. Doval HC, Nul DR, Grancelli HO, et al: Randomised trial of low dose amiodarone in severe congestive heart failure. Lancet 344:493–498, 1994.
16. Singh SN, Fletcher RD, Fisher SG, et al: Amiodarone in patients with congestive heart failure and asymptomatic ventricular arrhythmia. N Engl J Med 333:77–82, 1995.

17. Sim I, McDonald KM, Lavori PW, et al: Quantitative overview of randomized trials of amiodarone to prevent sudden cardiac death. Circulation 96:2823–2829, 1997.
18. Amiodarone Trials Meta-Analysis Investigators: Effect of prophylactic amiodarone on mortality after acute myocardial infarction and congestive heart failure: Meta-analysis of individual data from 6500 patients and randomised trials. Lancet 350:1417–1424, 1997.
19. Goldschlager N, Epstein AE, Naccarelli G, et al: Practical guidelines for clinicians who treat patients with amiodarone. Arch Intern Med 160:1741–1748, 2000.
20. The Antiarrhythmics versus Implantable Defibrillators (AVID) Investigators: A comparison of antiarrhythmic-drug therapy with implantable defibrillators in patients resuscitated from near-fatal ventricular arrhythmias. N Engl J Med 337:1576–1583, 1997.
21. Moss AJ, Hall WJ, Cannom DS, et al: Improved survival with an implanted defibrillator in patients with coronary disease at high risk for ventricular arrhythmia. N Engl J Med 335:1933–1940, 1996.
22. Buxton AE, Lee K, L, Fisher JD, et al: A randomized study of the prevention of sudden death in patients with coronary artery disease. N Engl J Med 341:1882–1890, 1999.
23. Kowey PR, Levine JH, Herre JM, et al: Randomized, double-blind comparison of intravenous amiodarone and bretylium in the treatment of patients with recurrent hemodynamically destabilizing ventricular tachycardia or fibrillation. Circulation 92:3255–3263, 1995.
24. Dorian P, Cass D, Schwartz B, et al: Amiodarone as compared with lidocaine for shock-resistant ventricular fibrillation. N Engl J Med 346:884–890, 2001.
25. Roy D, Talajic M, Dorian P, et al: Amiodarone to prevent recurrence of atrial fibrillation. N Engl J Med 342:913–920, 2000.
26. Giri S, White CM, Dunn AB, et al: Oral amiodarone for prevention of atrial fibrillation after open heart surgery, the atrial fibrillation suppression trial (AFIST): A randomized placebo-controlled trial. Lancet 357:830–836, 2001.
27. Singh BN: Antiarrhythmic actions of amiodarone: A profile of a paradoxical agent. Am J Cardiol 78:41–53, 1997.
28. Vorperian VR, Havighurst TC, Miller S, January CT: Adverse effects of low dose amiodarone: A meta-analysis. J Am Coll Cardiol 30:791–798, 1997.
29. Drouin E, Lande G, Charpentier F: Amiodarone reduces transmural heterogeneity of repolarization in the human heart. J Am Coll Cardiol 32:1063–1067, 1998.
30. Kharabsheh S, Abendroth CS, Kozak M: Fatal pulmonary toxicity occurring within two weeks of initiation of amiodarone. Am J Cardiol 89:896–898, 2002.
31. Siniakowicz RM: Diagnosis of amiodarone pulmonary toxicity with high-resolution computerized tomographic scan. J Cardiovasc Electrophysiol 12:431–436, 2000.
32. Jafari-Fesharaki M, Scheinman MM: Adverse effects of amiodarone. Pacing Clin Electrophysiol 21:108–120, 1998.
33. Goichot B, Grunenberger F, Schlienger J-L: Amiodarone-induced hyperthyroidism. Arch Intern Med 161:295, 2001.
34. Stanbury JB, Ermans AE, Bourdoux P, et al: Iodine-induced hyperthyroidism: Occurrence and epidemiology. Thyroid 8:83–100, 1998.
35. Harjai KJ, Licata AA: Amiodarone induced hyperthyroidism: A case series and brief review of the literature. Pacing Clin Electrophysiol 19:1548–1554, 1996.
36. High WA, Weiss SD: Pigmentation related to amiodarone. N Engl J Med 354:1464, 2001.
37. Pelosi F, Oral H, Kim MH, et al: Effect of chronic amiodarone therapy on defibrillation energy requirements in humans. J Cardiovasc Electrophysiol 11:736–740, 2000.
38. Lee KS, Lee EW: Ionic mechanism of ibutilide in human atrium: Evidence for a drug-induced Na^+ current through a nifedipine inhibited inward channel. J Pharmacol Exp Ther 286:9–22, 1998.
39. Sato N, Tanaka H, Habuchi Y, Giles WR: Electrophysiological effects of ibutilide on the delayed rectifier K^+ current in rabbit sinoatrial and atrioventricular node cells. Eur J Pharmacol 404:281–288, 2000.
40. Murray KT: Ibutilide. Circulation 97:493–497, 1998.
41. Ellenbogan KA, Stambler BS, Wood MA, et al: Efficacy of intravenous ibutilide for rapid termination of atrial fibrillation and atrial flutter: A dose-response study. J Am Coll Cardiol 28:130–136, 1996.
42. Stambler BS, Wood MA, Ellenbogen KA, et al: Efficacy and safety of repeated intravenous doses of ibutilide for rapid conversion of atrial flutter or fibrillation. Circulation 94:1613–1621, 1996.
43. Stambler BS, Wood MA, Ellenbogan KA: Comparative efficacy of intravenous ibutilide versus procainamide for enhancing termination
44. Oral H, Souza JJ, Michaud GF, et al: Facilitating transthoracic cardioversion of atrial fibrillation with ibutilide pretreatment. N Engl J Med 340:1849–1854, 1999.
45. Murdock DK, Schumock GT, Kaliebe J, et al: Clinical and cost comparison of ibutilide and direct current cardioversion for atrial fibrillation and flutter. Am J Cardiol 85:503–506, 2000.
46. Anderson JL, Prystowsky EN: Sotolol: An important new antiarrhythmic drug. Am Heart J 137:388–409, 1999.
47. Waldo AL, Camm AJ, deRuyter H, et al: Effect of d-sotalol on mortality in patient with left ventricular dysfunction after recent and remote myocardial infarction. The SWORD investigators. Survival With Oral d-Sotalol. Lancet 348:7–12, 1996.
48. Pacifico A, Hohnloser SH, Williams JH, et al: Prevention of implantable-defibrillator shocks by treatment with sotalol. N Engl J Med 340:1855–1862, 1999.
49. Dorian P, Newman D, Sheahan R, et al: d-Sotalol decreases defibrillation energy requirements in humans: A novel indication for drug therapy. J Cardiovasc Electrophysiol 7:952–961, 1996.
50. Gallik DM, Kim SG, Ferrick KJ, et al: Efficacy and safety of sotalol in patients with refractory atrial fibrillation or flutter. Am Heart J 134:155–160, 1997.
51. Benditt DG, Williams JH, Jin J, et al: Maintenance of sinus rhythm with oral d,l-sotalol therapy in patients with symptomatic atrial fibrillation and/or flutter. Am J Cardiol 84:270–277, 1999.
52. Tsikouris JP, Cox CD: A review of class III antiarrhythmic agents for atrial fibrillation: Maintenance of normal sinus rhythm. Pharmacotherapy 21:1514–1529, 2001.
53. Sung RJ, Tan HL, Karagounis L, et al: Intravenous sotalol for the termination of supraventricular tachycardia and atrial fibrillation and flutter: A multicenter, randomized, double-blind placebo-controlled study. Am Heart J 129:739–748, 1995.
54. MacNeil DJ: The side effect profile of class III antiarrhythmic drugs: Focus on d,l-sotalol. Am J Cardiol 80:90G–98G, 1997.
55. Chung MK, Schweikert RA, Wilkoff BL, et al: Is hospital admission for initiation of antiarrhythmic therapy with sotalol for atrial arrhythmias required? Yield of in-hospital monitoring and prediction of risk for significant arrhythmia complications. J Am Coll Cardiol 32:169–176, 1998.
56. Zimetbaum PJ, Schreckengost V, Cohen DJ, et al: Evaluation of outpatient initiation of antiarrhythmic drug therapy in patients reverting to sinus rhythm after an episode of atrial fibrillation. Am J Cardiol 83:450–453, 1999.
57. The Atrial Fibrillation Follow-Up Investigation of Rhythm Management (AFFIRM) Investigators: A comparison of rate control and rhythm control in patients with atrial fibrillation. N Engl J Med 347:1825–1833, 2002.
58. Dorian P, Paquette M, Newman D, et al: Quality of life improves with treatment in the Canadian Trial of Atrial Fibrillation. Am Heart J 143: 984–990, 2002.

第 102 章

腺苷与地高辛

John P. DiMarco

本章目录
- 腺苷 922
- 地高辛 926

一、腺苷

腺苷是一种内源性核苷,它是一种重要的生化介质,对许多器官起生理学调节作用,并且是一种具有很多临床用途的药剂[1-3]。本章讨论腺苷的细胞和临床电生理学效应以及它作为一种抗心律失常制剂的当代角色。

(一) 生理学

腺苷在心脏的生成有两条路径(图 102-1)。单磷酸腺苷(adenosine monophosphate,AMP)能通过 $5'$-核苷酸酶的作用经去磷酸化而生成腺苷。另一条路径为:在 S-高半胱氨酸腺苷水解酶的作用下使 S-高半胱氨酸腺苷与腺苷的可逆性转化。这两条路径对腺苷生成的作用,在不同的生理条件下有所不同。当心肌缺血或缺氧时使两条路径的活性增加。腺苷转运至细胞外以及从细胞间质的重摄取是由一个有效的转运系统介导的。腺苷通过脱氨化而降解为肌苷。

某些腺苷受体亚型已被识别:A_1、A_{2A}、A_{2B} 和 A_3。腺苷 A_1 受体看来像是负责腺苷的心脏电生理和变力效应的亚型。A_1 受体是一个 326-氨基酸多肽,其分子量为 36.6kD。业已证实:随着暴露于兴奋剂和阻断剂时间的延长,会发生腺苷受体上调和下调的反应。在人类心脏移植后,心脏对腺苷的敏感性增加已被证实[3-4]。

腺苷的电生理作用是由一个受体-效应器复合物介导的,该复合物包括 A_1 受体和一个鸟苷酸结合 G 蛋白(表 102-1)。腺苷受体激活时所产生的效应被定义为直接效应或间接效应。直接效应能使钾离子外流(I_{KAdo});间接效应是由抑制腺苷酸环化酶所介导的,可导致细胞内环磷酸腺苷(cAMP)浓度降低(表 102-1)。腺苷和乙酰胆碱对心脏产生相似的 G 蛋白介导效应,但乙酰胆碱是与一种不同的膜蛋白受体(M_2)相结合的。

腺苷的主要直接作用是激活钾离子外流(I_{KAdo}),这在窦房结、心房和房室结均有表现,但在心室肌细胞无此表现[1,5]。对窦房结和房室结细胞起搏离子流(I_f)的抑制以及对无刺激状态下基础钙离子内流(I_{Ca})的轻微抑制,也是腺苷对心房肌细胞的直接效应。钾离子外流的激活能导致心房肌动作电位的缩短和膜的超极化。对房室结细胞,腺苷直接减小房室结的动作电位峰值。对窦房结,腺苷直接减慢窦性心率,并引起起搏点替换以及窦房结细胞的超极化。

腺苷的间接作用是由于细胞内 cAMP 生成的抑制而产生的。这个因素会导致儿茶酚胺刺激的内向钙离子流(I_{Ca})和一过性内向离子流(transient inward current,I_{Ti})的减少。负性变时效应是通过抑制起搏离子流(I_f)而产生的。腺苷的这些抗肾上腺素能效应具有一些抗心律失常的作用,所有起搏点频率均被抑制,且受儿茶酚胺刺激的迟后除极和早后除极被抑制。在临床研究中,某些儿茶酚胺介导的房性和室性心律失常被终止或被抑制。其他由异丙肾上腺素刺激的离子流也同样被腺苷阻断。目前有许多将开发的腺苷类药物用于治疗的努力正在进行当中。其中,有一

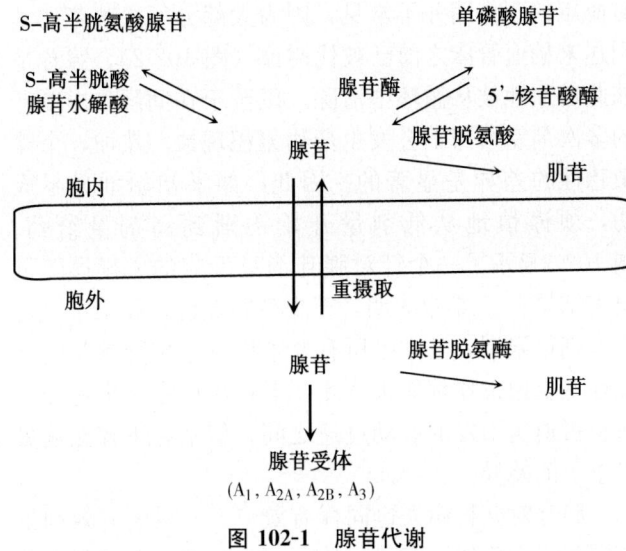

图 102-1 腺苷代谢

表 102-1　腺苷对离子流的效应

	主要	次要
直接作用*	↑I_{KAdo}	↓I_{Ca}
		↓I_f
间接作用*	↓I_{Ca}	↓I_{Cl}
	↓I_f	↓I_{Ks}
		↓I_{Ti}

*直接作用不要求儿茶酚胺刺激，而间接作用仅见于儿茶酚胺刺激；
↑I_{KAdo}在心室没有表现。

种合成物（CVT-510，Cardiovascular Theraputics Palo Alto，California 公司生产）作为房室结阻断剂已被用于动物实验和早期的临床研究[6,7]。

（二）临床电生理学

20 世纪初，腺苷就被证实有减慢房室传导的作用。在一些欧洲国家，由于错误地相信高能磷酸键的水解会给心脏传递一个化学性复律并重整窦性心律，因此三磷酸腺苷（adenosine triphosphate，ATP）也被用于终止阵发性室上性心动过速（paroxysmal supraventricular tachycardia，PSVT）[3]。有趣的是腺苷的电生理作用是由于腺苷聚积在缺氧和缺血的心肌组织而使房室结传导延长[1]。在离体猪心造成缺氧，由于组织氧分压减低，可发生房室结传导时间延长。如用双嘧达莫阻断腺苷重摄取可使细胞外腺苷增多而具有此效应，且该效应可被有阻断 A_1 受体作用的甲基黄嘌呤类药物或腺苷脱氨酶所逆转。此外，在一些临床试验中已经显示，氨茶碱逆转了一些前壁心肌梗死病人的持续性房室结阻滞，因此猜测这些腺苷的作用有临床相关性。

DiMarco 等[8]系统地研究了腺苷注射剂量对人体的效应。他们发现，给正在进行电生理检测的病人快速静脉注射腺苷，会导致一过性（小于 10s）窦性心率减慢，伴有或不伴有房室结阻滞，随之出现短阵（15～45s）窦性心动过速。如果在心房起搏时给予腺苷，可以观察到一个典型的 A-H 间期文氏延长而不伴有 HV 延长。窦性心率减慢和房室结阻滞的剂量要求是相似的。腺苷的负性变时和变导效应是由它的直接和间接作用引发的，因而也受自主神经张力的调节[9]。腺苷该效应对房室结双路径的病人，逆传快径不如前传慢径敏感[10,11]。腺苷对人类低位起搏点的作用是间接的，即对交界区和心室起搏点仅有次要效应。单相动作电位（monophasic action potential，MAP）记录能用于研究腺苷对心房和心室肌的效应。对心房，腺苷能缩短其 MAP 间期和有效不应期[12]。在心室则未见到 MAP 持续性改变。实际上，如果在 MAP 缩短期间导入单个房性早搏，所有病人都能诱发出心房颤动。预激综合征的病人可见几种不同的腺苷反应模式[13]。大部分旁路传导不被腺苷所阻断。如果在心房起搏下注射腺苷，由于房室结传导被选择性延长，体表心电图可以观察到预激成分的增加。但有一些旁路的有效不应期可以缩短。大多数伴有隐匿性旁路的病人，在给予腺苷后可见房室阻滞，但前向旁路传导可能被显露出来。也有报道，腺苷可阻断一些病人的旁路传导，大部分，但不是全部，这些腺苷敏感旁路或者有长的不应期或者表现为长的传导时间[13]。

当腺苷持续给药而不是快速注射时，可以观察到一个不同系列的作用[14,15]。腺苷注射会导致窦性心率的增快，并且由于降低舒张压而使脉压轻微增宽。窦性心率减慢和房室阻滞仅见于药物性或自发性自主神经阻滞或功能不全的背景下。窦性心动过速似乎是由肾上腺素能反射所引发，而肾上腺素能反射被认为是由于激活了主动脉弓化学感受器所致。可降低肺血管阻力和小范围的体循环血管阻力。

（三）临床药理学

一旦注射入血，腺苷能通过细胞吸收和酶的代谢而被迅速清除。但由于腺苷也可以由血小板产生和释放，所以很难测算其在血中的清除半衰期，估计在 0.5～5s 之间[1,3]。因此，从外周给予一次剂量的腺苷，在其到达心脏之前基本上已被清除。药剂的效应仅见于其首次通过循环的阶段。因为腺苷的清除速率如此迅速，相对来说，在注射部位和推注速度以及循环时间上的细微差异都会影响病人对所给药剂的反应。对同一病人进行序列剂量对比和对不同病人间的反应进行对比显示，这两者都是正确的。如果选择中心静脉作为注射部位，则对任何效应所要求的剂量都要更小一些[3]。临床上，相关的药物相互作用可见于双嘧达莫与甲基黄嘌呤类药物，其中双嘧达莫通过阻断腺苷的细胞吸收而使其产生腺苷样效应，而甲基黄嘌呤类药物则为腺苷受体 A_1 和 A_2 的阻滞剂。

（四）阵发性室上性心动过速：房室结折返和房室折返

因为阵发性室上性心动过速的两种常见类型——房室结折返和房室折返，都要求完整的房室结传导以使心动过速持续，所以阻断房室结的药物和生理性动作都能终止这些类型的心律失常。当腺苷的主要作用被认识后，它作为一种终止阵发性室上速急性发作的药物经受了检测。在一些地区，ATP 也被用于此目的，不过其主要作用是通过代谢为腺苷而产生的。

在房室结折返性心动过速，腺苷通常阻滞部位是在房室结前传慢径。此外，给予腺苷也常常能引发可以终止心动过速的房性和室性早搏。对房室结传导进行阻滞，也是终止房室折返性心动过速的通常机制。这与药物的已知药代动力学特性相吻合。通常阵发性室上性心动过速的终止发生在注射药物后 15~35s 时。

对血压的副作用并不常见，因为大部分所给腺苷在其到达末梢血管床之前已被代谢掉（图 102-2）。腺苷是如此迅速地被从循环中清除，以至于在间隔 30s 以上的多次剂量给药不会发生药物累积现象。然而，个体敏感性的差异是显著的。因此，如果初始剂量不成功，须谨慎地从低剂量开始逐渐到高剂量给药。图 102-3 显示了一个针对腺苷剂量反应的大规模随机研究结果[16]。结果表明，至少简明地说，如果不执行最大剂量限制，基本上所有要求房室结传导参与的阵发性室上速发作都能被终止。但在由房室结折返和由房室折返所引发的心动过速之间，似乎并不存在剂量要求上的差异。

腺苷对儿科病人也同样有效[3]。儿科的有效剂量范围与成人相似：37.5~300μg/kg。对婴儿和新生儿来说，腺苷的最大优点是不会发生血流动力学的降低，而这正是使用维拉帕米的潜在并发症。

（五）对比试验

有几项试验对比研究了腺苷和维拉帕米的功效[3,16]。其中，在一项随机试验中，对比研究了腺苷的两个序列剂量（6mg，12mg）和维拉帕米的两个序列剂量（5mg，然后 7.5mg），结果显示，腺苷的有效率为 57% 和 93%，而维拉帕米的有效率为 81% 和 91%[16]。阵发性室上速的再发在腺苷组稍显普遍（9% 比 3%，P 值无显著性差异）。

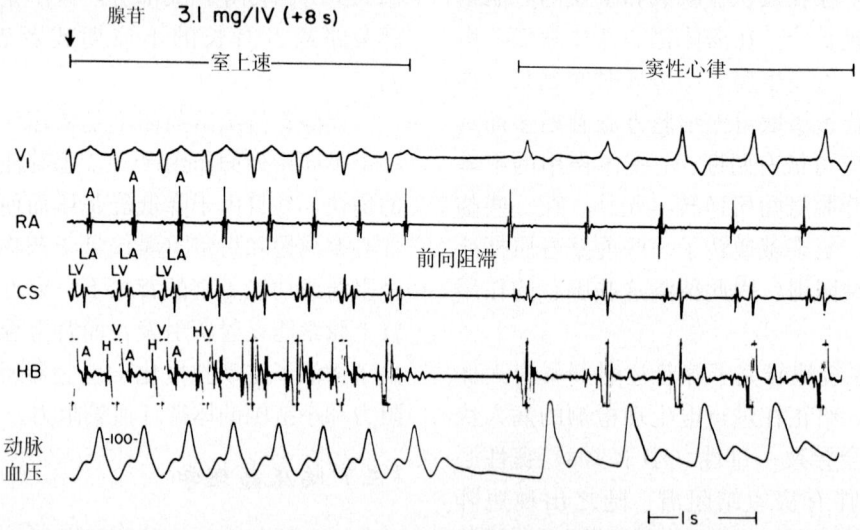

图 102-2　腺苷终止房室折返性心动过速　本图从上至下显示为体表 V_1 导联和心内记录的右心房（RA）、冠状窦（CS）标测的左心房（LA）和左心室（LV）信号、希氏束（HB）以及桡动脉压。腺苷通过阻断房室结传导而终止心动过速。当恢复正常窦性心律（NSR）时，可见血压升高和预激波出现。（引自 DiMarco JP, Sellers TD, Berne RM, et al: Adenosine: Electrophysiologic effects and therapeutic use for terminating paroxysmal supraventricular tachycardia. Circulation 68：1254-1263, 1983. Copyright 1983, American Heart Association.）

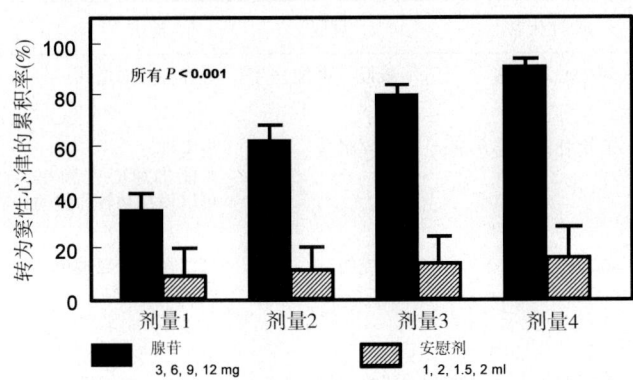

图 102-3 腺苷的剂量反应 所显示的资料来自于一个有四组腺苷剂量的安慰剂对照试验。（引自 DiMarco PJ，Miles W，Akhtar M，et al：Adenosine for paroxysmal supraventricular tachycardia：Dose ranging and comparison with verapamil in placebo-controlled，multicenter trials. Ann Intern Med 113：104-110，1990.）

这些对比试验资料提示：对于大多数病例，当终止阵发性室上速时，既可将腺苷作为首选也可将非二氢吡啶类钙通道阻滞剂作为首选（表 102-2）。对于严重左室功能不全、近期接受静脉 β 受体阻滞剂以及新生儿病人，偏向使用腺苷；而钙通道阻滞剂则偏向用于那些正在接受已知对腺苷的作用或代谢有干扰的药物治疗的病人，如活动性支气管痉挛的病人以及静脉通道不适合快速静脉注射的病人。对于疑诊为阵发性室上速但不确切的病人，假如心律失常持续，腺苷对血压的影响较小。然而，腺苷能诱发各种心律失常（见后讨论），因此，并不鼓励将其不加选择地用于诊断目的。如果在用腺苷终止后阵发性室上速再发，重复注射相同剂量的腺苷或者转而使用钙通道阻滞剂都是合适的。

（六）副作用

在使用腺苷后，很多病人有面部发热、胸痛或胸闷以及呼吸困难等不适。尽管受治病人中有 30%～50%有反应，但这些副作用都是剂量相关性的，典型

表 102-2 阵发性室上性心动过速的药物选择

倾向腺苷	中立	倾向维拉帕米/地尔硫䓬
低血压	通常 PSVT	静脉通道困难
新生儿		PSVT 再发
电生理检测		双嘧达莫
静脉使用 β 受体阻滞剂		茶碱
诊断不确定		支气管痉挛
心衰		

症状是短暂而轻微的，且仅在很少而有限的治疗中出现。这些副作用的产生可能有几种机制，毒蕈碱、β 肾上腺素能受体阻滞剂或者纳洛酮不能预防胸痛或胸闷。双嘧达莫能使疼痛增加而茶碱能使疼痛减弱，提示涉及对腺苷受体的直接效应。腺苷通过化学感受器的激活而使呼吸加快。吸入腺苷可以导致一些哮喘病人发生支气管痉挛。面部发热可能是由皮肤血管扩张所致，而这要部分归因于末梢交感神经释放的增加。

（七）致心律失常作用

阵发性室上速在被腺苷终止时，常常可以见到不明机制的频发房性或室性早搏，而这些早搏可能确实对心律失常的终止起部分作用。但更严重的致心律失常作用形式已经被报道。当腺苷终止阵发性室上速时，通常被注意到的是短暂的窦性心动过缓、窦性静止或房室阻滞。对存在心动过缓风险的心律失常患者，可以导致严重的后果。多形性室性心动过速在伴有或不伴有长 QT 间期的病人中都有报道[3]。

腺苷能缩短心房动作电位时间，而配对间期缩短的房性早搏或室性早搏逆传都能诱发心房颤动[12,13]。Glatter 等[13]报道，有 15% 的房室折返或房性心动过速的患者发生心房颤动，而房室结折返患者则未见发生。Strickberger 等[17]报道，在 200 例无显著性风险差异的房室结折返和房室折返性阵发性室上速患者中，心房颤动的发生率为 12%。而对于 WPW 综合征的患者，因为腺苷既不影响也不缩短旁道前传不应期，心房颤动的诱发只是潜在的危险。对于房性心律失常的患者，在继发性肾上腺素能张力增加期间，会发生加速性心室反应[13]。因为所涉及的传导路径的传导特性产生一过性不均衡，所以腺苷可以有效地激发诱发困难的房室结折返性心动过速[11]。

（八）其他房性心律失常

腺苷对其他房性心律失常的效应是不一致的[13,18]。在伴有心房颤动、心房扑动以及折返性房性心动过速的病人中，大部分对腺苷的反应是一过性房室阻滞。此外，还可以观察到有些心房周长的改变。而在窦房结折返的病例中，心动过速终止和伴随房室阻滞的心动过速持续，两者均有报道。对这些房性心动过速所显示的各种反应，既有一过性终止、伴随房室阻滞的心动过速持续，也可能无效[12,13]。腺苷对长

RP'型心动过速有效,此类心动过速既可用房室结慢径也可用慢传导旁道作为逆传支[13]。因为这两种心动过速的终止通常都发生在逆传阻滞,所以腺苷对区别这两种机制并无帮助。

(九) 室性心动过速

除了能确实抑制受儿茶酚胺刺激的钙离子流外,腺苷对人类心室肌细胞并无直接作用[1]。在先前的试验中,腺苷抑制由异丙肾上腺素导致的迟后除极和早后除极,但并不抑制由奎尼丁导致的早后除极和由哇巴因导致的迟后除极[1]。Lerman 等[19]首先描述了一组反复持续性室性心动过速的病人对腺苷有反应。这些病人的心动过速常与活动和精神紧张相关,且这些病人并无器质性心脏病。此类心律失常的典型 QRS 波群形态为左束支阻滞伴电轴不偏,但其他形态也有报道。在电生理检查中,心动过速既要求也可有效地被异丙肾上腺素所诱发。这些心动过速能被多种措施诱发及终止:程序刺激、使用腺苷或维拉帕米,以及迷走神经刺激等。基于这些观察,此类心动过速可被假设为:由源于 cAMP 介导的触发活动而产生的迟后除极所诱发。因此,此类心律失常能被细胞内钙超载所诱发,这就可以解释各种药理学反应和电生理学表现。现在还不清楚的是,为什么此类心动过速主要发生在心脏结构正常的个体,或者为什么大多数发生在右室流出道的一个相对小的解剖区域内。Lerman 等[20]在一位此型心动过速病人的组织标本中发现了体细胞突变。该突变位于一个抑制 G 蛋白($G_{\alpha i2}$)的三磷酸鸟苷结合区。

腺苷并不能终止陈旧性心肌梗死或其他类型器质性心脏病病人的反复性室性心动过速。

(十) 诊断性用途

宽 QRS 波群心动过速的误诊仍然是临床上的常见问题。因为腺苷的电生理作用范围具有良好的特征(表102-3),所以腺苷注射有助于诊断目的[21,22]。此用途的局限性包括:有导致房性心律失常引起快速心室反应的风险、诱发心房颤动的可能以及某些室性心动过速是腺苷敏感性的。尽管腺苷可能在某些情况下有助于临床鉴别诊断,但它并不能用以替代仔细的心电图分析和临床判断。经验丰富的心电图医师基本不用腺苷的诊断性帮助[21]。此外,腺苷对房性心律失常的作用可变性太大,以至于不能提供有关心律失常机制的确切信息。有报道提出,腺苷注射对窦房结功

表 102-3 各种心动过速对腺苷的反应

心律失常	反应	备注
窦性心动过速	减慢,可能房室阻滞	继发性心率增加
心房扑动、心房颤动	房室阻滞	继发性 可能加速心室频率、可以使扑动转为颤动
心房内折返	可变的	可以在一个缓慢传导区发生阻滞
房室结折返、房室折返、窦房结折返	终止	
其他房性心动过速	可变的	可能减慢、终止或者无影响,可见房室阻滞
预激性房性心律失常	增加预激	可能加速
室性心动过速 伴器质性心脏病 不伴器质性心脏病	无效 可变的	特发性右室流出道心动过速可终止

能不全的病人[23]以及对正在行直立倾斜试验的神经心源性晕厥病人[24,25]具有诊断价值。

二、地高辛

强心苷已经被医师使用了几个世纪。强心苷是一个与甾核相连接的环形分子——苷元和附着于一个内酯环上的 1/4 糖分子的结合物。糖分子和附着的氢氧基团决定其药代动力学特征,而其药理学效应则由苷元介导。地高辛是当代最常应用的强心苷制剂。尽管由于其他房室结阻滞剂的发展而使地高辛抗心律失常的作用变小,但它仍然有广泛的用途[26]。

(一) 生理学

多个研究业已证实了地高辛对心力衰竭病人的作用,即地高辛对死亡率无影响但降低住院率[27,28]。地高辛的主要抗心律失常作用是由其增加中枢和周围迷走神经张力的作用所介导的[28]。尽管对房室结和心房的直接作用已经被证实,但这些作用仅见于那些临床上所达到的药物浓度水平。在中毒浓度,地高辛增加交感神经张力并增加细胞内钙负荷,从而导致自律性和迟后除极增加。地高辛直接抑制钠-钾三磷酸腺苷泵,并能通过改变慢钙通道和抑制钠-钙交换而使细胞内钙浓度增加。这些作用改变了兴奋-收缩耦联并被认为是强心苷的正性肌力作用的机制。

（二）临床电生理学

地高辛的电生理作用源于迷走神经张力的增加[28]。在房室结，传导被减慢而有效不应期被延长。大多数个体的窦房结自律性不受影响或被轻微减慢，但有时窦房结功能不全的病人会表现出更显著的效应。在心房，迷走神经张力增加会导致不应期缩短和更快的传导。在中毒浓度，室上性组织和心室组织两者的自律性均被增加。地高辛缩短某些旁路的不应期，因而不建议用于显性预激病人。地高辛对持续性心房颤动的作用是有争议的。Duytschaever 等[29]发现，地高辛对山羊模型的心房颤动频率和稳定性没有影响。相反，Tieleman 等[30]在山羊模型中和 Sticherling 等[31]在病人中发现，地高辛加大了心房不应期的缩短程度，并使心房颤动倾向于再发。

在治疗性血浆浓度时，地高辛仅有轻微的电生理作用。除非存在窦房结和房室结疾病时，否则窦性周长、PR 间期和 QRS 间期通常保持不变。在心房颤动的病人中，平均 PR 间期增加、ST 段和 T 波电压降低[32]。对发生于地高辛中毒背景下的心律失常于本章稍后讨论。

（三）临床药理学

地高辛在胃和小肠被吸收[28]。标准片剂的口服生物利用度为 60%～80%。人们注意到凝胶或药液胶囊有更完全的吸收。一些药物，包括考来烯胺、考来替泊、抗酸剂、高岭土以及硫糖铝，通过在肠腔内与地高辛结合而降低其吸收率。肠道吸收网受多药物转运系统 P-糖蛋白的调控[33]。被吸收的地高辛再通过 P-糖蛋白被排泄回肠道。抑制此系统会导致生物利用度增加和中毒的可能，并从胃肠到组织的分布被延迟，且要达到血浆浓度和组织浓度间的平衡需 6～8h。因此，血浆浓度测定至少应在最后一次剂量的 6h 之后进行。地高辛的清除是通过肾排泄途径并再次涉及到 P-糖蛋白。肾功能正常病人的地高辛清除半衰期大约为 36h，而尿毒症病人的半衰期则为 3.5～5d。治疗要求的血浆浓度范围为 0.8～2.0ng/ml。

许多抗心律失常药都影响地高辛的药代动力学[28]。奎尼丁从组织结合部位置换地高辛。通过抑制 P-糖蛋白系统，奎尼丁能提高地高辛的生物利用度并降低肾清除，从而增加地高辛的血浆浓度。胺碘酮、普罗帕酮以及维拉帕米都降低其肾清除和非肾清除率。此外，环孢素、一些抗病毒药和抗真菌药以及苯二氮䓬类药物也能通过与 P-糖蛋白系统的相互作用而显著增加地高辛的血浆浓度。

（四）抗心律失常用途

地高辛作为一种抗心律失常药的主要作用是用于控制房性快速性心律失常的心室率。因为地高辛是通过增加基础副交感神经张力而发挥其主要效应的，所以在运动、生理性紧张以及其他交感神经张力增加的期间，地高辛的价值有限。

最多被描述的地高辛治疗的心律失常是心房颤动。Stafford 等[26]发现，地高辛的使用正在减少但仍然是主要的心率控制药物。在心律失常治疗的心房颤动随访调查（AFFIRM）的研究中[34]，地高辛作为用于心率控制目的的药物制剂的一部分，约有 70% 以上的病人服用地高辛。

地高辛如此广泛地被用于心房颤动的病人，并非因其优良的功效，而更多的是由于历史的因素和其有利的血流动力学一面。地高辛已经反复地被证实，对于心房颤动急性发作的病人转复为窦性心律的比率并无影响[35,36]。但对于急性心房颤动，有效的心率控制至少被推迟了 4～12h。不过钙通道阻滞剂和 β 肾上腺素能受体阻滞剂能提供更快更可靠的心率控制。联合应用地高辛和其中的一种制剂可能会有帮助，特别是对那些伴有收缩功能不全的病人[37]。缺镁的病人似乎有地高辛抵抗，而补镁对这些个体可能有帮助。

间歇发作的心房颤动病人常难以治疗，静息时窦性频率无法预测阵发性心房颤动时的心室率。心室率的范围可以从夜间的或迷走神经介导的缓慢到当肾上腺素能张力高时的非常快的情况。地高辛仅对快速心率产生控制，且从临床资料看，它对短阵心房颤动病人的用途并不合理[38]。

对伴有慢性持续性心房颤动的病人首选地高辛治疗。对持续性心房颤动的病人，控制心室率的治疗有以下目的：（1）避免由过度的心动过速而产生的症状；（2）避免可以产生心动过速性心肌病的持续心率增快；（3）允许分级运动时心率适应性增加。在处方治疗时，必须认识到无症状心房颤动病人通过控制心室率治疗后存在 24h 内心率波动范围较大的特点。RR 间期白天在 2.8s 以内而夜间在 4s 以内都被认为是正常的。

对老年人、相对久坐的持续性心房颤动病人，地高辛常常是唯一有效的控制心率药物。静息时心率低于 80～90 次/分和在适度步行时控制心率为 110

次/分或以下，这为治疗的力度提供了一个粗略的临床指南[34]。而对于伴有心悸、过度疲乏或运动受限症状的病人，心率控制的精确评估可能需要动态心电图监测或运动试验。

（五）副作用

一种更好地了解药代动力学并导入可替代的心率控制手段的方法是地高辛血浆浓度测定的应用。地高辛血浆浓度测定的应用已经降低了地高辛中毒发生的频率，但地高辛中毒仍然是一个重要的临床问题[39-41]。电解质异常、继发于年龄和疾病的肾功能改变、急性或慢性缺氧以及甲状腺疾病都是增加地高辛中毒风险的常见因素。地高辛中毒可能是心脏性或者是非心脏性的。

地高辛中毒的非心脏性表现有食欲减退、恶心和呕吐、头痛、抑郁以及包括视野缺失、散光和色盲在内的视力改变等。

心脏毒性可能由几种因素所致：对窦房结、房室结过度作用会导致心动过缓；细胞内钙超载会导致迟后除极和反复性发作；以及伴自主神经活性增加的中枢交感刺激。在高地高辛水平的病人中，几乎任何心律失常都发生过，但很多可能至少部分是由病人的基础疾病所致。有几种心律失常更特别地见于地高辛中毒。当发生高度房室阻滞伴加速性交界性心律失常或并行室性心动过速时强烈提示地高辛中毒。以往对伴有房室阻滞的房性心动过速被认为是地高辛中毒的诊断依据，但新近的研究提示，地高辛仅是多种原因中的一种。窦性心动过缓和室性异位心律是常发生在常规地高辛治疗的非特异性表现。

过量地高辛吸收伴很高的血浆浓度，会明显抑制钠-钾交换。这个问题会导致严重的有生命危险的电生理和血流动力学后果的高钾血症。

对明确或怀疑地高辛中毒病人的治疗基于其症状的严重性、当前血浆浓度、被吸收药物的量以及病人自己清除药物的能力。对无血流动力学后果的心律失常可以通过终止治疗和观察来处理。但应该纠正低钾血症和低镁血症。此外，利多卡因和苯妥英钠常被推荐使用是因为这些药对房室传导的影响有限，但并无对它们价值的系统研究。地高辛中毒背景下的电转复可以触发心室颤动，因而应避免对无生命危险的心动过速进行心脏转复。如果高钾血症存在于严重地高辛中毒的背景下，应避免使用钙剂，因为它可能因细胞内钙超载而引发心律失常。

大多数轻度或中度地高辛中毒的病人可以保守治疗，但对严重中毒病例，地高辛免疫Fab抗体治疗可能拯救生命[42,43]。特异性地高辛Fab片段是经山羊地高辛抗体的酶消化而产生的，且失活的复合物能从肾排泄。肾衰的病人不能自己清除该复合物并可以要求重复给药。由于地高辛的大量分布而使血浆置换作用有限[43]。抗体治疗后血浆地高辛监测是不可靠的，因为失活复合物能被大多数化验检测到。假如已经知道服用过量的严重意外或故意服用，则每吸收25片0.25mg片剂，应给予8~9小瓶地高辛特异片段。对慢性中毒状态，地高辛免疫片段的剂量，以38mg一小瓶的数量来表示，可以按以下公式估算：

$$被要求的瓶数 = \frac{稳态地高辛浓度（ng/ml）\times 体重（kg）}{100}$$

包括对地高辛Fab片段过敏反应在内的副作用都是不常见的。当地高辛的治疗作用被纠正时可见加速房室结传导。但用地高辛Fab抗体治疗非常昂贵，因此它的使用应该被限于明确的中毒情况下，这样它的使用才具有应有的价值。

（黄文新　译）

参考文献

1. Shyrock JC, Belardinelli L: Adenosine and adenosine receptors in the cardiovascular system: Biochemistry, physiology, and pharmacology. Am J Cardiol 79(12A):2–10, 1997.
2. Mubagwa K, Flameng W: Adenosine, adenosine receptors and myocardial protection: An updated overview. Cardiovasc Res 52:25–39, 2001.
3. Mangrum JM, DiMarco JP: Acute and chronic pharmacologic management of supraventricular tachyarrhythmias. In Antman EM (ed): Cardiovascular Therapeutics, 2nd ed. Philadelphia, WB Saunders, 2002, pp 423–444.
4. Bertolet BD, Eagle DA, Conti JB, et al: Bradycardia after heart transplantation: Reversal with theophylline. J Am Coll Cardiol 29:470–471, 1997.
5. Wang D, Shyrock JC, Belardinelli L: Cellular basis for the negative dromotropic effect of adenosine on rabbit single atrioventricular nodal cells. Circ Res 78:697–706, 1996.
6. Snowdy S, Liang HX, Blackburn B, et al: A comparison of the A_1 adenosine receptor agonist (CVT-510) with diltiazem for slowing of AV nodal conduction in guinea pig. Br J Pharmacol 126:137–146, 1999.
7. Lerman BB, Ellenbogen KA, Kadish A, et al: Electrophysiologic effects of a novel selective adenosine A_1 agonist (CVT-510) on atrioventricular nodal conduction in humans. J Cardiovasc Pharmacol Ther 6:237–245, 2001.
8. DiMarco JP, Sellers TD, Berne RM, et al: Adenosine: Electrophysiologic effects and therapeutic use for terminating paroxysmal supraventricular tachycardia. Circulation 68:1254–1263, 1983.
9. Kou WH, Man KC, Goyal R, et al: Interaction between autonomic tone and the negative dromotropic effect of adenosine in humans. Pacing Clin Electrophysiol 22:1792–1796, 1999.
10. Souza JJ, Zivin A, Fleming M, et al: Differential effect of adenosine on anterograde and retrograde fast pathway conduction in patients with atrioventricular nodal reentrant tachycardia. J Cardiovasc Electrophysiol 9:820–824, 1998.

11. Curtis AB, Belardinelli L, Woodard DA, et al: Induction of atrioventricular node reentrant tachycardia with adenosine: Differential effect of adenosine on fast and slow atrioventricular node pathways. J Am Coll Cardiol 30:1778–1784, 1997.
12. Tebbenjohanns J, Schumacher B, Pfeiffer D, et al: Dose and rate-dependent effects of adenosine on atrial action potential duration in humans. J Interv Card Electrophysiol 1:39–40, 1997.
13. Glatter KA, Cheng J, Dorostkar P, et al: Electrophysiologic effects of adenosine in patients with supraventricular tachycardia. Circulation 99:1034–1040, 1999.
14. Biaggioni I, Olafsson B, Robertson RM, et al: Cardiovascular and respiratory effects of adenosine in conscious man. Evidence for chemoreceptor activation. Circ Res 61:779–786, 1987.
15. Leppo J: Comparison of pharmacologic stress agents. J Nucl Cardiol 3:S22–S26, 1996.
16. DiMarco JP, Miles W, Akhtar M, et al: Adenosine for paroxysmal supraventricular tachycardia: Dose ranging and comparison with verapamil in placebo-controlled, multicenter trials. Ann Intern Med 113:104–110, 1990.
17. Strickberger SA, Man KC, Daoud EG, et al: Adenosine-induced atrial arrhythmia: A prospective analysis. Ann Intern Med 127:417–422, 1997.
18. Markowitz SM, Stein KM, Mittal S, et al: Differential effects of adenosine on focal and macroreentrant atrial tachycardia. J Cardiovasc Electrophysiol 10:489–492, 1999.
19. Lerman BB, Stein KM, Markowitz SM: Adenosine-sensitive ventricular tachycardia: A conceptual approach. J Cardiovasc Electrophysiol 7:559–569, 1996.
20. Lerman BB, Dong B, Stein KM, et al: Right ventricular outflow tract tachycardia due to a somatic cell mutation in G protein subunit$_{\alpha i2}$. J Clin Invest 101:2862–2868, 1998.
21. O'Rourke DJ, Palac RT, Schindler JT, et al: The clinical utility of adenosine in difficult to diagnose tachyarrhythmias. Clin Cardiol 22:633–636, 1999.
22. Bertolet BD, Hill JA: Adenosine: Diagnostic and therapeutic uses in cardiovascular medicine. Chest 104:1860–1871, 1993.
23. Burnett D, Abi-Samra F, Vacek JL: Use of intravenous adenosine as a noninvasive diagnostic test for sick sinus syndrome. Am Heart J 137:377–380, 1999.
24. Shen WK, Hamill SC, Munger TM, et al: Adenosine: Potential modulator for vasovagal syncope. J Am Coll Cardiol 28:146–154, 1996.
25. Mittal S, Stein KM, Markowitz SM, et al: Induction of neurally mediated syncope with adenosine. Circulation 99:1318–1324, 1999.
26. Stafford RS, Robson DC, Misra B, et al: Rate control and sinus rhythm maintenance in atrial fibrillation: National trends in medication use, 1980–1996. Arch Intern Med 158:2144–2148, 1998.
27. The Digital Investigation Group: The effect of digoxin on mortality and morbidity in patients with heart failure. N Engl J Med 336:525–533, 1997.
28. Eichhorn EJ, Gheorghiade M: Digoxin. Prog Cardiovasc Dis 2002:44:251–266.
29. Duytschaever MF, Garratt CJ, Allessie MA: Profibrillatory effects of verapamil but not of digoxin in the goat model of atrial fibrialltion. J Cardiovasc Electrophysiol 11:1375–1385, 2000.
30. Tieleman RG, Blaauw Y, Van Gelder I, et al: Digoxin delays recovery from tachycardia-induced electrical remodeling of the atria. Circulation 100:1836–1842, 1999.
31. Sticherling C, Oral H, Horrocks J, et al: Effects of digoxin on acute, atrial fibrillation-induced changes in atrial refractoriness. Circulation 102:2503–2508, 2000.
32. Hornestam B, Held P, Edvardsson N: Effects of digoxin on the electrocardiogram in patients with acute atrial fibrillation—a randomized, placebo-controlled study. Digitalis in Acute Atrial Fibrillation (DAAF) Trial Group. Clin Cardiol 22:96–102, 1999.
33. Kurata Y, Ieiri I, Kimura M, et al: Role of human MDR1 gene polymorphism in bioavailability and interaction of digoxin, a substrate of P-glycoprotein. Clin Pharmacol Ther 72:202–219, 2002.
34. The Atrial Fibrillation Follow-up Investigation of Rhythm Management (AFFIRM) Investigators: A comparison of rate control and rhythm control in patients with atrial fibrillation. N Engl J Med 347:1825–1833, 2002.
35. Digitalis in Acute Atrial Fibrillation Trial Group: Intravenous digoxin in acute atrial fibrillation. Results of a randomized, placebo-controlled multicentre trial in 239 patients. Eur Heart J 18:649–654, 1997.
36. Jordaens L, Trouerbach J, Calle P, et al: Conversion of atrial fibrillation to sinus rhythm and rate control by digoxin in comparison to placebo. Eur Heart J 18:643–648, 1997.
37. Farshi R, Kistner D, Sarma JSM, et al: Ventricular rate control in chronic atrial fibrillation during daily activity and programmed exercise: A crossover open-label study of five drug regimens. J Am Coll Cardiol 33:304–310, 1999.
38. Murgatroyd FD, Gibson SM, Baiyan X, et al: Double-blind placebo-controlled trial of digoxin in symptomatic paroxysmal atrial fibrillation. Circulation 99:2765–2770, 1999.
39. Marik PE, Fromm L: A case series of hospitalized patients with elevated digoxin levels. Am J Med 105:110–115, 1998.
40. Abad-Santos F, Carcas AJ, Ibanez C et al: Digoxin level and clinical manifestations as determinants in the diagnosis of digoxin toxicity. Ther Drug Monit 22:163–168, 2000.
41. Gittelman MA, Stephan M, Perry H: Acute pediatric drug ingestion. Pediatr Emerg Care 15:359–362, 1999.
42. Ward SB, Sjostrom L, Ujhelyi MR: Comparison of the pharmacokinetics and in vivo bioaffinity of DigiTAb versus Digibind. Ther Drug Monit 22:599–607, 2000.
43. Zdunek M, Mitra A, Mokrzycki MH: Plasma exchange for the removal of digoxin-specific antibody fragments in renal failure: Timing is important for maximizing clearance. Am J Kidney Dis 36:177–183, 2000.

第 103 章

非传统抗心律失常药物对心脏性猝死的影响

Jeffrey Goldberger, Kenneth M. Weinberg, and Alan H. Kadish

本章目录
- 病理生理学 ………………………… 930
- β受体阻滞剂 ………………………… 931
- 肾素-血管紧张素-醛固酮系统 ……… 934
- 调脂药和炎症 ………………………… 935
- 总结 …………………………………… 936

虽然在美国冠心病的死亡率下降了，但心脏性猝死仍然是一个主要临床问题，每年有30万人发生心脏性猝死。临床研究表明，减少猝死发生的策略包括预防基础心脏病、检出易发生猝死的遗传综合征患者、改进对发生猝死患者的急救（二级预防）或检出易发猝死的高危人群并适当干预。

对心脏性猝死可能有效的干预方法有改变生活方式、改变饮食结构、抗心律失常药物治疗、应用其他心血管药物治疗或植入式心脏复律除颤器（implantable cardioverter defibrillators, ICDs）治疗。但用钠或钾离子通道阻滞剂治疗心律失常来预防猝死的结果，从总体上来讲是令人失望的。和胺碘酮不同，这些药物对死亡率的影响是中性的甚至会增加死亡率。ICD 治疗可以预防部分高危患者发生猝死，但价格昂贵和一些并发症限制了 ICD 在预防心脏性猝死高危患者中的大规模应用。

抗心律失常药有几种不同的分类方法。其中，Vaughn-Williams 分类法是最古老也是目前应用最广的抗心律失常药分类方法，在这种分类法里，钠离子通道阻滞剂被分为 I 类抗心律失常药，β受体阻滞剂被分为 II 类抗心律失常药，钾离子通道阻滞剂被分为 III 类抗心律失常药，钙离子通道阻滞剂被分为 IV 类抗心律失常药。β 受体阻滞剂被认为是抗心律失常药物主要是因为它可以影响不同种类的心律失常。β受体阻滞剂还有其他作用包括预防心肌缺血，然而，那些主要阻滞钠和/或钾离子通道的药物，被认为是传统上的抗心律失常药。本章主要讨论那些非钠离子通道和非钾离子通道阻滞剂类药物（非传统抗心律失常药）对猝死的预防作用。

一、病理生理学

对临床研究的心脏性猝死结果难以解释的一个原因是死亡机制的分类不明确。在一些以往的研究中，所有在症状发生后 1～24 小时内的死亡都被划为心脏性猝死。这样的定义很明显对心律失常性心脏性猝死缺乏特异性，因为很多因心肌梗死（myocardial infarction, MI）在 24 小时内死亡患者的死因可能和心律失常无关。最近，临床试验中"终点事件"被用来对死因分类。因为很多这类试验都是大规模多中心研究，信息的质量和可信程度高，但根据终点事件也有其局限性，因为终点事件对死因的分类具有某些局限性。Epstein 评分系统[1]被用在一些临床研究中，这个评分系统不但强调病因，还考虑到这些因素的强弱。因此，在评价非传统抗心律失常药对猝死的影响时，还要考虑到它对总死亡率的影响，有时总死亡率的下降是由于猝死率的下降所致。

以往的研究表明，心脏性猝死的主要原因是室性心动过速和心室颤动。虽然心动过缓和电机械分离在充血性心力衰竭和长时间的心跳骤停中更常见，但权衡证据，室性心动过速和/或心室颤动仍是心脏性猝死的最主要原因。因此，评估对室性心动过速和心室颤动的治疗，可能会有益于降低心脏性猝死的发生率。

有证据证明，室性心动过速和心室颤动的危险性随着左室功能的变化而变化。此外，左室扩张时通过收缩-激动反馈改变了心脏的电生理特性，可能会产生心律失常。因此，改变心脏血流动力学的药物可以通过改善左室功能和左室直径起到抗心律失常作用，即使这些药物没有直接抗心律失常作用。

当描述非传统抗心律失常药对心脏性猝死的影响时，应考虑到心脏性猝死的病理生理分型和每种药物可能的作用机制。尽管对猝死进行了广泛的研究，仍没有一个被大家广泛接受的病理生理学分类。虽然大部分猝死患者有冠心病和心肌缺血病史，但非缺血性心肌病患者也有心脏性猝死的危险。此外，即使有冠心病的患者，也只有一小部分患者发生心脏性猝死同时伴有急性心肌梗死。另外，暂时的自律性和代谢性因素也可导致猝死。图103-1展示了一个猝死可能的病理生理模型。在这个结构里，短暂因素和自主节律以及基本解剖结构相互作用，导致了心脏性猝死。这个模型表明，触发心律失常的激动可能由于折返、异常自主激动或触发活动造成，其电生理学基础可能存在功能或解剖折返。因此，短暂的代谢和自主因素改变了电生理特性可以调整解剖特性从而导致猝死的发生。为鉴定这个模型的电生理特性，有必要（1）鉴定易于发生猝死的特殊的电生理机制和（2）鉴定在心律失常发生区域心肌内易诱发猝死的特殊离子通道，并确定这些离子通道的特性。目前，抗心律失常药作用于遍及心肌内的钠或钾离子通道，因此没有特异作用于心律失常的机制（局部或折返）或区域。因此，抗心律失常药对猝死问题没有特异性治疗作用。与此相反，假如猝死的诱因是由于精神紧张或运动后产生的肾上腺素高峰造成的，那么，阻滞这些机制的药物如β受体阻滞剂可能有效，这时，不需要抗心律失常的生理作用，同时，也不需要特殊的抗心律失常药治疗。非传统抗心律失常药和不加选择地阻滞心肌内离子通道的传统抗心律失常药相比，后者主要作用于心律失常的全身机制，因此，非传统抗心律失常药物对猝死的有效预防作用也就不足为奇了。综上所述，减少猝死治疗的潜在靶点如图103-1所示。表103-1列出了本章要讨论的可能降低心脏病死亡率的干预方法和可能降低猝死发生的药物。

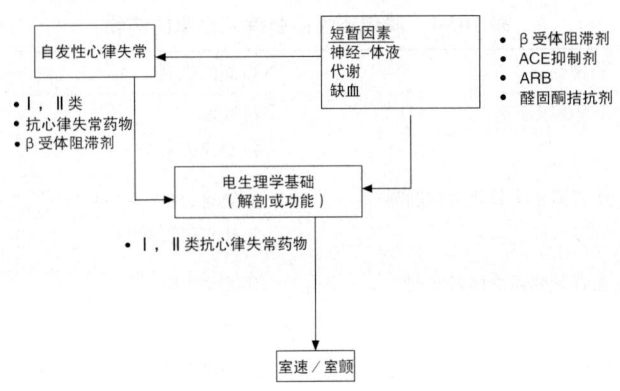

图 103-1　心律失常可能的机制和药物作用的可能部位
ACE：肾素血管紧张素转化酶；ARB：血管紧张素受体阻断剂。

二、β受体阻滞剂

β受体阻滞剂在心脏性猝死一级和二级预防中的作用越来越重视（表103-2）。β受体阻滞剂最初被用作预防心肌梗死后患者猝死的发生。最近，大规模临床实验证明β受体阻滞剂可以作为充血性心力衰竭患者猝死的一级预防药物。也有充分证据证明β受体阻滞剂可以预防室性心动过速再发。

（一）β受体阻滞剂在心肌梗死后患者中的作用

Freemantle等[2]分析了50 000多例心肌梗死患者，显示β受体阻滞剂治疗可以明显降低死亡率（相对危险性0.77；95%可信区间0.69～0.85）。另外，有一项大规模研究包括了医疗保险数据库内的200 000多例患者[16]。研究表明，β受体阻滞剂的有益治疗作用经受得住时间的考验，尽管当时已有了先进的治疗方法如溶栓治疗[20]。在CAPRICORN（Carvedilol Post-Infarct Survival Control in LV Dysfunction study，CAPRICORN）研究中，1 959名患心肌梗死后3～21天的患者，其左室射血分数小于等于40%，随机分为卡维地洛治疗组（n=975）和对照组（n=984）[17]。虽然，总死亡率不是最终终点，但在随访1.3年后治疗组和对照组的死亡率分别是12%和15%（降低死亡危险23%；95%可信区间2%～40%）。

（二）β受体阻滞剂在充血性心力衰竭患者中的作用

β受体阻滞剂也是预防充血性心力衰竭患者发生

表 103-1 降低慢性心脏病死亡率的药物

药物	可能的机制
β受体阻滞剂	抗缺血
	抗心律失常
血管紧张素转化酶抑制剂	血流动力学
	? 抗心律失常
血管紧张素受体阻滞剂	血流动力学
	? 抗心律失常
鱼油	抗心律失常
	抗动脉粥样硬化
安体舒通	抗心律失常
	血流动力学
阿司匹林	抗缺血
	抗炎
他汀类	抗动脉粥样硬化
胺碘酮	抗心律失常
	? 抗缺血
血管扩张剂（肼苯哒嗪/硝酸盐类）	血流动力学

猝死的有效药物。其中，卡维地洛可以降低心力衰竭患者的死亡率[21]，也可使总死亡率降低65%。在CIBIS-2（Cardiac Insufficiency Bisoprolol Study 2）研究中，2 657名心功能Ⅲ～Ⅳ级的患者，其左室射血分数小于35%，随机分成比索洛尔治疗组（n=1 327）和对照组（n=1 320）[19]。由于比索洛尔明显降低死亡率，本试验被提前终止。结果显示，比索洛尔组年死亡率为8.8%，而安慰剂组的年死亡率为13.2%（治疗组降低危险性34%；95%可信区间19%～46%）。美托洛尔也被证明可以提高充血性心力衰竭患者的生存率。在MERITHF（Metoprolol CR/XL Randomized Intervention Trial in Congestive Heart Failure）研究中，3 991名心功能Ⅱ～Ⅳ级（96%为Ⅱ和Ⅲ级）的心衰患者（左室射血分数<40%）被随机分为美托洛尔治疗组（n=1 990）和对照组（n=2 001）。这项试验也被安全委员会提前终止，因为β受体阻滞剂组明显获益。美托洛尔治疗组的年死亡率为7.2%，而对照组为11.0%（死亡率降低相对危险34%；95%可信区间19%～47%）。总之，在所有的试验中β受体阻滞剂都能减少猝死的发生率，降低死亡率。

（三）β受体阻滞剂对猝死的二级预防

有一些证据证明，β受体阻滞剂对室性心动过速有效。AVID（Antiarrhythmics Versus Implantable Defibrillators，AVID）研究的数据表明，β受体阻滞剂对治疗持续性室性心动过速有效[22]。这个研究共入选366名血流动力学受影响的室性心动过速或心室颤动患者，且没有接受过胺碘酮、索他洛尔或植入式心脏复律除颤器治疗。此外，对β受体阻滞剂的应用未作特殊要求。有150例患者接受了β受体阻滞剂治疗。213例患者未接受β受体阻滞剂治疗，只有50例患者接受了其他抗心律失常药治疗。结果表明，β受体阻滞剂治疗组的死亡率降低了50%。并且在植入式心脏复律除颤器患者中，β受体阻滞剂可减少室性心动过速的发作频率[23]。这项研究中绝大多数患者患有冠心病。根据有限的资料显示，β受体阻滞剂治疗可减少非缺血性扩张型心肌病患者需要ICD放电治疗的室性心动过速次数[24]。而且在这项研究的多因素分析中β受体阻滞剂治疗组需要ICD放电治疗的相对危险性是0.15（95%可信区间为0.05～0.45，$P<0.0007$）。除此，β受体阻滞剂对治疗长QT间期综合征也有效[25]。

虽然β受体阻滞剂可能是预防心脏性猝死的最有效的单剂药物，但值得注意的是在β受体阻滞剂治疗的基础上加上其他药物可使患者得到更多的益处。Steineck等[26]将115名有室性心动过速的患者随机分成β受体阻滞剂组或电生理测试指导治疗组。虽然两组的大体结果相似，但1年后β受体阻滞剂治疗组室性心动过速再发/猝死发生率超过40%，而室性心动过速再发/猝死在电生理检查指导下应用抗心律失常药物组的发生率仅为10%。在EMIAT（European Myocardial Infarct Amiodarone Trial）和CAMIAT（Canadian Amiodarone Myocardial Infraction Arrhythmia Trial）试验中发现，β受体阻滞剂和胺碘酮治疗有协同作用；同时，在接受β受体阻滞剂治疗的基础上加用胺碘酮可明显降低死亡率[27]。另外，在CAMIAT研究中，在β受体阻滞剂治疗的基础上加用胺碘酮较对照组明显降低相对危险性87%（$P=0.008$）。因此，虽然β受体阻滞剂是预防猝死的重要药物，但是单独应用β受体阻滞剂预防猝死往往是不够的。

（四）β受体阻滞剂获益的机制

在心肌梗死后应用β受体阻滞剂的试验中发现，β受体阻滞剂降低死亡率的主要原因是减少猝死的发生率。在7项猝死研究的荟萃分析中发现，β受体阻滞剂治疗能降低死亡率28%，猝死发生率降低33%，非

表 103-2 药物在降低死亡率和预防猝死中的作用

分类	药物	对照	研究	患者	数量（人）	随访	总死亡率（RR 或 HR）（95%CI）	SCD（RR 或 HR）（95%CI）
ACEI	雷米普利	安慰剂	AIRE[3]	MI 后+CHF	2 006	15 个月	RR 0.73 (0.60~0.89)	RR 0.70 (0.53~0.92)
	雷米普利	安慰剂	HOPE[4]	CV 病或 DM+CRF	9 297	5 年	RR 0.84 (0.75~0.95)	RR 0.62 (0.41~0.94)*
	卡托普利	安慰剂	SAVE[5]	MI 后+↓EF	2 231	42 个月	RR 0.81 (0.68~0.97)	NS
	依那普利	安慰剂	CONSENSUS I[6]	AMI	6 090	6 个月	RR 1.01 (0.93~1.29)	NS
	依那普利	安慰剂	SOLVD-P[7] Prevention	↓EF	4 228	37 个月	RR 0.92 (0.79~1.08)	RR 0.93 (0.71~1.22)
	依那普利	水合氯醛/异山梨醇	V-Helft[8]	CHF	804	2.5 年	RR 0.72	RR 0.65
	佐诺普利	安慰剂	SMILE[9]	AMI	1 556	6 周	RR 0.78 (0.52~1.12)	RR 0.37 (0.11~1.02)
	群多普利	安慰剂	TRACE[10]	MI 后+↓EF	1 749	24~50 个月	RR 0.78 (0.67~0.91)	RR 0.76 (0.59~0.89)
ARB	撷沙坦	安慰剂	Val-Helft[11]	CHF	5 010	23 个月	RR 1.02 (0.88~1.18) 98%CI	NS
	氯沙坦	卡托普利	ELITE[12]	CHF	722	48 周	RR 0.54 (0.31~0.95)	RR 0.36 (0.14~0.97)
	氯沙坦	卡托普利	ELITE II[13]	CHF	3 152	1.5 年	HR 1.13 (0.95~1.35) 95.7%CI	HR 1.30 (1.00~1.69)
	氯沙坦	阿替洛尔	LIFE[14]	HTN+LVH	9 193	4.8 年	HR 0.90 (0.78~1.03)	HR 1.91 (0.64~5.72)+
	氯沙坦	卡托普利	OPTIMAAL[15]	MI 后+CHF	5 477	2.7 年	RR 1.33 (0.99~1.28)	RR 1.19 (0.99~1.43)‡
β受体阻滞剂	未分类	安慰剂	1999 荟萃分析[2]	MI 后	24 974		RR 0.77 (0.69~0.85)	
	未分类	安慰剂	医疗保险资料[16]	MI 后	201 752	2 年	RR 0.60 (0.57~0.63)	
	卡维地洛	安慰剂	CAPRICORN[17]	MI 后+↓EF	1 959	1.3 年	HR 0.77 (0.60~0.98)	HR 0.74 (0.51~1.06)
	美托洛尔	安慰剂	MERIT-HF[18]	CHF	3 991	1 年	RR 0.66 (0.53~0.81)	RR 0.59 (0.45~0.78)
	比索洛尔	安慰剂	CIBIS-II[19]	CHF	2 657	1.3 年	HR 0.66 (0.54~0.81)	HR 0.56 (0.39~0.80)

*心脏骤停；+心脏骤停复苏。‡猝死+心脏骤停复苏。
ACEI，血管紧张素转化酶抑制剂；AMI，急性心肌梗死；ARB，血管紧张素受体阻断剂；CHF，充血性心力衰竭；CI，可信区间；CRF，心脏危险因素；CV，心血管；DM，糖尿病；EF，射血分数；HR，危害比；HTN，高血压；LVH，左室肥厚；MI，心肌梗死；NS，无显著性；RR，相对危险度；SCD，心脏性猝死。

猝死率降低 20%[28]。此外，β受体阻滞剂降低充血性心力衰竭患者的死亡率也是由于减少猝死发生体现的[18]。

β受体阻滞剂治疗的临床益处可能是由于β肾上腺素受体信号在控制健康或疾病状态下的心血管系统起着重要的作用。由于β肾上腺素受体在心脏内无处不在的特性和心脏交感神经系统的病理生理变化，心脏对交感神经刺激发生反应，循环中的儿茶酚胺可以出现在心脏病变部位，产生不利的电生理影响，易于发生威胁生命的室性心动过速[29]。例如，心肌梗死后出现局部去神经支配[30,31]，这可能导致梗死区去神经支配过敏高峰。除此，心肌梗死后心率变异的变化和压力感受器敏感性的变化也反映了交感神经和副交感神经张力的异常，有一些学者发现室性心律失常发生前先有心率和心率变异的变化，提示自主神经张力的改变可能会触发心律失常。

三、肾素-血管紧张素-醛固酮系统

（一）血管紧张素转化酶抑制剂

血管紧张素转化酶（angiotensin-converting enzyme，ACE）抑制剂在心脏性猝死的高危人群中，包括充血性心力衰竭和心肌梗死患者中被广泛研究。虽然研究涉及的 ACE 抑制剂可明确降低总死亡率（降低危险 8%～40%）和/或心血管死亡率，但极少有研究发现 ACE 抑制剂对心律失常死亡也有相似作用。

ACE 抑制剂有几个可能的抗心律失常作用。除了心肌梗死后期，ACE 抑制剂被发现有直接抗心律失常作用，但也有一些矛盾的地方[33,34]。如在有或没有心衰的患者中低钾血症是室性心律失常的一个重要危险因素。ACE 抑制剂可以升高血钾水平，可能对心肌结构产生有益的影响[35]。这个结果和其他研究并不一致。虽然这样，ACE 抑制剂对自主神经系统有直接和间接的影响，可改变室性心律失常的危险性[36]。ACE 抑制剂能提高压力感受器的敏感性，因此，减低交感神经张力、增加副交感神经张力、改善血流动力学状态也使循环中儿茶酚胺浓度降低。左室重构是一个涉及到衰竭心脏纤维化和扩张的复杂过程，并对心脏电传导系统有着不利的影响，如能减少左室扩张就能减少室性心律失常[37]。ACE 抑制剂治疗可以逆转左室重构，因此，可减少心律失常发作从而减少猝死的发生率。

AIRE（Acute Infarction Ramipril Efficacy study）和 TRACE（Trandolapril Cardiac Evaluation）试验是证明 ACE 抑制剂能减少心脏性猝死发生仅有的两项随机双盲试验[3,10]。这两项试验入选的都是近期心肌梗死患者，其中在 AIRE 试验中 2006 例近期患心肌梗死合并有临床心衰证据的患者被随机分成雷米普利治疗组（5mg/d）和对照组。在 15 个月的随访期内雷米普利组的总死亡率降低了 27%，减少了 30%猝死的发生率（12.3%～8.9%）。在 TRACE 试验中 1749 位急性心肌梗死患者，其左室射血分数小于等于 35%，随机分成群多普利治疗组和对照组，在 24～50 个月的随访期内，治疗组心血管死亡率降低了 25%，心脏性猝死降低了 26%（15.2%～12.0%）。另外，一个包括 AIRE 和 TRACE 在内的心肌梗死后 ACE 抑制剂治疗的中长期疗效荟萃分析包括了 15,104 名患者，所有的大规模临床试验中应用 ACE 抑制剂组的猝死率都有降低的趋势（相对危险性 0.80，95%可信区间 0.70～0.92），总死亡率也有相应的明显降低[38]。

在 HOPE（Heart Outcomes Prevention Evaluation）研究中，9000 多名有血管疾病或糖尿病和具有一个心血管危险因素的患者被随机分为雷米普利治疗组和对照组[4]，经过 5 年的临床观察，结果发现治疗组降低了 26%心血管死亡率，降低 37%心脏骤停，但本试验对心脏性猝死未作特殊分析。

但还没有随机双盲试验来证明 ACE 抑制剂较安慰剂能降低慢性心衰患者猝死的发生率。不过，有三项主要临床试验 CONSENSUS（Cooperative New Scandinavian Enalapril Survival Study），SOLVD-治疗（Studies of Left Ventricular Dysfunction）和 SOLVD-预防报告了猝死的结果[6,7]。另外，在 V-Heft 2（Second Veterans Administration Vasodilator-Heart Failure Trial）研究中，804 名纽约心功能分级Ⅱ和Ⅲ级心衰男性患者被随机分为依那普利（20mg/d）治疗组、合用盐酸肼苯哒嗪（300mg/d）组和硝酸异山梨酯（160mg/d）组[8]，在两年的随访中，结果显示依那普利组总死亡率降低了 28%，这是因为猝死发生率降低了 38%，结果显现出有益作用可能是由于硝酸异山梨酯组的猝死率上升所造成的。虽然这样，在 V-Heft 1（小样本）研究中，对照组的心脏性猝死发生率高于硝酸异山梨酯组，也高于 V-Heft 2 的硝酸异山梨酯组。然而，综上所述，随机双盲试验没有证明降低猝死的发生率是由 ACE 抑制剂所致。

（二）血管紧张素受体阻断剂

在生理水平上，血管紧张素-2 是一种有力的血管收缩物质，长期应用 ACE 抑制剂类药物情况下血管紧张素也可以通过在非 ACE 依赖途径合成。血管紧张素-2 可能的致心律失常作用包括激活神经激素介质（去甲肾上腺素、醛固酮和内皮素）、加快传导速度和缩短心肌的不应期[39]。此外，和 ACE 抑制剂不同，血管紧张素受体-2 阻滞剂（angiotensin 2 receptor blockers，ARBs）不升高因去甲肾上腺素水平升高的缓激肽水平[40]。但升高儿茶酚胺水平在理论上可导致更多的室性心律失常和猝死。因此，直接阻断血管紧张素-2 受体可以进一步减少需要阻滞肾素-血管紧张素-醛固酮系统患者的猝死发生率和死亡率。但 RALES（Randomized Aldactone Evaluation Study）研究对血管紧张素-2 受体阻断剂的这些保护作用提出了疑问（见下一节）。此外，对用 ACE 抑制剂治疗的充血性心力衰竭患者被随机分到安体舒通治疗组，尽管血浆中血管紧张素-2 水平明显升高，但猝死发生率却明显降低[41]。和 ACE 抑制剂一样，ARB 可以提高血钾浓度，可能对心脏有潜在的保护作用。

ARB 主要在几个心衰和高血压的试验中与 ACE 抑制剂进行比较。重要的是，有一项配对分析显示，两类药物的总死亡率相似[42]。其中，只有一项试验显示，ARB 和 ACE 抑制剂比较前者可以降低猝死发生率，但大规模试验的结果却与此相反。在 ELITE（Evaluation of Losartan in the Elderly）研究中，722 名心功能 Ⅱ～Ⅳ 级患者，其左室射血分数小于等于 40%，随机分为氯沙坦和卡托普利治疗组[12]，结果表明，在 48 周氯沙坦组总死亡率下降了 45%，其中猝死患者减少（5 比 14 人，相对危险性降低 36%）是导致总死亡率下降的一个原因。但是，在更大规模的 ELITE2 试验中，3 152 名左室射血分数小于 40% 的心衰患者入选，随机分为氯沙坦和卡托普利治疗组[13]，随访 1.5 年后显示，卡托普利组的猝死率和总死亡率较氯沙坦组明显降低。此外，OPTIMAAL（Optimal Trial in Myocardial Infarction with the Angiotensin 2 Antagonist Losartan）试验在心肌梗死后伴有心衰的患者中比较氯沙坦和卡托普利的疗效，其结果和 ELITE 2 试验相似，也得出了对卡托普利有利的结果[15]。

（三）醛固酮受体拮抗剂

ACE 抑制剂对肾素-血管紧张素-醛固酮系统的神经激素抑制是不完全的。因此，醛固酮能对心衰患者的心血管系统有持续的损害。醛固酮促进钠潴留、镁和钾外流、激活交感神经、抑制副交感神经、导致心肌和血管纤维化、压力感受器功能失常、损害血管和影响动脉顺应性。

安体舒通作为醛固酮受体拮抗剂和保钾利尿剂被广泛应用于严重充血性心力衰竭患者中。如在 RELES 试验中，1 663 名纽约心功能分级 Ⅲ～Ⅳ 级、左室射血分数小于等于 35% 的心衰患者被随机分为安体舒通（25mg/d）治疗组和对照组[43]，随访 24 个月后发现，心血管死亡率降低了 31%，这是通过进展性心衰死亡率降低了 36% 和心脏性猝死发生率降低了 29% 所体现的。

对安体舒通抗心律失常机制的一个解释是醛固酮可能会促进左室重构，特征是成纤维和炎性细胞进入受损血管的血管间隙导致纤维化。这些变化对机械功能、血管扩张储备和心脏电传导系统都有不利影响[44]。最近对 RALES 试验亚组分析表明、胶原蛋白合成的血清标记物和心脏纤维化和形态学证据相关[45]。在应用安体舒通 6 个月后这些标记物水平降低，而在对照组中水平不变。安体舒通能轻度升高血钾水平而具有心脏保护作用，但持续利尿时易发生低钾血症。在 RALES 研究的安体舒通组其血钾水平较对照组高 0.3mEq/L。还有一些研究表明，非保钾利尿剂能增加心脏性猝死并且有明显的量效关系。其中有一个病例分析显示，应用噻嗪类利尿剂能增加心脏性猝死的危险性，当合用保钾利尿剂时可使危险降低[46]。

四、调脂药和炎症

（一）3-羟基-3-甲基-辅酶还原酶抑制剂

众多的大规模随机双盲试验都证明了 3-羟基-3-甲基-辅酶还原酶抑制剂，即他汀类药物对心血管的保护作用。虽然，他汀类药物被广泛用来预防冠心病死亡和心肌梗死，但还不清楚这类药物在冠状动脉作用外是否有抗心律失常作用。他汀类药物可以通过减轻缺血负担来发挥抗心律失常作用，很多研究都发现他汀类药物可减少缺血和梗死。但是，他汀类的降脂作用还有除了防止动脉粥样硬化斑块进展外的保护作用，因为，在开始应用他汀 16 周时就可以降低临床事件的发生率。对内皮功能的作用、抗炎、稳定斑块、对血小板的作用等可能是他汀早期起作用的原因。但现在还不知道他汀类药物的有益作用中是否有直接的电生理作用。

在两个他汀类药物的二级预防试验中有潜在抗心律失常作用的线索。在 4S（Scandinavian Simvastatin Survival Study）试验中，4 444 名有高脂蛋白血症的冠心病患者被随机分成辛伐他汀治疗组和对照组[47]，5.4 年后，治疗组的总死亡率降低了 30%。本试验给出了发病后立刻死亡和发病后 1 小时内死亡患者的数据，但没有做统计学分析，但在对照组有 63 例死亡，治疗组有 37 例死亡。另外，在 LIPID（Long-term Intervention with Pravastatin in Ischemic Heart Disease）试验中，9 014 名有高脂蛋白血症的冠心病患者被随机分为普伐他汀治疗组和对照组[48]。6.1 年后，普伐他汀组的总死亡率降低了22%，对照组中211例发生了猝死，治疗组中有182例，对这个结果也没有做统计学分析。虽然，这可能提示有抗心律失常益处，但是，这两个试验观察期长，猝死发生率的不同可能是由于他汀防止了动脉粥样硬化斑块的进展体现的。

在一项78名植入ICD的冠心病患者的回顾性研究中[49]，应用调脂药物（59%他汀类，41%贝特类）治疗在随访中可减少ICD放电次数，只有22%患者发生放电治疗，而非调脂治疗组有57%的患者在随访中发生放电治疗，其机制是他汀治疗减轻动脉粥样硬化可能导致了以上作用。还有一项入选200名植入ICD患者用阿洛伐他汀或安慰剂治疗的前瞻性研究正在进行，预计2003年将会发表结果。

（二）多不饱和脂肪酸

n-3多不饱和脂肪酸（polyunsaturated fatty acids，PUFAs）对心血管系统的保护作用最初是在爱斯基摩人和地中海地区人群的流行病学研究中发现的。通常这些人的饮食富含多脂鱼类，其中富含以N端的双键三碳结构命名的分子。重要的是n-3 PUFAs中包含二十碳五烯酸和α-亚麻酸。n-3 PUFAs的心血管保护机制还在阐明中。潜在的有益因素包括抑制室性心律失常、有益于脂代谢、降低血压、抗炎作用、稳定血小板和抗凝作用。已有很多研究都发现食入鱼油和冠心病的负相关关系。有几项试验指出，PUFAs的主要作用可能是减少心脏性猝死的发生。此外，离体心肌细胞、动物实验和对人的初步研究的证据指出，n-3 PUFAs可能有直接抗心律失常作用。研究表明，制成犬心肌梗死模型后喂食n-3 PUFAs可以明显减少心肌缺血诱发的心室颤动[50]。n-3 PUFAs通过作用于I_{Na}和$I_{Ca,L}$通道，使静止的膜电位轻度超极化，导致刺激阈值升高，不应期延长[51]。这些特性有助于解释在缺血和中毒区域提高电稳定性的原因。

有几项前瞻性序列研究发现，n-3 PUFAs可减少有或无冠心病患者猝死的发生率。其中，在DART试验中，心肌梗死后生存的男性患者被分成8个饮食干预组[52]。在饮食富含多脂鱼类组，2年后，冠心病死亡率降低了33%，非致死性心肌梗死有所增加但没有达到统计学差异。对死亡率的降低在6个月时最明显。另外，在里昂心脏饮食研究中也有相似发现，被随机分到地中海饮食组的患者其饮食中富含α-亚麻酸，降低了73%包括心脏死亡和非致死性MI在内的联合终点事件[53]。试验组有8例心脏性猝死，对照组中无心脏性猝死发生。

在最近，大规模临床试验有足够的统计学证据来特别研究那些没有被作为一级终点事件的心脏性猝死。其中，GISSI-预防研究是一项多中心、开放式、随机试验，共入选了11 323名近期心肌梗死患者[54]，被随机分成2×2因子设计、接受n-3 PUFAs（1mg/d）、维生素E（300mg/d）组，两组都服用或都不用治疗，所有患者都接受标准治疗，即食用鱼类和橄榄油含量比美国饮食高的地中海饮食。共有265例猝死，其中146例立即死亡，103例发生在症状发作后1小时内死亡，10例被证实为心律失常死亡，6例死亡时无人在现场。在42个月的随访期内，对照组的猝死发生率为2.7%，而接受n-3 PUFAs组死亡率为2.0%（$P<0.001$），并可降低59%总死亡率。重要的是，在随访3个月时，血脂还没有变化，但猝死的降低已接近出现统计学差异。Bucher等[55]对n-3 PUFAs预防冠心病的随机试验作了荟萃分析。在他们的分析结果中，总死亡率、致死性心肌梗死和猝死发生率在n-3 PUFAs组都明显降低，且有减低非致死性心肌梗死的趋势。

五、总结

和阻滞钠或钾离子通道的传统的抗心律失常药物不同，抗肾上腺素作用和神经激素作用可以降低器质性心脏病患者的总死亡率和猝死发生率。虽然在一些试验中胺碘酮被证实可以降低猝死的发生率，但对此似是而非的假定是胺碘酮的抗肾上腺素作用导致了以上结果，因为其他钠或钾离子通道阻滞剂对猝死是中性影响或增加猝死率。

我们从预防猝死的药物试验中得出两个重要结论，其一，致死性心律失常总体上来说是散发的，至少决定其发生的一系列心脏外部复杂变化能被改变肾上腺素和肾素-血管紧张素-醛固酮系统的药物调整；其二，主要激活心脏离子通道的非特异性药物不减低猝死的发生率。这个报告说明，尽管我们关于心律失常基础机制的认识在加深，但目前我们对猝死机制的认识还不足以区分出特殊的离子通道来预防猝死。不过，在开发出明显减少猝死发生的抗心律失常药物前，还需要进一步研究局部离子通道特性的变异和基因相互作用。此外，还需要进行进一步的基础研究，以便更全面地了解猝死的发生机制。

（温尚煜　译）

参 考 文 献

1. Epstein A, Carlson M, Fogoros R, et al: Classification of death in anti-arrhythmia trials. J Am Coll Cardiol 27:433–442, 1996.
2. Freemantle N, Cleland J, Young P, et al: Beta blockade after myocardial infarction: Systematic review and meta regression analysis. BMJ 318:1730–1737, 1999.
3. Cleland J, Erhardt L, Murray G, et al: Effect of ramipril on morbidity and mode of death among survivors of acute myocardial infarction with clinical evidence of heart failure. Eur Heart J 18:41–51, 1997.
4. Yusuf S, Sleight P, Pogue J, et al: Effects of an angiotensin-converting-enzyme inhibitor, ramipril, on cardiovascular events in high-risk patients. Heart Outcomes Prevention Evaluation Study Investigators. N Engl J Med 342:145–153, 2000.
5. Pfeffer M, Braunwald E, Moye L, et al: Effect of captopril on mortality and morbidity in patients with left ventricular dysfunction after myocardial infarction: Results of the Survival and Ventricular Enlargement Trial. N Engl J Med 327:669–677, 1992.
6. CONSENSUS Trial Study Group: Effects of enalapril on mortality in severe congestive heart failure: Results of the Cooperative North Scandinavian Enalapril Survival Study (CONSENSUS). N Engl J Med 316:1429–1435, 1987.
7. SOLVD Investigators: Effect of enalapril on mortality and the development of heart failure in asymptomatic patients with reduced left ventricular ejection fractions. N Engl J Med 327:685–691, 1992.
8. Cohn J, Johnson G, Ziesche S et al: A comparison of enalapril with hydralazine-isosorbide dinitrate in the treatment of chronic congestive heart failure. N Engl J Med 325:303–310, 1991.
9. Ambrosioni E, Borghi C, Magnani B: The effect of the ACE inhibitor zofenopril on mortality and morbidity after anterior myocardial infarction. The Survival of Myocardial Infarction Long-Term Evaluation (SMILE) Study Investigators. N Engl J Med 332:80–85, 1995.
10. Kober L, Torp-Pedersen C, Carlsen J, et al: A clinical trial of the angiotensin-converting enzyme inhibitor trandolapril in patients with left ventricular dysfunction after myocardial infarction. N Engl J Med 333:1670–1676, 1995.
11. Cohn J, Tognoni G, Valsartan Heart Failure Trial Investigators: A randomized trial of the angiotensin-receptor blocker valsartan in chronic heart failure. N Engl J Med 345:1667–1675, 2001.
12. Pitt B, Segal R, Martinez F, et al: Randomised trial of losartan vs. captopril in patients ≥ 65 with heart failure (Evaluation of Losartan in the Elderly study, ELITE). Lancet 349:747–752, 1997.
13. Pitt B, Poole-Wilson P, Segal R, et al: Effect of losartan compared with captopril on mortality in patients with symptomatic heart failure: Randomized trial—the Losartan Heart Failure Survival Study, ELITE II. Lancet 355:1582–1587, 2000.
14. Dahlof B, Devereux R, Kjeldsen S, et al: Cardiovascular morbidity and mortality in the Losartan Intervention For Endpoint Reduction in Hypertension study (LIFE): A randomised trial against atenolol. Lancet 359:995–1003, 2002.
15. Dickstein K, Kjekshus J, OPTIMAAL Steering Committee of the OPTIMAAL Study Group: Effects of losartan and captopril on mortality and morbidity in high-risk patients after acute myocardial infarction: The OPTIMAAL randomised trial. Lancet 360:752–760, 2002.
16. Gottlieb S, McCarter R, Vogel R: Effect of beta-blockade on mortality among high-risk and low-risk patients after myocardial infarction. N Engl J Med 339:489–497, 1998.
17. Dargie HJ: Effect of carvedilol on outcome after myocardial infarction in patients with left-ventricular dysfunction: The CAPRICORN randomised trial. Lancet 357:1385–1390, 2001.
18. Effect of metoprolol CR/XL in chronic heart failure: Metoprolol CR/XL randomised Intervention Trial in Congestive Heart Failure (MERIT-HF). Lancet 353:2001–2007, 1999.
19. Lechat P, Brunhuber K, Hofmann R, et al: The cardiac insufficiency bisoprolol study II (CIBIS-II): A randomized trial. Lancet 353:9–13, 1999.
20. Pfisterer M, Cox J, Granger C, et al: Atenolol use and clinical outcomes after thrombolysis for acute myocardial infarction: The GUSTO-I experience. J Am Coll Cardiol 32:634–640, 1998.
21. Packer M, Bristow M, Cohn J, et al: The effect of carvedilol on morbidity and mortality in patients with chronic heart failure. N Engl J Med 334:1349–1355, 1996.
22. Exner D, Reiffel J, Epstein A, et al: Beta-blocker use and survival in patients with ventricular fibrillation or symptomatic ventricular tachycardia: The Antiarrhythmics versus Implantable Defibrillators (AVID) trial. J Am Coll Cardiol 34:325–333, 1999.
23. Seidl K, Hauer B, Schwick N, et al: Comparison of metoprolol and sotalol in preventing ventricular tachyarrhythmias after the implantation of a cardioverter/defibrillator. Am J Cardiol 82:744–748, 1998.
24. Rankovic V, Karha J, Passman R, et al: Predictors of appropriate implantable cardioverter-defibrillator therapy in patients with idiopathic dilated cardiomyopathy. Am J Cardiol 89:1072–1076, 2002.
25. Moss A, Zareba W, Hall W, et al: Effectiveness and limitations of beta-blocker therapy in congenital long-QT syndrome. Circulation 101:616–623, 2000.
26. Steinbeck G, Andresen D, Bach P, et al: A comparison of electrophysiologically guided antiarrhythmic drug therapy with beta-blocker therapy in patients with symptomatic, sustained ventricular tachyarrhythmias. N Engl J Med 327:987–992, 1992.
27. Boutitie F, Boissel J, Connolly S, et al: Amiodarone interaction with beta-blockers: Analysis of the merged EMIAT (European Myocardial Infarct Amiodarone Trial) and CAMIAT (Canadian Amiodarone Myocardial Infarction Trial) Databases. Circulation 99:2268–2275, 1999.
28. Panidis I, Morganroth J: Initiating events of sudden cardiac death. Cardiovasc Clin 15:81–92, 1985.
29. Gersh B, Braunwald E, Rutherford J: Chronic coronary artery disease. In Braunwald E (ed): Heart Disease: A Textbook of Cardiovascular Medicine, 5th ed. Philadelphia, WB Saunders Company, 1997, pp 1289–1365.
30. Inoue H, Zipes D: Time course of denervation of efferent sympathetic and vagal nerves after occlusion of the coronary artery in the canine heart. Circ Res 62:1111–1120, 1988.
31. Minardo J, Tuli M, Mock B, et al: Scintigraphic and electrophysiological evidence of canine myocardial sympathetic denervation and reinnervation produced by myocardial infarction or phenol application. Circulation 78:1008–1019, 1988.
32. Shusterman V, Aysin B, Weiss R, et al: Dynamics of low-frequency R-R interval oscillations preceding spontaneous ventricular tachycardia. Am Heart J 139:126–133, 2000.
33. Van Gilst W, DeGraeff P, Wesseling H, et al: Reduction of reperfusion arrhythmia in the ischemic isolated rat heart by angiotensin converting enzyme inhibitors: A comparison of captopril, enalapril, and HOE 498. J Cardiovasc Pharmacol 8:722–728, 1986.
34. DeLangen D, DeGraeff P, Van Gilst W, et al: Effects of angiotensin II and captopril on inducible sustained ventricular tachycardia two weeks after myocardial infarction in the pig. J Cardiovasc Pharmacol 13:186–191, 1989.
35. Cleland J, Dargie H, Ball S, et al: Effects of enalapril in heart failure: A double-blind study of effects on exercise performance, renal function, hormones, and metabolic state. Br Heart J 54:305–312, 1985.
36. Grassi G, Cattaneo B, Seravalle G, et al: Effects of chronic ACE inhibition on sympathetic nerve traffic and baroreflex control of circulation in heart failure. Circulation 39:463–470, 1997.
37. Pogwizd S: Focal mechanisms underlying ventricular tachycardia during prolonged ischemic cardiomyopathy. Circulation 90:1441–1458, 1994.
38. Domanski M, Exner D, Borkowf C, et al: Effect of angiotensin converting enzyme inhibition on sudden cardiac death in patients following acute myocardial infarction: A meta-analysis of randomized clinical trials. J Am Coll Cardiol 33:598–604, 1999.
39. Gavras I, Gavras H: The antiarrhythmic potential of angiotensin II antagonism: Experience with losartan. Am J Hypertens 13:512–517, 2000.
40. Minisi A, Thames M: Distribution of left ventricular sympathetic afferents demonstrated by reflex responses to transmural myocardial ischemia and to intracoronary and epicardial bradykinin. Circulation 87:240–246, 1993.
41. Rousseau M, Gurne O, Duprez D, et al: Beneficial neurohormonal profile of spironolactone in severe congestive heart failure. J Am Coll Cardiol 40:1597–601, 2002.
42. Jong P, Demers C, McKelvie R, et al: Angiotensin receptor blockers in heart failure: Meta-analysis of randomized controlled trials. J Am Coll Cardiol 39:463–470, 2002.
43. Pitt B, Zannad F, Remme W, et al: The effect of spironolactone on morbidity and mortality in patients with severe heart failure. N Engl

J Med 341:709-717, 1999.
44. Weber K, Brilla C, Janicki J: Myocardial fibrosis: Functional significance and regulatory factors. Cardiovasc Res 27:341-348, 1993.
45. Zannad F, Alla F, Dousset B, et al: Limitation of excessive extracellular matrix turnover may contribute to survival benefit of spironolactone therapy in patients with congestive heart failure: Insights from the Randomized Aldactone Evaluation Study (RALES). N Engl J Med 102:2700-2706, 2000.
46. Siscovick D, Raghunathan T, Psaty B, et al: Diuretic therapy for hypertension and the risk of primary cardiac arrest. N Engl J Med 330:1852-1857, 1994.
47. Scandinavian Simvastatin Survival Study Group: Randomized trial for cholesterol lowering in 4444 patients with coronary heart disease: The Scandinavian Simvastatin Survival Study (4S). Lancet 344:1383-1389, 1994.
48. The Long-Term Intervention with Pravastatin in Ischaemic Disease (LIPID) Study Group: Prevention of cardiovascular events and death with pravastatin in patients with coronary heart disease and a broad range of initial cholesterol levels. N Engl J Med 339:1349-1357, 1998.
49. DeSutter J, Tavernier R, DeBuyzere M, et al: Lipid lowering drugs and recurrences of life-threatening ventricular arrhythmias in high-risk patients. J Am Coll Cardiol 36:766-772, 2000.
50. Billman G, Kang J, Leaf A: Prevention of ischemia induced cardiac sudden death by n-3 polyunsaturated fatty acids. J Lipids 32:1161-1168, 1997.
51. Leaf A: The electrophysiological basis for the antiarrhythmic actions of polyunsaturated fatty acids. Eur Heart J 3(suppl D):D98-D105, 2001.
52. Burr M, Fehily A, Gilbert J, et al: Effects of changes in fat, fish, and fiber intakes on death and reinfarction: Diet and reinfarction trial (DART). Lancet ii:757-761, 1989.
53. deLorgeril M, Renaud S, Mamelle N, et al: Mediterranean alpha-linolenic acid-rich diet in secondary prevention of coronary heart disease. Lancet 343:1454-1459, 1994.
54. Marchioli R, Barzi F, Bomba E, et al: Early protection against sudden death by n-3 polyunsaturated fatty acids after myocardial infarction. Circulation 105:1997-1903, 2002.
55. Bucher H, Hengstler P, Schindler C, et al: N-3 polyunsaturated fatty acids in coronary heart disease: A meta-analysis of randomized controlled trials. Am J Med 2002 112:298-304, 2002.

第 104 章

新的抗心律失常药物

N. A. Mark Estes III

本章目录

- 阿齐利特 ······················· 940
- 阿齐利特与室性心律失常 ········ 941
- 决奈达隆 ······················· 941
- 替地沙米 ······················· 942
- 曲西利特 ······················· 942
- 艾生利特 ······················· 942
- 氨巴利特 ······················· 942
- 阿莫兰特 ······················· 943
- 司美利特 ······················· 943
- 总结 ··························· 943

在过去的20年里，抗心律失常药物的发展经历了相当大的变化。基于恰当设计的随机前瞻性试验的结果，对抗心律失常药临床应用的危害和益处进行了重新的评价。室上性和室性心律失常的治疗已经很少依赖药物治疗。导管射频消融术治愈了大多数室上性心律失常。对于室性心律失常的高危患者，ICD已经证明在降低猝死率和总死亡率中优于抗心律失常药。

20世纪70~80年代发展起来的药物，利用钠通道阻滞的效应抑制室性早搏。这些药物包括美西律、妥卡胺、氟卡胺、恩卡胺、普罗帕酮、莫雷西嗪。由于它们的主要效应是阻滞钠通道，因而被分为Ⅰ类抗心律失常药。不幸的是，这些药物的临床应用增加了无症状心律失常和缺血性心脏病患者的死亡率[1,2]。试验证实Ⅰ类药物增加了心梗后患者的死亡率后，基础和临床的研究者加深了对Ⅲ类药物的研究[2-4]。基于溴苄胺的实验和临床经验，研究者的兴趣转向了延长动作电位时间（APD）的钾通道阻滞剂，甲氧苯汀（meobentine），N-乙酰基普鲁卡因酰胺（NAPA），口服溴苄胺（bretylium）和d-索他洛尔[2]。重点集中在Ⅲ类药物对室颤的阻滞效应。自从发现了d-索他洛尔增加心梗患者的死亡率，降低射血分数后，应用分子量较小的单纯Ⅲ类阻滞剂受到质疑。这从很多方面影响了抗心律失常药物的设计。药物如具有抗肾上腺素能延长复极及阻断I_{Kr}的d,l-索他洛尔和胺碘酮等以及阻断I_{Kr}和I_{Ks}的多非利特成为药物设计和发展的焦点。

基础的电生理研究者目前认定钾通道至少有9个区。已经很明显，许多阻断I_{Kr}和I_{Ks}的抗心律失常药对不同钾通道的作用有重复[2]。药厂也把重点放在治疗室性心律失常的I_{Kr}和I_{Ks}阻断剂上，上述离子流主要参与心室复极[2]。在心房，复极不连续的离子流，包括一过性的外向电流（I_{to}）和超快的I_K（I_{Kur}）。这些参与心房和心室复极的离子流的不同可以产生选择性治疗的房性和室性心律失常的药物。同样，选择性阻断钾通道的药物被低浓度的三磷酸腺苷（ATP）激活，已知的I_{K-ATP}可以作为缺血引起的心律失常治疗的目标。

钾通道阻滞剂的任何抗心律失常益处必须衡量其延长动作电位引起的尖端扭转型室速的危险[2]。阻断延迟整流钾通道（I_{Kr}），延长复极和不应期的Ⅲ类药物被认为与潜在的致命性尖端扭转型室速有关[1-5]。动作电位时程（APD）延长与尖端扭转型室速之间的关系是明确的。由于纯I_{Kr}阻滞剂有延长心室肌不应期和引起尖端扭转型室速的趋势，尽管动物模型中的电生理的研究出现有希望的结果，但它还是没有进入临床研究。I_{Kr}和

I_{Ks}阻滞剂多非利特引起尖端扭转型室速的发生率低（见18章的讨论）。它已经获准在美国用于临床治疗房颤和房扑，而有些药厂已经因为单纯阻断I_{Kr}的Ⅲ类药物引起尖端扭转型室速的发生率较高终止了临床试验。

对植入ICD的原发性室性心律失常患者，药物治疗被用作减少ICD放电[6]。Ⅲ类抗心律失常药d,l-索他洛尔最近被证明在减少植入ICD患者快速心律失常的发生中有效[6]。阿齐利特也在植入ICD患者中有相似的疗效。另一种Ⅲ类药物，即静脉使用的胺碘酮，在院外心脏骤停时紧急使用治疗不稳定的室性心律失常可以降低死亡率[7,8]。虽然如此，与安慰剂相比，胺碘酮这个多通道阻滞剂还是没有降低心梗和充血性心衰患者的总死亡率[1,2]。Ⅲ类药物是有吸引力的，它没有负性血流动力学作用，对心房和心室组织都有作用，可以静滴也可以口服。

在对理想的新型抗心律失常药物特征的描述中，对健康的组织没有影响应当首先考虑[2,3]。新型抗心律失常药应当改变心律失常的基质、抑制心律失常的触发、表现为正性频率依赖、适当的药代动力学、口服和静脉使用效果相当[2,3]。另外，理想的抗心律失常药应当副作用少，表现为正性频率阻滞作用，心脏选择性的离子通道阻滞作用[2,3]。在本章讨论的新型抗心律失常药包括：阿齐利特，决奈达隆，替地沙米，曲西利特，艾生利特，氨巴利特，阿莫兰特，司美利特（表104-1）。多非利特和依布利特是更新的抗心律失常药，已经在美国应用于临床，将在别处讨论。

一、阿齐利特（azimilide）

阿齐利特是一种新型Ⅲ类药物，阻断延迟整流钾电流中的I_{Kr}和I_{Ks}通道，临床研究相对较多[2-17]。结构上阿齐利特是氯苯基呋喃化合物，与其他Ⅲ类药物不同，没有甲基磺胺。最初的研究表明，它通过阻断I_{Kr}和I_{Ks}延长动作电位，避免了频率依赖效应[4,58-10]。在临床前和临床研究中，阿齐利特以剂量依赖方式延长心脏不应期[8-10]。表现为APD、QTc间期、有效不应期延长[2,15]。阿齐利特不影响PR间期或QRS时限，对血流动力学影响很小[2,15]。它的电生理效应不是频率依赖的，而且在缺血或缺氧状况下仍能维持[2,15]。

在动物研究中，对APD的作用不影响频率[2,10-12]。这个效应在心率增快时维持药物诱导APD延长的情况下也可以增强。在动物模型中，阿齐利特

表104-1 新的抗心律失常药

抗心律失常药	细胞膜作用
阿齐利特（Azimilide）	阻断I_{Kr}和I_{Ks}
决奈达隆（Dronedarone）	阻断I_{Kr}，I_{Ks}，β_1
	钙通道
替地沙米（Tedisamil）	阻断I_{Kr}，I_{to}，I_{Katp}
艾生利特（Ersentilide）	阻断I_{Kr}，β_1
曲西利特（Tercetilide）	激活I_{NA-S}
	阻断I_{Kr}
氨巴利特（Ambasilide）	阻断I_{Kr}和I_{Ks}
阿莫兰特（Almokalant）	阻断I_{Kr}
司美利特（Sematilide）	阻断I_{Kr}

已经表现出对室上性心律失常的抑制作用[2,4,5,9]。在狗心肌梗死模型中，它抑制了缺血诱发的室性心律失常，减低了猝死模型的死亡率[2,15]。基础的电生理研究表明，阿齐利特阻断I_{Kr}和I_{Ks}和β肾上腺素受体。阿齐利特的这种对钾通道慢和快成分以及β受体的理论上的阻滞，很少用于逆转交感刺激期间的电生理效应[2,5]。

阿齐利特的药代动力学表明，口服后几乎被完全吸收，给药后2h血浆中达到峰值[2,15,18,19]。吸收的程度不受食物影响。94%与蛋白质结合在肝脏清除，大约10%通过肾脏代谢[2,15,18,19]。不像其他Ⅲ类药物，d,l-索他洛尔、多非利特、阿齐利特已经用于院外患者的临床试验，甚至用于那些有器质性心脏病的患者[20,21]。不同年龄、性别、肝肾功能及是否合用地高辛或华法林时，不必调整剂量。它的半衰期较长为4天[13,14,16,17]。因此，每天一次即可。最初的研究表明，其对充血性心衰患者是安全的[15]。

阿齐利特已经在房颤、房扑及室上性心动过速（PSVT）的治疗中进行了系统的研究[2,4,9,13,14,16,17]。在多个临床试验中，阿齐利特的剂量达到每天200mg时，QTc间期延长4%~42%[2,3,13,14,16,17,19]。该药对室上性心律失常的安全性和有效性已经进行了研究。在这些研究中，超过1000例的房颤、房扑及PSVT患者被随机地分为接受安慰剂组和剂量逐步增加的口服阿齐利特组[5,13-17]。房颤、房扑及PSVT患者随机地分为安慰剂组（$n=87$），阿齐利特50mg/d（$n=99$），或100~125mg/d（$n=181$）组。心律失常复发的平均时间在高剂量组显著延长（60∶17天；$P<0.005$）[2,13,14]。合并3个临床试验的906例房颤、房扑患者，阿齐利特显著延长了房颤、房扑的复发时间，给予100mg/d时复发危险率为1.32，$P=0.02$，

123mg/d 时复发危险率 1.81，$P<0.01$[17]。

在一项 133 例 PSVT 患者的研究中，50 例服用安慰剂，83 例服用阿齐利特[16]。阿齐利特显著延长了无心律失常时间（危险率为 2.4，阿齐利特剂量 100mg/d，$P=0.01$）[16]。重要的是，在这些 PSVT 的研究中，尖端扭转型室速的总发生率少于 0.8%[5,13,17]。在房颤的研究中，严重副作用的发生率没有明显超过安慰剂（阿齐利特 8.5%，安慰剂 6.4%，统计学差异不显著）[5,13,17]。在 0.39% 的患者中观察到可逆的中性粒细胞减少[5,13,17]。在室上性心律失常的研究中，与安慰剂相比阿齐利特没有增加死亡率[5,13,17]。

在阿齐利特和室上性心律失常的研究中，针对 193 例有症状的 PSVT 患者的实验设计是双盲、随机及安慰剂对照的[16]。这些研究也包括一些房颤和房扑患者。患者接受了阿齐利特或安慰剂（在 SVA-1, 100mg/d；在 SVA 2＋3，35mg/d 或 70mg/d；在 SVA-4, 125mg/d）。在这 4 个分别的研究中，患者被分为房颤/房扑或阵发性室上性心律失常分别分析有效性。初步终点是远程的心电事件记录器首次记录到症状性室上性心律失常（PSVT，房颤或房扑）。初步的结果显示，复发时间以剂量相关的方式延长了[16]。在分析阿齐利特和室上性心律失常治疗的剂量相关性时，在所有的研究中，随着剂量的增加心律失常复发时间延长[16]。有趣的是，最大剂量 125mg/d 的阿齐利特与安慰剂相比并未显示出明显的改善[16]。但当 125mg/d 和 100mg/d 两组合并与安慰剂组相比时，则显示显著延长首次复发时间[16]。

在这些研究中，阿齐利特组报告的副作用比例高于安慰剂治疗组（67%：59%，$P=0.002$）。服用 100mg/d 或 125mg/d 阿齐利特的患者最常出现的副作用包括（阿齐利特：安慰剂）头痛（12%：16%），虚弱（9%：11%），恶心（10%：10%）。研究中没有死亡病例，有 1 例接受 100mg/d 阿齐利特的患者出现尖端扭转型室速。

二、阿齐利特与室性心律失常

阿齐利特已经在近期心梗患者中进行了评价[22]。阿齐利特梗死后评价试验（ALIVE）是一项国际性研究，对比观察了阿齐利特和安慰剂降低近期心梗（21 天）和左室射血分数在 15%～35% 患者死亡率[22]。它是一项双盲安慰剂对照的多中心研究，用 LVEF 和心率变异性作为确定心梗后患者高心脏性猝死危险的方法[22]。ALIVE 的试验设计参照以前有关心梗患者抗心律失常药物的试验，包括心律失常抑制试验（CAST），口服 d-索他洛尔存活试验（SWORD）及欧洲心梗胺碘酮试验（EMIAT）[1,22]。样本量是基于假设 1 年后，猝死高危患者（心率变异性≤20）服用安慰剂总死亡率降低 15%，而服用阿齐利特总死亡率至少降低 45%。三组患者随机地分为 75mg/d，100mg/d 及安慰剂组。共有 3 381 例患者入选，用总死亡率作为初步终点，阿齐利特的疗效是中性的（$P=0.739$）。在心率变异性<20 单位的亚组分析中（$n=1264$），高危组 1 年存活率明显低于低危组（死亡率 15% 比 9.5%，$P=0.0005$）。在房颤患者中阿齐利特组转复为窦律的更常见。目前，使用阿齐利特减少 ICD 放电正进入 II 期临床实验，研究显示与安慰剂相比阿齐利特可显著减少 ICD 放电及抗心律失常起搏[5]。

三、决奈达隆（dronedarone）

决奈达隆是胺碘酮（amiodarone）的非碘衍生物，其心肌细胞的电生理作用与胺碘酮相同[22-27]。决奈达隆是一种非碘的苯丙呋喃衍生物 SR33589，发展这种药物的目的是保留胺碘酮的抗心律失常作用，而降低它的副作用[22-27]。除了具有 III 类抗心律失常药物的钾通道阻滞及延长 APD 的作用外，胺碘酮还具有抗肾上腺活性、抑制快慢钙通道的作用[22-27]。由于它是一种碘化合物，它摄入后的主要副作用可能由碘引起[28]。研究表明眼睛、肺和甲状腺的副作用可由碘引起[28]。

与胺碘酮相比尽管决奈达隆是肝代谢的，但它的半衰期短[2,5,22-27]。它的电生理和药理作用时间较胺碘酮短[2,5,22-27]。在最初的研究中，引起减低同样心率和体表心电图 QT-QTc 间期变化的剂量较胺碘酮大[2,5,22-27]。在动物模型中它有抗肾上腺作用[26-28]。也延长房室传导时间，增加 QRS 时限及延长心房和心室不应期[28,29]。

决奈达隆的负性作用主要是影响心房和心室肌的有效不应期，显著降低心率[20]。在动物模型中，它能够减少心肌缺血引起的室性心律失常[25]。已有的资料显示，该药物对复极的影响受服药率的影响。与胺碘酮相同，它能使复极同步化，抑制由阿莫兰特诱发的尖端扭转型室速[22]。在心梗大鼠模型中，它减少室性早搏，没有促心律失常作用[24]。离体心肌组织灌注实验结果表明，像胺碘酮一样，决奈达隆缩短了APD，降低了ADP升支的最大速度[22,24]。相反，用决奈达隆预处理3周的动物组织，窦房结的自律性降低的同时，显著增加APD50和APD90，延长窦房结的APD[22,24,28]。因此，决奈达隆降低心率，延长体表心电图的QT-QTc间期的作用比胺碘酮要强。

从现有的资料看，尽管决奈达隆的分子结构上没有碘，但它的电生理特性与胺碘酮相似[22-28]。然而，还需要更多的有关其疗效和毒性的临床资料。目前有关的临床研究集中在房颤和植入ICD的患者。

四、替地沙米（tedisamil）

替地沙米是一种早期快速复极时I_{to}和I_{Kr}通道阻滞剂[2,5,30-34]。可能还有ATP钾通道（I_{K-ATP}）阻滞作用。它已经成为一种抗心肌缺血和心动过缓的制剂。由于它阻断了心肌复极的多种离子流，并且有减慢心率的作用，使它在电生理作用方面与多非利特，d-索他洛尔及其他Ⅲ类抗心律失常药物不同[1,2]。人体观察显示，静脉给予替地沙米（0.3mg/kg）减慢心率12%，伴有QT间期延长而对QRS时限无影响[30]。QTc和左室单相动作电位时程延长可被增快的心房起搏消除，因此，提示它对左室复极和不应期延长有反向功能依赖作用[30]。

在犬的心梗模型中，替地沙米抑制了10条犬中的8条的诱发性室性心律失常。与对照组比较，它能减少急性后侧壁心肌缺血引起的致命性缺血性心律失常的发生率（$P=0.027$）[31]。在离体的兔心缺氧、再氧化及吡那地尔诱发室颤的实验中，与对照组相比替地沙米降低了室颤的发生率（6个中的5个比6个中的0个；$P=0.007$）[32]。替地沙米抗室颤的作用可能是通过阻断I_{to}和I_{Kr}通道，但对I_{K-ATP}通道的抑制也起了一定作用[31-34]。

替地沙米的血流动力学效应表明它不损害左室功能或收缩性[33]。替地沙米降低平均心率，但并不损害心室的泵功能或收缩性。在动物模型中，尽管心率下降，但左室充盈压和dp/dt不变，LVEF及充盈量仅轻微降低（3%～13%）[33]。左室容积增加，其中舒张末容积增加6%，收缩容积增加23%[33]。已经证明替地沙米具有反向功能依赖作用。目前的研究正在评价它对房颤和房扑的治疗作用[33,34]。

五、曲西利特（trectilide）

曲西利特对心肌的作用与依布利特相似，正在成为口服制剂[35,36]。曲西利特是依布利特的一系列类似物中的一种，氟代替了庚基侧链，具有Ⅲ类药物的抗心律失常活性、代谢稳定性及潜在的促心律失常作用。氟替代后使侧链的氧化代谢稳定。有了这种替代，曲西利特有能力在快速和慢速起搏的情况下增加不应期。兔模型的多形性室速的产生依赖于苯甲基碳。其对称对应体的促心律失常作用较它的外消旋物少。这个系列的化合物中，曲西利特抗心律失常活性较强，代谢稳定。最初的研究表明，在兔模型中曲西利特没有促心律失常作用。在这个研究基础上，曲西利特被选作进一步评价。

与依布利特不同，曲西利特具有很好的口服生物利用度[3]。除了阻断I_{Kr}外，还通过其他未知的机制延长不应期[35,36]。目前，它正被发展为口服和静脉制剂，可能在终止房颤和房扑中有价值。

六、艾生利特（ersentilide）

艾生利特是一种I_{Kr}阻断剂和选择性β_1肾上腺素受体阻断剂。这一方面它与d,l-索他洛尔相似。它延长APD并且具有反向功能依赖作用[2,5,37-40]。在犬的浦氏纤维及心房肌和心室肌，艾生利特对最大舒张电位、动作电位的振幅或最大速度无影响[37-40]。它对三氟溴氯乙烷麻醉下肾上腺素诱导的室性心律失常及心梗后3～8天程序刺激诱发的室性心律失常有效[38]。艾生利特延长了动作电位时程（APD）、有效不应期及钙依赖的慢反应动作电位时间[37]。已经注意到艾生利特可以增加洋地黄产生的犬的除极后延迟的量，但不增加也不降低洋地黄诱发的心律失常的发生率[37]。艾生利特可以用于治疗房颤、室速及预防心脏性猝死。目前临床资料尚不充分，因此这种药物潜在的毒性和作用还不十分清楚。然而，从它的电生理特性来看，它对通道活性的影响范围与d,l-索他洛尔相似[2,5,37-40]。

七、氨巴利特（ambasilide）

氨巴利特是一种更新型抗心律失常药，它非选择性阻断延迟整流钾电流的I_{Kr}和I_{Ks}通道，及其他复极

钾电流的 I_{to}、I_K、I_{Kach} 及 I_{Kur} 通道[20,41-45]。氨巴利特在动作电位的快速偏移过程中阻断快钠通道[41]。在人和动物的心房细胞中已经证实，氨巴利特以剂量依赖方式延长心房 APD 和有效不应期[20,41-45]。在犬房颤模型中，氨巴利特和 d,l-索他洛尔的作用进行了比较[42]。氨巴利特 100% 终止心律失常，83% 的犬不能诱发[42]。相反 d,l-索他洛尔只阻断了 12% 的房颤，而且没有 1 例能阻止房颤诱发（$P<0.02$）[42]。目前该药已经进入三期临床试验，但还没临床资料。

八、阿莫兰特（almokalant）

阿莫兰特是另一种正在临床研究的选择性阻断 I_{Kr} 的Ⅲ类抗心律失常药。静脉制剂有很高的诱发尖端扭转型室速的发生率[20,46]。在兔动物模型中，阿莫兰特可延长浦肯野纤维和心室肌的动作电位时间。它还被证明可以产生早期除极后除极[20,46]。在连续 100 例，维持时间 8 ± 12 个月的房颤[95]或房扑[5]患者中，6h 内滴入阿莫兰特（$25\pm4mg$）。转复率 32%，平均转复时间 $3.5\pm2.2h$。经食管心房电图确定，心房率从 425 ± 30 次/分降到 284 ± 44 次/分。QTc 从 $425\pm30ms$ 延长到 $487\pm44ms$（$P<0.001$）。T 波振幅从 $0.31\pm19mV$ 降到 $0.23\pm16mV$（$P<0.001$）。T 波振幅的降低预示房颤会转为窦率。尖端扭转型室速的发生率为 4%[46]。目前没有临床研究的计划。

九、司美利特（sematilide）

司美利特是另一种已经在动物实验模型中评价的纯的 I_{Kr} 通道阻滞剂。它具有阻断离体的豚鼠心室肌和兔心房肌的内向整流钾电流的作用[47,48]。与其他阻断内向整流钾电流的制剂类似，这种药物延长动作电位时程和不应期。用两步结扎冠状动脉法、洋地黄、肾上腺素、冠状动脉结扎、再灌注及程序电刺激诱发的犬室性心律失常模型中，司美利特仅对程序刺激诱发的心律失常有作用[47,48]。而对其他方法诱发的心律失常无效[47-50]。像其他 I_{Kr} 阻断剂一样，司美利特具有潜在的延长复极及引起尖端扭转型室速的作用。司美利特还没有进入到临床研究。

十、总　结

在过去数年中，药物在心律失常治疗中的地位经历了很大变化。有很多药物特别是延长心房有效不应期和激动波长的Ⅲ类药物应用于房颤治疗的疗效正处于评价中[46,47]。最近的实验研究结果表明，某些制剂仅选择性延长心房复极而不延长心室复极[46,47]。与此同时，对有关房颤节律控制、心室率控制及抗凝药物的益处和危害进行了再评价。由于导管和外科方法用于治愈房颤，抗心律失常药物的地位削弱了。用β受体阻滞剂和钙通道阻滞剂控制心室率加抗凝剂，或用射频消融可能是将来治疗房颤更好的方法。对大多数室上性心律失常患者，目前室上性心动过速的射频消融优于药物治疗。

多项临床对照试验证明，抑制无症状和左室功能不良患者的室性心律失常可能增加死亡率[1]。同时，对比研究的结果表明，ICD 在延长有持续性室速或室颤危险或有病史的患者的生存时间上优于药物。尽管非药物策略在这类心律失常的治疗中占主导地位，但抗心律失常药物在植入 ICD 患者的治疗中继续有用，它可减少室性心律失常的发作频率从而减少了 ICD 的放电[6]。抗心律失常药物也可降低除颤阈值、降低心动过速的频率因而增加了抗心动过速起搏治疗的疗效。在将来，单独使用抗心律失常药物治疗室性心律失常还会继续减少。尽管研发对健康组织无作用、价格便宜、有效安全的理想药物的努力还将继续，因此心律失常治疗的基本策略正面对心律失常药物治疗地位的重新评价。

（王　龙译）

参 考 文 献

1. Camm AJ, Yap YG: Clinical trials of antiarrhythmic drugs in post-myocardial infarction and congestive heart failure patients. J Cardiovasc Pharm Ther 6:99-106, 2001.
2. Woolsey RL: New Antiarrhythmic drugs. In Zipes DP (ed): Cardiac Electrophysiology: From Cell to Bedside. Philadelphia, WB Saunders, 2000, pp 939-943.
3. Camm AJ, Yap YG: What should we expect from the next generation of antiarrhythmic drugs? J Cardiovasc Electrophysiol 10:307-317, 1999.
4. Singh BN: Current antiarrhythmic drugs: An overview of mechanisms of action and potential clinical utility. J Cardiovasc Electrophysiol 10:283-301, 1999.
5. Sager PT: New advances in class III antiarrhythmic drug therapy. Curr Opin Cardiol 15:41-53, 2000.
6. Pacifico A, Hohnloser SH, William JH, et al: Prevention of implantable defibrillator shocks by treatment with sotalol. d,l-sotalol Implantable Cardioverter Defibrillator Study Group. N Engl J Med 340:1855-1862, 1999.
7. Dorian P, Cas D, Schwartz B, et al: Amiodarone as compared with lidocaine for shock resistant ventricular fibrillation. N Engl J Med 346:884-890, 2002.
8. Kudenchuk PJ, Cobb LA, Copass MK, et al: Amiodarone for resuscitation after out-of-hospital cardiac arrest due to ventricular fibrillation. N Engl J Med 341:871-878, 1999.
9. Nattel S, Liu L, St. Georges D: Effects of the novel antiarrhythmic agent azimilide on experimental atrial fibrillation and atrial electro-

physiologic properties. Cardiovasc Res 37:627–635, 1998.
10. Fermini B, Jurkiewicz NK, Jow B, et al: Use-dependent effects of the class III antiarrhythmic agent NE-10064 (azimilide) on cardiac repolarization: Block of delayed rectifier ptoassium and L-type calcium currents. J Cardiovasc Pharmacol 26:259–271, 1995.
11. Salata J, Brooks R: Pharmacology of azimilide dihydrochloride (NE-10064), A Class III antiarrhythmic agent. Cardiovasc Drug Rev 15:137–156, 1997.
12. Nair LA, Grant AO: Emerging class III antiarrhythmic agents: mechanism of action and proarrhythmic potential. Cardiovasc Drugs Ther 11:149–167, 1997.
13. Pritchett ELC, Page RL, Connolly S, et al: Antiarrhythmic effect of azimilide in atrial fibrillation. J Am Coll Cardiol 36:794–802, 2000.
14. Pritchett E, Page P, Connelly S, et al: Azimilide treatment in atrial fibrillation. Circulation 98(Suppl):I633, 1999.
15. Karam R, Marcello S, Brooks R, et al: Azimilide hydrochloride, a novel antiarrhythmic agent. Am J Cardiol 84:40D–46D, 1998.
16. Page RL, Connolly SJ, Wilkinson WE, et al, and the Azimilide Supraventricular Arrhythmia Program (ASAP) Investigators. Antiarrhythmic effects of azimilide in paroxysmal supraventricular tachycardia: Efficacy and dose-response. Am Heart J 143:643–649, 2002.
17. Connolly S, Schnell D, Page R, et al: Dose-response relations of azimilide in the management of symptomatic, recurrent atrial fibrillation. Am J Cardiol 88:974–979, 2001.
18. Corey A, Agnew J, Bao J, et al: Effect of age and gender on azimilide pharmacokinetics after a single oral dose of azimilide dihydrochloride. J Clinical Pharm 37:946–953, 1997.
19. Corey A, Al-Khalidi H, Brezovic C, et al: Azimilide pharmacokinetics and pharmacodynamics upon multiple oral dosing. Biopharm Drug Dispos 20(2):59–68, 1999.
20. Castro A, Bianconi L, Santini M: New antiarrhythmic drugs for the treatment of atrial fibrillation. Pacing Clin Electrophysiol 25:249–259, 2002.
21. Camm AJ, Karam R, Pratt CM: The Azimilide Post-infarct Survival Evaluation (ALIVE) Trial. Am J Cardiol 81:35D–39D, 1998.
22. Verdyin SC, Vos MA, Leunissen HDM, et al: Evaluation of the acute electrophysiologic effect of intravenous dronedarone, an amiodarone-like agent, with special emphasis on ventricular repolarization and acquired torsades de pointes arrhythmias. J Cardiovasc Pharmacol 33:212–222, 1999.
23. Manning AS, Bruyninckx C, Ramboux J, Chatelain P: SR33589. A new amiodarone-like agent: effect on ischemia and reperfusion-induced arrhythmias in anesthetized rats. J Cardiovasc Pharmacol 26:453–461, 1995.
24. Aimond F, Beck L, Gautier P, et al: Cellular and in vivo electrophysiological effects of dronedarone in normal and postmyocardial infarcted rats. J Pharmacol Exp Ther 292:415–424, 2000.
25. Fiance O, Manning A, Chatelain P: Effects of a new amiodarone-like agent, SR 33589, in comparison to amiodarone, D,L-sotalol and lignocaine, on ischemic-induced ventricular arrhythmias in anesthetized pigs. J Cardiovasc Pharmacol 26:570–576, 1995.
26. Chatelain P, Meysmans L, Matteazzi JR, et al: Interaction of the antiarrhythmic agents SR 33589 and amiodarone with beta-adrenoceptor and adenylate cyclase in rate heart. Br J Pharmacol 116:1949–1956, 1995.
27. Hodeige D, Heyndrickx JP, Chatelain P, Manning A: SR 33589, a new amiodarone-like antiarrhythmic agents: Antiadrenoceptor activity in anaesthetized and conscious dogs. Eur J Pharmacol 279:25–32, 1995.
28. Sun W, Sarma J, Singh B: Electrophysiological effects of dronedarone (SR33589), a noniodinated benzofuran derivative, in the rabbit heart: Comparison with amiodarone. Circulation 100:2276–2281, 1999.
29. Manning A, Thisse V, Hodeige D, et al: SR 33589, a new amiodarone-like antiarrhythmic agent: Electrophysiological effects in anesthetized dogs. J Cardiovasc Pharmacol 25:252–261, 1995.
30. Bargheer K, Bode F, Klein HU, et al: Prolongation of monophasic action potential duration and the refractory period in the human heart by tedisamil, a new potassium-blocking agent. Eur Heart J 15:1409–1414, 1994.
31. Wallace AA, Stupienski RF, Baskin EP, et al: Cardiac electrophysiologic antiarrhythmic actions of tedisamil. J Pharmacol Exp Ther 273:168–175, 1995.
32. Chi L, Park JL, Friedrichs GS, et al: Effects of tedisamil (KC-8857) on cardiac electrophysiology and ventricular fibrillation in the rabbit isolated heart. Br J Pharmacol 117:1261–1269, 1996.
33. Thormann J, Mitrovic V, Riedel H, et al: Tedisamil (KC 8857) is a new specific bradycardic drug: Does it also influence myocardial contractility? Analysis by the conductance (volume) technique in coronary artery disease. Am Heart J 125:1233–1245, 1993.
34. Wettwer E, Himmel HM, Amosg L, et al: Mechanism of block by tedisamil of transient outward in human ventricular subepicardial myocytes. Br J Pharmacol 125:659–666, 1998.
35. Hester JB, Gibson JK, Buchanna LV, et al: Progress toward the development of a safe and effective agent for treating reentrant cardiac arrhythmias: Synthesis and evaluation of ibutilide analogues with enhanced metabolic stability and diminished proarrhythmic potential. J Med Chem 44:1099–1115, 2001.
36. Buist SC, Hsu CY, Walters RR: Sensitive determination of a new antiarrhythmic agent, trecetilide, in plasma by high-performance liquid chromatography with fluorescence detection. J Chromatogr 828(1-2):259–265, 1998.
37. Lee JH, Rosenshtraukh L, Beloshapko G, et al: The electrophysiologic effects of ersentilide on canine hearts. Eur J Pharmacol 285:25–35, 1995.
38. Argentieri TM, Troy HH, Carroll MS, et al: Electrophysiologic activity and antiarrhythmic efficacy of CK-3579, a new antirrhythmic agent with B-adrenergic blocking properties. J Cardiovasc Pharmacol 21:647–655, 1992.
39. Weyerbrock S, Schreieck J, Karch M, et al: Differential class III antiarrhythmic effects of ambasilide and dofetilide at different extra-cellular potassium and pacing frequencies. J Cardiovasc Pharmacol 28:314–320, 1999.
40. Adamson BP, Vanoli E, Hull SS, et al: Antifibrillatory efficacy of ersentilide, a novel betaadrenergic and I_{KR} blocker, in conscious dogs with a healed myocardial infarction. Cardiovasc Res 40:56–63, 1998.
41. Gijni V, Korth M, Schreieck J, et al: Differential class III antiarrhythmic effects of ambasilide and dofetilide at different extra-cellular potassium and pacing frequencies. J Cardiovasc Pharmacol 28:314–320, 1999.
42. Wang Z, Feng J, Nattel S: Class III antiarrhythmic drug action in experimental atrial fibrillation. Differences in reverse use dependence and effectiveness between d-sotalol and the new antiarrhythmic drug ambasilide. Circulation 90:2032–2040, 1994.
43. Yue L, Feng J, Wang Z, et al: Effects of ambasilide, quinidine, flecainide, and verapamil on ultra-rapid delayed rectifier current in canine atrial myocytes. Cardiovasc Res 46:151–161, 2000.
44. Feng J, Wang Z, Li GR, et al: Effects of class III antiarrhythmic drugs on transient outward and ultrarapid delayed rectifier currents in human atrial myocytes. Pharmacol Exp Ther 281:383–392, 1997.
45. Bosch RF, Milek IV, Popovic K, et al: Ambasilide prolongs the action potential and blocks multiple potassium currents in human atrium. J Cardiovasc Pharmacol 762–771, 1993.
46. Houlz B, Darpo B, Swedberg IC, et al: Almokalant and predictors of chronic atrial tachyarrhythmias to sinus rhythm. A prospective study. Cardiovasc Drugs Ther 13:329–338, 1999.
47. Ishii Y, Muraki K, Kurihara A, et al: Effects of sematilide, a novel class III antiarrhythmic agent, on membrane currents in rabbit atrial myocytes. Eur J Pharmacol 331(2-3):295–302, 1997.
48. Takai H, Sato R, Katori R: Sematilide blocks the inward rectifier potassium channel in isolated guinea pig ventricular myocytes. Gen Pharmacol 28:665–670, 1997.
49. Yue L, Feng J, Li GR, Natlel S: Characterization of ultra rapid delayed rectifier potassium channel involved in canine atrial repolarization. J Physiol 496:647–662, 1996.
50. Feng J, Xu D, Wang Z, Natlel S: Ultra rapid delayed rectifier current inactivation in human atrial myocytes properties and consequences. Am J Physiol 225:1717–1725, 1998.

第 105 章

经胸心脏复律与电除颤

Richard E. Kerber

本章目录

- 电除颤的概念 945
- 电复律与除颤的能量选择 945
- 适应证、准备和操作 945
- 电极 946
- 把除颤器的应用范围从床旁扩大到社区 ... 947

一、电除颤的概念

经胸电除颤（体外除颤）终止心律失常是一种有效的、快速安全的操作，已经在全世界广泛应用多年。

二、电复律与除颤的能量选择

电除颤（终止室速）或转复（终止房颤、房扑、室速）所需的能量大小通常用单位——焦耳或瓦特表示，过大的能量和电流有潜在的心脏毒害性，可引起形态学损伤，表现为心肌坏死、功能受损、房室传导障碍，这种除颤介导的损伤机制尚不明确，可能与心肌内温度上升及过氧化物脂、自由基产生相关[2]。因此，早期低能量除颤及转复是既有效又可能减少损伤的办法。根据传统的单相衰减正弦波，首次电除颤的能量推荐为 200J，如不能转复，第 2 次能量应为 200J，第 3 次 300J、甚至 360J[3]。

双相波除颤应用于植入式除颤器已经很多年了，现已应用于经胸除颤器（图 105-1）。双相波除颤比传统的单相衰减正弦波更有效，用低能量即能更好地终止心动过速[4]。能够自动调整电压和脉宽是这种除颤器的特点。AHA 推荐双相波电除颤首次能量应≤200J[3]，许多病人能量是否可以大于 200J 目前还不清楚，对于房颤复律，双相波能量应≤150J[5,6]。

室颤在儿童是不常见的，儿科心脏骤停常继发于呼吸骤停。如果室颤持续，双相波除颤能量为 2J/kg，首次不成功则能量加倍[3]，儿童双相波除颤最适合的能量值尚不清楚。

三、适应证、准备和操作

在房性心律失常，心律失常的持续时间、心房纤维化程度、左房的大小对于复律的成功及成功复律后窦性心律的维持均是重要的决定因素。然而，偶尔有左房大、持续时间长的房颤在复律后能够维持窦性心律。在心脏复律前，常常使用胺碘酮以达到除颤后维持窦性心律的目的。

在电复律前 3 周传统推荐使用抗凝药物以避免栓塞事件发生，以下为血栓形成的高危患者：（1）二尖瓣狭窄；（2）任何原因导致的左房大；（3）慢性、长期性房颤；（4）以往发生过血栓栓塞事件；（5）糖尿病；（6）高血压。尽管经胸心脏超声能够很好的反映左房容量，但常不能准确反映左房内附着物、大多数左房内血栓大小。新近发展起来的经食管超声（TEE）能很好地反映左房内附着物，而且对血栓的存在高度敏感。Manning 及其同事[7]报道当经食管超声显示左房内无附壁血栓时，在房颤患者复律前 2 天静脉使用肝素，行心脏复律术后无栓塞事件发生。然而，也有报道，尽管经食管超声证实左房内无附壁血

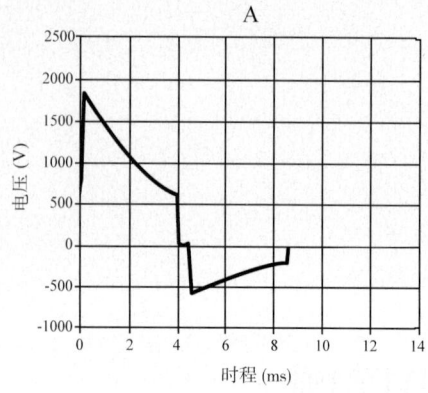
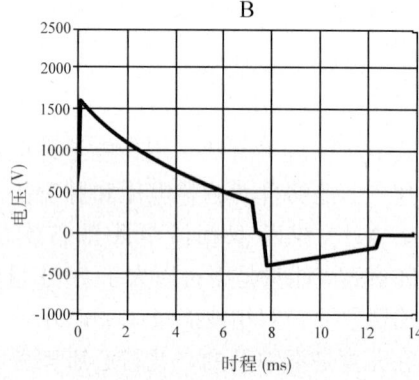
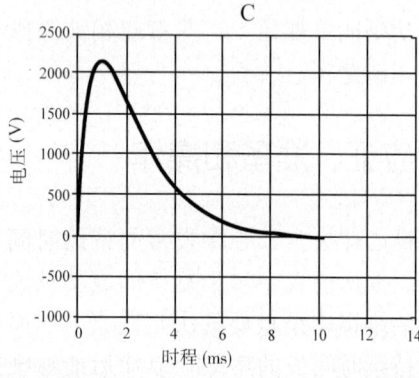

图 105-1 经胸电除颤时的减震正弦曲线同两种新型双向波的比较　同减震正弦曲线相比，双向波除颤终止室颤所用能量较小。

栓，患者复律后未经抗凝治疗3周，复律后仍有栓塞事件发生[8]。经食管超声指导心脏复律目前推荐使用肝素（或华法林达到治疗化的国际标准化比值）达到短期抗凝（24～48h）。在经食管超声证实无左房附壁血栓，心脏复律后，即使经食管超声阴性，仍推荐4周的抗凝治疗。如果经食管超声证实有血栓存在，心脏复律应该延迟直到完成3周的抗凝治疗，应重复经食管超声检查证实是否有血栓存在。尽管房扑心脏复律后血栓形成少见，但仍有报道[9]血栓事件发生与经食管超声显示左房内存在云雾状血栓有关，因此在房扑心脏复律前应考虑更短期抗凝治疗[10]。

在心脏复律当天一般禁止使用洋地黄制剂，因为洋地黄增加心肌自律性，当达到中毒剂量时，易于室性心律失常或室颤的发生，洋地黄中毒时应避免进行电复律。心脏复律的患者必须麻醉，因为经胸的电流会引起疼痛性强直性收缩，仅仅镇静是不够的，在某些情况下患者可能需要气管内插管。

必须与QRS波群的R波同步放电，如果除颤落在心动周期的易损期易诱发室颤（图105-2）。根据作者的经验，这是房性心律失常电复律最常见的严重并发症，经常由于操作者没有适当的同步化或选择的ECG导联R波没有达到被同步器识别的足够高度，也可能是因为心律失常形成时，室速的R波识别有时比较困难所致。如果患者因为快速室性心动过速导致血流动力学不稳定，非同步电除颤可能优于过多花费时间进行同步电除颤。

四、电　极

经胸电流模式取决于电极放置的位置，不正确的位置可能导致电除颤失败[11]。多种放置模式已被成功应用，包括心尖-心底位（右胸骨旁上），心前-心后位（左或右肩胛骨），心尖右肩胛骨位。心尖-心底位在反复电除颤时是最方便的体位。令人惊讶的是几乎没有电流经过心脏。Lerman和Deale[12]报道仅有4%的经胸电流是经过心脏的，其余的经心外途径通过。

电极的大小决定经胸电阻和电流，高等医疗建议协会推荐每个电极的面积不小于$50cm^2$，两个电极的总面积不小于$150cm^2$[13]。尽管更小的儿童电极已经为儿童产生，在10kg（大约1岁）以上儿童应该使用成人电极以减少经胸阻抗[14]。

在电极板金属表面使用耦合剂（通常是凝胶）是非常重要的。不这样做会导致高阻抗和低电流，必须注意避免在两个电极之间涂抹凝胶或导电糊，因为电流可能沿着有导电糊介导的低阻抗通道流过，而偏离了心脏的电流[11]。在女性患者，心尖电极应放在乳房旁或乳房下，放在乳房上会导致高阻抗和电流衰减[15]。

大的自粘式的除颤电极板是传统手握电极的有用补充，经常装备于自动体外除颤器（AEDs）。经胸直流电除颤后一度皮肤烧伤是常见的[16]，因为电流在电极边缘通过，可见典型的电极形状的烧伤轮廓。

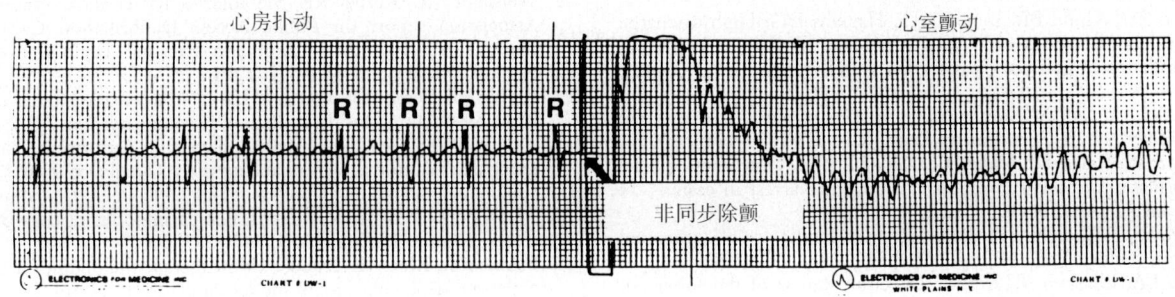

图 105-2 一个可以避免的电转复并发症：非同步电除颤意外地在 T 波易损期放电诱导的室颤（箭头所示） 正确的同步放电应确保在 R 波上放电，从而避免这种并发症。（引自 Tacker W/A：Defibrillation of the Heart：ICDs，AEDs and Manual. St. Louis，Mosby-Year Book，1994.）

五、把除颤器的应用范围从床旁扩大到社区

早期的除颤器用于抢救心脏骤停患者。AHA 定义"生存链"为：急诊医疗系统的早期行为（通过拨打就近的 911 电话）；旁观者实行早期的心肺复苏；早期进行电除颤；早期严密的心脏监护。

自动体外除颤器是新发展起来的一项重要技术，尤其应用于院外心脏骤停的抢救。救助者仅需培训如何开启设备，如何使用电极，对于室颤（与其他不需要除颤的心律失常鉴别）判断必须准确。由第一个发现者诸如消防员、警察、保安等使用自动体外除颤器已经显著提高了院外心脏骤停患者的生存率，明显地缩短了援助者从到达到转运到接受电除颤的时间[17]。最近报道由于广泛放置和使用自动体外除颤器使得高危地区诸如飞机场等地心脏骤停患者的生存率大大提高[18-20]，AHA 强烈推荐使用，这种方法被称为"公众除颤"[22,23]。

大多数心脏骤停发生在家里[24]，对于已知心脏病的患者家中备有 AEDs 进行家庭除颤是否有效？其限制是必须有人目击到患者心脏骤停发生。而且目击者能够拿到自动体外除颤器，能够正确地应用和使用它。出于这种考虑，佩带式的除颤器应运而生，它能持续佩带在患者身上，监视其心电图，当判断有室颤发生时自动电除颤，不需要其他援助者。这种装置适合于已知有心脏病具有一定致死心律失常危险（但并非高危患者）的患者使用（高危患者应佩带植入式除颤器），最初的结论已经令人鼓舞[25]。

这些新技术的发展及进行的社区教育计划对心肌梗死的早期识别和广泛的心肺复苏的技术培训，使得心脏骤停者存活率增加。

（张 灵 译）

参 考 文 献

1. Tacker WA: Defibrillation of the Heart: ICDs, AEDs and Manual. St. Louis, Mosby-Year Book, 1994.
2. Caterine MR, Spencer KT, Pagan-Carlo LA, et al: Direct current shocks to the heart generate free radicals: An electron paramagnetic resonance study. J Am Coll Cardiol 28:1598–1609, 1996.
3. American Heart Association guidelines 2000 for CPR and emergency cardiac care. Circulation 102:1–1, 2000.
4. Bardy GH, Marchlinski FE, Sharma AD, et al: Multicenter comparison of truncated biphasic shocks and standard damped sine waveform modified shocks for transthoracic ventricular defibrillation. Circulation 94:2507–2514, 1996.
5. Mittal S, Ayati S, Stein KM, et al: Transthoracic cardioversion of atrial fibrillation: Comparison of rectilinear biphasic vs. damped sine wave monophasic shocks. Circulation 101:1282–1287, 2000.
6. Page RL, Kerber RE, Russell JK, et al: Biphasic vs. monophasic shock waveform for conversion of atrial fibrillation: The results of an international randomized, double-blind multicenter trial. J Am Coll Cardiol 39:1956–1963, 2002.
7. Manning WJ, Silverman DI, Gordon SPF, et al: Cardioversion from atrial fibrillation without prolonged anticoagulation with use of transesophageal echocardiography to exclude the presence of atrial thrombi. N Engl J Med 328:750–755, 1993.
8. Black I, Hopkins AP, Lee CLL, Walsh W: Evaluation of transesophageal echocardiography before cardioversion of atrial fibrillation and atrial flutter in nonanticoagulated patients. Am Heart J 126:375–381, 1993.
9. Irani WN, Grayburn PA, Afridi I: Prevalence of thrombus, spontaneous echo contrast, and atrial stunning in patients undergoing cardioversion of atrial flutter: A prospective study using transesophageal echocardiography. Circulation 95:962–966, 1997.
10. Olshansky B, Kerber RE: Cardioversion of atrial flutter. In Waldo AL, Touboul P (eds): Atrial Flutter: Advances in Mechanisms and Management. Armonk, NY, Futura Publishing, 1996, pp 387–409.
11. Caterine MR, Yoerger DM, Spencer KT, et al: Effect of electrode position and gel-application technique on predicted transcardiac current during transthoracic defibrillation. Ann Emerg Med 29:588–595, 1997.
12. Lerman BB, Deale OS: Relation between transcardiac and transthoracic current during defibrillation in humans. Circ Res 67:1420–1426, 1990.
13. Association for the Advancement of Medical Instrumentation: American National Standard: Cardiac Defibrillator Devices. ANSI/AAMI DF2–1996. Arlington, VA, AAMI, 1996.
14. Atkins DL, Kerber RE: Pediatric defibrillation: Current flow is improved by using "adult" paddle electrodes. Pediatrics 94:90–93, 1994.
15. Pagan-Carlo LA, Spencer KT, Robertson CE, et al: Transthoracic defibrillation: Importance of avoiding electrode placement directly on the female breast. J Am Coll Cardiol 27:449–452, 1996.
16. Pagan-Carlo LA, Stone MS, Kerber RE: Nature and determinants of skin burns after transthoracic cardioversion. Am J Cardiol

79:689–691, 1997.
17. White RD, Asplin BR, Bugliosi TF, Hankins DG: High discharge survival rate after out-of-hospital ventricular fibrillation with rapid defibrillation by police and paramedics. Ann Emerg Med 28:480–485, 1996.
18. Page RL, Joglar JA, Kowal RC, et al: Use of automated external defibrillators by a US airline. N Engl J Med 343:1210–1216, 2000.
19. Valenzuela T, Roe DJ, Nichol G, Clark LL, et al: Outcomes of rapid defibrillation by security officers after cardiac arrest in casinos. N Engl J Med 343:1206–1209, 2000.
20. Caffrey S, Willoughby PJ, Pepe PE, et al: Public use of automated external defibrillators. N Engl J Med 347:1242–1247, 2002.
21. Cobb LA, Eliastam M, Kerber RE, et al: Report of the American Heart Association Task Force on the Future of Cardiopulmonary Resuscitation. Circulation 85:2346–2355, 1992.
22. Weisfeldt ML, Kerber RE, McGoldrick RP, et al: American Heart Association report on Public Access Defibrillation Conference, December 8–10, 1994: Automatic External Defibrillation Task Force. Circulation 92:684–692, 1995.
23. Kerber RE, Becker LB, Bourland JD, et al: Automatic external defibrillators for public access defibrillation: Recommendations for specifying and reporting arrhythmia analysis algorithm performance, incorporating new waveforms and enhancing safety. Circulation 95:1677–1682, 1997.
24. Weaver DL, Peberdy MA: Defibrillation in public places—one step closer to home. N Engl J Med 347:1233, 2002.
25. Feldman A, Klein H, Tchou P: New therapeutic option for patients with time-dependent risk of sudden cardiac death. J Am Coll Cardiol 39:101A, 2002.

第 106 章

植入式心脏复律除颤器：技术与现状

Bruce L. Wilkoff

本章目录

- 系统组成 ················· 949
- 心动过速治疗 ············· 954

植入式心脏复律除颤器（ICD）技术的发展已经超过了对其临床应用的理解。尽管如此，该技术仍然是不成熟的，电池、电容器、导线、算法发展的速度使该治疗方法整合入临床实践更具挑战性。ICD 有两项基本任务：心动过速的识别与终止。本章主要介绍这两项功能的现状与发展前景。

本章同时还将介绍与 ICD 技术发展相关的其他内容。最容易被忽略的技术包括程控仪、诊断程序及遥测技术，对于这些功能的临床影响及其相关内容做再多强调也不过分。

一、系统组成

ICD 的组成包括 ICD 脉冲发生器、起搏与感知电极，以及一根或多根高能电极。ICD 脉冲发生器的外壳通常包含多根高能电极中的一根。与起搏导线类似，ICD 电极，或称导线，通过密封的接口与脉冲发生器顶盖相连，感知与起搏导线使用 IS-1 心动过缓接口标准。高能导线接口由 1 个直径 3.2mm 的带短柄的绝缘器构成，称为 DF-1 接口。ICD 导线通常分成 3 支，通过 1 个 IS-1（心动过缓）和 2 个 DF-1（高能）接口插入 ICD 脉冲发生器。在不久的将来，1 个新的接口标准——IS-4，将把心动过缓与心动过速电极组合成单个 3.2mm 4 极接口，改变目前使用的 ICD 导线三分叉与顶盖相连的现状。

（一）ICD 脉冲发生器

与早期型号相比，目前的 ICD 脉冲发生器的体积显著下降。早期的脉冲发生器大（160～190cm^3）而重（>200g），必须植入于腹壁皮下或腹直肌下。现在，这些不能程控的机器已经让位于更小的、可程控的仪器。早期的 ICD 仅仅针对室速或室颤发放电击，而现在可通过单腔或双腔频率应答起搏器及再同步化治疗来处理心动过缓。最新一代的 ICD 增加了通过电话问询的识别标准、治疗参数及诊断信息。其他改进包括针对室速的附加治疗、心动过速鉴别诊断算法的改进、抗心动过速与心动过缓起搏、非侵入性程序刺激、快速心率计数器或腔内电图的储存、双相波除颤。目前的 ICD 都具备以上功能，而脉冲发生器大小降至约 35cm^3。ICD 脉冲发生器体积的下降将其植入胸前皮下筋膜处成为可能，与目前普通起搏器的植入部位相同。与非开胸电极（NTL）的发展一起，ICD 体积变小显著降低了植入手术操作过程的复杂程度，也使手术可以在严重心脏病患者中进行。

ICD 脉冲发生器的外壳由不锈钢或钛制成。鉴于强度、在体液中不发生反应及重量轻，钛被认为是更为合适的材料。外壳主要用于保护电路免受体液腐蚀，但在目前许多 ICD 型号中，外壳也作为一个主动电极。顶盖通常由透明的多聚甲基丙烯树脂制成，所以在植入过程中与导线的连接可以直观得到确认，一旦部件异常或可能发生故障需要启动 ICD 故障排除系统时，可以直接检测到。电极连接通过导线穿过外壳上密封的开孔接入 ICD 电路。

ICD 内部是由电池、电容器、DC-DC 转换器和微处理器、遥测通信线圈及相互连接组成的复合体[1]。感知到的心室信号，振幅一般在 5~25mV 之间，通过导线进入脉冲发生器，然后经过过滤，由 ICD 已设置好的算法进行分析。电路经特殊设计、经硅胶包埋，用于室速或室颤的分析与识别。一旦达到识别标准，ICD 就对患者进行高能除颤和除颤后起搏治疗。

（二）电池

早期 ICD 脉冲发生器使用锂五氧化钒电池，储存大约 8 000J 的能量，相当于大约 150 次最大能量的除颤。现在大多数 ICD 脉冲发生器使用的电池是锂银钒氧化电池，包含约 18 000J 的能量[2,3]。在充足电的情况下，该电池可释放约 3.2V 的能量。由于每个 ICD 脉冲发生器通常使用 2 个串联的电池，所以开始时充足电压是 6.4V。大多数除颤器使用同一个电池系统执行所有功能，除了给用于高能除颤的电容器充电，还包括心动过缓起搏、低电压维持功能如记忆、遥测，以及为关键性电路供电。

电池状态取决于测得的电压。从 ICD 获得的遥测信息一定包括电池电压的指示。与永久起搏器一样，当电池耗竭的特定指示即择期更换指征（elective replacement indicator，ERI）出现时，就需要对脉冲发生器进行更换。当电池电压降至约 2.6V 时，通常会出现 ERI，此时需要在几个月内择期进行脉冲发生器的更换，具体时间取决于 ICD 发放治疗的频率。当电池电压低至约 2.2V 时，提示脉冲发生器的更换更加紧迫，因为为取得合适的除颤能量，电容器需要更长的充电时间，此时称为电池的耗竭期（end of life，EOL）。此外，将电容器充足电所需的时间也可作为电池状态的一个指标，当所需时间超过某一特定值，就需要进行更换。

（三）电容器

电池本身无法释放除颤所需的高能量。目前的 ICD 电池不能以除颤必需的高电压形式贮存能量。因此，通过 DC-DC 转换器，电容器可以从 6.4V 的电池中贮存 30~40J 的能量，然后在 10~20ms 的时间内，向心脏释放接近 750V 的高电压。为便于除颤，与电池一样对电容器有特定的要求[3,4]。电容器必须能在临床允许的时间范围内（<10~30s）充电至 10~30J。由于只有符合识别标准并且对除颤治疗完成程控后，电容器才能充电，因此一旦充电时间延长，将使患者处于血流动力学停滞状态的时间延长。动物实验显示，当室颤持续时间超过 20s 时，除颤所需能量将增加[5]。由于能够在规定的时间内完成充电，铝电解电容器已被广泛使用。大多数电容器开始并不是为 ICD 专门设计的，也没有考虑到它的大小与形状。圣犹达公司使用的一款铝电解电容器（Flatcaps）是特意为它的 ICD 脉冲发生器设计的，因此更薄、更适于植入胸前。

（四）电极

除颤系统有 3 个主要功能：识别心动过速、起搏和除颤。电极是实现这些功能的导线中非绝缘部分。电极的感知与起搏技术与永久起搏器相似。然而，感知与起搏的双极是从心室导线顶端到远端除颤电极，而不是从心室导线顶端到环状电极。这称为集成双极（integrated bipolar），而不是真双极（true bipolar）系统。双室 ICD 的心室起搏是从左室和右室导线顶端到环状电极或者远端除颤电极，而某些 ICD 的感知可仅仅局限于右室。识别功能一般通过一个双极电极系统完成，使检测到的腔内电图局限于心室。

然而高能量除颤需要特殊电极，该电极能够将高能电流传导到心脏，并以一种恰当的方式分配至心室供除颤。早期 ICD 系统使用心外膜片状电极，而近年来使用经静脉安置于心内膜的电极系统（the NTL）。

（五）非开胸电极

非开胸电极（NTLs）最早由 CPI（Cardiac Pacemakers Inc）公司生产，称为 Endotak 导线。这些导线是集成双极双线圈导线的原型，包括一个感知/起搏顶端电极和两个大的线圈电极用于高能除颤。远端线圈位于导线顶端附近，因此能够定位于右室。右室线圈位于右室心尖部对除颤效果很重要[6,7]。近端线圈常位于上腔静脉或锁骨下静脉（左侧多见）。心室电图记录来自电极顶端与远端线圈电极之间的信号。此类感知方式称为集成双极。第二个非开胸电极由美敦力公司生产（Medtronic Transvene），包括用于感知（真双极感知）的顶端电极和环状电极，以及两个感知电极近端的单个导体线圈。

当这些非开胸电极刚出现时，ICD 脉冲发生器的大小并不能供大多数患者进行胸前区植入。因此这些电极经左侧锁骨下或头静脉植入，通过皮下隧道与脉冲发生器相连。然后将脉冲发生器埋置于腹直肌表面皮下，偶尔在体瘦的患者中植于腹直肌下面。

所有的非开胸电极都有一个高能线圈靠近电极远

端,并位于右室腔。其他厂商生产的非开胸电极都有类似的结构,尽管有些细节不同(表106-1)。然而,直流电的物理特性需要至少另一个电极以完成除颤回路。在胸前植入ICD广泛开展之前,第二根高能电极常常是另一根经静脉线圈电极,或是皮下片状电极,或是两者兼有。第二根经静脉线圈电极常安置于左锁骨下静脉或上腔静脉。偶尔有高能线圈电极被放置在冠状窦,并与右室线圈电极构成除颤电路的成功报道[8]。第二根血管内电极的主要缺点是需要静脉路径的第二个穿刺点(除非两个线圈位于同一根导线上),并增加血管并发症的潜在危险。皮下或肌肉下片状电极不需要额外的血管路径,可以避免血管并发症。不幸的是,这些片状电极需要皮下组织的大块分离,增加出血、疼痛和感染的危险。

随着体积更小的ICD脉冲发生器的发展,胸前区植入成为可能,脉冲发生器的外壳就可作为第二个电极(即"热机壳")[9]。动物实验将热机壳ICD系统分别埋置于左胸前区或腋下区、右胸前区、左或右侧腹部这3个部位的除颤效果进行比较。结果显示,左胸前区和腋下部位优于所有其他位置,右胸前区优于腹部位置。这些结果提示,当左锁骨下静脉堵塞或由于其他原因不能使用左胸前区时,也可以将ICD植入其他位置[10]。

(六)心动过速的识别

ICD识别快速心律失常是一系列复杂的过程。然而,更加复杂的是,ICD必须也能识别快速心律失常不发作的状态。这是非常重要的,因为除了一小部分时间,患者大部分时间处于非心动过速状态,识别非心动过速状态就像识别致命性心律失常同样重要。因此,假设起搏与除颤治疗有效,对心律的正确识别既要考虑到患者的生活质量,还要考虑到患者的生命安全。

ICD能正确识别心律并非都受ICD技术的潜在影响。最值得注意的是,心律失常的频率与机制和ICD的程控是心律识别的主要决定因素,也是与技术方法几乎完全无关的因素。然而,通过分析传递到ICD的信号本质、使ICD正确识别这些信号、限制程控选项,常常可以使ICD正确发挥功能。

(七)感知

治疗是建立在对传递到脉冲发生器的信号进行分析的基础上的。所有目前使用的ICD将心室率作为识别心动过速的基础变量。然而为确定心率,必须对每个心室除极间期进行测量。ICD通过感知和分析患者的腔内电图事件,该过程始于感知导线的放置,腔内

表106-1 目前临床使用的非开胸电极的特征

生产商	型号	导体起搏:感知/线圈	电极起搏:感知/线圈	线圈数目	感知方式
CPI Guidant, St. Paul, Minn.	所有	钴-铬-镍合金/拉制的黄铜股	铂-铱合金/铂包裹的钛	1或2	集成双极
Medtronic Minneapolis, Minn.	Quattro	钴-铬-镍合金/钴-铬镍合金,银核心	铂-铱合金/铂-铱合金镀过的钽	2	真双极
Medtronic	所有	钴-铬-镍合金/钴-铬镍合金,银核心	镨-铱合金/铂-铱合金	1或2	真或集成双极
St. Jude Medical, Sylmar, Calif.	Riata/TVL-ADX	钴-铬-镍合金/钴-铬-镍合金	氮化钛包裹的铱合金/铂-铱合金	1或2	真双极
St. Jude Medica	所有	钴-铬-镍合金/钴-铬-镍合金	铂-铱合金/铂-铱合金	1或2	集成双极
Biotronik, Portland, Ore.	Kentrox	钴-铬-镍合金/钴-铬-镍合金	铂-铱均分包裹/铂-铱均分包裹	1或2	集成双极
ELA(Investigational), Plymouth, Minn.	Swift	钴-铬-镍合金/钴-铬-镍合金,银核心	镨-铱合金/铂-铱合金	1	集成双极

电图取决于与导线紧密接触的心肌是否处于正常状态，同时也取决于横膈、心房的结构，以及诸如起搏器、移动电话等仪器和其他电磁干扰源。腔内电图事件的识别完全依赖于信号质量的好坏，而信号质量在导线安放时就已经确定了。由于除颤效果几乎总是在右室心尖部最佳，有时感知功能就受导线在心尖部安置的影响[11]。其他受电极位置潜在影响的方面还有腔内电图的形态，如腔内电图事件的宽度。将心房导线信息传入脉冲发生器，使心律失常的准确识别更加复杂。虽然将导线安放在可以获得最大腔内电图波形的位置，不会减少误计心律失常的机会，但心房电极的植入部位必须不出现心室电图。感知功能不仅是心室的信号/噪声比值问题，也要使心房导线去除所有非心房事件。

（八）带通滤波器（band pass filtering）

感知放大器对从导线获取、传到脉冲发生器的信号进行处理。放大器将特定频率的信号传递到识别区，而其他信号均被过滤掉。带通滤波器由一个高频、低频临界点和一条包含真正信号事件的频率带区间组成，目的是防止无关信号干扰导致 ICD 误识别快速心律失常。遗憾的是，在复极与除极波之间、心房与心室事件之间、心室起搏后极化与除极之间、肌电位与心肌除极之间、环境信号与心脏事件之间，都存在一些频率重叠区。

（九）频率与振幅

传到带通滤波器的信号的振幅与信号包含的频率之间存在明显关系。通过将频谱移至带通滤波器的频率中心，增大的信号常能提高腔内电图事件识别的特异性。某些相对弱（如 4~6mV）但频率合适的信号，表现为在起搏系统分析仪上测得的斜率超过 1V/s，可能优于强（8~10mV）而斜率低于 0.1V/s 的信号[12]。

（十）自动增益与自动阈值调整（autogain and autothreshold）

ICD 识别算法遇到的一个重要问题是必须被准确识别的信号振幅存在明显波动。常见的例子有通过希氏束-浦肯野系统自然下传的心搏振幅有 10mV，每个起搏尖峰后极化电压的振幅有 5 000mV，室性早搏与室速的振幅在 2~25mV 之间，心搏停止的腔内电图振幅为 0~0.15mV，室颤的振幅在 0.2~20mV 之间。以上任何一种心律失常间的转换必须得到正确处理。

最困难的两个问题是区分从低振幅到高振幅和从高振幅再回到低振幅的腔内电图事件引起的频率波动，同时不过度感知信号。解决方法是分别使用自动增益与自动阈值调整。自动增益技术使用固定振幅电压阈值，根据各种算法对增益连续变化的信号进行放大，对强弱信号单次计数。自动阈值调整技术使用一个放大增益和一个连续变化的阈值来完成相同的任务。在一个心动周期中阈值常发生变化，即使对信号振幅进行成比例的调整，在每次感知或起搏事件后仍会发生衰减。有时可以对电压下限进行程控调整，以区分信号上的噪声与低振幅的室颤信号。

（十一）合适振幅的估算

心室感知电极是在非心动过速状态下安置的。因此，在进行除颤阈值（DFT）测试诱发室颤前，必须确定安置是否合适。尽管室颤连续发作与单个室颤事件时平均腔内电图事件振幅明显不同，但在窦性心律时腔内电图的振幅与随后诱发出的心律失常的平均、最小、最大室颤腔内电图事件之间存在一定关系。幸好为了识别快速心律失常，不必识别每个腔内电图事件。作为合适的估计，窦性心律时腔内电图 5mV 的振幅可以预测未被感知的腔内电图事件发生率低于 10%，快速心律失常不被识别的可能性可以排除。虽然在窦性心律腔内电图振幅低于 5mV 时识别失败的发生率也很低，但是室颤的振幅更低，识别失败的几率将显著增加[13]。

（十二）识别算法（detection algorithm）

一旦检测到一个腔内电图事件，识别算法就对事件之间的波形进行解释。算法试图对检测到的需要不同治疗方法的心律失常进行分级，如心动过缓、需要抗心动过速起搏的室速、需要低能电击的室速、需要高能除颤的室颤。排除与室性心律失常频率重叠的窦性心动过速和房颤特别困难。为了区分这些心律，在心室率标准外增加了心律失常的时限、心率加快的突发性、心动周期中每个心搏间的变化。从腔内电图形态衍生来的有模板、时限、向量关系，随着心房电极的增加，心房与心室事件之间的关系进一步提高了心律失常识别的特异性。需要注意的是这些新的算法损失的检测敏感性有多大。重要的是，这些算法主要针对非常快的心动过速发放电击，而不管它们起源于心房还是心室。

（十三）敏感性与特异性（房性室性心律失常）

威胁生命的心律失常必须得到识别和终止。然而，心律失常的发生机制与频率并不总是与其血流动力学影响相关。患者可因 1∶1 的房扑或频率 110 次/分的单形性室速而死亡。将心率识别的临界点设得越低，敏感性越高，但对真正致命性心律失常检测的特异性就越差。最早由 Intec 公司研制的 AID-B 心律转复除颤器，以及随后由 CPI 公司研制的 AICD，均使用相对低的心率识别临界点，对窦速、房颤、室速、室颤都一视同仁。患者接受电击的次数与心律失常的类型无关，而与机器出厂时设定的无法程控的心率识别临界点多低直接相关。新的识别算法和多种治疗方法有可能延迟对患者发放本来不应耽搁的治疗。目前面临的挑战是使用一些可以避免发生不恰当治疗的算法，以便 ICD 更好地适应，同时改善患者的生活质量。

（十四）频率与时限

需要治疗的室性心律失常的主要特征是心律失常的频率与时限。频率慢的、时限短的心律失常不需要治疗。而心率快时，等着观察心律失常是否结束而 ICD 不加干预，将可能导致不良后果。不能识别低振幅的腔内电图事件引起干预延迟或识别被阻止都将导致严重后果。结果就是心率越快，留给识别的时间就越短。室速识别时，连续心律失常事件频率快于某一程控的频率就可确定；而室颤时，大量连续的心动间期中出现几个短的心动间期，将有助于室颤的识别。这个算法很重要，因为室颤时腔内电图的振幅与间期变化多端。

（十五）突发性（sudden onset）

折返性室性心动过速和一些机制不明的折返性心律失常开始发生时，频率突然加快，与发生前的非心动过速心律明显不同。心动周期的突然缩短有时在区分窦性心动过速与缓慢的室性心动过速时有用。窦速时防止误识别为室速的最好方法是程控一个更快的室速检测频率，然而，如果该方法不可能，使用突发的标准有一定但有限的作用。不幸的是，当室速由窦速或运动引发时，使用突发的标准将增加心律失常得不到处理的危险。

（十六）周期稳定性（cycle length stability）

与房颤时的心室反应不同，大多数室速的心动周期稳定，每个心动周期间的差值<40ms。虽然这并不总是正确的，但与发作不频繁的房颤伴快速心室率鉴别时，以上标准适用。对持续性房颤或频繁发作的阵发性房颤，尤其在需要处理的缓慢性室速时，行房室结消融术后安置一个频率应答起搏器是更好的选择。随着新的频率应答、单腔、双腔、双室起搏器与 ICD 的组合，这将是一个更常见的选择。把心房与心室心动周期整合在一起，将极大地提高房颤识别的特异性，但也使房颤时发生室速的双重性心动过速的识别更加复杂。

（十七）再识别与再确认

与任何其他方法一样，心动过速也是根据贝氏统计法识别的。真正阳性结果的可能性直接与治疗人群中该现象的发生率成比例。一旦某个心律被严格的标准识别为室速或室颤并被治疗，有可能符合频率标准的心律失常未停止，很快需要再次治疗，以防止晕厥。再识别时通过减少需要检测的心动周期的数目、取消其他识别标准，增强处理的快速性与敏感性。相反，ICD 电容器充电需要时间，这个过程中心律失常可能已经终止。因此，在发放治疗前，需要对心动过速进行再确认，防止对非持续性心动过速患者在窦性心律情况下进行电击。危险在于，在血流动力学进行性衰竭时，自动增益或自动阈值调整算法不能识别振幅非常低的室颤波。因此，对室颤识别区的心律进行再确认时要小心。某些机器允许在室颤或室速和室颤识别区进行约定式与非约定式除颤。

（十八）波形与 QRS 波宽度

早期由 Mirowski 设计的除颤器（AID），基于心室电图电压从基线偏移的时间百分比，采用概率密度函数（probability density function）计算，只能识别室颤。在使用该机器的早期就已明确，如果没有频率标准，敏感性、特异性、快速性都是不够的[14]。此后，腔内电图宽度测量、波形标准，以及最近的波形模板配对和向量相关技术已被用于增强心动过速识别的快速性与特异性，且已取得一些成功。

（十九）心房电极标准

植入心房电极后，就可获取心房与心室活动的关系供分析。如果数据准确，在前文提到的远场信号的警告下，快速室性心律失常时发生房室分离就可确诊为室速。如果是 1∶1 的房室关系，是室速还是室上速取决于 AV 间期与 VA 间期的比值。但仍有可能房性心动过速与室速同时发生。心房电极能减少但不能完全防止不恰当的治疗,因为一切算法结果总有偏倚,因此即使室颤不能完全得到识别,但很少会被漏诊。

二、心动过速治疗

(一) 起搏治疗

所有ICD为心动过缓提供单腔、双腔或三腔起搏。在一次高能除颤对心律失常进行超速抑制后,起搏模式、频率、刺激输出常常是单独可程控的。尽管大多数植入ICD的患者可以进行双腔频率应答起搏,但这些人中只有极少数有起搏治疗的适应证。双腔与单腔可植入型除颤器(DAVID)研究,针对已植入ICD但无起搏适应证的患者,与心室备用起搏相比,观察DDDR模式起搏的效果。结果显示,DDDR起搏增加心衰住院或死亡的联合终点事件。因此,对没有明确抗心动过缓起搏适应证的患者,需要设置为心室备用起搏模式[15]。对心室失同步化和纽约心功能分级Ⅲ或Ⅳ级的充血性心力衰竭患者,双室起搏是合适的;但对心衰程度不严重或需要抗心动过缓起搏的患者来说,合适的治疗方法还不清楚。

此外,目前所有ICD都具备抗心动过速起搏功能。抗心动过速起搏是指ICD发放短阵快速刺激终止室速,刺激频率快于ICD所识别的室速的频率。抗心动过速起搏技术有多种,包括固定频率的短阵快速刺激(burst)与自动递减扫描刺激,即随后每一个起搏间期较前一个间期逐渐缩短(即频率逐渐加快)。经验性地程控ICD的抗心动过速起搏功能,终止室速的成功率可达90%,而在放电前先进行抗心动过速起搏测试,可将成功率提高到95%[16]。

抗心动过速起搏的缺点是,在某些患者,有可能加快心动过速的频率或使之转变成室颤,以致需要高能量除颤。至少有5%的患者经历过抗心动过速起搏引起的心动过速频率加快。一般针对室速,根据患者的耐受性,先程控一个或多个抗心动过速起搏程序,再进行除颤治疗。在治疗算法中加入一些安全措施,在抗心动过速起搏或低能量转复时,如治疗时间延长、无效,就开始采用更积极的治疗(如高能量除颤)。一旦抗心动过速起搏不能终止快速心律失常,就发放除颤治疗。

(二) 除颤治疗

ICD发放的电除颤来自于电容器的放电,通过高能电极进入心脏。电容器放电以指数形式衰减(图106-1),取决于两个变量:机器的总电容与电极系统的阻抗。任何一个变量增加,电压与电流放电衰减更慢,形成一个平坦的波形。每个脉冲发生器常使用两个电容器,每个电容器的电容约240~300μF,最高电压可达350~375V[4]。两个电容器常常并联充电,直到可程控的最大电压值。但放电时,两个电容器以串联形式排列,因此总电压是加倍的(即最大电压可达700~750V)。虽然串联时电压加倍,但电容减少一半。因此目前大多数临床使用的机器,系统的电容为120~150μF(表106-2)。由于大多数电极阻抗在40~70欧姆之间,这导致电压在20ms内降低60%~90%。电容器放电形成的除颤波形通过电极系统传给患者。

(三) 除颤阈值和安全界限

衡量除颤效率最简单的方法是测量除颤阈值(DFT),除颤阈值是除颤需要的最低能量强度(常以能量表示)[17]。除颤阈值是通过逐级下调的方式测试确定,诱发室颤后,释放的除颤强度逐步降低,最低的成功除颤强度即为除颤阈值。同样,除颤也可从低能量开始,以一种能量逐步增加的方式释放。但是,该方法开始时的除颤都是失败的,患者循环骤停的时间较长。第三种确定DFT的方法是,在心动周期的易损期发放除颤测试,即靠近体表心电图T波顶点处[18]。理论上,在此复极期发放低能电击,由于复极时间的离散,将诱发室颤。如果此期发放的除颤测试不能诱发室颤,就认为电击强度高于除颤阈值,随后可降低除颤测试的强度,直至室颤发生。这个概念称为易损性的上限(upper limit of vulnerability),优点是在测试期仅需诱发1次室颤。未能诱发出室颤的最低电击能量被认为等同于除颤阈值。该方法的缺点是ICD正确识别室颤的能力及随后采样除颤治疗的决策能力无法得到测试。

由于电除颤用S形概率函数描述最佳(图106-2)[19],用除颤阈值进行衡量显得过于简单。尽管如此,逐级下调测试除颤阈值法是植入手术时便于操作的测定方法,成功率一般能达到70%~80%左右[20,21]。这种方法有重要的临床意义,因为ICD正确植入需要对第一次除颤成功有足够信心。根据以往经验,10J的安全界限(除颤阈值与ICD最大输出能量之间的范围)被认为是最低的植入标准。因此,考虑到大多数机器30~35J的输出能量,最大可接受除颤阈值就定为20~25J。这个安全界限是根据使用心外

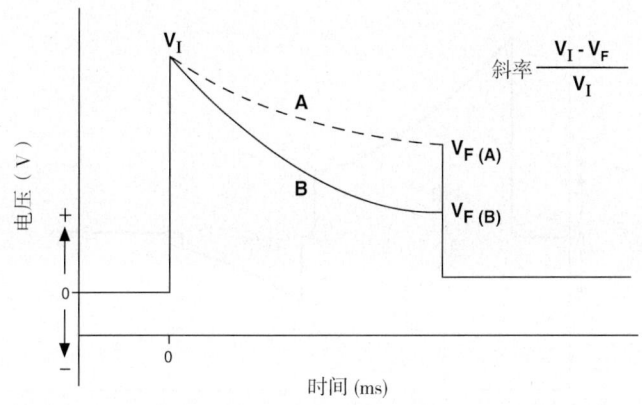

图 106-1 电容器放电反转形成单相波,也是最简单的 ICD 波形 初始电压(V_I)取决于电容器的充电。一段时间(取决于 ICD 的不同型号)后,当达到特定的终末电压(V_f)时,波形反转。电压衰减的速度(斜率)与电极系统阻抗和 ICD 总电容成反比。斜率根据图上的公式计算出来。波形 A 的斜率低于 B。

(四)单相波

最简单的除颤波是单相波,由于终末电压可能有致心律失常作用,因此电容器在完全放电之前发生反转[24]。早期的 ICD 脉冲发生器使用单相波,且在心外膜系统有效。单相或双相除颤波的大小一般用波的振幅(峰电压或电流)与电压衰减的速度(斜率)描述(图 106-1)。比如某个波形的振幅降低到初始值的一半,则斜率是 50%。

当非开胸电极首次用于临床并使用单相波时,右室线圈电极作为阴极,上腔静脉线圈电极或皮下片状电极作为阳极。这个约定是根据起搏需要确定的,因为与阳极相比,阴极端兴奋心脏所需电压与电流更低。随后的基础与临床研究比较了右室阴极图形与右室阳极图形。令人惊讶的是,右室阳极电极导致患者除颤阈值显著降低,且减少了对辅助电极的需求[25]。尽管在动物研究中也得到证实,以上极性差别的发生机制尚不完全清楚[26]。虽然单相波极性合适时有额外益处,但有时所需要的除颤能量太高,以致不能确信室颤一定可被成功处理[25]。双相波的提出就可基本解决这个问题。

膜电极和单相波确定的。最近研究提示,使用双相波除颤和非开胸电极,采用除颤阈值 1.9 倍的能量就可取得 95% 的成功率[22]。心外膜片状电极可以为单相波常规提供合适的除颤阈值,并可取得 10J 的安全界限。然而,使用单相波时,为了保证合适的安全界限,非开胸电极常需要额外的导线或皮下电极,或两者兼备[23]。

表 106-2 目前使用的 ICD 双相波的特征

生产商	型号	电容	第一相特征	第二相特征	单相
CPI Guidant	PrizmⅡ	158μF	60%斜率(不能程控)	50%斜率(不能程控)	67%
CPI Guidant	所有其他	100~124μF	60%斜率(不能程控)	50%斜率(不能程控)	67%
Medtronic	GEM	130μF	65%斜率(不能程控)	65%斜率(不能程控)	无
Medtronic	GEM Ⅲ AT	118μF	50%斜率(可程控)*	50%斜率(可程控)*	无
Medtronic	所有其他	118~130μF	50%斜率(不能程控)	50%斜率(不能程控)	无
St. Jude Medical	Photon/Atlas	116~126μF	65%斜率(可程控)或 5.5 ms 脉宽(可程控)	65%斜率(可程控)或 5.5 ms 脉宽(可程控)	65%(可程控)
St. Jude Medical	Epic/Photon	99~102μF	65%斜率(可程控)或 5.5 ms 脉宽(可程控)	65%斜率(可程控)或 5.5 ms 脉宽(可程控)	65%(可程控)
Ela	所有	105~120μF	50%斜率(不能程控)	50%斜率(不能程控)	无
Biotronik	所有	130~150μF	60%斜率,16ms 最大脉宽	50%斜率,10ms 最大脉宽	无

斜率:电压衰减的速度。同一厂家不同型号的电容该值可能变化。在时相参数可程控的型号,表中数值是出厂时的默认值。有区间的数值表示同一厂家不同型号产品的参数。

* 只适用于心房除颤斜率,心室除颤斜率不能程控。

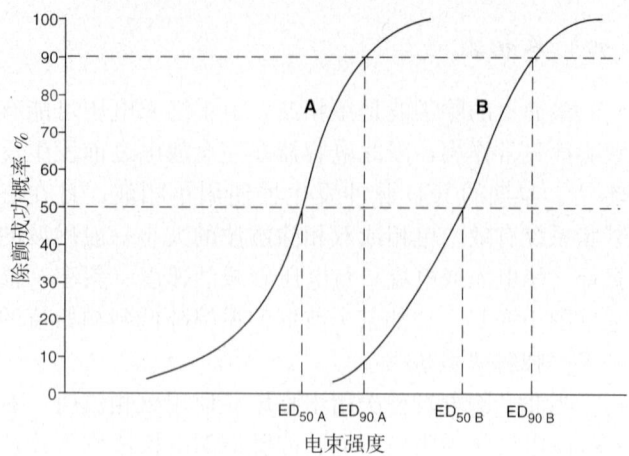

图 106-2 图示除颤成功可能性与电击强度的关系，即电除颤能量强度越大，成功率越高 ED_{50} 与 ED_{90} 分别代表除颤成功率达50%与90%时的除颤能量强度。曲线A与B代表不同除颤效果的波形。A的成功率较B高（波形A的 ED_{50} 与 ED_{90} 较B的低）

（五）双相波

从降低除颤阈值的角度，ICD最有益的创新就是提出双相除颤波（图106-3）[27,28]。该波形由电容器放电后极性相反的两个时相组成。在电容器放电反转前，第一相与单相波相同，但时程较短。随后，脉冲发生器内的电连接在 $2\sim3\mu s$ 内迅速反转，以相反的极性释放第二相，需要 $3\sim6ms$。表106-2列出了目前临床使用的ICD双相波的特征。

已有许多研究通过双相波的调整来降低除颤阈值能量。早期的研究使用心外膜电极或心脏组织标本的局部刺激[29,30]。这些研究结果不完全适用于使用心内膜电极系统时的除颤[31]。最近的一个研究将双相波的特征测试扩展到动物，发现两个可以降低心内膜除颤阈值的条件：（1）第一相的时间必须长于第二相；（2）仅在第一相时限超过10ms或当第二相时间超过第一相时，第一相的极性才显得重要[31]。

另外一些研究针对其他时相特征的有效性。其中一个有趣的改进是通过在第一与第二相之间将电容器由串联改为并联，把第二相初始电压加倍[32]。这也可将第二相的电容降低一半，导致斜率增加，电压衰减加速。动物试验已证明以上方法可以降低除颤阈值。

（六）展望

双相波、热机壳与低极化电极的组合已将许多ICD系统的平均除颤阈值降至10J以下。这也使最大输出降至 $20\sim25J$，以便为大多数患者提供足够的安

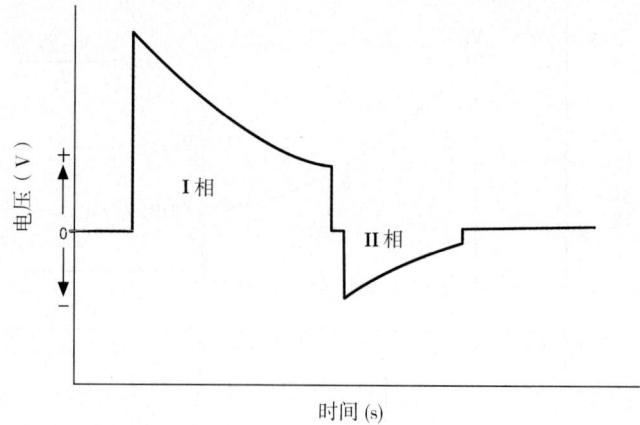

图 106-3 目前所有ICD使用的双相波。电容器放电被分成极性相反的两个时相。每个时相的时限取决于ICD的不同型号，某些机器可以程控。第二相的初始电压等于第一相反转后电容器的剩余电压

全界限。此外，最新的铝电解电容器（St. Jude公司产品）已允许高能密度，使电容器在ICD脉冲发生器中所占体积更小，为胸前植入和最大输出 $25\sim30J$ 提供方便。最后，通过降低除颤阈值，开发更有效的除颤波形，使最大输出更低，最终缩小脉冲发生器的体积。

未来在识别算法方面的改进，将区分可能与室速重叠的快速室上性心律失常。如果采用心率作为唯一标准，这些患者将因室上性心律失常而接受室速治疗。某些厂家已经采用心室电图波形算法，根据识别的腔内电图的时限和形态正确区分室上速与室速。心房电极正开始被用于抗心动过速起搏和房性心律失常的抑制。一些厂家现在生产的ICD能进行心房与心室起搏，将来还会有更多产品。心房信号正开始被识别算法使用。

最后，用于房颤的ICD和联合对心室与心房除颤的ICD已经生产出来，正在进行临床观察，以便将治疗范围扩大到心房。以往对心房进行除颤治疗有顾虑，因为有潜在的诱发室颤的危险。到目前为止的临床研究显示尽管患者可能有不适感，但均能有效地终止房颤[33]。有关心房除颤仪的识别、治疗、硬件与软件可能是重要的，但不在本章讨论范围之内。但是，有一种趋势，即使用非药物方法治疗心律失常（ICD与射频消融），而且前景无限。

（王建安　蔡思宇　译）

参 考 文 献

1. Bach SM, Monroe P: High power circuitry. In Kroll MW, Lehmann MH (eds): Implantable Cardioverter Defibrillator. Norwell, MA, Kluwer Academic Publishers, 1996, pp 257–273.
2. Holmes D, Curtis F: The battery. In Kroll MW, Lehmann MH (eds): Implantable Cardioverter Defibrillator. Norwell, MA, Kluwer Academic Publishers, 1996, pp 205–221.
3. Mehra R, Cybulski Z: Tachycardia termination: Lead systems and hardware design. In Singer I (ed): Implantable Cardioverter Defibrillator. Mount Kisco, NY, Futura, 1994, pp 109–133.
4. Ennis JB, Kroll MW: The high voltage capacitor. In Kroll MW, Lehmann MH (eds): Implantable Cardioverter Defibrillator. Norwell, MA, Kluwer Academic Publishers, 1996, pp 223–239.
5. Echt DS, Barby JT, Black JN: Influence of ventricular fibrillation duration on defibrillation energy in dogs using bidirectional pulse discharges. Pacing Clin Electrophysiol 11:1315–1323, 1988.
6. Usui M, Walcott GP, KenKnight BH, et al: Influence on defibrillation efficacy of the malpositioning of transvenous leads with and without a subcutaneous array. Pacing Clin Electrophysiol 17:784, 1994.
7. Strajdur KC, Ott GY, Kron J, et al: Optimal electrode position for transvenous defibrillation: A prospective randomized study. J Am Coll Cardiol 27:90–94, 1996.
8. Bardy GH, Allen MD, Mehra R, Johnson G: An effective and adaptable transvenous defibrillation system using the coronary sinus in humans. J Am Coll Cardiol 16:887–895, 1990.
9. Bardy GH, Johnson G, Poole JE, et al: A simplified, single-lead unipolar transvenous cardioversion-defibrillation system. Circulation 88:543–547, 1993.
10. Yamanouchi Y, Mowrey KA, Niebauer MJ, et al: Additional lead improves defibrillation efficacy with an abdominal "hot can" electrode system. Circulation 96:4400–4407, 1997.
11. Fotuhi PC, Kenhight BH, Melnick SB, et al: Effect of a passive endocardial electrode on defibrillation efficacy of a nonthoracotomy lead system. J Am Coll Cardiol 29:825–830, 1997.
12. Ellenbogen KA, Wood MA, Stambler BS, et al: Measurement of ventricular electrogram amplitude during intraoperative induction of ventricular tachyarrhythmias. Am J Cardiol 70:1017–1022, 1992.
13. Michelson BI, Igel DA, Wilkoff BL: Adequacy of ICD lead placement for tachyarrhythmia detection by sinus rhythm electrogram amplitude. Am J Cardiol 76:1162–1166, 1995.
14. Mirowski M, Mower MM: The automatic implantable defibrillator: Some historical notes. In Brugada P, Wellens H (eds): Cardiac Arrhythmias: Where to Go from Here? Mount Kisco, NY, Futura, 1987, pp 655–662.
15. The DAVID Investigators: Dual-chamber pacing or ventricular backup pacing in patients with an implantable defibrillator. JAMA 288:3115–3123, 2002.
16. Schaumann A, Von zur Mühlen F, Herse B, et al: Empirical versus tested antiachycardia pacing in implantable cardioverter defibrillators: A prospective study including 200 patients. Circulation 97:66–74, 1998.
17. Rattes MF, Jones DL, Sharma AD, Klein GJ: Defibrillation threshold: A simple and quantitative estimate of the ability to defibrillate. Pacing Clin Electrophysiol 10:70–77, 1987.
18. Hwang C, Swerdlow CD, Kass RM, et al: Upper limit of vulnerability reliable predicts the defibrillation threshold in humans. Circulation 90:2308–2314, 1994.
19. McDaniel WC, Schuder JC: The cardiac ventricular defibrillation threshold: Inherent limitations in its application and interpretation. Med Instrum 21:170–176, 1987.
20. Singer I, Lang D: The defibrillation threshold. In Kroll MW, Lehmann MH (eds): Implantable Cardioverter Defibrillator. Norwell, MA, Kluwer Academic Publishers, 1996, pp 89–129.
21. Lawton JS, Ellenbogen KA, Wood MA, et al: Clinical experience with nonthoracotomy cardioverter defibrillators. Ann Thorac Surg 59:1092–1099, 1995.
22. Strickberger SA, Daoud EG, Davidson T, et al: Probability of successful defibrillation at multiples of the defibrillation energy requirement in patients with an implantable defibrillator. Circulation 96:1217–1223, 1997.
23. Mitrana RD, Klein LS, Rardon DP, et al: Current trends in the implanyable cardioverter-defibrillator. In Zipes DP, Jalife J (eds): Cardiac Electrophysiology: From Cell to Bedside, 2nd ed. Philadelphia, WB Saunders, 1995, pp 1393–1403.
24. Geddes LA, Tacker WA: Engineering and physiological considerations of direct capacitor-discharge ventricular defibrillation. Med Biol Eng 9:185–199, 1971.
25. Strickberger SA, Hummel J, Horwood L, et al: The effect of shock polarity on ventricular defibrillation threshold using a transvenous lead system. J Am Coll Cardiol 24:1069–1072, 1994.
26. Usui M, Walcott GP, Strickberger SA, et al: Effects of polarity for monophasic and biphasic shocks on defibrillation efficacy with an endocardial system. Pacing Clin Electrophysiol 19:65–71, 1996.
27. Bardy GH, Ivey TD, Allen MD, et al: A prospective randomized evaluation of biphasic vs. monophasic waveform pulses on defibrillation efficacy in humans. J Am Coll Cardiol 14:728–733, 1989.
28. Block M, Hammel D, Böcker D, et al: A prospective randomized cross-over comparison of mono- and biphasic defibrillation using nonthoracotomy lead configurations in humans. J Cardiovasc Electrophysiol 5:581–590, 1994.
29. Tang ASL, Yabe S, Wharton M, et al: Ventricular defibrillation using biphasic waveforms: The importance of phasic duration. J Am Coll Cardiol 13:207–214, 1989.
30. Feeser SA, Tang ASL, Kavanaugh KM, et al: Strength-duration and probability of success curves for defibrillation with biphasic waveforms. Circulation 82:2128–2141, 1990.
31. Huang J, KenKnight BH, Walcott GP, et al: Effect of electrode polarity on internal defibrillation with monophasic and biphasic waveforms using an endocardial lead system. J Cardiovasc Electrophysiol 8:161–171, 1997.
32. Yamanouchi Y, Mowrey KA, Nadzam GR, et al: Large change in voltage at phase reversal improves biphasic defibrillation thresholds: Parallel-series mode switching. Circulation 94:1768–1773, 1996.
33. Jung W, Lüderitz B: Performance of the lead system for the Metrix automatic implantable atrial defibrillator [abstract]. J Am Coll Cardiol 31(Suppl A):513, 1998.

第 107 章

植入式心脏复律除颤器的临床应用

Charles D. Swerdlow and Kalyanam Shivkumar

本章目录

- 植入方法 ········· 958
- 植入时测试 ········· 958
- 高除颤阈值患者的处理 ········· 961
- 植入式心脏复律除颤器的程控 ········· 962
- 常见临床表现 ········· 966
- 室速与室上性快速心律失常 ········· 968
- 特殊问题 ········· 969
- 选择合适的植入式心脏复律除颤器 ········· 969
- 展望 ········· 970

对多数心室颤动（简称室颤）或致命性室性心动过速（简称室速）的高危患者，应选择植入式心脏复律除颤器（implantable cardioverter defibrillator，ICD）治疗。前瞻性随机试验已证实，对心脏骤停幸存者或室速伴低血压者，ICD 治疗优于抗心律失常药物[1]；在严重缺血性心肌病患者中，在最佳药物治疗基础上应用 ICD 能进一步减少总病死率[2]。对初级医疗计划和老年医疗计划数据库的分析[3]显示，根据现行的指南[4]ICD 仍然未得到很好的应用。

一、植入方法

经静脉植入 ICD 导线，在胸前放置脉冲发生器的方法与植入起搏器相似。因为 ICD 的脉冲发生器的机壳通常作为一个除极电极（"热壳"），故应放置在左前胸以保障电击除颤的向量最佳（图 107-1）。单腔 ICD 围手术期主要并发症的发生率约为 5%[5]。双腔 ICD 还有心房导线脱位的并发症，约为 3%[6]。室速/室颤复苏成功后患者，30 天手术病死率不足 3%，与用抗心律失常药物治疗的患者前 30 天内病死率相近[5]。最早的心外膜植入方法仅用于年幼儿童（经静脉导线不能适应其生长发育的变化）以及先天性心脏病伴中央型分流、静脉途径受限和少数除颤阈值（DFT）较高而不适于经静脉植入导线的患者。

二、植入时测试

ICD 植入时测试旨在确认：（1）导线和脉冲发生器的电连接是否完好；（2）在窦性心律时感知和起搏功能正常；（3）可靠的室颤感知、识别和再识别功能；（4）设置最佳或至少足够的电击强度；（5）脉冲发生器的功能正常[7]。

（一）感知

ICD 自动调整增益或自动调节感知灵敏度（见第 106 章和图 107-2）以确保房颤和室颤时 ICD 能对电图振幅低而变化大的房颤波和室颤波的正常感知，同时避免 T 波感知过度（图 107-2）。为了感知频率较快的电活动，每个心腔的空白期设置较短，交叉心腔空白期较短或为零。但这样设置易引起感知过度。应检查窦性和起搏心律时标记通道，以观察有无 P 波、R 波和 T 波的感知过度（见后文"感知过度"）。心房导线的定位应使感知到的远场 R 波最小。

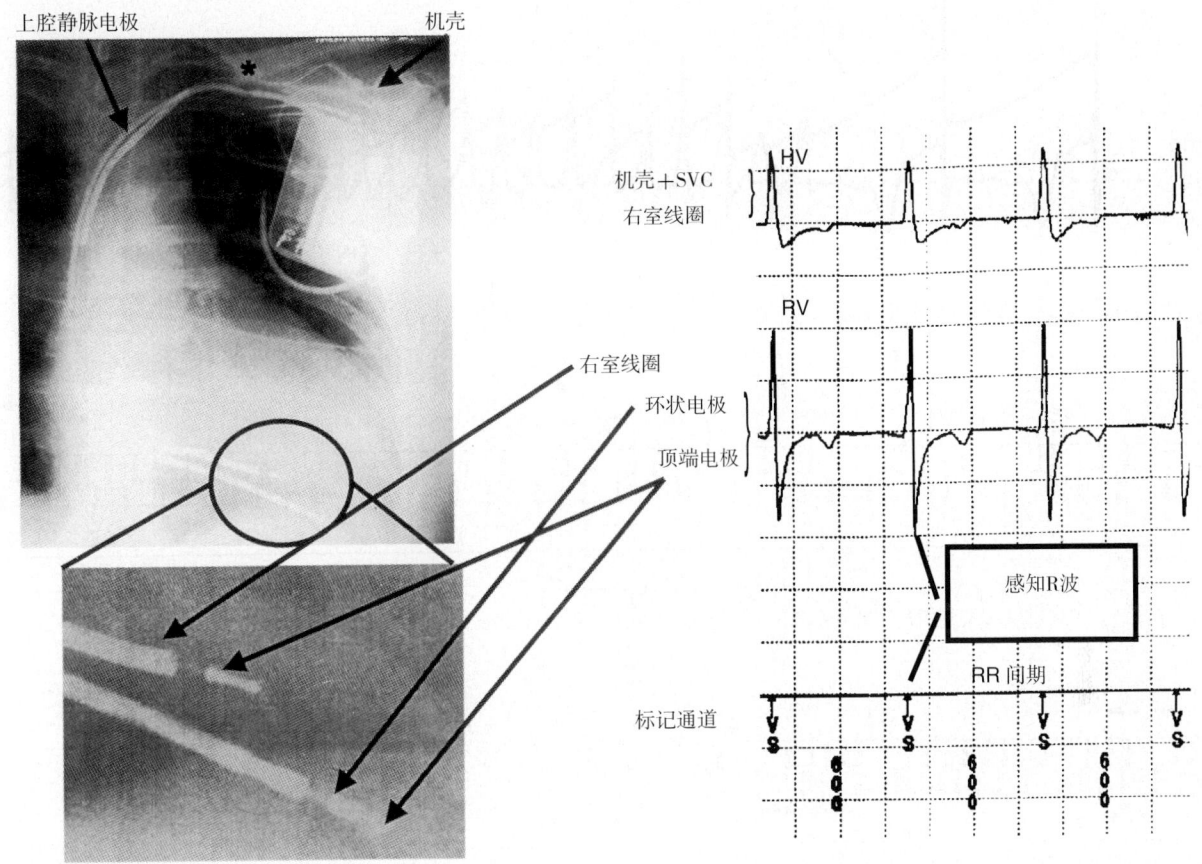

图 107-1 ICD 导线和心内电图 左上图显示 ICD 系统，包括左前胸的机壳和 2 根右心室导线。右图显示遥测的电图。左上图 X 线影显示单腔 ICD 与一根双线圈导线相连，还有一根被"锁骨下挤压"损伤而已废弃的单线圈导线（*）。与 ICD 相连的导线定位较佳，其顶部定位在右室（RV）心尖部，而近侧线圈的远端位于右心房与上腔静脉（SVC）连接处。废弃导线的定位欠佳。左下图显示废弃导线为集成双极导线，其在远端线圈和顶部电极间感知。与 ICD 相连的双线圈导线采用的是真正双极感知，在顶端电极和环状电极间感知。右图显示高压电图、感知电图和标记通道。标记通道上心室感知（VS）指从右室电图感知 R 波、现导线的环-端电极或废弃导线的顶端-右室线圈的计时。ICD 从该电图上测量所有的心室计时间期。高压电图是右室线圈至热壳和 SVC 电极。这些较大的、间距较宽的电极可全面展示心电活动，有利于形态分析，但易受到体外电磁干扰。

（二）室颤的感知和识别

为测试室颤的识别功能，将最大感知灵敏度调整至不敏感范围（~1mV）以保证在指定的灵敏度（~0.3mV）时感知室颤"细颤波"的安全范围。如果 ICD 应用的是早期顶端至线圈间距窄的（6mm）集成双极导线，则需测试电击后室颤的再识别功能，因为这些导线易发生电击后感知不良[8]。随着双腔 ICD 的问世，少有患者另需植入起搏器。对已植入了起搏器的患者，需进行特殊测试以避免装置间干扰[9]，其中最严重的是起搏器发放脉冲时由于 ICD 感知灵敏度的自动调整或增益的自动控制功能的重新设置，不能感知室颤。在双腔 ICD 中，"装置内"干扰可导致室颤识别延迟或不能识别，如室颤波落入与起搏频率平滑作用有关的心室空白期内[10]。

（三）评估除颤效果的方案

ICD 植入的标准就是除颤能力的水平，就是预计能对自发性室颤有足够高的除颤成功率。如果除颤能力不能符合该植入标准，需要重新检查该系统。要权衡预测植入标准患者的比例数与随后自发性室颤除颤成功率[11]。

评估 ICD 除颤效果可采取"患者个体化方案"和"安全范围"方案。患者个体化方案旨在找到能可靠除颤的最低除颤能量。安全范围方案仅测试在连续除颤所需的电击强度和 ICD 最大输出之间是否有足够的安全范围。

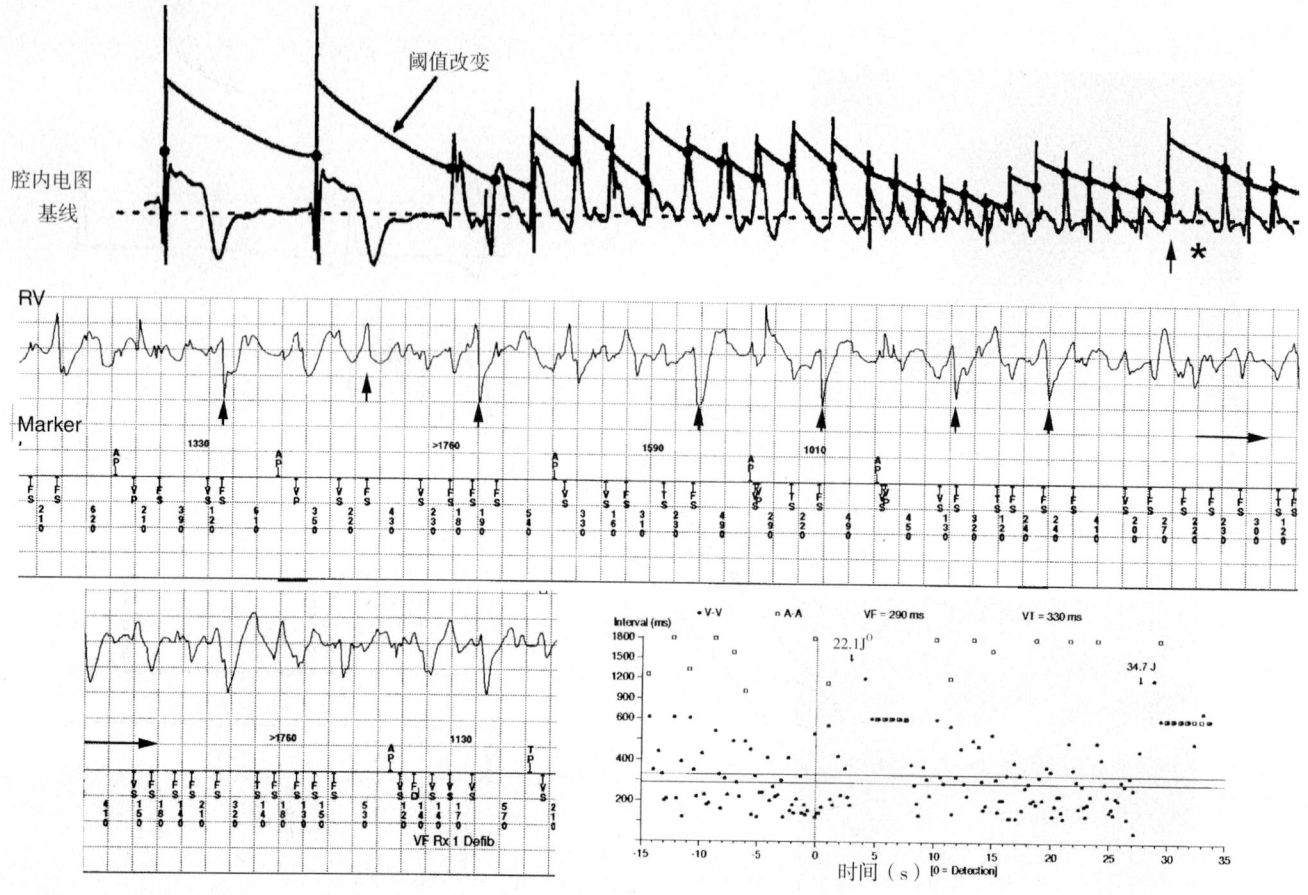

图 107-2　上图：自动调整感知灵敏度　图中分别显示在窦性心律时（前2个心搏）和自发性室颤时（VF）的实时双极心室电图（EGM）和感知阈值。图中圆点表示感知，此处信号处于阈值变化中。可以选择自动调整感知灵敏度的时间常数，以防止在窦性心律时或起搏心律时T波感知过度，同时要求在室颤时能安全可靠地感知到心室电图。星号所示为高振幅电图（箭头所示）之后立即出现室颤的低振幅波，引起感知不良。（引自 Olson WH. Tachyarrhythmia sensing and detection. In Singer I : Implantable Cardioverter Defibrillator. Armonk, NY, Futura, 1994, pp 71-107.）。下图：尽管感知不良，仍检测到室颤　图中显示心室感知电图及双腔起搏标记通道，从中图至下图为连续的心室电图。由于心室电图振幅和斜率变化较快，发生了感知不良，在每次高振幅电图（箭头）之后就会发生低振幅电图感知不良，直至感知灵敏度自动增加。在下面电图的末端，当18/24个间期短于室颤识别间期（290ms）时，ICD识别到室颤（VF Rx 1 Defib）。如要求感知这些室颤电图以及尽管有感知不良仍要可靠识别室颤，则可能在其他情况下发生感知过度而误识别室速/室颤。右侧的间期散点图显示，RR间期差异较大，很多间期比室颤间期长。图中"22.1J"所示的电击后，恢复了6个房室周期（房室起搏），随后室颤复发。ICD将这次电击定义为不成功，因为重识别"窦性"心律需要8个连续的"窦性"间期。因此，用最大输出电击（34.7J）治疗第2次室颤，室颤终止，进行房室起搏。FS、TS和VS分别表示室颤、室速、"窦性"心律区的间期。AP和VP分别代表心房和心室起搏，后者由于心室感知不良和AP后立即感知到心室电位（心室"安全"起搏）。

（四）除颤测试

患者个体化方案的目的是准确估计达到95%～99%成功概率（DFT_{95}～DFT_{99}）所需的电击能量。测定每个患者完整的除颤成功概率曲线（第46章）需要多次诱发室颤，然后除颤，这对人体不适用，也不安全。故常采用除颤阈值测试（DFT）方法，此处"阈值"的概念代表患者除颤成功概率曲线的点估计。通过快速起搏，直流电或T波电击方法几次诱发室颤，在设定的等待期后应用不同的能量进行电击除颤测试。如果测试的电击能成功除颤，则下一次放电测试降低能量。如未能成功除颤，加大能量补救电击，下次放电测试也要增加能量。在成功除颤概率曲线上点估计的误差与电击次数和曲线上的点呈非线性函数关系。应用优化的序列电击能量，当电击次数从2增加到6时，误差的均方根降低45%～65%；而电击次数从6增加到10时，误差的均方根只降低21%～25%[12]。

不同的测试除颤阈值方法接近除颤成功概率曲线

上不同的点。应用多次反向测试方案可估计 DFT_{50}。普遍应用的级降电击能量的除颤阈值根据初始的电击能量和级差的不同，约在 $DFT_{50} \sim DFT_{70}$ 之间[11]。其他的方案要求 2 次或 3 次连续的除颤成功以确定"增强测试的"阈值，分别表示为 DFT+和 DFT++[13]。这些点在除颤成功概率曲线上比 DFT 高。Bayes 方案最适于估计曲线上任意点[12]。

（五）易损性测试

易损性上限（ULV）是在易损期内放电不能诱发室颤的最弱的电击强度。ULV 与可靠除颤的最低电击强度相关（第 46 章）。为了测量 ULV，必须在易损期内最易受损的时间发放 T 波电击（T-wave shock）。该易损区的"峰值"在时间上与最近的单向 T 波锋值密切相关。由于在体表心电图与易损期峰值的精确时间关系的差异，故在测试放电时要在几个不同的耦联间期扫描 T 波[14]。

（六）植入测试方案和方法的选择

除颤和易损性测定方法均适于患者个体化方案或安全范围方案。两种方法对自发性室速/室颤的转复率都很高[7,11,13,15]。除颤方法最常用，该方法很直观，而且不需记录 6~12 导联心电图。ULV 测试方法可直接测定除颤成功曲线的高点[16]，比逐步降低 DFT 法重复性好[17]。易损性测试方法减少了植入测试中发生室颤或其他不可电击的循环骤停的危险，如顽固性室颤、脑灌注不足、心肌缺血等。

患者个体化方案可减少因电击强度过大引起的长期副作用，如心肌抑制。这对于患者由于室速/室颤"风暴"、ICD 故障、误识别快速室上性心律失常（supraventricular tachyarrhythmia，SVT）而在短期内多次放电（ICD 电风暴）尤为重要。因为所需的电击能量越大，ICD 电容器充电的时间就越长，因此在首次电击设置患者个体化的低能量比设置最大能量输出者发生晕厥及其导致的外伤危险要低。如果患者经常发生自行终止的室速，引起电容器充电而未放电，则该方案可延迟电池消耗。为设置首次电击能量，可逐渐增加除颤阈值或易损性上限，增加强度可根据除颤成功概率曲线的点估计及估计的准确度而变化。推荐的患者个体化首次电击程序包括 10J+DFT[18]、2×DFT[19]、5J+DFT++[13]、100V+DFT_{80}[20]、5J+ULV[15]等。

安全范围方案可减少电击以及诱发室颤-除颤测试的危险。例如，体外除颤不可靠的患者、冠状动脉严重狭窄或近期冠脉介入治疗者。然而，在自主心律 R 波<5~7mV[7]或已植入了起搏器的患者，易损性安全范围测试法不能确保识别室颤，必须进行室颤检测测试。建议的安全范围测试包括用比最大输出低 10J 能量成功电击 2 次[11]、用比最大输出至少低 5J 的 T 波电击扫描 4 次未诱发室颤[7]。安全范围测试后，首次电击强度设置为最大输出或 T 波电击能量+5J。

多数患者双相波除颤的 ICD 的慢性除颤阈值较稳定[13]，但在设置为 10J 安全范围的患者[21]，尤其是长期应用胺碘酮[22]或急性心肌缺血的患者（高达 15%）存在除颤阈值升高。除颤有效性降低的可能。

三、高除颤阈值患者的处理

植入双线圈导线和植入胸前的 ICD 患者中 90% 以上除颤阈值<15J[23]。左室重量[23]和长期胺碘酮治疗[24]与经静脉除颤阈值高相关；但没有一项临床、超声心动图或 X 线指标是较强的预测因子。因此，在植入前很难识别除颤阈值高的患者[23]。患者病情相关的以及 ICD 系统相关的一些因素可能与除颤阈值高相关。除颤阈值增高的患者在组织水平的相关因素包括高钾血症、应用某些抗心律失常药、心肌缺血[25]。胸腔积液和心包积液产生了胸腔内并行的电流路径，可使电流从心脏分流。遗留的旧导丝或电极碎片也可能导致电流分流。

ICD 系统相关的因素包括电击向量和波形。理想情况下，三维的电击向量使穿过左室的电场均一（第 46 章）。该向量取决于高压线圈和热壳相对于心脏的位置。右室线圈应送到心尖部。如果在心尖部感知不良，应在右室另一位置放置频率感知导线。在近端的线圈（上腔静脉，SVC）如果位置较高，可以防止电流从右房血池中分流，通常可以降低除颤阈值[26]（图 107-1）。若其必须定位在低位右房，则近端线圈不应设置在除颤环路中。如在右侧植入 ICD，则机壳不应设置在除颤环路中，可用无名静脉放置线圈代替。也可以选用皮下阵列式电极以降低除颤阈值[27]。

对于固定斜率波形的 ICD，波形宽度取决于输出容量和放电路径的阻抗（第 47 章）。对可程控波形、波形宽度和斜率的 ICD，可优化波形参数，与路径阻抗无关。缩短波形宽度可降低高除颤阈值[28]。

表 107-1　药物-ICD 相互作用

室速/室颤的频度
　增高
　　抗心律失常药
　　促心律失常作用的药物
　　与促心律失常药相互作用的药物
　降低
室速/室颤的识别
　程控频率范围
　　室速频率（降低——Ⅰc类药、胺碘酮）
　　SVT 的心室率
　　　降低（β受体阻滞剂、胺碘酮、索他洛尔）
　　　增高（服用Ⅰc类药，房扑1∶1传导）
　ICD 对室上速-室速鉴别方法
　　室速间期稳定性（服用Ⅰc类药、胺碘酮更不规整）
　　心内电图形态改变
室速/室颤的治疗
　除颤能量要求
　　增加（Ⅰb类药、Ⅰc类药、长期服用胺碘酮、维拉帕米）
　　降低（Ⅲ类药，但胺碘酮除外）
　对起搏器的影响
　　阈值升高（Ⅰc类）
　　抗心动过缓起搏
　　抗心动过速起搏时的药物使用依赖性
　　药物引起的窦性心动过缓或房室阻滞，导致起搏增多，增加电池消耗

缩短双相波形中的2相波形宽度可降低长期口服胺碘酮患者的除颤阈值[24]。上腔静脉或皮下电极降低了除颤阈值可能部分由于路径阻抗减少引起的固定斜率波形时程的缩短。在第1相右室线圈应为阳极，如为双极电击，则逆转极性对除颤阈值影响甚小[29]。

操作时间过长或室颤事件过多可能会使除颤阈值升高。在一些病例中，最好的方法是择日再测试一次。高除颤阈值的逐步解决方法见表 107-1。

四、植入式心脏复律除颤器的程控

（一）感知和识别

感知是 ICD 通过分析双极电图确定每个心房波和心室波的计时过程。识别是 ICD 处理（即计数、测量、分类）感知到的信号以将心律分类并决定是否放电的算法。ICD 对室颤和血流动力学不稳定的室速应当高度敏感，能正确识别。这种灵敏度有时会将室上速误识别为室速。识别血流动力学稳定的室速应更有特异性，识别时可允许一定的时间延迟。

（二）灵敏度

如果植入时窦性心律的 R 波振幅大于或等于 7mV[7]，设置最大灵敏度 0.3mV 左右通常可适当感知室颤。如果设置过于灵敏，则易对 T 波或膈肌电位感知过度，而降低灵敏度会增加对室颤感知不良的风险。为了对房颤时心房电位能正确感知，应当设置心房通道的感知灵敏度最大，心室后空白期最短，以预防对远场 R 波发生感知过度。

（三）识别时间

识别时间过短或识别间期数过少增加了非持续性室速或室上速引起电容器误充电，导致不必要的电池消耗及不放电或误放电。识别时间过长可能增加晕厥危险，患者个体化方案中晕厥的发生率约为 1%[7,15]。仅当没有其他方法可以可靠识别时，才缩短室颤的识别时间。血流动力学稳定的室速的识别间期不应缩短。对于非持续性室速发作时间长的患者（如长 QT 综合征），设置的参数值应该增加。电击治疗后再识别时间应当设置足够长，以防止如果初次放电后室速/室颤延迟终止而使 ICD 发放不必要的电击（而且具有促心律失常作用）。如果患者对室速能很好地耐受，室速的再识别应延长到指定值以外，以减少不必要的电击治疗，但抗心动过速起搏不能推迟。如果电击后发生明显的感知不良，再检测时间应当缩短。

（四）分区范围

ICD 有3个识别区，以便针对每个区设置特定治疗方案和室上速-室速鉴别条件。通常至少应设置2个区，即使临床上只表现为室颤。大多数室颤是从室速转变而来的[30,31]，而多数快速性室速可以通过抗心动过速起搏终止，减少了发生晕厥的危险[30,31]。设3个区可以：（1）对2种频率截然不同的室速采用不同的抗心动过速起搏方法（ATP）或不同的 ATP 治疗次数；（2）对2种频率截然不同的室速采用不同的室上速-室速鉴别方法；（3）对周长与多形性室速有重叠的单形性室速进行抗心动过速起搏治疗。

最慢室速频率区的下限应比预计室速的周长至少长 40ms，以防止 ICD 不能识别不规则室速。如果不太可能发生室上速或室上速-室速鉴别较可靠时，下限频率应更慢些。对于心衰晚期患者，应设置较长的室速识别间期，如果 ICD 不能识别慢频率室速，可能会引起严重后果[32]（图 107-3）。若开始应用抗心律失常

药治疗，则室速识别间期应该延长。

采用不同的抗心动过速起搏方法或室上速-室速鉴别方法通常根据周长划分出室速区中的"快频率室速"区的界限。"快频率室速"区-室颤区的界限通常也是根据心动过速的周长划分的，周长小于此界限，不能发放抗心动过速起搏治疗。这3个频率区界限常常分别设置为360～500ms、340～300ms、280～240ms。在选择分区界限时应考虑间期计数的类型（连续计数与X/Y计数，见第106章）。例如12/16个间期<330ms用于识别室颤，快速房颤可能被误识别成为室颤，即使平均周长和周长中位数远慢于330ms（图107-4D）。

如果未设置对慢频率室速的治疗，可将最慢频率区设置为仅监测区，将检测设置为"开"、治疗设置为"关"。在这种情况下，仅监测区的计数器与快频率区的计数器的相互作用可能会减少识别心动过速所需的间期数，快频率室速区将出现识别功能增强。一些ICD可设置独立的仅监测区以避免上述现象。

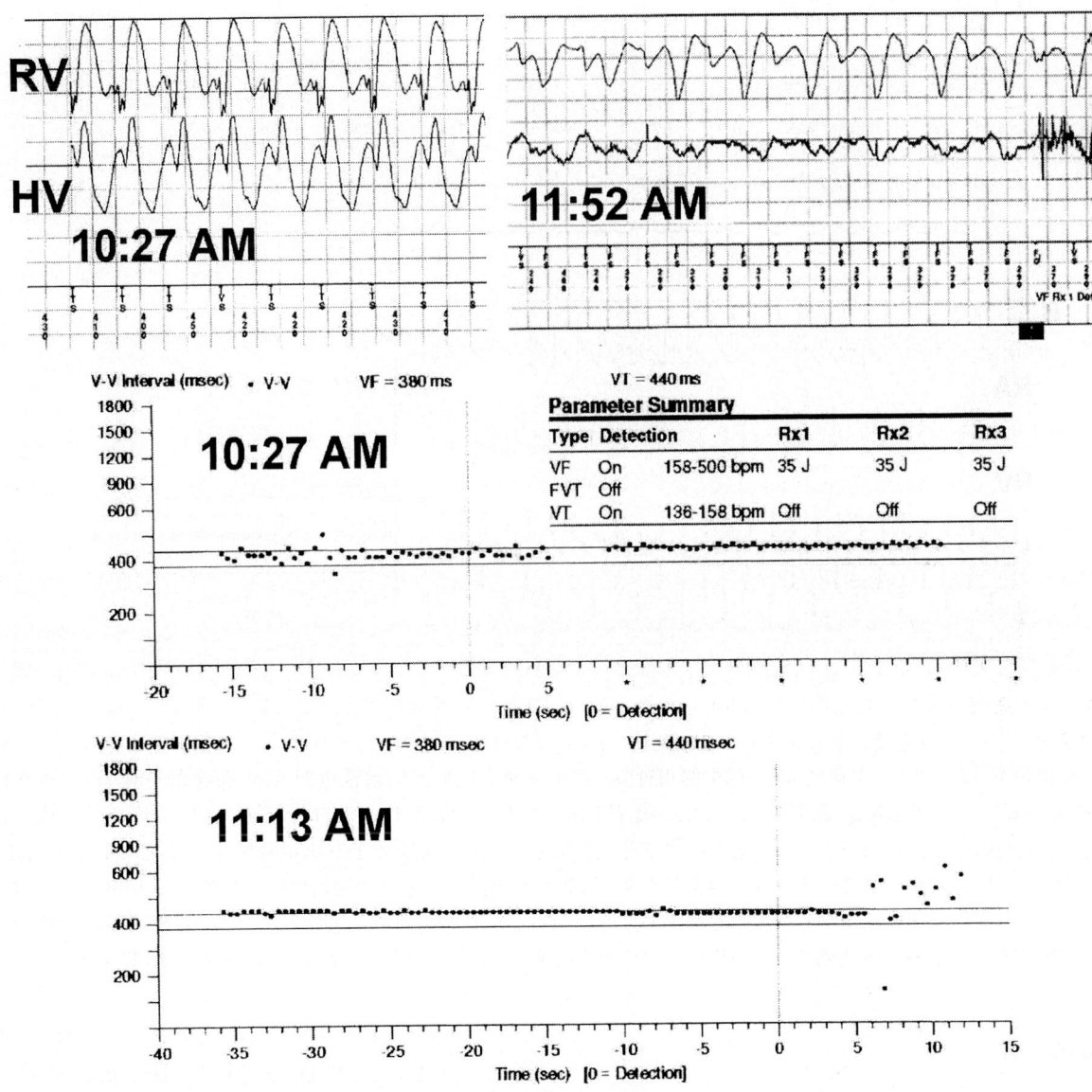

图107-3 比设置的治疗界限频率低的慢频率致命性室速 图中心室通道显示感知电图和高压电图（HV）。参数小结（parameter summary）显示室速识别设置为"开"，频率136～158次/分（周长440～380ms），但室速治疗设置为"关"。因此室速区作为"仅监测"区。左上图中，10:27AM检测到周长为420ms的室速，中图为间期散点图，显示在识别到440～450ms的室速周长后不久，室速周长增加，以至5s后在仅监测区不能识别到室速。在11:13AM，在仅监测区再次识别到室速，因为其逐渐加速至周长低于室速识别间期（下图），但未发放治疗，直至11:52AM（右上图）对T波感知过度导致ICD误识别室速为室颤（室颤）（VF Rx 1 Defib）。注意室速的周长在识别的临界范围，甚至在仅监测区。

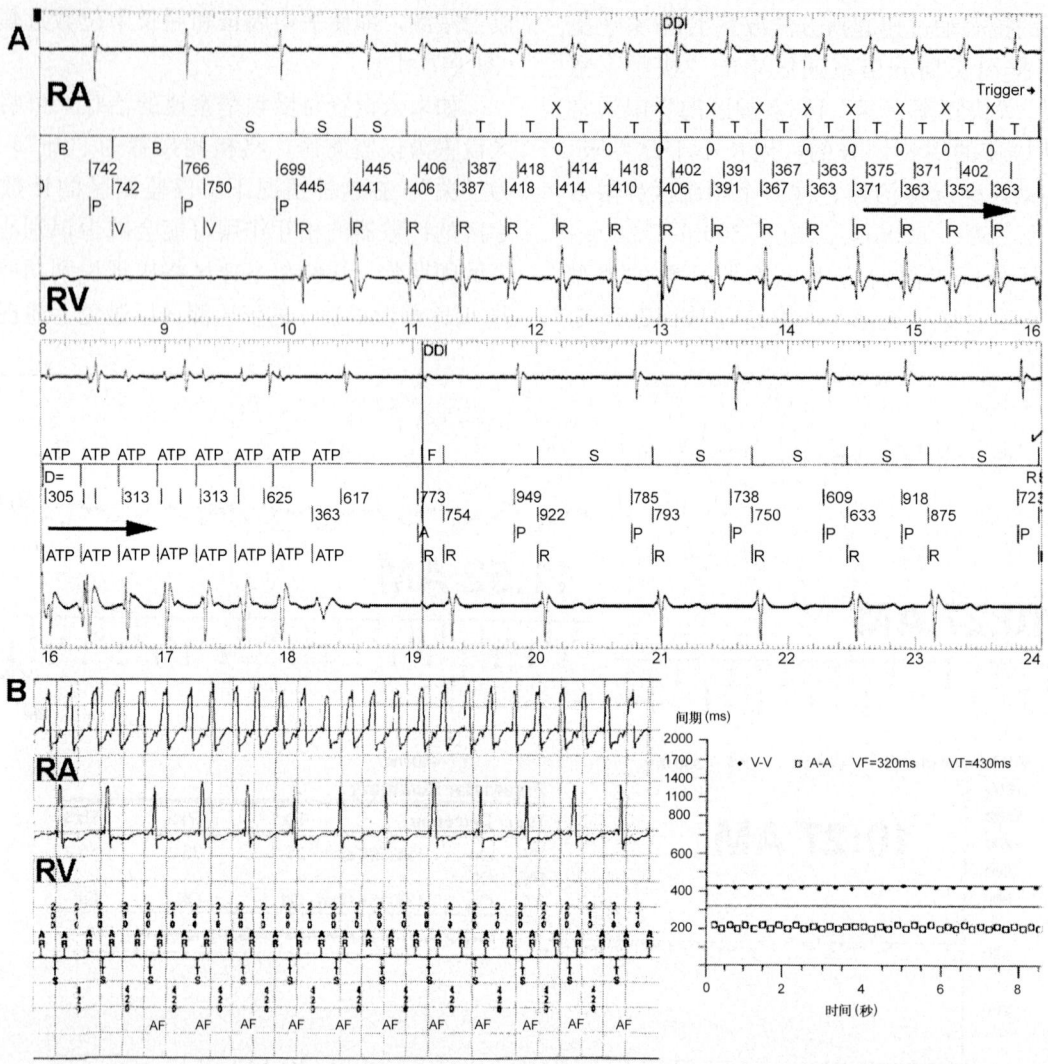

图 107-4　室上速-室速鉴别　每图均显示双极心房电图（RA）、双腔标记通道和频率感知（RV）或高压（HV）电图。A图：正确检测室速伴1∶1室房逆传。在心房感知、心室起搏（PV）时发生室速。通过心内电图的形态鉴别室速与室上速。右下方可见在标记通道下方的"0"与室速区（T）的电图相对应，提示室速电图形态与窦性电图（R）形态的符合率为0。在标记通道的上方相对应的"X"表示形态学算法将该心律归类为室速。在左下方猝发抗心动过速起搏（ATP）终止了室速，右上图"trigger"表示识别到室速。左下方"D="表示心房率等于心室率。S代表间期处于室速识别区400ms之上的窦性心律区内，时间刻度为秒。B图：正确识别快速的心房扑动为室上速。因为心房节律和心室节律均较规整，存在2∶1房室关系，因此房扑被ICD识别。图中标注"AF"（房颤）指示在室速频率区的间期数已达到所需检测的间期数（16个），但因诊断为房扑，故未发放治疗。间期散点图显示房室比例2∶1。AR代表起搏不应期中的心房间期。TS代表室速区中的心室间期（继续）

（五）治疗

递增（ramp）和猝发（burst）抗心动过速起搏两者临床结果相近，有效性高（80%～90%）而使室速加速率低（～5%）[30,31]。开始起搏周长设置为室速周长的百分数：慢频率室速设为70%～80%，快频率室速设置为80%～90%。至少应设置1次抗心动过速起搏以减少电击的次数。应根据植入时的测试设置室颤首次电击强度。随后的电击输出能量应该较高。室速时，一个心动周期的易损区还可能长达下一个R波，因此，室速电击应大于或等于易损性上限以防诱发室颤。

（六）识别快速室上性心律失常

增强识别或室上速-室速鉴别算法是识别算法中可程控的一部分，可在识别到心动过速后进一步鉴别室

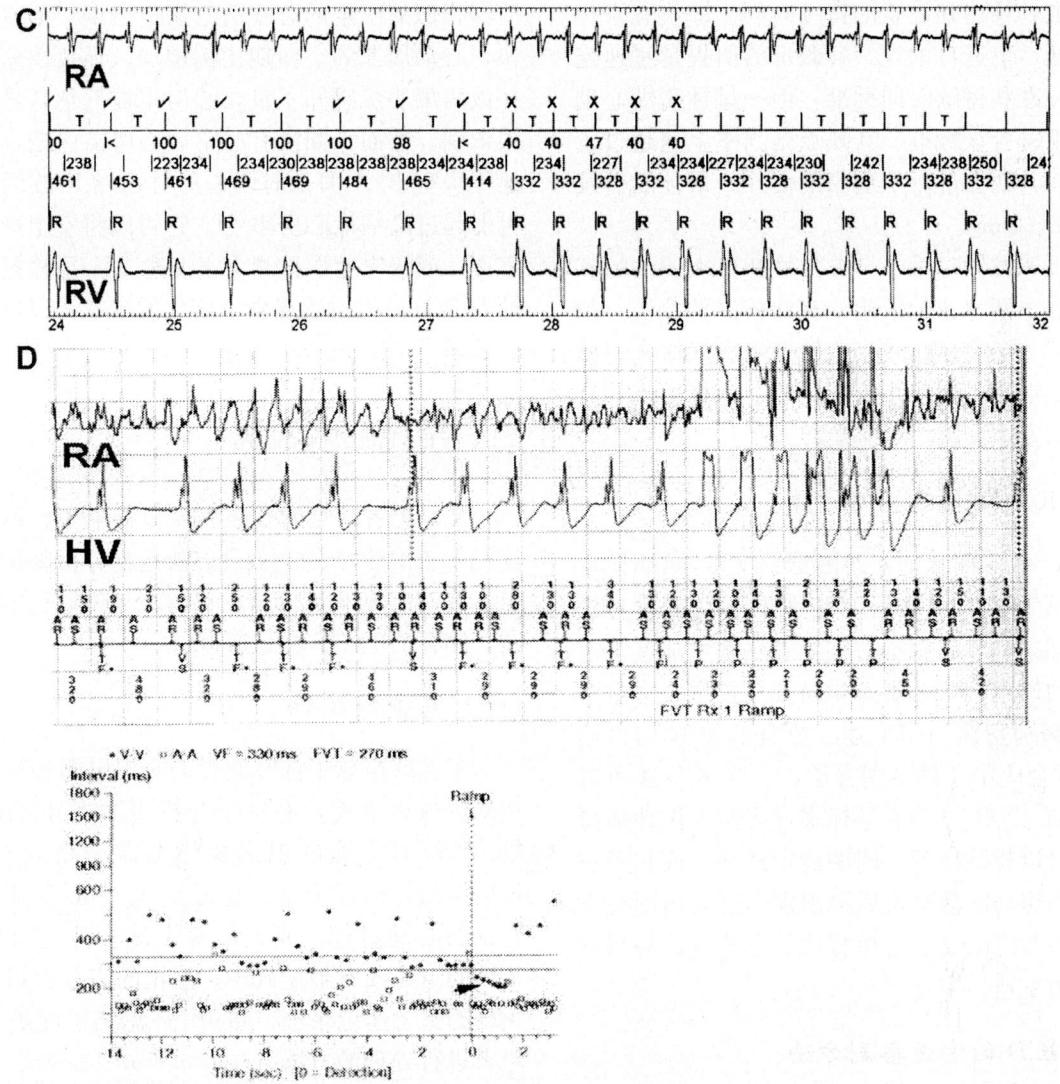

图 107-4 C图：心房扑动伴室速。房扑伴 2∶1 房室传导时发生室速。时间刻度线表明在图的开始部分心室率在室速区达 24s。由于 2∶1 房室传导关系，而且心室电图与窦性心律的心内电图（图中未显示）形态相似，标记通道显示房扑时形态相符率 98%～100%，而与室速相符率为 40%～47%。"<"表示心室率低于心房率。通过房室分离、形态匹配率＜60%，识别为室速。标记通道上方表明每个心搏形态学上归类为室上速（√）或室速（X）。D图：误识别心室率在室颤区的快速房颤。在快频率室速区（FVT）检测到房颤，FVT是室颤区的较慢部分。快频率室速区设置为12/16个间期＜室速检测间期 330ms。在电图的右侧，发生了首次不恰当治疗（递减抗心动过速起搏）(Rx 1 Ramp)，图中标有 TP。室颤识别间期相对长以及识别时间比指定值短，增加了误识别快速下传的房颤的可能性。在室颤区，可以用形态学标准识别房颤，但不能应用周期稳定性，因为室颤间期可以是不规则的。间期散点图显示 RR 间期变异较大，很多长于室颤检测间期。箭头所示为抗心动过速起搏。长的 AA 间期与间歇性心房感知不良有关。AS 代表感知的心房间期。VS 代表"窦性心律区"的心室间期。

速与室上速[33]。其目的是防止对室上速按室速误治疗，后者可能致痛或引发新的心律失常[33,34]（第104章）。ICD 设置多个识别区使缓慢室速和室上速重叠概率很高。当 ICD 仅根据频率标准识别室速时，12个月内 45% 的患者发生对室上速按室速/室颤误治疗[35]。然而，室上速-室速鉴别可能延迟或不能识别室速。对血流动力学稳定的室速发生短暂延迟不会造成太大影响，但延迟时间过长或不能识别到室速可能会引起严重后果（图 107-3）。

人们设计了两个"防止漏检"（fail-safe）的安全算法来确保室速的检测。"室上速范围"算法是设置一个周长范围，在此范围以下不进行室上速-室速鉴别。其可以与其中一个室速/室颤频率区范围相连。如果单独程控，应该设置此功能以防止识别血流动力学不稳定的室速的时间过长。"超长持续时间"（sustained-duration override）算法是指如果心动过速符合室速频率标准，且达到设置的持续时间，即使鉴别标准提示室上速，也进行治疗。其假定的前提是室速连续符合频率标准和持续时间标准，但一过性窦性心动过速或房颤不符合该标准。其缺点是当室上速超过了设置的时间时，就会进行不适当的治疗。最佳的持续时间可能为2～3min。

在心动过速发作时对心律失常诊断再次评估的算法可以减少漏识别室速的危险。有些较好的算法，如"突然发作性"或"起源心腔"，如果初次评估未正确鉴别室上速或室速，则停止治疗。后一种算法仅与持续时间过长的安全算法一起设置。

（七）单腔ICD的室速鉴别方法

单腔ICD有3种鉴别室速方法：（1）间期稳定性：根据心室节律的规整程度鉴别单形性室速与房颤；（2）突然发作性：根据心率是否逐渐增加鉴别室速与窦性心动过速；（3）形态学特征：根据心室电图的形态特征鉴别室速与室上速。所有的ICD均可选"AND"以联合应用几种鉴别方法，一些ICD还可以选"AND"或"OR"。形态学标准或突然发作性加持续时间标准可以排除窦速。间期稳定性和（或）形态学标准可鉴别房扑。但电击后再识别不能应用形态学标准鉴别，因为电击可引起短暂性形态改变，易将室上速误识别为室速。

（八）双腔ICD的室速鉴别方法

双腔ICD的室速鉴别算法结合了单腔ICD的室速鉴别算法和心房节律分析。如果ICD能正确识别心房电图，比较心房率和心室率是一个简单而有效的鉴别室上速和室速的方法。在双腔ICD室速区中90%以上的室速心室率大于心房率[36]。因此，对不足10%的室速需再加上其他鉴别方法，以减少漏识别室速的危险。双腔ICD的算法也可包括测量稳定的1：1或N：1房室关系（图107-4B）。"起源心腔"（加速）、"过早刺激"和心室电图的形态（图107-4A和4C）可鉴别窦速或房速伴1：1房室传导与室速伴1：1室房传导[33]。若心房导线不稳定，则不能设置房室关系参数。如心房率超过心室率则双腔ICD不发放室速治疗，以防止心房导线脱位至心室，引起严重后果。

不能准确识别心房电图是引起ICD误识别的重要原因。常见原因有心房导线脱位、心房感知过度、由于心房电图振幅低或空白期导致感知不良等。为了防止对远场R波的感知过度，一些双腔ICD采用了与起搏器相似的固定的心室后心房空白期。随着心室率增快，心动周期的空白期比例增加，导致快速下传的房扑或房颤心房感知不良，心房率被低估，导致室速的误识别。然而，如没有心室后心房空白期，在心动过速伴房室1：1关系时因心房对远场R波的感知过度可引起过高估计心房率[36]。这可以将室上速误识别为室速，或将室速误检测为室上速[33]。可程控心房空白期的ICD可以设置患者个体化的参数，以优化检测心房节律。

五、常见临床表现

ICD患者常见的临床表现包括电击、不能发放治疗、无效治疗等[37]。处理方法包括分析临床资料（病史、胸片）和ICD资料（程控、导线阻抗值和趋势图、储存的电图、标记通道）。

（一）电击的诊断

室速或室颤事件时储存的心内电图和标记通道提供的资料很重要，有助于分析ICD放电的原因和结果。ICD对室速的识别和分类方法并不十分完美：ICD检测并储存为室上速或室速/室颤事件并不代表真正的心动过速；真正的室上速事件也可能储存在ICD的室速或室颤记录中；真正的室速也可能储存在ICD的室上速记录中。图107-5总结了经历ICD电击患者进行处理的方法。

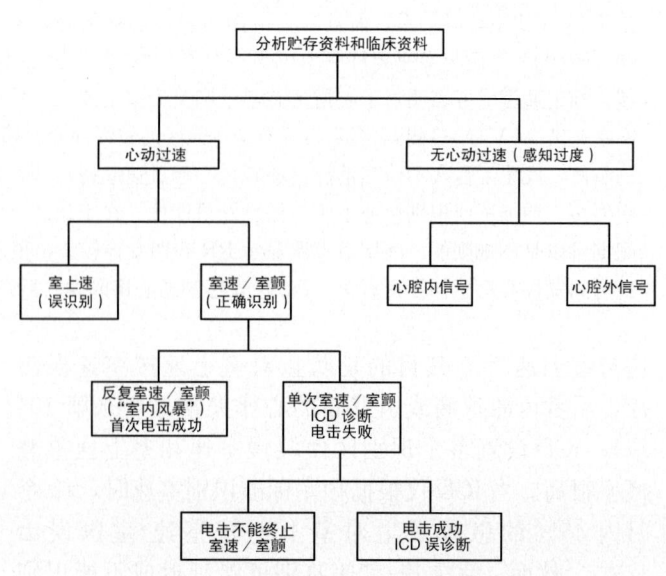

图107-5 经历ICD电击患者的处理方法

(二) 感知过度

若 ICD 对并不是心律失常的生理性或非生理性信号感知过度并识别为心律失常，则在无心律失常时也会发生放电[37,38]。非生理性信号通常是心腔外的信号。生理性信号可以是心腔内的信号（P 波、R 波、T 波等），也可以是心腔外的信号（肌电信号）（图 107-6）。

对生理性心腔内信号的感知过度，会导致 ICD 在每个心动周期 2 次检测到 R 波。对 P 波感知过度和 R 波双重计数表现为心动周长的交替。对 T 波感知过度表现为心内电图形态的交替[38]。如果集成双极导线的远端线圈太靠近三尖瓣，就容易发生对 P 波的感知过度。如果所感知心内电图的时限超过 120~140ms 的心室空白期，可能会发生 R 波双重计数。应用钠通道阻滞剂可能会使 R 波更加增宽，尤其是在心率快时，频率依赖性钠通道阻滞作用增强。R 波双重计数导致所有的室速都在室颤区中检测到。这在双心室 ICD 在左心室和右心室电极末端之间感知室速或室上速下传到心室时较常见[39]。因此此时 ICD 对所有室速，不论周长如何，均不进行抗心动过速起搏治疗。T 波感知过度通常发生在 R 波振幅较低时。T 波感知过度除了引起误治疗外，还可误抑制抗心动过缓起搏或发放不正确频率起搏治疗。

发生对心腔外信号感知过度的标志是等电位线消失，代之以高频噪声，与心动周期无固定关系[37]。体

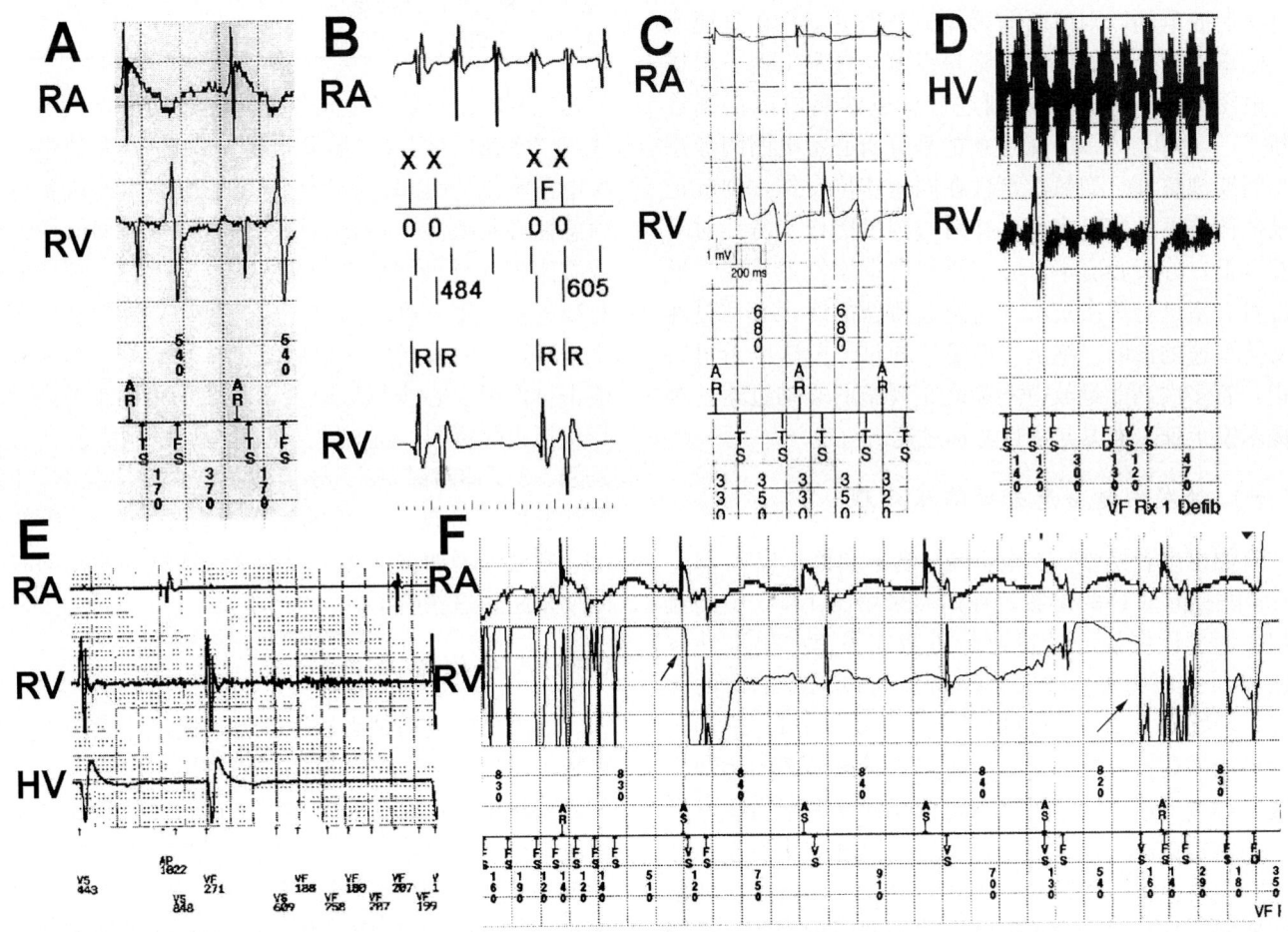

图 107-6 ICD 对生理性心腔内信号（A~C）或心腔外信号（D~F）的感知过度导致误识别为室颤（VF） A 图：窦性心律时 ICD 对 P 波的感知过度，导线为集成双极导线，远端线圈在三尖瓣附近。B 图：双心室感知 ICD 在房颤时对下传的 R 波双重计数。C 图：ICD 对低振幅 R 波患者（注意 1mV 标高）T 波感知过度。D 图：动力钻引起的电磁干扰，在电极间距宽的高压电图上的振幅比在真正的双极感知电图（电极间距较窄）上要高。E 图：膈肌电位的感知过度。患者在右室（RV）心尖部的电极为集成双极电极。注意噪声水平较固定，但感知过度到自动增益调整增加到一定的程度后才发生，约在感知到 R 波后 600ms。F 图：导线断裂引起电位间歇性超出放大器范围（箭头所示）。

外电磁干扰通常是连续的[37,38]，从极间距较宽的电极记录的高压电图上其信号振幅要比极间距较小的电极记录的感知电图的振幅大。由于导线或连接器（连接头、适配器或螺钉部分）的问题引起的感知过度通常是间歇性的，仅出现在一小部分心动周期，通常伴有起搏导线阻抗的异常。在感知电图上能记录到导线/连接器信号，可能超出了放大器范围。肌电位感知间期变化大。胸部肌电位通常在高压电图上表现明显，而膈肌电位通常在感知电图上表现明显。膈肌电位感知过度主要发生在右室心尖部为集成双极导线、脉冲发生器应用自动调整增益的男性患者[40]。

六、室速与室上性快速心律失常

如果储存的心内电图提示 ICD 是在真正发生心动过速后放电的，则诊断的第 2 步是确定储存在室速或室颤事件记录中的心律失常是室速还是室上速。根据心电图和心内电图的原则进行分析常能得出正确诊断[37]。对单腔 ICD，最主要的是分析心室电图的形态和间期规整性。如每次事件在同一体位发作，则应记录该体位下的实时窦性心律时心内电图作参考。对双腔 ICD，分析心房率、心室率和房室比例最重要。通过对心室进行单次抗心动过速起搏就能终止心动过速支持室速的诊断。绝大多数室速通过一两次电击可终止，若多次高能量放电不能终止规整的心动过速，则提示室上速，尤其是窦性心动过速。

（一）对发生电击患者的临床处理

如果患者经受一次电击或电击不频繁，应在 24～48h 内查询 ICD 的参数，查询应采用图 107-5 中的流程。通过设置抗心动过速起搏治疗快速的单形性室速[31]，或应用抗心律失常药物[41]可以减少电击的频度。药物与 ICD 之间的相互作用见表 107-1。感知过度可能需要再程控、调整导线位置或更换新的感知导线。对室上速误治疗可能需要重新程控频率区或室上速的鉴别算法。也可以选择药物或消融方法治疗室上速。通常通过重新程控以预防对窦速的误治疗。其他快速室上性心律失常可能需要结合这两种方法。重新程控可能影响到对室速的识别。

频繁或反复发生 ICD 电击者需要紧急处理。如果是室上速或窦性心律时感知过度引起反复误放电，则需立即用程控仪或磁铁关闭室速/室颤检测功能。可以采用解决单腔 ICD 误放电的方法解决这些问题。对

表 107-2 高除颤阈值患者的处理步骤

第 1 步：找出并纠正可逆性因素
生理性因素：高钾血症、药物、低氧血症、心肌缺血
电流分流
  胸腔积液或心包积液
  残留的钢丝
  原心腔内或血管内电极碎片
多次诱发室颤-除颤引起测试时间过长

第 2 步：优化经静脉电击的向量
右心室电极顶端置于心尖部
近端线圈置于高位右房（如位置太低则不用近端线圈*）
右侧植入：除颤环路不用机壳* 或用冷壳
如果除颤环路不用机壳或近端线圈，在无名静脉/上腔静脉再放一个线圈

第 3 步：优化电击波形（如可程控）
缩短波形宽度，尤其是当阻抗＞60Ω
长期服用胺碘酮者，缩短第 2 相波形宽度

第 4 步：植入皮下阵列电极

第 5 步：考虑植入心外膜电极

室速反复电击可能是电击终止室速成功后再次发作室速（"室速风暴"/"集束放电"）或一次室速事件多次电击不成功引起，其治疗方案迥异。室速风暴可能由急性心肌缺血、心衰加重、代谢异常（如低钾血症或胺碘酮介导的甲状腺功能亢进）、药物影响（如促心律失常作用、更改药物、未遵医嘱）等引起。在发生室速风暴时诊断急性冠脉综合征较困难，因为多次电击可以引起心肌复极改变、血肌钙蛋白 I 增高。治疗包括去除诱因、抗心律失常药物（索他洛尔[41]、胺碘酮、β 受体阻滞剂）、导管消融。少见情况下，ICD 对复发的、可自行终止的室速反复进行不必要的放电，则通过增加识别和再识别室速或室颤所需的时间期来防止这些电击。

（二）无效放电

因为除颤成功是必然性事件，偶尔的除颤不成功可随机发生，但若安全范围适当，用大于或等于 2 倍的最大输出仍不成功非常罕见。植入时间较长的 ICD 放电未终止室速或室颤，可能是因为病人自身的原因或 ICD 的原因所致（见前文中高除颤阈值患者的处理）。ICD 相关的原因包括设置的电击能量不足、电池耗竭、脉冲发生器故障、导线故障或脱位、ICD 与导线连接故障（包括适配器）。

若在 ICD 检测到电击后的窦性心律之前室速复发，ICD 有可能将有效电击误判为无效电击（图 107-2 中的间期散点图）。这可以通过缩短对窦性心律的再识别时间间隔来纠正，也可以通过延长室速的再识别时间

来防止对电击后非持续性室速的误判断。如果电击后心律是在室速频率区的室上速（儿茶酚胺介导性窦速或电击介导的房颤），ICD 也可能将电击误判为无效电击。这可以通过室上速-室速鉴别算法来再识别室速、增加电击能量以防止发生电击介导性房颤或给予β受体阻滞剂减慢电击后室上速的频率来纠正。

（三）不能发放治疗或延迟治疗

这两种情况可能由 ICD 参数设置问题（包括人为错误）、ICD 系统本身问题或两者共存。如果 ICD 失灵、室速频率慢于所设置的识别间期、室上速-室速鉴别算法诊断为室上速、装置间干扰或装置内干扰影响了感知功能等，则不能识别室速或室颤。导线、连接器或脉冲发生器故障，可导致感知不良或不能发放有效治疗。室颤时可能由于参数设置（感知灵敏度、频率范围、持续时间）、心内电图振幅低而变异大、药物影响、电击后组织变化等因素导致感知不良。

七、特殊问题

（一）社会心理问题

ICD 患者可能因意外电击而感到焦虑，但也可能感觉到 ICD 保护自己免遭猝死危险。致命性室速/室颤患者中 ICD 治疗组和抗心律失常药治疗组的生活质量相似，但 ICD 电击与生活质量降低相关[43]。咨询、教育和支持组织可使 ICD 患者获益。

目前已制订了 ICD 患者驾驶和飞行的指南[44]，主要根据心律失常的症状和频度进行限制。作为一级预防植入 ICD 的患者可以不必限制驾驶个人小汽车（但不能驾驶商用汽车）。指南建议每次电击后 6 个月或因症状性室速/室颤植入 ICD 后 6 个月内不应驾驶[44]。但大多数患者提前恢复驾驶。然而 ICD 患者发生交通事故率要低于普通驾驶员[45]。

（二）电磁干扰

电磁波无处不在，其可影响 ICD 的功能。电磁干扰可导致 ICD 短暂性或永久性失活（这样就不能发放对室速/室颤的治疗）、误识别室速/室颤、误起搏或抑制起搏[46,47]。电磁干扰对真正的双极感知的影响要比对集成双极电极感知的影响小。

1. 非医源性电磁干扰

除了工业和军用设施干扰外，日常生活中有临床意义的电磁干扰十分罕见，但偶有引起严重后果的干扰的报告[46,47]。常规应用家用电器不会干扰 ICD 功能。开机状态的数字式手机不应放在植入侧的胸部口袋中，建议将手机放到 ICD 脉冲发生器对侧的耳旁接听。ICD 患者可以步行走过机场金属探测器和正常距离的电子监视器，但暴露在磁场中时间过长，可能抑制起搏和对室速/室颤的识别，误识别室速/室颤，在一些 ICD 中还可使室速/室颤识别功能关闭。一些工业干扰也有危险（如电弧焊接、电动工具、大型磁铁），应在工作环境中测定场强。患者在操作这些设备时，应记录 ICD 电图和标记通道，最好将 ICD 设在"仅监测"模式。

2. 医源性电磁干扰

磁共振成像对 ICD 患者具有多种危险，因此该检查属禁忌证。如果外科手术应用电刀等器械需用接地电极，应当关闭 ICD 室速/室颤识别功能。手术完毕应立即查询 ICD 并打开识别功能。放射治疗可损伤 ICD 电路，应将 ICD 遮挡或移到对侧。在行射频消融时应关闭室速/室颤识别能力。消融应尽可能远离电极，并经静脉放置临时起搏器。因为在消融后 24h 起搏阈值达到高峰，起搏器的输出应加大设置，数天后再次检查阈值。

八、选择合适的植入式心脏复律除颤器

（一）双腔与单腔 ICD

双腔 ICD 能进行双腔起搏，有室上速-室速的鉴别算法，而单腔 ICD 则没有。一些双腔 ICD 还可有监测与治疗房性心律失常的功能（第 106 章）。双腔 ICD 的缺点包括太复杂、费用高、心房导线的并发症、使用寿命短、由于心室起搏和室速/室颤识别图形间的相互影响而引起的强制心室起搏。现行的指南指出"尽管双腔 ICD 广泛应用，但其长期的益处尚无充分的资料证实"[4]。

大约 10% 的 ICD 患者有双腔起搏的绝对适应证（Ⅰ类），大约 30% 为相对（Ⅱ类）适应证[48]。一项随机的、前瞻性研究比较了 DDDR 起搏（70 次/分）和 VVI 起搏（40 次/分）在 ICD 患者无特定起搏适应证的应用效果[49]。DDDR 组比 VVI 组更多达到联合终点（死亡和住院），提示在这些患者中自身房室传导优于以心房同步的右室起搏。

到目前为止，关于确定仅为提高室上速-室速的鉴别程度而植入双腔 ICD 尚没有公认的标准。与单腔 ICD 相比，双腔 ICD 贮存的心内电图增加了诊断准确度。一些双腔 ICD 算法中将设置指定为"ON"是安全的[33,36]，这比单腔 ICD 患者个体化方案更简单。双腔 ICD 可能包括冗余的单腔和双腔算法，其有特殊的优点，如鉴别不规整且心室率大于心房率的室速与快速下传的房颤。双腔 ICD 的算法几乎可识别所有的心室率大于心房率的室速，检测室速的敏感度高达 99% 以上[33,36]。为达到相似的敏感度，单腔 ICD 算法需延长持续时间，这必然会降低特异度。然而，若经过优化设置，甚至旧式单腔 ICD 算法，对在缓慢室速区的室速检测的阳性预测值约达 90%，对几乎所有的在室颤区中占 5%～10% 的室上速，单腔和双腔 ICD 算法均不能正确检测[33,36]。早期的研究表明，第一代双腔 ICD 算法的阳性预测值与单腔 ICD 算法相似，但前者对室速漏检的可能性较小[50]。

（二）再同步化治疗

晚近，双室再同步化起搏（第 108 章）已与 ICD 结合在一起治疗心室间收缩不同步患者的心力衰竭。一项随机化、前瞻性研究比较了单纯药物治疗与药物治疗加再同步化起搏或再同步化 ICD 治疗心力衰竭（但无室速/室颤）患者的疗效[51]。初期结果表明单纯药物治疗组比再同步治疗组患者更多达到联合终点（死亡和住院）。同步化两亚组住院率相近，ICD 组比起搏器组病死率低，但差异无统计学意义。对终止室速双心室抗心动过速起搏略优于单纯右心室起搏[52]。未来 ICD 应用左心室除颤导线可望大大降低除颤阈值[53]。基于晚期心衰患者心律失常性死亡的危险性很高，一些学者建议所有的再同步化装置均为 ICD，但是用低阻抗的双心室导线持续起搏会影响 ICD 使用寿命；且再同步化 ICD 有其独特的左心室导线带来的并发症。现行的再同步化 ICD 不论双室感知[39]还是集成双极感知均还有感知和检测问题的风险。

九、展望

今后，ICD 功能将增强，其复杂性也呈增加的趋势。自动化、自检、自行调整功能将会不断更加实用，减少人工误差。ICD 功能从单纯治疗室速/室颤扩展到同时有双腔起搏、监测和治疗房性心律失常、心脏再同步化治疗等强大功能。仍在研发中的 ICD 功能包括监测心力衰竭，未来的 ICD 可能监测其他伴随疾病如心肌缺血。通过 Internet 网远程下载 ICD 的资料会涉及：（1）监测能力超过资料储存和处理能力；（2）监测伴发疾病可为医务工作者提供有价值的资料，后者可以通过远程获得数据；（3）从 ICD 下载的复杂数据可以远程处理，其数据应表达为有用的临床知识，而不是工程学数据。但 ICD 的一些进展方向尚不确定：可靠地预测室速/室颤、预防室速/室颤、对室颤无痛性治疗等。

同复杂性和费用增加的主流相反，有一种使 ICD 更加简单化的趋势，强调降低费用[54]，这会使更多患者从应用 ICD 作为一级预防而获益。一些学者支持开发功能较少的 ICD 作为一级预防，甚至可能不需要心腔内电极。

不论 ICD 如何发展，新型 ICD 的功能和设计必须注意安全性（包括人们不期望发生的事件如起搏的副作用[49]、装置内相互干扰[10]）以及保证临床有益。

（孙宝贵　译）

参 考 文 献

1. Connolly SJ, Hallstrom AP, Cappato R, et al: Meta-analysis of the implantable cardioverter defibrillator secondary prevention trials. AVID, CASH and CIDS studies. Antiarrhythmics vs Implantable Defibrillator study. Cardiac Arrest Study Hamburg. Canadian Implantable Defibrillator Study. Eur Heart J 21:2071–2078, 2000.
2. Moss AJ, Zareba W, Hall WJ, et al: Prophylactic implantation of a defibrillator in patients with myocardial infarction and reduced ejection fraction. N Engl J Med 346:877–883, 2002.
3. Ruskin JN, Camm AJ, Zipes DP, et al: Implantable cardioverter defibrillator utilization based on discharge diagnoses from Medicare and managed care patients. J Cardiovasc Electrophysiol 13:38–43, 2002.
4. Gregoratos G, Abrams J, Epstein A, et al: ACC/AHA/NASPE 2002 guideline update for implantation of cardiac pacemakers and antiarrhythmia devices: A report of the American College of Cardiology/American Heart Association Task Force on Practice Guidelines (ACC/AHA/NASPE Committee on Pacemaker Implantation), 2002: Available at www.acc.org/clinical/guidelines/pacemaker/pacemaker.pdf.
5. A comparison of antiarrhythmic-drug therapy with implantable defibrillators in patients resuscitated from near-fatal ventricular arrhythmias: The Antiarrhythmics versus Implantable Defibrillators (AVID) Investigators. N Engl J Med 337:1576–1583, 1997.
6. Schoels W, Swerdlow CD, Jung W, et al: Worldwide clinical experience with a new dual-chamber implantable cardioverter defibrillator system. J Cardiovasc Electrophysiol 12:521–528, 2001.
7. Swerdlow CD: Implantation of cardioverter defibrillators without induction of ventricular fibrillation. Circulation 103:2159–2164, 2001.
8. Natale A, Sra J, Axtell K, et al: Undetected ventricular fibrillation in transvenous implantable cardioverter-defibrillators: Prospective comparison of different lead system-device combinations. Circulation 93:91–98, 1996.
9. Glikson M, Trusty JM, Grice SK, et al: A stepwise testing protocol

for modern implantable cardioverter-defibrillator systems to prevent pacemaker-implantable cardioverter-defibrillator interactions. Am J Cardiol 83:360–366, 1999.
10. Shivkumar K, Feliciano Z, Boyle NG, Wiener I: Intradevice interaction in a dual chamber implantable cardioverter defibrillator preventing ventricular tachyarrhythmia detection. J Cardiovasc Electrophysiol 11:1285–1288, 2000.
11. DeGroot PJ, Church TR, Mehra R, et al: Derivation of a defibrillator implant criterion based on probability of successful defibrillation. Pacing Clin Electrophysiol 20:1924–1935, 1997.
12. Li H, Malkin RA: An approximate bayesian up-down method for estimating a percentage point on a dose-response curve. J Appl Stat 27:579–587, 2000.
13. Gold MR, Higgins S, Klein R, et al: Efficacy and temporal stability of reduced safety margins for ventricular defibrillation: Primary results from the Low Energy Safety Study (LESS). Circulation 105:2043–2048, 2002.
14. Swerdlow C, Martin D, Kass R, et al: The zone of vulnerability to T-wave shocks in humans. J Cardiovasc Electrophysiol 8:145–154, 1997.
15. Swerdlow C, Peter C, Hwang C, et al: Programming of implantable defibrillators based on the upper limit of vulnerability rather than the defibrillation threshold. Circulation 95:1497–1504, 1997.
16. Swerdlow C, Ahern T, Kass R, et al: Upper limit of vulnerability is a good estimator of shock strength associated with 90% probability of successful defibrillation in humans with transvenous implantable cardioverter defibrillators. J Am Coll Cardiol 27:1112–1117, 1996.
17. Swerdlow C, Davie S, Ahern T, Chen PS: Comparative reproducibility of defibrillation threshold and upper limit of vulnerability. Pacing Clin Electrophysiol 19:2103–2111, 1996.
18. Marchlinski FE, Flores B, Miller JM, et al: Relation of the intraoperative defibrillation threshold to successful postoperative defibrillation with an automatic implantable cardioverter defibrillator. Am J Cardiol 62:393–398, 1988.
19. Strickberger SA, Man KC, Souza J, et al: A prospective evaluation of two defibrillation safety margin techniques in patients with low defibrillation energy requirements. J Cardiovasc Electrophysiol 9:41–46, 1998.
20. Malkin RA, Herre JM, McGowen L, et al: A four-shock Bayesian up-down estimator of the 80% effective defibrillation dose. J Cardiovasc Electrophysiol 10:973–980, 1999.
21. Tokano T, Pelosi F, Flemming M, et al: Long-term evaluation of the ventricular defibrillation energy requirement. J Cardiovasc Electrophysiol 9:916–920, 1998.
22. Pelosi F Jr, Oral H, Kim MH, et al: Effect of chronic amiodarone therapy on defibrillation energy requirements in humans. J Cardiovasc Electrophysiol 11:736–740, 2000.
23. Hodgson DM, Olsovsky MR, Shorofsky SR, et al: Clinical predictors of defibrillation thresholds with an active pectoral pulse generator lead system. Pacing Clin Electrophysiol 25:408–413, 2002.
24. Merkely B, Lubinski A, Kiss O, et al: Shortening the second phase duration of biphasic shocks: Effects of class III antiarrhythmic drugs on defibrillation efficacy in humans. J Cardiovasc Electrophysiol 12:824–827, 2001.
25. Dorian P: Amiodarone and defibrillation thresholds: A clinical conundrum. J Cardiovasc Electrophysiol 11:741–743, 2000.
26. Gold MR, Olsovsky MR, DeGroot PJ, et al: Optimization of transvenous coil position for active can defibrillation thresholds. J Cardiovasc Electrophysiol 11:25–29, 2000.
27. Gradaus R, Block M, Seidl K, et al: Defibrillation efficacy comparing a subcutaneous array electrode versus an "active can" implantable cardioverter defibrillator and a subcutaneous array electrode in addition to an "active can" implantable cardioverter defibrillator: Results from active can versus array trials I and II. J Cardiovasc Electrophysiol 12:921–927, 2001.
28. Mouchawar G, Kroll M, Val-Mejias JE, et al: ICD waveform optimization: A randomized, prospective, pair-sampled multicenter study. Pacing Clin Electrophysiol 23:1992–1995, 2000.
29. Shorofsky SR, Gold MR: Effects of waveform and polarity on defibrillation thresholds in humans using a transvenous lead system. Am J Cardiol 78:313–316, 1996.
30. Schaumann A, von zur Muhlen F, Herse B, et al: Empirical versus tested antitachycardia pacing in implantable cardioverter defibrillators: A prospective study including 200 patients. Circulation 97:66–74, 1998.
31. Wathen MS, Sweeney MO, DeGroot PJ, et al: Shock reduction using antitachycardia pacing for spontaneous rapid ventricular tachycardia in patients with coronary artery disease. Circulation 104:796–801, 2001.
32. Bansch D, Castrucci M, Bocker D, et al: Ventricular tachycardias above the initially programmed tachycardia detection interval in patients with implantable cardioverter-defibrillators: Incidence, prediction and significance. J Am Coll Cardiol 36:557–565, 2000.
33. Swerdlow CD: Supraventricular tachycardia-ventricular tachycardia discrimination algorithms in implantable cardioverter defibrillators: State-of-the-art review. J Cardiovasc Electrophysiol 12:606–612, 2001.
34. Pinski SL, Fahy GJ: The proarrhythmic potential of implantable cardioverter-defibrillators. Circulation 92:1651–1664, 1995.
35. Dorian P, Newman D, Thibault B, et al: A randomized clinical trial of a standardized protocol for the prevention of inappropriate therapy using a dual chamber implantable cardioverter defibrillator [abstract]. Circulation 1:I–786, 1999.
36. Wilkoff BL, Kuhlkamp V, Volosin K, et al: Critical analysis of dual-chamber implantable cardioverter-defibrillator arrhythmia detection: Results and technical considerations. Circulation 103:381–386, 2001.
37. Lloyd M, Hayes D, Friedman P: Troubleshooting. In Hayes D, Lloyd M, Friedman P: Cardiac Pacing and Defibrillation: A Clinical Approach. Armonk, NY, Futura, 2000, pp 347–452.
38. Gunderson B, Patel A, Bounds C: Automatic identification of implantable cardioverter-defibrillator lead problems using intracardiac electrograms. Comput Cardiol 29:121–124, 2002.
39. Schreieck J, Zrenner B, Kolb C, et al: Inappropriate shock delivery due to ventricular double detection with a biventricular pacing implantable cardioverter defibrillator. Pacing Clin Electrophysiol 24:1154–1157, 2001.
40. Sweeney MO, Ellison KE, Shea JB, Newell JB: Provoked and spontaneous high-frequency, low-amplitude, respirophasic noise transients in patients with implantable cardioverter defibrillators. J Cardiovasc Electrophysiol 12:402–410, 2001.
41. Pacifico A, Hohnloser SH, Williams JH, et al: Prevention of implantable-defibrillator shocks by treatment with sotalol. d,l-Sotalol Implantable Cardioverter-Defibrillator Study Group. N Engl J Med 340:1855–1862, 1999.
42. Goldschlager N, Epstein A, Friedman P, et al: Environmental and drug effects on patients with pacemakers and implantable cardioverter/defibrillators: A practical guide to patient treatment. Arch Intern Med 161:649–655, 2001.
43. Schron EB, Exner DV, Yao Q, et al: Quality of life in the antiarrhythmics versus implantable defibrillators trial: Impact of therapy and influence of adverse symptoms and defibrillator shocks. Circulation 105:589–594, 2002.
44. Epstein AE, Miles WM, Benditt DG, et al: Personal and public safety issues related to arrhythmias that may affect consciousness: Implications for regulation and physician recommendations—A medical/scientific statement from the American Heart Association and the North American Society of Pacing and Electrophysiology. Circulation 94:1147–1166, 1996.
45. Akiyama T, Powell JL, Mitchell LB, et al: Resumption of driving after life-threatening ventricular tachyarrhythmia. N Engl J Med 345:391–397, 2001.
46. Pinski SL, Trohman RG: Interference in implanted cardiac devices, part II. Pacing Clin Electrophysiol 25:1496–1509, 2002.
47. Pinski SL, Trohman RG: Interference in implanted cardiac devices, Part I. Pacing Clin Electrophysiol 25:1367–1381, 2002.
48. Best PJ, Hayes DL, Stanton MS: The potential usage of dual chamber pacing in patients with implantable cardioverter defibrillators. Pacing Clin Electrophysiol 22:79–85, 1999.
49. Wilkoff BL, Cook JR, Epstein AE, et al; Dual Chamber and VVI Implantable Defibrillator Trial Investigators: Dual-chamber pacing or ventricular backup pacing in patients with an implantable defibrillator: The Dual Chamber and VVI Implantable Defibrillator (DAVID) Trial. JAMA 288:3115–3123, 2002.
50. Hügl B, Ziegenbalg K, Grosse A, et al: Are enhanced dual chamber detection algorithm superior to single chamber algorithm? Long term results of the multicenter ICD-Trial DETECT. Circulation 106:II–321, 2002.
51. The Companion Trial Investigators. To be presented at ACC Meeting 2003. J Am Coll Cardiol 2003.
52. Kuhlkamp V: Initial experience with an implantable cardioverter-

defibrillator incorporating cardiac resynchronization therapy. J Am Coll Cardiol 39:790–797, 2002.

53. Butter C, Meisel E, Tebbenjohanns J, et al: Transvenous biventricular defibrillation halves energy requirements in patients. Circulation 104:2533–2538, 2001.

54. Zipes DP: Implantable cardioverter-defibrillator: A Volkswagen or a Rolls Royce—how much will we pay to save a life? Circulation 103:1372–1374, 2001.

55. Olson WH: Tachyarrhythmia Sensing and Detection. In Singer I: Implantable Cardioverter Defibrillator. Armonk, NY, Futura, 1994, PP 71–107.

第 108 章

植入式心房除颤器治疗心房颤动

Samuel Lévy

本章目录

- 前言 ……………………………… 973
- 心房除颤器的发展历程 ………… 973
- 植入式除颤器 …………………… 974
- 心房除颤器的临床应用 ………… 975
- 患者选择 ………………………… 976
- 亟待解决的问题 ………………… 976

一、前言

心房颤动（房颤）是临床上常见的心律失常，常发生于器质性心脏病患者和老年人，是当今临床治疗实践中的一项重大挑战。许多房颤患者服用抗心律失常药物后可能疗效不佳或者出现无法耐受的副作用。对于这些患者，可以考虑非药物治疗。房颤的非药物治疗主要包括外科消融、导管消融、房室交界区消融后植入永久起搏器以及起搏器预防房颤和植入式心房除颤器。

植入式转复除颤器（ICDs）的成功应用促进了植入式心房除颤器的发展，这种装置能够识别和转复房颤。植入式心房除颤器是将转复和维持窦性心律作为房颤治疗需要达到的终点而研发的，可使一些阵发性房颤患者反复转复为窦性心律，而无需药物和住院治疗。尽早迅速除颤可以预防快速心房率导致的电生理重构，而后者可以进一步促进房颤的维持（图108-1）。

二、心房除颤器的发展历程

本节阐述植入式心房除颤器的相关问题，主要包括心房除颤的可行性、耐受性和安全性[1]。

（一）低能量心房除颤的可行性

低能量转复房颤的可重复性是开发植入式心房除颤器的先决条件。在对绵羊进行的实验性工作后[2]，许多研究[3-9]显示，在右房和冠状静脉窦之间释放的160～400V（1～6J 能量峰前电压）双相波电击可以终止90%的阵发性或起搏诱发的房颤，以及75%的持续性房颤。终止持续性房颤所需的能量明显高于阵发性或起搏诱发的房颤[6]。

许多患者电击后可能出现胸部不适，因此在转复前需要应用镇静药物。尽管峰前电压或能量的大小与胸部不适的程度有关，但是仍有较大的个体差异[5-8]。因此，在植入前对低能量转复装置进行测试时评价患者对电击的耐受性是很重要的。由于电除颤可以将房颤转复为窦性心律，尽管有不适症状，许多患者都能够耐受电击。

（二）低能量心房除颤的安全性

单独心房除颤器（无心室除颤器）的一个重要特点是保证适当地发放心房电击而不引起室性心律失常。在一项多中心体外除颤器研究中[6]，1700多次R波同步电击均没有促室性心律失常的情况发生。应该注意的是，当电击前的RR间期短于500ms时，将不会发放心房电击[9]。一项动物模型研究显示，R波同步电击是很重要的，要求电击至少落在前一个R波后

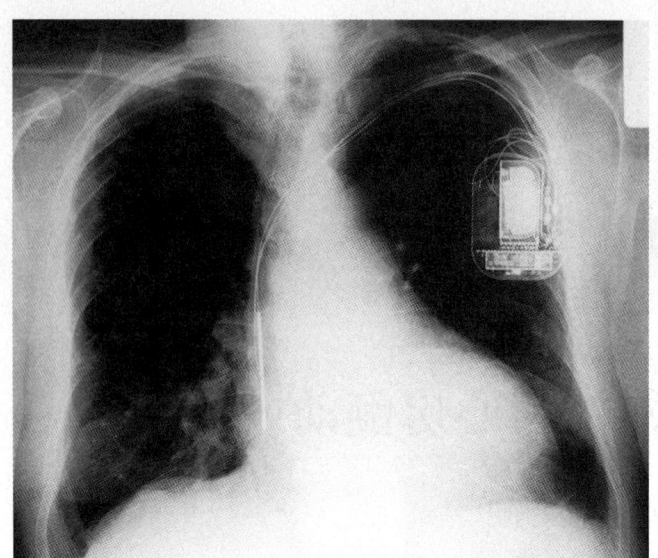

图 108-1 胸部 X 线显示胸前植入的心房除颤装置和 3 根电极 2 根心房电极用于心房感知和心房除颤，1 根心室电极用于心室感知和心室起搏。

300ms 内，否则就可能重叠在前一个 T 波上[9]。目前已有 2 例[7,10]在应用体外除颤器发放低能量心房电击时触发室性心律失常的病例报道。在这两例中，电击前的 RR 间期都短于 300ms，且其中 1 例为非 R 波同步电击[7]。

三、植入式除颤器

应用装置描述

目前已成功开发两种类型的装置用于研究和临床。

1. 单独心房除颤器

Metrix 3020（InControl，Redmond，WA）是一种单独心房除颤器，大小 53cc，重 82g，可以使用与植入起搏器相似的技术植入在胸前区。它可以发放脉宽为 6ms，最大电压为 300V（能量 6J）的双相波电击。Metrix 3020 能够程控为以下两种模式：自动模式或患者（医生）激活模式[12,13]。该除颤器有睡眠设置，其持续时间可以程控（1min～2h）。当患者醒来后，装置分析心脏节律确定患者为窦性心律还是房颤。当识别到房颤时，心房除颤器由医生（开始植入时推荐）、患者（多数应用模式），或已经程控为自动模式（少见）激活，发放 R 波同步电击。此装置使用复杂的识别规则（静息间期和跨基线）[12]，特异度可

达 100%，敏感度可达 93%。如果出现电击后停搏，此装置将起搏右室直至心室率大于程控的起搏低限频率。这个装置共连接 3 根电极：2 根电极用于心房感知和除颤，1 根电极用于心室感知和起搏。1 根心房电极使用带有非伸缩圈的主动固定电极固定于右房，1 根电极放置在冠状静脉窦。为了保持电极的稳定性，在导丝撤出后电极导管的末端均保持螺旋形状。

2. 双腔除颤器

ICD 的 1 次电击可能诱发房颤。1 次非同步（在 R 波上）的心房除颤可以导致室颤。因此，对于一些患者，1 个能够进行心房和心室除颤且能准确鉴别这两种心律失常的装置是十分有用的。目前有两种双腔除颤器可供临床和研究应用：Medtronic 7250（也称为 Jewel-AF）和 Guidant Prism-AVT。

Medtronic 7250 或 Jewel-AF（AMD 7250，Medtronic，Minneapolis，MN）是一种双腔除颤器，开始用于需要植入心室除颤器且反复发作房颤的患者[11,14-16]。其大小为 55cc，重 96g，植入胸前区。该型心房除颤器可在脉冲发生器机壳（Acitve Can）和心内电极导线之间发放双相电击波，能量可控范围是 0.4～27J。它最少使用 2 根导线（心房和心室），最多使用 3 根，其中第 3 根导线放置在冠状静脉窦中。此装置有多种抗心动过速功能，可以使用心房短促刺激（burst，最快频率为 50Hz）和连续递增起搏刺激（ramp pacing）起搏方式终止心房颤动和扑动。Medtronic 7250 可被程控为 2 种模式：自动模式或患者（医生）激活模式。

心房除颤器可以利用两个程控的重叠区和心动周期的规律性区分房性心动过速和房颤。如果周长持续时间在重叠区内是规则的，这种心律被定义为房性心动过速，如果是不规则的，则为房颤[15]。Medtronic 7250 也可以储存发作持续时间、使用的治疗方式和治疗结果等信息。它可以储存治疗前 5s 的心电图，治疗前标记的 60 个事件和终止后标记的 60 个事件。

心房除颤器使用分层治疗预防和终止房性心律失常。当合用药物治疗或患者自发心动过缓时，心房除颤器可以及时进行心房起搏，因此减少了心动过缓诱发房颤的可能。如果发生了房性心律失常，快速心房起搏可被程控为终止房性心动过速和心房扑动的初级治疗。高能量电击是终止房颤的最高级治疗。

Guidant Prism AVT（Guidant，Minneapolis，MN）在许多方面与 Jewel-AF 相似。但是，它使用了

另一个识别规则且包括许多与房颤预防有关的特点。一项相关的多中心试验正在进行中,其结果将在不久发表。

四、心房除颤器的临床应用

(一) Metrix 系统

Wellens 及其同事详细报道了 Metrix 系统临床评价结果的详细内容[12]。该型心房除颤器在开始阶段均被医生激活以评价其安全性和疗效。在 3719 次发放的治疗或测试电击中,未发现促室性心律失常现象的发生。已证明该装置能有效识别房颤,特异性可达 100%,可成功终止 96% 的房颤发作。最初的经验是在无明显器质性心脏病患者中使用医生激活模式。患者激活模式的应用经验证实了医生激活模式所取得的结果。房颤的早期复发率为 27%,51% 的患者需要通过心房除颤器激活进行重复转复,在一些病例是由于继发电击失败引起的。

今后心房除颤器可能需要改进的内容中,增加双腔起搏功能和多部位起搏预防和终止房颤似乎是最实用的。

单独心房除颤器已不再应用于临床,并非因为其疗效和安全性。InControl 作为 Guidant 公司的产品,已经改进为双腔除颤器。

(二) 双腔除颤器的应用经验

据我们所知,目前仅有 Medtronic 7250 型双腔除颤器的临床应用报道。

世界 Jewel AF 研究组的最初应用经验是由 Gold 及其同事报道的[14],研究共入选药物难治性房颤患者 144 例,平均随访 12±6 年。结果显示双腔除颤器识别房性心律失常的阳性预测值为 99%,使用快速起搏可以终止 40% 的心律失常,应用电击可以终止 87% 的发作。Adler 及其同事[15]报道了世界 Jewel AF 研究组起搏疗法的疗效,共包括 537 例患者,平均随访 11.4±8.2 月。所有患者都有植入 ICD(心室)的临床适应证。起搏治疗成功终止 127 例患者 1500 次自发性房性心动过速发作中的 59%,及 101 例患者 880 次房颤发作中的 30%(图 108-2)。后一种情况可作如下解释:30% 的房颤发作开始为有规律的房性心律失常,并能被心房快速起搏终止。起搏治疗房性心动过速/房颤的总体疗效为 48%,平均时间为 1.1min。25% 的病例出现早期复发(1min 内)。Friedman 及其同事[16]分析了世界 Jewel AF 研究组在 30 天或以上随访中出现房性快速性心律失常的 269 例患者的资料,观察了心房除颤器治疗对这些患者心律失常负荷的影响。起搏和电击治疗可以将心律失常负荷由每月

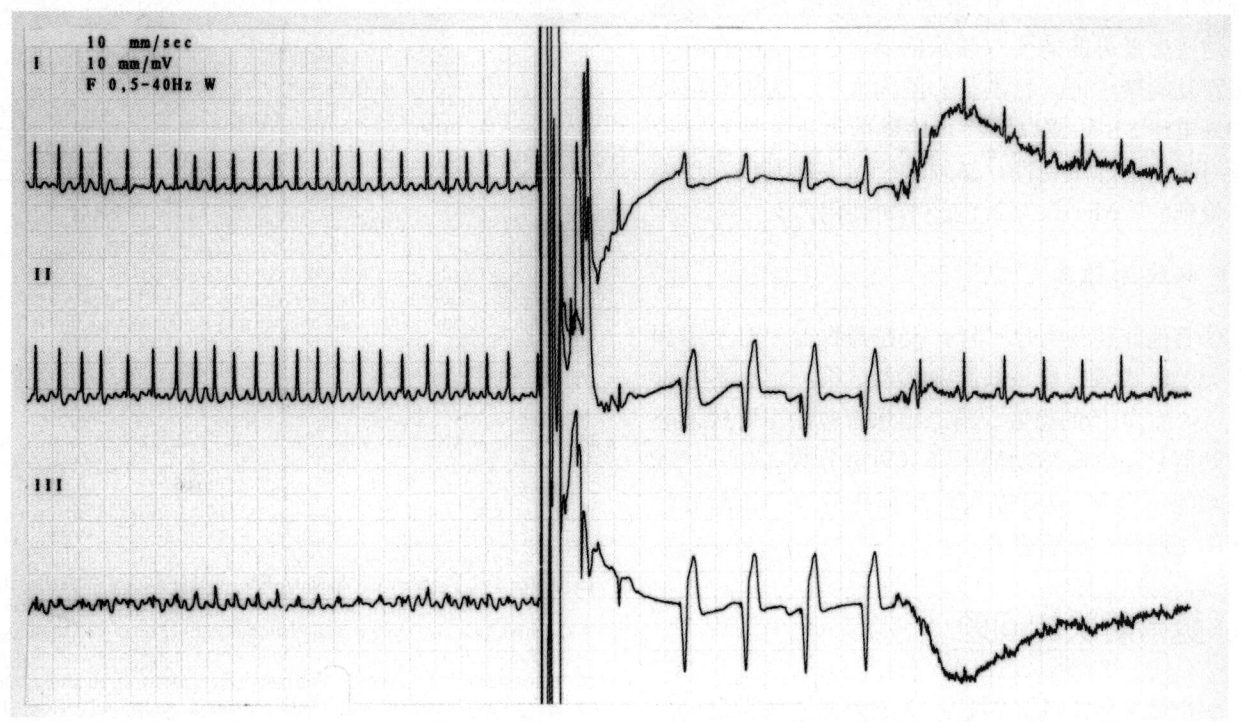

图 108-2 医生激活模式下记录的房颤终止　注意电击后和恢复窦性心律前的短暂心室起搏。

58.5h减少为7.8h，差异有显著性。有趣的是心律失常负荷的下降仅出现在使用起搏治疗时。

五、患者选择

（一）可能从植入式心房除颤器获益的房颤患者

目前尚无植入式心房除颤器适应证的共识。根据我们的经验，心房除颤器适用于以下3类患者，这些患者均经抗心律失常药物钠通道或钾通道阻滞剂预防房颤复发无效。

1. 房颤发作持续24h或以上，或在这段时间内需要接受药物或电转复的患者。

2. 成功转复的持续性房颤（≤7d）患者出现晚期复发（>1个月且<12个月）需要再次转复。

3. 患者十分需要转复和维持窦性心律（例如尽管进行了抗凝治疗仍出现缺血性脑卒中或栓塞危险很高的患者）。同样，很难耐受房颤或出现血流动力学恶化的患者也可能从心房除颤器获益。

反之，阵发性、自行终止的房颤（<24h）患者应当排除。

（二）单独心房除颤器

在对单独心房除颤器（Metrix系统）的最初评估中，急性心肌缺血、近期心肌梗死史（<3个月）、射血分数下降（≤40%）的患者不考虑植入心房除颤器。这些患者可能需要双腔除颤器[14-16]。应检查有无反复转复的禁忌证，特别是心腔内血栓。为了验证导线边缘电压240V或以下终止房颤的可重复性和评价患者对于电击的耐受性，必须进行植入前测试。正如刚才提到的，Metrix系统已经不再使用。

（三）双腔除颤器[11,14-16]

像其他非药物治疗一样，仅在药物治疗对于房颤患者无效时才考虑植入双腔除颤器。第一组患者包括应植入心室ICD的患者。第二组患者包括需要植入心房除颤器且左室收缩功能下降（射血分数<40%）或舒张功能不全和/或可能有较高猝死危险，如部分经选择的肥厚型心肌病患者。

六、亟待解决的问题

一个尚未解决的问题是心房除颤器应作为最后的治疗手段还是应作为一线或二线治疗。植入式心房除颤器与房室交界区消融比较有一定优势，房室交界区消融可产生不可逆的解剖病变及起搏器依赖。多数房颤患者需要联合药物治疗，目的是减少发作次数和尽量避免植入心房除颤器干预治疗。

双腔除颤器作为目前仅有的植入式心房除颤器，其主要局限性是费用昂贵，已经超过了本已很贵的心室ICD。能够支付如此高昂费用来治疗房颤这样一个常见而非致命性心律失常的医疗保健体系不多。如果其费用降低及其他治疗房颤的非药物手段的长期结果未达到治疗要求，植入式心房除颤器将吸引心脏病医生和厂家的注意。

（李广平 刘彤 译）

参 考 文 献

1. Lévy S, Camm AJ: An implantable atrial defibrillator: An impossible dream? Circulation 87:1769–1772, 1993.
2. Cooper RA, Alferness CA, Smith WN, Ideker RE: Internal cardioversion of atrial fibrillation in sheep. Circulation 87:1673–1686, 1993.
3. Keane D, Sulke N, Cooke R, et al: Endocardial cardioversion of atrial flutter and fibrillation. Pacing Clin Electrophysiol 16:928, 1993.
4. Murgatroyd F, Slade AK, Sopher M, et al: Efficacy and tolerability of transvenous low energy cardioversion of paroxysmal atrial fibrillation in humans. J Am Coll Cardiol 25:1347–1353, 1995.
5. Alt E, Schmitt C, Ammer R, et al: Initial experience with intracardiac atrial defibrillation in patients with chronic atrial fibrillation. Pacing Clin Electrophysiol 17:1067–1078, 1994.
6. Lévy S, Ricard P, Lau CP, et al: Multicenter low energy transvenous atrial defibrillation (XAD) trial: Results in different subject of atrial fibrillation. J Am Coll Cardiol 29:750–755, 1997.
7. Lévy S, Ricard P, Guenoun M, et al: Low-energy cardioversion of spontaneous atrial fibrillation: Immediate and long-term results. Circulation 96:253–259, 1997.
8. Saksena S, Prakash A, Mangeon L, et al: Clinical efficacy and safety of atrial defibrillation using biphasic shocks and current non-thoracotomy endocardial lead configurations. Am J Cardiol 76:913–921, 1995.
9. Ayers GM, Alferness CA, Ilina M, et al: Ventricular proarrhythmic effects of ventricular cycle length and shock strength in a sheep model of transvenous atrial defibrillation. Circulation 89:413–422, 1994.
10. Barold H, Warton JM: Ventricular fibrillation resulting from synchronized internal defibrillation in a patient with ventricular preexcitation. J Cardiovasc Electrophysiol 8:436–440, 1997.
11. Jung W, Luderitz B: Implantation of an arrhythmia management system for ventricular and supraventricular tachyarrhythmias. Lancet 349:853–854, 1997.
12. Wellens HJ, Lau CP, Lüderitz B, et al: Atrioverter: An implantable device for the treatment of atrial fibrillation. Circulation 98:1651–1656, 1998.
13. Josephson ME: New approaches to the management of atrial fibrillation: The role of the atrial defibrillator. Circulation 98:1594–1596, 1998.
14. Gold MR, Sulke N, Schwartzman DS, et al: Clinical experience with a dual-chamber defibrillator to treat atrial tachyarrhythmias. J Cardiovasc Electrophysiol 12:1247–1252, 2001.
15. Adler SW, Wolpert C, Warman EN, et al: Efficacy of pacing therapies for treating atrial tachyarrhythmias in patients with ventricular arrhythmias receiving a dual-chamber defibrillator. Circulation 104:887–892, 2001.
16. Friedman PA, Dijkman B, Warman EN, et al: Atrial therapies reduce arrhythmia burden in defibrillator patients. Circulation 104:1023–1028, 2001.

第 109 章

植入式起搏器

David L. Hayes

本章目录

- 起搏治疗的历史 ………………… 977
- 起搏器命名 ……………………… 977
- 起搏适应证 ……………………… 978
- 起搏模式的合理选择 …………… 979
- 电磁干扰 ………………………… 986
- 总结 ……………………………… 986

自从 1958 年首次植入心脏起搏器以来，永久性心脏起搏器的植入数量逐步增加且高科技含量日益增多。由于技术的进步，起搏器的适应证已经拓宽，它已经成为治疗学的中流砥柱。参与治疗心律失常的医生必须对心脏起搏器有深入的理解。

一、起搏治疗的历史

1958 年第一个心外膜起搏系统植入后，起搏器技术得到飞速发展。随着复杂而精细的感知电路的进展，1963 年单腔按需型起搏系统问世。尽管在 20 世纪 50 年代已经有心房同步起搏系统和双腔起搏系统的报告，但在其后的很多年，这些装置并没有应用于临床。70 年代出现了锂电池和起搏器程控技术。80 年代的里程碑包括双腔起搏系统得到广泛认同和频率适应性起搏系统的推广。90 年代见证了诸多传感器技术的进展和可程控起搏器的自动化功能参数的增多。

二、起搏器命名

1974 年首次提出用一个由 3 个英文字母所组成的代码来描述各种起搏系统的基本功能。从那时起，由北美心脏起搏和电生理学会以及英国心脏起搏和电生理工作组（NASPE/BPEG）所组成的委员会定期更新此代码。这种代码被指定为北美心脏起搏和电生理学会和英国心脏起搏和电生理工作组代码（NBG 代码），用于心脏起搏器命名（表 109-1）。最近一次修订该代码是在 2001 年[1]。其由 5 位通用代码组成，其中并未对每种起搏器的特殊或独特的功能特征进行描述。

第 1 位字母表示起搏心腔："A"表示心房，"V"表示心室，"D"表示双腔（心房和心室）。

第 2 位字母表示感知心腔。字母的意思和第 1 位相同。在第 1 位和第 2 位使用"S"表示为单腔起搏器，可用于起搏心房或心室任一心腔。

第 3 位字母表示感知模式或起搏器对感知信号的反应。"I"表示感知信号抑制起搏器脉冲发放，并且使计时周期进行一次或多次重整。"T"表示感知信号触发起搏器发放脉冲。"D"表示同时具有抑制和触发两种功能。这种设定仅限于双腔起搏系统。当感知一个心房事件时会抑制心房起搏，但会触发心室起搏。单腔触发模式（VVT 或 AAT）在感知后会立即触发脉冲发放，与此不同，双腔起搏器系统在感知心房事件和触发心室输出之间有一个延迟，模拟了正常的 PR 间期。若感知来自心室信号或 R 波则抑制心室输出，甚至可能会抑制心房输出，这取决于感知发生的部位。

第 4 位字母仅表示频率应答（或适应）模式。"R"表示起搏器和内置的传感器共同控制起搏器脉冲

表 109-1 修订的 NASPE/BPEG 抗心动过缓起搏的通用代码

	Ⅰ	Ⅱ	Ⅲ	Ⅳ	Ⅴ
位置	起搏	感知	感知	频率	多部位
分类	心脏	心脏	后反应	应答	起搏
	O=无	O=无	O=无	O=无	O=无
	A=心房	A=心房	T=触发	R=频率应答	A=心房
	V=心室	V=心室	I=抑制		V=心室
	D=双腔	D=双腔	D=双重反应		D=双腔
	(A+V)	(A+V)	(T+I)		(A+V)
	S=单腔（A 或 V）	S=单腔（A 或 V）			
	（仅是制造商的设计）	（仅是制造商的设计）			

引自 Bernstein AD, Daubert JC, Fletcher RD, et al: The revised North American Society of Pacing and Electrophysiology (NASPE) / British Pacing and Electrophysiology Group (BPEG) generic code for antibradycardia, adaptive-rate, and multisite pacing. Pacing Clin Electrophysiol 25: 260-264, 2002. With permission from Futura Publishing.

发放频率，而不依赖于心脏固有节律。

第 5 位字母表示是否存在多部位起搏，"O"表示无多部位起搏，"A"表示心房多部位起搏，"V"表示心室多部位起搏，"D"表示心房和心室均为多部位起搏。多部位起搏是指在双心房、双心室起搏和在任一心腔中多于一个以上的部位起搏或这几种情况的任意组合。

三、起搏适应证

美国心脏病学会和美国心脏协会（ACC/AHA）的联合委员会制定的标准已经将心脏起搏适应证分为Ⅰ类，绝对适应证；Ⅱ类，相对适应证；Ⅲ类，非适应证[2]。Ⅱ类适应证中又进一步分为ⅡA 和ⅡB，ⅡA 指一致认为是起搏器适应证，但公布的资料有限；ⅡB 指存在分歧，但一些专家认为是起搏器适应证。尽管一些起搏器适应证是相对肯定和明确的，但有些情况需要有经验的专家进行鉴定和判断。临床心内科医师应该掌握起搏适应证及其相关争议。

有关植入起搏器的临床需要和适当的客观资料，例如心电图，必须清楚地以医疗记录文件的方式加以证明，以便提供给医疗保险或其他付款人。

（一）获得性房室阻滞

最常见的获得性房室阻滞（AVB）是特发性 AVB，并和年龄相关，此外还有许多潜在的原因。获得性 AVB 病人永久性起搏的Ⅰ类适应证包括任何有症状的 AVB，以及射频消融后的 AVB 或心外科手术后永久性 AVB。ⅡA 类适应证包括无症状的三度和二度Ⅱ型 AVB，以及无症状的位于 His 束内或 His 束下的二度Ⅰ型 AVB[2]。一度 AVB 伴有血流动力学损害的病人为ⅡA 类适应证[2]。一度 AVB 伴有左心功能不全及充血性心力衰竭的病人，优化 AV 间期可使其血流动力学得到改善则为ⅡB 类适应证[2]。

心肌梗死后有持续的症状性二度或三度 AVB，位于希浦系统内的持续性二度 AVB，有双侧束支阻滞或希浦系统内或以下的三度 AVB 者，一般认为是起搏器适应证[2]。位于房室结以下的一过性高度 AVB 和伴有束支阻滞也是Ⅰ类适应证[2]。位于房室结水平的持续性二度或三度 AVB 是ⅡB 适应证[3]。

（二）先天性三度房室阻滞

虽然三度房室阻滞病人植入起搏器的最佳时间仍存在争议，但是目前愈来愈倾向于在这些病人中早期、常规应用起搏器。儿科病人如出现下述情况推荐植入起搏器：充血性心力衰竭、严重室性逸搏或运动耐力下降；婴儿清醒状态下平均心室率低于 50bpm 或者有晕厥或先兆晕厥病史[4]。因为不可预期的高致死性晕厥、心率逐渐降低和继发性二尖瓣关闭不全的高发生率，所以，一般认为，即使没有症状，在成年人中预防性植入起搏器也是合适的[3]。

（三）慢性双分支和三分支阻滞

双分支和三分支阻滞伴有症状或一过性三度房室阻滞是植入起搏器的明确适应证。如伴有无症状的高度 AVB 也应植入起搏器。ACC/AHA Ⅱ类适应证包括慢性双分支和三分支阻滞病人不能证明晕厥是由于高度 AVB 引起，也不能用其他的任何原因解释，HV 间期＞100ms，或电生理检查发现有起搏诱发的 His 束下阻滞病人。这些病人植入起搏器可能是必要的[2]。

（四）窦房结功能不良

窦房结功能不良包括不同的亚型：慢-快综合征、

病态窦房结综合征、症状性窦性心动过缓、窦性静止（sinus arrest）与窦性停搏（或称窦性间歇 sinus pause；译者注：sinus arrest 和 sinus pause 汉译通常混用，但是英语用法是不完全相同的）、变时功能不全。这些术语常常用作同义词来使用。心动过缓的定义是不同的，但通常是认为在清醒状态下心率低于40bpm。对于需要治疗的心律绝对周期长度仍有不同意见。尽管对每一位病人需要个体化考虑，但是大多数医生赞同在清醒时窦性间歇（sinus pause）大于3s应该考虑为异常，行起搏治疗是合理的。睡眠过程中出现的间歇很难加以归类。由于迷走神经的影响，临床上正常人可在睡眠中出现长于3s的间歇，或在清醒时出现，但无症状或心律不齐乱，或者上述两种情况并存，然而这些情形不需要起搏治疗。对于病因不可逆转的任何症状性缓慢性心律失常的病人，应行永久性起搏治疗。

心肌梗死后窦房结功能不良的病人如果出现症状性心动过缓，需要植入永久性起搏器。如果药物治疗造成症状性心动过缓应考虑行永久性起搏治疗。

（五）神经心源性晕厥

某些类型的神经介导性晕厥可能是永久性起搏治疗的适应证。最近的 ACC/AHA 指南建议刺激颈动脉窦反复诱发的晕厥为Ⅰ类适应证[2]。在这些病人中，未使用任何抑制传导系统药物的情况下，轻微的颈动脉窦按摩会诱发3s以上的心室停搏。无明确刺激因素而反复发作晕厥者，颈动脉窦按摩呈阳性者是ⅡA类适应证[2]。自发性或直立倾斜试验诱发的伴有明显心脏抑制的神经心源性晕厥是ⅡA类适应证[2]。

尽管多数神经介导性晕厥病人可能不需要起搏治疗，但一些药物治疗无效的晕厥和有明显心动过缓参与的特殊病人可从永久性双腔起搏治疗中明确获益。一些随机试验的结果支持在特殊亚组病人中行起搏治疗[5,6]。

（六）非心动过缓起搏适应证

因非心动过缓适应证接受起搏器治疗的病人人数日益增加。非心动过缓起搏适应证主要包括心脏再同步治疗难治性充血性心力衰竭、药物治疗无效的症状性肥厚型梗阻性心肌病的双腔起搏治疗、起搏治疗预防心房颤动。

四、起搏模式的合理选择

选择最佳起搏模式时，除应考虑潜在的节律紊乱，同时还应考虑病人的全身情况、伴随的医疗问题、运动能力和对运动的变时功能的反应[7]。

心室按需抑制型起搏（VVI）具有心室感知通道，当起搏器感知到一次心室活动时则抑制起搏器输出（图109-1）。在起搏或感知心室事件后 VVI 起搏器进入心室不应期。在不应期内发生的任何心室事件都不能感知，而且起搏器也不会重设计时周期。

单腔频率适应性起搏模式（AAIR，VVIR）的计时周期和非频率适应的其他起搏模式无明显区别。区别在于潜在的起搏频率的可变性。根据起搏器内置的传感器和病人的运动水平，基础起搏周期从所程控的低限起搏频率的基础上开始缩短，缩短程度受程控的上限起搏频率所允许的最短计时间期所限定。

对于慢性心房颤动和缓慢心室率的病人应行 VVIR 起搏。尽管 VVI 起搏的适应证有一定的局限性，但它仍然是世界范围内最常用的起搏模式。VVI 起搏可保护病人免受致死性心动过缓的伤害；其局限性包括不能恢复或维持房室同步和对变时功能不良的病人不能提供频率应答功能。此外，VVI 起搏在心室起搏时可能造成患者出现症状性血流动力学恶化。如果起搏系统功能正常，仍然导致明显症状或限制病人

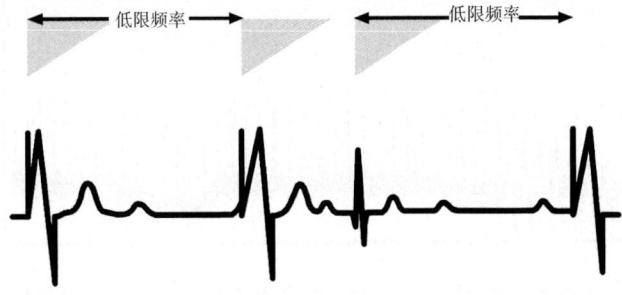

图109-1　心室按需抑制型起搏（VVI）计时周期由确定的低限频率（LRL）和心室不应期组成（VRP，由三角代表）LRL 计时结束时，如未感知自身心室事件则发放起搏脉冲。如果其结束前起搏器感知自身心室事件，则从该点开始 LRL 计时。VRP 开始于任何感知或起搏活动。（引自 Hayes DL, Levine PA：Pacemaker timing cycles. In Ellenbogen KA (ed)：Cardiac Pacing. Boston, Blackwell Scientific Publications, 1992，pp263-308.）

达到最佳的功能状态时，这种血流动力学恶化称起搏器综合征（图 109-2）。

起搏器综合征最初是在 VVI 起搏中被认识的，但是如果患者存在房室分离，任何起搏模式中都会出现该综合征。起搏器综合征的发生率取决于所采用的定义。如果条件限定在任何起搏模式造成的房室分离而使病人出现临床症状，那么在 VVI 或 VVIR 起搏的病人中起搏器综合征的发生率约 7%~10%[8]。在一项研究中，将植入 DDD 起搏器的病人随机分组为 DDD 或 VVI 起搏模式，83% 的病人出现了某种程度的起搏器综合征[9]。据报道，最常见的症状是气短、头晕、疲劳、颈部或腹部搏动、咳嗽和焦虑不安。如果存在房室分离，在任何起搏模式下都可能会发生起搏器综合征，认识到这一点是很重要的。

心房按需抑制型起搏（AAI）具有相同的计时周期，区别在于起搏和感知均发生在心房，起搏器感知自身心房波后抑制起搏脉冲发放（图 109-3）。心房起搏或感知事件启动不应期，在不应期内起搏器不感知任何事件。心房起搏过程中，当多个心室激动出现时可能会导致节律紊乱。例如，除心房起搏下传后产生的自身 QRS 波外，在其后跟随一个室性早搏，那么它不会抑制心房脉冲发放。心房计时周期结束时，无论是否有心室激动都将发放心房起搏脉冲，因为 AAI 起搏器感知不到任何心室事件。如果心室信号被心房电极不恰当地感知（远场感知），心房计时周期将被重置。这种异常情况可通过降低心房感知灵敏度或延长心室不应期而被纠正。

对于窦房结功能不全的病人选择 AAIR 起搏是合适的（AAI 起搏，即没有频率适应性心房起搏，是一个很少选择的起搏模式。如果考虑病人可能是单纯的窦房结功能不全，仅需要心房起搏，那么应该提供频率适应性起搏）。心房起搏明显的缺点是在出现房室阻滞时缺乏心室起搏支持。如果在窦房结功能不全的病人植入起搏器时，能仔细评价是否存在房室结疾病，那么有临床意义的房室结疾病的发生率很低，每年小于 2%。通过临床长期随访病人的结果表明，经严格选择的适合 AAI（R）起搏病人进展为房室阻滞的忧虑已有所消释[10]。AAI 起搏器植入前的评价应包括递增性心房起搏，要求 1:1 房室结下传的心率达到 120~140bpm。

房室顺序、非 P 波同步心室起搏、双腔感知

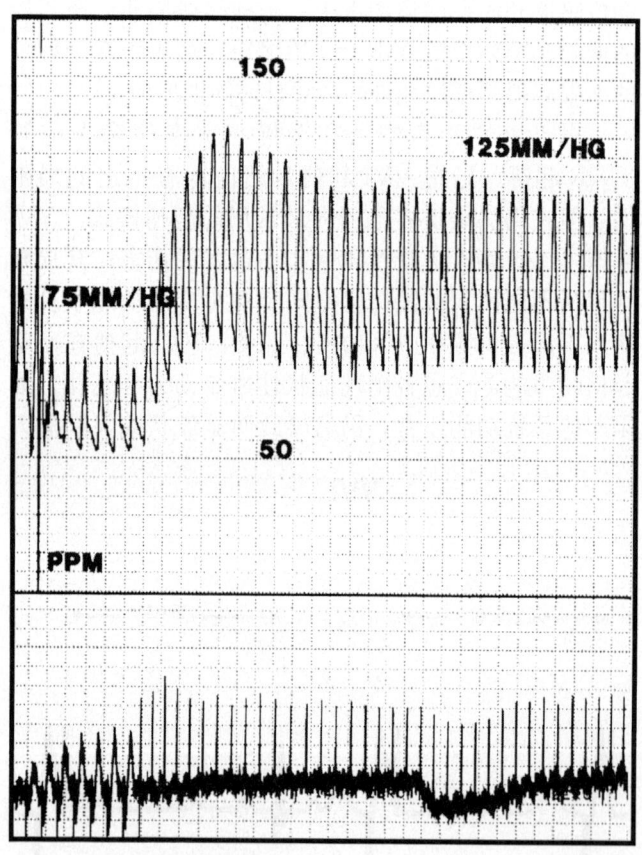

图 109-2　起搏器综合征病人的血流动力学描记　描记的开始部分显示心室起搏时收缩期动脉压约 75mmHg。病人自身窦性节律抑制心室起搏时，收缩期动脉压上升至约 125mmHg。（引自 Hayes DL, Holmes DR Jr: Hemodynamics of cardiac pacing. In Furman S, Hayes DL, Holmes DR Jr (eds): A Practice of Cardiac Pacing, 3rd ed. Mount Kisco, NY, Futura Publishing, 1993, pp 195-218. By permission of Mayo Foundation.）

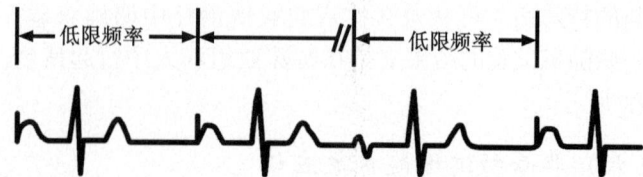

图 109-3　心房按需抑制型起搏（AAI）计时周期由确定的低限频率（LRL）和心房不应期组成　LRL 计时结束时，如未感知自身心房事件则在心房发放起搏脉冲。如果出现自身 P 波，则从该点开始 LRL 计时。心房不应期开始于任何感知或起搏活动。（引自 Hayes DL, Levine PA: Pacemaker timing cycles. In Ellenbogen KA (ed): Cardiac Pacing. Boston, Blackwell Scientific Publications, 1992, pp263-308.）

(DDI) 是没有心房跟踪的 DDD 起搏。DDI 是起搏器植入前很少选择的模式，但植入后，它仍然是很多双腔起搏器的一种可程控的模式。DDI 具有心房和心室感知功能，可以预防竞争性心房起搏，这种竞争性心房起搏可发生在 DVI 起搏中。DDI 模式的感知反应类型仅仅有抑制功能，即没有 P 波跟踪功能。因此，程控的起搏心室率不会超过程控的基础起搏频率。

心房同步（P 波跟踪）心室起搏方式（VDD）具有单心室起搏和双腔感知功能，因而通过感知自身心室活动抑制心室起搏脉冲和感知心房 P 波而发生心室跟踪反应。VDD 起搏适用于窦房结功能正常而有房室传导异常的病人。这个系统的主要局限性是如果这些病人出现窦房结功能不全则缺乏心房起搏支持。由于是单电极导线起搏系统，VDD 模式已变得越来越有用。在这个系统中，一个单独的电极能在心室起搏，并通过位于心房内的电极感知心房活动。

在 VDD 模式中，感知心房事件启动房室间期（AVI）。如果自身心室事件在 AVI 结束前出现，心室

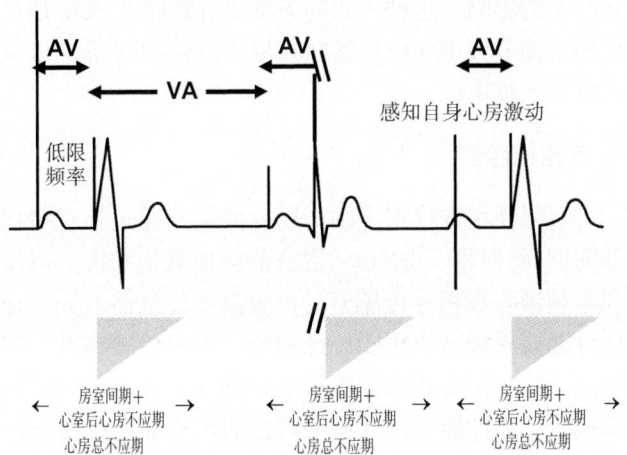

图 109-4 DDD 计时周期包括低限频率（LRL）、房室间期（AVI）、心室后心房不应期（PVARP）和高限频率　AVI 和 PVARP 组成心房总不应期（TARP）。DDD 计时周期有 4 种变化。如果自身心房和心室活动在 LRL 结束前出现，房室双起搏脉冲输出通道被抑制，无起搏出现。如果没有自身心房和心室活动出现，则发生房室顺序起搏（第一顺序）。如果在 VA 间期结束前没有感知到心房活动，则发放心房起搏脉冲，并启动 AVI。如果在 AVI 结束前出现自身心室活动，起搏器的心室输出被抑制，即心房起搏（第二顺序）。如果在 VA 间期结束前感知到 P 波，则心房起搏脉冲发放被抑制。AVI 启动，如果在 AVI 结束前没有心室活动被感知，则发放心室起搏脉冲，即 P 波同步心室起搏（第三顺序）。（引自 Hayes DL, Levine PA: Pacemaker timing cycles. In Ellenbogen KA（ed）: Cardiac Pacing. Boston, Blackwell Scientific Publications, 1992, pp263-308.）

起搏脉冲被抑制，并且低限频率计时周期将重设。如果在 AVI 结束时出现心室起搏，那么从这一次起搏重新开始低限频率起搏。如果没有心房事件，起搏器以低限频率起搏心室，即在没有感知心房事件时，起搏器表现为 VVI 模式起搏。

DDD 起搏和感知的机制是容易理解的。和低限频率相关的基本计时周期被分为两部分：室房（VA）间期和房室间期（AVI）。AVI 可以通过房室顺序起搏确定，例如心房起搏后相继出现自身的心室传导或由感知自身 P 波触发随后的心室起搏（图 109-4）。起搏器的最大跟踪频率由心房总不应期确定，心房总不应期由 AVI 和心室后心房不应期（PVARP）组成。

从正常 DDD 的功能，可以看到 4 种不同的心律：(1) 正常窦性心律；(2) 心房起搏；(3) 房室顺序起搏；(4) P 波同步心室起搏。DDD 起搏模式最适合窦房结功能正常的房室阻滞病人。DDDR 起搏器具有 DDD 起搏器全部功能。此外，P 波同步心室起搏可以作为一种增加心率的模式，而内置传感器的起搏器也可使心率增加。由此可见，起搏器所产生的节律可以是窦性激动所驱动的（也可称为心房驱动或 P 波同步心室起搏）或传感器驱动的两种。

DDDR 起搏适用于窦房结功能不全和房室传导异常的病人。如果植入起搏器的医师对 AAIR 起搏的安全性存在疑虑，那么 DDDR 起搏也适合于单纯窦房结功能不全的病人。

(一) 起搏模式对发病率和死亡率的影响

过去已证明，AAI 起搏病人比 VVI 起搏病人心脏事件的发病率和死亡率明显降低。回顾性研究已广泛复习和评论了起搏模式对死亡率的影响。虽然回顾性分析有其内在的欠缺，但是不能因此而否定这些研究所得出的相近结果。

此后，一些大型随机对照试验相继完成。Andersen 及其同事[10] 公布了起搏模式和生存率的前瞻性资料，在这个研究中 225 名窦房结功能不全的病人被随机分为 AAI 或 VVI 起搏组。结果证明，AAI 组较 VVI 组有较低的心房颤动和血栓栓塞发生率。加拿大生理性起搏试验（CTOPP）[11] 将 2568 名病人随机分为生理性起搏（双腔或 AAIR）组或心室起搏组（VVI），结果两组病人的死亡率和生活质量没有差别。但是，心房颤动的相对危险下降 18%。作为主要研究者，Lamas 已经完成了两项试验：PASE（pacing mode selection in the elderly, 老年病人起搏模式的选

择)[12] 和 MOST (mode selection trial，模式选择试验)[13]。PASE 未能证明生理性起搏比心室起搏获益。当按基础心律失常分类将病人分为窦房结功能不全和房室传导阻滞两类时，结果表明窦房结功能不全组有一定生活质量的改善。此外，心室起搏的病人有 26% 起搏模式的改变，原因是这些病人不能耐受心室起搏。和 CTOPP 一样，MOST 研究在死亡率方面也未证明有任何差异，但是确实证明了生理性起搏降低了心房颤动的发生率，减少了心力衰竭的症状和体征，并轻度改善了患者的生活质量。该研究结论认为，和心室起搏相比，所有双腔起搏均显示出有益的改善[13]。

(二) 为频率适应性起搏选择合适的传感器

各种用于频率适应性起搏的传感器已经取得了长足的发展，图 109-5 列出了传感器的一些生理反应的变化终点。

1. 体动传感器

体动传感器通过感知振动（压电晶体或加速度计）控制起搏器输出频率，由于它简单，易于临床应用和启动频率应答反应的速度快，所以它是最广泛应用于频率适应性起搏的传感器方式。

压电晶体和加速度计之间最大的区别是压电晶体感知上下运动的振动，而加速度计还感知前后运动[14]。某些研究者认为基于加速度计的起搏器比基于压电晶体的起搏器趋向于更具生理性的心率变化，而对局部的拍打或压力变化较少发生反应，所以加速度计已成为主要应用的体动传感器。

2. 分钟通气量传感器

分钟通气量（呼吸频率×潮气量）与代谢需求有着良好的相关性。由于胸阻抗随呼吸变化而发生变化，测量胸阻抗可以用于测定分钟通气量，通过分钟通气量变化就可用来改变起搏频率。因为分钟通气量可以预测代谢需求状况，故测定每个病人分钟通气量数值的大小可以确定该病人休息和不同的活动状态的水平[15]。分钟通气量传感器长期应用的可靠性已得到充分的肯定。

3. QT 间期传感器

用起搏的 QRS 波起点到 T 波终点的间期调节起搏频率已经应用多年。脉冲-T 波结束间期受自主活动和心率的影响，这种一致的关系使得脉冲-T 波间期可以用来调节频率。QT-感知频率适应性起搏系统已成功应用于临床。

4. 其他传感器

有限使用或仅用于临床研究的传感器包括有射血前间期/每搏量、dP/dt、混合静脉血氧饱和度、温度和电刺激除极积分传感器。内置温度传感器的频率适应性起搏系统已应用于临床多年。这种传感器有一些优点，但它需要特殊的热敏电极导线，并且在劳动负荷低时工作性能欠佳（有关其他的传感器已有很好的文献报告[16,17]，具体细节不在此赘述）。上述某些传感器可应用于组合成多传感器的频率适应性起搏器。某些频率适应性传感器可用于其他目的，而不限于调整起搏频率，例如用来优化 AV 间期或减少特殊的与节律相关的症状[18]。

5. 双传感器联合

性能良好的传感器应该能够对抗所有非生理性干扰刺激。一种多传感器的频率适应性起搏系统可以通过一个传感器对另一个传感器进行核查，或者相互之间的验证而提高特异性[19,20]。目前，植入的多传感器的频率适应性起搏器的数量相对较少。应用最广泛的传感器组合包括：加速度计-分钟通气量传感器和加速

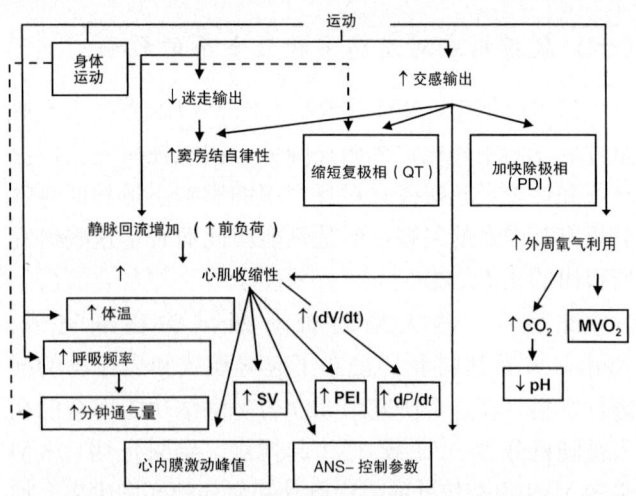

图 109-5　已经研究或临床应用的频率适应性永久性心脏起搏器生理反应　方框内的术语代表用于频率适应性起搏器的各种终点。虚线连接的传感器已经应用于双传感器频率适应性起搏系统。ANS：自主神经系统；MVO_2：最大静脉氧饱和度；PDI：起搏除极间期；PEI：射血前间期；SV：每搏量。

表 109-2　起搏器植入和元件相关因素所致并发症

通常早期发现的并发症	通常晚期发现的并发症	早期或晚期均可能发生的并发症
疼痛或瘀斑	皮肤溃烂	电极脱位
气胸	皮肤粘连	起搏器相关心律失常
血肿	血栓	Twiddler 综合征
心外刺激	电极断裂或绝缘不良	感染
电极穿孔		起搏器综合征
手术中电极损伤		电路失灵
皮下气肿		电极或连接器连接松动
损伤胸导管		输出阻滞
气体栓塞		对起搏器过敏
臂丛神经损伤		
误穿锁骨下动脉		

度计-QT 间期传感器。

6. 起搏器并发症

并发症可以由植入技术直接造成，或者由起搏器系统的元件故障造成。许多并发症与植入者的经验直接有关。表 109-2 列举了最常见的并发症，这些并发症可能见于起搏器植入后早期或者晚期。

7. 心电图异常的释义

起搏器病人心电图异常可以被归纳为以下几个种类：失夺获、无输出、感知不良和不恰当的频率改变[21,22]。

失夺获表现为起搏信号后无心脏除极（图 109-6，表 109-3）。无输出有时被错误地理解为失夺获的同义词。

无输出通常是由于超感知和输出抑制引起，但也可以由于起搏器本身确实无输出或电路中断导致电信号不能到达心脏引起（图 109-7，表 109-3）。

失夺获的鉴别诊断与无输出的鉴别诊断有所重叠。例如，螺旋导线断裂的心电图现象可以包括失夺获，原因是在导线不全断裂处明显的漏电，残余的电流不足以产生对心肌的有效刺激而不起搏，在心电图上只出现起搏信号。另一方面，泄露的电流可以被起搏器感知从而抑制了起搏器输出。如果导线完全断裂导致电路中断，心电图则无法检测到起搏器输出脉冲，继发的感知异常也会出现。

虽然多数绝缘不良表现为感知异常，但有时也可以表现为超感知和无输出或失夺获。此外，分辨不清的起搏心电图波形可以由心电图记录系统本身的原因而引起。对数字电路的心电记录系统而言，起搏器信号的大小并不重要，也不是总能记录到可见的起搏信号。这样看上去就像是无输出，实际上，如果应用有脉冲信号通道的动态心电图或心内电图就可以记录出发放的脉冲信号。

起搏器电池耗竭时，既可以因为输出电压下降而

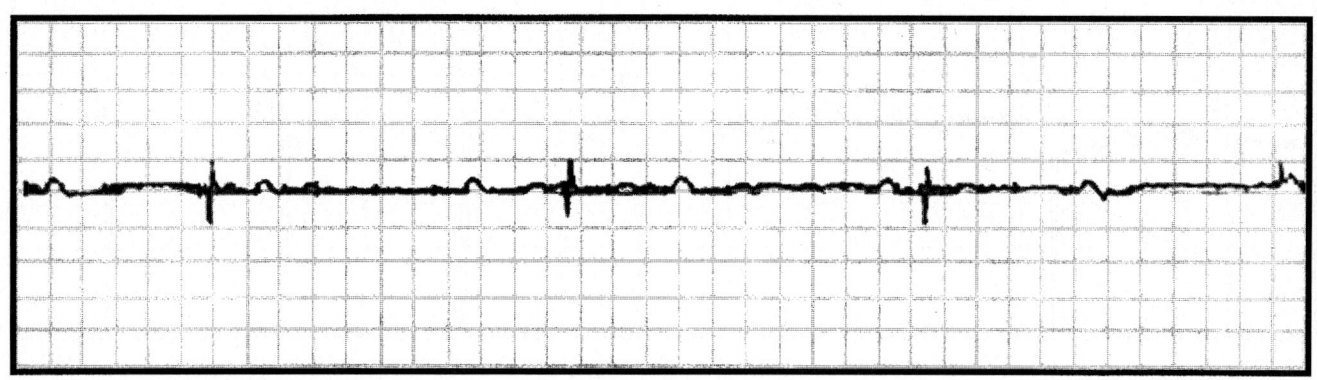

图 109-6　起搏器病人的心电图描记，心脏电复律前程控为 VVI 模式 50bpm　描记显示约 80bpm 的正常窦性心律。但是 4 次心室起搏输出均未夺获心室。在电复律后 24h 内，心室起搏阈值恢复至基线。

表 109-3　起搏器功能障碍

失夺获	无输出	感知异常	起搏频率改变
高阈值伴不适当的程控输出不足	电路失灵	自主心搏形态与幅度和植入时测量不同	电路失灵
电路部分断路	完全或间断的电极导线断裂	电极脱位或电极接触不良	电池耗竭
绝缘不良	间断或永久性起搏器固定螺丝松动	电极绝缘不良	应用磁铁
电极脱位或穿孔	电池全部耗竭	电路失灵	滞后功能开启
电池接近完全耗竭	电极内部绝缘不良（双极电极）	应用磁铁	交叉感知
功能性失夺获	超感知各种心外干扰	弹簧开关工作失灵	超感知
电极连接器与起搏器不全或完全连接不良	起搏器阳极接触失灵*	电磁干扰	起搏器再次程控时未记录
电路失灵		电池耗竭	起搏器奔放
单极起搏器囊袋内有气体			心电记录仪器失灵（如纸速改变）

* 例如：双极发生器中应用单极电极，双极电极起搏器程控为单极，单极系统囊袋内有气体，单极起搏器未在囊袋中。

导致失夺获，也可以因为电池完全耗竭而造成无输出。电池耗竭的程度可以通过适时的随访而避免。需要注意的是起搏器信号落在自主心搏的不应期内也可引起失夺获，这种情况称为功能性失夺获。

感知异常可以分为真性感知异常和功能性感知异常（后者见表 109-3）。真性感知异常包括感知不良，即不能感知正常的自主心电活动（图 109-8）；感知过度，即感知不应该感知到的内在或外在电信号（图 109-7）。人工伪差也可造成感知过度和无输出的表现（图 109-9）。真正的感知不良最常见于电极脱位或电极位置不适当。感知异常也常常继发于绝缘不良，但少见于间歇的连接系统断裂。

工作正常的起搏系统有时不能检测到心房或心室的期前收缩。植入起搏器时，感知阈值是通过电极头端测量该局部的自主心搏的心内电图所得到的。如果期前收缩发生在心脏的其他部位，感知到的心电向量可能会和局部测量的自主心搏的向量不同，其所产生的电压可能过小不足以为起搏器所感知到。这种情况是事先无法预见的，除非术后的期前收缩与植入时的期前收缩的形态相同，并且植入时可以测量到。这种情况下就需要重新程控起搏器的感知灵敏度，以感知期前收缩，但即使程控后还不能解决这一感知异常，也极少为此重置电极。

如果自主的心搏落在起搏器的不应期内也会表现为功能性感知不良。例如，一个自主的心房搏动落在心室后心房不应期，起搏器就不会感知这个心搏。因此如果不完整地了解计时周期，就容易误以为是真的感知不良。

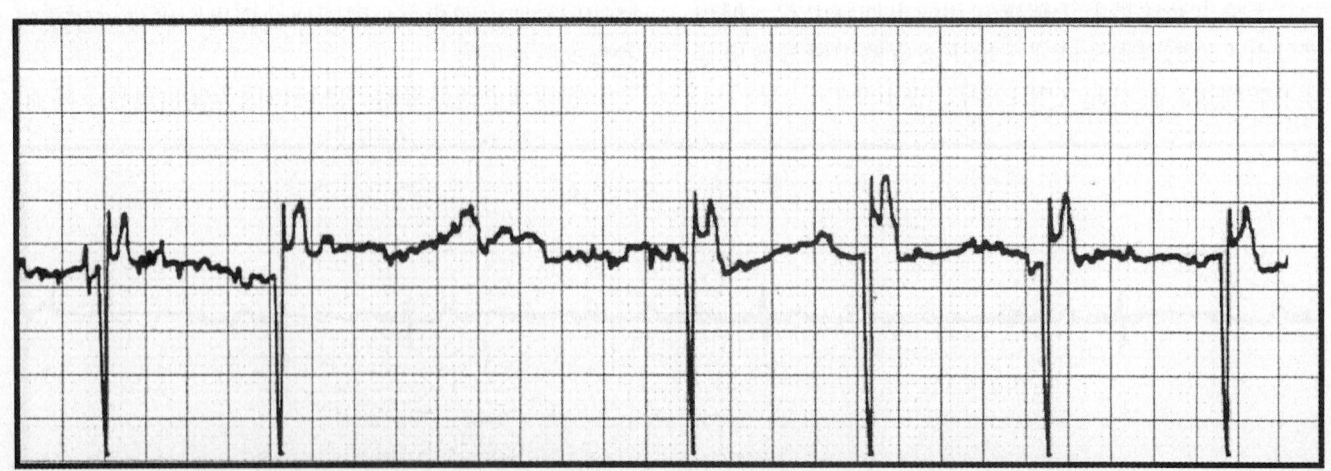

图 109-7　起搏器以 VVI 模式工作，基础频率 70bpm　患者全部心室激动均为起搏节律，呈起搏器依赖状态，心电图记录中有基线不稳。起搏器对肌电干扰超感知，抑制了心室输出，造成第 2、3 个 QRS 波群之间的长 RR 间期。

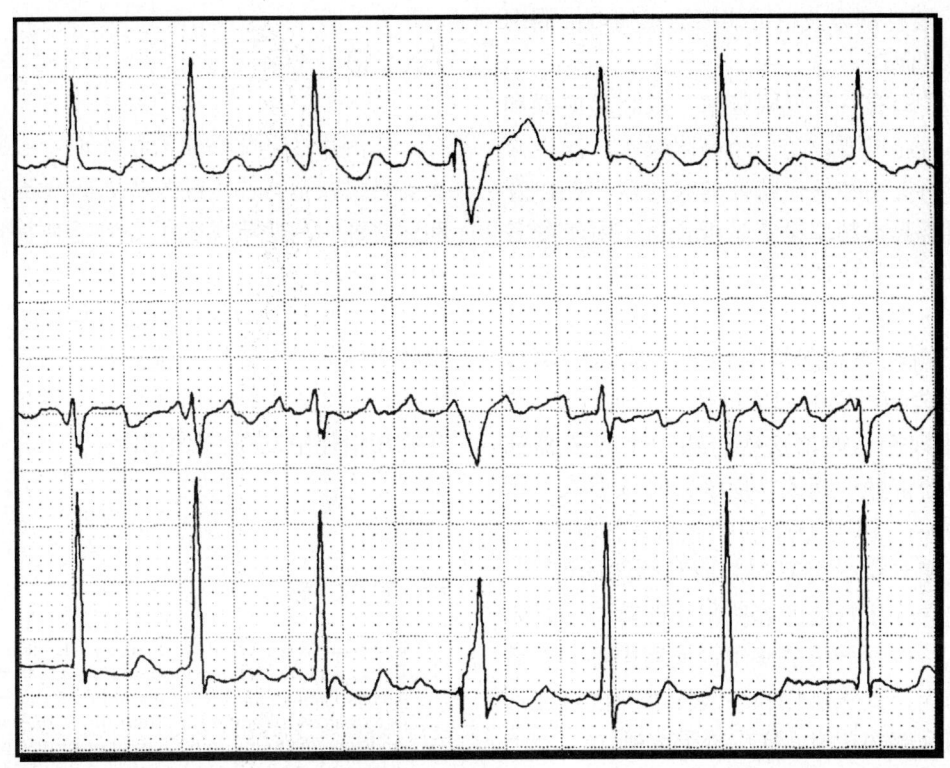

图 109-8　VVI 起搏器病人的心电图描记，程控为 85bpm（周长 705ms）　基础节律是心房颤动。单个的心室起搏事件出现在前面自身心室事件之后，周长短于 705ms，和间歇性心室感知不良是一致的。

融合和假性融合波的产生是由于无效起搏脉冲信号重叠于自身 P 波或 QRS 波上。融合波是指心搏的形态介于自主心律与起搏心律的形态之间。假性融合波是指起搏信号发出太晚，心脏搏动的形态完全呈自主心搏的形态。这通常是由于在自主心搏产生足够的电压振幅之前，感知线路不能感知到自主心搏，起搏器就发放脉冲落在心房活动或心室活动的不应期内。当自主节律与起搏频率相近时就可能发生这种情况。

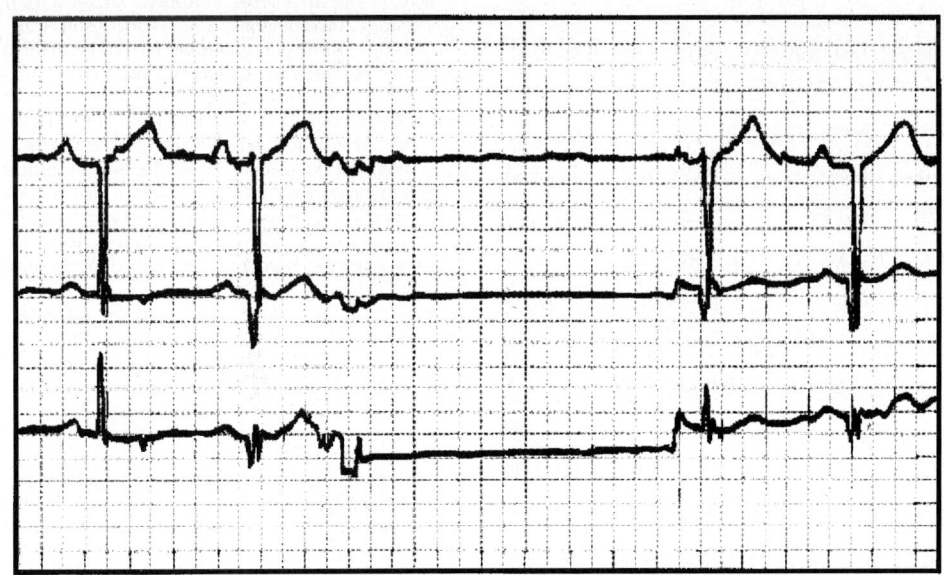

图 109-9　DDD 起搏器病人的动态心电图，低限频率程控为 60bpm　图中起搏器以 P 波同步模式工作，即跟踪自身心房频率，当自身心房率大于起搏器设置的低限频率 60bpm 时，心室率亦大于 60bpm。第 1 个 QRS 波群是自身下传的，第 2、4 个 QRS 波群是经起搏器下传的，第 3 个 QRS 波群是经起搏下传和自身 QRS 波群的融合波。第 2、3 个 QRS 波群之间的长间期大于起搏器设置的基础起搏周长，是第 3、4 个 QRS 波群周期的倍数。而此时（包括以后记录到长间期时）患者无不适症状。该长间歇属于动态心电图描记过程中的人工伪差，起搏器功能是正常的。

在 VVI 起搏器，假性融合波也可能因为感知电极周围心室肌电传导延迟而产生。

每个起搏模式均有一个低限频率，双腔起搏器和频率适应性起搏器还需要设定一个高限频率。医生必须熟知该起搏器的类型和任何特殊起搏器功能以及计时周期，以判断起搏频率设定是否合适。由于受各种各样原因的影响，起搏器程控的频率可能和最初设定的不同（表 109-3）。

药物可以影响感知和起搏阈值而造成心电图异常[23]。尽管许多药物可影响起搏阈值，但通常仅ⅠC类药物引起临床问题。如果这些药物用于起搏器病人，尤其是起搏器依赖的病人，应该监测该病人是否有起搏器阈值增加。ⅠC类药物亦可造成感知异常。

电解质和代谢异常也可影响起搏和感知阈值[23]。高钾血症是引起有临床意义的起搏器功能障碍的最常见的电解质紊乱，但是严重的酸中毒或碱中毒、高碳酸血症、高血糖症、低氧血症和黏液性水肿也可能影响起搏器的起搏和感知功能，亦应给予重视。

五、电磁干扰

电磁干扰（EMI）是指任何在一定频率范围起搏器感知电路检测到的生物或非生物信号。电磁干扰能导致起搏器频率变化、感知异常、磁铁模式反应或需要重新程控起搏器。

生物信号可能会引起超感知，包括 T 波、肌电干扰、延迟后电位和 P 波。等电位的期外收缩（isoelectric extrasystoles）可表现为超感知[23,24]。

医院的仪器设备可能会干扰起搏器功能，包括外科电凝术、电复律、电除颤、核磁共振检查、超声碎石术、射频消融术、电休克疗法和电热疗法。

潜在的电磁干扰可来源于医院以外相对少见的环境，包括一些电焊设备、消磁设备、传导加热器、移动（蜂窝式）电话和防盗装置。模拟电路移动式电话对起搏器病人是安全的。数字移动式电话有较大的潜在电磁干扰的可能性，所以依赖起搏器的病人使用数字移动电话要加以小心[25]。病人尽量避免将电话放在起搏器上，即不在起搏器或 ICD 上面的衣服口袋里携带开机的电话，即可以避免有害的临床事件。

某些防盗装置对起搏器有潜在的干扰，可导致起搏器抑制、感知异常和诱发期外收缩[26]。然而，从实践观点看，如果病人以规则的步伐快步走过防盗门，一般不会引起起搏器起搏和感知功能异常[27]。

六、总 结

在治疗缓慢性心律失常方面，心脏起搏术已经融入高科技技术，并不断发展。最近有关起搏器命名[1]和适应证[2]的变革代表了心脏起搏治疗学和临床试验在起搏领域的进展。今后起搏器的自动化和自我管理程度一定会日益增加。虽然人们可以期盼通过基因工程技术修复心脏传导系统异常来治疗缓慢性心律失常疾病，但在未来很长时期里，心脏植入装置仍会继续在临床治疗中发挥重要作用。

（万 征 译）

参 考 文 献

1. Bernstein AD, Daubert JC, Fletcher RD, et al: The revised NASPE/BPEG generic code for antibradycardia, adaptive-rate, and multisite pacing. Pacing Clin Electrophysiol 25:260–264, 2002.
2. Gregoratos G, Abrams J, Epstein AE, et al: ACC/AHA/NASPE 2002 guideline update for implantation of cardiac pacemakers and antiarrhythmia devices: Summary article: A report of the American College of Cardiology/American Heart Association Task Force on Practice Guidelines (ACC/AHA/NASPE Committee to Update the 1998 Pacemaker Guidelines). Circulation 106:2145–2161, 2002.
3. Michaelsson M, Jonzon A, Riesenfeld T: Isolated congenital complete artrioventricular block in adult life: A prospective study. Circulation 92:442–449, 1995.
4. Serwer GA, Dorostkar PC, LeRoy SS: Pediatric pacing and defibrillator usage. In Ellenbogen KA, Kay GN, Wilkoff BL (eds): Clinical Cardiac Pacing and Defibrillation, 2nd ed. Philadelphia, WB Saunders, 2000, pp 953–989.
5. Connolly SJ, Sheldon R, Roberts RS, Gent M, the Vasovagal Pacemaker Study Investigators: The North American Vasovagal Pacemaker Study (VPS): A randomized trial of permanent cardiac pacing for the prevention of vasovagal syncope. J Am Coll Cardiol 33:16–20, 1999.
6. Sutton R, Brignole M, Menozzi C, et al, Vasovagal Syncope International Study (VASIS) Investigators: Dual-chamber pacing in the treatment of neurally mediated tilt-positive cardioinhibitory syncope: Pacemaker versus no therapy: A multicenter randomized study. Circulation 102:294–299, 2000.
7. Hayes DL, Friedman PA: Generator and lead selection. In Hayes DL, Lloyd MA, Friedman PA (eds): Cardiac Pacing and Defibrillation: A Clinical Approach. Armonk, NY, Futura Publishing, 2000, pp 125–157.
8. Janosik DL, Ellenbogen KA: Basic physiology of cardiac pacing and pacemaker syndrome. In Ellenbogen KA, Kay GN, Wilkoff BL (eds): Clinical Cardiac Pacing and Defibrillation, 2nd ed. Philadelphia, WB Saunders, 2000, pp 333–382.
9. Heldman D, Mulvihill D, Nguyen H, et al: True incidence of pacemaker syndrome. Pacing Clin Electrophysiol 13:1742–1750, 1990.
10. Andersen HR, Nielsen JC, Thomsen PE, et al: Long-term follow-up of patients from a randomised trial of atrial versus ventricular pacing for sick-sinus syndrome. Lancet 350:1210–1216, 1997.
11. Connolly SJ, Kerr CR, Gent M, et al, the Canadian Trial of Physiologic Pacing Investigators: Effects of physiologic pacing versus ventricular pacing on the risk of stroke and death due to cardiovascular causes. N Engl J Med 342:1385–1391, 2000.
12. Lamas GA, Orav EJ, Stambler BS, et al, the Pacemaker Selection in the Elderly Investigators: Quality of life and clinical outcomes in elderly patients treated with ventricular pacing as compared with dual-chamber pacing. N Engl J Med 338:1097–1104, 1998.
13. Lamas GA, Lee KL, Sweeney MO, et al, the Mode Selection Trial in Sinus-Node Dysfunction: Ventricular pacing or dual-chamber pacing for sinus-node dysfunction. N Engl J Med 346:1854–1862, 2002.

14. Millerhagen JO, Combs WJ: Activity sensing and accelerometer-based pacemakers. In Ellenbogen KA, Kay GN, Wilkoff BL (eds): Clinical Cardiac Pacing and Defibrillation, 2nd ed. Philadelphia, WB Saunders, 2000, pp 249-270.
15. Pioger G, Geroux L, Limousin M, the French Group of Investigation of Chorum: Automatic basic rate variation algorithm driven by a minute-ventilation sensor: Clinical results [abstract]. Pacing Clin Electrophysiol 20:1445, 1997.
16. Salo R, O'Donoghue S, Platia EV: The use of intracardiac impedance-based indicators to optimize pacing rate. In Ellenbogen KA, Kay GN, Wilkoff BL (eds): Clinical Cardiac Pacing. Philadelphia, WB Saunders, 1995, pp 234-249.
17. Boute W, Feith F, Leunk S-K, Lau C-P: Evoked QT interval-based and intracardiac impedance-based pacemakers. In Ellenbogen KA, Kay GN, Wilkoff BL (eds): Clinical Cardiac Pacing and Defibrillation, 2nd ed. Philadelphia, WB Saunders, 2000, pp 293-306.
18. Deharo JC, Peyre JP, Chalvidan T, et al: Continuous monitoring of an endocardial index of myocardial contractility during head-up tilt test. Am Heart J 139:1022-1030, 2000.
19. Barold SS, Barold HS: Optimal cardiac pacing in patients with coronary artery disease. Pacing Clin Electrophysiol 21:456-461, 1998.
20. Lau CP, Leung SK, Lee IS: Delayed exercise rate response kinetics due to sensor cross-checking in a dual sensor rate adaptive pacing system: The importance of individual sensor programming. Pacing Clin Electrophysiol 19:1021-1025, 1996.
21. Love CJ, Hayes DL: Evaluation of pacemaker malfunction. In Ellenbogen KA, Kay GN, Wilkoff BL (eds): Clinical Cardiac Pacing. Philadelphia, WB Saunders, 1995, pp 656-683.
22. Hayes DL: Pacemaker timing cycles and pacemaker electrocardiography. In Hayes DL, Lloyd MA, Friedman PA (eds): Cardiac Pacing and Defibrillation: A Clinical Approach. Armonk, NY, Futura Publishing Company, 2000, pp 201-245.
23. Atlee JL, Bernstein AD: Cardiac rhythm management devices (part II): Perioperative management. Anesthesiology 95:1492-1506, 2001.
24. Hayes DL: Electromagnetic interference with implantable cardiac devices. In Barold SS, Mugica J (eds): The Fifth Decade of Cardiac Pacing. Oxford, UK, Blackwell Publishing, 2003.
25. Hayes DL, Wang PJ, Reynolds DW, et al: Interference with cardiac pacemakers by cellular telephones. N Engl J Med 336:1473-1479, 1997.
26. McIvor ME, Reddinger J, Floden E, Sheppard RC: Study of Pacemaker and Implantable Cardioverter Defibrillator Triggering by Electronic Article Surveillance Devices (SPICED TEAS). Pacing Clin Electrophysiol 21:1847-1861, 1998.
27. Groh WJ, Boschee SA, Engelstein ED, et al: Interactions between electronic article surveillance systems and implantable cardioverter-defibrillators. Circulation 100:387-392, 1999.

第110章

起搏器的新应用

Michael R. Gold and Robert W. Peters

本章目录

- 起搏改善心衰血流动力学 ………… 988
- 心率 ………………………………… 988
- 房室同步 …………………………… 989
- 右室激动 …………………………… 989
- 双室起搏（心脏再同步化治疗）…… 989
- 心房颤动 …………………………… 990
- 肥厚型心肌病 ……………………… 991
- 神经心源性晕厥 …………………… 991
- 长QT综合征 ……………………… 992
- 总结 ………………………………… 992

自从20世纪60年代最早应用永久起搏器以来，起搏技术已经发生翻天覆地的变化。从最初使用的原始的固定频率单腔起搏器起，起搏器在性能和复杂程度方面已经历了巨大转变。最初，永久起搏器主要用于有症状的窦房结功能障碍及高度房室阻滞（AVB）病人，为这些有症状的心动过缓病人提供心率支持。随着技术进步及对病理生理学认识的深入，永久起搏器已被建议作为其他多种疾病的治疗手段。其中许多情况并不存在心动过缓，而是通过起搏来改变心肌激动方式，以抑制心动过速或改善血流动力学。本章着重介绍永久起搏的一些新应用。

一、起搏改善心衰血流动力学

现在的美国正处于充血性心力衰竭（CHF）发病较高的年代，每年新增病人数达55万。尽管药物治疗心力衰竭已有了很大进展，但令人失望的是死亡率仍很高。由于供体缺乏，心脏移植严重受限，而左室辅助装置虽然前景看好，但价格高昂，其功效和总的适用性有待于进一步探讨。很久以来已经被人们认可的右室心尖部起搏已非最佳选择，特别是在伴随室内传导障碍的病人和一些血流动力学异常（"起搏器综合征"）的病人。因此，特别是对有左室功能减低的病人，重新评估起搏治疗已引起较大的兴趣。

二、心 率

永久起搏可以调整心率的快慢，患者可以直接从中受益。如果已明确病人心排血量的降低是由于静息时心动过缓或心脏变时性降低引起，通过增加起搏频率或再加上频率适应功能可能会缓解或部分缓解病人症状。然而，更多的心衰病人存在心动过速。心率对心脏血流动力学的影响是复杂的问题，总的说来所知甚少，甚至在充血性心力衰竭的情况下也没弄清楚多少。可能的情况是，由于左（和右）室功能、房室传导特性、自主神经功能、心脏病的病因、心脏活性药物、血压状态以及其他多种因素间复杂的相互作用，心衰病人的最佳心率和变时反应因人而异，在对这个领域的问题进一步阐明之前，单靠调整起搏频率不大可能在心衰病人群体中适用。

三、房室同步

据估计，适时的心房收缩在健康人可以增加 15%～30% 的心排血量。尽管对此仍有异议，但是心房收缩对心衰病人尤其重要，特别是有左室舒张功能下降者。正常房室同步的丧失会造成许多负面影响，包括心房在房室瓣关闭时收缩而造成肺和静脉系统淤血，由于正常瓣膜受干扰而引起收缩期二、三尖瓣反流，房室瓣延迟关闭引起的舒张期反流，以及由于心房扩张造成了自主神经系统激活，并进一步引起不适当的血管舒张。"起搏器综合征"最早用于上述多种因素共同引起的心排血量下降和低血压病人。

由此，有人建议重建合适的房室传导（程控起搏器的房室间期）会改善心衰病人的血流动力学异常。早期进行的没有对照组的研究显示，短的房室间期（或房室延迟）可以使双腔起搏病人获益，推测是通过减少舒张期二尖瓣反流实现的。但这些结果并没有被随后进行的随机试验证实[1,2]。事实上，双腔（DDD）与单腔（VVI）除颤器（DAVID）的研究显示，在可能的情况下应尽量避免右室心尖部起搏。对植入双腔 ICD 的病人进行评估，这些病人有左室收缩功能障碍，但窦房结与房室结功能正常。所有病人植入双腔 ICD 后，随机分为 DDDR 起搏组或备用 VVI 起搏组。因为没有标准的起搏适应证，VVI 起搏组作为对照组，并最大可能地减少起搏。主要的终点为病人死亡或因 CHF 入院。结果 DDDR 组更早达到这个终点[3]。

虽然短房室间期双腔起搏可能对经过筛选的病人亚组仍然有益，但目前人们一般不再将其用于改善患者的血流动力学。事实上，基于 DAVID 结果，应用起搏器或 ICD 的可程控性将起搏器设置为房室搜索滞后、长房室间期，或 AAI 模式，以最大限度减少心室起搏。这种程控策略与没有左室收缩功能障碍或传导延迟病人的起搏器程控是一致的。在随后的分组研究中，与没有或最小限度右室起搏组相比，正常右室起搏组病人血流动力学状态较差，而且心衰恶化的机会增加[4,5]。

四、右室激动

永久起搏的最早设计就是从右室心尖部起搏，因为导线容易到达该部位，而且较少移位。大量证据表明右室心尖起搏并不理想，其中包括室间隔矛盾运动和对二尖瓣附属装置的干扰。操控性更好的导管、主动和被动固定电极的发展为永久起搏提供了更多可选择的部位。一项新起搏技术从希氏束旁部位起搏特殊传导系统，但还未观察到这种起搏对心衰病人的长期作用。右室流出道或右室间隔部位起搏的初步研究显示，短房室间期起搏具有改善血流动力学的可能。但是，这些结果未能在随后进行的随机双盲试验中得到证实[6]，因此，这方面的应用几乎被放弃。近期报道，持续性间隔起搏比心尖起搏对左室功能的损害小，尽管这个作用可能要在 18 个月后才能显现出来[7]。越来越清楚的是在左心衰竭的病人应尽量避免右室心尖部起搏，因为其有加重原有心力衰竭或引发新的心力衰竭的危险。在此考虑之下，在提供应有的心率支持条件下，通过延长房室间期以最大可能减少右室起搏，比缩短房室间期模仿房室结生理状态更会使病人获益。

五、双室起搏（心脏再同步化治疗）

据估计，高达 50% 的充血性心衰患者存在室内传导障碍。这些传导障碍会造成心室运动不协调，并因此引起进一步的血流动力学障碍[8]。值得注意的是，虽然并非所有的传导障碍病人都表现出运动不协调，但一般来说，心室运动不协调的发生机会随着传导障碍严重程度的增加而增加。事实上，已有的资料显示，心衰的死亡率与 QRS 波群时限相关[9,10]。心房同步双室起搏（心脏再同步化治疗，CRT）能协调左右室收缩，增强心室的收缩力，改善心功能。动物研究和心衰病人急性试验证实了此假设[11-14]。

在此背景下，开始了几个大型临床试验以评价 CRT 的长期作用（表 110-1）。使用随机单盲交叉设计，Cazeau 和心肌病多部位起搏（MUSTIC）研究者发现，CRT 改善了 67 名心功能 III 级（NYHA 心功能分级）和 QRS 时限大于 150ms 的病人的运动耐量、生活质量，减少了住院次数[15,16]。与此相似，PATH-CHF 试验的研究者报道，CRT 改善了运动能力和功能状态[17]。近来，Abraham 及同事[18]报道了多中心 INSYNCH 随机临床评估试验（MIRACLE）结果。在 453 名左室射血分数（LVEF）小于 36% 的中重度心衰伴 QRS 时限大于 129ms 的病人中，CRT 治疗改善了运动耐量及生活质量，减少了因心衰住院的次数，同时 QRS 时限缩短，平均左室射血分数相应提高，

表 110-1　充血性心力衰竭心脏再同步化治疗的长期随机临床试验

研　究	入组患者	结　果
PATH-CHF	42 名由于收缩功能不良和室内传导不良导致的心功能 Ⅲ～Ⅳ级的患者	CRT 可以长期改善运动耐量；左室游离壁的同步化优于前壁
MUSTIC	48 名心功能Ⅲ级和 IVCD 的患者	CRT 可以改善运动耐量和生活质量
MIRACLE	453 名患者心功能Ⅲ～Ⅳ级，EF≤35%，QRS≥130ms	CRT 可以改善运动耐量、生活质量、射血分数和再住院率
COMPANION	1670 名患者心功能Ⅲ～Ⅳ级，EF≤35%，QRS≥120ms	CRT 可以降低死亡率和再住院率，CRT-D 可以降低死亡率

左室舒张末期室径下降。

许多心衰病人有植入 ICD 的典型指征。此外，心衰人群中猝死的危险很高。因此，ICD 和 CRT 结合的装置（CRT-D）应运而生以同时解决这些问题[19]。对这些设备进行的随机对照试验证实了 CRT 的益处，特别是对心功能Ⅲ、Ⅳ级（NYHA 分级）的病人。心力衰竭的药物、起搏和除颤治疗比较研究（COMPANION 试验）的初步结果显示，CRT（单独，或与 ICD 联合应用）能使心功能Ⅲ～Ⅳ级、左室射血分数小于 34%、QRS 时限大于 120ms（任何原因）病人因任何原因导致的死亡率与住院次数明显降低。进一步分析提示植入 CRT-D 与最佳药物治疗方案相比降低了死亡率。

总体来说，CRT 已被证实可改善一些进展性心力衰竭病人（主要合并左束支型室内阻滞者）的心功能。这项技术还在不断改进，早期试验中的许多困难，如左室入路的安全性和有效性问题现已改进（现在左室起搏常规通过冠状窦和心脏静脉系统完成）。电极技术和输送系统的改进缩短了植入时间，提高了成功率。正在进行的和未来的 CRT 和 CRT-D 试验有望帮助识别能从心脏再同步化治疗中获益的病人（如基线 QRS 波群增宽的幅度或起搏后 QRS 波群变窄程度迄今还不能成功地预测治疗效果）。近来研究显示，CRT 对有慢性房颤的心衰病人情况的改善可与正常窦律的 CHF 病人相媲美[20]。正在评估其他定量测量左室非同步情况的方法，包括超声心动图和其他影像学方法，以筛选双室起搏能为其带来最佳血流动力学效应的病人[21,22]。其中一组是进行右室起搏的假性左束支阻滞病人，但研究资料尚不充分。

可以预期，将来 CRT 技术的改进将有助于提供更多的关于最佳房室间期[23]、心房起搏与自身房室传导对比以及左室最有效的起搏部位等特异性信息[24]，甚至还包括减少因心房超感知造成的不恰当电击治疗。

六、心房颤动

在美国，房颤是临床最常见的持续性心律失常，患病的人数超过 200 万。房颤的发生频率随着年龄增加而增加，据估计超过 4% 的 60 岁以上老年人患房颤。虽然一些病人对房颤有很好的耐受性，但房颤与卒中、心力衰竭的住院和死亡风险性增加相关[26]。房颤的基础治疗包括抗凝、心率控制（联合应用 β 受体阻滞剂、洋地黄、钙拮抗剂）以及抗心律失常药控制心律（维持窦性心律）。不幸的是，药物治疗会产生耐药性、毒性反应，而且复发率高，使得人们对其他替代治疗方法产生兴趣。而且，近来房颤节律控制随访研究（AFFIRM）显示最初用抗心律失常药物控制节律的治疗策略不能降低死亡率。

有持续性或慢性房颤伴缓慢心室率的病人应植入永久起搏器。有证据表明在这些人群中永久起搏治疗可以预防房颤，可能的机理包括有效地协调心房活动，降低心房压并因此而降低心房扩张程度，降低心房不应期的离散度，避免具有潜在致心律失常作用的心脏停搏和抑制异位心房搏动[28]。几个大型随机临床试验证明，永久起搏，特别是双腔起搏，可减少窦房结功能低下病人心房颤动的发生率[29-31]。与双腔起搏相比，单纯心房起搏使这些病人获益最大。

对于没有窦房结功能低下的病人，用起搏器预防房颤是否有效尚不清楚，正处于积极研究中。有人建议，采用比窦率稍快的频率进行永久起搏可能有助于预防房颤发作，机理包括抑制异位心房活动，降低心房不应期的离散度，尤其是在房性早搏之后[32]。目前，已应用多种算法确保持续心房起搏。一个有前景的方法是动态心房超速起搏，该方法可以持续监测窦房结的自主心率，并用稍快的心率持续起搏心房。其可以减少病人发生有症状房颤的天数。还需要解决的其他问题包括起搏对房颤复发、致死率、慢性充血性心力衰竭发生率和血栓栓塞事件的作用。

另一种方法是在不同部位起搏心房。有病变的心房经常有散在的瘢痕组织，从而干扰激动从右房向左房的传播。在室间隔、冠状窦或房间束（Bachmann束）部位起搏时冲动可同时传向左右房，缩短了P波时限，可能会降低房颤的发生率[33,34]。

心房双部位起搏提供了另一个或许更有效的心房收缩同步化方法。双部位起搏常常指同时起搏右心耳和冠状窦。虽然仍然存在一些问题，包括需要放置两个心房导线、自身窦性节律的双感知以及其他问题等，但初步的结果仍令人振奋[35]。随后进行的大型随机临床研究提示，仅少数病人能从此方法中获益。这项技术特别适合的人群是接受冠状动脉搭桥手术的病人，因为其房颤发生率高达40%[36]。而且，在手术中可直接将电极放在左心房，这种方法比冠状窦起搏更有效。尽管受心外膜导线寿命限制，但其初步结论令人振奋。

七、肥厚型心肌病

肥厚型心肌病以心肌纤维与肌丝排列紊乱为特征，并引起过度的、不适当的左室肥厚，以室间隔为常见。肥厚心肌影响心室舒张，在超过25%的病人会导致动力性左室流出道梗阻。造成心室容量下降、心肌收缩力增加和影响心室舒张的因素都会造成临床表现恶化。典型症状包括：胸部不适（可能与心肌肥厚造成的血流相对减少、心肌缺血有关）、肺淤血、晕厥，甚至心源性猝死，后者常由室颤引起。

有症状的肥厚型心肌病病人的初始治疗一般是药物治疗，包括β受体阻滞剂、非二氢吡啶类钙通道阻滞剂或丙吡胺。病人如有持续性或特别严重的症状可行外科心肌切开术或心肌切除术，有时需同时进行二尖瓣置换。作为替代疗法，室间隔化学消融也可采用，通常直接将无水乙醇注入冠状动脉左前降支的一个室间隔支中。虽然手术和化学消融方法对药物抵抗的病人相对有效，但也有较高的并发症和一定的致死率。有过室颤而存活的肥厚型心肌病病人常需植入自动转复除颤器。

永久起搏器治疗肥厚型心肌病的方法源于观察到右室心尖部起搏造成了心室运动不协调、室间隔矛盾运动和随后的心室扩张，使跨左室流出道压力梯度降低（本质上，这种状况下起搏治疗的效果与扩张型心肌病病人起搏的治疗作用刚好相反）。

一些早期的病例报告和小规模无对照的系列研究提示起搏治疗使血流动力学改善，特别是采用非常短AV间期的双腔起搏，使肥厚部位的室间隔提前激动。在一个来源于国家心肺血研究所的大型无对照组的梗阻型心肌病病人群中，Fananapazir和同事[39]报道短AV间期双腔起搏戏剧性改善病人临床症状。重要的是他们发现了左室肥厚局部消退的证据，提示起搏与心肌重构相关。这一观点在他们的进一步观察中得到证实，即起搏停止后很长时间临床症状仍然持续改善。

这些有希望的观察结果促使了有对照的临床试验的进行（表110-2）。Nishimura和同事[40]在19例肥厚型心肌病病人的双盲交叉研究中报道，与AAI（安慰剂组）起搏比较，双室起搏降低左室流出道压力阶差，但临床症状改善不明显。在肥厚型心肌病起搏器治疗研究（PIC）中[41]，双腔起搏改善了83例耐药的肥厚型心肌病患者的生活质量和运动耐量，尽管在临床症状改善和基础状态下的压力阶差没有关联。在对48例人群中进行的研究（M-PATHY研究）发现[42]，虽然左室流出道压力阶差明显降低，但临床上主观和客观症状改善不明显。Linde和同事报道的永久起搏器明显的安慰剂作用对这些表面上的矛盾现象作出了解释[43]。

总之，已经证实永久起搏器可以降低肥厚型心肌病患者左室流出道压力阶差，但这个结果与临床症状的改善之间缺乏必然的联系。虽然初步研究结果令人振奋，但起搏的益处很难进行客观验证。此外，永久起搏治疗不能改善生存率，虽然到目前为止已进行的研究可能在例数上尚不足以检测出死亡率的差别。现在，植入永久起搏器应该作为肥厚型心肌病的辅助治疗手段，主要用于标准治疗不能改善病情的有症状患者。酒精消融治疗是可选择的非药物治疗方式。

八、神经心源性晕厥

晕厥是一个常见的问题，在美国占每年入院患者的比例大约6%。虽然改进了诊断技术，但原因不明的晕厥仍占全部晕厥病例的50%。其中许多病例可能是神经介导的。名词神经心源性晕厥（也称血管迷走性晕厥或神经介导性晕厥）常被用来描述一组相关的

表 110-2 肥厚型心肌病永久起搏治疗的主要临床试验

研 究	人群及设计	结 果
Fananapazir[39]	开放式、无对照的研究 84 例药物治疗效果不好的肥厚型梗阻性心肌病（静息或激发试验下的压力阶差）	平均随访 2.3 年，90% 病人运动耐量和生活质量改善，左室肥厚消退，并持续到停止起搏以后
Nishimura[40]	随机、双盲、交叉研究，安慰起搏，每一种模式 3 个月，19 例肥厚型梗阻性心肌病病人	压力阶差显著降低，在起搏组和对照组症状分别改善 63% 和 42%，运动耐量没有明显的客观改善
起搏治疗肥厚型心肌病的多中心研究 (M-PATHY)[42]	随机、双盲、交叉研究，安慰起搏，每一种模式 3 个月，48 例药效不好的肥厚型心肌病病人，压力阶差 > 49mmHg	压力阶差显著降低，但心血管功能没有明显的客观改善
心肌病起搏治疗（PIC）[41]	随机、双盲、交叉研究，安慰起搏，81 例药效不好的肥厚型梗阻性心肌病病人	压力阶差降低和症状改善没有明显关系，甚至安慰起搏也能降低压力阶差

情况，包括颈动脉窦高敏、咳嗽性晕厥、排尿性晕厥等。其确切的机理尚未完全阐明，但这些病理状态似乎均具有共同的特点：自主神经系统的过度反应，最初是交感神经的激活，以后随着交感神经激活的消退而出现迷走神经张力增高。许多健康人在一生中作为对特别强刺激（经常包括中枢神经系统）如剧痛、惊恐和生气等反应可能出现晕厥或先兆晕厥。神经心源性晕厥适用于没有明显诱因的复发性晕厥。

直立倾斜试验的出现为评价神经心源性晕厥病人提供了重要的诊断工具。直立倾斜试验阳性包括两种情况：血管抑制反应（最初的事件是血管扩张，引起症状性低血压）和心脏抑制反应（主要表现为症状性心动过缓或心脏停搏）。常见的情况是，这种反应是两种类型的结合（复合反应），难以决定低血压和心动过缓哪个是始动因子。

虽然神经心源性晕厥的首要治疗方法一般是药物治疗，但人们对永久起搏器寄予很大希望，特别是心动过缓是主要症状之一时。早期使用单-双腔起搏器的研究结果是令人失望的。最近，起搏器"频率骤降反应"功能的出现重新唤起了人们对永久起搏器的兴趣，该功能可在心率突然下降时启动相对短暂（1～2min）的快速起搏（100～120ppm）。北美迷走性晕厥起搏器研究（VPS）显示，使用心率骤降功能可使晕厥发作事件下降 85%[44]。虽然试验是随机的，但设计是开放的，因此起搏器的安慰剂作用会使结论出现偏倚。欧洲神经心源性晕厥研究（VASIS）报道显示与此相似的晕厥发生率明显下降，但也存在相似的设计缺陷[45]。北美血管迷走性晕厥起搏器研究 II（VPS-II）的设计克服了这一问题，该研究设置了有安慰性起搏的对照组（DDD 起搏频率设置在 45ppm，同时关闭频率骤降功能），从而达到双盲研究设计。两组之间晕厥的发生率没有明显差异。

总之，虽然早期的临床研究结果令人鼓舞，但起搏用于防止神经心源性晕厥的有效程度还没有得到证实。

九、长 QT 综合征

长 QT 综合征可由不同的病因引起，其共同特点是 QT 间期延长，可发展成特殊类型的多形性室性心动过速（尖端扭转型室速）和心源性猝死。这种病人的先天异常与特定基因的染色体异常相关，获得性长 QT 综合征常常因使用能延长 QT 间期的药物引起（如奎尼丁、三环类抗抑郁药等），而且这些药物的数目还在增加。也可能先天与后天长 QT 综合征其实是一个连续的整体，只是有些人在基础状态下出现异常，而另外一些需要激发因子才能诱发 QT 间期延长。在此综合征中室性心律失常的发病机理尚未完全阐明，但似乎与交感神经激活和早后除极有关。

长 QT 综合征的治疗通常是首先选择药物治疗（β 受体阻滞剂），也可以建议采用左星状神经节切除和永久心脏起搏治疗。有效的起搏治疗的机制尚不清楚，但可能与以下原因有关：防止尖端扭转型室速发生前的特征性的心脏长间歇，消除早后除极和降低不应期离散度。现在 ICD 常规用于已证明有心脏骤停、持续性室性心动过速、β 受体阻滞剂治疗无效的复发性晕厥的长 QT 综合征患者。

十、总 结

随着技术进步，永久起搏器的适应证无疑也会不断增加。本章介绍了永久起搏器的 4 个新应用，但其基本的作用仍是改善血流动力学或抑制心律失常，或两者都有。虽然在特定的人群中起搏器的有效性已得到证实（如双腔起搏用于防止有潜在窦房结功能低下病人的房颤，双室起搏用于有严重左室收缩功能障碍和左束支阻滞的病人），但是多数情况下，治疗结果仍然是不确定的或非结论性的。如果将起搏治疗与近来出现的其他新技术相结合，如 ICD、持续体内药物泵入、射频消融治疗和其他技术等，可能具有更大的应用价值，其潜在的应用领域也将继续扩大。

（王 斌 译）

参 考 文 献

1. Gold MR, Feliciano Z, Gottlieb SS, et al: Dual-chamber pacing with a short atrioventricular delay in congestive heart failure: A randomized study. J Am Coll Cardiol 26:967–973, 1995.
2. Linde C, Gadler F, Edner M: Results of atrioventricular synchronous pacing with severe congestive heart failure. Am J Cardiol 75:919–923, 1995.
3. The DAVID Trial Investigators: Dual-chamber pacing or ventricular backup pacing in patients with an implantable defibrillator: The Dual Chamber and VVI Implantable Defibrillator (DAVID) Trial. JAMA 288:3115–3123, 2002.
4. Rosenqvist M, Isaaz K, Botvinick EH, et al: Relative importance of activation sequence compared to atrioventricular synchrony in left ventricular function. Am J Cardiol 67:148–156, 1991.
5. Sweeney M, Hellkamp A, Greenspon A, et al: Baseline QRS duration > 120 milliseconds and cumulative percent time ventricular paced predicts increased risk of heart failure, stroke, and death in DDDR-paced patients with sick sinus syndrome in MOST [abstract]. Pacing Clin Electrophysiol 25:690, 2002.
6. Victor F, Leclerq C, Mabo P, et al: Optimal right ventricular pacing site in chronically implanted patients: A prospective randomized cross-over comparison of apical and outflow tract pacing. J Am Coll Cardiol 33:311–316, 1999.
7. Tse HF, Lau CP: Long-term effect of right ventricular pacing on myocardial perfusion and function. J Am Coll Cardiol 15:744–749, 1997.
8. Grines CL, Bashore TM, Boudoulas H, et al: Functional abnormalities in isolated left bundle branch block: The effect of interventricular synchrony. Circulation 79:845–853, 1989.
9. Aaronson KD, Schwartz JS, Chen TM, et al: Development and prospective validation of a clinical index to predict survival in ambulatory patients referred for cardiac transplant evaluation. Circulation 95:2660–2667, 1997.
10. Shamin W, Francis DP, Yousufuddin M, et al: Intraventricular conduction delay: A prognostic marker in chronic heart failure. Int J Cardiol 70:171–178, 1999.
11. Blanc JJ, Etienne Y, Gilard M, et al: Evaluation of different ventricular pacing sites in patients with severe congestive heart failure: Results of an acute hemodynamic study. Circulation 96:3273–3277, 1997.
12. Kass DA, Chen CH, Curry C, et al: Improved left ventricular mechanics from acute VDD pacing in patients with dilated cardiomyopathy and ventricular conduction delay. Circulation 99:1567–1573, 1999.
13. Auricchio A, Stellbrink C, Block M, et al: Effect of pacing chamber and atrioventricular delay on acute systolic function of paced patients with congestive heart failure. The Pacing Therapies for Congestive Heart Failure Study Group. Circulation 99:2993–3001, 1999.
14. Nelson GS, Berger RD, Fetics BJ, et al: Left ventricular or biventricular pacing improves cardiac function at diminished energy costs in patients with dilated cardiomyopathy and left bundle branch block. Circulation 102:3053–3059, 2000.
15. Cazeau S, Leclercq C, Lavergne T, et al: Effects of multisite biventricular pacing in patients with heart failure and intraventricular conduction delay. N Engl J Med 344:873–880, 2001.
16. Linde C, Leclercq C, Rex S, et al: Long-term benefits of biventricular pacing in congestive heart failure: Results from the Multisite Stimulation in Cardiomyopathy study. J Am Coll Cardiol 40:111–118 2002.
17. Auricchio A, Stellbrink C, Sack S, et al: Long-term clinical effect of hemodynamically optimized cardiac resynchronization therapy in patients with heart failure and ventricular conduction delay. J Am Coll Cardiol 39:2026–2033, 2002.
18. Abraham WT, Fisher WG, Smith AL, et al: Cardiac resynchronization in chronic heart failure. N Engl J Med 346:1845–1853, 2002.
19. Kuhlkamp V: Initial experience with an implantable cardioverter-defibrillator incorporating cardiac resynchronization therapy. J Am Coll Cardiol 39:790–797 2002.
20. Leon AR, Greenberg JM, Kanuru N, et al: Cardiac resynchronization in patients with congestive heart failure and chronic atrial fibrillation. J Am Coll Cardiol 39:1258–1263, 2002.
21. Aranda JM, Schofield RS, Leach D, et al: Ventricular dyssynchrony in dilated cardiomyopathy: The role of biventricular pacing in the treatment of congestive heart failure. Clin Cardiol 25:357–362, 2002.
22. Breithardt OA, Stellbrink C, Kramer AP, et al: Echocardiographic quantification of left ventricular asynchrony predicts an acute hemodynamic benefit of cardiac resynchronization therapy. J Am Coll Cardiol 40:536–545, 2002.
23. Stellbrink C, Breithardt OA, Franke A, et al: Impact of cardiac resynchronization therapy using hemodynamically optimized pacing on left ventricular remodeling in patients with congestive heart failure and ventricular conduction disturbances. J Am Coll Cardiol 38:1957–1965, 2001.
24. Butter C, Auricchio A, Stelbrink C, et al: Effect of resynchronization therapy stimulation site on the systolic function of heart failure patients. Circulation 104:3026–3029, 2001.
25. Roelke M: Atrial oversensing in biventricular devices: Shocked? (or inhibited?). Pacing Clin Electrophysiol 25:1411–1412, 2002.
26. Benjamin EJ, Wolf PA, D'Agostino RB, et al: Impact of atrial fibrillation on the risk of death: The Framingham Heart study. Circulation 98:946–952, 1998.
27. Wyse DG, Waldo AL, DiMarco MJ, et al, for the Atrial fibrillation Follow-Up Investigation of Rhythm Management (AFFIRM) Investigators: A comparison of rate control and rhythm control in patients with atrial fibrillation. N Engl J Med 347:1825–1833, 2002.
28. Cooper JM, Katcher MS, Orlov MV: Implantable devices for the treatment of atrial fibrillation. N Engl J Med 346:2062–2068, 2002.
29. Connolly SJ, Kerr C, Gent M, et al: Comparison of the effects of physiologic pacing versus ventricular pacing versus ventricular pacing on cardiovascular death and stroke. N Engl J Med 342:1385–1391, 2000.
30. Skanes AC, Krahn AD, Yee R, et al: Progression to chronic atrial fibrillation after pacing. J Am Coll Cardiol 38:167–172, 2001.
31. Lamas GA, Orav J, Stambler BS, et al: Quality of life and clinical outcomes in elderly patients treated with ventricular pacing as compared with dual-chamber pacing. N Engl J Med 338:1097–1104, 1998.
32. Garrigue S, Barold SS, Cazeau S, et al: Prevention of atrial arrhythmias during DDD pacing by atrial overdrive. Pacing Clin Electrophysiol 21:1751–1759, 1998.
33. Bailin SJ, Adler S, Giudici M, et al: Prevention of chronic atrial fibrillation by pacing in the region of Bachmann's bundle: Results of a multicenter randomized trial. J Cardiovasc Electrophysiol 12:912–917, 2001.
34. Padeletti L, Pieragnoli P, Ciapetti C, et al: Randomized crossover comparison of right atrial appendage pacing versus interatrial septum pacing for prevention of atrial fibrillation in patients with sinus bradycardia. Am Heart J 142:1047–1055, 2001.
35. Saksena S, Prakash A, Hill M, et al: Prevention of recurrent atrial fibrillation with chronic dual-site right atrial pacing. J Am Coll Cardiol 28:687–694, 1996.
36. Daubert JC, Mabo P: Atrial pacing for the prevention of postoperative atrial fibrillation: How and where to pace. J Am Coll Cardiol 35:1423–1427, 2000.
37. Daoud E, Dabir R, Achambeau M, et al: Randomized, double-blind trial of simultaneous right and left atrial epicardial pacing for prevention of post-open heart surgery atrial fibrillation. Circulation 102:761–765, 2000.

38. Crystal E, Connolly SJ, Sleik K, et al: Interventions of prevention of postoperative atrial fibrillation in patients undergoing heart surgery: A meta-analysis. Circulation 106:75-80, 2002.
39. Fananapazir L, Epstein ND, Curiel RV, et al: Long-term results of dual-chamber (DDD) pacing in obstructive cardiomyopathy: Evidence for progressive symptomatic and hemodynamic improvement and reduction of left ventricular hypertrophy. Circulation 90:2731-2742, 1994.
40. Nishimura RA, Trusty JM, Hayes DL, et al: Dual-chamber pacing for hypertrophic cardiomyopathy: A randomized double-blind crossover study. J Am Coll Cardiol 29:435-441, 1997.
41. Kappenberger L, Linde C, Daubert C, et al: Pacing in hypertrophic cardiomyopathy: A randomized crossover study: PIC Study Group. Eur Heart J 18:1249-1256, 1997.
42. Maron BJ, Nishimura RA, McKenna WJ, et al: Assessment of permanent dual-chamber pacing as a treatment for drug-refractory symptomatic patients with obstructive hypertrophic cardiomyopathy: A randomized, double-blind, crossover study (M-PATHY). Circulation 99:2927-2933, 1999.
43. Linde C, Gadler F, Kappenberger L, et al: Placebo effect of pacemaker implantation in obstructive hypertrophic cardiomyopathy. Am J Cardiol 83:903-907, 1999.
44. Connolly SJ, Sheldon R, Roberts RS, et al: The North American Vasovagal Pacemaker Study (VPS): A randomized trial of permanent cardiac pacing for the prevention of vasovagal syncope. J Am Coll Cardiol 33:16-20, 1999.
45. Sutton R, Brignole M, Menozzi C, et al: Dual-chamber pacing in the treatment of neurally mediated tilt-positive cardioinhibitory syncope: Pacemaker versus no therapy: A multicenter randomized study. Circulation 102:294-299, 2000.
46. Connolly SJ, Sheldon R, Thorpe KE, et al: Pacemaker therapy for prevention of syncope in patients with recurrent severe vasovagal syncope: Second vasovagal pacemaker study (VPS II): A randomized trial. JAMA 289:2224-2229, 2003.

第111章

射频导管消融术中损伤形成的生物物理学及病理生理学基础

David E. Haines

本章目录

- 心脏射频加热的生物物理学 ………… 995
- 射频能量介导心肌损伤的机制 ………… 997
- 射频消融的组织效应 ………… 998
- 射频消融的细胞学效应 ………… 1000
- 总结 ………… 1002

消融的基本原理是，对于每一种心律失常来说，这种心律失常在临床上得以维持必须有一个异常冲动形成和传导的关键解剖部位，如果这一基质受到不可逆的改变或毁损，那么心律失常就不再自然发生或是被诱发。若通过导管达到此目的，则必须满足几个条件。这项技术需要产生边界清楚的局部损伤，需要控制损伤范围的大小，既要包含靶点，即：关键解剖部位，又要对邻近组织的损伤最小，并且这项技术能够常规在电生理室配备和使用。尽管对于多种不同的导管消融技术有相当多的经验及实践，但使用射频（RF）电能的消融技术脱颖而出并备受偏爱。对于射频能量加热以及组织对损伤反应机制的研究有助于帮助我们认识这样那样的现象，并且可使手术操作者优化手术操作结果。

本章的目的是回顾心脏射频导管消融术的生物物理学特性，回顾相关的重点以及释放的能量、系统阻抗、电极的几何形状、导管的接触压力、电极-组织界面的温度、微循环的对流冷却、循环血液、电极头端的灌注之间的相互关系。电流及高热对心肌细胞及心肌组织的病理生理学效应将在本章的第二部分讨论。通过这些资料可完整构建出一个关于患者的射频导管消融损伤的框架。

一、心脏射频加热的生物物理学

当电流通过导电介质时，在介质中会有电阻损耗，这样当射频电流经过组织时就以热能的形式消散了。加热能量的大小与组织中功率密度成正比[1]，与辐射半径的四次方成反比[2]。由于电介质阻抗加热的物理学特征，直接阻抗组织加热或是体积加热的深度是很小的（大多数情况下小于2mm），所有发生在较深层水平组织的加热都是热量传导的结果。用于心脏射频消融的射频电流频率一般在300～1000kHz之间。任何一种低频的交流电以及直流电，对于任何一个组织会产生一个相似程度的加热，但是较低的频率会使骨骼肌及心肌产生兴奋激动。相反，高频电流的射频消融一般是无痛的而且很少会诱发快速的多形性心律失常，但这种心律失常在60Hz频率的低频电流下常常可以看到。频率超过1000kHz（1MHz）对于组织产生加热是有效的，但是随着频率的提高沿着传导线的能量损失也增加，而且热能的形式也由阻抗加热变为介质加热。因此，为了便于临床应用安全及患者舒适，300～1000kHz之间的频率是理想的。

射频电流通常以单极形式从电极导管的顶端电极释放到放置于患者皮肤上的无关电极上。因为射频电流是交流电，所以从电极到发生器之间的线路连接的极性并不重要。标准消融电极的表面积（大约12mm²）明显小于无关电极的表面积（100～250cm²），因而在电极-组织接触点的功率密度和造成的组织加热是巨大的，而无关电极的皮肤表面接触点却没有任何能量产生。无关电极可以放置在任何方便部位的皮肤表面，因为无论无关电极位置如何，能量在距离消融电极的 2~3mm 范围内的分布是相当一致的。无关电极的位置与消融电极直接相对可增加射频加热的功效，并且可造成稍大一点的损伤[3]，但这一理论上的优势从未被临床证实。当射频发生器的功率输出是损伤形成的制约因素时，一个较大表面积的无关电极放置于患者胸部可以降低系统阻抗，从而增加射频能量释放的功效[4]。

用于开胸线性心房消融的双极消融系统用另一种形式释放射频能量。两个线性电极被安装在一个钳夹样装置上，当钳夹合拢时，心房组织被压缩在钳夹装置中，射频能量在电极间以双极形式释放使组织干燥及消融。最初的电流强度分布是不均匀的，随着夹闭组织的部分变干，电传导下降，射频电流被分流向那些未消融的组织。以这种形式，射频过程将继续，直至整个消融线全长的电传导下降到一个阈值水平，消融才完成[5]。虽然这套装置系统在某些方面比单极消融优越，但它目前需要经过外科途径，不适合于导管为基础的消融途径。一个独特的射频能量释放方式是通过为线性消融而设计的多极电极导管来完成的，射频电流可以以任意一个单极形式从全部的电极释放到皮肤上的无关电极，或以双极形式在任意两个电极间释放。因为射频电流是以连续正弦波形式传导的，所以，单极和双极能量传导形式的混合可以通过在相邻电极间转换射频波形的相位来完成，射频能量从导管到皮肤以单极的形式传导，但是邻近电极之间的相位不同也可以使电流以双极形式传导[6]。如果电极与组织间的接触良好，就可以改善线性消融过程中损伤的连续性。

虽然所有射频电流传导的电学参数已经用于监控射频导管消融[1]，但由电能转换为组织热的功效变化非常大，因此，在射频导管消融过程中应该持续监测组织温度。组织内热能传导的动力学已经被制成模型，考虑到了所有的因素，比如新陈代谢的热产物、组织灌注的冷却对流和通过组织的热传导等。传统射频消融术的体积加热的深度很小（小于 2mm），多数对于深部组织产生的组织加热都是热能传导的结果，所以，可以认为射频电极产生的热量与从一个纯粹的热源产生的传导热相同。为了射频导管消融术的目的，即：热量暴露的持续时间短暂，温度相对较高，在体外试验中，一个简单的在均一介质中热能传导的分析模型准确地描述了稳态环境[2]。在这个模型中，组织温度的降低与热源的距离成反比，这一模型还预测当功率调整到能在电极-组织接触面维持一个恒定的温度时，损伤的大小在一定程度上应该与这一温度呈线性正比关系，也和电极的半径呈这一关系。由于这一简单的模型假定的是相同的电和热的传导率以及稳态的环境，所以它在体内射频消融术中的应用受到限制。特别是，电极几何形状的改变和来自循环血流的对流冷却的变化改变了由这一模型得出的预测值。

热力学模型预测，温度越高、电极的尺寸越大则会产生更大的射频损伤。因为更大的损伤面积包含心律失常传导的关键解剖部位的可能性就越大，所以会提高手术操作的有效性。这种电极-组织接触面温度与手术操作的有效性的关系已经被临床证实[8]，同样消融导管顶端电极越大，射频导管消融的有效性也就越大[9]。非常重要的是，增加电极表面积需要相应地增加射频功率，以便射频能量强度持续恒定。如果相对于已有的射频功率来说，电极的尺寸太大，那么能量强度会减低，结果是损伤的区域面积不会增加，甚至会缩小[10]。理论上，在电极-组织接触面上很高的温度应该会造成非常大的损伤，而实际上，在高温情况下电传导率下降时，这一结果是有限的[11]。当电极-组织接触面温度达到或超过 100℃ 时，电极表面的血浆沸腾，凝固的血浆和干燥的组织在传导面形成一个绝缘的薄膜[11]，有效的电极表面积随之减少，导致电流强度的增加，更多的组织加热，更多的"凝固物"形成，从而最终释放能量减少。单一的温度传感器会经常低估电极-组织接触面温度的峰值，这通常发生在远离电极顶端传感器的电极基底部[12]。由于这个原因，电极顶端的温度峰值应该被限定在 70℃ 或 80℃ 之内以避免超过 100℃ 的温度峰值。

一些减少组织加热的因素，比如循环血液的对流作用可使热量丧失，如果消融的能量受到限制会导致损伤面积的缩小。射频消融损伤在心内膜表面的损伤直径通常要小于在心内膜下的损伤，这是因为在心内膜表面的对流作用使热量丧失的效果。如果导管的位置不稳定，组织接触压低，或是导管位于血流速度较快的部位，那么，对流冷却的作用将会非常大，而损伤就会缩小[13,14]。然而，如果有足够的能量传输到电极顶端，对流冷却作用反而可以造成较大的损伤面积。当导管顶端在心内膜表面被冷却时，可以传输非常高的能量，而没有凝固物形成和电阻抗突然增加的危险。当非常高的能量释放时，直接加热体积的深度和直径增加，因此增加了消融损伤的大小（图 111-1）。高能量及导管顶端对流冷却的射频消融可以产生深度大于 10mm 的损伤。可以通过导管顶端及心内膜之间的滑动，或是通过冷盐水循环或灌注冷却电极顶端以达到导管顶端的对流冷却的目的[15,16]。大的射频消融电极除了提供更大的电极-组织接触面积外，还增大了循环血流冷却电极顶端的表面积，从而增加了损伤范围[10]。虽然顶端冷却增大了损伤范围，但却丧失了监控损伤形成区域的能力，应用大的电极导管或是盐水灌注导管，电极顶端的对流冷却作用影响了电极顶端温度的测量。在这种情况下，测量损伤范围不能依靠温度测量，最好用调节输出功率的办法逐渐增加损伤范围[10]。由于主动或被动冷却的最高组织温度发生在心内膜表面以下，有可能心内膜下的组织温度已经非常高而导管顶端的温度感受器测量到的温度是低的。最坏的情况是，心内膜下组织温度超过100℃，造成快速的蒸汽膨胀及凹痕形成，常可听到"嘭"的一声。这种爆裂损伤可以造成血栓形成，引起像心房样的薄壁结构破裂，但是应用这种技术达到增加损伤的深度和宽度的目的，可能在消融难治性的心律失常基质时有用，比如折返性的室性心动过速的基质。

电极-组织接触面的心肌加热速度非常快，而热量向深部组织层传导却相对缓慢。一项射频导管消融使心肌损伤形成的研究报道，在体外应用一个很小顶端的电极消融时，损伤形成一半的时间是8s，只有消融40s以后才能达到稳定的损伤范围[13]。在一项应用传统导管的体内研究中，在距消融电极3mm处，心肌内温度在10、20、30s时分别增加为60s时最终消融温度的32%、48%、和63%[17]。热力学模型提示，损伤形成在第一个20s速度最快，在恒定温度消融100s时达到稳定状态[3]。因此如果操作者想要达到一个稳定的状态，射频能量释放应至少持续60s，如果希望达到最大的损伤范围应持续120s。热能从表面向深层的传导有温度和时间依赖性。如果在短暂的射频脉冲释放之后，心内膜的表层达到高温，即使射频能量停止释放，深层心肌的组织温度还会持续增加[18]。这种热量的延迟现象在临床射频消融中具有很重要的意义，即：即使迅速停止能量的释放，还可能会产生一些不希望发生的作用（如：房室结传导阻滞）。

为了优化射频导管消融的结果，操作者必须有很高的技术水平和对心律失常的基质有透彻了解，这样导管才能到位准确而且位置稳定。应该使用顶端大的电极导管，能量应该调整到电极-组织接触面的温度至少达到70℃但不超过85℃的水平，这样阻抗增加的危险性才最小。如果能量释放至少60s和电极-组织接触很好，就会达到最好的损伤结果，即使电极与组织滑行接触，有高能量射频输出，也会形成有意义的损伤。重要的是，技术和工艺增加了组织加热和损伤范围，提高了射频消融手术的有效性，但是不能避免不良结果，游离壁穿孔、冠状动脉损伤、肺静脉狭窄等并发症会随着组织加热的增加而增加。虽然这些并发症发生的危险性很小，但是的确存在，所以应该与损伤加深带来的潜在益处相权衡。

二、射频能量介导心肌损伤的机制

假定射频导管消融造成心肌损伤的机制是热量介导的。除了电能转换成热能以外，电活动的震荡也可能对心肌细胞产生某些直接的作用，特别是对肌纤维膜。虽然在导管消融损伤的中央区域主要是组织的热凝固物，但是热能及电能损伤对损伤的边缘区域的影响尚未可知。

肿瘤学的高温治疗对不同组织的热能损伤时间和温度的关系做了详细的研究。对于持续20min、温度大于45℃的高热，多数细胞易受损伤。较低的温度需要较长的暴露时间而且细胞死亡的比率较低，并依赖于组织的热敏感性。在体外的心肌射频和微波导管消融术，对损伤的边缘区域不可逆组织损伤的温度（组织损伤的等温线）做了研究。尽管消融时间在1~10min之间变化，但是测量的重复性好的等温线位于52~55℃之间[19]。如前面章节所述，在导管消融试验中损伤的范围与电极-组织接触面的温度有关[2]。在临床射频导管消融术中，达到有意义的组织加热，消融中测量的组织温度的最大值与临床结果相关[8]。

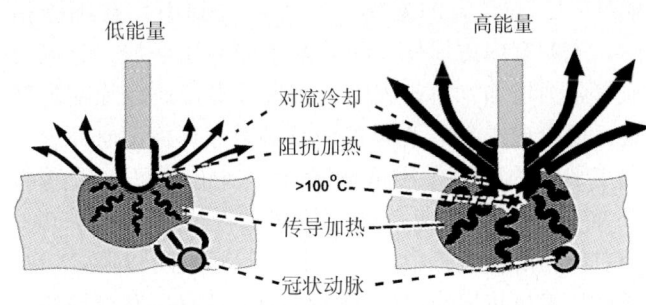

图111-1 射频导管消融过程中直接阻抗加热（容积加热）和传导加热的分布示意图 左侧：对流冷却较小，低能量输出就能达到预期的电极-组织接触面温度，阻抗加热的深度小（小于2mm），损伤的大小有限。右侧：对流冷却较大，高能量输出可能达不到预期的电极-组织接触面温度，然而，阻抗加热的深度大（大于3mm），损伤的范围也大。遗憾的是，心内膜下温度超过100℃，会造成突然气体膨胀和凹痕形成，而且透壁的心肌加热可潜在增加冠状动脉损伤的危险。

在一项患者接受房室交界区消融的研究中，在51±4℃观察到出现加速性的交界区心律而没有房室阻滞，而在58±6℃时则可以看到房室阻滞。因此，在较低温度时可以观察到高热的生理学效应，但是要造成不可逆的组织损伤则需要较高的温度[20]。

尽管一些证据支持高热是射频导管消融时不可逆心肌损伤的机制，但还是应该考虑直接电损伤对于细胞死亡的作用。对细胞膜进行电刺激可以引起电介质破坏和细胞除极。但是在没有组织加热时，评价射频电场的生理学效应面临技术问题而且从未被研究过。在射频导管消融过程中电损伤对热能损伤的作用还需要进一步研究。下面的章节将回顾一些关于高热和电流对不同组织和离体标本的病理生理学效应的资料。通过这些资料，可构建一个关于心脏射频导管消融的病理生理学理论框架。

三、射频消融的组织效应

（一）射频导管消融损伤的病理学

当射频能量释放到体外的离体灌注或是新鲜的组织时，组织会立即明显变色。组织苍白变色标志着肌细胞蛋白的变性，主要是肌红蛋白，是红色素脱失的结果。虽然在体外或体内射频介导损伤的总体表现是损伤后立即会呈现这种大体上的表现，但它会低估实际的损伤范围，因为边界组织变色的等温线大约是60℃，而在50℃时细胞就产生了显著的生理学变化（见后文）。体内心内膜表面的急性损伤通常是灰白色的，表面覆盖薄层的纤维素膜，有时会有附壁血栓，当射频能量传导过程中电阻抗突然升高和温度升高超过100℃时，这种情况非常常见，组织的表面会被明显烧焦[11]，在与导管接触的心内膜表面可观察到损伤的核心部位体积减少而表现为小小的凹陷。

由于心内膜表面的对流冷却减少了有效的加热和浅表组织坏死，所以在横断面上，损伤通常是泪滴状的。损伤的中心是灰白色的，损伤的边缘有时候会出血。在体内射频消融的数小时内可观察到急性的组织学改变，包括在损伤中心区域早期典型的凝固坏死、细胞核固缩及提示细胞内钙超载的嗜碱性点染。在细胞结构明显破坏的区域之外是一条过渡区域带，有出血及单核炎性细胞浸润的表现（图111-2）[1,20]，可以观察到急性组织水肿，在体内用心腔内超声心动图检查可以观察到很明显的室壁增厚及组织异常回声[21]。

在导管消融后的4~5天，损伤中心区域呈明显凝固坏死及早期脂肪变性的表现。过渡区域消失，存活及坏死组织之间有明显的界限[1,20]。在临床射频消融成功后，射频能量释放停止的数分钟后或是数周之后，心律失常基质的功能有可能再次恢复[22]。推测消融后有炎症的过渡区域可能是电生理功能晚期恢复的原因（即有少量坏死组织的过渡区域炎症消退）。相反，已观察到在临床明显不成功的导管消融术后数小时，心律失常也可以永久性地消失[23]。同样，炎症也可以引起迟发的电生理效应（即在炎症区域坏死的进展）。

射频导管消融的慢性病理学与其他类型的损伤修复相似。第一周发生脂肪变性，损伤完全被纤维化代替需要8周时间[24]。慢性损伤表现为明显的收缩和体积减少。损伤的边缘区域边界清楚，没有任何片状坏死及损伤区域岛状心肌存活的表现。导管消融术后晚期心律失常复发很少可能是因为损伤都有相同的性质。

（二）射频导管消融术与冠脉血流

射频电流在没有高热时对微血管灌注的影响还不清楚。但是，微循环对高热产生反应时的变化已有大量的研究。目前的很多资料来源于对实体肿瘤血液循环的研究，一小部分来源于心肌微灌注术。在所有组织中微循环的损伤都有时间和温度依赖性。大鼠的骨骼肌暴露在45℃的温度，持续20min时，立刻观察到水肿、充血和出血，经过48小时，进展为血管内皮和实质组织的损伤[25]。培养的人内皮细胞的热敏感性，在42~45℃的范围内持续30min时表现出剂量依赖性[26]。在高温的暴露下，可以见到中性粒细胞粘附，表明有内皮损伤，随后发生静脉压增加、分流及血管阻力增加、血管收缩、血液淤滞，而后红细胞聚集，血栓形成[27]。在体的兔耳部微循环标本研究表明内皮细胞的屏障作用遭到破坏，当组织在50℃暴露1h时，与对照相比，有6倍多的荧光标记的150kD的右旋糖酐从血管中渗漏出来[28]。这就可以假定，在微循环发生热损伤后引起缺血是早发或迟发组织坏死的原因。

为了评价射频导管消融对于心肌微循环的影响，在开胸犬左前降支供血区域的心肌标本上造成心内膜的射频消融损伤，左前降支通过颈动脉的体外泵进行灌注。用实时的高分辨率二维超声心动图观察损伤形成。射频消融60s后，经动脉注射白蛋白微泡，测定超声造影剂通过心肌微循环的传送速度。与正常对照

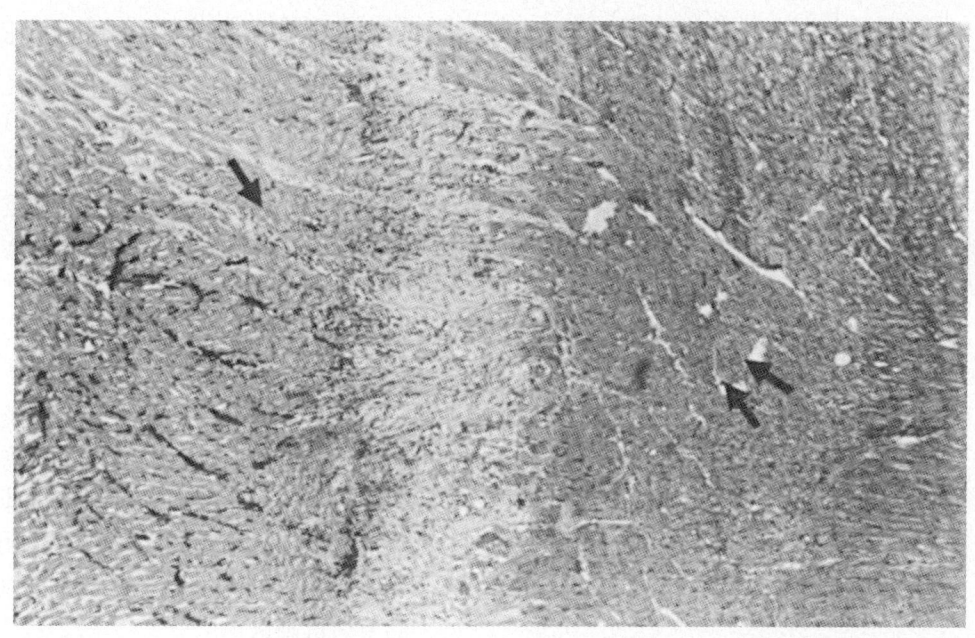

图 111-2　射频导管消融术后 5 天左心室的显微照片可见心内膜的坏死　（苏木精及伊红染色，40 倍放大）。坏死心肌（单箭头）和正常心肌（双箭头）之间的分界很明显，间杂有颗粒状的组织。（引自 Huang SK，Graham AR，Wharton K：Radiofrequency catheter ablation of the left and right ventricles：Anatomic and electrophysiologic observations. Pacing Clin Electrophysiol 11：449-459，1988.）

相比，测量的病理损伤边界内的传导率是 25%±12%（均值±标准差），在损伤边界以外 3mm 的周边范围内的传导率是正常的 48%±27%，在损伤边界以外 3～6mm 的周边范围内的传导率是 82%±28%（相互比较 $P<0.05$）[29]。电子显微照片显示这些灌注受损的区域有明显的浆膜及基底膜破坏伴红细胞渗出（图 111-3）。这些包绕急性病理损伤的组织存在潜在的损伤，在消融后数日可能进展或是恢复。

虽然在肿瘤的高热治疗中，微循环引起的组织冷却是一个重要的因素，但是在射频导管消融中的作用却不大[2]。这是因为射频能量释放持续时间短，心肌层中小动脉和小静脉的热耦联紧密，以及消融组织的微血管灌注减少。相反，在房室瓣环射频消融旁路的过程中，心外膜的冠状动脉对于局部的冷却有很重要的意义。一般认为在高热治疗中不均匀的组织冷却是不好的，但心外膜冠状动脉血流的这种"热消退"（heat sink）效应却起到了意外的自我保护作用。在冠状动脉中高速的血流大大防止了任何对血管内皮的加热作用，即使是在射频电极离血管很近时。

虽然在体内还没有测量冠状动脉的对流冷却作用，但许多其他的试验支持这一假设[30]。热消退作用可以解释为什么文献报道的冠状动脉并发症极少或是射频导管消融术前和术后冠状动脉造影未显示可测量的变化，即便是在消融旁道时消融电极会离这些血管很近的情况下[31,32]。然而，亚临床的冠状动脉损伤是可能的，特别是在对年轻及年龄较小患者的心脏进行消融时[33]。射频导管消融术后随访时间最长的是 18 年，大多数患者随访的时间是 15 年或稍短一些。不可能在术后几十年还会观察到射频消融的后遗症，比如早期的冠状动脉疾病，而且也得不到这些资料。

（三）射频能量介导的血栓形成

与射频消融相关的一个重要危险因素是有血栓栓塞风险的血栓及焦痂形成。栓塞物质形成的潜在机理包括与消融相关的血栓形成普遍增加，血液成分的热变性使血栓形成，内皮破坏使血栓形成，及过度加热导致焦痂、凝固物和血栓形成。研究表明在电生理检查过程中导管的放置与凝血酶-抗凝血酶Ⅲ及 d-二聚体水平的升高有关，值得注意的是射频消融并不额外增加升高的凝血酶-抗凝血酶Ⅲ及 d-二聚体水平。在操作过程中使用肝素抗凝可以减少血栓的形成[34]。在体外测试射频电流加热对非肝素化血循环的影响，表明能量释放 60s 后，尽管最高温度并未超过 80℃，但在消融电极上粘附聚集着一些变性的半固体样的蛋白质团块[35]。然而这个体外研究处于非生理状态，在抗凝患者体内进行射频消融时，应用心脏内超声从未发现这种低温度状态下的软血栓，因此，这种软血栓形成的现象似乎只是发生在体外。而当电极-组织接触面温度

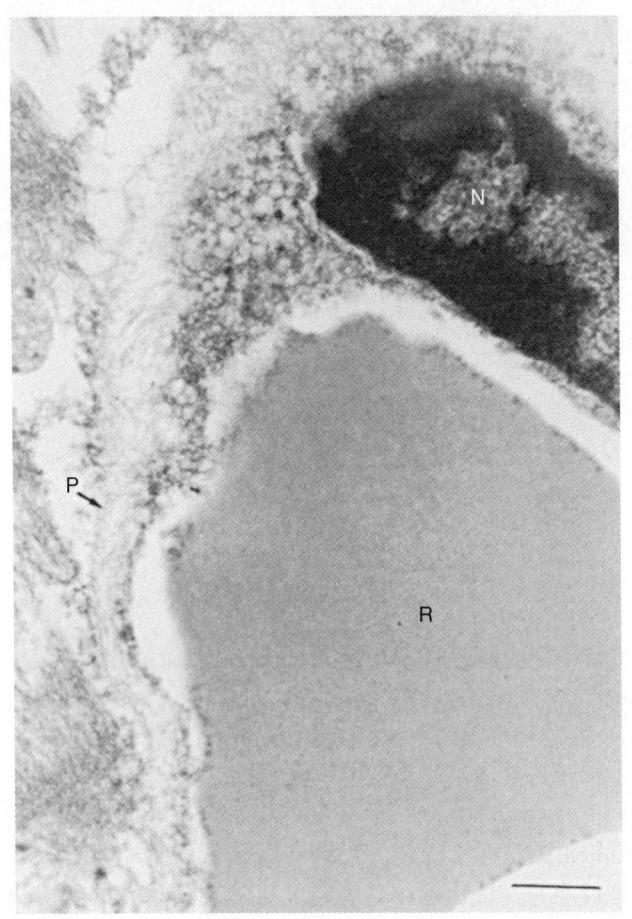

图111-3 位于射频导管消融试验急性损伤可存活边界区域内的一条小动脉的电子显微图 血管内皮有明显的损伤，伴浆膜破坏，基底膜破损，循环红细胞淤滞。N，内皮细胞核；P，浆膜；R，红细胞；比例尺＝0.5mm，放大55 000倍。

峰值超过100℃时，可以形成炭化干燥的凝固物及血栓[11]，而且测量的温度肯定要低于消融过程中的峰温度。所幸的是血液循环的冲洗效应、温度反馈调节的功率控制以及常规使用静脉肝素使得与射频导管消融相关的血栓并发症发生率很低[31]。

四、射频消融的细胞学效应

（一）电穿孔

使用高压电休克可达到导管消融的目的，在电休克后可观察到暂时的心肌顿抑。试验表明高压电休克破坏磷脂双分子层，并在肌纤维膜形成孔隙。这些孔隙是可逆性的，允许电解质和微粒自由通过直至自发性地孔隙关闭。短时间的孔隙形成可能是电除颤机制[36]，这一现象被称作电穿孔（electroporation）。描述细胞膜对射频电流反应的资料很有限，但是在低强度的射频能量场中（50～200V/cm）长时间的暴露（1～100s），DNA质粒已经成功地转染到大肠杆菌[37]。另外，众所周知高热增加浆膜的流动性（见后）。这样，射频电流的电动力和细胞加热的共同协同作用可以使肌纤维膜的孔隙形成。

（二）细胞器反应

活细胞的所有组成结构都有一定程度的热敏感性。热损伤对不同细胞结构和细胞功能成分的相对影响最终取决于高热造成的损伤是可逆的、部分可逆的，还是不可逆的。在加热情况下个体细胞的生存能力可能取决于细胞结构和功能链的薄弱连接。通过研究高热时亚细胞单位的个体成分，可以获得对于细胞死亡的复杂机制认识。

肌纤维膜首先接触受传导热影响的细胞，在维持细胞稳定性及兴奋性上起重要作用。改变或破坏细胞膜将会对细胞存活产生深远的影响。典型的肌纤维膜是由双层磷脂组成，亲水端构成了膜的表面，疏水的尾端构成了膜的中心部分。磷脂的饱和程度决定它们在不同温度下的状态和流动性。一般来说，在低温下纯净的磷脂双层结构是半固体的。从0～37℃它们经过一个或多个状态的改变，它们呈相对的流体状态。虽然在46～50℃时细胞膜有显著的变化，如流动性增加，但不会发生更进一步的状态改变。已经证实培养的细胞在43～44℃之间的温度下长时间的加热会增加细胞膜的流动性和渗漏[38]。膜流动性的增加可以引起肌纤维膜蛋白动力学的变化。在一条离体的心肌标本上，在38～45℃高温下只暴露1min就可以记录到dV/dt_{max}的增加。在更高的温度下（45～50℃），dV/dt_{max}下降并降至基线水平以下[39]。提示在较低高温温度范围内dV/dt_{max}的增加是钠通道的动力学温度依赖性增加的结果。随后数值的下降可能归因于温度使钠通道失活或（更可能是）电压依赖的钠通道失活，与静息膜电位温度依赖性的除极一致（见后文）。当然，在高温暴露下观察到的膜通透性的增加应该是增加的膜流动性与电穿孔共同协同作用的结果。

所有哺乳动物的细胞都由结构蛋白来构成微丝、微管和中间丝的丝状结构。微丝组成胞浆束（cytoplasmic bundles）称为张力丝（stress filaments）。张力丝主要成分是肌动蛋白，还有肌球蛋白、α辅肌动蛋白、原肌球蛋白。这个蛋白丝结构被统称为细胞骨架，它们用于维持细胞的大小、形态和细胞膜的稳定性。细胞骨架在肌细胞中尤其重要，因为它们是收缩蛋白向细胞外传导收缩力的结构成分。已经证实在不同的培养细胞株中这些组成细胞骨架的蛋白有不同的热敏感性，这些结构的破坏造成细胞结构缺失、起泡，及细胞外形与形态学上的改变[40]。然而还未研究高热对心肌细胞骨架的特殊影响。

如果在一定的温度下可以使细胞核遭受明显的破坏，那么高热对细胞核结构及功能的影响可能与肌细胞在高热下的生存能力有关，但这还未被验证。不同的细胞株中可以观察到加热至44℃超过10min会引起DNA碎裂和凋亡[41]。其他研究显示高热可以抑制DNA合成和损伤细胞核蛋白质。因为成人的肌细胞不能主动复制，所以加热对细胞复制的影响虽然在肿瘤学中重要，但在射频消融的病理生理学中不那么重要。

（三）代谢及电生理学

高热可以对暴露细胞的代谢产生很广泛的影响。在稍低的高热范围内可以增加某些生化反应的动力学，但是较高的温度会使关键的酶学系统失活。40~42℃的温度时，收缩力下降（是正常体温时的38%），耗氧量增加[42]。代谢蛋白质，如肌酸激酶，是温度敏感性的，但是它会在62.5℃时失活，所以不可能在细胞死亡中起重要作用。

高热对细胞膜的许多成分有很重要的影响，因为心肌细胞的电生理及收缩功能全部依赖于肌纤维膜和细胞内成分如肌浆网、线粒体的功能完整，这些结构的热破坏会削弱细胞的兴奋性及兴奋-收缩耦联。高热对细胞膜的损伤可能是细胞在射频导管消融术时存活的限制因子。在表面灌流的犬的心外膜心肌条带模型上研究了射频导管消融对局部动作电位的影响。在距损伤边缘6~8mm的范围内观察到静息膜电位的负值减小、dV/dt 值的下降以及动作电位时程缩短等异常，但是只在一个2mm的范围内记录到严重异常[44]。

为了进一步明确射频导管消融对细胞的影响，测定了豚鼠右室乳头肌细胞在高温下的电生理反应[39]。直径小于1mm的乳头肌在高流速的组织腔内表面灌流，头端连接一个能量传感器，常规微电极刺入表面的细胞，在静息和起搏状态下测量跨膜电压（V_m）、动作电位增加的最大速率（dV/dt_{max}）。动作电位（AP）振幅，50%（APD_{50}）及90%（APD_{90}）的动作电位时程。对高温灌注液的快速温度变化（在组织测量的温度改变的 $t_{1/2}$ 小于1s）维持60s，之后将温度迅速恢复至37℃。在高热暴露下，可重复观察到一些现象，静息跨膜电压只是轻度增加，直到温度达到45℃时，一些标本才开始明显除极。在温度超过50℃时，最终所有的细胞均除极，并且大部分表现为挛缩状态（图111-4）。同时观察到高温引起动作电位与温度相关的显著变化，包括动作电位时程缩短及动作电位振幅减小。在大约45℃时，dV/dt_{max} 增加，然后在舒张期 V_m 变化后经历平台期和再下降。在中值温度48℃时（42.7~51.3℃范围）高温介导的兴奋性丧失是可逆性的，在大于50℃时则是不可逆的，并在温度超过45℃时介导产生异常的自律性[39]。因为未发现刺入微电极部位的正常细胞有自律性，因此认为高温引起的自律性是来源于部分损伤或缺血的细胞。在Langendorff液灌注的兔心脏标本上行光学AP标测证实了这些资料。在心肌消融开始后APD快速缩短，数分钟后在损伤边界以外超过1mm处APD完全恢复，而在损伤边界以内并未恢复，在损伤边界以外1mm范围内，观察到APD部分恢复[45]。一个在细胞内记录动作电位的相似研究显示APD及AP振幅在损伤边缘的2.5mm范围内急性下降，在损伤边界区域传导时间减慢，而 dV/dt_{max} 无变化。慢性损伤（消融后22天）并未显示边界区域AP或传导时间持续异常[46]。

假定肌细胞的高温除极是由于非特异的阳离子进入细胞造成的，而不是由于特异的离子通道电导的变化。在豚鼠乳头肌标本上，通过间接测量收缩力及直接测量fluo-3 AM（分子探针，Eugene Ore）的染色荧光发现高温时钙离子进入肌细胞。在稍低的高温范围内（小于45℃）变化极少。在中等高温的范围（45~50℃），收缩力和钙离子内流进入细胞增加。这一结果不会被镉或是维拉帕米削弱，说明钙离子进入细胞并不通过特异的通道。当细胞钙负荷的缓冲能力被thapsigargen削弱时（thapsigargen是一种选择性的肌浆网的钙离子泵阻滞剂），这种现象增强。在高温范围时（大于50℃）细胞收缩并且死亡[47]。由此可见钙离子进入细胞和细胞超载可能是高温介导肌细胞损伤和死亡的机制。

Simmers和他的同事[48]完成了一些补充研究，把犬心室心肌标本表面灌流到37℃，利用片状电极测量表面传导速度。灌注液的温度在38.5~54.4℃范围内不断增加。观察到传导速度在较低温度范围时（38.5~45.4℃）增加；在中等温度时（45.4℃到大约50℃）传导减慢；在大于49.5~51.5℃的温度范围时，可以发现暂时的传导阻滞及自律性；温度在51.7

~54.4℃时，发生永久性的传导阻滞（图111-5）。在随后的研究中使用了类似的标本，但在这一研究中，测量是通过一个外科手术造成的峡部的传导情况，在测量部位正下面的组织被一个片状电极释放的射频能量加热。通过这项技术，作者再次观察到，短暂传导阻滞发生在50.7±3.0℃的温度，在58.0±3.4℃时发生永久性传导阻滞[49]。因为无论是经纯粹的热能源或是射频电能源加热，传导阻滞的阈值是相似的，所以作者[48]认为射频能量释放对心肌组织的主要消融作用可能是热能，而直接的电损伤对最终损伤形成只有很小的作用甚至并无作用。

五、总 结

在射频导管消融术中，射频电流通过与电极紧密接触的组织时，这些组织就被阻抗加热了。损伤边缘的组织温度在50~55℃之间，而且有可重复性。虽然试验表明电场可以依靠电场强度顿抑和杀死细胞，但心肌损伤的主要方式可能是热损伤。基于对心肌损伤的观察，损伤区域组织表现为干燥、炎症、微血管损伤，最终导致缺血。在损伤边缘区域的组织发生晚期损伤或是修复可能是炎症反应或内皮损伤进展或消退的结果。在细胞学水平，肌细胞损伤存在许多可能的机制，但是细胞膜受损可能是其主要机制。这可能导致细胞除极，细胞内钙离子超载和细胞死亡。长时间暴露在高温下，在较低的温度时可发生细胞骨架、细胞代谢和细胞核的进一步损伤。射频导管消融已经被证明是有效的治疗心律失常的临床方法，但是这一经验性的治疗手段在组织和细胞水平的许多基本的病理生理学效应还有待于进一步探讨。

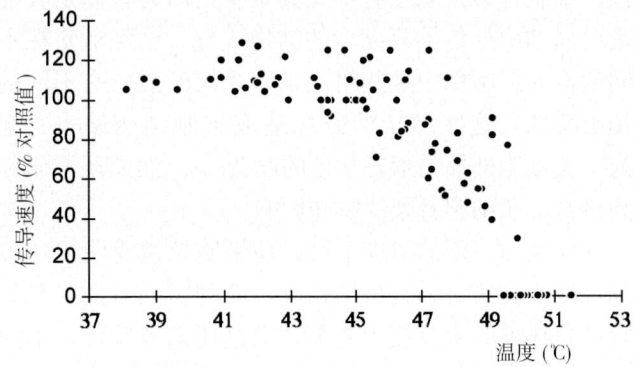

图111-5 在体外犬右室心肌标本上，传导速率与表面灌注液温度的关系 在高温后30s测量传导速率，并以标化值与先前的对照值比较来表示。所有标本的基线传导速率是0.35±0.13m/s。（引自 Simmers TA, de Bakker JM, Wittkampf FH, Hauer RN: Effects of heating on impulse propagation in superfused canine myocardium. J Am Coll Cardiol 25: 1457-1464, 1995. Reprinted with permission from the American College of Cardiology。）

（杨俊娟 译）

参 考 文 献

1. Wittkampf FH, Hauer RN, Robles de Medina EO: Control of radiofrequency lesion size by power regulation. Circulation 80:962-968, 1989.
2. Haines DE, Watson DD: Tissue heating during radiofrequency catheter ablation: A thermodynamic model and observations in isolated perfused and superfused canine right ventricular free wall. Pacing Clin Electrophysiol 12:962-976, 1989.
3. Jain MK, Wolf PD: Temperature-controlled and constant-power radiofrequency ablation: What affects lesion growth? Trans Biomed Eng 46:1405-1412, 1999.
4. Tungjitkusolmun S, Woo EJ, Cao H, et al: Finite element analyses of uniform current density electrodes for radio-frequency cardiac ablation. IEEE Trans Biomed Eng 47:32-40, 2000.
5. Nath S, DiMarco JP, Gallop RG, et al: Effects of dispersive electrode position and surface area on electrical parameters and temperature during radiofrequency catheter ablation. Am J Cardiol 77:765-767, 1996.
6. Prasad SM, Maniar HS, Schuessler RB, Damiano RJ Jr: Chronic transmural atrial ablation by using bipolar radiofrequency energy on the beating heart. J Thorac Cardiovasc Surg 124:708-713, 2002.
7. Haines DE, Watson DD, Verow AF: Electrode radius predicts lesion radius during radiofrequency energy heating: Validation of a proposed thermodynamic model. Circ Res 67:124-129, 1990.
8. Wagshal AB, Crystal E, Katz A: Patterns of accelerated junctional rhythm during slow pathway catheter ablation for atrioventricular nodal reentrant tachycardia: Temperature dependence, prognostic value, and insights into the nature of the slow pathway. J Cardiovasc Electrophys 11:244-254, 2000.
9. Tsai CF, Tai CT, Yu WC, et al: Is 8-mm more effective than 4-mm tip electrode catheter for ablation of typical atrial flutter? Circulation 100:768-771, 1999.
10. Hogh Petersen H, Chen X, Pietersen A, et al: Lesion dimensions during temperature-controlled radiofrequency catheter ablation of left ventricular porcine myocardium: Impact of ablation site, electrode size, and convective cooling. Circulation 99:319-325, 1999.

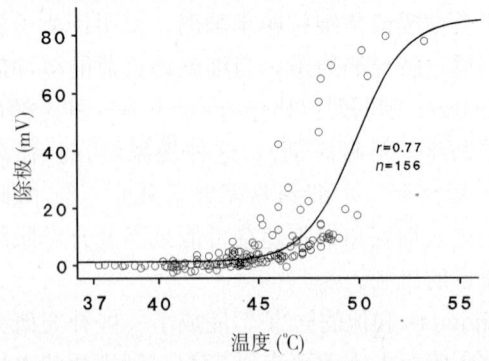

图111-4 豚鼠右室乳头肌标本从37℃基线水平暴露在高温灌注液60s，在不同温度时静息跨膜电压的变化 跨膜电压在温度小于45℃时保持相对恒定。在较高温度下肌细胞开始除极，并在超过50℃时发生不可逆的挛缩。

11. Haines DE, Verow AF: Observations on electrode-tissue interface temperature and effect on electrical impedance during radiofrequency ablation of ventricular myocardium. Circulation 82:1034–1038, 1990.
12. McRury ID, Mitchell MA, Panescu D, Haines DE: Non-uniform heating during radiofrequency ablation with long electrodes: Monitoring the edge effect. Circulation 96:4057–4064, 1997.
13. Haines DE: Determinants of lesion size during radiofrequency catheter ablation: The role of electrode-tissue contact pressure and duration of energy delivery. J Cardiovasc Electrophysiol 2:509–515, 1991.
14. Simmers TA, de Bakker JM, Coronel R, et al: Effects of intracavitary blood flow and electrode-target distance on radiofrequency power required for transient conduction block in a Langendorff-perfused canine model. J Am Coll Cardiol 31:231–235, 1998.
15. Nakagawa H, Yamanashi WS, Pitha JV, et al: Comparison of in vivo tissue temperature profile and lesion geometry for radiofrequency ablation with a saline-irrigated electrode versus temperature control in a canine thigh muscle preparation. Circulation 91:2264–2273, 1995.
16. Soejima K, Delacretaz E, Suzuki M, et al: Saline-cooled versus standard radiofrequency catheter ablation for infarct-related ventricular tachycardias. Circulation 103:1858–1862, 2001.
17. Wittkampf FH, Simmers TA, Hauer RN, Robles de Medina EO: Myocardial temperature response during radiofrequency catheter ablation. Pacing Clin Electrophysiol 18:307–317, 1995.
18. Wittkampf FH, Nakagawa H, Yamanashi WS, et al: Thermal latency in radiofrequency ablation. Circulation 93:1083–1086, 1996.
19. Whayne JG, Nath S, Haines DE: Microwave catheter ablation of myocardium in vitro: Assessment of the characteristics of tissue heating and injury. Circulation 89:2390–2395, 1994.
20. Nath S, DiMarco JP, Mounsey JP, et al: Correlation of temperature and pathophysiological effect during radiofrequency catheter ablation of the AV junction. Circulation 92:1188–1192, 1995.
20. Huang SK, Graham AR, Wharton K: Radiofrequency catheter ablation of the left and right ventricles: Anatomic and electrophysiologic observations. Pacing Clin Electrophysiol 11:449–459, 1988.
21. Ren JF, Callans DJ, Schwartzman D, et al: Changes in local wall thickness correlate with pathologic lesion size following radiofrequency catheter ablation: An intracardiac echocardiographic imaging study. Echocardiography 18:503–507, 2001.
22. Langberg JJ, Calkins H, Kim YN, et al: Recurrence of conduction in accessory atrioventricular connections after initially successful radiofrequency catheter ablation. J Am Coll Cardiol 19:1588–1592, 1992.
23. Takahashi M, Mitsuhashi T, Hashimoto T, et al: Transient complete atrioventricular block occurring 1 week after radiofrequency ablation for the treatment of atrioventricular nodal re-entrant tachycardia. Circulation J 66:1073–1075, 2002.
24. Huang SK, Bharati S, Lev M, et al: Electrophysiologic and histologic observations of chronic atrioventricular block induced by closed-chest catheter desiccation with radiofrequency energy. Pacing Clin Electrophysiol 10:805–816, 1987.
25. Ferguson MK, Seifert FC, Replogle RL: Leukocyte adherence in venules of rat skeletal muscle following thermal injury. Microvasc Res 24:34–41, 1982.
26. Fajardo LF, Schreiber AB, Kelly NI, Hahn GM: Thermal sensitivity of endothelial cells. Radiat Res 103:276–285, 1985.
27. Reinhold HS, van den Berg AP: Effects of hyperthermia on blood flow and metabolism. In Field SB, Hand JW (eds): An Introduction to the Practical Aspects of Clinical Hyperthermia. London, Taylor and Francis, 1990, pp 77–107.
28. Gerlowski LE, Jain RK: Effect of hyperthermia on microvascular permeability to macromolecules in normal and tumor tissues. Int J Microcirc Clin Exp 4:363–372, 1985.
29. Nath S, Whayne JG, Kaul S, et al: Effects of radiofrequency catheter ablation on regional myocardial blood flow: Possible mechanism for late electrophysiological outcome. Circulation 89:2667–2672, 1994.
30. Huang HW, Chen ZP, Roemer RB: A counter current vascular network model of heat transfer in tissues. J Biomech Eng 118:120–129, 1996.
31. Hindricks G: The Multicentre European Radiofrequency Survey (MERFS): Complications of radiofrequency catheter ablation of arrhythmias. Eur Heart J 14:1644–1653, 1993.
32. Chatelain P, Zimmermann M, Weber R, et al: Acute coronary occlusion secondary to radiofrequency catheter ablation of a left lateral accessory pathway. Eur Heart J 16:859–861, 1995.
33. Bokenkamp R, Wibbelt G, Sturm M, et al: Effects of intracardiac radiofrequency current application on coronary artery vessels in young pigs. J Cardiovasc Electrophysiol 11:565–571, 2000.
34. Dorbala S, Cohen AJ, Hutchinson LS, et al: Does radiofrequency ablation induce a prethrombotic state? Analysis of coagulation system activation and comparison to electrophysiologic study. J Cardiovasc Electrophys 9:1152–1160, 1998.
35. Demolin JM, Eick OJ, Munch K, et al: Soft thrombus formation in radiofrequency catheter ablation. Pacing Clin Electrophysiol 25:1219–1222, 2002.
36. Al-Khadra A, Nikolski V, Efimov IR: The role of electroporation in defibrillation. Circ Res 87:797–804, 2000.
37. Xie TD, Tsong TY: Study of mechanisms of electric field-induced DNA transfection: II. Transfection by low-amplitude, low-frequency alternating electric fields. Biophys J 58:897–903, 1990.
38. Nishida T, Akagi K, Tanaka Y: Correlation between cell killing effect and cell membrane potential after heat treatment: Analysis using fluorescent dye and flow cytometry. Int J Hypertherm 13:227–234, 1997.
39. Nath S, Lynch C III, Whayne JG, Haines DE: Cellular electrophysiologic effects of hyperthermia on isolated guinea pig papillary muscle: Implications for catheter ablation. Circulation 88:1826–1831, 1993.
40. Coss RA, Linnemans WA: The effects of hyperthermia on the cytoskeleton: A review. Int J Hypertherm 12:173–196, 1996.
41. Nakano H, Kurihara K, Okamoto M, et al: Heat-induced apoptosis and p53 in cultured mammalian cells. Int J Radiat Biol 71:519–529, 1997.
42. Saeki A, Goto Y, Hata K, et al: Negative inotropism of hyperthermia increases oxygen cost of contractility in canine hearts. Am J Physiol 279:H2855–H2864, 2000.
43. Haines DE, Whayne JG, Walker J, et al: The effect of radiofrequency catheter ablation on myocardial creatine kinase activity. J Cardiovasc Electrophysiol 6:79–88, 1995.
44. Ge YZ, Shao PZ, Goldberger J, Kadish A: Cellular electrophysiological changes induced in vitro by radiofrequency current: Comparison with electrical ablation. Pacing Clin Electrophysiol 18:323–333, 1995.
45. Wu CC, Fasciano RW, Calkins H, Tung L: Sequential change in action potential of rabbit epicardium during and following radiofrequency ablation. J Cardiovasc Electrophys 10:1252–1261, 1999.
46. Wood MA, Fuller IA: Acute and chronic electrophysiologic changes surrounding radiofrequency lesions. J Cardiovasc Electrophys 13:56–61, 2002.
47. Everett TH, Nath S, Lynch C, et al: Role of calcium in acute hyperthermic myocardial injury. J Cardiovasc Electrophysiol 12:563–569, 2001.
48. Simmers TA, de Bakker JM, Wittkampf FH, Hauer RN: Effects of heating on impulse propagation in superfused canine myocardium. J Am Coll Cardiol 25:1457–1464, 1995.
49. Simmers TA, de Bakker JM, Wittkampf FH, Hauer RN: Effects of heating with radiofrequency power on myocardial impulse conduction: Is radiofrequency ablation exclusively thermally mediated? J Cardiovasc Electrophysiol 7:243–247, 1996.

第 112 章

心房颤动触发灶和基质的导管射频消融术

Michel Haïssaguerre, Prashanthan Sanders, Pierre Jais, Mélèze Hocini, Dipen C. Shah, and Jacques Clémenty

本章目录

- 触发灶的导管消融 ················ 1004
- 导管消融改良房颤基质 ············ 1008
- 总结 ·························· 1013

心房颤动（房颤）是人类最常见的持续性心动过速，普通人群的发病率为2%，年龄每增长10岁，发病率随之增加，在65岁以上的老年人其发病率可达5.9%。房颤可以导致血栓性脑血管意外、心房收缩功能下降、心动过速相关的心房与心室肌的病理改变，因而导致较高的死亡率和明显的致残率[1]。治疗策略包括两方面：控制心室率并抗凝治疗或者恢复并维持窦性节律。目前研究证据显示药物维持窦性节律，至少在老年患者和那些有永久性房颤或器质性心脏病的患者，其有效性和价值具有一定的局限性[2-4]。因此，使用非药物治疗、导管介入治疗来维持窦性节律的方法受到越来越多的关注。本章重点讨论目前标测技术和导管消融技术在针对房颤触发灶和维持基质方面的治疗现状和利弊。

一、触发灶的导管消融

房颤多由来自肺静脉（PVs）[5-8]、Marshall 韧带[9]、冠状窦[7,10]、界嵴[7,10]、上腔静脉和下腔静脉的自发激动或期前收缩所引发，其中绝大多数的自发电活动来源于肺静脉[5-7]。这些肺静脉的电活动在对房颤的维持以及慢性房颤电复律后的复发中也起着重要的作用[11-13]。来源于肺静脉的自发性电活动可表现为多种房性心律失常。单一的电活动表现为单独的期前收缩，周期长的反复电活动表现为较慢的心房节律（甚至类似于窦性节律），而周期短的反复电活动表现为房性心动过速。对存在房颤维持基质的某些患者，快速的持续性局灶电活动（有时为几小时、几天，甚至更长）可以引起驱动性持续房颤（即局灶性房颤，是指触发和维持机制均为局灶起源，图112-1A），而短阵快速电活动可以引起触发性房颤（局灶触发性房颤；图112-1B）[6]。这些局灶电活动还可以引起峡部依赖性房扑。目前针对这些触发灶的消融已经成为导管消融治疗房颤广受关注的课题。

（一）肺静脉触发性房颤的局灶消融

最初导管消融的靶点为记录到自发异位激动时的最早心内电图部位，因此称为房颤的局灶消融[6]。对房颤发作频繁（每天发作）和伴有频发早搏而药物治疗无效的45例患者进行标测研究，结果显示其中94%的异位冲动来源于肺静脉。标测到的最早局灶电活动主要位于肺静脉开口及其分支的2～4cm内，其局灶电活动引起的尖峰样电位（肺静脉电位）较心房电位提前35～45ms。对最早心内电活动的部位进行射频消融可消除房性异位激动，随访8±6个月，在未使用抗心律失常药物的情况下有62%的患者未再发生房颤。

很多患者由于手术中很少甚至无自发的异位激动

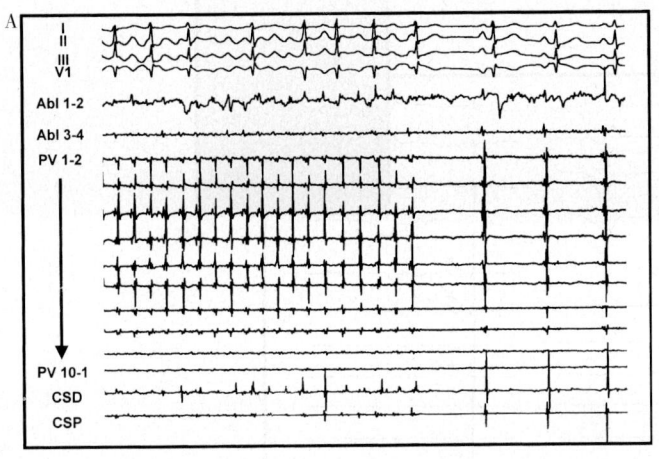

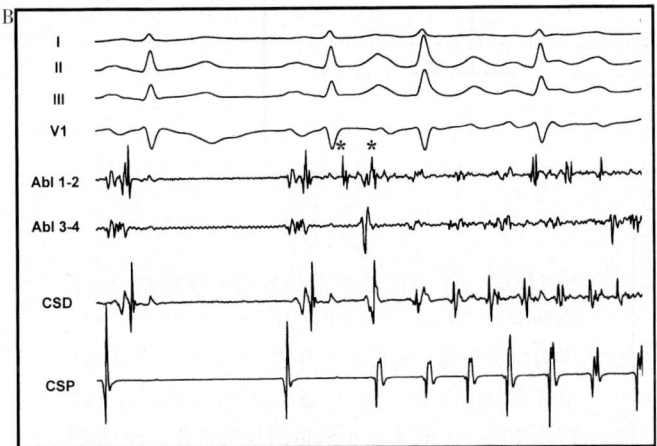

图112-1 A：为一例持续6个月的慢性房颤患者，在肺静脉口部的消融中心内电图逐步变为规则，随后房颤终止，说明肺静脉在房颤维持中起了重要作用。该例随之进行了所有肺静脉的电隔离。B：来源于右上肺静脉局灶性房颤，＊显示在消融导管顶端记录的局灶电活动。

出现，而使这种治疗方法的应用受到了限制。可使用几种方法试图去克服，包括在异位冲动时观察右心房心内膜的电活动顺序；通过去除或不去除相关QRS-T波群的方法来显示"P on T"中P波形态，然后根据这种异位P波形态去推测心律失常起源的肺静脉；使用多极标测导管以增加异位激动时的标测点，以及进行电转复后房颤即刻复发时的心内标测等[11]。越来越多的证据显示在房颤易于发作的患者，其自发电激动可来自多根静脉以及某一根静脉的多个局灶起源点[14]，而这些异位灶也同样需要进一步的干预[15,16]。因此，目前局灶消融的方法已经逐步被以电隔离所有肺静脉为终点的肺静脉口部消融所取代。

（二）肺静脉电隔离

随着环状标测电极导管的应用，可以确定肺静脉活动在静脉口部分布情况以及活动的序列[17]。这种标测已经证明，反映局部肌束的肺静脉电位在周径上呈现出一定程度的变化（在不同的静脉变化不同），以及肺静脉心肌的电活动经常由最早活动的节段区域开始呈现一种顺序性激动。因此，在肺静脉口部行节段性消融可使肺静脉和左房产生电隔离（图112-2和112-3）。在消融后4±5个月随访期间，73％的患者在未用抗心律失常药物的情况下未再发作房颤。而其他一些研究报道成功率仅接近50％，尤其对只进行过一次消融的患者。

尽可能在肺静脉的近端（口部）消融有利于减少肺静脉狭窄的发生风险。应用选择性肺静脉造影或者结合心腔内超声有利于口部消融的定位。这两种方法也有助于检测肺静脉狭窄的发生。然而确定肺静脉的开口部并不容易，因为左房和肺静脉连接部多呈漏斗形。在左肺静脉的前壁和下壁的消融中，要获得导管的稳定性经常会损伤肺静脉。而且，由于在肺静脉和左房连接部位的心肌组织较厚，因此在口部消融进行电隔离多更加困难。此外，在12％阵发性房颤和50％的慢性房颤患者中应用通常30W的消融能量达不到电隔离的目的，可能是由于局部血液降温的不充分所致。这些问题可以通过使用8mm的消融电极或者通过盐水灌注消融导管以增加能量输出的方法来解决[18]。

1. 肺静脉电图

由于左房和肺静脉彼此邻近，因此两者的电位在环状电极标测中常常呈现融合状态。在环状标测电极上没能辨别出远场心房电位的存在是消融过程中经常遇到的难题，从而增加了消融时间。这种现象在窦性心律下标测左肺静脉时尤为明显，即左肺静脉电位与左房或左心耳电位同步出现。冠状窦远端或左心耳起搏夺获左房能使左肺静脉电位与远场心房电位分开，从而使肺静脉电位在消融中容易被辨认（图112-2A）[19]。

变化起搏位置（冠状窦、左心耳或左房后壁）可以使这些电位的远场成分提前激动，由此可判断其心房起源性质。在标测左上肺静脉时由于位于前壁的电极对记录到的肺静脉电位与左心耳后壁的电激动在时间上同步，因此这一融合现象更为常见[20]。在左下

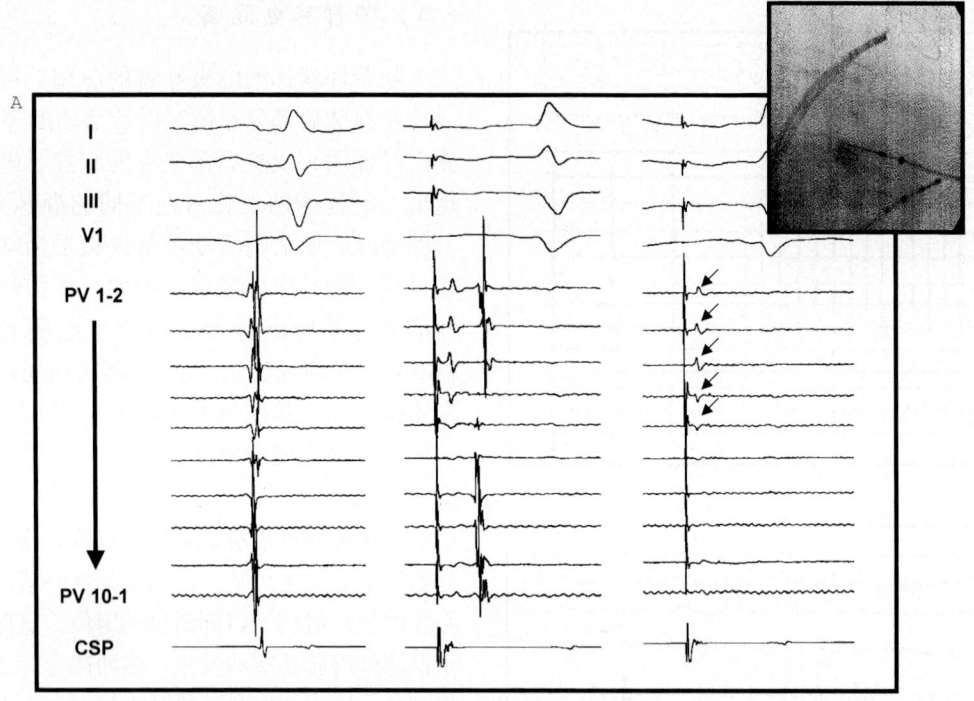

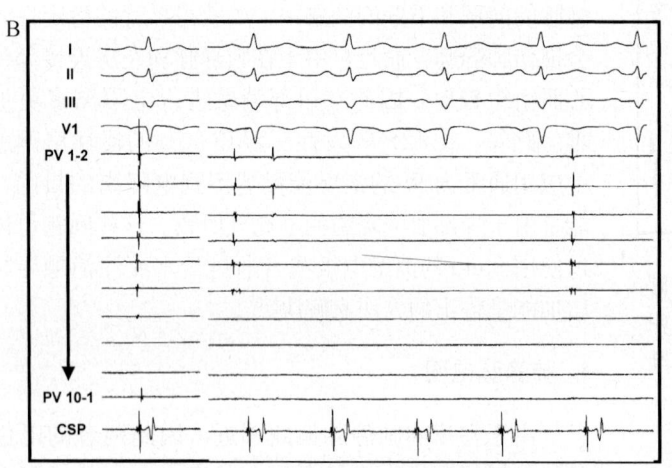

图 112-2　A：在左上肺静脉环状电极标测的心房远场电位。左组图显示窦性节律时融合电位。中间组图显示在冠状窦远端起搏时左心耳电位从肺静脉电位中分离出来。右组图显示肺静脉电隔离后残留的远场电位。箭头表示残留的远场电位。B：肺静脉电活动的分离。显示窦性节律下右上肺静脉环状标测的心内电图。随着肺静脉电隔离可观察到肺静脉自主节律与窦律分离。

肺静脉，其环状标测电极的上部或前部电极对也常记录到与左房前壁电位一致的电位。在右上肺静脉前壁经常记录到相似的两重或三重成分的电位。根据对不同周围结构进行的三维电解剖激动标测研究，显示右上肺静脉记录到的最初成分与 P 波的起始相一致，在时间上与相邻的上腔静脉电位同步。后面的成分与房间隔上部的电活动相一致，并在静脉内向远端发生传导延迟。这些电位不能被低位右房或右房侧壁起搏所提前。

左房到肺静脉的优势传导区（由消融确定）常位于上肺静脉的底部（发生率 85%）和下肺静脉的顶部（发生率 75%）[21]。电图的极性反转（定义为在相邻的两个电极间出现相反的极性）结合最早的激动部位是另一种有效判断消融靶点的标准，它确定优势传导区的敏感性为 88%，特异性为 91%（图 112-3）。发生极性反转的电极数明显少于能够记录到最早激动的电极数（2.0±0.4 极 vs 3.4±2.0 极）。使用极性反转的方法来确定消融靶点，比传统应用最早激动点的方法所需要的射频消融放电时间更短（10.3±3.0min vs 12.3±3.4min）[21]。

2. 消融的终点

肺静脉的电隔离（肺静脉电位的消失或分离；图112-2）为导管消融提供了明确的终点，随着对环状标测电图判读水平的不断提高，达到这一终点并不需要很长的消融操作时间以及 X 线曝光时间[18]。将来新的消融设备可能会进一步缩短手术时间。经球囊环状超声消融系统用于肺静脉隔离在动物模型上似乎可复，70%则来源于非肺静脉病灶，其中一半病灶主要位于左心房（后壁）靠近肺静脉口部附近，其余的病灶距消融部位则较远，包括冠状窦、上腔静脉和右心房。在术中对这些部位补充进行射频消融能够减少房颤的早期复发。

在不应用抗心律失常药物的情况下，肺静脉电隔离的长期成功率可达 70%，Oral 等报道成功率则达 85%[12]。

3. 肺静脉消融的风险及局限性

与肺静脉消融最相关的并发症是肺静脉狭窄[26]。在早期的系列研究中，使用经食道超声心动图，42%消融的肺静脉血流>80cm/s[8]。目前在有症状的大部分患者中，血管造影显示肺静脉狭窄（静脉直径缩小>50%）的发生率<2%。随着应用较低能量的口部消融和手术经验的积累，肺静脉狭窄的发生率明显减少。在我们超过 1800 例接受肺静脉隔离患者中仅有 2 例需进行肺静脉球囊成型和植入支架的治疗。

一些患者肺静脉隔离后可观察到左心房内存在大折返。在 100 例进行肺静脉电隔离的阵发性房颤患者中，5 例患者发展为持续性左房扑动，其中 4 例为二尖瓣周折返，1 例围绕右肺静脉折返。连接左下肺静脉到二尖瓣环的消融线可成功地消除围绕二尖瓣环的折返，连接两上肺静脉间的消融线可打断围绕右肺静脉的折返。

大多数临床研究显示尽管肺静脉消融对阵发性房颤患者是有益的，但对慢性房颤患者则存在一定的局限性。在一项 15 例（7 例器质性心脏病）持续性房颤患者（5±4 个月）的研究中，根据电转复后频发的早搏为基础，隔离心律失常源性肺静脉，随访 11±8 个月，在未用抗心律失常药物的情况下，60%的患者维持窦性心律[13]。随着时间延长这个结果可能有所降低。一项仅对持续性房颤患者进行右和左上肺静脉的经验性电隔离的系列研究显示，随访 29±8 个月，在未服用抗心律失常药物的情况下，仅 21%的患者维持窦性心律[27]。其他的系列研究已经证实肺静脉电隔离后 5 个月，仅 22%的慢性房颤患者症状未再发作[25]。

现已清楚显示，在大部分慢性房颤患者和 30%的阵发性房颤患者中，仅进行肺静脉电隔离以维持窦性心律是不够的。因此，为进一步提高导管消融的长期成功率需要提高对非肺静脉病灶的标测技术或改良房颤本身的基质。

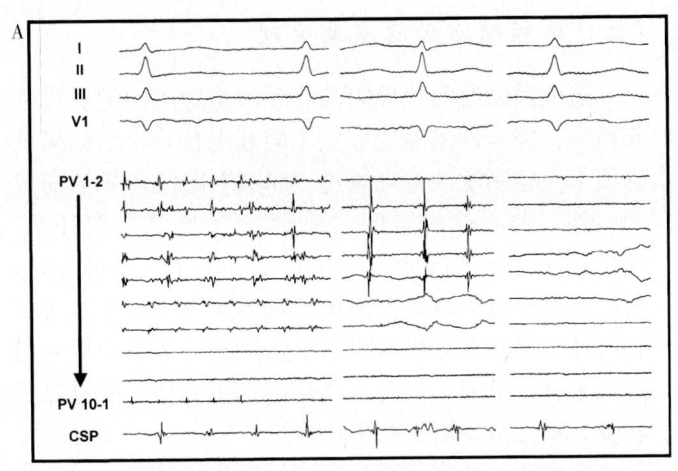

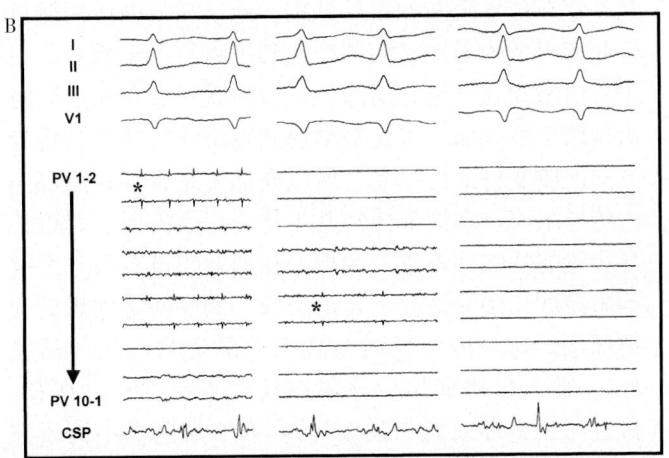

图 112-3　房颤中的肺静脉电隔离　A：患者最初的靶点位于肺静脉（PV）的上部，它产生相对规则的肺静脉活动（第 2 组图）。在最早肺静脉电活动的部位进行消融产生电隔离（第 3 组图）。B：患者最初的靶点位于环状标测导管极性反转的部位（第 1 组图中＊）。在第二个极性反转的部位再次进行消融（第 2 组图中＊）达到肺静脉的电隔离（第 3 组图）。

行，但是临床上仍存在一些问题，目前临床上仍处于研究阶段[22,23]。解剖标测或导管跟踪系统的应用也便于进行肺静脉电隔离，其操作时间以及长期成功率相似，但 X 线曝光时间明显减少。已有报告显示单纯应用解剖消融而不必行肺静脉电隔离治疗阵发性房颤的成功率，在不使用抗心律失常药物的情况下为 38%[23]～80%[24]。

房颤消融报道的即刻成功率在 94%～100%不等[18,25]，然而，多达 48%的患者在消融的几天内出现房颤的早期复发。复发时频发的异位激动有利于早期行二次介入治疗中的标测，否则这种有利条件将不存在。其中 30%的复发是由于已隔离肺静脉电位的恢

二、导管消融改良房颤基质

房颤的发生依赖于多个复杂机制的相互作用，这些机制大致分为触发作用和基质两方面[28]，即使改良房颤的基质时也要强调治疗触发机制的重要性。目前证据显示房颤发生的基质可能与心房的结构重构及其电生理结果有关。

同很多心律失常一样，外科治疗一直是导管消融治疗房颤的基础。根据房颤多子波折返假说，Cox等[29]研究出了一种双心房外科手术治疗房颤（Maze手术），这种手术将心房进行分割以使折返活动不再可能发生。这种手术以及其他类似的分割手术已被不断改进，现在主要围绕左心房进行，并证实了具有较高的恢复窦性节律的成功率（在应用抗心律失常药物的情况下房颤的长期治愈率达80%～99%）[29]。这些结果唤起了对发展以导管技术来改变房颤基质的更大兴趣，并为勿需开胸手术从而达到相似的长期治愈房颤提供了希望。由于不断进行技术上的改进和完善，现在以导管为基础的线性消融已被认为是"闭式心脏外科手术"。

（一）线性消融的导管技术

很多实验室正在进行形成连续、透壁线性损伤技术的研究。这些技术包括应用普通的导管在不同形状外鞘的导引下通过逐步回撤的方法行顺序点消融，也可以通过多电极同步放电或长电极消融（应用或不用导引鞘）。为达到这种消融的目的，已经研究了多极、间隙紧密的环状电极、螺旋状、带状以及球囊状电极导管，以及一些像盐水灌注、同时多极能量发放以"覆盖"电极间的区域，或者不同的能量模式等其他多种技术[30,31]。然而要设计出一种理想的多极消融导管并非易事，因为这种导管必须既易于操控和固定，又能确保电极与心内膜紧密接触，既能够通过电极释放足够的能量以保证消融的连续性和透壁性，同时又没有血栓及焦痂的危险。目前这些技术仍处于研究阶段，还未应用于临床。

比较起来，行点状消融的导管技术已经明显改进，特别是应用盐水灌注系统，可允许发放更大的能量，并同时减少在电极和心内膜产生焦痂或血凝块的危险，因而降低了左房消融时血栓事件的危险性。我们实验室常规使用盐水灌注消融导管行左和右心房房扑以及房颤的消融。当然，应用解剖标测或导管跟踪系统，以及通过心内超声也有助于指导线性消融[32]。

（二）线性消融的临床电生理

造成消融线的传导阻滞是预测消融成功的关键临床指标。完全性阻滞能够完全阻断电传导，而如果消融线不完整则激动波可通过"间隙"跨线传导从而成为另外一种心律失常的"基质"，主要是心房扑动。评价线性传导情况的电生理标准有多个。在房颤时，可以通过评价阻滞线两侧电活动的关系来证实是否存在线性传导阻滞，也可根据沿消融线局部电图振幅的降低来进行推测，但是这些标准都不确切，所以需要转复为窦性节律后进一步评价。

心房激动波阵面遇到阻滞线后的传导变化是证实是否存在传导阻断的重要证据。通过在消融线两侧进行起搏以增加激动时间的变化程度将有助于判断。由于心房激动在二维心房组织呈放射状扩布，从而同时出现两个波阵面，因此最早遇到阻滞线的波阵其传导方向的改变将最为显著。所以要证实是否存在局部房内传导阻滞，窦性节律经常不适合，而需要在邻近传导径线的特殊部位进行起搏。在消融线没有与一个解剖阻滞区连接的情况下，消融线一侧中间是理想的起搏部位。如果传导径线与较大的障碍物连接（房室环），那么起搏部位应该移向这个连接部位（例如，接近三尖瓣环或者二尖瓣环），右心房明显不同于左心房，右心房预先存在由界嵴形成较长的缓慢传导区，由于其他的传导径线的参与从而扩展了电活动的绕行路径。通过在传导线路上或其周围进行标测，使用不同标准可以确定线性传导阻滞的发生。

1. 心房激动的绕行

由线性传导阻滞产生电活动的绕行依赖于以下几个因素：(1) 电活动的起源部位；(2) 线性传导径线的长度或与其他传导径线间的相互连接；(3) 传导径线与解剖障碍物连接；以及 (4) 沿绕行路径不同部分的传导速度。

使用同步记录比序列记录能更容易进行全面的等时标测。传统的多极导管、篮状导管或三维标测系统均能用于标测，但需要覆盖所有的电活动绕行路径，以便能根据特征性的电传导变化来判断是否出现线性阻滞。然而，如果标测电极的部位远离了消融线，则可能标测不到，通常必须邻近消融线才能够标测到传导"缝隙"。

记录最早和最晚电活动发生的两个部位，可以简

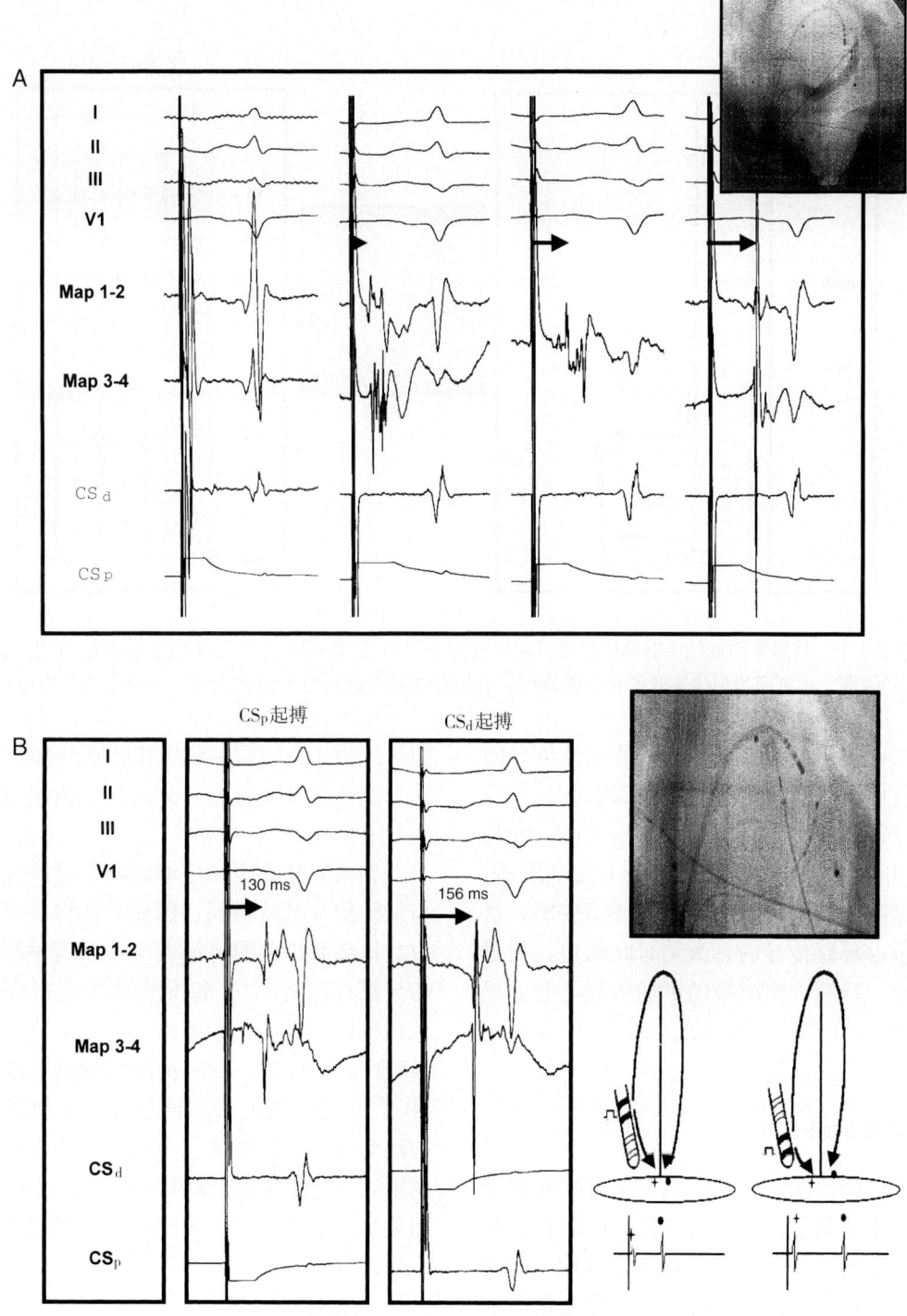

图 112-4　二尖瓣峡部消融中确定线性传导阻滞的特征　A：在二尖瓣峡部消融中，冠状窦近端（CS$_p$）起搏下可见心内膜标测导管电图以及心外膜的冠状窦远端（CS$_d$）电图有传导的逐步延迟。B：显示冠状窦起搏时不同部位的图形变化情况（见正文）。（接下页）

单估计电活动的绕行路径。可以通过测量阻滞线两侧的局部电图与参照点（如人工刺激信号）的距离加以判断，也可用跨阻滞线的多极导管，或者位于阻滞线上的双极导管进行标测和判断。在左房，冠状窦对于判断与二尖瓣环相连接阻滞线的传导情况最为重要（图 112-4）。如果多极导管覆盖传导线路，只要在术中监测阻滞线近端的局部电图动态变化即可推测消融线的阻滞情况。

经传导径线绕行的电活动与通过传导径线间缝隙传导的电活动，两者的传导时间是不同的（图 112-4）。

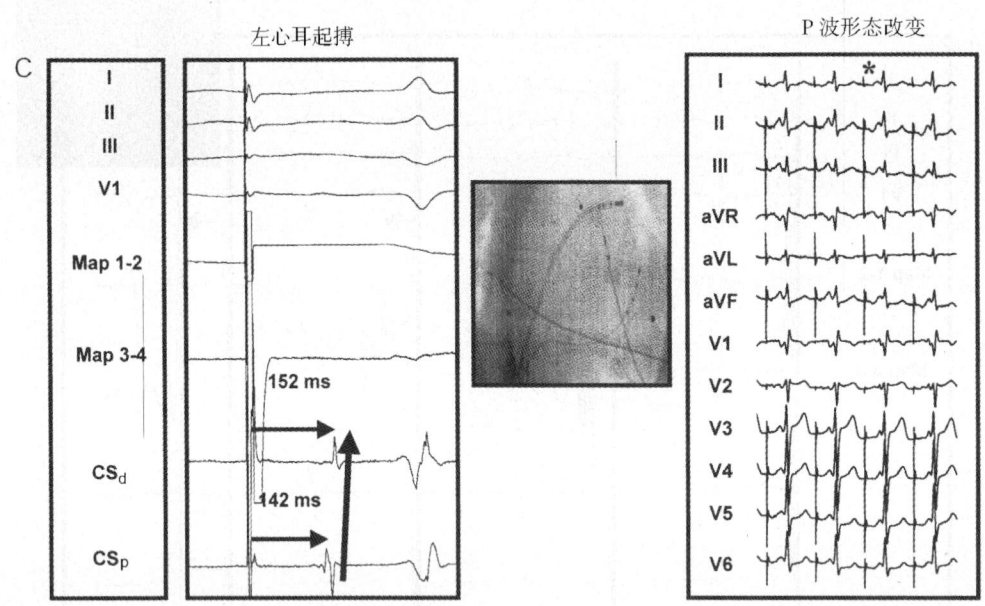

图 112-4 （续上页）C：从阻滞消融径线的侧壁起搏（此例在左心耳），导致冠状窦由近端到远端的电活动，意味着在二尖瓣峡部出现双向峡部阻滞。也证明当二尖瓣峡部传导阻滞时，在冠状窦近端起搏时 P 波的变化。＊显示传导阻滞时 P 波的变化。

传导时间短于某一数值说明存在不完全的线性传导阻滞；例如，阵发性房颤患者在二尖瓣峡部消融后产生消融线完全传导阻滞的传导时间为 153 ± 27 ms，如低于 100ms 则说明阻滞线不完全，即存在不完全阻滞。消融径线上有缝隙存在能使激动的折返环路变短，从而造成环绕该折返环路传导的总激动时间缩短，如果起搏部位邻近这一缝隙，则缩短的更加明显，而如果起搏部位远离这一缝隙，这种判断标准则缺少特异性。

2. 局部电图和向量标测

在传导径线两侧记录到的电位形态可为判断激动的传导方向提供重要信息。在径线上进行单极和双极标测也可判断激动的传导是绕行还是跨线进行。一个完全绕行的电活动在起始点起搏时为一个完全负向的单极电图，在终点起搏则为完全正向的单极电图。如果激动传导方向不变以及双极记录电极连接的顺序不变，则双极电图可见极性的反转。

双电位的出现被证明是解剖或功能上存在线性传导阻滞的标志。双电位之间的等电位间期等于电活动从一端到另一端的传导时间。因而，双电位发生间期较窄或碎裂的电图可以确定线性消融不完整。通过在消融线上行双电位标测能揭示在传导径路上应用其他判断标准易被遗漏的呈缓慢传导的缝隙（有时这一间隙可以很小）。在心房组织最厚的部分，缝隙可能与深部的解剖裂隙有关，此时在心内膜也能记录到宽大的双电位。

如果缝隙间传导足够缓慢，其跨线传导时间可以与绕线传导时间相同。因而，选择一个理想的起搏部位并仔细分析电图特征对于识别缓慢跨线传导和绕线传导很有意义[33]。将导管放置在可疑缝隙附近能够识别缓慢传导和单向阻滞，依次从远端向近端进行双极顺序心房起搏，同时记录传导路上的电位（图 112-4B）。从远端到近端起搏增加了从刺激到第一个电位的活动时间。如果第二个电位由于慢传导发生，那么到第二个电位的传导时间也增加（有相似的增加），如果第二个电位是由于线性传导阻滞而绕行产生，那么传导时间减少。

3. 心电图变化

与房扑消融一样（图 112-4C）[34]，房颤所需的消融径线也经常很长，以至于可改变体表心电图的 P 波形态。此外，激动起源点与消融径线的距离对体表心电图 P 波的影响非常重要。三尖瓣峡部或左房侧壁（例如左下肺静脉到二尖瓣环）的消融径线一般不能改变窦性心律的 P 波，因为两个径线的位置均与窦性心律的起源点较远，传导的波阵面在各自的心腔形成融合，因此需要行起搏以判断消融线。消融径线与初始心房激动波阵的相互干扰，如上腔静脉到右房前壁三尖瓣环以及到 Bachmann 束左房终端的消融，会造成窦性节律时 P 波形态的改变。如果消融径线方向垂直于三尖瓣或二尖瓣环，则心电图Ⅱ、Ⅲ和 aVF 导联的 P 波形态变化最明显。在形成完全线性传导阻滞时多会伴有 P 波的快速而明显的变化，然而，如果为持续的缓慢传导则 P 波的变化往往不明显或没有变化。因此，需要结合心电生理指标进一步确认线性阻滞发生与否。一旦能够确定 P 波形态的改变，即使没有心内记录，也能通过对 P 波形态的监测来证实线性传导阻滞的稳定性。

（三）心房线性消融的临床经验

人们一直尝试通过几种消融径线的组合来找出一种既简单又安全，既适用于多数患者又能达到根治房颤目的的消融方案。

1. 右心房线性消融隔离的效果

鉴于安全因素，线性消融最初应用于右心房。有 3 个系列研究对 45 例患者进行了复杂的右心房线性消融（图 112-5A）[5]。右心房消融使得局部心房电活动变为规律，其中的 18 例患者（40%）在术中恢复稳定的窦性节律。然而，90 条消融线中仅 4 条（5%）达到了线性传导阻滞，这是线性消融存在的主要问题。45 例持续性房颤患者中 40 例仍然可诱发房颤。70% 的病例发现了以前未曾诊断的典型房扑，并需要进一步以三尖瓣峡部为靶点继续进行消融。尽管 24 例患者（53%）在中期得到一些改善，但在 26±5 个月的随访中，仅 11% 在未用药物控制下无房颤的发作[35]。然而有趣的是，其中 4 例复发的患者在进一步的观察中没有再次发作的症状。对 10 例有症状的复发患者进行了左心房消融[5]，从而第一次发现了肺静脉触发灶的存在，以及认识到除了线性消融外还应该对触发的局灶进行消融，但使用传统的导管并不能达到完全的线性阻滞。

Gaita 等[36]报道了进行右心房线性消融的 16 例阵发性房颤患者，结果在消融后随访 11±4 个月 56% 没有房颤复发。Garg 等[37]对 12 例阵发性房颤患者进行右房线性消融，在随访 12.6±13 个月中仅 1 例未复发房颤。Ernst 等[38]对 32 例患者在电解剖标测指导下进行右房线性消融。术后对 27 例患者的消融线效果进行统计，证明 16 例（59%）产生完全峡部消融线，12 例产生前壁消融线，4 例产生腔静脉间消融线。32

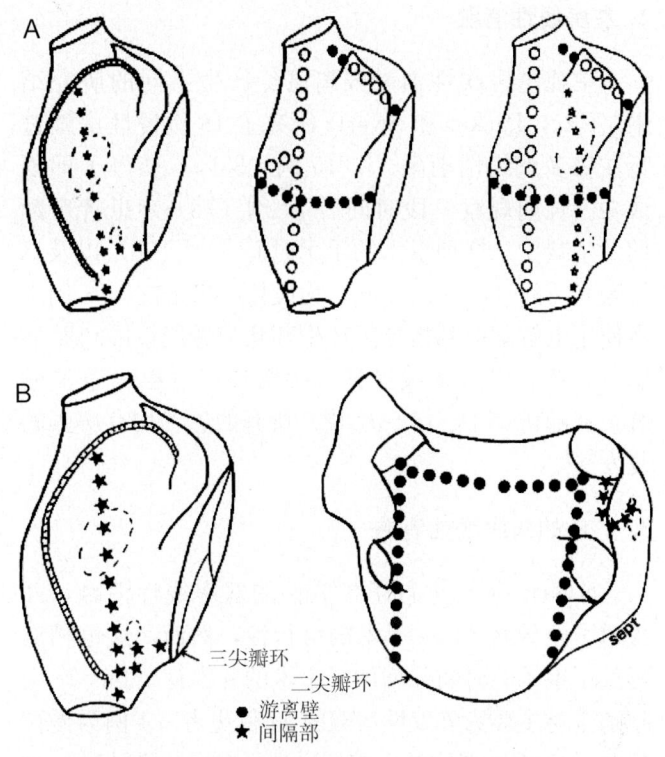

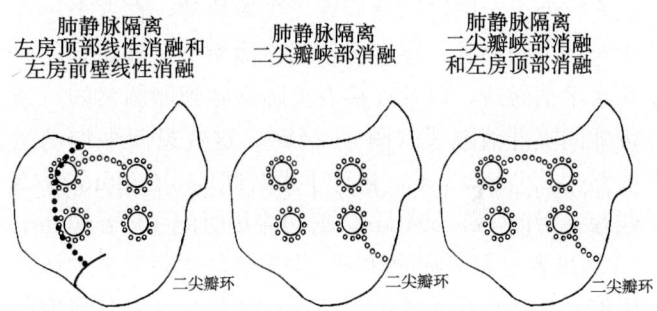

图 112-5　Bordeaux 研究的线性消融序列　A：复杂的右房消融隔离。B：扩大的双房消融。C：结合右房三尖瓣峡部消融的局限性双房消融。

例中除 2 例外包括右房水平消融的患者均出现了房颤的复发。

尽管这些研究已经清楚地显示了右房线性消融隔离治愈房颤的益处是有限的，但是能够辨别出发生房颤的基质可能位于右房内的一些患者，例如界嵴[39]，或者在左房消融后房颤复发时右房可能是额外触发因素的一些患者，以及可能受益于局限于右房内消融的一些患者，这一点很重要。一些研究也已显示在三尖瓣峡部成功消融后，随后的房颤发生率降低，意味着房扑促进房颤的发生，而且是由于经峡部颤动波样的传导形成的微折返环所致。

2. 左房线性消融

单纯左房线性消融隔离已经产生不同的研究结果。Kay，Packer和Swartz研究了18例慢性房颤进行左房多重线性消融[40]。15例（83%）获得了即刻成功。长期观察一段时间后14例（78%）患者房颤的发生减少。这种手术的手术时间（8~15h）以及X线曝光时间（30~210min）均很长。相比较，13例患者使用电解剖标测指导下产生环状消融线以隔离肺静脉口，然后将这条线连到二尖瓣环产生第二条消融线，在随访26天（1~47周）所有的患者均有房颤的复发[38]。

3. 广泛的双房线性消融

Swartz等[40]进行了扩展性的双房线性消融，并报道了经导管Maze手术的可行性，然而，这也相应延长了手术的时间并增加了手术的并发症。Jais等[41]报道了对主要为阵发性房颤的44例患者（4例为慢性房颤，11例有器质性心脏病）进行双房线性消融。在右房，消融仅限于间隔部和三尖瓣峡部。在左房消融线连接两个上肺静脉然后到二尖瓣峡部，在这个过程中包括下肺静脉、在左房顶部连接两个上肺静脉的一条水平消融线，以及连接右上肺静脉到卵圆窝的一条额外间隔部消融线（图112-5B），这些患者平均消融线路为2.7±1.3条，累计手术时间615±345min，X线曝光时间171±94min，射频应用时间104±56min。13例患者由右上肺静脉到二尖瓣峡部达到完全的线性阻滞，4例患者经过了顶部，1例患者为左上肺静脉到二尖瓣间的消融线。31例患者可观察到左心房房扑，主要由于通过不完全的消融线而传播的微折返。29例患者由局灶触发，主要来源于肺静脉。使用这种方法，不用药物情况下维持窦性节律的成功率达57%，而再次应用以前无效的抗心律失常药物其成功率则增加到84%。然而，术中可观察到明显的并发症，5例患者发生心包积液，1例发生肺静脉血栓，1例发生下壁心肌梗死，1例发生左肺静脉阻塞，1例发生可逆转的脑卒中。

Pappone等[42]应用电生理标测行3条右房消融线（三尖瓣峡部、腔静脉间和前壁至房间隔）结合环肺静脉的一个长消融线。手术时间为312±103min，X线曝光时间107±44min。随访10±3个月后，27例患者中16例无症状发作（4例应用抗心律失常药物）。Ernst等[38]对12例患者使用电解剖标测和相似的线性消融路径没有产生相似的结果，仅1例患者产生完全的线性传导阻滞，所有的患者均有房颤的复发。

对广泛的双房线性消融的这些研究已经证明很难产生完全的线性消融阻滞，同时手术及X线曝光时间过长。患者由于不完全的消融线产生左房扑动，从而需要频繁的进一步消融手术治疗。最终，这种消融产生了明显的手术并发症。

4. 有限性的双房线性消融

为提高临床结果并使房颤导管消融更多地应用于临床，我们实验室除彻底行肺静脉电隔离外，对不同的线性消融路径和三尖瓣峡部消融进行了评价。

前壁心房间连接的水平消融线：动物模型显示心房间连接在房颤发生的基质中起着关键的作用[43,44]。对24例阵发性房颤（16例）或者慢性房颤患者（8例）前壁心房间连接（Bachmann束）的水平消融线进行评价。连接两上肺静脉间进行线性消融，然后这条消融线再连接到前壁二尖瓣环以打断整个前壁房间传导束（图112-5C）。并同时进行肺静脉电隔离和三尖瓣峡部消融。通过证实电活动经过后壁到达后侧壁，最后到达左房的前壁来确定线性阻滞。20例患者在房颤发生中进行消融，12例患者在进行前壁房间水平消融时房颤终止。然而，仅在14例患者（58%）中证实达到了完全的线性消融，手术时间为187±102min，X线曝光时间为54±26min，包括42±16min的射频能量应用时间。在24±4个月的随访中，14例患者（58%）需要进一步的消融，16例患者（67%）未用抗心律失常药物的情况下维持窦性节律。

尽管这种方法对中止房颤是有效的，但其局限性是有较高的复发率及线性消融的不完全性，与窦律时体表心电图观察到的一样，可产生左房电活动的不一致性以及活动延迟，这可能导致血流动力学的不稳定。

二尖瓣峡部消融：二尖瓣峡部（左下肺静脉或心耳到二尖瓣环）是改变基质很重要的靶点，因为它的长度很短并接近于冠状窦使导管容易定位从而易达到线性传导阻滞。对复发的163例房颤患者进行二尖瓣峡部的消融，最初应用在肺静脉隔离后的房颤复发患者，然后在手术中常规加入。对所有的患者进行肺静脉电隔离和三尖瓣峡部消融。在连接左下肺静脉到二尖瓣环的侧壁进行二尖瓣峡部消融（图112-5C）[45]。在二尖瓣环的消融以电图1∶1到2∶1的房室比例开始，然后在心内膜拖拽到左下肺静脉口（图112-4A）。

最初的心内膜消融能量在40~60W间进行，但是考虑安全的因素在后来的系列研究中减少到最大为42W。为确保理想的能量发放将导管灌注增加到60ml/min。当接近肺静脉口部或左心耳时仔细操作以避免导管误入这些结构。通过双电位的出现（在冠状窦起搏中，发生电位的逐渐延迟，图112-4A）来监测消融，并在传导路的一侧起搏或通过不同的起搏技术来确定电活动的绕行（图112-4B和C）。在52例患者（32％）中，21±11min的心内膜消融达到了二尖瓣峡部传导阻滞。对遗留持续的峡部传导患者中，106例患者（64％）在冠状窦内标测显示有心外膜传导的证据，消融能量为20~30W，流速为30~60ml/min。在心外膜应用5±4min的射频消融，使93例患者发生传导阻滞。5例患者心内膜消融后没有达到传导阻滞，心外膜消融未能进行，因为导管不能在冠状窦的远端进行消融操作。89％的二尖瓣峡部消融病例被证实成功地产生了传导阻滞，手术时间为176±61min，X线曝光时间为51±21min，包括65±26min的射频能量应用时间。在随访7±3个月中，133例患者（82％）在未用抗心律失常药物的情况下没有房颤发作，应用以前无效的药物则成功率可达到85％。

重要的是，尽管在冠状窦起搏中有明显的电活动绕行，在窦律下二尖瓣峡部消融的结果没有使心房电活动发生变化。然而，这个手术明显的并发症是心包填塞，6例患者（3.6％）在术中需要心包引流。其中2例患者在左房的导管操作中发生，3例患者在二尖瓣峡部心内膜高能量的消融中发生（2例可听见爆裂声），1例患者发生在三尖瓣峡部消融的过程中。随着心内膜发放最大能量的减低，并发症没有进一步发生。在冠状窦内的消融已引起重视，尤其是对冠状动脉的损害，但所有的患者需经最大运动负荷试验或者冠状动脉造影筛选除外有狭窄的迹象。世界范围的报道显示心包填塞的危险因素明显与心房线性消融相关（6.1％）[40]，对技术重要性的不断强调和导管技术的发展可能有助于将来的治疗。

根据应用这种治疗的30例慢性房颤（79±57个月）的初步数据显示，在6±5个月的短期随访中，24例患者（80％）维持窦性心律，其中18例没有应用抗心律失常药物。应用解剖标测系统指导消融便于这种手术进行，可减少手术时间（40±18min、62±36min）、X线曝光时间（9±4min、19±10min）以及射频能量应用时间（20±12min、30±15min）。

基质改良的合理方法： 由于心房线性消融在技术上存在挑战，不完全的消融可能导致心律失常的产生，因此需要我们术前来判断哪些病例能从基质改良的治疗中受益。我们已经发现尽管进行了成功的肺静脉隔离，但房颤发作持续时间＞24h以及心房较大（纵行直径＞57mm）的患者更容易出现房颤的复发。此外，在肺静脉电隔离后持续性房颤的可诱发性与临床近50％的房颤复发相关。这些患者为达到房颤的临床治愈需要进一步改良基质的治疗。相反，术中不能诱发房颤的患者其复发率仅为20％，且主要是由于肺静脉传导的恢复。根据正在进行的前瞻性研究认为，预测需进一步改良基质的合理方法是肺静脉隔离后持续性房颤的可诱发性，消融术后房颤的不能诱发是判断房颤消融手术终点的有效办法。

三、总　结

近10年来，我们对房颤的理解已经有了明显的发展，导管消融技术已经证明可治愈房颤。局限于肺静脉和可标测的非肺静脉病灶的消融能使阵发性房颤的治愈成功率接近70％，在慢性房颤患者则较低一些，这一结果因附加基质改良的治疗而得到了进一步的改善。尽管许多患者在未用抗心律失常药物的情况下仍可维持窦性节律，症状因此减轻，然而为了进一步增加适应证和使得这一技术得到更大发展，还需要进一步的研究以证实是否能够降低血栓事件的风险，或者与其他治疗方法相比能否进一步提高生存率。

（杨延宗　刘　莹　译）

参考文献

1. Benjamin EJ, Wolf PA, D'Agostino RB, et al: Impact of atrial fibrillation on the risk of death: The Framingham Heart Study. Circulation 98:946-952, 1998.
2. Hohnloser SH, Kuck KH, Lilienthal J, for the PIAF investigators: Rhythm or rate control in atrial fibrillation—pharmacological intervention in atrial fibrillation (PIAF): A randomised trial. Lancet 356:1789-1794, 2000.
3. The atrial fibrillation follow-up investigation of rhythm management (AFFIRM) investigators: A comparison of rate control and rhythm control in patients with atrial fibrillation. N Engl J Med 347:1825-1833, 2002.
4. Van Gelder IC, Hagens VE, Bosker HA, et al, for the rate control versus electrical cardioversion for persistent atrial fibrillation study group. A comparison of rate control and rhythm control in patients with recurrent persistent atrial fibrillation. N Engl J Med 347:1834-1840, 2002.
5. Haissaguerre M, Jais P, Shah DC, et al: Right and left atrial radiofrequency catheter therapy of paroxysmal atrial fibrillation. J Cardiovasc Electrophysiol 7:1132-1144, 1996.
6. Haissaguerre M, Jais P, Shah DC, et al: Spontaneous initiation of atrial fibrillation by ectopic beats originating in the pulmonary veins.

N Engl J Med 339:659–666, 1998.
7. Jais P, Haissaguerre M, Shah DC, et al: A focal source of atrial fibrillation treated by discrete radiofrequency ablation. Circulation 95:572–576, 1997.
8. Chen SA, Hsieh MH, Tai CT, et al: Initiation of atrial fibrillation by ectopic beats originating from the pulmonary veins: Electrophysiological characteristics, pharmacological responses, and effects of radiofrequency ablation. Circulation 100:1879–1886, 1999.
9. Hwang C, Wu TJ, Doshi RN, et al: Vein of Marshall cannulation for the analysis of electrical activity in patients with focal atrial fibrillation. Circulation 101:1503–1505, 2000.
10. Chen SA, Tai CT, Yu WC, et al: Right atrial focal atrial fibrillation: Electrophysiologic characteristics and radiofrequency catheter ablation. J Cardiovasc Electrophysiol 10:328–335, 1999.
11. Lau CP, Tse HF, Ayers GM: Defibrillation-guided radiofrequency ablation of atrial fibrillation secondary to an atrial focus. J Am Coll Cardiol 33:1217–1226, 1999.
12. Oral H, Knight BP, Özaydin M, et al: Segmental ostial ablation to isolate the pulmonary veins during atrial fibrillation: feasibility and mechanistic insights. Circulation 106:1256–1262, 2002.
13. Haissaguerre M, Jais P, Shah DC, et al: Catheter ablation of chronic atrial fibrillation targeting the reinitiating triggers. J Cardiovasc Electrophysiol 11:2–10, 2000.
14. Hocini M, Haissaguerre M, Shah D, et al: Multiple sources initiating atrial fibrillation from a single pulmonary vein identified by a circumferential catheter. Pacing Clin Electrophysiol 23:1828–1831, 2000.
15. Gerstenfeld EP, Guerra P, Sparks PB, et al: Clinical outcome after radiofrequency catheter ablation of focal atrial fibrillation triggers. J Cardiovasc Electrophysiol 12:900–908, 2001.
16. Sanders P, Morton JB, Deen VR, et al: Immediate and long-term results of radiofrequency ablation of pulmonary vein ectopy for cure of paroxysmal atrial fibrillation using a focal approach. Intern Med J 32:202–207, 2002.
17. Haissaguerre M, Shah DC, Jais P, et al: Electrophysiological breakthroughs from the left atrium to the pulmonary veins. Circulation 102:2463–2465, 2000.
18. Macle L, Jais P, Weerasooriya R, et al: Irrigated-tip catheter ablation of pulmonary veins for treatment of atrial fibrillation. J Cardiovasc Electrophysiol 13:1067–1073, 2002.
19. Hocini M, Shah DC, Jais P, et al: Concealed left pulmonary vein potentials unmasked by left atrial stimulation. Pacing Clin Electrophysiol 23:1832–1835, 2000.
20. Shah D, Haissaguerre M, Jais P, et al: Left atrial appendage activity masquerading as pulmonary vein potentials. Circulation 105:2821–2825, 2002.
21. Yamane T, Shah DC, Jais P, et al: Electrogram polarity reversal as an additional indicator of breakthroughs from the left atrium to the pulmonary veins. J Am Coll Cardiol 39:1337–1344, 2002.
22. Natale A, Pisano E, Shewchik J, et al: First human experience with pulmonary vein isolation using a through-the-balloon circumferential ultrasound ablation system for recurrent atrial fibrillation. Circulation 102:1879–1882, 2000.
23. Stabile G, Turco P, La Rocca V, et al: Is pulmonary vein isolation necessary for curing atrial fibrillation? Circulation 108:657–660, 2003.
24. Pappone C, Rosanio S, Augello G, et al: Mortality, morbidity, and quality of life after circumferential pulmonary vein ablation for atrial fibrillation: outcomes from a controlled nonrandomized long-term study. J Am Coll Cardiol 42:185–197, 2003.
25. Oral H, Knight BP, Tada H, et al: Pulmonary vein isolation for paroxysmal and persistent atrial fibrillation. Circulation 105:1077–1081, 2002.
26. Robbins IM, Colvin EV, Doyle TP, et al: Pulmonary vein stenosis after catheter ablation of atrial fibrillation. Circulation 98:1769–1775, 1998.
27. Kanagaratnam L, Tomassoni G, Schweikert R, et al: Empirical pulmonary vein isolation in patients with chronic atrial fibrillation using a three-dimensional nonfluoroscopic mapping system: Long-term follow-up. Pacing Clin Electrophysiol 24:1774–1779, 2001.
28. Allessie MA, Boyden PA, Camm AJ, et al: Pathophysiology and prevention of atrial fibrillation. Circulation 103:769–777, 2001.
29. Cox JL, Ad N, Palazzo T, et al: Current status of the Maze procedure for the treatment of atrial fibrillation. Semin Thorac Cardiovasc Surg 12:15–19, 2000.
30. Mackey S, Thornton L, He DS, et al: Simultaneous multielectrode radiofrequency ablation in the monopolar mode increases lesion size. Pacing Clin Electrophysiol 19:1042–1048, 1996.
31. Nakagawa H, Yamanashi WS, Pitha JV, et al: Comparison of in vivo tissue temperature profile and lesion geometry for radiofrequency ablation with a saline-irrigated electrode versus temperature control in a canine thigh muscle preparation. Circulation 91:2264–2273, 1995.
32. Olgin JE, Kalman JM, Chin M, et al: Electrophysiological effects of long, linear atrial lesions placed under intracardiac ultrasound guidance. Circulation 96:2715–2721, 1997.
33. Shah D, Haissaguerre M, Takahashi A, et al: Differential pacing for distinguishing block from persistent conduction through an ablation line. Circulation 102:1517–1522, 2000.
34. Hamdan MH, Kalman JM, Barron HV, Lesh MD: P-wave morphology during right atrial pacing before and after atrial flutter ablation—a new marker for success. Am J Cardiol 79:1417–1420, 1997.
35. Jais P, Shah DC, Takahashi A, et al: Long-term follow-up after right atrial radiofrequency catheter treatment of paroxysmal atrial fibrillation. Pacing Clin Electrophysiol 21:2533–2538, 1998.
36. Gaita F, Riccardi R, Calo L, et al: Atrial mapping and radiofrequency catheter ablation in patients with idiopathic atrial fibrillation. Electrophysiological findings and ablation results. Circulation 97:2136–2145, 1998.
37. Garg A, Finneran W, Mollerus M, et al: Right atrial compartmentalization using radiofrequency catheter ablation for management of patients with refractory atrial fibrillation. J Cardiovasc Electrophysiol 10:763–771, 1999.
38. Ernst S, Schluter M, Ouyang F, et al: Modification of the substrate for maintenance of idiopathic human atrial fibrillation: Efficacy of radiofrequency ablation using nonfluoroscopic catheter guidance. Circulation 100:2085–2092, 1999.
39. Liu TY, Tai CT, Chen SA: Treatment of atrial fibrillation by catheter ablation of conduction gaps in the crista terminalis and cavotricuspid isthmus of the right atrium. J Cardiovasc Electrophysiol 13:1044–1046, 2002.
40. Packer DL: Linear ablation for atrial fibrillation: The pendulum swings back. In Zipes DP, Haissaguerre M (eds): Catheter Ablation of Atrial Arrhythmias. Armonk, NY, Futura Publishing, 2002, pp 107–128.
41. Jais P, Shah DC, Haissaguerre M, et al: Efficacy and safety of septal and left-atrial linear ablation for atrial fibrillation. Am J Cardiol 84:139R–146R, 1999.
42. Pappone C, Oreto G, Lamberti F, et al: Catheter ablation of paroxysmal atrial fibrillation using a 3D mapping system. Circulation 100:1203–1208, 1999.
43. Kumagai K, Uno K, Khrestian C, Waldo AL: Single site radiofrequency catheter ablation of atrial fibrillation: Studies guided by simultaneous multisite mapping in the canine sterile pericarditis model. J Am Coll Cardiol 36:917–923, 2000.
44. Betts TR, Roberts PR, Morgan JM: Feasibility of a left atrial electrical disconnection procedure for atrial fibrillation using transcatheter radiofrequency ablation. J Cardiovasc Electrophysiol 12:1278–1283, 2001.
45. Jais P, Hocini M, Weerasooriya R, et al: Left atrial isthmus ablation: Technique and results in patients with atrial fibrillation [abstract]. Circulation 106(Suppl II):II-501, 2002.

第 113 章

心房颤动的肺静脉隔离

Carlo Pappone，*Salvatore Rosanio*

本章目录

- 组织学背景 …………………… 1015
- 适于导管消融的病理生理基质 …… 1016
- 消融技术 ……………………… 1020
- 结果 …………………………… 1024
- 讨论 …………………………… 1025
- 总结 …………………………… 1026
- 致谢 …………………………… 1027

正如 AFFIRM 试验（持续性心房颤动节律控制的随访研究）和 RACE 试验（心房颤动室率控制和电转律治疗的比较研究）[1,2]研究结果所显示的，尽管不断有新的具有更高选择性的药物[3,4]研发出来，通过目前现有的药物治疗心房颤动（房颤）安全而有效地获得并维持窦性心律仍十分困难。药物治疗房颤的相对无效性、抗心律失常药物致心律失常的副作用，以及对房颤恶化健康效应的进一步认识[5]，均推动了寻找能够彻底恢复窦性心律、根治房颤方法的研究。

因此，目前对这种心律失常的治疗变得更加积极，而且治疗方法转向了非药物手段，包括对心律失常发生和维持基质的适度改良——即所谓的消融治疗[6-9]。

对心律失常发生和维持机制的不断深入认识，以及标测和成像技术的不断改进和提高，使得目前关注的方向集中在对消融靶点的选择和确定上。其目的是希望最终将所有症状性和耐药性房颤全部划归在适于导管消融治疗的范围内。

肺静脉（PV）消融根治房颤有多种导管消融方法和消融能量可以采用[10-17]，但在本章中我们主要介绍应用射频能量的环肺静脉消融[16,17]，并总结我们中心成功消融治疗 2000 例房颤的方法和经验。

一、组织学背景

在过去的 10 年里，房颤导管治疗方法持续而稳步地改进更新。线性射频消融治疗房颤的最初概念来源于 Moe 的早期观察[18]。在 20 世纪 50 年代末，Moe 强调了多子波折返在房颤维持中的作用，认为心房组织的大小是颤动波能够维持的关键因素。这一理论学说由 Allessie 及其同事进一步发展，并提出一个重要概念——折返波长[19]。

这些电生理概念最初推动了外科在进行二尖瓣病变手术同时进行房颤的恢复窦律治疗技术的开展。迷宫术[20]即是由 Cox 及其合作者在 1987 年设计出来的，试图用外科途径将心房分割成多个豆腐块，使颤动波无法维持下去。这一术式经过不断改良、简化，手术疗效不断提高，有报道 98% 以上的患者长期随访无房颤复发。

因此，有人开始尝试在心内膜复制类似外科迷宫手术的射频能分割心房——导管迷宫术，通过点-点消融连线来治疗对药物无效的房颤[21-23]。

考虑到右房风险小于左房，消融方法最开始仅限于右房，但这一术式并未能得到广泛应用[21,22]。一些研究显示折返环或异位病灶大多位于左房后壁，并不在右房。基于左房作为房颤的主要电主导腔的假设，那么应该通过导管穿间隔技术在左房的这一区域进行消融。结果表明，在左房这一区域消融，成功率可达到60%以上[23]。

近5年在房颤病理生理方面的一个重要进展为发现并证实部分阵发性房颤患者的心律失常起源于肺静脉内的类似心房肌的组织，同时强调左房是房颤的主导腔（driving chamber）[24,25]。

认识到肺静脉内存在房颤的触发源，并可能同时起着维持房颤的作用，那么将肺静脉从左房内电隔离出来的治疗技术继之开展起来，而且获得了成功。单纯阻断肺静脉电连接治疗阵发性房颤的成功率约为70%。目前已经清楚地认识到房颤是左房疾病，左房后壁关键部位更广泛的消融策略不仅使阵发性房颤而且使慢性房颤的消融治疗也获得成功[10-17]。表113-1总结了不同试验中房颤消融的结果。

二、适于导管消融的病理生理基质

关于目前已迅速成为心律失常领域中研究热点的房颤病因，在本书其他章节中有更深入的讨论，不是本章阐述的范围。但为了阐明这一疾病的病理发生过程，在此作一简述。

自1994年陆续有几个报道证实起源于局灶的小而快速的异位激动可以触发阵发性房颤的理论[24,25]。这些触发灶大多位于肺静脉内，虽然肺静脉在整个心脏的轮廓之外，但其内壁上却有延伸出来的心肌袖；这些触发灶是阵发性房颤的主要原因，它可以通过一个小折返环机制也可能是通过其他非折返机制触发房颤。这些病灶的电活动可以直接表现为类似体表ECG上房颤的无规律颤动，或者更为常见，由一阵短阵的超速异位活动蜕变成或触发出经典的房颤[24,25]。

肺静脉-左房交界部位的解剖和电生理特点可以解释房颤病理机制许多方面的问题[26,27]。正常的左房心肌纤维可以以环状、螺旋状或斜形延伸进入肺静脉内几厘米，上肺静脉较下肺静脉多见。延伸进入肺静脉的心肌组织在直径、厚度、延伸或环绕肺静脉的程度上（即肌袖长度）均有显著差异，肌袖间为纤维组织缝隙。另外，肺静脉内的心肌结构也具有很大差异，

表113-1 心房颤动的导管消融研究

作者	年份	例数	AF类型	指导仪器	消融方法	总的无AF发生率（%）*	随访时间（月）
Haissaguerre 等[22]	1996	45	PAF	Fluoro	线性消融		11±4
					RA	33	
					双房	60	
Maloney 等[21]	1998	15	CAF	Fluoro	线性消融		23±10
					RA	81	
Haissaguerre 等[14]	1998	45	PAF	Fluoro	局灶性PV消融	62	8±6
Papponne 等[22]	1999	27	PAF	CARTO	线性消融		11±3
					RA	50	
					LA	60	
					双房	85	
Ernst 等△	1999	45	PAF	CARTO	线性消融		1±1
					LA	0	
					双房	0	
Haissaguerre 等[15]	2000	70	PAF	Fluoro	节段性PV消融	73	4±
Papponne 等[16]	2000	26	PAF和CAF	CARTO	环PV消融	85	9±3
Papponne 等[17]	2001	251	PAF和CAF	CARTO	环PV消融	80	10±5
Oral 等[10]	2002	70	PAF和CAF	Fluoro	节段性PV消融	63	6±3

* 无房颤复发患者的比例为报道的最大成功率，伴或不伴抗心律失常药物治疗。

△ Ernst S, Schluter M, Ouyang F, et al. Modification of the substrate for maintenance of idiopathic human atrial fibrillation. Circulation 100: 2085-209, 1999.

AF, 心房颤动（房颤）；CAF, 慢性房颤；Fluoro, 透视；PAF, 阵发性房颤；PV, 肺静脉；RA, 右房；LA, 左房。

其复杂的网络状交错排列、牵张、纤维化的增加，均可导致显著非均一的、各向异性的电生理特性。因此，环肺静脉的心肌纤维的几何排列，或者由于血管平滑肌上覆盖的心肌组织耦联较差，以及这些心房肌袖组织不同部位不应期的差异，均使肺静脉成为折返活动形成的有利地带。纤维化改变更常见于老年患者，可以引起传导阻滞、折返和缓慢传导。所有这些特点可以导致波阵面的不连续扩布，是肺静脉内早搏和心动过速频繁出现传出阻滞的前提。房颤可以由肺静脉内的快速房性心动过速开始，后者导致的重构促进了心动过速向多环路折返的演变。近来已证实肺静脉内的快速电活动可以由房性心动过速的重构效应进一步强化而具有维持房颤（不仅仅是触发房颤）的作用[28]。

需要指出，所有 4 个肺静脉均可成为异位激动的灶源而触发房颤，而且在 14% 的患者中可以发现不同肺静脉间存在着电连接[29]。事实上肺静脉的解剖检查证实，同侧肺静脉口之间的心房肌长度可为 7.3mm，也可短至 3mm 以下，且约有 40% 小于 3mm。这一发现提示相邻肺静脉间的心肌可以是连续的，因为组织学检查证实上肺静脉和下肺静脉之间的肺静脉肌束存在相互交叉[26]现象，尤其是在肺静脉口之间有较窄峡部的患者中。这一发现可以解释肺静脉间传导的解剖学基础[29]。

而且，组织学、电生理以及免疫组织学方法均提示肺静脉-左房交界部位存在具有起搏功能特征的心肌细胞[30,31]。胚胎学家对静脉窦段（sinus venosus segment）在肺静脉形成时的作用有争议。有研究显示结样细胞存在于环肺静脉的心肌中。这一区域的起搏电活动在荷兰猪试验中已得到证实。HNK-1 抗原是用于人类胚胎发育过程中显示心脏传导系统的标记物，在肺静脉共干（common PV）周围心肌组织有这一标记物的一过性表达。尽管这些发现提示肺静脉内或环肺静脉区域可能存在起搏细胞的电活动，但问题是为什么这一区域的起搏细胞在人类心脏保持休眠状态如此之久？为什么异位活动仅在有限数量的患者中表现出来？事实上，这些心肌袖的致心律失常特性可能由于或者部分由于它们的胚胎来源与传导系统具有相同的基质，因而容易出现异常的自律性。但是，目前尚不清楚肺静脉起源的心律失常是由自律性、折返还是触发活动所引起，而且很可能是多种机制在这些心律失常的发生中共同起着作用。

标测并选择性地消融这些快速发放电活动的心律失常病灶则有可能治愈房颤，尽管理论上很诱人，但是这种局灶点消融是一种非常困难的方法，其手术时间和射线曝光时间均延长，常需二次消融，手术中常没有足够的心房异位激动可供标测，而且可发生严重并发症，最常见为肺静脉狭窄。因此，尽管这种方法消融结果令人鼓舞，但准确标测肺静脉内的靶点比较困难，阻碍了这一方法的广泛应用，目前这一方法不再常规采用[14,24,25]。

有人指出，尽管肺静脉肌袖覆盖肺静脉周围较大范围，但在左房内有特殊的突破口，仍可以通过最小范围的消融获得肺静脉口部的电隔离[15]。窦性心律时，肺静脉内心肌组织从不以环形同步激活，提示激动是从周边突破口进入静脉内。左房-肺静脉的突破口可以通过标测肺静脉口周围激动顺序来确定。通过标测和评价肺静脉电位的分布和激动顺序，可以进行肺静脉口部最早激动点的节段性消融，其隔离终点为在窦性心律或左房起搏时肺静脉电位消失[10,11,15]。但是，这一终点判定标准忽略了肺静脉口部由肺静脉向左房的传导阻滞情况，因而肺静脉口部节段性消融的范围小于实际心肌袖所覆盖的范围。

肺静脉口部节段性消融的主要局限在于，肺静脉不规则的几何结构使导管很难在口部同一基线上进行标测，这对解释所记录到的电图是一个挑战。而且，导管漂移有时可以误导术者对肺静脉口位置的判定。另外，这一术式不适用于在肺静脉口外的射频消融，因为后者要求做到完整的环形消融才能达到在远处隔离肺静脉。最后，肺静脉间电连接的存在、肺静脉口部周边新出现或暴露的局部病灶均是获得肺静脉彻底隔离所面临的挑战。

尽管房颤常起源于肺静脉已经得到清楚证实，但对持续性和永久性房颤的起源和维持仍是悬而未决的问题。这比局灶性或局灶诱发的房颤（易于消融，如阵发性房颤）复杂得多，目的仅在于隔离肺静脉的导管消融方法存在明显不足[10,11]。肺静脉隔离治愈慢性房颤的成功率因确立的消融靶点不同而差异较大[10,11,16,17]。外科研究显示肺静脉隔离可以治愈房颤，但这些术式的隔离范围大多远远超过隔离肺静脉本身。慢性房颤是一种非常复杂的疾病，不同机制或者多种机制同时存在于不同的患者。尚需对所有这些因素进一步认识才能研发出更加有效、合理的治疗方法，目前我们至少已经清楚房颤是一种左房疾病，尤其是左房后壁[28,32,33]。

已经有充足的证据证实左房后壁是消融治疗恢复

窦性心律的关键区域,这里包含了导管消融治疗的靶部位。房颤时的主导频率几乎总是在这一区域里标测到[16,28]。

在持续快速心房起搏制成的慢性房颤狗模型,以及孤立的二尖瓣疾病患者中发现,其左房激动频率快于右房。而且,在其左房后壁上可识别出许多小的明显的快速激动区域。标测研究显示肺静脉的激动频率快于左房,而左房快于右房,提示肺静脉可能是持续性房颤的一个快速激动源。事实上,阻断肺静脉/Marshall 韧带(LOM)与左房之间,以及左房和右房之间的传导,可以导致这些区域内激动频率梯度的形成[28,32,33]。

因此,我们对房颤患者进行了标测并评价其心内电活动的分布和类型(图 113-1)。局部波长经自动分析以直方图显示,心内电活动分型如下:A 型,定义为相对规律的电活动,可以清楚看到等电位线;B 型,不规则的电活动,基线消失和/或高度碎裂电图;C 型,A 型和 B 型电图交替出现。A 型电图为快速的高频活动,房颤时在肺静脉区域可以持续描记到,但在左房的其他部位并未记录到。Jais 及其同事最近证实肺静脉内心肌细胞的有效不应期短[34],这可以部分解释这种 A 型电图的分布现象。

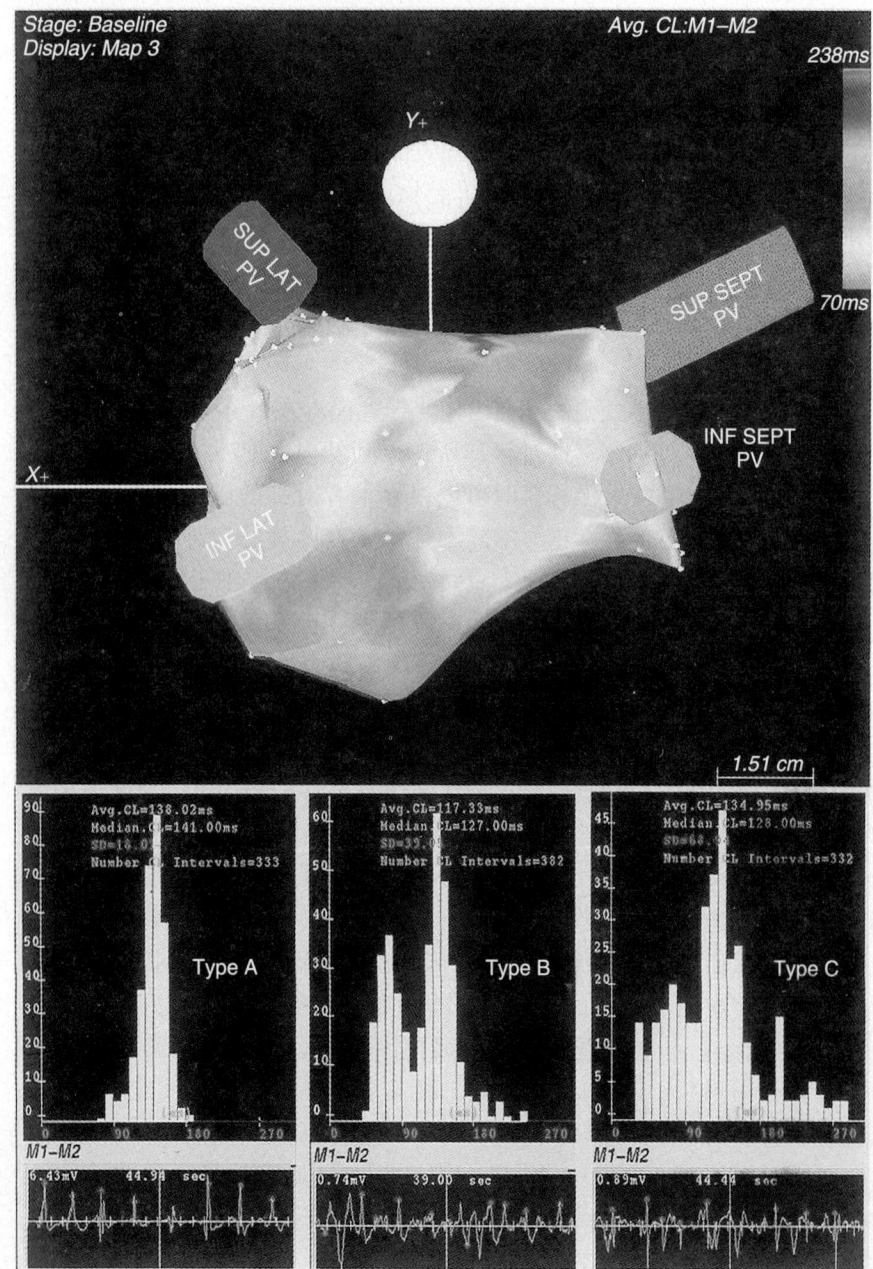

图 113-1　**左房电图**　上图:房颤时的左房电解剖图(后前位),每点采样时间为 45s。电生理信息以不同色彩显示,红色代表最短环长(CL),紫色为最长环长。注意,较短的环长多聚集在肺静脉周围。下图:A 型、B 型、C 型局部双极电图及相应的环长直方图。(见彩图 45)

持续性房颤时在肺静脉口或附近可以记录到反复性电活动，呈连续、间断或交替活动。在反复电活动最早激动部位记录到的双极电图显示为复杂的电活动，与阵发性房颤时肺静脉部位记录到的相似。一定基质条件下的多波折返是慢性房颤的一个重要机制，如果这一理论得到普遍认同，那么由肺静脉局灶释放快速冲动所产生的反复电活动，如在阵发性房颤中观察到的，或由肺静脉-左房交界部位的折返波阵引起的反复电活动，也可能同样具有重要意义；它提示出一个令人兴奋的可能性，即慢性房颤同样，或者至少部分，是由肺静脉发放的快速反复电活动所产生。有意思的是，曾有人认为肺静脉组织的重构可以产生这种反复电活动[28]。

在房颤开始时，反复电活动可由房性早搏开始，而以起源部位出现最早的颤动活动为终止，最早的颤动活动可以在房颤反复复发的同一部位重复诱发出来。颤动活动从这些起源区域不断向邻近区域扩布。有趣的是，这些起源区域大多可在左房后壁标测到[32]。因此，肺静脉反复发放颤动样电活动在房颤的发生和维持中起着重要作用，在这一部位可标测到围绕微小核心的旋转子或旋涡状的折返环[32]。因此，单纯消融房性早搏的治疗策略其有效性将会有限，因为其他触发因素，例如规则的房性心律失常（房扑或房速）甚至室性早搏均可以激活起源区域而诱发房颤。因而对这些起源区域进行标测并划入消融策略是合理的，同时可将房性早搏触发灶也同时纳入消融靶目标中。如果左房后壁参与慢性房颤的维持，那么为治愈慢性房颤而设计的消融策略里必须包括左房后壁的一部分，而不仅仅是单纯隔离肺静脉。

实际上，尽管房颤是由房性早搏诱发的，房颤的维持仍需初始易患基质的存在，冲动的传导需要一定先决条件才能演变成房颤。在肺静脉-左房交界区[35,36]，由于存在房间隔下、后部位连接左右两心房的心肌束传导不良，异位冲动可以演变为房颤。这一房间传导肌束早在200年前Bourgery即已描述过[37]。促进这种冲动发生演变的情况包括缓慢传导、波阵面的分离、不应期离散度的增加，尤其当这些因素同时发生在一个小区域内时。房颤时常伴发房间传导障碍[35]。这种相关性进一步在孤立性房颤患者心内电生理检查中得到证实。连接左右心房的房间束差异较大，可由邻近心房壁的几个细纤维组成（≈1mm厚），或由明显可辨的纤维束构成，后者走行在覆盖于冠状静脉窦上的心外膜脂肪层中或贴靠在心房壁上[36]。根据其与心房壁的关系可将位于后部的双心房间的心肌束分成两组：一组为通路型，完全走行在心外膜脂肪层下，贴靠在心房壁，肌束与心房肌并行；另一组为桥型，连接心房后壁的两个部位，肌束与心房肌之间有心外膜脂肪组织相隔。正如早先 Mikhailov 和 Chukbar 所报道的，双房间的前通路（如 Bachmann 束等）并不是普遍存在的结构；他们在 77 例人心脏尸检中发现，仅有 55％的组织切片上可见到 Bachmann 束，仅在 29％的大体标本见到前通路。最近，采用新的非接触性标测技术进行左房标测研究，其结果进一步支持这一观察发现。这一研究发现窦性心律下，左房激动主要通过后间隔纤维，提示 Bachmann 束并不如以往所认为的那样重要[36]。在房间沟心外膜脂肪层中发现的细小连接纤维提示，这些结构潜在易损性的增加均可导致房颤的发生。可以认为，前、后心房间连接纤维在形态和功能上的特点更适于右向左激动的均衡传导，从而降低"触发"折返活动的可能性，反之亦然。在一些房颤患者中可见到 P 波异型，提示在后间隔区域存在传导延迟和冠状窦存在逆向激动。孤立性房颤患者在冠状窦口和后间隔区域存在显著的传导延迟，这可能是其房颤发生的机制之一。

因此，房颤的发生与左房下、后部位明显的冲动传导延迟相关。Platonov 等[36]的有创研究证实在这一部位存在左右心房间的传导障碍，而且在此附近可以记录到自发或起搏诱发的房颤发作的初始颤动样电活动。房间传导延迟常见于阵发性和慢性房颤患者中，那么通过对房间隔的阻断术完全阻断房间传导则有可能消除房颤。环右下肺静脉的消融可能确实打断了左侧肺静脉和 Bourgery-Platonov 束之间的关键连接，或者改良了这一肌束的电生理特性。

我们很早以前就认识到自主神经系统在房颤发生中具有潜在的重要意义。过去称之为迷走性房颤或交感介导性房颤，以表明哪种自主神经在房颤发生中占主导地位[37]。这两种房颤均夸大了交感或迷走神经活动对心房动作电位时程和传导速度的影响，进而产生促心律失常的作用，它们主要发生于无明显器质性心脏病证据的患者中[37]。

有意思的是，房颤触发灶的空间分布与压力敏感性受体的分布明显一致，表现为肺静脉消融时可以通过迷走神经纤维引起 Bezold-Jarisch 样反射现象[38-42]。在静脉-心房交界部位存在丰富的自主神经系统的神经和神经节，在这一区域进行消融可以改变房颤发生中交感和迷走神经的调节机制。Randall 和 Ardell[39] 以及 Marron 等[40] 均证实左、右两侧迷走神经在心包内走行于窦房结区域，由肺静脉共干区域进入心外膜；在同一区域，左房顶部和 4 个肺静脉周围已发现存在广泛分布的特殊的神经末梢和大群的无髓鞘的 C 纤维末梢，可能参与心脏抑制性压力反射活动。迷走传入神经末梢多在环肺静脉消融的有限区域内分布，而交感神经分支则弥漫分布于整个左心房，因此更广范围的左房消融多影响的是交感神经末梢[39,40]。心率变异性分析证实环肺静脉消融术后迷走交感神经的平衡更偏向于副交感，提示消融导致的一些结构的损害，如心内膜神经末梢和/或 Marshall 韧带，可能影响了自主神经调节功能[16]。

最后，我们提出的"电解剖重构"一词来源于随访中观察到的有效环肺静脉消融可以使左房大小显著回缩以及左房功能显著改善这一事实[17]。最近一项大规模的前瞻性研究提出了左房大小在房颤发生中重要地位的证据。因此，左房扩大应视为房颤发生的一个强力而主要的危险因素。随访观察到心房电学和解剖学的恢复，表明环肺静脉消融是能够改良房颤维持的一个重要决定因素。

总之，确定肺静脉起源或左房后壁起源是个关键。因此，为根治慢性房颤而设计的消融术必须包括左房后壁的一部分，将线性消融和肺静脉隔离两种方法成功而可行地融合在一起。相反，不包括心房组织的非常局限的消融方法，如节段性肺静脉隔离，则具有许多局限性，可能无法治愈慢性房颤[33]。

毋庸置疑，快速节律刺激下的心房组织的解剖和电学重构在慢性房颤的维持中起着重要作用，即我们常常引用的"房颤致房颤"（AF begets AF）效应[19]。房颤可引起钙超载[43]，进而诱导心房肌细胞对房颤这一"电学风暴"产生"生存适应性"的去分化改变，包括钾离子通道表达、缝隙连接以及收缩环节的改变。电生理和结构异常的结果导致动作电位时程和房颤波长的缩短、频率适应性的丧失以及肌浆网的破坏。如果能够在房颤发生几小时或几天内迅速逆转这种电生理的异常重构，那么解剖重构就会明显延迟发生和不发生，这也表明控制房颤更加积极的态度应该是寄希望于能够防止房颤的进行性重构效应。有趣的是，重构同样可以累及肺静脉组织，导致冲动的持续发放。房颤持续时间较长的患者其主导房颤环长度非常短，而且其主导环长的自发性昼夜变异率极小，钙通道阻滞剂对主导房颤环长的延长作用微弱，这些改

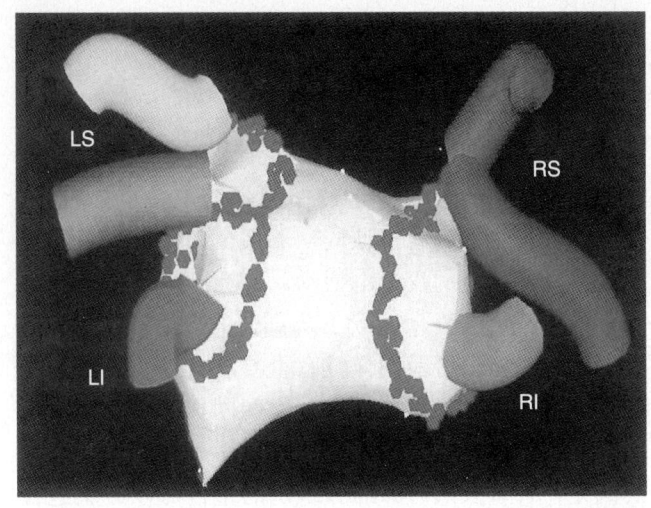

图 113-2　左房和肺静脉的三维标测图　实心灰色的左房标测图，后前位。红色圆点为射频消融靶点，彩色管道为肺静脉。注意，左上肺静脉有早期分支，右上肺静脉恰好位于开口上，右侧消融线环绕所有静脉。LI：左下肺静脉；LS：左上肺静脉；RI：右下肺静脉；RS：右上肺静脉。（见彩图46）

变均提示这些患者所发生的重构是不可逆的。对这种患者，应该在其房颤出现耐药性和影响其生活质量之前进行消融治疗。

三、消融技术

（一）导管放置

分别在冠状窦、右房和右室心尖部放置一个 4 极 6F 导管，通过房间隔穿刺术标测左房和肺静脉。

（二）标测方法

应用非射线电解剖标测系统（CARTO，Biosense Webster，Diamond Bar，Calif），通过穿间隔途径实时构建左房和肺静脉的三维图像，重建静脉-心房交界部位的解剖。根据肺静脉-左房交界部位的复杂结构，我们制定出每例患者的消融线路和范围（图 113-2）[16,17]。

采用特殊标测和消融导管重新构建的三维电解剖图像，以一个固定电极作参照，可以显示局部心肌激动时间（LATs）的空间分布。标测导管深入到每个肺静脉内 2～4cm，而后慢慢回撤。在回撤过程中进行多部位记录以标测肺静脉轮廓。当透视下观察到导管尖端进入心脏轮廓内，同时伴有阻抗的降低和心房电位的出现，则确定为肺静脉入口。在二尖瓣环上记录 3 个部位，标测出二尖瓣环。顺序标测至少 50 个位

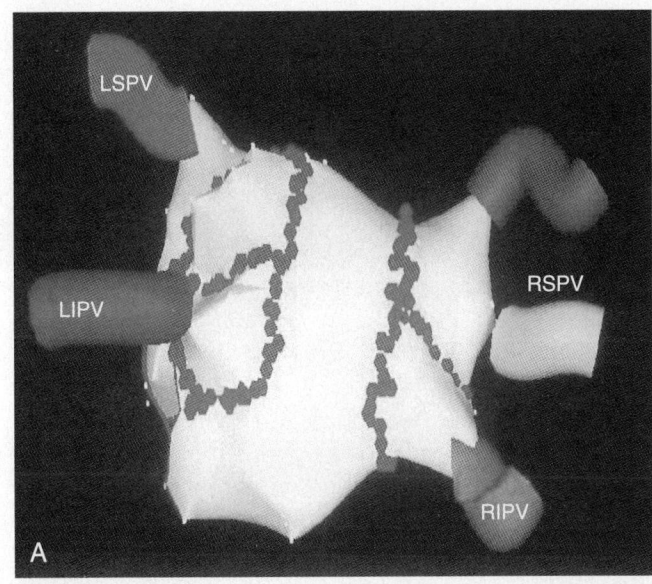 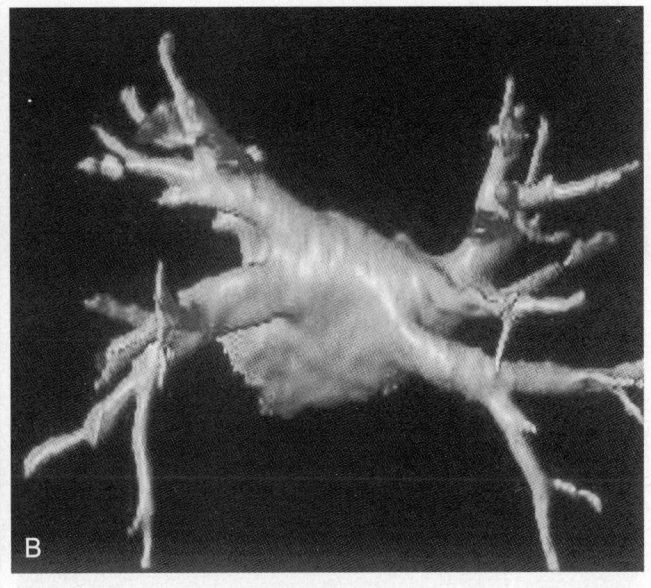

图 113-3 三维重建肺静脉-左房交界区 CARTO 重建的肺静脉-左房交界区三维图像（B）与磁共振血管成像（A）的比较。注意，两种成像技术所显示的左房和肺静脉在形态和大小上具有高度的相似性。LIPV：左下肺静脉；LSPV：左上肺静脉；RIPV：右下肺静脉；RSPV：右上肺静脉。（见彩图 47）

点获得左房图形。对手术时为窦性心律者，在冠状窦或右心耳处以 600ms 周长起搏标测获得上述各部位图形。每一位点的电图均在导管位置稳定时进行记录，导管位置的稳定性由舒张末期的稳定性（连续记录的两个舒张期时的导管位置相差小于 2mm）和局部心肌激动时间的稳定性（连续记录的两个 LAT 时间差小于 2ms）来评价。当记录电位为两个分离的碎裂电位时，选择较陡峭的一个测量局部心肌激动时间。

（三）标测系统

CARTO 系统通过持续记录标测导管的每次标测位置，使每个记录部位的电生理特性与其心内解剖位点一一对应起来[44,45]。CARTO 重建的左房解剖是非常可靠的，其构型和大小与磁共振成像所获得指标相一致（图 113-3）。采用此系统的远端和近端有两个记录电极的标测导管，可以经皮在左房内进行单极和双极电图的记录。导管位置以患者后背部固定贴片为参照，因此即使患者有所活动，标测部位的相对位置也不受影响。标测导管在心内膜进行不同部位的顺序标测，完成整个标测程序。在每一位点，当电极与心内膜接触稳定，同时记录电极尖端的位置和这一部位的心内电图。以体表心电图或心内一个固定电极为参照，测量获得局部心肌激动时间。CARTO 系统通过持续监测导管与组织接触情况和局部心肌激动时间的稳定性来保证每一部位测量的真实性和可重复性。而后，所获得的信息以不同色彩对应展现出来。每获得一个新的标测位点，系统就会实时刷新、重建三维解剖图像，以色彩对应的激动时间梯度图展现出来。除激动时间梯度图外，在计算机工作站还可以动态演示激动顺序和传导扩布的影片。另外，根据所获得的数据还可以显示电压梯度图（基质图），以三维模型展示局部峰电压的大小。这些均有助于确定瘢痕和电异常的组织区域。这一系统可以精确指导导管顶端回到曾经标测过的有意义的位点，确定出消融靶点所在部位，或标记出静脉和瓣环的位置，且具有高度空间定位的准确性（＜1mm）。这种三维的电解剖重建所标测的心房以及导管导航功能简化了线性消融手术，只需在重建图上完成消融线即可，但是导管的"到位"操作仍是一个挑战。另一个技术挑战是如何确定消融线的真正完成，因为相邻消融点之间的缝隙会使冲动得以传导而具有致心律失常作用，导致围绕手术区域的心房扑动。电解剖标测可以确定消融线的完整性，但整个消融线必须通过导管逐一标测确定有无可以传导电激动的部位。

（四）消融步骤

标测出肺静脉口后，通过 CARTO 导管顶端电极和经皮穿刺部位电极夹以单极模式释放射频能量制造环形传导阻滞线。这些线由一个个消融点连续而成，各点距肺静脉口部至少 5mm。最高消融温度设定在 60℃，射频能量（最高达 50W）释放 30～60s 直到局部电图振幅降低 80%。如果出现阻抗增高或患者出现

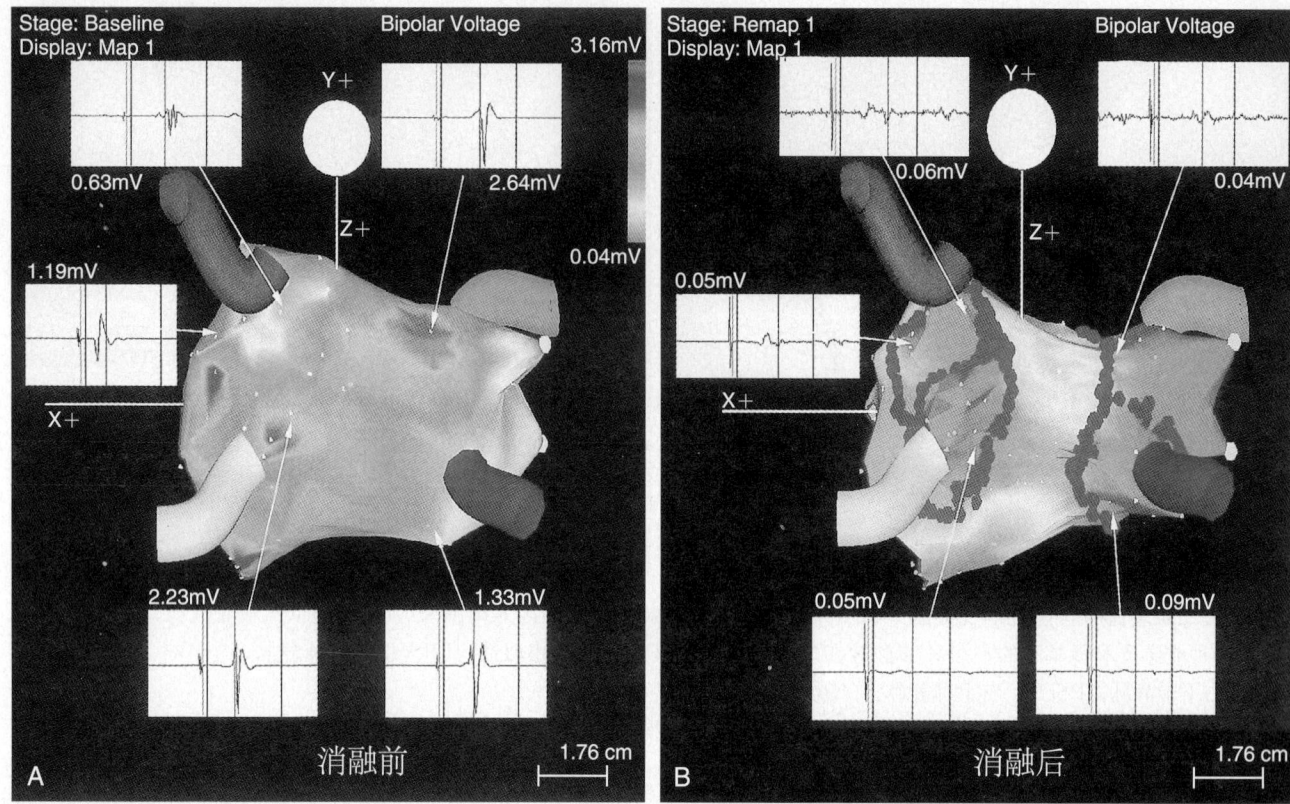

图 113-4 三维左房电压图 后前位（A：消融术前；B：消融术后），显示峰-峰双极电图振幅。红色代表最低电压，紫色为最高电压。紫红色圆点为射频消融靶点。术后，在消融线内及其周围区域，包括一定范围的左房后壁，显示低振幅（<0.1mV）电图（电解剖重构）。术前电图可见肺静脉口部电位，提示此处肌纤维具有将冲动传出和传入静脉的传导功能。经环每根肺静脉射频消融之后，可见术前口部同一部位的肺静脉电位消失（术后电图），即心房静脉间电连接阻断。（见彩图 48）

咳嗽、烧灼痛或严重的心动过缓，则终止射频能量的释放。

大多数患者均清晰地标测出 4 根肺静脉口，并围绕每一根肺静脉分别进行环形消融。在某些情况下，当外侧和/或间隔侧两个肺静脉口间相距小于 20mm，或有一个提早分支的共同开口，或存在一个单独分支的肺静脉时，则围绕同侧两个肺静脉做一条环形消融线（图 113-2）。因此，消融线是根据肺静脉-左房交接部位的特点制定的，不同于目前新出来的事先即已设定大小和形状的环形消融，后者较难适用于开口较大的、开口偏心形状的，或者近端分支复杂的肺静脉消融[26,27]。在窦性心律或房颤时均可进行消融，不需反复施行电转律，24% 的房颤患者可即刻转为窦性心律。

在这种基本的消融设计基础上，对于阵发性房颤患者可以进一步加做线性消融，以预防左房消融线介导的切口性心动过速的发生。这种心动过速并发症发生率在 2% 以内，是绝大多数患者需再次消融治疗的主要原因。这一线性消融线加做在右下肺静脉和二尖瓣环之间（图 113-4）。对于慢性 AF 和具有复发危险因素的患者（包括左房直径 > 55mm，射血分数 < 40%，合并器质性心脏病和年龄 > 65 岁），分别在右、左下肺静脉和二尖瓣环之间，两上肺静脉以及两下肺静脉之间额外加做线性消融。

如果阻抗增加、导管移位，或出现任何并发症征象时，立即停止射频能量的释放。操作过程中持续动态监测心电图和血压，注意有无自主神经刺激引起的 Bezold-Jarisch 样反射发生。

（五）再次标测及消融部位的确认

对于窦性心律的患者，消融术后再次进行标测，并与消融前的解剖标测图相对照，精确比较消融前后激动顺序的变化，以发现有无新的靶点。对于房颤患者，恢复窦性心律后，在术前房颤时的解剖标测图上进行再次标测，保留相同的标记和消融靶点，以保证确认消融靶点的可靠性。我们发现在心脏舒张期末期进行记录的房颤时无心房收缩下的解剖标测图和起搏下的标测图之间无显著差异。

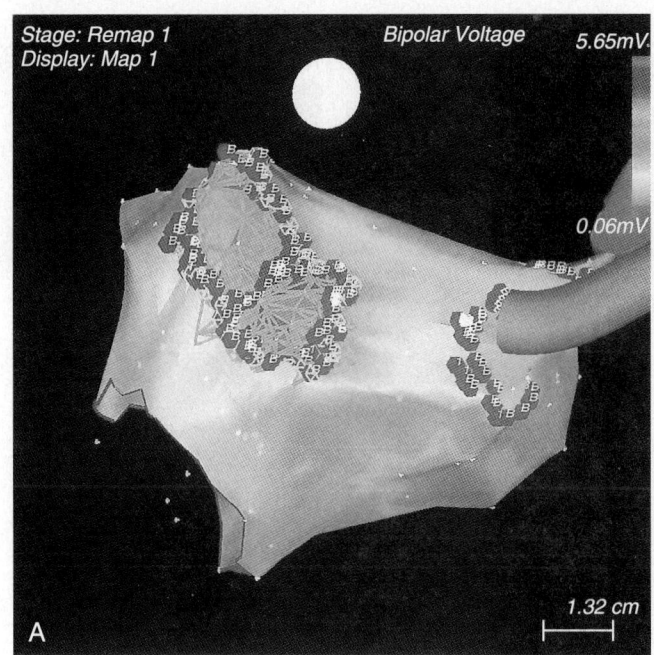 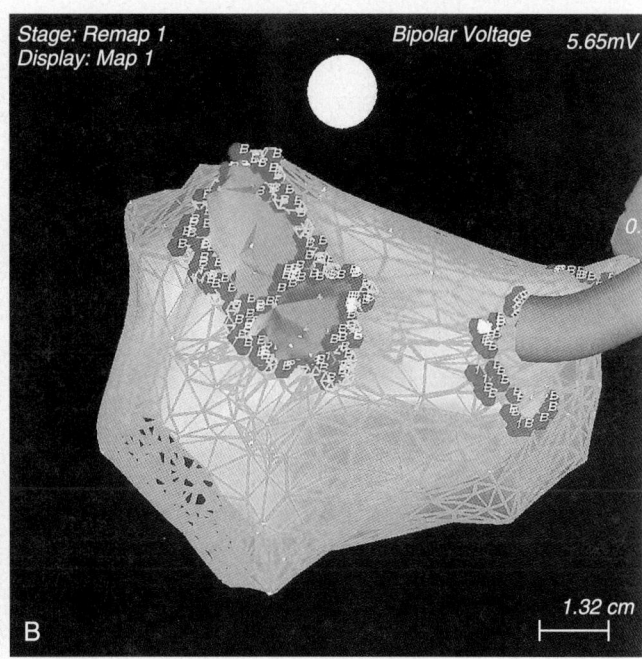

图 113-5　利用 CARTO 软件定量测量环肺静脉口部低电压区域的面积　环形的低电压区域是指最外侧的低于 0.1mV 双极电压位点所围成区域内的表面积，这些最外侧的低电压位点是通过手动选择的（A）。在环形区域外任意点击一处，左房剩余表面积即可自动计算得出（B）。（见彩图 49）

消融靶点的确认首先要分别获得在冠状窦和右房起搏下的外侧和间隔侧肺静脉的两份标测图。这种做法的理由是，在消融靶点附近起搏可以缩短激动至消融靶点的传导时间，利于发现环形消融线内有无延迟的电活动。消融线完整性的判断标准如下：（1）消融环内双极电图峰-峰振幅的降低（< 0.1mV），通过局部电图分析和电压图确定；（2）消融环外和内同一轴线上相邻点之间的局部心内膜激动时间延迟 > 30ms，通过激动顺序图进行评价。激动传导的变化同样也可以从激动动态扩布图进行评价。消融线两侧出现骑跨消融线的双电位图，则认为存在传导或消融缝隙。

关于传导阻滞的评价，确定无冲动穿过消融线的标准是消融环内电图的振幅 < 0.1mV。理论上，如果达到消融完全则消融环内不应出现电活动，这种低振幅的电信号很可能是标测系统感知的远场信号，显示为类似激动信号，而实际上并不是传导过来的电位。再者，消融线确认的标准现已修改，电活动延迟这一标准已被废弃[17]。只有通过消融术后标测的电压图才能确认消融靶点情况：如果消融线内双极电图峰-峰振幅 < 0.1mV，则认为消融是完全的或阻滞是彻底的，因为在不同部位起搏时消融环内局部信号的振幅是相似的（图 113-5）。促使我们重新评价肺静脉从左房内有效隔离终点的最适宜标准源于一个重要发现，即消融环内电压的降低与肺静脉电位的消失是相关的

（图 113-5）。这一发现提示，通过一个非常简单而迅速的方法就可以获得肺静脉的电隔离，不需费时而又费力的标测检查[17]。

环肺静脉口的低电压（双极幅度 < 0.1mV）和消融环外的左房面积可以通过电压图进行定量分析；常规/定做设计的软件可应用于标准 CARTO 参照系统（图 113-6）。为了计算消融环内低电压区域的大小，必须仔细回顾每一个标测位点，证实消融环内及消融部位所有标测位点的双极电位小于 0.1mV。选择出振幅小于 0.1mV 的位点并进行标记，软件可以在三维重建的解剖图上以 mm^2 为单位计算出标记区域的面积，消融环外的左房面积则可自动确定[17]。

（六）围消融期的处理

抗心律失常药物（除胺碘酮）和地高辛停用至少 5 个半衰期。对于没有采取长期抗凝治疗的患者，为预防卒中和其他栓塞事件的发生，应用组织多普勒经食道超声（TEE）指导下的短期抗凝治疗方法进行替代 3 周的常规抗凝治疗。根据此方法，心房内有血栓的患者，必须接受常规抗凝治疗，并经过经食道超声检查确切除外心脏内血栓后才可进行消融治疗。

消融期间，应用肝素维持部分凝血酶原时间在 60~90s。

环肺静脉消融术后，患者需接受 48h 的遥测监

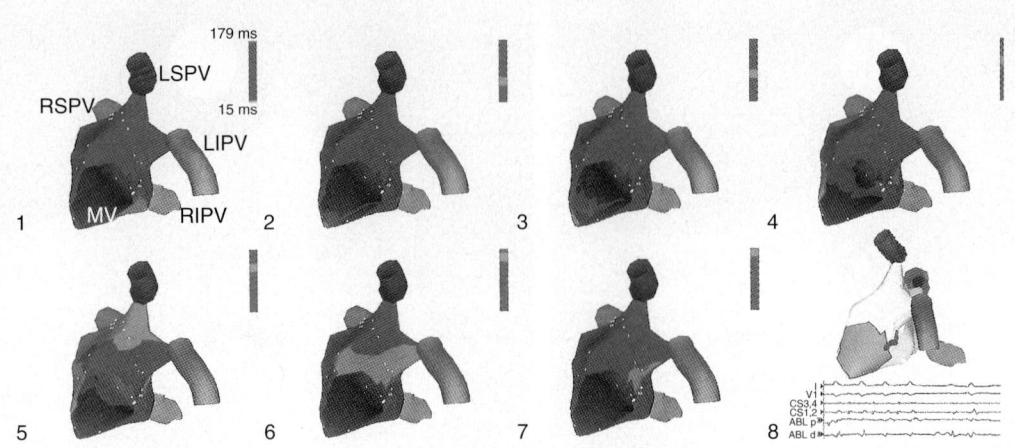

图 113-6　环肺静脉消融后的左房心动过速时的激动扩布图　第 1～7 幅为动态顺序播放中的冻结图像（左侧观）。蓝色背景下的红色阴影代表局部心内膜激动时间，范围 30ms（时程的红色图标在各图的右侧）。注意，激动波阵围绕二尖瓣环进行环形运动。如心内电生理标测所示，心律失常在射频消融（紫红色圆点）左下肺静脉和二尖瓣环之间的峡部时终止（第 8 幅）。CS：冠状窦；LSPV：左上肺静脉；MV：二尖瓣；RIPV：右下肺静脉；RSPV：右上肺静脉。（见彩图 50）

控。出院时患者通常为窦性心律，对于住院期间房颤复发或消融术未行电复律者，需继续服用其术前即已应用的Ⅰ类或Ⅲ类抗心律失常药物。这些措施有利于术后最初几周内电重构的逆转。对于所有没有症状性房颤发作的患者，1 个月后不再接受抗心律失常药物治疗。对于无房颤复发和心脏超声显示左房机械功能恢复的患者，标准化比值维持在 2.5（2～3 之间）的抗凝治疗可以在消融术后 1 个月安全停用。阿司匹林（250mg）也可以服用数周。消融术后 1 个月和 3 个月时，常规行超声和 Holter 监测的 24h 心电图检查。

在某些中心，消融术后 2 周内复发的房颤（ER-AF）可早期再次行消融治疗，但根据我们的经验，短期的药物治疗可能更为合适。

四、结　果

这一部分将介绍我们中心采用这一方法治疗连续收治的房颤患者，平均随访 2 年以上的（31±19 个月）的临床结果。

（一）消融

自 1998 年至 2002 年，共有 1211 例阵发性房颤患者和 776 例慢性房颤患者在我们中心接受消融治疗。在这些患者中，有 1.5% 以前曾接受过局灶或节段性肺静脉隔离治疗，但未能成功。包括复发的再次手术一共进行了 2029 次消融手术，其中 42 例患者接受即时再次消融治疗。操作和标测时间分别为 162±32min 和 75±27min，透视时间为 29±11min。因此，操作时间是可以接受的，大多数患者在 ≤2h 完成，所有患者透视时间均少于 30 min。消融面积为 4.9±0.5cm²，占整个左房标测表面的 28%±9%。有 32% 的房颤患者在消融过程中恢复窦性心律。98.5% 的患者消融成功。在消融放电过程中有 71 例（3.6%）患者出现 Bezold-Jarish 样反射表现，如一过性的高度或完全房室传导阻滞、严重的心动过缓、窦性停搏或收缩压降低（＜90mmHg），尤其在进行环间隔侧上肺静脉消融时（17 例）。这些患者在后来的遥测监控期间未记录到缓慢性心律失常。

手术过程中，在肺静脉口周围进行放电消融时，有 7.2% 的患者出现了难以忍受的疼痛或严重咳嗽。

（二）生存率

至分析时，有 115 例（5.8%）患者死亡，其中 61 例死于心血管原因（心衰，$n=41$；心肌梗死，$n=11$；卒中，$n=7$；猝死，$n=2$），死亡时 31 例（50.8%）患者为房颤和 30 例为窦性心律，其中 16 例（55%）出现多次房颤复发。值得注意的是，死于心衰的 41 例患者中有 29 例为房颤心律。

与意大利人群年龄和性别特异死亡率为基础计算出的预期死亡率相比，我们观察到的死亡率与预期死亡率并无显著差别。在基础特征中，缺血性心脏病史、射血分数 ＜45%、以及左室质量指数 ＞125g/m² 是死亡的独立预测因素。

（三）复发及其预测

平均随访 29 个月，总的无房颤复发者占 80%，且在阵发性（81%）和慢性（76%）房颤患者中无显著差别。15% 的患者有早期（2 周内）的房颤复发，但其中 78% 的患者在长期随访中未再有房颤发作，且未服用抗心律失常药物治疗。慢性房颤患者有较高的早期复发倾向（22% vs 11% 阵发性房颤）。尽管如此，在此短暂的时间窗内复发的房颤，不论在慢性房颤还是阵发性房颤患者中，均不能预测消融的远期效果，在长期的随访中 77% 的这类患者未再出现症状性房颤。

绝大多数环肺静脉消融术后早期复发的患者，在长期随访中获得最终成功的临床效果，表明房颤早期复发是个短暂现象，并不能作为长期消融失败的预测因素。其原因可能是由于射频热能损伤导致的急性炎症改变，和/或射频能量的延迟治疗效应。事实上，有一些研究已经报道了炎症与房颤相关。大约 33% 的开胸手术患者可出现短暂的术后房颤，可能就是由心房内的炎症反应所触发。射频能量的延迟治疗效应可能是由于消融术后最初几天消融病灶的扩大，而界限清晰的坏死区域要在术后 2 周才能形成[11]。

消融过程中我们也观察到 Bezold-Jarish 样反射表现，其中射频热能刺激迷走神经末梢可能起着重要作用[46]。而且，在早期房颤复发的这组患者中，相对局灶性肺静脉消融[38]，环肺静脉消融可以导致一过性和短期（1 个月内自行恢复）的心率变异性（HRV）频域的降低，这表明交感迷走神经失衡更趋向交感神经激活和/或迷走神经活性降低。

关于消融过程中出现的心动过缓-低血压，比较统一的解释为可能与短暂地刺激了迷走传入纤维、神经节后的副交感纤维，或左房后壁特殊的神经末梢有关，这些神经具有刺激窦房结的作用[11]。这些相似的传入纤维的有限损伤，可引起短暂的副交感神经减弱或抑制/去神经化效应，或相应的交感神经传入通路的短暂兴奋，这些可能在早期房颤复发（ERAF）患者心率变异性（HRV）的变化方面起着重要作用。心房局部纤维化可破坏交感和/或副交感神经纤维的连续性，导致局部区域的副交感或交感神经的抑制，因而具有一过性的神经抑制的高敏性。因此，消融后 1~6 个月如果确定有心率变异性的异常、高频的副交感神经成分再次出现，提示神经调节作用的恢复。最后，一过性自主神经纤维的水肿也可能在窦房结神经调节功能不良中起了一定作用。相反，自主神经功能的短暂改变，包括交感神经活性的增强或副交感神经功能的减退或两者兼有，可以通过细胞内钙超载直接或间接地触发房性早搏或改变心房电活动特性，而易于心律失常的发生，阵发性房颤患者自发转律前后心率变异性（HRV）的分析也提示同样的结论[47,48]。

最后，既往被房颤所诱导的电学和解剖的重构，其逆转是一个缓慢但却不断进展的过程。对于 B 型和 C 型房颤患者（表 113-1），我们认为对既往未应用抗心律失常药物治疗者应给予一定疗程的（1~2 个月）抗心律失常药物治疗，来加速心房电重构的逆转。

无房颤复发的 Kaplan-Meier 可能性在阵发性和慢性房颤患者之间的差别在 6 个月时最大（永久性房颤为 97% vs 阵发性房颤为 87%），在 1 年（84% vs 83%）和 2 年（75% vs 82%）时最小。78% 的复发患者对抗心律失常药物治疗有效，且与房颤类型和复发的时间无关。

在单变量分析中，倾向于恢复窦性心律的独立预测因素为左房大小和消融术后低电压区域的面积，即左房扩大患者需要更大面积的隔离才能消除房颤。随访中无房颤复发的患者可观察到其左房内径变小（从 45±7mm 缩小至 39±9mm），消融前左房扩大及消融后低电压区域面积较小（<15% 整个左房内膜面积）是房颤复发的独立预测因素。随访中通过二尖瓣血流多普勒检查发现，所有无房颤复发患者的左房收缩功能均得到保留和/或改善。这一终点的评价（心房收缩力的恢复）是非常重要的，因为这一治疗较之于简单的消融阻断房室结并起搏治疗的长处即在于此。

（四）安全性

房颤的射频导管消融危险性相对较低；在我们的系列治疗中未出现严重的并发症，包括死亡、卒中或其他血栓栓塞事件。少量心包积液发生率（4%）与既往穿间隔操作的报道相似。有 5 例患者因心包填塞行心包穿刺术。

消融术后 3 天和 1~3 个月时行经食道超声检查未发现肺静脉口处有提示狭窄的高速血流，这可能是因为消融线远离肺静脉口 5mm 以上，因而避免了热能损害引起瘢痕和静脉壁的挛缩。而且，为了进一步降低损伤肺静脉的危险性，我们避免了在未明确记录到心房电位的部位进行射频消融。

五、讨 论

对于阵发性房颤消融治疗的各种不同方法均已有

描述[10-17]。不同术式对阵发性房颤消融治疗的成功率（>70%）无明显差别，这表明没有哪一种消融方法优于另外一种。实际上，环肺静脉消融在消除房颤方面高度有效且具有较低风险，因而被建议作为症状性、药物难治性房颤患者和不能接受长期药物治疗的症状性房颤患者的治疗选择。

环肺静脉消融是一种解剖消融方法，即在CARTO指引下围绕每一根肺静脉口作环形传导阻滞线，目的是将这些静脉从左房中隔离出来，同时能够降低肺静脉狭窄的风险[16,17]。这一方法是基于实验数据和临床外科手术观察得出的，它支持肺静脉-左房交界区是触发和维持房颤的关键部位这一观点。这种基于解剖的消融技术摒除了标测自发性或诱发性心律失常的必要性，而且可以有效预防由于存在多个肺静脉触发灶而导致的房颤复发，即使将来出现新的触发灶也可以有效预防。

电压图定量分析得出的重要结果提供了一个从生理病理方面解释这种解剖消融方法成功的原因。虽然结果显示消融线的完整性（定义为消融环内双极电图振幅小于0.1mV）和临床结果之间无相关性，但射频消融术后消融环内低电压区域的面积占整个左房面积的比例在无房颤复发患者中大于复发者，因此这是消融成功的唯一预测指标[17]。

然而，另一个重要发现也使我们重新评价将肺静脉有效隔离出左房的最准确的终点判定指标，即消融环内电压的降低与肺静脉电位的消失以及A型房颤（即肺静脉心动过速）的消除是同步相关的。

环肺静脉消融对阵发性和慢性房颤同样有效，表明这种纯粹的解剖消融方法或者导致心房-静脉间的电连接中断，如肺静脉口电位的消失以及消融线外起搏时消融环内未记录到可辨认的电活动所证实，或者导致心房复杂的电解剖重构，如消融环内以及消融部位周边区域（累及部分左房后壁）电压的降低所显示[17]。

实际上，环肺静脉口消融面积的减小是一种较强的预测房颤复发的因素。因此，临床结果和消融线完整性之间缺乏相关性这一结果表明，肺静脉灶的隔离不是房颤根除的唯一机制；房颤的根除可能是有效消融造成的累及部分左房后壁的复杂心房电解剖重构，即房颤的维持基质不再存在。

肺静脉口周围靶区域的消融可以阻断肺静脉内心肌袖和心房肌之间的连接，使之无法形成折返环路，破坏房颤维持的局部主导旋转子，和/或诱导去神经效应。关于后者，心率变异性分析证实环肺静脉消融术后迷走交感神经的平衡更偏向于副交感，提示消融导致的一些结构损害，如心内膜神经末梢和/或Marshall韧带，可能影响了自主神经的调节功能。

这也许可以解释为什么这种消融方法治疗这两种类型房颤的成功率高于不干预任何心房肌的在口部进行肺静脉隔离的标测消融方法[10-15]。

如果说以前房颤的局灶假说已经引起了我们的重视，那么新近的外科手术和标测研究是人们寻找更合理的消融治疗方法的动力。外科手术治疗房颤同样需要重新关注心房大小在房颤中的作用，这表明心房的回缩不仅仅是一个相关的变量，而且是房颤永久消除的一个重要机制和关键的决定因素，它可诱导解剖重构的逆转[49]。在房颤起源部位之外颤动波传导区域，可产生新的折返源并发展成为另一个主导环，因此，心房越大发展成颤动源的数目就越多，房颤持续的可能性就越大。事实上，术后为窦性心律的患者其术后心房相对较小。这些数据表明，减小心房的大小联合迷宫术可以提高手术的成功率，这与我们观察到的消融隔离区域的大小是消融成功的强有力的预测因素这一结果相一致。环肺静脉消融不仅隔离了肺静脉内房颤的局部起源灶，而且类似外科手术减小了具有"电活性"的心房面积，对包括左房后壁相当一部分组织在内的左房的30%进行了消融隔离。它保留了心房的机械功能却改变了房颤维持所必需的解剖面积。此外，消融线外电压幅度的降低现象可能是一个鉴别因素。

当前具有肺静脉隔离经验的中心只有很少几个。这里存在一个明显学习曲线，与最初肺静脉隔离手术操作相比，我们后期手术的透视、标测和消融时间均明显降低，两者存在显著差异，整个手术时间平均缩短了60%。现在我们消融方法的可行性逐渐显现出来，采用最初描述的技术，手术操作时间显著缩短，房颤时仅依据简单的解剖标测图即可进行消融。虽然临床经验仍有限，但是这种方法已经显示出其有效性，随着这种方法的不断成熟，其应用将逐渐扩大到其他中心。

六、总　结

目前射频导管消融技术已广泛开展，并成功地治疗了许多心律失常。由于药物治疗的不理想和选择性消融治疗令人鼓舞的结果，不难理解我们努力的重点转向发现一种可行的、能够广泛应用且具有高度安全

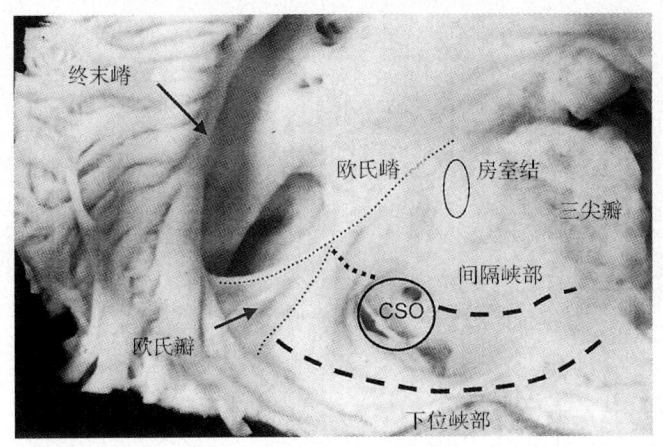

图 114-1　右前斜位下人体右心房内腔模拟图　下位峡部自三尖瓣环下方延伸至下腔静脉（下方虚线），间隔峡部位于三尖瓣环和冠状窦口（CSO）间（上方虚线），并向欧氏嵴延伸（点虚线）。注意漂浮的欧氏瓣呈三角形结构。（引自 Courtesy of Yen Ho，National Heart & Lung Institute and Royal Brompton Hospital，London，UK.）（见彩图 51）

择 7F 消融导管（图 114-2）。冠状窦导管可以稳定地进行起搏，记录冠状窦口（靠近消融线）电活动。当迷走神经亢进致心动过缓或房室阻滞时，右室心尖部导管可以安全地进行心室起搏，导管上端还可间接提示希氏束区域（图 114-2）。在我们实验中心，不需额外常规使用 20 极标测导管（见"峡部消融终点"）。

三、峡部消融

手术开始时为窦性心律时，在冠状窦口以 500～600ms 周期起搏，并在此起搏心律下，完成整个消融过程。手术开始为持续房扑心律时，可直接开始消融；终止房扑后，在冠状窦口起搏。虽然消融靶点有赖于解剖定位，但除此以外，通常还需要电生理指引，也就是通过消融导管标测记录心电图进行定位。我们一般在 6 点处开始消融（三尖瓣环在左前斜 60 度时被看作是一个钟表）（图 114-2B），要求记录到大而尖锐的心室波，而心房波较小（在心电图上电位幅度比为 3:1～5:1）。有时候，需要使用较大弧度的消融导管或较长的鞘以到达并稳定置于邻近三尖瓣环的峡部远端。消融过程中，逐步回撤消融导管直到导管到达下腔静脉边缘、下位峡部近端。在放电中，我们不拖拽导管。每次放电后，重新分析心电图。典型改变表现为双极记录心电图波幅轻度降低，常呈相邻紧密而小的双电位（图 114-3～5），提示局部阻滞（并非峡部完全阻滞！），而在单极记录心电图表现为波幅降低，这是消融靶点的局部反应。然而，生物物理学参数或电生理参数都不能明确地反映透壁损伤。峡部厚度，特别是导管放置的稳定性都是透壁损伤的影响因素。峡部平均长度 3cm，我们经常沿着峡部进行 5～7 次放电。除了要求透壁外，消融线必须连续致密，避免产生裂隙。传统的方法为右前斜 30 度和左前斜 60 度投照下逐步回撤消融导管（图 114-2）。右前斜 30 度有利于控制导管从峡部远端向近端移动，左前斜 60 度有利于充分显现三尖瓣环下方，从而沿着三尖瓣环"钟表"放置导管（如 6 点位置），也有利于控制导管前向或后向移动。应用电解剖标测系统（CARTO）能够在非 X 射线照射下，更加精确地标测和消融定位（图 114-4）[11]。

四、消融工具和生物学参数

在我们研究中心，我们不用 4mm 头端消融导管，而常规使用 8mm 头端导管进行峡部消融[12]。在一些有经验的电生理研究中心[13]，主要使用盐水灌注导管进行消融，后者在我中心仅在 8mm 头端导管消融不能奏效时使用（见"并发症"）。我们应用 8mm 头端导管，在温控能量（目标 70℃）下对每个靶点（非拖动中）消融 90s，最大功率为 50～70W。与 4mm 头端导管相比，应用 8mm 头端电极导管和我们设置的参数消融，会使更多患者感到明显的疼痛。因此，我们在很多患者峡部消融时，同时使用咪达唑仑和芬太尼镇痛。

五、峡部消融终点和残存裂隙标测

普遍认为，房扑终止和不能诱发不是消融成功的可靠标志，因为以上现象不能证实达到完全透壁的峡部传导阻滞。目前广泛使用分析起搏中 20 极标测导管所示三尖瓣侧壁激动次序的改变，从而评估峡部阻滞（图 114-3）[14]。消融前冠状窦口起搏导致顺钟向激动和逆钟向激动在三尖瓣侧壁 10～11 点钟处融合（20 极标测导管第 5～6 对电极处）。峡部不完全阻滞时，可经峡部缓慢传导，这样导致两种波形在更低的部位（图 114-3，8 点钟处，第 3 对电极位置）融合。最终，冠状窦口起搏，在右房前下壁产生的完全头尾向激动，最迟激动出现在 20 极标测导管的第 1 对电极处，这意味着峡部完全阻滞（图 114-3）。可通过

第 114 章

心房扑动的导管消融

Hans Kottkamp and Gerhard Hindricks

本章目录

- 解剖结构 ·········· 1029
- 峡部消融电生理特点和导管放置 ··· 1029
- 峡部消融 ·········· 1030
- 消融工具和生物学参数 ······ 1030
- 峡部消融终点和残存裂隙标测 ···· 1030
- 非典型右心房和左心房房扑的消融
  ·················· 1032
- 并发症和临床转归 ········ 1032

在过去几年中，精确的电生理标测技术清楚地揭示了典型心房扑动（房扑）和非典型房扑的折返环路[1-3]。导管标测显示峡部（位于三尖瓣环下方和下腔静脉之间）是典型房扑折返环路必需的一部分。射频消融通过产生线性损伤在峡部造成电隔离从而治愈典型房扑[4]，因此，与旁路局灶消融不同，峡部消融采用线性消融。目前在各个心电生理中心，房扑已成为消融的最常见适应证。新近调查显示，这种心律失常在美国每年新增病例 200 000 例，远远超过预先估计[5]。一项前瞻性随机试验比较了房扑病人接受抗心律失常药物与射频消融治疗，结果显示，射频消融成功率更高，且改善生活质量，并使心房颤动发生率下降，随访中再住院率低，可以作为一线治疗[6]。在我们研究中心，再发有症状的房扑或血流动力学显著异常的房扑都是消融的适应证。

一、解剖结构

典型房扑消融靶点仅由解剖结构决定（图 114-1）。在大多数心电生理中心，消融靶点是所谓从三尖瓣环延伸至下腔静脉口的下位峡部，也可选用位于三尖瓣环和冠状窦口之间，并进一步延伸至欧氏嵴[7]的间隔峡部作为消融靶点。下位峡部不同部位存在不同形态的组织：后方靠近下腔静脉处通常为纤维组织，中间往往是肌小梁，前方靠近三尖瓣环是光滑的前庭壁[8]。右心房造影显示，下位峡部长 17~54mm，平均 31mm[9]。峡部许多解剖结构形态特点可影响消融过程：分布广泛的、较厚的梳状肌侵入峡部，使得消融难以产生连续的线性透壁损伤；欧氏嵴下较深的凹陷使得导管很难探及；下腔静脉瓣（位于下腔静脉入口）的解剖变异使得导管很难置于靠近下腔静脉口的峡部后方（图 114-1）。

二、峡部消融电生理特点和导管放置

逆钟向折返的典型房扑患者，体表心电图下壁导联负向锯齿状扑动波强烈提示下位峡部是消融靶点目标。因此，依据我们的经验，对于心电图呈典型房扑的患者不需起搏拖带，可直接开始消融。对于所有其他类型的房扑，包括心电图提示可能是呈顺钟向折返的典型房扑或非典型房扑患者，均需要起搏拖带以判断是否为峡部依赖，或折返环路依赖于右心房或左心房的其他峡部[2,3,10]。

在我们研究中心，通常把 6F 多极导管置于冠状窦，近端电极靠近窦口，4F 导管置于右室心尖部，选

39. Randall WC, Ardell JL: Nervous control of the heart: Anatomy and pathophysiology. In: Zipes DP, Jalife J (eds): Cardiac Electrophysiology, from Cell to Bedside. Philadelphia, WB Saunders, 1990, pp. 291–299.
40. Marron K, Wharton J, Sheppard MN, et al: Distribution, morphology, and neurochemistry of endocardial and epicardial nerve terminal arborizations in the human heart. Circulation 92:2343–2351, 1995.
41. Kocovic DZ, Harada T, Shea JB, et al: Alterations of heart rate and of heart rate variability after radiofrequency catheter ablation of supraventricular tachycardia. Delineation of parasympathetic pathways in human heart. Circulation 88:1671–1681, 1993.
42. Doshi RN, Wu TJ, Yashima M, et al: Relation between ligament of Marshall and adrenergic atrial tachycardia. Circulation 100:876–883, 1999.
43. Van Wagoner DR, Pond AL, Lamorgese M, et al: Atrial L-type Ca^{2+} currents and human atrial fibrillation. Circ Res 85:428–436, 1999.
44. Ben-Haim SA, Osadky D, Shuster I, et al: Non fluoroscopic, in vivo navigation and mapping technology. Nat Med 2:1393–1395, 1996.
45. Smeets JLRM, Ben-Haim S, Rodriguez LM, et al: New method for non fluoroscopic endocardial mapping in humans: Accuracy assessment and first clinical results. Circulation 97:2426–2432, 1998.
46. Tsai CF, Chen SA, Tai CT, et al: Bezold-Jarisch-like reflex during radiofrequency ablation of the pulmonary vein tissues in patients with paroxysmal focal atrial fibrillation. J Cardiovasc Electrophysiol 10:27–35, 1999.
47. Kanaoupakis EM, Manios EG, Mavrakis HE, et al: Relation of autonomic modulation to recurrence of atrial fibrillation following cardioversion. Am J Cardiol 86:954–958, 2000.
48. Lombardi F, Colombo A, Basilico B, et al: Heart rate variability and early recurrence of atrial fibrillation after electrical cardioversion. J Am Coll Cardiol 37:157–162, 2001.
49. Schuessler RB: Does size matter? J Cardiovasc Electrophysiol 12:875–876, 2001.
50. Wellens HJJ: Pulmonary vein ablation in atrial fibrillation. Hype or hope? Circulation 102:2562–2564, 2000.
51. Wellens HJJ: Atrial fibrillation: The last big hurdle in treating supraventricular tachycardias. N Engl J Med 331:944–945, 1994.

性的方法来治疗房颤。房颤的射频消融治疗已经成为心律失常研究的前沿，目前仍被认为是一种探索性技术，但全球多个中心临床经验表明这一技术已经比较成熟，可以作为一种临床常规的治疗。

未来的研究方向，为提高这一技术的可行性，应该包括开发新的肺静脉隔离的消融术式，简化导管设计确保电极与组织接触的稳定性。我们希望通过更深地认识房颤发生的基本机制，开发出更安全而有效的针对发病机制的治疗方法。另外，采用温控装置或其他能量的消融方法应该进一步提高其操作的安全性及定位技术的精确性。最后，需要对导管消融治疗患者进行长期的前瞻性随机调查研究，来评价这一方法的长期安全性和有效性，从而战胜房颤这一"室上性心律失常治疗的最后堡垒"[51]。

七、致　谢

感谢 Giuseppe Augello 医生为本文所作的数据收集工作，还有 Filippo Gugliotta 校正排版工作。

（杨延宗　李　真　译）

参 考 文 献

1. The Atrial Fibrillation Follow-up Investigation of Rhythm Management (AFFIRM) Investigators: A comparison of rate control and rhythm control in patients with atrial fibrillation. N Engl J Med 347:1825–1833, 2002.
2. Van Gelder I, Hagens VE, Bosker HA, et al: A comparison of rate control and rhythm control in patients with recurrent persistent atrial fibrillation. N Engl J Med 347:1834–1840, 2002.
3. Roy D, Talajic M, Dorian P, et al: Amiodarone to prevent recurrence of atrial fibrillation. N Engl J Med 342:913–920, 2000.
4. Falk RH: Atrial fibrillation. N Engl J Med 344:1067–1078, 2001.
5. Wolf PA, Mitchell JB, Baker CS, et al: Impact of atrial fibrillation on mortality, stroke, and medical costs. Arch Intern Med 158:229–234, 1998.
6. Guerra PG, Lesh MD: The role of nonpharmacologic therapies for the treatment of atrial fibrillation. J Cardiovasc Electrophysiol 10:450–460, 1999.
7. Scheinman MM, Morady F: Non-pharmacologic approaches to atrial fibrillation. Circulation 103:2120–2125, 2001.
8. Calkins H: Progress continues in the quest to cure atrial fibrillation with catheter ablation techniques. Eur Heart J 22:2038–2040, 2001.
9. Asirvatham SJ, Friedman PA: Ablation for atrial fibrillation: Is the cure at hand? J Cardiovasc Electrphysiol 12:909–911, 2001.
10. Oral H, Knight BP, Tada H, et al: Pulmonary vein isolation for paroxysmal and persistent atrial fibrillation. Circulation 105:1077–1081, 2002.
11. Oral H, Knight BP, Ozaydin M, et al: Clinical significance of early recurrences of atrial fibrillation after pulmonary vein isolation. J Am Coll Cardiol 40:100–104, 2002.
12. Natale A, Pisano E, Shewchik J, et al: First human experience with pulmonary vein isolation using a through-the-balloon circumferential ultrasound ablation system for recurrent atrial fibrillation.
13. Saliba W, Wilber D, Packer D, et al: Circumferential ultrasound ablation for pulmonary vein isolation. J Cardiovasc Electrophysiol 13:957–961, 2002.
14. Haissaguerre M, Jais P, Shah DC, et al: Spontaneous initiation of atrial fibrillation by ectopic beats originating in the pulmonary veins. N Engl J Med 339:659–666, 1998.
15. Haissaguerre M, Shah DC, Jais P, et al: Electrophysiological breakthroughs from the left atrium to the pulmonary veins. Circulation 101:1409–1417, 2000.
16. Pappone C, Rosanio S, Oreto G, et al: Circumferential radiofrequency ablation of pulmonary vein ostia. Circulation 102:2619–2628, 2000.
17. Pappone C, Oreto G, Rosanio S, et al: Atrial electroanatomical remodeling after circumferential radiofrequency pulmonary vein ablation. Circulation 104:2539–2544, 2001.
18. Moe GK: On the multiple wavelet hypothesis of atrial fibrillation. Arch Int Pharmacodyn Ther 140:183–188, 1962.
19. Allessie MA, Konings K, Kirchhof CJHJ, Wijffels M: Electrophysiologic mechanisms of perpetuation of atrial fibrillation. Am J Cardiol 77:10A–23A, 1996.
20. Cox JL, Sundt TM: The surgical management of atrial fibrillation. Annu Rev Med 48:511–523, 1997.
21. Maloney JD, Milner L, Barold S, et al: Two-staged biatrial linear and focal ablation to restore sinus rhythm in patients with refractory chronic atrial fibrillation. Pacing Clin Electrophysiol 21:2527–2532, 1998.
22. Haissaguerre M, Jais P, Shah DC, et al: Right and left atrial radiofrequency catheter therapy of paroxysmal atrial fibrillation. J Cardiovasc Electrphysiol 7:1132–1144, 1996.
23. Pappone C, Oreto G, Lamberti F, et al: Catheter ablation of paroxysmal atrial fibrillation using a 3D mapping system. Circulation 100:1203–1208, 1999.
24. Chen SA, Hsieh MH, Tai TC, et al: Initiation of atrial fibrillation by ectopic beats originating from the pulmonary veins. Circulation 100:1879–1866, 1999.
25. Haissaguerre M, Jais P, Shah DC, et al: Catheter ablation of chronic atrial fibrillation targeting the reinitiating triggers. J Cardiovasc Electrophysiol 11:2–10, 2000.
26. Ho SY, Sanchez-Quintana D, Cabrera JA, Anderson RH: Anatomy of the left atrium: Implication for radiofrequency ablation of atrial fibrillation. J Cardiovasc Electrophysiol 10:1525–1533, 1999.
27. Weiss C, Gocht A, Willems S, et al: Impact of the distribution and structure of myocardium in the pulmonary veins for radiofrequency ablation of atrial fibrillation. PACE 25:1352–1356, 2002.
28. Wu TJ, Doshi RN, Huang BS, et al: Simultaneous biatrial computerized mapping during permanent atrial fibrillation in patients with organic heart disease. J Cardiovasc Electrophysiol 13:571–577, 2002.
29. Takahashi Y, Iesaka Y, Takahashi A, et al: Electrical connections between pulmonary veins. Circulation 105:2998–2903, 2002.
30. Bloom NA, Gittenberger-de Groot AC, DeRuiter MC, et al: Development of the cardiac conduction tissue in human embryos using HNK-1 antigen expression: Possible relevance for understanding of abnormal atrial automaticity. Circulation 99:800–806, 1999.
31. Cheung DW: Electrical activity of the pulmonary vein and its interaction with the right atrium in the guinea pig. J Physiol 314:445–456, 1981.
32. Ndrepepa G, Karch MR, Schneider AE, et al: Characterization of paroxysmal and persistent atrial fibrillation in the human left atrium during initiation and sustained episodes. J Cardiovasc Electrophysiol 13:525–532, 2002.
33. Kadish AH: Mechanism(s) of chronic atrial fibrillation. J Cardiovasc Electrophysiol 13:578–579, 2002.
34. Jais P, Hocini M, Macle L, et al: Distinctive electrophysiological properties of pulmonary veins in patients with atrial fibrillation. Circulation 106:2479–2485, 2002.
35. Olsson SB: Atrial fibrillation—Where do we stand today? J Intern Med 250:19–28, 2001.
36. Platonov PG, Mitrofanova LB, Chireikin LV, Olsson SB: Morphology of interatrial conduction routes in patients with atrial fibrillation. Europace 4:183–192, 2002.
37. Coumel P: Autonomic arrhythmogenic factors in paroxysmal atrial fibrillation. In: Olsson SB, Alessie MA, Campbell RW (eds): Atrial Fibrillation: Mechanism and Therapeutic Strategies. Armonk, NY: Futura, 1994, pp. 171–184.
38. Hsieh MH, Chiou CW, Wen ZC, et al: Alterations of heart rate variability after radiofrequency catheter ablation of focal atrial fibrillation originating from pulmonary veins. Circulation 30:2237–2243, 1999.

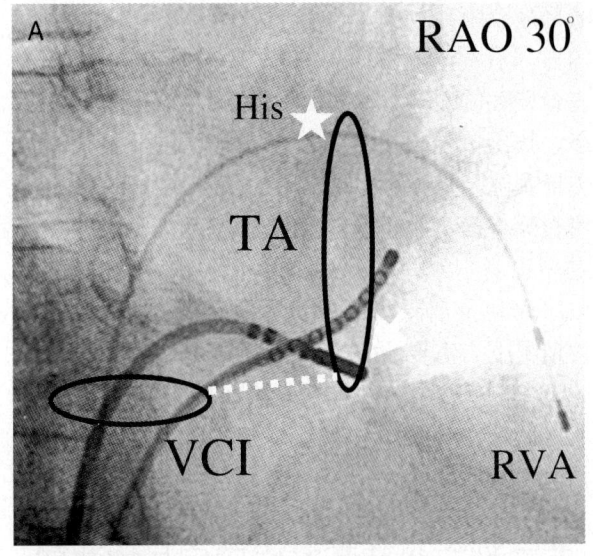
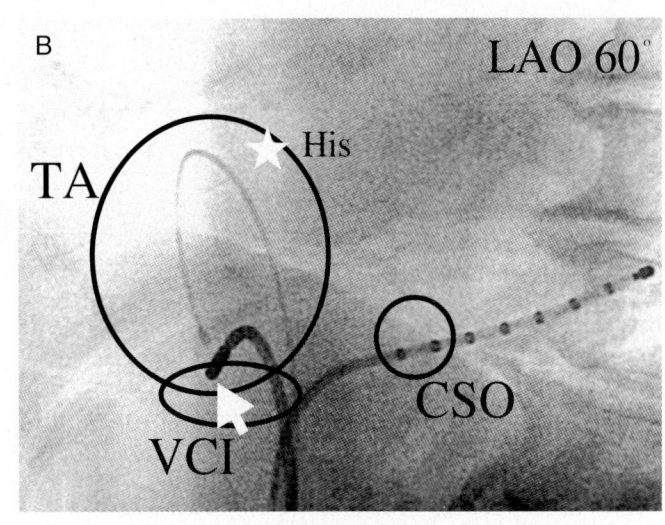
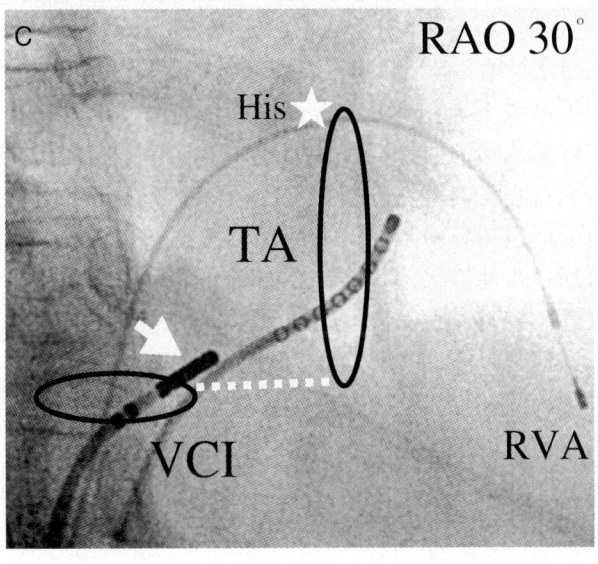
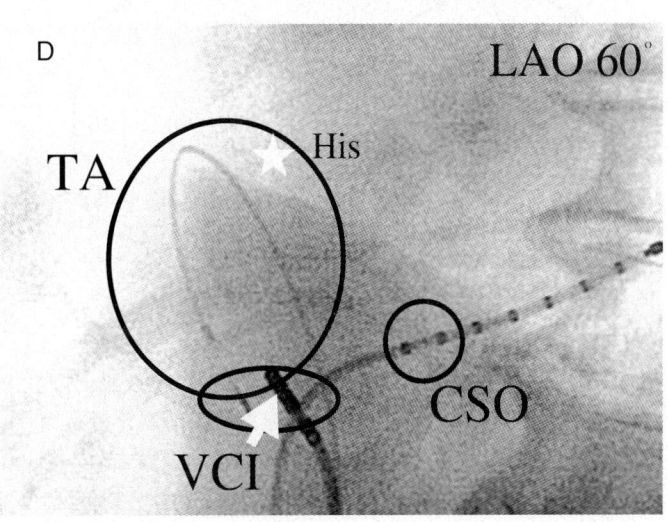

图 114-2　右前斜 30 度和左前斜 60 度投照角度进行下位峡部消融（白点为消融线）　8 极导管置于冠状窦，2 极导管置于右室心尖部。解剖结构投影定位：三尖瓣环（TA）、下腔静脉（VCI）、冠状窦口（CSO）和希氏束（HIS）（星号）。A 图和 B 图，8mm 头端消融导管（白箭头所指）置于峡部远端、三尖瓣环下方 6 点位置（左前斜 60 度，三尖瓣环恰似一钟表）。在消融过程中消融导管逐步回撤直到下腔静脉口的峡部近端（图 C 和 D）（图中未显示）。

右房前下方，亦即 20 极标测导管的第 1 对电极处起搏证实双向阻滞。然而，20 极标测导管正确放置是至关重要的，就是要将远端电极置于靠近消融线（图 114-3）。不足的是，应用这种间接标准，20 极标测导管中只有 1 对电极直接邻近峡部消融区，不能用这种标测导管定位残存的峡部裂隙。

与 20 极标测导管根据右房激动分析间接判断峡部阻滞相比，直接标准即冠状窦口或右心房前下方起搏，沿消融线分析心电图，可以更加精确地判断峡部部分阻滞或完全阻滞，包括峡部靶点区域对裂隙进行三维精确定位[15-17]。在峡部完全阻滞之后，冠状窦口起搏，直接记录消融线部位的电图显示消融线两侧激动不同步，导致出现两个有等电位线相间的心房电位，即双电位（图 114-4、图 114-5）。应用这种技术，消融导管再次标测完整的消融线，沿峡部消融线均可记录到双电位，并对此分析。首先，记录到具有平行双电位的完整通道，沿着消融线记录到的双电位间隔相等，无先后次序之分。其次，双电位宽而分离，典型的宽而分离的双电位间隔大于 100ms[17]。此外，冠状窦口起搏时，记录到消融线上方前向顺序传导波，加上 20 极标测导管提供的间接信息，可证实峡部完全阻滞（图 114-4）。当单一或狭窄的消融线就可达到确认峡部完全阻滞。

同样，沿着消融线标测的技术可用于定位峡部消融不完全残存的裂隙（图114-5）。比较双电位间期找出趋势，找出单个碎裂电位或分裂最窄的双电位就可定位传导裂隙。典型的传导裂隙，直接在靶点放电就可关闭裂隙，而不必再次消融整个峡部。在一些峡部完全阻滞患者，经过界嵴横向传导可以导致提前激动，顺序激动至消融线远端，类似跨峡部的慢传导。在这种情况下，需要更加完整的峡部电生理标测（图114-6）或动态起搏技术[18-20]，从而验证峡部完全阻滞。消融后观察30min有助于检测和治疗早期出现的裂隙，防止房扑复发。

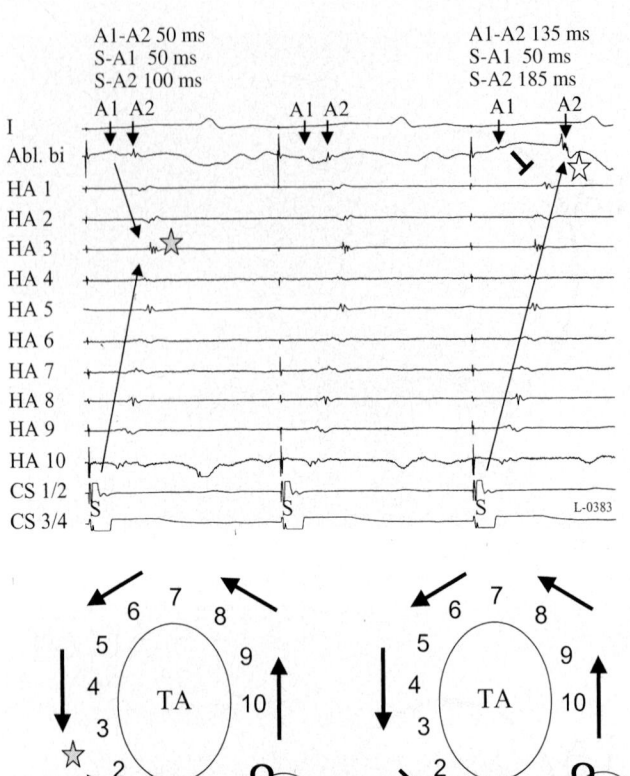

图114-3 峡部消融时，使用20极标测导管（10个双极记录：HA1～HA10）记录冠状窦口（CSO）起搏的激动图分析及简明示意图 消融下位峡部（黑色环）的远端和中段之后，仍可通过靠近下腔静脉残存的心肌束向前传导（曲线），在3极处（灰色星号）（三尖瓣环8点处），两个传导波融合（箭头）。消融导管置于邻近下腔静脉（VCI）处，标测到间隔紧密的双电位（A1和A2）。第三跳刺激（S）后，传导顺序发生改变，即靠近下腔静脉的传导裂隙被成功消融（灰色圆圈），这样造成峡部完全传导阻滞，在右房前壁记录到头尾向的先后激动模式，没有融合。20极标测导管标测，最迟的激动出现在HA1（白色星号）（三尖瓣环6点处），从冠状窦口起搏点看，恰在峡部消融线远端。在第三跳刺激后，消融导管记录到宽而分离的双电位（A1-A2间期>100ms）。

峡部完全阻滞时，双电位记录和分析技术较为简便，但是当需要在较大范围放电消融时，应用该技术分析心电图较为困难[18]。然而，在后者情况下，顺序标测记录可得到消融区直接信息，即导管首先置于消融线旁近冠状窦口记录到第一个心房电位波A1，然后导管顺时针缓慢移动到达消融线的另一侧，记录到第二个心房电位波A2。另外，冠状窦口起搏时，记录到消融线上方前向顺序传导波，可进一步通过间接信息

六、非典型右心房和左心房房扑的消融

对于所有沿着三尖瓣环顺钟向或逆钟向折返的房扑，可消融下位峡部或间隔峡部治疗。消融非典型，即非峡部依赖的房扑，需要通过起搏拖带标测定位左心房或右心房内折返的关键部位。与左心房房扑有关的折返环包括心房阻滞区域或电静止区域，大多数病例可通过线性消融治疗[2]。右心房非典型房扑常见于先天性心脏病外科修补术后（切口性心动过速）。常在心房切开术瘢痕和解剖屏障（如三尖瓣环下方或下腔静脉）间进行线性消融或标测出低电压区域形成的狭窄通道后进行局部消融[3]。

七、并发症和临床转归

正如以上描述，峡部消融相对安全。轻微并发症与股静脉穿刺有关。严重并发症罕见，如间隔峡部消融造成完全房室阻滞。我们最近观察到一位患者，冷盐水灌注消融下位峡部时出现严重的右冠脉狭窄，需要支架植入。

有了峡部完全阻滞的判断标准，峡部消融后复发房扑而需要二次消融的发生率已骤降到不足10%[11,13,18]。然而，部分有基础心脏病的房扑，在消融后的长期随访中，一些患者会发展为房颤。

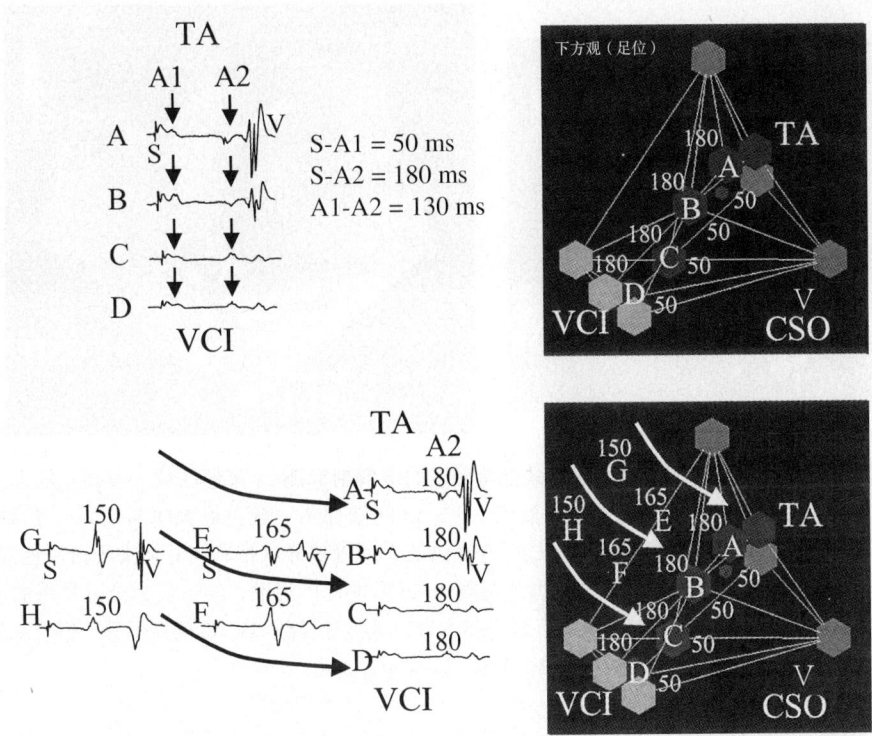

图 114-4　验证消融后峡部传导完全阻滞　左上图：消融三尖瓣环（TA）和下腔静脉（VCI）之间峡部后，冠状窦口（CSO）起搏，沿着整个峡部的 4 个点（A~D）都可标测到双电位。右上图：从下方看峡部电生理标测的解剖结构：3 个点代表三尖瓣环下方（中间的不代表 6 点位置），3 个点代表下腔静脉，深红点代表 5 个消融点。沿着整个消融线记录到宽而分离的双电位（A1 和 A2），A1-A2 间期均为 130ms。下图：除了标测到双电位，冠状窦起搏首先记录到向前上方传导的电位进一步证实峡部完全阻滞，而前方游离壁下传波（箭头）最迟激动点恰位于消融线（峡部消融线电图 A2），可以排除跨间隔的慢传导。此后，通过从消融线另一侧起搏可证实双向阻滞。（见彩图 52）

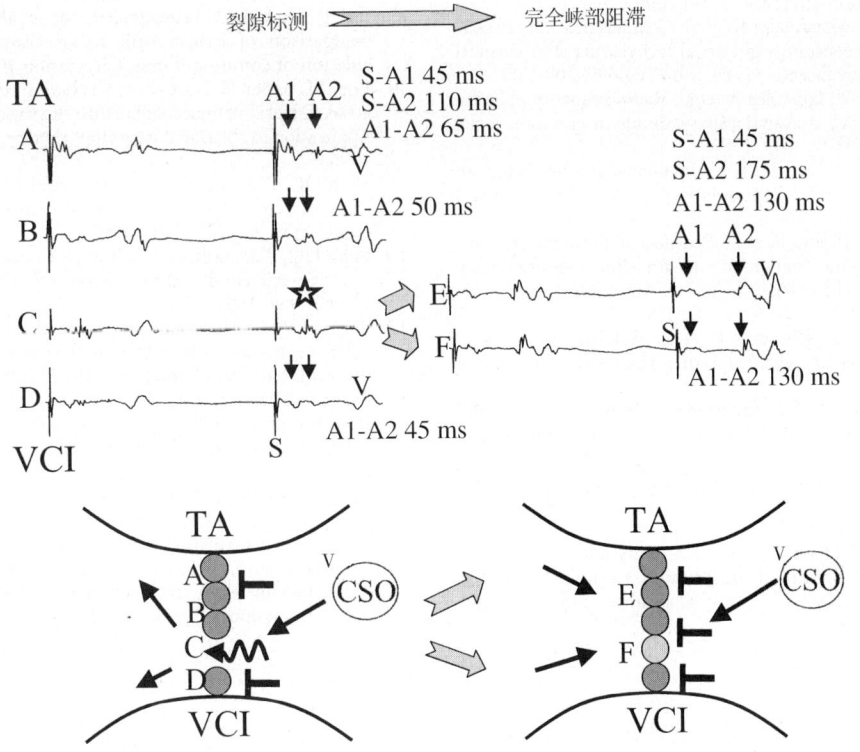

图 114-5　首次峡部线性消融后标测传导裂隙　左图：从三尖瓣环（TA）到下腔静脉（VCI）沿着峡部消融线重新标测（A~D）。靠近三尖瓣环处（A），标测到相距紧密的双电位，A1-A2 间距 65ms。在峡部中央（B）、靠近下腔静脉处（D）出现更加紧密的双电位，间期仅分别为 50ms（B）和 45ms（D）。C 点记录到连接 A1 和 A2 的心房碎裂电位，即所谓的裂隙电位（星号）。右图：额外进行一次点消融（灰色圆圈）导致完全传导阻滞。沿着整条消融线重新记录到分离显著的双电位，A1-A2 间期均为 130ms（图例 E 和 F）。

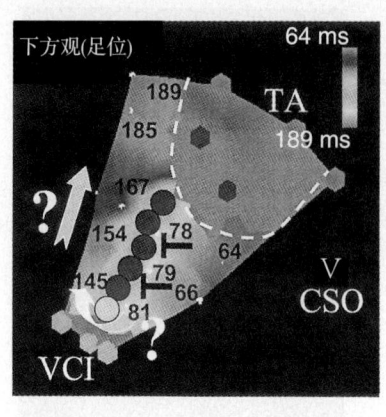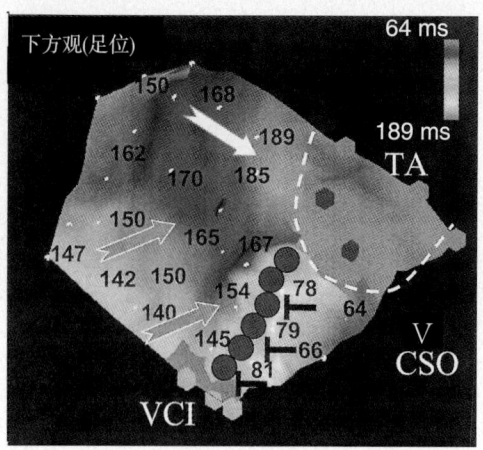

图 114-6 消融后，冠状窦口（CSO）起搏，重新进行峡部消融线的电解剖标测　灰色区域（虚线）代表三尖瓣环下方没有传导能力的纤维组织。左图：沿着消融线记录双电位，然而，A1-A2 间期并不一致。最大间期 89ms，消融线中部 A1-A2 间期 75ms，近端仅有 64ms，因此假设靠近下腔静脉处（VCI）存在跨峡部的慢传导（带有问号箭头所指灰色圆圈）。右图：进一步的再次标测证实峡部完全传导阻滞（靠近下腔静脉的黑色圆圈），不需进行再消融。经证实为经过界嵴的下端传导回路（灰色箭头），与三尖瓣环（TA，白箭头）前向传导波融合。经过界嵴较快地传导导致 A1-A2 间期不等，但最晚的激动仍然位于消融线（峡部消融线电图 A2 波），因此证实为峡部完全传导阻滞。（见彩图 53）

（高连君　译）

参 考 文 献

1. Shah DC, Jais P, Haissaguerre M, et al: Three-dimensional mapping of the common atrial flutter circuit in the right atrium. Circulation 96:3904–3912, 1997.
2. Jais P, Shah D, Haissaguerre M, et al: Mapping and ablation of left atrial flutters. Circulation 101:2928–2934, 2000.
3. Nakagawa H, Shah N, Matsudaira K, et al: Characterization of reentrant circuit in macroreentrant right atrial tachycardia after surgical repair of congenital hert disease. Circulation 103:699–709, 2001.
4. Cosio FG, Lopez-Gil M, Goicolea A, et al: Radiofrequency ablation of the inferior vena cava-tricuspid valve isthmus in common atrial flutter. Am J Cardiol 71:705–709, 1993.
5. Granada J, Uribe W, Chyou PH, et al: Incidence and predictors of atrial flutter in the general population. J Am Coll Cardiol 36:2242–2246, 2000.
6. Natale A, Newby KH, Pisano E, et al: Prospective randomized comparison of antiarrhythmic therapy versus first-line radiofrequency ablation in patients with atrial flutter. J Am Coll Cardiol 35:1898–1904, 2000.
7. Nakagawa H, Lazzara R, Khastgir T, et al: Role of the tricuspid annulus and the Eustachian valve/ridge on atrial flutter. Circulation 94:407–424, 1996.
8. Ho SY, Anderson RH, Sanchez-Quintana D: Atrial structures and fibres: Morphologic bases of atrial conduction. Cardiovasc Res 54:325–336, 2002.
9. Heidbüchel H, Willems R, van Rensburg H, et al: Right atrial angiographic evaluation of the posterior isthmus. Circulation 101:2178–2184, 2000.
10. Morton JB, Sanders P, Deen V, et al: Sensitivity and specificity of concealed entrainment for the identificaion of a critical isthmus in the atrium: Relationship to rate, antomic location and antidromic penetration. J Am Coll Cardiol 39:896–906, 2002.
11. Kottkamp H, Hügl B, Krauss B, et al: Electromagnetic versus fluoroscopic mapping of the inferior isthmus for ablation of typical atrial flutter. A prospective randomized study. Circulation 102:2082–2086, 2000.
12. Tsai CF, Tai CT, Yu WC, et al: Is 8-mm more effective than 4-mm tip electrode catheter for ablation of typical atrial flutter? Circulation 100:768–771, 1999.
13. Jais P, Shah DC, Haissaguerre M, et al: Prospective randomized comparison of irrigated-tip versus conventional-tip catheters for ablation of common flutter. Circulation 101:772–776, 2000.
14. Poty H, Saoui N, Nair M, et al: Radiofrequency catheter ablation of atrial flutter. Further insights into the various types of isthmus block: Application to ablation during sinus rhythm. Circulation 94:3204–3213, 1996.
15. Shah DC, Haissaguerre M, Jais P, et al: Simplified electrophysiologically directed catheter ablation of recurrent common atrial flutter. Circulation 96:2505–2508, 1997.
16. Shah DC, Takahashi A, Jais P, et al: Local electrogram-based criteria of cavo-tricuspid isthmus block. J Cardiovasc Electrophysiol 10:662–669, 1999.
17. Tada H, Oral H, Sticherling C, et al: Double potentials along the ablation line as a guide to radiofrequency ablation of typical atrial flutter. J Am Coll Cardiol 38:750–755, 2001.
18. Anselme F, Savoure A, Cribier A, et al: Catheter ablation of typical atrial flutter: A randomized comparison of 2 methods for determining complete bidirectional isthmus block. Circulation 103:1434–1439, 2001.
19. Chen J, de Chillou C, Basiouny T, et al: Cavotricuspid isthmus mapping to assess bidirectional block during common atrial flutter radiofrequency ablation. Circulation 100:2507–2513, 1999.
20. Shah D, Haissaguerre M, Takahashi A, et al: Differential pacing for distinguishing block from persistent conduction through an ablation line. Circulation 102:1517–1522, 2000.

第 115 章

房性心动过速的导管消融

Chin-Feng Tsai，*Ching-Tai Tai*，and *Shih-Ann Chen*

本章目录

- 房性心动过速的电生理诊断 ········· 1035
- 局灶性房性心动过速 ··············· 1036
- 局灶性房速的标测和消融 ··········· 1036
- 大折返性房性心动过速 ············· 1038
- 大折返性房速的标测和消融 ········· 1039
- 总结 ···························· 1042

房性心动过速是起源于心房的一种心律失常，在电生理实验室中占有症状的室上性心动过速的比例低于10%。有些房速病人可有频发的房性早搏，且对抗心律失常药物治疗无效。因此，导管消融治疗房性心动过速的重要作用日趋显现，在有经验的中心甚至已经成为房性心动过速的一线治疗手段。

房性心动过速传统的定义仍依据心率＜240bpm，P波之间有等电位线的心电图标准。然而，心率和是否存在等电位线对房性心动过速机制的判定缺乏特异性。新近，有人提出房性心动过速的发生机制上分为"基质"机制、局灶起源性机制和大折返机制[1]。这种分类有利于采用不同的治疗策略和对发病机制的判定。局灶性房速常起源于心房的某一区域并向两心房扩布，对房速起源的局部行导管消融可成功治愈心动过速，该心动过速的可能机制包括自律性异常、触发活动和微折返。大折返性房性心动过速是由围绕固定的和功能性解剖屏障发生的一个或多个折返环折返激动形成的，对折返环路的关键峡部等区域的线性消融可治愈这种心动过速。其临床特点是心房激动的折返环路涵盖了整个心动过速的周长，并可以被心房起搏拖带。从消融的治疗角度上，房性心动过速可以是局灶性，也可以是大折返性房性心动过速。本章主要回顾与不同类型房性心动过速导管消融相关的治疗技术的目前状况、消融结果和并发症等问题。

一、房性心动过速的电生理诊断

在电生理实验室，符合下列条件可诊断为房性心动过速：（1）心动过速时心房激动顺序既与窦性心律不同，也与心室起搏时心房的激动顺序不同；（2）房室阻滞不影响心动过速的发作；（3）心动过速时A-A间期变化，V-V间期也随之发生改变[1-3]。然而，有时房性心动过速与某些房室结折返性心动过速或隐匿性间隔旁路参与的房室折返性心动过速也很难鉴别。有几种起搏方法有助于对心动过速机制的判定：第一，可以在心动过速时给予一心室刺激，如果室性早搏落入希氏束不应期内，心房激动出现提前或室性早搏尽管未逆传至心房，但终止了该心动过速，可排除房速（考虑为房室折返性心动过速）。第二，应用比心动过速周期更短的频率连续起搏右心室，如果室房分离可排除房室旁路。如果该超速起搏呈室房1∶1逆传，但心房激动顺序发生改变，最大可能为房性心动过速，但需要排除存在另一条旁观旁路参与了逆传。若心室刺激时心动过速未终止，且心房激动顺序也未发生改变，停止心室起搏后出现V-A-A-V现象，支持房性心动过速的诊断。第三，采用同样频率进行心房刺激，如果心动过速即刻终止，或发生在房室阻滞后终止，不支持房速的诊断。第四，在心动过速下应用超速心房刺激，当心房刺激停止后，心动过速不

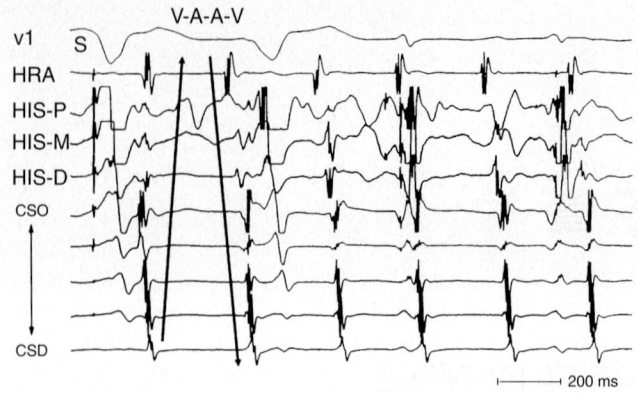

图 115-1 电极导管放置在高位右房（HRA）、希氏束（HIS）和冠状静脉窦（CS） 心室起搏后出现不同程度的房室阻滞和典型 V-A-A-V 现象，支持房速的诊断。

终止，而 VA 间期基本保持不变（变化幅度小于10ms），不支持房性心动过速的诊断。若 VA 间期总是在变化，支持房速的诊断（图 115-1）。

二、局灶性房性心动过速

局灶性房性心动过速可起源于心房的任何部位，既往的研究认为局灶性房性心动过速的特点是有起源的好发部位，右房房速最常起源于接近功能学和解剖学特殊变化的部位，如界嵴、三尖瓣环、冠状窦口、包括接近房室结区域附近的房间隔和右心耳[2-9,11-13]。左房局灶性房速最常见的好发部位为肺静脉内或肺静脉口周围和左心耳，以及二尖瓣瓣环的附近[2-4,9,10,12-15]。从心动过速好发部位所提示的这些特殊的解剖结构上告诉我们应注意心脏各向异性在其中的作用，如细胞间连接不良和胚胎发育异常在心律失常起源中的作用[5,11]。

最近，有一个重要的发现：起源于肺静脉内、上腔静脉和冠状窦的局灶性房性心律失常是引起所谓的局灶性房颤和某些阵发性房颤的原因。通过解剖学和电生理学研究已经证实，这些静脉在结构上具有从心房向静脉内延伸的肌袖组织。这些附着在血管壁上的肌肉组织在某些特定状况下可具有致心律失常的特征[16]。从局灶起源的这种出现得早的快速异位激动可发生传出阻滞或不均匀地传导至心房引起房颤样特征的心电图表现[17,18]。这些快速触发灶也可作为阵发性房颤的驱动机制，之后被多子波折返得以维持[19-21]。对这些静脉异位灶局灶性消融可成功地根治这种类型的心房颤动，详细的讨论请参考第 111 章和 112 章。

三、局灶性房速的标测和消融

在电生理实验室，一旦局灶起源的机制被确定，在心动过速发作时或频发房性早搏的情况下，通过心内膜详细标测通常可找到消融靶点。另外，这种成串反复发作局灶起源的房性心动过速的特点和 P 波形态可为标测和消融提供有利的帮助。

（一）P 波极性

通常，局灶起源的房性心动过速在所有导联上 P 的特点是 P 波之间有等电位线。然而，一些 P 波节律紊乱、等电位线消失者也可见于一些局灶起源性房性心动过速的病人[17,18,22]。另一方面，心动过速时 P 波和 T 波的融合也会影响 P 波的形态。在某些病例，心动过速发作时，可给予心室早搏刺激或颈动脉窦按压以及应用腺苷药物引起一过性房室阻滞使 P 波显露，通过分析 P 波形态可对心动过速的起源部位进行大致定位。

区别左、右心房的房性心动过速常采用 aVL 和 V_1 导联[23]。aVL 导联 P 波呈负向或等电位线和 V_1 导联呈正向提示为左房房速。反之，aVL 导联正向或呈正负双向，而 V_1 导联呈负向或正负双向提示为右房房速。另外，在下壁导联 P 波直立提示房速起源于心房上部或前壁，P 波呈正负双向或负向提示房速起源于心房的后壁或心房下部。其他利用 P 波极性预测房速起源的方法有：（1）aVR 导联 P 波负向通常提示为右房局灶起源性房速[24]；（2）胸前和下壁导联均负向提示为三尖瓣瓣环下方起源的房速[11]；（3）V_6 导联 P 波负向，V_1 导联 P 波正向，3 个下壁导联均呈负向提示后间隔房速或冠状窦口下方的房速[8]；（4）V_1 导联 P 波直立可以是房室结周围和房间隔左侧起源的房速[9,10]；（5）界嵴上部的房速与窦性心动过速和窦房折返性心动过速时的 P 波形态几乎相同[5]。

（二）心内膜激动标测

心内膜标测应首先按常规方法放置电极导管分别至高位右心房、冠状窦和希氏束部位，为心动过速下心房激动的标测提供一基本的激动顺序，精确的标测仍需要应用一消融电极导管以 P 波的起点作参考，在房速起源的可能部位再进行细致的标测，寻找最早激动点，或者以与 P 波有固定关系的冠状窦电图或高位右房电图作为参考电极，寻找最早激动点。成功消融的靶点要求比P波的起点提前大于30ms。但对不同病例可能有一些差别。人们已经认识到这种常规的标测技术也存在一定的局限性。

首先，在心房内从一点到另一点的标测可能需要花费很多的时间，在技术上也存在一定的困难。因此常需要采用不同类型的标测导管放置在相应的特殊部位以标测心动过速的激动起源。如且放置界嵴导管至右房界嵴三尖瓣瓣环附近（Cordis-Webster导管）。一种可伸缩的多极篮状电极（EPT导管）为快速确定在整个心房中房速的起源提供帮助。即使这样也不可能完全涵盖整个心房，尤其心耳部和峡部，对有血栓的病人，左房的标测也会受到限制。另外，为缩短标测时间，也常采用两根电极导管技术进行标测，先通过移动消融电极导管粗略标测到最早心房激动的区域，然后固定其中一根导管为参考电极，另一根导管在其周围缓慢移动，直至标测到最早的心房激动。

其次，左房房速也并不那么简单，因为对左房的标测常需要穿刺房间隔，而且再冠状窦的激动仅是一粗略的标测。有几种不同起源部位的早搏容易误导人的判断，如右上肺静脉起源的激动，其远场电位可以在邻近的右心房区域被记录到，且其在这两个部位起源的房性心律失常P波形态又非常相似。因此，当房性心动过速表现为界嵴上部或窦房交界区起源时，应考虑右上肺静脉起源的可能[5,26]。在右心房中部偏后的上方记录到肺静脉的远场电位被确定后强烈提示右肺静脉起源的可能。

其他起源于静脉系统的局灶性房速是起源于上腔静脉的房速，对于考虑为高位右心房的房速应包括上腔静脉内的仔细标测，另外还要考虑左侧间隔部房速。局灶性房速可起自房间隔邻近房室结的任何一侧，在该区域消融有损伤房室结的危险。如果最早的心房激动位于房间隔右侧，但心动过速时心房激动比P波起点提前不足15ms，或V_1导联呈直立向上，或推断其起源位于Bachmann束区域时，在右房间隔消融前应考虑先进行左房标测[9,10]。另外，已明确发现心外膜结构也可以致心律失常，且其可与肺静脉、左房肌或冠状窦远端存在电的连接。因此，若最早的心内膜激动位于二尖瓣环的后侧区域或在左上或左下肺静脉附近，需要通过冠状窦远端详细的心外膜标测，以确定是否为起源于心外膜的局灶起源性房速[27,28]。

当最早的激动部位被确定后，局部电图的特点可以为确定靶点提供一些信息，可利用单极电图记录显示出局部电图为完全负向的波形，其波形的起始为快速陡直向下时提示为心动过速的起源部位，局部的碎裂电位和尖峰电位（spike电位）也常常提示为成功消融的靶点，但其缺乏敏感性和特异性[5]。另外，导管压迫引起间歇性终止心动过速的部位也是预示成功消融的有效靶点[29]。但应当注意这种机械损伤确定的心动过速起源部位可能存在一定问题，因为该损伤也可能仅持续几小时。

（三）起搏激动顺序标测

起搏激动顺序标测也常用来确定房性心动过速的起源部位，尤其是该心动过速不能持续或很难诱发时。心房起搏标测是把消融导管放置在可能为最早异位激动的部位，起搏下比较心内膜心房激动的顺序，并用心房起搏下P波的形态与心动过速时的P波形态进行比较。但是，该标测在空间上可以相差达1.7cm，这种心内膜起搏标测技术仅属于附加的参考标测。

（四）新的标测系统

心腔内超声已经应用于常规多极电极标测中，该技术使我们在对相应的心内膜解剖结构了解的情况下较容易进行激动标测，并通过超声指导这种特殊的电极导管到达消融部位，为提高成功率提供了可能[5]。三维（3D）标测技术（非接触和接触标测系统）提供了非常好的空间结构，极大地加强了标测的精确性[25,31-34]。电解剖标测系统（CARTO系统，Biosense Webster，Diamond Bar，CA）建立在能对心脏的几何结构和电激动顺序进行细致重建的一种连续标测技术上。在心动过速时，在心内膜最早激动点进行高精度的标测可以细致地标测出心动过速灶，因而，若对可能的好发区域未能细致完整标测可能会导致误判和消融失败。该系统的最大局限性是对非持续性心动过速和不能诱发的心动过速的标测。对一些短阵发作的房速，非接触标测系统或多极篮状电极是可供选择的方法，比激动顺序标测有一定的优势。其特点是通过一跳激动信号可同时获得多个电极信号（图115-2）。

（五）局灶消融

一旦消融部位被确定，可应用25～50W的消融能量放电30～60s，放电中心动过速出现加速的现象，常提示该点对热量有反应，可成功消融这种自律性心律失常。放电10s内心动过速很快终止多表明该靶点十分有效和较低的复发率。是否被成功消融可通过手

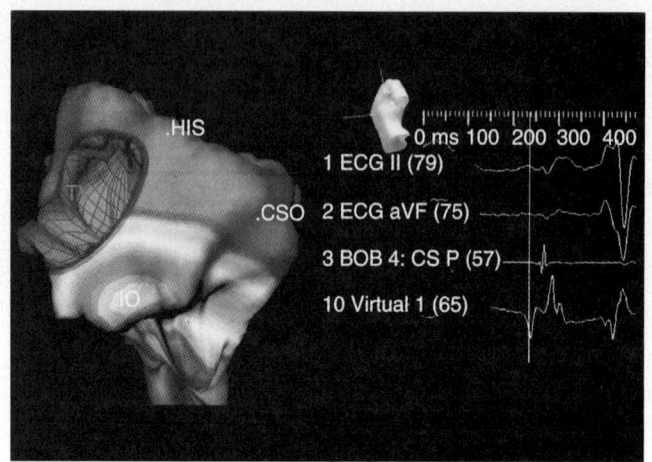

图 115-2 等时图标测显示心房最早激动部位于三尖瓣环下缘 最早激动点比 P 波提前 10ms。CSP，冠状窦近端。（见彩图 54）

术前后的诱发和静点异丙肾上腺素来证实。

对消融过程的有效性和安全性中的几个问题值得关注。第一，对不适宜的窦性心动过速治疗的改良问题[35]。对窦房结的导管消融首先从界嵴的上部开始，并沿界嵴逐渐向下消融，在静点异丙肾上腺素或阿托品后较术前心率下降 25%～30% 为有效消融的终点。过度的或不适当的能量释放可引起窦房结功能受损而需要植入永久起搏器，也可因窦房结周围局部的狭窄引发上腔静脉阻塞综合征，也有膈神经受损的报道。第二，需要注意房间隔或 Koch 三角房速有引起房室阻滞的危险。消融部位能记录到希氏束电位不是射频能量释放的禁忌，可采用滴定法消融（从低能量 10W 开始，逐渐递增，每次 5～10W，最大能量可达 40W），消融中需严密监测房室传导，预防意外的房室阻滞。第三，瓣环周围的房速其成功消融的心内电图同旁道消融特点相似，为大 V 小 A 的图形。第四，应当注意心脏静脉起源的房速心房激动和 P 波前的高频 spike 电位的特点。温控法消融（不超过 50～55℃）可以避免血栓形成，以及导管结痂和静脉狭窄的风险。

（六）导管消融的结果

导管消融局灶起源性房速的消融结果已经有几项研究报告发表，同时作者也对其进行过综述报道[5]。从相关报道的 252 例消融的病例中表明其成功率为 93%，复发率 7%。左房房速较右房房速成功率低，多部位起源的房速比单部位起源的房速复发率明显增高。值得注意的是，病人年龄是存在多源性房速和成功消融后房速复发的独立预测指标。这些发现提示心房退行性改变导致的病理学变化在致心律失常方面起重要作用（图 115-3、图 115-4）。对药物治疗无效的多源性房速，房室结消融可以作为改善症状的一种治疗手段[36]。

四、大折返性房性心动过速

大折返性房性心动过速是围绕一"大的"屏障形成的折返环路进行折返的一种心动过速，它既可见于正常的心脏患者（如围绕界嵴的折返），也可见于有心房组织病理改变的患者。根据激动的传播是否经过三尖瓣到下腔静脉之间的下部（三尖瓣-下腔静脉峡部）把具有典型大折返房速分为峡部依赖性房速和非峡部依赖性房速。峡部依赖性大折返性心动过速包括逆钟向典型性心房扑动、顺钟向典型性心房扑动和低环折返性心房扑动。非峡部依赖性大折返心动过速包括围绕心房切口瘢痕和围绕病理性损害区的大折返性心动过速。这种切口性大折返的频率范围可以很宽，有一定的交叉。即使既往有心房切开术病史者典型性心房扑动仍是最常见的大折返性房速[37]。非峡部依赖性大折返性心动过速常见于先天性心脏病外科修补术后或二尖瓣疾病外科术后[38-45]。大折返环的中心屏障可以是心房切口的瘢痕，也可以是间隔修补的补片、缝合线和瘢痕的边缘部位的相关部位。由于这些复杂的解剖、折返环路的易变性和多环折返的多个出口，

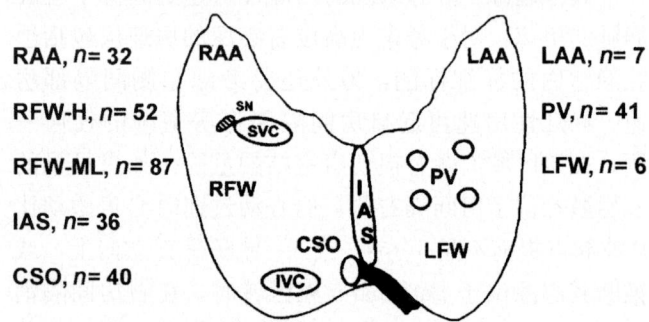

图 115-3 房速起源的分布 CSO：冠状窦口；IAS：房间隔；IVC：下腔静脉；LAA：左心耳；LFW：左侧游离壁；PV：肺静脉；RAA：右心耳；RFW-H 和 RFW-W：右房游离壁上部和中下部；SN：窦房结；SVC：上腔静脉。（引自 Chen SA, Tai CT, Chiang CE, et al: Focal atrial tachycardia: Reanalysis of clinical and electrophysiologic characteristics and prediction of successful radiofrequency ablation. J Cardiovasc Electrophysiol 9: 335-365, 1998.）

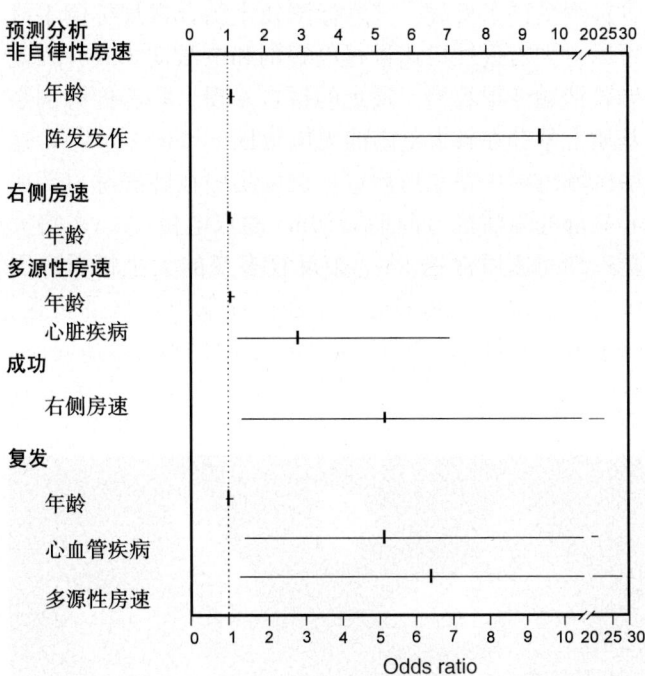

图 115-4 对自律性房速（AT），右房房速，多源性房速成功消融和消融后复发的独立预测因素分析 （引自 Chen SA，Tai CT，Chiang CE，et al：Focal atrial tachycardia：Reanalysis of clinical and electrophysiologic characteristics and prediction of successful radiofrequency ablation. J Cardiovasc Electrophysiol 9：335-365，1998.）

使得标测和消融显得非常困难。无外科手术史的右房游离壁大折返是通过界嵴上的间隙造成的折返，而无手术瘢痕者可能是围绕病理性损害区形成的折返。左房大折返性心动过速提示左心房参与了整个大折返的环路[45,48-50]。根据初始的标测在整个心动过速中右心房内未见折返激动，因而可以排除右房房速。心房大折返的环路的数目、环的大小和折返部位可有很多变化和不固定。应用碎裂电位标测来确定解剖屏障和折返环路的关键峡部对指导靶点消融至关重要。本章的重点是讨论非峡部依赖性大折返性房性心动过速，其他问题请参考其他章节（见第113章）。

五、大折返性房速的标测和消融

（一）P 波极性

心电图对大折返性房速的定位更加复杂，可靠性更低。临床上多种不同折返环周长和不同P波形态的房速，可能是由于房内不同的折返环独自形成，也可能是不同折返环同时激动所形成的。例如，左房大折返环房速在心电图上可以表现为典型房速的特点，如P波独立存在、P波间有等电位线、典型的房扑图形，也可表现为V$_1$导联P波直立向上的非典型房扑的图形[1,48,50]。另外，表现为典型性房扑体表心电图的患者可以是右房游离壁和峡部依赖参与的大折返性房扑，或者是局部孤立的异位激动，或者下腔三尖瓣峡部只是旁观者，或者是由包括冠状窦心房肌参与的左房大折返所形成[1,41,43,46,48,50]。这就意味着即使对表现为典型性房扑的患者也必须行下腔三尖瓣峡部拖带标测，以确定消融靶点对彻底根治心动过速是必需的。

（二）激动和拖带常规标测技术

常规标测技术包括激动标测和起搏拖带标测，该方法常用于确定传导障碍区或阻滞区，以判定消融导管是否在折返环路上来指导消融[1,37-40,42,43,46,50]。首先，典型的房内折返性心动过速可通过激动顺序标测寻找到最早和最晚的激动顺序而明确诊断，心房激动的标测范围应达到整个折返周长的90%以上。标测电极导管不容易到达的一些复杂的解剖部位可能会导致通过心动过速折返环路的激动未被完全标测出来。可通过标测低电位区、碎裂电位、瘢痕或补片上的电位消失或由于通过阻滞区的各不相同的激动顺序而形成的双电位等电传导特点，来确定传导阻滞和传导延缓区域。电极导管的轻微移动导致电信号振幅和时限的显著变化，也是确定典型解剖障碍区传导的重要手段。在大多数围绕损伤区的大折返性房速的病人中，这些异常的区域常为相应的心房切口或补片的部位，认识这些区域有助于我们对可能的解剖环路的判定。其次，结合舒张期电位和起搏后间期与心动过速周长相差小于20ms的隐匿性拖带可确定折返环内的"保护性峡部"。

（三）三维标测

最近，三维标测系统作为一项新的技术不仅应用于电生理和解剖标测，也为复杂的大折返性心动过速的消融提供了有益的帮助。它们能够准确地确定心房大折返的折返环路的各个部分，其中包括致密区、补片瘢痕区，并能够重建激动模板的等时图和电压图。等时激动标测的分析也可以快速确定缓慢传导区以指导拖带起搏和导管消融的部位。三维电解剖标测可以使瘢痕和补片区以及解剖障碍区清晰显示出来，使我们很容易对折返环的峡部进行横向线性损伤。另外，对所有消融过的部位进行定位和储存，并可检验消融线路上有无可传导间隙。

既往的研究表明,以前有瘢痕史的峡部依赖性房扑和大折返性房扑是瘢痕性大折返房速的最常见机制,通常为房内的两个折返环路向两个方向折返,最后通过一共同通道单向激动传导[39,41-43]。消融其中的一个折返环路常可显露出另一折返环路。这就要求我们必须仔细观察心房激动顺序和心电图形的变化。因此两个环路的消融对消融手术的成功显得尤为重要。

最近 Nakagawa 及其同事[44]对患先天性心脏病外科修补术后的 16 例患者行电解剖标测,以确定其是否存在独立的通路,他们声明该研究的目的就是要证实"没有独立存在的异常通路就没有大折返性心动过速"。结果发现在所有的病人中均有一较大面积的低电压区(≤0.5mV)。该区域内均存在一条狭窄的通道(其宽度≤2.7cm)。该通路可以是小的瘢痕之间的独立通路,也可以是正常心肌之间的异常通道。该通道可经过在折返环内起搏拖带被证实。不论是心电图图形、心动周期,还是起搏拖带,在狭窄的通道内外都是截然不同的。在该通道内局灶消融或较短的线性消融替代了对心房切口和解剖屏障之间峡部所进行的长线性损伤,可成功地治愈这种大折返性房性心动过速。他们还发现用常规标测技术无法找到所有的通道,因此消融成功率较低,尤其对那些施行过 Fontan 手术的病人。Delacretaz 及其同事[42]也有发现,在某些病例中,当确定了某一较窄的峡部后,对其进行局灶消融就可终止心动过速。

最近我们实验室对非切口性和非峡部依赖性右房大折返性房速的发生机制有了一些新的发现。我们通过应用非接触标测系统发现右房大折返房速可以是激动从界嵴中间的缝隙传导而形成的心房上部环形折返,其折返环路可以围绕中心屏障,其既可以顺钟向折返,也可以形成逆钟向折返,其折返环路是由界嵴、功能性阻滞区和上腔静脉构成的。在界嵴上更低的缝隙突破点也被发现(图 115-5),这可能是由于界嵴上缓慢的各向异性传导在该区域进一步受损形成了房内折返性心动过速的基础。通过对该传导缝隙(折返环路上最窄的部位)进行线性消融即可终止这种右房游离壁的大折返房速。

左房大折返性房速可表现为两个或三个折返环路的折返。由于这种复杂的折返环路、多种电位折返环、碎裂电位的存在以及低电压区限制了起搏拖带标测等因素,在技术上操作十分困难,使得应用常规导管标测受到了挑战。三维标测技术结合常规标测手段可以对大折返性房速进行电解剖和电激动重建,因此导管消融变得容易。最近的报告发现,心房的解剖学基质上常存在较大范围的无电位区(<0.05mV),这些区域可集中在左房后壁,也可集中在肺静脉口部或心耳部的阻滞区(间期≥50ms的双电位)[48]。左房大折返性房速通常是 1~3 个反复多变的大小折返环围绕着二尖瓣环、肺静脉、阻滞区或低电压区的折返。Ouyang 及其同事[49]进一步阐明了两种不同基质间保

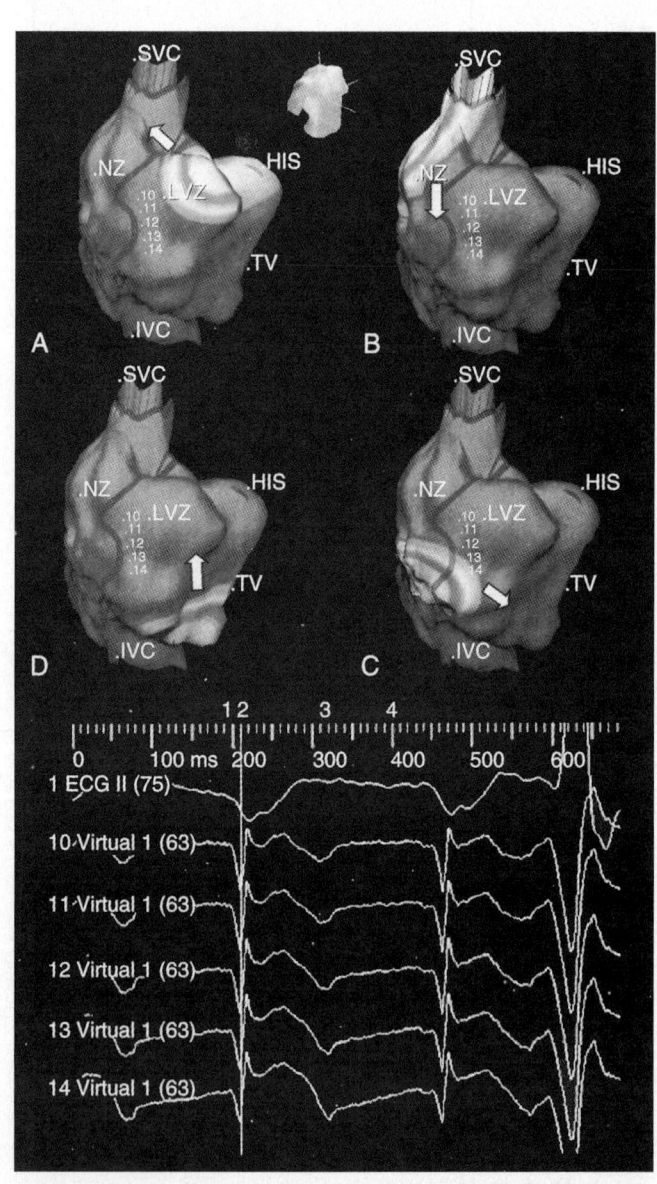

图 115-5 等电位图表示位于右房前游离壁低电压区或瘢痕处的大折返环 白色标尺代表最大负极电位,蓝色代表次级负电位,黄色箭头代表大折返心动过速的激动方向。中心阻滞区的实际单极电图代表双电位(从 10 到 14)。A~D 是按时间顺序排列的。(见彩图 55)

表 115-1 大折返性房速的标测和导管消融

第一作者（年）	病例数	类型	折返环或通道数量	折返周长（ms）	标测技术	消融模式	即刻成功率	复发率	随访期（月）	并发症
Triedman (1995)[38]	10	切口性 (RA)	30	323±14	激动 拖带	局部	8 (80%)	4/8 (50%)	4	无
Kalman (1996)[39]	18	切口性 (RA)	26	316±59	拖带	线性	15 (83%)	2/15 (13%)	17±8	无
Baker (1996)[40]	14	切口性 (RA)	31	314±88	激动	线性	13 (93%)	1/13 (7.7%)	7.5±5.3	大腿假性动脉瘤
Chan (2000)[37]	19	切口性 (RA)	21	293±73	拖带	线性	18 (95%)	7/18 (39%)	48	无
Akar (2001)[43]	16	切口性 (RA)	24	308±105	激动 拖带	线性	14 (87.5%)	1/14 (7%)	24±21	无
Delacretaz (2001)[42]	20	切口性 (RA)	47	315±79	拖带 (7) CARTO (13)	线性	18 (90%)	2/18 (11%)	19±4	无
Shah (2000)[41]	5	切口性 (RA)	6	262±40	CARTO	线性	5 (100%)	0	19±6	无
Nakagawa (2001)[44]	16	切口性 (RA)	29	NA	CARTO	局灶（短线）	15/16 (100%)	3/16 (19%)	13.5	无
Markowitz (2002)[45]	10	切口性（三尖瓣术后）(RA: 3, LA: 3)	6	344±110	CARTO	线性	3/5 (60%)	NA	NA	NA
Kall (2000)[46]	6	非切口性 (RA)	6	264±43	拖带 (6) CARTO (3)	线性	6 (100%)	0 (0%)	18±17	无
Tai (2002)[47]	8	非切口性 (RA) (3)	8	214±20	EnSite	线性	6/6 (100%)	0 (0%)	3.2±1.1	无
Jais (2000)[48]	22	切口性 (4) (LA)	17	303±78	CARTO	线性	20 (91%)	3/20 (15%)	15±7	无
Ouyang (2002)[49]	28	非切口性 (19) 切口性 (9) (LA)	42	337±82	CARTO	线性	25 (89%)	0 (0%)	14	腹股沟血肿 (2)

护性峡部在大折返性房速中的重要性。Nakagawa 也有类似的结果，他们发现关键峡部相对较窄，更适合于局部或较短的线性消融。Markowitz 及其同事[45]认识到了在左房大折返性房速的发生中左房间隔和右肺静脉之间峡部的作用。对关键峡部的传导进行阻滞可成功治愈这种心动过速和预防复发。

（四）导管消融的结果

导管消融可在电生理指导下对具有缓慢传导的关键峡部的出口和入口部进行消融，也可以通过解剖学标测对两个瘢痕之间或瘢痕与邻近的解剖学屏障区之间最窄的部位进行线性消融。成功消融的终点是指消融放电中心动过速终止、心动过速不能被诱发和消融后消融线两侧出现双向阻滞。表 115-1 汇总了关于非峡部依赖性大折返性房速导管消融的最新报告。通过随访认为解剖标测法消融优于电生理常规标测法。房速复发的原因是发生新的心动过速，或由于峡部宽而厚未形成彻底阻断所致，也可能是因为未诊断出可能存在的其他各种折返路径。8mm 大头导管和冷盐水灌注导管对可能较厚或有瘢痕的心房壁的消融成功率很高。

六、总　结

在心脏介入的电生理时代可通过常规电生理技术和新的三维标测系统明确房速的诊断，对房速机制和局部激动或者折返环的详细研究表明大多数房速可被成功治愈，且有较低的并发症和复发率。

（李学斌　译）

参 考 文 献

1. Saoudi N, Cosio F, Waldo A, et al: Classification of atrial flutter and regular atrial tachycardia according to electrophysiologic mechanism and anatomic bases: A statement from a joint expert group from the working group of arrhythmias of the European Society of Cardiology and the North American Society of Pacing and Electrophysiology. J Cardiovasc Electrophysiol 12:852–866, 2001.
2. Chen SA, Chiang CE, Yang CJ, et al: Sustained atrial tachycardia in adults: Electrophysiologic characteristics, pharmacologic responses, possible mechanisms, and results of radiofrequency ablation. Circulation 90:1262–1278, 1994.
3. Knight BP, Zivin A, Souza J, et al: A technique for the rapid diagnosis of atrial tachycardia in the electrophysiology laboratory. J Am Coll Cardiol 33:775–781, 1999.
4. Chen SA, Tai CT, Chiang CE, et al: Focal atrial tachycardia: Reanalysis of clinical and electrophysiologic characteristics and prediction of successful radiofrequency ablation. J Cardiovasc Electrophysiol 9:355–365, 1998.
5. Kalman JM, Olgin JE, Karch MR, et al: "Cristal tachycardias:" Origin of right atrial tachycardias from the crista terminalis identified by intracardiac echocardiography. J Am Coll Cardiol 31:451–459, 1996.
6. Iesaka Y, Takahashi A, Goya M, et al: Adenosine-sensitive atrial reentrant tachycardia originating from the atrioventricular node transitional area. J Cardiovasc Electrophysiol 8:854–864, 1997.
7. Lai LP, Lin JL, Chen TF, et al: Clinical, electrophysiological characteristics, and radiofrequency catheter ablation of atrial tachycardia near the apex of Koch's triangle. Pacing Clin Electrophysiol 21:367–374, 1998.
8. Chen CC, Tai CT, Chiang CE, et al: Atrial tachycardias originating from the atrial septum: Electrophysiologic characteristics and radiofrequency ablation. J Cardiovasc Electrophysiol 11:744–749, 2001.
9. Frey B, Kreiner G, Gwechenberger M, Gossinger HD: Ablation of atrial tachycardia originating from the vicinity of the atrioventricular node: Significance of mapping both sides of the interatrial septum. J Am Coll Cardiol 38:394–400, 2001.
10. Marrouche NF, SippensGroenewegen A, Yang Y, et al: Clinical and electrophysiologic characteristics of left septal atrial tachycardia. J Am Coll Cardiol 40:1133–1139, 2002.
11. Morton JB, Sanders P, Das A, et al: Focal atrial tachycardia arising from the tricuspid annulus: Electrophysiologic and electrocardiographic characteristics. J Cardiovasc Electrophysiol 12:653–659, 2001.
12. Nogami A, Sugut M, Tomita T, et al: Novel form of atrial tachycardia originating at the atrioventricular annulus. Pacing Clin Electrophysiol 21:2691–2694, 1998.
13. Matsuoka K, Kasai A, Fujii E, et al: Electrophysiological features of atrial tachycardia arising from the atrioventricular annulus. Pacing Clin Electrophysiol 25:440–445, 2002.
14. Mallavarapu C, Schwartzman D, Callans DJ, et al: Radiofrequency catheter ablation of atrial tachycardia with unusual left atrial sites of origin: Report of two cases. Pacing Clin Electrophysiol 19:988–992, 1996.
15. Hatala R, Weiss C, Koschyk DH, et al: Radiofrequency catheter ablation of left atrial tachycardia originating within the pulmonary vein in a patient with dextrocardia. Pacing Clin Electrophysiol 19:999–1002, 1996.
16. Chen YJ, Chen SA, Chang MS, Lin CI: Arrhythmogenic activity of cardiac muscle in pulmonary veins of the dog: Implication for the genesis of atrial fibrillation. Cardiovasc Res 48:265–273, 2000.
17. Jais P, Haissaguerre M, Shah DC, et al: A focal source of atrial fibrillation treated by discrete radiofrequency ablation. Circulation 95:572–576, 1997.
18. Mecca AL, Guo H, Telfer A, Olshansky B: Atrial tachycardia originating from a single site with exit block mimicking atrial fibrillation eliminated with radiofrequency applications. J Cardiovasc Electrophysiol 9:1100–1108, 1998.
19. Haissaguerre M, Jais P, Shah DC, et al: Spontaneous initiation of atrial fibrillation by ectopic beats originating in the pulmonary veins. N Engl J Med 339:659–666, 1998.
20. Chen SA, Hsieh MH, Tai CT, et al: Initiation of atrial fibrillation by ectopic beats originating from the pulmonary veins: Electrophysiological characteristics, pharmacological responses, and effects of radiofrequency ablation. Circulation 100:1879–1886, 1999.
21. Tsai CF, Tai CT, Hsieh MH, et al: Initiation of atrial fibrillation by ectopic beats originating from the superior vena cava: Electrophysiological characteristics and results of radiofrequency ablation. Circulation 102:67–74, 2000.
22. Goya M, Takahashi A, Nuruki N, et al: A peculiar form of focal atrial tachycardia mimicking atypical atrial flutter. Jpn Circ J 64:886–889, 2000.
23. Tang CW, Scheinman MM, Van Hare GF, et al: Use of P wave configuration during atrial tachycardia to predict site of origin. J Am Coll Cardial 26:1315–1324, 1995.
24. Tada H, Nogami A, Naito S, et al: Simple electrocardiographic criteria for identifying the site of origin of focal right atrial tachycardia. Pacing Clin Electrophysiology 21(Pt II):2431–2439, 1998.
25. Schmitt C, Zremmer B, Schneider M, et al: Clinical experience with a novel multielectrode basket catheter in right atrial tachycardia. Circulation 99:2414–2422, 1999.
26. Soejima K, Stevenson WG, Delacretaz E, et al: Identification of left atrial origin of ectopic tachycardia during right atrial mapping: Analysis of double potentials at the posteromedial right atrium. J Cardiovasc Electrophysiol 11:975–980, 2000.
27. Katritsis D, Giazitzoglou E, Korovesis S, et al: Epicardial foci of atrial arrhythmias apparently originating in the left pulmonary veins. J Cardiovasc Electrophysiol 13:319–323, 2002.

28. Volkmer M, Antz M, Hebe J, Kuck KH: Focal atrial tachycardia originating from the musculature of the coronary sinus. J Cardiovasc Electrophysiol 13:68–71, 2002.
29. Pappone C, Stabile G, De Simone A, et al: Role of catheter-induced mechanical trauma in localization of target sites of radiofrequency ablation in automatic atrial tachycardia. J Am Coll Cardiol 27:1090–1097, 1996.
30. Man KC, Chan KK, Kovack P, et al: Spatial resolution of atrial pace mapping as determined by unipolar atrial pacing at adjacent sites. Circulation 94:1357–1363, 1996.
31. Natale A, Breeding L, Tomassoni G, et al: Ablation of right and left atrial tachycardias using a three-dimensional nonfluoroscopic mapping system. Am J Cardiol 82:989–992, 1998.
32. Hoffmann E, Reithmann C, Nimmermann P, et al: Clinical experience with electroanatomic mapping of ectopic atrial tachycardia. Pacing Clin Electrophysiol 25:49–56, 2002.
33. Wetzel U, Hindricks G, Schirdewahn P, et al: A stepwise mapping approach for localization and ablation of ectopic right, left, and septal atrial foci using electroanatomic mapping. Eur Heart J 23:1387–1393, 2002.
34. Schmitt H, Weber S, Schwab JO, et al: Diagnosis and ablation of focal right atrial tachycardia using a new high-resolution, non-contact mapping system. Am J Cardiol 87:1017–1021, 2001.
35. Lee RJ, Kalman JM, Fitzpatrick AP, et al: Radiofrequency caheter modification of the sinus node for "inappropriate" sinus tachycardia. Circulation 92:2919–2928, 1995.
36. Ueng KC, Lee SH, Wu DJ, et al: Radiofrequency catheter modification of atrioventricular junction in patients with COPD and medically refractory multifocal atrial tachycardia. Chest 117:52–59, 2000.
37. Chan DP, Van Hare GF, Mackall JA, et al: Importance of atrial flutter isthmus in postoperative intra-atrial reentrant tachycardia. Circulation 102:1283–1289, 2000.
38. Triedman JK, Saul JP, Weindling SN, Walsh EP: Radiofrequency ablation of intra-atrial reentrant tachycardia after surgical palliation of congenital heart disease. Circulation 91:707–714, 1995.
39. Kalman JM, Van Hare GF, Olgin J, et al: Ablation of "incisional" reentrant atrial tachycardia complicating surgery for congenital heart disease: Use of entrainment to define a critical isthmus of conduction. Circulation 93:502–512, 1996.
40. Baker BM, Lindsay BD, Bromberg BI, et al: Catheter ablation of clinical intraatrial reentrant tachycardias resulting from previous atrial surgery: Localizing and transecting the critical isthmus. J Am Coll Cardiol 28:411–417, 1996.
41. Shah D, Jais P, Takahashi A, et al: Dual-loop intra-atrial reentry in humans. Circulation 101:631–639, 2000.
42. Delacretaz E, Ganz LI, Soejima K, et al: Multiple atrial macro-reentry circuits in adults with repaired congenital heart disease: Entrainment mapping combined with three-dimensional electroanatomic mapping. J Am Coll Cardiol 37:1665–1676, 2001.
43. Akar JG, Kok LC, Haines DE, et al: Coexistence of type I atrial flutter and intra-atrial re-entrant tachycardia in patients with surgically corrected congenital heart disease. J Am Coll Cardiol 38:377–384, 2001.
44. Nakagawa H, Shah N, Matsudaira K, et al: Characterization of reentrant circuit in macroreentrant right atrial tachycardia after surgical repair of congenital heart disease: Isolated channels between scars allow "focal" ablation. Circulation 103:699–709, 2001.
45. Markowitz SM, Brodman RF, Stein KM, et al: Lesional tachycardias related to mitral valve surgery. J Am Coll Cardiol 39:1973–1983, 2002.
46. Kall JG, Rubenstein DS, Kopp DE, et al: Atypical atrial flutter originating in the right atrial free wall. Circulation 101:270–279, 2000.
47. Tai CT, Huang JL, Lin YK, et al: Noncontact three-dimensional mapping and ablation of upper loop re-entry originating in the right atrium. J Am Coll Cardiol 40:746–753, 2002.
48. Jais P, Shah DC, Haissaguerre M, et al: Mapping and ablation of left atrial flutters. Circulation 101:2928–2934, 2000.
49. Ouyang F, Ernst S, Vogtmann T, et al: Characterization of reentrant circuits in left atrial macroreentrant tachycardia: Critical isthmus block can prevent atrial tachycardia recurrence. Circulation 105:1934–1942, 2002.
50. Olgin JE, Jayachandran JV, Engesstein E, et al: Atrial macroreentry involving the myocardium of the coronary sinus: A unique mechanism for atypical flutter. J Cardiovasc Electrophysiol 9:1094–1099, 1998.

第 116 章

房室结折返性心动过速的导管消融

Jonathan M. Kalman

本章目录

- 适应证 ·· 1044
- 导管治疗 AVNRT 的发展史：直流电消融和快径消融 ······························ 1044
- 慢径消融 ·· 1045
- 慢径消融的终点 ···································· 1046
- 慢径消融中发生房室阻滞的危险 ··· 1047
- 房室传导损伤情况下房室结折返的消融 ··· 1048
- 伴有上部共径阻滞的 AVNRT 的消融··· 1048
- 慢径消融后的不适宜性窦速 ·········· 1048
- 慢径消融：相关的解剖异常 ·········· 1048
- 射频的生物物理学因素 ··················· 1048
- 不可诱发的 AVNRT ······················· 1049
- 合并有其他心律失常的 AVNRT：心动过速诱发的心动过速 ···················· 1049
- 不典型 AVNRT 的消融治疗 ··········· 1049
- 总结 ··· 1049

一、适应证

射频消融（RF）治疗房室结折返性心动过速（AVNRT）已成为反复发作或有明显症状的 AVNRT 患者的首选治疗方法，美国心脏病学会（ACC）和美国心脏协会（AHA）在关于导管消融临床应用指南中建议"伴有临床症状的持续的 AVNRT 患者，药物不能缓解或患者不能耐受药物、不希望长期服用药物者"为射频消融治疗的 I 类指征。在我们的经验中，大多数年轻的有症状的 AVNRT 患者宁愿选择根治疗法而不愿意长期服药。而且，近年来的资料显示，即使心室功能正常的年轻患者，AVNRT 也不像以往认为是完全良性的疾病。Wood 等[1]报道至少 2% 的非致命性心脏骤停和 20% 的晕厥发作与室上性心动过速有关，75% 的患者心动过速发作时伴有明显的头晕。

二、导管治疗 AVNRT 的发展史：直流电消融和快径消融

自从 Roos 等[2]首次报道通过选择地阻断结周的心房组织并保留正常的房室传导治疗 AVNRT 以来，不断发展到目前的经皮技术进行治疗。最初导管治疗方法是利用直流电击来改变快径传导。Haissaguerre 等[3]报道采用这种方法治疗了 21 例顽固性 AVNRT 患者，他们将消融导管定位在心动过速时最早的心房激动部位，距可记录的最大 His 电位 5～10mm。释放 160 或 240J 电能导致房室结逆向传导的损伤，前向传导被改良，但有 2 例患者出现完全性心脏阻滞。

此后，AVNRT 的导管治疗采用射频电流消融快径。Lee 等[4]采用了同以上相似的技术，用射频能量行消融治疗。在此处导管记录到最大的房室电图，伴有一个小的希氏束电图。消融的终点为出现一度房室阻滞或出现室房传导损伤和 AVNRT 不能诱发。结果 39 例患者中成功 32 例（82%），3 例患者（8%）出现完全性房室阻滞需安置永久起搏器。Langberg 等[5]进行了快径和慢径消融治疗的随机对照研究，发现两种方法的有效性和安全性相似。这些研究采用能量递增的方法，开始时给予较低的能量以避免在消融快径

时造成房室阻滞[6]。然而，大系列研究显示快径消融成功率低且房室阻滞的发生率高。而且，行快径消融的患者，无论术中是否出现一过性的房室传导阻滞，均有出现迟发房室阻滞的可能[7]。因此，大多数电生理室选择消融慢径的方法治疗 AVNRT。

三、慢径消融

1992 年，Jackman 等[8]首次发表了具有里程碑意义的慢径射频消融文章，Broadly 认为，此方法将电生理的慢径电位标测与解剖定位两种技术相结合用于慢径消融。最初的报道采用电生理的方法记录"慢径"电位[8,9]，尽管此方法有很高的成功率但这种电位差异很大。Jackman 等[8]在冠状窦口（CSO）与三尖瓣环之间记录到高振幅高频电位（图 116-1 和 116-2）。在逆向慢径传导期间，这些高频电位在低频的心房电位前，而在窦性心律时顺序相反。以此作为靶点，作者消融治疗 AVNRT 的成功率达 100%。Haissaguerre 等[9]继而报道了慢径电位是一个在房室结后下和 CSO 前部的低频低振幅电位（图 116-1 和 116-2）。这些电位位于 Koch 三角内跨越肌性房室间隔处，其邻近三尖瓣环。在此靶点处消融治疗典型 AVNRT 也可得到 100% 的成功率。

然而，这些电位是否真正代表慢径电位目前仍有争议。McGuire 等[10]使用 60 极片状电极在外科手术治疗 AVNRT 时标测 Koch 三角区，结果显示在慢径逆向传导时，在最早的心房激动上方 16mm 以内均能记录到低频和高频电位。Niebauer 等[11]对在 AVNRT 患者后间隔部位邻近 CSO 处记录的心内电图与无 AVNRT 者记录的心内电图进行比较，并同时记录了 3 个其他心房部位心内电图，结果显示，AVNRT 患者后间隔区慢径电位的阳性率与对照组相比无明显差异（68%：70%）。然而在其他的心房部位，只有 6%～25% 能记录到慢径电位。提示这些电位可能反映了后壁过渡区的传导特性，它们与 AVNRT 的存在无关。此外，在已经成功的慢径消融后，许多患者仍有慢径电位存在。

在一项利用微电极技术对犬和猪心脏的研究中，McGuire 等发现，在 CSO 和三尖瓣环之间可记录到由于冠状窦口上方和下方两组大的肌束不同步激动所产生的低频和高频电位[12]。相反，在冠状窦的上方和前方可记录到由心房细胞和类结细胞束的不同步激动所产生的高频和低频电位，后者被认为是慢径的解剖基质。

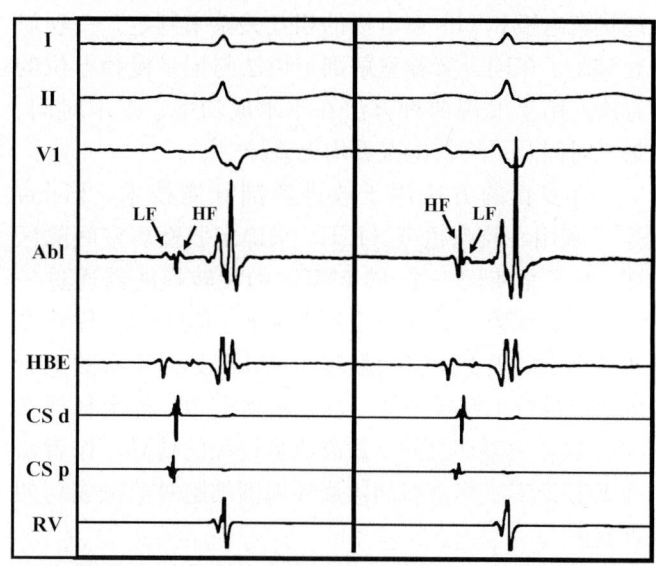

图 116-1　左侧为消融导管在冠状窦口（CSO）和三尖瓣环之间记录的电图　这些低频（LF）电位后跟随一高频电图（HF）构成 Jackman 等[8]描述的慢径电位。右侧显示消融导管位于 CSO 上方，肌性房室（AV）间隔邻近三尖瓣环处记录的电图，这里一个 HF 电位后紧随一个 LF 电位构成 Haissaguerre 等[9]描述的慢径电位，此患者在此处消融成功。

利用解剖定位进行慢径消融已成为目前的主要方法。这种方法基于慢径的解剖部位位于三尖瓣环和 CSO 下部连线及三尖瓣环与 Todaro 韧带所构成的三角区内，利用这种技术，导管被置于 CSO 和三尖瓣隔瓣之间三尖瓣环的心房面，在此区域内，可记录到高频的心房电图，而且心房与心室电图振幅比小于 0.5。如果此区域消融不成功，导管可逐渐向上进行消融，直至达到终点。解剖定位可以通过投影时消融导管与

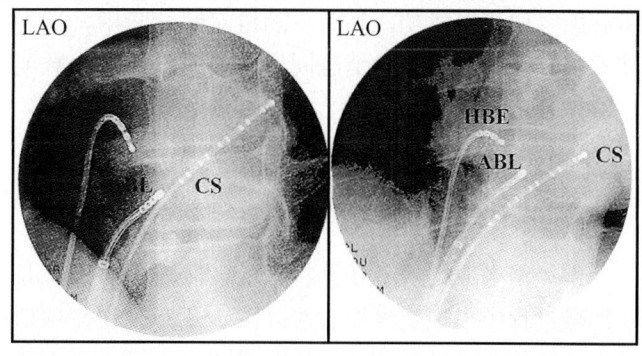

图 116-2　2 例患者左前斜位导管消融成功的部位　此投照角度有助于确认消融导管的位置与冠状窦口（CSO）的关系。左图显示消融导管位置在 CSO 和三尖瓣环之间（CS 导管的正上方），右图显示消融导管位于 CSO 肌性房室（AV）间隔的上方。注意导管在 CS 5，6 对电极的上方，$CS_{5,6}$ 位于 CSO。

冠状窦电极和His束电极的相互关系来判定。一项研究对比了在同一实验室解剖定位法与记录慢径电位的方法，结果发现两种方法在手术成功率、手术时间、曝光时间及平均放电次数均无差异[13]。

许多新的方法用于改进解剖标测技术，Fisher等[14]利用心腔内超声（ICE）来确定肌性房室间隔区域。ICE是使用一个12.5MHz的旋转换能器通过一个长的静脉鞘，引导导管到Koch三角区[14]，导管在肌性房室间隔上距三尖瓣环2~7mm处对所有的患者成功地进行了慢径消融。在这项研究中，能量释放在CSO和三尖瓣环之间，没有改良慢径的传导。作者认为ICE证实了房室肌间隔瓣环周围细胞对消融成功的重要性。

另一项改进慢径消融解剖标测技术的方法是在三尖瓣环通过Koch三角的后下部到CSO之间造成"拖带"损伤，尽管这种方法已被用于疑难的患者，但导管的稳定性、接触情况及心内电图信号的判定都很困难，故不推荐常规使用这种方法。

综合上述方法，目前慢径消融建议采用解剖影像结合心内电生理标测确定慢径区域指导消融。Sra等[15]采用单个程序期前刺激在慢径区域内打入AVNRT周期发现，能终止心动过速的最长配对间期的部位预示慢径消融的成功部位，其成功率达95%（18/19）。另一种确定慢径的方法是通过阈下刺激[16]，采用这种方法，用单极模式通过消融导管的远端电极，从1.0mA开始给予5s直流电脉冲，然后每次增加1.0mA直到心动过速终止或局部夺获。Willems等[16]在对50例患者进行的研究显示，47例患者阈下刺激仅仅在慢径区域内能终止AVNRT，而且在此处消融所有患者均获得成功。在另一随机对照试验中，这种技术与标准技术对慢径消融同样有效而且放电次数明显减少。

四、慢径消融的终点

慢径消融成功的一个非特异的，但敏感的标志是在消融过程中出现交界性心律（图116-3）。在一项研究中，成功消融的患者100%出现结性心律，而不成功的患者仅65%出现结性心律[17]，如果结性心律越多时间越长，消融可能越有效。有趣的是，Hsieh等[18]发现在成功施行了慢径消融的患者中，有很少一部分患者没有出现结性心律，他们报告在一组353例连续的AVNRT患者中，有20例（5.7%）没有出现结性心律。其原因可能有消融的位置偏后，心内电图心房振幅/心室振幅小（环周部位），缺少慢径电位成为快-慢型AVNRT。

在消融慢径时结性心律的来源仍有争议，一项细致的标测研究显示，这种心律来自于房室结移行区细胞的自律性增高，而不是通过一个分离的慢路径直接刺激房室结。然而，另一项研究认为当慢径活动完全阻断时往往伴有加速性结性心律反应的消失[20]，因而作者认为交界性心律对慢径损伤具有特异性。

消融时出现交界性心律后，须确认慢径消融是否成功。最常用的终点通常为在异丙肾上腺素输注前或输注中不能再次诱发心动过速。但是，与心动过速虽不能诱发但仍存在房室结双径电生理现象和单个回波相比，是否所有慢径传导的消除预示了晚期更低的复发率仍存在争议[21,22]。目前大多数电生理实验室都认为出现单个回波而不出现持续性心动过速（出现于异丙肾上腺素使用前和使用中）是明确的治疗终点[8,9]。据报道，在成功患者的长期随访中，多达65%的人会持续存在房室结双径电生理并伴有单个回波[8]（图116-4）。另外，近期资料表明，只有消融前要用儿茶酚胺诱发心动过速的患者才需在术后应用儿茶酚胺来评估消融终点[23]。

慢径消融成功的另一个指标是快径不应期的缩短[24]（图116-4）。尽管不是所有的研究都能观察到这一现象，Strickberger等[25]最近证实这可能取决于慢径是否完全消除。消融后持续性双路径存在并伴有单个回波的患者，没有观察到有效不应期的缩短，这与慢径对快径有电张力抑制有关。

有趣的是，对那些AVNRT伴有平滑房室结功能曲线的患者，不能以房室结双径电生理的丧失作为手术终点。虽然这些患者慢径的成功消融的确会导致代表慢径的曲线"尾巴"的丧失[26]。同样，在消融后心房起搏时，AH最大间期的显著缩短也表明具有平滑房室结功能曲线的AVNRT患者消融成功[27]。可见，貌似平滑的房室结功能曲线确实是由代表快径和慢径两部分组成，即便典型的"跳跃"并没出现。最近，Kou等[28]证实，在大多数A1A2/A2H2曲线平滑的患者，使用A1A2A3能暴露出A2A3/A3H3曲线的不连续性。此外，消融成功后"跳跃"的消失和最大A3H3间期的缩短表明可将其视为具有平滑房室结功能曲线患者的补充或附加治疗终点。

另一部分患者则是伴有多重前传慢径的患者，其证据是在房室结传导曲线中出现了多处中断[29]。在这

1. 一项研究发现，在消融过程中出现快速的交界性心律提示将可能发生房室阻滞[30]，但其他研究并未证实此观点。重要的是如果在消融过程中出现短周长的交界性心动过速，应立即终止放电以确定 1 : 1 房室传导，并且无 PR 间期延长。

2. 消融中解剖定位非常重要。通常在较前位置的消融发生房室阻滞的几率较高。但是，在一些病例中快路径位于非常靠后的位置，这可能是在后位消融术中造成房室阻滞的原因。Engelstein 等[31]发现 7 例 AVNRT 患者在 CSO 附近有后位的快通道，在此位置消融导致 6 例患者快通道顺向及逆向传导受损。这一研究强调在对 AVNRT 患者消融前，对快通道逆传出口位置的精细标测及定位的重要性。

3. 也许最有价值的指标是在消融过程中交界性心律出现不同程度的室房阻滞（图 116-3）[17,30]。因此，在消融过程中需严密监测 VA 关系，如出现 VA 间隔延长或突然出现 VA 阻滞提示即将发生心脏传导阻滞。

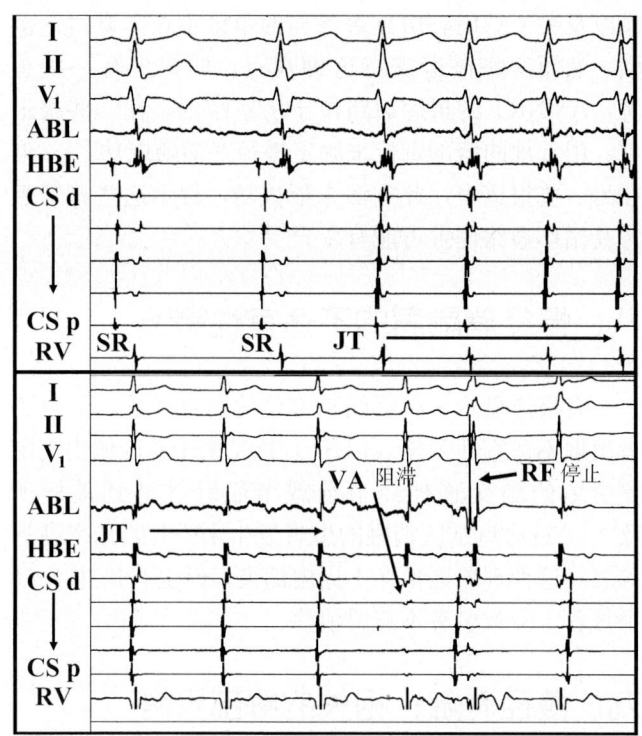

图 116-3 上图示射频消融（RF）术中加速性结性心律（JT）的出现。下图显示一单个室房阻滞（VA）（如箭头所示），370ms 后消融终止。室房传导阻滞通常提示应立即终止射频消融，并密切观察。SR，窦性心律。

组患者中，多数仅一条慢径与心动过速的发作有关，尽管在以往的报道中，有的多达 3 条慢径。在这些患者中，一半以上单一位点的射频消融即可以完全消除所有的慢径传导，而另一半患者则需多点位消融。慢路径多位于较后的位置。在多数患者以不能诱发心动过速（伴有或不伴有房室结双径电生理）为终点达到长期临床治愈。

五、慢径消融中发生房室阻滞的危险

在已报道的各组中，慢径消融中发生房室阻滞的比例不同，但总的来讲不超过 1%[5,6,8,9]。在早期的报道中应用前位消融法，其 AV 阻滞发生率较高为 3%，这在今天来说是不能接受的。对那些慢、快径间距很小或导管固定困难、稳定性难以达到的患者，可采取一些方法避免快路径损伤以免影响房室结传导。在一些病例中我们倾向应用长血管鞘并使用全身麻醉使肌肉松弛、呼吸平稳。此方法已证实非常有效，在一些困难病例中可确保导管的稳定性。

尽管有很多征象提示将出现房室阻滞的可能，但并未得到普遍认可。

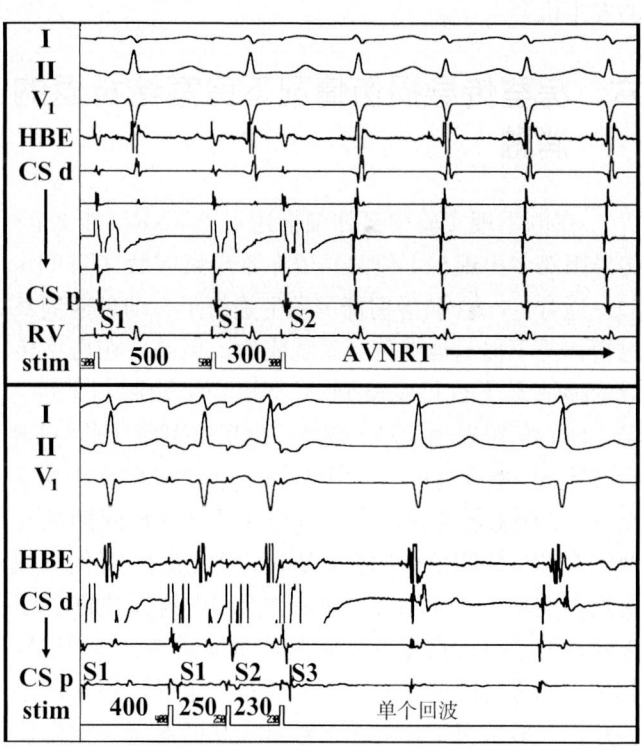

图 116-4 上图示室上心动过速（SVT）反复发作的一位 26 岁女性患者，通过刺激周期为 500ms、S2 间期为 300ms 诱发典型 AVNRT 发作。下图示消融术后，仅可激发单个回波。以其为治疗终点，治疗后 1 年 SVT 未复发。注意，消融术后仅可通过刺激周期为 400ms、S2 间期为 250ms、S3 间期为 230ms 引出慢径传导（单个回波），表明了快径有效不应期（ERP）的缩短。

4. 最后，Hintringer 等[32]应用一种新的方法，即观察消融导管标测的心房激动时间与希氏束记录的心房激动时间两者的相互关系来预测 AV 阻滞的发生。

尽管大多数 AV 阻滞出现在消融过程中，但也有的慢径消融后 9~15 个月才出现 AV 阻滞的报道[33]。

最近，Skanes 等[34]报道在 18 例 AVNRT 患者中冷冻消融的应用。在冷冻标测中可逆性慢路径传导的消失已得到证实，18 例患者中 17 例消融成功，在其后 5 个月的随访中未出现复发。需要注意的是，在冷冻消融过程中，即使在有效部位亦不会出现交界性心动过速。因此，交界性心动过速不能用于评估损伤的疗效。但是，在冷冻消融术中因导管头部的粘附作用，可减少所需的曝光时间，并提高导管的稳定性，以便在消融过程中进行心房起搏来检测慢径传导。2 例患者在 Koch 三角区前部冷冻消融过程中出现快路径的损伤，但随后立即加温均完全恢复。此项技术令人振奋，因为它能在某一特殊标测部位进行永久性损伤之前先评估其电生理结果，这可能会减少房室阻滞的发生机会。

六、房室传导损伤情况下房室结折返的消融

在电生理实验中已详细描述了 AVNRT 伴 2∶1 传导阻滞多出现在下位共径或在希氏束区域（图 116-5）。通常，2∶1 传导阻滞的发生是由于心动过速周长过短，并不提示远端传导系统疾病。但是，在房室传导受损情况下也可观察到 AVNRT 的发生（图 116-5）。Sra 等[35]描述了对 7 例伴一度房室阻滞（平均 PR=237ms）患者进行 AVNRT 消融治疗的有效性及安全性。7 例患者均消融成功并且未出现 PR 间期延长及完全性房室阻滞。同样，Basta 等报道了 18 例长快通道不应期（>500ms）患者中有 16 例成功进行了 AVNRT 消融，且未发生永久性房室阻滞[36]。但是，其中 1 例患者因反复出现暂时性房室阻滞而终止消融治疗。一般情况下，对大多数有症状的患者，如有快路径传导受损的证据，慢路径消融需谨慎进行，因有导致房室阻滞的风险。

七、伴有上部共径阻滞的 AVNRT 的消融

最近几个报道描述了 AVNRT 伴有不同程度的上部共径阻滞现象，尽管对 AVNRT 环路的解剖参数回顾以及关于结周心房是否参与的争论不在本章讨论范围，然而这些报道支持这种观点，即至少有一些患者，AVNRT 的折返通路位于房室结内。在一些报道中，用常规的解剖定位来确定慢径并消融成功[37]。但在另一些报道中，此方法未能成功，提示这些特殊患者其循环通路位置可能有变异[38]。

八、慢径消融后的不适宜性窦速

有报道显示，在后间隔部位的消融术后，部分患者出现不适宜性窦速（IAST）这是由于此区域内支配窦房结的副交感神经节前或节后纤维遭到破坏所致[39]。行房室结区消融的患者发生 IAST 的几率高达 10%。这种现象通常在 1 周内消失，但也有长达 1~6 个月者。多数患者不需要治疗。

九、慢径消融：相关的解剖异常

已有大量研究评价有典型 AVNRT 发作的患者其冠状窦畸形的发生情况，但结果不同。Doig 等[40]发现，AVNRT 患者与对照者相比，其冠状窦近端较大并形如袜套状，而对照组的冠状窦通常是管状的。有作者认为此项发现可能与心律失常的发生机制有关。但 Hummel 等[41]未发现两组间冠状窦大小有差异。研究表明正常冠状窦口直径和形态变异较大，其与 AVNRT 的发生与否无关。有报道称，在有左上腔静脉和显著扩张的冠状窦患者，在冠状窦口内进行标测能成功消融 AVNRT[42]，但在这些患者中显著扩张的冠状窦与其心律失常发生间的关系尚不清楚。

十、射频的生物物理学因素

早期 AVNRT 消融研究显示温控（T=60℃）消融与能量（P=35W）消融相比效率提高，而且慢径完全消融成功率较高[43]。Strickberger 等报道在后间隔部位消融热效率较低，这可能是由于此区域血流较多，因而导致消融导管温度下降。此区域消融通常需要较高的能量以便达到目标温度，因而温控消融是最佳选择。而且，温控 48℃与温控 60℃相比，即时成功率较低（75%∶100%），但在交界性心律出现室房阻滞的比例亦显著性降低[44]，而两者间出现房室阻滞不得不安置起搏器的几率无显著性差异。我们的方法是应用温控消融至 60℃，同时严密监控 VA 间期变化。

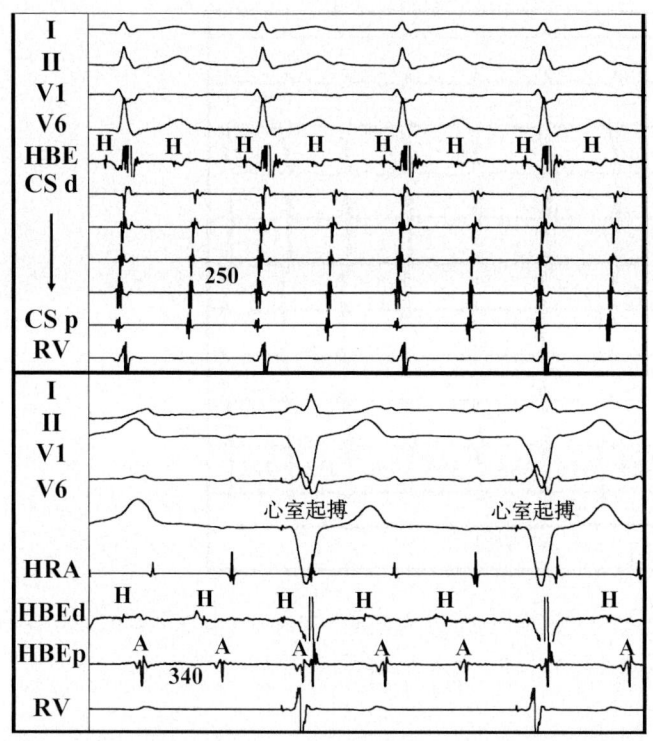

图 116-5 上图显示一个 18 岁男性患者无远端传导疾病的证据，在 AVNRT 发作时出现 2∶1 功能性 His 内阻滞。远端阻滞发生在心动过速发作时，原因是心动过速的周长过短（250ms）。下图显示一个 74 岁伴有完全心脏阻滞并安置永久起搏器的女性患者发生持续性的 AVNRT，H-A 间期固定，单一的心房期前刺激不能终止，此患者心动过速周长是 340ms，远端阻滞是由于远端 HV 阻滞，患者诉颈部有快速跳动感，起搏器储存电图显示一个快速的房性心率，慢径消融后症状消失。

很少有资料研究射频消融所需的时间长度。尽管通常情况下消融旁道需要 60s，但在正确的靶点及温度下大多数慢径消融 30s 即已足够[20]。

十一、不可诱发的 AVNRT

有大约 10% 的患者，在常规方法或应用异丙肾上腺素、阿托品后仍难以诱发 AVNRT[45]。导致难以诱发的基本原因包括：不能达到临界性 AH 间期、快通道阻滞及慢通道阻滞。在一些病例中，异丙肾上腺素通过缩短快径 ERP 可改变 AVNRT 的不可诱发特性，而它显然阻止了慢径传导[46]。在已证实有 SVT 发作、实验室检查有房室结双路径但未能诱发心动过速的患者，可行经验性的慢径消融，多数患者可临床治愈。

十二、合并有其他心律失常的 AVNRT：心动过速诱发的心动过速

据报道，AVNRT 可合并有其他心律失常，包括 AVRT、房速和房扑[48,49]。高达 15% 的 AVNRT 患者可通过心房起搏来诱发房速。他们中的大多数，AVNRT 的消融成功足以治愈临床上的心动过速并消除症状。然而，当房速在电生理室持续发作时，手术则应进行直到两种心律失常成功消融为止。有些患者，房速的短阵发作的确可引发持续性 AVNRT（图 116-6）。当合并存在的心动过速周期相近时，经常发生相互转换[48]。

十三、不典型 AVNRT 的消融治疗

不典型 AVNRT 是另外一组少见的心律失常，曾被命名为后位 AVNRT、快-慢 AVNRT 或慢-慢 AVNRT。尽管近期的资料已描绘了一些不典型的 AVNRT 环路[50]，但它们不都是典型 AVNRT 环路的反相，而更倾向于利用了两条分离的"慢"径。据报道，不典型 AVNRT 可发生于在电生理室对典型的 AVNRT 慢径消融治疗后，这种情况被认为是慢径传导改良的结果。多数患者可利用解剖手段消融慢径或标测心动过速发作中最早的逆行房性激动点来消融不典型 AVNRT[51]。有时，不典型 AVNRT 可具有貌似偏心的逆行激动顺序（似左侧旁路），最早逆行激动点在后侧冠状窦电极甚或冠状窦的侧壁，反映出环路的解剖定位[52]。此时，在常规的解剖学慢径区进行消融即可获得成功。

十四、总 结

AVNRT 的射频消融治疗具有成功率高、并发症少和手段不同、结果相似的特点。它应被视为反复发作室上速的一线治疗。对多数患者，射频消融可作为日常手术来进行[53]。

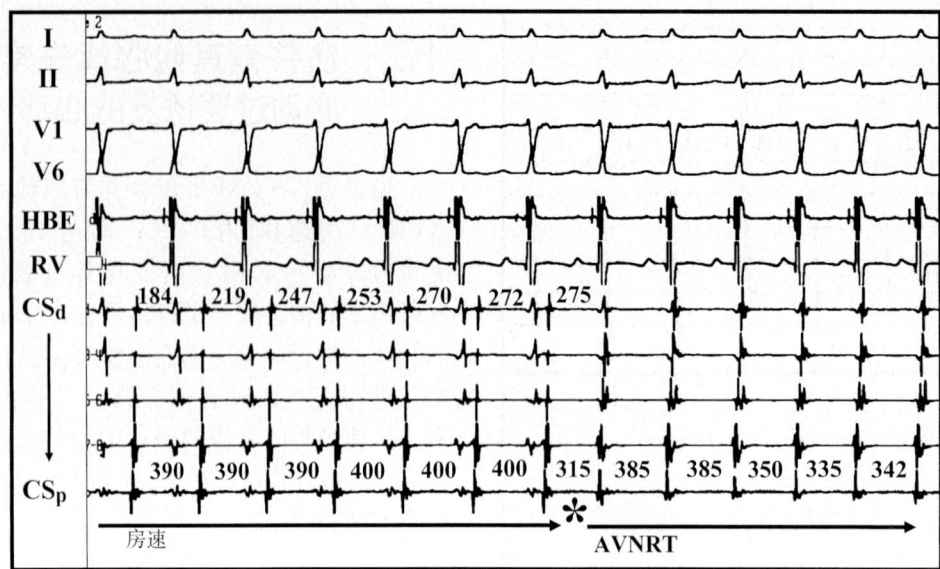

图 116-6 同时具有房速和 AVNRT 的患者 左侧为房速，CS_d 中的数字指逐渐增加的房室间期。同时要注意室房关系（V-A）不固定。CS_p 中的数字指房-房（A-A）间期。注意其后部尽管心动过速频率增加，但室房关系固定。这时，房速引发了 AVNRT，分别对慢径消融和在界嵴中部对房速消融获得了成功。

（许 静 译）

参 考 文 献

1. Wood KA, Drew BJ, Scheinman MM: Frequency of disabling symptoms in supraventricular tachycardia. Am J Cardiol 79:145–149, 1997.
2. Ross DL, Johnson DC, Denniss AR, et al: Curative surgery for atrioventricular junctional ("AV nodal") reentrant tachycardia. J Am Coll Cardiol 6:1383–1392, 1985.
3. Haissaguerre M, Warin JF, Lemetayer P, et al: Closed-chest ablation of retrograde conduction in patients with atrioventricular nodal reentrant tachycardia. N Engl J Med 320:426–433, 1989.
4. Lee MA, Morady F, Kadish A, et al: Catheter modification of the atrioventricular junction with radiofrequency energy for control of atrioventricular nodal reentry tachycardia. Circulation 83:827–835, 1991.
5. Langberg JJ, Leon A, Borganelli M, et al: A randomized, prospective comparison of anterior and posterior approaches to radiofrequency catheter ablation of atrioventricular nodal reentry tachycardia. Circulation 87:1551–1556, 1993.
6. Kalbfleisch SJ, Morady F: Catheter ablation of atrioventricular nodal reentrant tachycardia. In Zipes DP, Jalife J (eds): Cardiac Electrophysiology: From Cell to Bedside. Philadelphia, WB Saunders, 2002, pp 1477–1487.
7. Jazayeri MR, Hempe SL, Sra JS, et al: Selective transcatheter ablation of the fast and slow pathways using radiofrequency energy in patients with atrioventricular nodal reentrant tachycardia. Circulation 85:1318–1328, 1992.
8. Jackman WM, Beckman KJ, McClelland JH, et al: Treatment of supraventricular tachycardia due to atrioventricular nodal reentry, by radiofrequency catheter ablation of slow-pathway conduction. N Engl J Med 327:313–318, 1992.
9. Haissaguerre M, Gaita F, Fischer B, et al: Elimination of atrioventricular nodal reentrant tachycardia using discrete slow potentials to guide application of radiofrequency energy. Circulation 85:2162–2175, 1992.
10. McGuire MA, Bourke JP, Robotin MC, et al: High resolution mapping of Koch's triangle using sixty electrodes in humans with atrioventricular junctional (AV nodal) reentrant tachycardia. Circulation 88:2315–2328, 1993.
11. Niebauer MJ, Daoud E, Williamson B, et al: Atrial electrogram characteristics in patients with and without atrioventricular nodal reentrant tachycardia. Circulation 92:77–81, 1995.
12. McGuire MA, de Bakker JM, Vermeulen JT, et al: Origin and significance of double potentials near the atrioventricular node: Correlation of extracellular potentials, intracellular potentials, and histology. Circulation 89:2351–2360, 1994.
13. Kalbfleisch SJ, Strickberger SA, Williamson B, et al: Randomized comparison of anatomic and electrogram mapping approaches to ablation of the slow pathway of atrioventricular node reentrant tachycardia. J Am Coll Cardiol 23:716–723, 1994.
14. Fisher WG, Pelini MA, Bacon ME: Adjunctive intracardiac echocardiography to guide slow pathway ablation in human atrioventricular nodal reentrant tachycardia: Anatomic insights. Circulation 96:3021–3029, 1997.
15. Sra J, Jazayeri M, Natale A, et al: Termination of atrioventricular nodal reentrant tachycardia by premature stimulation from ablating catheter: A reliable guide to identify site for slow-pathway ablation. Circulation 91:1095–1100, 1995.
16. Willems S, Weiss C, Shenasa M, et al: Optimized mapping of slow pathway ablation guided by subthreshold stimulation: A randomized prospective study in patients with recurrent atrioventricular nodal reentrant tachycardia. J Am Coll Cardiol 37:1645–1650, 2001.
17. Jentzer JH, Goyal R, Williamson BD, et al: Analysis of junctional ectopy during radiofrequency ablation of the slow pathway in patients with atrioventricular nodal reentrant tachycardia. Circulation 90:2820–2826, 1994.
18. Hsieh MH, Chen SA, Tai CT, et al: Absence of junctional rhythm during successful slow-pathway ablation in patients with atrioventricular nodal reentrant tachycardia. Circulation 98:2296–2300, 1998.
19. Boyle NG, Anselme F, Monahan K, et al: Origin of junctional rhythm during radiofrequency ablation of atrioventricular nodal reentrant tachycardia in patients without structural heart disease. Am J Cardiol 80:575–580, 1997.
20. Wagshal AB, Crystal E, Katz A: Patterns of accelerated junctional rhythm during slow pathway catheter ablation for atrioventricular nodal reentrant tachycardia: Temperature dependence, prognostic value, and insights into the nature of the slow pathway. J Cardiovasc Electrophysiol 11:244–254, 2000.
21. Manolis AS, Wang PJ, Estes NA III: Radiofrequency ablation of slow pathway in patients with atrioventricular nodal reentrant tachycardia: Do arrhythmia recurrences correlate with persistent slow pathway conduction or site of successful ablation? Circulation 90:2815–2819, 1994.

22. Tebbenjohanns J, Pfeiffer D, Schumacher B, et al: Impact of the local atrial electrogram in AV nodal reentrant tachycardia: Ablation versus modification of the slow pathway. J Cardiovasc Electrophysiol 6:245–251, 1995.
23. Weismuller P, Kuly S, Brandts B, et al: Is electrical stimulation during administration of catecholamines required for the evaluation of success after ablation of atrioventricular node re-entrant tachycardias? J Am Coll Cardiol 39:689–694, 2002.
24. Natale A, Klein G, Yee R, et al: Shortening of fast pathway refractoriness after slow pathway ablation: Effects of autonomic blockade. Circulation 89:1103–1108, 1994.
25. Strickberger SA, Daoud E, Niebauer M, et al: Effects of partial and complete ablation of the slow pathway on fast pathway properties in patients with atrioventricular nodal reentrant tachycardia. J Cardiovasc Electrophysiol 5:645–649, 1994.
26. Sheahan RG, Klein GJ, Yee R, et al: Atrioventricular node reentry with 'smooth' AV node function curves: A different arrhythmia substrate? Circulation 93:969–972, 1996.
27. Tai CT, Chen SA, Chiang CE, et al: Complex electrophysiological characteristics in atrioventricular nodal reentrant tachycardia with continuous atrioventricular node function curves. Circulation 95:2541–2547, 1997.
28. Kuo CT, Lin KH, Cheng NJ, et al: Characterization of atrioventricular nodal reentry with continuous atrioventricular node conduction curve by double atrial extrastimulation. Circulation 99:659–665, 1999.
29. Tai CT, Chen SA, Chiang CE, et al: Multiple anterograde atrioventricular node pathways in patients with atrioventricular node reentrant tachycardia. J Am Coll Cardiol 28:725–731, 1996.
30. Thakur RK, Klein GJ, Yee R, et al: Junctional tachycardia: A useful marker during radiofrequency ablation for atrioventricular node reentrant tachycardia. J Am Coll Cardiol 22:1706–1710, 1993.
31. Engelstein ED, Stein KM, Markowitz SM, et al: Posterior fast atrioventricular node pathways: Implications for radiofrequency catheter ablation of atrioventricular node reentrant tachycardia. J Am Coll Cardiol 27:1098–1105, 1996.
32. Hintringer F, Hartikainen J, Davies DW, et al: Prediction of atrioventricular block during radiofrequency ablation of the slow pathway of the atrioventricular node. Circulation 92:3490–3496, 1995.
33. Elhag O, Miller HC: Atrioventricular block occurring several months after radiofrequency ablation for the treatment of atrioventricular nodal re-entrant tachycardia. Heart 79:616–618, 1998.
34. Skanes AC, Dubuc M, Klein GJ, et al: Cryothermal ablation of the slow pathway for the elimination of atrioventricular nodal reentrant tachycardia. Circulation 102:2856–2860, 2000.
35. Sra JS, Jazayeri MR, Blanck Z, et al: Slow pathway ablation in patients with atrioventricular node reentrant tachycardia and a prolonged PR interval. J Am Coll Cardiol 24:1064–1068, 1994.
36. Basta MN, Krahn AD, Klein GJ, et al: Safety of slow pathway ablation in patients with atrioventricular node reentrant tachycardia and a long fast pathway effective refractory period. Am J Cardiol 80:155–159, 1997.
37. Morady F: Ventriculoatrial block during a narrow-QRS tachycardia: What is the tachycardia mechanism?—IV. J Cardiovasc Electrophysiol 7:174–177, 1996.
38. Calo L, Lamberti F, Ciolli A, et al: Atrioventricular nodal reentrant tachycardia with ventriculoatrial block and unsuccessful ablation of the slow pathway. J Cardiovasc Electrophysiol 13:705–708, 2002.
39. Kocovic DZ, Harada T, Shea JB, et al: Alterations of heart rate and of heart rate variability after radiofrequency catheter ablation of supraventricular tachycardia: Delineation of parasympathetic pathways in the human heart. Circulation 88:1671–1681, 1993.
40. Doig JC, Saito J, Harris L, et al: Coronary sinus morphology in patients with atrioventricular junctional reentry tachycardia and other supraventricular tachyarrhythmias. Circulation 92:436–441, 1995.
41. Hummel JD, Strickberger SA, Man KC, et al: A quantitative fluoroscopic comparison of the coronary sinus ostium in patients with and without AV nodal reentrant tachycardia. J Cardiovasc Electrophysiol 6:681–686, 1995.
42. Okishige K, Fisher JD, Goseki Y, et al: Radiofrequency catheter ablation for AV nodal reentrant tachycardia associated with persistent left superior vena cava. Pacing Clin Electrophysiol 20:2213–2218, 1997.
43. Strickberger SA, Daoud EG, Weiss R, et al: A randomized comparison of fixed power and temperature monitoring during slow pathway ablation in patients with atrioventricular nodal reentrant tachycardia. J Interv Card Electrophysiol 1:299–303, 1997.
44. Strickberger SA, Tokano T, Tse HF, et al: Target temperatures of 48 degrees C versus 60 degrees C during slow pathway ablation: A randomized comparison. J Cardiovasc Electrophysiol 10:799–803, 1999.
45. Strickberger SA, Daoud EG, Niebauer MJ, et al: The mechanisms responsible for lack of reproducible induction of atrioventricular nodal reentrant tachycardia. J Cardiovasc Electrophysiol 7:494–502, 1996.
46. Hatzinikolaou H, Rodriguez LM, Smeets JL, et al: Isoprenaline and inducibility of atrioventricular nodal re-entrant tachycardia. Heart 79:165–168, 1998.
47. Bogun F, Knight B, Weiss R, et al: Slow pathway ablation in patients with documented but noninducible paroxysmal supraventricular tachycardia. J Am Coll Cardiol 28:1000–1004, 1996.
48. Kuo JY, Tai CT, Chiang CE, et al: Mechanisms of transition between double paroxysmal supraventricular tachycardias. J Cardiovasc Electrophysiol 12:1339–1345, 2001.
49. Sticherling C, Tada H, Greenstein R, et al: Incidence and clinical significance of inducible atrial tachycardia in patients with atrioventricular nodal reentrant tachycardia. J Cardiovasc Electrophysiol 12:507–510, 2001.
50. Yamabe H, Shimasaki Y, Honda O, et al: Demonstration of the exact anatomic tachycardia circuit in the fast-slow form of atrioventricular nodal reentrant tachycardia. Circulation 104:1268–1273, 2001.
51. Strickberger SA, Kalbfleisch SJ, Williamson B, et al: Radiofrequency catheter ablation of atypical atrioventricular nodal reentrant tachycardia. J Cardiovasc Electrophysiol 4:526–532, 1993.
52. Hwang C, Martin DJ, Goodman JS, et al: Atypical atrioventricular node reciprocating tachycardia masquerading as tachycardia using a left-sided accessory pathway. J Am Coll Cardiol 30:218–225, 1997.
53. Man KC, Kalbfleisch SJ, Hummel JD, et al: Safety and cost of outpatient radiofrequency ablation of the slow pathway in patients with atrioventricular nodal reentrant tachycardia. Am J Cardiol 72:1323–1324, 1993.

第 117 章

房室折返性心动过速的导管消融

Sabine Ernst, Feifan Ouyang, Matthias Antz, Riccardo Cappato, Karl-Heinz Kuck

本章目录

- 解剖学 1052
- 旁路的标测和消融技术 1052
- 单个心内膜旁路的射频消融 1053
- 房室多旁路 1056
- 具有递减慢传导特性的房室旁路 ... 1057
- 旁路患者射频消融的有效性 1058
- 复发 1058
- 与旁道位置有关的并发症 1058
- 射频导管消融时的危害 1058
- 总结 1058

射频导管消融术自其应用于临床以来已成为房室折返性心动过速患者的治疗选择之一（见第58章）[1,2]。对旁路消融可以防止 WPW 综合征患者发生猝死（因为房颤可沿旁路前传）[3]。此外，因为导管消融的并发症发生率很低，并在绝大多数治疗中心其远期成功率超过95%，所以现在越来越少采用手术治疗[4,5]。本章主要讨论旁路的导管消融术，特别强调一些疑难病例并分析了房室旁路的不同类型。

本章所使用的术语包括正确的解剖学术语（方括号中）和目前所使用的术语[6]。

一、解剖学

导管消融包括采用沿房室瓣环的电活动来定位房室旁路（标测，见后文），以及其后使用特殊的消融电极导管在旁路靶点发放射频电流。为了使心脏组织达到足够的温度，需要在发放射频电流时保证导管稳定充分的接触（见第 111 章）。

二、旁路的标测和消融技术

（一）确定房室沟

在不需要考虑心律的情况下可以通过使用心房和心室的双极/单极记录来定位导管在瓣环上的位置。2个电位的振幅与瓣环在心房侧和心室侧以及激动波阵的方向和高低有关（如当波阵与电极平行时记录到最大的波形）。

（二）导管途径

1. 左侧旁路

两个途径可供选择。多数情况下选择逆行法，导管经股动脉通过主动脉瓣在二尖瓣下到达心室面或向前推送至心房面消融旁路的心房插入端。如果导管在二尖瓣瓣叶下（心室端），那么导管头端的运动与心室的运动一致。在这个位置，房室电位振幅（A/V）比值小于 1（0.05~0.7）。当在连续的心脏搏动时，心房电位振幅的改变小于20%表明导管在二尖瓣环接触牢固。相反，在房室瓣环的心房面，导管头端的摆动常与心室运动脱节。此时 A/V 比值为 1 或更大，并且当导管进一步推送远离瓣环时此比值更大。心房电位振幅变化超过 20% 时说明导管的稳定性减低[7]。另一种方法是经静脉送入消融导管通过房间隔消融旁路的心房端，当使用长鞘时导管的稳定性提高。

2. 右侧旁路

除了前间隔旁路［上位间隔］（使用经颈静脉途径）外，消融导管可经股静脉途径（图117-1）。右侧旁路的消融常常是在瓣环的右房侧，而不用考虑 A/V 比值。如果需要可使用长鞘送至下腔静脉口以提高消融导管的稳定性。为了达到所需的消融温度可能需要增加放电时间。

（三）确认旁路

插入位点

为了确认旁路的解剖学位置可能需要参考下述的电生理学参数：（1）预先激动的局部心室或心房时间，或二者的时间；（2）局部房室或室房间期，或二者的间期；（3）旁路电位的直接记录。

最早心室和心房电位：在常见病例中，提前出现的最早局部心室和心房电位（显性旁路）可确认旁路的心室和心房插入点[8]。在窦性心律或心房起搏时，最早心室激动位点可确定能够前传旁路的心室插入点。同样的，在逆传旁路的顺向型房室折返性心动过速或心室起搏时可以确定最早心房激动位点。在最早心室激动点使用单极记录时的 QS 型局部单极电位波可证实预激波的心内膜突破点[9]。

房室和室房间期：在双极记录时可以最佳分辨局部房室或室房间期，且在最早激动点位置二者相互邻近。然而，应当注意间期可能会受到旁路走行、传导特性以及激动波阵方向与消融电极走行的关系等影响。

房室旁路电位的记录：在前传时，如果在局部心房波之后可以记录到明显的双极电位，并在体表心电图的 delta 波之前出现且其后有心室波，即认为其为旁路电位。而在逆传时，常常不能明确确认旁路电位[10]，可能是因为心室电位叠加在上面的原因（大概30%）。在绝大多数的病例中，旁路电位多紧随在心室电位 15～30ms 以后或与其起始部位重合。除此，还可以通过心房和心室起搏来使心房和心室电位与可能的旁路电位分离以确认旁路电位。

三、单个心内膜旁路的射频消融

（一）右或左侧游离壁的房室旁路

可以通过在本节所介绍的方法来定位和消融心内膜游离壁旁路。旁路的标测和消融并不在本章讨论。

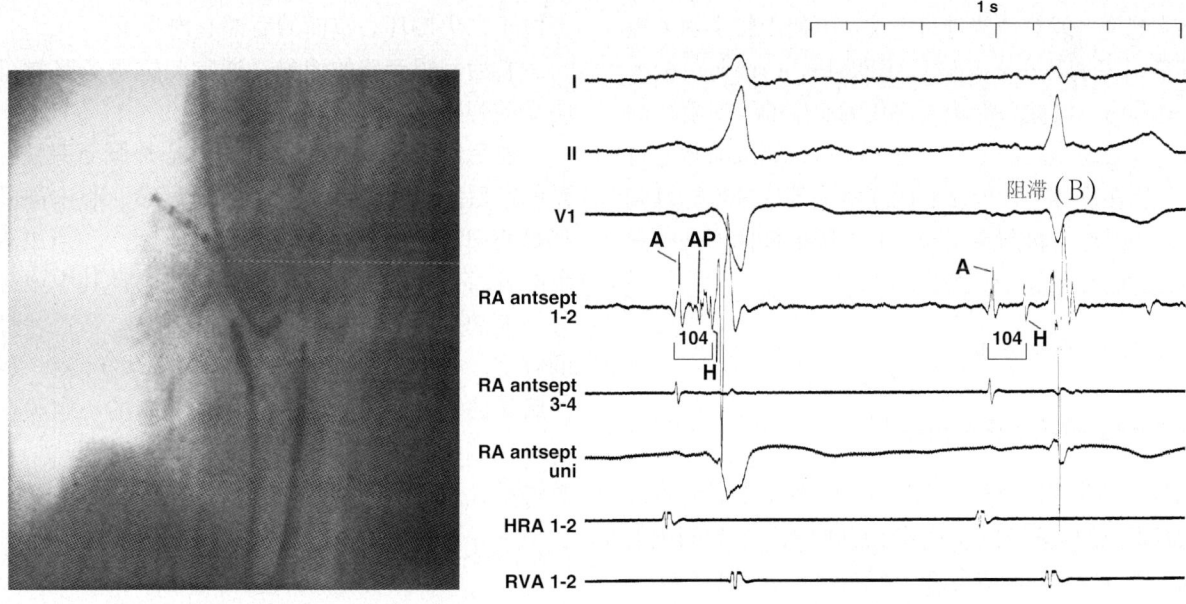

图117-1 左图：前间隔旁路经颈静脉途径的典型方法（左前斜位），图中加标注部位是希氏束多极导管、高位右房（HRA）4 极导管和右室心尖部（RVA）导管。右图：预激波（A）和非预激波（B）的 3 个体表心电图导联和心腔内电图。注意第一跳的旁路电位和希氏束（H）电位，而在旁路阻滞后的旁路电位消失而希氏束电位仍存在。

（二）Ebstein 畸形患者的右侧房室旁路消融

Ebstein 畸形的特点为三尖瓣的间隔瓣和后瓣在房室瓣环的附着点下移而产生了不同程度的心房化心室。

25%～30%的 Ebstein 畸形患者可能发生阵发性房室折返性心动过速，5%～25%的体表心电图可见预激波。房室旁路常常位于不正常瓣环的同样位置，其中在 50% 患者中可见多旁路。在所有旁路患者中与此疾病有关的旁路大约占 2%，而在右侧旁路中占 9%[11]。

发育异常瓣环中的标测和消融技术

Ebstein 畸形患者由于存在多旁路以及由于其位于发育异常的三尖瓣环上，所以精确的旁路定位可能受到影响，但在 50% 的病例中可见能记录到碎裂心内膜电位的区域（持续超过 50ms 的多个尖峰电位）[11]。其碎裂电位说明局部传导延缓可能是体表心电图上右束支阻滞图形的原因。为了区分心房和心室激动，常在邻近的心房位置发放期前刺激以使心房波与心室波分开。在窦性心律时，应提前发放心房期前刺激以进入旁路不应期，从而发现预激时的最早心室激动。当逆向型房室折返性心动过速发作时，心房期前刺激可使局部心房电图与心动过速脱节而确认沿房室瓣环的最早激动点。

如果起搏不能对旁路进行定位，可使用较小的多极电极导管（2F；Pathfinder，CARDIMA，Canada）送入右冠状动脉内，以提高沿着心房化的心室的房室瓣环的心外膜侧电激动标测的效果（图 117-2）。如果动脉走行的解剖位置在房室沟，可在心内膜对应部位进行标测和消融，该消融点与解剖定位和从心外膜电极标测到的旁路电位得到的心电图定位能很好地匹配。

（三）间隔部房室旁路

1. 房室瓣环部位的房间隔解剖[12]

间隔部旁路的传统分类法考虑到旁路与房室结/希氏束和冠状窦口的空间关系，可分为前间隔[上位间隔]、中间隔[间隔]和后间隔旁路[下位间隔]（图 117-3）。

2. 前间隔[上位间隔]房室旁路

定义：如果在希氏束区域的导管可以同时记录到旁路电位和希氏束电位则旁路为希氏束旁/前间隔旁路。

消融技术：将希氏束电极放置到位后，射频消融的理想靶点是同时可以记录到心房和心室电位以及旁路电位，但只有很小的希氏束电位的位置（图 117-1）。虽有几项技术用来定位旁路，但依我们的经验最有用的方法是通过上位途径（经颈静脉或锁骨下静脉）将消融导管置于三尖瓣环心室面。旁路位置常常较靠上，因此应注意不要机械性损伤阻断旁路，因为这可能延长手术时间并降低远期成功率[13]。

3. 中间隔[间隔]房室旁路

定义：中间隔旁路位于房间隔的左侧或右侧，前为希氏束，后为冠状窦口（以冠状窦导管为标志）的这一区域内能记录到旁路电位的旁路[14,15]。

右中间隔旁路的消融技术：因为房室结可能很邻近旁路的心房插入端，所以消融时导管应放置在房室瓣环的心室面，其标志为 A/V 比值大于 1。

左中间隔旁路的消融技术：通过逆行途径或穿间隔途径，使消融导管位于希氏束和冠状窦所标志的二尖瓣环的区域内[14]。

4. 后间隔[下位间隔]房室旁路

定义：穿行过后间隔三角形区域的旁路进一步分为右后间隔旁路和左后间隔旁路。右后间隔旁路紧邻冠状窦口沿三尖瓣环走行。左后间隔旁路走行邻近冠状窦口部，位于冠状窦近端的心外膜或心中静脉，或者位于二尖瓣环心室面的后部心内膜下。

右后间隔旁路的消融：通常此位置旁路常可通过明显的旁路电位来识别。

左后间隔旁路的消融：(1) 心外膜下旁路：心外膜的左后间隔旁路常常与冠状窦近端、心中静脉或冠状窦心中静脉的憩室有关（图 117-4）[16]。当放置冠状窦导管后，将消融导管送入冠状窦内在其中或分支内寻找大的旁路电位。冠状窦造影可以显示冠状静脉窦的解剖。右颈内静脉途径有助于憩室的标测。(2) 心内膜旁路：左后间隔沿二尖瓣环分布的心内膜旁路常常可在二尖瓣环的心室面或心房面消融成功，且大多数均是经过逆行途径消融的。

（四）心外膜房室旁路

1. 右侧心外膜房室旁路

旁路消融患者中有 0.5% 为右侧心外膜旁路。通常在前传时有最早心室激动点和逆传时有最早心房激动点，但只有较小的或甚至不能记录到旁路电位。如

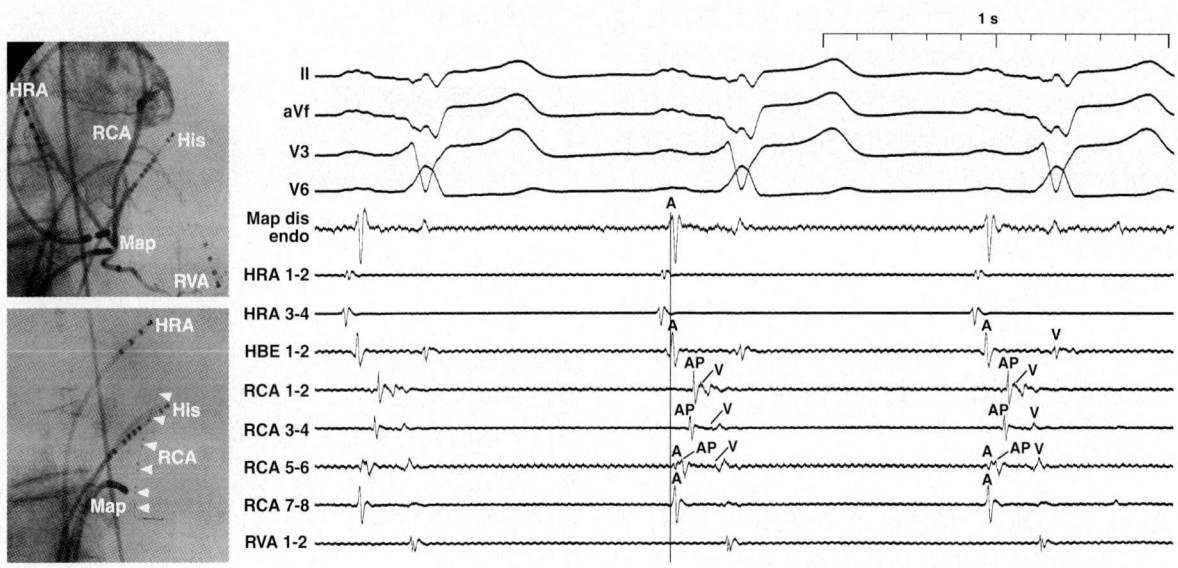

图 117-2 左图：使用多极 2F 导管送至右冠状动脉（RCA）后在右室游离壁的心外膜标测。上面的影像为 RCA 造影，下图显示在右前斜位心外膜导管的位置（箭头示心外膜电极对）。三尖瓣环心房面的消融导管（Map）显示了相应的心内膜位置。其他导管包括希氏束（His）导管和高右房（HRA）导管。右图：4 个导联的体表心电图和消融导管的心内电图。注意 RCA1~6 的旁路电位。消融导管上并无旁路证据（与 RCA 电极 3-4 相对应）。

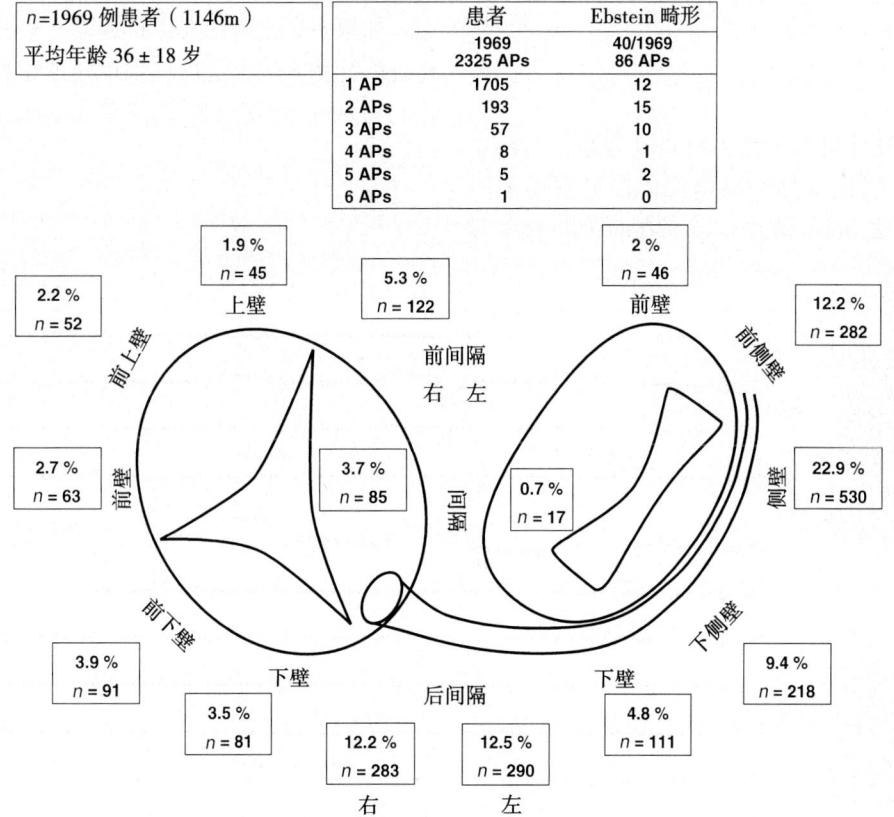

图 117-3 左前斜位显示 2 个房室瓣环，有 1969 例连续消融患者的旁路电位 在相应的房室瓣环位置显示旁路的绝对数值和百分比（使用的是由 Cosio 及其同事所制定的解剖术语[6]）。表中给出了每种旁路的数量并特别强调了 Ebstein 畸形患者的数量。

前所述，直径较小的多极导管（2-Fr）可以送入右冠状动脉进行心外膜标测（图117-2）。心外膜导管可以定位和指引心内膜导管消融。此外，已有报道通过经皮穿刺心包腔进行心外膜消融的报道[18]，但因其邻近右冠状动脉且在房室沟旁有心外膜脂肪组织所以会有困难。此外，在心外膜记录的指引下用冷灌注导管在心房面可以取得消融成功。

2. 左侧心外膜房室旁路

沿左侧房室瓣环分布的心外膜旁路其特点为可在冠状窦或其分支内记录到明显的旁路电位，大约占4%的患者，可在冠状窦或其分支内安全有效地射频消融[19,20]。

3. 心耳-心室连接

旁路的心房插入端有时会在左或右心耳内(0.4%)[21]。这些旁路的传导是双向的：在左侧，最早的前传和逆传激动常可从冠状窦的心室分支中记录到，然而右侧的旁路的最早心室激动或者其振幅较低或可从瓣环外的10mm记录到。虽然射频消融在瓣环上常无效或其仅能一过性阻断旁路传导，但在心耳深处消融可阻断旁路传导。

4. 左前房室旁路

大约0.5%的显性房室旁路为前间隔旁路，但在希氏束区域常常并不能记录到旁路电位，仅见到局部心室电位但并不比体表delta波提前。而在心大静脉中标测可见到明显的旁路电位且心室电位比体表心电图提前20～30ms。可从静脉系统或经主动脉逆行途径在此位置成功消融[22]。

四、房室多旁路

多旁路的发生率在5%～33%之间（外科手术患者）[23,24]。在我们的患者中多旁路发生率为12%（除外Ebstein畸形患者）。

除外Ebstein畸形患者，多旁路患者与单旁路患者相比，其右侧游离壁旁路发生率更高（23%：10%），而左侧游离壁旁路发生率较低（44%：56%）[23]。多旁路患者的隐匿性旁路的总体发生率为45%（单旁路患者的发生率为24%）。最引人注目的就是右侧游离壁旁路的增加，其发生率为39%，而单旁路患者中此发生率为9%[23]。

标测和消融技术

多旁路的标测和消融大体上与单旁路相同。但如果逆传同时经2条旁路可能会使旁路的定位发生困难。然而，如果多旁路患者发生折返性心动过速时，那么使用传统的标测方法也足以识别可能的组合方式。对每条旁路的射频电流发放次数与单旁路患者并没有显著差异[23]。

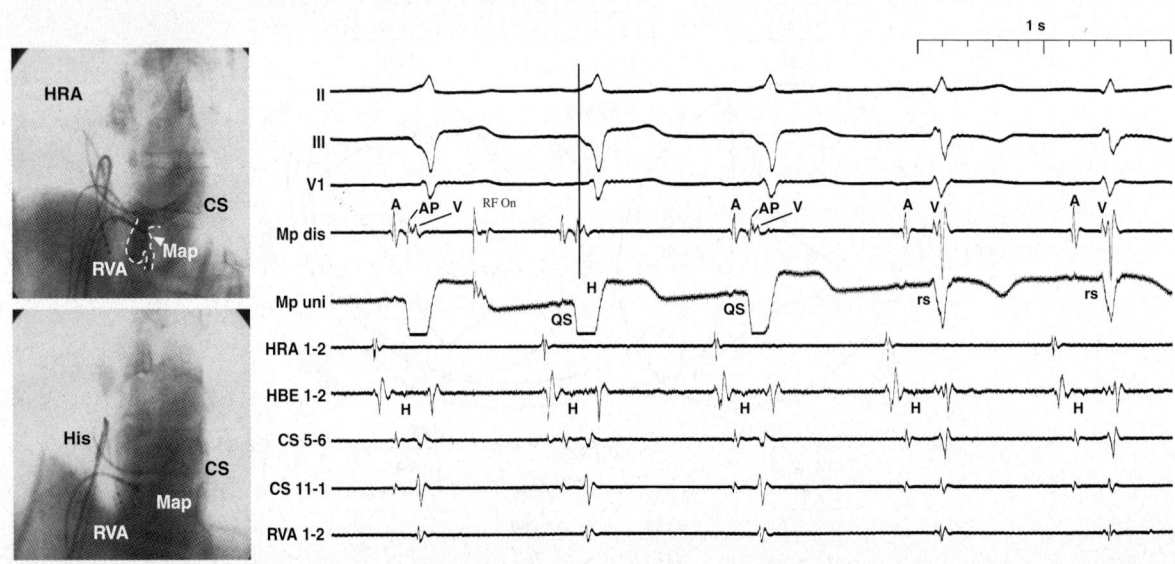

图117-4　左图：在冠状窦憩室部位标测后间隔旁路（左前斜位）。上图显示使用Amplatzer导管行冠状窦（CS）近端造影。白色箭头显示在憩室颈部的标测导管头部（下图显示更清楚）。右图：在发放射频电流时3个体表心电图和标测电极（Mp单极和双极）以及高位右房（HRA）、希氏束（His）、右室心尖部（RVA）和冠状窦电极记录的电图。注意在体表心电图上比delta波提前的旁路电位。预激波上单极记录时呈QS形态，而当旁路阻滞时变为rS形。

五、具有递减慢传导特性的房室旁路

（一）Mahaim 样预激旁路

Mahaim 样预激旁路发生率较低（约为 2%），其特点是前向递减传导并在窦性心律时体表心电图上仅可见到较小的预激波或无预激波。该条旁路常常仅有前传功能（但在很少情况下也证实有逆传功能）。

心动过速时典型特点为左束支传导阻滞型的宽 QRS 波心动过速。

根据上位和下位的插入点不同，旁路可分为房室旁路、房束旁路（如果旁路的低位插入点位于右束支的浦肯野纤维附近）、结室束和结束束。通常，旁路的低位插入点位于心室的深部，但有时也会在三尖瓣环的心室面[25]。

标测和消融技术

当满足下述标准时可以鉴别结室束（或束室束）与房室或房束纤维：（1）心动过速时晚发的右房期前刺激（在希氏束和冠状窦口在没有先前心房激动的情况下给予提前 40ms 的刺激[25]）可以使心室激动提前（图 117-5A）；（2）右房起搏时可以拖带心动过速并出现心房融合波[25]；（3）起搏右房比起搏冠状窦更易于出现心室预激[26]。

（二）房室/房束纤维

1. 心房插入端

在表现为 Mahaim 样预激患者中常用 3 种标测技术来确定旁路的心房插入端：记录局部的旁路电位[27]；导管在三尖瓣环操作时出现旁路的机械性阻断；在三尖瓣环以固定频率起搏时出现最大预激波时测定最短的刺激信号至 QRS 波间期[28]。

2. 心室插入端

低位房室插入端的消融标准包括：在最大预激情况下确认最早心室激动点、有局部旁路激动电位或起搏时 QRS 波形态与心动过速时 QRS 形态在 12 导联上均一致，或这两个条件均符合。虽然这些纤维的低位插入端常常位于瓣环上方 2～3cm，但也有在瓣环下方的报道[26,28]。

房束束患者前向传导慢且其远端心室插入点在右束支远端，并在窦性心律和心动过速情况下于整个瓣环上记录的局部心房和心室电位是明确分离的（图 117-5B），可用来指导消融。

此外，在心房面导管操作可一过性引起旁路的机械性前传阻滞，并可简单重复出现。这种现象可经常在房束束患者中出现并提示其为心内膜走行，可用来指导消融[26]。

（三）结室/结束纤维

在右中间隔的心室面消融 Mahaim 旁路，说明旁路可能是结室/结束走行。少见病例中预激时最早心室激动可在瓣环或紧邻瓣环处记录到，表明可能是心室而不是束支为低位插入点。在这些患者中房室结折返性心动过速也很常见。在消融旁路时，房室结慢径可消融有时也可不消融。目前并不清楚是否这些纤维起自房室结，如 Mahaim 所描述的那样，或纤维在经房室瓣环走行时邻近于房室结。

（四）持续性交界性心动过速

持续性（大于 12h）交界性折返性心动过速（PJRT，见第 58 和 94 章），其特点为窄 QRS 波，诱发时并不需要有 PR 间期延长，房室 1:1 关系，且 RP 间期大于 PR 间期，在体表心电图上逆行 P 波为负向[30]。这种心动过速常在婴儿和儿童中发生并持续至成年。药物治疗常无效[31]。虽然 PJRT 常常并没有症状或临床症状较轻，但可引起心动过速性心肌病。

研究显示，顺向型房室折返性心动过速的基础是传导呈慢递减的逆向传导的旁路。偶尔前向递减传导可引起程度不同的预激[30]。在 80% 以上的患者中，旁路靠近或刚好位于冠状窦口，少数患者可位于右或左侧游离壁。

标测和消融技术

下述方法可鉴别 PJRT 与不典型（快慢型）的房室结折返性心动过速，当心动过速时在希氏束不应期发放心室早搏刺激：（1）产生提前的逆传房波而激动顺序不变；（2）无逆传房波时，心动过速可终止；（3）使 VA 间期显著延长（大于 50ms）。

最早逆传心房波处为消融靶点并可记录到明显的旁路电位（在心动过速或心室起搏时）。间隔部旁路多数使用右侧导管途径在冠状窦近端消融成功（70% 患者）。而当最早心房激动在冠状窦口内 1cm 或更远处记录到旁路电位时建议采用左侧心内膜消融。

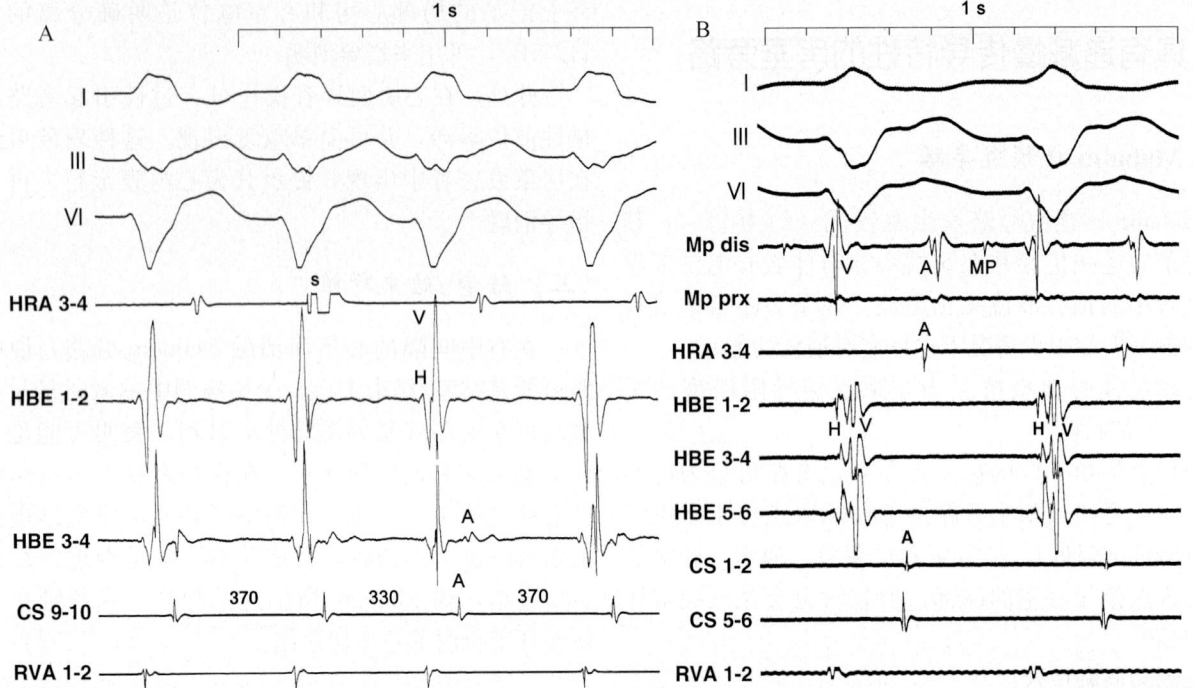

图 117-5 A：房束型 Mahaim 纤维患者的心内膜记录电图，在心动过速时发放晚发心房刺激〔并不比希氏束和冠状窦（CS）区域的房波提前〕并使心室激动提前。注意下一个心房波在提前的心室波之后。B：在 Mahaim 纤维房室折返性心动过速时体表导联和心内膜导联显示典型的左束支阻滞形态。注意在三尖瓣环远端双极标测电极显示典型的高尖频低电压的 Mahaim 电位（mp）。标测电极在右室心尖部记录的心室激动比三尖瓣环记录到的略早，与房束相符。

六、旁路患者射频消融的有效性

近来有经验的消融中心对于由旁路所引起的房室折返性心动过速的消融成功率高于 95%[4,5,32]。我们对 1969 例患者的消融经验，根据旁路插入点的不同消融成功率在 95%～99%（结果总结见图 117-3）。

七、复　发

消融后有临床症状的患者房室折返性心动过速的复发并需要再次消融的比例为 5%～10% 之间[33]。近来报道这部分患者中的一小部分为以前未注意的旁路引起的症状再发（静止型旁路）。

欧洲多中心射频消融研究的综合结果显示，消融总的并发症发生率为 4.4%（MERFS）[34]。其中有生命危险的并发症如心包填塞和血栓分别为 0.7% 和 0.6%。

八、与旁路位置有关的并发症

在消融中间隔部旁路时有产生不可逆的房室结阻滞的报道。下述措施可减少这种危险：（1）选择最佳导管稳定性的静脉途径；（2）使用温控电极消融；（3）当发放射频电流时如出现交界区心律伴逆传阻滞时应立即停止放电；（4）如不能及时阻断旁路应尽早停止放电。

九、射频导管消融时的危害

对于患者和术者的潜在危害是射线照射。在美国，平均每例消融术的曝光量在乳房部位 2.5REM（roentgen equivalent man = 0.1J/kg）、骨髓部位 2.0REM、肺部为 7.5REM[35]。研究显示，在每 100 万个射线量超过 60min 的人群中可能引起下述终身的危险性：150 例乳腺恶变（仅限女性）；120 例骨髓恶变；710 例肺部恶变（由射线引起的致死性恶变的危险性为 0.07%）。

十、总　结

20 世纪 80 年代晚期开始的旁路的射频消融术已经成为这部分患者的首选治疗手段。因为其成功率高而危险性小且患者负担轻，所以消融术可以用于症状轻微的患者，即使是儿童患者也可使用。由于消融能量技术的提高仍需在不同的中心以验证其优越性。最后，影像技术仍需提高以减少患者和术者的射线曝光量。

（李学斌 译）

参 考 文 献

1. Jackman WM, Wang X, Friday KJ, et al: Catheter ablation of accessory atrioventricular pathways (Wolff-Parkinson-White syndrome) by radiofrequency current. N Engl J Med 324:1605–1611, 1991.
2. Kuck KH, Schlüter M, Geiger M, et al: Radiofrequency current catheter ablation of accessory atrioventricular pathways. Lancet 337:1557–1561, 1991.
3. Antz MR, Weib C, Volkmer M, et al: Risk of sudden death after successful accessory atrioventricular pathway ablation in resuscitated patients with Wolff-Parkinson-White Syndrome. J Cardiovasc Electrophysiol 13:231–236, 2002.
4. Calkins H, Yong P, Miller JM, et al: Catheter ablation of accessory pathways, atrioventricular nodal reentrant tachycardia, and the atrioventricular junction: Final results of a prospective, multicenter clinical trial. Circulation 99:262–270, 1999.
5. Dagres N, Clague JR, Kottkamp H, et al: Radiofrequency catheter ablation of accessory pathways: Outcome and use of antiarrhythmic drugs during follow-up. Eur Heart J 20:1826–1832, 1999.
6. Cosio FG, Anderson RH, Kuck KH, et al: Living anatomy of the atrioventricular junctions: A guide to electrophysiologic mapping. Circulation 100:e31-e37, 1999.
7. Cappato R, Schlüter M, Mont L, Kuck KH: Anatomic, electrical, and mechanical factors affecting bipolar endocardial electrograms: Impact on catheter ablation of manifest left free-wall accessory pathways. Circulation 90:884–894, 1994.
8. Bashir Y, Heald SC, Katritsis D, et al: Radiofrequency ablation of accessory atrioventricular pathways: Predictive value of local electrogram characteristics for the identification of successful target sites. Br Heart J 69:315–321, 1993.
9. De Bakker JMT, Hauer RNW, Simmers TA: Activation mapping: Unipolar versus bipolar recording. In Zipes DP, Jalife J (eds): Cardiac Electrophysiology: From Cell to Bedside. Philadelphia, WB Saunders, 1995, pp 1068–1078.
10. Villacastin J, Almendral J, Medina O, et al: "Pseudodisappearance" of atrial electrogram during orthodromic tachycardia: New criteria for successful ablation of concealed left-sided accessory pathways. J Am Coll Cardiol 27:853–859, 1996.
11. Cappato R, Schlüter M, Weiss C, et al: Radiofrequency current catheter ablation of accessory atrioventricular pathways in Ebstein's anomaly. Circulation 94:376–383, 1996.
12. Anderson R, Ho SW: Structure and location of accessory muscular atrioventricular connections. J Cardiovasc Electrophysiol 10:1119–1123, 1999.
13. Belhassen B, Ciskin S, Fish R, et al: Catheter-induced mechanical trauma to accessory pathways during radiofrequency ablation: Incidence, predictors and clinical implications. J Am Coll Cardiol 33:767–774, 1999.
14. Kuck KH, Ouyang F, Cappato R, et al: Ablation of septal accessory pathways. In Zipes DP (ed): Catheter Ablation of Arrhythmias. Armonk, NY, Futura, 2001, pp 305–320.
15. Tai CT, Chen SA, Chiang CE, Chang MS: Characteristics and radiofrequency catheter ablation of septal accessory atrioventricular pathways. Pacing Clin Electrophysiol 22:500–511, 1999.
16. Omran H, Pfeiffer D, Tebbenjohanns J, et al: Echocardiographic imaging of coronary sinus diverticula and middle cardiac veins in patients with preexcitation syndrome: Impact on radiofrequency catheter ablation of posteroseptal accessory pathways. Pacing Clin Electrophysiol 18:1236–1243, 1995.
17. Sapp J, Soejima K, Couper GS, Stevenson WG: Electrophysiology and anatomic characterization of an epicardial accessory pathway. J Cardiovasc Electrophysiol 12:1411–1414, 2001.
18. Yamane T, Jais P, Shah DC, et al: Efficacy and safety of an irrigated tip catheter for the ablation of accessory pathways resistant to conventional radiofrequency catheter ablation. Circulation 102:2565–2568, 2000.
19. Haissaguerre M, Gaita F, Fischer B, et al: Radiofrequency catheter ablation of left lateral accessory pathways via the coronary sinus. Circulation 86:1464–1468, 1992.
20. Giorgberidze I, Saksena S, Krol RB, Mathew P: Efficacy and safety of radiofrequency catheter ablation of left-sided accessory pathways through the coronary sinus. Am J Cardiol 76:359–365, 1995.
21. Soejima K, Mitamura H, Miyazaki T, et al: Catheter ablation of accessory atrioventricular connection between right atrial appendage to right ventricle: A case report. J Cardiovasc Electrophysiol 9:523–528, 1998.
22. Kuck KH, Schlüter M, Cappato R, et al: Left anterior accessory pathways mimicking a right anteroseptal location: Implications for catheter ablation [abstract]. Circulation 92:I-212, 1995.
23. Schlüter M, Cappato R, Ouyang F, et al: Clinical recurrences after successful accessory pathway ablation: The role of "dormant" accessory pathways. J Cardiovasc Electrophysiol 8:1366–1372, 1997.
24. Huang JL, Chen SA, Tai CT, et al: Long-term results of radiofrequency catheter ablation in patients with multiple accessory pathways. Am J Cardiol 78:1375–1379, 1996.
25. Tchou P, Lehman MH, Jazayeri M, Akhtar M: Atriofascicular connection or a nodofascicular Mahaim fiber? Electrophysiologic elucidation of the pathway and associated reentrant circuit. Circulation 77:837–848, 1988.
26. Cappato R, Schlüter M, Weiss C, et al: Catheter-induced mechanical conduction block of right-sided accessory fibers with Mahaim-type preexcitation to guide radiofrequency ablation. Circulation 90:282–290, 1994.
27. McClelland J, Wang X, Beckman KJ, et al: Radiofrequency catheter ablation of right atriofascicular (Mahaim) accessory pathways guided by accessory pathway activation potentials. Circulation 89:2655–2666, 1994.
28. Klein LS, Hackett FK, Zipes DP, Miles WM: Radiofrequency catheter ablation of Mahaim fibers at the tricuspid annulus. Circulation 87:738–747, 1993.
29. Grogin HR, Randall JL, Kwasman M, et al: Radiofrequency catheter ablation of atriofascicular and nodofascicular Mahaim tracts. Circulation 90:272–281, 1994.
30. Gaita F, Haissaguerre M, Giustetto C, et al: Catheter ablation of permanent reciprocating tachycardia with radiofrequency current. J Am Coll Cardiol 25:655–664, 1995.
31. Lindinger A, Heisel A, von Bernuth G, et al: Permanent junctional re-entry tachycardia: A multicenter long-term follow-up study in infants, children and young adults. Eur Heart J 19:936–942, 1998.
32. Kay GN, Epstein AE, Dailey SM, et al: Role of radiofrequency ablation in the management of supraventricular arrhythmias: Experience in 760 consecutive patients. J Cardiovasc Electrophysiol 4:371–389, 1993.
33. Calkins H, Prystowsky E, Berger RD, et al: Recurrence of conduction following radiofrequency catheter ablation procedures: Relationship to ablation target and electrode temperature. J Cardiovasc Electrophysiol 7:704–712, 1996.
34. Hindricks G: The Multicentre European Radiofrequency Survey (MERFS): Complications of radiofrequency catheter ablation of arrhythmias. Eur Heart J 14:1644–1653, 1993.
35. Calkins H, Niklason L, Sousa J, et al: Radiation exposure during radiofrequency catheter ablation of accessory atrioventricular connections. Circulation 84:2376–2382, 1991.

第 118 章

室性心动过速的导管消融

William G. Stevenson and Kyoto Soejima

本章目录

- 瘢痕区域相关的折返环 ……………… 1060
- 导管消融靶点的定位 ………………… 1061
- 瘢痕相关性室速的消融方法 ………… 1066
- 特殊类型的瘢痕相关性室速 ………… 1068
- 总结 …………………………………… 1069

经导管消融对反复发作性室性心动过速（简称室速，VT）患者是一种有效的治疗方法，标测和消融的具体方法取决于室速的类型（表118-1）。一般来讲，适于消融的室速大部分是单形的、具有重复一致的心室除极顺序，并表明该心律失常产生的基础相对稳定，因而可作为消融的靶点。而少部分多形性室速或心室颤动（简称室颤，VF）可能是由局灶异位激动所诱发，通过消融致这些心律失常的局灶位点也可有效预防多形性室速或室颤的反复发作[1]。对发生于结构正常心脏的特发性室速（见第72章）的病灶因相对较小且孤立，可以通过起搏标测或激动顺序标测来识别，并通过局灶的消融以阻止室速的发作。对束支折返性室速，右束支通常是折返环的关键峡部，可以被识别和消融（见第73章）。

心肌梗死等原因造成的心肌瘢痕所引起的室速（表118-1）通常是折返机制，其折返环有时难以准确定位[2]。标测和消融方法取决于室速的稳定性、室速的发作次数以及心肌瘢痕的位置。如果室速发作时伴有血流动力学不稳定时需要频繁被终止，或室速时的QRS波形状有变化，或心动过速不能被诱发，都使得标测难以进行。拖带标测对于指导稳定型室速的消融十分有用，而通过分析窦性心律和起搏标测时的心内和体表心电图，有利于在窦性心律下识别可能的消融部位，从而有助于不稳定型室速的消融。

一、瘢痕区域相关的折返环

一般来说，引起室速的心肌瘢痕区多具有多个潜在的传导通路（图118-1），因此，瘢痕所形成的折返环在大小、形状、位置等方面表现不同[2,3]（见第61、62、63和66章）。折返环路的形成受以下因素的影响：一是波阵面碰撞或组织不应性导致的功能性传导阻滞；二是致密而不可兴奋瘢痕或纤维环引起的病理性固定的传导阻滞[4,5]；再者存活的心肌细胞被纤维化的组织分隔而导致折返环路的某些部分传导缓慢，从而使折返更容易形成[6]。

为了便于标测，折返环被模式化为具有不同的节段（图118-1）。许多折返环路存在一个传导的峡部，它的除极在体表心电图上检测不到。当激动的波阵面通过峡部从出口出现，并沿着心室扩展，就可以记录到QRS波（图118-1 A和B）。出口前的峡部区域一般称为折返环的中部和近端，离开出口以后，折返的波阵面经过一个环型传播后回到峡部的近端区域。外环是沿着瘢痕边缘的一定范围内的心肌传导的折返环（图118-1 A和C），该环通过入口进入位于瘢痕内的内环（图118-1B）。折返环路可以是一个或多个，例如在图118-1A中的8字型折返。位于折返环路外的心肌是旁观者。

经导管射频消融引起典型损伤的直径一般小于

表 118-1 室性心动过速的标测和消融

局灶起源室速	可能的机制	典型的 QRS 波群形态	通常消融位点	消融成功率
特发性右室流出道 VT	A	LBBB，电轴向下	RVOT	85%～90%
左室流出道 VT	A，R	电轴向下 $V_1=RS$ 或 R， $V_2\sim V_5=R$	近主动脉瓣	高
二尖瓣环 VT	A，R	RBBB，电轴向下	近二尖瓣环	可能很高
涉及希浦系统的 VT				
束支折返	R	LBBB，很少 RBBB	左或右束支	>95%
左室维拉帕米敏感性	R	RBBB，电轴偏左上或右	左室中间隔偏下	>90%
瘢痕相关性 VT				
既往有 MI	R，A 少见	不定	MI 边缘，峡部，二尖瓣环	60%～80%
RV 发育不良	R	LBBB	RVOT，近三尖瓣环	姑息性
Chagas 病	R	不定	近 LV 瘢痕，心外膜	未知
法洛四联症	R	LBBB 或 RBBB	RVOT 或间隔	80%
结节病	R	不定	不定	不定/姑息性

A，自律性；LBBB，左束支阻滞；LV，左室；MI，心肌梗死；R，折返；RBBB，右束支阻滞；RV，右室；RVOT，右室流出道；VT，室性心动过速。

1cm，因此为了阻断宽的通路常常需要多点消融[3,7]。通常，折返环的出口、中部和近端区域往往构成所谓的峡部，较少的靶点即可使折返环中断。有研究发现，稳定型室速的峡部通常位于心内膜，长和宽大约为 30mm（18～41mm）和 16mm（6～36mm）[3]。心梗瘢痕引起的室速，其峡部通常位于心内膜下，但也有可能在心内膜深部或在心外膜下。对于心梗患者，多种形态的单形性室速常常并存，它们可以起源于完全不同的区域，也可能共用一个峡部，在这种情况下在一个区域消融就可以消除多种形态的室速[3,5,7-9]。

二、导管消融靶点的定位

(一) 室速的 QRS 波群形态

局灶起源的室速其 QRS 波群形态主要由心律失常病灶的位置来决定的，因此，评价和对比起搏与室速时的 QRS 波群形态是一种十分有效的标测方法（表 118-1 和第 72 章）。与瘢痕相关的折返性室速，其 QRS 波群形态在一定程度上表明折返环出口的位置，但也可能是一种假象而引起误导[10]。一般来说，V_1 导联表现为类左束支阻滞形态的室速，其出口在右室或室间隔；而 QRS 波的平均电轴左偏通常提示室速折返环的出口在下壁，电轴不偏或右偏则说明出口在前（上）壁。在 $V_2\sim V_4$ 导联，以 S 波为主时通常表明出口靠近心尖；以 R 波为主表明出口靠近心室基底部（房室瓣环）。

(二) 电极导管的记录和起搏：技术方面的考虑

心室肌激动起源的部位和记录的技术决定了所记录腔内心电图的特征。单极心内电图是通过在心肌上的电极和另一个远场参考电极之间记录获得的，参考电极通常为 Wilson 中心电端或置于下腔静脉的电极[11]。当滤波较少时，通常称作未滤波（高通滤波频率≤0.5Hz），除极波阵面到达记录电极引起正向波，当波阵面经过电极和向远处传播引起负向波。最大负向斜率与局部心肌除极时间一致。起源于正常心肌的局灶性室速，其室速起源部位未滤波的心内单极电图呈 qS 波形，单极心内电图最初的降支与同步记录的双极心电图的第一个波锋一致[11]。未滤波单极信号的大部分是远离电极的心肌除极引起的远场信号。在瘢痕区，远场信号常使得形成峡部的少量肌束的低振幅电位变得模糊（图 118-3A 和 B）[12]。通过高通滤波或电极间距较小的双极记录，可以衰减掉大量的远场信号。在心腔内双极记录时，双极电图的波锋与局部心

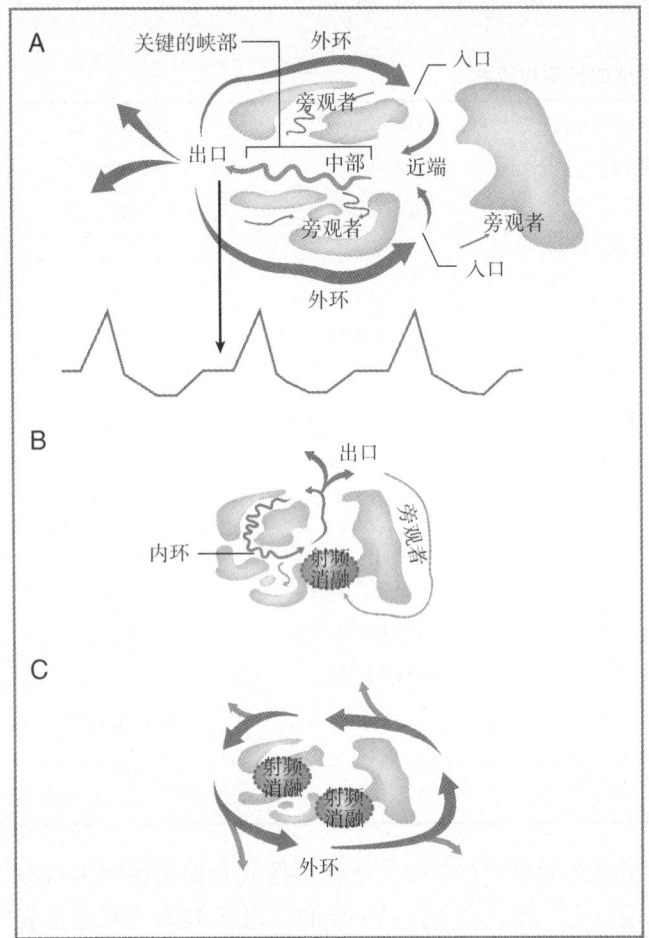

图118-1 在相同的瘢痕区域有3种理论上的折返环和射频消融的可能效果 图中有些区域是电静止的心肌瘢痕,它决定了多个通过瘢痕的潜在通道,这些通过瘢痕区域的传导通道构成了折返环中的峡部。A:双环折返(8字折返)包括了一个关键的峡部和两个外环。峡部的除极(从近端通过中部至出口)发生在心动周期的舒张期,在体表心电图上不能检测到。当激动波阵面从出口出现后QRS波的起始才出现。它通过外环传播经入口到达峡部的近端,从而回到峡部。旁观者(Bys)不在环路内。B:如A所示,在折返路的入口之一消融后,形成了中部、出口和内环区域的单环折返。C:尽管消融了折返环关键的峡部,仍可形成包括单个外环构成的折返环路。

肌的除极时间一致,但所记录到的心电信号可能来自两个记录电极中的任何一极,并通过同步的单极记录可以证实这一现象[11]。

通过标测导管发放电刺激可进行起搏和拖带标测,或用于评价电极与组织之间是否接触良好,也可以用来评价消融的效果[2,4]。心肌电刺激有单极和双极两种发放方式。双极刺激是指两个电极都在心脏内,激动源于其中一个或两个电极,这可能使对起搏效果的解释变得复杂化。单极起搏可以避免这个问题,单极起搏的一个电极为标测导管的远端电极,另一个电极是位于下腔静脉内或位于体表的电极,但是这种方式可以引起相对较大的人工刺激信号,使得起搏时体表心电图变形(图118-3)。

(三) 通过起搏标测来确定出口、电静止瘢痕和缓慢传导区域

窦性心律下以标测导管起搏的标测方法称为起搏标测(图118-2,左底部)[4,10,13](局灶性室速见第72章)。对于特发性室速,在室速起源部位起搏所形成的QRS波形态与室速发作时相同。但对瘢痕相关的折返性室速,如在折返环峡部出口进行起搏标测也会形成与室速相似的QRS波形,但是在出口附近相对较大区域起搏可能均可见到与室速QRS波形一致或相近的图形。此外,有时即便是起搏的部位在折返环上,所形成的QRS波形与室速的QRS波形也可能相差较大,因为起搏时心室肌的激动波阵面可以通过另外一个不同于室速时的通路传导[10,14],因此,不排除在与室速的QRS波形态不一致的起搏标测部位消融成功。

利用消融导管起搏的方法还可以用来识别心肌电静止区(electrically unexcitable scar,EUS),该区界定了折返环路的部位和走行(图118-2)[4]。心肌梗死造成的瘢痕区域其局部电位振幅小,起搏阈值高。例如有研究发现,在有心梗病史的14例患者中,窦性心律下双极电图振幅小于1.5mV的1641个部位中,有12%的部位起搏阈值(脉宽2ms)超过10mA。左心室的三维标测亦显示电静止区存在多个可构成和参与折返的潜在峡部,这些部位可以作为消融的靶点[4]。但是单纯依赖电压图(见后文)并不能准确识别这些峡部,因为它常常存在于振幅极低的区域。

起搏标测也可以识别一些传导缓慢的部位,在12导联心电图上表现为从刺激信号到QRS波群起始(S-QRS)有超过40ms以上的延迟(图118-2)[4,10],这些缓慢传导部位可能是折返环的一部分,也可能是旁观者。

(四) 窦性心律下标测与基质标测

应用电极间距为1mm的射频消融导管,滤波范围在10~400Hz,在心脏结构正常的成年人窦性心律下标测,所记录的心内电图平均振幅为4.8±3.1mV,其中超过95%的部位超过1.55mV。在右心室平均振

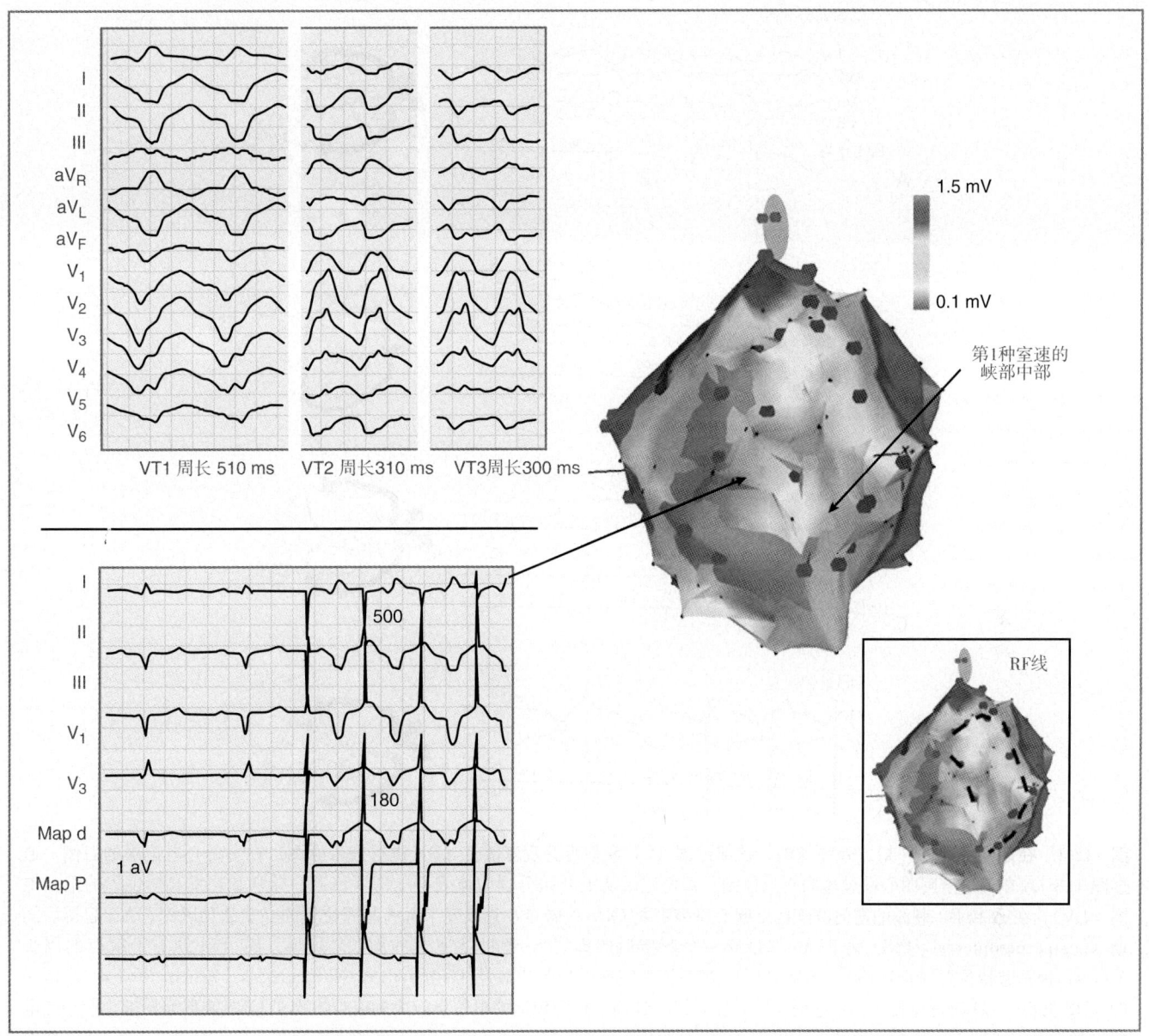

图 118-2 既往有前壁心梗病史室速患者的标测 左上，12 导联心电图显示 3 种不同形态的室速（VT），其中两种室速的血流动力学不稳定。右侧是左心室的三维标测电位图。以不同的颜色表示不同的电位振幅，超过 1.5mV 用紫色表示，电静止瘢痕（起搏阈值>10mA）以灰色表示。左下，如箭头所示，窦性心律时所记录部位的局部电图振幅低，起搏时 S-QRS 间期为 180ms，提示存在传导延迟。起搏时的 QRS 波群形态与第 1 种室速（VT1）相似，提示刺激的部位在第 1 种室速的出口区域。该例在瘢痕区并沿着电压低振幅区的边缘进行射频（RF）消融（红圈），消除了所有的室速。（彩图 56）

幅为 3.7±1.7mV，超过 95% 的部位振幅超过 1.44mV[9]。心室的三维解剖重建，以标测点逐峰的电压振幅重建的图通常被称作电压图，在此图上以低电压界定瘢痕或心梗区域（图 118-2）[4,9]。

多个肌束非同步激动导致心内电图增宽或有多个快速激动成分，被称作碎裂电位（见图 118-3 中的左室电图）[6]。窦性心律下，在 QRS 波群终末出现的电位是晚电位。碎裂电位和晚电位均与心肌的异常传导有关，这些传导异常的心肌可能参与了心动过速的折返，也可能仅仅是旁观者[14-16]。

（五）室速时心内电图和激动顺序标测

QRS 波群的起始通常被用作室速激动顺序标测的参考。在局灶性室速（见第 72 章），室速起源部位的激动常常早于体表 QRS 波群，一般在 QRS 波群之前 15ms 或更多。对于瘢痕相关的折返性室速，收缩期前的电活动存在于折返环的出口，而更早的舒张期活动可以在出口、中间和近端部位记录到[14,17,18]，但是

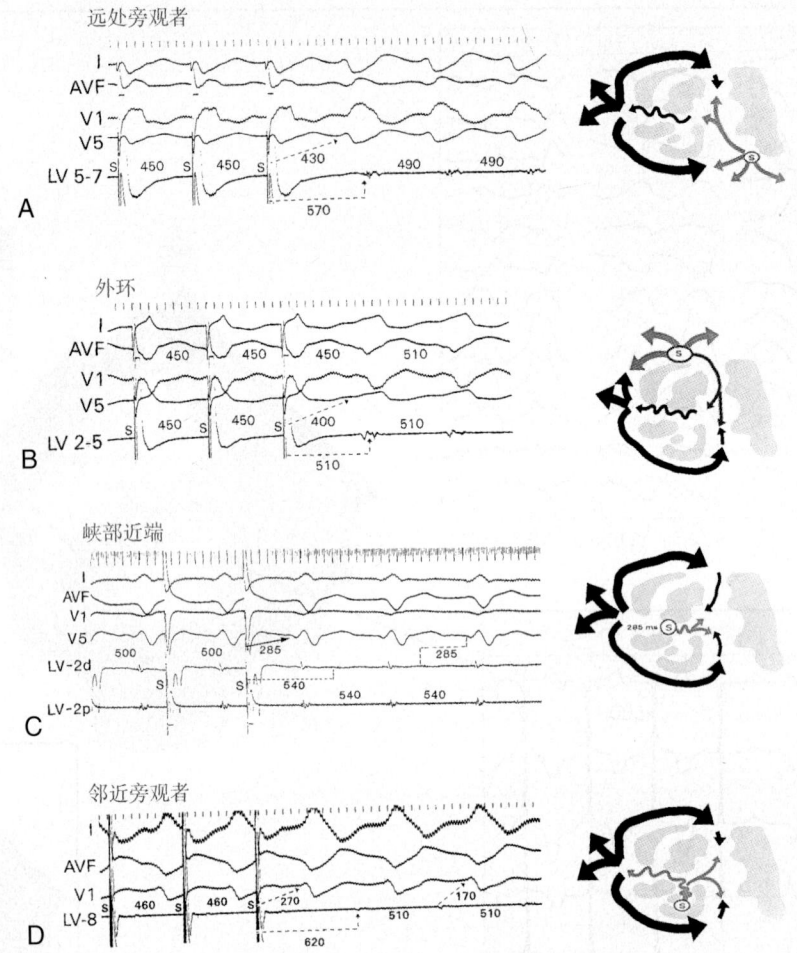

图 118-3 在远处旁观者（A）、外环（B）、峡部近端（C）和邻近旁观者部位（D）进行拖带标测 在每份心电记录的右侧，通过图 118-1A 在理论上阐明心动过速的折返机制。每份记录从上开始分别为体表心电图（ECG）导联和左室起搏位置的记录电图（LV）。在 A 和 B，刺激的逆向波阵面引起心室拖带及 QRS 波融合，且改变了远离起搏位置的心室激动顺序。A：起搏后间期（postpacing interval，PPI）为 570ms（最后一个刺激后的虚线），超过了室速的周长 490ms。B：PPI 约等于室速的周长 510ms，提示起搏位置在折返环上。在 C 和 D，起搏拖带室速伴隐匿性融合（entrainment with concealed fusion，ECF），起搏时的 QRS 波群与室速时相同。C：室速时 LV2d 导联记录到两个相距较远的电位。较大的电位出现于 QRS 波群起始部，较小的电位出现于电舒张期。拖带时较大的电位出现于刺激信号前，表明它不是直接夺获，而是一个远场电位。较小的电位是局部电位，是刺激直接夺获局部组织所致，在起搏时看不到。当 PPI 测量至局部电位（虚线），并约等于室速的周长时，提示起搏点位于折返环中。S-QRS 285ms 表示激动从起搏位置到出口的传导时间（从最后一个刺激信号开始的实心箭头），约等于同一心内电图通道上记录到的局部电位到体表 QRS 起始处的传导时间（E-QRS 间期）（到最后一个 QRS 起始处的虚线）。S-QRS 285ms 是室速周长的 52%，提示位于折返环近端。D：存在 ECF，PPI 620ms 超过了室速的周长 510ms，且 S-QRS 270ms 超过了 E-QRS 间期 170ms，均说明起搏位置是折返的旁观者。时间以毫秒计。（引自 Stevenson WG, Friedman PL, Sager PT, et al: Exploring post-infarct reentrant VT with entrainment mapping. J Am Coll Cardiol 29：1180-1189，1997. Reprinted with permission from the American College of Cardiology.）

这些电位的出现时间有时可造成误导。另外，收缩期前和舒张期电活动也常在旁观者区域记录到。且在折返环的近端区域记录到的电活动有时也可出现于 QRS 波群终末，而不是在舒张期[19]。单纯的舒张期电位是发生在心脏舒张期的低振幅电位，在 QRS 波群之间（图 118-3B 和 C）。它们常起源于折返环的峡部，但也可以出现在旁观者区域[15,17,19]。

（六）拖带标测

绝大部分瘢痕相关的稳定型单形性室速是由折返机制引起的，这样的环形折返激动如果存在一个可兴奋性间隙，则适时的起搏即可重整折返激动（图 118-4）。拖带是指一系列的刺激持续地使折返激动重整[2,20]，即在心动过速时以超过室速的频率起搏，可以使所有 QRS 波群和心内电图加速至起搏的频率

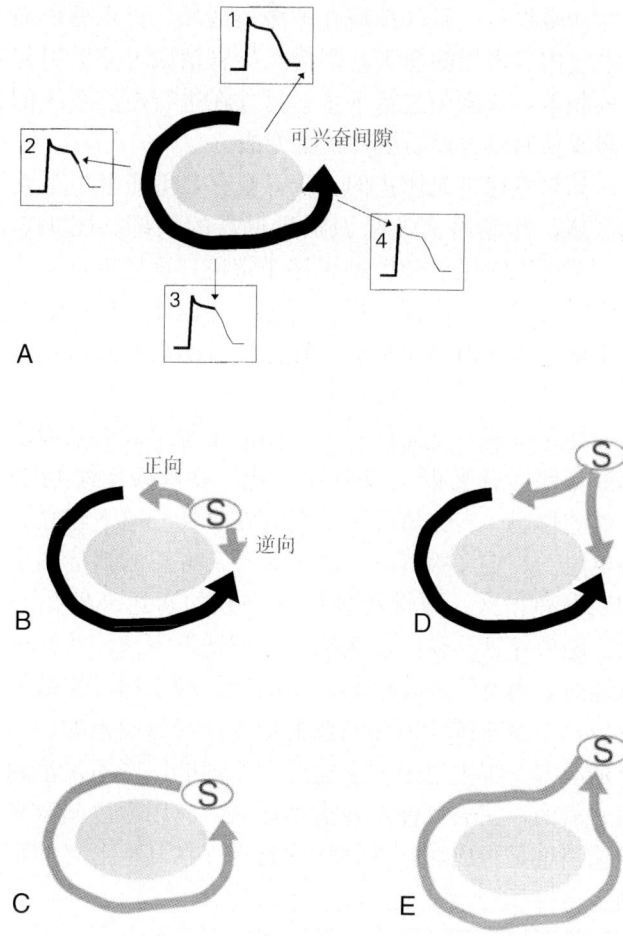

图 118-4 伴有可兴奋间隙的折返激动、重整和起搏后间期 (PPI) 折返激动的波阵面（实心箭头）沿着未兴奋区域（灰色）传播。心肌每一部位除极后都在一段时间内处于不应期。图 A 中的小框是不同部位心肌处于动作电位除极和复极过程中的不同时期（1，2，3，4）。如果完成折返激动 1 周所需要的时间（即室速的周长）超过心肌所有部位的不应期，则在一次除极恢复后和下一个除极波阵面到达之前产生一个可兴奋间隙。图 B 显示一个刺激夺获了折返环中某一部位的心肌引起心动过速重整，该刺激（S）产生了正向和逆向的两个波阵面（灰色箭头）。逆向的波阵面与返回的上一激动周期的正向波阵面相撞。图 C 示刺激产生的正向波阵面通过环路向前传播，并使心动过速重整，从起搏部位发出的由刺激引起的正向波阵面在沿折返环激动 1 周后回到起搏部位所需要的时间，即为起搏后间期 PPI。图 D 和 E 示在旁观者部位起搏引起心动过速重整，一个夺获的刺激产生波阵面传播至环路，并在环路内沿着正向和逆向传播。逆向的波阵面与前一个正向的波阵面相撞而消失，而刺激引起的正向波阵面沿着环路继续向前传播，并回到起搏部位（图 E）。PPI 是从起搏部位到环路，并通过环路回到起搏部位的传导时间，它超过了室速的周长。（引自 Stevenson WG, Friedman PL, Sager PT, et al: Exploring post-infarct reentrant VT with entrainment mapping. J Am Coll Cardiol 29: 1180-1189, 1997. Reprinted with permission from the American College of Cardiology.）

（图 118-2），当起搏终止后原来的室速仍然继续。起搏时 QRS 波群的形态介于室速与起搏 QRS 波群之间，即为融合的 QRS 波群，提示室速已被拖带（图 118-3A 和 B）。拖带技术可用来对心动过速进行标测，但如果室速不稳定或室速被起搏所终止，则无法进行拖带标测。而一个刺激终止室速又不产生相应的 QRS 波群是不常见的，但可能表明起搏的部位是在折返环上，可能是由于刺激夺获局部心肌后形成的波阵面传导阻滞所致。

1. 应用起搏后间期确定折返环的位置

起搏后间期（PPI）是从拖带或重整室速的最后一个刺激信号至起搏部位心肌的下一次除极间的时间[2,20,21]。如果起搏部位在折返环上，则 PPI 约等于室速的周长（误差在 30ms 以内；图 118-3B 和 C）；与此相反，如果起搏部位在旁观者位置，PPI 比室速的周长要长 30ms 以上（图 118-3D）。在进行拖带标测时，起搏的频率应当比室速稍快一点，以避免缓慢传导或改变折返路径从而延长 PPI。因为 PPI 不能区别狭窄的峡部和宽阔的折返路径（例如外环的位点），因此，PPI 不能作为选择消融靶点的唯一标准。

当起搏标测电极可以记录到多个电位时，PPI 的测量应该是起搏电极所在部位的局部电位，而不是远场心电信号（图 118-3C）[12]。测量到远场电位是一个常见的错误，由于远场电位是由远离起搏位点的心肌除极引起，因此，常常导致 PPI 短于心动过速的周长。而在起搏拖带标测过程中，如果远场电位明显并位于起搏刺激信号标记之前时，常常可以被识别出来（图 118-3C）；与此相反，局部电位受起搏刺激信号的影响而变得模糊不清。如果起搏电极的远端和近端所记录到的电位在时间上一致，在刺激信号引起的电噪声使远端电极所记录到的局部电位不易识别时，可以从起搏标测导管近端电极所记录到的心内电图测量 PPI[21]。PPI 减去室速周长的差值也可以用相应电位与稳定的参考电位（如 QRS 波群）之间的关系来评价。

2. 隐匿拖带识别峡部

一般情况下，由于拖带刺激产生的波阵面改变了远离起搏部位的心室激动顺序，所以会出现 QRS 波群融合（图 118-3A 和 B），对没有改变心室激动顺序和室速发作时的 QRS 波群形态的起搏拖带称为隐匿性融合拖带（ECF），是隐匿拖带的一种形式（图

118-3C 和 D)[2,18,23]。如果起搏的部位在折返环上狭窄的峡部，则起搏产生的波阵面在某些方向上的传播受到限制，只可能沿着折返环传播，与室速的波阵面具有相同的传播路径（图 118-3），则产生隐匿性拖带。刺激到 QRS 波群起始部的间期（S-QRS）约等于激动从起搏部位到折返环出口的传导时间，在折返环的出口、中间、近端和内环等部位起搏时，S-QRS 间期会依次逐渐延长（图 118-2）。如果起搏部位在折返环上，S-QRS 间期等于室速时该部位局部心电信号到 QRS 起始部的传导时间，而在旁观者部位却并非如此。最长的 S-QRS 间期，可在内环和一些旁观者部位记录到，最长可达心动过速周长的 70%，在这些部位消融常常是无效的。与此相反，在峡部的出口、中间和近端等部位进行射频消融，终止室速的可能性超过 70%，特别是当消融部位存在孤立的电位时；如果峡部较宽，则需要进行线性消融[2,18,23]。

三、瘢痕相关性室速的消融方法

对于瘢痕相关性室速的消融，术前首先需要明确基础心脏疾病的严重程度，同时要充分考虑和评价室速是否与严重的心肌缺血有关。心脏超声下室壁运动异常通常提示心肌存在潜在的瘢痕区域。对于超声显示左室内有血栓的患者，因为经导管消融可能会引起血栓脱落，应避免进行手术，另外在进行左心系统的消融操作时应遵循系统性抗凝方法。

如果室速是无休止的，应寻找存在舒张期电活动的区域，并应用拖带来识别折返环的峡部（图 118-5）。并可以应用射频消融来终止室速，这样可进一步证实消融靶点是否位于折返环上。室速终止后应继续在该低电压区消融，最后以靶点区域的起搏阈值超过 10mA 作为充分消融的指标[8]。

如果室速不是无休止的，则应用程序刺激来明确诊断，评估有无束支折返性室速，并观察室速 QRS 波群的形态。多数情况下应首先在窦性心律下建立心室电压图、定义瘢痕区（图 118-2），并以起搏标测来识别电静止区、缓慢传导区和潜在的折返环路出口处。随后导管放在可能的靶点区域诱发室速，并评价室速时心内及体表心电图图形的特征和室速对拖带的反应，于室速持续下在满意的靶点区行射频消融。完整的心室三维重建图和室速时的激动顺序图不是消融所必需的。完成目标室速的消融后，应用程序刺激来确认消融是否成功，并且评估是否存在其他形态的室速。

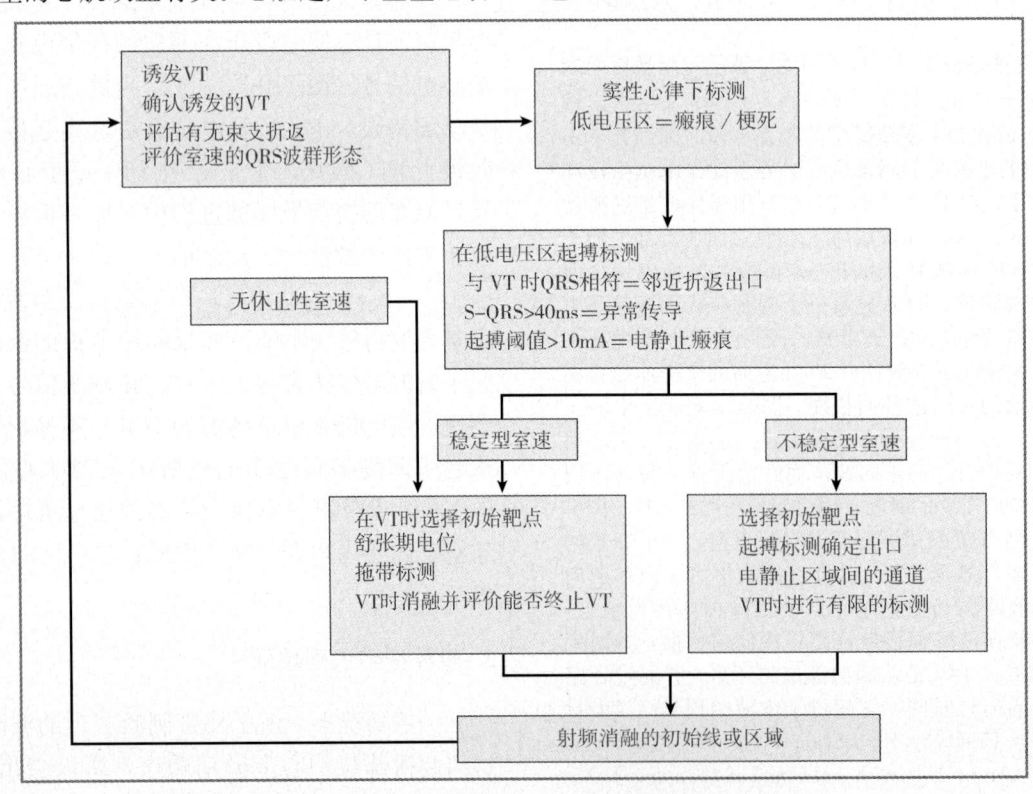

图 118-5 瘢痕相关性室速的标测和消融方法流程图

（一）多形性和不稳定型室速的消融

有一些患者在进行心内电生理检查时可以诱发出3种到4种不同形态的室速，其中与平时自行发作者的QRS波群形态一致者被称为临床型室速，但由于在临床情况下室速可被ICD迅速终止，有时临床型室速并不易定义[7,8]。有人尝试在窦性心律下进行基质标测（见后文）或以多极电极对室速时的心室激动顺序进行标测来确定靶点，并行线性消融来治疗多形性和不稳定型室速[4,7,9]。用完整的环形消融来隔离异常区域可以在一些病人身上实现，但是对大片的区域就难以完成，并且也不是成功消融所必需的，更确切的方法是确定位于瘢痕区域室速的关键部位并进行消融[4,7,9]。在消融与瘢痕相关的室速时，消融部位应尽量局限于瘢痕低电压区以避免损伤正常的心室肌。通常情况下，房室瓣环是室速折返环路峡部的边界之一，尤其是瘢痕区位于下壁或后壁邻近二尖瓣环的部位[5,24]，因此，心室基底部的消融线通常应延伸到二尖瓣环。因为室速出口的常见部位在瘢痕的边缘，因此消融线通常至少包括边界区域的一部分，应用起搏标测来确定折返环出口在瘢痕边缘的部位。

Marchlinski和他的同事对16例不稳定型室速的患者行线形消融治疗[9]，其消融线包括从低电压区通过经起搏标测确定为折返环路潜在出口的瘢痕边缘区到房室环或正常电压心肌区，平均55个射频靶点构成1~9条消融线（平均4条），每条消融线的平均长度为3.9cm。对既往有心梗病史并能诱发出室速的9例患者中，消融后有3例患者的室速不能再被诱发，4例改善；而在7例非缺血性心肌病患者中，4例患者的室速被成功消融，1例改善。与手术相关的并发症包括1例患者发生脑卒中。经过平均8个月的随访，15例室速患者中4例复发，但仅1例患者的室速发作频繁。该研究证明了在窦性心律下定义电静止瘢痕区，并对确定的折返环峡部进行消融治疗不稳定型室速的可行性（图118-2）[4]。

如果室速发作时血流动力学不稳定，也可以应用拖带标测方法来确认折返环的位置[4,7]，先在窦性心律下确定可能参与折返激动的某些心肌部位，然后诱发室速，完成标测后则迅速终止室速。以这样的方法对既往有心梗病史的40例室速患者中，25例（63%）发现了参与折返的峡部，其中包括60%不稳定型室速患者。对可以确定折返环峡部的25例室速患者中，成功消融了18例（72%）患者的所有可诱发的室速，消融线的平均长度为4.3cm，随访10个月，无室速发作。在峡部没有确定的15例室速患者中，消融线平均长度为6.6cm，消除了33%患者的所有可诱发室速，这15例患者中有47%在随访中没有室速发作。不管术中是否准确定义了峡部的部位或室速是否稳定，消融后ICD放电治疗从每月12次显著地减少到每月0.04次，并且无手术相关严重并发症发生。

应用带有球囊的电极阵列导管可以采集反映远离球囊的心脏电激动（Endocardial Solutions，St. Paul, MN），并对"真实"电信号进行数学重建，从而以诱发室速的单个心跳获得的心室激动顺序信息来指导消融[25-27]。在超过90%的室速，最早的心内膜激动可能位于折返环的出口附近，另外，大约有三分之二的病例可以发现舒张期电活动。因为折返环的一部分可能位于心内膜深部或峡部的电压振幅过低，应用非接触球囊标测技术对室速进行标测时很少能定义出完整的心动过速折返环。在3个系列的76例患者中，有32例为不稳定型室速，经导管消融能成功消除目标室速的70%以上；经过1~18个月的随访，58%~71%的患者未再有室速发作。但有6例患者发生了严重的并发症，包括脑梗死、心包填塞和血流动力学恶化。

（二）心外膜折返环的消融

导管消融失败常常是由于室速峡部的位置位于心内膜的深部，通过冠状静脉系统可对室速进行有限的心外膜标测，而更进一步的心外膜标测和导管消融治疗可以通过把电极导管置入心包腔来完成[28]。在没有心包粘连的情况下，导管可以在心包内自由移动。有研究发现，在14例下壁心梗导致的室速患者中，30个室速中有7个折返环的一部分从心外膜被识别和消融[28]。心外膜的环路也可以发生在非缺血性心肌病和Chagas病的患者。在心包腔内进行心外膜消融时，放电之前需要行冠脉造影以避免紧靠冠状动脉进行放电。经心包腔进行心外膜消融治疗室速的主要并发症是血性心包积液和心包炎。

（三）冷盐水灌注射频消融

用冷盐水灌注消融电极导管治疗室速，可以应用更大的消融能量来增加消融损伤的范围，且消融电极远端没有焦痂的形成。与标准4mm射频消融电极导管相比，冷盐水灌注消融电极导管能更有效地终止室速[29,30]。虽然在消融时组织被过度加热到超过100℃时会形成蒸汽而引起爆裂（pops），并可以导致在某些区域心肌穿孔和发生心包填塞,但是在瘢痕区的消融显示了相当好的安全性[31]。开放的灌注系统允许盐水经消融电极导管远端的小孔流进体内,因而应重视额外增加的液体量对患者心功能产生的可能影响[4,29]。

有一项入选了 146 例有器质性心脏病室速患者的多中心临床试验研究,评估了一种闭合的冷盐水灌注消融电极导管的有效性和安全性(Boston Scientific, Inc., Boston, Massachusetts)[31]。该项研究应用该导管进行消融,消除了 75% 的患者所有可标测到的室速,消融后有 46% 患者的室速不能再被诱发。在平均 8 个月的随访中,54% 的患者没有室速发作。12 例患者(8%)出现严重的并发症,包括脑卒中或一过性脑缺血发作(2.7%)、心包填塞(2.7%)、完全性房室阻滞(1.4%)、1 例心梗和 1 例主动脉瓣叶损伤,其中与手术操作相关的总死亡率为 2.7%。

(四) 导管消融结果的评价和消融后的处理

程序刺激可以用于评价消融治疗的即刻效果:(1)室速不能诱发;(2)改良:可以诱发出单形性室速,但与先前的室速形态和周长不同;(3)临床心动过速可被持续诱发。在一组既往有心梗病史的室速患者的 18 个月随访中,消融治疗后在不能诱发室速、改良的可诱发室速和可诱发临床型室速 3 组患者中,室速的复发率分别为 16%、13% 和 83%[8]。如果在左室进行较多的线性消融,建议术后用华法林进行抗凝治疗至少 6~8 周;如果应用华法林进行抗凝治疗有禁忌,则可考虑每日服用阿司匹林。

(五) 安全性

对于心脏疾病相关室速的消融,与操作有关的死亡率在 1%~2.7% 的范围内。在已发表的 393 例伴有基础心脏病接受室速消融治疗的患者中,严重并发症的发生率为 5%,包括脑卒中(1.7%)、房室阻滞(1.3%)、心包填塞(1.7%)[32]。大约 10% 的患者在随访过程中死于心衰,这部分患者平均左室射血分数在 0.22~0.33 之间。消融室速时对心肌收缩功能的损伤是可能的,应尽量避免和减少,并严格把消融部位限制在低电压的瘢痕区[9,32-35]。

四、特殊类型的瘢痕相关性室速

(一) 心梗后室速

选择经导管消融的心梗后室速患者一般是对抗心律失常药疗效不满意、室速仍反复发作者[3,4,7-9,18,27,32,35,36],每个患者通常可诱发出 3~4 种不同形态的室速。通常与下壁心梗相关的折返环位于梗死心肌的基底侧,其峡部与二尖瓣环平行[3,5,24],少数情况下折返环可涉及右室或右室间隔[4]。20%~30% 心梗后室速患者的折返环在心内膜深部或心外膜下[28]。

如以临床记录到的稳定型室速为目标,71%~79% 患者的室速消融可以取得成功[32,33,35-37]。在即刻消融成功后,在 9 至 25 个月的随访中,约 31% 的患者其室速复发,其中有些复发的室速在消融过程中被认为是 "非临床型" 而没有消融。对于血流动力学稳定的室速患者的临床治疗原则目前尚无共识,这些患者是否应接受 ICD 治疗亦存在争议[35,37]。Della Bella 和同事们[35]对 124 例此类患者进行了经导管消融治疗,其中 73% 患者的室速消除,术后 86% 的患者需继续服用胺碘酮或 β 受体阻滞剂,仅 11 例接受了 ICD 治疗。这项研究发现,在消融成功患者中室速的复发率为 27%,其他患者室速的复发率为 60%,而且仅有 3 例患者(2.5%)在平均 45 个月的随访期内猝死。在该研究的入选患者中尽管大多数复发病例的室速是非致命的,但这些患者在植入 ICD 后,可以通过抗心动过速起搏来终止反复发作的室速[35,37]。

对于控制无休止性室速或需要 ICD 终止的反复发作的症状性室速,经导管消融治疗具有明显的优势[4,7,9,36]。消融后超过 70% 的患者其室速的发作次数可以减少到每月少于 1 次,从而明显改善患者的生活质量,对不稳定型室速经导管消融治疗也有效[4,7,9,36]。

(二) 其他瘢痕相关性室速

对于反复发作的致心律失常性右室发育不良心肌病引起的室速,经导管消融治疗有助于减少室速的发作次数,但是由于这些心脏疾病本身呈进行性发展,所以经导管消融治疗被认为是姑息性的治疗手段[27,37,38]。此类室速的折返环通常位于右室流出道或沿着三尖瓣环分布。

法洛四联症修补术后的室速通常由折返机制引

起，可能与心肌修补引起的瘢痕相关，室速的起源部位大多在右室流出道、室间隔，少数情况下在左室流出道[39]。消融可以成功，但经验有限。

在非缺血性心肌病中20%～30%患者的持续性单形性室速是由束支折返引起，偶尔是局灶自律性增高引起的[40]。少数情况下，心肌病是无休止的特发性室速引起的心动过速性心肌病。其余三分之二的持续单形性室速是由与瘢痕相关的折返引起的[40]。此类室速消融的即刻成功率似乎低于心梗后室速，因为室速可能是多形性的，折返环路可能位于心外膜下。一项包括26例非缺血性心肌病室速患者的临床研究中，经导管消融消除了53%患者的所有可诱发室速；其中60%的患者在平均11±12个月的随访中没有室速发作。

五、总　结

经导管消融对于局灶性、心内膜起源或束支折返机制引起的室速十分有效，而对瘢痕相关性室速的治疗则相对较困难，但可以在大部分患者有效地控制无休止性室速的发作，并减少ICD的放电治疗次数。窦性心律时通过对瘢痕区域的心电生理特征进行标测和评价，有利于指导多形性和不稳定型室速的消融。

（刘少稳　译）

参 考 文 献

1. Haissaguerre M, Shoda M, Jais P, et al: Mapping and ablation of idiopathic ventricular fibrillation. Circulation 106:962-967, 2002.
2. Stevenson WG, Friedman PL, Sager PT, et al: Exploring postinfarction reentrant ventricular tachycardia with entrainment mapping. J Am Coll Cardiol 29:1180-1189, 1997.
3. de Chillou C, Lacroix D, Klug D, et al: Isthmus characteristics of reentrant ventricular tachycardia after myocardial infarction. Circulation 105:726-731, 2002.
4. Soejima K, Stevenson WG, Maisel WH, et al: Electrically unexcitable scar mapping based on pacing threshold for identification of the reentry circuit isthmus: Feasibility for guiding VT ablation. Circulation 106:1678-1683, 2002.
5. Wilber DJ, Kopp DE, Glascock DN, et al: Catheter ablation of the mitral isthmus for ventricular tachycardia associated with inferior infarction. Circulation 92:3481-3489, 1995.
6. de Bakker JM, van Capelle FJ, Janse MJ, et al: Fractionated electrograms in dilated cardiomyopathy: Origin and relation to abnormal conduction. J Am Coll Cardiol 27:1071-1078, 1996.
7. Soejima K, Suzuki M, Maisel WH, et al: Catheter ablation in patients with multiple and unstable VTs after myocardial infarction: Short ablation lines guided by reentry circuit isthmuses and sinus rhythm mapping. Circulation 104:664-669, 2001.
8. Stevenson WG, Friedman PL, Kocovic D, et al: Radiofrequency catheter ablation of ventricular tachycardia after myocardial infarction. Circulation 98:308-314, 1998.
9. Marchlinski FE, Callans DJ, Gottlieb CD, et al: Linear ablation lesions for control of unmappable VT in patients with ischemic and nonischemic cardiomyopathy. Circulation 101:1288-1296, 2000.
10. Stevenson WG, Sager PT, Natterson PD, et al: Relation of pace mapping QRS configuration and conduction delay to VT reentry circuits in human infarct scars. J Am Coll Cardiol 26:481-488, 1995.
11. Delacretaz E, Soejima K, Gottipaty VK, et al: Single catheter determination of local electrogram prematurity using simultaneous unipolar and bipolar recordings to replace the surface ECG as a timing reference. Pacing Clin Electrophysiol 24:441-449, 2001.
12. Tung S, Soejima K, Maisel WH, et al: Recognition of far-field electrograms during entrainment mapping of ventricular tachycardia. J Am Coll Cardiol 42:110-115, 2003.
13. van Dessel PF, de Bakker JM, van Hemel NM, et al: Pace mapping of postinfarction scar to detect VT exit sites and zones of slow conduction. J Cardiovasc Electrophysiol 12:662-670, 2001.
14. Bogun F, Bahu M, Knight BP, et al: Response to pacing at sites of isolated diastolic potentials during VT in patients with previous myocardial infarction. J Am Coll Cardiol 30:505-513, 1997.
15. Harada T, Tomita Y, Nakagawa T, et al: Pace-mapping conduction delay at reentry circuit sites of ventricular tachycardia after myocardial infarction. Heart Vessels 12(Suppl):232-234, 1997.
16. Brunckhorst CB, Stevenson WG, Jackman WM, et al: Ventricular mapping during atrial and ventricular pacing. Relationship of multipotential electrograms to VT reentry circuits after myocardial infarction. Eur Heart J 23:1131-1138, 2002.
17. Kocovic DZ, Harada T, Friedman PL, et al: Characteristics of electrograms recorded at reentry circuit sites and bystanders during VT after myocardial infarction. J Am Coll Cardiol 34:381-388, 1999.
18. El-Shalakany A, Hadjis T, Papageorgiou P, et al: Entrainment/mapping criteria for the prediction of termination of VT by single RF lesion in patients with coronary artery disease. Circulation 99:2283-2289, 1999.
19. Bogun F, Knight B, Goyal R, et al: Discrete systolic potentials during ventricular tachycardia in patients with prior myocardial infarction. J Cardiovasc Electrophysiol 10:364-369, 1999.
20. Delacretaz E, Stevenson WG: Catheter ablation of ventricular tachycardia in patients with coronary heart disease: Part I: Mapping. Pacing Clin Electrophysiol 24:1261-1277, 2001.
21. Hadjis TA, Harada T, Stevenson WG, et al: Effect of recording site on postpacing interval measurement during catheter mapping and entrainment of postinfarction VT. J Cardiovasc Electrophysiol 8:398-404, 1997.
22. Soejima K, Stevenson WG, Maisel WH, et al: The N + 1 difference: A new measure for entrainment mapping. J Am Coll Cardiol 37:1386-1394, 2001.
23. Bogun F, Bahu M, Knight BP, et al: Comparison of effective and ineffective target sites that demonstrate concealed entrainment in patients with coronary artery disease undergoing RF ablation of VT. Circulation 95:183-190, 1997.
24. Hadjis TA, Stevenson WG, Harada T, et al: Preferential locations for critical reentry circuit sites causing VT after inferior wall myocardial infarction. J Cardiovasc Electrophysiol 8:363-370, 1997.
25. Strickberger SA, Knight BP, Michaud GF, et al: Mapping and ablation of VT guided by virtual electrograms using a noncontact, computerized mapping system. J Am Coll Cardiol 35:414-421, 2000.
26. Schilling RJ, Peters NS, Davies DW: Feasibility of a noncontact catheter for endocardial mapping of human ventricular tachycardia. Circulation 99:2543-2552, 1999.
27. Della Bella P, Pappalardo A, Riva S, et al: Non-contact mapping to guide catheter ablation of untolerated ventricular tachycardia. Eur Heart J 23:742-752, 2002.
28. Sosa E, Scanavacca M, d'Avila A, et al: Nonsurgical transthoracic epicardial catheter ablation to treat recurrent VT occurring late after myocardial infarction. J Am Coll Cardiol 35:1442-1449, 2000.
29. Soejima K, Delacretaz E, Suzuki M, et al: Saline-cooled versus standard radiofrequency catheter ablation for infarct-related ventricular tachycardias. Circulation 103:1858-1862, 2001.
30. Nabar A, Rodriguez LM, Timmermans C, et al: Use of a saline-irrigated tip catheter for ablation of VT resistant to conventional RF ablation: Early experience. J Cardiovasc Electrophysiol 12:153-161, 2001.
31. Calkins H, Epstein A, Packer D, et al: Catheter ablation of ventricular tachycardia in patients with structural heart disease using cooled radiofrequency energy: Results of a prospective multicenter study. J Am Coll Cardiol 35:1905-1914, 2000.
32. Delacretaz E, Stevenson WG: Catheter ablation of VT in patients with coronary heart disease. Part II: Clinical aspects, limitations, and

recent developments. Pacing Clin Electrophysiol 24:1403–1411, 2001.
33. Nabar A, Rodriguez LM, Batra RK, et al: Echocardiographic predictors of survival in patients undergoing radiofrequency ablation of postinfarct clinical ventricular tachycardia. J Cardiovasc Electrophysiol 13:S118–S121, 2002.
34. Khan HH, Ho C, Maisel WH, et al: Effect of radiofrequency ablation for ischemic ventricular tachycardia on left ventricular function. Pacing Clin Electrophysiol 24(II):545, 2001.
35. Della Bella P, De Ponti R, Uriarte JA, et al: Catheter ablation and antiarrhythmic drugs for haemodynamically tolerated post-infarction VT. Eur Heart J 23:414–424, 2002.
36. Strickberger SA, Man KC, Daoud EG, et al: A prospective evaluation of catheter ablation of VT as adjuvant therapy in patients with coronary artery disease and an ICD. Circulation 96:1525–1531, 1997.
37. van der Burg AE, de Groot NM, van Erven L, et al: Long-term follow-up after radiofrequency catheter ablation of VT: A successful approach? J Cardiovasc Electrophysiol 13:417–423, 2002.
38. Ellison KE, Friedman PL, Ganz LI, et al: Entrainment mapping and radiofrequency catheter ablation of ventricular tachycardia in right ventricular dysplasia. J Am Coll Cardiol 32:724–728, 1998.
39. Gonska BD, Cao K, Raab J, et al: Radiofrequency catheter ablation of right ventricular tachycardia late after repair of congenital heart defects. Circulation 94:1902–1908, 1996.
40. Delacretaz E, Stevenson WG, Ellison KE, et al: Mapping and radiofrequency catheter ablation of the three types of sustained monomorphic ventricular tachycardia in nonischemic heart disease. J Cardiovasc Electrophysiol 11:11–17, 2000.

第 119 章

儿童患者的导管消融

John D. Kugler

本章目录

- 儿童患者及其家属的术前教育和心理准备 ………… 1071
- 消融步骤 ………………………………… 1071
- 儿童患者消融治疗的效果 …………… 1074
- 适应证 …………………………………… 1075
- 致谢 ……………………………………… 1075

虽然儿童患者的导管消融与成人患者有许多相同之处，但是也有许多不同的特点，具体的不同之处在本书的第二版第 133 章[1]和第三版的第 114 章[2]均有很详尽的说明，本章不再详细讨论，而只重点说明一些最重要的特点。与本书的前几版一样，本章将加入一些儿童患者射频消融登记（pediatric RCA registry）资料的新数据。

一、儿童患者及其家属的术前教育和心理准备

与儿童患者及其家属的第一次、最细致的谈话最好由儿科电生理医生和护士一起进行，此后，儿科电生理护士可以再次强调谈话的一些重点，以加强患者及家属的理解。预先针对儿童患者及其家属印制的宣传小册子对于术前教育是很好的参考资料。消融步骤的讨论中也包括了消融前后的电生理检查步骤。大多数与患者及其家属的谈话内容中应包括儿童患者的消融过程中有哪些情况是已知并可以解决的，哪些是目前不能解决的。谈话内容也应该包括简单的消融发展历史、消融的危险性、成功率、可能的长期预后和消融应该进行的术后随访。此外，谈话内容中还应当包括 X 射线的已知和未知的效应，射线暴露可能出现的远期不良后果。

谈话内容涉及患者的特定心动过速的治疗历史也非常重要[1-3]，尤其是对于患者及其家属要在射频消融和其他可能的治疗方法之间作出更合适的选择。在目前消融很受欢迎的情况下，很容易忘记告诉患者及其家属还有其他可能的选择，而在权衡消融治疗的利弊的同时，让患儿及家属了解其他治疗方法是非常有必要的。

二、消融步骤

（一）镇静/麻醉

事实上对于所有的儿童患者均需要镇静和/或麻醉。持续静脉注射异丙酚来深度镇静（低剂量）或者全身麻醉（高剂量）后，后续的镇静效应较少，患者恢复较快，而且与麻醉剂或其他药物相比，停药后的恶心、呕吐等反应大大降低，所以提高了患者对消融的接受程度[4]。恶心和呕吐发生率的降低也减少了 Valsalva 动作诱发的导管穿刺部位的出血和血肿。虽然有麻醉作用的镇静药可以用作异丙酚的替代药，但使用时必须考虑有可能出现的电生理作用，必要时，可以用咪达唑仑来代替地西泮，部分原因是前者对电生理的影响较小[1,2]。异丙酚的使用也有局限性，特别是对于心房异位起搏点兴奋性增加的心动过速（atrial ectopic tachycardia，AET），因为有资料表明异丙酚对 AET 有抑制作用[5]。异氟烷和恩氟烷麻醉也被证

实对患儿的旁道不应期（refractory periods，RPs）有延长作用[6,7]，Chang等作出了使用上述两个麻醉剂的患儿测定旁道前传有效不应期的回归模型[7]，该组研究者强调，如果结合旁道不应期来权衡是否进行消融治疗，同时考虑麻醉剂的作用是非常重要的。

全身麻醉使用人工控制通气，因此对于维持消融稳定性更有优势[8]。如果消融过程中没有麻醉师在场，可以和成人患者一样，根据患儿的体重给予镇静药物，但是，处理儿童患者的难度更高，因为患者往往更加焦虑，需要更频繁地使用低剂量药物，也需要更细致和密切的监护和观察，以免在耗时较长的操作过程中出现镇静药物过量。同时有一位有儿科工作经验的护士在场，对于给予患儿更多的心理支持和安慰、降低镇静药用量和药物过量的危险都有好处。

（二）儿童患者在导管室的术前准备

儿科护士对于患儿刚进导管室时，用与患儿年龄相称的方式迎接患儿，并进行术前准备，也是非常有价值的。患儿体位的选择应该根据年龄而定，并且以约束带进行可靠而不过分的固定。由于操作过程可能很长，应当避免长时间将患儿的手臂固定于头上，以免造成臂丛神经的损伤。将手臂固定于胸外侧会影响侧位透视，但是可以通过以较小角度的左前斜位（10°～20°）透视来避免手臂对透视的影响。

（三）鞘管置入和导管选择及导管置入路径

鞘管置入和导管选择的细节问题，如其中的经皮穿刺技术、鞘管的数目、大小、血管的选择、心腔内的位置、是否抗凝等问题，已经在本书的第二版中有详尽的叙述[2]。

儿科射频消融登记资料和一个电生理中心分别总结和报告了儿科患者左侧旁道的导管置入路径[9,10]。经调查儿科射频消融登记的各成员的常用和惯用方式，各种左侧旁道的导管置入路径均在登记资料中得到了分析。

本书第三版（Kugler所写的第114章）总结了登记资料的结果，主要的结论包括：(1) 无论选择何种方法，医生经验对于提高成功率、降低透视时间和合并症都很重要；(2) 试用多种方法有助于提高成功率；(3) 为了提高后间隔旁道的消融成功率，应当使用冠状窦内消融。Law等研究发现[10]，房间隔穿刺和经主动脉逆行进入左心室的合并症发生率类似，但是房间隔穿刺需要使用的导管更少，透视时间更短，因此效果更好些。

（四）透视

双球管X光机（biplane fluoroscopy）对于年龄较小的患儿（尽管心脏结构正常）和年龄较大的先天性心脏病患儿都是很必要的，导管操作过程中只需要踩一下脚踏板，便可以立即得到垂直平面（或类似平面）的导管位置影像，对提高安全性很有帮助。而使用单球管X光机（single-plane fluoroscopy），由于转动球管需要耗费时间，所以容易忽视其他投照位置的影像。

双球管X光机的缺点是总的放射暴露有可能增加，因为操作过程中容易更多地使用透视。尽管直接检测放射剂量很重要[11]，但另外一个包括859例儿童和成人患者放射暴露的多中心研究估测了皮肤的放射暴露量[12]，根据估测进行计算所得的结果表明，儿童受到的射线照射明显低于成年人，而且儿童患者和成年患者中分别有11%和22%所受放射超过了引起皮肤损伤的阈值（2 Sievert或200REM）。大剂量照射的独立预测因子包括患者年龄、男性、消融失败，以及所在医学中心的经验。该组研究者还估计了患者死于恶性肿瘤的危险性大约增加2/1000[12]。

有研究比较了儿科射频消融登记资料中没有器质性心脏病的阵发性室上性心动过速消融的放射暴露时间，发现以2年为一个周期，平均放射暴露时间呈现逐渐下降的趋势。此外，比较早期（1991－1995年）和晚期（1996－1999年），也是呈逐渐下降的趋势[13,14]。这些登记资料显示，在最初的2年中，平均透视时间为60±44min（中位数为36min，90%百分位数为97min，10%百分位数为10min），其后1995－1996年2年的平均透视时间为40±35min。消融早期和晚期的平均透视时间分别是50.9±39.9min和40.1±35.1min。消融失败和消融成功的病例相比，前者的透视时间总是长于后者。多因素分析表明，较长的透视时间主要与右侧游离壁旁路、后间隔旁路、前间隔旁路和体重增加有关系，较短的透视时间与经验多、房室结折返性心动过速（AVNRT）消融有关。有器质性心脏病或者血流动力学异常的消融登记资料显示，该组患者透视时间较长[2]。研究表明，比较早期和晚期的消融资料后显示，除了AET以外的所有室上性心动过速（SVT）患者的透视时间均缩短了[14]。

几个很有可能在将来进一步缩短射频消融透视时

间的因素包括：设备的不断更新，如脉冲式透射［可变焦距采集图像（acquisition zoom）等技术可能进一步优化设备］、替代影像技术的进步和操作经验的不断积累[3,15-17]。而且，登记资料的分析还有可能影响病人的选择，例如，由于右侧游离壁旁路、前或者后间隔旁路和体重增加均与增加透视时间有关，也许某些病人或者家属会选择非消融的其他替代治疗方式。另外，北美起搏与电生理协会（NASPE）专家共识和美国心脏病学会（ACC）关于心脏疾病诊治过程中放射安全的专家共识中，均强调指出，虽然儿童接受心导管检查和治疗的放射暴露似乎是可以接受的低危险，但是在操作中尽最大的努力减少放射剂量是非常重要的[3,16]。

（五）心电图记录、刺激、射频电流的应用

与成人患者相比，儿童患者的心电图记录、刺激和射频电流的发放均没有什么差别。由于儿童的心率较快，为了更好地在标测过程中分辨和评价心电图，应当使用更快的走纸速度（≥200mm/s）来记录、显示和分析心电图（图119-1）。射频能量的发放本身也与成人患者类似，但是也有一些研究者发现对于AVNRT，使用较低温度消融（平均47.9±2.7℃）和减慢房室结传导的方法在儿童患者中可成功消融[18]。另外有人主张对于有旁路的儿童患者，先用50℃消融，旁路阻断后升温至70℃[19]继续消融。Laohaprasitiporn等分析了58例儿童和青少年患者，发现如果放电数秒内旁路没有被阻断，即停止放电，是比较好的方法。所有上述技术手段的目的是一样的：成功消融治疗心律失常的同时，尽量减少对正常心肌组织的永久损伤。

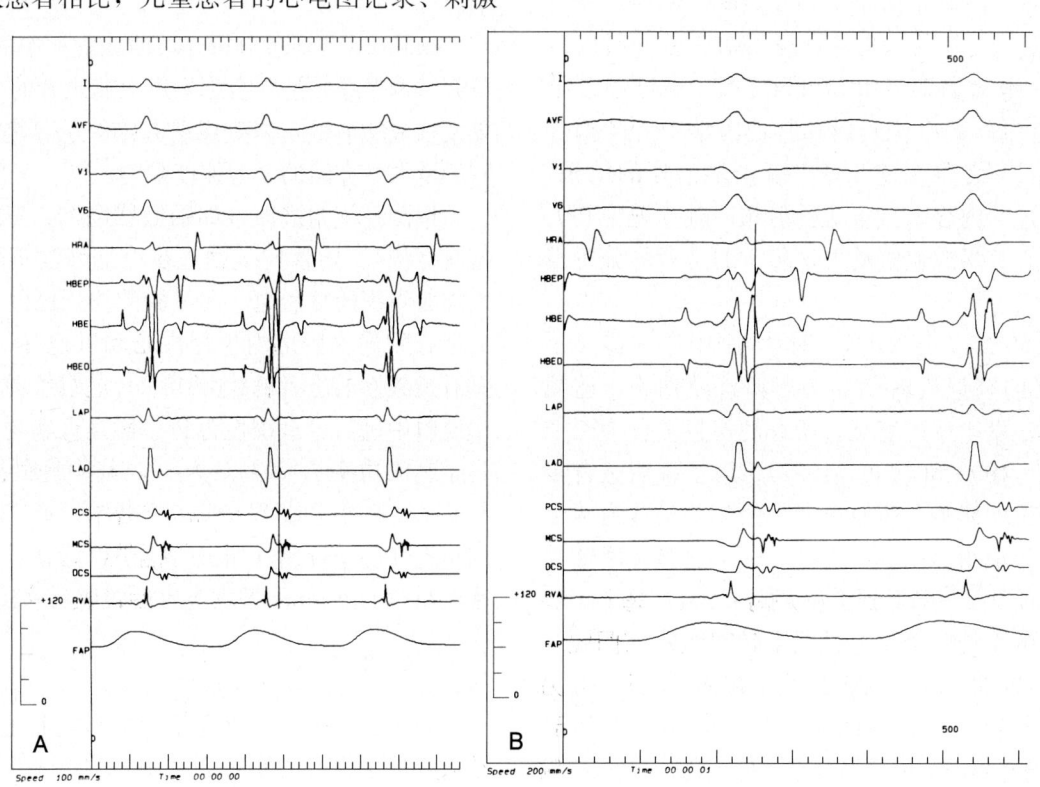

图119-1 不同走纸速度的心电图记录（A：100mm/s；B：200mm/s）显示标测过程中快速记录的优势　13岁男孩的左侧房室旁路仅有逆传功能，100mm/s的记录速度很难看出心动过速（周期为310mm/s）时最早的心房激动位置（A）。当记录速度增加到200mm/s时（B），将一竖标记线置于远端左心房，可以很快判断出最早的心房激动部位。穿刺房间隔，将标测电极跨过二尖瓣瓣环，置于侧游离壁，电极即可记录到远端左心房的电图。FAP，股动脉压力；Ⅰ、AVF、V_1、V_6，体表心电图；HBEP、HBE、HBED，近端、中段和远端希氏束电图；HRA，高位右心房；LAP and LAD，置于二尖瓣环处左侧心房游离壁的4mm标测导管的近端和远端电极记录的心电图；PCS、MCS、DCS，近、中和远端冠状窦电图；RVA，右心室心尖部电图。

(六) 消融治疗所需要的时间

1997年对PSVT登记资料的分析显示，消融治疗所需要的平均时间（从置入第一个鞘管到消融结束后拔除所有鞘管的时间）为 257 ± 157 min（中位数为240min)[13]，如果以每2年为一个周期进行分析，成功消融病例的平均时间和总消融病例的平均时间均显著下降，而消融失败病例的平均时间没有变化。消融时间延长与右侧游离壁旁路、后或者前间隔旁路以及体重增加有关，AVNRT消融所需要的时间往往较短。除了医生经验与较短的消融治疗时间无关外，影响消融时间的因素与影响透视时间的因素是类似的。

三、儿童患者消融治疗的效果

自从早期一些单个医学中心发表的病例回顾分析和1994年第一次发表了儿科射频消融登记资料以后（上述报告在本书的第二版[1]和第三版[2]中已经总结过），不断有更新的登记资料和其他医学中心的报告发表[14,21-25]。下文将综述儿童患者消融治疗的结果，这部分更新过的内容来自于儿科射频消融登记中心关于无器质性心脏病或血流动力学异常的患者的分析报告[14]。

截止1999年3月24日，有48个中心共递交了7600例患者的登记资料[14]，为了评价成功率、透视时间和合并症发生率的变化，所有的资料被分为两个时期（1991－1995和1996－1999）；为了说明患者年龄对消融效果的影响，所有患者根据年龄又分为两个亚组，即低年龄组（<5岁）和5～21岁组。消融失败率从早期的9.6%降低到了晚期的4.8%，每个年龄组的消融失败率均降低了。虽然不同时期的前间隔旁路（83%变为86%）和AET的消融成功率（均为89%）没有提高，但是后间隔旁路（从87%增加到93%）、右侧游离壁旁路（从85%增加到95%）、左侧游离壁旁路（从94%增加到97%）和AVNRT（从95%到99%）的成功率均提高了。不同年龄组的分析中，只有高年龄组的右侧和左侧游离壁旁路、后间隔旁路和AVNRT的成功率提高了。

另外有两个登记资料的报告，着重研究某个特别有挑战性的问题。Reich等分析了Ebstein畸形患者的登记资料（$n=65$)[22]，Blaufox等分析了射频消融治疗中有争议的问题（137例≤18个月的婴幼儿的资料）。

Ebstein畸形患者右侧游离壁（79%）、右间隔（89%）和其他部位（75%）的急性期成功率，与Hebe等人所报告的先天性心脏病中的一组Ebstein畸形的效果类似（26/30，急性期成功率为86%)[25]。Reich等还发现消融成功的患者可有轻度的三尖瓣反流（而不是严重程度的），体表面积为 $1.7m^2$ 或更少[22]。

婴儿患者的登记资料与非婴儿患者的登记资料相比，有两个主要的不同[23]。第一，婴儿患者中器质性心脏病患者占36%，而非婴儿患者中仅有11.2%；第二，更多的婴儿患者因为危及生命的心律失常或药物疗效差行射频消融治疗；另外，还有些中心不为婴儿作射频消融，这些中心的病人登记例数往往少于可以为婴儿患者行射频消融的中心的登记例数。婴儿或非婴儿患者的总成功率或某种心律失常的成功率没有差别。

Danford等通过分析学习曲线过程中的登记资料，研究了术者经验是否会影响室上速患者的疗效[26]，结果发现成功消融左侧游离壁旁路的学习速度最快，而右侧游离壁旁路的学习速度最慢。

标测系统的进展（如网篮状电极、三维标测、非接触标测）、导管技术的进步（如灌注消融导管可以增加对组织的穿透力）和经验的积累已经提高了对先天性心脏病术后房内折返性心动过速（IART）这组具有挑战性的患者的疗效[27-31]。这组患者并没有在登记资料中进行过系统性分析，但是近来有几个中心报告了其成功率为70%～85%，其中房间隔手术（如Mustard修补术或Senning修补术）或"切口性"房内折返性心动过速（如房间隔缺损修补术后）的成功率较高，而Fontan型吻合术后的成功率较低。

(一) 合并症

登记资料中对于所有年龄组和室上速的病例，操作过程的主要合并症的发生率为0.106%，涉及患者的主要合并症的发生率为0.117%[14]。此外，分析不同时期的资料发现，早期合并症发生率为4.2%，晚期降为3.0%[14]，其中所有年龄组的左室游离壁（从4%到3%）和后间隔旁路（从4%到2%）的合并症发生率均下降了，高年龄组后间隔旁路和AVNRT的合并症减少了，但低年龄组（5岁以下）各种旁路的消融合并症发生率均未下降。其中比较3个最主要的合并症：二度或者三度房室阻滞、导管穿孔/心包积液和血栓/栓塞，结果显示两个年龄组的发生率均无变化。早期有3例死亡（2例旁路，1例AET），后期仅有1例死亡（旁路）。Schaffer等[32]进一步调整了登记资料中的死亡病例发现，死亡病例更多地伴有基础心脏病、体重较低、放电次数较多，多为左侧病变，他们也发现术者的经验看起来与死亡率高无关。

由于总是有合并症的报告，所以仍有新的研究资料不断发表[33-38]。研究者认为消融游离壁和后间隔旁路时，必须同时考虑有无冠状动脉的病变。有一项包括29个中心、1749例射频消融的登记资料的分析显示，存在由于操作不够谨慎而引起房室阻滞的危险[39]，其中中间隔旁路（10.4%）的危险性最高，后间隔旁路和AVNRT的危险性最低（1.0%～1.6%）。

（二）随访

与有关射频消融的其他问题相比，很少有关于随访的报告发表。Johnson等报告了31例儿童患者的Holter随访结果[40]，发现偶尔有房性早搏/心动过速发生，与术前的Holter相比，没有发现新的心律失常。Atakr多中心研究发现，远程心电监测对于判断患者有症状时是否有心律失常非常有价值，而通过重复电生理检查进行随访是没有必要的[41]。

登记资料中关于随访的数据主要集中于发现无基础心脏病的阵发性室上速消融术后与消融操作相关的合并症、心律失常和/或相关基础病变的复发（如预激）[13]。通过分析有相应随访资料的这组病人（2578例射频消融中76.3%符合随访条件），1%的患者在随访过程中出现了另外的合并症，最严重的是3例死亡（见"合并症"一节）。Kaplan-Meier分析（用Wilcoxon检验进行比较）显示，射频消融术后3年中77%的旁路和71%的AVNRT没有复发，而且这两组病人没有显著性差异。不同部位旁路的复发情况也进行了比较，结果显示左侧游离壁旁路较右侧游离壁和间隔旁路均有较低的复发率。射频消融后数年，一些复发病例被认识到，这是否代表了对晚期复发时程的精确估计，或者仅是延迟检出和报告了实际上早期即出现的复发，目前尚不清楚。

较高的复发率令人失望，但这有可能是自愿递交的登记资料的偏倚造成的[13]，本随访研究仅包括了登记资料中无基础心脏病的阵发性室上速消融后病例的76.3%，这个随访率相对较低，那些完全或者几乎没有症状的患者相信自己被治愈了，不愿意再来随诊，而回来随诊的病人则可能主要是复发的病人，因此，据此可以推测，实际的复发率很可能更低。有一项前瞻性的多中心研究（由大多数的登记资料的成员中心组成）目前正在进行中，目的是确切了解真实的复发率和晚期合并症的发生率。本临床研究没有包括更具有挑战性的房内折返性房速和伴有基础心脏病的患者，所以后两种情况的数据只能来自于回顾性研究或者单中心的报告。截止现在，据报告房内折返性房速的复发率较高（大约40%～60%）[3,31]。Ebstein畸形患者的登记资料显示，右侧游离壁、右侧间隔和其他部位旁路的复发率分别是32%、29%和7%[22]。

四、适应证

事实上，当讨论某种治疗措施的适应证时，多种因素需要考虑，包括客观资料报告、主观的个人经验和专家的意见[1-3,13,23-25,42-44]。与讨论和最终的建议相关的是治疗措施的发展历史、病人的症状/临床表现、治疗措施的近期和远期的风险/收益比较、可能的最糟糕的情况、医生和病人及其家属的个人经验、治疗的花费。本书的前几版详尽地讨论了这些问题，NASPE关于儿童射频消融的专家共识也有相关的说明[1-3]。

儿童患者射频消融的适应证

基于前文所述的多种因素和已有资料，似乎有理由相信儿科患者的射频消融适应证与年龄和症状相关。在Van Hare建议的方法基础上[42]，2002年NASPE专家共识采用了美国心脏病学会用于其他已发表适应证指南的定义方式，对儿童射频消融的适应证进行了分类：Ⅰ类即广泛同意行射频消融治疗的适应证；Ⅱ类即进行射频消融治疗，但有不同意见存在的适应证；Ⅲ类即不需要行射频消融治疗的适应证（表119-1）。

五、致 谢

感谢 Kris Houston, R.N.B.S.N., M.A. 和 Gary Felix, B.A. 帮助分析资料数据；感谢 David Danford, M.D. 审稿和提出修改意见；感谢 Deb Hanson 为书写本章而做的准备工作。

表 119-1 儿童射频消融的适应证

I 类适应证
1. 预激综合征的猝死存活者
2. 预激综合征合并晕厥，且晕厥发生时心房颤动伴旁道前传，RR 间期缩短（小于 250ms，或者心房程序刺激时心房的有效不应期小于 250ms）
3. 慢性或者反复发作的 SVT 伴心室功能异常
4. 反复发作室速，伴血流动力学异常，导管消融有效

II A 类适应证
1. 反复发作和/或药物治疗无效的有症状的 SVT，并且年龄大于 4 岁
2. 拟作先天性心脏病手术治疗，术后导管进入血管或者心腔将受到影响
3. 心室功能正常的慢性（首次发作后持续 6～12 个月）或者无休止的 SVT
4. 慢性或者反复发作的 IART
5. 心悸伴心脏电生理检查中可以诱发持续性 SVT

II B 类适应证
1. 无症状的预激综合征，ECG 显示为 WPW 综合征，大于 5 岁，没有明确的心动过速史，消融治疗和心律失常本身的利弊均已经解释清楚
2. SVT，大于 5 岁，长期口服抗心律失常药有效，消融可以作为另外一种替代药物的治疗手段
3. SVT，小于 5 岁（包括婴儿），包括胺碘酮和索他洛尔在内的抗心律失常药的疗效不好或者出现了不能耐受的不良反应
4. 每年发作 1～3 次、需要药物治疗的 IART
5. 反复发作、治疗困难的 IART，可以选择房室结消融加起搏器植入作为替代的治疗方法
6. 发作一次伴有血流动力学异常的室速，导管消融有效

III 类适应证
1. 无症状的 WPW 综合征，年龄小于 5 岁
2. 抗心律失常药有效的 SVT，年龄小于 5 岁
3. 非持续性阵发性室速，不是无休止性（一次数小时的心电监测或者任何 1h 的心电监测均可以记录到），不伴有心室功能的异常
4. 非持续 SVT 多次发作，但不需要药物治疗，或者症状很轻

SVT，室上性心动过速；VT，室性心动过速；WPW，预激综合征。

（引自 Friedman RA, Walsh EP, Silka MJ, et al: NASPE Expert Consensus Conference: Radiofrequency catheter ablation in children with and without congenital heart disease. Report of the Writing Committee. Pacing Clin Electrophysiol 25：1000，2002.）

（丁燕生 译）

参 考 文 献

1. Kugler JD: Catheter ablation in pediatric patients. In Zipes DP, Jalife J (eds): Cardiac Electrophysiology: From Cell to Bedside, 2nd ed. Philadelphia, WB Saunders, 1995, pp 1524–1537.
2. Kugler JD: Catheter ablation in pediatric patients. In Zipes DP (ed): Cardiac Electrophysiology: From Cell to Bedside, 3rd ed. Philadelphia, WB Saunders, 2000, pp 1056–1064.
3. Friedman RA, Walsh EP, Silka MJ, et al: NASPE Expert Consensus Conference: Radiofrequency catheter ablation in children with and without congenital heart disease. Report of the Writing Committee. Pacing Clin Electrophysiol 25:1000, 2002.
4. Lavoie J, Walsh EP, Burrows FA, et al: Effects of propofol or isoflurane anesthesia on cardiac conduction in children undergoing radiofrequency catheter ablation for tachydysrhythmias. Anesthesiology 82:884, 1995.
5. Lai L-P, Lin J-L, Wu M-H, et al: Usefulness of intravenous propofol anesthesia for radiofrequency catheter ablation in patients with tachyarrhythmias: Infeasibility for pediatric patients with ectopic atrial tachycardia. Pacing Clin Electrophysiol 22:1358, 1999.
6. Chang R-K R, Wetzel GT, Shannon KM, et al: Age- and anesthesia-related changes in accessory pathway conduction in children with Wolff-Parkinson-White syndrome. Am J Cardiol 76:1074, 1995.
7. Chang R-K R, Stevenson WG, Wetzel GT, et al: Effects of isoflurane on electrophysiological measurements in children with the Wolff-Parkinson-White syndrome. Pacing Clin Electrophysiol 19:1082, 1996.
8. Vazir-Marino F, Young M-L, Kohli V, et al: Controlled ventilation enhances catheter stability during radiofrequency ablation. Pacing Clin Electrophysiol 22:86, 1999.
9. Kugler JD, Danford DA, Houston K, et al: Radiofrequency ablation of left free wall accessory pathways: Transatrial, retrograde, or coronary sinus approach? In Singer I (ed): Nonpharmacological Therapy of Arrhythmias for 21st Century: The State of the Art. Armonk, NY, Futura, 1998, pp 73–87.
10. Law LH, Fischbach PS, LeRoy S, et al: Access to the left atrium for delivery of radiofrequency ablation in young patients: Retrograde aortic *vs.* transseptal approach. Pediatr Cardiol 22:204, 2001.
11. Geise RA, Peters NE, Dunnigan A, et al: Radiation doses during pediatric radiofrequency catheter ablation procedures. Pacing Clin Electrophysiol 19:1605, 1996.
12. Rosenthal LS, Mahesh M, Beck TJ, et al: Predictors and risk of radiation exposure during catheter ablation procedures: Results of a multicenter study. Am J Cardiol 82:451, 1998.
13. Kugler JD, Danford D, Houston K, et al: Radiofrequency catheter ablation for paroxysmal supraventricular tachycardia in children and adolescents without structural heart disease. Am J Cardiol 80:1438, 1997.
14. Kugler, JD, Danford DA, Houston K, Felix G: Pediatric radiofrequency catheter ablation registry success, fluoroscopy time, and complication rate for supraventricular tachycardia: Comparison of early and recent eras. J Cardiovasc Electrophysiol 13:336, 2002.
15. Ross RD, Joshi V, Carravallah DJ: Reduced radiation during cardiac catheterization of infants using acquisition zoom technology. Am J Cardiol 79:691, 1997.
16. Limacher MC, Douglas PS, Germano G, et al: Radiation safety in the practice of cardiology. J Am Coll Cardiol 31:892, 1998.
17. Drago F, Silvetti MS, DiPino A, et al: Exclusion of fluoroscopy during ablation treatment of right accessory pathway in children. J Cardiovasc Electrophysiol 13:778, 2002.
18. Vega-Arrillaga F, Young M-L, Wu J-M, Wolff GS: Initial low temperature setting in radiofrequency catheter ablation of Wolf-Parkinson-White syndrome. Pacing Clin Electrophysiol 23:2097, 2000.
19. Rhodes LA, Wieand TS, Vetter VL: Low temperature and low energy radiofrequency modification of atrioventricular nodal slow pathways in pediatric patients. Pacing Clin Electrophysiol 22:1071, 1999.
20. Laohaprasitiporn D, Walsh EP, Saul JP, et al: Predictors of permanence of successful radiofrequency lesions created with controlled catheter tip temperature. Pacing Clin Electrophysiol 20:1283, 1997.
21. Berul GI, Hill SL, Wang PJ, et al: Neonatal radiofrequency catheter ablation of junctional tachycardias. J Interv Card Electrophysiol 2:91, 1998.

22. Reich JD, Auld D, Hulse JE, et al: The Pediatric Radiofrequency Ablation Registry's experience with Ebstein's anomaly. J Cardiovasc Electrophysiol 9:1371, 1998.
23. Blaufox AD, Felix GL, Saul JP: Radiofrequency catheter ablation in infants ≤ 18 months old. Circulation 104:2803, 2001.
24. Iturralde P, Colin L, Kershenovich S, et al: Radiofrequency catheter ablation for the treatment of supraventricular tachycardias in children and adolescents. Cardiol Young 10:376, 2000.
25. Hebe J, Hansen P, Ouyang F, et al: Radiofrequency catheter ablation of tachycardia in patients with congenital heart disease. Pediatr Cardiol 21:557, 2000.
26. Danford DA, Kugler JD, Deal BJ, et al: The learning curve of radiofrequency ablation of tachyarrhythmias in pediatric patients. Am J Cardiol 75:587, 1995.
27. Zrenner B, Ndrepepa G, Schneider AE, et al: Mapping and ablation of atrial arrhythmias after surgical correction of congenital heart disease guided by a 64-electrode basket catheter. Am J Cardiol 88:573, 2001.
28. Kanter RJ, Papagiannis J, Carboni MP, et al: Radiofrequency catheter ablation of supraventricular tachycardia substrates after Mustard and Senning operations for d-transposition of the great arteries. J Am Coll Cardiol 35(2):428, 2000.
29. Collins KK, Love BA, Walsh EP, et al: Location of acutely successful radiofrequency catheter ablation of intraatrial reentrant tachycardia in patients with congenital heart disease. Am J Cardiol 86:969, 2000.
30. Paul T, Windhagen-Mahnert B, Kriebel T, et al: Atrial reentrant tachycardia after surgery for congenital heart disease: Endocardial mapping and radiofrequency catheter ablation using a novel, non-contact mapping system. Circulation 103:2266, 2001.
31. Triedman JK, Alexander ME, Love BA, et al: Influence of patient factors and ablative technologies on outcomes of radiofrequency ablation of intra-atrial re-entrant tachycardia in patients with congenital heart disease. J Am Coll Cardiol 39:1827, 2002.
32. Schaffer MS, Gow RM, Mooak JP, Saul JP: Mortality following radiofrequency catheter ablation (from the Pediatric Radiofrequency Ablation Registry). Am J Cardiol 86:639, 2000.
33. Paul T, Bokenkamp R, Trappe HJ: Coronary artery involvement early and late after radiofrequency current application in young pigs. Am Heart J 133:436, 1997.
34. Windhagen-Mahnert B, Bokenkamp R, Bertram H, et al: Radiofrequency current application on immature porcine atrial myocardium: No evidence of areas of slow conduction after 12-month follow-up. J Cardiovasc Electrophysiol 9:1305, 1998.
35. Bokenkamp R, Wibbelt G, Sturm M, et al: Effects on intracardiac radiofrequency current application on coronary artery vessels in young pigs. J Cardiovasc Electrophysiol 11:565, 2000.
36. Khanal S, Ribeiro PA, Platt M, et al: Right coronary artery occlusion as a complication of accessory pathway ablation in a 12-year-old treated with stenting. Catheter Cardiovasc Interv 46:59, 1999.
37. Strobel GG, Trehan S, Compton S, et al: Successful pediatric stenting of a nonthrombotic coronary occlusion as a complication of radiofrequency catheter ablation. Pacing Clin Electrophysiol 24:1026, 2001.
38. Bertram H, Kokenkamp R, Peuster M, et al: Coronary artery stenosis after radiofrequency catheter ablation of accessory atrioventricular pathways in children with Ebstein's malformation. Circulation 103:538, 2001.
39. Schaffer MS, Silka MJ, Ross BA, et al: Inadvertent atrioventricular block during radiofrequency catheter ablation: Results of the Pediatric Radiofrequency Ablation Registry. Circulation 94:3214, 1996.
40. Johnson TB, Varney FL Jr, Gillette PC, et al: Lack of proarrhythmia as assessed by Holter monitor after atrial radiofrequency ablation of supraventricular tachycardia in children. Am Heart J 132:120, 1996.
41. Wagshal AB, Pires LA, Yong PG, et al: Usefulness of follow-up electrophysiologic study and event monitoring after successful radiofrequency catheter ablation of supraventricular tachycardia. Am J Cardiol 75:50, 1995.
42. Van Hare GF: Indications for radiofrequency ablation in the pediatric population. J Cardiovasc Electrophysiol 8:952, 1997.
43. Kugler JD: Indications for catheter ablation of accessory pathways and typical atrioventricular nodal tachycardia in infants and children. In Walsh EP, Saul EP (eds): Cardiac Arrhythmias in the Pediatric Patient: Evolving Concepts in Clinical Management. Philadelphia, Lippincott Williams & Wilkins, 2001, pp 445–459.
44. Bromberg BI, Lindsay BD, Cain ME, et al: Impact of clinical history and electrophysiologic characterization of accessory pathways on management strategies to reduce sudden death among children with Wolff-Parkinson-White syndrome. J Am Coll Cardiol 27:69, 1996.

第 120 章

心律失常的外科治疗

Pierre L. Pagé

本章目录

- 室性心动过速 1078
- 室上性心律失常 1082
- 心房颤动 1082
- 房室旁路 1085
- 总结 1087

对于几乎所有的室上性或室性心动过速目前已设计出相应的外科手术方案（表 120-1），这些手术方法是在特定的年代中产生的，该时期临床上主要关注单形性折返性心律失常，因此该类心律失常也是临床心脏电生理研究的一个重要的类型[1]。由于恰如其分的手术方案应根据心律失常的机制来加以选择，因此术中电生理标测是手术成功的基本要素。本章介绍外科治疗心律失常的方法以及在当前经皮介入技术和可植入装置迅速发展的年代，外科治疗心律失常的新角色。

一、室性心动过速

1959 年 Couch 及同事首次明确提出反复发作的室性心动过速是左心室室壁瘤切除的指征，尽管这只是一种相对有效的方法，但直到 Guiraudon 等强调对于室性心动过速应直接消除产生心律失常的基础，并在窦性心律标测引导下施行单纯心室切除术治疗不伴有冠状动脉疾病的室性心动过速以前，这种简单的室壁瘤切除使用了 15 年。到了 20 世纪 70 年代，随着程序刺激技术应用于临床和在动物模型上的完美试验，证明了单形性室性心动过速的基础是折返机制。由于这种折返的稳定性，理论上讲有可能确定心动过速的激动部位，而且可通过切除或消融予以根除。1979 年 Josephson 及同事进一步深化了这一理论，提出对经心内膜标测明确的心动过速起源处采用心内膜切除术[1]，即切除约 2mm 厚、3~5cm² 面积大小的心内膜瘢痕。这种首次采用非药物性治疗手段的早期成功激发了研究者们极大的热情，从此涌现出不少外科手术方法。但是尽管手术的成功率接近 85% 以及死亡率在 5%~10% 之间，在此后的 10 年期间外科治疗室性心动过速的病例数量还是大大地下降，这是因为外科手术的复杂性和植入性抗心动过速装置的开展，使得适合于外科手术的病人转为非手术治疗[2]。而且随着术中电生理标测技术在几个医疗中心的广泛应用，对心律失常机制的认识更为深入，使之能够确定并采用微创的方法消融引起心律失常的部位[1,3]，因此可采用经皮导管消融技术来治疗选择性病人（第 117 章）。与此同时，其他新的非药物治疗手段在不断发展，更好的药物治疗方法也在探索之中。尽管抗心律失常药物在安全性和有效性方面不可能与非药物手段相比，但对于急性心梗的治疗（如溶栓和经皮冠状动脉内介入）肯定能减少因大片心肌瘢痕所引起的室性心律失常发病率。不论怎样，尤其对于频繁反复发作的室性心动过速以及需要干预治疗心室再灌注和心室重塑方面，外科手术仍然占有重要地位。

对于伴有冠状动脉疾病的室性心动过速，有几种不同的外科治疗方法[1,4]。所有的这些方法都是基于相同理论，即这类室性心动过速都源于不可逆性损伤的心肌内（如慢性已愈合的梗死心肌），因此任何原因引起的心室弥漫性病理状态，如扩张性心肌病、瓣

表 120-1　外科治疗的心律失常

心律失常类型	手术方法
1. 室性心动过速（伴有冠状动脉疾病）	心室心内膜环状切除* 广泛性心内膜切除 心内膜切除±冷冻消融 局部心内膜切除＋冷冻消融*
2. 室性心动过速（不伴有冠状动脉疾病）	单纯心室切除 局部冷冻 右心室分离手术*
3. 折返性室上性心动过速（WPW）	旁路切断
4. 房性心动过速	局部冷冻
5. 心房扑动	广泛性心房切开 局部冷冻
6. 房室结折返性心动过速	房室结周围冷冻*
7. 阵发性心房颤动	改良 Cox-迷宫-Ⅲ式手术* 左房隔离术* 左房消融术* 肺静脉隔离术
8. 慢性持续性心房颤动	改良 Cox-迷宫-Ⅲ式手术* 左房隔离术* "走廊"手术* 左房消融术*

* 可以不需术中标测。

膜性心肌病都不适合外科治疗。遵循这一原则，对于非冠状动脉疾病的室性心动过速，只有当存在孤立性病灶时才适合于外科手术，如 Chagas 病、结节病及特发性瘤。起源于右心室发育不良的心律失常具有以上这两种损伤的特征：心律失常的起源部位通常局限于右心室，但这种多发性散在分布的致心律失常病灶却使得分散消融效果不好。因此 Guiraudon 等提出了右心室分离术，其目的在于将左心室与产生心律失常的病灶分隔开以消除心律失常。

长期以来一直在研究外科治疗室性心动过速的策略，其焦点在于如何平衡既要消除足够的心肌组织以控制心律失常而又要保护左心室功能，尤其是当室性心动过速伴有心肌梗死时。在未充分认识到左心室重建以前这是很现实的，例如左心室心内膜环切除后的高死亡率正是因为左心室功能恶化引起的。此后一些作者相继报告心内膜切除术后可以改善左心室射血指数和心功能，其主要原因是切除了室壁瘤和对远离梗死瘢痕区的心肌血管重建。最近一个时期手术的方式由对左心室的电生理纠正向几何重建的模式转变[5-9]。近来认为电生理标测图对于手术成功并非很重要，因为根据多年来标测所获得的经验已能用于辨别解剖部位。Dor 及同事强调左心室几何形态的重要性[10]，并提出采用心内膜圆形补片以重建心室来维持左心室的椭圆形状。这类手术还包括其他所有能影响左心室功能因素的手术，如心肌血运重建、通过减小房室环以纠正二尖瓣反流、室间隔的心内膜切除和冷冻。笔者认为成功来源于两方面的结合：一方面是基于对左心室功能的解剖学认识，另一方面是对室性心律失常的电生理机制理解，从这个角度出发，应全面复习过去 25 年来所获取的术中电生理标测经验。

（一）术中标测：技术和知识

心脏标测是一种直接记录、分析心肌电活动并以类似几何图像显示出来的方法，其概念和技术已在有关章节中详细描述[1,3,4,11]。逐点标记是最为简便的方法，但也具有明显缺点，其中主要问题之一是不稳定和不能诱发出能持续足够长时间的心动过速，以容许采集到最低限度部位的心电活动。为了克服这些局限性，多点标测系统随之问世。用于心外膜标测的是一种可膨胀的带有多个探头的网罩，而心内膜标测采用固定有多个电极的充气球囊，这个球囊可从左心房经二尖瓣入左心室，或送入右心室。笔者的研究部门已将该系统广泛应用于伴有冠心病的室性心律失常病人，结果显示 100% 的患者在术中均能诱发出心动过速。笔者体会必须将心外膜与心内膜标测相结合并采用三维图像进行分析，以充分评估产生心律失常的基础。

据认为陈旧性心肌梗死伴心动过速的折返环位于左心室梗死区域心内膜内，这是第一类被大家所接受的能用外科治疗的室性心动过速，与此相应术中电生理标测主要集中在左心室心内膜，这是指导手术的标准方法。尽管标测的最终目的是要明确引起临床或潜在的室性心动过速的折返环部位，但要想能准确无误记录到全部折返环是不可能的，因为大部分的折返环可能存在于心肌内或甚至于心外膜下，而所用的探查电极仅能覆盖大部分心内膜或心外膜。根据左心室心内、外膜标测的全部数据，作者在研究中按照以下标准将心动过速分为 5 类，其标准为：（1）心内膜和心外膜最早激动的相对时间；（2）找出一个完整的折返模式，这种折返模式能解释实际记录到的 90% 或更多心动过速周期的长度，而且最早激动与最晚激动点相邻；（3）左、右心室心外膜发生激动的部位。这种分析方法提示仅采用左心室心内膜标测的准确性可能低于与心外膜标测联合应用。采用这种方法可将心动过速分为以下几类：Ⅰ. 完全性（≥90%室性心动过速的折返长度）心内膜下折返，占室性心动过速的 15%

（病人的 25%，图 120-1A）；Ⅱ．完全性心外膜下折返，占室性心动过速的 9%（病人的 14%，图 120-1B）；Ⅲ．标测的折返不完全，其左心室心内膜激动多于心外膜激动，占心动过速的 53%（病人的 75%，图 120-1C）；Ⅳ．标测的折返不完全，其左心室心外膜激动多于心内膜激动，占心动过速的 6%（病人的 11%）[11]；Ⅴ．右心室心外膜激动多于左心室心内膜激动，占心动过速的 17%（病人的 25%，图 120-1D）。左心室心内膜下折返（Ⅰ和Ⅲ型）与传统的起源于左心室心内膜下激动相似，占室性心动过速的 68%，但起源于心外膜下（Ⅱ及Ⅳ型）和间隔深处（Ⅴ型）可高达室性心动过速的 32%，这种发生率高于过去所采用的心外膜移动式电极标测的数据，这种心外膜移动式电极标测往往是不完全的。

作者的资料证实了这种观点，即室性心动过速的激动部位最常见于左心室心内膜，也有少数位于心外膜下或心肌内，尽管数量不多，但毕竟有室性心动过速发源于此。应注意的是这里所提出的将室性心动过速分成 5 类，并不意味着存在不同的发病机制，提出这种分类的目的是为了提高心外膜/心内膜标测的使用，以便更好拟定外科手术计划。

（二）手术策略

从标测得到的经验所知，在多数情况下心外膜和心内膜最早激动的部位在解剖上是与此相符的，事实上心外膜标测都能判明所有起源于心室游离壁的室性心动过速。在此种情况下，笔者推荐采用冷血心肌保护液使心脏停跳，局部冷冻心肌消融（温度 -60℃，每个点 1.5cm，持续 2min）。对于间隔部的心动过速，左心室的心外膜与心内膜的关系要复杂得多，在作者的病例中占 76%，这类情况下可能还伴有远处心外膜的激动点[3]。作者将这类病人再分为两个亚组研究，第一组为术前未归为Ⅴ型室间隔深部的室性心动过速而手术；第二组是术前已明确为Ⅴ型而采用了间隔心内膜切除加心肌冷冻（在完成心内膜切除后于左室间隔面进行冷冻）。术中电生理研究结果显示第一组中 38% 的病人能诱发出室性心动过速，而在第二组只有 4%（$P < 0.05$），推测其原因可能第一组仅仅消融了左心室的间隔面。Ⅴ型心动过速的特性是心外膜的激动发生于右心室的游离壁，而且要先于左心室心内膜的最早激动点[3]。对动物模型的全面标测和临床上采用右心室心内膜标测球囊对间隔性室性心动过速病人的研究支持这种发现，即间隔性室性心动过速存在几种类型，其折返可能：（1）完全位于左心室间隔的心内膜下；（2）累及间隔内（图 120-1C）；（3）完全位于右心室间隔的心内膜下（图 120-1D）[3]。因此，右心室心外膜和左心室心内膜激动部位两点相关的时间可以间接提示折返存在的深度，从而避免了右心室心内膜标测。此外，因为右心室间隔的心动过速往往在体表心电图（ECG）上表现为左束支阻滞图形，当临床上出现心动过速而 ECG 有此图像时应考虑起源于间隔，外科方案应因此而定。基于这些原则，对于左心室前壁室壁瘤的患者可避免标测，而对于间隔性室性心动过速中 76% 的病人，可根据此原则而常规采用间隔心内膜切除加冷冻治疗[6]。

尽管在非开胸置入 ICD 以前（1990 年前）外科手术的平均死亡率为 23%，但近十年来大多数外科中心死亡率已低于 5%[4-9]。van Hemel 等将残留的左心室功能定量并作为能否手术的指标，其住院死亡率已降为 1.3%，4 年的实际生存率为 85%。Rastegar[5] 等报告 25 例在标测引导下心内膜切除及室壁瘤切除左心室成形术，手术死亡率为零，而采用植入心脏除颤器的 5 年猝死率为 4%～17%[12]。笔者[4] 和 Rastegar[5] 所报告的 5 年猝死率（2.5%）均优于 ICD，心律失常的再复发率也明显低于 ICD 组。这些结果显示对于合适的病人采用外科手术是一种可接受的选择方法。尽管不可忽视在手术后一部分病人仍可诱发出室性心动过速（2%～20%，但包括作者在内大多数专家的研究报告中都 <15%）。外科手术对室性心动过速来讲远期效果是显著的[4-9]。van Hemel 已证明左心室 3 个以上节段的室壁运动正常者预后较好。Nath 在术前采用右前斜位心室造影，根据中心弧线的运动计算室壁活动，认为 16% 或以上是预后好坏的分界线，Di Donato[6] 等采用心室内补片成形和室间隔冷冻消融治疗可诱发性室性心律失常的患者，5 年无事件发作的生存率为 82%。在作者的研究中发现，仅仅在Ⅴ型室性心动过速亚组中一小部分病人，因间隔消融不完全而抗心律失常的效果不好[3,4]。

外科手术指征

目前已知，作为最后的手段外科手术不一定就有很好的效果，对于陈旧性心梗伴有单形性室性心动过速或可诱发出室性心动过速的心室颤动患者，应首先仔细研究左心室造影图。图 120-2 列举出不同的心室造影图像，对于图 120-2A～D 的情况，笔者毫不犹豫都采用手术治疗，但如果梗死区域运动度很小（图

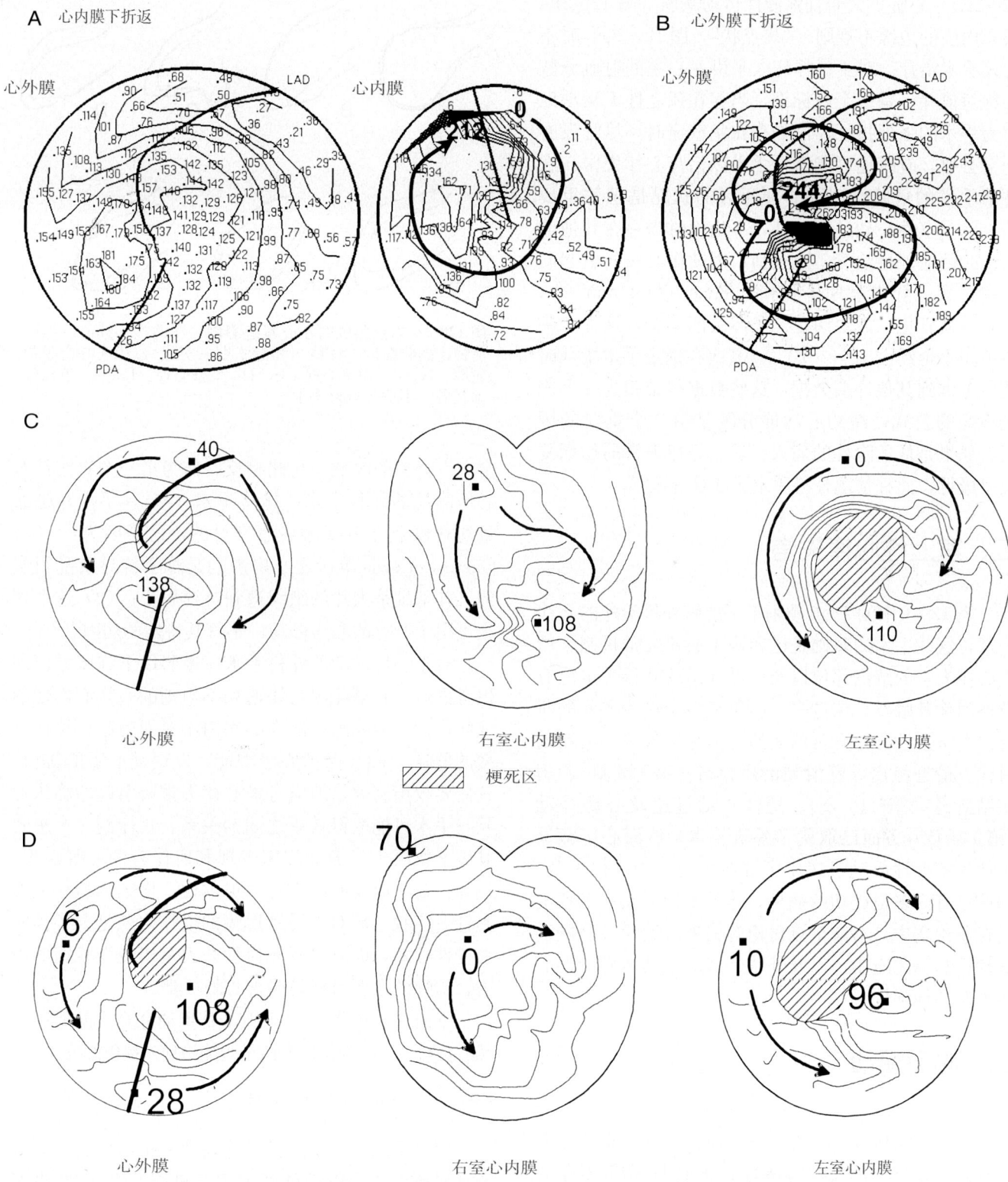

图 120-1 心外膜和心内膜顺序激动图 图中的方格坐标代表一个极的心脏图像,此时心脏的底部位于圆形的外围,心尖部位于中心,每隔 20ms 画等容线,图中的小字代表激动时间。A:完全性心内膜下折返,符合 I 型激动类型。心内膜图显示激动波以单向的逆时钟环状前向性扩散,最后的激动时间(212ms)与最早的激动时间相邻,其折返环在前间隔与左心室前游离壁之间完成。心外膜图(左图)显示从左心室前游离壁向右心室后壁的被动激动。B:完全性心外膜下折返(如 II 型激动类型),表现出 8 字形的折返环,通常激动波横行朝向梗死区(200~244ms)然后向后蔓延到心内膜激动部位(0 点)。C:A 型的侧面图,中间的图显示半环状向上传播,在右心内膜的方格坐标表示右心流出道的延迟。是左间隔的 III 型心动过速。D:V 型心动过速,典型的右侧间隔型。(引自 Pagé PL:Surgical treatment of ventricular tachycardia. Indications and results. Arch Mal Coeur 89(1):115-121,1996.)

120-2E)、心脏扩大而且弥漫性运动减弱（图 120-2F）或心内膜的边缘不规则（"斑点状"，图 120-2G）时不建议手术治疗。对于选择病人来讲左心室的射血分数的绝对值并不是一个好标准，当存在孤立性无运动区时为手术的强烈指征，而如存在室壁瘤时，尽管没有绝对必要，有时也可能需要手术以治疗心律失常。在评估手术的危险性时，非梗死区的状况是至关重要的。除了室性心动过速以外，不论何时当存在其他的指征时都应外科治疗，这包括：因缺血心肌病引起的心室扩大、舒张末期容积指数超过 100ml/min[6,10]；需要再血管化；需要纠正二尖瓣关闭不全，这种二尖瓣关闭不全约占 10%～20%。其次在确定手术指征时还应考虑到其他许多数据，这些数据很难归为一个固定不变的公式，纽约心功能分级是第二个重要的因素。如果是低危险性的病人，加之心律失常的远期复发率极低，此种情况外科手术或许是首选[4]。

二、室上性心律失常

表 120-1 中的 1～6 项列举了能够外科治疗的心律失常，这些手术的基础是已明确了心律失常机制、产生心律失常的解剖部位以及所设计出的外科手术能有效地消除其触发。在过去十多年来由于这些方面的研究使得室上性心律失常的非药物治疗进入了一个新的时代，最近经皮导管射频治疗旁路（第 115 章）、房室结折返（第 116 章）、房性心动过速及心房扑动（第 114 章）方面已取代了外科手术。然而心房颤动仍然是室上性心动过速中了解最少的一种心律不齐，即使已有许多很成功的病例，其手术指征及手术方法仍在争论之中。本章重点讨论有关外科治疗心房颤动的理论和临床应用，以及外科手术对于其他室上性心律失常的局限性。

三、心房颤动

由于心房颤动的高发生率和所伴随的严重临床并发症，以及抗心律失常药物的作用有限，因此对于心房颤动的治疗来讲，外科手术已成为诱人的主要手段。心律失常的外科治疗开始于 1968 年，当时采用的方法是在一个小的限定区域内切割以治疗房室旁道，随后此种方法相继应用于其他几种心律失常（表 120-1，1～6 项），其目的是消融一个特定的与心律失

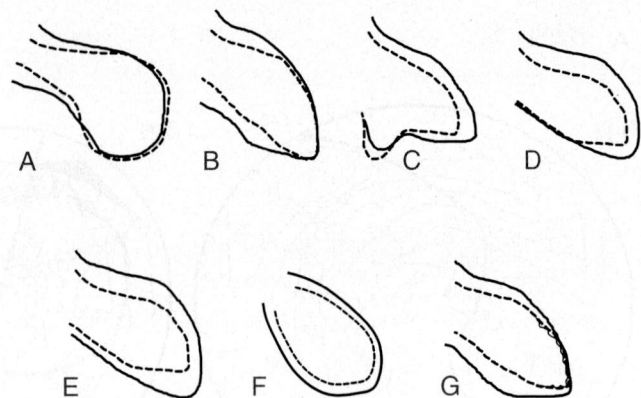

图 120-2 右前斜位的左心室造影图 在两次连续心跳期间所描记的收缩期（虚线）和舒张期（实线），代表心内膜的轮廓。A、B：前壁心梗。C、D：下壁心梗。E～G：节段运动减弱，不适合外科手术。

常产生有关的区域。与此相反，作为第一个直接针对心房颤动的外科手术，迷宫手术（Maze 手术）是通过切割整个心房以达到治疗目的，这是因为：（1）Garrey、Lewis 等认为心房颤动是整个传导紊乱引起的，其基础是大片的组织遭到持续病变；（2）这个理论可用于所有的心房颤动，不管其特殊的病因[13]。

对于心房颤动的外科手术应遵照以下临床方面加以考虑：（1）消除因为快速和不规则的心律而出现的症状；（2）消除因血液在心房内淤滞而引起血栓性栓塞的危险；（3）保护心房功能，以保证心脏的排血。这需要权衡利弊，即应考虑心律失常所引起的临床症状与手术可能取得效果之间的关系，具体到一个患者其因素取决于房颤的临床表现和所伴有的心脏疾患。例如：对于偶发的阵发性"孤立性"房颤的治疗主要是针对症状，而对于慢性房颤的治疗主要是为了预防血栓性栓塞，而对伴有充血性心力衰竭或瓣膜病的患者，治疗的主要目标是改善心脏功能。

下面首先复习与外科治疗心房颤动有关的病理生理，然后再讨论这种创伤性方法是否能给病人提供好处。

(一) 外科治疗的合理性

因自主激动产生的异常冲动和因折返引起的异常激动传播为心房颤动的两大主要机制，但在 20 世纪并未意识到这两种因素的相互作用，反而认为这是两种相互竞争的机制[13]。因此，如何走出这一困境，以解释越来越多临床上所遇到的问题，对于治疗至关重要。事实上如果主要是因异位病灶引起，则控制自主兴奋性的药物应该有效，相反如因折返环引起，则应

阻断其组织间的相互连接，如外科手术。在20世纪的后半时期，多折返学说成为心房颤动的主要理论，Allessie及同事们对此特别感兴趣，他们的研究证实折返激动可发生于传导阻滞的功能区，而不是在解剖上的梗阻区[13]。对心房颤动探索的第三个主要进步来自于近期的基础研究，这些研究显示细胞的激动是由于几种跨膜离子电流所控制。这些发现有助于理解临床上所观察到的现象，即心房颤动一旦发生，其电生理的特性随之即发生了变化，从而可再激活和维持心律紊乱，这个过程称之为电生理重构，而且不论房颤持续多久，这在临床上具有重要意义[14]。此外，Haissaguerre等[15]发现引起心房颤动的异位电活动起源于肺静脉的开口处，这对临床治疗房颤产生了极大的影响。这种观点不仅为导管介入消融这些病灶提供了理论依据，而且在此基础上可设计出新的手术方案。

面对上述复杂的情况，应该赞扬华盛顿大学专家们所作出的先驱性工作，因为他们提出了一个能导致外科手术成功的理论[16]。其依据是假设心房内有多种电生理机制共存，因此需要有一种针对各种病理基础的标准手术方式，其设计包括：(1) 根据Garey[13]提出的观点，将心房组织切割为小块状，使得多个折返不能维持；(2) 为了保证心房的收缩、传送功能以及减少血栓性栓塞的发生，所有切成小块的心房组织应重新缝在一起；使整个心房能够除极以维持其收缩性，而又不会发生折返；(3) 基于前面的两种假设，心房上的这些多条切口可以中断任何可能存在的大折返通路。自从1987年以来，这些理论已应用于临床实践，取得了非常好的效果[17-19]。

最后一种改良的迷宫手术称之为Cox-迷宫-Ⅲ (Cox-Maze-Ⅲ) 式手术，该手术已成为外科治疗房颤的标准术式[16]，圣路易斯州Barnes医院报告的结果显示，术后14年无房颤率为93%，其中既不需药物治疗也无房颤的比例为80%[17]。尽管有如此好的效果，但该手术并未被所有外科医生接受，其原因是：大家认为这种手术不易掌握，此外该手术还有一些缺陷，如主动脉阻断和体外循环时间过长；还存在体液潴留、心房功能改变、由于去自主神经引起的心房变时性不全等并发症以及高达15%的患者需要安装起搏器。由于这些问题，不少学者开始探索更为简化的手术而且已在小宗病例中取得可比性结果。应该提到的是，在评估外科治疗心房颤动的合理性时，应考虑到近来对肺静脉与左心房连接处新的认识。

（二）迷宫-Ⅲ式的手术方法

关于改良迷宫-Ⅲ式手术的方法已在其他章里详细描述，此处仅作简要介绍（图120-3）[17,20]。该手术采用胸部正中切口在体外循环下进行，由于需要在左心房内手术，故建议使用冷血停跳液保护心脏。先在右心房的游离壁做切口并向下延至三尖瓣环，在靠近三尖瓣瓣环处冷冻消融以保证能达到完全阻滞的目的。然后于房间沟切开左心房，将全部肺静脉口环状切开，该切线连接于二尖瓣环，在靠近二尖瓣瓣环及冠状窦处用冷冻消融，最后在卵圆窝水平横行切开房间隔，两个心耳亦应同时切除。

（三）改良迷宫-Ⅲ式手术的临床结果

自1987年9月25日迷宫手术首次施行以来，Cox等已完成346例手术[17]。依据不同病人的情况，手术死亡率为2%～3%之间，其中包括了同时施行其他高危险心脏手术的病人。总的房颤手术成功率已达到99%，就手术本身来讲不会引起永久性窦房结功能障碍，术后左心房的长期功能维持率在93%，右心房为99%。在日本，对2500多例病人实施了几种不同的迷宫手术[19]，其中房颤伴有先心病组施行右心房迷宫手术和其他相关手术，成功率约50%，明显低于其他手术的成功率（$P<0.005$），而其他手术的成功率超过70%，在这几种手术方式中成功率没有明显的差别。从1993到1999年Mayo医院共完成221例Cox-迷宫手术[18]，其中有75%以上的患者因伴有心脏病而同时施行其他心脏手术，总的早期死亡率为1.4%，术后3.2%需安装永久性起搏器，81%病人的房颤得以控制。他们认为心室功能低下不是手术的禁忌证，而且多数病人在Cox-迷宫手术后由于恢复窦性心律改善了左心室的射血功能。克里夫兰医院为100例病人施行了迷宫-Ⅲ式手术，平均随访3年，90.4%的病人能维持窦性心律（或心房起搏）[21]。

（四）外科手术的评估

早年对心房颤动治疗的目标是减慢快速的心室率，因此最早的手术方式是切断房室结的传导同时置入永久性起搏器[22]。第二类手术是左心房隔离术，Williams等在动物上实验，Graffigna等在为病人施行瓣膜手术的同时首次完成，长期随访结果显示70%的病人术后维持窦性心律。为了保证窦性冲动能传到心

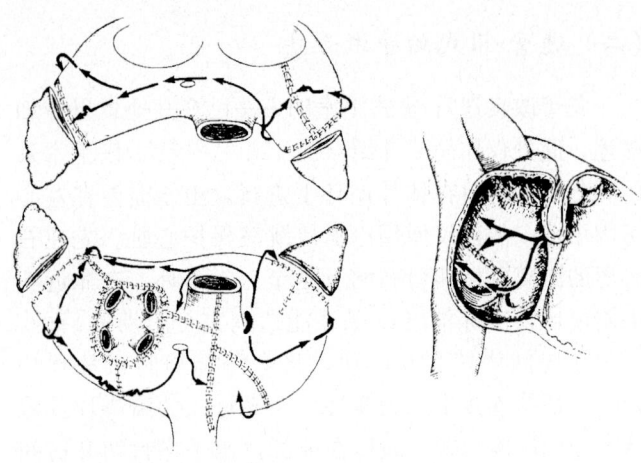

图120-3 迷宫-Ⅲ手术 心房的后面观,显示左心房(左)与右心房(右),向上展开心房的前部,心耳部分已切除。环状切割、缝合肺静脉,在上腔静脉后方做切口,并向房间隔下延直达冠状静脉窦口。(引自 Cox JL: Evolving application of the maze procedure for atrial fibrillation. Ann Thorac Surg 55; 578-580, 1993. Reprinted with permission from the Society of Thoracic Surgenons)

室,Guiraudon 等[23]设计出了一种称为"走廊"的手术,即在窦房结与房室结之间建立一条游离肌束,长期随访30例,结果显示在"走廊"内可发生心房颤动,在维持窦性心律的病人中,有31%的患者心房功能降低,此后有两例病人出现了脑卒中。因此上述这3种手术都不能很好地预防血栓性栓塞,而且并不优于内科治疗。分析 Ad 及 Cox 所施行迷宫手术12年的结果显示,在所有主要的术式中迷宫手术发生脑卒中的几率是最低的[24]。

近年来在技术和理论方面外科治疗的策略都发生了很大变化,包括术式的简化和更为微创的手术入路。如果这些理念都能达到而又不影响其效果,外科治疗心房颤动的并发症势必更加降低,从而能更广泛地开展。因此在评价外科手术时,应考虑以下几个策略:(1)用不同能量对心肌组织进行线条状的消融而替代传统外科的切口("切割、缝合"技术),以避免典型迷宫手术时所采用的广泛切割和缝合;(2)只对肺静脉开口处进行游离、消融,而保持了静脉口之间左心房体部心肌的活性及功能;(3)在可选择性的情况下,减少或避免在右心房上做多个切口;(4)根据临床情况制定消融范围及方法。

目前已有许多技术能满足这些要求并正在使用(表120-2)。这包括线状的或尖部能冷却的单极射频能、双极射频能、冷冻消融、微波以及两极红外激光。所有这些能量都已用于临床并取得了满意的效果,而且大多数也与 Cox 等所报告的迷宫-Ⅲ手术的结果相似[17]。采用这些不同能量的治疗器械具有相同

的目的,即造成细胞死亡,有些是用50℃以上的温度加热使组织凝固性坏死,或以-60℃的温度破坏细胞膜。绝大多数这些技术也具有相应的缺点,包括在每个点需要两分钟以上的消融时间、因高温引起局部组织炭化、因能量的意外扩散或难以把握的透壁性损伤而造成心脏本身或心外的副损害。此外,如在心脏表面用温度消融,其消融点难以稳定。

Sie 等[25]所采用的消融线路与迷宫-Ⅲ手术采用的切割线类似(图120-4),他们采用带有一个灌注头的单极射频棒,消融的同时可向心房内膜注水。他们共为122例病人施行了手术,这些病人都因器质性心脏病而同时接受其他心脏手术,其中主要是二尖瓣成形术,因附加的在左心房行改良迷宫射频消融术,主动脉阻断时间需延长 $14\pm3\min$,住院死亡率为4.1%,39个月的总存活率为90%,术后无房扑或房颤率为 $78.5\%\pm5.1\%$。对其中窦性、房性心律或房-室顺序起搏的89例患者做超声多普勒心动图检查,显示83%的右心房具有传输功能,77%左心房具有传输功能。Mohr 等[26]所采用的方法与改良迷宫-Ⅲ式大不一样(图120-5)。首先避免了对右心房的切割;其次左心房的消融范围包括了肺静脉口与二尖瓣环之间的连线;第三,射频消融是使用一个线状的导管。术后12个月随访,总共有72%的病人维持窦性心律,然有4例发生食管穿孔,他们将此归之于应用经食道超声心动图检查所致。

目前也正在评价其他可使用的能量,其中已允许使用的能量之一是微波。微波(电磁)是水分子去电子而产生热能,这种能量比传统所用的技术(如射频消融术)可以更深、更可靠地消融心房组织,Williams 等[27]的研究证实可以通过调整微波的能量及消融时间而控制穿透深度,前期的临床经验已证明采用这种输出装置可以将微波安全和成功地应用于对心脏组织的消融[28]。

就理想的消融部位来讲还存在着争论(图120-5),最主要的焦点是避免对右心房的消融。对慢性房颤和器质性心脏病手术的电生理标测资料显示左心房可能是颤动波发生的部位,而右心房为被动激动[29,30]。这些资料支持更为局限性消融的概念,至少有一组报告了双房消融与左心房消融的对比研究,其结果证明手术后两组间在房颤发生率上无差别[31]。为了保持更多的生理激动顺序和心房的传输功能,Nitta 及同事们[32]设计出不同类型的手术方式,这些术式是从迷宫手术衍生而来并有所发展,从窦房结朝向房室环缘做放射状的切口,并与冠状动脉平行,他们发现

表 120-2 心房颤动的外科治疗

能量种类	设备
切割法	标准外科设备*
射频法	单极： 线状消融头*△▲（Cobra，Boston Scientific，Natick，Massachusetts）；尖部带灌注的消融头*△▲（Cardioblate，Medtronic，Inc.） 双极：（Cardioblate Bipolar®，Medtronic, Inc., Minneapolis, Minnesota）；双极止血*△▲（Atricure）
微波法	可弯曲性线状消融头*△▲（Flex 4，AFx，Freemont，California） 导管电极△☆#¥（Flex 10，AFx）
激光法	线状消融头*△▲ （Edwards Life Sciences，Irvine，California）

入路：△心内膜；▲心外膜；*开胸；☆胸部小切口；#胸腔镜；¥机器人辅助。

这种放射切口比迷宫手术容易，因为这种切口在左心房内更呈线状，在左房内没有隔离切口或"T形"切口。经胸超声多普勒心动图检查发现放射状的切口（RIA）在保护左心房的传输功能方面优于迷宫手术，而在保护右心房的传输功能方面则两者相同，术后的无房颤率相似（92%），他们认为放射状切口的方法对于心房颤动外科手术来讲或许提供了一种更符合生理的选择。

尽管最近几组的报告中所使用的技术、手术切口以及设备各不相同，但术后1年的无房颤发生率都在50%～85%之间[25-28,33-36]，而且无血栓性栓塞的比例也非常高，不管怎样仍需仔细评估术后的远期效果，尤其是开展微创的方法治疗心房颤动还需要新的资料。

四、房室旁路

1968年5月28日Sealy WC在Duke大学医院首次手术切断导致WPW综合征的房室旁路，此后发表了许多有关房室旁路解剖和电生理特征的论文。作为另外一类的室上性心律不齐，目前导管消融已成为对其永久性根治的首选方法（第115章）。Duke大学最后1例采用外科手术切断单纯性房室旁路是在1992年[37]。目前需要外科治疗的WPW综合征指征包括：（1）至少两次以上射频消融失败；（2）伴有需要外科手术纠正的器质性心脏病，尤其是Ebstein畸形和二

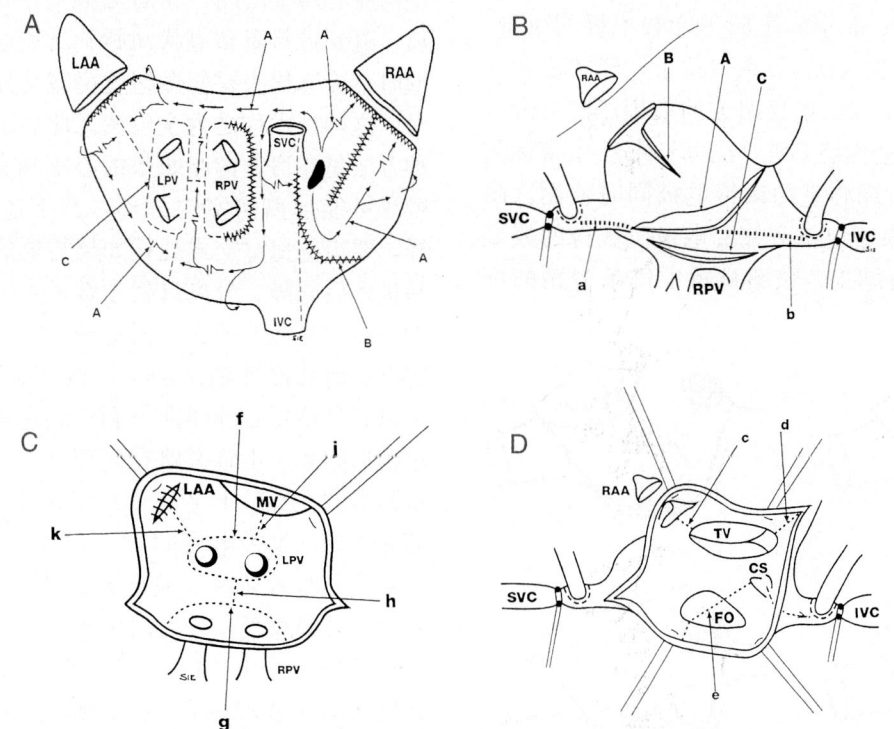

图120-4 A：改良的射频消融迷宫手术：（A）电活动线路；（B）锯齿状线：表示心房上的切口；（C）点状线：表示心内膜消融线路。B：心房侧面观：（A）右心房侧面切口；（B）右心房前面切口；（C）房间沟的左心房切口，腔静脉间的心内膜消融线路以a，b表示。C：房内面观：牵引线显露左心房，虚线表示消融线路（f，g，h，j和k）。D：房内面观：牵引线显露右心房，虚线表示消融线路（c，d和e）。CS：冠状静脉窦；FO：卵圆窝；IVC：下腔静脉；LAA：左心耳；LPV：左肺静脉；RAA：右心耳；RPV：右肺静脉；SVC：上腔静脉；TV：三尖瓣。（引自参考文献25）。

尖瓣病变。从1985～1991年，笔者共施行了65例WPW综合征手术，而1991年后仅有6例，其中2例为导管消融失败，包括1例Ebstein畸形；1例在消融过程中引起二尖瓣后瓣穿孔而接受手术；1例为主动脉瓣接受猪生物瓣置换术后，因退行性衰变需二次手术；1例因肥厚型心肌病需要切除部分室间隔；1例为需要外科手术纠正的Ebstein畸形，所有这些病人均采用心外膜途径成功切断旁路，关于其方法在下面予以介绍。

手术方法

有两种切断房室旁道的基本手术途经：Sealy及同事首先提出，后由Cox等完善的心内膜途径；由Guiraudon等提出的心外膜途径[20,37-39]。根据旁路的特殊部位这两种手术途经有所不同，按照解剖分为：（1）左侧游离壁，（2）右侧游离壁，（3）后间隔，（4）前间隔。变异性预激的部位包括非典型间隔旁路、结室旁路、房束旁路及结束旁路。手术切断旁路时通常需要在术中标测指引下完成，笔者的中心采用两种记录设备来标测旁路：（1）带电极的袜套状标测装置，该装置包括一条分布着63个单极电极的束带，每个电极的间距为0.5cm，该束带位于袜套状装置的底部；（2）由63个双极电极组成的束带；该束带可以在心外膜房室沟处围绕心脏，也可与袜套-束带标测装置或另外一条围绕心室的束带电极同时使用。图120-6为采用心室束带电极和袜套电极所获得的典型前向性激动的分析结果，该图显示了每条旁路的部位。术前往往难以辨认多发性旁路，笔者发现经计算机处理的多点标测图对此尤其有用，因为房颤时体表心电图QRS的形态变化可反映出各个旁路的传导。

心外膜或心内膜途径都需要胸骨正中切口，不需在体外循环下即可以完成电生理标测，当采用心外膜途径切断旁道时这点更具优势，因为这样可以在非体外循环下完成手术[38,39]。然而对于左侧旁路，若经心内膜途径则需要阻断主动脉，使用含血心肌停跳液，在左心房内二尖瓣环的上方做切口。对于跨行于三尖瓣环的旁路，需要在窦性心律、体外循环下在右心房内手术，其分离面沿着心室肌的顶点向下到心外膜返折。对于后间隔的旁路，要在希氏束的后方做切口，逆时针向于右心房游离壁内分离，然后与三尖瓣环平行直到二尖瓣环、左心室的后上面和室间隔的顶端，再解剖出锥形间隙。对于前间隔的旁路，应在右冠状动脉、希氏束的上方、右心室漏斗部的下面和右心房壁的前中份之间的纤维三角内进行分离。

心外膜途径不需要切开心腔，可以在常温非体外循环、心脏跳动下完成。最早的手术方法是在左心房游离壁房室沟脂肪垫上心外膜的顶端做切口，在脂肪垫与左心房壁之间，朝向房室交界处左心室的底部分离，直到冠状窦和冠状动脉旋支的返折处。冷冻心房壁时，冷冻探头要稍微超过房室交界区与左心室壁接触，这种技术称之为全位法。此后出现了直接法，这种方法是在房室沟脂肪垫的心室端做一切口，沿心室壁尽可能远离房室沟分离，与上述全位冷冻技术一样，要冷冻房室交界处，如果需要的话其分离面很容易进入后间隔。分离过程中常常可以看到在离断旁路的一瞬间预激波消失，但这种情况并不意味着不需要完全分离和冷冻消融房室沟区。对于后间隔的旁道，可以容易地将心外膜向下剥离到左室后、上方而显露出锥形间隙。不管旁路在何部位，只要心外膜标测显示预激波在心脏十字交叉处即为后旁路。右心室的膈面先激动（束带电极的第30～35点）或与十字交叉的左侧同时激动时（最常见的部位，图120-6D），如采用心外膜途径，分离面应限制于后间隔间隙（束带电极的第25～40点，图120-6）；如十字交叉的左侧首先激动（第35～40点），则心外膜的分离面应延续到左心室的钝缘。因此采用心外膜途径可以很容易分离出所有部位，而经心内膜分离左、右心房，分离面可能更为广泛和更具危险性。

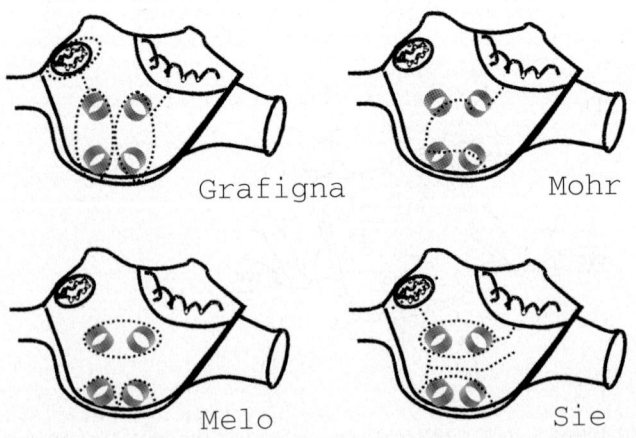

图120-5 射频消融和微波消融术时，左心房内的不同消融线路
注意Sie医生对于大心房，在左心房后壁所增加的切割线。后者代表了多数中心所采用的左心房消融方式，即使已隔离右心房。

五、总　结

外科手术治疗 WPW 综合征的成功为非药物性的电生理方法分离房室交界区及其异常连接提供了一种方法，但是因开胸手术具有潜在并发症、住院费用高、住院时间以及恢复到正常活动所需要的时间长等因素，促使了经皮技术的发展。房颤治疗也遵循了同样的发展道路，目前针对不同的解剖部位及发生机制已设计出了相应的消融技术，尽管微创的方法在临床效果上还不尽如人意，但由于其对患者的损伤程度及住院费用方面要小于创伤性手术，因此往往总能"存在"下去。对于导管难以消融或伴有其他需外科手术的心脏病患者，外科手术仍然不失为一个重要选择。

心房扑动、房性心动过速、房室结折返

对于这类折返性质的心动过速已设计出行之有效的手术方法[20,38,39]，然而由于导管介入治疗已替代了外科手术，因此目前不再认为外科手术是必不可少的方法。

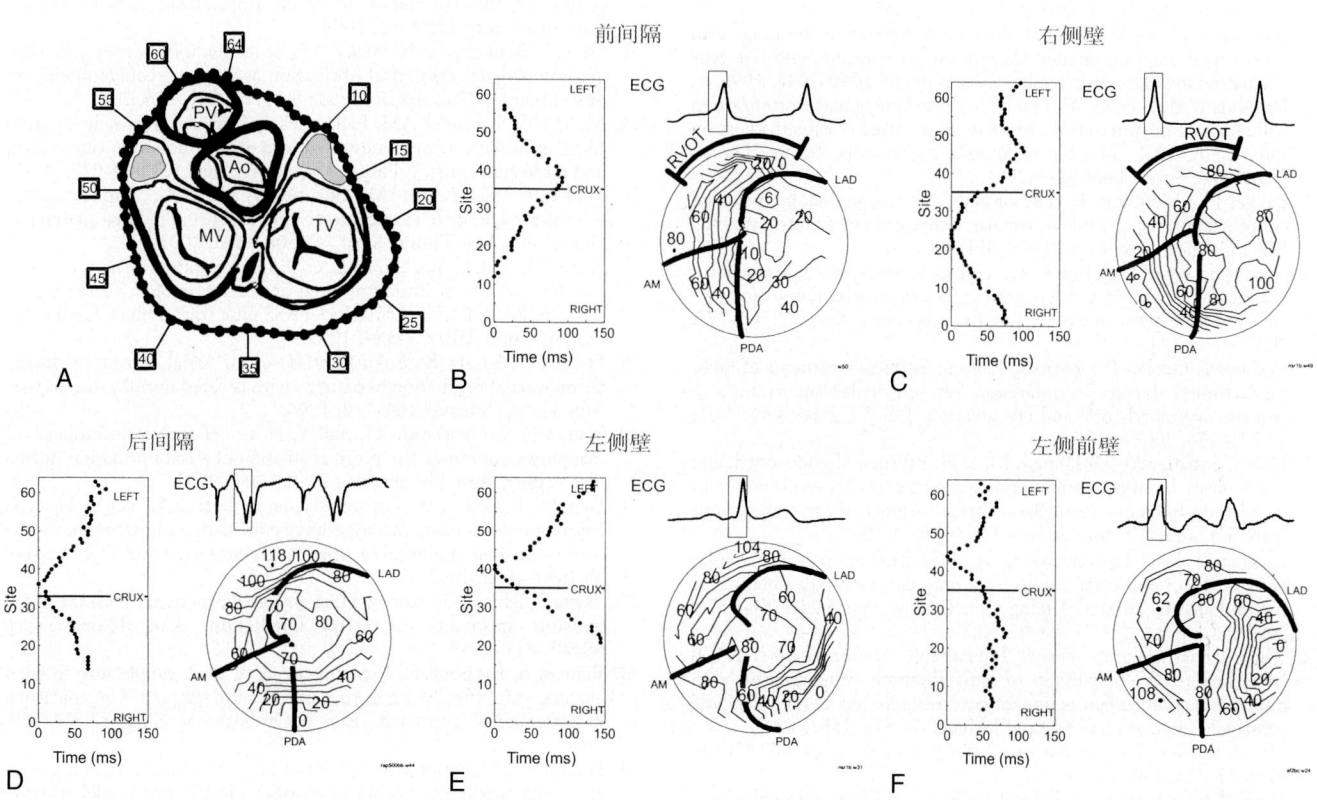

图 120-6　不同部位旁路的典型心外膜顺序激动范例　A：心底部观，圆点代表带状电极所记录的心外膜 1~63 个点。标准的第 35 点为十字交叉，第 10~34 点为心脏的右侧（1~9 点通常不能与心脏接触，因此可省略），第 36~63 点为心脏的左侧。注意心房的电极带应在主动脉的后方穿过横窦，以与心房内的电极带接触。旁路的定位：第 10~15 点为前间隔，第 16~29 点为右游离壁，第 30~39 点为后间隔，第 40~55 点为左游离壁。B~F：为各个旁路的情况，每个图的左边标记方格为心室的前向性激动数据，右边为心外膜标测的全貌。心外膜图用一个极图表示，心尖部位于圆圈的中央，心底部位于外周。心电图 QRS 波上的矩形框为标测窗，表示相应的心外膜标记时间。圆圈内的数字为等时线，每间隔 10ms 记录一次。0 点为最早激动的部位，此点即为旁路进入心室的部位。图 E 为最常见的左侧旁路，而图 F 为左前侧旁路，因为 "0" 点位于左前降支附近。注意心室标记格的 "V" 波形态，尖形的 "V" 波表示插入心室的旁路窄，而扁平的 "V" 波表示插入心室的旁路宽。Ao：主动脉瓣；AM：心脏锐缘；ECG：体表心电图；LAD：冠状动脉前降支；MV：二尖瓣；PDA：冠状动脉后降支；PV：肺动脉瓣；RVOT：右室流出道；TV：三尖瓣。（引自 Pagé PL: Surgery for atrial fibrillation and other supraventricular arrhythmias. In Zipes and Jalife (eds): Cardiac Electrophysiology, from cell to bedside. Philadelphia, WB Saunders, 2000, pp 1107-1165.）

（解基严　译）

参 考 文 献

1. Miller JM, Rothman SA, Addonizio VP: Surgical techniques for ventricular tachycardia ablation. In Singer I (ed): Interventional Electrophysiology. Baltimore, MD, Williams and Wilkins, 1997, pp 641–684.
2. Gregoratos G, Cheitlin MD, Conill A, et al: ACC/AHA Guidelines for implantation of cardiac pacemakers and antiarrhythmia devices: Executive summary—a report of the American College of Cardiology/American Heart Association Task Force on Practice Guidelines (Committee on Pacemaker Implantation). Circulation 97:1325–1335, 1998.
3. Kawamura Y, Pagé PL, Cardinal R, et al: Mapping of septal ventricular tachycardia: Clinical and experimental correlations. J Thorac Cardiovasc Surg 112:914–925, 1996.
4. Pagé PL: Surgical treatment of ventricular tachycardia. Indications and results. Arch Mal Coeur 89(I):115–121, 1996.
5. Rastegar H, Link MS, Foote CB, et al: Perioperative and long-term results with mapping-guided subendocardial resection and left ventricular endoaneurysmorrhaphy. Circulation 94:1041–1048, 1996.
6. Di Donato M, Sabatier M, Dor V: Surgical ventricular restoration in patients with postinfarction coronary artery disease: Effectiveness on spontaneous and inducible ventricular tachycardia. Semin Thorac Cardiovasc Surg 13:480–485, 2001.
7. Bakker PFA, de Lange F, Hauer RNW, et al: Sequential map-guided endocardial resection for ventricular tachycardia improves outcome. Eur J Cardiothorac Surg 19:448–454, 2001.
8. Otto von Oppell U, Milne D, Okreglicki A, Millar RNS: Surgery for ventricular tachycardia of left ventricular origin: Risk factors for success and long-term outcome. Eur J Cardiothorac Surg 22:762–770, 2002.
9. Wellens F, Geelen P, Demirsoy E, et al: Surgical treatment of tachyarrhythmias due to postinfarction left ventricular aneurysm with endoaneurysmorrhaphy and cryoablation. Eur J Cardiothorac Surg 22:771–776, 2002.
10. Dor V, Sabatier M, Di Donato M, et al: Efficacy of endoventricular patch plasty in large postinfarction akinetic scar and severe left ventricular dysfunction: Comparison with a series of large dyskinetic scars. J Thorac Cardiovasc Surg 116:50–59, 1998.
11. Lacroix D, Klug D, Marquié C, et al: Identification of ventricular tachycardia of epicardial origin from unipolar potentials obtained at the endocardial surface. Pacing Clin Electrophysiol 25:1561–1570, 2002.
12. The Antiarrhythmics Versus Implantable Defibrillators (AVID) Investigators: A comparison of antiarrhythmic-drug therapy with implantable defibrillators in patients resuscitated from near-fatal ventricular arrhythmias. N Engl J Med 337:1576–1583, 1997.
13. Nattel S: New ideas about atrial fibrillation 50 years on. Nature 415:219–226, 2002.
14. Wijffell MC, Kirchhof CJ, Dorland R, et al: Electrical remodeling due to atrial fibrillation in chronically instrumented concious goat: Role of neurohumoral changes, ischemia, atrial stretch, and high rate electrical activation. Circulation 96:3710–3720, 1997.
15. Haissaguerre M, Jais P, Shah DC, et al: Spontaneous initiation of atrial fibrillation by ectopic beats originating in the pulmonary veins. N Engl J Med 339:659–666, 1998.
16. Cox JL, Jaquiss RDB, Schuessler RB, Boineau JP: Modification of the maze procedure for atrial flutter and atrial fibrillation. II. Surgical technique of the maze III procedure. J Thorac Cardiovasc Surg 110:485–495, 1995.
17. Cox JL, Ad N, Palazzo T, et al: Current status of the Maze procedure for the treatment of atrial fibrillation. Semin Thorac Cardiovasc Surg 12:15–19, 2000.
18. Schaff HV, Dearani JA, Daly RC, et al: The Cox-Maze procedure for atrial fibrillation: The Mayo Clinic experience. Semin Thorac Cardiovasc Surg 12:30–37, 2000.
19. Kosakai Y: Treatment of atrial fibrillation using the Maze procedure: The Japanese experience. Semin Thorac Cardiovasc Surg 12:44–52, 2000.
20. Ferguson TB Jr: Surgery approach to atrial flutter and atrial fibrillation. In Singer I (ed): Interventional Electrophysiology. Baltimore, MD, Williams and Wilkins, 1997, pp 595–639.
21. McCarthy PM, Gillinov AM, Castle L, et al: The Cox-Maze procedure: The Cleveland Clinic experience. Semin Thorac Cardiovasc Surg 12:25–29, 2000.
22. Proclemer A, Della BP, Tondo C, et al: Radiofrequency ablation of atrioventricular junction and pacemaker implantation versus modulation of atrioventricular conduction in drug refractory atrial fibrillation. Am J Cardiol 83:1437–1442, 1999.
23. van Hemel NM, Defauw JJ, Guiraudon GM, et al: Long-term follow-up of corridor operation for lone atrial fibrillation: Evidence for progression of disease? J Cardiovasc Electrophysiol 8:967–973, 1997.
24. Ad N, Cox JL: Stroke prevention as an indication for the Maze procedure in the treatment of atrial fibrillation. Semin Thorac Cardiovasc Surg 12:56–62, 2000.
25. Sie HT, Beukema WP, Misier AR, et al: Radiofrequency modified maze in patients with atrial fibrillation undergoing concomitant cardiac surgery. J Thorac Cardiovasc Surg 122:249–256, 2001.
26. Mohr FW, Fabricius AM, Falk V, et al: Curative treatment of atrial fibrillaiton with intraoperative radiofrequency ablation: Short-term and midterm results. J Thorac Cardiovasc Surg 123:919–927, 2002.
27. Williams MR, Knaut M, Bérubé D, Oz MC: Application of microwave energy in cardiac tissue ablation: From in vitro analyses to clinical use. Ann Thorac Surg 74:1500–1505, 2002.
28. Knaut M, Spitzer SG, Karoli L, et al: Intraoperative microwave ablation for curative treatment of atrial fibrillation in open heart surgery. The MCRO-STAF and MICRO-PASS pilot trial. Thorac Cardiovasc Surg 47(Suppl III):379–384, 1999.
29. Harada A, Sasaki K, Fukushima T, et al: Atrial activation during chronic atrial fibrillation in patients with isolated mitral valve disease. Ann Thorac Surg 61:104–112, 1996.
30. Yamauchi S, Ogasawara H, Saji Y, et al: Efficacy of intraoperative mapping to optimize the surgical ablation of atrial fibrillation in cardiac surgery Ann Thorac Surg 74:450–457, 2002.
31. Deneke T, Khargi K, Grewe PH, et al: Left atrial versus bi-atrial Maze operation using intraoperative cooled-tip radiofrequency ablation in patients undergoing open-heart surgery. J Am Coll Cardiol 39:1644–1650, 2002.
32. Nitta T, Ishii Y, Ogasawara H, et al: Initial experience with the radial incision approach for atrial fibrillation. Ann Thorac Surg 68:805–811, 1999.
33. Benussi S, Pappone C, Nascimbene S, et al: A simple way to treat chronic atrial fibrillation during mitral valve surgery: The epicardial radiofrequency approach. Eur J Cardiothorac Surg 17:524–529, 2000.
34. Hoenicke EM, Strange RG Jr, Patel H, et al: Initial experience with epicardial radiofrequency ablation catheter in an ovine model: Moving towards an endoscopic Maze procedure. Surg Forum 51:79–82, 2000.
35. Raman JS, Ishikawa S, Power JM: Epicardial radiofrequency ablation of both atria in the treatment of atrial fibrillation: Experience in patients. Ann Thorac Surg 74:1506–1509, 2002.
36. Guden M, Akpinar B, Sanisoglu I, et al: Intraoperative saline-irrigated radiofrequency modified Maze procedure for atrial fibrillation. Ann Thorac Surg 74:S1301–S1306, 2002.
37. Lowe JE: Arrhythmia surgery: Then and now. Pacing Clin Electrophysiol 20(2 pt 2):585–599, 1997.
38. Guiraudon GM, Klein GJ, Yee I (ed): Surgical techniques in supraventricular arrhythmias. In Singer I (ed): Interventional Electrophysiology. Baltimore, MD, Williams and Wilkins, 1997, pp 565–593.
39. Guiraudon GM, Klein GJ, Yee R, Guiraudon CM: Surgery for supraventricular tachycardia. Archives des Maladies du Coeur et des Vaisseaux 89(Spec No 1):123–127, 1996.

索 引

2 相折返　587
4,5-二磷酸磷脂酰肌醇（PIP2）　29
8 字折返　487,494,1061
AED　883
AH 间期　499
Andersen 综合征　464
anrep 效应　242
ATP 敏感 K^+ 电流　110
ATP 试验　803
AVID　905
Bachmann 束　367,499
Brugada 诊断流程　743,744
Brugada 综合征　81,147,295,435,463,587,714,748,753,871,885
CARTO 系统　846
CASQ2 缺陷　628
CAST 试验　820
Ca^{2+}/CaM　38
Ca^{2+}-ATP 酶　43
Ca^{2+} 释放通道　51,52
Ca^{2+} 瞬变　192
Cl^- 通道　57
Cx40　73
Cx43　69,155
DNA 损伤　718
Duchenne 和 Becker 型肌营养不良　633
Ebstein 畸形　854,1053,1086
EGTA 或 BAPTA　15,16
Fontan 手术　552
Friedreich 共济失调　637
GPCRs　33
GTP　33

G_α 亚基　33
G 蛋白　33,390
G 蛋白调控的内向整流性钾通道（GIRK）　34
G 蛋白耦联受体　285
G 蛋白耦联受体激酶　286
HB-RB 夺获　548
HCN1　63
HCN2　63
HCN4　63
HCN 通道　60,103
HERG　29,92
IA 类抗心律失常药物　595,893
I_{Ca}　16
$I_{Ca,L}$　10
$I_{Ca,T}$　10
IDS　905
IP_3R　51
I 间碘苄胍（Meta-$[^{131}I]$ iodobenzylguanidine,MIBG）　294
Jervell-Lange-Nielsen 综合征　681
Kapan-Meier 生存分析　828
KCNE1　142
KCNH2　24
KCNH2（HERG）　37
KCNQ1　24,90,142
KCNQ1/KCNE1-I_{ks}　36
Kearns-Sayre 综合征　456
Kir1　29
Kir2.x 通道　390
Kir7　29
Koch 三角　200,498,531
Kv1.5　88

索 引

KvLQT1　24
Kv 通道　19
Kv 通道相互作用蛋白（KChIPs）　26，171
Lenègre 病　463
LocaLisa　848
LQT1　148
LQT3　80
LQT-5　142
L-型（长时间开放）钙通道（LTCC）　131
L 型二氢吡啶敏感性钙电流　373
L 型钙通道　36，190，238，602
Mahaim 旁路　844
Mahaim 样预激旁路　1057
Maze 术　506
Mink　28
minK　89
MscL　96
MscS　96
Mustard 手术　552
M 细胞　148，230
Na^+-Ca^{2+} 交换　46
Na^+-K^+-ATP 酶　42，43
NBG 代码　977
NCX1.1　47
NHE1　45
NO　56
PAAs　134
pH 门控　73
PJRT 综合征　857
PR 间期　481
P-环　3
P 波形态　496
QRS 波电交替　742
QRS 波宽度　953
QRS 波群电交替　522
QRS 波群反正常化　724
QRS 波心动过速　736
QT/T 交替　688
QT 间期　647
QT 间期传感器　982
QT 间期延长　705
QT 离散度　573，750
ryanodine　54

RyR2　51，140
RyR2 突变　628
RyRs　104
S4　3
S6　4
SACs　96
SCN5A　38，78，699
Senning 手术　552
Southern 印迹分析　431
SR　16，57
SR 连接蛋白　53
S-亚硝　55
Todaro　531
Todaro 腱　204
TTX　5
TTX/STX　5
T-型（短暂开放）钙通道（TTCC）　131
T 波　646
T 波电交替　573，687，750
T 波基底增宽　646
T 波双峰　646
Uhl 畸形　589
Valsalva 动作　738
Vasalva 动作　748
VA 间期　499
Wolff-Parkinson-White（WPW）预激综合征　447
X-连锁遗传　453
X-连锁遗传疾病　442
X 连锁性状遗传　567
X 连锁遗传　441
X 线影像　842
X 综合征　764
ZO-1　161
"大炮"音　738
"推拉"概念　222
"心脏表面"等效发生器　790
HERG 基因　645
I_f　102
I_f 电流　60
I_{Ca-L}　133
$I_{K,ACh}$　110
$I_{K,ATP}$　110
I_{kr}　28，88

索 引

I_{Kr} 149
I_{ks} 28, 88
I_{kur} 28, 88
$I_{K.ACh}$ 33
I_{Na} 77, 125
KCNE1 140
KCNQ1 140
LQTS1 658
LQTS2 658
LQTS3 658
minK 基因 645
KCNE1 基因 644
SCN5A 645
IC 类药物 492
Ⅰ型房扑 488
Ⅱ型房扑 488
Ⅲ类抗心律失常药物 492, 913
β-AR 信号 140
β-肾上腺素受体 601
β肾上腺素能受体 136
β肾上腺素能受体阻滞剂 513
β受体阻滞剂 548, 605, 631, 651, 656, 709, 900, 931
β受体阻滞剂治疗 829
β亚基 6
^{123}I-间碘苄胍成像 588
阿莫兰特 943
阿齐利特 940
阿替洛尔 901
艾-德肌营养不良 635
艾伯斯坦畸形 451
艾生利特 942
安全系数（safety factor） 213
安全性 1025
氨巴利特 942
胺碘酮 913, 914
靶点 1061
斑块不稳定 716
斑块破裂 760
瘢痕 502, 1060, 1066
瘢痕心肌 820
背景电流 388
背景钾电流通道 19

被动倾斜试验 801
比索洛尔 901, 903
编码离子通道 718
变异型心绞痛 764
标测 347, 1036
表达差异 167
表面等效电源 791
表现度 442
丙吡胺 893
并发症 511, 1032, 1058
并行心律 728
并行心律的异化现象 734
病态窦房结综合征 197
波锋 424
波锋碰撞 854
波形 953
不典型的癫痫 777
不典型房扑 550
不均匀性传播 216
不明原因的晕厥 783
不适宜性窦速 499, 1048
不适宜性窦性心动过速 476
不应期 332, 483, 506
不应期回剥 723
布新洛尔 903
餐后低血压 868
侧面平均 212
测试 958
颤动样传导 508
颤动组织 506
长 QT 综合征 80, 254, 432, 459, 644, 704, 748, 753, 839, 992
长短周期现象 686
长间歇 484
常染色体显性遗传 568, 618, 628
常染色体遗传 441
常染色体隐性遗传 567, 628
超常传导 723
超极化 405
超极化激活环化核苷酸门控 60, 190
超极化激活离子流 189
超敏 296
超射期 820

索引

超声心动图　477
超速延迟整流钾电流　372
沉默遗传变异　718
陈旧性心肌梗死　561
程序刺激　676
迟后除极　376
持久性房颤　374
持续性单形性室性心动过速　593
持续性房颤　351
持续性交界性心动过速　1057
持续性室性心动过速　561
持续性室性心律失常　622
充血性心力衰竭　505，570
除颤　413
除颤测试　959
除颤阈值　422，919，954
除极　332
除极化　406
触发　494
触发活动　305，351，518，570，821
触发性心律失常　662
触发因素　509，705
触发灶　1004
穿膜膜片钳　432
传出阻滞　723
传导间期　622
传导衰竭　205
传导速度　506
传导延迟　482
传导延缓　676
次级起搏点　484
猝发　964
猝发刺激　499
猝死　570
猝死的一级预防　700，890
猝死危险性　565
醋丁洛尔　901
错义突变　441，708
大折返性反复单形性室速　675
大折返性房性心动过速　494，550，1038
带通滤波器　952
单倍体不足　460
单独心房除颤器　974，976

单个电偶　790
单个移动电偶　790
单个折返环　509
单光子发射计算机断层成像　835
单核苷酸多态性　468
单环路折返　508
单基因遗传病　441
单链构象多态性　445
单腔 ICD　966
单细胞链　210
单相波　955
单相动作电位　238，433，495，817，820
单向传导阻滞　602
单向阻滞　309，313
单形室性心动过速持续　824
单形性室性心动过速　330，377
单一折返环　494
胆碱能性房颤　300
蛋白激酶 C　137
导管射频消融术　301，518
导管消融　492，677
导航系统　556
等电位线　495
等积分图　788
等率性房室分离　484
等时图逆解法　790
等时性标测　502
等位基因　440
等位基因性疾病　628
等效电源逆解法　790
低回声区　477
低振幅信号　780
地尔硫䓬　134，907－909
地高辛　513，922，926
地高辛特异片段　928
递增　964
颠换（transversion）　441
典型房扑　487
点突变　441
电极　946
电-机械脱耦联　420
电不均一性　587
电场　403

电池　950
电除颤　945
电穿孔　1000
电磁干扰　969，986
电复律　877
电话传输　872
电恢复　232
电极　950
电交替　242
电解剖标测系统　1020，1037
电解质失衡　519
电解质紊乱　570，698
电紧张　196
电流接收器　current sink　220
电耦联　195
电容器　950
电生理　571
电生理基质　277，561，621
电生理检查　665，873
电生理重构　371
电势梯度　423
电压调节内向整流钾电流　29
电压门控 K^+（voltage-gated K^+，Kv）通道　165
电压门控 K^+ 通道相关蛋白（K^+ channel accessory protein，KChAP）　171
电压门控钾通道　19
电压敏感染料荧光成像技术　202
电压依赖性钠电流　373
电源　220
电源-电流接收器　208
电张性调整　728，729
电重构　173
电转复　277
动态心电图　594，759
动作电位　251，475
动作电位时程　230，239，297
窦房传导时间　477
窦房结　188，475
窦房结本身　478
窦房结不应期　873
窦房结功能不良　477，615，978
窦房结功能障碍　862
窦房结恢复时间　477

窦房折返性心动过速　476，499
窦房结周围　478
窦房折返　479
窦性夺获　517
毒碱受体密度　841
毒碱乙酰胆碱受体　840
毒蕈碱受体　834
毒蕈碱样的 K^+ 外向电流　305
短程频谱分析　816
短联律间期性尖端扭转型室速　630
短暂性脑灌注不足　798
多巴胺试验　764
多不饱和脂肪酸　936
多电极矩阵　847
多非利特　688
多环路折返　505，507
多聚腺苷尾巴　429
多旁路　523，1056
多态性　468
多形室速家族性　768
多形性室速　330，376，597，621，679
多源性房性心动过速　511
多中心非持续性心动过速试验（MUSTT）　898
多子波　229
多子波假说　360
多子波折返　351
儿茶酚胺　570
儿茶酚胺敏感　476
儿茶酚胺敏感性 I_{Ks} 通道　755
儿茶酚胺敏感性多形性室速　465，619，626，694，753
儿童　1071
二度　481
二度Ⅰ型房室阻滞　482
二级预防　596，700，890
二尖瓣反流　576
二尖瓣环　498
二尖瓣脱垂　587，768
二氢吡啶［DHPs］　132
法洛四联症　611
法洛四联症手术　519，552
反复房速　300，302
反复心律　302

反义寡核苷酸　172
房颤　489，502，639
房颤波长　506
房颤样传导　823
房颤诱发房颤　864
房间隔　498
房间隔缺损　552
房内折返性心动过速　551
房室/房束纤维　1057
房室传导　489
房室分离　481，738，740
房室间隔缺损修补术　519
房室结　481
房室结双径路　530
房室结消融　519
房室结折返性心动过速　530，1044
房室旁路　853
房室同步　988
房室折返性心动过速　1052
房室阻滞　481，615，864，978，1047
房束束折返性心动过速　677
房性心动过速　315，494，1035
非Q波型心肌梗死　788
非持续性室性心动过速　594，784，886
非电张性调整　728
非接触标测　666，1074
非接触式标测系统　847
非接触式球囊导管　847
非均质躯干电阻率　791
非开胸电极　950
非缺血性心肌病　576
非同义多态性　709
非外科方法的标测　849
非峡部依赖的房扑　502，1032
非致心律失常型右室发育不良　587
肥厚型心肌病　446，593，714，875，991
肺动脉瓣关闭不全　612
肺静脉　302，1017
肺静脉电隔离　1005
肺静脉电图　1005
肺静脉畸形引流矫正术　552
分支性室速　672
分支折返性室速　675

分钟通气量传感器　982
分子流行病学　710
分子生物学　878
缝隙连接　67，177，251，332，726，825
缝隙连接蛋白　159，398，586
缝隙连接通道　118，154
氟卡胺　893，896
父母猝死病　717
复发　1024，1058
复极　332
复极等时线（repolarization isochrone line　231
复极交替　231，688
复极异常　766
副交感神经　475，664
傅立叶谱分析　811
钙超载　374
钙调蛋白　55
钙调控耦联　720
钙离子通道　484
钙瞬变（Ca^{2+} transient）　197
钙瞬变时程　239
钙通道阻滞剂　513，548
钙网织蛋白　437
钙运作（Ca^{2+} Handling）　196
感知　951，958
感知过度　966
刚度矩阵　271
高除颤阈值　961
高度房室阻滞　483，492
高分辨心电图　778
高危婴儿猝死综合征　704
格林-巴利综合征　639
各向异性折返　229
梗死边缘区　698
功率频谱　816
功率频谱密度　810
功能性差异性传导　736
功能性阻滞线　487
孤立性心肌炎　588
固有心率　475
冠状动脉性心脏病　714
冠状动脉粥样硬化　714
冠状静脉窦　503

光电二极管光学标测系统　182
光刻技术　222
光学标测　275
光学相干断层成像　200，203
过表达　429
过度反应　801
汉堡心律失常抑制试验（CASH）　897
核磁共振显像　582
核素冲刷率　839
后除极　242，821
后间隔　1054
呼吸暂停假说　703
环肺静脉消融　1015
环核苷酸门控通道（CNG）　60
环核苷酸门控通道基因（HCN）　36
环磷腺苷-蛋白激酶 A（PKA）　33
环路的大小　506
环行运动　359
环形波　263
环状回旋波　341
缓慢传导　498，602
缓慢传导区　590
缓慢的反复心律　300
缓慢外向钾离子电流（I_{Ks}）　142
缓慢性回返心律　302
缓慢性心律失常　478
磺酰脲类受体　174
恢复窦性心律　512
恢复曲线　232
回波　306
回旋波　334，340
回旋波折返　340
混沌　242
获得性长 QT 综合征　690，706
获得性功能突变　510
机械电的离散　245
机械电转换　238
机械感受器　798
机械交联系统　240
肌集钙蛋白　465
肌浆网（SR）　131
肌浆网钙泵　197
肌浆网离子通道　51

肌膜 Ca^{2+}-三磷酸腺苷酶　42
肌袖　354
肌营养不良　633
基础自主神经调节　811
基因的多态性　440
基因连锁分析　444
基因特异性治疗　658
基因突变　704
基因图距　444
基因位点　440
基因携带者　648
基因遗传缺陷　881
基因转录　440
基因作图　444
基质　502，507，1004，1007，1013，1016，1062
激动标测　666
激动波锋　789
激动顺序标测　844
激动延迟　576
急性风湿性心脏炎　520
急性冠脉综合征　764
急性脑血管病　640
急性心肌梗死　484，697
脊髓肌萎缩　639
脊柱横断　640
计算机断层扫描　833，874
继发性交界区心律　520
加速性室性　692
家族肥厚型心肌病　620
家族聚集性　717
家族性长 QT 综合征　170，441
家族性房颤　510
家族性肥厚型心肌病　442
家族遗传性疾病　706
甲状腺功能亢进　510
假神经递质　835，837
尖端扭转型室速　147，330，376，587，679，698，821，894
尖峰电位　1037
间歇性并行心律　732
间质纤维化　509
减数分裂　444
交感神经　293，475，482，584，664，814

交界区 484
交界区异位心动过速 517，521
交替的心跳 232
交替性心动过缓 197
接触电极记录技术 817
接头蛋白 286
节段性运动障碍 588
节律控制 514
结-束旁路 521
结-希区 201
结室/结束纤维 1057
结束旁路 854
结细胞 201
截断突变 441
解剖屏障 487
解剖学基质 410，561，669
解剖学屏障 502
解剖学阻滞 502
解剖障碍区 698
界嵴 181，475，495
紧密连接蛋白-1 177
颈动脉窦按摩 738，748，776，870
颈动脉窦过敏 868
颈动脉窦综合征 798
静脉-小动脉反射 798
局部微折返 305
局灶点 301
局灶消融 1004
局灶型房颤 303
局灶性 494，1036
局灶性房颤 351
局灶性房速 494
聚合酶链反应 429，444
卷形波 320
决奈达隆 941
均匀的电偶 790
卡维地洛 901，903
抗胆碱能药物 640
抗凝治疗 492，512
抗栓治疗 880
抗心动过速起搏器 492
抗心律失常药物 492，574，606
抗血栓 606

可激动间隙 327，823
可耐受室速 565
控制心室率 492，513，879
跨壁复极离散 601
跨壁复极离散度 648
跨壁复极离散度 TDR 147
跨膜电位 420，422
跨膜动作电位上升支速率变化（dV/dt$_{max}$） 212
快-慢型 542，1049
快-慢综合征 551
快径路和慢径路 531
快频率室速 963
快速心室率 511
快速荧光成像 200
奎尼丁 893
扩张型心肌病 452，567，714
兰尼定右室心肌病 585
兰尼定受体 192
篮状电极导管 849
累积生存曲线 650
冷灌注导管 556
冷却 732
冷却现象 494
冷盐水灌注 1067
离体灌流模型 400
离子交换器 238
离子通道 251，602
利多卡因 893，896
连接伴侣 161
连接蛋白 69，120，182
连接蛋白 37（Cx37） 118
连接蛋白 40（Cx40） 118
连接蛋白 43（Cx43） 68，118，177
连接蛋白 45（Cx45） 118
连接子 184
连缀现象 864
裂隙现象 724
磷酸二酯酶抑制剂 624
磷酸化 7
磷酸腺苷活化蛋白激酶基因 451
铝电解电容器 956
螺旋波 340
螺旋式扩展 793

慢-快型	536，539	旁路	521
慢-慢型	539，1049	旁路电位	523
慢传导旁路	527	胚胎干细胞	431
慢节律	300	佩带式的除颤器	947
慢径消融	1045	偏差标测图	788
慢快综合征	513，862	频率控制	514
慢性肺动脉瓣关闭	612	频谱相关性	812
慢性冠状动脉疾病	564	平面波	264
慢性疲劳综合征	805	浦氏纤维电位	672
慢性心肌缺血	697	普拉洛尔	903
盲径	845	普鲁卡因胺	893
美托洛尔	901，903	普罗帕酮	893，896
美西律	893，896	普萘洛尔	900，901，903
孟德尔遗传定律	441	期前刺激	495，562
弥散张量	274	奇异相	216
迷宫手术	1083	启动子	429
迷走风暴	804	起搏标测	666
迷走神经张力	482	起搏点的湮灭	731
密码子	440	起搏点复合体	301
膜电位	251，371，403	起搏器	657，977
膜片钳	388	起搏器并发症	983
纳多洛尔	901	起搏器综合征	980
纳克索斯病	585	起搏阈值	422
钠-钙交换	42	起搏治疗	654
钠-氢交换	42	器官镶嵌现象常见	443
钠钙交换泵	602	器质性心脏病	492
钠钙交换体	601	牵张激活通道	238，399
钠离子通道阻滞剂	621	前间隔	1054
钠通道	1，77，125	强直性肌营养不良	634
脑血管痉挛	798	桥粒斑蛋白右室心肌病	585
脑血流自动调节反射	798	切口性房速	550
内向整流 K^+ 电流	29，372	球-链结合作用	156
内向整流电流	388	球-链样	73
内向整流性钾通道	19	曲西利特	942
逆传希氏束电位	541	全位法	1086
逆解法	790	全细胞透析技术	432
逆向刺激	204	醛固酮受体拮抗剂	935
逆向舒张期电位	673	缺血总负荷	761
逆向型房室折返性心动过速	857	人类基因组计划	440
逆钟向折返	486	溶栓时代	782
盘状球蛋白	586	融合波	742，985
庞加莱散点图	811	闰盘	177
旁观细胞致死	154	噻吗洛尔	901，903

索 引

三度房室阻滞　481，483，484，519
三尖瓣环　498
三尖瓣峡部区域　823
三磷酸腺苷　923
三磷酸腺苷（ATP）依赖的 K^+ 电流　168
三维标测　556，1039，1074
三维电解剖标测　666
散点图　811
散发长 QT 综合征　706
散漫光断层成像　202
丧失　29
色原烷醇 293B　297
射频消融　368，476，564，998
神经介导性晕厥　797，870，991
神经新生　293
肾上腺素能受体阻滞剂　574
肾上腺素受体　285
肾上腺素受体阻滞剂　640
渗出性出血　519
生物利用度　469
生物振荡　731
识别算法　952
实时定位系统　849
使用依赖性　127
始动因素　509
示踪剂　834
事件记录仪　750
试验　905
适应证　978，1075
室壁瘤　1078
室颤　597，639
室颤持续　824
室颤阈值　760
室房阻滞　517
室间隔缺损修补术　519
室内差异性传导　736
室上速伴差异性传导　738
室性心动过速　294，376，639，1060，1078
室性心律失常　277，567，941
室性早搏　244，376
收缩功能　576
手术后交界区异位心动过速　519
受体防卫模型　127

舒张功能　576
舒张期充盈不良　511
舒张期电位　672
舒张期自发除极　628
束支折返性室速　570，675
束支阻滞　570
数学模型　254
双传感器联合　982
双电位　502，1031
双腔 ICD　966
双腔除颤器　974，976
双室起搏　989
双室再同步化起搏　970
双相波　955
双相波电除颤　945
双相波转复　878
双向性室速　626，693
双心室起搏　576
双域模型　264
顺向型房室折返性心动过速　451，521
顺钟向　486
顺钟向型和逆钟向型房扑　788
瞬时外向 K^+ 电流（I_{to}）　166，602
瞬时外向电流 I_{to}　26
司美利特　943
丝裂原活化蛋白激酶　285
丝裂原激活蛋白激酶　603
斯里兰卡肉桂碱　825
随访　1075
碎裂电位　1037
损伤　519
损伤电位　817
索他洛尔　901，903，913，918
他汀类药物　935
糖基化　7
特发性室颤　627
特发性室性心动过速　662
梯形图　724
体表电位图　788
体动传感器　982
体外循环　615
替地沙米　942
通道　190

同步心脏电复律 564	细胞骨架 1000，1001
同源重组 431	细胞间隙 405
头部外伤 640	细胞内钙超载 507，628
突变 468	峡部 487，1029
突发性 953	峡部依赖 502
突破点 789	下壁心肌梗死 779
拖带 487，563，1039	先天性长 QT 综合征 681，752，825
拖带标测 502，1064	先天性房室阻滞 484
脱氧核糖核酸 429	先天性缺陷 853
瓦氏变性 293	先天性三度房室阻滞 978
外科 1078，1082	先天性心脏病 550，611
外科 Maze 术 507	先心病修补术 615
外科标测 849	先兆性心律失常 698
外膜远场反射 793	先兆晕厥 762
外显率 442	显性负相 429
晚电位 242	显性旁路 521
晚电位检测 766	显性遗传 441，442
晚电位阳性 829	线粒体脑肌病 638
晚后除极 355	线性损伤 477
晚期复极 166	线性消融 1008，1011
危险分层 649，761	线性张量 270
危险性 657	腺苷 494，671，922
威尼斯心肌病 585	腺苷敏感性室性心动过速 662
微伏级 T 波电交替 824，825	腺苷酸环化酶 662
微折返 309，376，413，494	腺嘌呤核苷酸 53
维持窦性心律 512	消融 995，1036，1071
维持因素 509	消融靶点 672
维拉帕米 495，900，907，908	消融后间隔 519
伪超常传导 723	消融终点 1030
温醒 494，732	校正 477
文氏现象 482	心率 988
无辜的旁观者 844	心电图 571
无休止性 495，517	心电图筛查 709
无义突变 441	心动过缓 558
无症状心肌缺血 761	心动过速 330
西北象限电轴 739	心动过速的识别 951
吸附电极 817	心动过速性心肌病 511，521，927
希浦氏系统 519	心房 481
希浦系统 481，484	心房颤动 359，505，990，1004，1015，1082
希氏束电位 517	心房的大小 506
希氏束夺获时 523	心房钙代谢障碍 509
希氏束旁起搏 522	心房激动顺序 499
细胞电容 189	心房扑动 486，1029

心房起搏　　490，495
心房颤动　　300
心房重构　　507
心房最早激动部位　　531
心肺感受器　　798
心肌瘢痕　　714
心肌瘢痕组织　　714
心肌电静止区　　1062
心肌梗死　　1060
心肌缺血　　395，520
心肌细胞离子通道遗传变异　　759
心肌重塑　　727
心力衰竭　　600
心律失常　　694
心律失常抑制试验（CAST）　　886，897
心率变异性　　242，573，750，760，766，809
心率振荡　　767
心率振荡现象　　761
心内膜电图　　572
心内膜旁道　　1053
心室颤动　　278，695，697
心室程序刺激　　572，622
心室晚电位　　779
心室重塑　　600
心外膜　　1067，1086
心外膜边缘带　　296
心外膜房室旁道　　1054，1056
心外膜封套　　791
心源性猝死　　715
心源性晕厥　　873
心脏标测技术　　842
心脏传导系统疾病　　568
心脏电交替　　824
心脏肥大　　600
心脏基质　　759
心脏记忆　　788
心脏离子通道　　709
心脏内向整流钾（Kir）通道　　110
心脏事件　　649
心脏停搏　　639，718
心脏性猝死　　623，712，781，824，930
心脏骤停　　564，577
心脏骤停幸存者　　596

新霉素抗性基因　　431
新生儿狼疮综合征　　484
新生突变　　708
信号平均心电图　　572，664，829
信号通路　　275
信号噪声比　　781
信使核苷酸　　440
兴奋收缩耦联　　247
兴奋性介质　　314
星状神经节阻滞　　640
幸存者　　657
胸前导联同向性　　740
胸腺嘧啶核苷激酶　　431
旋转子　　333，334
漩涡波　　327
血管紧张素受体阻断剂　　934
血管紧张素转换酶抑制剂　　605，886，934
血管扩张和心动过缓-血管迷走性反射　　798
血管扩张剂　　573
血管迷走事件　　797
血管迷走性晕厥　　621，797，875
血流动力学稳定　　565
血流动力学异常　　611
血栓　　397，999
血栓栓塞性　　511
血栓形成瀑布激活　　719
血小板聚集　　760
循环前清除　　469
压力反射　　812
压力反射调节　　812
压力反射敏感性　　809
压力感受器对压力　　798
压力敏感的离子通道　　95
延迟后除极　　507，628，663，694
延迟钠电流（late I_{Na}）　　148
延迟外向整流 K^+ 电流（I_k）　　166
延迟整流 K^+ 电流　　189
延迟整流 K^+ 电流（I_k）　　166
延迟整流钾电流　　602
延迟整流钾电流（I_{Kur}）　　24
延伸突变　　441
炎症标志物　　715
炎症反应　　519

索 引

阳性区逆钟向旋转　793
洋地黄中毒　520，693
洋地黄中毒　693
氧烯洛尔　903
药代动力学　468
药物　506
药物复律　877
药物基因组学　468
一度　481
一度房室阻滞　481
一过性房室阻滞　490
依布利特　490，913，917
遗传标记　444
遗传连锁　444
遗传性长QT综合征　170
遗传性疾病　714
遗传性心律失常　759
遗传性心律失常性　710
遗传学　620
乙酰胆碱 K^+ 电流　372
异丙肾上腺素　494，517，588
异位激动　354
异位心房激动　478
异型缝隙连接通道　196
易损性上限　961
逸搏　300
吲哚洛尔　903
隐匿传导　723
隐匿性房室旁路　855
隐匿性融合拖带　1065
隐匿性拖带　488，495，503，845，1066
隐性遗传　441，442
应激活化　185
婴儿猝死综合征　618，703，705
永久性　505
永久性起搏器　519
永久性心脏起搏器　479
有效不应期　371，676，821
右侧交感神经节切除　706
右侧旁道　1052
右房房速　496
右冠状动脉窦　667
右室激动　989

右室流出道　584
右室流出道室速　295，663
右室心力衰竭　581
右束支阻滞　673，675
右向左分流　615
预测因素　571
预防性干预措施　715
预激综合征　521，768，855，871
运动负荷试验　750
运动平板　831
运动性心律失常　752
运动员晕厥　875
晕厥　775，867
杂合　440
再确认　953
再识别　953
暂时外向钾电流　373
早后除极　147，355，376
早期复极　166
早期后除极　242，435，507，663，681，819
噪音刺激　649
增强拮抗　286
窄QRS波心动过速　517
粘合膜连接　182
张力激活的离子通道　95
张力丝　1000
张力整合体　240
折返　277，360
折返环　229，487
折返活动　283
折返机制　562
折返激动　340
折返性房速　495
折返周期　313
阵发性　505，517
阵发性房颤　304，351
真超常传导　723
振荡学说　732
震荡电场　419
整倍性　441
正电子发射断层扫描　664
正电子发射计算机断层成像　835
肢带型肌营养不良　636

肢体导联同向性　740
脂肪分裂综合征　587
脂肪组织　582
直接法　1086
直立倾斜试验　621,750,775,776,797,872
直流电复律　492
直流电消融　1044
植入式"Holter"　773
植入式心房除颤器　973
植入式心脏复律除颤器　564,594,624,652,657,718,949,958
植入型心脏复律除颤器　454,883
植物碱　56
致命室性心律失常　890
致命性事件　705
致命性心律失常　776
致死性　596
致死性室性心律失常　596
致心律失常性　414
致心律失常性右室发育不良　580,699,714,752,754,784
致心律失常性右室心肌病　295
致心律失常作用　894
中间隔　1054
中间耦联电导　196
重度心力衰竭　885
重构　371,509
重合角　793
重整　538
重整反应　562
重整心动过速　538
重症肌无力　639
重组　444
周期稳定性　953
周期性麻痹　637
轴突的再生　294
蛛网膜下腔出血　640
主导起搏位点　188
主动的膜特性　220
转复窦律　877
转换　441
转基因　429
转基因小鼠　429

转子　387
自动除颤　874
自动调节感知灵敏度　958
自动调整增益　958
自动体外除颤器　718,889,947
自动阈值调整　952
自动增益　952
自发心电图异常　623
自发性　518
自发性室性心律失常　571,831
自发性晕厥　775
自律性　354,570
自律性房速　495
自律性异常　494
自律性增强　507
自身拖带　732
自旋波　388
自主神经　399
自主神经成像　833
自主神经的张力变化　729
自主神经调节　814
自主神经系统　495
自主神经系统功能障碍　800
自主神经张力　705,759
总死亡率　571
阻滞部位　481
阻滞区　483
阻滞线　487
组织重构　825
最大舒张电位　188
最早的心房激动点　519
最早心房逆传激动点　541,788
左侧颈胸交感神经节切除术　655
左侧旁道　1052
左房房速　496
左冠状动脉窦　667
左后分支　675
左后分支阻滞　673
左前分支　675
左室辅助装置　577
左室流出道室性心动过速　666
左室射血分数　828,830
左星状神经节切除　992

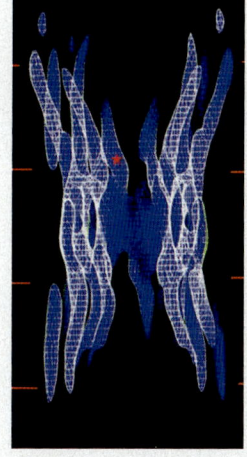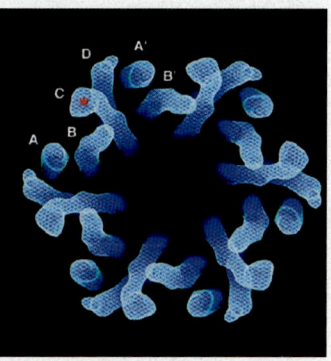

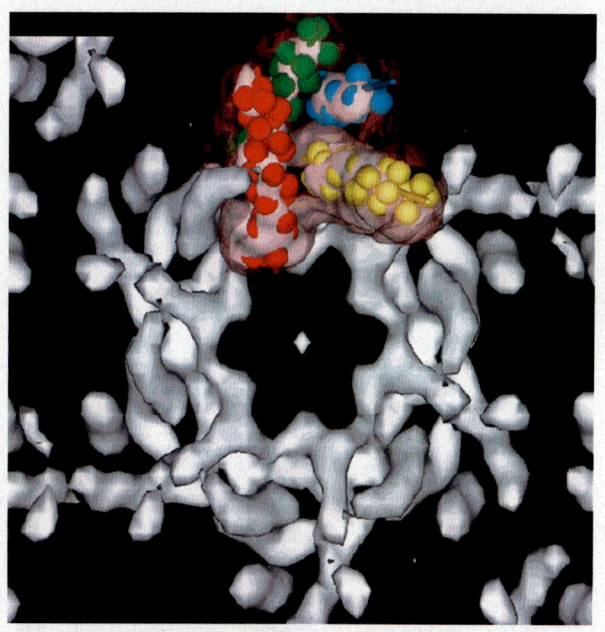

彩图1（图8-3） 通过电子晶体学得到的Cx43超微结构 平面距离是7.5Å，垂直距离是21Å。左图显示的是整个通道的侧面观，红线代表脂质双分子层，红星代表那些孔径被估计最小的点。右图代表横切面的形状，通道由六个面组成，每个面又由四个相同密度区组成，每个密度区代表一个转膜区（引自 Unger VM, Kumer NM, Gilula NB, Yeager, MR: Three_dimensional structure of a recombinant gap junction membrane channel. Science 283:1176-1180, 1999）

彩图2（图8-4） Cx43通道的分子模型 以电子晶体光谱获得的Cx43通道超微结构为基础（图8-3），将主要序列的氨基酸排列成超微结构确定的跨膜域。模型构建了低能量构型，根据这一模型，Unger26确定的主要序列与α螺旋间的关系是：TM4，螺旋C（绿色）；TM1，螺旋D（红色）；TM2，螺旋B′（黄色）；TM3，螺旋A′（蓝色）。然而，这一模型仍存在局限性，一些特殊点似乎不合理（引自 Nunn RS, Macke TJ, Olson AJ, Yeager M: Transmembrane alpha-helices in the gap junction membrane channel: Systematic search of packing models based on the pair potential function. Microsc Res Tech 52:344-351, 2001.）

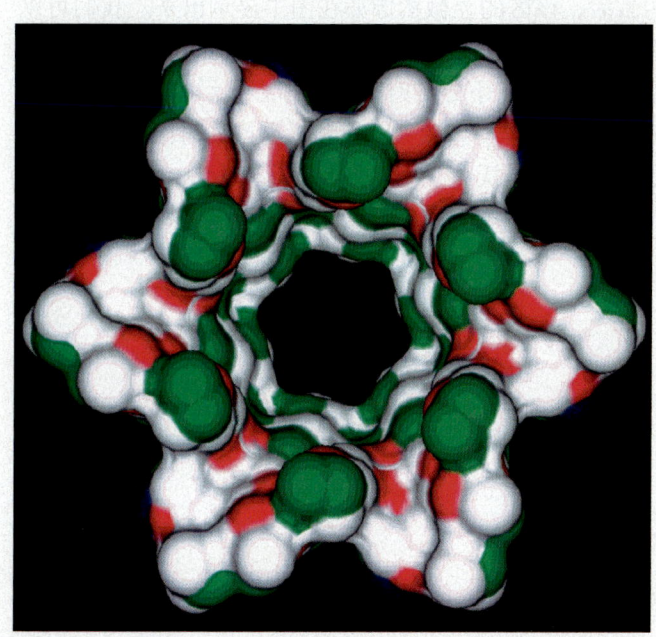

彩图3（图8-5） 连接子模型的上面观 球代表氨基酸，直径10Å。排列颜色如下：红色，Asp Glu；蓝色，Arg Lys；绿色，Tyr Phe Trp；黄色，Met Cys；白色，Gly Ala Val Leu Ile Pro。这一模型代表了低能量构型。然而，特征仍不合理，例如，充电残基与脂质相连（引自Nunn RS, Macke TJ, Olson AJ, Yeager M: Transmembrane alpha-helices in the gap junction membrane channel: Systematic search of packing models based on the pair potential function. Microsc Res Tech 52: 344-351,2001.）

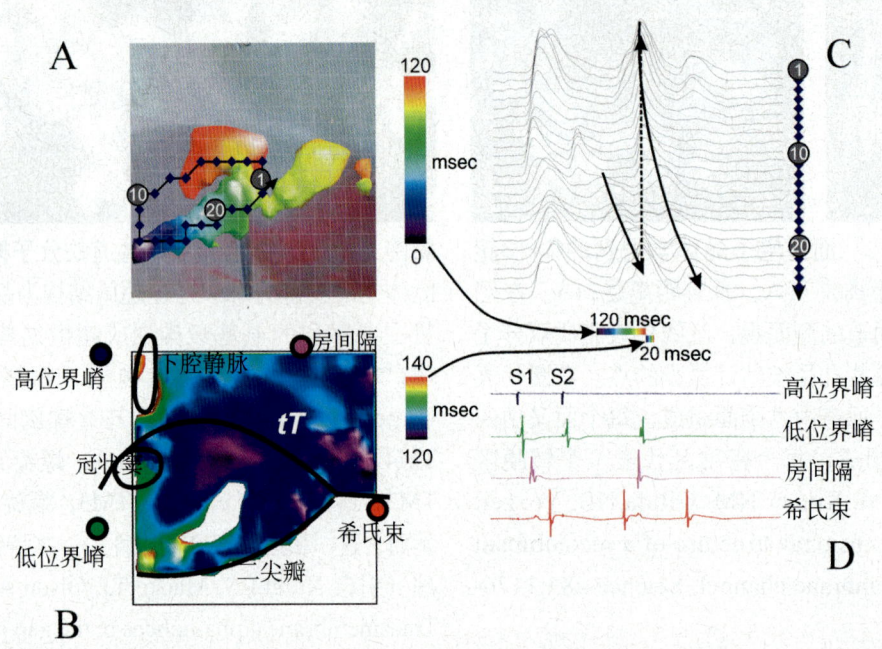

彩图 4（图 23-2）　来自界嵴的早搏刺激引起的典型（慢-快）房室结折返　A：单个早搏冲动引起的折返时的传导彩图。它只显示了折返的前 120 ms，描绘了结后延伸部，致密房室结，以及快径路的激活。该图是与标本图像重叠在一起的（见图 B 相应标志）。蓝色菱形指示的位点，其相应光学记录见图 C。B：折返传导的延续部分：过渡区房结层 20 ms 的激活。该区的显微图像亦在图中显示出来。我们可以发现 A、B 两图的激活时间有明显差别。C：折返通路上的动作电位光学记录：实线箭头指示的是慢径路和快径路的传导。虚线箭头指示的是表面过渡层的快传导。下方的时间尺度标志显示的是 A、B 两幅传导图中相应的时间间隔。D：于最后一次基本刺激（S1）、早搏刺激（S2）和折返搏动时记录到的传统的双极电描记图。记录了从高位界嵴、低位界嵴、房间隔到希氏束（引自 Nikolski VI, Jones SA, Lancaster MK, Boyett MR, Efimov IR：Cx43 and dual-pathway electrophysiology of the atrioventricular node and atrioventricular nodal reentry. Cir Res 2003;92：469-475.）

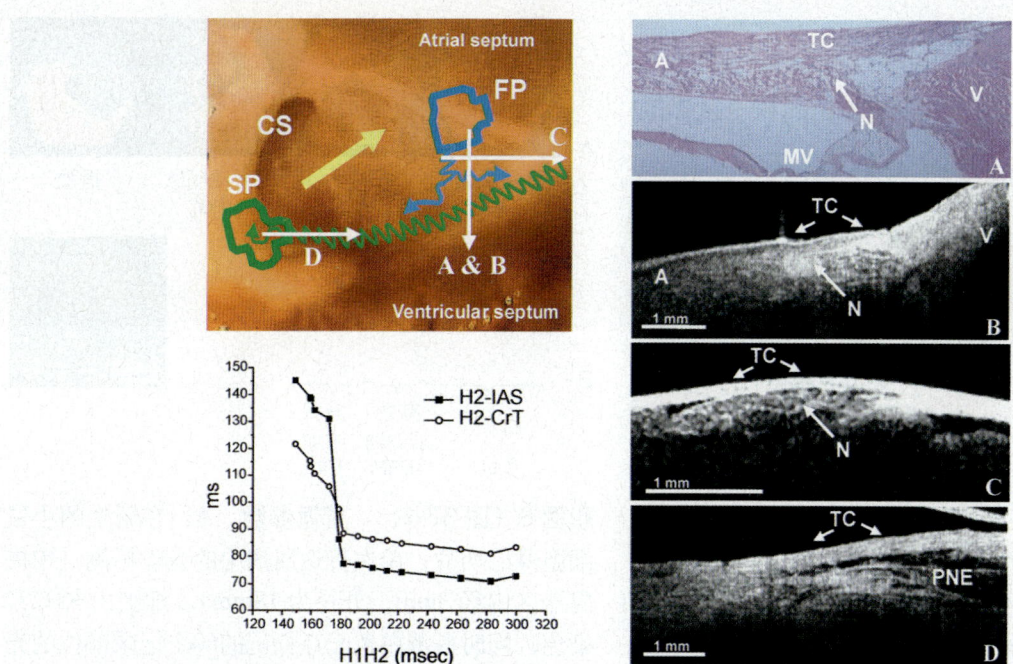

彩图 5（图 23-5） 光学相干断层（Optical Coherence Tomography，OCT）成像显示了在早搏刺激下（具有不同代偿间歇，表现在传导曲线上是呈"跳跃性"的改变），突破点发生转移的双径路传导 左上图：标本图像以及对应于慢（SP）快（FP）径传导的不同代偿间歇时的突破位点图像。双径路是由荧光成像来确定的。左下图：由希氏束产生逆向刺激时的传导曲线，表现了早搏刺激H2和房间隔（IAS）及界嵴区（CrT）的激动（双极电极记录）之间存在延迟。我们注意到传导曲线中存在明显的跳跃，尤其是黑色曲线，它反映的是希氏-隔传导延迟。这种传导曲线中的跳跃，反映了从快路径到慢路径突破位点的转移。右图：沿着左图所示标本的纵切面图，包括从上到下组织的组织学（彩色）和OCT（灰色）图像。A：房间隔；CS：冠状窦；N：致密房室结；PNE：结后延伸部；TC：过渡区细胞；V：室间隔（引自 Gupta M, Rolins AM, Izatt JA, Efimov IR: Imaging of the atrioventricular node using optical coherence tomography. J Cardiovasc Electrophysiol 2002;13:95.）

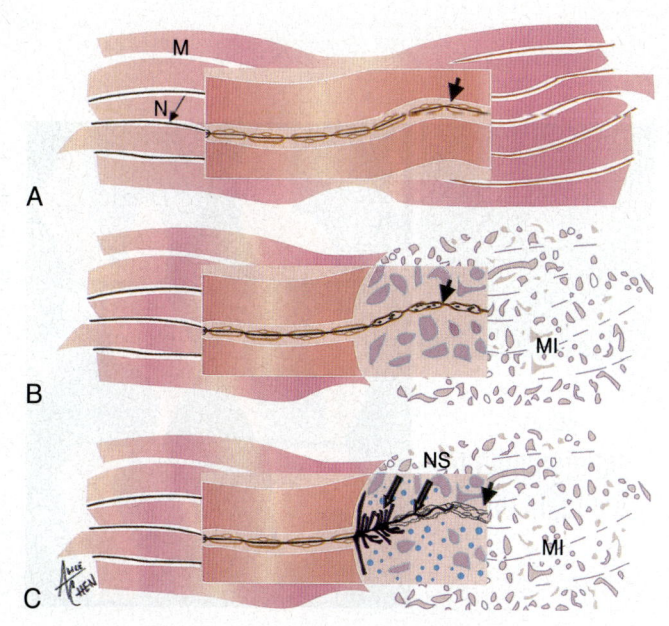

彩图 6（图 33-1） 心肌梗死后的神经芽生 A：分布于血管周围及心肌细胞之间的交感神经，神经纤维沿着心肌细胞的长轴定向分布（实心箭头所示）。B：心肌梗死后梗死部位的神经纤维受到损伤。远端的残干发生了瓦氏变性（图B和C中的实心箭头所示）。C：邻近损伤的地方有神经纤维的轴突芽生（空心箭头所示）。M：心肌细胞；N：神经纤维；MI：心肌梗死；NS：神经芽。

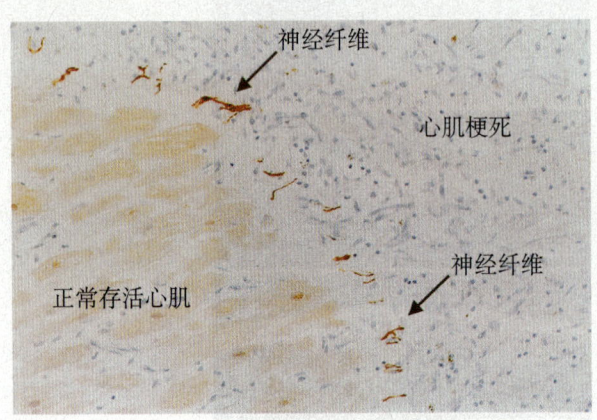

彩图7（图33-2） 心肌梗死后区域性的神经高支配 神经纤维（箭头）在梗死外围最丰富。相比之下，梗死的坏死区及纤维化区无神经纤维。心肌梗死后的去神经支配及神经芽生可导致心脏交感神经的不均匀性分布（摘自 Chen P-S et al. Sympathetic nerve sprouting, electrical remodeling and the mechanisms of sudden cardiac death. Cardiovasc Res 2001；50：409-416.）

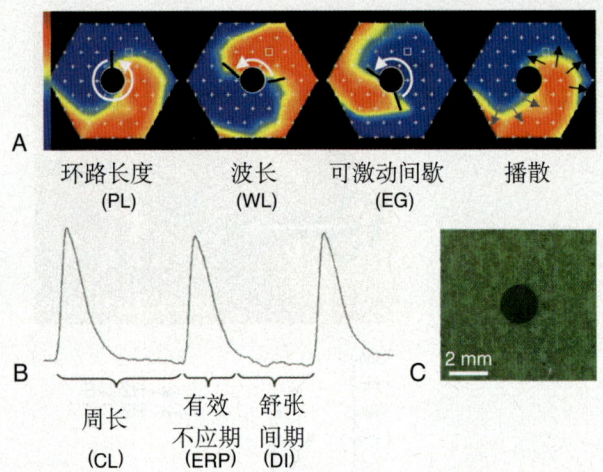

彩图8（图37-1） 折返参数 A：在新生的小鼠细胞薄层切片，单次折返周期中的光学标测（中央阻滞区内径3mm，外径为18mm）。细胞由RH237染色，同时监测白色光点标记的60个记录部位的光学动作电位。左侧的彩条表示相对电压，蓝色代表静息细胞或完全复极化的细胞。红色代表完全除极化的细胞。数字表示时间，并以毫秒为计量单位。前三个图形表示了在障碍物的周长所测量出的环路长度（PL）、波长（WL）以及可激动间隙（EG）。在右侧的最后一个图形显示出波峰（用黑色箭头表示）和波尾（用灰色箭头表示）扩布的方向。B：在同一次折返中，对某个记录部位通过光学过滤记录到的动作电位。图中显示出了三个参数：环路长度（CL）、有效不应期（ERP）以及舒张间期。C：另外一个通过培养的显微结构的显微照片。环形解剖阻滞的直径为2mm。细胞肌动蛋白通过荧光染色得以显现（引自Y.Nabutovsky, N, Bursac, and L, Tung, 未公开不发表的资料）。

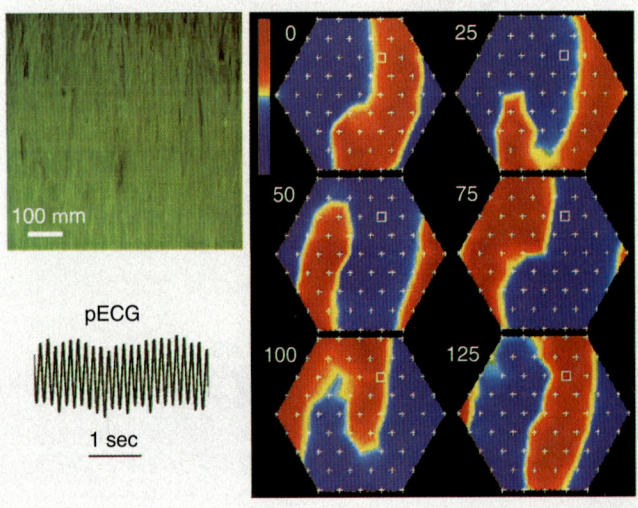

彩图9（图37-3） 各向异性单层构筑可通过florescinphalloids染色显示肌动蛋白纤维 右侧图显示单个顺时针方向旋转的转子。彩色棒状线表示正常电压水平；如图37-1所示，从左向右、从顶端至底部阅读该幅图，数字表示时间，单位ms。折返环长度135ms。伪心电图（PECG）在左下图显示，呈单形性。

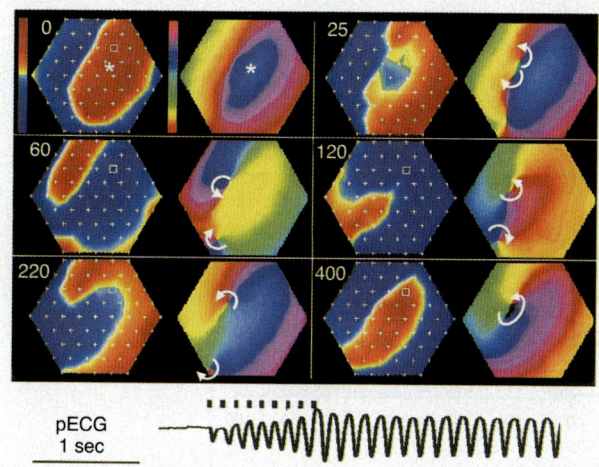

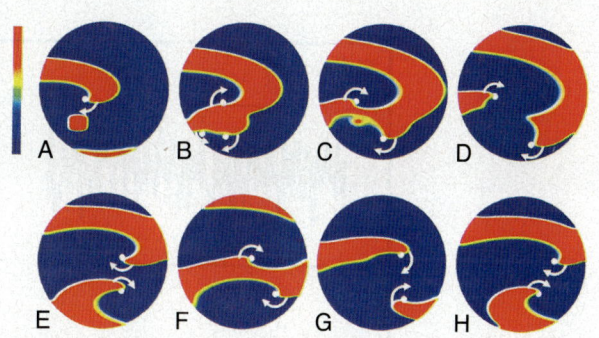

彩图 10（图 37-4） 通过单一的点电极的快速起搏所诱发的单环折返：通过开始时的电压所致的电压和相应的时相点 左图显示的电压彩条和图 37-3 中的相同。第一时相左侧的彩条显示从 $-\pi$（0%）到 $+\pi$（100%）。图形阅读从左到右，从上到下。数字显示为 ms。星号显示起搏位点。箭头显示转子的方向。稳定的快速起搏导致 25ms 时波的碎裂。

彩图 11（图 37-5） 计算机模拟双支螺旋波的起始和维持 A 到 D，在螺旋波上发放单个 S3 刺激，导致了新的双支螺旋波。每个图形之间的间距为 50ms。白色的标记表示单相波的时相。E 到 H，完整的双支螺旋波。图形之间的间距为 100ms。

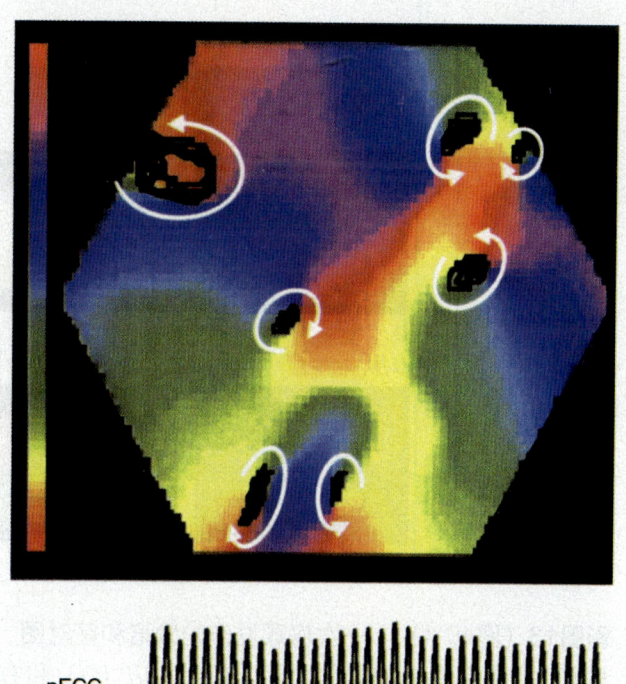

彩图 12（图 37-6） 复杂但稳定的静态的 7 个转子组成的折返的示意图，彩条和图 37-4 相同 白色箭头表示 7 个并存的、频率和时相相同的转子的旋转方向。在 5s 的活动中，旋转轨道的尖端用黑色表示。时相心电图是单相的。

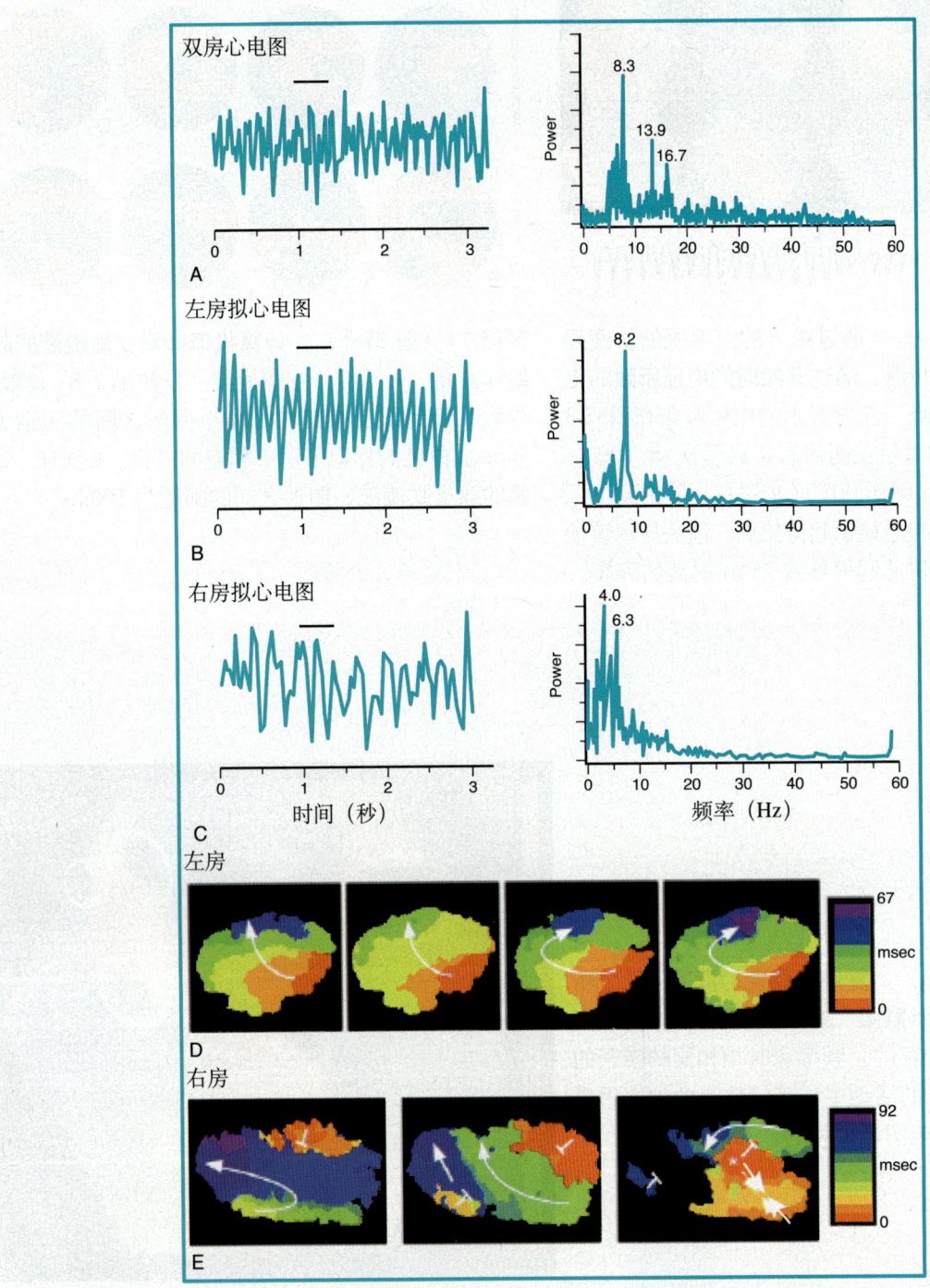

彩图13（图40-1） 一次房颤发作的频谱和等时图 A：双房整体活动的双极电图记录及相应能谱。B和C：左房和右房及相应能谱。连续 左房（D）和右房（E）同步记录等时图。等时图时间由水平标尺指示（改自 Skanes A，Mandapati R，Berenfekl O，等：Spatiotemporal periodicity during atrial fibrillation in the isolated sheep heart.Circulation 98:1236-1248，1998.）

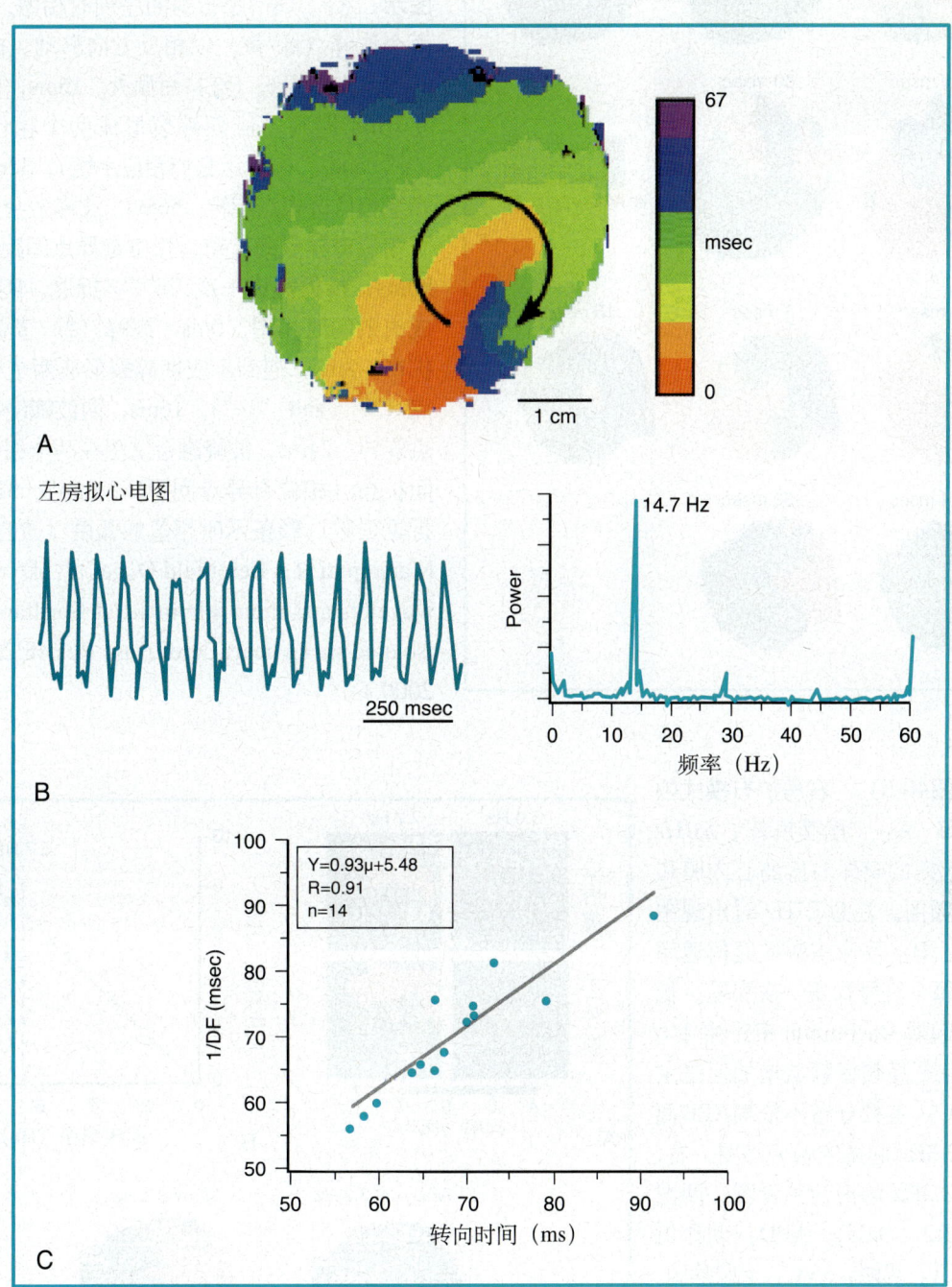

彩图14（图40-2） 房颤的折返源 A：持续房颤时左房游离壁的光标测等时图，示顺时针折返。B：同次发作的左房拟心电图及相应能谱。C：全部视频记录拟心电图的主频倒数同房颤折返周期的相关性（改自 Mandapati R，Skanes A，Chen J，et al：Stable microreentrant sources as a mechanism of atrial fibrillation in the isolated sheep heart.Circulation 101:194-199，2000.）

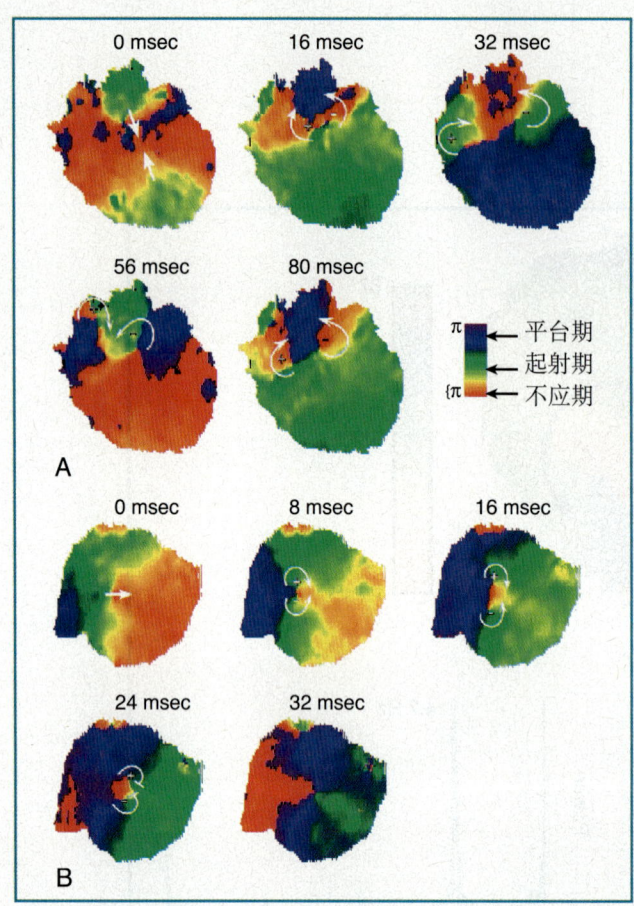

彩图15（图40-3） 波动碎裂和折返形成时相图示 A："8"字折返的序列时相图。在0ms，两个波峰（绿/黄）以相反方向移动。向下的波遇到不应期组织（红）而湮灭。16ms，向上的波在0ms遇到不应期碎裂形成两个相位奇异点（"+"and"-"示它们相应手性）。32ms，两波峰绕相位奇异点旋转。56ms，波峰融合开始在两个相位奇异点间扩布（相位奇异点间距6.8mm）。80ms，折返完成一次"8"字折返。B：折返形成失败的时相图。0ms，波峰（绿/黄）左向右扩布。8ms，遇到不应期碎裂形成两个相位奇异点（"+"and"-"）。16ms，两波峰绕相位奇异点旋转。24ms，波峰融合试图在两个相位奇异点间扩布（相位奇异点间距3.3 mm）。32ms时，折返失败。彩条示时相值的弧度（改自Chan J, Mandapati R, Berenfeld O, et al: Dynamics of wavelets and their role in atrial fibrillation in the isolated sheep heart.Cardiovasc Res 48:220-232, 2000.）

彩图16（图40-5） 右房扩布模式依赖起搏频率 A："崩溃频率"。5.0Hz和7.7Hz起搏的离体右房的心内膜和心外膜主频图。注意7.7Hz时出现主频域异质。B：反应主频域起搏速率（n=5）。每个符号代表一次实验。低于6.7Hz起搏Bachmnnn束产生1：1激动。在更高频率频域增加但是主频下降。C：主频分布不依赖APD离散。左，3.3Hz起搏的APD75图；右，同一标本8.3Hz起搏的主频图。两图无相关（R2 = 0.05）。APD：动作电位时程；CT：界嵴；SVC：上腔静脉。(改自Berenfeld O, Zaitsev AV, Mironov AF, et al: Frequency-dependent breakdown of wave propagation into fibrillafory conduction across the pectinate muscle network in the isolated sheep right atrium.Circ Res 90:1173-1180, 2002.)

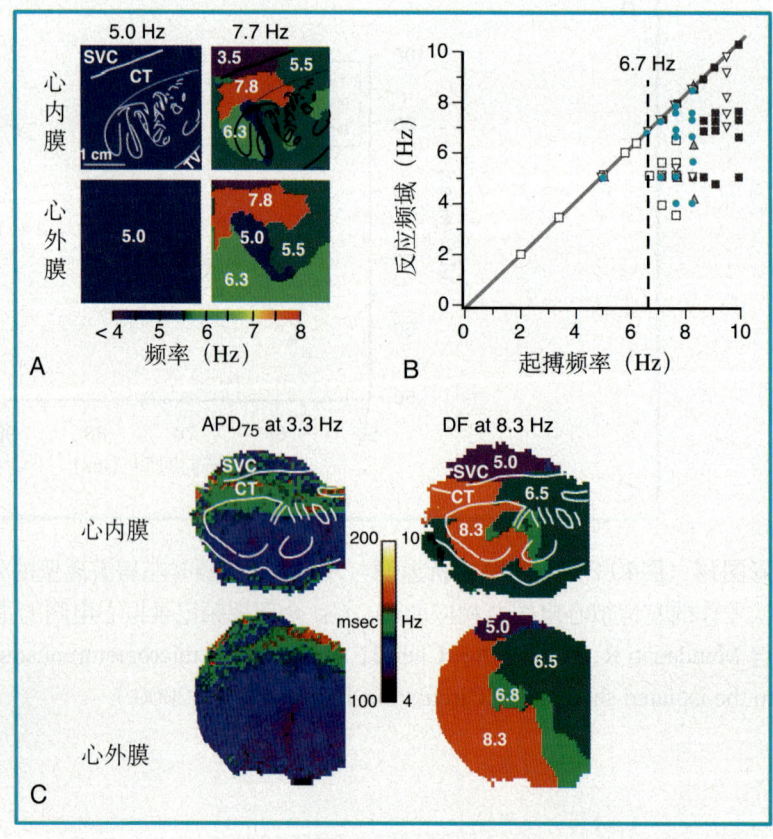

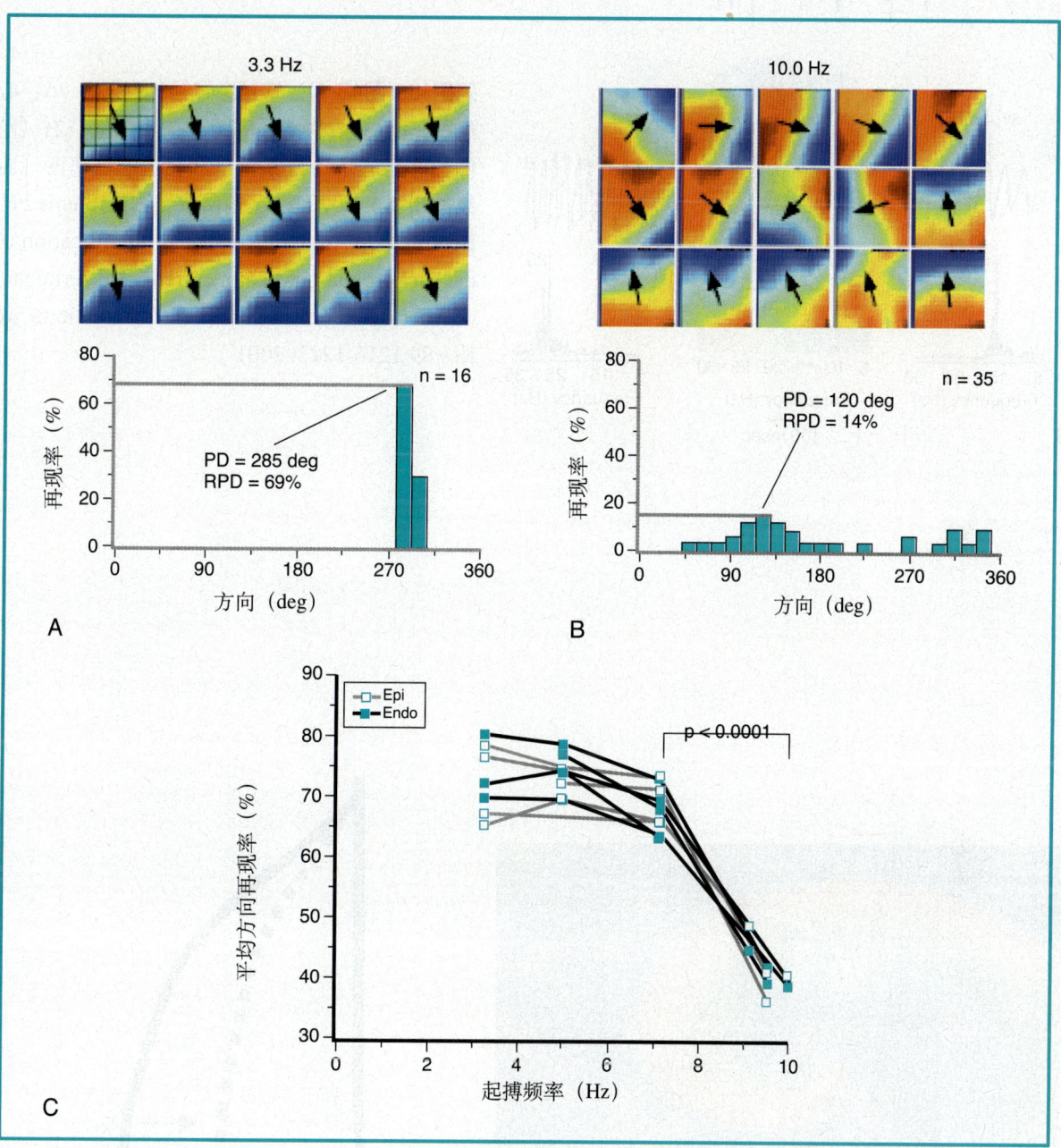

彩图17（图40-6） 优势传导方向（PD）的频率依赖 上图，心内膜同一位置3.3Hz（A）和10Hz（B）起搏的15幅连续的等时图。两图的色价以红比蓝标准化。下图，既定方向主导扩布再现率（RPD）的直方图。C，5次实验中心内膜（Endo）和心外膜（Epi）平均RPD的起搏频率依赖。注意超过6.7Hz起搏时RPD突然下降。（改自 Berenfeld O, Zaitsev AV, Mironov AF, et al: Frequency-dependent breakdown of wave propagation into fibrillatory conduction across the pectinate muscle network in the isolated sheep right atrium.Circ Res 90:1173-1180, 2002.）

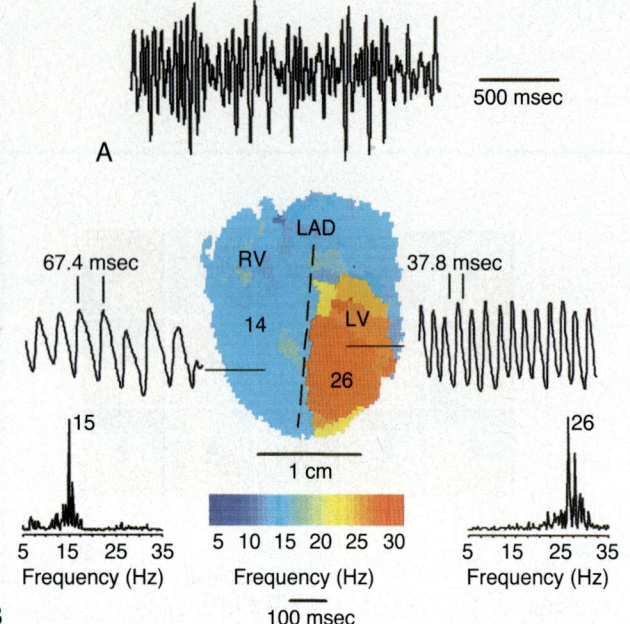

彩图18（图43-1） 室颤主导频率的分析 A：心电图，B：主导频率标测图与左（右侧）、右（左侧）心室的单一像素记录和相应的功率谱（曲线的下面）。LAD，左前降支（引自Samie FH, Berenfeld O, Anumonwo J, et al: Rectification of the background potassium current: A determinant of rotor dynamics in ventricular fibrillation.Circ Res 89:1216-1223, 2001.）

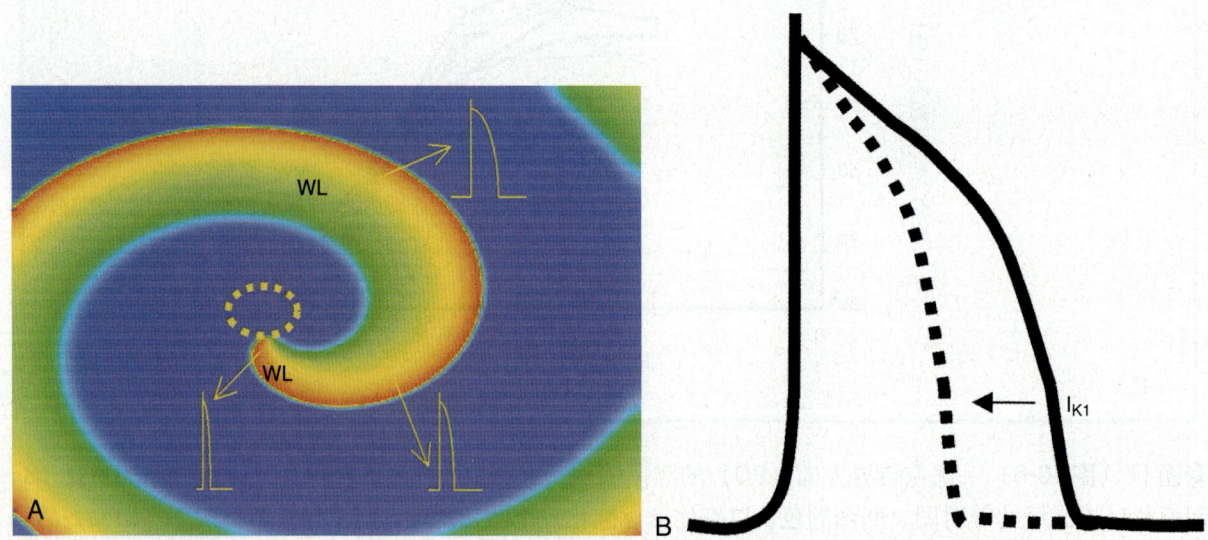

彩图19（图43-2） 核心对波长和动作电位时程的作用 A：在 2×2 cm 的各向异性（长与宽速度之比为4：1）心脏组织中的自旋波活动，遵照Luo与Rudy修正的全动作电位模型建立的方法（技术细节见Gilmour等[26]）。波锋为红色，波尾为绿色，静息组织为兰色。注意波锋曲度沿转动中心方向增大（核心为虚线圈）。随曲度增大传导速度减慢。波长定义为兴奋状态的空间范围，从中心到周边增长。其原因是由于核心的电张作用，动作电位时程从中心到周边增长（局部波长等于传导速度×动作电位时程）。B：功能性折返中 I_{K1} 导致动作电位时程缩短的示意图。

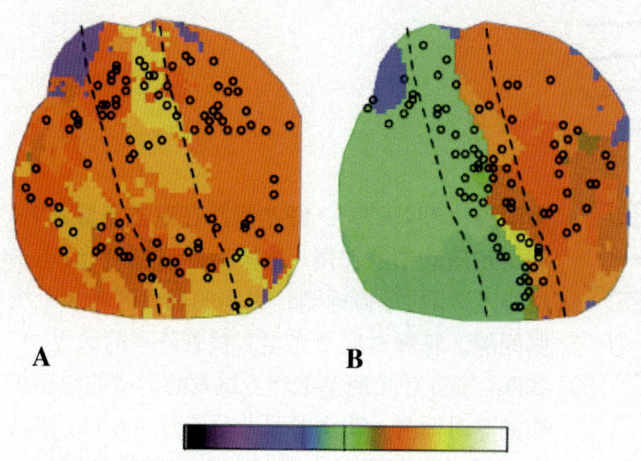

彩图20（图44-2） 心脏区域性缺血引发室颤时在缺血边缘带小波的形成增加 彩图代表室颤时主导兴奋频率（DF）的空间分布。DF与局部冲动的周长成反比，周长与局部不应期相关[16]。圆圈标注波的碎裂位置，导致室颤时的小波形成。A与B图中，波碎裂分布与围缺血期室颤（A）和缺血室颤（B）的DF标测图。注意跨缺血的边缘带的不应期较大梯度区与密集的波碎裂区相连。（引自 Zaitsev AV, Sarmast F, Kolli A, et al: Wave break formation during ventricular fibrillation in the isolated, regionally ischemic pig heart. Circ Res 92:546-553, 2003.）

彩图21（图44-3） 离体灌注猪心整体的缺血和高血钾的抗颤作用 A：室颤（VF）时平均兴奋主导频率（DF）与波碎裂（WB）的密度作为细胞外钾（K^+）的函数。随着$[K^+]_o$的升高，室颤波变得更有周期性和更加有序，直至$[K^+]_o$浓度相当于12.5mM时变为室速。B：室颤时心肌整体缺血前后2min时左室前壁心外膜的标测。箭头指示波锋的扩布，圆圈表示新生小波的位点。在正常灌注的心脏，标测区域最多同时存在5个小波。而整体缺血后2min，观察区仅见单一的自旋波。

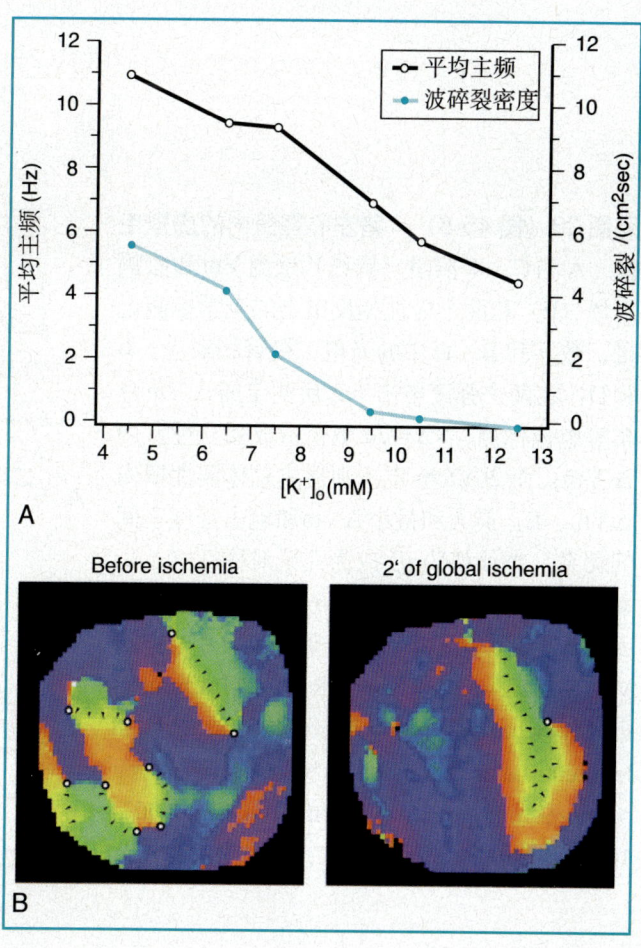

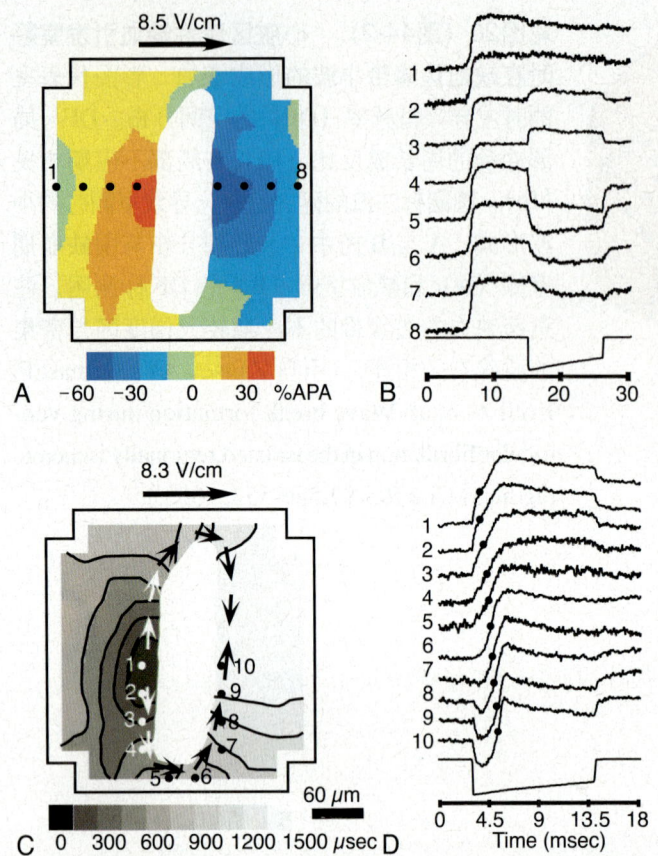

彩图22（图45-2） 细胞间隙在电击诱导ΔVm和组织激动中的作用　A和B：极性相反时电击诱导ΔVm的等势标测。中间的白色区域表示细胞间隙。轮廓对应于光电二极管阵列的边界。C和D：来自舒张期电击产生继发源形成的激动扩布的等时标测。箭头提示激动扩布的方向。激动时间通过标测区域中最早激动的时间来确定。（引自Fast VG, Rohr S, Gillis AM, Kleber AG: Activation of cardiac tissue by extracellular clefts in monolayers of cultured myocytes. Cir Res 82: 375-385, 1998.）

彩图23（图45-6） 猪左心室壁内的虚拟电极　A和C：对照组（黑线）壁内Vm和除颤电场（E）和两个极性相反电击的光学标测记录。数字和B、D中的光电二极管相对应。B和D：在两个强度电击9ms后测定的ΔVm分布等电位标测。8.8V/cm电击造成孤立性壁内ΔVm，而26V/cm电击则造成总体阴性壁内ΔVm。E：最大和最小ΔVm和电击强度之间的关系。虚线将Vm反应为几乎对称性（Ⅰ）、非对称性孤立壁内ΔVm（Ⅱ）和总体阴性ΔVm（Ⅲ）这三个区域分隔开来（引自Fast VG, Sharifov OF, Cheek ER, et al: Intramural virtual electrodes during defibrillation shocks in left ventricular wall assessed by optical mapping of membrane potential. Circulation 106: 1007-1014, 2002.）

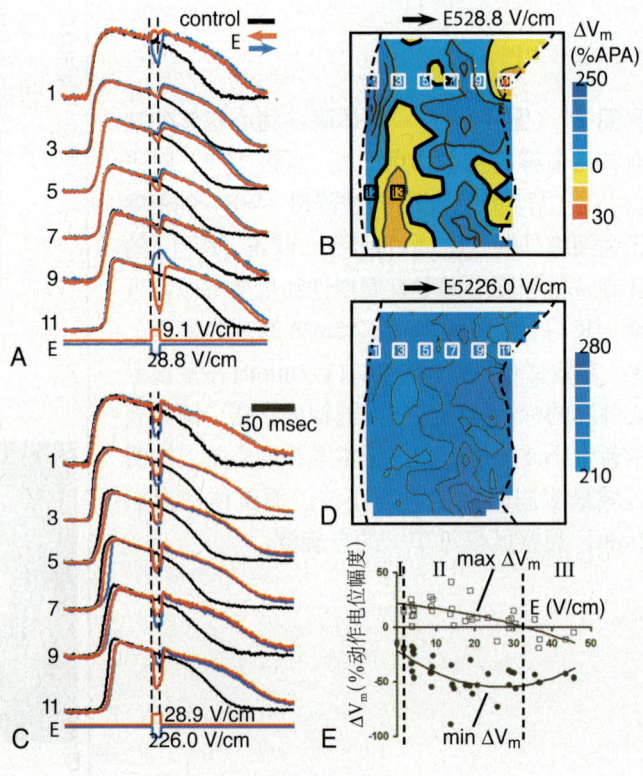

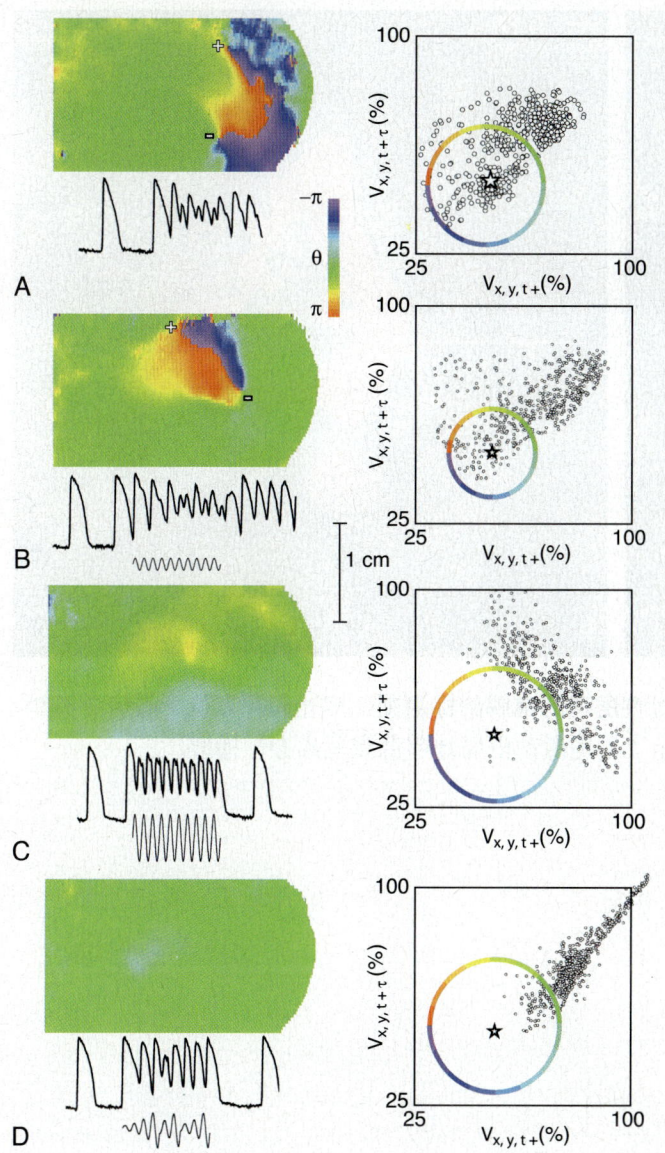

彩图24（图46-2） 室颤时的相位标测和散点图 室颤（A），时限1s，电压12V；频率10Hz的正弦曲线波形电击（B），时限1s，电压48V；频率10Hz正弦曲线波形电击（C）和时限1s；电压36V；频率10Hz混乱波形电击（D）期间的相位标测和散点图。来自一个部位的跨膜信号和刺激波形都显示在每幅位相图的下方。在12V正弦曲线波形电击期间（B），形成一对手性相反的位相奇点（+，顺时钟方向，-，逆时钟方向），从而诱发颤动。☆表示状态空间中的原点（V*，V*）。彩色圆圈代表由公式1计算的相角。

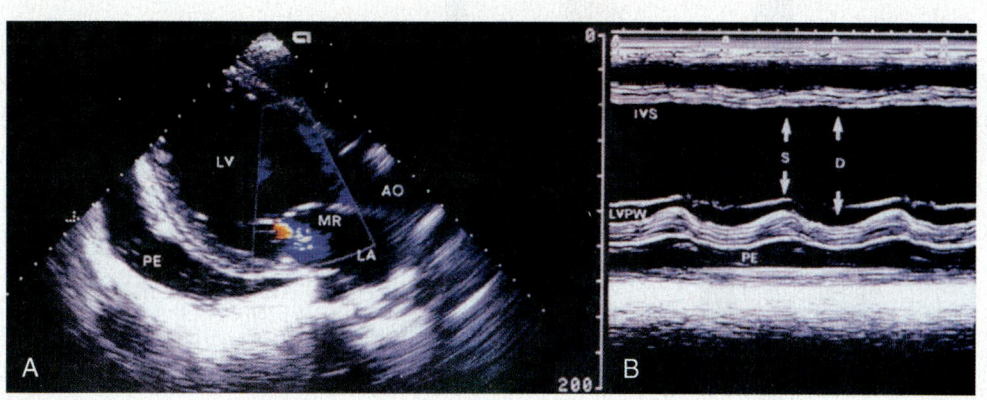

彩图25（图49-6） 扩张型心肌病超声心动图表现 左室长轴面显示左室（LV）扩大和二尖瓣返流（MR），而左房（LA）及主动脉根部（AO）大小正常，伴中等量心包积液（PE）。M型超声显示左室扩张伴收缩功能下降，以及心包积液。IVS：室间隔；LVPW：左室后壁；S：收缩期；D：舒展期

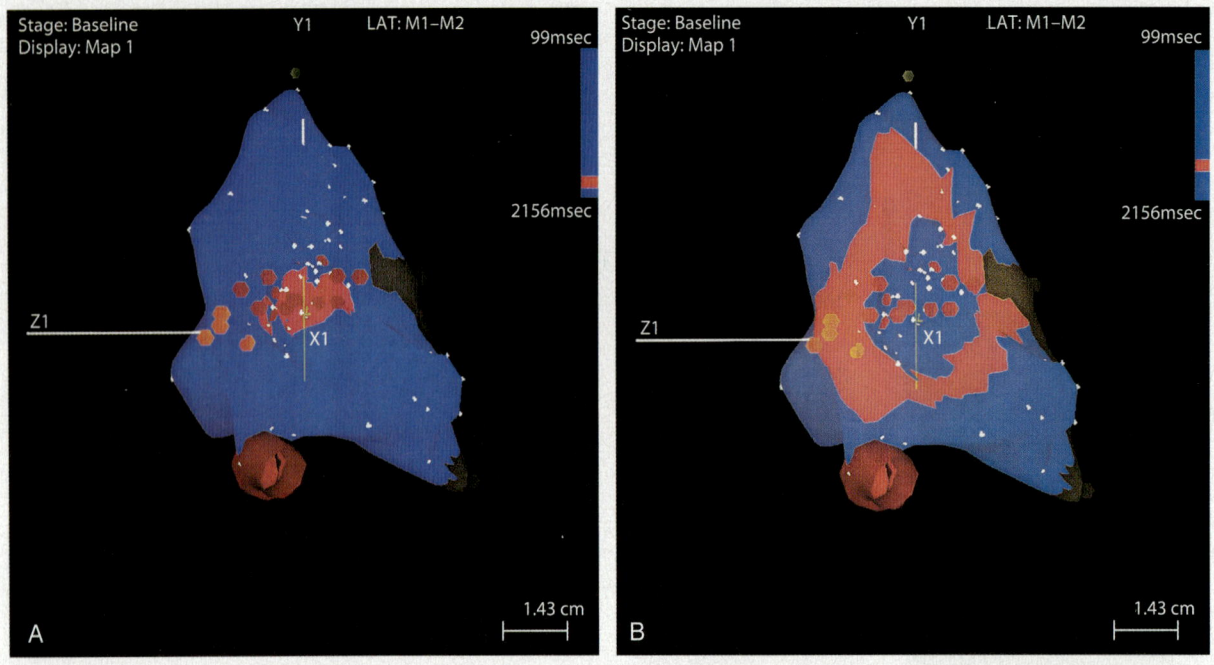

彩图26（图55-1） 开胸心脏手术后患者的局灶性房速的电解剖标测图 房速起源点位于右房游离壁，图中显示了房速时心房激动的顺序。标测图显示了心房激动由局灶起源点呈离心性播散。

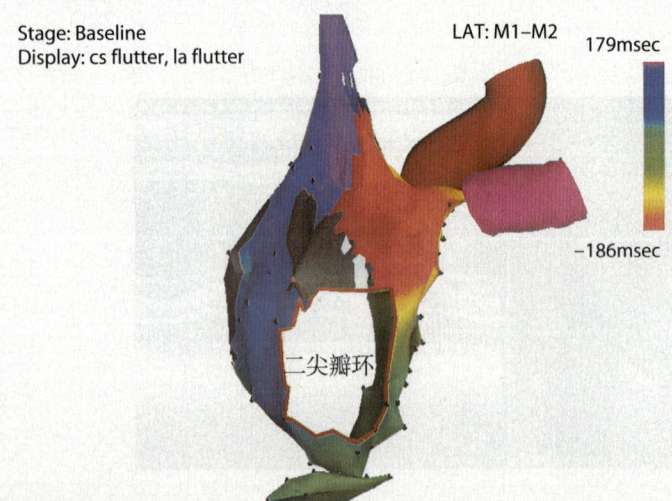

彩图27（图55-2） 大折返性房速的左房电解剖图 有二尖瓣疾病病史的患者发生了大折返性房速，电解剖图显示房速起源于临近左下肺静脉的折返环。使用由左下肺静脉至二尖瓣环的连续阻滞线成功消融了本例心动过速。

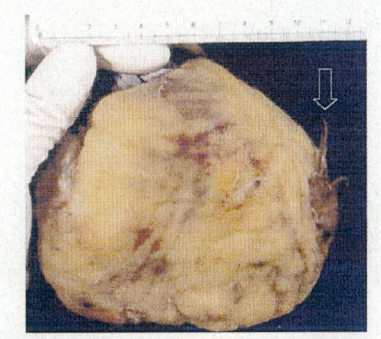
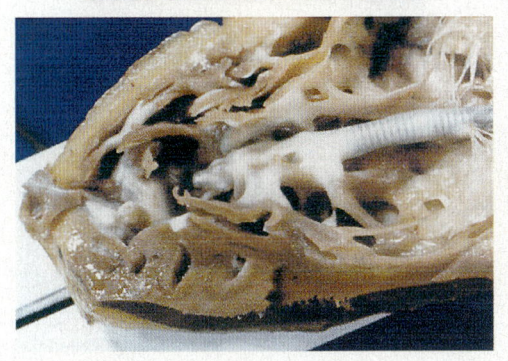
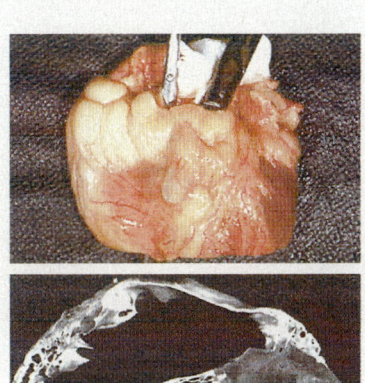
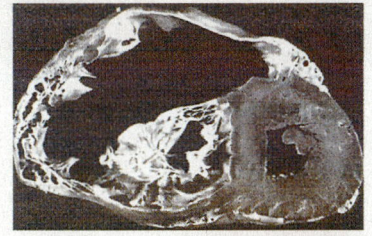
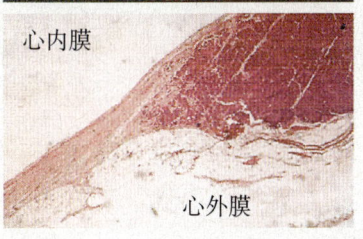

心内膜

心外膜

彩图 28（图 63-1） 右心室严重扩张 左图：一例典型致心律失常性右室发育不良患者进行心脏移植后切下的严重扩张的右心室。可见心肌被脂肪覆盖。箭头所示为因ICD心内膜电极感知不良而置入的心外膜电极。右图：感知不良系由于主动固定电极顶端已不再与心内膜接触，很可能是右心室扩张导致电极导管移位。ICD的"自动增益控制"功能导致不适当放电。

彩图29（图63-2） 成人典型的Uhl畸形 上图：肺动脉内插入剪刀，可见右心室呈透明状。中图：在另一例患者，沿三尖瓣水平切片。可见左心室大小及室壁厚度正常。右心室明显扩张，室壁极度变薄，间隔前部尤为明显。下图："心肌突然断续"，代之以纤维化和脂肪组织。

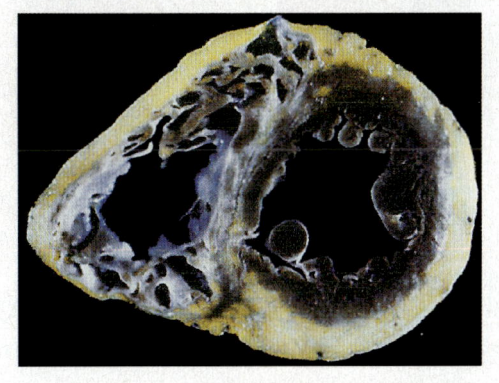

彩图 30（图 63-3） 双心室发育不良 患者左心室外壁与右心室一样，表现为同样的疾病过程，心肌被脂肪和纤维化所取代。在这些脂肪组织内可见存活的心肌细胞及纤维条索。

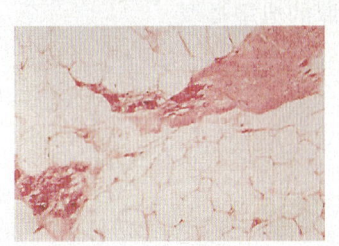
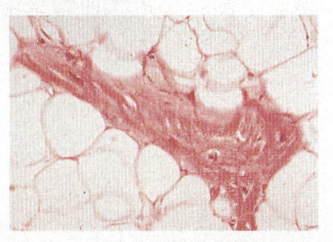

左室纤维组织　　　　左室心肌细胞

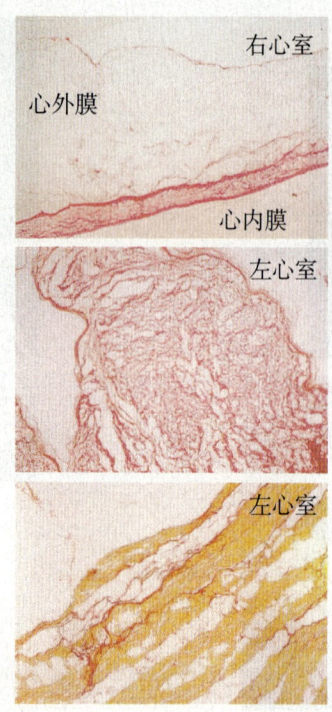

彩图 31（图 63-4）　双心室海绵样发育不良　上图：右心室壁完全被脂肪取代。两条纤维化线代表残存的心外膜和心内膜。中图：左室大部分心肌纤维被脂肪和小灶纤维化所分隔。下图：左心室游离壁高倍放大图。

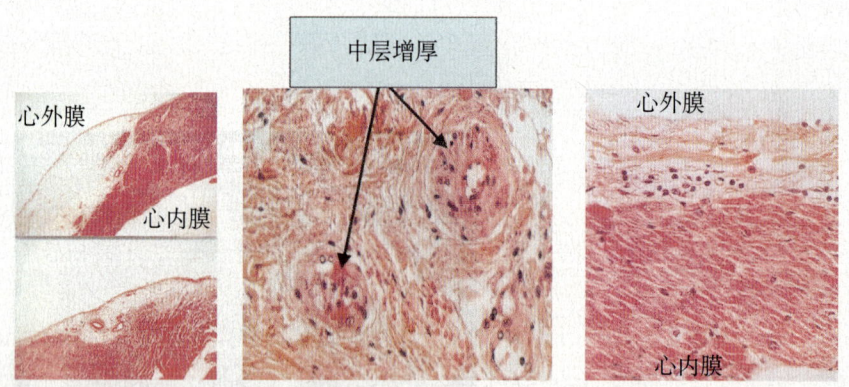

彩图 32（图 63-5）　一例既往无症状的 16 岁女孩发生猝死　上三幅图：漏斗部及其邻近的有肌小梁的区域可见心肌被大量脂肪细胞取代，夹以存活的心肌细胞带，提示为致心律失常性右室发育不良的局灶型。下图：小冠状血管壁增厚的典型类型。

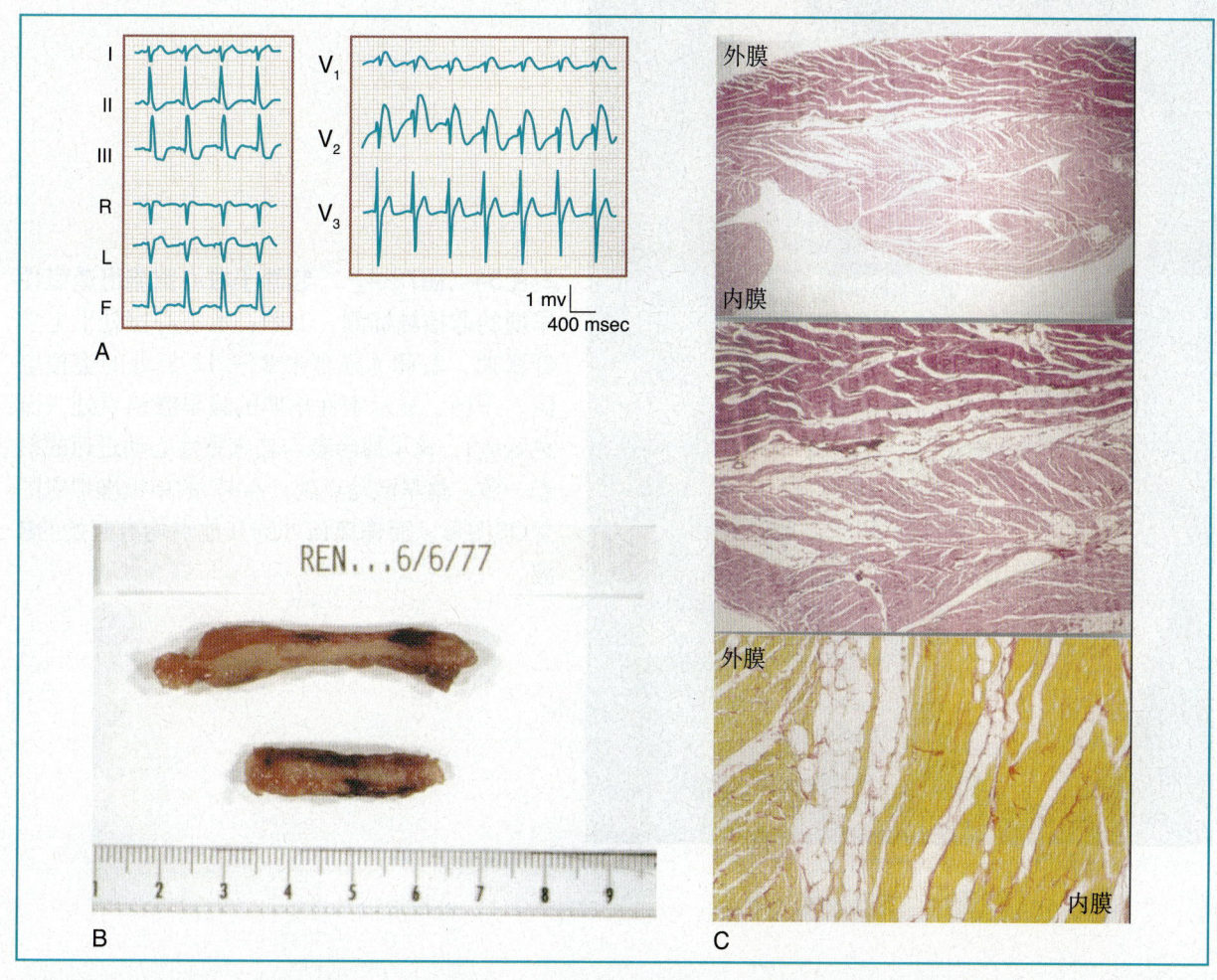

彩图33（图63-6） **具典型心电图特征的Brugada综合征** 右室游离壁可见心外膜与心内膜之间夹以脂肪组织，此类表现有可能不被常规的影像学检查检出。脂肪带与1977年手术治疗的典型致心律失常性右室发育不良患者相似。此患者在室速起源部位的右室呈"三明治"样结构，心外膜与心内膜两层间夹着厚厚的脂肪层。

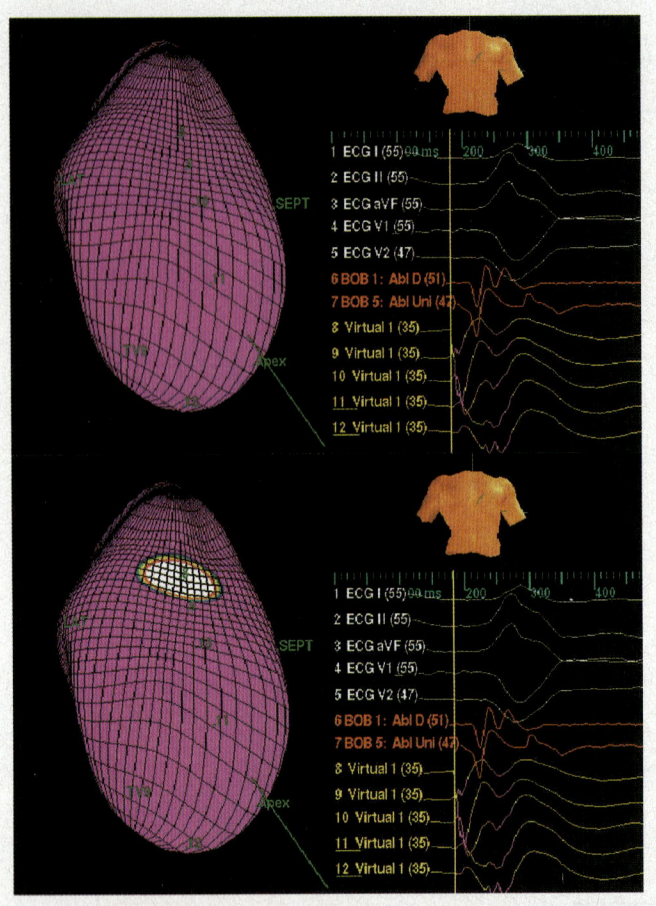

彩图34（图72-4）　起源于右心室流出道室性早搏的非接触标测　上图：示右心室处于电学舒张期，右侧为模型中8～12点处的虚拟电图。下图：显示室性早搏的最早激动点处（白色区域），该早搏形态与临床室性心动过速的形态一致。最早激动点处（点8）的单极虚拟电图呈QS图形，而偏离该处的其他点均有起始的R波。

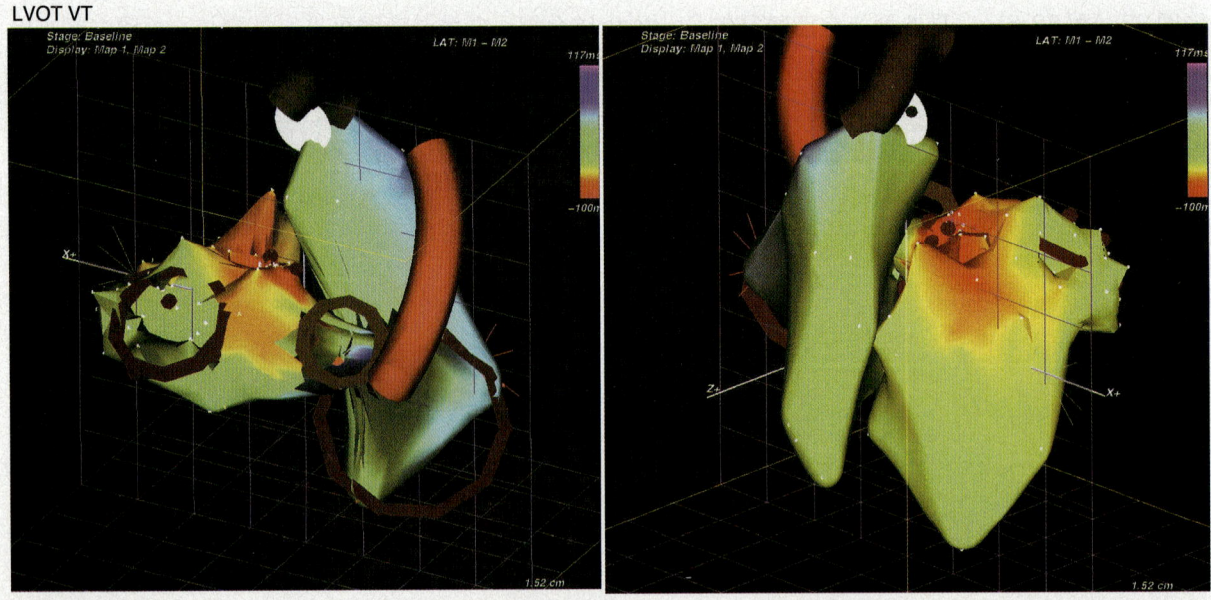

彩图35（图72-5）　起源于主动脉与二尖瓣连接处的左室流出道心动过速　左图为室性心动过速时电解剖标测图（后前位），三尖瓣环、二尖瓣环及主动脉瓣环均显示在模型中，红色管道为主动脉，灰色区域为肺动脉。心动过速的最早激动点呈红色。右图（前后位）显示消融点位于主动脉与二尖瓣连接处（暗红色点）。

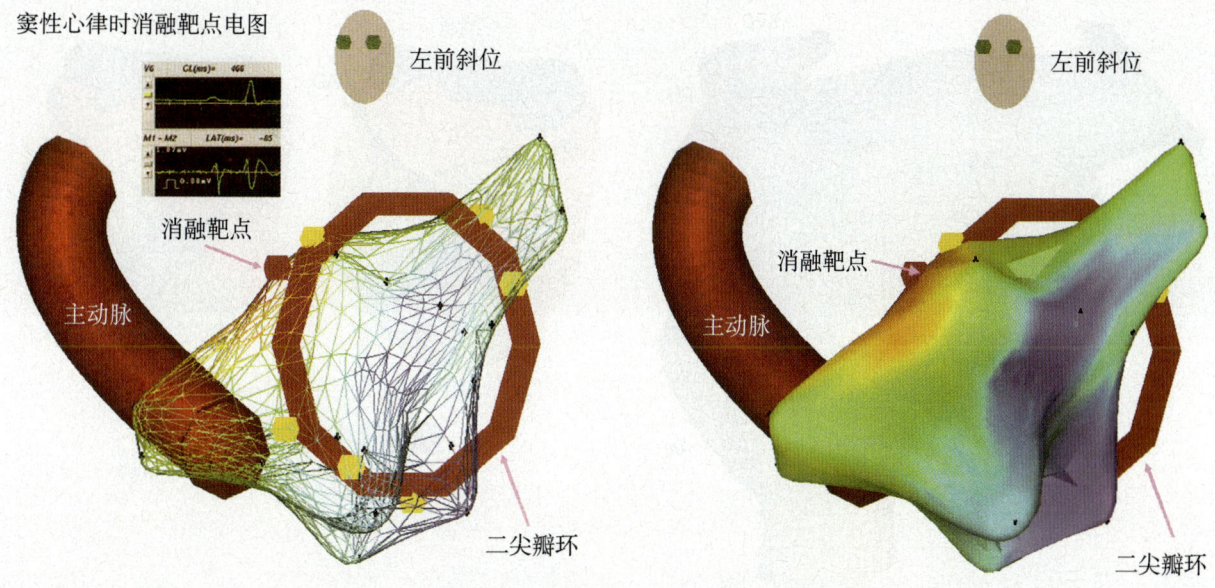

彩图 36（图 72-6） 起源于二尖瓣区域的左室室速 左图示窦律下构建的左室栅格状几何图形。成功靶点处的腔内电图显示在左上角，较大的心房和心室波提示该点邻近二尖瓣环。右图为心动过速时的激动顺序图。

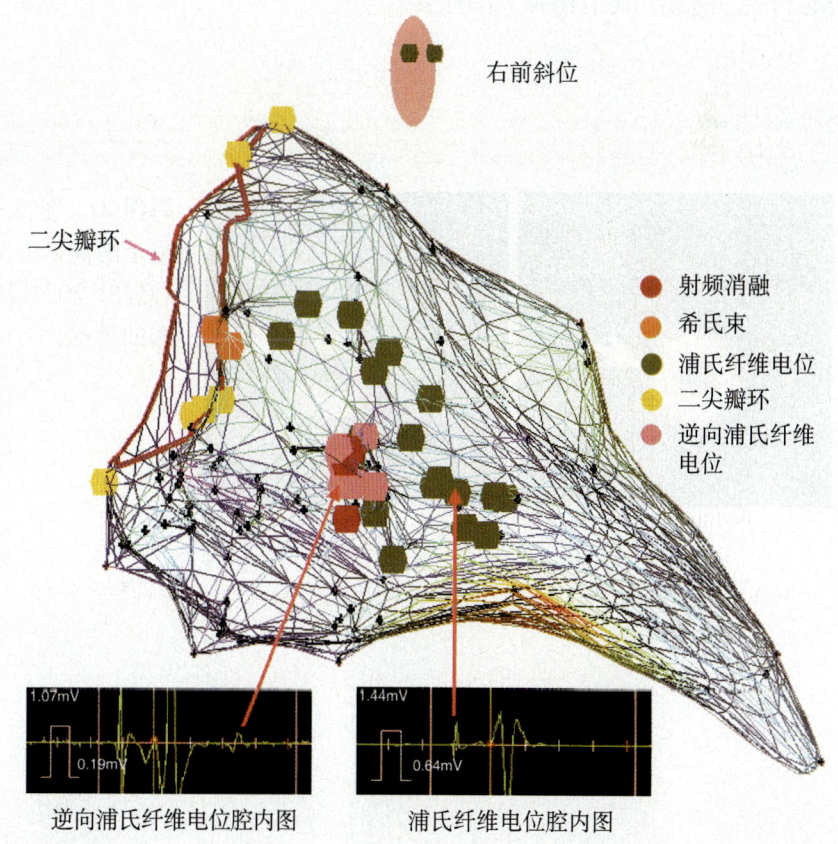

彩图 37（图 72-12） 分支性室速患者窦性节律下的浦氏纤维电位（PPs） 绿色标记表示左后分支区域可记录到浦氏纤维电位的点。右侧插图为该区域记录到的腔内电图，第一个棘波代表浦氏纤维激动，其后为心室激动波。粉红色标记为记录到逆向浦氏纤维电位的点（相当于心动过速时的舒张期电位）。左侧插图为该区域记录到的腔内电图，第一个棘波为浦氏纤维电位（PP），其后为心室激动波，最后为低频的逆向浦氏纤维电位。该点为最早的逆向浦氏纤维电位处，也是成功消融靶点。

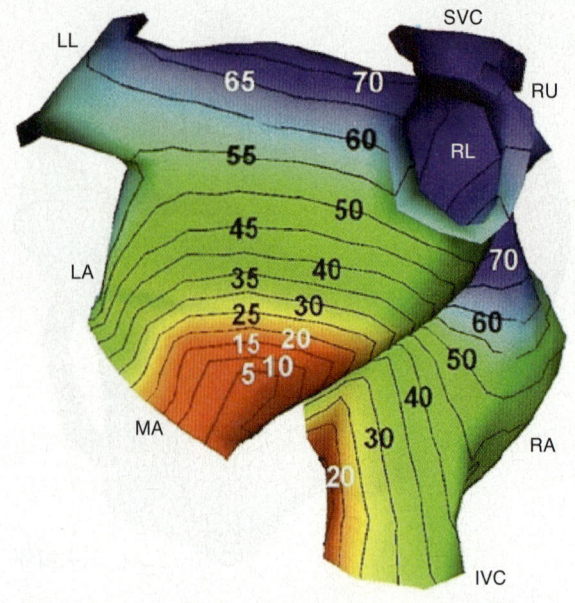
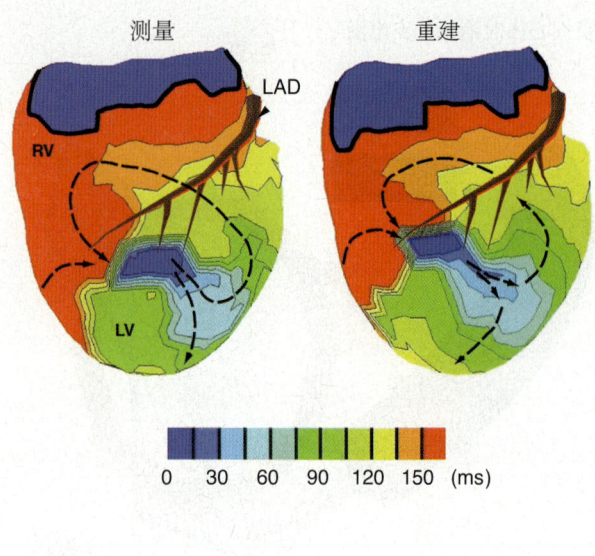

彩图 38（图 87-2） 一例正常人用导管在冠状窦进行刺激时用逆解法重建心内膜激动的时间图 图为后壁左侧观。IVC：下腔静脉；LA：左心房；LL：左下肺静脉；MA：二尖瓣环；RA：右心房；RL：右下肺静脉；RU：右上肺静脉；SVC：上腔静脉。（引自 Tilg B，Fischer G，Modre R，et al: Model-based imaging of cardiac electrical excitation in humans. IEEE Trans Med Imaging 21: 1031-1039，2003.）

彩图 39（图 87-4） 心肌梗死 5 天的心脏 程序刺激诱发了折返性的类单形性室速，在测量的心外膜等时图上（左图）和经计算机逆运算法重建的心外膜电图（右图）上清晰可见。（引自 Burnes JE，Taccardi B，Rudy Y: A noninvasive imaging modality for cardiac arrhythmias. Circulation 102: 2152-2158，2000.）

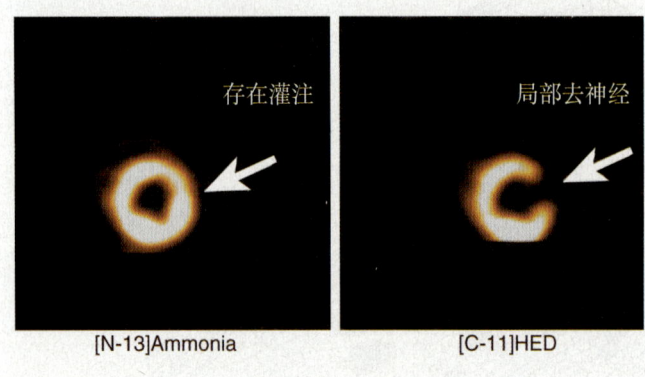

彩图40（图92-7） 犬去感神经 图像显示在用苯酚局部去交感神经后心室中部短轴面 NH_3（灌注）和对羟麻黄碱（HED）显示交感神经分布的情况。

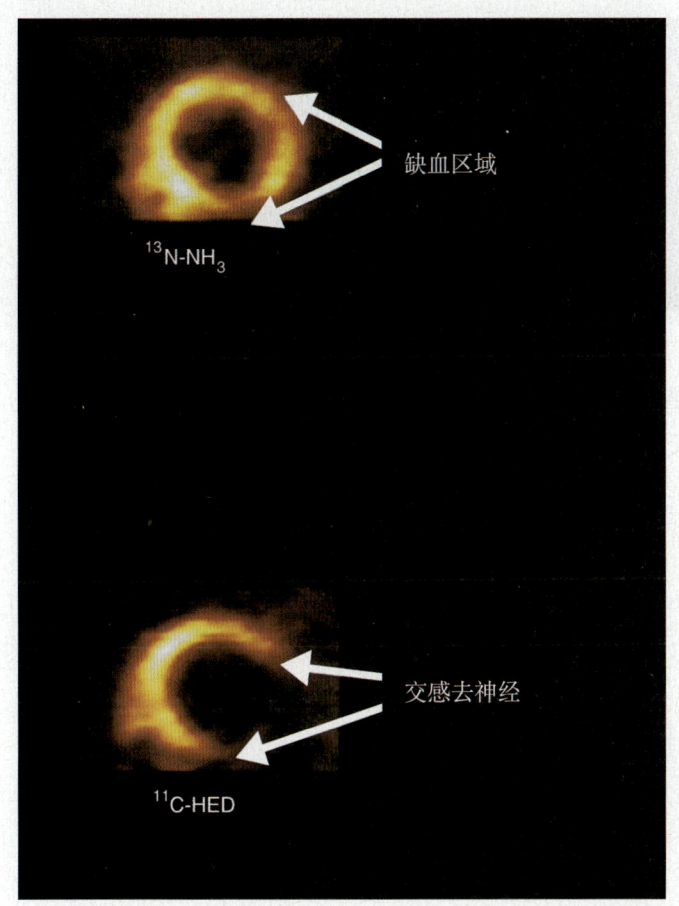

彩图 41（图 92-8） 冠心病患者去交感神经 图像显示心肌灌注（顶图）和交感神经分布（底图）情况。左室侧部有一相对较大的区域存在中等程度的灌注减少。对羟麻黄碱（HED）成像证实在左室相应的区域存在交感神经系统的受损。

彩图42（图93-2） 希氏束旁局灶起源的房性心动过速 图示后前位的左右心房的激动电图。淡黄色的六边形区域为希氏束，红色区域代表最先激动的区域，其位置邻近希氏束，紫色代表最晚激动的区域。

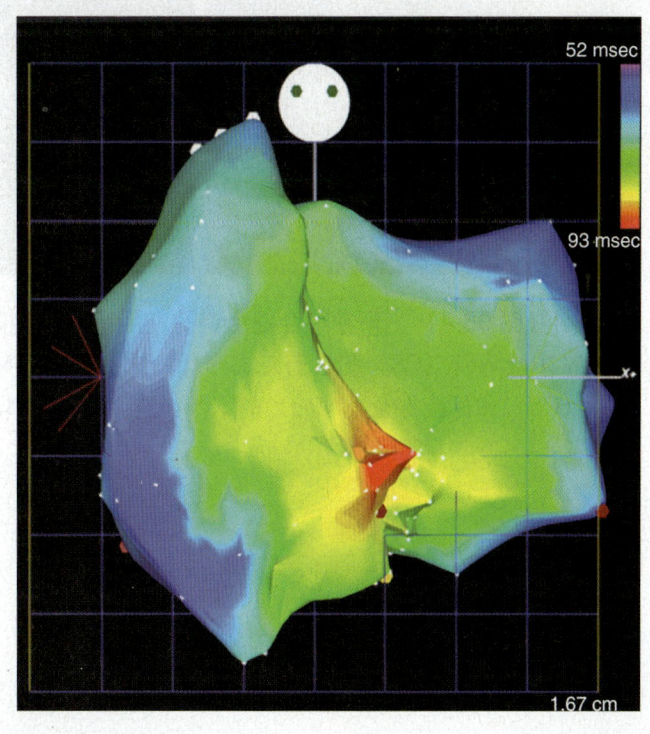

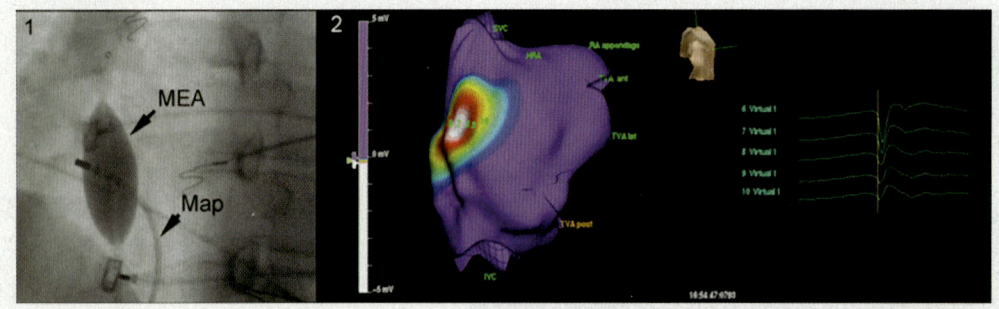

彩图43（图93-3）　使用非接触式标测对局灶性房性心动过速的标测和消融　1. 左前斜位下右房内的球囊多电极矩阵（MEA）和单个的标测大头导管（Map）。2. 右心房的等电位图（右侧位）。该等电位图显示局灶起源的右侧房速的心内膜的最早激动点（被其他颜色环绕的白色区域），这个区域被尚未除极的心内膜所包绕（用紫色代表）。放置于等电位图上局灶心律失常起源点位置的单极电图（图右侧）呈QS型。

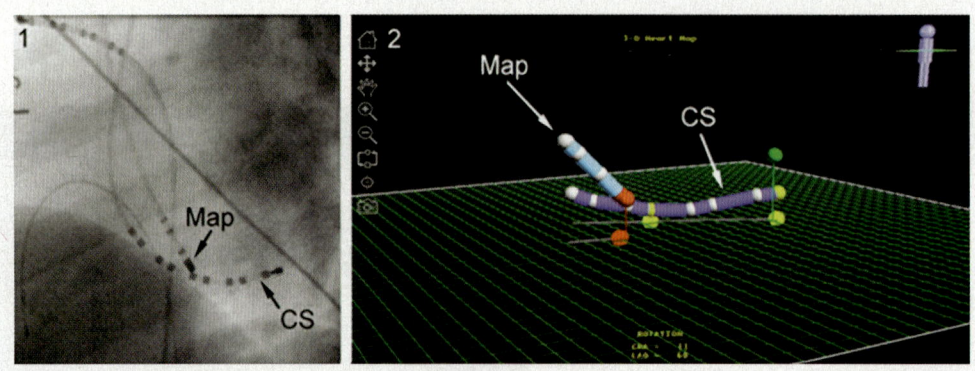

彩图44（图93-4）　预激综合征患者的左后旁路标测时导管的三维定位　1. 左前斜位时置于冠状静脉窦内的10极导管（CS）和沿着二尖瓣环的标测导管（Map）。2. 在LocaLisa的标测显示界面上的冠状窦导管（CS）和标测导管（Map）的三维位置。（感谢 Metronic 公司提供的样图）

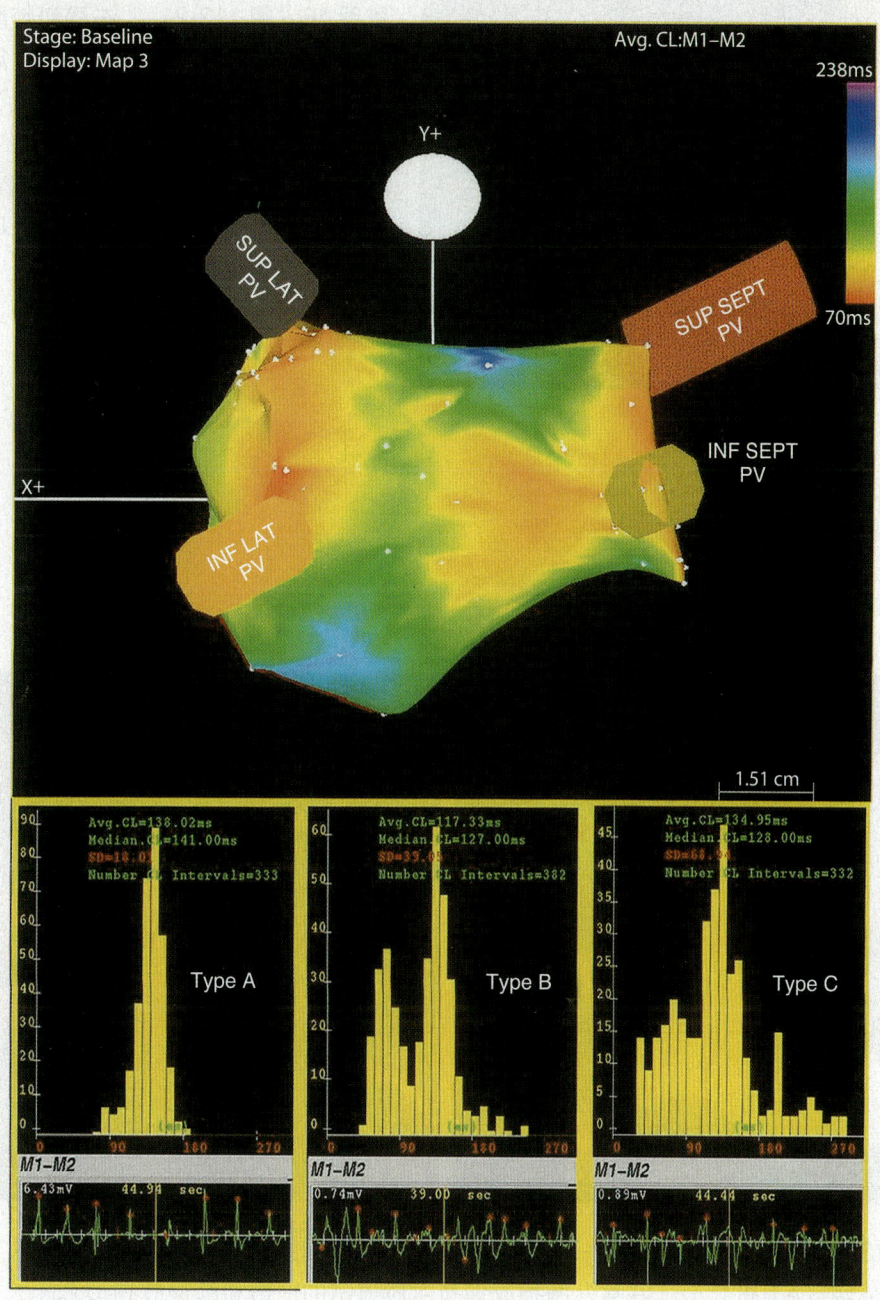

彩图45（图113-1） 左房电图 上图：房颤时的左房电解剖图（后前位），每点采样时间为45s。电生理信息以不同色彩显示，红色代表最短环长（CL），紫色为最长环长。注意，较短的环长多聚集在肺静脉周围。下图：A型、B型、C型局部双极电图及相应的环长直方图。

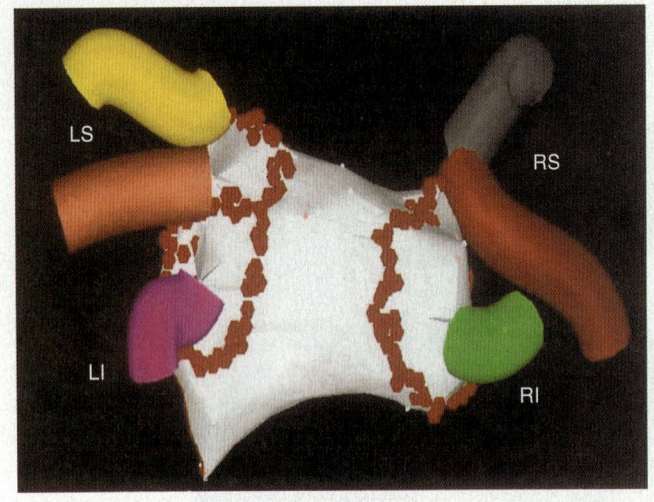

彩图46（图113-2） 左房和肺静脉的三维标测图 实心灰色的左房标测图，后前位。红色圆点为射频消融靶点，彩色管道为肺静脉。注意，左上肺静脉有早期分支，右上肺静脉恰好位于开口上，右侧消融线环绕所有静脉。LI：左下肺静脉；LS：左上肺静脉；RI：右下肺静脉；RS：右上肺静脉。

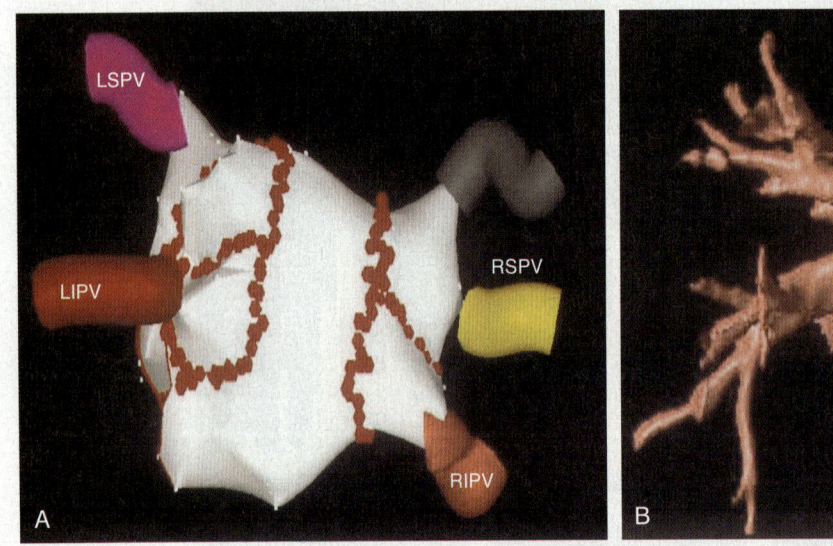 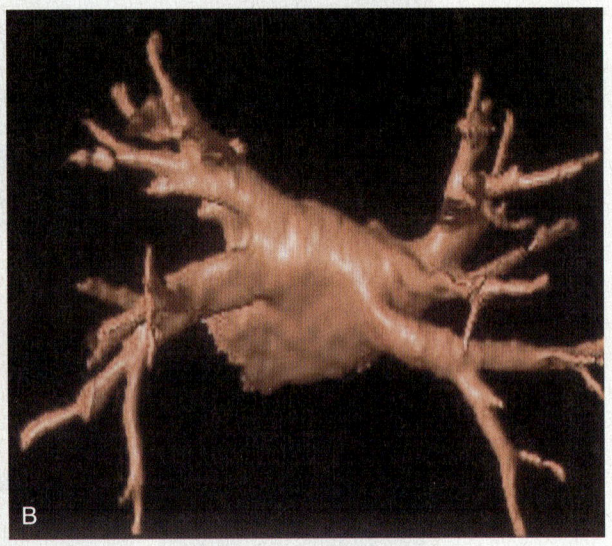

彩图47（图113-3） 三维重建肺静脉-左房交界区 CARTO重建的肺静脉-左房交界区三维图像（B）与磁共振血管成像（A）的比较。注意，两种成像技术所显示的左房和肺静脉在形态和大小上具有高度的相似性。LIPV：左下肺静脉；LSPV：左上肺静脉；RIPV：右下肺静脉；RSPV：右上肺静脉。

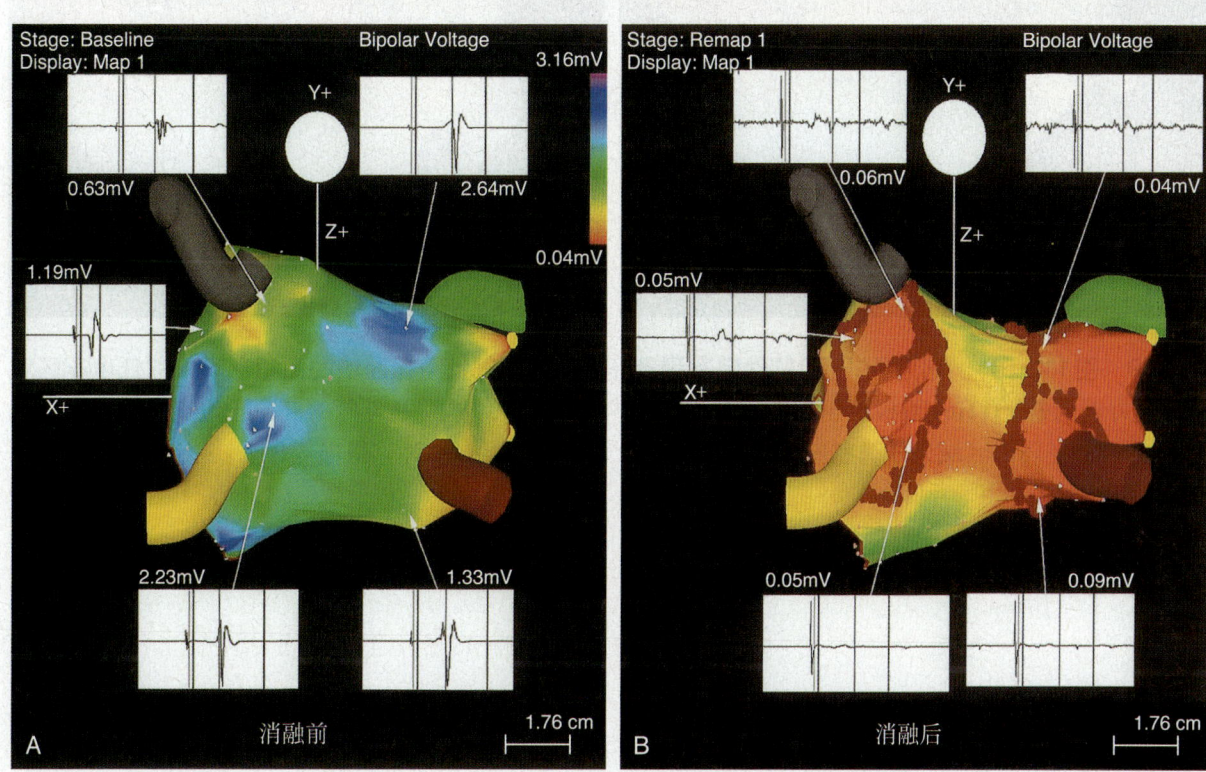

彩图48（图113-4） 三维左房电压图 后前位（A：消融术前；B：消融术后），显示峰-峰双极电图振幅。红色代表最低电压，紫色为最高电压。紫红色圆点为射频消融靶点。术后，在消融线内及其周围区域，包括一定范围的左房后壁，显示低振幅（<0.1mV）电图（电解剖重构）。术前电图可见肺静口部电位，提示此处肌纤维具有将冲动传出和传入静脉的传导功能。经环每根肺静脉射频消融之后，可见术前口部同一部位的肺静脉电位消失（术后电图），即心房静脉间电连接阻断。

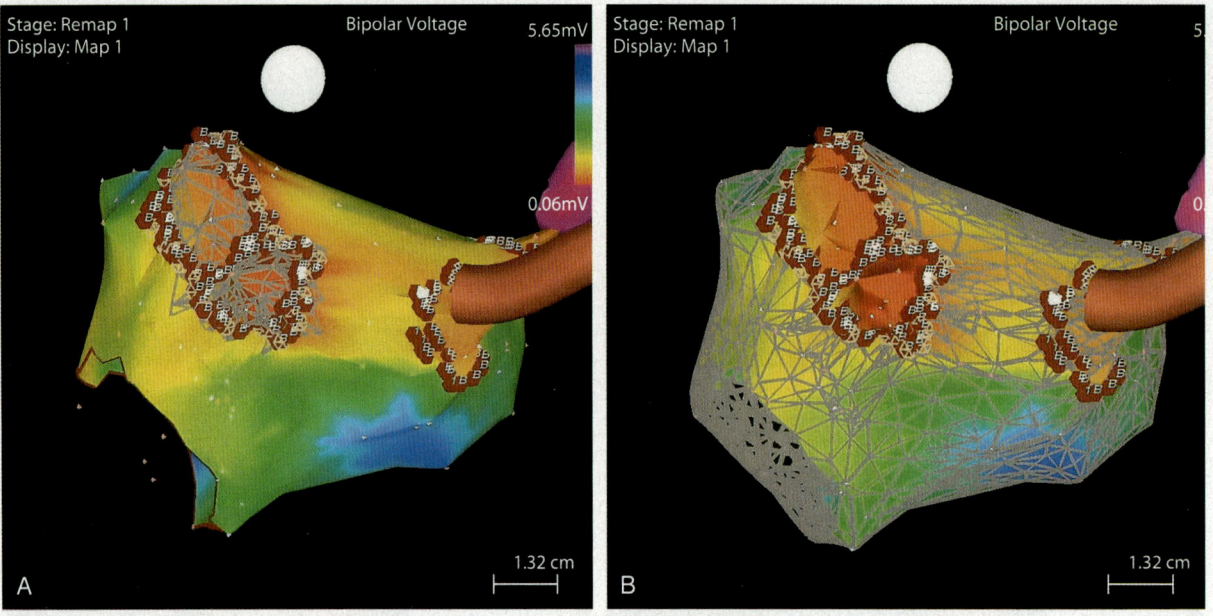

彩图49（图113-5）　利用CARTO软件定量测量环肺静脉口部低电压区域的面积　环形的低电压区域是指最外侧的低于0.1mV双极电压位点所围成区域内的表面积，这些最外侧的低电压位点是通过手动选择的（A）。在环形区域外任意点击一处，左房剩余表面积即可自动计算得出（B）。

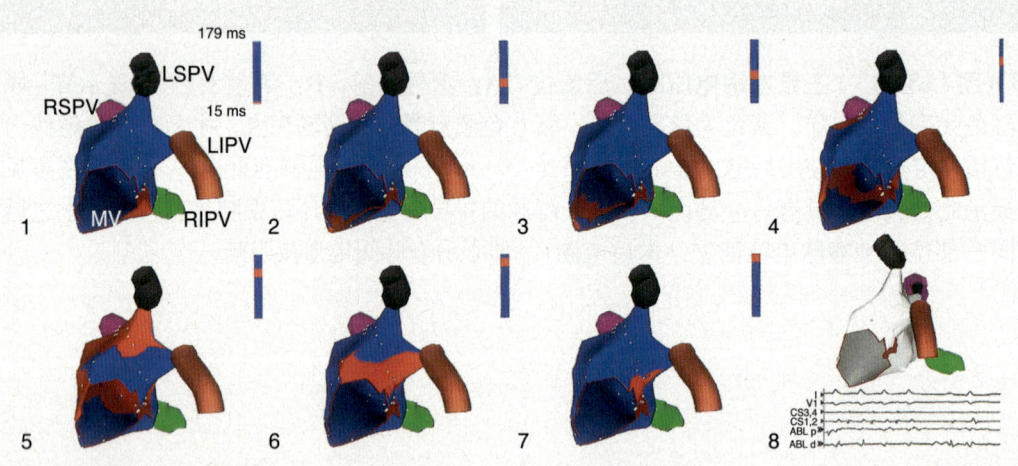

彩图50（图113-6）　环肺静脉消融后的左房心动过速时的激动扩布图　第1～7幅为动态顺序播放中的冻结图像（左侧观）。蓝色背景下的红色阴影代表局部心内膜激动时间，范围30ms（时程的红色图标在各图的右侧）。注意，激动波阵围绕二尖瓣环进行环形运动。如心内电生理标测所示，心律失常在射频消融（紫红色圆点）左下肺静脉和二尖瓣环之间的峡部时终止（第8幅）。CS：冠状窦；LSPV：左上肺静脉；MV：二尖瓣；RIPV：右下肺静脉；RSPV：右上肺静脉。

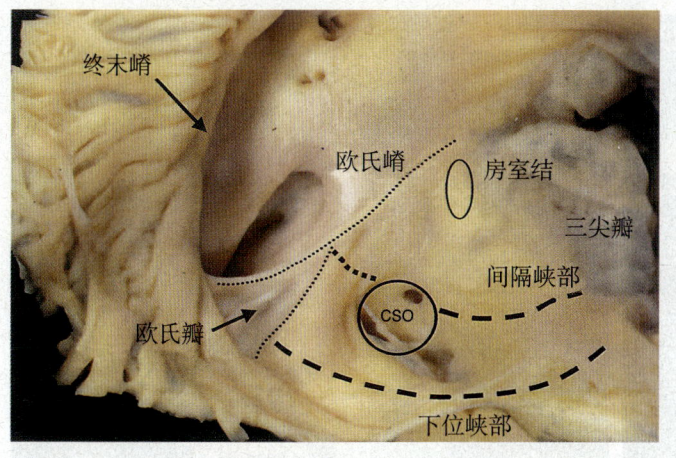

彩图51（图114-1） 右前斜位下人体右心房内腔模拟图 下位峡部自三尖瓣环下方延伸至下腔静脉（下方虚线），间隔峡部位于三尖瓣环和冠状窦口（CSO）间（上方虚线），并向欧氏嵴延伸（点虚线）。注意漂浮的欧氏瓣呈三角形结构。（引自Courtesy of Yen Ho, National Heart &Lung Institute and Royal Brompton Hospital, London, UK.）

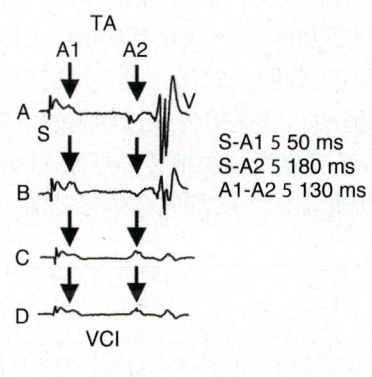
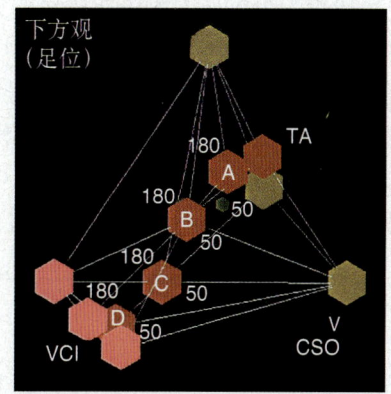

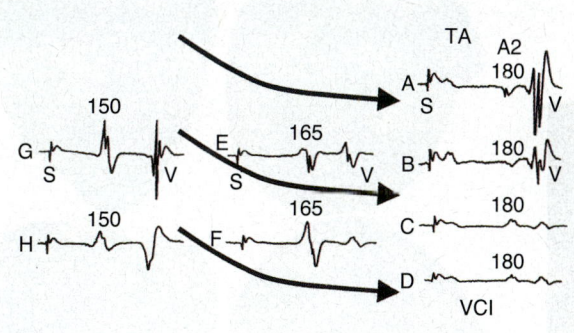
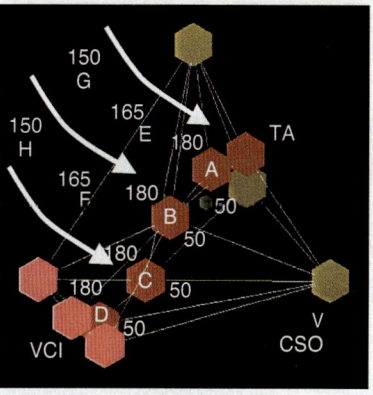

彩图52（图114-4） 验证消融后峡部传导完全阻滞 左上图：消融三尖瓣环（TA）和下腔静脉（VCI）之间峡部后，冠状窦口（CSO）起搏，沿着整个峡部的4个点（A～D）都可标测到双电位。右上图：从下方看峡部电生理标测的解剖结构：3个点代表三尖瓣环下方（中间的不代表6点位置），3个点代表下腔静脉，深红点代表5个消融点。沿着整个消融线记录到宽而分离的双电位（A1和A2），A1-A2间期均为130ms。下图：除了标测到双电位，冠状窦起搏首先记录到向前上方传导的电位进一步证实峡部完全阻滞，而前方游离壁下传波（箭头）最迟激动点恰位于消融线（峡部消融线电图A2），可以排除跨间隔的慢传导。此后，通过从消融线另一侧起搏可证实双向阻滞。

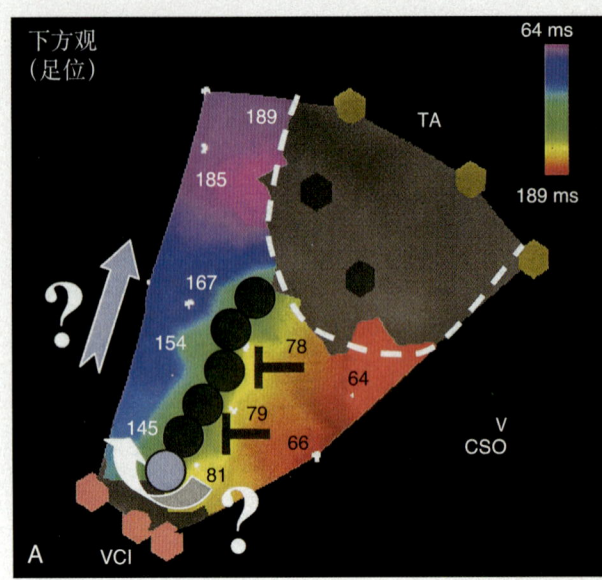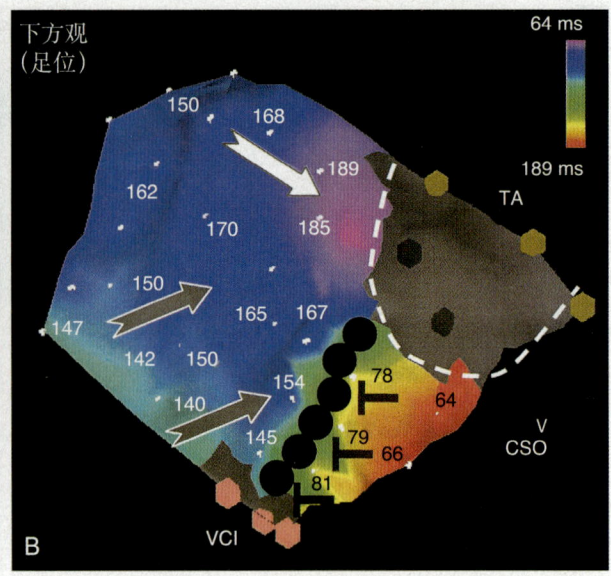

彩图53（图114-6） 消融后，冠状窦口（CSO）起搏，重新进行峡部消融线的电解剖标测 灰色区域（虚线）代表三尖瓣环下方没有传导能力的纤维组织。左图：沿着消融线记录双电位，然而，A1-A2间期并不一致。最大间期89ms，消融线中部A1-A2间期75ms，近端仅有64ms，因此假设靠近下腔静脉（VCI）处存在跨峡部的慢传导（带有问号箭头所指灰色圆圈）。右图：进一步的再次标测证实峡部完全传导阻滞（靠近下腔静脉的黑色圆圈），不需进行再消融。经证实为经过界嵴的下端传导回路（灰色箭头），与三尖瓣环（TA，白箭头）前向传导波融合。经过界嵴较快地传导导致A1-A2间期不等，但最晚的激动仍然位于消融线（峡部消融线电图A2波），因此证实为峡部完全传导阻滞。

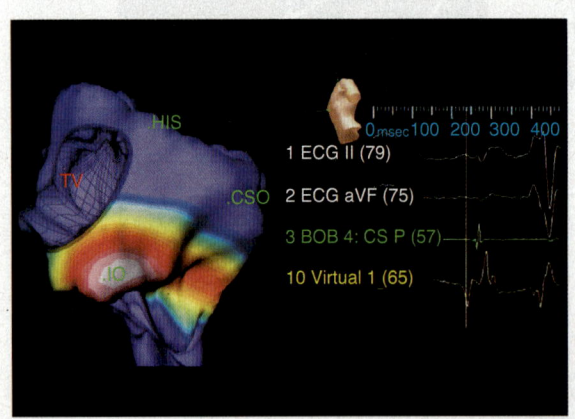

彩图54（图115-2） 等时图标测显示心房最早激动部位位于三尖瓣环下缘 最早激动点比P波提前10ms。CSP，冠状窦近端。

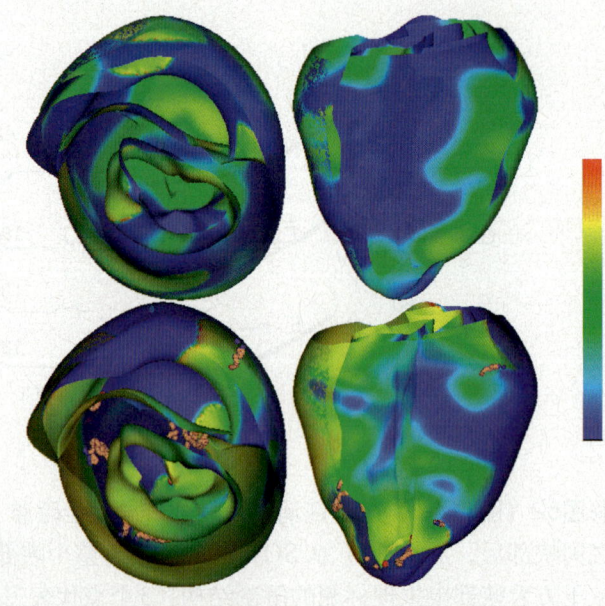

彩图57（图31-2） 猝发刺激诱发室颤时，兔心室模型基底部和正后壁在两个不同时间点跨膜电压图。

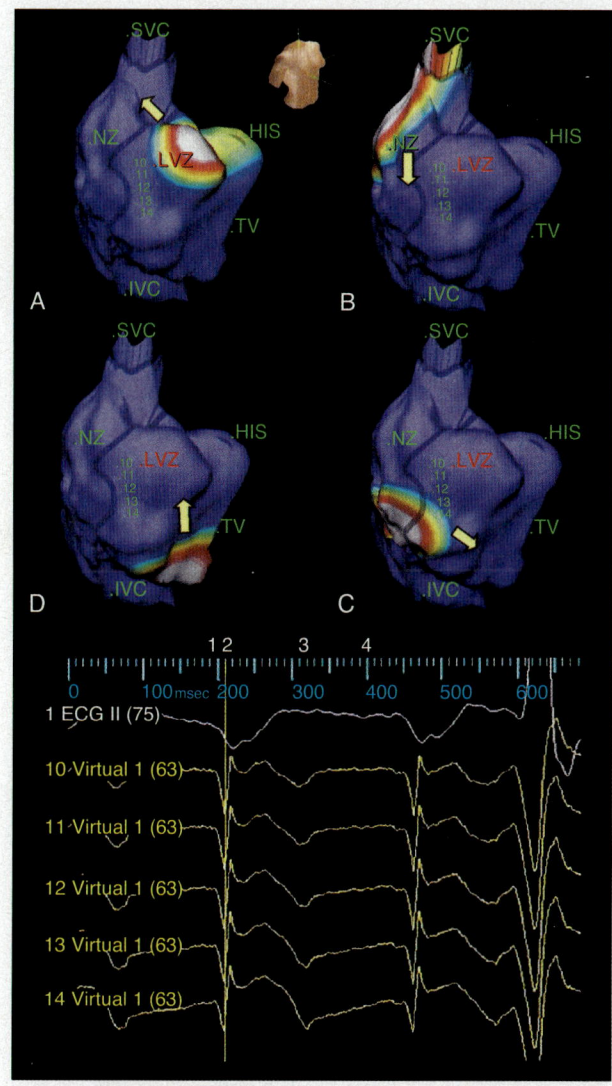

彩图55（图115-5） 等电位图表示位于右房前游离壁低压区或瘢痕处的大折返环 白色标尺代表最大负极电位，蓝色代表次级负电位，黄色箭头代表大折返心动过速的激动方向。中心阻滞区的实际单极电图代表双电位（从10到14）。A～D是按时间顺序排列的。

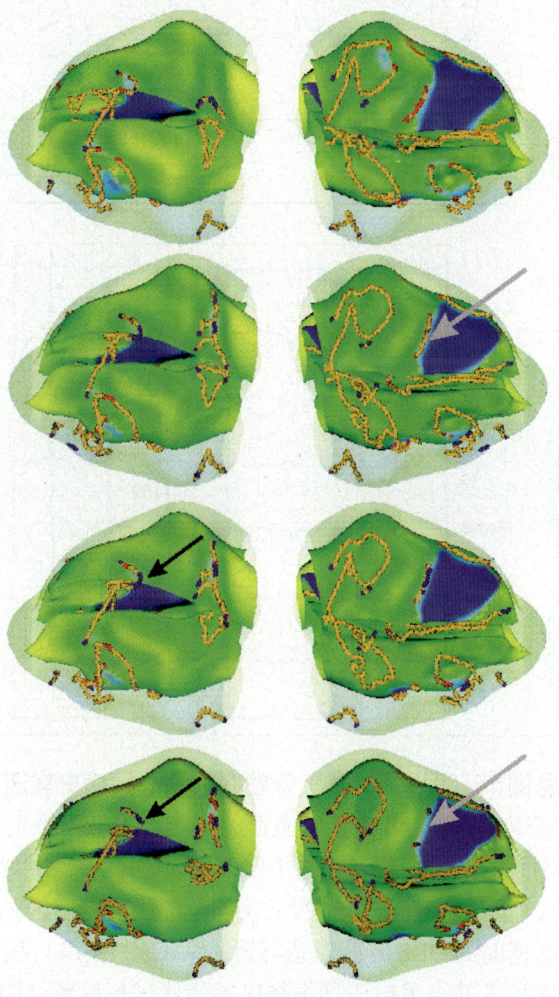

彩图58（图31-5） 电击除颤后30ms，心室模型中自旋波条纹的数量和分布左图为心室前壁，右图为心室后壁。条纹终点与心室的内膜面相连用红色表示，而条纹终点与外膜面相连则用紫蓝色表示，箭头所指详见本章内容。

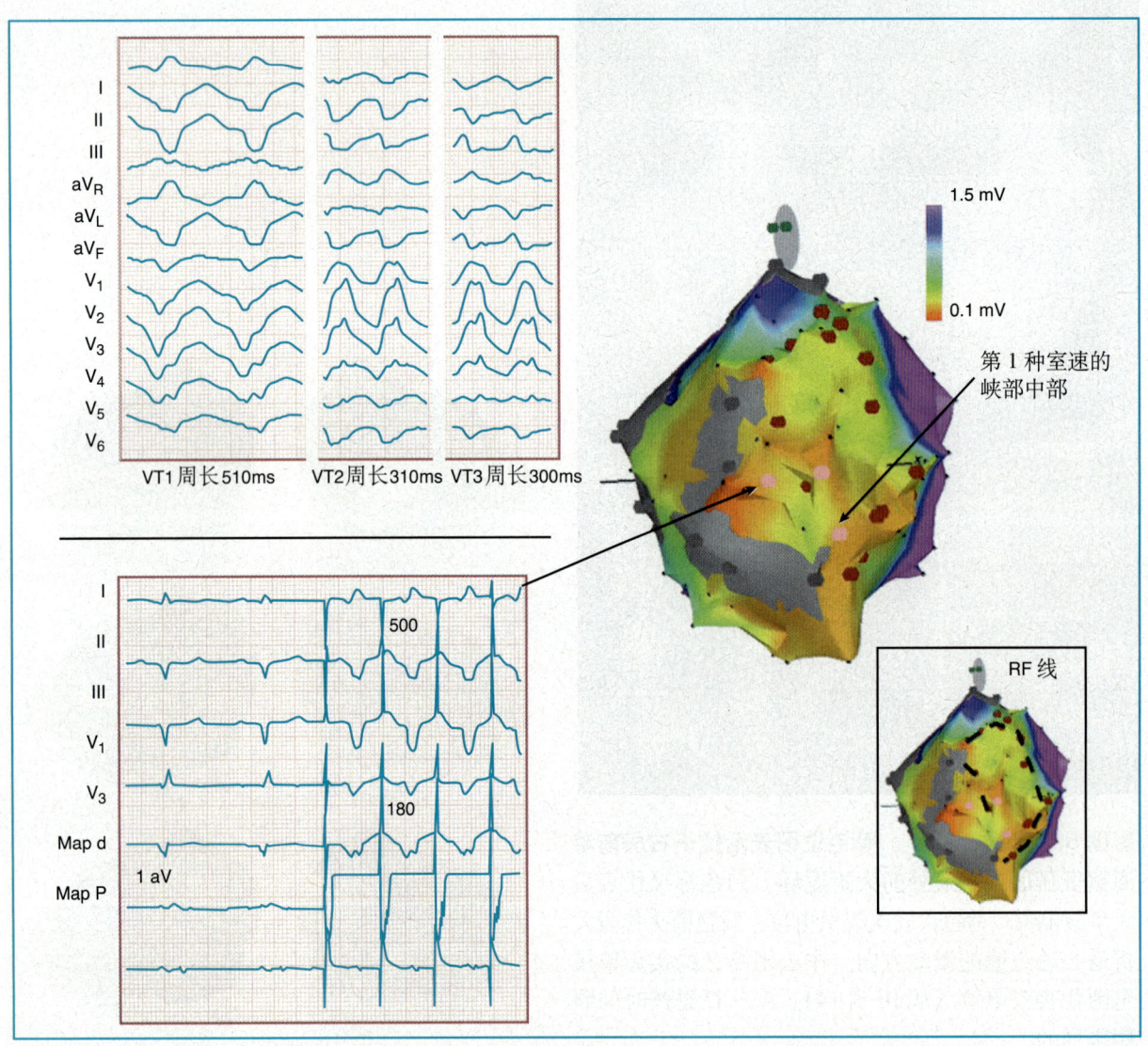

彩图56（图118-2） 既往有前壁心梗病史室速患者的标测 左上，12导联心电图显示3种不同形态的室速（VT），其中两种室速的血流动力学不稳定。右侧是左心室的三维标测电压图。以不同的颜色表示不同的电位振幅，超过1.5mV用紫色表示，电静止瘢痕（起搏阈值＞10mA）以灰色表示。左下，如箭头所示，窦性心律时所记录部位的局部电图振幅低，起搏时S-QRS间期为180ms，提示存在传导延迟。起搏时的QRS波群形态与第1种室速（VT1）相似，提示刺激的部位在第1种室速的出口区域。该例在瘢痕区并沿着电压低振幅区的边缘进行射频（RF）消融（红圈），消除了所有的室速。